Stahl's Essential Psychopharmacology
Third Edition

Stahl's Essential Psychopharmacology has become the definitive source of information on psychopharmacology and now continues as the established preeminent source of information in its field. This fully revised and expanded third edition enlists advances in neurobiology and recent clinical developments to explain with renewed clarity the concepts underlying drug treatment of psychiatric disorders. Clinical advances in antipsychotic and antidepressant therapy are discussed in detail; new, expanded material includes coverage of sleep disorders, obesity, addiction, chronic pain, and disorders of impulse control. The text also features four new chapters on psychiatric genetics, pain management, treatment of cognitive disorders, and treatment of sleep disorders. The text is also visually enhanced by art that has been increased by 100% and completely redrawn and a layout that has been completely redesigned for increased user friendliness. CME is also offered through questions available on the website of the Neuroscience Education Institute at neiglobal.com. *Stahl's Essential Psychopharmacology*, Third Edition, remains the essential text for students, scientists, psychiatrists, and other mental health professionals.

Stephen M. Stahl is Adjunct Professor of Psychiatry at the University of California at San Diego. He has conducted numerous research projects awarded by the National Institute of Mental Health, the Veterans Administration, and the pharmaceutical industry. Author of more than 350 articles and chapters, Dr. Stahl is an internationally recognized clinician, researcher, and teacher in psychiatry with subspecialty expertise in psychopharmacology.

Stahl's Essential Psychopharmacology

Neuroscientific Basis and Practical Applications

Third Edition

Stephen M. Stahl

University of California at San Diego

With Illustrations by
Nancy Muntner

Editorial Assistant
Meghan M. Grady

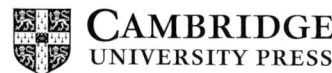

CAMBRIDGE UNIVERSITY PRESS
Cambridge, New York, Melbourne, Madrid, Cape Town, Singapore, São Paulo, Delhi

Cambridge University Press
32 Avenue of the Americas, New York, NY 10013-2473, USA

www.cambridge.org
Information on this title: www.cambridge.org/9780521673761

© Stephen M. Stahl 2008

This publication is in copyright. Subject to statutory exception
and to the provisions of relevant collective licensing agreements,
no reproduction of any part may take place without the written
permission of Cambridge University Press.

First published 2008
Reprinted 2009 (twice)

Printed in the United States of America

A catalog record for this publication is available from the British Library.

Library of Congress Cataloging in Publication Data

Stahl, S. M.
Stahl's essential psychopharmacology : neuroscientific basis and practical applications. – 3rd ed.
  p. ; cm.
Rev. ed. of: Essential psychopharmacology. Cambridge University Press. 2nd ed. 2000.
Includes bibliographical references and index.
ISBN 978-0-521-85702-4 (hardback) – ISBN 978-0-521-67376-1 (pbk.)
1. Mental illness–Chemotherapy. 2. Psychopharmacology. I. Essential
psychopharmacology. II. Title. III. Title: Essential psychopharmacology.
[DNLM: 1. Mental Disorders–drug therapy. 2. Central Nervous
System–drug effects. 3. Psychotropic Drugs–pharmacology. WM 402 S7811s 2008]
RC483.S67   2008
616.89'18–dc22   2007052875

ISBN 978-0-521-85702-4 hardback
ISBN 978-0-521-67376-1 paperback

Cambridge University Press has no responsibility for the persistence or
accuracy of URLs for external or third-party Internet Web sites referred to in
this publication and does not guarantee that any content on such Web sites is,
or will remain, accurate or appropriate. Information regarding prices, travel
timetables, and other factual information given in this work are correct at
the time of first printing, but Cambridge University Press does not guarantee
the accuracy of such information thereafter.

Every effort has been made in preparing this book to provide accurate and
up-to-date information that is in accord with accepted standards and
practice at the time of publication. Although case histories are drawn
from actual cases, every effort has been made to disguise the identities of
the individuals involved. Nevertheless, the authors, editors, and publishers
can make no warranties that the information contained herein is totally
free from error, not least because clinical standards are constantly
changing through research and regulation. The authors, editors, and
publishers therefore disclaim all liabilty for direct or consequential
damages resulting from the use of material contained in this book. Readers
are strongly advised to pay careful attention to information provided by
the manufacturer of any drugs or equipment that they plan to use.

In memory of Daniel X. Freedman, mentor, colleague, and scientific father.

To Cindy, my wife, best friend, and tireless supporter.

To Jennifer and Victoria, my daughters, for their patience and understanding of the demands of authorship.

Contents

Preface to the Third Edition	ix
CME Information	xiii

Chapter 1
Structure and Function of Neurons — 1

Chapter 2
Synaptic Neurotransmission and the Anatomically Addressed Nervous System — 21

Chapter 3
Signal Transduction and the Chemically Addressed Nervous System — 51

Chapter 4
Transporters and G Protein–Linked Receptors as Targets of Psychopharmacological Drug Action — 91

Chapter 5
Ion Channels and Enzymes as Targets of Psychopharmacological Drug Action — 123

Chapter 6
Psychiatric Genetics — 177

Chapter 7
Circuits in Psychopharmacology — 195

Chapter 8
From Circuits to Symptoms in Psychopharmacology — 223

Chapter 9
Psychosis and Schizophrenia — 247

Chapter 10
Antipsychotic Agents — 327

Chapter 11
Mood Disorders — 453

Chapter 12
Antidepressants — 511

Chapter 13
Mood Stabilizers — 667

Chapter 14
Anxiety Disorders and Anxiolytics — 721

Chapter 15
Pain and the Treatment of Fibromyalgia and Functional Somatic Syndromes — 773

Chapter 16
Disorders of Sleep and Wakefulness and Their Treatment — 815

Chapter 17
Attention Deficit Hyperactivity Disorder and Its Treatment — 863

Chapter 18
Dementia and Its Treatment — 899

Chapter 19
Disorders of Reward, Drug Abuse, and Their Treatment — 943

Suggested Readings — 1013
Index — 1057

Preface to the Third Edition

Stahl's Essential Psychopharmacology in its third edition has doubled in number of words and figures compared with the second edition and has almost quadrupled compared with the first edition. In this period of time, the field of psychopharmacology has experienced incredible growth; it has also experienced a major paradigm shift from a limited focus on neurotransmitters and receptors to an emphasis on brain circuits, neuroimaging, genetics, and signal transduction cascades. The third edition of *Stahl's Essential Psychopharmacology* attempts to reflect this transformation in the field, and elements of this paradigm shift are incorporated into every chapter of this new edition. Other changes in the third edition include discussions about how numerous neurotransmitter systems and their circuits are hypothetically linked to current treatments in psychopharmacology. In recent years, many new drugs have been introduced, and many more are now in clinical testing. These are covered in this new edition.

Specifically, the basic neuroscience section at the beginning of the book has expanded from four chapters in the second edition to eight chapters. The clinical section has expanded from ten chapters to eleven and has been extensively reorganized, rewritten, and illustrated with roughly twice the number of figures in every chapter. However, the didactic style of the first and second editions has not changed and continues in this third edition.

The text is purposely written at a conceptual level rather than a pragmatic level and includes ideas that are simplifications and rules, while sacrificing precision and discussion of exceptions to rules. Thus, this text is not intended for the sophisticated subspecialist in psychopharmacology. Also, this book is not extensively referenced to original papers but rather refers to textbooks, reviews, and a few selected original papers, with only a limited reading list for each chapter. For those of you who are interested in specific prescribing information about the most common 100 or so psychotropic drugs, this information is available in the companion textbook, *Essential Psychopharmacology Prescriber's Guide*.

Now, you also have the option of going to Essential Psychopharmacology Online at www.essentialpsych.org. We are proud to announce the launch of this new website, which is due to premiere in the fall of 2008. This website will allow you to search within the entire Essential Psychopharmacology series that includes not only this third edition of *Stahl's Essential Psychopharmacology* but also *Essential Psychopharmacology Prescriber's Guide*. This site will be updated regularly and should therefore provide an up-to-date source for what you need to know about the essentials of psychopharmacology between publication of subsequent editions of these books.

Much of the new content is based on updated lectures, courses, slides, and articles I have written. Many of the new illustrations are now available as animations on the Neuroscience Education Institute's website, as are the lectures, slides, articles, continuing medical education (CME) credits, tests, certifications, and much more. Explore this interactive reference by visiting the Neuroscience Education Institute's website at www.neiglobal.com. If you are interested in comprehensive materials, you can choose to have access to both websites.

In general, this text attempts to present the fundamentals of psychopharmacology in a simplified and readily readable form. Thus, this material should prepare the reader to consult more sophisticated textbooks as well as the professional literature. The organization of the information applies principles of programmed learning for the reader, namely, repetition and interaction, which has been shown to enhance retention.

Therefore, it is suggested that novices first review only the color graphics and the legends for these graphics. Virtually everything covered in the text is also covered in the graphics and icons. Next, read the text from the beginning, while reviewing the graphics at the same time. After the text has been read, the entire book can be rapidly reviewed by referring to the various color graphics in the book. Finally, as a member of the Neuroscience Education Institute, you can utilize the content available online at www.neiglobal.com to obtain continuing medical education credits for this activity or as a helpful interactive reference. Many of the graphics are animated and available on this site. Topics in the field covered in the Essential Psychopharmacology book series can be searched on Essential Psychopharmacology Online.

This mechanism of using the materials will create a certain amount of programmed learning because it incorporates the elements of repetition and interaction with visual learning through graphics. I hope that the visual concepts learned via graphics will reinforce abstract concepts learned from the written text, especially for "visual learners" (i.e., those who retain information better from visualizing concepts than from reading about them).

For those of you who are already familiar with psychopharmacology, this book should provide easy reading from beginning to end. Going back and forth between the text and the graphics should provide interaction. After the complete text has been read, reviewing the entire book by going through the graphics once again should be simple. In addition, the Neuroscience Education Institute's website further expands the *Essential Psychopharmacology* learning experience, and Essential Psychopharmacology Online allows quick searches of topics in this field.

For those of you who are interested in the specific updates made in the third edition, the first section on basic science expands its coverage of the structure and function of neurons, synaptogenesis, signal transduction cascades, ion channels, psychiatric genetics, brain circuits, neuroimaging, and disease models of malfunctioning brain circuits that result in psychiatric symptoms in psychiatric disorders.

The second section on clinical science has been extensively revised, with much expanded coverage of psychosis and antipsychotics, especially of the neurotransmitter glutamate, including the NMDA (N-methyl-d-aspartate) receptor hypofunction hypothesis of schizophrenia and genetic advances in schizophrenia. Several new antipsychotics are also included, as is extensive coverage of cardiometabolic risks and sedation related to antipsychotics.

The mood disorder chapter expands the descriptions of unipolar and bipolar disorders and discusses the entire bipolar spectrum. All clinical chapters include sections on matching the symptoms of the disorder under discussion to various hypothetically malfunctioning brain circuits. The antidepressant chapter includes extensive coverage not only of new drugs and several agents in late-stage testing, but also expanded coverage of "old" (and often neglected) drugs that remain valuable therapeutics but are off-patent and not promoted commercially. In this chapter are new sections on antidepressants and women; on trimonoamine modulators and brain stimulation therapies that may augment antidepressants; and a discussion of "symptom-based" antidepressant selection algorithms for combining antidepressants to treat residual symptoms and attain remission in major depressive disorder. A chapter specifically on mood stabilizers has been added and explains not only the mechanism of action of agents used to treat bipolar disorder but also the use of drugs in combinations to treat this disorder.

The chapter on anxiety disorders now includes coverage of fear conditioning, fear extinction, and stress biology as well as various anxiety disorders and their treatments with anxiolytics and with new drugs on the horizon that have novel mechanisms. Sleep disorders, including not only insomnia but also disorders of wakefulness (excessive daytime sleepiness) and their treatments, are now greatly expanded as a new, separate chapter, which also introduces histamine, a new neurotransmitter system.

A new chapter on chronic pain and fibromyalgia and their treatments has also been added. Attention deficit hyperactivity disorder, in both children and adults, covering both stimulants and nonstimulants, is now a separate chapter. Dementia is also a separate chapter and emphasizes disease-modifying treatments on the horizon. The final chapter is a greatly expanded chapter on reward, emphasizing drug abuse but also covering other disorders of reward, such as disorders of sexual function, eating disorders, and disorders of impulsivity.

This is an incredibly exciting time for the fields of neuroscience and mental health, creating fascinating opportunities for clinicians to utilize current therapeutics and to anticipate future medications that are likely to transform the field of psychopharmacology. Best wishes for your first step on your journey into this fascinating field of psychopharmacology.

Stephen M. Stahl, MD, PhD

CME Information

Release/Expiration Dates

Original release date: March 2008
CME credit expiration date: original expiration February 2011 (if this date has passed, please contact NEI for updated information)

Target Audience

This activity was designed for health care professionals, including psychiatrists, neurologists, primary care physicians, pharmacists, psychologists, nurses, and others, who treat patients with psychiatric conditions.

Statement of Need

The content of this educational activity was determined by rigorous assessment, including activity feedback, expert faculty assessment, literature review, and new medical knowledge, which revealed the following unmet needs:

- Psychiatric illnesses have a neurobiological basis and are primarily treated by pharmacological agents; understanding each of these, as well as the relationship between them, is essential in order to select appropriate treatment for a patient

- The field of psychopharmacology has experienced incredible growth; it has also experienced a major paradigm shift from a limited focus on neurotransmitters and receptors to an emphasis on brain circuits, neuroimaging, genetics, and signal transduction cascades

Learning Objectives

Upon completion of this activity, you should be able to:

- Apply neurobiologic and mechanistic evidence when selecting treatment strategies in order to match treatment to the individual needs of the patient

- Utilize new scientific data to modify existing treatment strategies in order to improve patient outcomes

Accreditation and Credit Designation Statements

The Neuroscience Education Institute is accredited by the Accreditation Council for Continuing Medical Education to provide continuing medical education for physicians.

The Neuroscience Education Institute designates this educational activity for a maximum of 90.0 *AMA PRA Category 1 Credits*™. Physicians should only claim credit commensurate with the extent of their participation in the activity.

Activity Instructions

This CME activity is in the form of a printed book and incorporates instructional design to enhance your retention of the information and pharmacological concepts presented. You are advised to go through the figures in this activity from beginning to end, followed by the text, and then complete the posttests and evaluations. The estimated time for completion of this activity is 90 hours.

Instructions for CME Credit

Certificates of CME credit or participation are available for each topical section of the book (total of twelve sections). To receive a section-specific certificate, please complete the relevant posttest (you must score at least 70% to receive credit) and section evaluation available online only at http://www.neiglobal.com/ep3. If a score of 70% or more is attained, you can immediately print your certificate. There is a fee for each certificate (varies per section).

NEI Disclosure Policy

It is the policy of the Neuroscience Education Institute to ensure balance, independence, objectivity, and scientific rigor in its educational activities. The Neuroscience Education Institute takes responsibility for the content, quality, and scientific integrity of this CME activity.

All faculty participating in any NEI-sponsored educational activity and all individuals in a position to influence or control content development are required by NEI to disclose to the activity audience any financial relationships or apparent conflicts of interest that may have a direct bearing on the subject matter of the activity. Although potential conflicts of interest are identified and resolved prior to the activity, it remains for the audience to determine whether outside interests reflect a possible bias in either the exposition or the conclusions presented.

Neither the Neuroscience Education Institute nor Stephen M. Stahl, MD, PhD has received any funds or grants in support of this educational activity.

Individual Disclosure Statements

Authors/Developers
Stephen M. Stahl, MD, PhD
Adjunct Professor, Department of Psychiatry
University of California, San Diego School of Medicine, San Diego, CA

Dr. Stahl has been a consultant, board member, or on the speakers bureau for the following pharmaceutical companies within the last three years: Acadia, Alkermes, Amylin, Asahi Kasei, Astra Zeneca, Avera, Azur, Biovail, Boehringer Ingelheim, BristolMyers Squibb, Cephalon, CSC Pharmaceuticals, Cyberonics, Cypress Bioscience, Dainippon,

Eli Lilly, Forest, GlaxoSmithKline, Janssen, Jazz Pharmaceuticals, Labopharm, Lundbeck, Neurocrine Biosciences, NeuroMolecular, Neuronetics, Novartis, Organon, Pamlab, Pfizer, Pierre Fabre, sanofi-aventis, Schering-Plough, Sepracor, Shire, SK Corporation, Solvay, Somaxon, Takeda, Tethys, Tetragenix, Vanda Pharmaceuticals, and Wyeth.

Meghan Grady
Director, Content Development
Neuroscience Education Institute, Carlsbad, CA
No other financial relationships to disclose.

Editorial and Design Staff
Nancy Muntner
Director, Medical Illustrations
Neuroscience Education Institute, Carlsbad, CA
No other financial relationships to disclose.

Disclosed financial relationships have been reviewed by the Neuroscience Education Institute CME Advisory Board to resolve any potential conflicts of interest. All faculty and planning committee members have attested that their financial relationships do not affect their ability to present well-balanced, evidence-based content for this activity.

Disclosure of Off-Label Use

This educational activity may include discussion of unlabeled and/or investigational uses of agents that are not approved by the U.S. Food and Drug Administration. Please consult the product prescribing information for full disclosure of labeled uses.

Disclaimer

Participants have an implied responsibility to use the newly acquired information from this activity to enhance patient outcomes and their own professional development. The information presented in this educational activity is not meant to serve as a guideline for patient management. Any procedures, medications, or other courses of diagnosis or treatment discussed or suggested in this educational activity should not be used by clinicians without evaluation of their patients' conditions and possible contraindications or dangers in use, review of any applicable manufacturer's product information, and comparison with recommendations of other authorities. Primary references and full prescribing information should be consulted.

Sponsorship Information

Sponsored by Neuroscience Education Institute

Support

This activity is supported solely by the sponsor, Neuroscience Education Institute.

CHAPTER 1

Structure and Function of Neurons

- Varieties of neurons
  - General structure
  - Structure of unique neurons
- Internal operations and the functioning of a neuron
  - Subcellular organelles
  - Protein synthesis
  - Neuronal transport: shipping and receiving molecules and organelles throughout the neuron
- Summary

Neurons are the cells of chemical communication in the brain. Human brains comprise tens of billions of neurons, each linked to thousands of other neurons. Thus, the brain has trillions of specialized connections known as synapses. Neurons have many sizes, lengths, and shapes, which determine their functions. Localization within the brain also determines function. When neurons malfunction, behavioral symptoms may occur. When drugs alter neuronal function, behavioral symptoms may be relieved, worsened, or produced. Thus, this chapter briefly describes the structure and function of normal neurons as a basis for understanding psychiatric disorders and their treatments.

Varieties of neurons

General structure

Although this textbook will often portray neurons with a generic structure (such as that shown in Figure 1-1A and B), the truth is that many neurons have unique structures (see Figures 1-2 through 1-8). All neurons have a cell body, known as the soma, and are set up structurally to receive information from other neurons through dendrites, sometimes via spines on the dendrites, and often through an elaborately branching "tree" of dendrites (Figure 1-1A and B). Neurons are also set up structurally to send information to other neurons via an axon, which forms presynaptic terminals as the axon passes by – "en passant" (Figure 1-1A) – or as it ends (in presynaptic axon terminals) (Figure 1-1A).

Structure of unique neurons

Many neurons in the central nervous system have unique structures. For example, each pyramidal cell has a cell body shaped like a triangular pyramid (Figure 1-2A is a somewhat

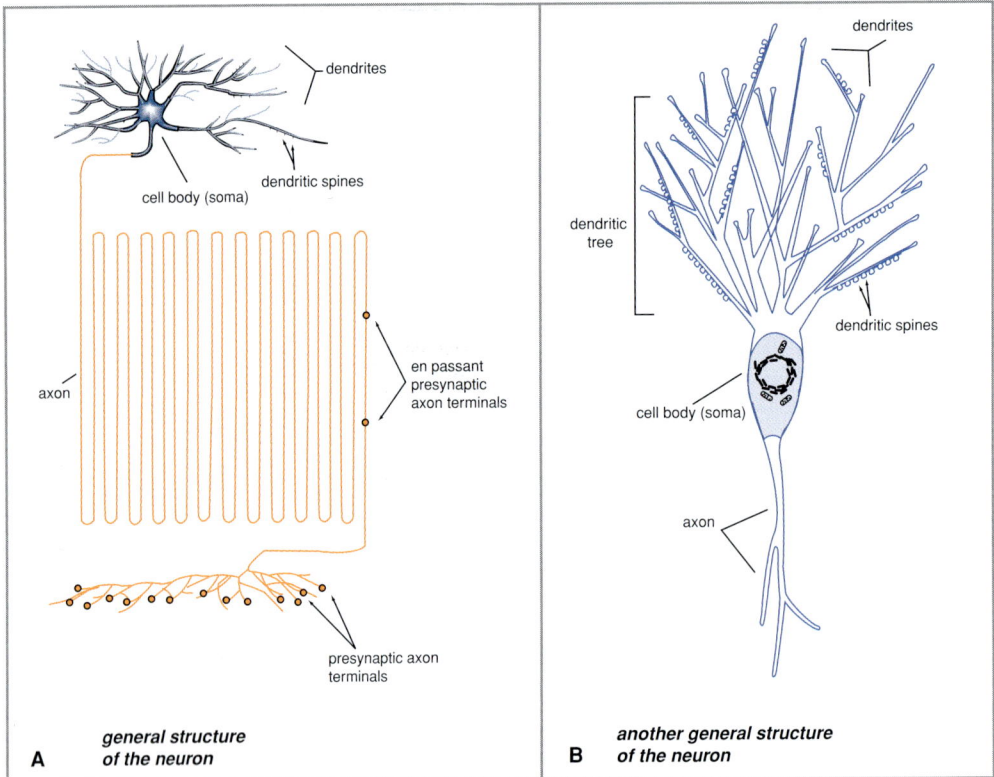

FIGURE 1-1A and B Generic structure of neuron. This is an artist's conception of the generic structure of a neuron. All neurons have a cell body known as the soma, which is the command center of the nerve and contains the nucleus of the cell. All neurons are also set up structurally to both send and receive information. Neurons send information via an axon, which forms presynaptic terminals as it passes by (en passant) or as it ends (**A**). Neurons receive information from other neurons through dendrites, sometimes via spines on the dendrites, and often through an elaborately branching tree of dendrites (**B**). Although all neurons share these properties, they can have unique structures that, in turn, dictate specialized functions.

realistic depiction and 1–2B is an icon of a pyramidal cell); each also has an extensively branched spiny apical dendrite and shorter basal dendrites (Figure 1-2B) as well as a single axon emerging from the basal pole of the cell body. Pyramidal neurons are discussed extensively in this textbook because they make up most of the neurons in the functionally important prefrontal cortex as well as elsewhere in the cerebral cortex. Several other neurons are named for the shape of their dendritic tree. For example, basket cells are so named because they have widely ramified dendritic trees that look rather like baskets (Figure 1-3A is a somewhat realistic depiction and 1–3B is an icon of a basket cell). Basket cells function as interneurons in the cortex, and the wide horizontal spread of their axons can make many local inhibitory contacts with the soma of other cortical neurons. Double bouquet cells are also inhibitory interneurons in the cortex and have a very interesting vertical bitufted appearance, almost like two bouquets of flowers (Figure 1-4A is a somewhat realistic depiction and 1–4B is an icon of a double bouquet cell). Each double bouquet cell has a tight bundle of axons that is also vertically oriented, with varicose collaterals that innervate the dendrites of other cortical neurons, including other double bouquet cells, and supply inhibitory input to those neurons. Spiny neurons, not surprisingly, have spiny-looking dendrites (Figure 1-5A

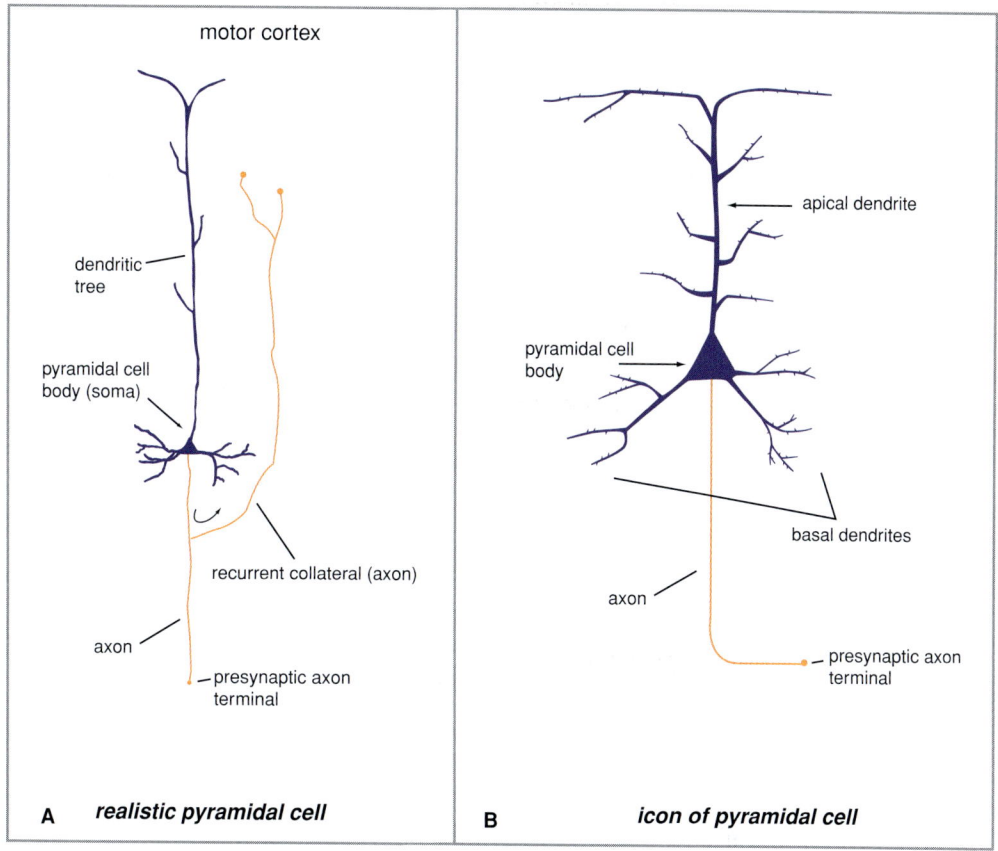

FIGURE 1-2A and B Pyramidal cells. Pyramidal cells (depicted somewhat realistically in **A** and iconically in **B**) have a cell body shaped like a triangular pyramid, an extensively branched spiny apical dendrite, shorter basal dendrites, and a single axon emerging from the basal pole of the cell body. The majority of the neurons in the cerebral cortex, particularly in the prefrontal cortex, are pyramidal neurons.

is a somewhat realistic depiction and 1–5B is an icon of a spiny neuron). Spiny neurons are located in the striatum in large numbers and have a highly ramified dendritic arborization that radiates in all directions and, of course, is densely covered with spines, which receive input from cortex, thalamus, and substantia nigra. Spiny neurons have long axons that either leave the striatum or circle back as recurrent collaterals to innervate neighboring spiny neurons. Finally, Purkinje cells from the cerebellum form a unique dendritic tree that, in fact, looks very much like a real tree (Figure 1-6). This dendritic tree is extensively branched and fans out from an apical position, with a single axon emerging from the basal pole of the cell.

At least one type of neuron is named for its unique axonal structure: the chandelier neuron (Figure 1–7A is a somewhat realistic depiction and 1–7B is an icon of a chandelier neuron). The axons of this cell look like an old-fashioned chandelier, with odd-appearing axon terminals shaped like vertically oriented cartridges, each consisting of a series of axonal swellings linked by thin connecting pieces. Chandelier neurons are yet another type of inhibitory interneuron in the cortex, where the characteristic "chandelier" endings of their axons have a specific function and location – namely, to serve as inhibitory contacts close to the initial segment of axons of pyramidal cells. Thus, chandelier neurons terminate in what

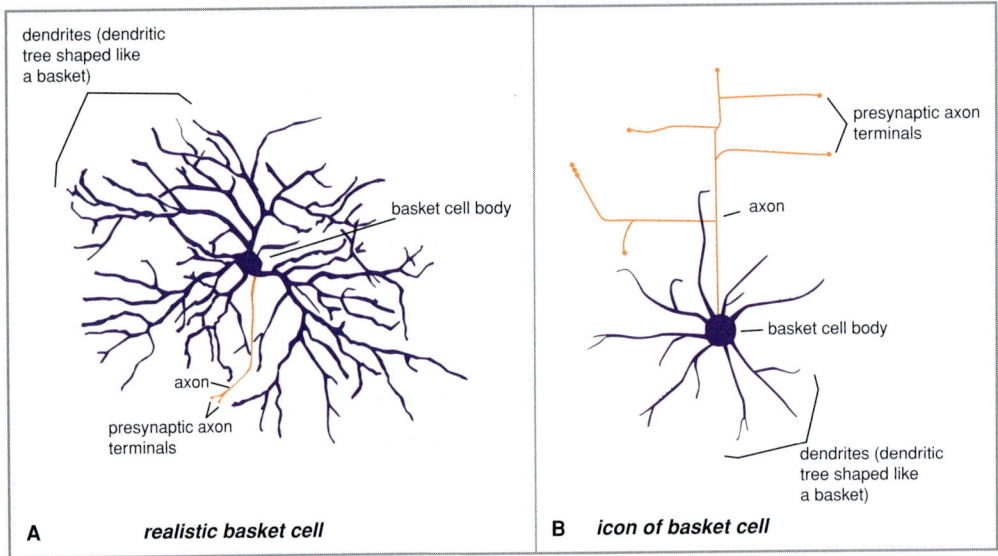

FIGURE 1-3A and B Basket neurons. Basket neurons are named for their widely ramified dendritic trees, which resemble baskets (depicted somewhat realistically in **A** and iconically in **B**). They are cortical interneurons with axons that spread horizontally to make many inhibitory contacts with the soma of other neurons.

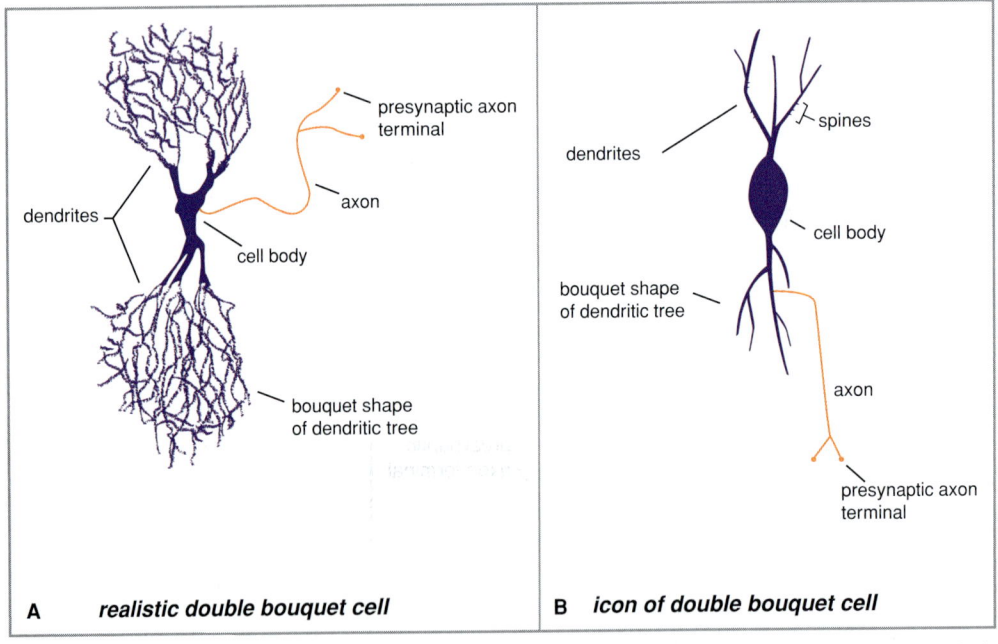

FIGURE 1-4A and B Double bouquet cells. Double bouquet cells are so called because of their vertical bitufted appearance, which resembles two bouquets of flowers (depicted somewhat realistically in **A** and iconically in **B**). Like basket neurons, double bouquet cells are inhibitory interneurons in the cortex. They have a tight bundle of axons that is oriented vertically, with varicose collaterals that innervate the dendrites of other cortical neurons, including other double bouquet cells.

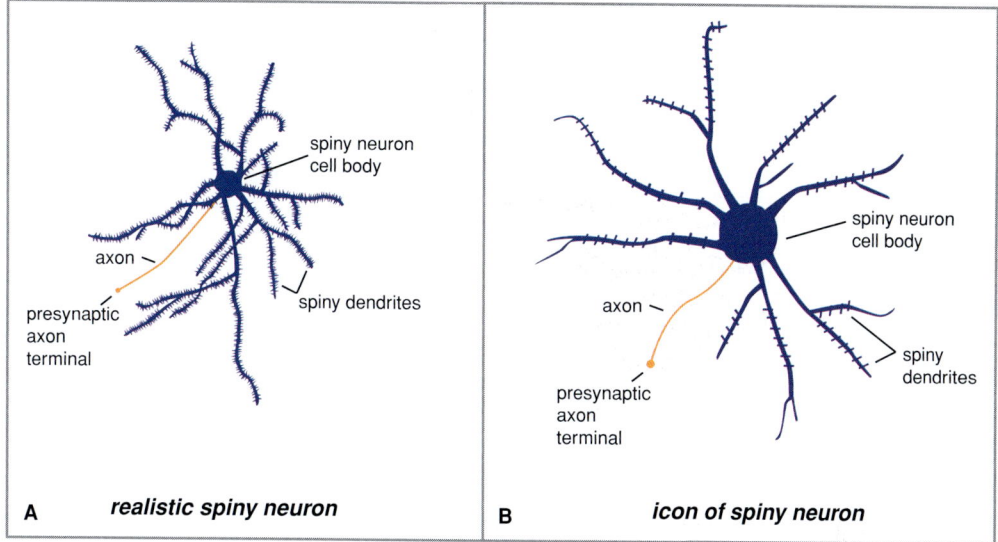

FIGURE 1-5A and B Spiny neurons. The dendrites of spiny neurons radiate in all directions and are densely covered with spines (depicted somewhat realistically in **A** and iconically in **B**). Spiny neurons are located in the striatum in large numbers and receive input from cortex, thalamus, and substantia nigra. The axons of spiny neurons are long and either leave the striatum or circle back as recurrent collaterals to innervate neighboring spiny neurons.

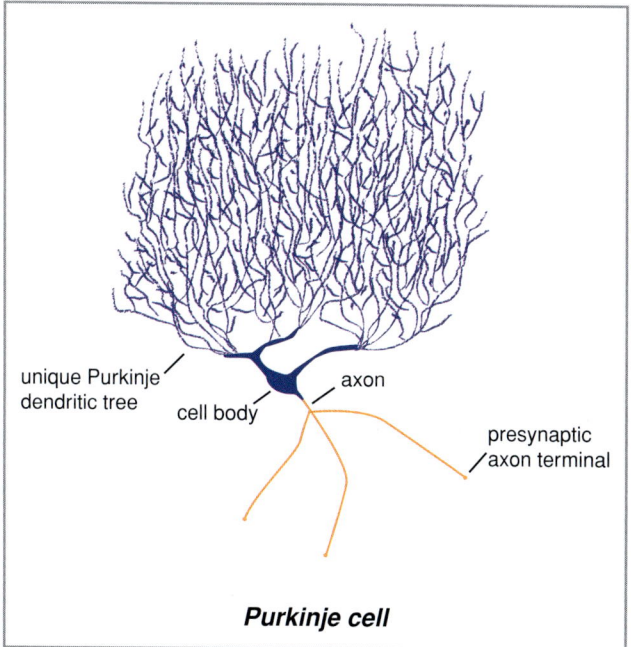

FIGURE 1-6 Purkinje cells. Purkinje cells from the cerebellum have extensively branched dendritic trees fanning out from an apical position, with a single axon emerging from the basal poll of the cell.

is called an axoaxonic synapse. Since the initial segment of a pyramidal cell's axon is the most influential location in determining whether that axon will fire or not, the chandelier neuron can potentially provide the most powerful inhibitory input to a pyramidal neuron, possibly even being able to completely shut down a pyramidal cell's firing. Many chandelier

Structure and Function of Neurons | 5

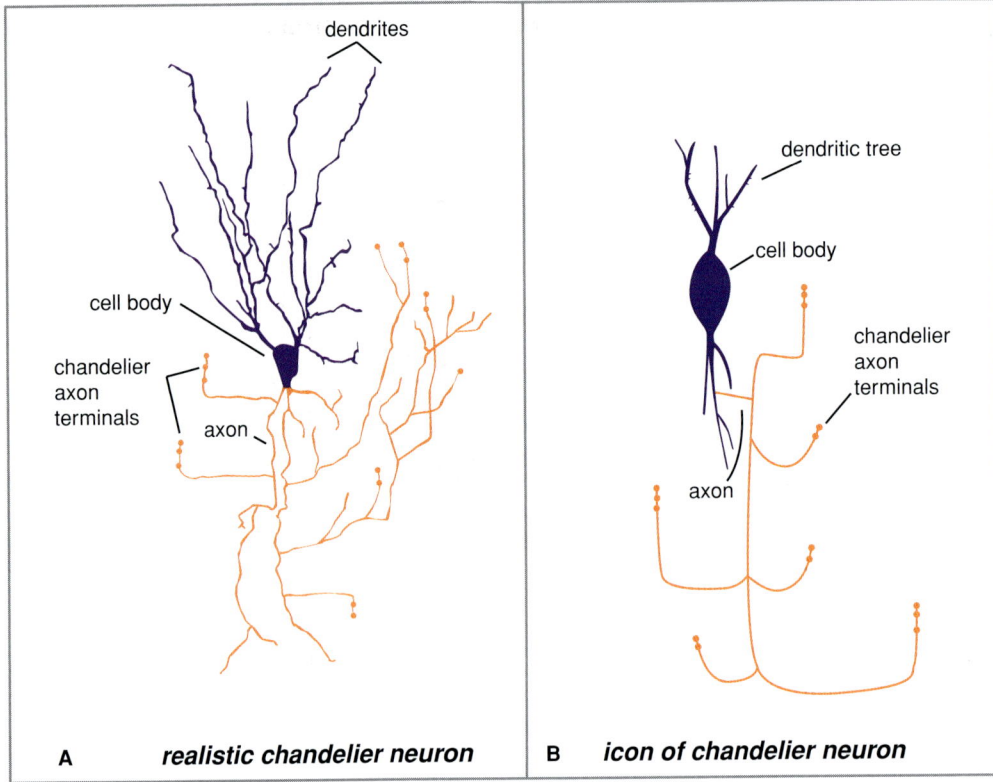

FIGURE 1-7A and B Chandelier neurons. The chandelier neuron is named for its unique axonal structure (depicted somewhat realistically in **A** and iconically in **B**). The axons resemble an old-fashioned chandelier with axon terminals shaped like vertically oriented cartridges, each consisting of a series of axonal swellings linked together by thin connecting pieces. Like basket neurons and double bouquet cells, chandelier neurons are inhibitory interneurons in the cortex. The "chandelier" endings of their axons come into close contact with the initial segments of pyramidal cell axons, forming what is called an axoaxonic synapse. The chandelier neuron can potentially provide powerful inhibitory input to a pyramidal neuron via this synapse, possibly even completely shutting down a pyramidal cell's firing. Many chandelier neurons provide input to a given pyramidal cell, and each chandelier neuron can provide input to several pyramidal cells.

neurons provide input to a given pyramidal cell, and each chandelier neuron can provide input to several pyramidal cells.

Internal operations and the functioning of a neuron

Subcellular organelles

In order to do its duties, the neuron contains various internal working parts that have specialized functions, from subcellular organelles and protein synthetic machinery to internal superhighways for transport of these materials into dendrites and axons on specialized molecular "motors." Specific neuronal functions are associated with each anatomical zone of a neuron (Figure 1-8). For example, the soma and dendrites together form the somatodendritic zone, which has the function of "reception." Neurons receive a wide variety of signals, sometimes simultaneously and sometimes sequentially, from other neurons, environment, chemicals, hormones, light, drugs, and so on. In addition to receiving this mass of incoming information, the somatic zone also serves as a "chemical integrator" of it all. It does this

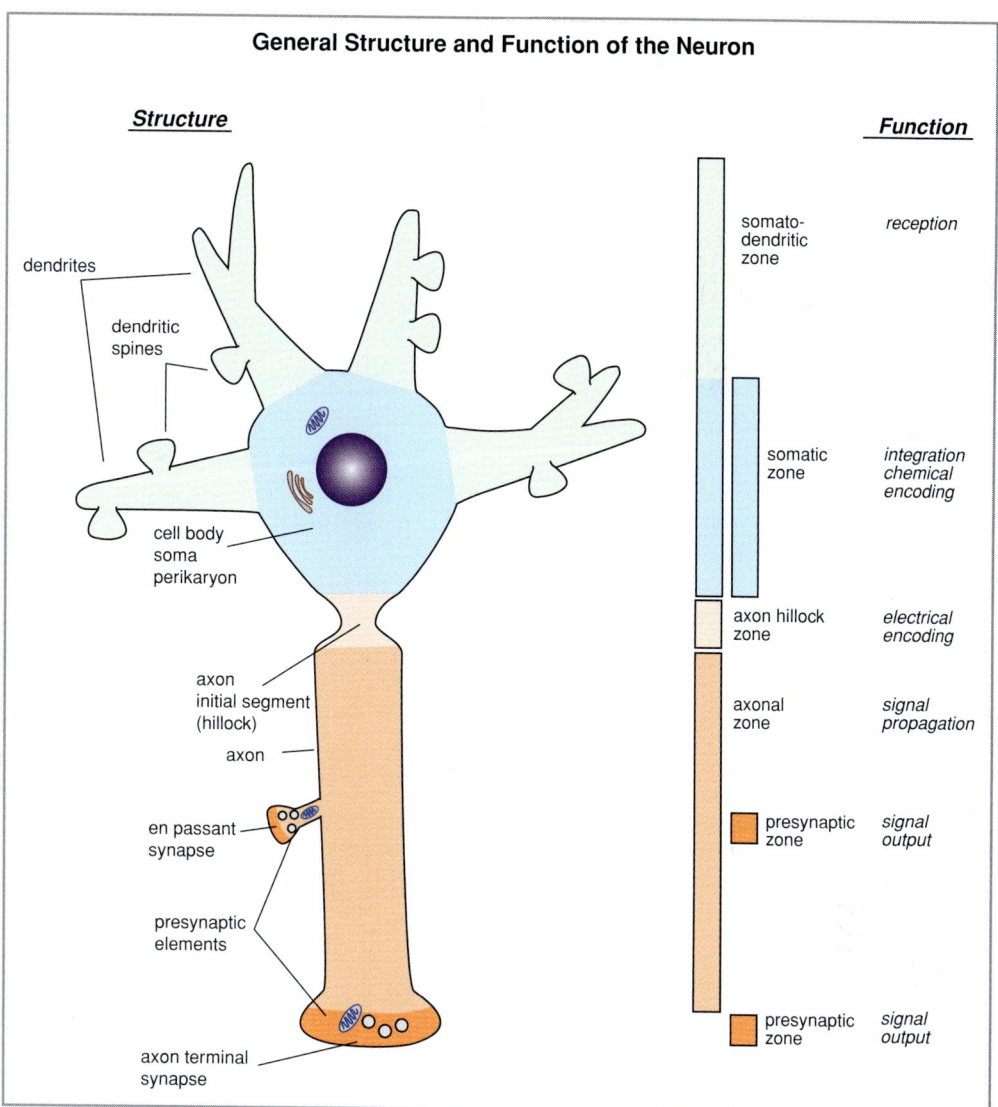

FIGURE 1-8 Anatomic zones of neurons. The different anatomic zones of neurons are associated with specific functions, as shown here. The soma and dendrites form the somatodendritic zone, which has the function of receiving a wide variety of signals from other neurons. The somatic zone also serves as a chemical integrator of incoming information: incoming signals from postsynaptic dendrites are decoded by the genome (located in the cell nucleus in the soma), which then encodes chemical signals destined for either internal or external communication. The initial segment of the axon, the axon hillock, serves as an electrical integrator, controlling whether or not the neuron will fire in response to incoming electrical information. The axon propagates these signals, with electrical signals traveling along the membrane of the axon and chemical signals traveling within its internal structural matrix. The presynaptic zone at the end of the axon contains unique structures that convert chemical and electrical signals into signal output.

by first generating cascades of incoming chemical signals from its postsynaptic dendrites, which speak directly with its genome, located in the cell nucleus in the soma (Figure 1-8). These incoming volleys of chemical information are then decoded and read by the genome, after which the genome adds its own reaction to this information by encoding chemical

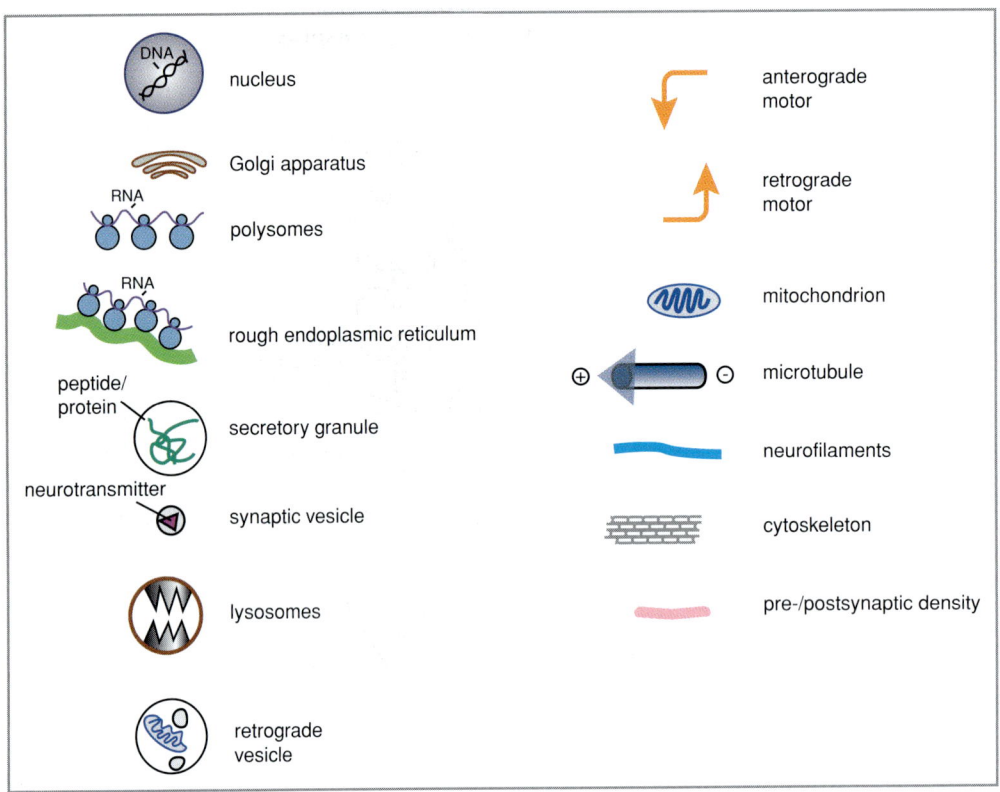

FIGURE 1-9 Neuronal components. Depicted here are many neuronal components manufactured by the cell nucleus, which contains the neuron's DNA. These components are located in specific locations within the neuron and have specific functions.

signals destined either for internal communication within its own neuronal boundaries or for external communication via its neuronal connections.

Another anatomical zone is that of the axon hillock, also called the axon's initial segment (Figure 1-8). Its job is to serve as an "electrical integrator" of all the incoming electrical information and decide whether or not to "fire" the neuron. Directly connected to the axon hillock is the axon itself, which propagates electrical signals along its membrane and chemical signals within its internal structural matrix. At the end of the axon is a specialized zone with unique structures that allow it to convert the chemical and electrical signals arriving there into signal output to the next neuron.

How does all of this happen? It is done by orchestrating many specialized neuronal instruments to work together in amazing functional harmony – at least when things are working normally. Many components of a functioning neuron are shown in Figure 1-9. A representation of where these components are localized within the neuron is shown in Figure 1-10. These specialized neuronal instruments are put into action in the remaining figures of this chapter (Figures 1-11 through 1-20). The specific roles that these specialized neuronal instruments play in neuronal functioning as shown in these figures are explained briefly here.

As already mentioned, the cell nucleus, containing the neuron's DNA, is located in the neuron's soma and is responsible for manufacturing essentially all the components shown

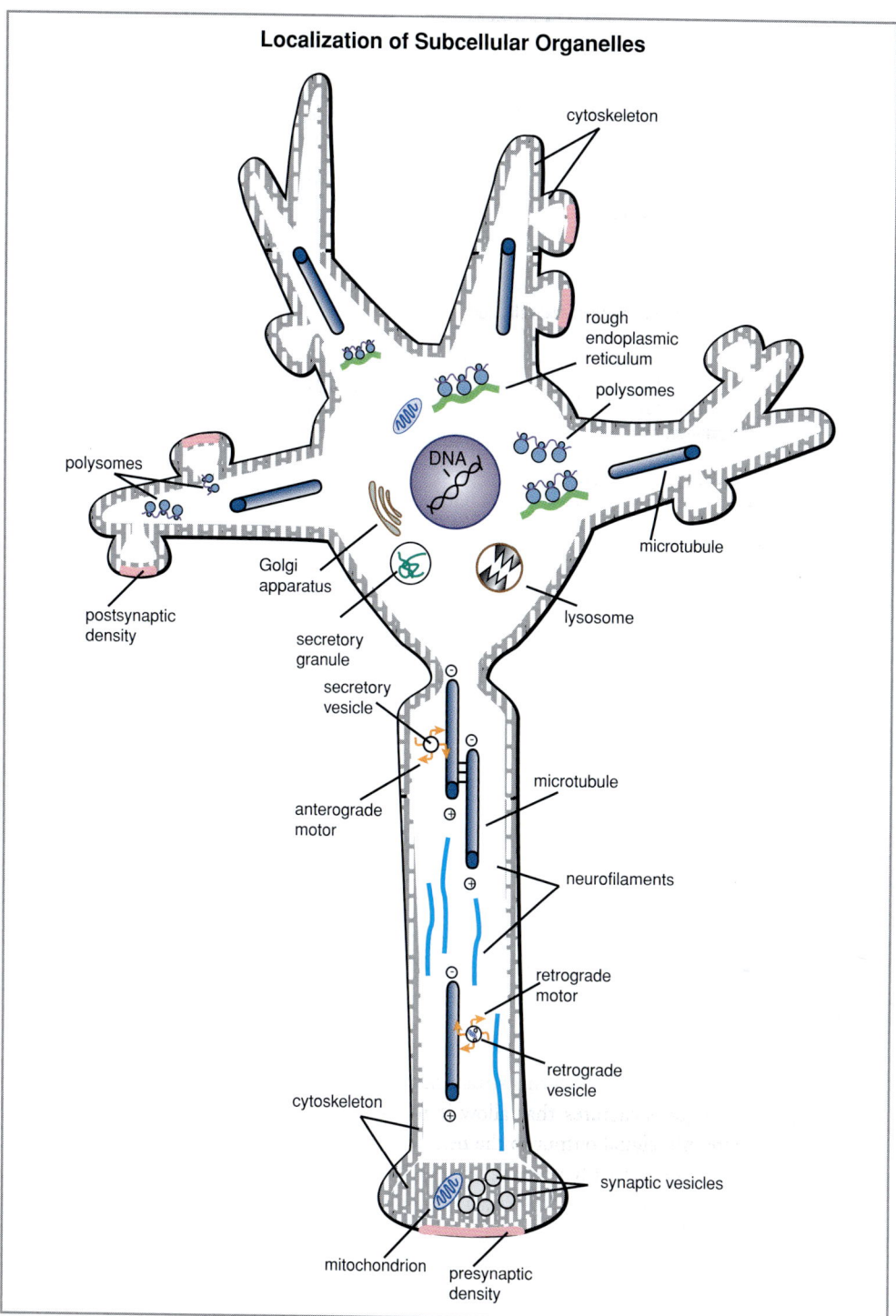

FIGURE 1-10 Localization of neuronal components. The function of each neuronal component is unique; in addition, each component is distributed differently throughout the neuron, as shown here. Thus, different parts of the neuron are associated with different functions. For example, DNA transcription occurs only in the soma, while protein synthesis, which involves polysomes and endoplasmic reticulum, occurs both in the soma and in dendrites.

Structure and Function of Neurons | 9

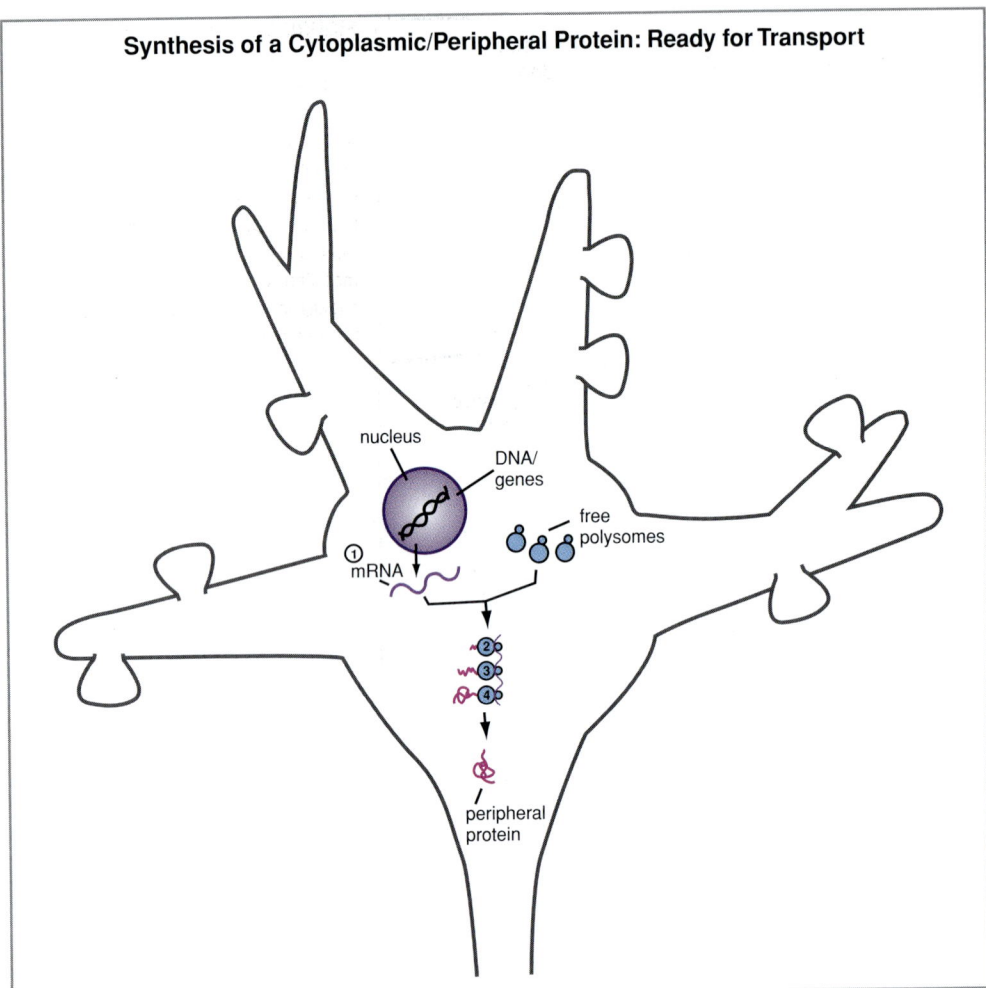

FIGURE 1-11 Protein synthesis. Most of the structural and regulatory molecules of a neuron are proteins. When DNA is transcribed into RNA, it is read by one of two types of ribosomes: free polysomes, which are not membrane bound, or rough endoplasmic reticula, which are membrane bound. Proteins are then synthesized on/within the ribosomes. Peripheral proteins, which are soluble and live in the cytoplasm, are synthesized on free polysomes and transported directly into the dendrites and axons.

in Figures 1-9 and 1-10. As can be seen from Figure 1-10, these components have specific locations within the neuron's specialized structure; therefore some functions occur in one part of the neuron but not another. For example, all the nuclear DNA is transcribed in the soma but all protein synthesis does not occur there, because the synthetic machinery of polysomes and endoplasmic reticulum exists in dendrites as well as the soma but not to any great extent in axons (Figure 1-10). The vital function of transport occurs in both axons and dendrites, but there are more microtubules for transport in dendrites and more neurofilaments for transport in axons (Figure 1-10). Cytoskeletal support proteins exist along the membranes of the entire neuron, but postsynaptic density proteins exist only in dendrites and soma membranes and at the beginning and end of axons, whereas presynaptic density proteins exist only in axon terminals (Figure 1-10).

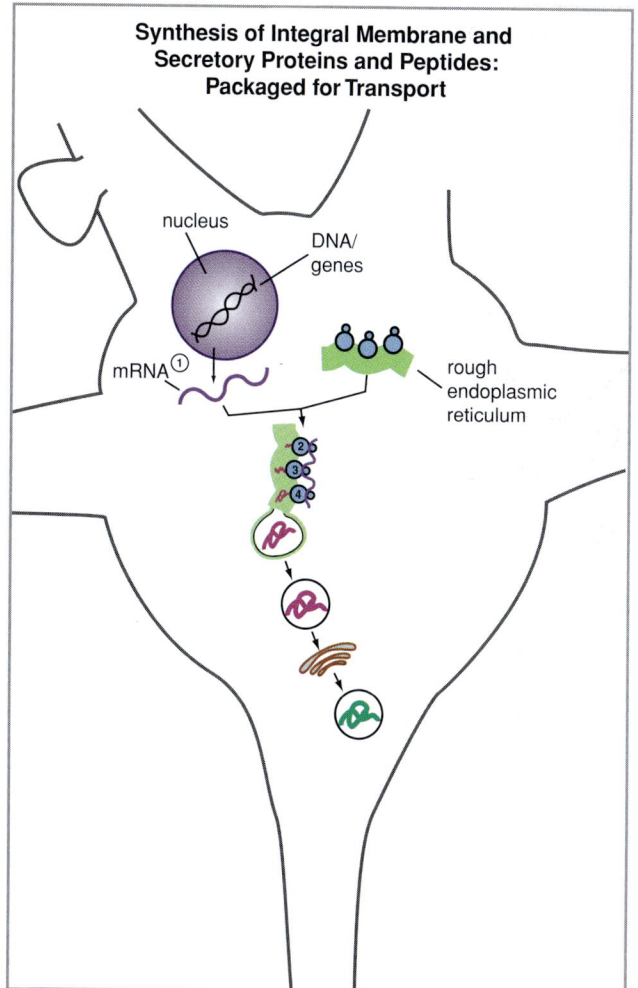

FIGURE 1-12 Peptide synthesis. Integral or secretory proteins, or peptides, are proteins that are inserted into a membrane. They are produced when mRNA is read by the rough endoplasmic reticulum, which synthesizes these proteins and packages them into vesicles to be sent to the Golgi apparatus. The proteins are then modified within the Golgi apparatus and packaged into secretory vesicles ready for transport.

Protein synthesis

Few neuronal functions are more important than the synthesis of proteins, which are produced as the result of gene activation. Because most of the important structural and regulatory molecules of a neuron are proteins, they functionally carry out orders from the genome. For example, proteins become the building blocks when the genome orders a new synapse to be made; proteins are the receptors and enzymes of the neuron; proteins can activate messengers or synthesize anything the neuron needs. Thus, it is no surprise that the neuron is organized so that high priority can be given to making and transporting various proteins.

Proteins are synthesized on a subcellular organelle known as a ribosome. When DNA is transcribed into RNA, the RNA can be read by either of two types of ribosomes in order for proteins to be synthesized. One type are called free polysomes, because they are not membrane-bound. The other type are membrane bound and are called rough endoplasmic reticulum, or "Nissl substance." Protein synthesis occurs predominantly in the soma (Figures 1-11 and 1-12). Proteins that are soluble, and thus live in the cytoplasm, are synthesized on

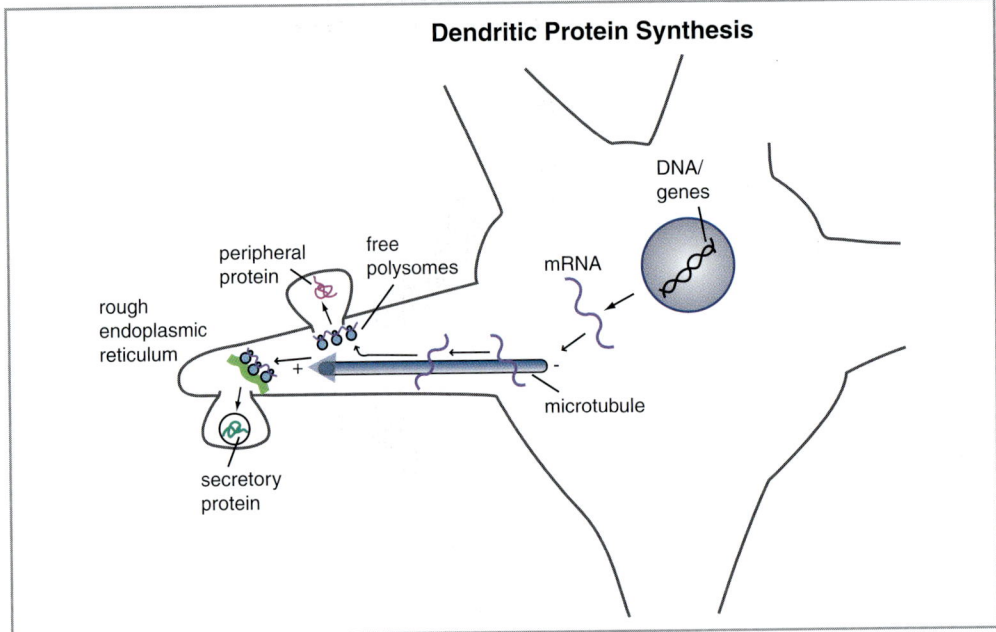

FIGURE 1-13 Dendrite protein synthesis. Most protein synthesis occurs in the soma; however, some protein synthesis occurs in dendrites. mRNA is somehow made accessible, perhaps via microtubules, to free polysomes and rough endoplasmic reticula located near dendritic spines, which then synthesize proteins locally.

free polysomes and then transported directly into dendrites and axons, wherever they are needed (Figure 1-11). These are called peripheral proteins. Proteins that are destined for insertion into a membrane, called integral or secretory proteins or peptides, are synthesized within the rough endoplasmic reticulum, packaged there into vesicles, and shipped to the Golgi apparatus, which modifies and molecularly "decorates" these proteins; finally, they exit the Golgi apparatus in secretory vesicles, ready for transport (Figure 1-12).

Some protein synthesis occurs in dendrites (Figure 1-13). Presumably these proteins are necessary for implementing those specialized functions unique to dendrites, such as receiving information, forming postsynaptic signal reception and signal transduction machinery, and the like. Polysomes are located in dendrites, often close to dendritic spines. RNA formed in the soma is somehow accessible to these polysomes in the dendrites, so that proteins can be synthesized locally where they would be ready for action immediately upon synthesis, as they would not need transport into the dendrite.

Neuronal transport: shipping and receiving molecules and organelles throughout the neuron

Much of the neuron functions like a busy depot. Following the manufacture of protein and organelles, these components must be packaged and shipped. Some must be dispatched with the speed of an "overnight" delivery system (fast transport), whereas others are sent with the deliberation of "snail mail" (slow transport). The various transport systems up and down axons and dendrites form a type of neuronal infrastructure of roads and bridges to get every component where it must go and when it must get there. For example, cytoplasmic proteins are sent into both axons and dendrites by a slow transport system (Figure 1-14). This system is really slow, moving only about 2 mm a day, or 50 to 100 μm an hour. Slow transport motors (indicated by a tortoise carrying the soluble proteins in Figure 1-14) crawl

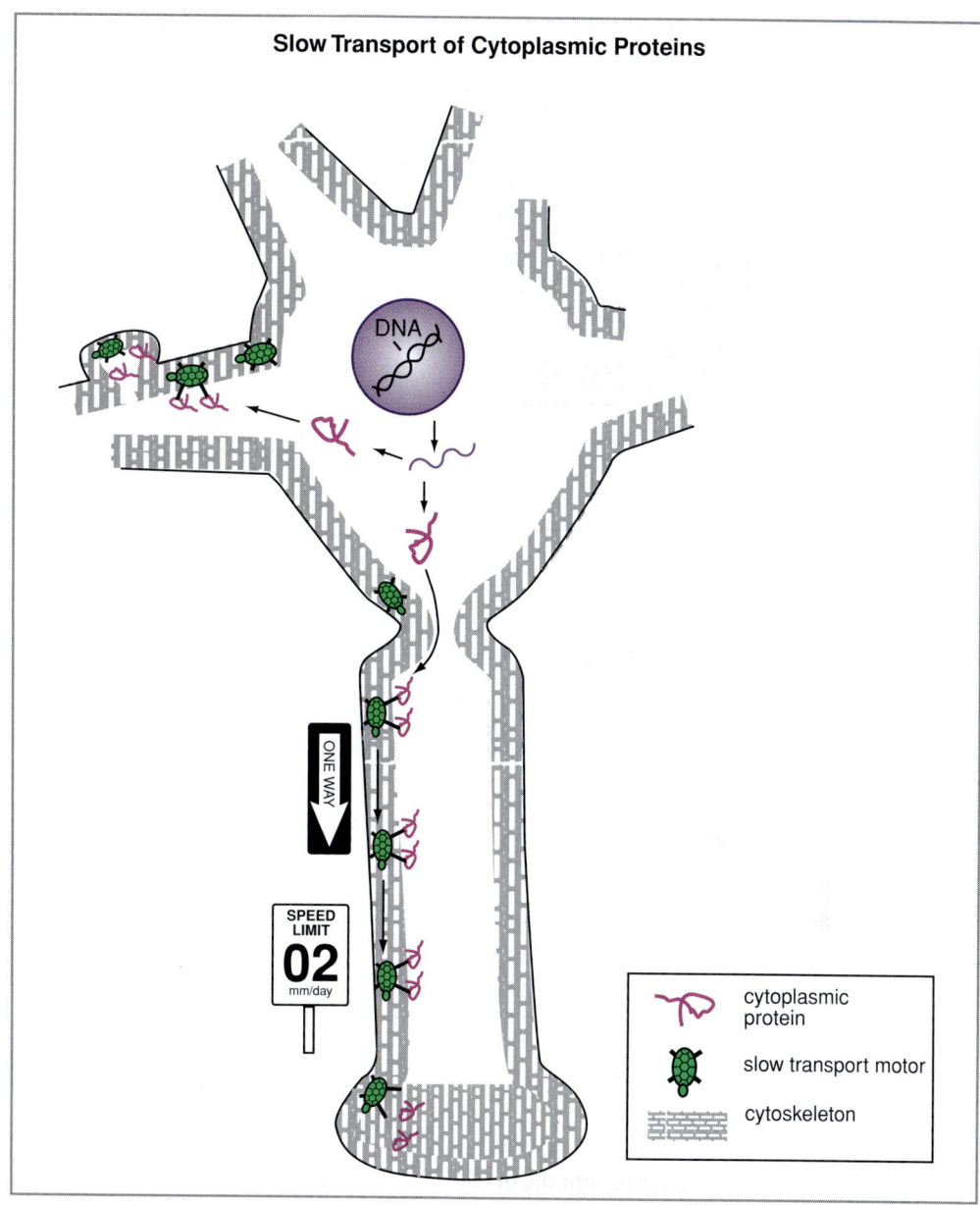

FIGURE 1-14 Slow transport of proteins. Once proteins and organelles have been made, they must be transported to their ultimate destination. This can occur via one of two delivery systems: slow transport or fast transport. Cytoplasmic proteins are sent via slow transport motors (depicted here as tortoises) that crawl along the cytoskeleton at a rate of 2 mm per day, or 50 to 100 μm an hour.

along the cytoskeleton and slowly yet inexorably deliver these proteins to both axonal and cytoplasmic destinations. Interestingly, the infrastructure system itself is also transported via this slow transport system (Figure 1-15). Thus, microtubules are transported slowly into dendrites and axons and neurofilaments are transported into axons (Figure 1-15) to form the very highways upon which other components are rapidly transported through the fast transport systems, which are shown in Figures 1-16 though 1-20.

Structure and Function of Neurons | 13

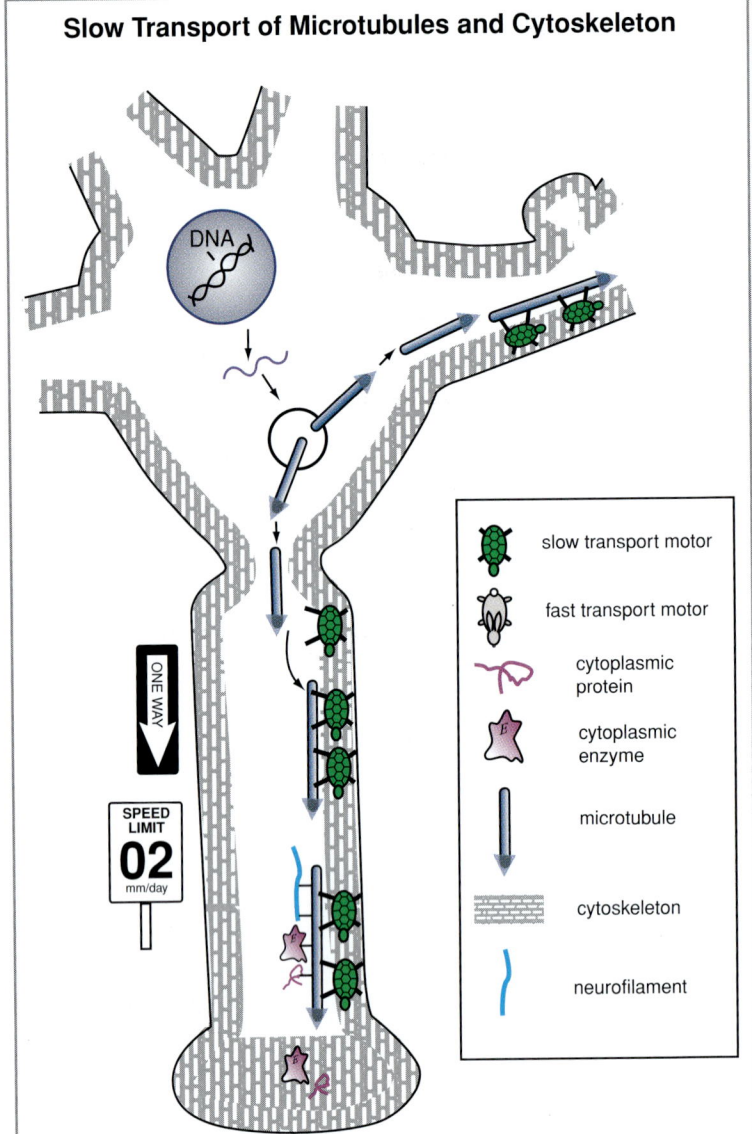

FIGURE 1-15 **Slow transport of microtubules and neurofilaments.** Slow transport is also the delivery system used for moving the organelles involved in fast transport. Thus, microtubules are delivered to dendrites and axons and neurofilaments are delivered to axons via slow transport.

Many neuronal materials are passengers that ride on fast transport systems with fast transport motors, which are shown as hares in Figure 1-17. Such passengers include mitochondria, synaptic vesicles containing neurotransmitters, secretory vesicles containing secretory proteins, and all sorts of other proteins, from receptors to enzymes to ion channels to transport pumps and many more. Transport of these materials allows supplies depleted during the normal conduct of neuronal business by dendrites and axons to be replenished. A fast transport system (indicated by "hares" in Figures 1-17 through 1-20) carries membrane-bound secretory vesicles full of secretory proteins at about 200 mm per day, but only from the soma to the axon terminal, a direction known as "anterograde" and designated in Figure 1-17 as "southbound lanes." There is also transport in the opposite direction, known as "retrograde" and designated in Figure 1-18 as "northbound lanes." However,

14 | Essential Psychopharmacology

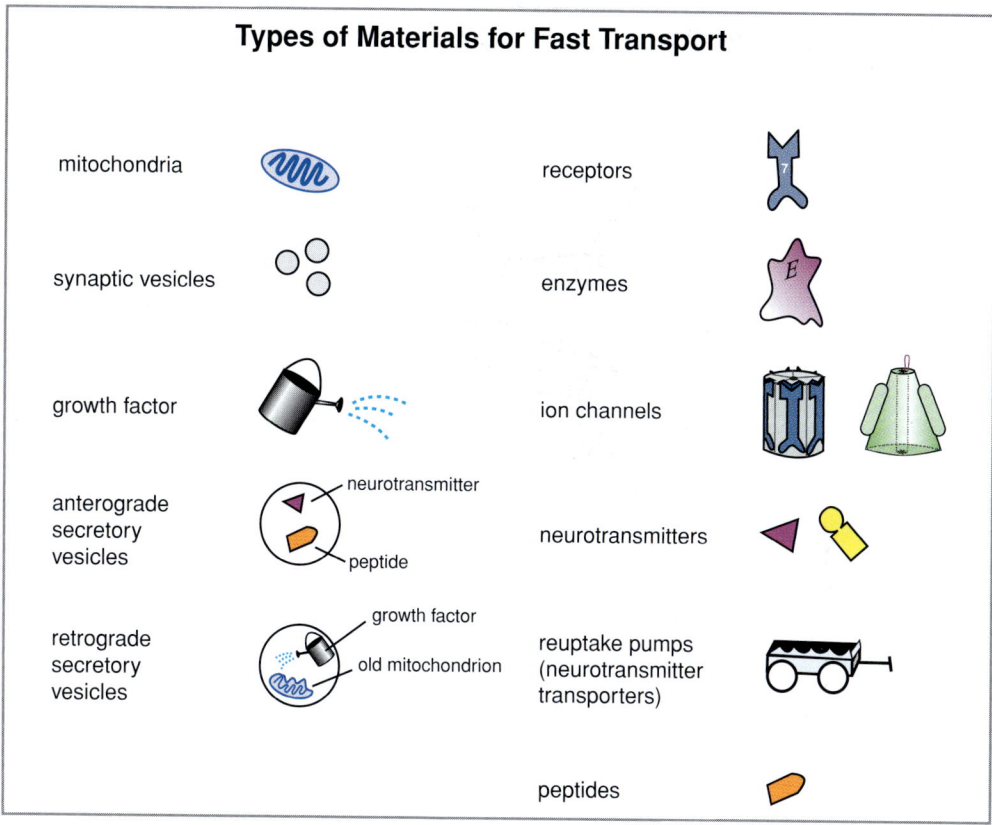

FIGURE 1-16 Materials for fast transport. Passengers of fast transport systems include mitochondria, synaptic vesicles containing neurotransmitters, secretory vesicles containing secretory proteins, receptors, enzymes, ion channels, reuptake pumps, and other proteins.

retrograde transport is about half as fast and includes the return of used and discarded proteins and organelles from the axon terminal, which are shipped up to the soma for destruction in lysosomes. Also, the retrograde system takes up growth factors and viruses from the synapse and sends them up to the soma, where they can signal the genome chemically (Figure 1-18).

Another fast transport system carries the machinery for synthesizing, metabolizing, and utilizing neurotransmitters. In the case of low-molecular-weight neurotransmitters such as monoamines, this includes all of their synthetic machinery, since these neurotransmitters are not only manufactured in the soma and shipped to the axon terminal but are also made locally in the axon terminal from synthetic enzymes shipped there (Figure 1-19). This is important, because the rate of utilization of these neurotransmitters can be greater than the rate at which they can be shipped all the way from the soma, even on a "fast" transport system. Neurotransmitter is thus packaged and stored in the presynaptic neuron in vesicles, like a loaded gun, ready to fire. Since a reuptake pump (monoamine transporter), which can recapture released monoamines, is present on the presynaptic neuron, monoamines used in one neurotransmission can be captured for reuse in a subsequent neurotransmission. This is in contrast to the way in which neuropeptides function in neurotransmission (Figure 1-20). That is, higher-molecular-weight peptides are synthesized only in the soma and are not taken back up into the presynaptic neuron by a reuptake pump. Fortunately, peptide

Structure and Function of Neurons | 15

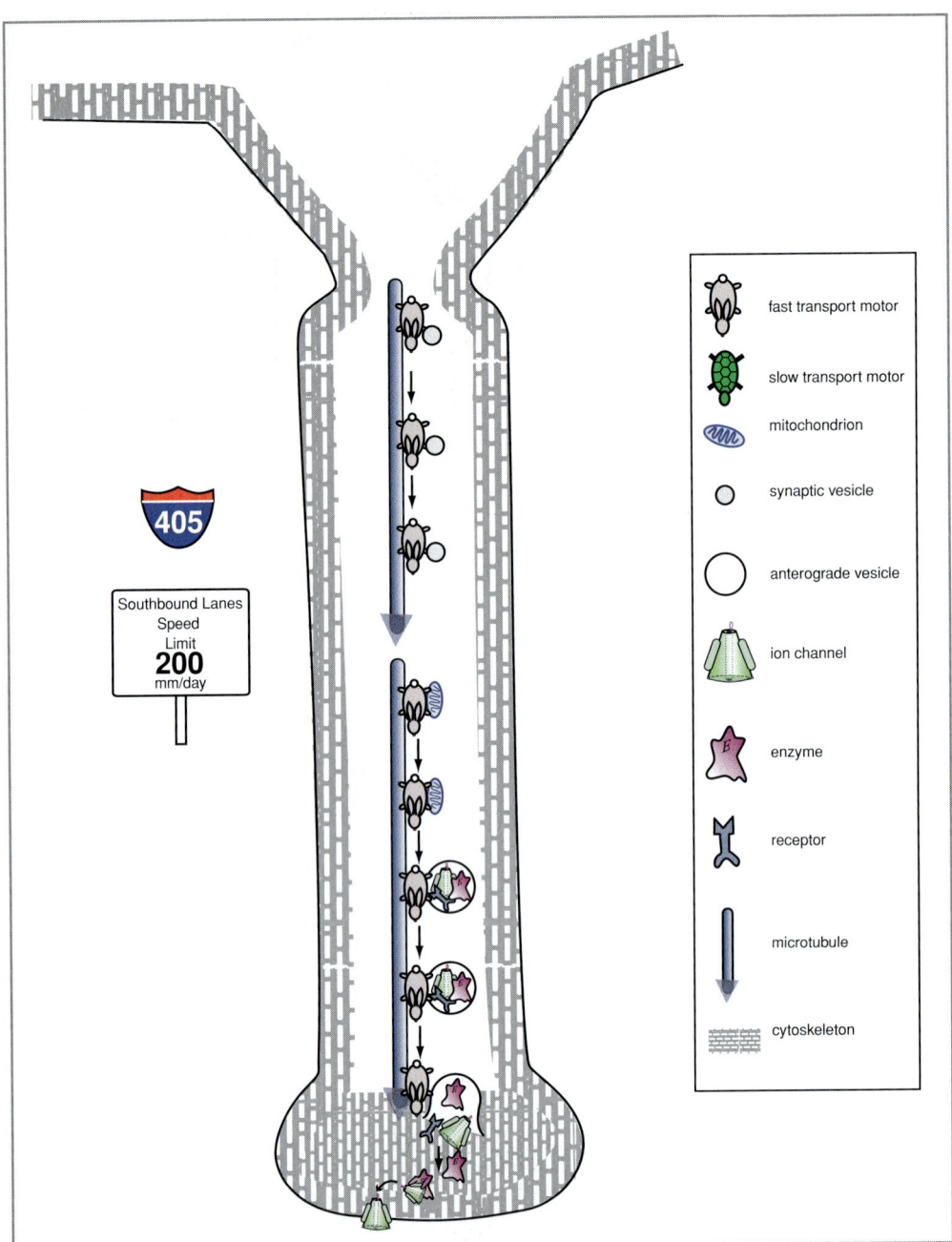

FIGURE 1-17 **Fast anterograde transport.** Shown here is delivery of various neuronal components to their axonal destinations via fast transport. Membrane-bound secretory vesicles full of secretory proteins are transported at a rate of 200 mm per day from the soma to the axon terminal in a direction known as anterograde (depicted here as southbound lanes).

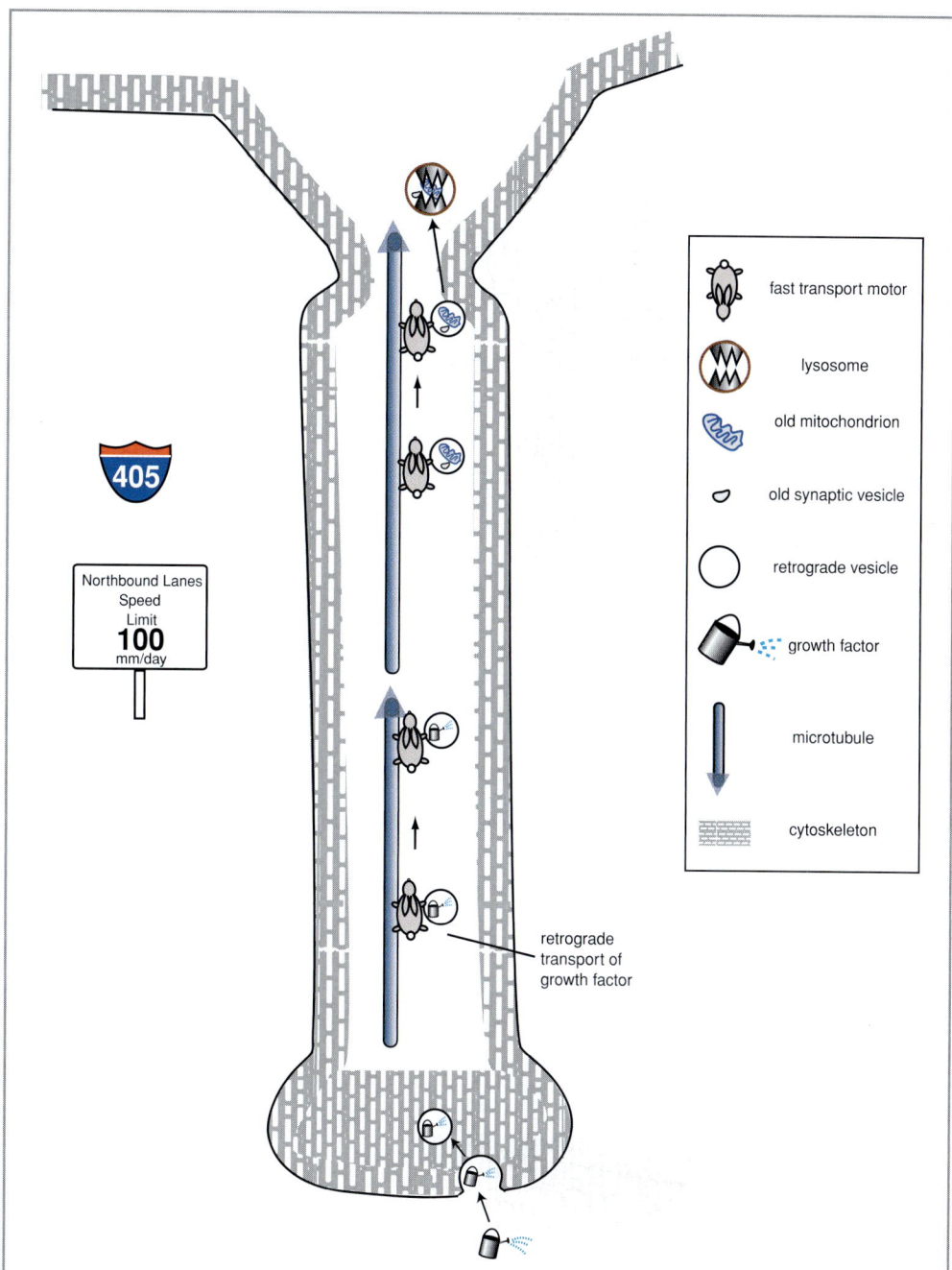

FIGURE 1-18 Fast retrograde transport. Fast transport also occurs in the opposite direction at 100 mm per day; this is known as retrograde transport (designated as northbound lanes here). With retrograde transport, used and discarded proteins and organelles are brought from the axon terminal to the soma, where they are destroyed by lysosomes. In addition, growth factors and viruses from the synapse are sent to the soma, where they can signal the genome chemically.

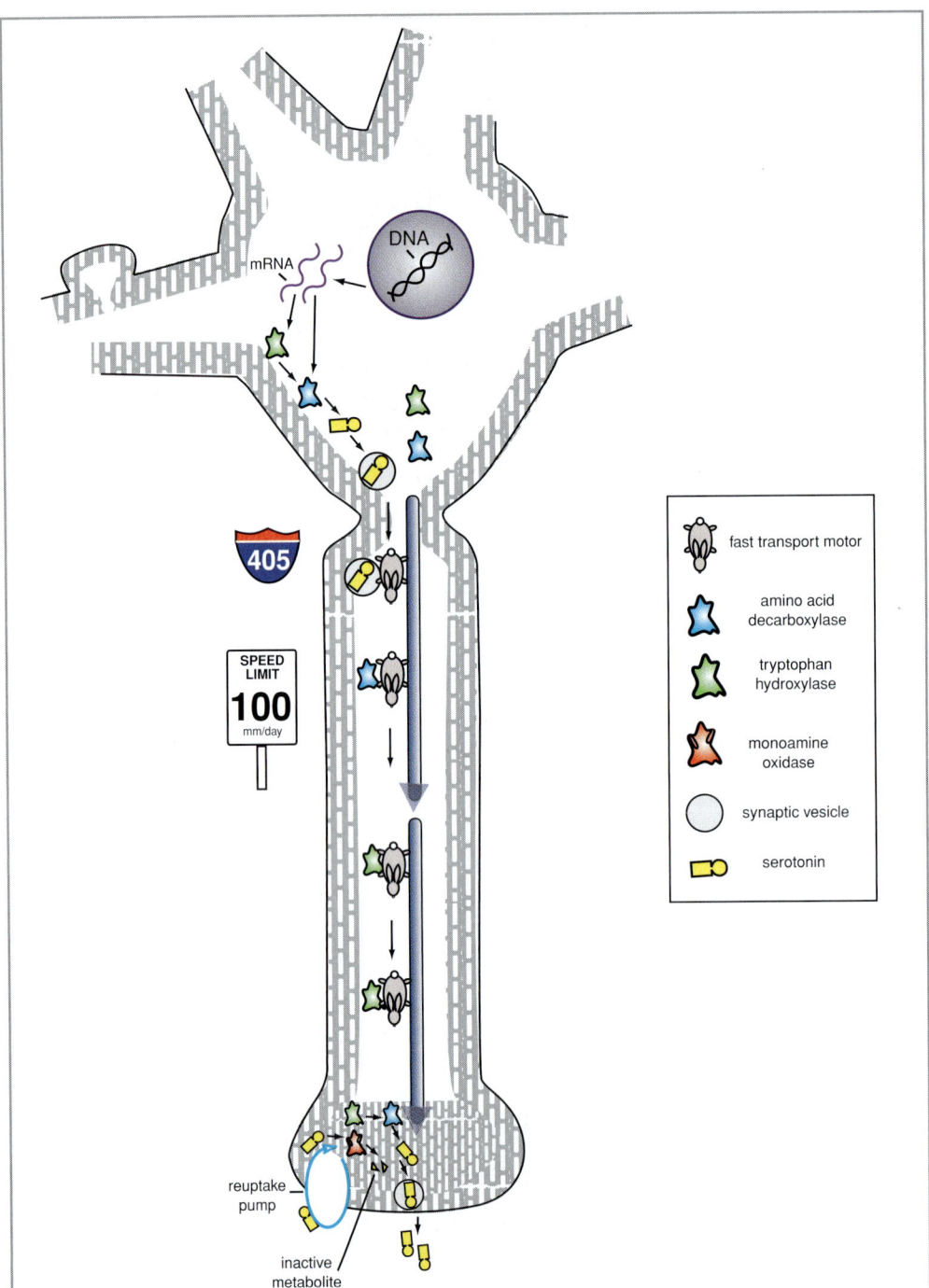

FIGURE 1-19 Fast transport: low-molecular-weight neurotransmitter machinery. Another fast transport system carries the machinery for synthesizing, metabolizing, and utilizing neurotransmitters. Because the synthetic enzymes involved in manufacturing low-molecular-weight neurotransmitters such as monoamines are transported to the axon terminal, these neurotransmitters can be made both in the soma and locally in the axon terminal. In addition, reuptake pumps can recapture released neurotransmitters for reuse in subsequent neurotransmission. This is important because the rate of utilization of these neurotransmitters can be greater than the rate at which they can be shipped from the soma.

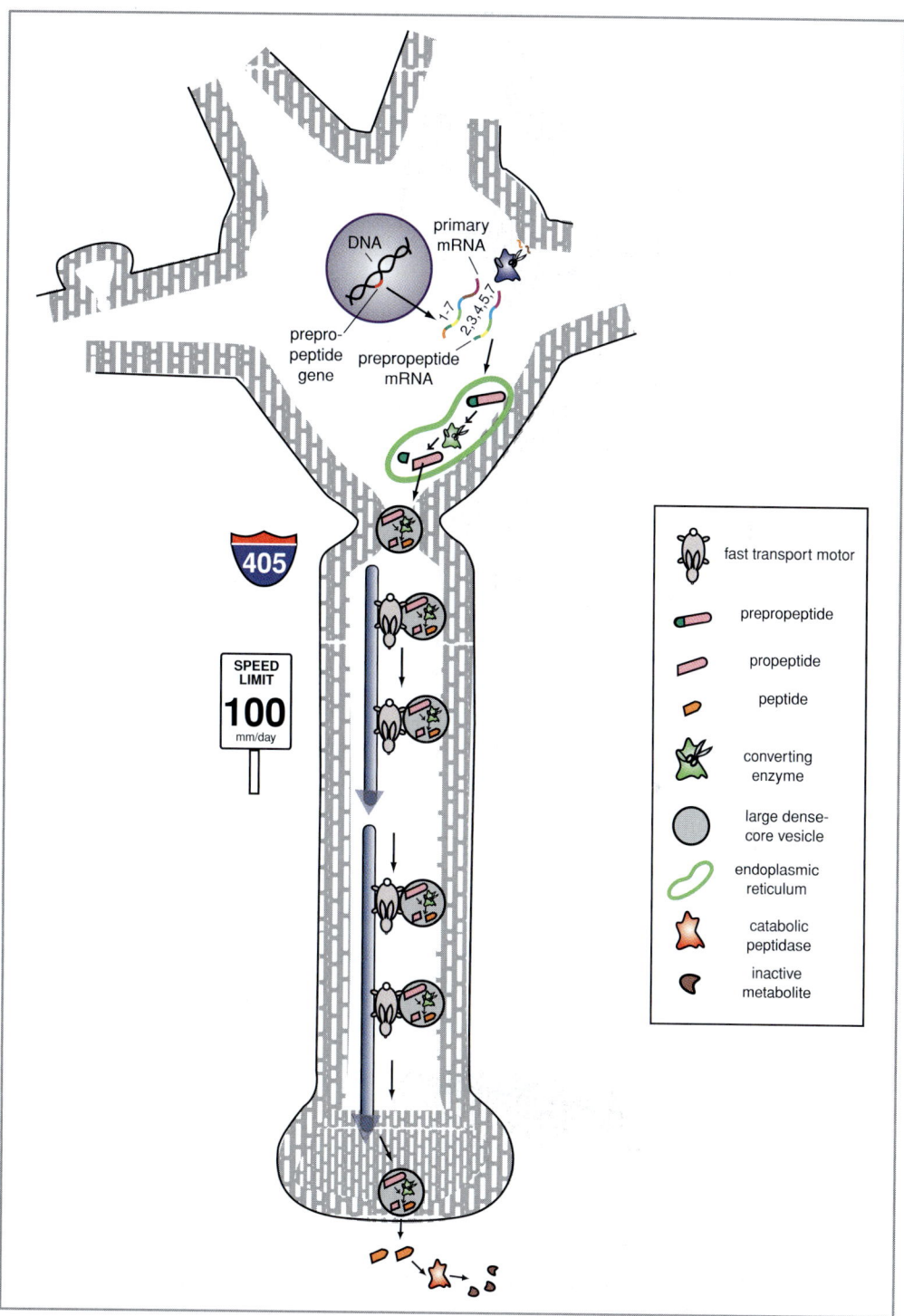

FIGURE 1-20 Fast transport: larger neuropeptide machinery. Unlike low-molecular-weight neurotransmitters, larger neuropeptides are synthesized only in the soma and are not taken back up into the presynaptic neuron by a reuptake pump. However, peptide neurotransmitters are generally released more slowly, allowing transport of these neurotransmitters from the soma in larger dense-core vesicles to keep up with demand.

Structure and Function of Neurons | 19

neurotransmitters are generally released more slowly, so that transport of these neurotransmitters from the soma in larger dense-core vesicles can keep up with demand (Figure 1-20).

Summary

This chapter has described the structure and function of various types of neurons. Although all neurons share some structural similarities, there are many unique aspects to some neurons, including the shapes of their somas, dendritic trees, and axons. This chapter has also reviewed how the various components of a neuron work together to carry out specialized functions, such as synthesis of important neuronal proteins and transport of proteins and other vital supplies throughout the neuron. An understanding of the structure and function of normal neurons can provide a good background for grasping what goes wrong with neurons in various psychiatric disorders and how drugs affect neurons to treat various psychiatric disorders.

CHAPTER 2

Synaptic Neurotransmission and the Anatomically Addressed Nervous System

- Neurodevelopment in the anatomically addressed nervous system
  - Time course of neurodevelopment
  - Neurogenesis
  - Neuronal selection
- Neuronal migration
- Synaptogenesis: directing the axons and arborizing the dendritic trees
- Synaptic plasticity
- Competitive elimination of synapses
- Summary

Modern psychopharmacology is largely the story of chemical neurotransmission. To understand the actions of drugs on the brain, to grasp the impact of diseases on the central nervous system, and to interpret the behavioral consequences of psychiatric medicines, one must be fluent in the language and principles of chemical neurotransmission. The importance of this fact cannot be overstated for the student of psychopharmacology. What follows in the next two chapters will form the foundation for the entire book and the road map for a journey through one of the most exciting topics in science today: the neuroscience of how drugs and disorders act on the central nervous system.

What is neurotransmission? It can be described in many ways: anatomically, chemically, electrically. This chapter (Chapter 2) describes the ***anatomical*** basis of neurotransmission by showing how neurons are the substrates of neurotransmission and how they develop, migrate, form synapses, and demonstrate "plasticity," or the ability to morph and change throughout life. Classically, the central nervous system has been envisioned as a series of "hard-wired" synaptic connections between neurons, not unlike millions of telephone wires within thousands upon thousands of cables. Building on the structural and functional description of neurons in Chapter 1, this chapter emphasizes what is called *the anatomically addressed nervous system*. The anatomically addressed brain is thus a complex wiring diagram, ferrying electrical impulses to wherever the "wire" is plugged in (i.e., at a synapse). Following this discussion, the next chapter (Chapter 3) describes the ***chemical*** basis of neurotransmission by demonstrating how chemical signals are coded, decoded, transduced, and sent along their way.

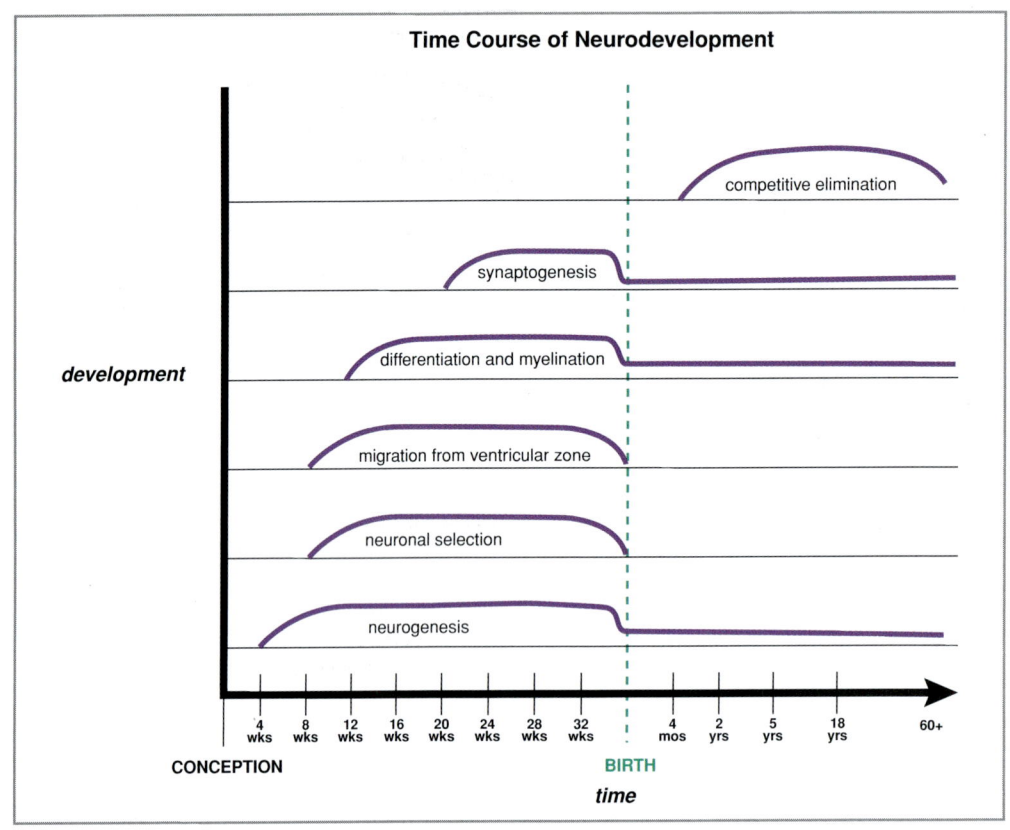

FIGURE 2-1 Time course of neurodevelopment. The time course of brain development is shown here. Most neurogenesis, neuronal selection, and neuronal migration occur before birth, although it has recently been discovered that new neurons can form in some brain areas even in adults. After birth, differentiation and myelination of neurons as well as synaptogenesis continue throughout a lifetime. Brain restructuring also occurs throughout life, but is most active during childhood and adolescence in a process known as competitive elimination.

Neurodevelopment in the anatomically addressed nervous system

Time course of neurodevelopment

Understanding of human brain development is advancing at a rapid pace. Most neurons are formed and the survivors selected by the end of the second trimester of prenatal gestation (Figures 2-1 and 2-2). Neuronal migration starts within weeks of conception and is largely complete by birth. Thus, human brain development is much more dynamic before than after birth, with the brain's volume reaching 95% of its adult size by age 5. On the other hand, several processes affecting brain structure persist throughout a lifetime. Myelination of axon fibers and branching or arborization of neurons into their treelike structures continue vigorously at least throughout adolescence and to a lesser degree throughout life. Brain restructuring also appears to occur throughout a lifetime, but it is most active during childhood and adolescence in a process known as competitive elimination of synapses (Figures 2-1 and 2-2). After an early burst, synaptogenesis seemingly occurs steadily thereafter. Recently, it has been discovered that the formation of new neurons also continues to occur in some brain areas (Figures 2-1 through 2-4). This is remarkable, since neurogenesis until recently was thought not to occur in adult humans. Both the neuron and its synapses are

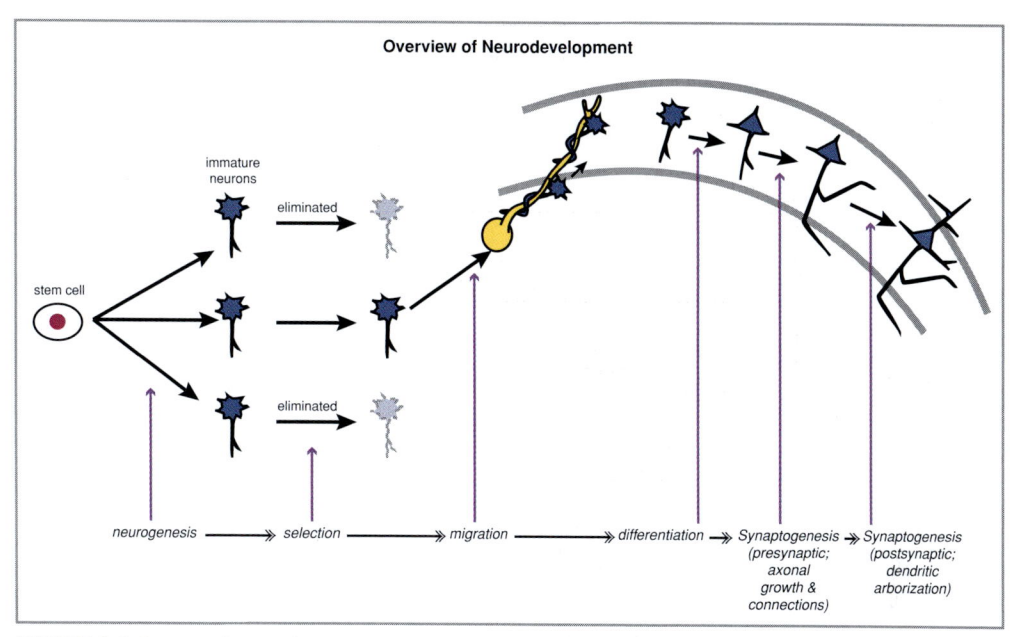

FIGURE 2-2 Process of neurodevelopment. The process of brain development is shown here. After conception, stem cells differentiate into immature neurons. Those that are selected migrate and then differentiate into different types of neurons, after which synaptogenesis occurs.

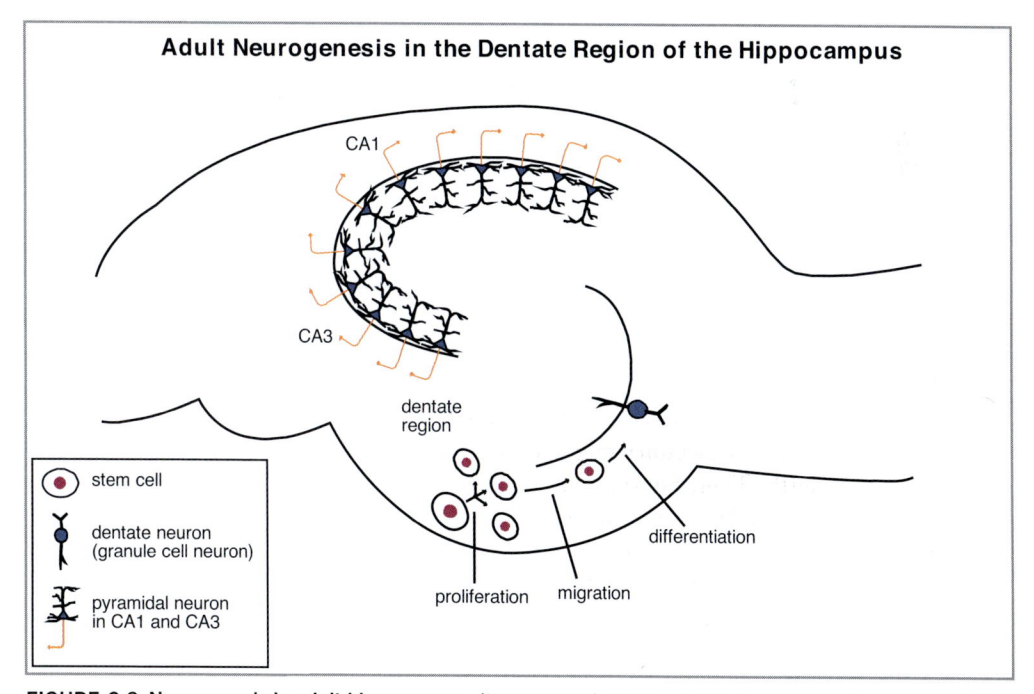

FIGURE 2-3 Neurogenesis in adult hippocampus. It was recently discovered that neurogenesis can occur in the adult brain. It occurs in two specific regions: the dentate gyrus of the hippocampus and the olfactory bulb. As shown here, neuronal precursors in the subgranular zone of the hippocampus proliferate, migrate, and differentiate into new functioning neurons.

Synaptic Neurotransmission and the Anatomically Addressed Nervous System | 23

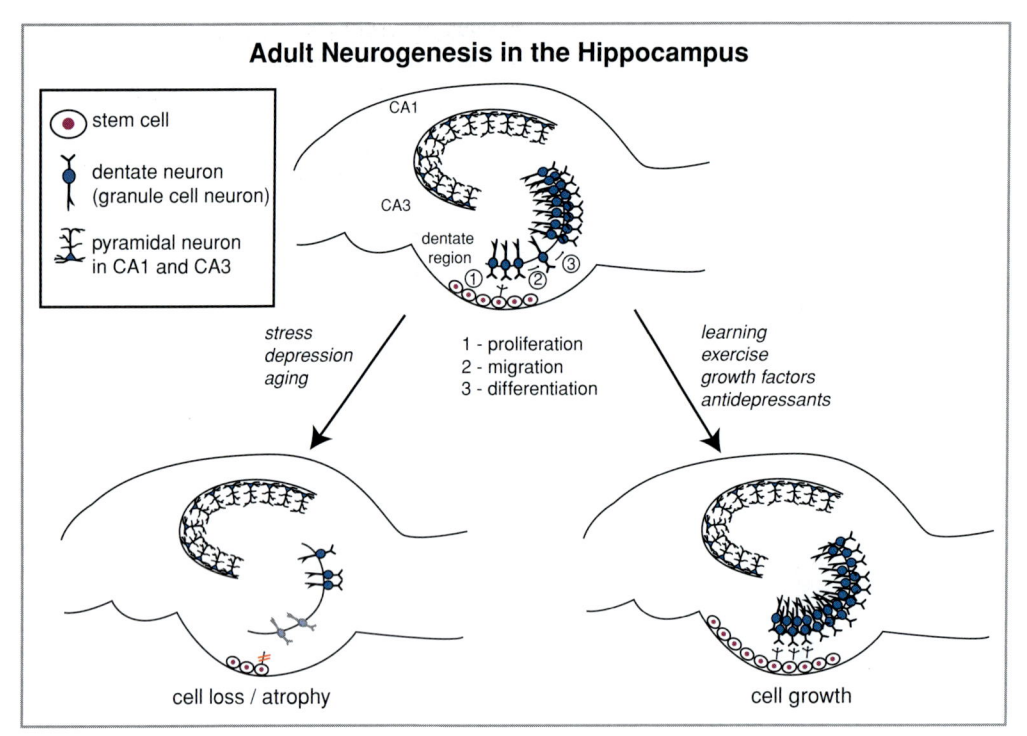

FIGURE 2-4 Neurogenesis in adult hippocampus. Learning, exercise, endogenous growth factors, psychotherapy, and even antidepressants and other psychopharmacological agents can help promote adult neurogenesis in the hippocampus. On the other hand, cell loss or atrophy may occur as a result of stress, depression, and aging.

quite "plastic" – changeable and malleable – more so earlier in life but to a certain extent forever.

Neurogenesis
Neurogenesis begins after conception with embryonic stem cells differentiating into immature neurons (Figures 2-1 and 2-2). In adults, this continues from adult stem cells, but only in two evolutionarily primitive regions: the hippocampal dentate gyrus from neuronal precursors in the subgranular zone (Figure 2-3) and the olfactory bulb from neuronal precursors in the subventricular zone. The hippocampus appears to be an area of the brain that is particularly sensitive and vulnerable to the ravages of stress, aging, and disease (Figure 2-4), so it is a good thing that this site is endowed with the ability to restore itself through the production, migration, and differentiation of precursor cells into new functioning neurons (Figures 2-3 and 2-4). Neurogenesis in the hippocampus may be stimulated through learning, psychotherapy, exercise, endogenous growth factors, and even certain psychopharmacologic agents (Figure 2-4).

The loss of synapses with or without the loss of neurons could also be triggered in other areas of the brain by the same factors that affect the hippocampus, such as stress, depression, aging, and neurodegeneration (compare Figures 2-5 and 2-6). One strategy to deal with this is to promote the production of endogenous growth factors to rescue ailing neurons before they actually die, and to do this with interventions such as learning, exercise, psychotherapy, and antidepressants and other psychopharmacologic drugs (Figure 2-7). If it

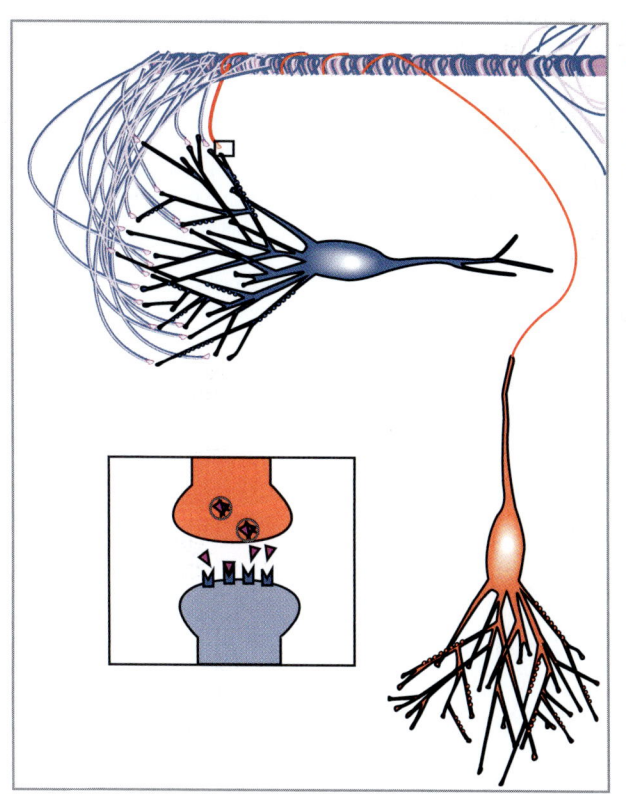

FIGURE 2-5 Normal synaptic connection. Shown here is a normal synaptic connection allowing normal communication between two healthy neurons, with the synapse between the red and blue neuron magnified.

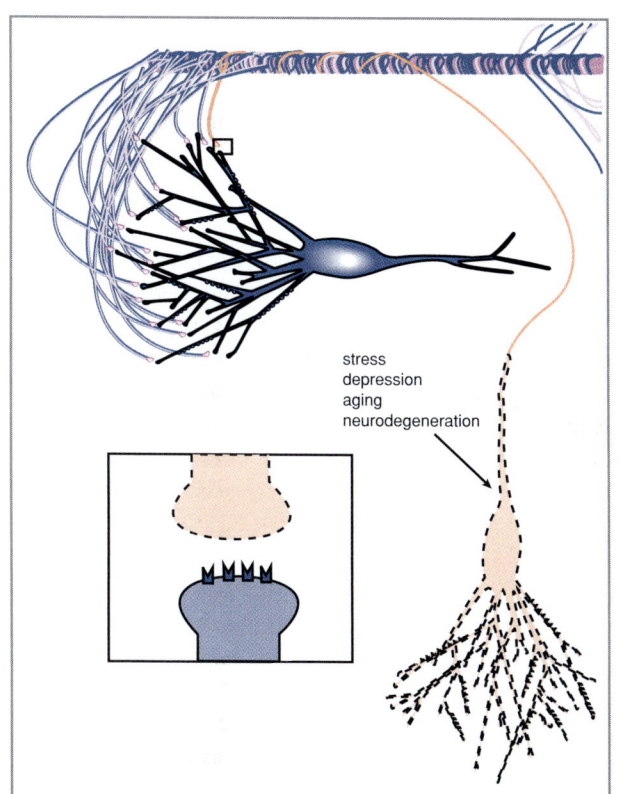

FIGURE 2-6 Synapse loss. Stress, depression, aging, and neurodegeneration can lead to the loss of synapses with or without the loss of neurons in any area of the brain. In contrast to the healthy neuron in Figure 2-5, the red neuron depicted here is no longer functioning to allow normal neurotransmission with the blue neuron (see box) and is about to die.

stress
depression
aging
neurodegeneration

Synaptic Neurotransmission and the Anatomically Addressed Nervous System

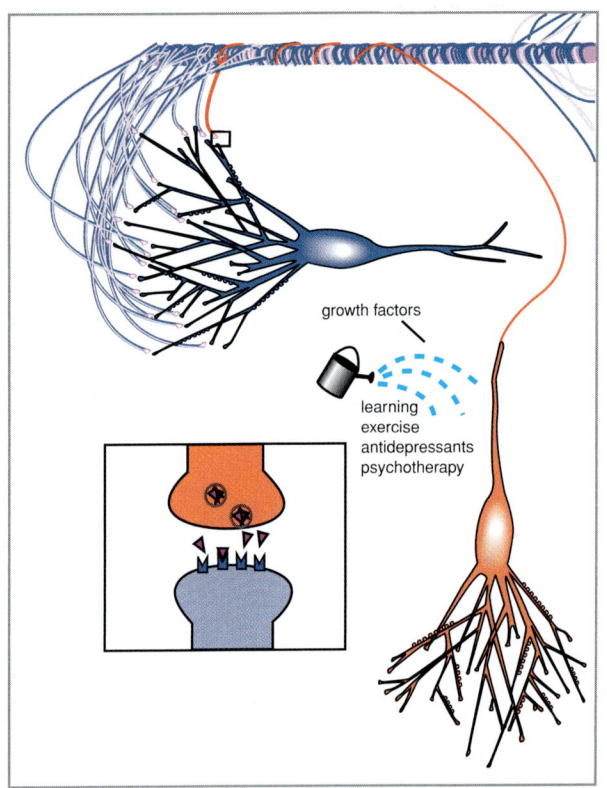

FIGURE 2-7 Restoration of neurons by growth factor. This figure demonstrates how a degenerating neuron might be rescued by a growth factor. In this case, the dying neuron of Figure 2-6 is salvaged by a growth factor, which restores the function of neurotransmission to reactivate normal communication between the red neuron and the blue neuron (see box). Promotion of endogenous growth factors can be achieved through learning, exercise, psychotherapy, or psychopharmacological agents.

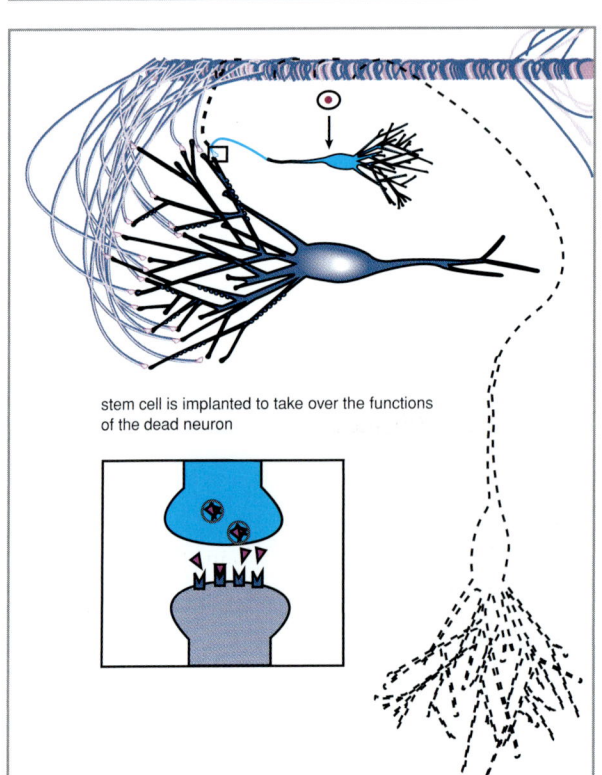

FIGURE 2-8 Transplantation of precursor stem cell. Transplantation of a precursor neuronal stem cell by neurosurgical techniques is another potential mechanism for replacing the function of a degenerated neuron. In this case, the transplanted stem cell differentiates into the turquoise neuron, which makes the same neurotransmitter that was formerly made by the red neuron (see Figure 2-5) prior to degenerating. Synaptic neurotransmission is theoretically restored when the transplanted neuron derived from the stem cell takes over the lost function of the degenerated neuron (see box). Transplantation of fetal substantia nigra cells has been performed in patients with Parkinson's disease and shown to improve motor functioning in some cases. Experimentation with the transplantation of both fetal and adult stem cells is ongoing and poses both technical and ethical issues that remain to be resolved.

26 | Essential Psychopharmacology

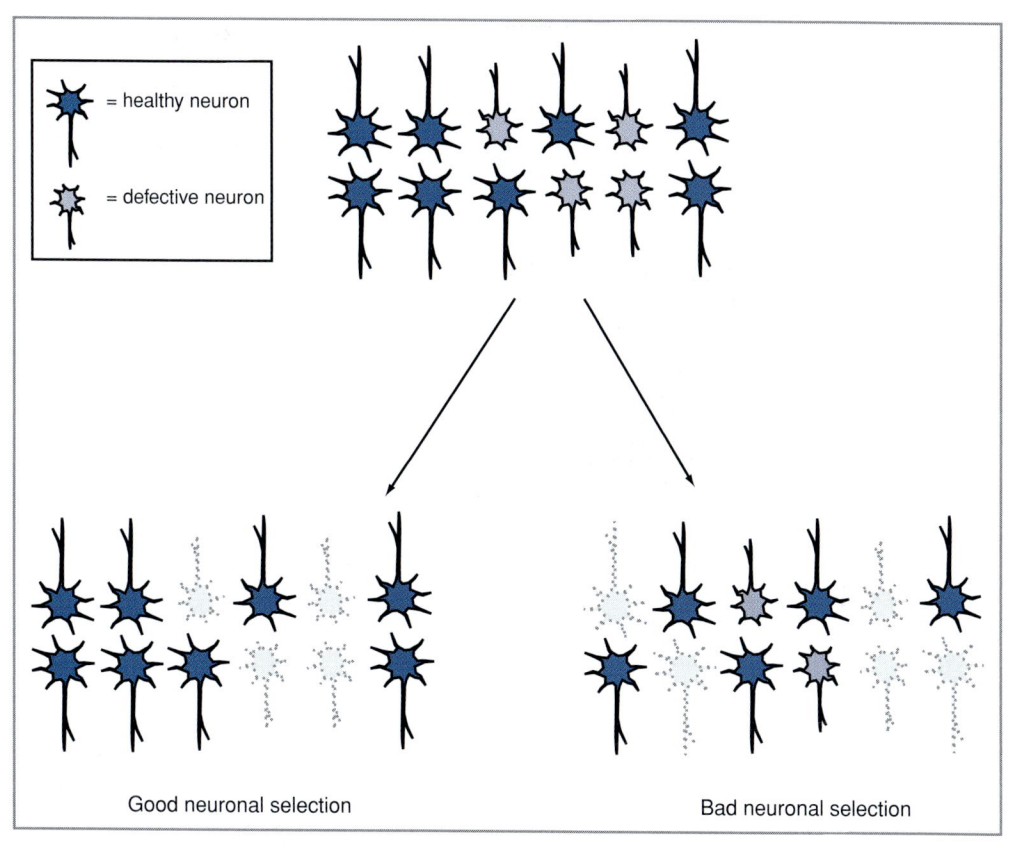

FIGURE 2-9 Neurodevelopment and neuronal selection. Neurons are formed in excess prenatally (top). Some are healthy and others may be defective. Normal neurodevelopment chooses the good neurons (left), but in a developmental disorder, some defective neurons may be chosen and thus cause a neurological or psychiatric disorder later in life when that neuron is called on to perform its duties (right).

is too late and neurons are already lost, it may be possible someday to replace the function of the dead neuron by transplanting a neuronal precursor stem cell where it is needed (Figure 2-8). Indeed, the recent identification of populations of neural precursors, or stem cells, in both embryonic and adult brains raises more than ever the possibility of future repair of neuronal loss from neurodegenerative diseases and from traumatic brain and spinal cord injuries – even from stroke. It might, in fact, be possible to substitute healthy neurons for defective ones in neurodevelopmental conditions (Figure 2-9).

Neuronal selection

If it is surprising that production of neurons (i.e., neurogenesis), as well as differentiation of neurons, can occur in mature human brains, it is perhaps equally shocking that – periodically throughout the life cycle and under certain specific conditions – neurons decide to kill themselves in a type of molecular hari-kari called apoptosis (Figures 2-1, 2-2, and 2-10). In fact, up to 90% of the neurons that the brain makes during fetal development commit "apoptotic suicide" before birth, particularly in some brain areas. Since the mature human brain contains approximately 100 billion neurons, whereas perhaps nearly a trillion are initially formed, this means that billions of neurons are apoptotically destroyed between conception and birth.

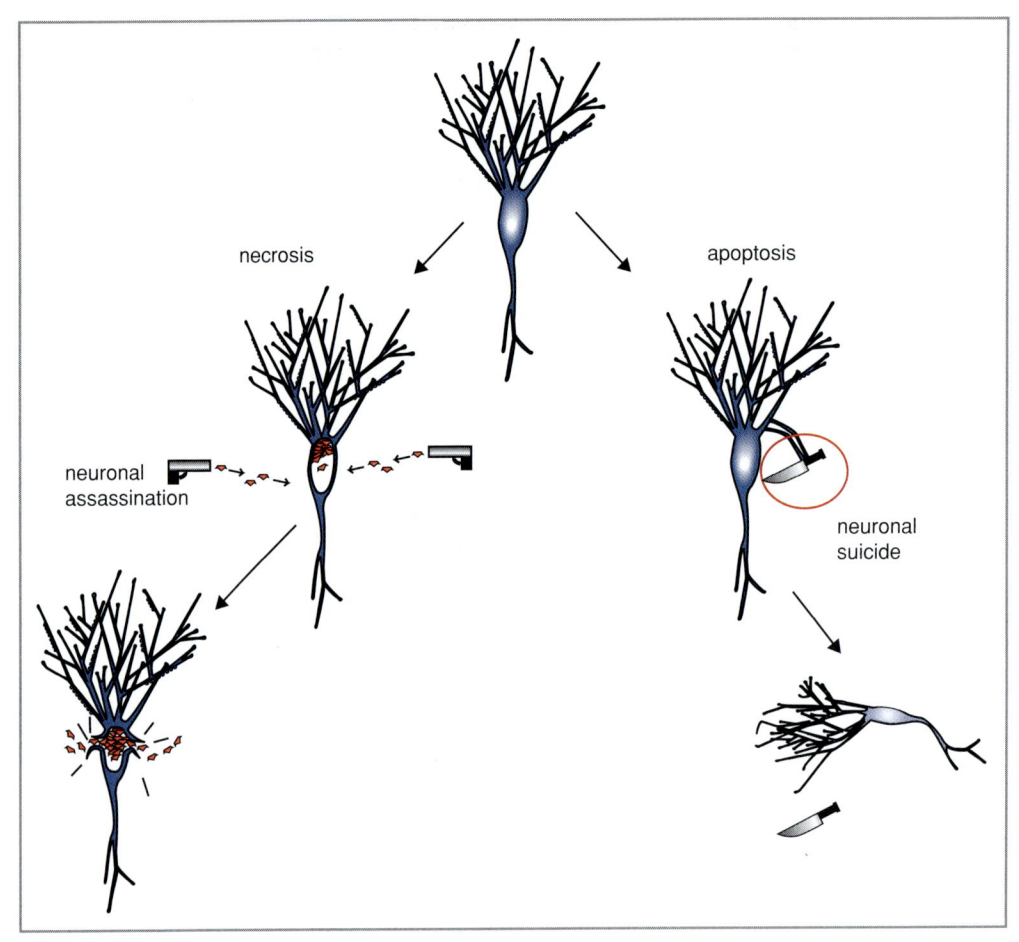

FIGURE 2-10 Necrosis and apoptosis. Neuronal death can occur by either necrosis or apoptosis. Necrosis is analogous to neuronal assassination, in which neurons, after being destroyed by poisons, suffocation, or toxins, explode and cause an inflammatory reaction. On the other hand, apoptosis is akin to neuronal suicide and results when the genetic machinery is activated to cause the neuron to literally "fade away" without causing the molecular mess of necrosis.

Why should a neuron purposely slit its own throat and commit cellular suicide? For one thing, if a neuron or its DNA gets damaged by a virus or a toxin, apoptosis destroys and silently removes these sick genes and their neurons, which may serve to protect surrounding healthy neurons. More importantly, apoptosis appears to be a natural part of development of the immature central nervous system. One of the many wonders of the brain is the built-in redundancy of neurons early in development. These neurons compete vigorously to migrate, innervate target neurons, and drink trophic factors necessary to fuel this process. Apparently there is survival of the fittest, because 50% to 90% of many types of neurons normally die at this time of brain maturation. Apoptosis is a natural mechanism to eliminate the unwanted neurons without making as big a molecular mess as would be involved in doing it via necrosis (Figure 2-10).

How do neurons kill themselves? Apoptosis is programmed into the genome of various cells, including neurons, and when activated, causes the cell to self-destruct. This is not the messy affair associated with cellular poisoning or suffocation known as necrosis

TABLE 2-1 Some selected neurotrophic factors: an alphabet soup of brain tonics

■ NGF	nerve growth factor
■ P75	proapoptotic receptors
■ TrkA	antiapoptotic receptors
■ GDNF	glial cell line–derived neurotrophic factors, which include neurturin, c-REF, and R-alpha
■ BDNF	brain-derived neurotrophic factor
■ NT-3, 4, and amp-5	neurotrophins 3, 4, and 5
■ CNTF	ciliary neurotrophic factor
■ ILGF I and II	insulin-like growth factors
■ FGF	fibroblast growth factor, which comes in both acidic and basic forms
■ EGF	epidermal growth factor

(Figure 2-10). Necrotic cell death is characterized by a severe and sudden injury associated with an inflammatory response. By contrast, apoptosis is more subtle, akin to fading away. Apoptotic cells shrink, whereas necrotic cells explode (Figure 2-10). The scientists who originally discovered apoptosis coined that term to rhyme with *necrosis*; it also means literally a "falling off," as the petals fall off a flower or the leaves fall from a tree. The machinery of cell death involves a set of genes that stand ever ready to cause self-destruction if activated.

Dozens of neurotrophic factors regulate the survival of neurons in the central and peripheral nervous systems (Table 2-1). A veritable alphabet soup of neurotrophic factors contributes to the brain broth of chemicals that bathe and nourish nerve cells. Some are related to nerve growth factor (NGF), others to glial cell line – derived neurotrophic factor (GDNF), and still others to various other neurotrophic factors (Table 2-1). A more comprehensive list of neurotrophins and growth factors is also given in Table 5-11. Some neurotrophic factors can trigger neurons to commit cellular suicide by making them fall on their apoptotic swords. The brain seems to choose which nerves live or die partially by whether a neurotrophic factor nourishes them or chokes them to death. That is, certain molecules (like NGF) can interact at proapoptotic "grim reaper" receptors to trigger apoptotic neuronal demise. However, if NGF decides to act on a neuroprotective "bodyguard" receptor, the neuron prospers.

Neuronal migration

Not only must the correct neurons be selected, but they must migrate to the right parts of the brain (Figures 2-1, 2-2, 2-11, and 2-12). While the brain is still under construction in utero, whole neurons wander (Figures 2-11 and 2-12). Improper migration of neurons can lead to a neurodevelopmental disorder later in life (Figure 2-12), such as epilepsy, mental retardation, psychosis, or possibly learning disabilities and various childhood-onset psychiatric disorders such as attention deficit hyperactivity disorder. Later, with the exception of those two areas of adult brain containing neuronal precursors and discussed above, only the axons of mature neurons can move.

Neurons are initially produced in the center of the developing brain. Consider that 100 billion human neurons, selected from nearly a trillion, must migrate to the right places in order to function properly. What could possibly direct all this neuronal traffic? It turns out that an amazing form of chemical communication calls forth the neurons to the right places and in the right sequences. At speeds up to 60 millionths of a meter per hour, they

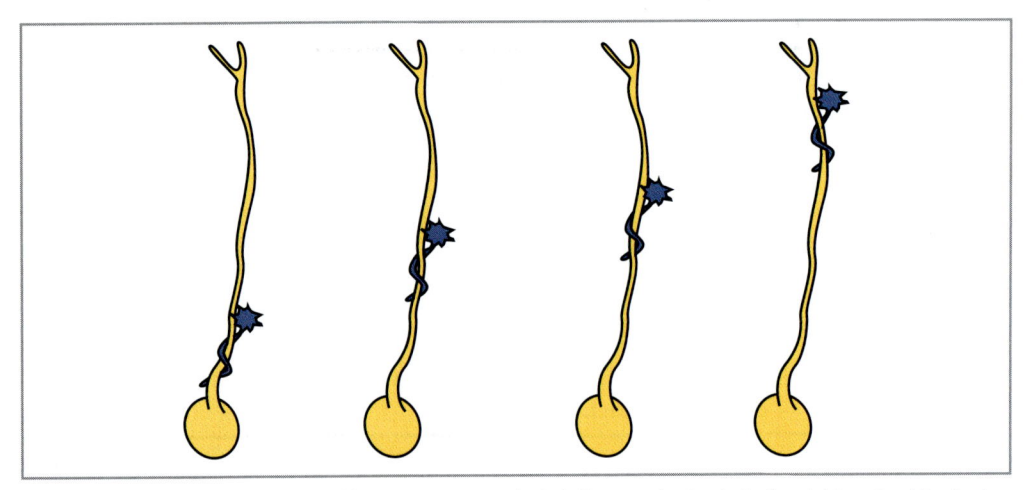

FIGURE 2-11 Neuronal migration. After neurons are selected, they must migrate to the right parts of the brain. Initially, neurons trace glial cells like a trail through the brain to their destinations. Adhesion molecules are coated on neuronal surfaces of the migrating neuron, while complementary molecules on the surface of glia allow the migrating neuron to stick there. Later, neurons can trace the axons of other neurons already in place.

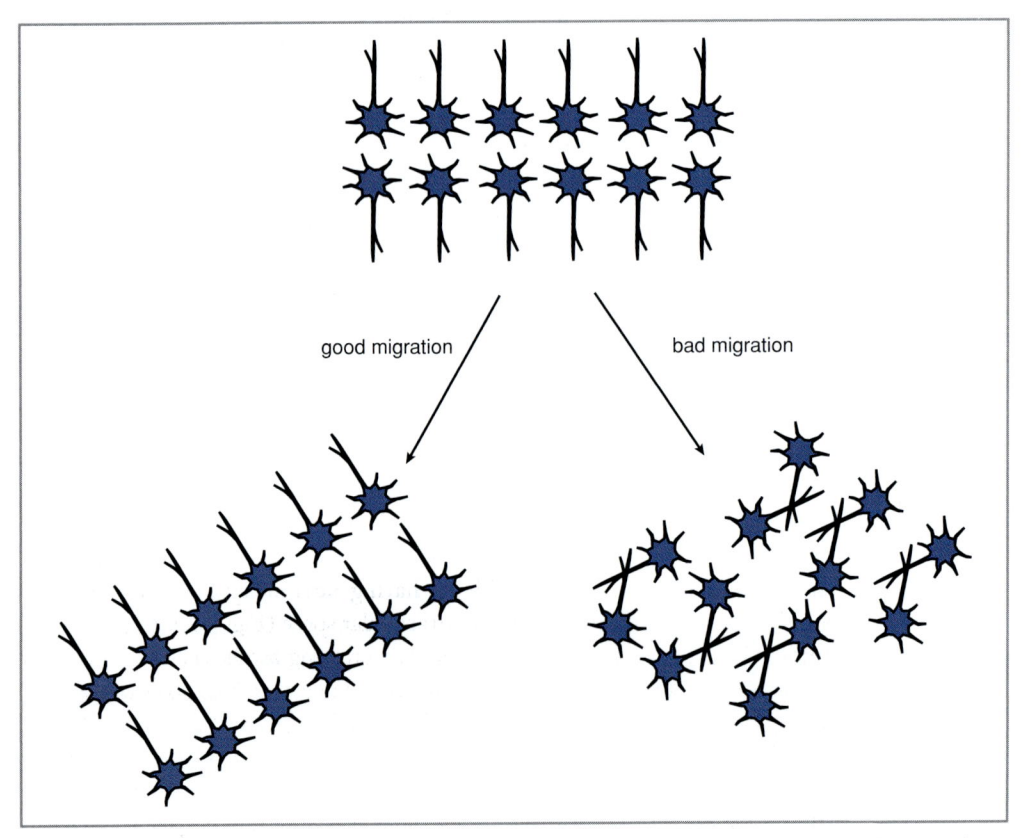

FIGURE 2-12 Neuronal migration. Neurons are formed in central growth plates (top) and then migrate out into the growing brain. If this is done properly (left), the neurons are properly aligned to grow, develop, form synapses, and generally function as expected. However, if there is abnormal migration of neurons (right), the neurons are not in the correct places and do not receive the appropriate inputs from incoming axons; therefore they do not function properly. This may result in a neurological or psychiatric disorder.

TABLE 2-2 Some selected recognition molecules

- PSA-NCAM — polysialic acid–neuronal cell adhesion molecule
- NCAM — neuronal cell adhesion molecules such as H-CAM, G-CAM, VCAM-1
- APP — amyloid precursor protein
- Integrin
- N-cadherin
- Laminin
- Tenscin
- Proteoglycans
- Heparin-binding growth-associated molecule
- Glial hyaluronate-binding protein
- Clusterin

travel to their proper destination, set up shop, and then send out their axons to connect with other neurons. These neurons know where to go because of a series of remarkable chemical signals, different from neurotransmitters, called adhesion molecules (Table 2-2). First, glial cells form a cellular matrix (Figures 2-2 and 2-11). Neurons can trace glial fibers like a trail through the brain to their destinations. Later, neurons can follow the axons of other neurons already in place and trace along the trail already blazed by the first neuron. Adhesion molecules are coated on neuronal surfaces of the migrating neuron, and complementary molecules on the surface of glia allow the migrating neuron to stick there. This forms a kind of molecular Velcro, which anchors the neuron temporarily and directs its walk along the route paved by the appropriate cell surfaces. Settlement of the brain by migrating neurons is complete by birth, but axons of neurons, upon activation, can grow for a lifetime.

Synaptogenesis: directing the axons and arborizing the dendritic trees

Once neurons settle down in their homesteads, their task is to form synapses. How do their axons know where to go? Neurotrophins regulate not only which neuron lives or dies but also whether an axon sprouts and which target it innervates. During development in the immature brain, neurotrophins can cause axons to cruise all over the brain, following long and complex pathways to reach their correct targets. Neurotrophins can induce neurons to sprout axons by having them form an axonal growth cone (Figures 2-13 and 2-14). Once the growth cone is formed, neurotrophins as well as other factors make various recognition molecules for the sprouting axon, presumably by having neurons and glia secrete these molecules into the chemical stew of the brain's extracellular space (Figures 2-13 and 2-14). These recognition molecules can either repel or attract growing axons, sending directions for axonal travel like a semaphore signaling a navy ship (Figure 2-13). Indeed, some of these molecules are called semaphorins to reflect this function. Once the axon growth tip reaches port, it is told to collapse by semaphorin molecules called collapsins, allowing the axon to dock into its appropriate postsynaptic slip and not sail past it (Figure 2-14). Other recognition molecules direct axons away by emitting repulsive axon guidance signals (RAGS) (Figure 2-13).

As brain development progresses, the distance that axonal growth cones can travel is greatly impeded but not completely lost. The fact that axonal growth is retained in the mature brain suggests that neurons continue to alter their targets of communication,

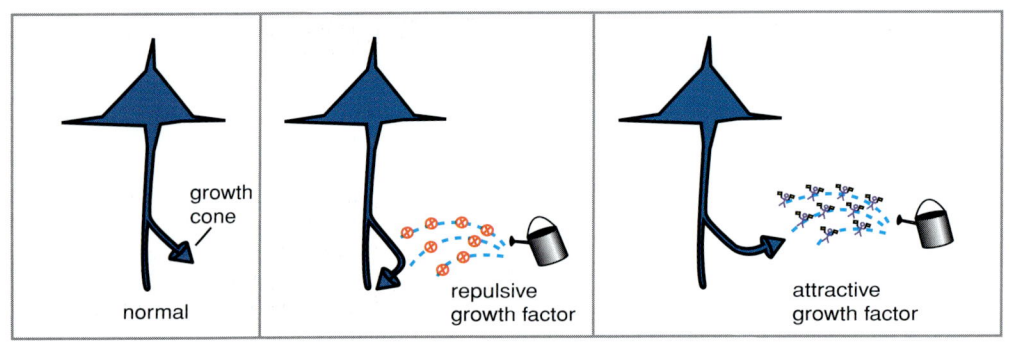

FIGURE 2-13 Axonal growth cones. Neurotrophins can induce neurons to sprout axons by having them form an axonal growth cone. Once the growth cone is formed, neurons or glia in the area make recognition molecules that are repulsive and cause axons to grow away from such molecules or that are attractant and encourage axonal growth toward such molecules. Neurotrophic factors thus direct axonal traffic in the brain and help determine which axons synapse with which postsynaptic targets.

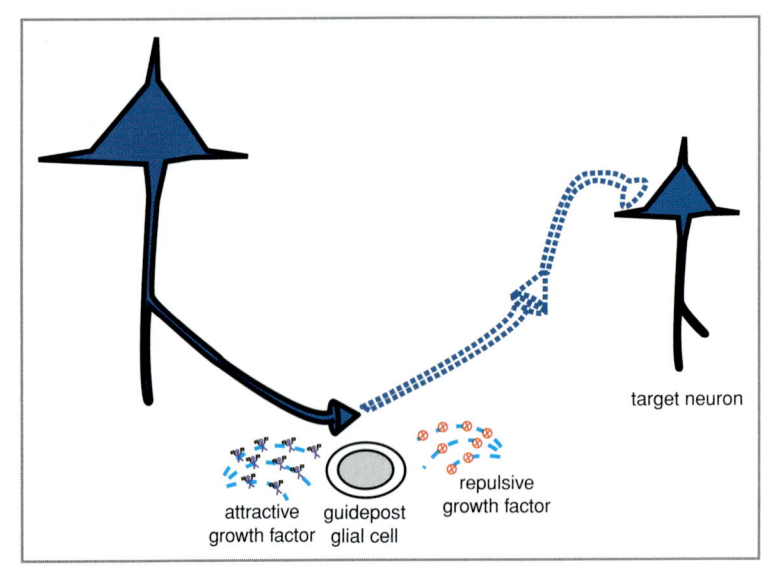

FIGURE 2-14 Axonal growth cone docking. This figure depicts the axonal growth cone "docking" at its neuronal destination with the guidance of various recognition molecules.

perhaps by repairing, regenerating, and reconstructing synapses as demanded by the evolving duties of a neuron. A large number of recognition molecules supervise this. Some of these include not only semaphorins and collapsins but also molecules such as netrins, neuronal cellular adhesion molecules (NCAMs), integrins, cadherins, and cytokines (Table 2-2). When things go right, innervation proceeds smoothly and the brain is correctly "wired" (Figure 2-15). However, if there is misdirection of synaptic formation, the wrong neurons can plug into the wrong places and leave the brain with the wrong wiring (Figure 2-16). It is difficult to conceptualize how to provide therapeutic agents that could correctly redirect these neurons. One possibility is that repetition of a good behavior, learning, or psychotherapy could all have the potential to restructure and thus rehabilitate the brain over long periods of time. Certainly having the best experiences and input from the environment during neurodevelopment seems to be a desirable goal, as this may lead to the proper direction of synapses to the correct target neurons and thus lead to the development of an appropriately arborized dendritic tree (Figures 2-17, 2-18, and 2-19). On the other hand, deprivation,

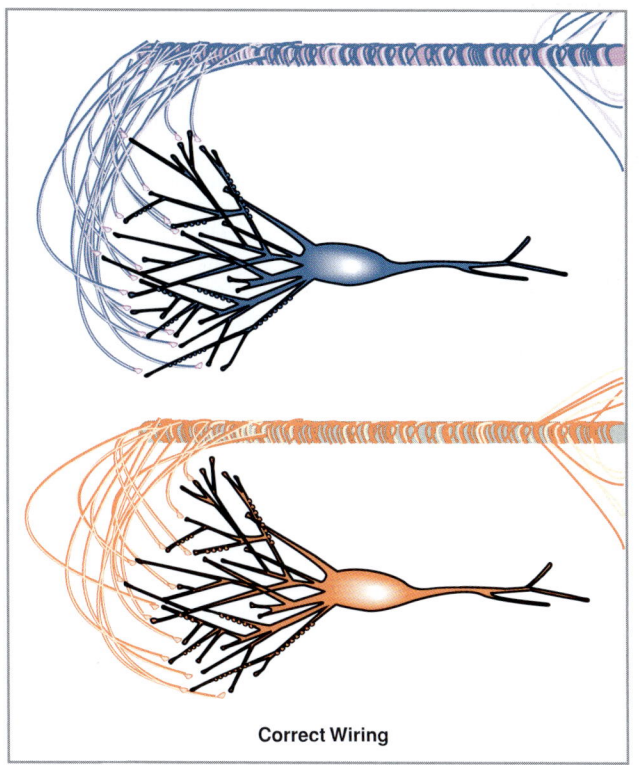

FIGURE 2-15 Correct wiring of neurons. This figure represents the correct wiring of two neurons. During development, the incoming blue axons from all different parts of the brain are appropriately directed to their appropriate target dendrites on the blue neuron. Similarly, the incoming red axons from various regions of the brain are appropriately paired with their correct dendrites on the red neuron.

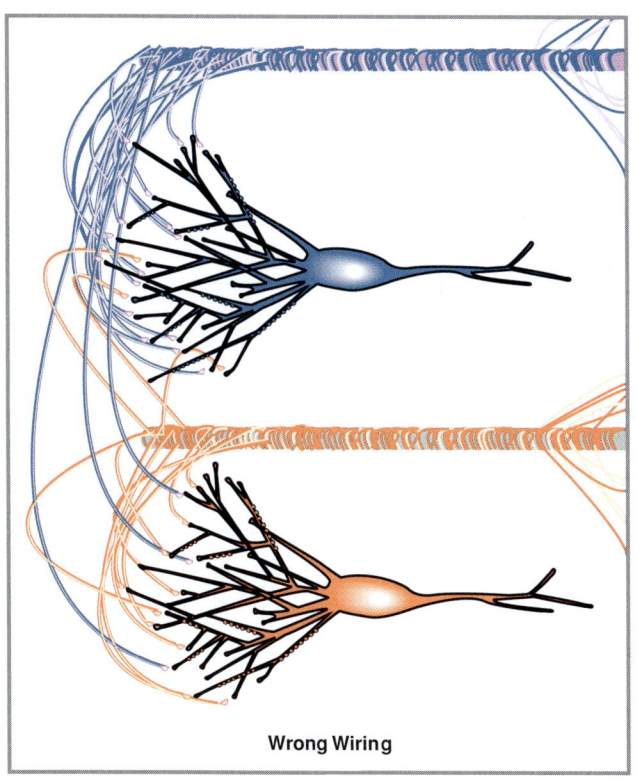

FIGURE 2-16 Wrong wiring of neurons. This figure represents simplistically a possible disease mechanism in neurodevelopment disorders. In this case, the neurons do not fail to develop connections, do not die, and do not degenerate. Rather, formation of the synapse is misdirected, resulting in the wrong wiring. This could lead to abnormal information transfer, confusing neuronal communications, and the inability of neurons to function; this is postulated to occur in schizophrenia, mental retardation, and other neurodevelopmental disorders. This state of chaos is represented here as a tangle of axons, where red axons inappropriately innervate blue dendrites and blue axons inappropriately pair up with red dendrites. This is in contrast to the organized state represented in Figure 2-15.

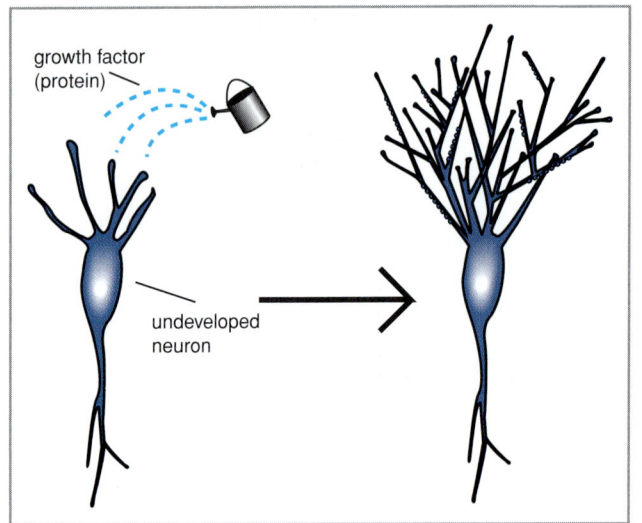

FIGURE 2-17 Dendritic tree. The dendritic tree of a neuron can sprout branches, grow, and establish a multitude of new synaptic connections throughout its life. The process of making dendritic connections on an undeveloped neuron may be controlled by various growth factors, which act to promote the branching process and thus the formation of synapses on the dendritic tree.

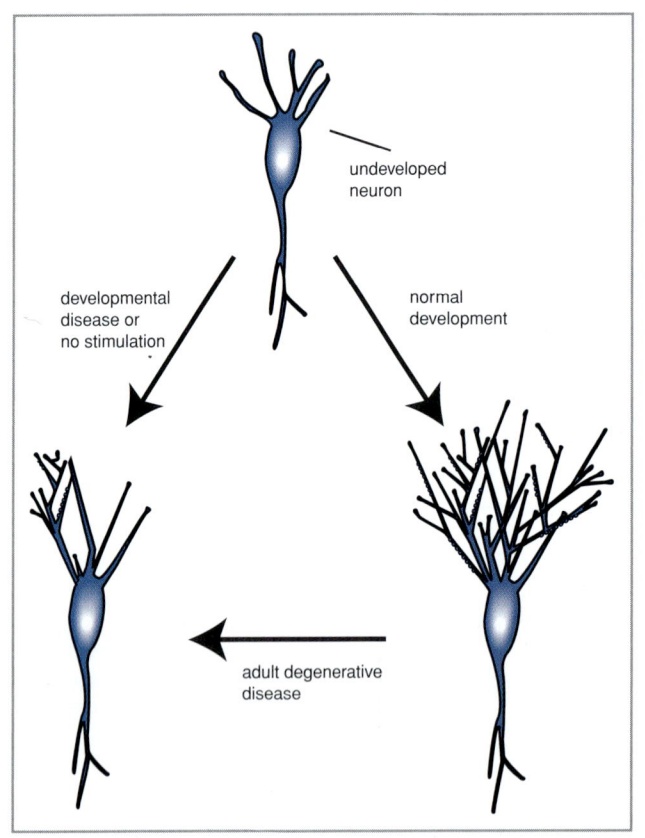

FIGURE 2-18 Neurodevelopment and neurodegeneration. An undeveloped neuron may fail to develop during childhood, either because of a developmental disease of some sort or the lack of appropriate neuronal or environmental stimulation for proper development (left arrow). In other cases, the undeveloped neuron does develop normally (right arrow), only to lose these gains when an adult-onset degenerative disease strikes it (bottom arrow).

emotional or physical abuse, or bad experiences during childhood while neurons are forming their synapses could potentially be associated with inadequate (Figures 2-18 and 2-19) as well as incorrect synaptogenesis (Figure 2-16), resulting in insufficient dendritic arborization (Figure 2-19). Contemporary theories suggest that failure to form the correct synapses or a rich, prosperous portfolio of synapses may be associated with neurodevelopmental

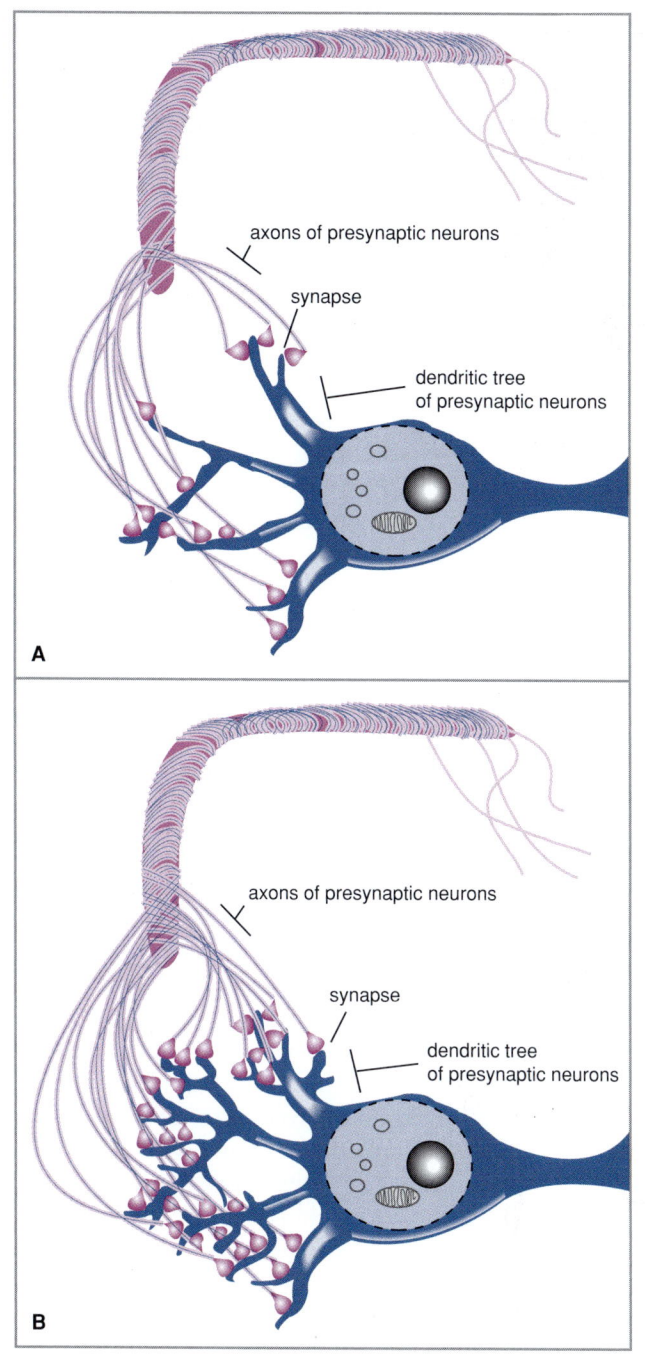

FIGURE 2-19 Neuronal arborization. This figure depicts a neuron with insufficient arborization (blue neuron, panel A); thus, there are few synaptic connections between its dendrites and the axons of other neurons. In contrast, the blue neuron in panel B is widely arborized and thus has many synaptic connections with other neurons.

disorders, whereas the hallmark of a neurodegenerative disorder is loss of the correct synapses once they have been developed in the right places (Figure 2-18).

Synaptic plasticity

Once the neurons have migrated to the right places and the axons grow into the proximity of the right dendrites, the next step is an elegant molecular structuring of the synaptic connections themselves. Synapses can form on many parts of a neuron, not just the dendrites as axodendritic synapses, but also on the soma as axosomatic synapses, and even at the beginning and at the end of axons (axoaxonic synapses) (Figure 2-20). Such synapses are said to be "asymmetric," since communication is structurally designed to be in one direction – i.e., anterograde from the axon of the first neuron to the dendrite, soma, or axon of the second neuron (Figures 2-20 and 2-21).

This means that there are presynaptic elements that differ from postsynaptic elements (Figure 2-21). Specifically, neurotransmitter is packaged in the presynaptic nerve terminal, like ammunition in a loaded gun, and then fired at the postsynaptic neuron to target its receptors.

How do synapses form? An overview of this process is shown in Figure 2-22. Many axons, long before they make any contact with a candidate postsynaptic site, have a few of the elements involved in making molecular contacts with postsynaptic elements already in place (Figures 2-22 and 2-23). Similarly, many potential postsynaptic sites, even when no axon is nearby, also express a few of the molecules that have the potential to link with presynaptic sites (Figures 2-22 and 2-23). Each of these constitutes a rudimentary hemisynapse that is capable of making a trial contact by linking prehemisynaptic molecules with posthemisynaptic molecules when the opportunity arises – that is, when one makes physical contact with the other. If the trial contact does not work out, the connection is never strengthened and is lost. However, much like dating, if the trial contact is successful, each hemisynapse works to improve the relationship with the other. That is, each element contributes more and more molecules to the connections they share with each other, eventually forming a fully functioning synapse (Figure 2-22).

Specifically, many specialized molecular components must be assembled to form a fully functional synapse from two rudimentary hemisynapses. These components are derived either from preformed supplies that are already waiting in an axon terminal's hemisynapse or a dendritic spine's hemisynapse or from newly synthesized synaptic molecules that are ordered by each hemisynapse chemically signaling its own genome, back in its corresponding cell nucleus, to make and then ship the necessary supplies to the site of the emerging synapse.

Just like a construction site, the area of new synapse formation is abuzz with activity, from ramping up the synthesis and delivery of supplies of some very specific proteins that are needed on each side of the synapse to actually erecting them into a structural and functional unit. Both pre- and postsynaptic hemisynapses contribute CAMs (cellular adhesion molecules) to their extracellular contact site, thus providing a type of "molecular glue" that solidifies the structural link they share (Figure 2-25 and Table 2-2). Both elements also need intracellular scaffolding proteins such as actin, the same protein that is in skeletal muscle, to support the shape and strength of the emerging pre- and postsynaptic elements (Figure 2-26). The presynaptic side needs some very specialized materials that are not present in the postsynaptic element, such as synaptic vesicles full of neurotransmitters, synthetic and catabolic enzymes, reuptake transporters, ion channels, and specialized proteins that constitute the active zone allowing neurotransmitter release (Figure 2-27). The postsynaptic side also requires specialized proteins not present on the presynaptic side, such as postsynaptic receptors matched to the neurotransmitter being used by the presynaptic neuron, signal cascade molecules, and specialized proteins constituting the postsynaptic density that allows signal detection from the presynaptic neuron (Figure 2-27).

Once the synapse is formed, it remains a dynamic area of intense molecular activity. In other words, the construction crew that ordered, manufactured, and received the shipped supplies of molecules and then assembled them into a working synapse are not dismissed as

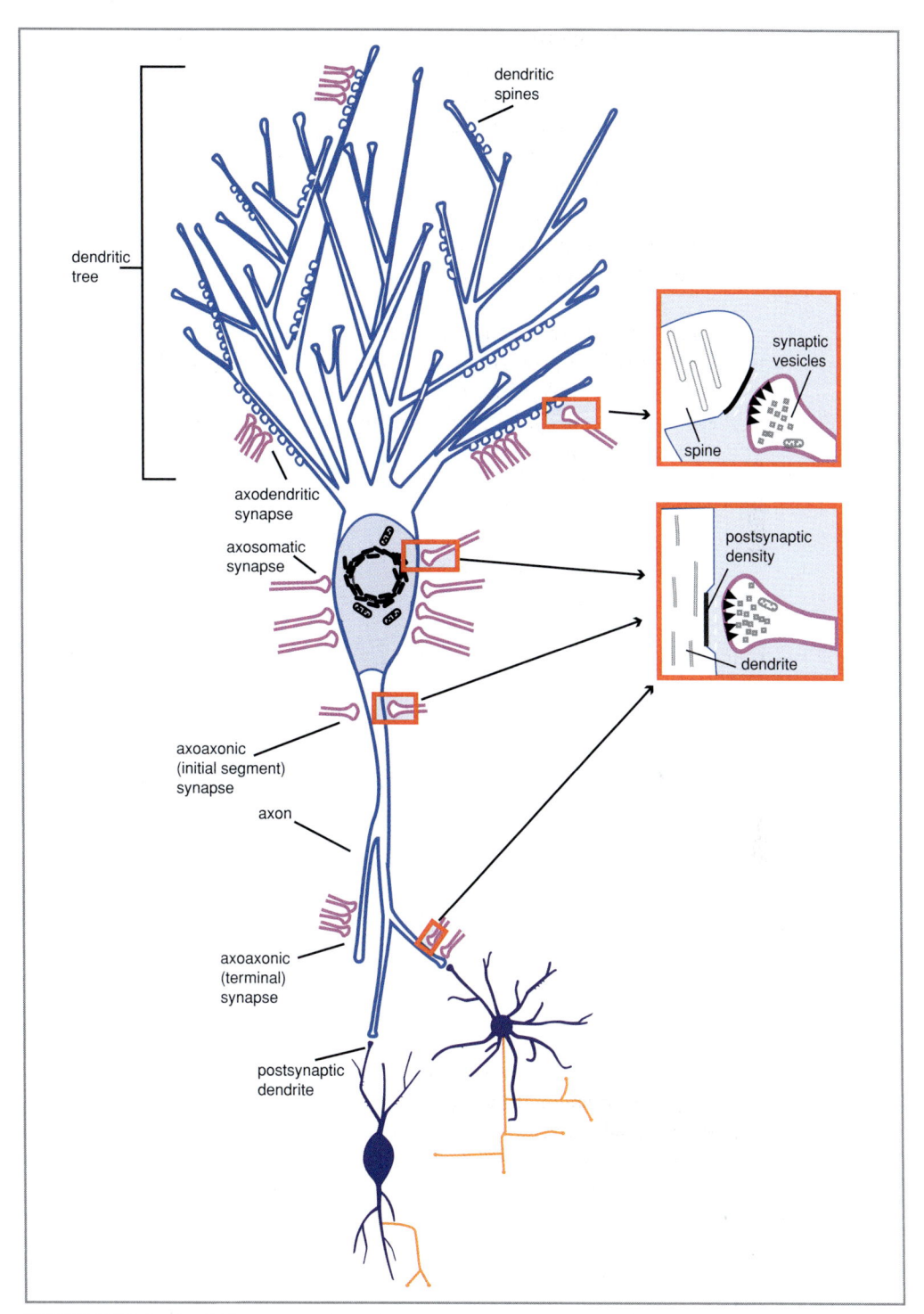

FIGURE 2-20 Axodendritic, axosomatic, and axoaxonic connections. After neurons migrate, they form synapses. As shown in this figure, synaptic connections can form not just between the axon and dendrites of two neurons (axodendritic) but also between the axon and the soma (axosomatic) or the axons of the two neurons (axoaxonic). Communication is anterograde from the axon of the first neuron to the dendrite, soma, or axon of the second neuron.

Synaptic Neurotransmission and the Anatomically Addressed Nervous System

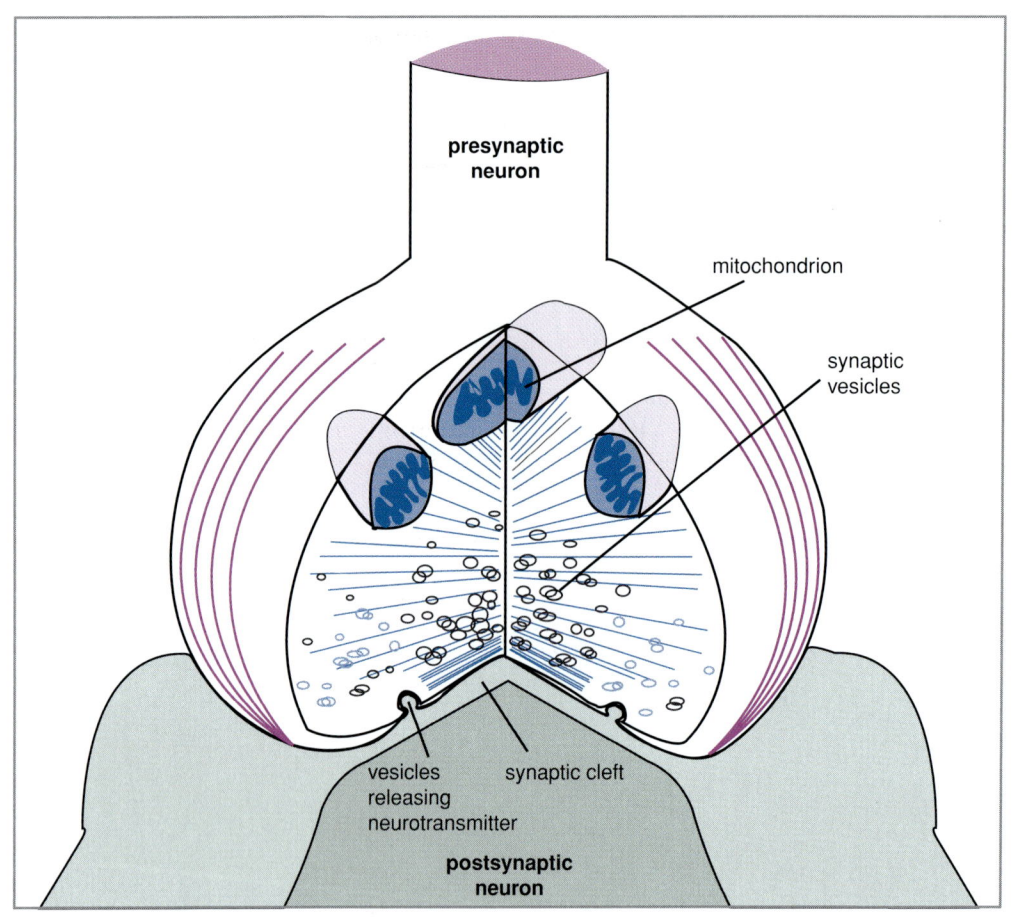

FIGURE 2-21 Enlarged synapse. The synapse is enlarged conceptually here showing the specialized structures that enable chemical neurotransmission to occur. Specifically, a presynaptic neuron sends its axon terminal to form a synapse with a postsynaptic neuron. Energy for neurotransmission from the presynaptic neuron is provided by mitochondria there. Chemical neurotransmitters are stored in small vesicles, ready for release upon firing of the presynaptic neuron. The synaptic cleft is the gap between the presynaptic neuron and the postsynaptic neuron; it contains proteins and scaffolding and molecular forms of "synaptic glue" to reinforce the connection between the neurons. Receptors are present on both sides of this cleft and are key elements of chemical neurotransmission.

soon as the synapse is functional. In many ways, a synapse is under constant revision as long as it is functional, with molecular maintenance and alterations constantly instituted to respond to changing conditions and its amount of use by the neurons it connects. For example, it has been said that "neurons that fire together wire together," and this is demonstrated not only by the construction of the synapse, shown in Figures 2-22 through 2-27, but also in the molecular changes shown in Figures 2-28 through 2-31. For example, as more neurotransmitter is released, it can change the number of pre- and postsynaptic receptors expressed at that synapse as well as the richness of the pre- and postsynaptic densities seen at the synapse (Figure 2-28). This presumably reflects adaptive molecular and structural changes that facilitate the ease of neurotransmission. Sometimes the changes instituted at a synapse in response to high degrees of utilization are not only on the molecular level but can lead to dramatic physical and structural alterations in the synapse. For example, the surface areas of both pre- and postsynaptic faces can increase, presumably to accommodate enriched

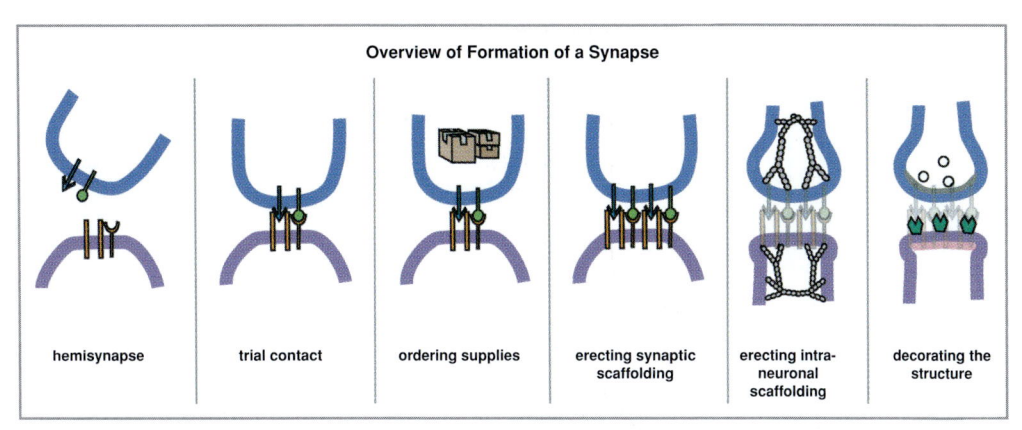

FIGURE 2-22 Synapse formation. This figure summarizes the process of synapse formation, which is depicted in more detail in Figures 2-23 through 2-27. Most pre- and postsynaptic sites already have some of the elements necessary for synaptic connections prior to physical contact; this is called a hemisynapse and allows the pre- and postsynaptic sites to make a trial contact with one another. In many cases, after trial contact, additional specialized molecular components are transported to the pre- and/or postsynaptic sites and assembled to form a fully functioning synapse.

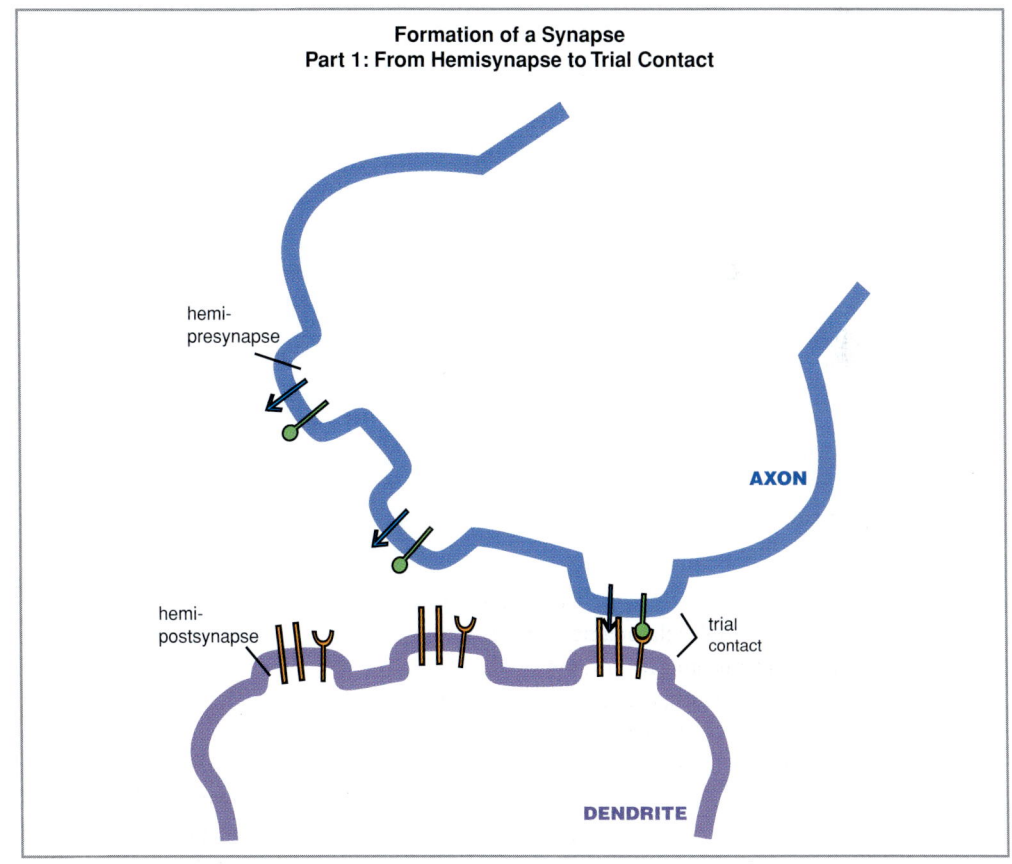

FIGURE 2-23 Formation of a synapse: trial contact. Formation of a synapse, part 1. Many presynaptic axons contain some of the molecular components necessary to form a synaptic connection even before making contact with a postsynaptic site; the same is true of postsynaptic sites (in this case, the site of a dendrite). Presynaptically, this is called a hemipresynapse, while postsynaptically it is called a hemipostsynapse. The pre- and postsynaptic sites are able to make a trial contact with one another by linking hemipresynaptic molecules with hemipostsynaptic molecules.

Synaptic Neurotransmission and the Anatomically Addressed Nervous System

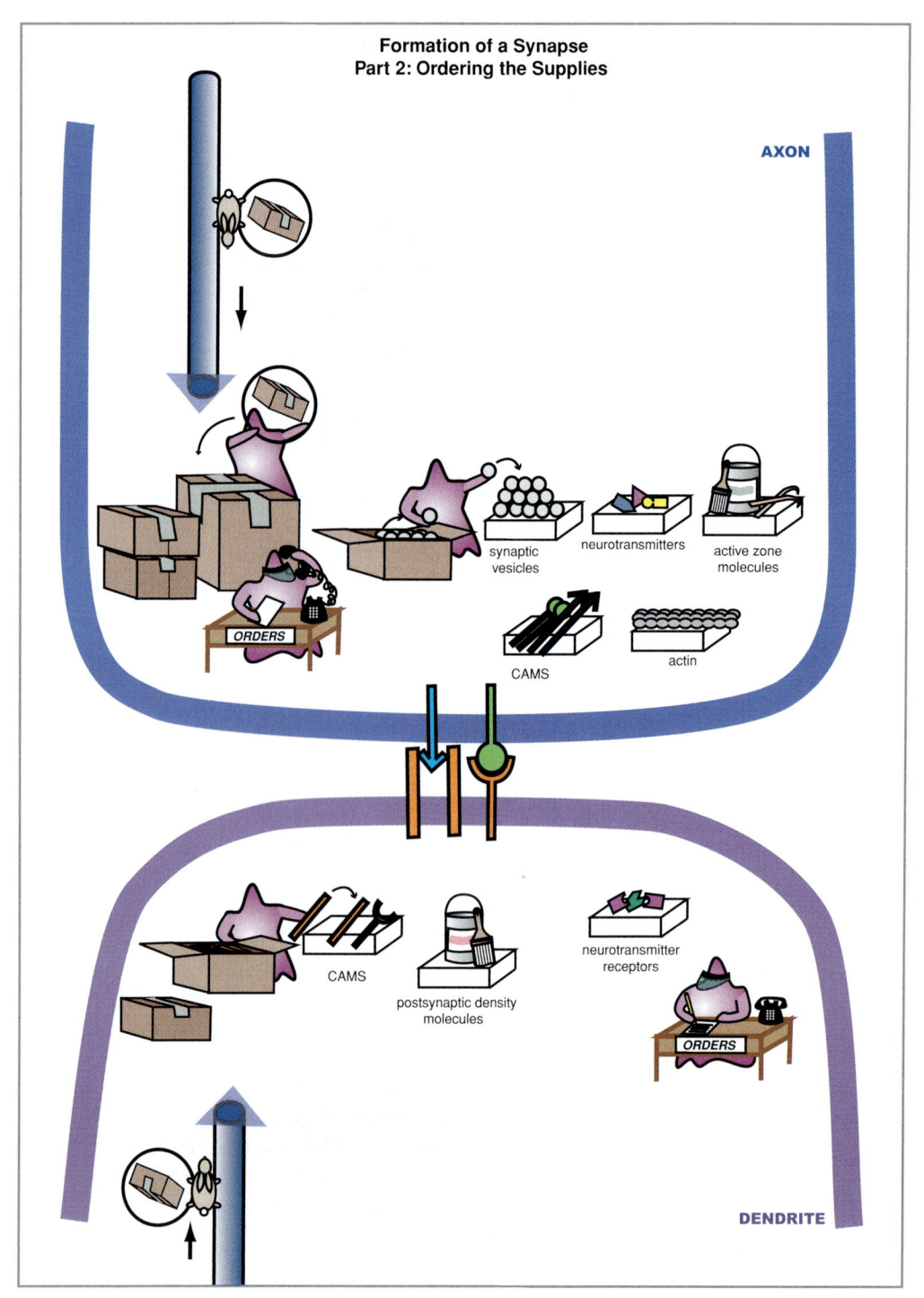

FIGURE 2-24 **Formation of a synapse: ordering supplies.** Formation of a synapse, part 2. In some cases, preformed molecular components needed to assemble a functioning synapse are already present in the pre- and posthemisynapses. In many cases, however, these supplies need to be ordered – that is, the hemisynapse signals the genome to synthesize and transport synaptic molecules to the emerging synapse.

Essential Psychopharmacology

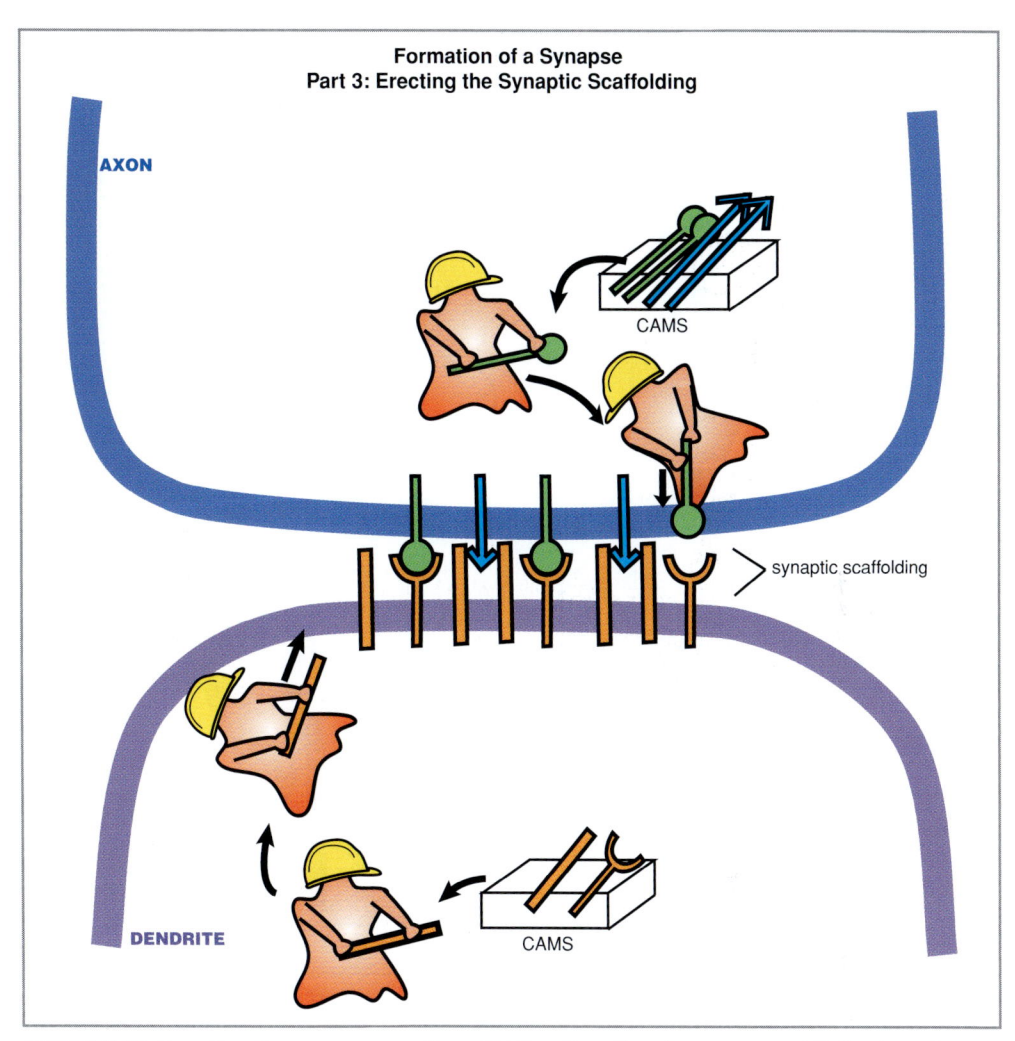

FIGURE 2-25 Formation of a synapse: synaptic scaffolding. Formation of a synapse, part 3. One type of molecule needed to form a functioning synapse is the cellular adhesion molecule (CAM). CAMs are "molecular glue" that solidify the structural link between the pre- and postsynaptic sites; they are required in both the pre- and posthemisynapses.

numbers and types of receptors that facilitate communication (Figure 2-29). Vigorous presynaptic messaging can also increase the postsynaptic response by inducing the formation of an entirely separate and adjacent postsynaptic structural element (Figure 2-30). Similarly, a postsynaptic hemisynapse in the area of a presynaptic neuron may be able to receive information from that neuron, initially by spillover of its neurotransmitter directed at a neighboring postsynaptic element. Over time, however, this arrangement can induce the sprouting of an axon collateral to construct a proper, fully functioning synapse (Figure 2-31).

Competitive elimination of synapses

After all of this elegant effort to create synapses, it may be surprising to learn that the neuron is equipped with mechanisms to eliminate synapses as well. Interestingly, more synapses are present in the brain by age 6 than at any other time in the life cycle (Figures 2-1 and 2-2).

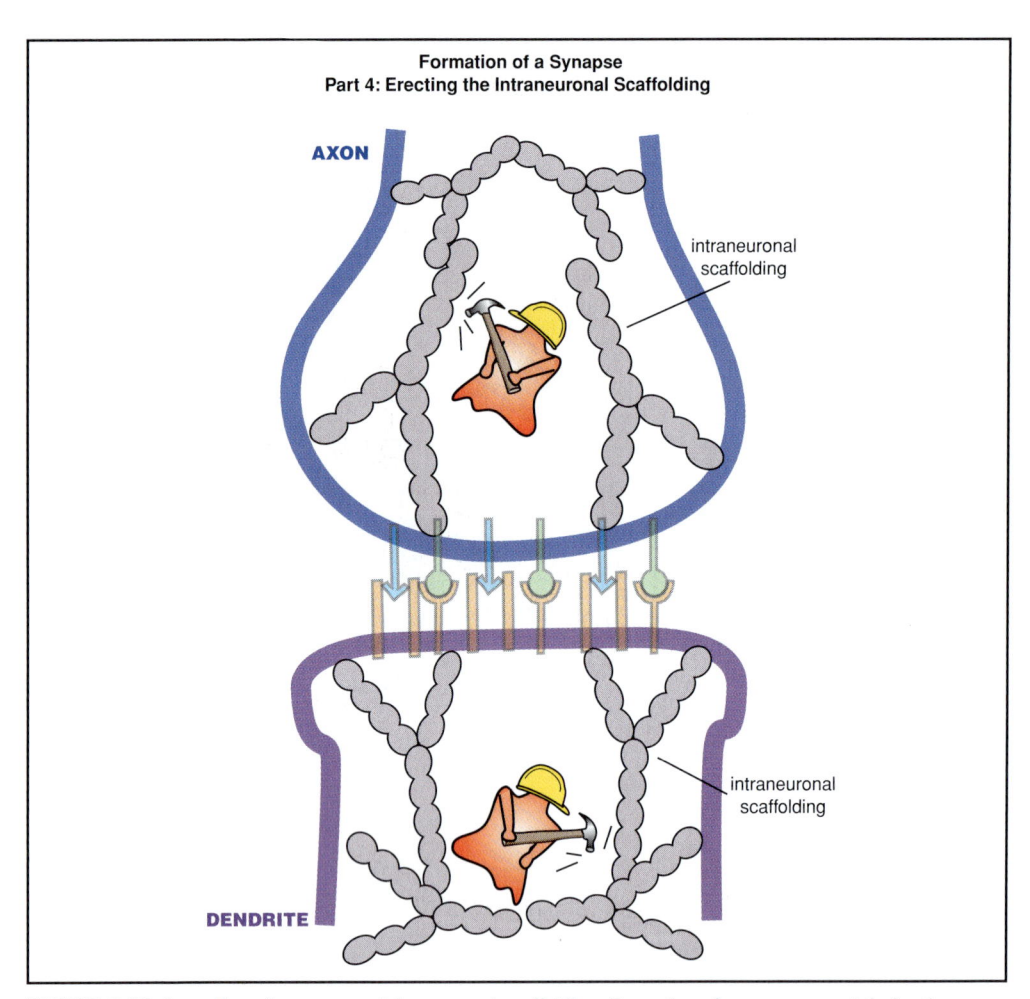

FIGURE 2-26 Formation of a synapse: intraneuronal scaffolding. Formation of a synapse, part 4. Another element needed by both the pre- and posthemisynapses for the formation of a functioning synapse is intracellular scaffolding protein (e.g., actin, the protein present in skeletal muscle). Actin and other intracellular scaffolding proteins help form the shape and strength of the emerging pre- and postsynaptic elements.

During the next 5 to 10 years and into adolescence, the brain systematically removes half of all synaptic connections present at age 6. This still leaves about 100 trillion synapses – up to 10,000 individual synapses for some neurons – and a massively restructured brain. At a lower level of activity, this same elimination of synapses (as well as formation of synapses) occurs over a lifetime.

How does the neuron eliminate synapses? Excitotoxicity may be the mechanism that mediates the pruning of synaptic connections. That is, just like a good gardener, the brain needs a mechanism to "prune" its dendritic tree of old, malfunctioning or unneeded synapses (Figure 2-32). Limited loss of synapses can provide a useful maintenance function. However, it is possible that this same mechanism gets turned on inappropriately or goes out of control in certain disease states (Figure 2-33) associated with excessive loss of synapses or even loss of neurons themselves (Figures 2-34 through 2-37).

Excitatory neurotransmission via the ubiquitous excitatory neurotransmitter glutamate is part of normal brain functioning; many key neurons utilize glutamate as their neurotransmitter and essentially all neurons can be excited by this neurotransmitter (Figure 2-34).

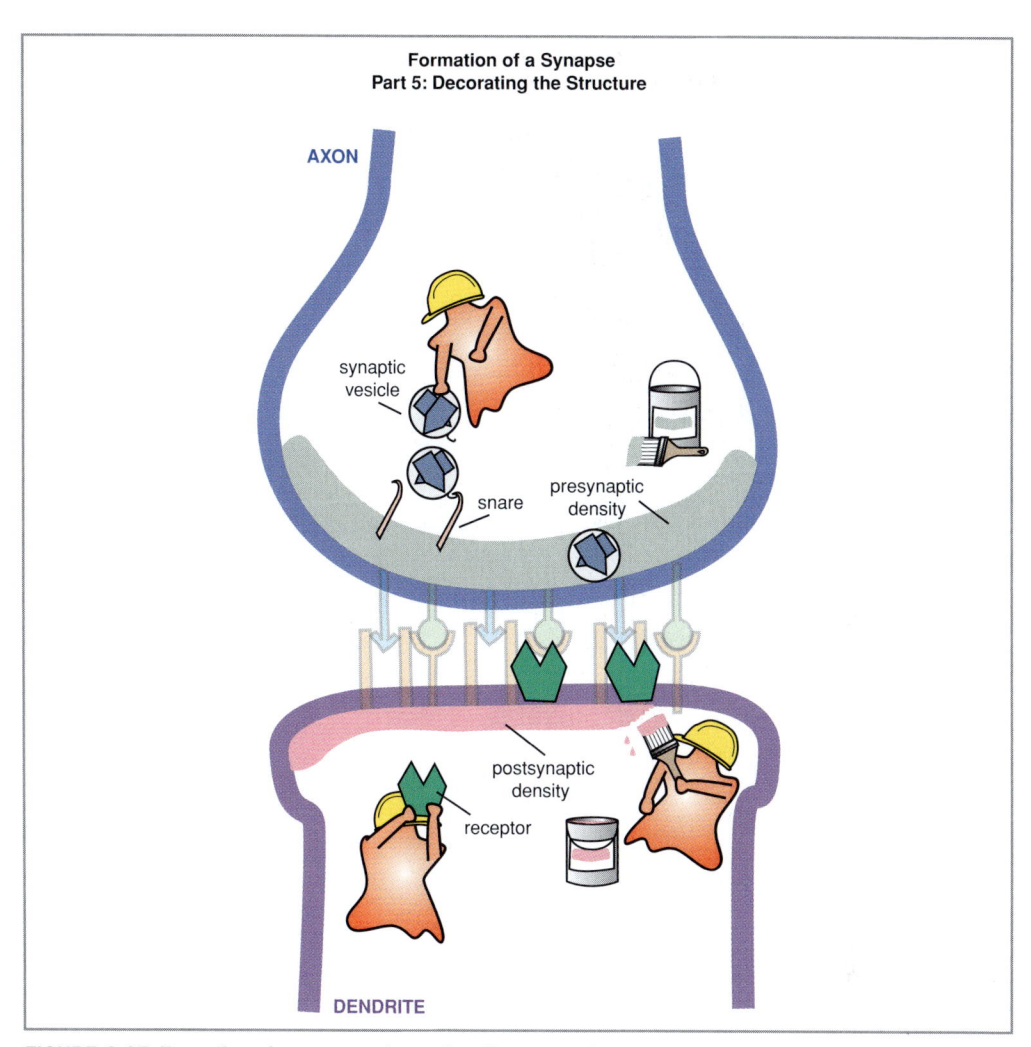

FIGURE 2-27 Formation of a synapse: decorating. Formation of a synapse, part 5. Some elements needed to form a synapse are unique to either the pre- or posthemisynapse. The prehemisynapse requires synaptic vesicles, neurotransmitters, synthetic and catabolic enzymes, reuptake transporters, ion channels, snare proteins, and other proteins that constitute the presynaptic density, which allows neurotransmitter release. The posthemisynapse requires postsynaptic receptors, signal cascade molecules, and specialized proteins constituting the postsynaptic density, which allows signal detection.

Hypothetically, some states of "overexcitation" may result in excessive excitatory neurotransmission and thus excessive neuronal activity in certain neuronal circuits. This process is theoretically associated with unwanted psychiatric or neurologic symptoms, such as panic, pain, or even a seizure (Figure 2-35). Following such a barrage of excessive excitatory neurotransmission and the associated symptoms, the brain may experience damage to the very synapses that mediated this process, to the point where parts of dendrites of the affected neurons are destroyed (Figure 2-36). Even greater degrees of excitation may hypothetically destroy entire neurons in some neurodegenerative conditions, such as schizophrenia (Figure 2-37). Thus, normal but limited excitotoxicity may be useful for routine pruning of neurons, but excitotoxicity run amok may be a mechanism for unwanted symptoms and even brain damage in certain pathological conditions.

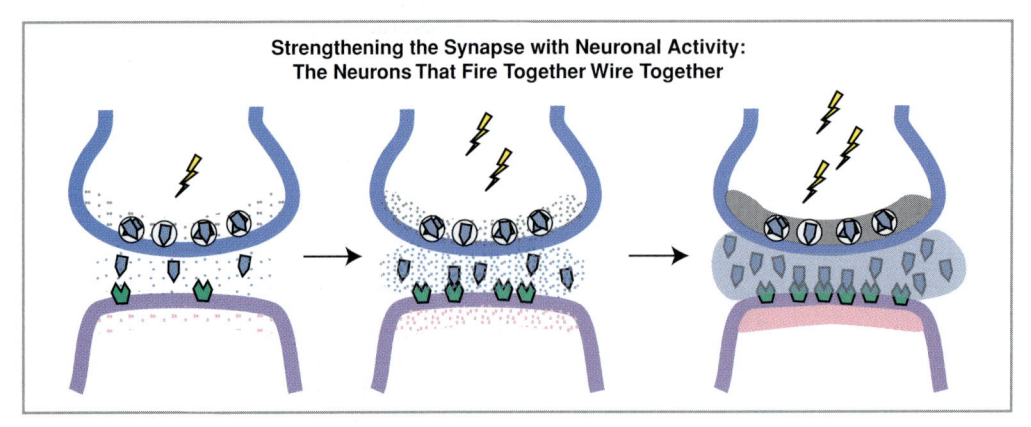

FIGURE 2-28 Strengthening the synapse. Functional synapses experience ongoing revision in response to changing conditions and the amount of use of a synapse by the neurons it connects. As depicted here, increased neurotransmitter release can alter the number of pre- and postsynaptic receptors expressed at a synapse (middle) as well as the richness of pre- and postsynaptic densities (right).

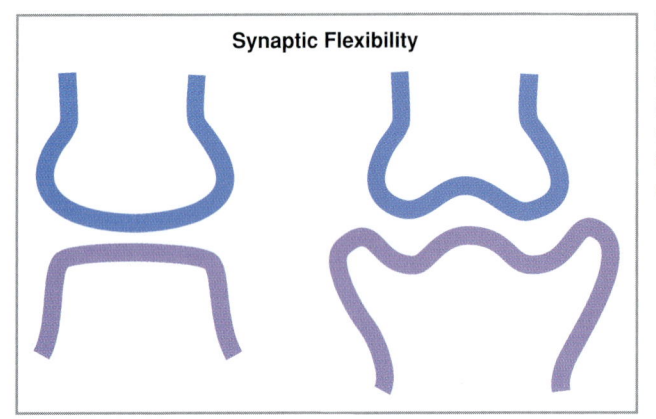

FIGURE 2-29 Synaptic flexibility. Increased utilization of a synapse can lead to adaptations on a structural level. As shown here, the surface area of both pre- and postsynaptic faces can increase to accommodate a greater number and array of receptors.

During neurodevelopment, perhaps some process like excitotoxicity is turned on in order to effect the dramatic restructuring of the brain that occurs in late childhood and adolescence (Figure 2-38). If all goes well, neurodevelopmental experiences and genetic programming will lead the brain to select wisely which connections to keep and which to destroy. Done appropriately, the individual prospers during this maturational task and advances gracefully into adulthood. Bad selections theoretically could lead to neurodevelopmental disorders such as schizophrenia or attention deficit hyperactivity disorder.

The growth of new synapses and the pruning of old synapses then proceeds throughout a lifetime, but at a much slower pace and over shorter distances than earlier in development. Thus the axons and dendrites of each neuron are constantly changing, establishing new connections and removing old ones. The brain never really stops developing; it only slows down. After dramatically reducing neurons before birth and then synapses during late childhood and early adolescence, this process calms down considerably in the mature brain, where maintenance and remodeling of synapses continue in modest amounts and over more limited distances. Although the continuous structural remodeling of synapses in the mature brain, directed by recognition molecules, cannot approximate the pronounced long-range growth of early brain development, this restriction can be beneficial, in part because it

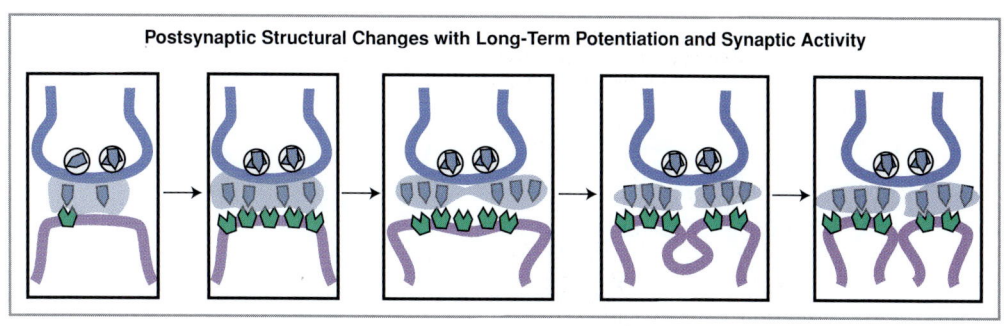

FIGURE 2-30 Formation of separate and adjacent postsynaptic site. Postsynaptic structural changes that can occur with long-term potentiation and synaptic activity are shown here. Increased neurotransmission may lead to an increased number of postsynaptic receptors (panel 2) as well as increased surface area of the postsynaptic face (panel 3), which may ultimately induce the formation of a separate and adjacent postsynaptic site (panels 4 and 5).

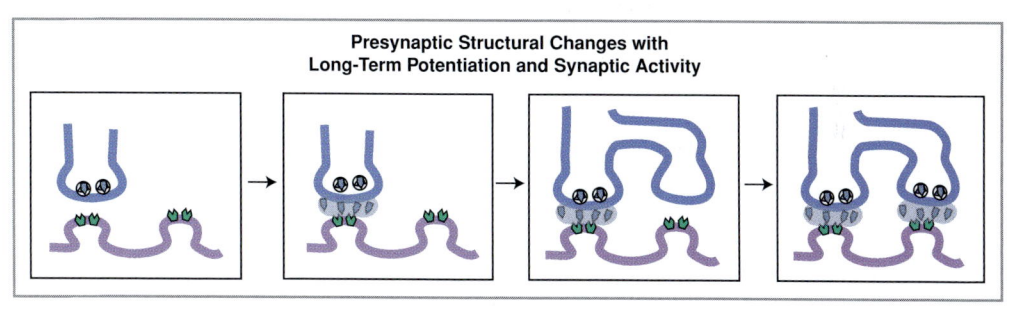

FIGURE 2-31 Formation of new functioning synapse. Presynaptic structural changes that can occur with long-term potentiation and synaptic activity are shown here. Formation of a new posthemisynapse (panels 1 and 2) may eventually lead to the formation of an axon collateral (panel 3) to construct a fully functioning synapse (panel 4).

simultaneously allows structural plasticity while restricting unwanted axonal growth. This would stabilize brain function in the adult and could, furthermore, prevent chaotic rewiring of the brain by limiting both axonal growth away from appropriate targets and ingrowth from inappropriate neurons. On the other hand, the price of such growth specificity becomes apparent when a long-distance neuron in the adult brain dies, thus making it difficult to reestablish original synaptic connections even if axonal growth is turned on.

As previously discussed, neurons and their supportive and neighboring glia elaborate a rich array of neurotrophic factors that either promote or eliminate synaptic connections. The potential for releasing growth factors is preserved forever, which contributes to the possibility of constant synaptic revision throughout the life of that neuron. Such potential changes in synaptogenesis may provide the substrate for learning, emotional maturity, and the development of cognitive and motor skills throughout life. However, it is not clear how the brain dispenses its neurotrophic factors endogenously during normal adult physiological functioning. Presumably, demand to use neurons is met by keeping them fit and ready to function – a task accomplished by salting the brain broth with neurotrophic factors that keep the neurons healthy. Perhaps thinking and learning provoke the release of neurotrophic factors. Maybe "use it or lose it" applies to adult neurons, with neurons being preserved and new connections being formed if the brain stays active. It is even possible that the brain could lose its "strength" in the absence of "mental exercise." Perhaps inactivity leads to pruning of unused, "rusty" synapses, even triggering apoptotic demise of entire inactive neurons. On

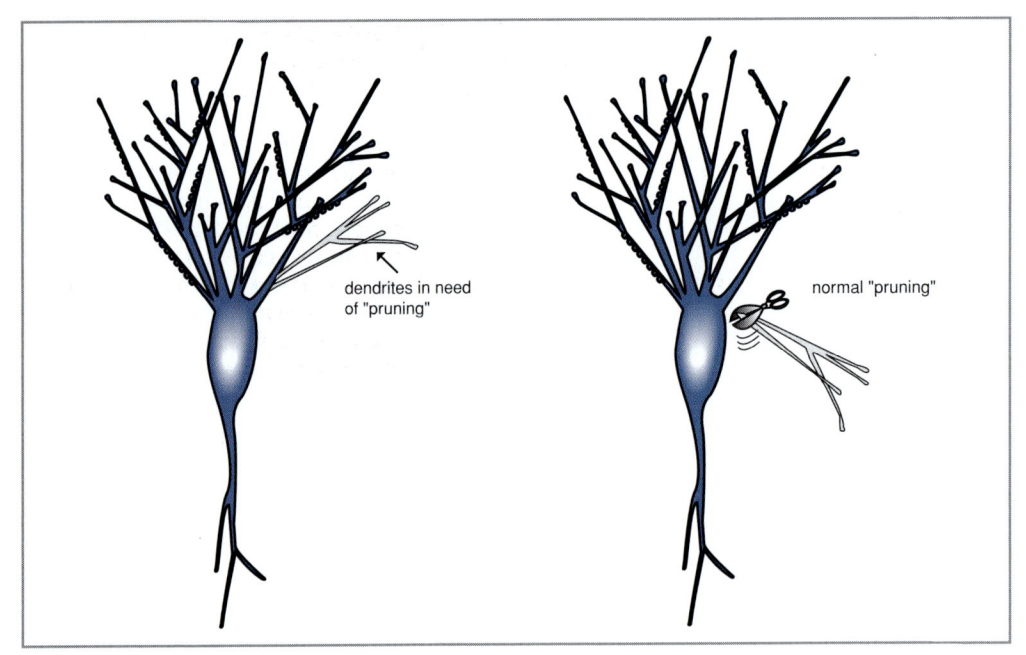

FIGURE 2-32 Normal dendritic pruning. The dendritic tree of a neuron not only sprouts branches, grows, and establishes a multitude of new synaptic connections throughout its life but can also remove, alter, trim, or destroy such connections when necessary. The process of dismantling synapses and dendrites may be controlled by removal of growth factors or by a naturally occurring destructive process sometimes called excitotoxicity. Thus, there is a normal "pruning" process for removing dendrites.

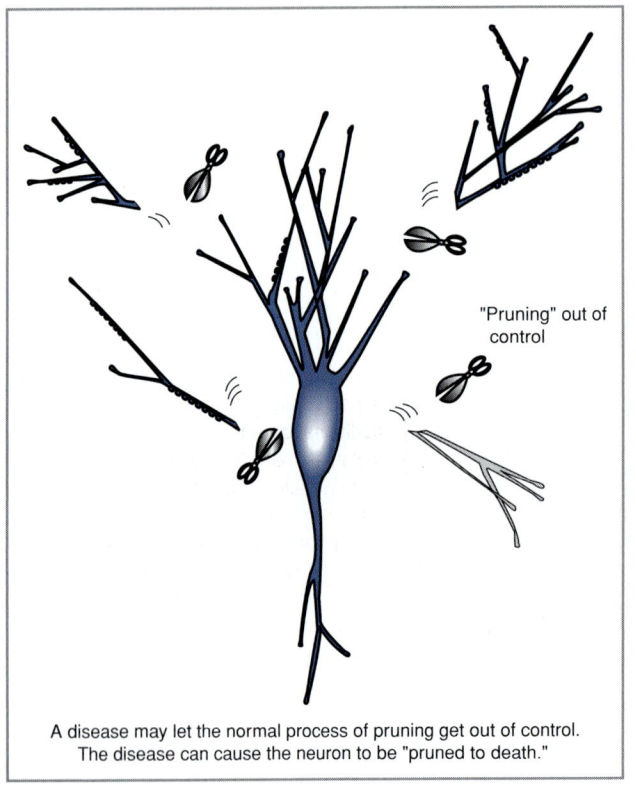

FIGURE 2-33 Out of control dendritic pruning. Neurons appear to have a normal maintenance mechanism for their dendritic tree by which they are able to prune or remove old, unused, or useless synapses and dendrites (shown in Figure 2-32). One postulated mechanism for some degenerative diseases is that this otherwise normal pruning mechanism may get out of control, eventually rendering the neuron useless or killing it by pruning it to death.

A disease may let the normal process of pruning get out of control. The disease can cause the neuron to be "pruned to death."

46 | Essential Psychopharmacology

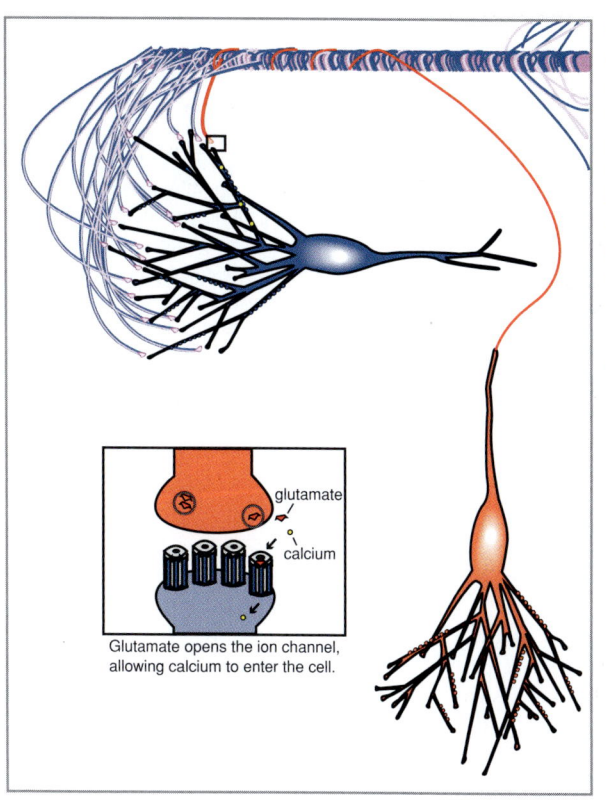

FIGURE 2-34 Glutamate opens the calcium channel. Shown here are details of calcium entering a dendrite of the blue neuron when the red neuron excites it with glutamate during normal excitatory neurotransmission. Glutamate released from the red neuron travels across the synapse, docks into its agonist slot on its receptor, and, as ionic gatekeeper, opens the calcium channel to allow calcium to enter the postsynaptic dendrite of the blue neuron to mediate normal excitatory neurotransmission (see box).

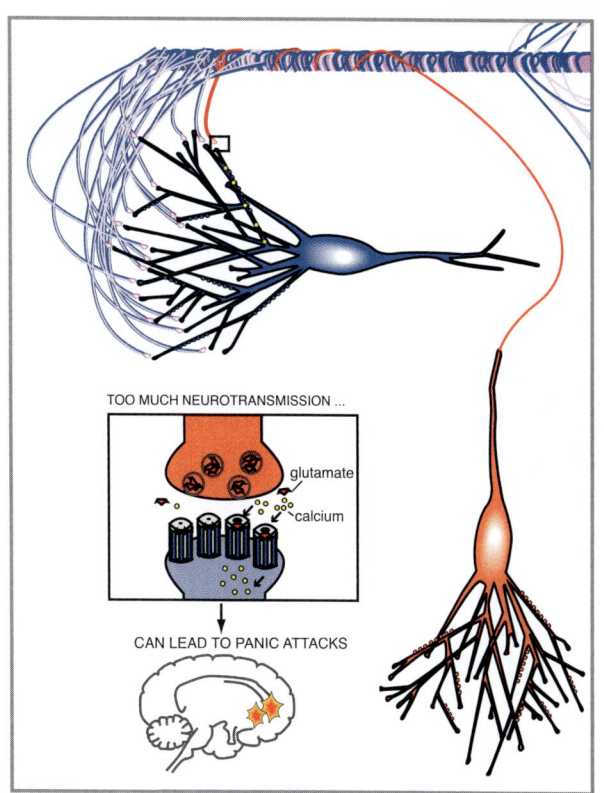

FIGURE 2-35 Too much neurotransmission can lead to symptoms. Shown here is what may happen when excitatory neurotransmission causes too much neurotransmission. This may possibly occur during the production of various symptoms mediated by the brain, including panic attacks. It could also occur during mania, positive symptoms of psychosis, seizures, and other neuronally mediated disease symptoms. In this case, too much glutamate is being released by the red neuron, causing too much excitation of the postsynaptic blue neuron's dendrite. Extra release of glutamate causes additional occupancy of postsynaptic glutamate receptors, opening more calcium channels and allowing more calcium to enter the blue dendrite (see box). Although this degree of excessive neurotransmission may be associated with psychiatric symptoms, it does not necessarily damage the neuron.

Synaptic Neurotransmission and the Anatomically Addressed Nervous System

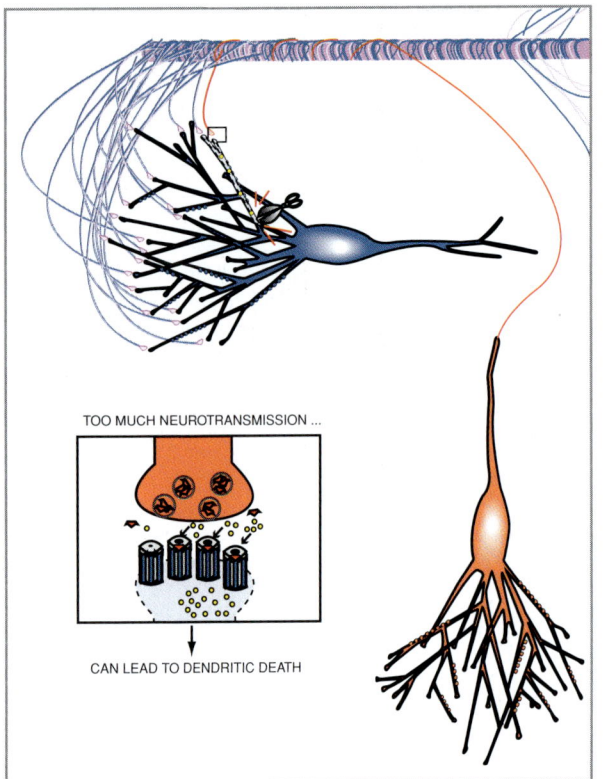

FIGURE 2-36 Too much neurotransmission can lead to dendritic death. If too much neurotransmission occurs for too long, it is hypothetically possible that this would lead to dendritic death. The mechanism for this may be tantamount to inappropriately activating the normal dendritic pruning process. Thus, far too much glutamate release can cause too much opening of the gates of the calcium channel, activating an excitotoxic demise of the dendrite (see box).

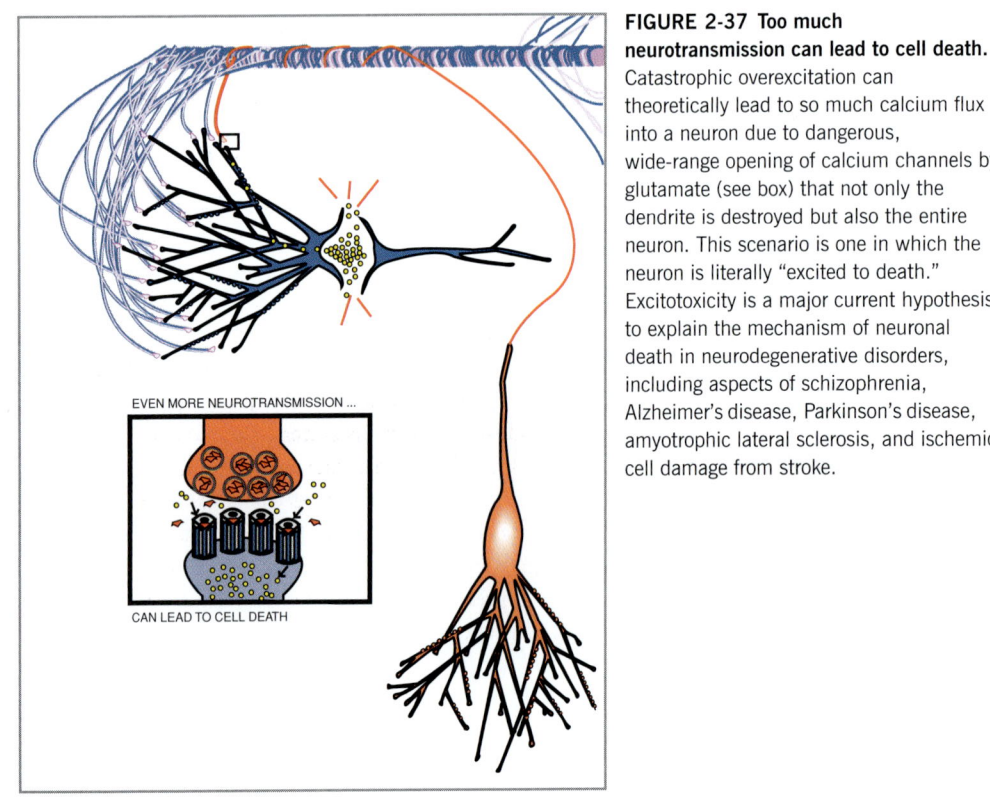

FIGURE 2-37 Too much neurotransmission can lead to cell death. Catastrophic overexcitation can theoretically lead to so much calcium flux into a neuron due to dangerous, wide-range opening of calcium channels by glutamate (see box) that not only the dendrite is destroyed but also the entire neuron. This scenario is one in which the neuron is literally "excited to death." Excitotoxicity is a major current hypothesis to explain the mechanism of neuronal death in neurodegenerative disorders, including aspects of schizophrenia, Alzheimer's disease, Parkinson's disease, amyotrophic lateral sclerosis, and ischemic cell damage from stroke.

48 | Essential Psychopharmacology

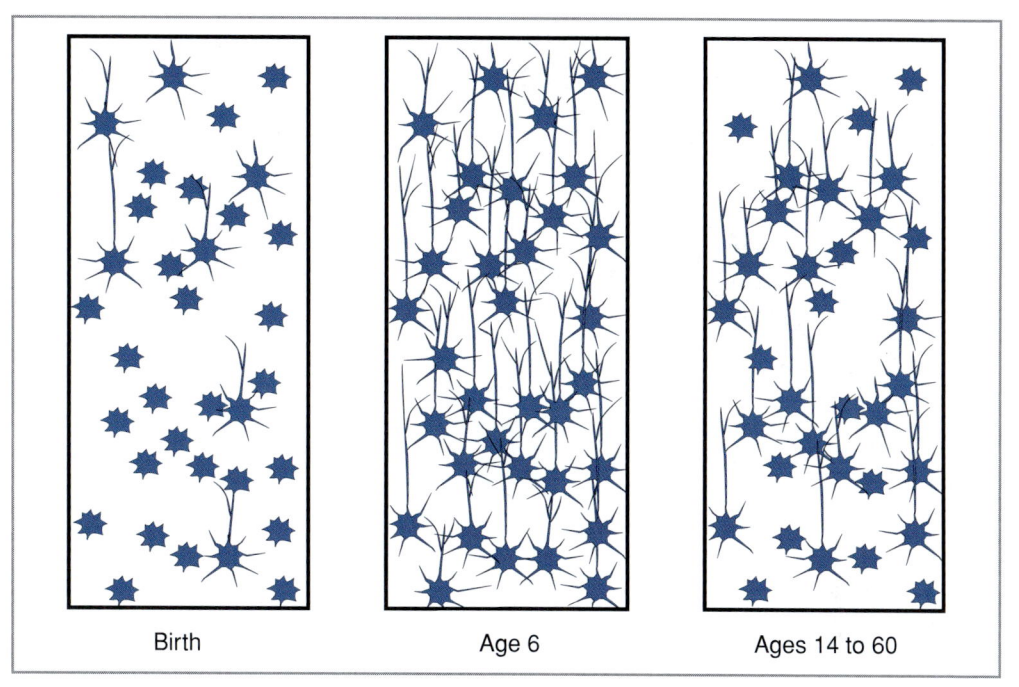

FIGURE 2-38 Synapse formation by age. Synapses are formed at a furious rate between birth and age 6. Competitive elimination and restructuring of synapses peaks during pubescence and adolescence, leaving about half to two-thirds of the synapses present in childhood to survive into adulthood.

the other hand, mental stimulation might prevent this, and psychotherapy may even induce neurotrophic factors to preserve critical cells and innervate new therapeutic targets leading to the alteration of emotions and behaviors. Only future research will clarify how to use drugs and psychotherapy to balance the seasonings in the tender stew of the brain.

Summary

The reader should now appreciate that synaptic neurotransmission is the foundation of psychopharmacology. Here we have described the "hard wiring" that supports chemical neurotransmission as the anatomically addressed nervous system. We have shown how neurons are formed, differentiate, migrate, are selected, and then form synapses. We have pointed out how normal functioning can go awry and cause neurodevelopmental or neurodegenerative disorders. The brain's neurons are largely selected before birth and its synapses by adolescence, but new neurons and new synapses are formed (and eliminated) at lower rates throughout life. Thus, the anatomically addressed nervous system, the structural substrate for synaptic neurotransmission as well as for psychiatric disorders and drug actions, is plastic, changing, and malleable. Coupling an understanding of concepts on the anatomical basis of normal synaptic neurotransmission described here, in Chapter 2, with knowledge about the chemical basis of normal neurotransmission discussed in Chapter 3 will lead to mastery of the many modern hypotheses underlying the biological basis of psychiatric disorders and their treatments, as described throughout the rest of this book.

CHAPTER 3

Signal Transduction and the Chemically Addressed Nervous System

- Principles of chemical neurotransmission
  - Neurotransmitters, cotransmitters, and natural polypharmacy
  - Neurotransmission: classic, retrograde, and volume
  - Excitation-secretion coupling
- Signal-transduction cascades
  - Overview
  - Forming a second messenger
  - Beyond the second messenger
  - Gene expression
- Summary

Neurotransmission has an **anatomical** infrastructure, but it is fundamentally a very elegant **chemical** operation. The discussions of the *anatomically addressed nervous system* and the structural basis of neurotransmission in the previous two chapters (Chapters 1 and 2) set the stage now, in Chapter 3, for describing the *chemically addressed nervous system* and the molecular basis of neurotransmission. An understanding of the principles of chemical neurotransmission is a fundamental requirement for grasping how psychopharmacological agents work via their actions upon key molecules involved in neurotransmission. Drug targeting of specific chemical sites that influence neurotransmission is discussed in the two chapters that follow (Chapters 4 and 5). An understanding of the chemically addressed nervous system is also a prerequisite for becoming a "neurobiologically informed" clinician, best able to translate exciting new findings on brain circuitry, functional neuroimaging, and genetics into clinical practice and potentially improving the manner in which psychiatric disorders and their symptoms are diagnosed and treated in the modern era. The chemistry of neurotransmission in specific brain regions is discussed in Chapter 6, and then these principles are applied to various specific psychiatric disorders throughout the rest of this book.

Principles of chemical neurotransmission

Neurotransmitters, cotransmitters, and natural polypharmacy

The known or suspected neurotransmitters in the brain already number several dozen (for a list of key neurotransmitters, see Table 3-1). Based on theoretical considerations of the

TABLE 3-1 Neurotransmitters in brain

Amines
   Serotonin
   Dopamine
   Norepinephrine/noradrenaline
   Epinephrine/adrenaline
   Acetylcholine
   Tyramine
   Octopamine
   Phenylethylamine
   Tryptamine
   Melatonin
   Histamine
   Agmatine

Pituitary peptides
   Corticotrophin (ACTH)
   Growth hormone (GH)
   Lipotrophin
   Alpha-methalocyte-stimulating hormone (alpha-MSH)
   Oxytocin
   Vasopressin
   Thyroid stimulating hormone (TSH)
   Prolactin

Circulating hormones
   Angiogensin
   Calcitonin
   Glucagon
   Insulin
   Leptin
   Atrial natriuretic factor
   Estrogens
   Androgens
   Progestins
   Thyroid hormones
   Cortisol

Hypothalamic releasing hormones
   Corticotrophin-releasing hormone (CRH)
   Gonadotropin releasing hormone (GnRH)
   Luteinizing hormone releasing hormone (LHRH)
   Somatostatin
   Thyrotropin releasing hormone (TRH)
   Growth hormone releasing hormone (GHRH)

Amino acids
   Gamma-aminobutyric acid (GABA)
   Glycine
   Glutamic acid (glutamate)
   Aspartic acid (aspartate)
   Gamma-hydroxy-butyrate
   d-serine

Gut hormones
   Cholecystokinin (CCK)
   Gastrin
   Motilin
   Pacreatic polypeptide
   Secretin
   Vasoactive intestinal peptide (VIP)

Opioid peptides
   Dynorphin
   Beta-endorphin
   Met-enkephalin
   Leu-enkephalin
   Kyotorphin
   Nociceptin (orphanin FQ)

Miscellaneous peptides
   Bombesin
   Bradykinin
   Carnosine
   Calcitonin G related peptide
   CART (cocaine and amphetamine related transcript)
   Neuropeptide Y
   Neurotensin
   Delta sleep factor
   Galanin
   Orexin/hypocretin
   Melanocyte concentration hormone

Gases
   Nitric oxide (NO)
   Carbon monoxide (CO)

Lipid neurotransmitter
   Anandamide

Neurokinins/tachykinins
   Substance P
   Neurokinin A
   Neurokinin B

Purines
   ATP (adenosine triphosphate)
   ADP (adenosine diphosphate)
   AMP (adenosine monophosphate)
   Adenosine

TABLE 3-2 Cotransmitter pairs

Amine/amino acid	Peptide
dopamine	enkephalin
dopamine	cholecystokinin
norepinephrine	somatostatin
norepinephrine	enkephalin
norepinephrine	neurotensin
epinephrine	enkephalin
serotonin	substance P
serotonin	thyrotropin releasing hormone
serotonin	enkephalin
acetylcholine	vasoactive intestinal peptide
acetylcholine	enkephalin
acetylcholine	neurotensin
acetylcholine	luteinizing hormone releasing hormone
acetylcholine	somatostatin
gamma-aminobutyric acid (GABA)	somatostatin
gamma-aminobutyric acid (GABA)	motilin

amount of genetic material in neurons, there may be several hundred to several thousand unique brain chemicals. In this book, however, only a half dozen or so particular neurotransmitters are emphasized, because psychotropic drugs utilized in clinical practice act largely on serotonin, norepinephrine, and dopamine as well as acetylcholine, glutamate, and GABA (gamma-aminobutyric acid). These six are sometimes considered the "classic" neurotransmitters because they were discovered first and also because they have developed into the major target systems for psychotropic drugs. Classic neurotransmitters are relatively low-molecular weight amines or amino acids. Other neurotransmitters, such as histamine and various neuropeptides and hormones, are also important neurotransmitters and neuromodulators and are mentioned in brief. Ultimately, many more neurotransmitters may become important in psychopharmacology as new drugs emerge (Table 3-1).

Some of the naturally occurring neurotransmitters may be similar to drugs; these have been called "God's pharmacopeia." For example, it is well known that the brain makes its own morphine (i.e., beta endorphin) and its own marijuana (i.e., anandamide). The brain may even make its own antidepressants, its own anxiolytics, and its own hallucinogens. Drugs often mimic the brain's natural neurotransmitters and the discovery of some drugs has preceded that of the natural neurotransmitters. Thus, morphine was used in clinical practice before the discovery of beta-endorphin; marijuana was smoked before the discovery of cannabinoid receptors and anandamide; the benzodiazepines diazepam (Valium) and alprazolam (Xanax) were prescribed before the discovery of benzodiazepine receptors; and the antidepressants amitriptyline (Elavil) and fluoxetine (Prozac) entered clinical practice before molecular clarification of the serotonin transporter site. This underscores the point that the great majority of drugs acting in the central nervous system act on the process of neurotransmission. Indeed, this apparently occurs, at times, in a manner that mimics the actions of the brain itself, when the brain uses its own chemicals.

It was originally thought that each neuron used only one neurotransmitter to send information and used that same neurotransmitter at all of its synapses. Today, however, we know that many neurons utilize more than one neurotransmitter at a single synapse (Table 3-2).

Thus, the concept of cotransmission at some synapses has arisen. This often involves a monoamine coupled with a neuropeptide. Under some conditions, the monoamine is released alone; under other conditions, both are released, adding to the repertoire of options for chemical neurotransmission by neurons that contain both neurotransmitters. Incredibly, therefore, the neuron's output may involve a certain "polypharmacy."

Furthermore, input to each neuron at various sites also involves many different neurotransmitters. An understanding of these inputs to neurons within functioning circuits can provide a rational basis for combining drugs to modify several neurotransmitters simultaneously. This theme is discussed in detail in Chapter 6 and throughout each of the chapters on various psychiatric disorders. The idea is that for the modern psychopharmacologist to influence abnormal neurotransmission in patients with psychiatric disorders, it may be necessary to target neurons in specific circuits. Since these networks of neurons send and receive information via a variety of neurotransmitters, it may therefore be not only rational but necessary to use multiple drugs with multiple neurotransmitter actions for patients with psychiatric disorders, especially if single agents with single neurotransmitter mechanisms are not effective in relieving symptoms. That is, if the neuron itself uses polypharmacy in sending information at individual synapses and in receiving information throughout its dendritic tree, perhaps so should the psychopharmacologist. With an understanding of the specific neurotransmitters that influence unique circuits in the brain – circuits thought to mediate specific symptoms in psychiatric disorders – a rationale is evolving for the use of drug combinations. In fact, this may explain why drugs with multiple mechanisms or multiple drugs in combination are the therapeutic rule in psychopharmacology practice rather than the exception. The trick is to be able to do this rationally.

Neurotransmission: classic, retrograde, and volume
Classic neurotransmission begins with an electrical process by which neurons send electrical impulses from one part of the cell to another part of the same cell via their axons (see neuron A of Figure 3-1). However, these electrical impulses do not jump directly to other neurons. Classic neurotransmission between neurons involves one neuron hurling a chemical messenger, or neurotransmitter, at the receptors of a second neuron (see the synapse between neuron A and neuron B in Figure 3-1). This happens frequently, but not exclusively at the sites of synaptic connections. In the human brain, a hundred billion neurons each make thousands of synapses with other neurons for trillions of chemically neurotransmitting synapses.

Communication *between* all these neurons at synapses is chemical, not electrical. That is, an electrical impulse in the first neuron is converted to a chemical signal at the synapse between it and a second neuron in a process known as excitation-secretion coupling, the first stage of chemical neurotransmission. This occurs predominantly in one direction, from the presynaptic axon terminal, to a second *postsynaptic* neuron (Figures 3-1 and 3-2 and the left panel of Figure 3-3). Finally, neurotransmission continues in the second neuron either by converting the chemical information from the first neuron back into an electrical impulse in the second neuron or, perhaps more elegantly, by the chemical information from the first neuron triggering a cascade of further chemical messages within the second neuron to change that neuron's molecular and genetic functioning (Figure 3-1).

An interesting twist to chemical neurotransmission is the discovery that postsynaptic neurons can also "talk back" to their presynaptic neurons. They can do this in at least two ways: indirectly via a third neuron circling back to the first neuron, in a long neuronal feedback loop as part of a neuronal circuit or network (Figure 3-2), and also directly via

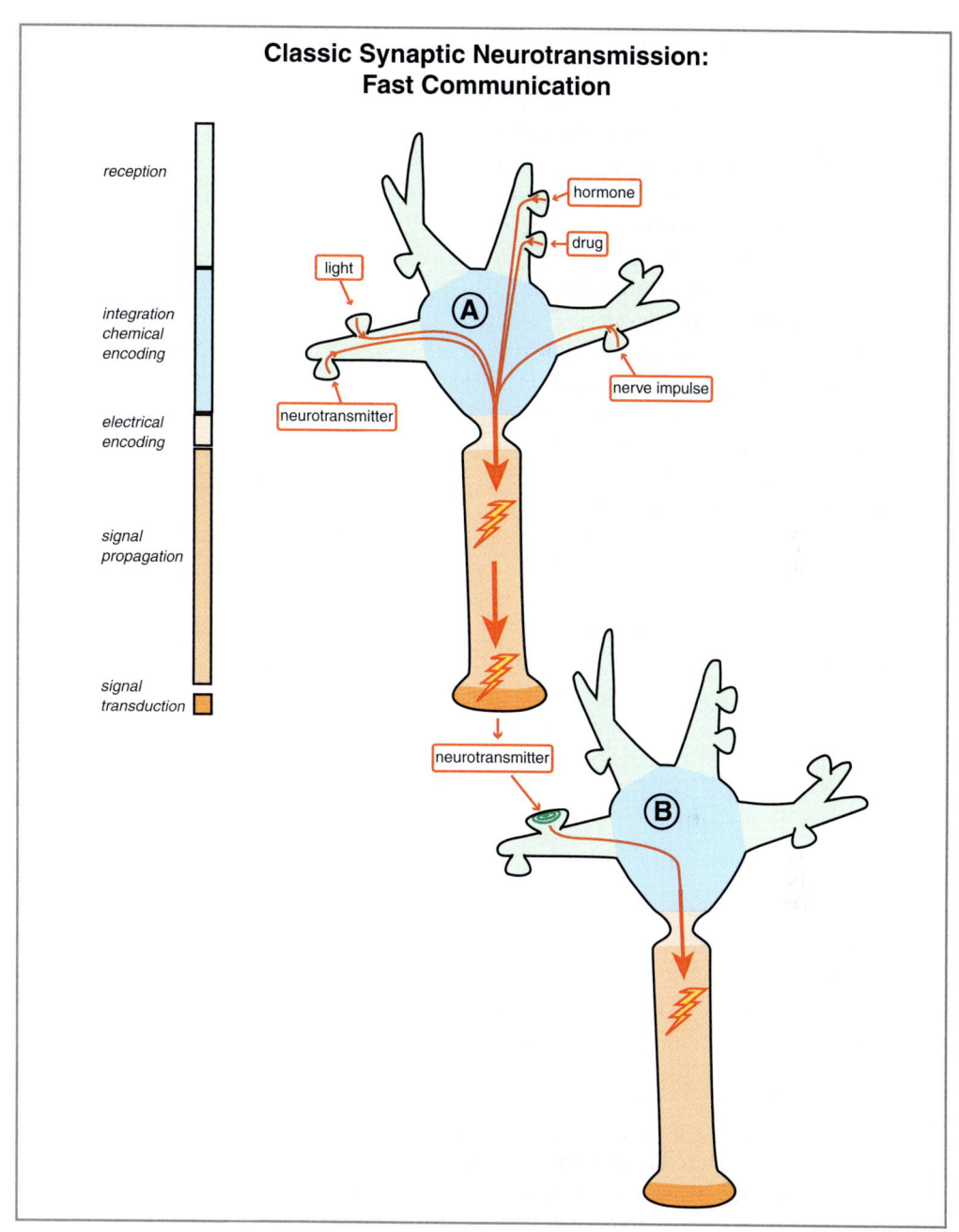

FIGURE 3-1 Classic synaptic neurotransmission. In classic synaptic neurotransmission, stimulation of a presynaptic neuron (e.g., by neurotransmitters, light, drugs, hormones, nerve impulses) causes electrical impulses to be sent to its axon terminal. These electrical impulses are then converted into chemical messengers and released to stimulate the receptors of a postsynaptic neuron. Thus, although communication *within* a neuron can be electrical, communication *between* neurons is chemical.

Signal Transduction and the Chemically Addressed Nervous System

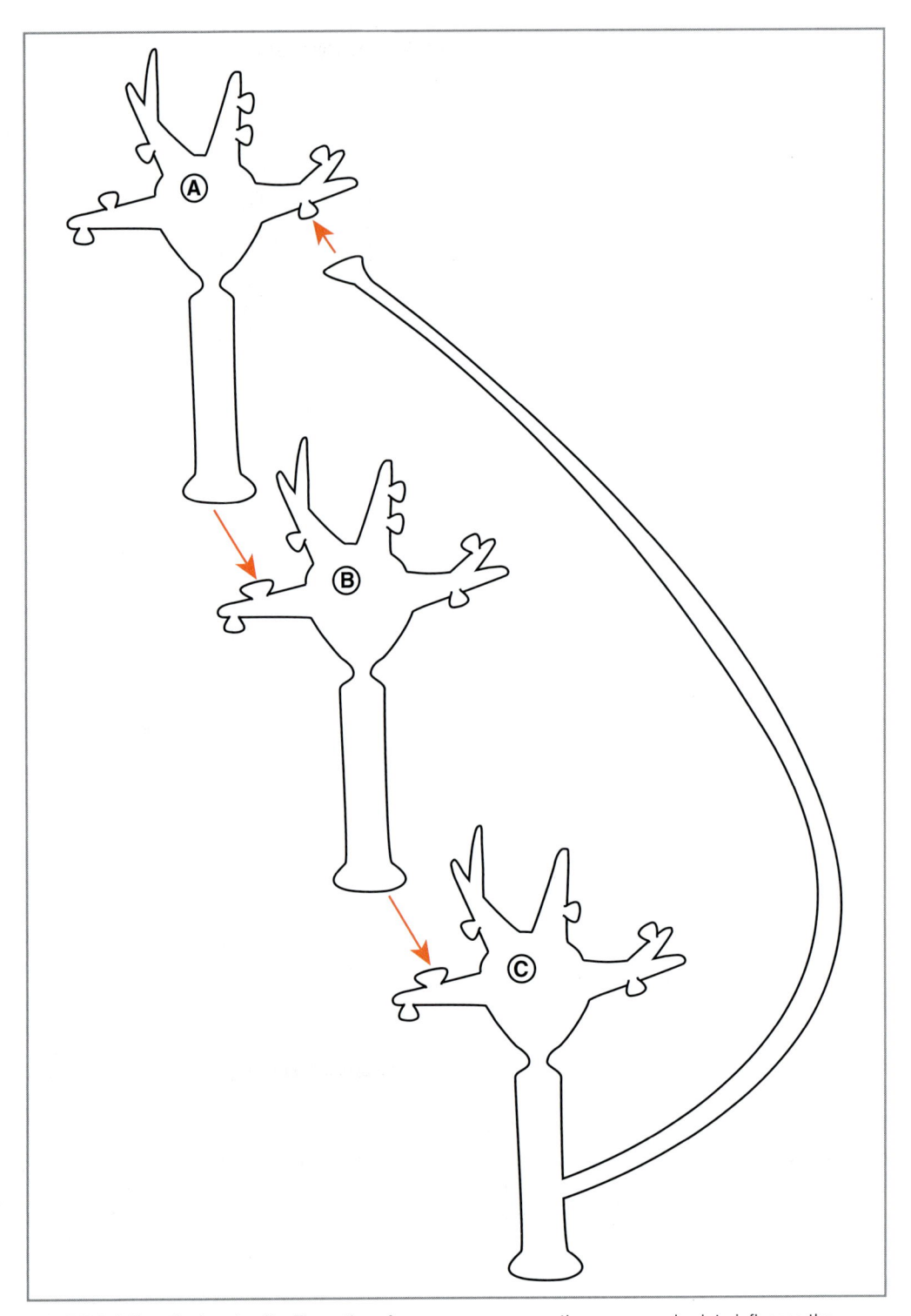

FIGURE 3-2 **Functioning circuits.** The action of one neuron upon another can come back to influence the original neuron by means of a third neuron wired into a loop or functioning circuit.

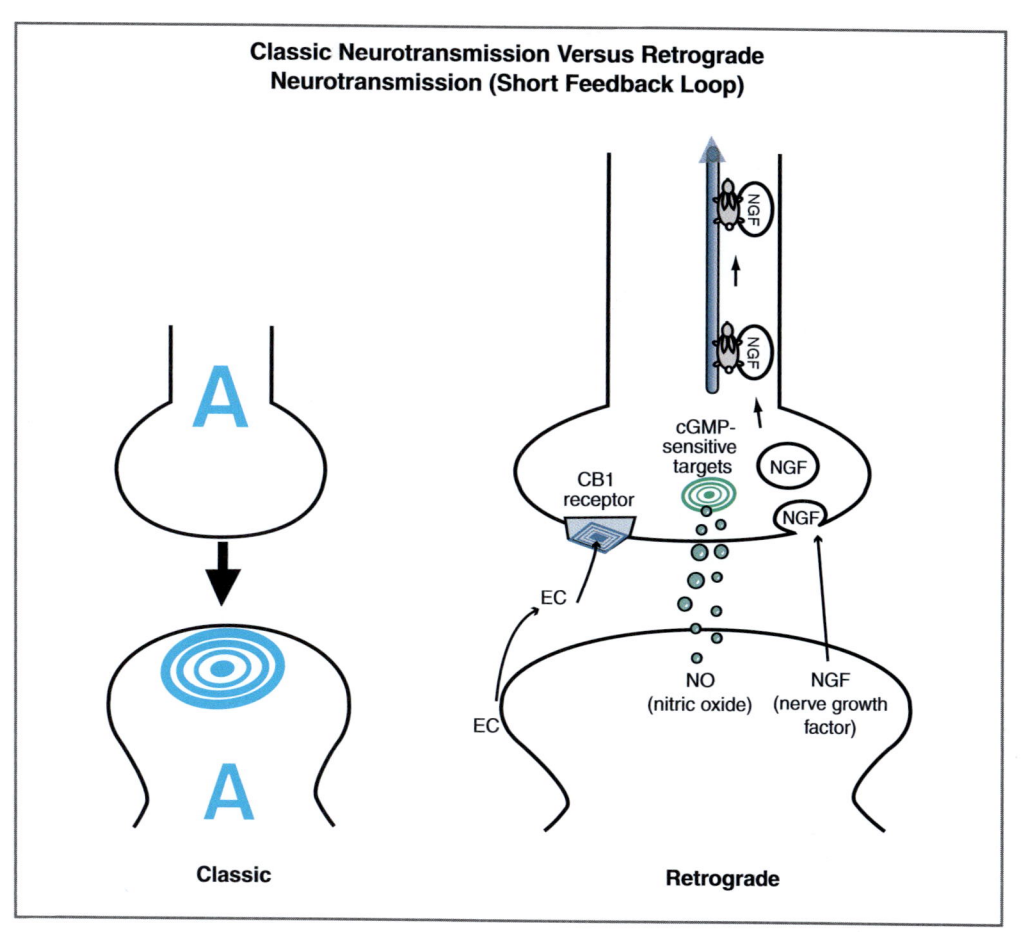

FIGURE 3-3 Retrograde neurotransmission. Not all neurotransmission is classic or anterograde or from top to bottom – namely, presynaptic to postsynaptic (left). Postsynaptic neurons may also communicate with presynaptic neurons from the bottom to the top via retrograde neurotransmission, from postsynaptic neuron to presynaptic neuron (right). Some neurotransmitters produced specifically as retrograde neurotransmitters at some synapses include the endocannabinoids (ECs, or endogenous marijuana), which are synthesized in the postsynaptic neuron, released, and diffuse to presynaptic cannabinoid receptors such as the cannabinoid 1 receptor (CB1); the gaseous neurotransmitter nitric oxide (NO), which is synthesized postsynaptically and then diffuses both out of the postsynaptic membrane and into the presynaptic membrane to interact with cyclic guanosine monophosphate (cGMP)-sensitive targets there; and neurotrophic factors such as nerve growth factor (NGF), which is released from postsynaptic sites and diffuses to the presynaptic neuron, where it is taken up into vesicles and transported all the way back to the cell nucleus via retrograde transport systems to interact with the genome there (see also Figure 1-18).

retrograde neurotransmission from the second neuron to the first at the synapse between them (right panel of Figure 3-3). Chemicals produced specifically as retrograde neurotransmitters at some synapses include the endocannabinoids (ECs, also known as "endogenous marijuana"), which are synthesized in the postsynaptic neuron; they are then released and diffuse to presynaptic cannabinoid receptors, such as the cannabinoid 1 receptor (CB1) (Figure 3-3, right panel). The gaseous neurotransmitter nitric oxide (NO) is synthesized postsynaptically and then diffuses out of the postsynaptic membrane and into the presynaptic neuron to interact with cyclic guanosine monophosphate (cGMP)–sensitive targets there (Figure 3-3, right panel). A third group of retrograde neurotransmitters are

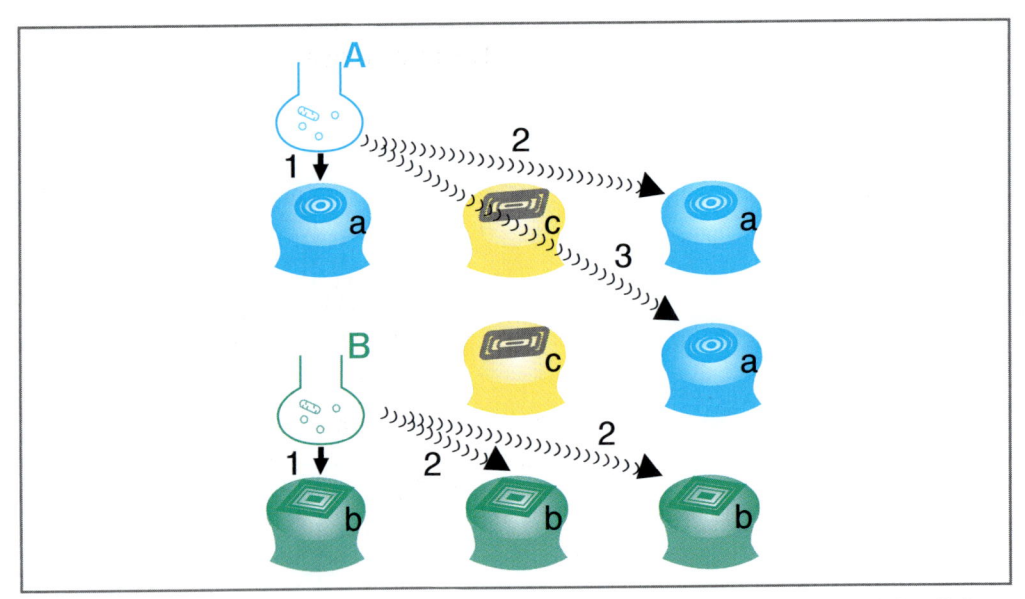

FIGURE 3-4 Volume neurotransmission. Neurotransmission can also occur without a synapse; this is called volume neurotransmission or nonsynaptic diffusion. In this figure, two anatomically addressed synapses (neurons A and B) are shown communicating (arrows 1) with their corresponding postsynaptic receptors (a and b). However, there are also receptors for neurotransmitter A, neurotransmitter B, and neurotransmitter C, which are distant from the synaptic connections of the anatomically addressed nervous system. If neurotransmitter A or B can diffuse away from its synapse before it is destroyed, it will be able to interact with other receptor sites distant from its own synapse (arrows 2). If neurotransmitter A or B encounters a different receptor not capable of recognizing it (receptor c), it will not interact with that receptor even if it diffuses there (arrow 3). Thus, a chemical messenger sent by one neuron to another can spill over by diffusion to sites distant from its own synapse. Neurotransmission can occur at a compatible receptor within the diffusion radius of the matched neurotransmitter. This is analogous to modern communication with cellular telephones, which function within the transmitting radius of a given cell. This concept is called the chemically addressed nervous system, in which neurotransmission occurs in chemical "puffs." The brain is thus not only a collection of wires but also a sophisticated "chemical soup."

neurotrophic factors such as nerve growth factor (NGF), which is released from postsynaptic sites and then diffuses to the presynaptic neuron, where it is taken up into vesicles and transported all the way back to the cell nucleus via retrograde transport systems to interact with the genome there (Figure 3-3, right panel; see also Figure 1-18). What these retrograde neurotransmitters have to say to the presynaptic neuron and how this modifies or regulates the communication between pre- and postsynaptic neuron are subjects of intense active investigation.

In addition to "reverse" or retrograde neurotransmission at synapses, some neurotransmission does not need a synapse at all! Neurotransmission without a synapse is called *volume neurotransmission*, or nonsynaptic diffusion neurotransmission; examples are shown in Figures 3-4 through 3-6. Chemical messengers sent by one neuron to another can spill over to sites distant to the synapse by diffusion (Figure 3-4). Thus, neurotransmission can occur at any compatible receptor within the diffusion radius of the neurotransmitter, not unlike modern communication with cellular telephones, which function within the transmitting radius of a given cell (Figure 3-4). This concept is part of the *chemically addressed* nervous system, and here neurotransmission occurs in chemical "puffs" (Figures 3-4, 3-5, and 3-6). The brain is thus not only a collection of wires but also a sophisticated "chemical soup." The

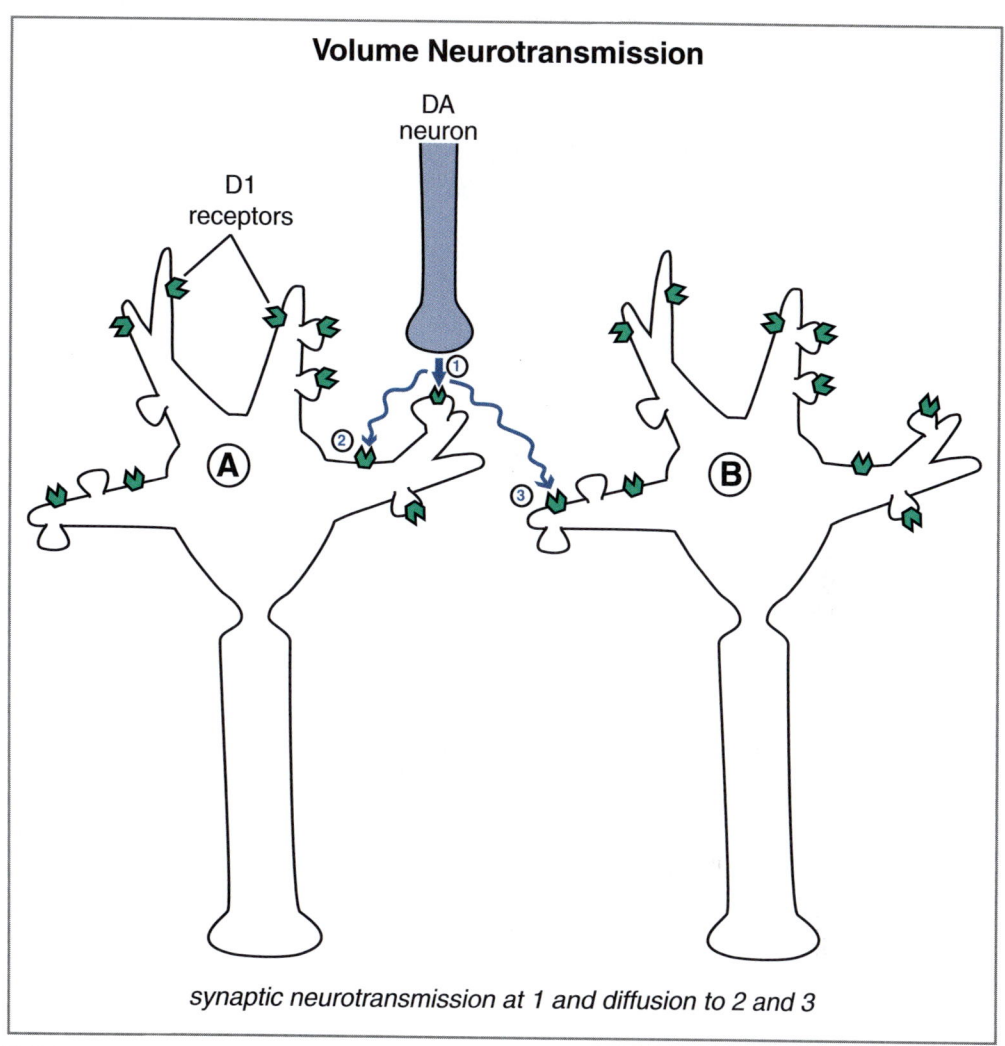

FIGURE 3-5 Volume neurotransmission: dopamine. An example of volume neurotransmission would be that of dopamine in the prefrontal cortex. Since there are few dopamine reuptake pumps in the prefrontal cortex, dopamine is available to diffuse to nearby receptor sites. Thus, dopamine released from a synapse (arrow 1) targeting postsynaptic neuron A is free to diffuse further in the absence of a reuptake pump and can reach dopamine receptors on that same neuron but outside of the synapse from which it was released, on neighboring dendrites (arrow 2). Shown here is dopamine also reaching extrasynaptic receptors on a neighboring neuron (arrow 3).

chemically addressed nervous system is particularly important in understanding the actions of drugs that act at various neurotransmitter receptors, since such drugs will act wherever there are relevant receptors, and not just where such receptors are innervated with synapses by the anatomically addressed nervous system.

In the case of dopamine neurotransmission in the prefrontal cortex, for example, there are very few dopamine reuptake transport pumps to terminate the action of dopamine released there by neurotransmission. This is much different from other brain areas such as the striatum, where dopamine reuptake pumps are present in abundance. Thus, when dopamine neurotransmission occurs at a synapse in the prefrontal cortex, dopamine is free

Signal Transduction and the Chemically Addressed Nervous System | 59

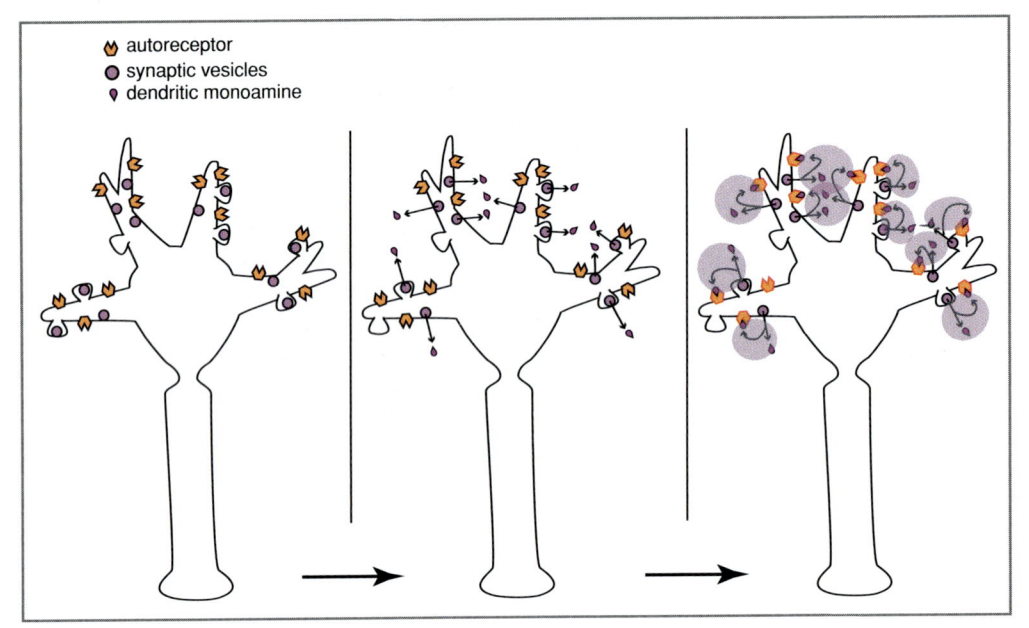

FIGURE 3-6 Volume neurotransmission: monoamine autoreceptors. Another example of volume neurotransmission could involve autoreceptors on monoamine neurons. Autoreceptors located on the dendrites and soma of a neuron (at the top of the neuron in the left panel) normally inhibit release of neurotransmitter from the axon of that neuron (at the bottom of the neuron in the left panel), and thus inhibit impulse flow through that neuron from top to bottom. Monoamines released from the dendrites of this neuron (at the top of the neuron in the middle panel) then bind to these autoreceptors (at the top of the neuron in the right panel) and would inhibit neuronal impulse flow in that neuron (from the bottom of the neuron in the right panel). This action occurs due to volume neurotransmission and despite the absence of synaptic neurotransmission in the somatodendritic areas of these neurons.

to spill over from that synapse and diffuse to neighboring dopamine receptors and stimulate them, even though there is no synapse at these "spillover" sites (Figure 3-5). Another important example of volume neurotransmission may be at the sites of autoreceptors on monoamine neurons (Figure 3-6). At the somatodendritic end of the neuron (top of the neurons in Figure 3-6) are autoreceptors that inhibit the release of neurotransmitter from the axonal end of the neuron (bottom of the neurons in Figure 3-6). Although some recurrent axon collaterals and other monoamine neurons may directly innervate somatodendritic receptors, these receptors may also receive neurotransmitter from dendritic release (Figure 3-6, middle and right panels). There is no synapse here, just neurotransmitter leaked from the neuron on its own receptors. The nature of a neuron's regulation by its somatodendritic autoreceptors is a subject of intense interest and may be linked to the mechanism of action of many antidepressants, as explained in Chapter 10. The take-home point here is that not all chemical neurotransmission occurs at synapses.

Excitation-secretion coupling

An electrical impulse in the first – or presynaptic – neuron is converted into a chemical signal at the synapse by a process known as *excitation-secretion coupling*. Once an electrical impulse invades the presynaptic axon terminal, it causes the release of chemical neurotransmitter stored there (Figure 3-1). Electrical impulses open ion channels – both *voltage-sensitive sodium channels* (VSSCs) and *voltage-sensitive calcium channels* (VSCCs) – by changing the ionic charge across neuronal membranes. As sodium flows into the presynaptic nerve through sodium channels in the axon membrane, the electrical charge of the action potential moves along the axon until it reaches the presynaptic nerve terminal, where it also opens calcium channels. As calcium flows into the presynaptic nerve terminal, it causes synaptic vesicles anchored to the inner membrane to spill their chemical contents into the synapse. The way is paved for chemical communication by previous synthesis of neurotransmitter and storage of neurotransmitter in the first neuron's presynaptic axon terminal.

Excitation-secretion coupling is thus the way in which the neuron transduces an electrical stimulus into a chemical event. This happens very quickly once the electrical impulse enters the presynaptic neuron. It is also possible for the neuron to transduce a chemical message from a presynaptic neuron back into an electrical chemical message in the postsynaptic neuron by opening ion channels linked to neurotransmitters there, especially by glutamate and GABA. This also happens very quickly when chemical neurotransmitters open ion channels that change the flow of charge into the neuron and, ultimately, action potentials in the postsynaptic neuron. Thus, the process of neurotransmission is constantly transducing chemical signals into electrical signals and electrical signals into chemical signals.

Signal-transduction cascades

Overview

Neurotransmission can be seen as part of a much larger process than just the communication of a presynaptic axon with a postsynaptic neuron at the synapse between them. That is, neurotransmission can also be seen as communication from the genome of the presynaptic neuron to the genome of the postsynaptic neuron (Figure 3-7) and then back from the genome of the postsynaptic neuron to the genome of the presynaptic neuron (Figure 3-8). Such a process involves long strings of chemical messages within both presynaptic and postsynaptic neurons (Figures 3-7 and 3-8). These are often called signal-transduction cascades. Signal transduction from the genome in the cell nucleus of neuron A begins with transcription of a gene into a protein (Figure 3-7). Signal transduction in neuron B begins with second messenger formation from chemical neurotransmission received from neuron A (Figure 3-7). Reverse signaling from neuron B begins with the transcription of genes triggered in the genome of neuron B owing to neurotransmission from neuron A (Figure 3-8). Ultimately, retrograde neurotransmission from neuron B to neuron A reaches the genome of neuron A, completing the round trip of information exchange between these two neurons.

The signal transduction cascades triggered by chemical neurotransmission thus involve numerous molecules, starting with neurotransmitter first messenger and proceeding to second, third, fourth, and more messengers (Figures 3-9 and 3-10). The initial events occur in less than a second, but the long-term consequences are mediated by downstream messengers that take hours to days to activate yet can last for many days or even for the lifetime of a synapse or neuron (Figure 3-9). Signal transduction cascades are somewhat akin to a molecular "pony express," with specialized molecules acting as a sequence of riders, handing off the message to the next specialized molecule, until the message has reached a functional destination, such as gene expression or activation of otherwise "sleeping" and inactive molecules (Figures 3-10 and 3-11).

An overview of such a molecular pony express, from first messenger neurotransmitter through several "molecular riders" to the production of diverse biological responses, is shown in Figure 3-10. Specifically, a first messenger neurotransmitter on the left activates

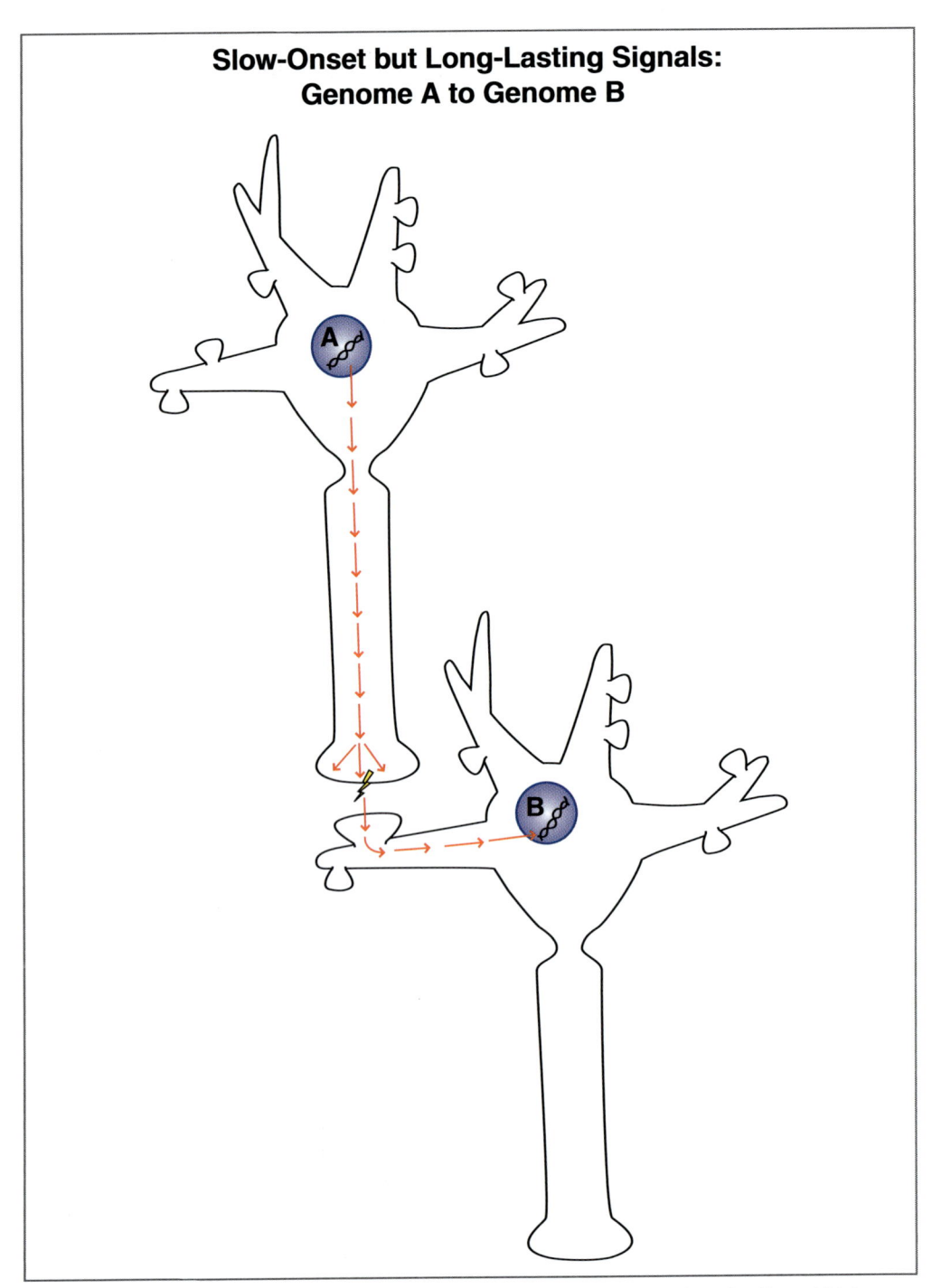

FIGURE 3-7 Slow-onset neurotransmitter signaling. Unlike fast-onset neurotransmitter signaling, which is depicted in Figure 3-1 and occurs from one side of a synapse to another, slow-onset long-lasting signaling from neurotransmission results from a signal arising from one genome that is able to get its message to another neuron's genome through a sequence of signal transduction cascades in both neurons. Such signal transduction cascades can take time, hours or days, to develop, but their consequences can be quite long-lasting, for many days, or almost permanently in the case of some structural changes.

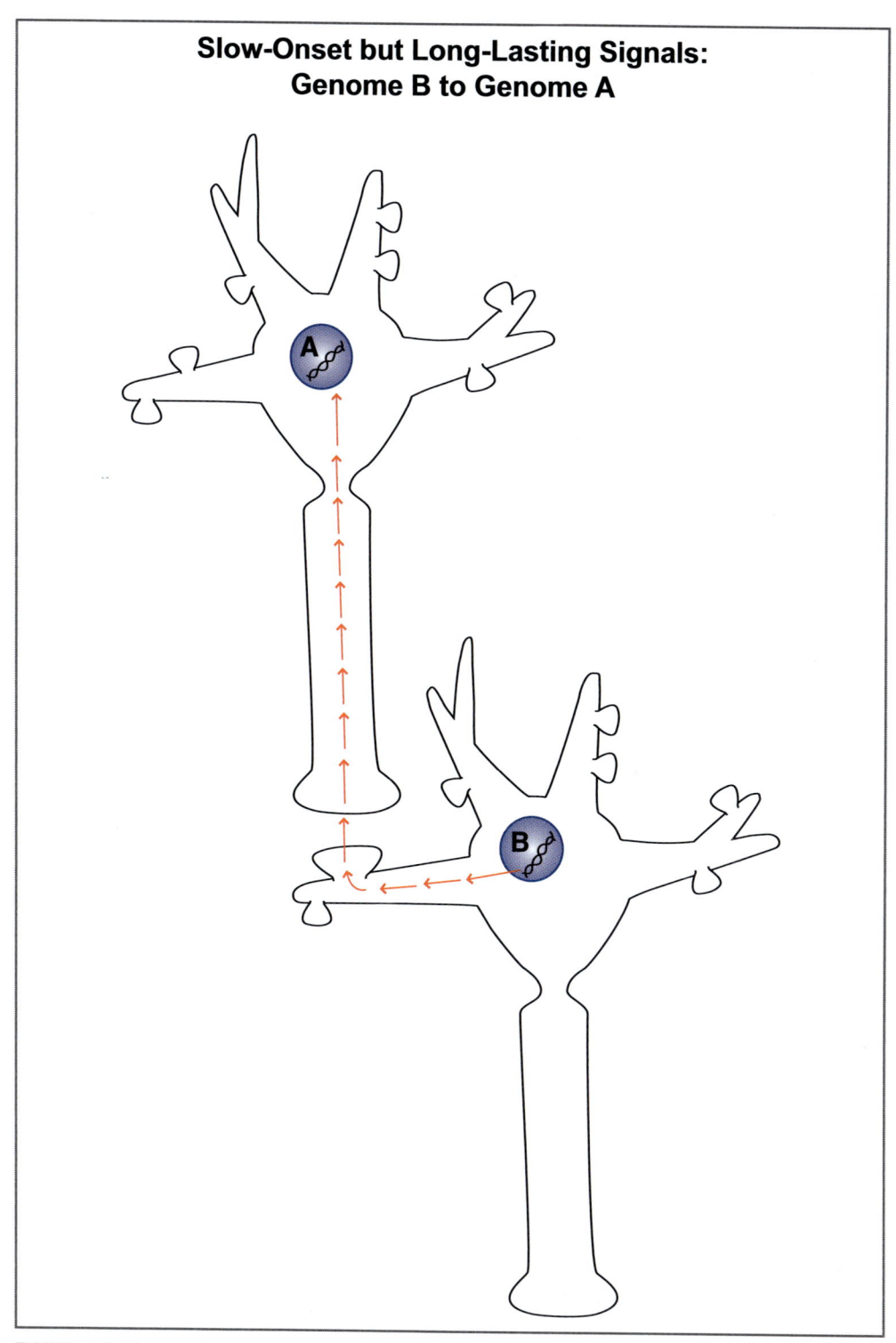

FIGURE 3-8 Slow-onset neurotransmitter signaling. Slow-onset long-lasting neurotransmission involves not only signaling from one genome to another, as shown in Figure 3-7, but can also involve signaling back from the second neuron to the first, as shown here.

Time Course of Signal Transduction

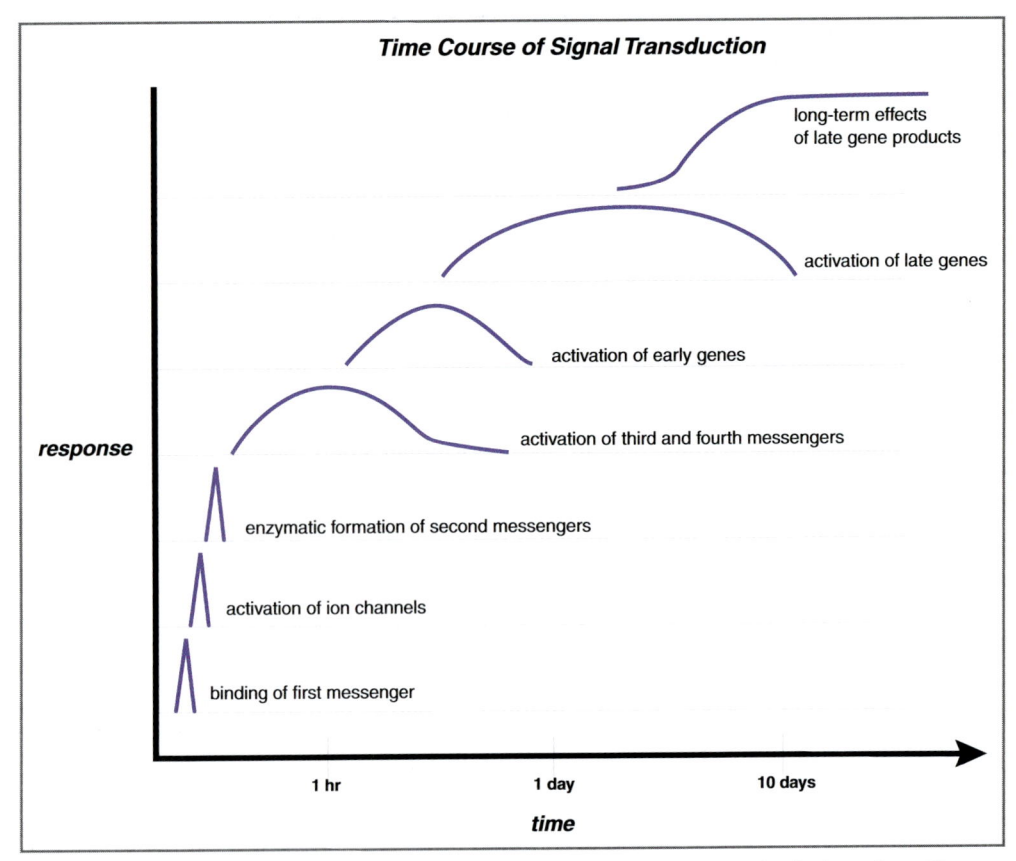

FIGURE 3-9 Time course of signal transduction. The time course of signal transduction is shown here. The process begins with binding of a first messenger (bottom), which leads to activation of ion channels or enzymatic formation of second messengers. This, in turn, can cause activation of third and fourth messengers, which are often phosphoproteins. If genes are subsequently activated, this leads to the synthesis of new proteins, which can alter the neuron's functions. Once initiated, the functional changes due to protein activation or new protein synthesis can last for at least many days and possibly much longer. Thus, the ultimate effects of signal transduction cascades triggered by chemical neurotransmission are not only delayed but also long-lasting.

the production of a chemical second messenger that in turn activates a third messenger – namely, an enzyme known as a kinase, which adds phosphate groups to fourth messenger proteins to create phosphoproteins (Figure 3-10, on the left). Another signal transduction cascade is shown on the right, with a first messenger neurotransmitter opening an ion channel, which allows calcium to enter the neuron and act as the second messenger for this cascade system (Figure 3-10, on the right). Calcium then activates a different third messenger on the right – an enzyme known as a phosphatase – which removes phosphate groups from fourth messenger phosphoproteins and thus reverses the actions of the third messenger on the left. The balance between kinase and phosphatase activity, signaled by the balance between the two neurotransmitters activating each, determines the degree of downstream chemical activity that gets translated into an active fourth messenger able to trigger diverse biological responses such as gene expression and synaptogenesis (Figure 3-10). Each molecular site within the cascade of transduction of chemical and electrical messages is a potential location for a malfunction associated with a mental illness; it is also

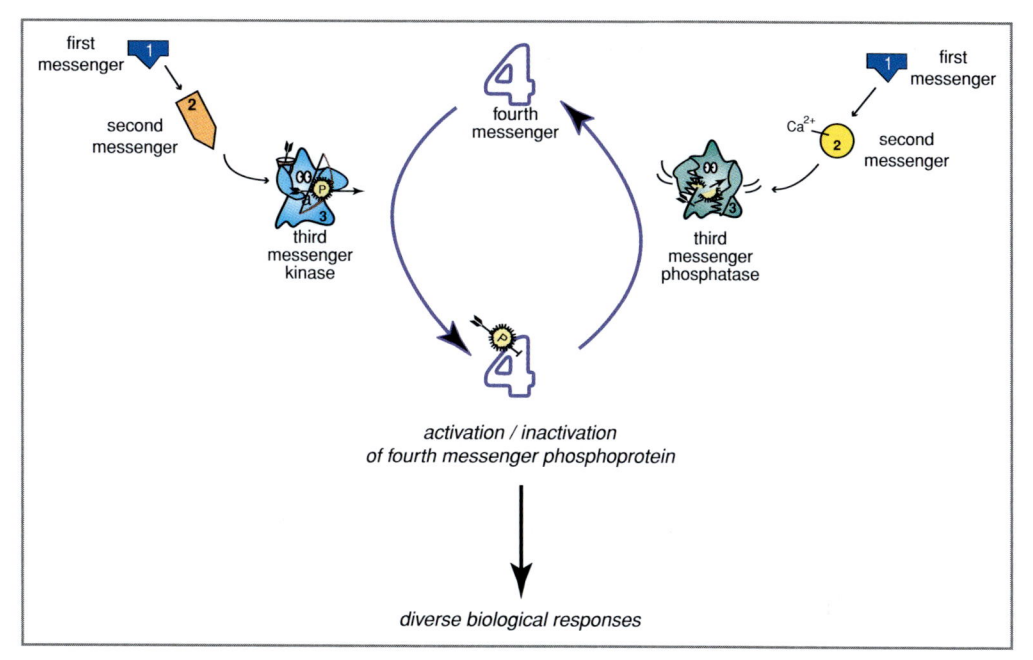

FIGURE 3-10 Signal transduction cascade. The cascade of events that occurs following stimulation of a postsynaptic receptor is known as signal transduction. Signal transduction cascades can activate third messenger enzymes known as kinases, which add phosphate groups to proteins to create phosphoproteins (on the left). Other signal transduction cascades can activate third messenger enzymes known as phosphatases, which remove phosphates from phosphoproteins (on the right). The balance between kinase and phosphatase activity, signaled by the balance between the two neurotransmitters that activate each of them, determines the degree of downstream chemical activity that gets translated into diverse biological responses, such as gene expression and synaptogenesis.

a potential target for a psychotropic drug. Thus, the various elements of multiple signal transduction cascades play very important roles in psychopharmacology.

Four of the most important signal transduction cascades in the brain are listed in Table 3-3 and shown in Figure 3-11. These include G protein–linked systems, ion channel–linked systems, hormone-linked systems, and neurotrophin-linked systems. There are many chemical messengers for each of these four critical signal transduction cascades; examples of first messengers for each are given in Table 3-4. Two of these cascades are triggered by neurotransmitters (Table 3-4): one system is G protein–linked and the other is ion channel–linked. Many of the psychotropic drugs used in clinical practice today target one of these two signal transduction cascades. Drugs that target the G protein–linked system are discussed in Chapter 4; drugs that target the ion channel–linked system are discussed in Chapter 5.

Forming a second messenger

Each of the four signal transduction cascades passes its message from an extracellular first messenger to an intracellular second messenger. Examples of key second messengers for each of the four critical families of signal transduction cascades are given in Table 3-5. In the case of G protein–linked systems, the second messenger is a chemical; but in the case of an ion channel–linked system, the second messenger can be an ion such as calcium (Figure 3-11 and Table 3-5). For hormone-linked systems, a second messenger is formed when the hormone finds its receptor in the cytoplasm and binds to it to form a

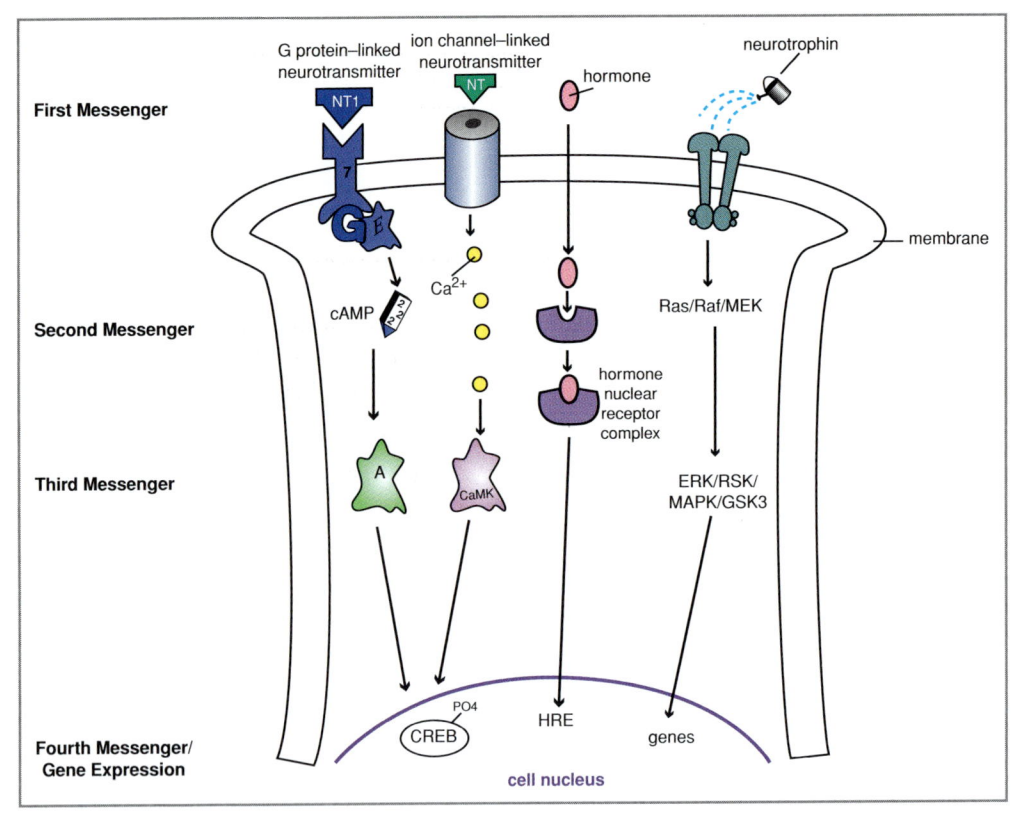

FIGURE 3-11 Different signal transduction cascades. Four of the most important signal transduction cascades in the brain are shown here. These include G protein–linked systems, ion channel–linked systems, hormone-linked systems, and neurotrophin-linked systems. Each begins with a different first messenger binding to a unique receptor, leading to activation of very different downstream second, third, and subsequent chemical messengers. Having many different signal transduction cascades allows neurons to respond in amazingly diverse biological ways to a whole array of chemical messaging systems. Neurotransmitters (NT) activate both the G protein–linked system and the ion channel–linked system on the left, and both of these systems activate genes in the cell nucleus by phosphorylating a protein there called cyclic AMP response element–binding protein (CREB). The G protein–linked system works through a cascade involving cyclic AMP (adenosine monophosphate) and protein kinase A, whereas the ion channel–linked system works through calcium and its ability to activate a different kinase called calcium/calmodulin kinase (CaMK). Certain hormones, like estrogen and other steroids, can enter the neuron, find their receptors in the cytoplasm, and bind them to form a hormone–nuclear receptor complex. This complex can then enter the cell nucleus to interact with hormone response elements (HRE) there to trigger activation of specific genes. Finally, the neurotrophin system on the far right activates a series of kinase enzymes, with a confusing alphabet soup of names, to trigger gene expression, which may control such functions as synaptogenesis and neuronal survival. Ras is a G protein, Raf is a kinase, and the other elements in this cascade are proteins as well (MEK stands for mitogen-activated protein kinase/extracellular signal–regulated kinase; ERK stands for extracellular signal–regulated kinase itself; RSK is ribosomal S6 kinase; MAPK is MAP kinase itself, and GSK3 is glycogen synthase kinase 3).

hormone–nuclear receptor complex (Figure 3-11). For neurotrophins, a complex set of various second messengers exists (Table 3-5 and Figure 3-11), including proteins that are kinase enzymes with an alphabet soup of complicated names.

The transduction of an extracellular first neurotransmitter from the presynaptic neuron into an intracellular second messenger in the postsynaptic neuron is known in detail for some second messenger systems, such as those that are linked to G proteins (Figures 3-12

TABLE 3-3

FOUR KEY SIGNAL TRANSDUCTION CASCADES

G protein–linked
ion channel–linked
nuclear hormone receptors
receptor tyrosine kinases

TABLE 3-4

EXAMPLES OF FIRST MESSENGERS FOR FOUR DIFFERENT SIGNAL TRANSDUCTION CASCADES

NEUROTRANSMITTERS (G PROTEIN–LINKED)	NEUROTRANSMITTERS (IONOTROPIC, ION CHANNEL–LINKED)
dopamine	glutamate (ionotropic)
serotonin	acetylcholine (nicotinic)
norepinephrine	GABA (GABA-A)
acetylcholine (muscarinic)	serotonin (5HT3)
glutamate (metabotropic)	
GABA (GABA-B)	
histamine	

HORMONES (NUCLEAR HORMONE RECEPTORS)	NEUROTROPIC FACTORS (RECEPTOR TYROSINE KINASES)
estrogen	BDNF
other gonadal steroids	NGF
glucocorticoids	many others
thyroid	

TABLE 3-5

EXAMPLES OF KEY SECOND MESSENGERS FOR FOUR DIFFERENT SIGNAL TRANSDUCTION CASCADES:
Generally lead to activation of protein kinases and thus phosphorylation cascades

G PROTEIN–LINKED	ION CHANNEL–LINKED
cAMP (cyclic AMP)	Ca^{2+} (calcium)
IP_3 (inositol 1,4,5, triphosphate)	

NUCLEAR HORMONE RECEPTORS	RECEPTOR TYROSINE KINASES
HORMONE –NUCLEAR RECEPTOR COMPLEX	ALPHABET SOUP
	Ras/Ras-GTP
	Raf (a protein kinase)
	MEK (**M**AP kinase **E** kinase **k**inase or MAP kinase)

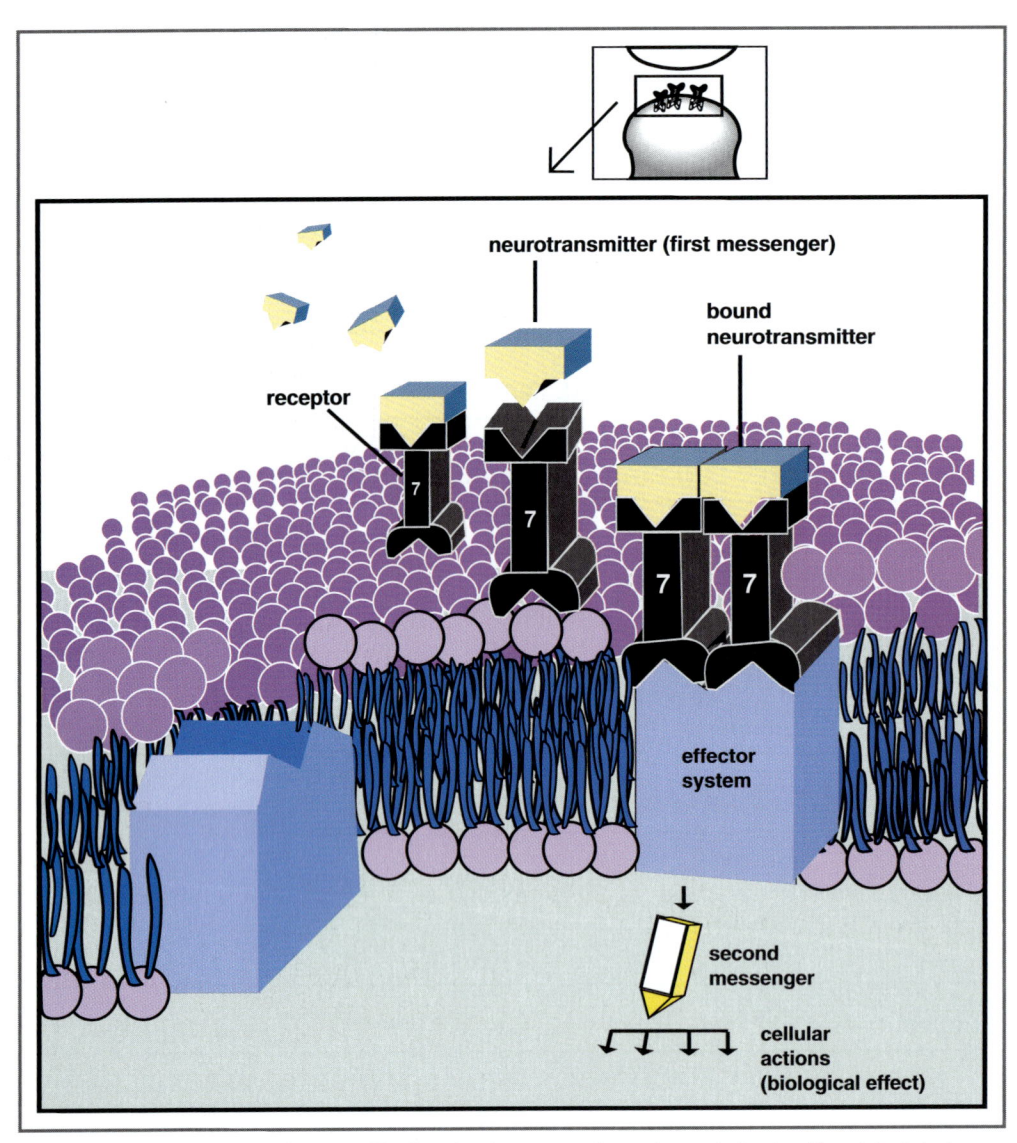

FIGURE 3-12 G protein-linked system. The functional outcome of neurotransmission in a G protein–linked system is depicted here in the postsynaptic neuron. Neurotransmitter released from the presynaptic neuron is considered the first messenger. It binds to its G protein–linked receptor (indicated here with 7 because it has seven transmembrane domains). The bound neurotransmitter causes an effector system, namely a G protein linked to an enzyme, to manufacture a second messenger. The second messenger is inside the postsynaptic neuron. It is this second messenger that then goes on to create cellular actions and biological effects by triggering, inside the neuron, further transduction of the signal it carries from the first messenger and passing it along to a third messenger. Examples of this are the neuron beginning to synthesize a chemical product, changing its firing rate, or constructing a synapse. Thus, information in the presynaptic neuron is conveyed to the postsynaptic neuron by a chain of events. This is how the brain is envisioned to do its work – thinking, remembering, controlling movement, etc. – through the synthesis of brain chemicals and the firing of brain neurons.

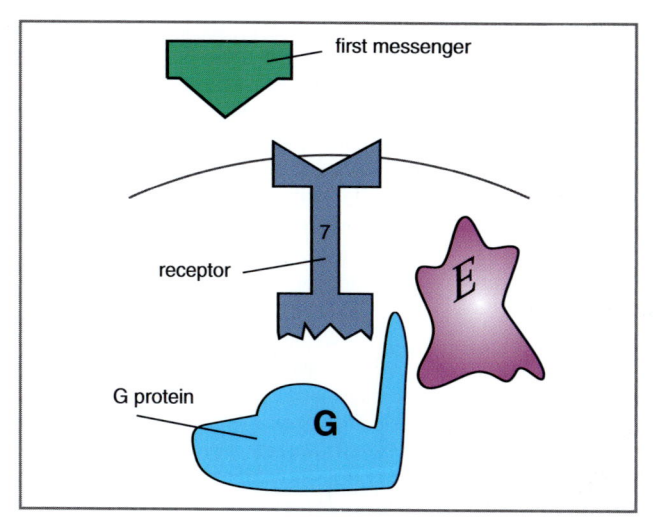

FIGURE 3-13 Elements of G protein-linked system. Shown here are the four elements of a G protein–linked second messenger system. The first element is the neurotransmitter itself, sometimes also referred to as the first messenger. The second element is the G protein–linked neurotransmitter receptor, which is a protein with seven transmembrane regions. The third element, a G protein, is a connecting protein. The fourth element of the second messenger system is an enzyme, which can synthesize a second messenger when activated.

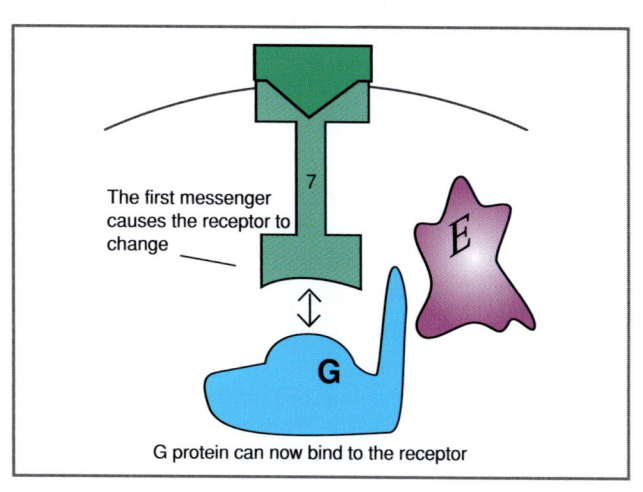

FIGURE 3-14 First messenger. In this figure, the neurotransmitter has docked into its receptor. The first messenger does its job by transforming the conformation of the receptor so that the receptor can bind to the G protein, indicated here by the receptor turning the same color as the neurotransmitter and changing its shape at the bottom in order to make it capable of binding to the G protein.

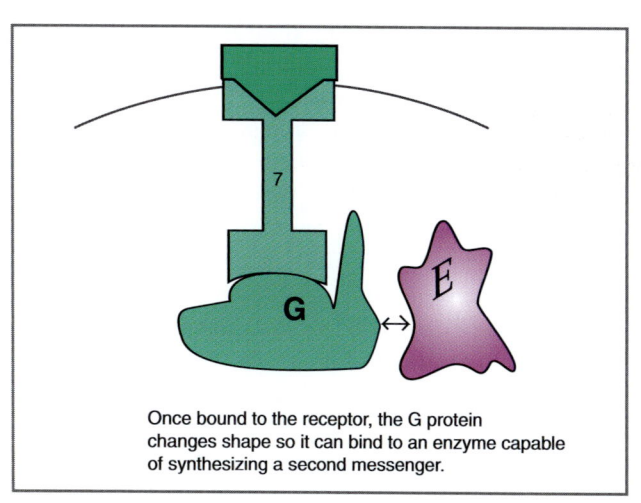

FIGURE 3-15 G protein. The next stage in producing a second messenger is for the transformed neurotransmitter receptor to bind to the G protein, depicted here by the G protein turning the same color as the neurotransmitter and its receptor. Binding of the binary neurotransmitter receptor complex to the G protein causes yet another conformational change, this time in the G protein, represented here as a change in the shape of the right-hand side of the G protein. This prepares the G protein to bind to the enzyme capable of synthesizing the second messenger.

Signal Transduction and the Chemically Addressed Nervous System

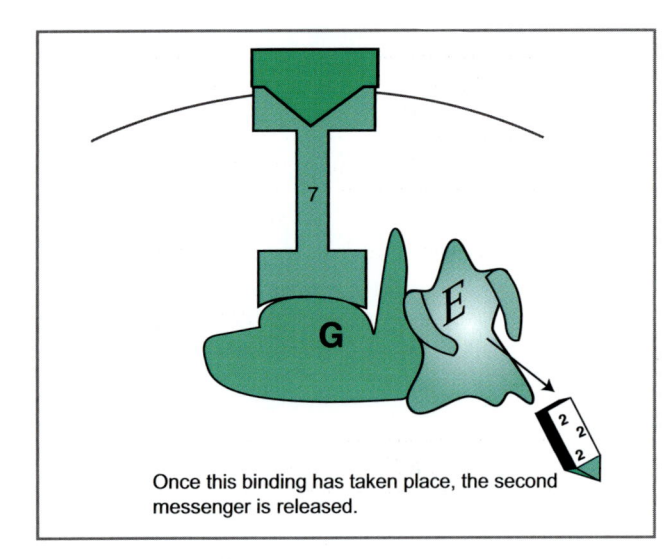

FIGURE 3-16 Second messenger. The final step in formation of the second messenger is for the ternary complex neurotransmitter-receptor-G protein to bind to a messenger-synthesizing enzyme, depicted here by the enzyme turning the same color as the ternary complex. Once the enzyme binds to this ternary complex, it becomes activated and capable of synthesizing the second messenger. Thus, it is the cooperation of all four elements, wrapped together as a quaternary complex, that leads to the production of the second messenger. Information from the first messenger thus passes to the second messenger through use of receptor–G protein–enzyme intermediaries.

Once this binding has taken place, the second messenger is released.

through 3-16). Specifically, chemical neurotransmission at G protein–linked receptors begins with receptor occupancy by the neurotransmitter – the *first messenger* binding to *highly specific sites* in the postsynaptic neuron (Figures 3-12 and 3-13). The neurotransmitter acts as a key that fits the receptor lock on the postsynaptic neuron quite selectively. The *first* messenger hands off its message to a second messenger, which is intracellular (Figure 3-12). It does this via an effector system that is able to synthesize an active second messenger (Figure 3-12).

There are four key elements to this second messenger system: the first messenger neurotransmitter; a receptor for the neurotransmitter that belongs to the receptor superfamily in which all have the structure of seven transmembrane regions (designated by the number 7 on the receptor in Figures 3-12 and 3-13); a G protein capable of binding both to certain conformations of the neurotransmitter receptor (7) and to an enzyme system (E) that can synthesize the second messenger; and finally the enzyme system itself for the second messenger (Figure 3-13). The first step is the binding of the neurotransmitter to its receptor (Figure 3-14). This changes the conformation of the receptor so it can now fit with the G protein; it is indicated by the receptor (7) turning green and its shape changing at the bottom. Next comes the binding of the G protein to this new conformation of the receptor-neurotransmitter complex (Figure 3-15). The two receptors cooperate with each other: namely, the neurotransmitter receptor itself and the G protein, which can be thought of as another type of receptor associated with the inner membrane of the cell. This cooperation is indicated in Figure 3-15 by the G protein turning green and its conformation changing on the right so that it is now capable of binding to an enzyme (E) that synthesizes the second messenger. Finally, the enzyme, in this case adenylate cyclase, binds to the G protein and synthesizes cyclic AMP (adenosine monophosphate), which serves as second messenger (Figure 3-16). This is indicated in Figure 3-16 by the enzyme turning green and generating cyclic AMP (cAMP) (the icon with number 2 on it).

There are several other examples of second messenger systems (Table 3-5) and many variations on the way that G proteins cooperate to affect the production of second messengers. Nevertheless, the principles for G protein–linked second messengers are all generally

TABLE 3-6

EXAMPLES OF KEY THIRD, FOURTH MESSENGERS (signal transduction proteins/phosphoproteins) FOR FOUR DIFFERENT SIGNAL TRANSDUCTION CASCADES

G PROTEIN–LINKED	ION CHANNEL–LINKED
activated phosphokinase A	CaMK
DAG (diacylglycerol)	(Calcium/calmodulin dependent protein kinase)
activated phosphokinase C	Calcineurin
activated phospholipase C	(Calcium/calmodulin dependent phosphoprotein phosphatase)
multiple phosphoproteins	
CREB	
(cyclic AMP response element binding protein)	

NUCLEAR HORMONE RECEPTORS	RECEPTOR TYROSINE KINASES
	ERK
	(extracellular signal regulated kinases)
HORMONE/NUCLEAR RECEPTOR COMPLEX	RSK
BINDING TO HORMONE RESPONSE ELEMENTS	(ribosome S6 kinase)
	MAPK
	(mitogen activated protein kinases)
	GSK-3
	(glycogen synthase kinase 3)

the same: the handing off of first messenger to second messenger by means of a molecular cascade, neurotransmitter to neurotransmitter receptor (Figure 3-13); neurotransmitter receptor to G protein (Figure 3-14); binary complex of two receptors to enzyme (Figure 3-15); and enzyme to second messenger molecule (Figure 3-16).

Beyond the second messenger

Recent research has begun to clarify the complex molecular links between the second messenger and its ultimate effects upon cellular functions. These links are specifically the third, fourth, and subsequent chemical messengers in the signal transduction cascades shown in Figures 3-10 and 3-11. Each of the four classes of signal transduction cascades shown in Figure 3-11 not only begins with a different first messenger binding to a unique receptor but also leads to activation of very different downstream second, third, and subsequent chemical messengers. Having many different signal transduction cascades allows neurons to respond in amazingly diverse biological ways to a whole array of chemical messaging systems. The first messengers for these cascades are listed in Table 3-4; the second messengers in Table 3-5; and examples of third, fourth, and subsequent messengers, generally an array of phosphoproteins, are listed in Tables 3-6 and 3-7.

What is the ultimate target of signal transduction? There are two major targets: phosphoproteins and genes. Many of the intermediate targets along the way to the gene are phosphoproteins (Figure 3-11). The targets of some signal transduction cascades are fourth messenger phosphoproteins lying dormant in the neuron until signal transduction wakes them up and they can spring into action (see Figures 3-17 through 3-21).

TABLE 3-7

ADDITIONAL EXAMPLES OF SIGNAL TRANSDUCTION PROTEINS/ PHOSPHOPROTEINS OFTEN USED AS THIRD, FOURTH AND SUBSEQUENT MESSENGERS BY VARIOUS SIGNAL TRANSDUCTION CASCADES

protein kinases
protein phosphatases
G protein coupled receptors (e.g., beta-adrenergic receptors; opioid receptors)
G protein alpha, beta, gamma subunits
Ras superfamily proteins
Voltage-gated calcium channels (alpha subunits)
Voltage-gated Na^+ channels
Caspases
Nuclear hormone receptors
DARPP-32 (**d**opamine and cyclic **A**MP **r**egulated **p**hospho**p**rotein)
neurotransmitter synthesizing enzymes (e.g., tyrosine hydroxylase; tryptophan hydroxylase)
neurotransmitter gated ion channels
GluR1 receptors (AMPA subunit)
NMDA-R1 receptors (NMDA subunit)
GABA-A receptors
Phospholipase C
IP_3 receptor
CaMK
TrK
Cytoskeletal proteins (e.g., MAP-2, Tau, myosin light chain)
synaptic vesicle proteins (e.g., synapsins)
transcription factors (e.g., CREB, STAT proteins)

The actions shown in Figure 3-10 on fourth messenger phosphoproteins as targets of signal transduction can be seen in more detail in Figures 3-17 through 3-21. Thus, one signal transduction pathway can activate a third messenger kinase through second messenger cAMP (Figure 3-17), whereas another signal transduction pathway can activate a third messenger phosphatase through second messenger calcium (Figure 3-18). In the case of kinase activation, two copies of the second messenger target each regulatory unit of dormant or "sleeping" protein kinase (Figure 3-17). When some protein kinases are inactive, they exist in dimers (two copies of the enzyme) while binding to a regulatory unit, thus placing them in a conformation that is not active. In this example, when two copies of cAMP bind to each regulatory unit, the regulatory unit dissociates from the enzyme and the dimer dissociates into two copies of the enzyme; the protein kinase is now activated – shown with bow and arrow – and ready to shoot phosphate groups into unsuspecting fourth messenger phosphoproteins (Figure 3-17).

Meanwhile, the nemesis of protein kinase is also forming in Figure 3-18 – namely, a protein phosphatase. Another first messenger is opening an ion channel here, allowing second messenger calcium to enter, which activates the phosphatase enzyme calcineurin. In the presence of calcium, calcineurin becomes activated; it is shown with scissors, ready to clip phosphate groups off fourth messenger phosphoproteins (Figure 3-18).

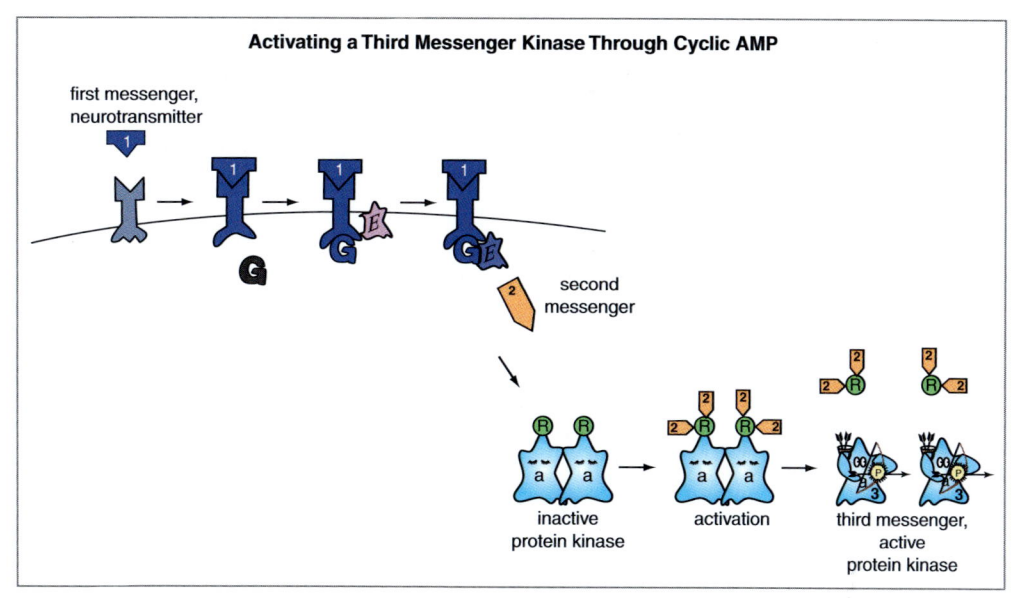

FIGURE 3-17 Third messenger protein kinase. This figure illustrates activation of a third messenger protein kinase through the second messenger cyclic AMP. Neurotransmitters begin the process of activating genes by producing a second messenger (cyclic AMP), as shown previously in Figures 3-12 through 3-16. Some second messengers activate intracellular enzymes known as protein kinases. This enzyme is shown here as inactive when it is paired with another copy of the enzyme plus two regulatory units (R). In this case, two copies of the second messenger interact with the regulatory units, dissociating them from the protein kinase dimer. This dissociation activates each protein kinase, readying this enzyme to phosphorylate other proteins.

The clash between kinase and phosphatase can be seen by comparing what happens in Figures 3-19 and 3-20. In Figure 3-19, third messenger kinase is putting phosphates onto various fourth messenger phosphoproteins, such as ligand-gated ion channels, voltage-gated ion channels, and enzymes; however, in Figure 3-20, third messenger phosphatase is taking those phosphates right off. Sometimes phosphorylation activates a dormant phosphoprotein; for other phosphoproteins, dephosphorylation can be activating. Figure 3-21, in the left panel, shows an example of an ion channel that is not active without a phosphate group but is then activated by a kinase that phosphorylates it, as shown in the right panel. Activation of fourth messenger phosphoproteins can change the synthesis of neurotransmitters, alter neurotransmitter release, change the conductance of ions, and generally maintain the chemical neurotransmission apparatus in either a state of readiness or dormancy. The balance between phosphorylation and dephosphorylation of fourth messenger kinases and phosphatases plays a vital role in regulating many molecules critical to the chemical neurotransmission process.

Gene expression

The ultimate cellular function that neurotransmission often seeks to modify is gene expression, either turning a gene on or turning one off. All four signal transduction cascades shown in Figure 3-11 end with the last molecule influencing gene transcription. Both cascades triggered by neurotransmitters are shown acting upon the CREB system, which is responsive to phosphorylation of its regulatory units (Figure 3-11 on the left). CREB stands for

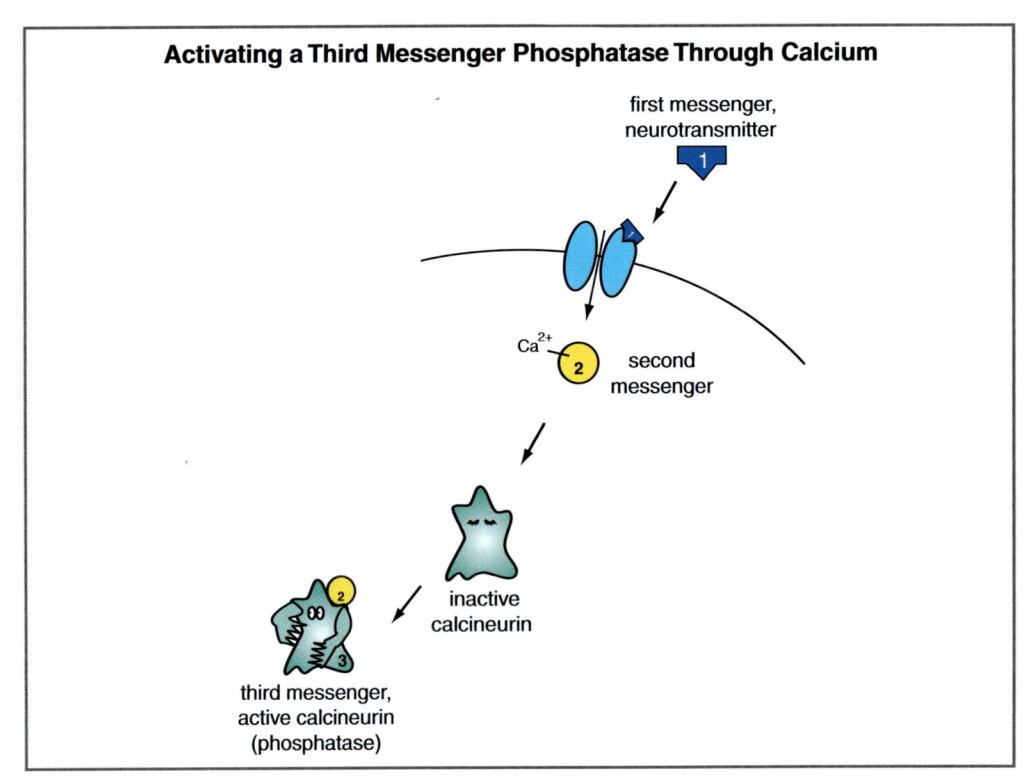

FIGURE 3-18 Third messenger phosphatase. This figure illustrates activation of a third messenger phosphatase through the second messenger calcium. Shown here is calcium binding to an inactive phosphatase known as calcineurin, thereby activating it and thus readying it to remove phosphates from fourth messenger phosphoproteins.

cAMP response-element binding protein, a transcription factor in the cell nucleus capable of activating the expression of genes, especially a group of genes known as immediate genes or immediate-early genes. When G protein–linked receptors activate protein kinase A, this activated enzyme can translocate or move into the cell nucleus and stick a phosphate group on CREB, thus activating this transcription factor and causing the nearby gene to become activated. This leads to gene expression first as RNA and then as the protein coded by the gene.

Interestingly, it is also possible for ion channel–linked receptors that enhance intracellular second messenger calcium levels to activate CREB by phosphorylating it. A protein known as calmodulin, which interacts with calcium, can lead to activation of certain kinases called calcium-calmodulin–dependent protein kinases (Figure 3-11). This is an entirely different enzyme than the phosphatase shown in Figures 3-10, 3-18, and 3-20. Here, a kinase and not a phosphatase is activated. When activated, this kinase can translocate into the cell nucleus and, just like the kinase activated by the G protein system, add a phosphate group to CREB and activate this transcription factor so that gene expression is triggered.

It is important to bear in mind that calcium is thus able to activate both kinases and phosphatases. There is a very rich and sometimes confusing array of kinases and phosphatases (see Tables 3-6 and 3-7), and the net result of calcium action is dependent upon which substrates are activated, because different phosphatases and kinases target

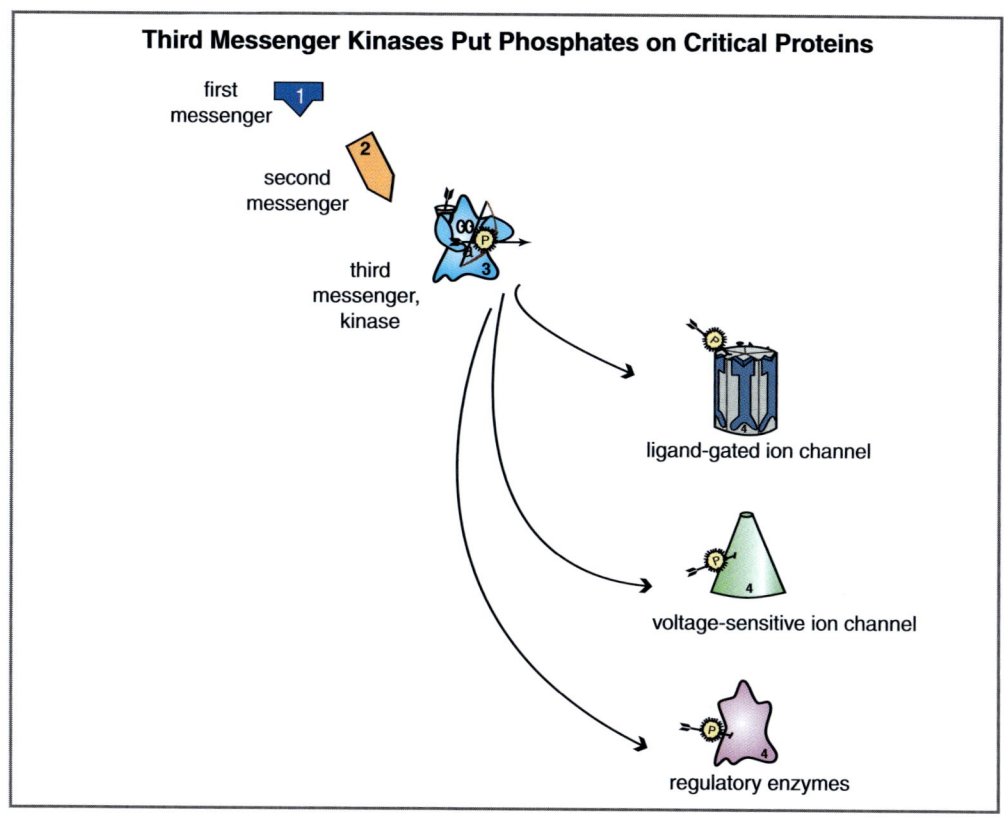

FIGURE 3-19 Third messenger kinase puts phosphates on critical proteins. Here the activation of a third messenger kinase adds phosphates to a variety of phosphoproteins, such a ligand-gated ion channels, voltage-gated ion channels, and various regulatory enzymes. Adding a phosphate group to some phosphoproteins activates them; for other proteins, this inactivates them.

very different substrates. Thus, it is important to keep in mind the specific signal transduction cascade under discussion – and the specific phosphoproteins acting as messengers in the cascade – in order to understand the net effect of various signal transduction cascades. In the case illustrated in Figure 3-11, the G protein system and ion channel system are working together to produce more activated kinases and thus more activation of CREB. However, in Figures 3-10 and 3-17 through 3-20, they are working in opposition.

Genes are also the ultimate target of the hormone signal transduction cascade in Figure 3-11. Some hormones – such as estrogen, thyroid, and cortisol (Table 3-4) – act at cytoplasmic receptors, bind them, and produce a hormone nuclear receptor complex that translocates to the cell nucleus, finds elements in the gene that it can influence (called hormone response elements, or HREs), and then acts as a transcription factor to trigger activation of nearby genes (Figure 3-11).

Finally, a very complicated signal transduction system with terrible-sounding names for its downstream signal cascade messengers is activated by neurotrophins and related molecules (Table 3-4). Activating this system by first messenger neurotrophins leads to activation of enzymes that are mostly kinases, one kinase activating another until finally one of them phosphorylates a transcription factor in the cell nucleus and starts transcribing

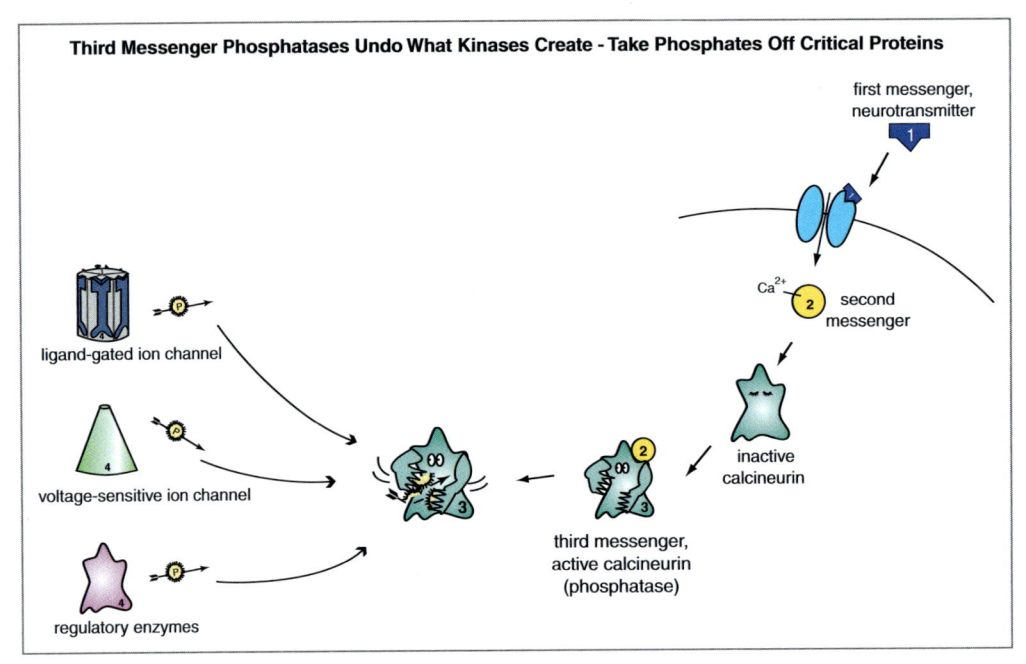

Third Messenger Phosphatases Undo What Kinases Create - Take Phosphates Off Critical Proteins

FIGURE 3-20 **Third messenger phosphatase removes phosphates from critical proteins.** In contrast to the previous figure, the third messenger here is a phosphatase; this enzyme removes phosphate groups from phosphoproteins such as ligand-gated ion channels, voltage-gated ion channels, and various regulatory enzymes. Removing a phosphate group from some phosphoproteins activates them; for others, it inactivates them.

genes (Figure 3-11). Ras is a G protein that activates a cascade of kinases with confusing names. For those who are good sports with an interest in the specifics, this cascade starts with Ras activating Raf, which phosphorylates and activates MEK (MAP kinase/ERK kinase or mitogen-activated protein kinase kinase/extracellular signal-regulated kinase kinase) which activates ERK (extracellular signal-regulated kinase itself), RSK (ribosomal S6 kinase), MAPK (MAP kinase itself), or GSK3 (glycogen synthase kinase), leading ultimately to changes in gene expression. Confused? It is actually not important to know the names; the take-away point is that neurotrophins trigger an important signal transduction pathway that activates kinase enzyme after kinase enzyme, ultimately changing gene expression. This is worth knowing because this signal transduction pathway may be responsible for the expression of genes that regulate many critical functions of the neuron, such as synaptogenesis and cell survival, as well as the plastic changes necessary for learning, memory, and even disease expression in various brain circuits. It is hoped that, someday, there will be psychopharmacological agents which target this system to attain therapeutic benefits for psychiatric disorders.

In the meantime, it is mostly important to realize that a very wide variety of genes are targeted by all four of these signal transduction pathways. Several examples of the key proteins made from these genes are listed in Table 3-8. They range from the genes that make synthetic enzymes for neurotransmitters, to growth factors, cytoskeleton proteins, cellular adhesion proteins, ion channels, receptors, and the intracellular signaling proteins themselves, among many others (Table 3-8). When genes are expressed by any of the signal transduction pathways shown in Figure 3-11, it can lead to making more

TABLE 3-8

EXAMPLES OF KEY PRODUCTS OF LATE GENES TARGETED BY ALL FOUR SIGNAL TRANSDUCTION CASCADES

Synthetic enzymes for neurotransmitters
(e.g., tyrosine hydroxylase; tryptophan hydroxylase)
Growth factors (e.g., BDNF)
Cytoskeleton proteins
Synaptic vesicle proteins
Ion channels
Receptors
Intracellular signaling proteins
Cellular adhesion molecules

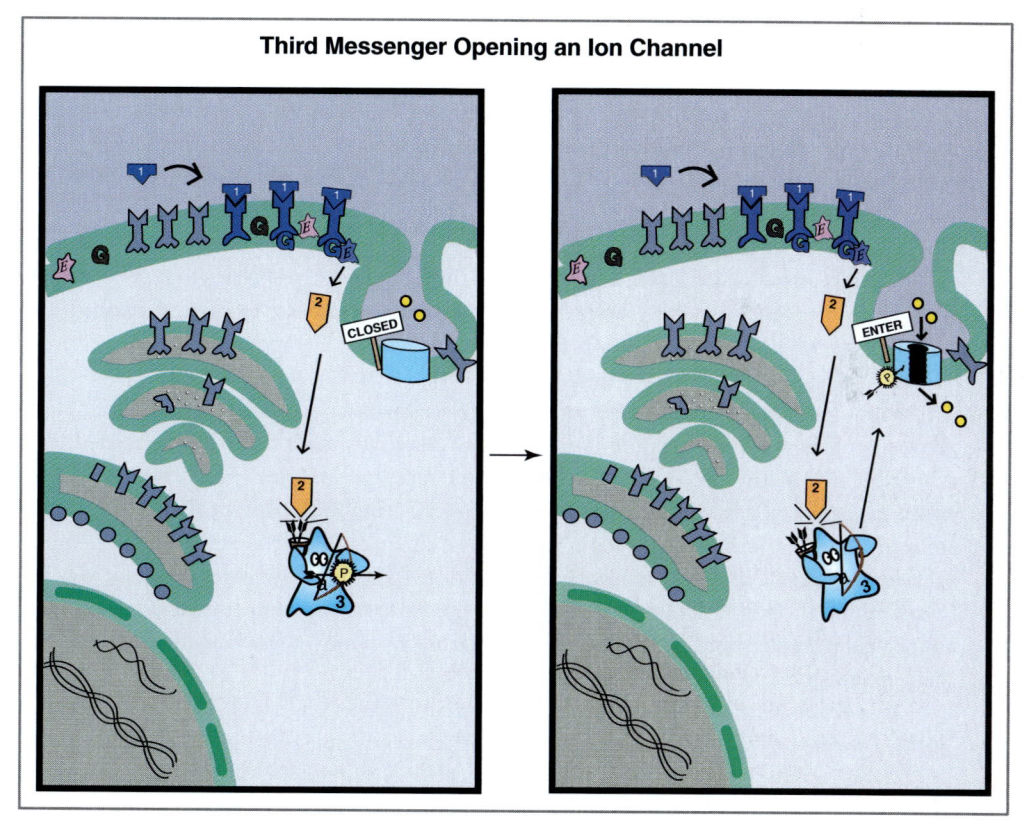

FIGURE 3-21 Third messenger opening an ion channel. An important function triggered by the signal transduction cascade is to change the membrane's permeability to ions. This can not only be mediated by neurotransmitters acting directly at ligand-gated ion channels as shown in Figure 3-18 but also indirectly through G protein–linked systems, as shown here. Thus, forming a second messenger through a G protein–linked system can activate a protein kinase (left panel). This protein kinase then phosphorylates a voltage channel, which in this case changes the permeability of that ion channel and allows ions to flow more readily through it (right panel).

TABLE 3-9

EXAMPLES OF DIVERSE BIOLOGICAL RESPONSES DUE TO LONG-TERM EFFECTS OF LATE GENE PRODUCTS FROM ALL FOUR SIGNAL TRANSDUCTION CASCADES

- synaptogenesis
- strengthen a synapse
- neurogenesis
- apoptosis
- neurodegeneration/atrophy
- learning
- memory
- antidepressant response
- psychotherapeutic response
- endocrine response
- increase the efficiency of information processing in circuits
- bias circuits towards decreased efficiency of information processing, especially under stress
- production of a mental illness (e.g., chronic pain; panic disorder)

or fewer copies of any of these proteins. Synthesis of such proteins is obviously a critical aspect of the neuron performing its many and varied functions. Numerous examples of the diverse biological responses effected in a neuron by gene expression triggered by the four major signal transduction cascades are listed in Table 3-9. These functions include synaptogensis, strengthening of a synapse, neurogenesis, apoptosis, learning, memory, antidepressant responses to antidepressant administration, behavioral responses to psychotherapy, increasing or decreasing the efficiency of information processing in cortical circuits, and possibly even the production of a mental illness as well as therapeutic responses to many different classes of psychotropic drugs (Table 3-9).

How does the gene express the protein it codes? That is, the discussion above has shown how the molecular "pony express" of signal transduction carries a message, encoded with chemical information from the neurotransmitter-receptor complex, which is passed along from molecular rider to molecular rider until it is delivered to the appropriate phosphoprotein mailbox (Figures 3-17 through 3-21) or DNA mailbox in the postsynaptic neuron's genome (Figure 3-11 and Figures 3-22 through 3-35). Since the most powerful way for a neuron to alter its function is to change the genes that are being turned on or off, it is important to understand the molecular mechanisms by which neurotransmission regulates gene expression.

It is estimated that the human genome contains approximately *25,000 to 30,000 genes* located within *3 billion base pairs* of DNA on 23 chromosomes. Incredibly, however, genes occupy only a few percent of this DNA. The other 97 percent of DNA is not well understood, but it is obviously there for some reason. Some scientists call it "junk" DNA, since it apparently has no coding function, but it is more likely that these segments have other important functions, such as whether or not a gene is expressed. It is not just the number of genes we have, it is whether and when and how often and under what circumstances they are expressed that seem to be the important factors in regulating neuronal function. These same factors of gene expression are now thought also to underlie the actions of psychopharmacological drugs and the mechanisms of psychiatric disorders within the central nervous system.

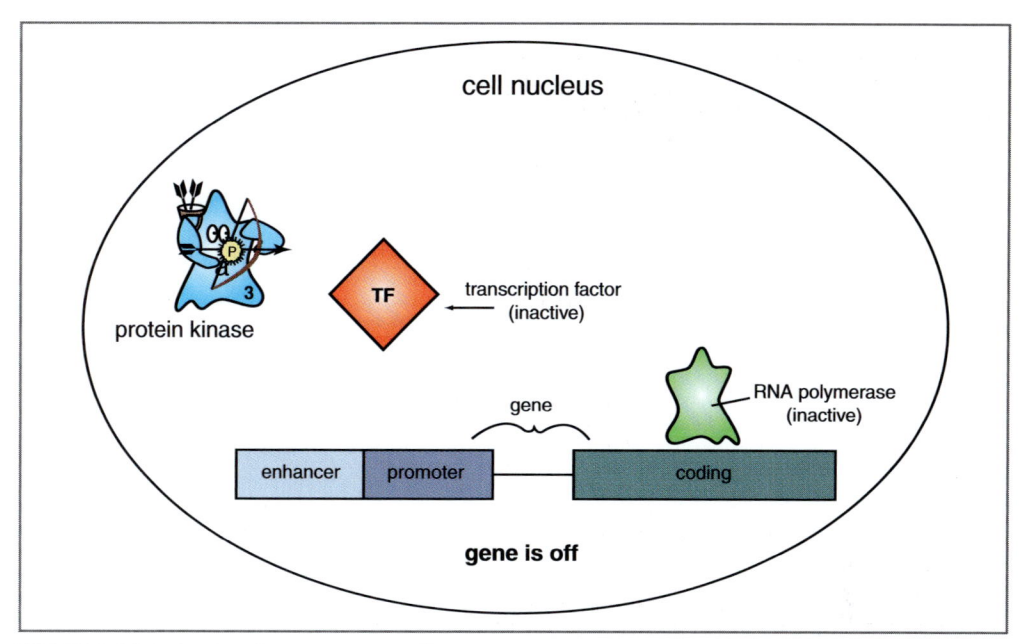

FIGURE 3-22 Activation of a gene: gene is off. Activation of a gene, part 1. Here the gene is "off." The elements of gene activation shown here include the enzyme protein kinase; a transcription factor, a type of protein that can activate a gene; RNA polymerase, the enzyme that synthesizes RNA from DNA when the gene is transcribed; the regulatory regions of DNA, such as enhancer and promoter areas; and finally the gene itself. This particular gene is off because the transcription factor has not yet been activated. The DNA for this gene contains both a regulatory region and a coding region. The regulatory region has both an enhancer element and a promoter element, which can initiate gene expression when they interact with activated transcription factors. The coding region is directly transcribed into its corresponding RNA once the gene is activated.

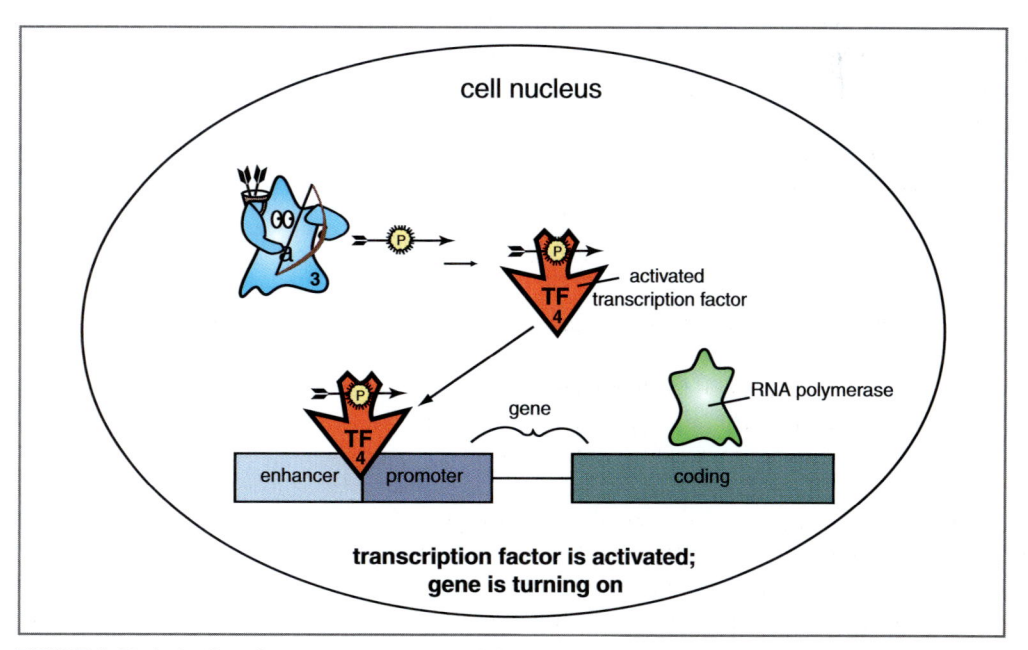

FIGURE 3-23 Activation of a gene: gene turns on. Activation of a gene, part 2. The transcription factor is now activated because it has been phosphorylated by protein kinase, allowing it to bind to the regulatory region of the gene.

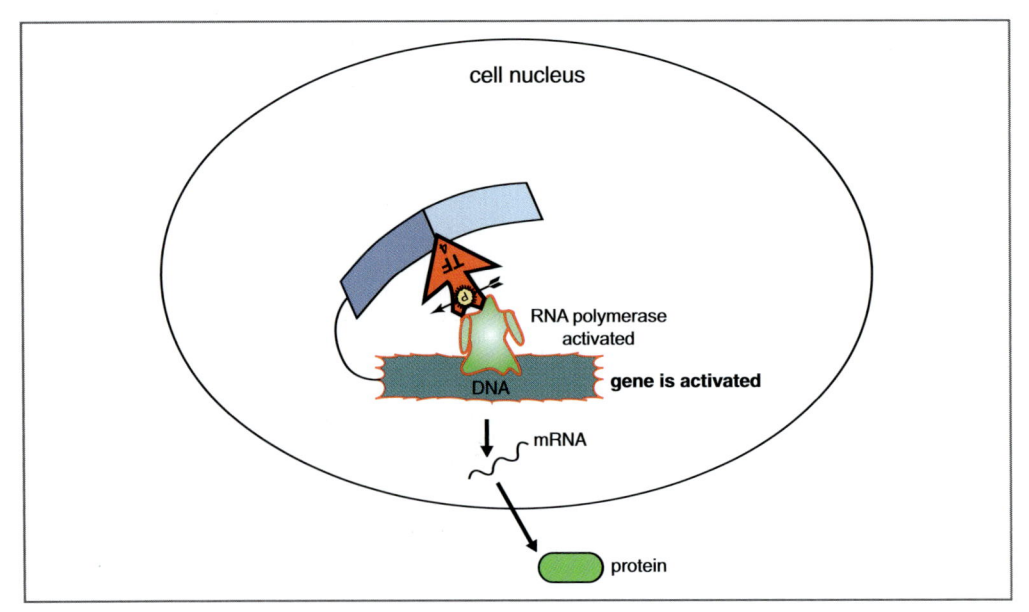

FIGURE 3-24 Activation of a gene: gene product. Activation of a gene, part 3. The gene itself is now activated because the transcription factor has bound to the regulatory region of the gene, in turn activating the enzyme RNA polymerase. Thus, the gene is transcribed into messenger RNA (mRNA), which in turn is translated into its corresponding protein. This protein is thus the product of activation of this particular gene.

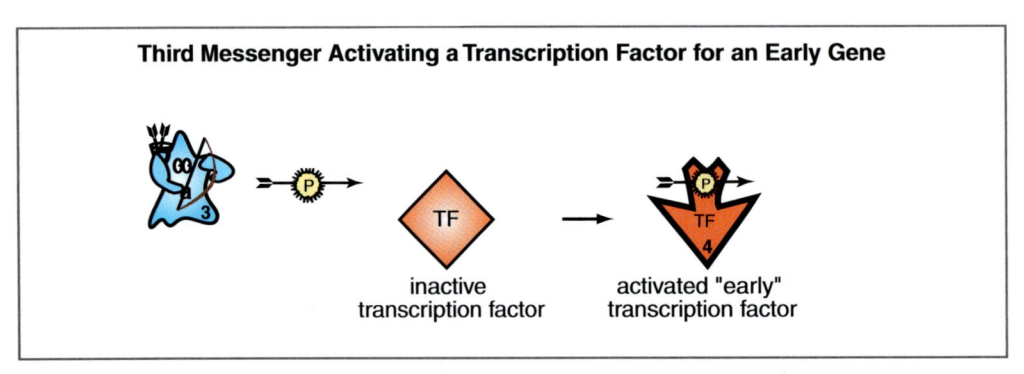

FIGURE 3-25 Immediate-early gene. Some genes are known as immediate-early genes. Shown here is a third messenger protein kinase enzyme activating a transcription factor, or fourth messenger, capable of activating, in turn, an early gene.

How does chemical neurotransmission regulate gene expression? It seems that chemical neurotransmission converts receptor occupancy by a neurotransmitter into the creation of third, fourth, and subsequent messengers that eventually activate the transcription factors that turn genes on (Figures 3-22 through 3-31). Most genes have two regions, a *coding region* and a *regulatory region*, with enhancers and promoters of gene transcription (Figure 3-22). The coding region is the direct template for making its corresponding RNA. This DNA can be transcribed into its RNA with the help of an enzyme called *RNA polymerase*. However, RNA polymerase must be activated or it won't work.

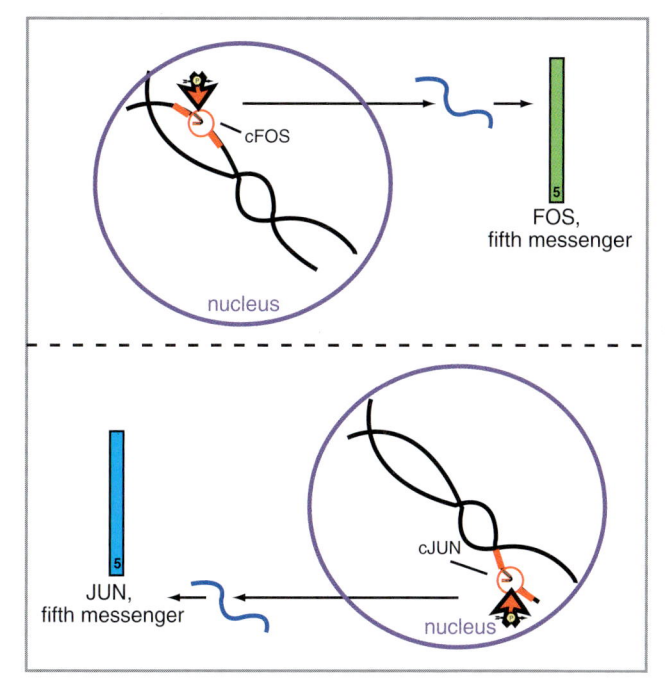

FIGURE 3-26 Early genes activate late genes. How early genes activate late genes, part 1. In the top panel, a transcription factor is activating the immediate-early gene cFos and producing the protein product Fos. While the cFos gene is being activated, another immediate-early gene, cJun, is being simultaneously activated and producing its protein, Jun, as shown in the bottom panel. Fos and Jun can be thought of as fifth messengers.

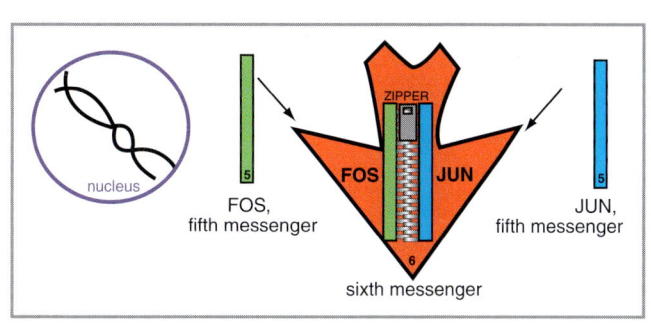

FIGURE 3-27 Fos-Jun combination protein. How early genes activate late genes, part 2. Once Fos and Jun proteins are synthesized, they can collaborate as partners and produce a Fos-Jun combination protein, which now acts as a sixth-messenger transcription factor for late genes.

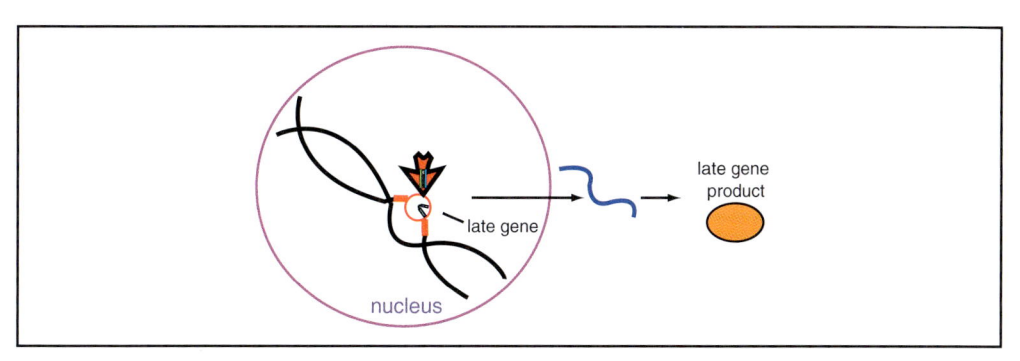

FIGURE 3-28 Leucine zipper transcription factor. How early genes activate late genes, part 3. The Fos-Jun transcription factor belongs to a family of proteins called leucine zippers. The leucine zipper transcription factor formed by the products of the activated early genes cFos and cJun now returns to the genome and finds another gene. Since this gene is being activated later than the others, it is called a late gene. Thus, early genes activate late genes when the products of early genes are themselves transcription factors. The product of the late gene can be any protein the neuron needs, such as an enzyme, a transport factor, or a growth factor.

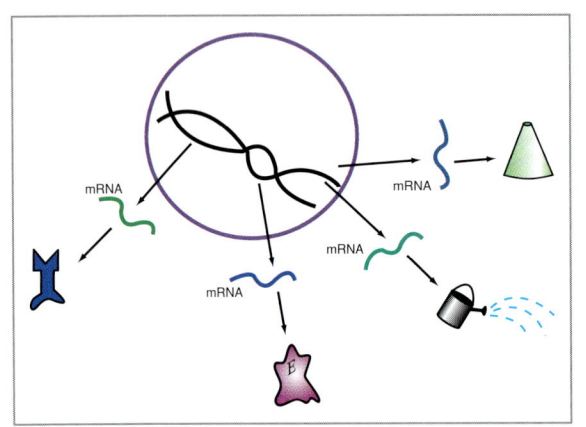

FIGURE 3-29 Late gene activation. Examples of late gene activation. Thus, a receptor, an enzyme, a neurotrophic growth factor, and an ion channel are all being expressed owing to activation of their respective genes. Such gene products go on to modify neuronal function for many hours or days.

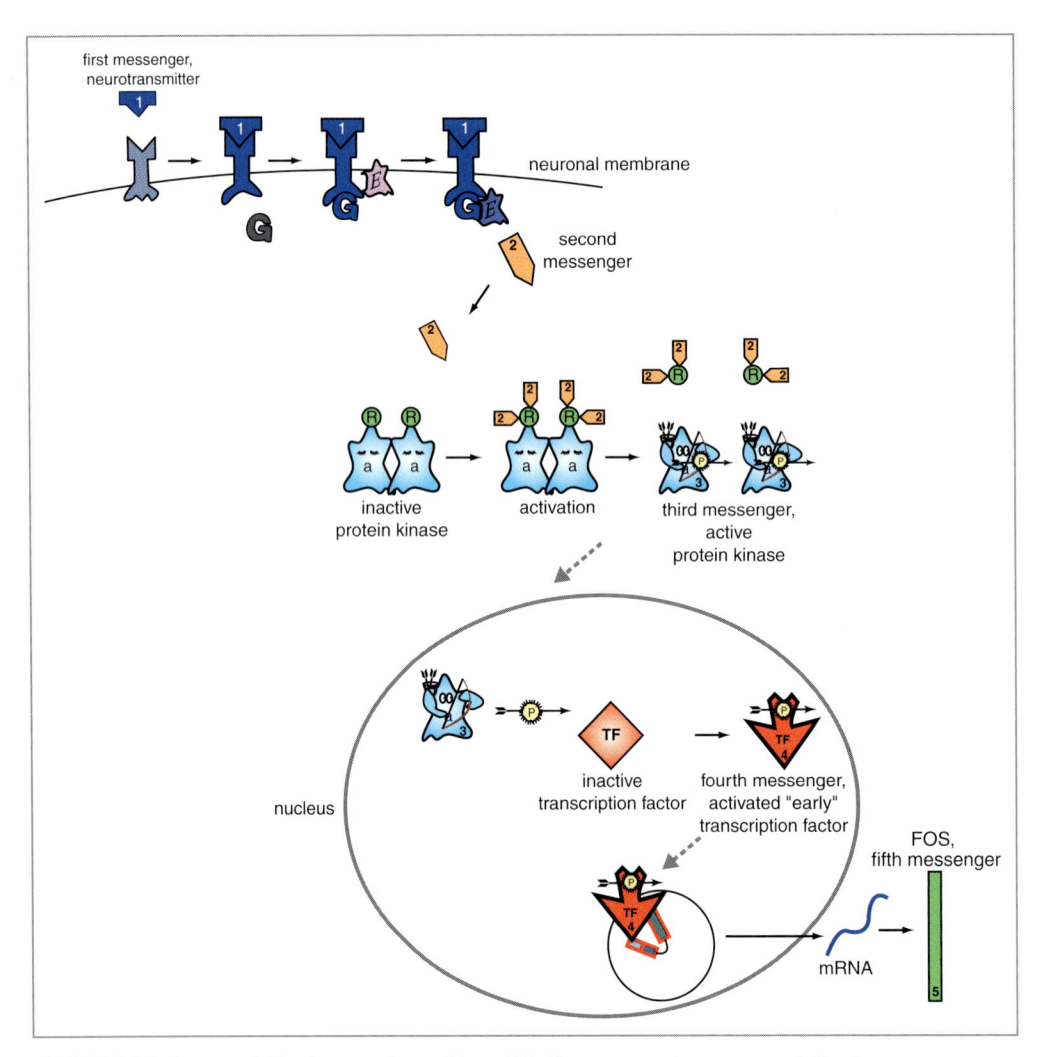

FIGURE 3-30 Gene regulation by neurotransmitters. This figure summarizes gene regulation by neurotransmitters, from first messenger extracellular neurotransmitter to intracellular second messenger, to third messenger protein kinase, to fourth messenger transcription factor, to fifth messenger protein, which is the gene product of an early gene.

82 | Essential Psychopharmacology

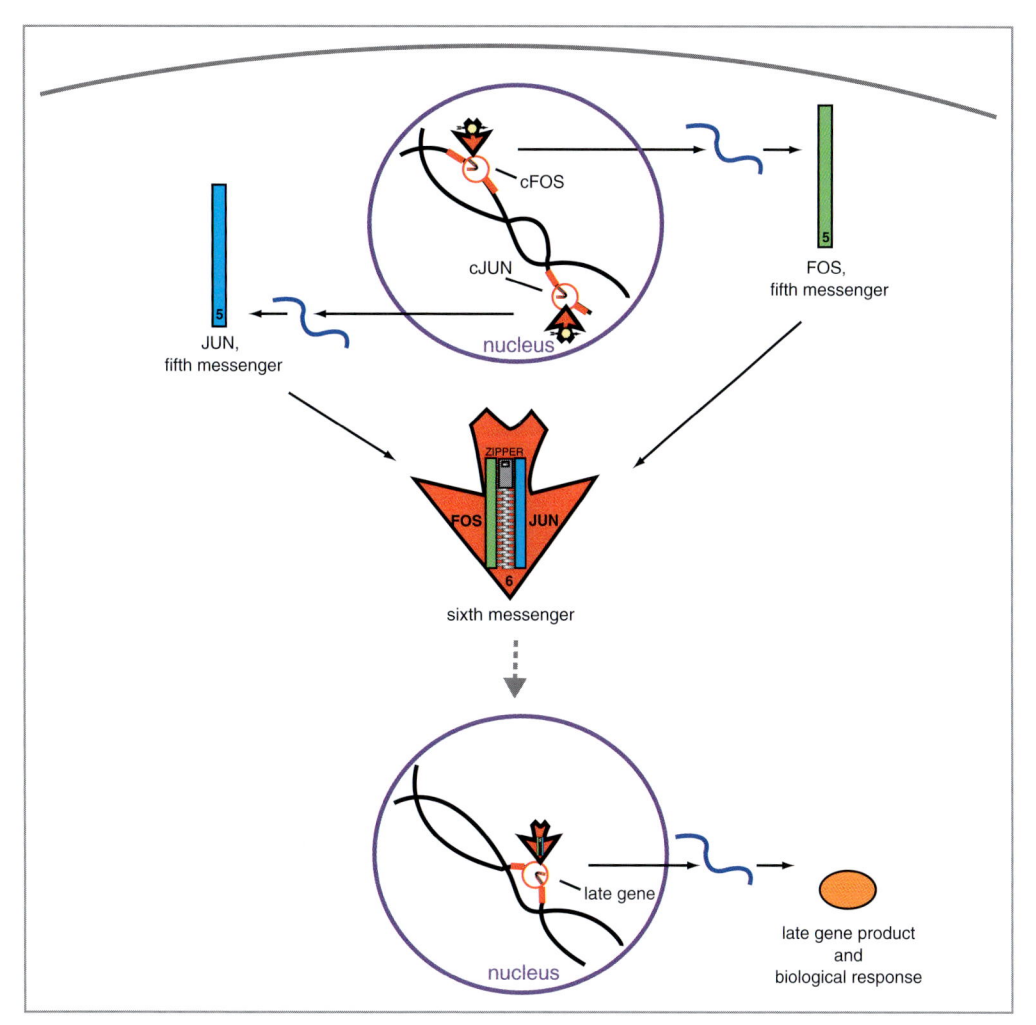

FIGURE 3-31 Activating a late gene. This figure summarizes the process of activating a late gene. At the top, immediate-early genes cFos and cJun are expressed and their fifth messenger protein products Fos and Jun are formed. Next, a transcription factor, namely a leucine zipper, is created by the cooperation of Fos and Jun together, combining to form the sixth messenger. Finally, this transcription factor goes on to activate a late gene, resulting in the expression of its own gene product and the biological response triggered by that late gene product.

Luckily, the regulatory region of the gene can make this happen. It has an *enhancer element* and a *promotor element* (Figure 3-22), which can initiate gene expression with the help of transcription factors (Figure 3-23). Transcription factors themselves can be activated when they are phosphorylated, which allows them to bind to the regulatory region of the gene (Figure 3-23). This, in turn, activates RNA polymerase, and off we go with the coding part of the gene *transcribing* itself into its mRNA (Figure 3-24). Once transcribed, of course, the RNA goes on to *translate* itself into the corresponding protein (Figure 3-24).

Some genes are known as immediate-early genes (Figure 3-25). They have weird names like cJun and cFos (Figures 3-26 and 3-27) and belong to a family called "leucine zippers" (Figures 3-28). These genes function as rapid responders to the neurotransmitter's input, like the first troops sent into combat once war has been declared. Such rapid deployment forces of immediate-early genes are the first to respond to the neurotransmission signal by

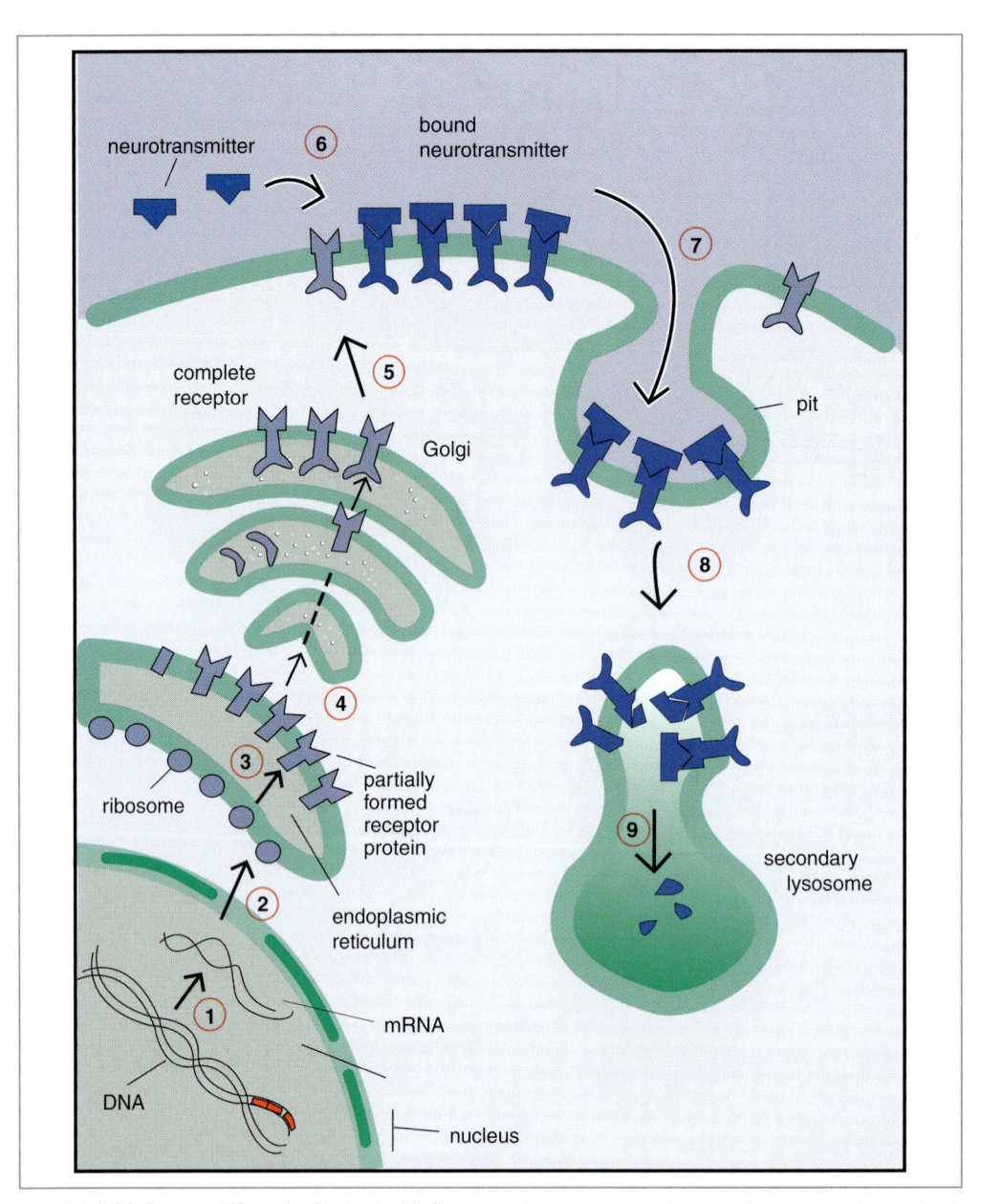

FIGURE 3-32 Receptor life cycle. Shown in this figure is the molecular neurobiology of a receptor life cycle from synthesis to destruction. The process begins in the cell nucleus, when a gene (red DNA segment) is transcribed into messenger RNA (arrow 1). Messenger RNA then travels to the endoplasmic reticulum (arrow 2), where ribosomes cause the messenger RNA to be translated into partially formed receptor protein (arrow 3). The next step is for partially formed receptor protein to be transformed into complete receptor molecules in the Golgi apparatus (arrow 4). Completely formed receptor molecules are proteins; these are transported to the cell membrane (arrow 5), where they can interact with neurotransmitters (arrow 6). Neurotransmitters can not only bind to the receptor, as shown in Figure 3-12, causing second messenger systems to be triggered, but the bound neurotransmitter may also reversibly cause the membrane to form a pit (arrow 7). This process takes the bound receptor out of circulation when the neuron wants to decrease the number of receptors available. This can be reversed or the receptor can progress from a pit into lysosomes (arrow 8), where receptors are destroyed (arrow 9). This helps to remove old receptors so that they can be replaced by new receptors coming from DNA in the cell nucleus.

Essential Psychopharmacology

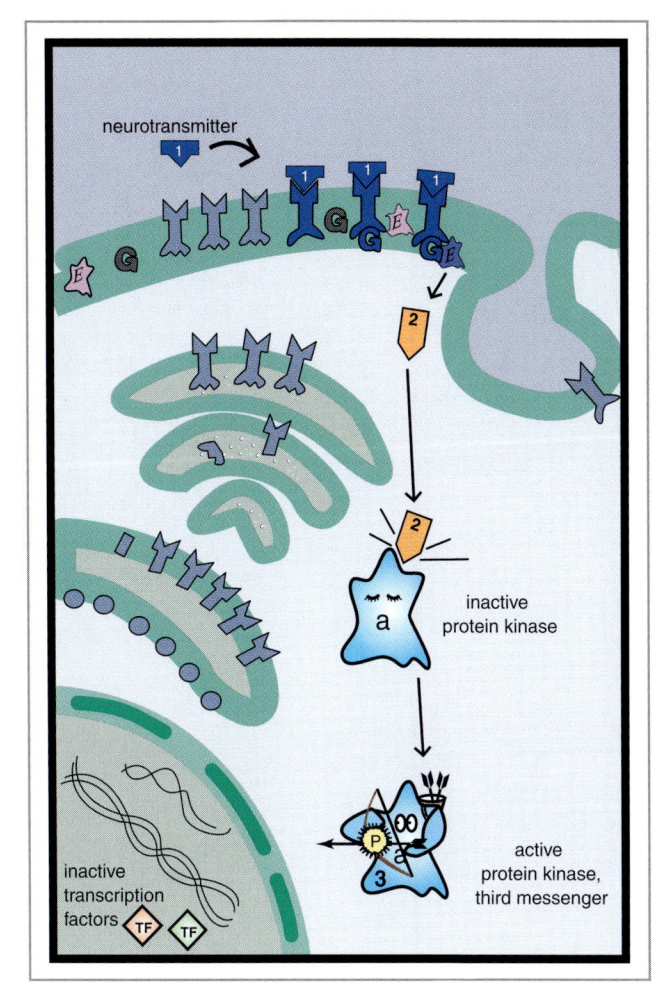

FIGURE 3-33 Receptor synthesis. Neurotransmitters can regulate the number of their own receptors. The production of chemical instructions by intracellular enzymes can include orders for the cell's DNA that regulate whether a greater or lesser number of its own receptors are synthesized. Shown here is the blue neurotransmitter cascade at the top, leading to formation of a second messenger, followed by second messenger activation of protein kinase. In this case, the kinase is targeting transcription factors that can turn on or off the synthesis of receptors for the neurotransmitter that triggered this whole cascade.

making the proteins they encode. In this example, it is Jun and Fos proteins coming from cJun and cFos genes (Figures 3-26). These are nuclear proteins; that is, they live and work in the nucleus. They get started within 15 minutes of receiving a neurotransmission but last for only a half hour to an hour (Figure 3-10).

When Jun and Fos team up, they form a leucine zipper–type of transcription factor (Figure 3-27), which in turn activates many kinds of later-onset genes (Figures 3-28 and 3-29). Thus, Fos and Jun serve to wake up the much larger army of inactive genes. Which individual soldier genes are so drafted to active gene duty depends on a number of factors, not the least of which is which neurotransmitter is sending the message, how frequently it is sending the message, and whether it is working in concert or in opposition with other neurotransmitters talking to other parts of the same neuron at the same time. When FOS and JUN partner together to form a leucine zipper–type of transcription factor, this can lead to the activation of genes to make anything you can think of, from enzymes to receptors to structural proteins (see Figure 3-29).

In summary, one can trace the events from neurotransmitting first messenger through gene transcription (Figures 3-30 and 3-31). Once the second messenger cAMP is formed

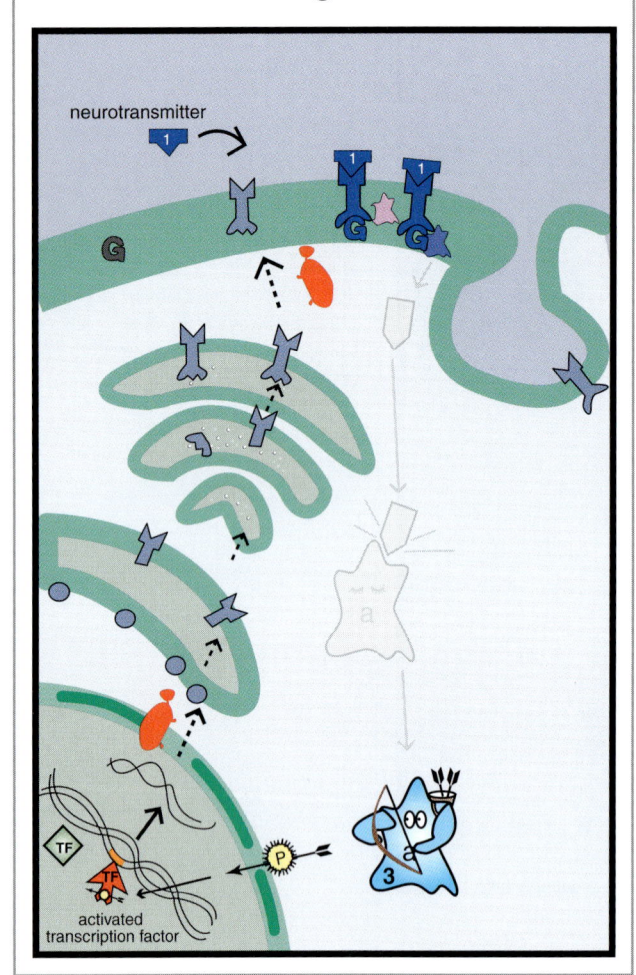

FIGURE 3-34 Receptor downregulation. The production of chemical instructions by intracellular enzymes can include orders for the cell's DNA to regulate the rate of synthesis of the neurotransmitter's own receptors. In this figure, protein kinase phosphorylates the transcription factor that tells the cell to slow down synthesis of the neurotransmitter's receptor. Thus, fewer blue neurotransmitter receptors are being formed, as represented by the tortoise on the arrows of neurotransmitter receptor synthesis. Such slowing of neurotransmitter receptor synthesis is called downregulation.

from its first messenger neurotransmitter (Figure 3-30), it can interact with a protein kinase third messenger. cAMP binds to the inactive or sleeping version of this enzyme, wakes it up, and thereby activates protein kinase. Once awakened, the protein kinase third messenger's job is to activate transcription factors by phosphorylating them (Figure 3-30). It does this by traveling straight to the cell nucleus and finding a sleeping transcription factor. By sticking a phosphate onto the transcription factor, protein kinase is able to wake up that transcription factor and form a fourth messenger (Figure 3-30). Once a transcription factor is aroused, it will bind to genes and cause protein synthesis – in this case, the product of an early-immediate gene, and this functions as a fifth messenger. Two such gene products bind together to form yet another activated transcription factor, the sixth messenger (Figure 3-31). Finally, the sixth messenger causes the expression of a late gene product, which could be thought of as a seventh messenger protein product of the activated gene. This late gene product then mediates some biological response important to the functioning of the neuron.

One common example of a biological response that is important to the functioning of the neuron is the ability of neurotransmitter-induced change to regulate the number of its

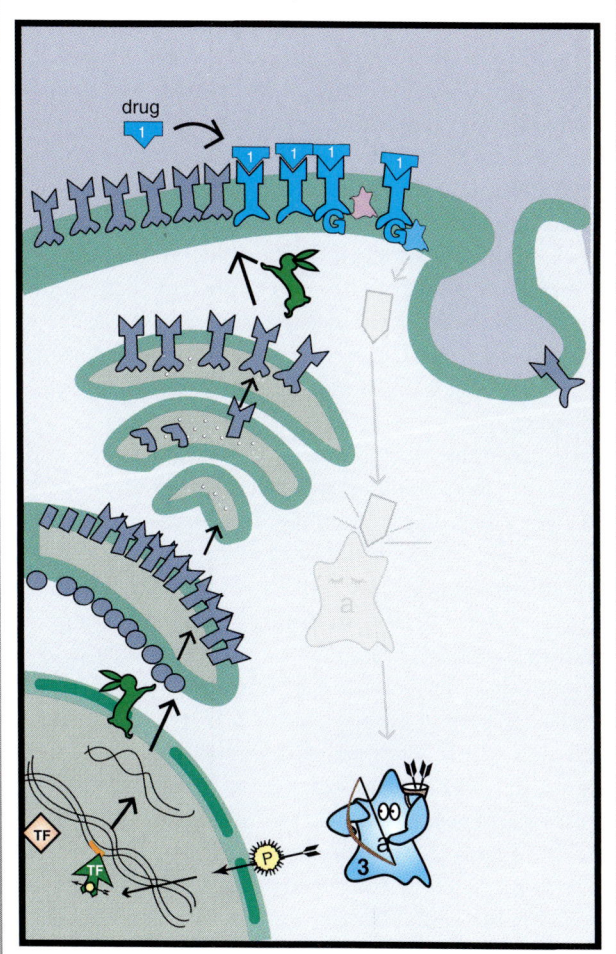

FIGURE 3-35 Receptor upregulation. In contrast to Figure 3-34, here phosphorylation of a different transcription factor causes the cell to speed up synthesis of the neurotransmitter's receptor. Thus a greater number of blue neurotransmitter receptors are being formed, as represented by the hare on the arrows of neurotransmitter receptor synthesis. Such an increase in neurotransmitter receptor synthesis is called upregulation.

own receptors (Figures 3-32 through 3-35). By asking for more copies or fewer copies of its own receptors, the neurotransmission process can therefore come full circle from receptor to gene and back to receptor again (Figure 3-32). The normal life cycle of a receptor is shown in Figure 3-32 and starts with synthesis from DNA to mRNA; it then goes on to partially formed receptor protein on ribosomes, to completed receptors in the Golgi apparatus, to insertion in the membrane. After use, receptors can be formed into a pit, which takes them out of functional action; this is then either reversed or the inactivated receptors progress to secondary lysosomes, where they are destroyed and degraded.

Receptor activation by neurotransmitter activates kinases, as shown earlier, but here this kinase is targeting transcription factors that regulate the rate of synthesis of the receptor itself (Figure 3-33). Theoretically, one targeted transcription factor (in red) might slow down the rate of protein synthesis (indicated by red tortoises on the synthetic arrows; Figure 3-34). This is called downregulation. Generally, downregulation of a receptor is caused by the neurotransmitter itself or by agonists that mimic the neurotransmitter at its receptor. Another targeted transcription factor (in green) might speed up the rate of synthesis of receptors

(Figure 3-35). This is called upregulation. Generally, upregulation of a receptor is caused by antagonists at the receptor.

This process of downregulation or upregulation takes days. Changes in the rates of receptor synthesis can powerfully modify chemical neurotransmission at the synapse. That is, a decreased rate of receptor synthesis results in less receptor being made and less transported down the axon to the terminal for insertion into the membrane. This would theoretically diminish the sensitivity of neurotransmission. Some neurotransmitters can cause a faster form of desensitization by activating an enzyme that phosphorylates the receptor, making the receptor immediately insensitive to its neurotransmitter. Receptors may be synthesized in excess under some conditions, especially if they are blocked by a drug for a long period of time. Too much receptor synthesis might not only increase the sensitivity of neurotransmission but also produce a disease. Exactly this is suspected to be the case for the condition known as tardive dyskinesia (see Chapter 10, on antipsychotics), which is apparently caused when dopamine receptor–blocking drugs cause abnormal changes in the number or sensitivity of dopamine receptors.

Of course, neurotransmitter-induced molecular cascades into the cell nucleus lead to changes not only in the synthesis of its own receptors but also in that of many other important postsynaptic proteins, including enzymes and receptors for other neurotransmitters. If such changes in genetic expression lead to changes in connections and in the functions that these connections perform, it is easy to understand how genes can *modify behavior*. The details of nerve functioning – and thus the behavior derived from this nerve functioning – are controlled by genes and the products they produce. Since mental processes and the behavior they cause come from the connections between neurons in the brain, genes exert significant control over behavior. But can behavior modify genes? Learning as well as experiences from the environment can indeed alter which genes are expressed and thus give rise to changes in neuronal connections. In this way, human experiences, education, and even psychotherapy may change the expression of genes that alter the distribution and "strength" of specific synaptic connections. This, in turn, may produce long-term changes in behavior caused by the original experience and mediated by the genetic changes triggered by that original experience. Thus, genes modify behavior and behavior modifies genes. Genes do not directly regulate neuronal functioning. Rather, they directly regulate the proteins that create neuronal functioning. Changes in function have to wait until the changes in protein synthesis occur and the events they cause start to happen.

Summary

The reader should now appreciate that chemical neurotransmission is the foundation of psychopharmacology. There are many neurotransmitters. Many neurons use a pair of cotransmitters and all neurons receive input from a multitude of neurotransmitters in classic presynaptic to postsynaptic asymmetrical neurotransmission. Such synaptic neurotransmission at the brain's trillion synapses is key to chemical neurotransmission, but some neurotransmission is retrograde from postsynaptic neuron to presynaptic neuron; other types of neurotransmission such as volume neurotransmission do not require a synapse at all.

The reader should also have an appreciation for elegant if complex molecular cascades precipitated by a neurotransmitter, with molecule-by-molecule transfer of that transmitted message inside the neuron receiving that message, eventually altering the biochemical machinery of that cell in order to carry out the message that was sent to it. Thus, the function of chemical neurotransmission is not so much to have a presynaptic neurotransmitter communicate with its postsynaptic receptors but to have a *presynaptic genome converse with a postsynaptic genome*: DNA to DNA – presynaptic "command center" to postsynaptic "command center" and back.

The message of chemical neurotransmission is transferred via three sequential "molecular pony express" routes: (1) a presynaptic neurotransmitter synthesis route from presynaptic genome to the synthesis and packaging of neurotransmitter and supporting enzymes and receptors; (2) a postsynaptic route from receptor occupancy through second messengers all the way to the genome, which turns on postsynaptic genes; and (3) another postsynaptic route starting from the newly expressed postsynaptic genes, which transfers information as a molecular cascade of biochemical consequences throughout the postsynaptic neuron.

It should now be clear that neurotransmission does not end when a neurotransmitter binds to a receptor or even when ion flows have been altered or second messengers have been created. Events such as these all start and end within milliseconds to seconds following release of presynaptic neurotransmitter. The ultimate goal of neurotransmission is to alter the biochemical activities of the postsynaptic target neuron in a profound and enduring manner. Since the postsynaptic DNA has to wait until molecular pony express messengers make their way from the postsynaptic receptors, often located on dendrites, to phosphoproteins within the neuron, or to transcription factors and genes in the postsynaptic neuron's cell nucleus, it can take a while for neurotransmission to begin influencing the postsynaptic target neuron's biochemical processes. The time it takes from receptor occupancy by neurotransmitter to gene expression is usually hours. Furthermore, since the last messenger triggered by neurotransmission – called a transcription factor – only initiates the very beginning of gene action, it takes even longer for the gene activation to be fully implemented via the series of biochemical events it triggers. These biochemical events can begin many hours to days after the neurotransmission occurred and can last days or weeks once they are put in motion.

Thus, a brief puff of chemical neurotransmission from a presynaptic neuron can trigger a profound postsynaptic reaction that takes hours to days to develop and can last days to weeks or even a lifetime. Every conceivable component of this entire process of chemical neurotransmission is a candidate for modification by drugs. Most psychotropic drugs act on the processes that control chemical neurotransmission at the level of the neurotransmitters themselves or their enzymes and especially their receptors. Future psychotropic drugs will undoubtedly act directly on the biochemical cascades, particularly on those elements that control the expression of pre- and postsynaptic genes. Also, mental and neurological illnesses are known or suspected to affect these same aspects of chemical neurotransmission. The neuron is dynamically modifying its synaptic connections throughout its life in response to learning, life experiences, genetic programming, drugs, and diseases; chemical neurotransmission is the key aspect underlying the regulation of these important processes.

CHAPTER 4

Transporters and G Protein–Linked Receptors as Targets of Psychopharmacological Drug Action

- Neurotransmitter transporters as targets of drug action
  - Classification and structure
  - Monoamine transporters (SLC6 gene family) as targets of psychotropic drugs
  - Other neurotransmitter transporters (SLC6 and SLC1 gene families) as targets of psychotropic drugs
  - Where are the transporters for histamine and neuropeptides?
  - Vesicular transporters: subtypes and function
  - Vesicular transporters (SLC18 gene family) as targets of psychotropic drugs
- G Protein–linked receptors
  - Structure and function
  - G Protein–linked receptors as targets of psychotropic drugs
- Summary

Psychotropic drugs have many mechanisms of action, but they all target specific molecular sites having profound effects upon neurotransmission. It is thus necessary to understand the anatomical infrastructure (Chapters 1 and 2) and chemical substrates of neurotransmission (Chapter 3) in order to grasp how psychotropic drugs work (included in this chapter and Chapter 5). Although over 100 essential psychotropic drugs are utilized in clinical practice today (see Stahl SM, *Essential Psychopharmacology: The Prescriber's Guide*), there are only a few sites of action for all these therapeutic agents. Specifically, about one-third of psychotropic drugs target one of the transporters for a neurotransmitter (Figure 4-1). Another third target receptors coupled to G proteins (also shown in Figure 4-1). Both of these sites of action are discussed here in Chapter 4.

The molecular sites of action for the other third of psychotropic drugs are discussed in Chapter 5. These include ligand-gated ion channels, voltage-sensitive ion channels, and various enzymes (Figure 4-2). Thus, mastering how just a few molecular sites regulate neurotransmission allows the psychopharmacologist to understand the theories about the mechanisms of action of virtually all psychopharmacological agents.

Major Targets of Psychopharmacologic Drug Action

12-transmembrane-
region transporter
~ 30% of psychotropic drugs

7-transmembrane-
region transporter
G protein–linked
~ 30% of psychotropic drugs

FIGURE 4-1 **G protein-linked receptors.** There are only a few major sites of action for the wide expanse of psychotropic drugs utilized in clinical practice. Approximately one-third of psychotropic drugs target one of the twelve transmembrane region transporters for a neurotransmitter (depicted by the icon on the left), while another third target seven transmembrane region receptors coupled to G proteins (depicted by the icon on the right).

Other Targets of Psychotropic Drug Action

4-transmembrane-region
ligand-gated ion channel
~ 20% of psychotropic drugs

6-transmembrane-region
voltage-sensitive ion channel
~ 10% of psychotropic drugs

Enzyme
~ 10% of psychotropic drugs

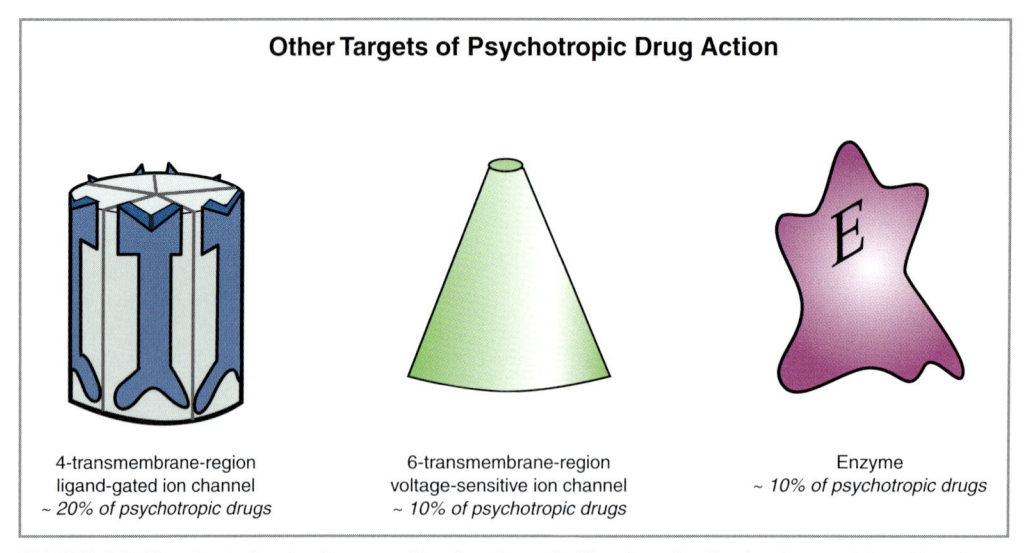

FIGURE 4-2 **Ligand-gated and voltage-sensitive ion channels.** The sites of action for the remaining third of psychotropic drugs (see Chapter 5) include four transmembrane region ligand-gated ion channels, six transmembrane region voltage-sensitive ion channels, and enzymes.

Neurotransmitter transporters as targets of drug action

Classification and structure

Neuronal membranes normally serve to keep the internal milieu of the neuron constant by acting as barriers to the intrusion of outside molecules and to the leakage of internal molecules. However, selective permeability of the membrane is required to allow discharge as well as uptake of specific molecules in response to the needs of cellular functioning. Good examples of this are neurotransmitters, which are released from neurons during neurotransmission and, in many cases, also transported back into presynaptic neurons as a recapture mechanism following their release. This recapture – or reuptake – is done in order for neurotransmitter to be reused in a subsequent neurotransmission. Also, once inside the neuron, most neurotransmitters are transported again into synaptic vesicles for storage, protection from metabolism, and immediate use during a volley of future neurotransmission.

TABLE 4-1 Presynaptic monoamine transporters

Transporter	Common Abbreviation	Gene Family	Endogenous Substrate	False Substrate
serotonin transporter	SERT	SLC6	serotonin	ecstacy (MDMA)*
norepinephrine transporter	NET	SLC6	norepinephrine	dopamine epinephrine amphetamine
dopamine transporter	DAT	SLC6	dopamine	norepinephrine epinephrine amphetamine

*MDMA = 3.4-methylene dioxy methamphetamine.

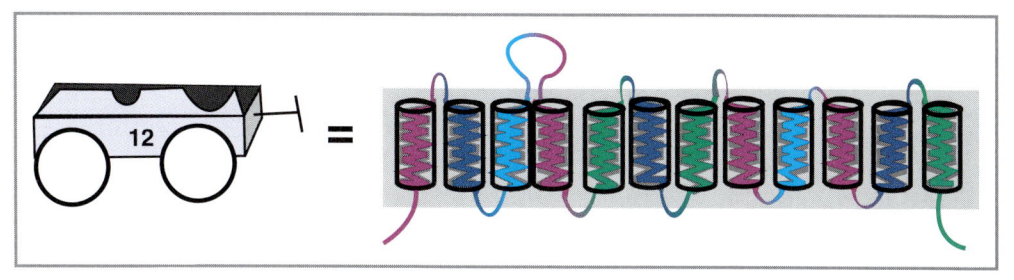

FIGURE 4-3 Neurotransmitter transporters. Neurotransmitter transporters are receptors that bind to neurotransmitter and then transport it across the membrane and back into the presynaptic neuron. Neurotransmitter transporters weave in and out of the neuronal membrane twelve times and thus are twelve transmembrane region receptors.

Both types of neurotransmitter transport – presynaptic reuptake as well as vesicular storage – utilize a molecular transporter belonging to a "superfamily" of 12 transmembrane region proteins (Figure 4-3). That is, neurotransmitter transporters have in common the structure of going in and out of the membrane 12 times (Figure 4-3). These transporters are receptors of a type that binds to the neurotransmitter prior to transporting that neurotransmitter across the membrane.

Recently, details of the structures of neurotransmitter transporters have been revealed based on modeling from crystallizations of bacterial homologues, and this has led to a proposed subclassification of neurotransmitter transporters. That is, there are two major subclasses of *plasma membrane transporters* for neurotransmitters (Tables 4-1 and 4-2). Some of these transporters are presynaptic and others are on glial membranes. The first subclass comprises sodium/chloride-coupled transporters, called the solute carrier SLC6 gene family, and includes transporters for the monoamines serotonin, norepinephrine, and dopamine (Table 4-1) as well as for the neurotransmitter gamma aminobutyric acid (GABA) and the amino acid glycine (Table 4-2). The second subclass comprises high-affinity glutamate transporters, also called the solute carrier SLC1 gene family (Table 4-2).

In addition, there are three subclasses of *intracellular synaptic vesicle transporters* for neurotransmitters: the SLC 18 gene family made up of both vesicular monoamine transporters (VMATs) for serotonin, norepinephrine and dopamine, as well as the vesicular

TABLE 4-2 Neuronal and glial GABA and amino acid transporters

Transporter	Common Abbreviation	Gene Family	Endogenous Substrate
GABA transporter 1 (neuronal and glial)	GAT-1	SLC 6	GABA
GABA transporter 2 (neuronal and glial)	GAT-2	SLC 6	GABA beta alanine
GABA transporter 3 (mostly glial)	GAT-3	SLC 6	GABA beta alanine
GABA transporter 4 also called betaine transporter (neuronal and glial)	GAT-4 BGT-1	SLC 6	GABA betaine
glycine transporter 1 (mostly glial)	GlyT-1	SLC 6	glycine
glycine transporter 2 (neuronal)	GlyT-2	SLC 6	glycine
excitatory amino acid transporters 1-5	EAAT-1-5	SLC 1	L-glutamate L-aspartate

TABLE 4-3 Vesicular neurotransmitter transporters

Transporter	Common Abbreviation	Gene Family	Endogenous Substrate
Vesicular monoamine transporters 1 and 2	VMAT 1 VMAT 2	SLC 18	serotonin norepinephrine dopamine
Vesicular acetylcholine transporter	VAChT	SLC 18	acetylcholine
Vesicular inhibitory amino acid transporter	VIAAT	SLC 32	GABA
Vesicular glutamate transporters 1-3	VGlut 1-3	SLC 17	glutamate

acetylcholine transporter (VAChT); the SLC32 gene family and their vesicular inhibitory amino acid transporters (VIAATs); and finally the SLC17 gene family and their vesicular glutamate transporters, such as VGlut 1–3 (Table 4-3).

Monoamine transporters (SLC6 gene family) as targets of psychotropic drugs
Reuptake mechanisms for monoamines utilize unique presynaptic transporters in each different monoamine neuron but the same vesicular transporter in the synaptic vesicle membranes of all three monoamine neurons (Figure 4-4). That is, for the monoamine serotonin, the unique presynaptic transporter is known as SERT; for norepinephrine, it is known as NET; and for dopamine, it is DAT (Table 4-1 and Figure 4-4). All three of these monoamines are then transported into synaptic vesicles of their respective neurons by the same vesicular transporter, known as vesicular monoamine transporter 2 (VMAT2) (Figure 4-4 and Table 4-3).

Although the presynaptic transporters for these three neurotransmitters – SERT, NET, and DAT – are unique in their amino acid sequences and binding affinities for monoamines, each presynaptic monoamine transporter nevertheless has appreciable affinity for amines other than the one matched to its own neuron (Table 4-1). Thus, if other transportable neurotransmitters or drugs are in the vicinity of a given monoamine transporter, they may also be transported into the presynaptic neuron by hitch-hiking a ride on certain transporters that can carry them into the neuron.

For example, the norepinephrine transporter NET has high affinity for the transport of dopamine as well as for norepinephrine; the dopamine transporter DAT has high affinity

Monoamine Transporters

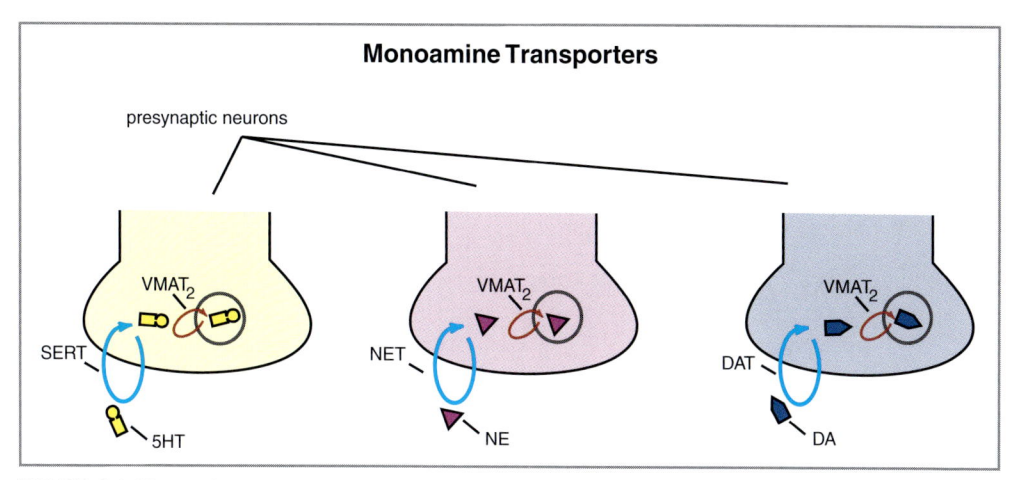

FIGURE 4-4 Monoamine transporters. Once neurotransmitter has been transported back into the presynaptic neuron, it can either be metabolized or repackaged into synaptic vesicles and thus readied for future neurotransmission. Although each of the monoamines has a unique presynaptic transporter (SERT for serotonin, NET for norepinephrine, and DAT for dopamine), they all utilize the same vesicular transporter, known as VMAT2 (vesicular monoamine transporter 2).

for the transport of amphetamines as well as for dopamine; the serotonin transporter SERT has high affinity for the transport of "ecstacy" (the drug of abuse 3,4-methylenedioxymethamphetamine, or MDMA) as well as for serotonin (Table 4-1).

How are neurotransmitters transported? Monoamines are not passively shuttled into the presynaptic neuron because it requires energy to concentrate monoamines into a presynaptic neuron. That energy is provided by transporters in the SLC6 gene family coupling the "downhill" transport of sodium (down a concentration gradient) with the "uphill" transport of the monoamine (up a concentration gradient) (Figure 4-5). Thus, the monoamine transporters are really sodium-dependent cotransporters; in most cases, this involves the additional cotransport of chloride and in some cases the countertransport of potassium. All of this is made possible by coupling monoamine transport to the activity of a sodium potassium ATPase (adenosine triphosphatase), an enzyme sometimes called the "sodium pump," which creates the downhill gradient for sodium by continuously pumping sodium out of the neuron (Figure 4-5).

The structure of a monoamine neurotransmitter transporter from the SLC6 family has recently been proposed to have binding sites not only for the monoamine but also for two sodium ions (Figures 4-6 and 4-7). In addition, these transporters may exist as dimers, or two copies working together with each other; however, the manner in which they cooperate is not yet well understood and is not shown in the figures. There are other sites on this transporter – not well defined – for drugs such as antidepressants, which bind to the transporter and inhibit reuptake of monoamines but do not bind to the substrate site and are not transported into the neuron; thus they are allosteric (i.e., "at another site") (Figure 4-7).

In the absence of sodium, the monoamine transporter has low affinity for its monoamine substrate and thus binds neither sodium nor monoamine. An example of this is shown for the serotonin transporter SERT in Figure 4-7A, where the transport "wagon" has flat tires, indicating no binding of sodium as well as absence of binding of serotonin to its substrate binding site, since the transporter has low affinity for serotonin in the absence of sodium.

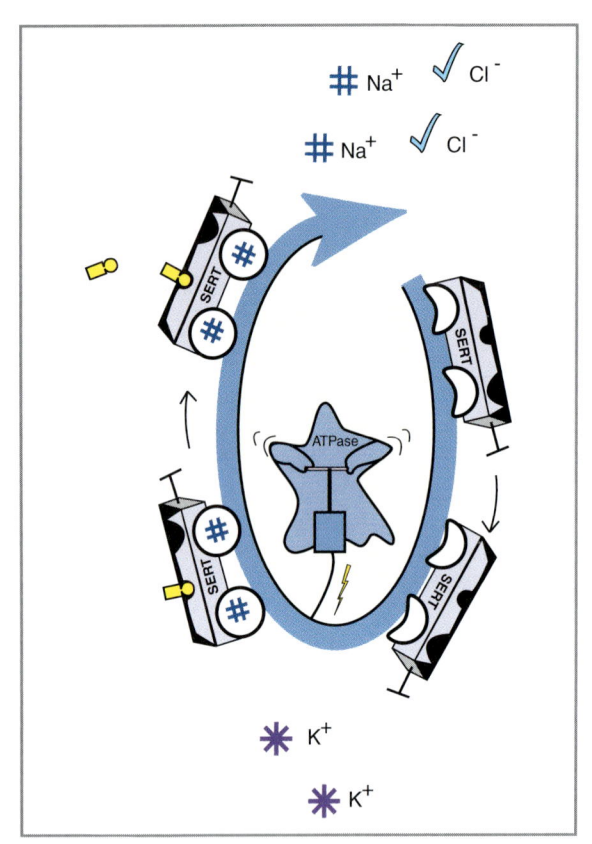

FIGURE 4-5 Sodium potassium ATPase. Transport of monoamines into the presynaptic neuron is not passive, but rather requires energy. This energy is supplied by sodium potassium ATPase, an enzyme that is also sometimes referred to as the sodium pump. Sodium potassium ATPase continuously pumps sodium out of the neuron, creating a downhill gradient. The "downhill" transport of sodium is coupled to the "uphill" transport of monoamines. In many cases this also involves cotransport of chloride and in some cases countertransport of potassium.

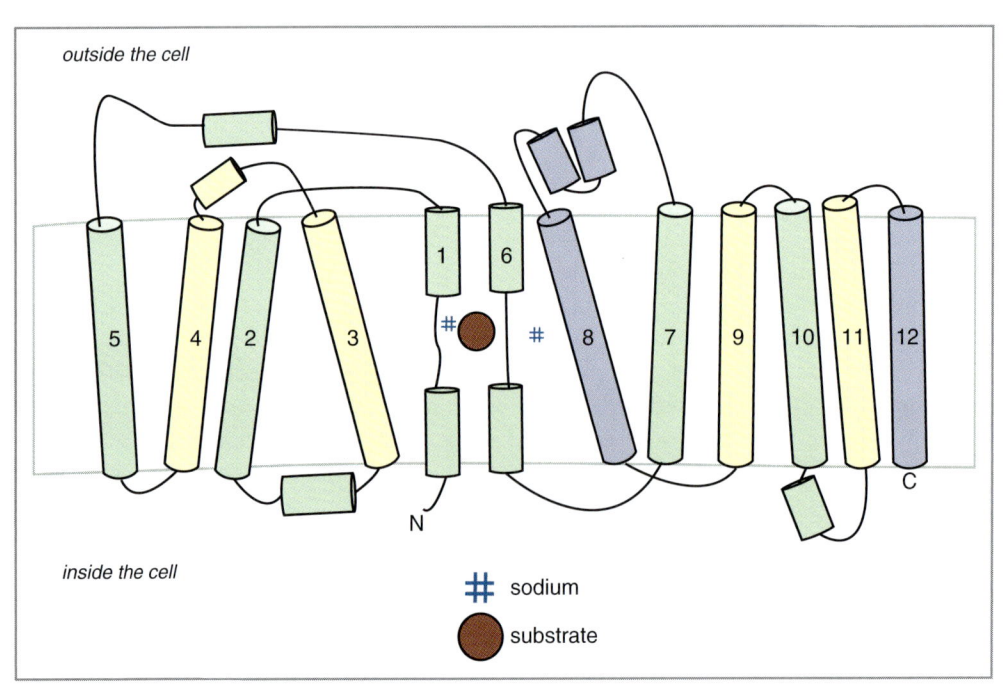

FIGURE 4-6 Monoamine transporter binding sites. The twelve transmembrane region monoamine transporter is believed to have binding sites not only for the monoamine (substrate) but also for two sodium ions.

96 | Essential Psychopharmacology

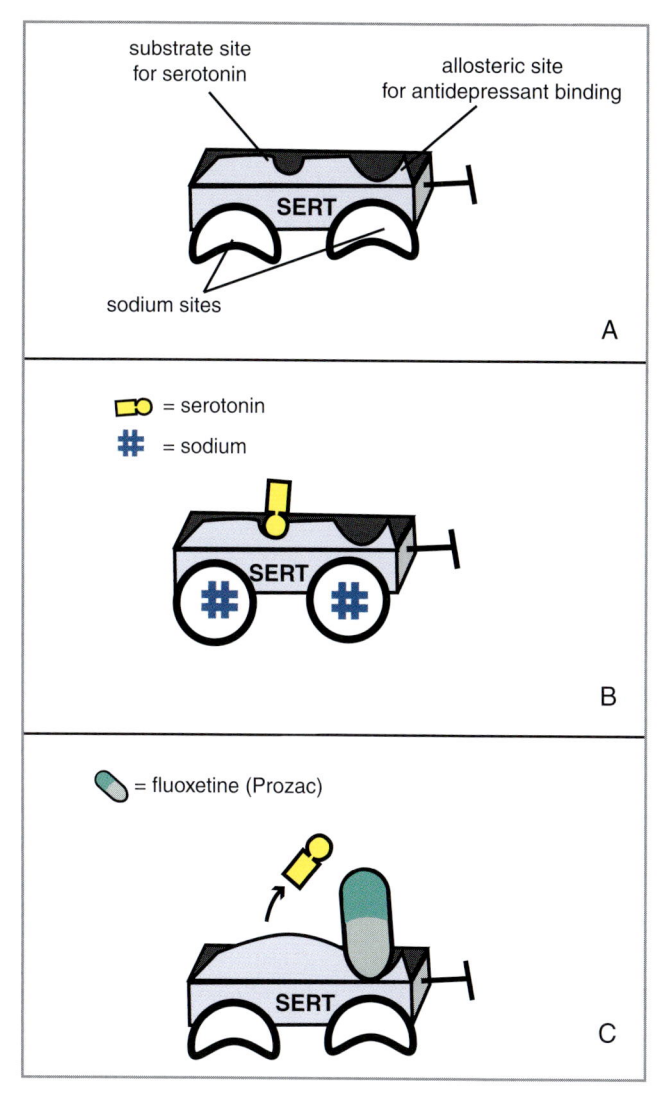

FIGURE 4-7A, B, and C Monoamine transporter binding sites. In addition to binding sites for monoamine and sodium ions, monoamine transporters may have allosteric binding sites, meaning sites at which molecules (e.g., an antidepressant) may bind to affect transport without themselves being transported into the neuron. An example of this is shown here for the serotonin transporter SERT. In panel A, the transport "wagon" has flat tires and no binding or transport of serotonin. In panel B, neurotransmitter is bound to transporter sites, ready for a trip inside the neuron. Serotonin is bound because sodium ions are also bound, which increases the transporter's affinity for serotonin, resulting in the tires being pumped up and full of air, ready for transport. In panel C, binding of the serotonin reuptake inhibitor fluoxetine to its allosteric site essentially bumps serotonin neurotransmitter molecules out of their seats on the transporter. This causes inhibition or blockade of neurotransmitter transport into the neuron. Sodium binding is also decreased, and the tires go flat, so that transport is halted.

The allosteric site for antidepressant binding is also empty in Figure 4-7A. However, in Figure 4-7B, in the presence of sodium ions, the tires are "inflated" by sodium binding and serotonin can now also bind to its substrate site on SERT. This situation is primed for serotonin transport back into the serotonergic neuron, along with cotransport of sodium and chloride down the gradient and into the neuron and countertransport of potassium out of the neuron (Figure 4-7B). If a drug binds to an inhibitory allosteric site on SERT, as the antidepressant fluoxetine (Prozac) is doing in Figure 4-7C, this reduces the affinity of the serotonin transporter SERT for its substrate serotonin, and serotonin binding is prevented (Figure 4-7C).

Why does this matter? Blocking the presynaptic monoamine transporter has a huge impact on neurotransmission at any synapse utilizing that monoamine. The normal recapture of serotonin in Figure 4-8A keeps the levels of this neurotransmitter from accumulating in the synapse. Normally, following release from the presynaptic neuron, serotonin has time only for a brief dance on the synaptic receptors; the party is soon over because

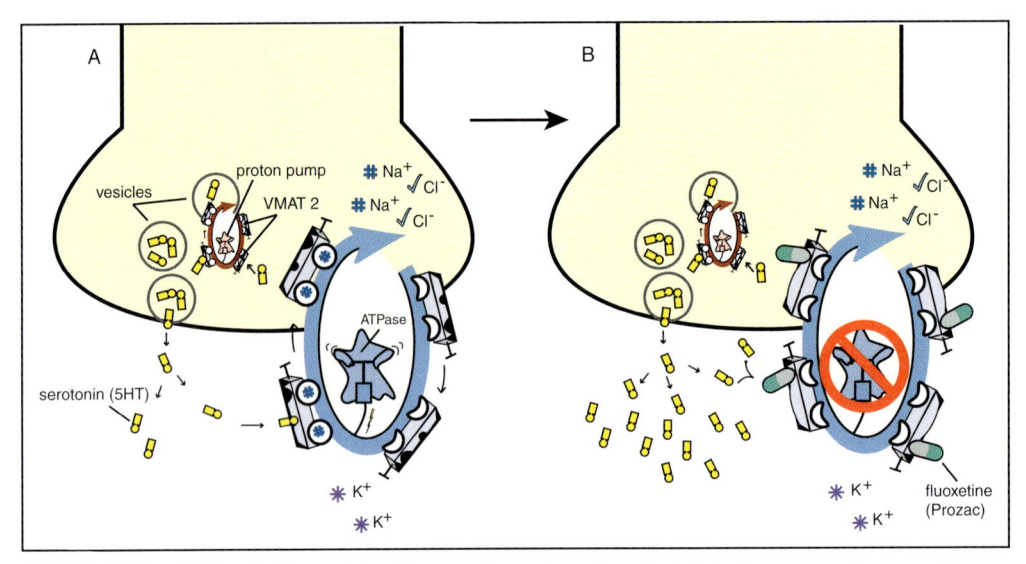

FIGURE 4-8A and B Serotonin reuptake. The normal recapture of serotonin into the presynaptic neuron is shown on the left (**A**). Once the neurotransmitter molecules are released by the neuron, they can be snatched by the transporter, given a seat on the shuttle, and driven into the cell on the track created by the transport carrier, using energy provided by ATPase (the sodium pump). Once inside the cell, the neurotransmitter gets out of its seat on the shuttle and can be stored again in synaptic vesicles via the actions of the vesicular transporter VMAT2. This allows the neurotransmitter to be reused in a subsequent neurotransmission. Shown on the right (**B**) is how the antidepressant fluoxetine (Prozac) prevents neurotransmitter from shuttling into the neuron. In this case, binding of the transport carrier by fluoxetine prevents serotonin neurotransmitter molecules from taking a seat on the shuttle. Thus, there is no ride for the serotonin into the neuron. This means that the neurotransmitter serotonin remains in the synapse until it diffuses away or is destroyed by enzymes.

serotonin climbs back into the presynaptic neuron on its transporter SERT. If one wants to enhance normal synaptic activity of serotonin or restore diminished synaptic activity of serotonin, this can be accomplished by blocking SERT, as shown in Figure 4-8B. Although this might not seem to be a very dramatic thing, the fact is that this alteration in chemical neurotransmission − namely, the enhancement of synaptic monoamine action − is thought to underlie the clinical effects of all the agents that block monoamine transporters, including most known antidepressants and stimulants. Specifically, many antidepressants enhance serotonin, norepinephrine, or both due to actions on SERT and/or NET. Some antidepressants act on DAT, as do stimulants. Also, recall that many antidepressants that block monoamine transporters are also effective anxiolytics, reduce neuropathic pain, and have additional therapeutic actions as well. Thus, it may come as no surprise that drugs that block monoamine transporters are among the most frequently prescribed psychotropic drugs.

A list of various antidepressants that block one or more of the presynaptic monoamine transporters is given in Table 4-4, along with a list of stimulants that are either substrates or inhibitors of presynaptic monoamine transporters. Many of the agents that act on monoamine transporters are more selective for one transporter than for another, but selectivity is dose-dependent, and many agents with predominant actions on one transporter have clinically relevant secondary actions on another transporter, particularly when drugs are administered at high doses. This will be discussed in further detail in later chapters on antidepressants and on stimulant use and abuse. The point to be appreciated here is that

TABLE 4-4 Monoamine transporters as targets of antidepressants and stimulants

Transporter	Antidepressant	Stimulant
SERT	SSRIs (6 drugs) SNRIs (3 drugs) TCAs (>12 drugs; some only at high doses) Trazodone, nefazodone (high doses)	cocaine
NET	SNRIs (3 drugs) TCAs (>12 drugs) NRIs (atomoxetine, reboxetine) NDRIs (bupropion)	cocaine amphetamine methylphenidate
DAT	NDRI (bupropion) Some TCAs (high doses)	cocaine modafinil amphetamine methylphenidate

SSRI = serotonin selective reuptake inhibitor (e.g., fluoxetine, sertraline, paroxetine, citalopram, escitalopram, fluvoxamine)
SNRI = serotonin norepinephrine reuptake inhibitor (e.g., venlafaxine, duloxetine, milnacipran)
TCA = tricyclic antidepressant (many)
NRI = norepinephrine selective reuptake inhibitor (e.g., reboxetine, atomoxetine)
NDRI = norepinephrine dopamine reuptake inhibitor (e.g., bupropion)

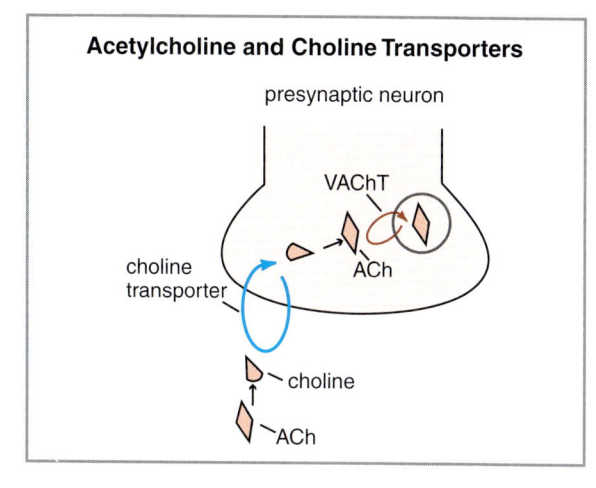

FIGURE 4-9 Acetylcholine and choline transporters. Presynaptic transporters exist for many neurotransmitters in addition to the monoamines. Shown here is the presynaptic transporter for choline, the precursor to the neurotransmitter acetylcholine, as well as the vesicular transporter for acetylcholine, known as VAChT.

about one-third of the currently prescribed essential 100 psychotropic drugs act by targeting one or more of the three monoamine transporters.

Other neurotransmitter transporters (SLC6 and SLC1 gene families) as targets of psychotropic drugs

In addition to the three transporters for monoamines discussed in detail above, there are several other transporters for various different neurotransmitters or their precursors. Although this includes a dozen additional transporters, there is only one psychotropic drug used clinically that is known to bind to any of these transporters. Thus, there is a presynaptic transporter for choline, the precursor to the neurotransmitter acetylcholine (Figure 4-9), but no known drugs target this transporter. There are also several transporters for the ubiquitous

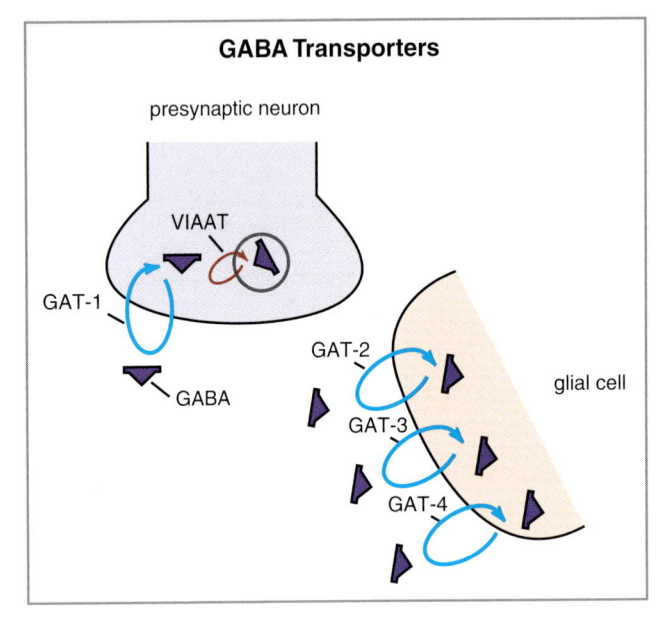

FIGURE 4-10 GABA transporters. Transporters for the inhibitory neurotransmitter gamma-aminobutyric acid (GABA) are known as GAT1-4. The localizations of the subtypes of the GAT transporter are not definitely known, but GAT1 has been identified as a presynaptic transporter, while GAT2-4 may exist on glial cells. The vesicular transporter for GABA is called VIAAT (vesicular inhibitory amino acid transporter).

inhibitory neurotransmitter GABA, known as GAT1–4. Although debate continues about the exact localization of these subtypes to presynaptic neurons, neighboring glia, or even postsynaptic neurons, it is clear that a key presynaptic transporter of GABA is the GAT1 transporter (Figure 4-10). The anticonvulsant tiagabine is a selective inhibitor of GAT1, and when GAT1 is blocked by tiagabine, synaptic GABA concentrations are increased. In addition to anticonvulsant actions, this increase in synaptic GABA may have therapeutic actions in anxiety, sleep disorders, and pain. No other inhibitors of this transporter are available for clinical use.

Finally, there are multiple transporters for two amino acid neurotransmitters, glycine and glutamate. No drugs utilized in clinical practice are known to block glycine transporters. The glycine transporters, along with the choline and GABA transporters, are all members of the same gene family as the monoamine transporters (SLC6) and have a similar structure (Figures 4-4 and 4-6 and Tables 4-1 and 4-2). However, the glutamate transporters belong to a unique family, SLC1, and have a unique structure and somewhat different functions compared to those transporters of the SLC6 family.

Specifically, there are several transporters for glutamate, known as excitatory amino acid transporters 1-5, or EAAT1-5 (Table 4-2). The exact localization of these various transporters to presynaptic neurons, postsynaptic neurons, or glia is still under investigation, but the uptake of glutamate into glia is well known to be a key system for recapturing glutamate for reuse once it has been released (Figure 4-11). Transport into glia results in the conversion of glutamate to glutamine; then glutamine enters the presynaptic neuron for reconversion back into glutamate (Figure 4-11). No drugs utilized in clinical practice are known to block glutamate transporters.

One difference between transport of neurotransmitters by the SLC6 gene family and transport of glutamate by the SLC1 gene family is that glutamate does not seem to cotransport chloride with sodium when it also cotransports glutamate. Also, glutamate transport is almost always characterized by the countertransport of potassium, whereas this is not always the case with SLC6 gene family transporters. The specific structural differences

Glutamate Transporters

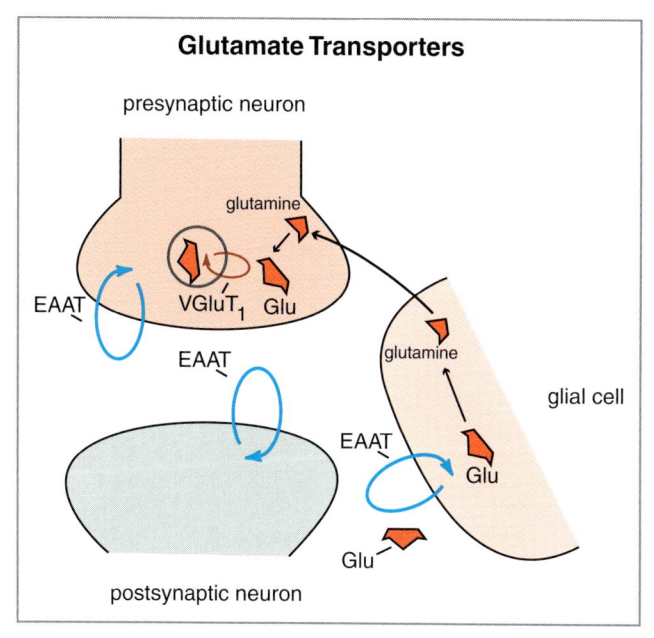

FIGURE 4-11 Glutamate transporters. There are several transporters for the excitatory neurotransmitter glutamate. These transporters are known as excitatory amino acid transporters 1 to 5, or EAAT1-5. The localizations of the subtypes of the EAAT transporter are not definitely known, although uptake into glia is known to occur. Vesicular transporters for glutamate are called vGluT1-3.

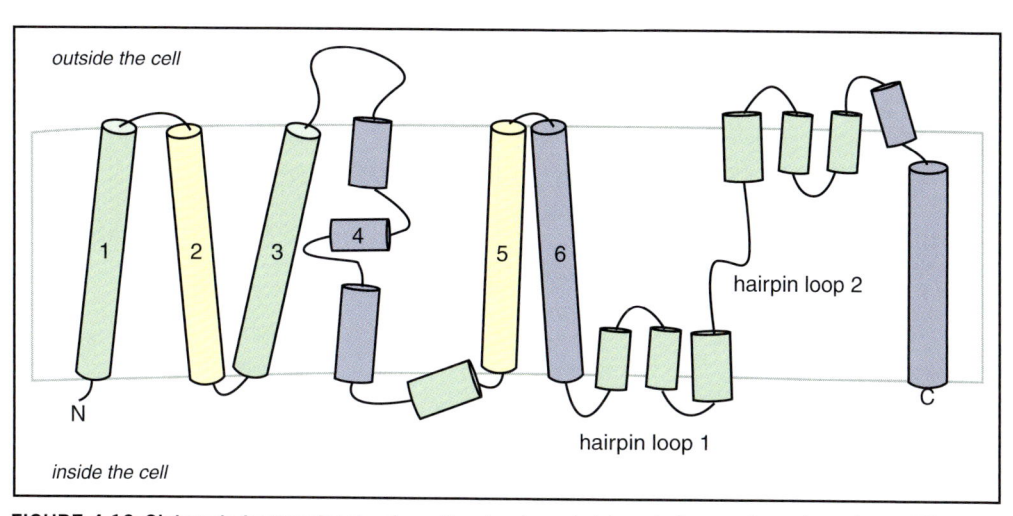

FIGURE 4-12 Glutamate transporter structure. The structure of glutamate transporters, shown here, differs from that of monoamine transporters. Glutamate transporters may be described as consisting of six transmembrane domains plus two hairpin turns.

between glutamate transporters and members of the SLC6 gene family are shown in Figure 4-12 and can be contrasted with Figure 4-6. Although the glutamate transporters can still be characterized as having twelve transmembrane domains, it might be more accurate to describe these transporters as having six transmembrane domains plus two hairpin turns (Figure 4-12). Furthermore, glutamate transporters may work together as trimers rather than dimers, as the SLC6 transporters seem to do. The functional significance of these differences remains obscure but may become more apparent if clinically useful psychopharmacological agents that target glutamate transporters are discovered. Since it may often be desirable to diminish rather than enhance glutamate neurotransmission (see Figures 2-35 through 2-37), the future utility of glutamate transporters as therapeutic targets is also unclear.

Where are the transporters for histamine and neuropeptides?

It is an interesting observation that apparently not all neurotransmitters are regulated by reuptake transporters. The central neurotransmitter histamine apparently does not have a transporter for it presynaptically. Its inactivation is thus thought to be entirely enzymatic. The same can be said for neuropeptides, since reuptake pumps and presynaptic transporters have not been found and are thus thought to be lacking for this class of neurotransmitter. Inactivation of neuropeptides is apparently by diffusion, sequestration, and enzymatic destruction but not by presynaptic transport. It is always possible that a transporter will be discovered in the future for some of these neurotransmitters, but at present there are no known presynaptic transporters for either histamine or neuropeptides.

Vesicular transporters: subtypes and function

Vesicular transporters for the monoamines – members of the SLC18 gene family and known as VMATs – have already been discussed above. They are shown in Figure 4-4 and listed in Table 4-3. The vesicular transporter for acetylcholine – also a member of the SLC18 gene family but known as VAChT – is shown in Figure 4-9 and listed in Table 4-3. The GABA vesicular transporter is a member of the SLC32 gene family and is called vesicular inhibitory amino acid transporter (VIAAT); it is shown in Figure 4-10 and Table 4-3. Finally, vesicular transporters for glutamate, called vesicular glutamate transporters 1, 2, and 3 (vGluT 1-3), are members of the SLC17 gene family; they are shown in Figure 4-11 and listed in Table 4-3. A novel twelve-transmembrane region synaptic vesicle transporter of uncertain mechanism and with unclear substrates is mentioned briefly in Chapter 5 and shown in Figure 5-35. It is localized within the synaptic vesicle membrane and is called the SV2A transporter. Levetiracetam, one of the anticonvulsants, binds selectively and uniquely to this site, perhaps to interfere with neurotransmitter release and thereby reduce seizures.

How do neurotransmitters get inside synaptic vesicles? In the case of vesicular transporters, storage of neurotransmitters is facilitated by a proton ATPase, known as the "proton pump," which utilizes energy to pump positively charged protons continuously out of the synaptic vesicle (Figure 4-13). The neurotransmitters can then be concentrated against a gradient by substituting their own positive charge inside the vesicle for the positive charge of the proton being pumped out. Thus, neurotransmitters are not so much transported as they are "antiported" – i.e., they go in while the protons are actively transported out, keeping charge inside the vesicle constant. This concept is shown in Figure 4-13 for the VMAT transporting dopamine in exchange for protons. Contrast this with Figure 4-5, where a monoamine transporter on the presynaptic membrane is cotransporting a monoamine along with sodium and chloride, but with the help of a sodium potassium ATPase (sodium pump) rather than a proton pump.

Vesicular transporters (SLC18 gene family) as targets of psychotropic drugs

Vesicular transporters for acetylcholine (SLC18 gene family), GABA (SLC32 gene family), and glutamate (SLC17 gene family) are not known to be targeted by any drug utilized by humans. However, vesicular transporters for monoamines in the SLC18 gene family, or VMATs, particularly those in dopamine and norepinephrine neurons, are potently targeted by amphetamine. Thus amphetamine has two targets: monoamine transporters and

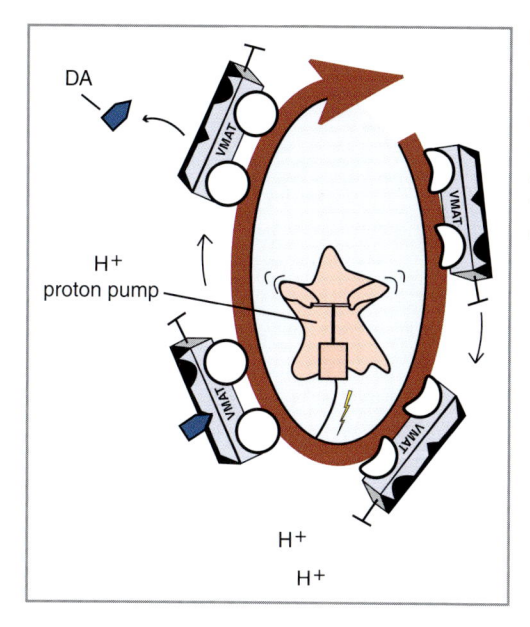

FIGURE 4-13 Vesicular transporters. Vesicular transporters package neurotransmitters into synaptic vesicles through the use of a proton ATPase, or proton pump. The proton pump utilizes energy to pump positively charged protons continuously out of the synaptic vesicle. Neurotransmitter can then be transported into the synaptic vesicle, keeping the charge inside the vesicle constant.

VMATs. In contrast, other stimulants such as methylphenidate and cocaine target only the monoamine transporter, and in much the same manner as described for antidepressants targeting SERT and shown in Figures 4-7 and 4-8.

In order to understand the differences in mechanism of action of various stimulants, it is therefore important to grasp the differences in their actions on monoamine transporters versus VMATs. Normally, dopamine is released (arrow 1 in Figure 4-14), then taken back up into the dopaminergic neuron by DAT (arrows 2 in Figure 4-14) and finally stored in the synaptic vesicle by VMAT (arrows 3 in Figure 4-14). Some antidepressants, such as bupropion as well as certain experimental "triple" reuptake inhibitors (for serotonin, norepinephrine, and dopamine) in clinical testing, block DAT allosterically and stop reuptake of dopamine via DAT. This is the same action on DAT as already shown for fluoxetine (Prozac) acting on SERT in Figure 4-8.

It might be surprising to know that several stimulants, including methylphenidate and cocaine, also block DAT in this manner. The difference between a stimulant and an antidepressant when both act at DAT may be largely that stimulants act much faster and occupy a greater number of transporters than do antidepressants acting at DAT. Stimulants might also act at sites on DAT that differ from those where certain antidepressants act. Rapid onset of action and a high degree of transporter occupancy by stimulants may be facilitated as well by the fact that stimulants are often snorted, injected, or smoked rather than ingested. Rapid and high degrees of DAT occupancy may cause euphoria and lead to abuse, whereas slow onset and lower degrees of DAT occupancy may be consistent with antidepressant actions and improvement in attention in attention deficit hyperactivity disorder (ADHD). These actions and hypotheses are discussed in further detail in the chapters on antidepressants, cognitive enhancers, and substance abuse.

Other stimulants, such as amphetamine and its derivatives, also act at DAT, but as competitive inhibitors of dopamine they act directly at dopamine substrate binding sites on DAT (Figure 4-15). The consequence of acting at the substrate site is

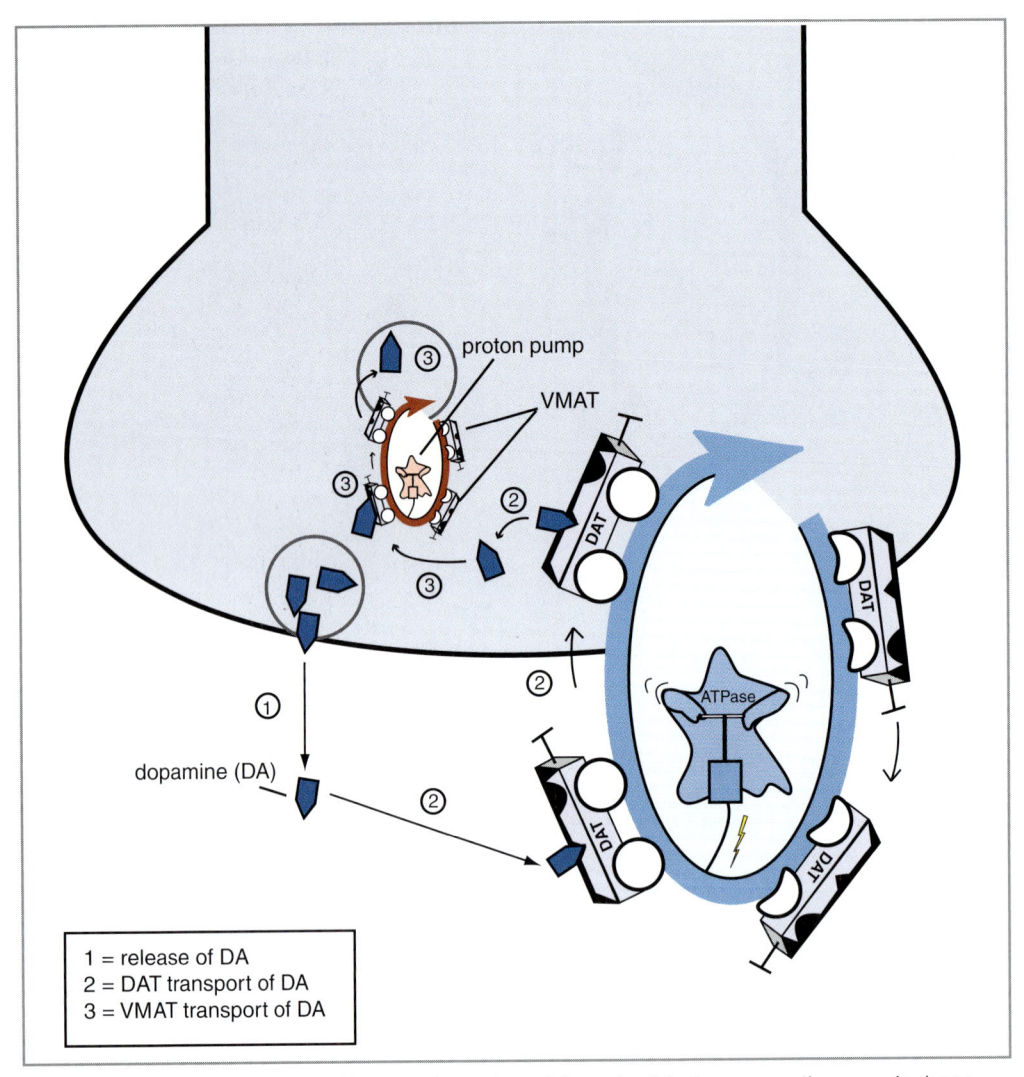

FIGURE 4-14 Dopamine reuptake. The normal recapture of dopamine into the presynaptic neuron is shown here. Once the neurotransmitter molecules are released by the neuron (arrow 1), they can be taken back up into the neuron by the dopamine transporter (arrows 2), using energy provided by ATPase (the sodium pump). Once inside the cell, dopamine can be stored again in synaptic vesicles via the actions of the vesicular transporter (arrows 3), allowing it to be reused in a subsequent neurotransmission.

that not only dopamine transport is blocked but also that of the antidepressants and methylphenidate, both of which act elsewhere on DAT. Amphetamine is actually also transported into the neuron as a hitch-hiking pseudosubstrate (Figure 4-15). Once inside the neuron, amphetamine has additional actions that nontransported stimulants and antidepressants lack, particularly when amphetamine is present suddenly and in high amounts.

Notably, amphetamine also competitively inhibits dopamine at the VMAT as well as DAT and thus is also transported into the synaptic vesicle (Figure 4-15). This causes the displacement of dopamine from synaptic vesicles (Figure 4-15). Soon, massive intracellular amounts of dopamine are available; this has two important consequences, both

104 | Essential Psychopharmacology

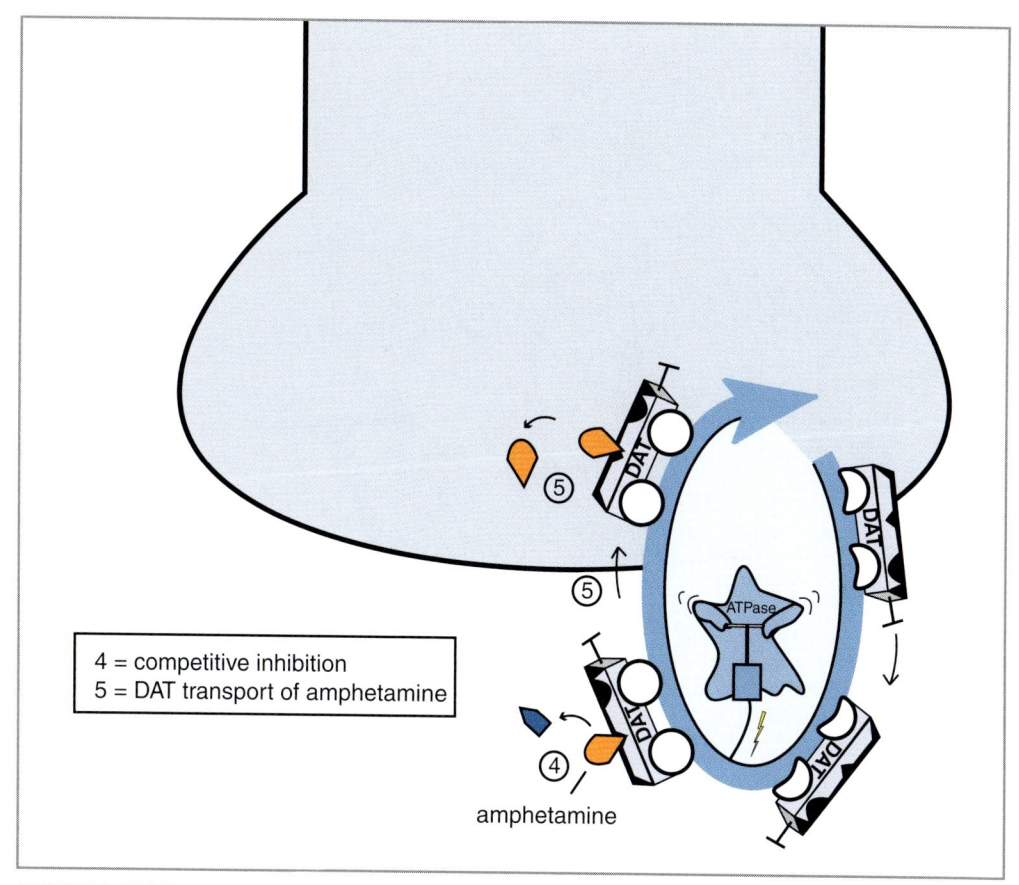

FIGURE 4-15A Dopamine transporter uptake of amphetamine. Several psychotropic drugs, such as the antidepressant bupropion and the stimulants methylphenidate and amphetamine, have actions at the dopamine transporter (DAT); however, the specific actions at DAT may differ for different agents. Unlike antidepressants and methylphenidate, which block the DAT allosterically, amphetamine is a competitive inhibitor of dopamine, acting directly at dopamine substrate binding sites on DAT (arrow 4). Thus, amphetamine not only blocks reuptake of dopamine into the neuron but is also actually transported into the neuron itself (arrows 5).

of which lead to all of this dopamine being dumped into the synapse. High concentrations of intracellular dopamine cause channels to open and release dopamine into the synapse (Figure 4-15D). High concentrations of intracellular dopamine also cause a reversal of the DAT, so that dopamine is now pumped out of the neuron instead of into the neuron, resulting in another way for dopamine to be released into the synapse (Figure 4-15D). All of these mechanisms of amphetamine are not well characterized yet; they may only become activated at high doses of amphetamine. Nevertheless, it is clear that the actions of amphetamine both at DAT and at VMAT differ from actions of antidepressants and stimulants that are not transported by DAT or VMAT, such as bupropion and methylphenidate.

G Protein–linked receptors

Structure and function

Another major target of psychotropic drugs is the class of receptors linked to G proteins. These receptors all have the structure of seven transmembrane regions, meaning

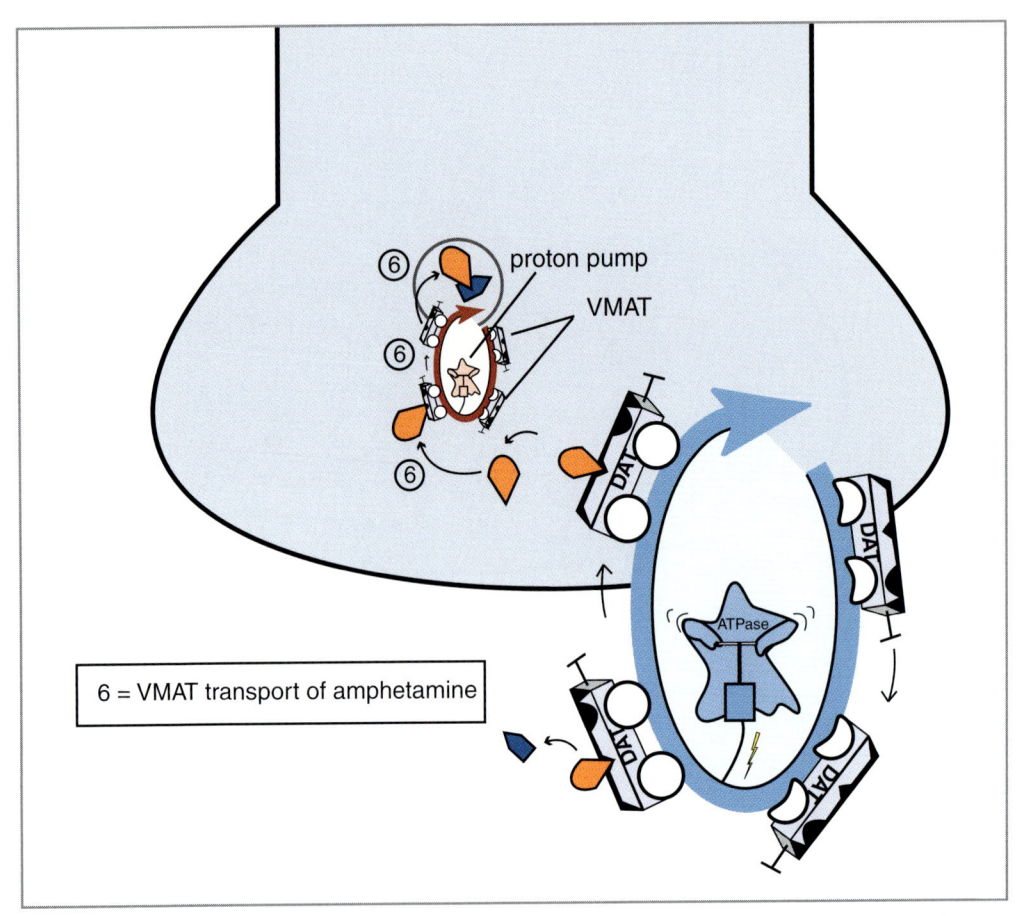

FIGURE 4-15B VMAT transport of amphetamine. In addition to its actions at DAT, amphetamine has unique actions on the vesicular transporter. Amphetamine competitively inhibits dopamine at the VMAT, and thus can itself be transported into the synaptic vesicle (arrows 6).

that they span the membrane seven times (Figure 4-16). Each of the transmembrane regions clusters around a central core which contains a binding site for a neurotransmitter (side view shown in Figure 4-17 and top view shown in Figure 4-18). Drugs can interact at this neurotransmitter binding site or at other sites (allosteric sites) on the receptor. This can lead to a wide range of modifications of receptor actions due to mimicking or blocking, partially or fully, the neurotransmitter function that normally occurs at this receptor. Such drug actions can thus determine downstream molecular events, such as which phosphoproteins are activated or inactivated and therefore which enzymes, receptors, or ion channels are modified by neurotransmission. Such drug actions can also change which genes are expressed and thus which proteins are synthesized and which functions are amplified, from synaptogenesis, to receptor and enzyme synthesis, to communication with downstream neurons innervated by the neuron with the G protein–linked receptor.

All of these actions on neurotransmission by G protein–linked receptors are described in detail in Chapter 3 on signal transduction and chemical neurotransmission. The reader should have a good command of the function of G protein–linked receptors and their role in signal transduction from specific neurotransmitters, as described in Chapter 3, in order to

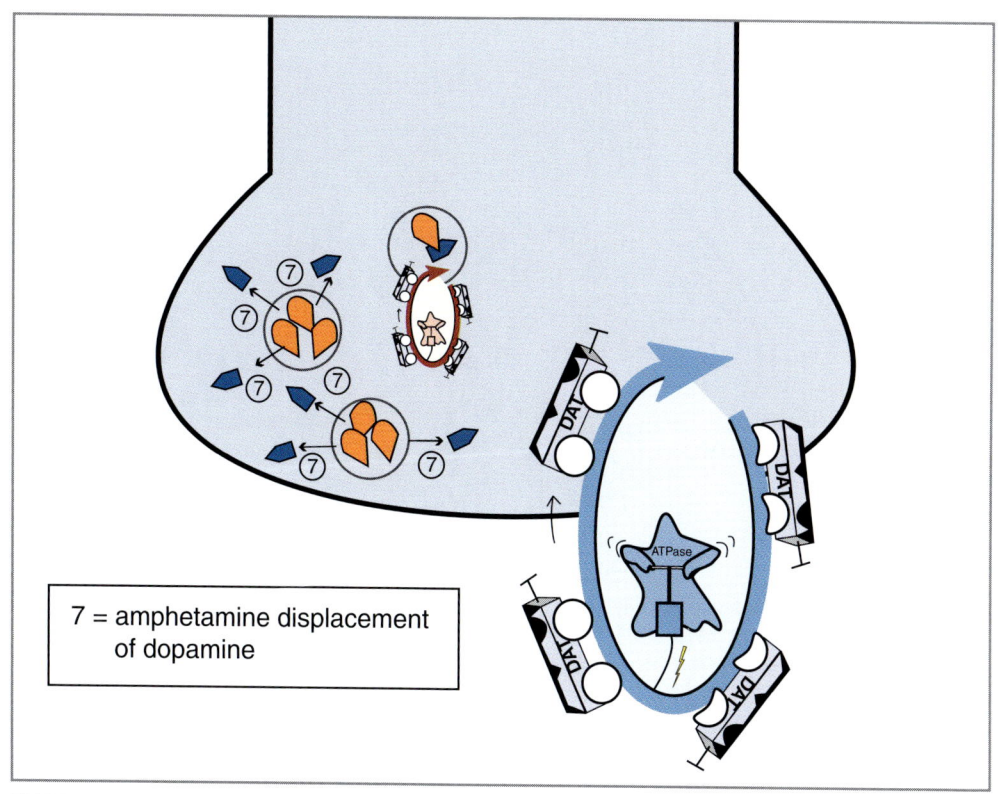

FIGURE 4-15C Amphetamine displacement of dopamine. Competitive inhibition of dopamine at the VMAT and transport of amphetamine into the synaptic vesicles causes the displacement of dopamine from synaptic vesicles (arrows 7).

understand how drugs acting at G protein–linked receptors modify the signal transduction arising from these receptors. This is important to understand because such drug-induced modifications in signal transduction from G protein–linked receptors can have profound effects on psychiatric symptoms. In fact, the single most common action of psychotropic drugs utilized in clinical practice is to modify the actions of G protein–linked receptors, resulting in either therapeutic actions or side effects. Here we will describe how various drugs stimulate or block these receptors, and throughout this book we will show how specific drugs acting at specific G protein–linked receptors have specific actions on specific psychiatric disorders.

G Protein–linked receptors as targets of psychotropic drugs

G protein–linked receptors are a large superfamily of receptors that interact with many neurotransmitters and many psychotropic drugs (Figure 4-19). There are many ways to subtype these receptors (Table 4-5). Genetic, molecular, G-protein, and second messenger subtypes of G protein–linked receptors were already discussed in Chapter 3 and will be further discussed in later chapters dealing with specific drug actions at various G-protein receptor subtypes. Pharmacological subtypes are perhaps the most important to understand for clinicians who wish to target specific receptors with psychotropic drugs utilized in clinical practice. That is, the natural neurotransmitter interacts at all of its receptor subtypes, but many drugs are more selective than the neurotransmitter itself for just certain receptor

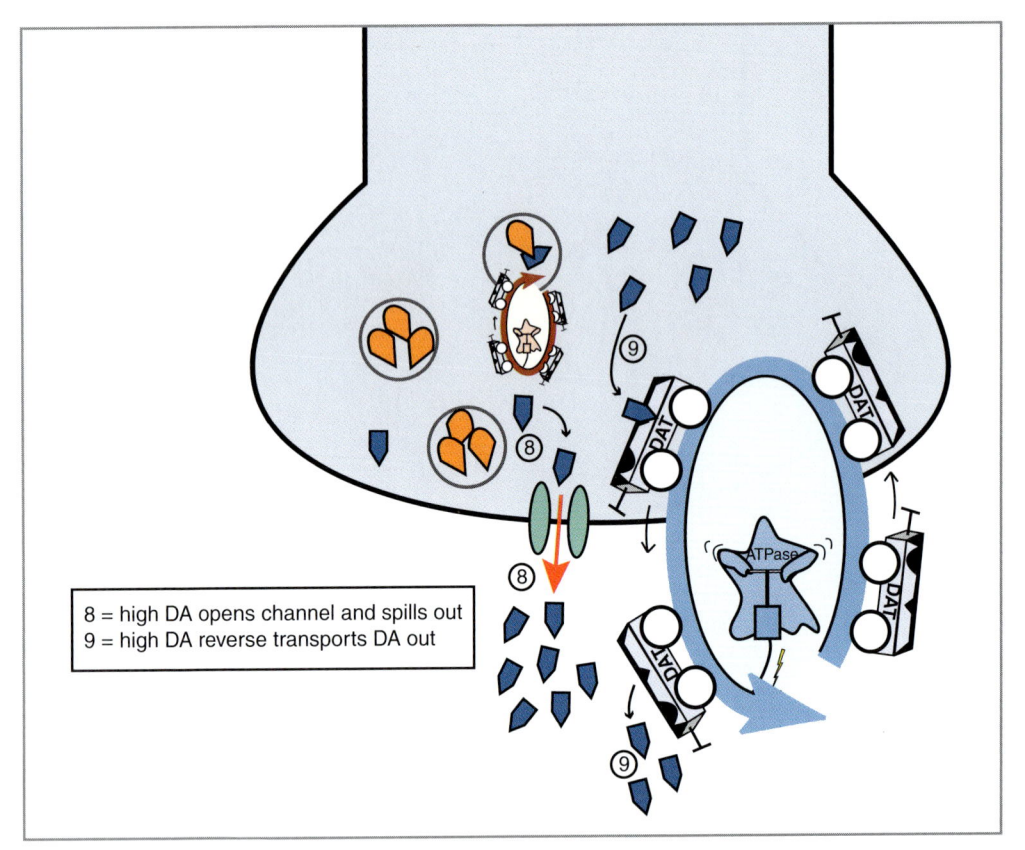

FIGURE 4-15D Reversal of dopamine transporter. Displacement of dopamine from synaptic vesicles causes intracellular dopamine to accumulate, leading channels to open and release dopamine into the synapse (arrows 8). It also causes a reversal of DAT, so that dopamine is pumped out of the neuron instead of into the neuron (arrows 9).

subtypes and thus define a pharmacological subtype of receptor at which they specifically interact. This is not unlike the concept of the neurotransmitter being a master key that opens all the doors and drugs that interact at pharmacologically specific receptor subtypes functioning as a specific key opening only one door (Figure 4-20). Here we will develop the concept that drugs have many ways of interacting at pharmacological subtypes of G protein–linked receptors across an agonist spectrum (Figure 4-21).

No agonist
An important concept for the agonist spectrum is that the absence of agonist does not necessarily mean that nothing is happening with signal transduction at G protein–linked receptors. Agonists are thought to produce a conformational change in G protein–linked receptors that leads to full receptor activation and thus full signal transduction. In the absence of agonist, this same conformational change may still be occurring at some receptor systems, but only at very low frequency. This is referred to as "constitutive activity," which may be present especially in receptor systems and brain areas where there is a high density of receptors. Thus, when something occurs at very low frequency but among a high number of receptors, it can still produce detectable signal transduction output. This is represented as a small amount – but not absent – signal transduction in Figure 4-22.

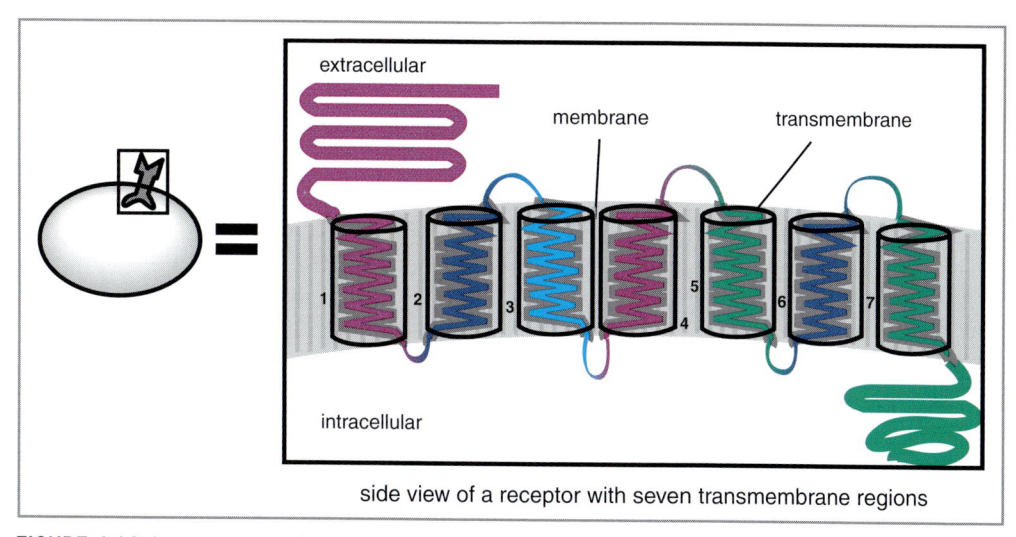

FIGURE 4-16 Seven transmembrane region receptors. Receptors linked to G proteins all have a seven transmembrane structure. That is, the string of amino acids goes in and out of the cell seven times to create three portions of the receptor: first, the part that is outside the cell (called the extracellular portion); second, the part that is inside the cell (called the intracellular portion); and third, the part that traverses the membrane (called the transmembrane portion).

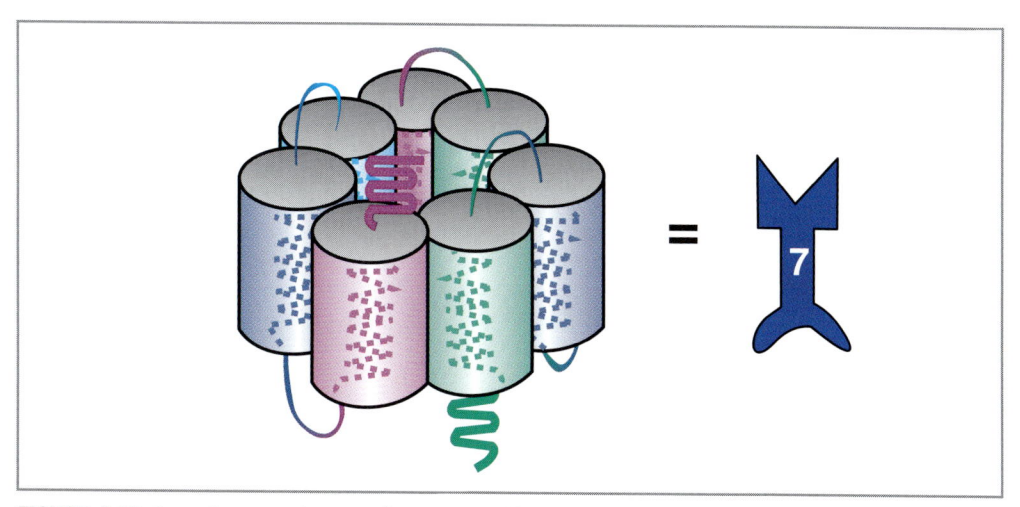

FIGURE 4-17 Seven transmembrane region receptor side view. The side view of a seven transmembrane receptor is shown here. The seven transmembrane regions are not arranged in a line but rather in a circle. In the middle of this circle is the central core, where neurotransmitters find their binding sites. This figure depicts each transmembrane region as a spiral, since each is actually an alpha helix. Also shown is how these spirals are arranged, so that the seven of them form a circle. In the middle of the circle is the binding site for the neurotransmitter. Since there are seven transmembrane regions (left), the icon representing this will have the number 7 on it (right).

Transporters and G Protein–Linked Receptors as Targets of Psychopharmacological Drug Action

TABLE 4-5 Many G protein receptor subtypes for each neurotransmitter

Subtype	
genetic	encoded by slightly different forms of the same gene
molecular	encoded by entirely different genes
pharmacologic	usual definition used for clinical practice; defined by different agonists and antagonists
G proteins	linked to different types of G proteins
second messenger	linked to different second messengers
anatomic	located in different brain regions or on different parts of the neuron (presynaptic axon terminal, presynaptic somatodendritic area, postsynaptic)
functional	inhibit neurotransmitter release (autoreceptors or heteroreceptors); trigger different signal transduction cascades (to activate or inactivate critical phosphoproteins or genes)

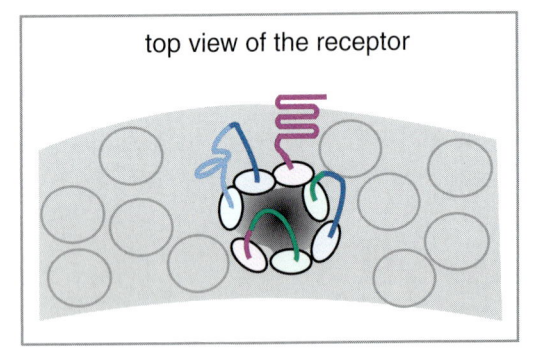

FIGURE 4-18 Seven transmembrane region receptor top view. This figure shows a top view of the seven transmembrane receptor. All that is seen are the extracellular portions of the receptor sticking out of the membrane. These regions connect the various transmembrane regions to each other. In the center of the bits of receptor is the central core, where the neurotransmitter for that receptor binds.

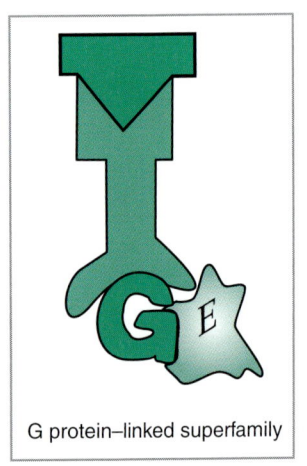

FIGURE 4-19 G protein-linked superfamily. G protein–linked receptors are part of a large superfamily of receptors (the G protein–linked receptor superfamily) which interact with many neurotransmitters and many psychotropic drugs. Each member of this family has a receptor containing seven transmembrane regions, represented here as a simple receptor icon. Each receptor in this family is linked to a G protein and also uses a second messenger system triggered by a cooperating enzyme. A more detailed breakdown and explanation of this superfamily with a series of icons was given in Figures 3-13 through 3-16.

Agonists

An agonist produces a conformational change in the G protein–linked receptor that turns on the synthesis of second messenger to the greatest extent possible (i.e., the action of a *full* agonist) (Figure 4-23). The full agonist is generally represented by the naturally occurring neurotransmitter itself, although some drugs can also act in as full a manner as the natural neurotransmitter itself. What this means from the perspective of chemical

Pharmacological Receptor Subtypes

Neurotransmitter (master key)

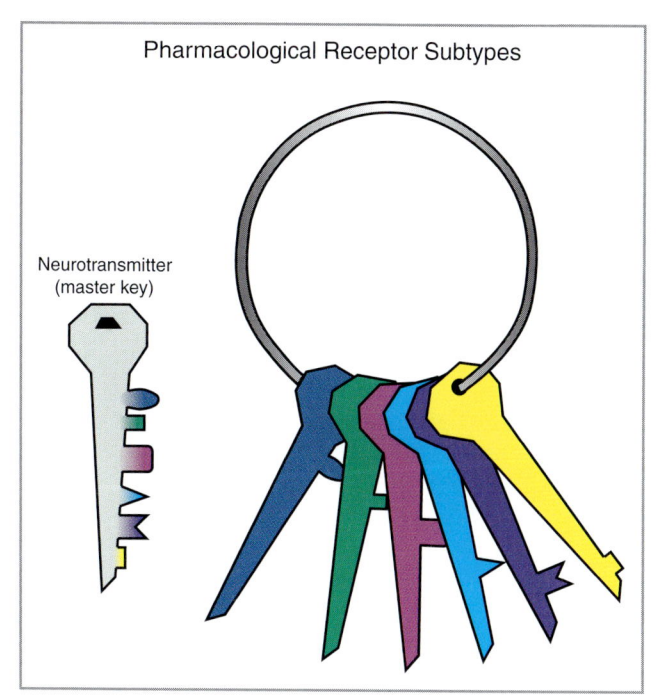

FIGURE 4-20 Multiple receptor subtypes. Neurotransmitters have multiple receptor subtypes with which to interact. It is as though the neurotransmitter were a master key capable of unlocking each of the multiple locks of receptor subtypes. Drugs can be made that mimic the neurotransmitter, but many are more selective than the natural neurotransmitter, thus defining a pharmacological subtype at which they specifically interact. This figure shows a neurotransmitter capable of binding to several different receptor subtypes (i.e., the master key). Also shown are several different drugs on a key chain. Each of these drugs is selective for a single subtype of the neurotransmitter receptors.

The Agonist Spectrum

antagonist
partial agonist
agonist
inverse agonist

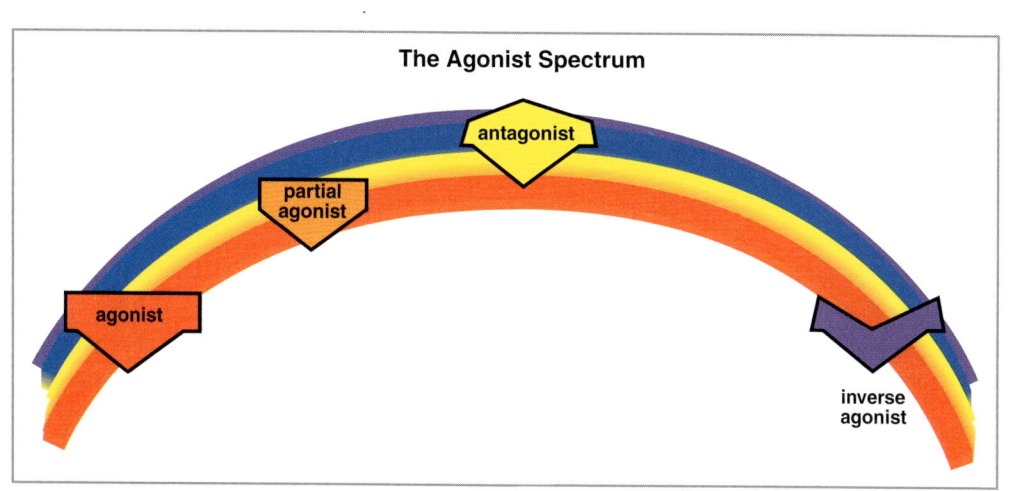

FIGURE 4-21 Agonist spectrum. Shown here is the agonist spectrum. Naturally occurring neurotransmitters stimulate receptors and are thus agonists. Some drugs also stimulate receptors and are therefore agonists as well. It is possible for drugs to stimulate receptors to a lesser degree than the natural neurotransmitter; these are called partial agonists or stabilizers. It is a common misconception that antagonists are the opposite of agonists because they block the actions of agonists. However, although antagonists prevent the actions of agonists, they have no activity of their own in the absence of the agonist. For this reason, antagonists are sometimes called "silent." Inverse agonists, on the other hand, do have opposite actions compared to agonists. That is, they not only block agonists but can also reduce activity below the baseline level when no agonist is present. Thus, the agonist spectrum reaches from full agonists to partial agonists through to "silent" antagonists and finally inverse agonists.

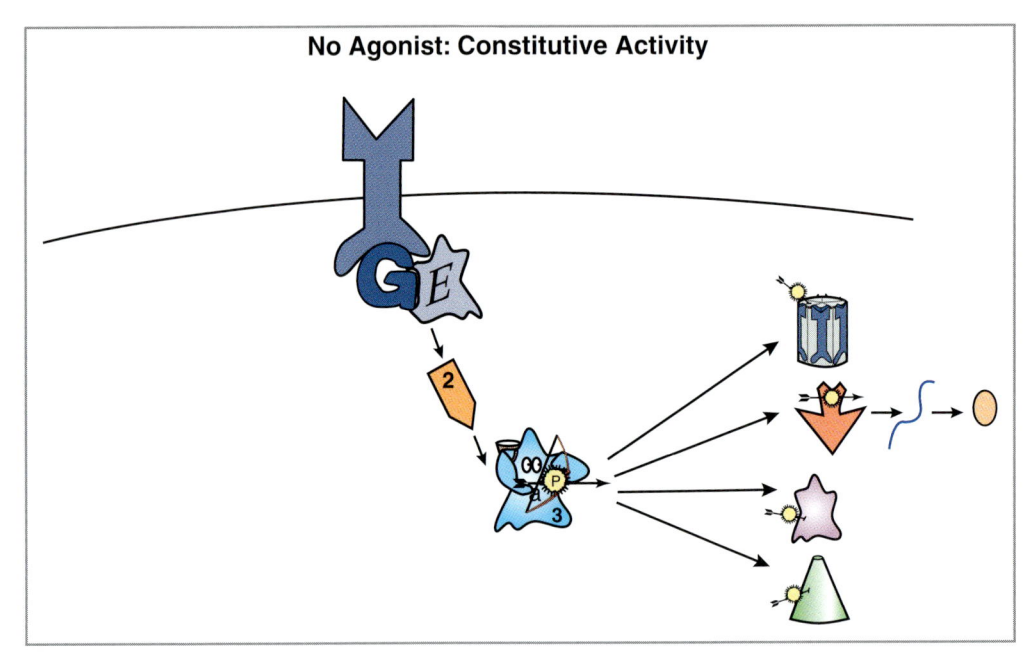

FIGURE 4-22 Constitutive activity. The absence of agonist does not mean that there is no activity related to G protein–linked receptors. Rather, in the absence of agonist, the receptor's conformation is such that it leads to a low level of activity, or "constitutive activity." Thus, signal transduction still occurs, but at a low frequency. Whether this constitutive activity leads to detectable signal transduction is affected by the receptor density in that brain region.

neurotransmission is that the full array of downstream signal transduction is triggered by a full agonist (Figure 4-23). Thus, downstream proteins are maximally phosphorylated and genes are maximally affected. Loss of the agonist actions of a neurotransmitter at G protein–linked receptors, due to deficient neurotransmission of any cause, would lead to the loss of this rich downstream chemical tour de force. Thus, agonists that restore this natural action would be potentially useful in states where reduced signal transduction leads to undesirable symptoms.

There are two major ways to stimulate G protein–linked receptors with full agonist action. First, there are several examples of drugs that *directly* bind to the neurotransmitter site and produce the same array of signal transduction effects as a full agonist (see Table 4-6). These are direct-acting agonists. Second and more importantly, there are many other drugs that can *indirectly* act to boost the levels of the natural full agonist neurotransmitter itself (Table 4-7). This happens when neurotransmitter inactivation mechanisms are blocked. The most prominent examples of indirect full agonist actions have already been discussed above, namely inhibition of the monoamine transporters SERT, NET, and DAT and the GABA transporter GAT1. Another way to accomplish indirect full agonist action is to block the enzymatic destruction of neurotransmitters (Table 4-7). Two examples of this, namely inhibition of the enzymes monoamine oxidase (MAO) and acetylcholinesterase, are discussed in Chapter 5.

Antagonists

On the other hand, it also is possible that full agonist action can be too much of a good thing and that maximal activation of the signal transduction cascade may not always be

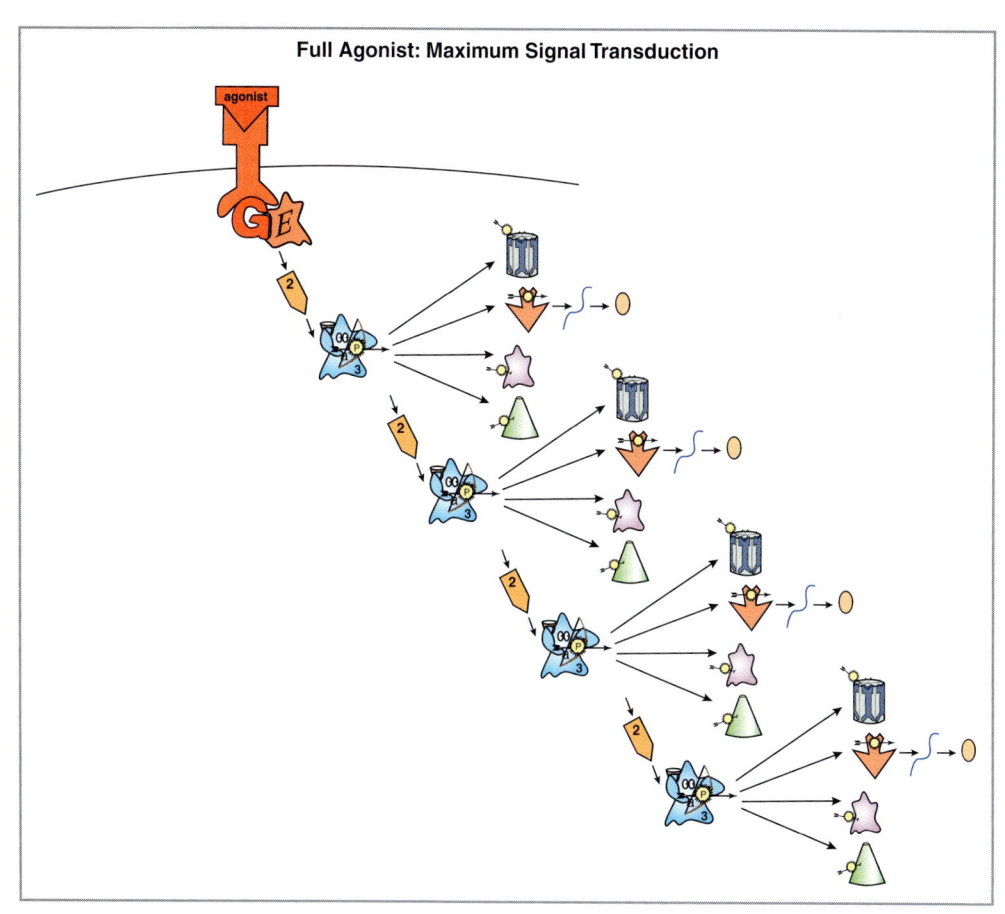

FIGURE 4-23 Full agonist: maximum signal transduction. When a full agonist binds to G protein–linked receptors, it causes conformational changes that lead to maximum signal transduction. Thus, all the downstream effects of signal transduction, such as phosphorylation of proteins and gene activation, are maximized.

desirable, as in states of overstimulation by neurotransmitters. In such cases, blocking the action of the natural neurotransmitter agonist may be desirable. This is the property of an antagonist. Antagonists produce a conformational change in the G protein–linked receptor that causes no change in signal transduction – including no change in whatever amount of any "constitutive" activity that may have been present in the absence of agonist (compare Figure 4-22 with Figure 4-24). Thus, true antagonists are "neutral," and since they have no actions of their own, they are also called "silent."

There are many more examples of important antagonists of G protein–linked receptors than there are of direct-acting full agonists in clinical practice (see Table 4-6). Antagonists are well known both as the mediators of therapeutic actions in psychiatric disorders and as the cause of undesirable side effects (Table 4-6). Some of these may prove to be inverse agonists (see below), but most antagonists utilized in clinical practice are characterized simply as "antagonists."

Antagonists block the actions of everything in the agonist spectrum (Figure 4-21). In the presence of an agonist, an antagonist will block the actions of that agonist but do nothing itself (Figure 4-24). The antagonist simply returns the receptor conformation back to the same state as exists when no agonist is present (Figure 4-22). Interestingly, an antagonist

TABLE 4-6 Key G protein–linked receptors directly targeted by psychotropic drugs

Neurotransmitter	G Protein Receptor and Pharmacologic Subtype Directly Targeted	Pharmacologic Action	Drug Class	Therapeutic Action
Dopamine	D_2	antagonist or partial agonist	conventional antipsychotic; atypical antipsychotic	antipsychotic; antimanic
Serotonin	$5HT_{2A}$	antagonist or inverse agonist	atypical antipsychotic	reduced motor side effects; possible mood stabilizing & antidepressant actions in bipolar disorder
			antidepressant, hypnotic	Improve mood and insomnia
	$5HT_{1A}$ $5HT_{1B/1D}$ $5HT_{2C}$ $5HT_6$ $5HT_7$	antagonist or partial agonist	atypical antipsychotic	unknown secondary receptor actions, possibly contributing to efficacy and tolerability
	$5HT_{1A}$	partial agonist	anxiolytic	anxiolytic; booster of antidepressant action
Norepinephrine	alpha 2	antagonist	antidepressant	antidepressant
		agonist	antihypertensive	cognition and behavioral disturbance in attention deficit hyperactivity disorder
	alpha 1	antagonist	many antipsychotics and antidepressants	side effects of orthostatic hypotension and possibly sedation
GABA	GABA-B	agonist	gamma hydroxy butyrate/sodium oxybate	cataplexy, sleepiness in narcolepsy; possible enhanced slow wave sleep and pain reduction
Melatonin	MT1	agonist	hypnotic	improve insomnia
	MT2	agonist	hypnotic	improve insomnia

(*Continued*)

TABLE 4-6 *(Continued)*

Neurotransmitter	G Protein Receptor and Pharmacologic Subtype Directly Targeted	Pharmacologic Action	Drug Class	Therapeutic Action
Histamine	H_1	antagonist	Many antipsychotics and antidepressants; some anxiolytics	Therapeutic effect for anxiety and insomnia; side effect of sedation and weight gain
Acetylcholine	M_1	antagonist	Many antipsychotics and antidepressants	Side effects of memory disturbance, sedation, dry mouth, blurred vision, constipation, urinary retention
	M_3/M_5	antagonist	Some atypical antipsychotics	May contribute to metabolic dysregulation (dyslipidemia and diabetes)

will also block the actions of a partial agonist. Partial agonists are thought to produce a conformational change in the G protein–linked receptor that is intermediate between a full agonist and the baseline conformation of the receptor in the absence of agonist (Figures 4-25 and 4-26). An antagonist reverses the action of a partial agonist by returning the G protein–linked receptor to that same conformation as exists (Figure 4-24) when no agonist is present (Figure 4-22). Finally, an antagonist reverses an inverse agonist. Inverse agonists are thought to produce a conformational state of the receptor that totally inactivates it and even removes the baseline constitutive activity (Figure 4-27). An antagonist reverses this back to the baseline state that allows constitutive activity (Figure 4-24), the same as exists for the receptor in the absence of the neurotransmitter agonist (Figure 4-22).

It is easy to see, therefore, that true antagonists, by themselves, have no activity, which is why they are sometimes referred to as "silent." Silent antagonists return the entire spectrum of drug-induced conformational changes in the G protein–linked receptor (Figures 4-21 and 4-28) to the same place (Figure 4-24) – i.e., the conformation that exists in the absence of agonist (Figure 4-22).

Partial agonists

It is possible to produce signal transduction that is something more than an antagonist yet something less than a full agonist. Turning down the gain a bit from full agonist actions, but not all the way to zero, is the property of a partial agonist (Figure 4-25). This action can also be seen as turning up the gain a bit from silent antagonist actions but not all the way to a full agonist. The relative closeness of this partial agonist to a full agonist or to a

TABLE 4-7 Key G protein–linked receptors indirectly targeted by psychotropic drugs

Neurotransmitter	G Protein Receptor and Pharmacologic Subtype Indirectly Targeted	Pharmacologic Action	Drug Class	Therapeutic Action
Dopamine	D_1 and D_2 (possibly D_3, D_4)	agonist via increasing dopamine itself at all dopamine receptors	stimulant (actions at dopamine and/or synaptic vesicle transporters DAT and $VMAT_2$)	Improvement of attention deficit hyperactivity disorder (ADHD)
		antidepressant	antidepressant; actions at dopamine and/or norepinephrine transporters (DAT and/or NET)	antidepressant; ADHD
			MAO inhibitor (reducing dopamine metabolism)	antidepressant
Serotonin	$5HT_{1A}$ (presynaptic somatodendritic autoreceptors) $5HT_{2A}$ (postsynaptic receptors; possibly $5HT_{1A}$, $5HT_{2C}$, $5HT_6$, $5HT_7$ postsynaptic receptors	agonist via increasing serotonin itself at all serotonin receptors	antidepressant; actions at serotonin transporters (SERT)	antidepressant; anxiolytic
			MAO inhibitor (reducing serotonin metabolism)	antidepressant
Norepinephrine	$beta_1$ postsynaptic; possibly alpha 2 presynaptic and postsynaptic	agonist via increasing norepinephrine itself at all norepinephrine receptors	Antidepressant; neuropathic pain actions at norepinephrine transporter (NET)	antidepressant; ADHD; neuropathic pain (when combined with SERT inhibition)
			MAO inhibitor (reducing norepinephrine metabolism)	antidepressant

(*Continued*)

TABLE 4-7 *(Continued)*

Neurotransmitter	G Protein Receptor and Pharmacologic Subtype Indirectly Targeted	Pharmacologic Action	Drug Class	Therapeutic Action
GABA	GABA-A; GABA-B	agonist via increasing GABA itself at all GABA receptors	Anticonvulsant; actions at the GABA GAT1 transporter	Anticonvulsant; possibly anxiolytic, for chronic pain, for slow wave sleep
Acetylcholine	M_1 (possibly M_2-M_5)	Agonist via increasing acetylcholine itself at all acetylcholine receptors	Acetylcholinesterase inhibitor (reducing acetylcholine metabolism	Slowing progression in Alzheimer's Disease

DAT = dopamine transporter
NET = norepinephrine transporter
SERT = serotonin transporter
MAO = monoamine oxidase
VMAT = vesicular monoamine transporter

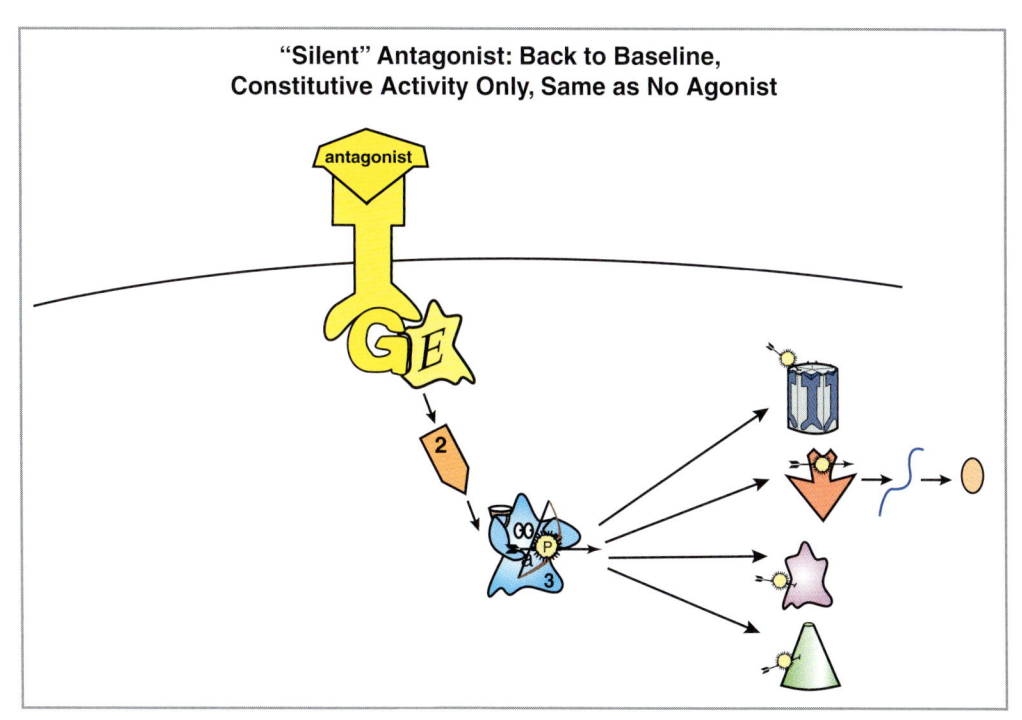

FIGURE 4-24 "Silent" antagonist. An antagonist blocks agonists (both full and partial) from binding to G protein–linked receptors, thus preventing agonists from causing maximum signal transduction and instead changing the receptor's conformation back to the same state as exists when no agonist is present. Antagonists also reverse the effects of inverse agonists, again by blocking the inverse agonists from binding and then returning the receptor conformation to the baseline state. Antagonists do not have any impact on signal transduction in the absence of an agonist.

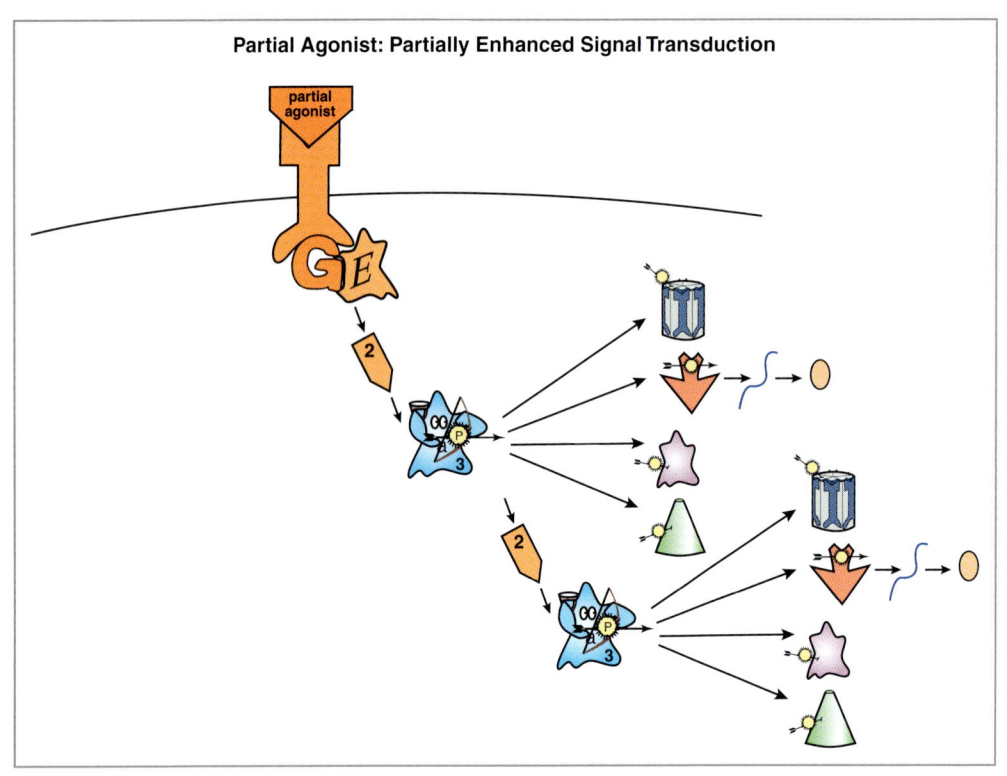

FIGURE 4-25 Partial agonist. Partial agonists stimulate G protein–linked receptors to enhance signal transduction but do not lead to maximum signal transduction the way full agonists do. Thus, in the absence of a full agonist, partial agonists increase signal transduction. However, in the presence of a full agonist, the partial agonist will actually turn down the strength of various downstream signals. For this reason, partial agonists are sometimes referred to as stabilizers.

silent antagonist on the agonist spectrum will determine the impact of a partial agonist on downstream signal transduction events.

The amount of "partiality" that is desired between agonist and antagonist – that is, where a partial agonist should sit on the agonist spectrum – is both a matter of debate as well as trial and error. The ideal therapeutic agent may have signal transduction through G protein–linked receptors that is not too "hot" yet not too "cold" but "just right"; this is sometimes called the "Goldilocks" solution (Figure 4-25). Such an ideal state may vary from one clinical situation to another, depending on the balance between full agonism and silent antagonism that is desired.

In cases where there is unstable neurotransmission throughout the brain, as when pyramidal neurons in the prefrontal cortex are out of "tune" (see Figures 2-19A and B and 2-20), it may be desirable to find a state of signal transduction that stabilizes G protein–linked receptor output somewhere between too much and too little downstream action. For this reason, partial agonists are also called "stabilizers," since they have the theoretical capacity to find a stable solution between the extremes of too much full agonist action and no agonist action at all (Figure 4-25).

Since partial agonists exert an effect less than that of a full agonist, they are also sometimes called "weak," with the implication that partial agonism means partial clinical

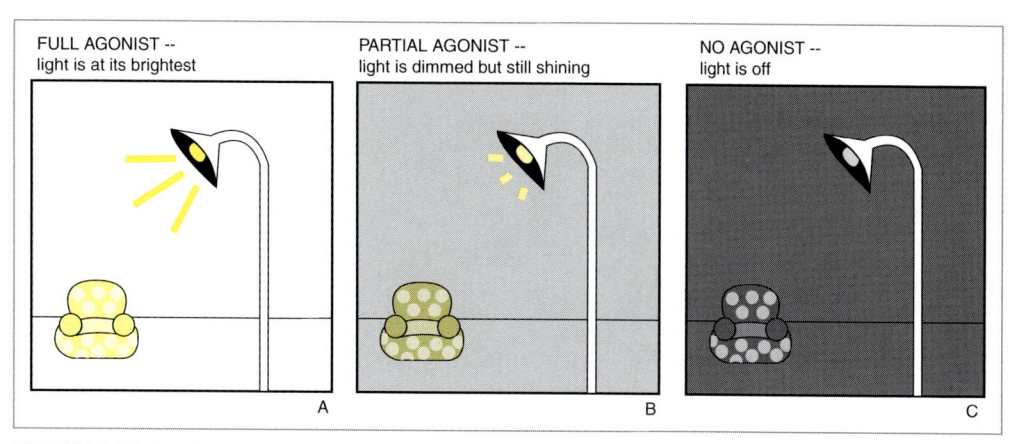

FIGURE 4-26 Agonist spectrum: rheostat. A useful analogy for the agonist spectrum is a light controlled by a rheostat. The light will be brightest after a full agonist turns the light switch fully on (left panel). A partial agonist will also act as a net agonist and turn the light on, but only partially, according to the level preset in the partial agonist's rheostat (middle panel). If the light is already on, a partial agonist will "dim" the lights, thus acting as a net antagonist. When no full or partial agonist is present, the situation is analogous to the light being switched off (right panel).

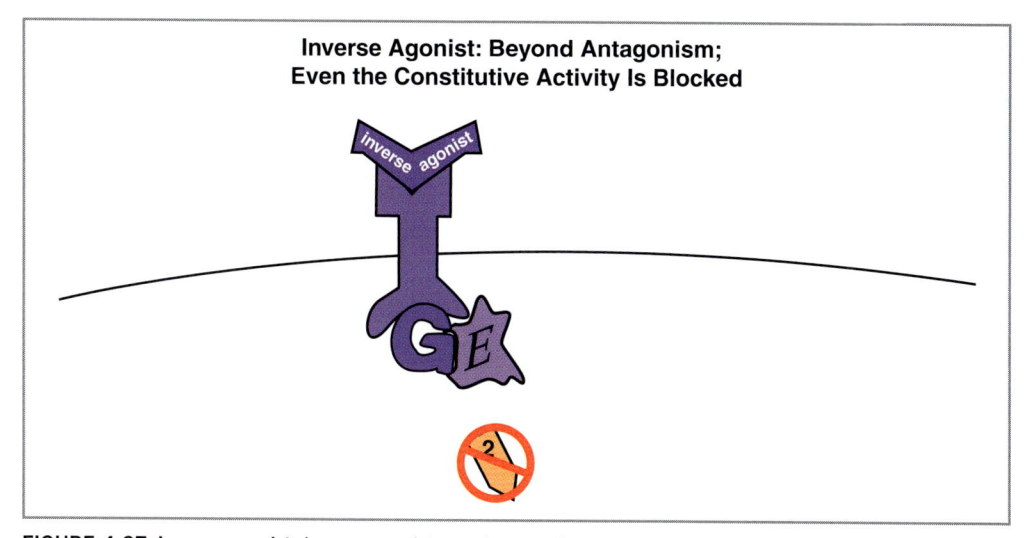

FIGURE 4-27 Inverse agonist. Inverse agonists produce conformational change in the G protein–linked receptor that renders it inactive. This leads to reduced signal transduction as compared not only to that associated with agonists but also that associated with antagonists or the absence of an agonist. The impact of an inverse agonist is dependent on the receptor density in that brain region. That is, if the receptor density is so low that constitutive activity does not lead to detectable signal transduction, then reducing the constitutive activity would not have any appreciable effect.

efficacy. That is certainly possible in some cases, but it is more sophisticated to understand the potential stabilizing and "tuning" actions of this class of therapeutic agents, and not to use terms that imply clinical actions for the entire class of drugs which may apply only to some individual agents. A few partial agonists are utilized in clinical practice (Table 4-6) and more are in clinical development.

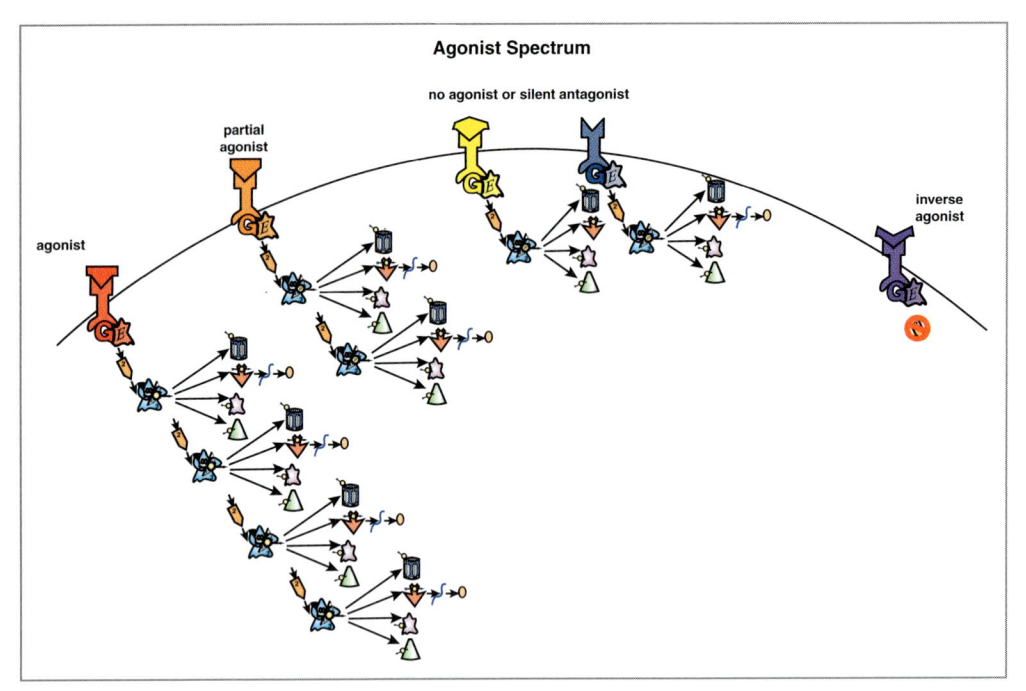

FIGURE 4-28 Agonist spectrum. This figure summarizes the implications of the agonist spectrum. Full agonists cause maximum signal transduction, while partial agonists increase signal transduction compared to no agonist but decrease it compared to full agonist. Antagonists lead to constitutive activity and thus, in the absence of an agonist, have no effects; in the presence of an agonist, they lead to reduced signal transduction. Inverse agonists are the functional opposites of agonists and actually reduce signal transduction beyond that produced in the absence of an agonist.

Light and dark as an analogy for partial agonists

It was originally conceived that a neurotransmitter could only act at receptors like a light switch, and turn things on when the neurotransmitter was present and off when the neurotransmitter was absent. We now know that many receptors, including the G protein–linked receptor family, can function rather more like a rheostat. That is, a full agonist will turn the lights all the way on (Figure 4-26A), but a partial agonist will turn the light on only partially (Figure 4-26B). If neither full agonist nor partial agonist is present, the room is dark (Figure 4-26C).

Each partial agonist has its own set point engineered into the molecule, such that it cannot turn the lights on brighter even with a higher dose. No matter how much partial agonist is given, only a certain degree of brightness will result. A series of partial agonists will differ one from the other in the degree of partiality, so that, theoretically, all degrees of brightness can be covered within the range from "off" to "on," but each partial agonist has its own unique degree of brightness associated with it.

What is so interesting about partial agonists is that they can appear as a net agonist or as a net antagonist, depending on the amount of naturally occurring full-agonist neurotransmitter present. Thus, when a full-agonist neurotransmitter is absent, a partial agonist will be a net agonist. That is, from the resting state, a partial agonist initiates somewhat of an increase in the signal transduction cascade from the G protein–linked second messenger system. However, when a full-agonist neurotransmitter agonist is present, the same partial agonist will become a net antagonist. That is, it will decrease the level of full signal output to a lesser level but not to zero. Thus, a partial agonist can simultaneously *boost* deficient neurotransmitter activity yet *block* excessive neurotransmitter activity—another reason that partial agonists are called stabilizers.

Returning to the light switch analogy, a room will be dark when agonist is missing and the light switch is off (Figure 4-26C). A room will be brightly lit when it is full of natural full agonist and the light switch is fully on (Figure 4-26A). Adding partial agonist to the dark room where there is no natural full agonist neurotransmitter will turn the lights up, but only to the degree that the partial agonist works on the rheostat (Figure 4-26B). Relative to the dark room as a starting point, a partial agonist therefore acts as a net agonist. On the other hand, adding a partial agonist to the fully lit room will have the effect of turning the lights down to the intermediate level of lower brightness on the rheostat (Figure 4-26B). This is a net antagonistic effect relative to the fully lit room. Thus, after adding partial agonist to the dark room and to the brightly lit room, both rooms will be equally bright. The degree of brightness is that of being partially turned on, as dictated by the properties of the partial agonist. However, in the dark room, the partial agonist has acted as a net agonist, whereas in the brightly lit room, the partial agonist has acted as a net antagonist.

An agonist and an antagonist in the same molecule is quite a new dimension to therapeutics. This concept has led to proposals that partial agonists could treat not only states that are theoretically deficient in full agonist but also states that are theoretically with an excess of full agonist. An agent such as a partial agonist may even be able to treat simultaneously states that are mixtures of both excess and deficiency in neurotransmitter activity.

Inverse agonists

Inverse agonists are more than simple antagonists and are neither neutral nor silent. These agents have an action that is thought to produce a conformational change in the G protein–linked receptor that stabilizes it in a totally inactive form (Figure 4-27). Thus, this conformation produces a functional reduction in signal transduction (Figure 4-27) that is even less than that produced when there is either no agonist present (Figure 4-22) or a silent antagonist present (Figure 4-24). The result of an inverse agonist is to shut down even the constitutive activity of the G protein–linked receptor system. Of course, if a given receptor system has no constitutive activity, perhaps in cases when receptors are present in low density, there will be no reduction in activity and the inverse agonist will look like an antagonist.

In many ways, therefore, inverse agonists do the *opposite* of agonists. If an agonist increases signal transduction from baseline, an inverse agonist decreases it, even below baseline levels. In contrast to agonists and antagonists, therefore, an *inverse agonist* neither increases signal transduction like an agonist (Figure 4-23) nor merely blocks the agonist from increasing signal transduction like an antagonist (Figure 4-24); rather, an inverse agonist binds the receptor in a fashion to provoke an action opposite to that of the agonist, namely causing the receptor to *decrease* its baseline signal transduction level (Figure 4-27). It is unclear from a clinical point of view what the relevant differences are between an inverse agonist and a silent antagonist. In fact, some drugs that have long been considered to be silent antagonists may turn out in some areas of the brain actually to be inverse agonists. Thus, the concept of an inverse agonist as clinically distinguishable from a silent antagonist remains to be proven. In the meantime, inverse agonists remain an interesting pharmacological concept.

In summary, G protein–linked receptors act along an agonist spectrum, and drugs have been described that can produce conformational changes in these receptors to create any state from full agonist, to partial agonist, to silent antagonist, to inverse agonist (Figure 4-28). When one considers the spectrum of signal transduction in this way (Figure 4-28), it is easy to understand why agents at each point along the agonist spectrum differ so much from each other, and why their clinical actions are so different.

Summary

About one-third of psychotropic drugs in clinical practice bind to a neurotransmitter transporter and another third bind to G protein–linked receptors. These two molecular sites of action, their impact upon neurotransmission, and various specific drugs that act at these sites have all been reviewed in this chapter.

Specifically, there are two subclasses of plasma membrane transporters for neurotransmitters and three subclasses of intracellular synaptic vesicle transporters for neurotransmitters. The monoamine transporters for serotonin, known as SERT, for norepinephrine, known as NET, and for dopamine, known as DAT, are key targets for most of the known antidepressants. In addition, stimulants target DAT. The vesicular transporter for all three of these monoamines is known as VMAT2 (vesicular monoamine transporter 2) and is also a target of the stimulant amphetamine.

G-protein receptors are the most common targets of psychotropic drugs, and their actions can lead to both therapeutic effects and side effects. Drug actions at these receptors occur in a spectrum, from full agonist actions, to partial agonist actions, to antagonism and even to inverse agonism. Natural neurotransmitters are full agonists, and so are some drugs used in clinical practice. However, most drugs that act directly on G protein–linked receptors act as antagonists. A few act as partial agonists and some as inverse agonists. Each drug interacting at a G protein–linked receptor causes a conformational change in that receptor that defines where on the agonist spectrum it will act. Thus, a full agonist produces a conformational change that turns on signal transduction and second messenger formation to the maximum extent. One novel concept is that of a partial agonist, which acts somewhat like an agonist but to a lesser extent. An antagonist causes a conformational change that stabilizes the receptor in the baseline state and thus is "silent." In the presence of agonists or partial agonists, an antagonist causes the receptor to return to this baseline state as well and thus reverses their actions. A novel receptor action is that of an inverse agonist, which leads to a conformation of the receptor that stops all activity, even baseline actions. An understanding of the agonist spectrum can lead to the prediction of downstream consequences of signal transduction, including clinical actions.

CHAPTER 5

Ion Channels and Enzymes as Targets of Psychopharmacological Drug Action

- Ligand-gated ion channels as targets of psychopharmacological drug action
  - Ligand-gated ion channels, ionotrophic receptors and ion channel–linked receptors: different terms for the same receptor/ion channel complex
  - Ligand-gated ion channels: structure and function
  - Pentameric subtypes
  - Tetrameric subtypes
  - The agonist spectrum
  - Different states of ligand-gated ion channels
  - Allosteric modulation: PAMs and NAMs
  - GABA, glutamate, and regulation of ligand-gated ion channels
- Voltage-sensitive ion channels as targets of psychopharmacological drug action
  - Structure and function
  - Voltage-sensitive sodium channels (VSSCs)
  - Voltage-sensitive calcium channels (VSCCs)
- Ion channels and neurotransmission
- Enzymes as sites of psychopharmacological drug action
- Other novel or potential targets of psychopharmacological drug action
- Summary

Many important psychopharmacological drugs target ion channels or enzymes. The roles of ion channels and enzymes as important regulators of synaptic neurotransmission have been covered in previous chapters (Chapters 1, 2, and 3). Here we discuss how the targeting of these molecular sites causes alterations in synaptic neurotransmission that are linked, in turn, to the therapeutic actions of various psychotropic drugs. Specifically, we will cover ligand-gated ion channels and voltage-sensitive ion channels as well as enzymes as targets of psychopharmacological drug action. We will also briefly mention a few additional novel or potential targets of drug action.

Ligand-gated ion channels as targets of psychopharmacological drug action

Ligand-gated ion channels, ionotrophic receptors and ion channel–linked receptors: different terms for the same receptor/ion channel complex

Ions (Figure 5-1) normally cannot penetrate membranes because of their charge. In order to selectively control access of ions into and out of neurons, their membranes are decorated

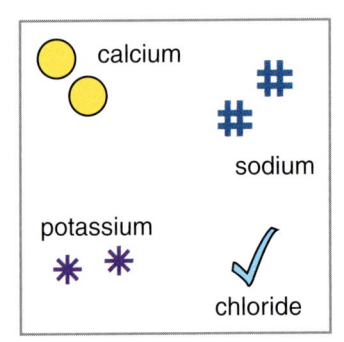

FIGURE 5-1 Calcium, sodium, chloride, potassium. Various ions are represented here. Channels for one ion are unique from channels for other ions. The ions shown here include calcium, sodium, chloride, and potassium.

with all sorts of ion channels. The most important ion channels in psychopharmacology regulate calcium, sodium, chloride, and potassium (Figure 5-1). Many can be modified by various drugs, and this will be discussed throughout this chapter.

There are two major classes of ion channels, and each class has several names. One class of ion channels is opened by neurotransmitters and goes by the names "ligand-gated ion channels," "ionotrophic receptors," and "ion channel–linked receptors." These channels and their associated receptors will be discussed next. The other major class of ion channel is opened by the charge or voltage across the membrane and is called either a "voltage-gated" or a "voltage-sensitive" ion channel; these will be discussed later in this chapter.

Ion channels that are opened and closed by actions of neurotransmitter ligands at receptors acting as gatekeepers are shown conceptually in Figures 5-2A and B. When a neurotransmitter binds to a gatekeeper receptor on an ion channel, that neurotransmitter causes a conformational change in the receptor that opens the ion channel (Figure 5-2A and B). A neurotransmitter, drug or hormone that binds to a receptor is sometimes called a "ligand" (meaning "that which ties"). Thus, ion channels linked to receptors that regulate their opening and closing are often called "ligand-gated ion channels." Since these ion channels are also receptors, they are also sometimes called "ionotrophic" receptors or "ion channel–linked" receptors. These terms will be used interchangeably with "ligand-gated ion channels" here.

Numerous drugs act at many sites around such receptor/ion channel complexes, leading to a wide variety of modifications of receptor/ion channel actions. These modifications not only immediately alter the flow of ions through the channels, but with a delay can also change the downstream events that result from transduction of the signal that begins at these receptors. The downstream actions have been extensively discussed in Chapter 3 and include both activation and inactivation of phosphoproteins, shifting the activity of enzymes, the sensitivity of receptors, and the conductivity of ion channels. Other downstream actions include changes in gene expression and thus determine which proteins are synthesized and which functions are amplified. Such functions can range from synaptogenesis, to receptor and enzyme synthesis, to communication with downstream neurons innervated by the neuron with the ionotrophic receptor, and many more. The reader should have a good command of the function of signal transduction pathways described in Chapter 3 in order to understand how drugs acting at ligand-gated ion channels modify the signal transduction that arises from these receptors.

Drug-induced modifications in signal transduction from ionotrophic receptors can have profound effects on psychiatric symptoms. About one-fifth of psychotropic drugs currently utilized in clinical practice, including many drugs for the treatment of anxiety and insomnia

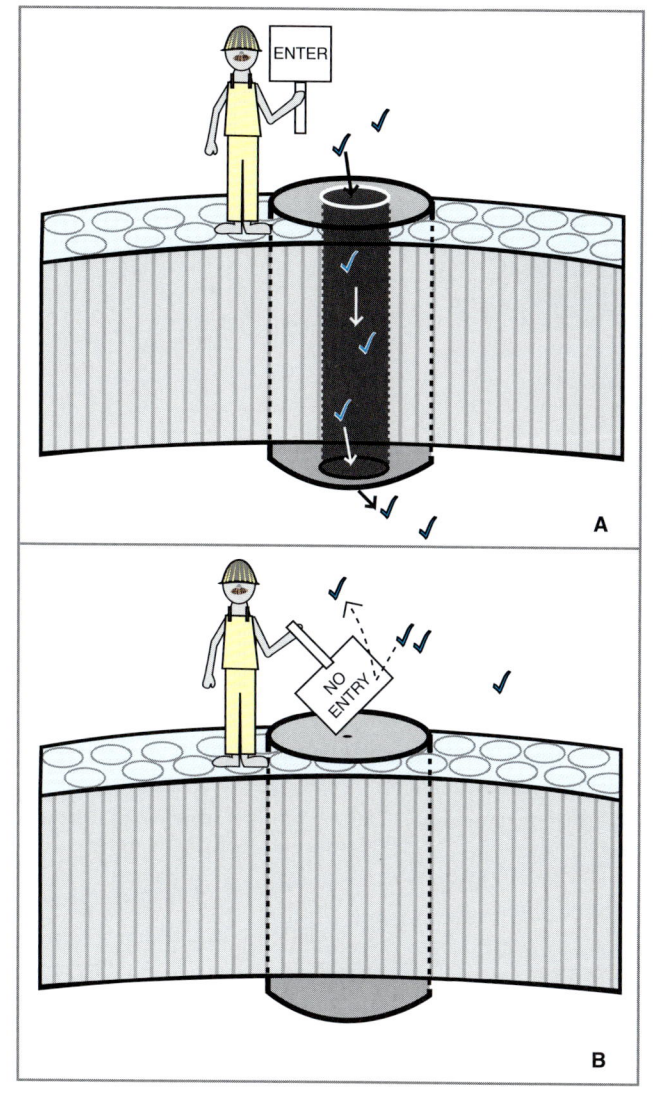

FIGURE 5-2 Ligand-gated ion channel gatekeeper. This schematic shows a ligand-gated ion channel. In panel A, a receptor is serving as a molecular gatekeeper that acts on instruction from neurotransmission to open the channel and allow ions to travel into the cell. In panel B, the gatekeeper is keeping the channel closed so that ions cannot get into the cell. Ligand-gated ion channels are a type of receptor that forms an ion channel and are thus also called ion channel–linked receptors or ionotrophic receptors.

such as the benzodiazepines, are known to act at these receptors. Because ionotrophic receptors immediately change the flow of ions, drugs that act on these receptors can have an almost immediate effect, which is why many anxiolytics and hypnotics acting at these receptors may have immediate clinical onset. This is in contrast to the actions of many drugs at G protein–linked receptors described in Chapter 4, some of which have clinical effects, such as antidepressant actions, that may occur with a delay necessitated by awaiting initiation of changes in cellular functions activated through the signal transduction cascade. Here we will describe how various drugs stimulate or block various molecular sites around the receptor/ion channel complex. Throughout this book we show how specific drugs acting at specific ionotrophic receptors have specific actions on specific psychiatric disorders.

Ligand-gated ion channels: structure and function

Are ligand-gated ion channels receptors or ion channels? The answer is yes – ligand-gated ion channels are both a type of receptor and they form an ion channel. That is why they

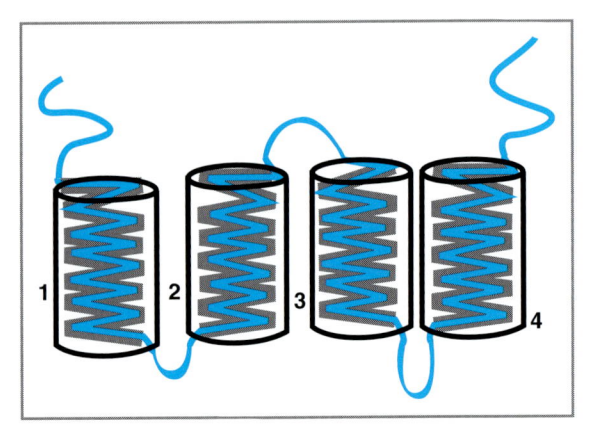

FIGURE 5-3 Four transmembrane region receptor. Shown here is a four transmembrane subunit of a pentameric ligand-gated ion channel. There are five copies of these subunits in a fully constituted receptor. Each subunit weaves in and out of the membrane four times and thus has four transmembrane regions.

are called not only a channel (ligand-gated ion channel) but also a receptor (ionotrophic receptor and ion channel–linked receptor). These terms try to capture the dual function of these ion channels/receptors and may explain why there is more than one term for this receptor/ion channel complex.

Ligand-gated ion channels comprise several long strings of amino acids assembled as subunits around an ion channel. Decorating these subunits are also multiple binding sites for everything from neurotransmitters to ions to drugs. That is, these complex proteins have several sites where some ions travel through a channel and others also bind to the channel; where one neurotransmitter or even two cotransmitters act at separate and distinct binding sites; and where numerous allosteric modulators – i.e., natural substances or drugs that bind to a site different than where the neurotransmitter binds – increase or decrease the sensitivity of channel opening.

Pentameric subtypes

Many ligand-gated ion channels are assembled from five protein subunits; that is why they are called pentameric. The subunits for pentameric subtypes of ligand-gated ion channels each have four transmembrane regions (Figure 5-3). These membrane proteins go in and out of the membrane four times (Figures 5-3 and 5-4A). When inserted into the neuronal membrane, the four transmembrane regions of these subunits are actually clustered together, as shown in Figure 5-4A, rather than stretched out, as shown in Figure 5-3. When five copies of these subunits are selected (Figure 5-4B), they come together in space to form a fully functional pentameric receptor with the ion channel in the middle (Figure 5-4C). The receptor sites are in various locations on each of the subunits; some binding sites are in the channel, but many are present at different locations outside the channel.

This pentameric structure is typical for GABA-A receptors, nicotinic cholinergic receptors, serotonin 5HT3 receptors, and glycine receptors (Table 5-1). Drugs that act directly on pentameric ligand-gated ion channels are listed in Table 5-2, and those that have indirect agonist or antagonist actions at these receptors are listed in Table 5-3.

If this structure were not complicated enough, pentameric ionotrophic receptors actually have many different subtypes. Subtypes of pentameric ionotrophic receptors are defined based upon which forms of each of the five subunits are chosen for assembly into a fully constituted receptor. That is, there are several subtypes for each of the four transmembrane subunits, making it possible to piece together several different constellations of fully constituted receptors. Although the natural neurotransmitter binds to every subtype of

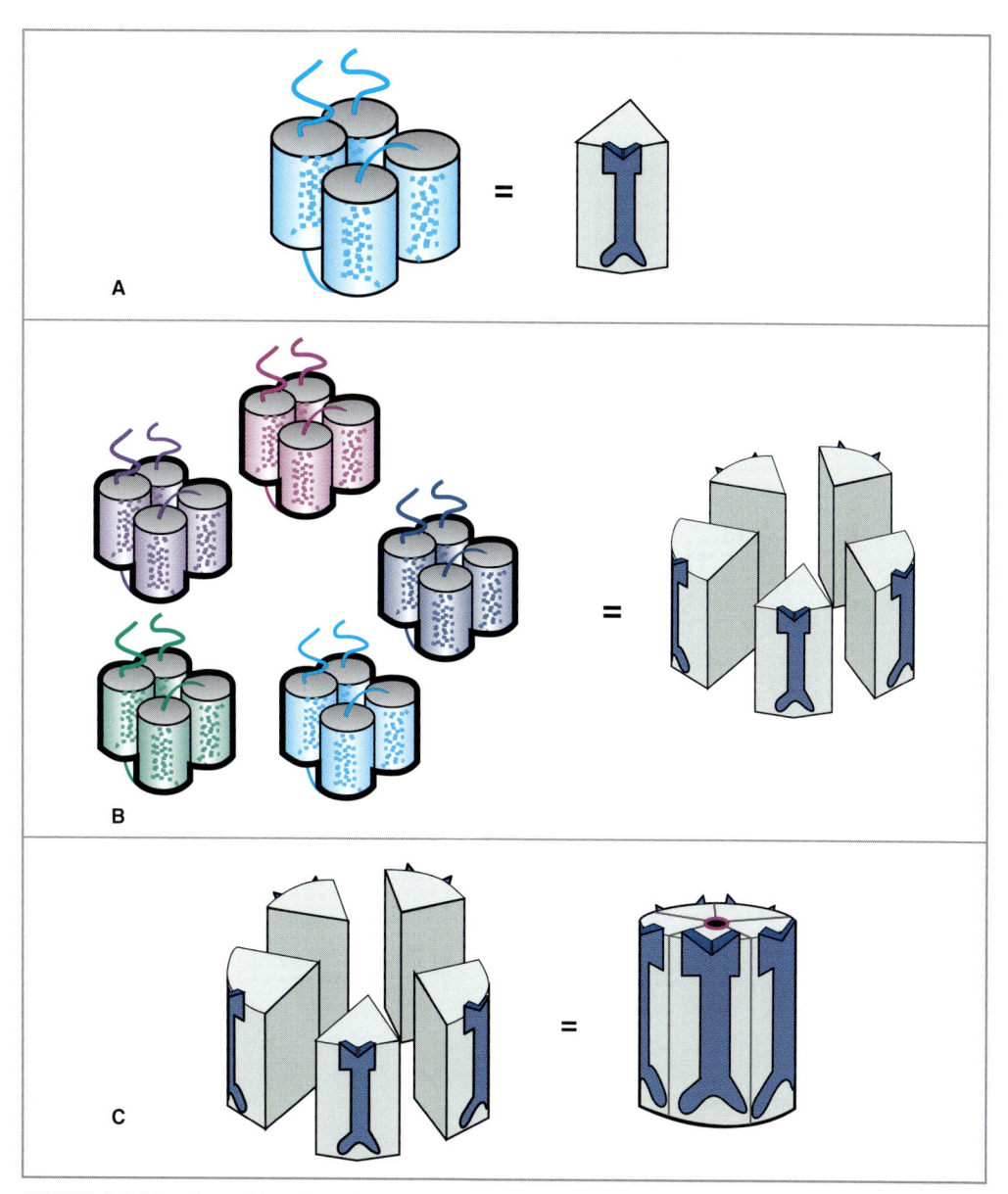

FIGURE 5-4 Ligand-gated ion channel structure. The four transmembrane regions of a single subunit of a pentameric ligand-gated ion channel form a cluster, as shown in panel A. An icon for this subunit is shown on the right in panel A. Five copies of the subunits come together in space (panel B) to form a functional ion channel in the middle (panel C). Ligand-gated ion channels have receptor binding sites located on all five subunits, both inside and outside the channel.

ionotrophic receptor, some drugs used in clinical practice and many more in clinical trials are able to bind selectively to one or more of these subtypes but not to others. This may have functional and clinical consequences. Specific receptor subtypes and the specific drugs that bind to them selectively are discussed in chapters that cover their specific clinical use. Some of these subtype-selective agents are listed in Table 5-2.

TABLE 5-1 Pentameric ligand-gated ion channels

4 transmembrane regions
5 subunits

Neurotransmitter	Receptor Subtype
acetylcholine	nicotinic receptors (e.g. alpha$_7$ nicotinic receptors; alpha$_4$ beta$_2$ nicotinic receptors)
GABA	GABA-A receptors (e.g. alpha$_1$ subunits)
glycine receptors	strychnine sensitive glycine
serotonin	5HT$_3$ receptors

TABLE 5-2 Key ligand-gated ion channels directly targeted by psychotropic drugs

Neurotransmitter	Ligand Gated Ion Channel Receptor Subtype Directly Targeted	Pharmacologic Action	Drug Class	Therapeutic Action
acetylcholine	alpha$_4$ beta$_2$ nicotinic	partial agonist	nicotinic receptor partial agonist (NRPA) (varenicline)	smoking cessation
GABA	GABA-A benzodiazepine receptors	full agonist	benzodiazepines	anxiolytic
	GABA-A non benzodiazepine PAM sites	full agonist	"Z DRUGS"/ hypnotics (zolpidem, zaleplon, zopiclone, eszopiclone)	improve insomnia
glutamate	NMDA NAM channel sites/Mg^{++} sites	antagonist	NMDA glutamate antagonist (memantine)	slowing progression in Alzheimer's disease
	NMDA open channel sites	antagonist	PCP/phencyclidine ketamine	hallucinogen anesthetic
serotonin	5HT$_3$	antagonist	antidepressant (mirtazapine)	unknown; reduce nausea
	5HT$_3$	antagonist	anti-emetic	reduce chemotherapy-induced emesis

PAM = positive allosteric modulator
NAM = negative allosteric modulator
NMDA = N-methyl-d-aspartate
Mg = magnesium

Tetrameric subtypes

Ionotrophic glutamate receptors have a different structure from the pentameric ionotrophic receptors just discussed. These ligand-gated ion channels for glutamate comprise subunits that have three full transmembrane regions and a fourth reentrant loop (Figure 5-5), rather than four full transmembrane regions as shown in Figures 5-3 and 5-4. When inserted into the neuronal membrane, the three transmembrane segments plus the reentrant loop of these glutamate subunits are actually clustered together, as shown in Figure 5-6, rather

TABLE 5-3 Key ligand gated ion channels indirectly targeted by psychotropic drugs

Neurotransmitter Therapeutic Action	Ligand Gated Ion Channel Receptor Subtype Indirectly Targeted	Pharmacologic Action	Drug Class
acetylcholine slowing progression in Alzheimer's disease	all nicotinic receptor subtypes	agonist via increasing acetylcholine itself at all acetylcholine receptors	acetylcholinesterase inhibitor (reducing acetylcholine metabolism)
GABA anticonvulsant, possibly anxiolytic, chronic pain, for slow wave sleep	GABA-A agonist sites	agonist via increasing GABA itself at all GABA receptors	anticonvulsant; actions at GABA transporter
glutamate	all glutamate receptor subtypes	possible inhibition of glutamate resulting in lack of glutamate at receptors, and thus functional antagonism	anticonvulsant, mood stabilizers (e.g., pregabalin, gabapentin, lamotrigine, riluzole)

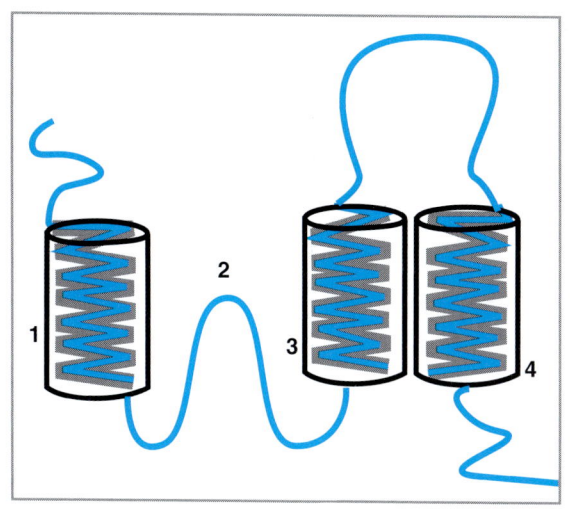

FIGURE 5-5 Subunit of tetrameric ligand-gated ion channel. Another type of ligand-gated ion channel comprises subunits that have three full transmembrane regions (numbers 1, 3, and 4) and a fourth reentrant loop (number 2). Since four copies of these subunits are required to form a fully functional receptor, they are called subunits of a tetrameric ligand-gated ion channel.

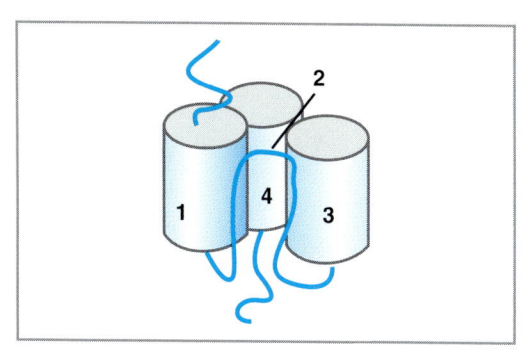

FIGURE 5-6 Subunit of tetrameric ligand-gated ion channel. The three transmembrane regions plus the reentrant loop of a single subunit of a tetrameric ligand-gated ion channel cluster together, as shown here.

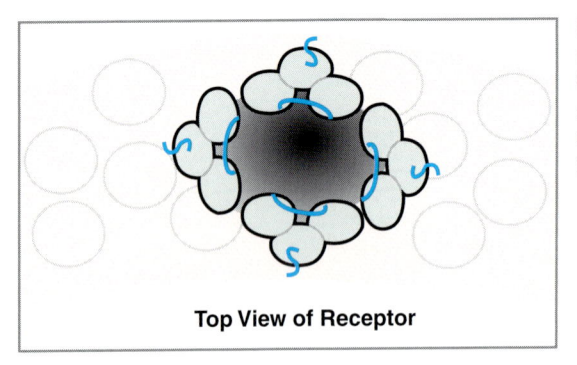

FIGURE 5-7 Tetrameric ligand-gated ion channel top view. Four copies of the three transmembrane region subunits come together in space to form a fully functional ion channel in the middle, with the four reentrant loops lining the ion channel. The top view of this is shown here.

Top View of Receptor

than stretched out, as shown in Figure 5-5. When four copies of these subunits are selected, they come together in space to form a fully functional ion channel in the middle with the four reentrant loops lining the ion channel, as seen from a top view in Figure 5-7. Icons for the subunits are shown in Figure 5-8A, with selection of four copies of these subunits, in Figure 5-8B, coming together to form a fully functional tetrameric receptor with the ion channel in the middle (Figure 5-8C). Thus, tetrameric subtypes of ion channels (Figure 5-8) are analogous to pentameric subtypes of ion channels (Figure 5-4) but have just four subunits rather than five. Receptor sites are in various locations on each of the subunits; some binding sites are in the channel, but many are present at different locations outside the channel.

This tetrameric structure is typical of the ionotrophic glutamate receptors known as AMPA (alpha-amino-3-hydroxy-5-methyl-4-isoxazole-priopionic acid), kainate, and NMDA (N-methyl-d-aspartate) subtypes (Table 5-4). Drugs that act directly at tetrameric ionotrophic glutamate receptors are listed in Table 5-2 and those that act indirectly at these receptors in Table 5-3. Receptor subtypes for glutamate, according to the selective agonist acting at that receptor as well as the specific molecular subunits that comprise that subtype, are listed in Table 5-4. Subtype-selective drugs for ionotrophic glutamate receptors are under investigation but not currently used in clinical practice.

The agonist spectrum

The agonist spectrum for G protein–linked receptors discussed extensively in Chapter 4 and illustrated in Figures 4-21 through 4-28 is the very same for ligand-gated ion channels (compare Figures 5-9 and 4-28). Thus, *full agonists* change the conformation of the receptor to open the ion channel to the maximal amounts and frequencies allowed by that binding site (Figure 5-9 and Figure 5-10A and B). This then triggers the maximal amount of downstream signal transduction that can be mediated by this binding site. The ion channel can open to an even greater extent and even more frequently than with a full agonist alone, but this requires the help of a second receptor site, that of positive allosteric modulator (PAM).

Antagonists stabilize the receptor in the resting state (Figure 5-11B), which is the same as the state of the receptor in the absence of agonist (Figures 5-10A and 5-11A). Since there is no difference between the presence of antagonist (Figure 5-11B) and the absence of agonist (Figure 5-11A), the antagonist is said to be neutral or silent. The resting state is not a fully closed ion channel, so there is some degree of ion flow through the channel even in the absence of agonist (Figures 5-10A and 5-11A) and even in the presence of antagonist (Figure 5-11B). This is due to occasional and infrequent opening of the channel even when an agonist is not present and even when an antagonist is present. This is called

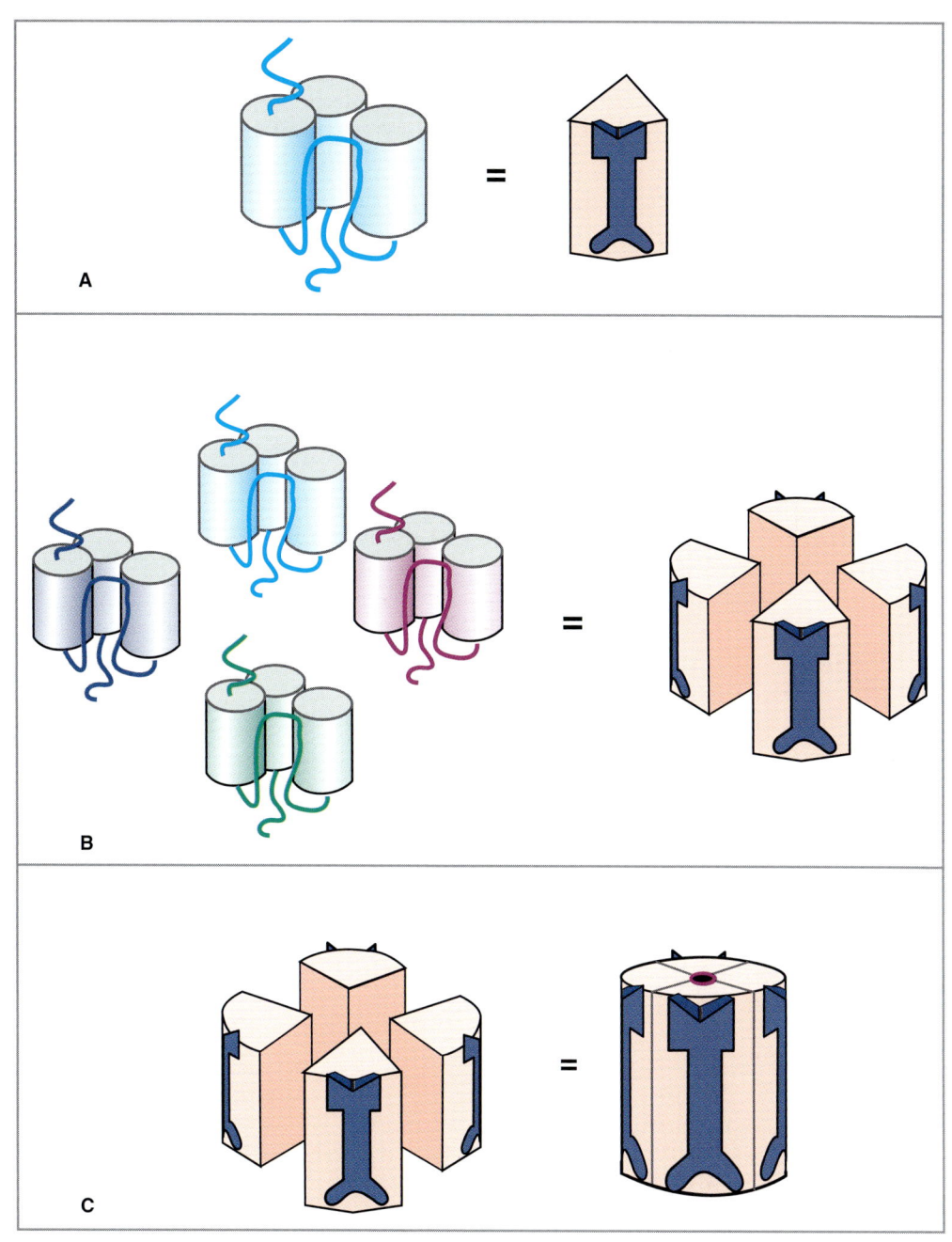

FIGURE 5-8 Tetrameric ligand-gated ion channel structure. A single subunit of a tetrameric ligand-gated ion channel is shown to form a cluster in panel A, with an icon for this subunit shown on the right in panel A. Four copies of these subunits come together in space (panel B) to form a functional ion channel in the middle (panel C). Ligand-gated ion channels have receptor binding sites located on all four subunits, both inside and outside the channel.

Ion Channels and Enzymes as Targets of Psychopharmacological Drug Action | 131

TABLE 5-4 Tetrameric ligand-gated ion channels

3 transmembrane regions and one reentrant loop
4 subunits

Neurotransmitter	*Receptor Subtype*
Glutamate	AMPA (e.g., $GluR_{1-4}$ subunits)
	KAINATE (e.g., $GluR_{5-7}$, KA_{1-2} subunits)
	NMDA (e.g., $NMDAR_1$, $NMDAR_{A-D}$, $NMDAR_{3A}$ subunits)

AMPA = alpha-amino-3-hydroxy-5-methyl-4-isoxazole-priopionic acid
NMDA = N-methyl-d-aspartate

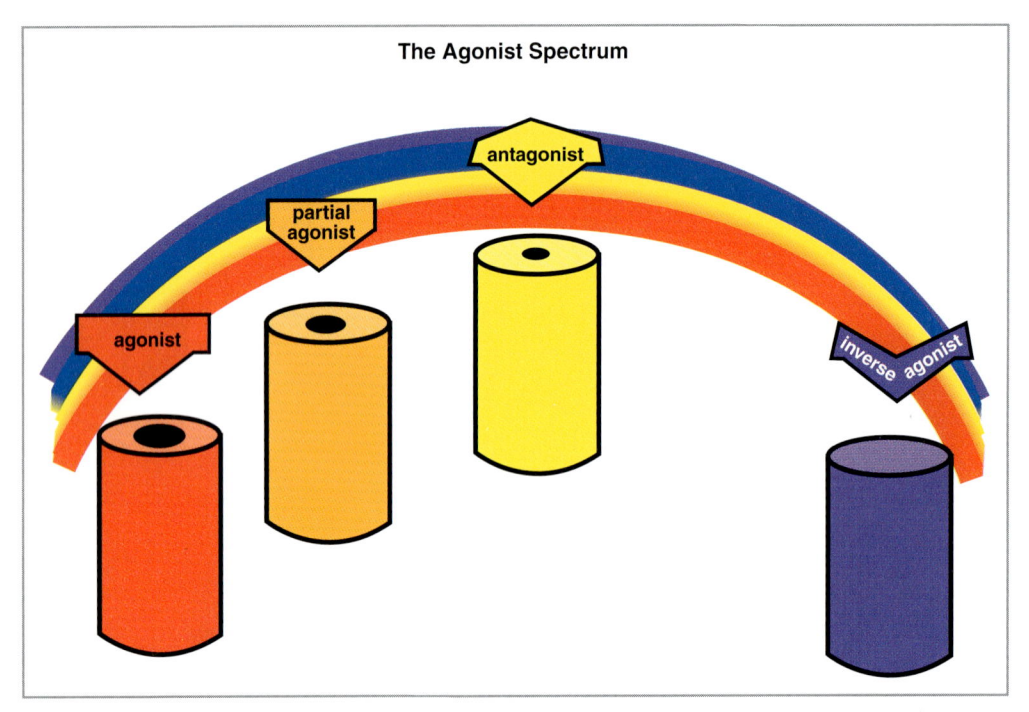

FIGURE 5-9 Agonist spectrum. The agonist spectrum and its corresponding effects on the ion channel are shown here. This spectrum ranges from agonists (on the far left), which open the channel the maximal amount and frequency allowed by that binding site, through antagonists (middle of the spectrum), which retain the resting state with infrequent opening of the channel, to inverse agonists (on the far right), which put the ion channel into a closed and inactive state. Between the extremes of agonist and antagonist are partial agonists, which increase the degree and frequency of ion channel opening as compared to the resting state, but not as much as a full agonist. Antagonists can block anything in the agonist spectrum, returning the ion channel to the resting state in each instance.

constitutive activity; it is also discussed in Chapter 4 for G protein–linked receptors and illustrated in Figure 4-22. Antagonists of ion channel–linked receptors reverse the action of agonists (Figure 5-12A and B) and bring the receptor conformation back to the resting baseline state but do not block any constitutive activity.

Partial agonists produce a change in receptor conformation such that the ion channel opens to a greater extent and more frequently than in its resting state but less than in the

Channel in its resting state in the absence of agonist.	Agonist binds to the receptor, and the channel is more frequently open.
A	B

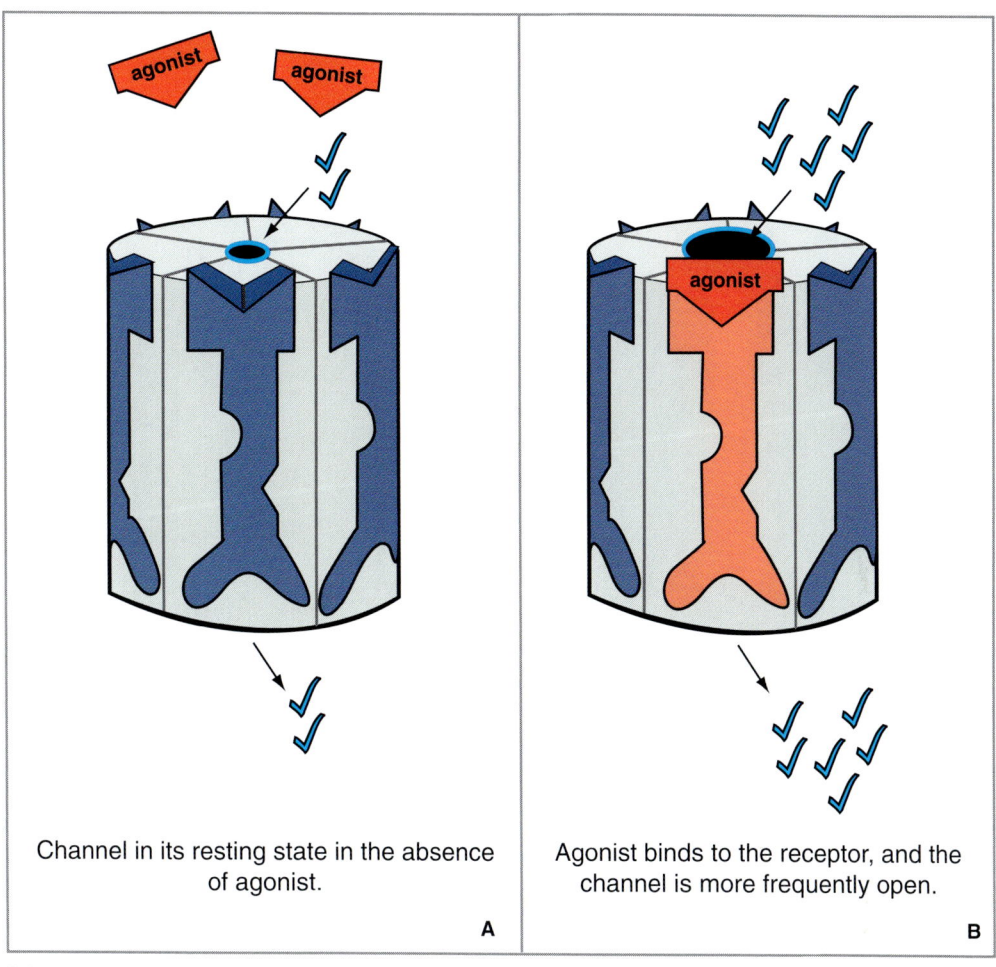

FIGURE 5-10 Actions of an agonist. In panel A, the ion channel is in its resting state, during which the channel opens infrequently (constitutive activity). In panel B, the agonist occupies its binding site on the ligand-gated ion channel, increasing the frequency at which the channel opens. This is represented as the red agonist turning the receptor red and opening the ion channel.

presence of a full agonist (Figure 5-13A and B and Figure 5-14). An antagonist reverses a partial agonist, just like it reverses a full agonist, returning the receptor to its resting state (Figure 5-15A and B). Partial agonists thus produce ion flow and downstream signal transduction that is something more than an antagonist (Figure 5-15B) yet something less than a full agonist (Figures 5-10B and 5-14). Just as in the case of G protein–linked receptors, the degree of closeness of this partial agonist to a full agonist or to a silent antagonist on the agonist spectrum will determine the impact of a partial agonist on downstream signal transduction events.

The ideal therapeutic agent should have ion flow and signal transduction that is not too hot, yet not too cold, but just right; this is called the "Goldilocks" solution in Chapter 4 (Figure 4-25) – a concept that can apply here to ligand-gated ion channels as well. Such an ideal state may vary from one clinical situation to another, depending on the balance between full agonism and silent antagonism that is desired. In cases where there is unstable neurotransmission throughout the brain, finding such a balance may stabilize receptor

Ion Channels and Enzymes as Targets of Psychopharmacological Drug Action

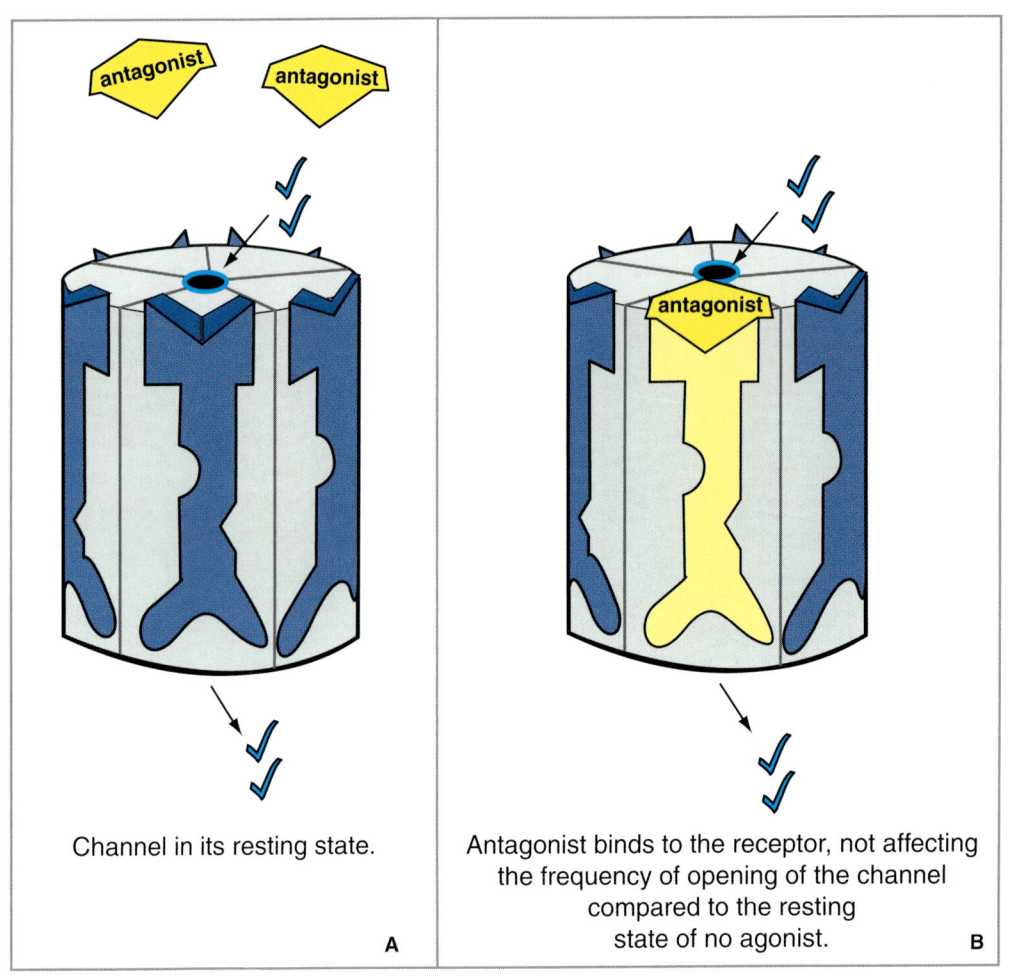

FIGURE 5-11 Antagonists acting alone. In panel A, the ion channel is in its resting state, during which the channel opens infrequently. In panel B, the antagonist occupies the binding site normally occupied by the agonist on the ligand-gated ion channel. However, there is no consequence to this, and the ion channel does not affect the degree or frequency of opening of the channel compared to the resting state. This is represented as the yellow antagonist docking into the binding site and turning the receptor yellow but not affecting the state of the ion channel.

output somewhere between too much and too little downstream action. For this reason, partial agonists are also called "stabilizers," since they have the theoretical capacity to find the stable solution between the extremes of too much full agonist action and no agonist action at all (compare Figures 4-25 and 5-14).

Just as is the case for G protein–linked receptors, partial agonists at ligand-gated ion channels can appear as net agonists or as net antagonists, depending on the amount of naturally occurring full agonist neurotransmitter present. Thus, when a full agonist neurotransmitter is absent, a partial agonist will be a net agonist (Figure 5-14). That is, from the resting state, a partial agonist initiates somewhat of an increase in the ion flow and downstream signal transduction cascade from the ion channel–linked receptor. However, when full agonist neurotransmitter agonist is present, the same partial agonist will become a net antagonist (Figure 5-14). That it, it will decrease the level of full signal output to

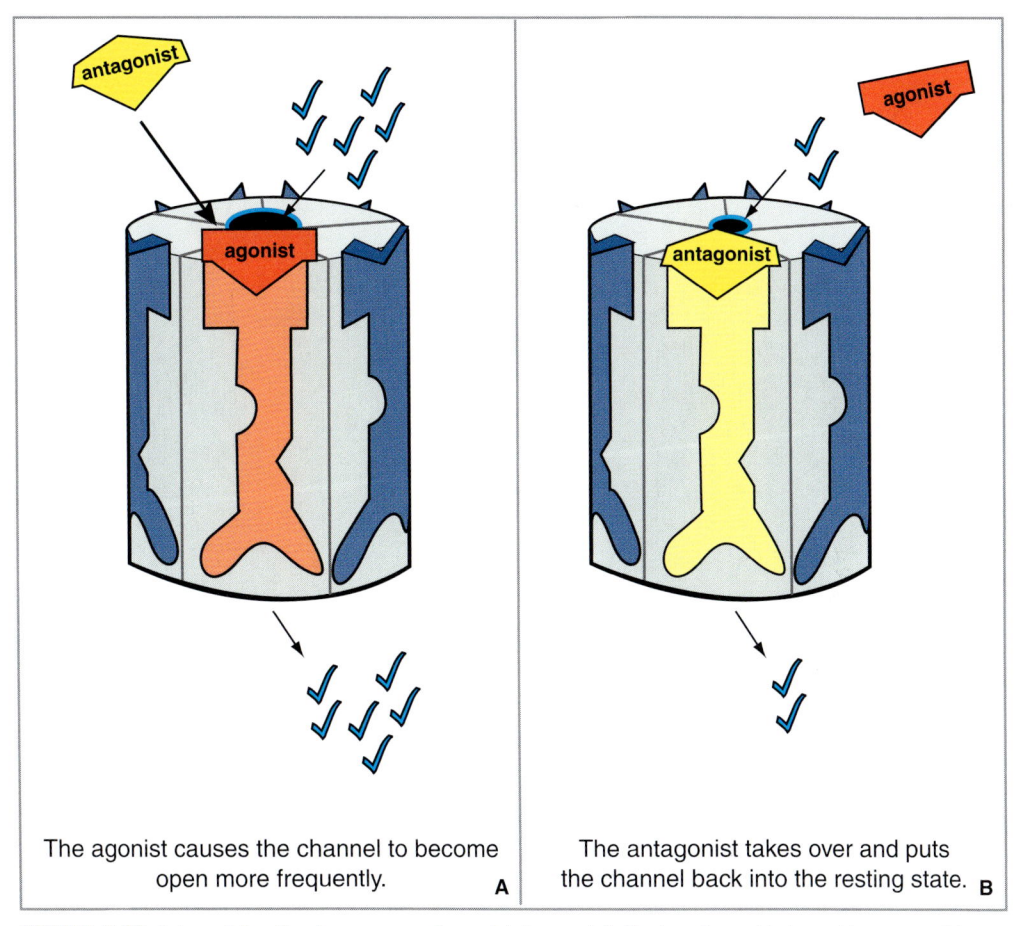

FIGURE 5-12 Antagonist acting in presence of agonist. In panel A, the ion channel is bound by an agonist, which causes it to open at a greater frequency than in the resting state. This is represented as the red agonist turning the receptor red and opening the ion channel as it docks into its binding site. In panel B, the yellow antagonist prevails and shoves the red agonist off the binding site, reversing the agonist's actions and restoring the resting state. Thus, the ion channel has returned to its status before the agonist acted.

a lesser level but not too zero. Thus, a partial agonist can simultaneously *boost* deficient neurotransmitter activity yet *block* excessive neurotransmitter activity – another reason that partial agonists are called stabilizers. An agonist and an antagonist in the same molecule acting at ligand-gated ion channels is quite an interesting new dimension to therapeutics. This concept has led to proposals that partial agonists could treat not only states that are theoretically deficient in full agonist but also those that are theoretically in excess of full agonist. As mentioned in the discussion of G protein–linked receptors in Chapter 4, a partial agonist at ligand-gated ion channels could also theoretically treat states that are mixtures of both excessive and deficient neurotransmitter activity. Partial agonists at ligand-gated ion channels are just beginning to enter use in clinical practice (Table 5-2), and several are in clinical development.

Inverse agonists at ligand-gated ion channels are different from simple antagonists and are neither neutral nor silent. Inverse agonists are explained as well in Chapter 4 in relation to G protein–linked receptors (Figure 4-27). Inverse agonists at ligand-gated ion

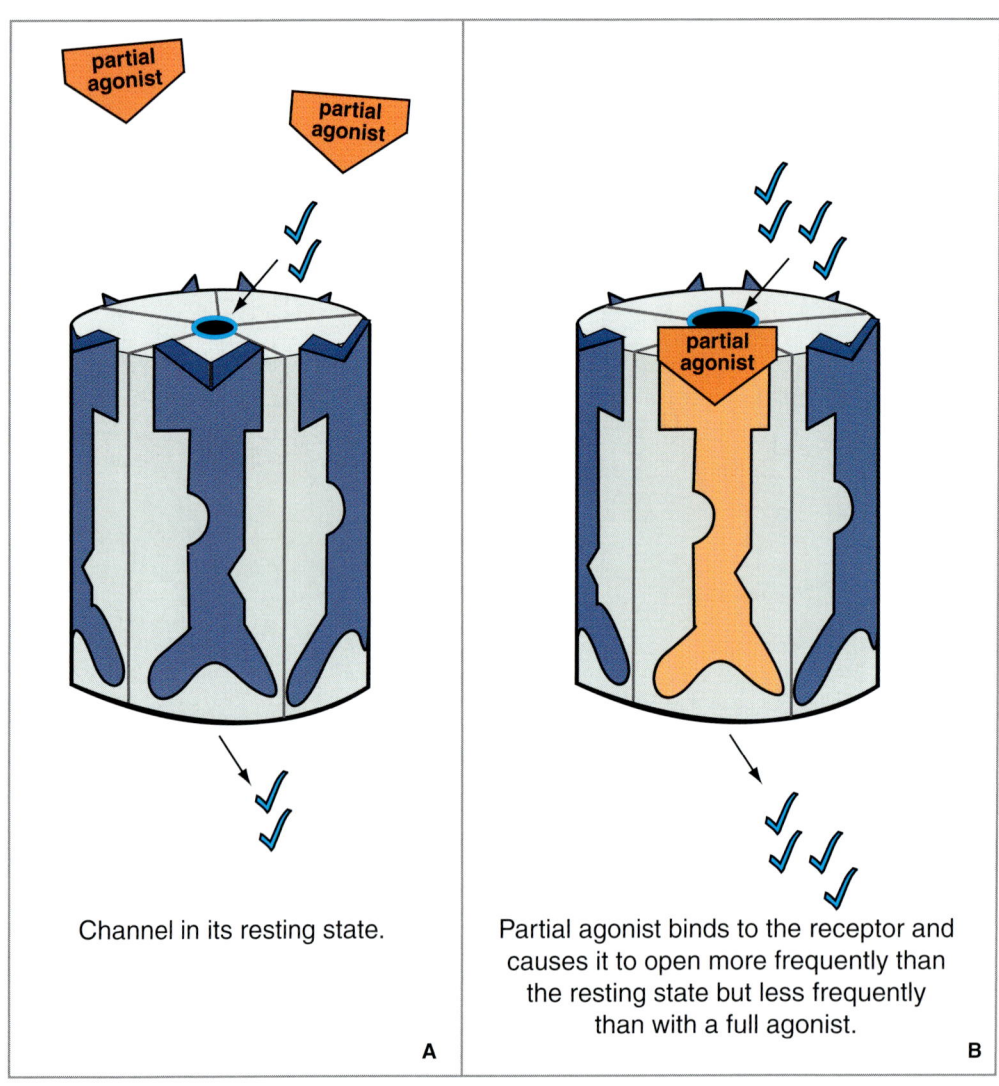

FIGURE 5-13 Actions of a partial agonist. In panel A, the ion channel is in its resting state and opens infrequently. In panel B, the partial agonist occupies its binding site on the ligand-gated ion channel and produces a conformational change such that the ion channel opens to a greater extent and at a greater frequency than in the resting state, though less than in the presence of a full agonist. This is depicted by the orange partial agonist turning the receptor orange and partially but not fully opening the ion channel.

channels are thought to produce a conformational change in these receptors that first closes the channel and then stabilizes it in an inactive form (Figure 5-16B). Thus, this inactive conformation (Figure 5-16B) produces a functional reduction in ion flow and in consequent signal transduction compared to the resting state (Figure 5-16A) that is even less than that produced when there is either no agonist present (Figure 5-16A) or when a silent antagonist is present (Figures 5-11B and 5-17B). Antagonists reverse this inactive state caused by inverse agonists, returning the channel to the resting state (Figure 5-17B). The result of an inverse agonist (Figures 5-16B and 5-17A) is to shut down even the constitutive activity of the ligand-gated ion channel.

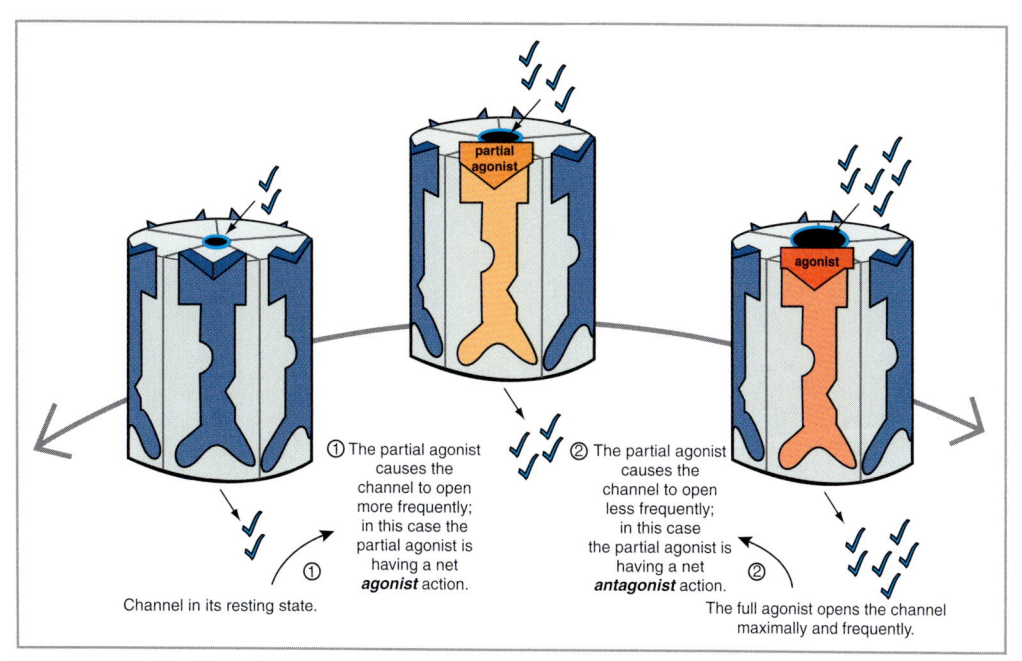

FIGURE 5-14 Net effect of partial agonist. Partial agonists act either as net agonists or as net antagonists, depending on the amount of agonist present. When full agonist is absent (on the far left), a partial agonist causes the channel to open more frequently as compared to the resting state; thus, the partial agonist is having a net agonist action (moving from left to right). However, in the presence of a full agonist (on the far right), a partial agonist decreases the frequency of channel opening in comparison to the full agonist and thus acts as a net antagonist (moving from right to left).

In many ways, therefore, an inverse agonist does the *opposite* of an agonist. If an agonist increases signal transduction from baseline, an inverse agonist decreases it, even below baseline levels. Also, in contrast to antagonists, which stabilize the resting state (Figures 5-17B and 5-18), inverse agonists stabilize an inactivated state (Figures 5-16B and 5-18). It is not yet clear if the inactivated state of the inverse agonist can be distinguished clinically from the resting state of the silent antagonist at ionotrophic receptors (Figure 5-18). In the meantime, inverse agonists remain an interesting pharmacological concept.

In summary, ion channel–linked receptors act along an agonist spectrum, and drugs have been described that can produce conformational changes in these receptors to create any state from full agonist, to partial agonist, to silent antagonist, to inverse agonist (Figure 5-9). When one considers the spectrum of signal transduction in this way (Figure 5-9), it is easy to understand why agents at each point along the agonist spectrum differ so much from each other and why their clinical actions are so different.

Different states of ligand-gated ion channels

There are even more states of ligand-gated ion channels than those determined by the agonist spectrum discussed above and shown in Figures 5-9 through 5-18. The states discussed so far are those that occur predominantly with acute administration of agents which work across the agonist spectrum. These range from the maximal opening of the ion channel from conformational changes caused by a full agonist (Figure 5-10B) to the maximal closing of the ion channel caused by an inverse agonist (Figure 5-16B). Such changes in conformation caused by the acute action of agents across this spectrum are

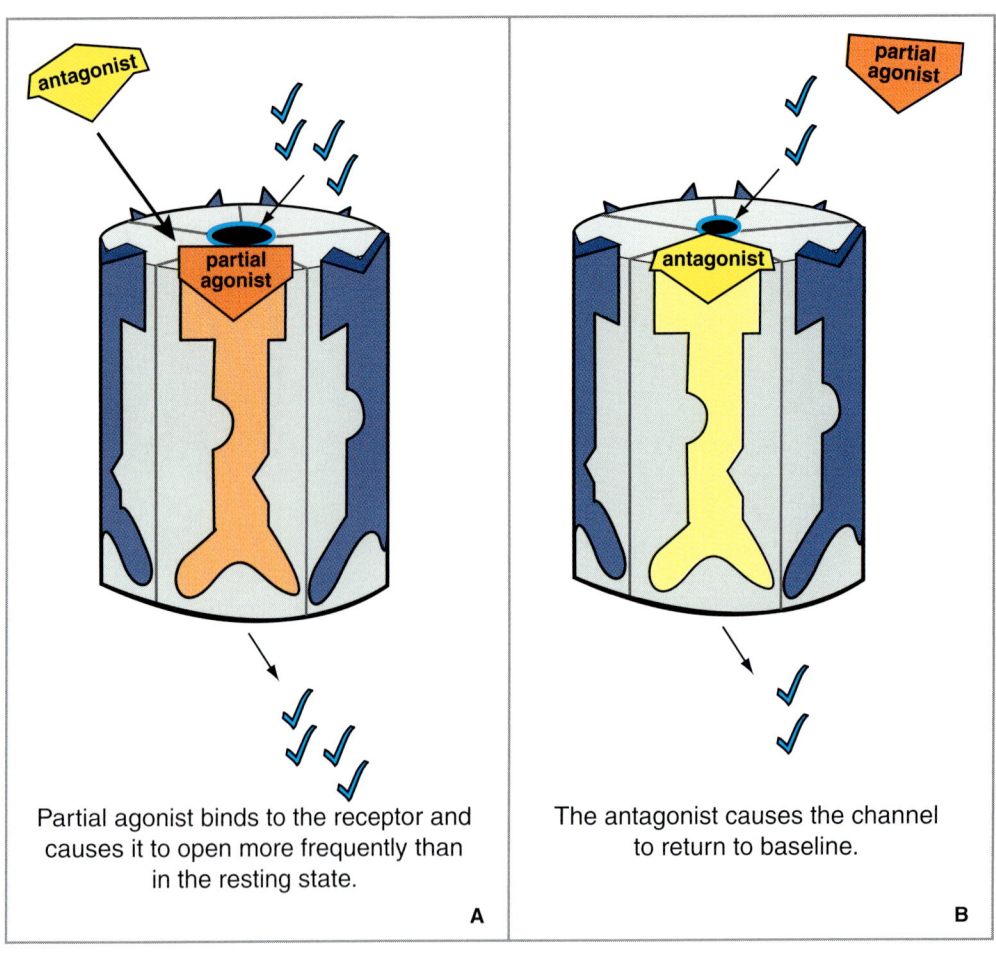

FIGURE 5-15 Antagonist acting in presence of partial agonist. In panel A, a partial agonist occupies its binding site and causes the ion channel to open more frequently than the resting state. This is represented as the orange partial agonist docking to its binding site, turning the receptor orange, and partially opening the ion channel. In panel B, the yellow antagonist prevails and shoves the orange partial agonist off the binding site, reversing the partial agonist's actions. Thus the ion channel is returned to its resting state.

subject to change over time, since these receptors have the capacity to adapt, particularly when there is chronic or excessive exposure to them.

We have already discussed the resting state, the open state, and the closed states shown in Figure 5-19. The best known adaptive states are those of desensitization and inactivation, also shown in Figure 5-19. We have also briefly discussed inactivation as a state that can be caused by acute administration of an inverse agonist, beginning with a rapid conformational change in the ion channel that first closes it but over time stabilizes the channel in an inactive conformation that can relatively quickly be reversed by an antagonist, which then restabilizes the ion channel in the resting state (Figures 5-16, 5-17, and 5-18).

Desensitization is yet another state of the ligand-gated ion channel shown in Figure 5-19. Ion channel–linked receptor desensitization can be caused by prolonged exposure to agonists (Figure 5-20) and may be a way for receptors to protect themselves from overstimulation. An agonist acting at a ligand-gated ion channel first induces a change in receptor conformation that opens the channel, but with the continuous presence of the agonist, over

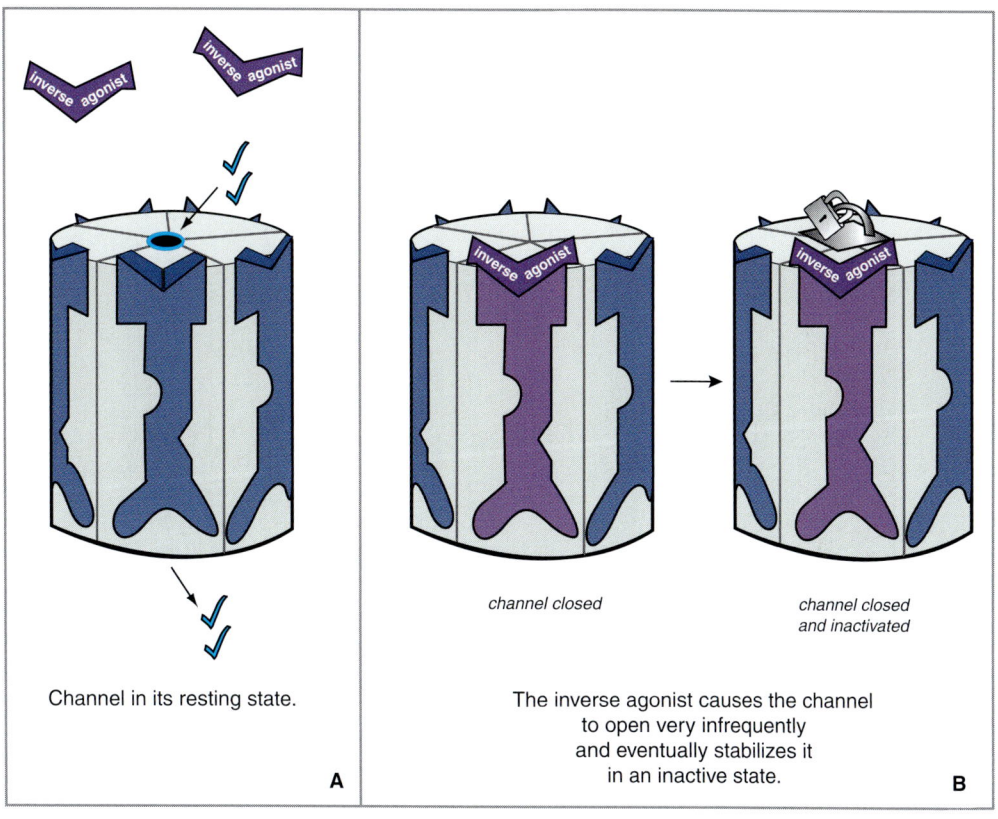

FIGURE 5-16 Actions of an inverse agonist. In panel A, the ion channel is in its resting state and opens infrequently. In panel B, the inverse agonist occupies the binding site on the ligand-gated ion channel and causes it to close. This is the opposite of what an agonist does and is represented by the purple inverse agonist turning the receptor purple and closing the ion channel. Eventually, the inverse agonist stabilizes the ion channel in an inactive state, represented by the padlock on the channel itself.

time leads to another conformational change where the receptor essentially stops responding to the agonist even though the agonist is still present (Figure 5-20). This receptor is then considered to be desensitized (Figures 5-19 and 5-20). This state of desensitization can at first be reversed relatively quickly by removal of the agonist (Figure 5-20). However, if the agonist stays much longer, on the order of hours, the receptor converts from a state of simple desensitization to one of inactivation (Figure 5-20). This state does not reverse simply upon removal of the agonist, since it also takes hours in the absence of agonist to revert back to the resting state, where the receptor is again sensitive to new exposure to agonist (Figure 5-20).

The state of inactivation may be best characterized for nicotinic cholinergic receptors – ligand-gated ion channels that are normally responsive to the endogenous neurotransmitter acetylcholine. Acetylcholine is quickly hydrolyzed by an abundance of the enzyme acetylcholinesterase, so it rarely gets the chance to desensitize and inactivate its nicotinic receptors. However, the drug nicotine is not hydrolyzed by acetylcholinesterase and is famous for stimulating nicotinic cholinergic receptors so profoundly and so enduringly that the receptors are not only rapidly desensitized but also enduringly inactivated, requiring hours in the absence of agonist to get back to the resting state. These transitions among

Ion Channels and Enzymes as Targets of Psychopharmacological Drug Action

The inverse agonist causes the channel to stabilize in an inactive form.

A

The antagonist returns the channel to the resting state.

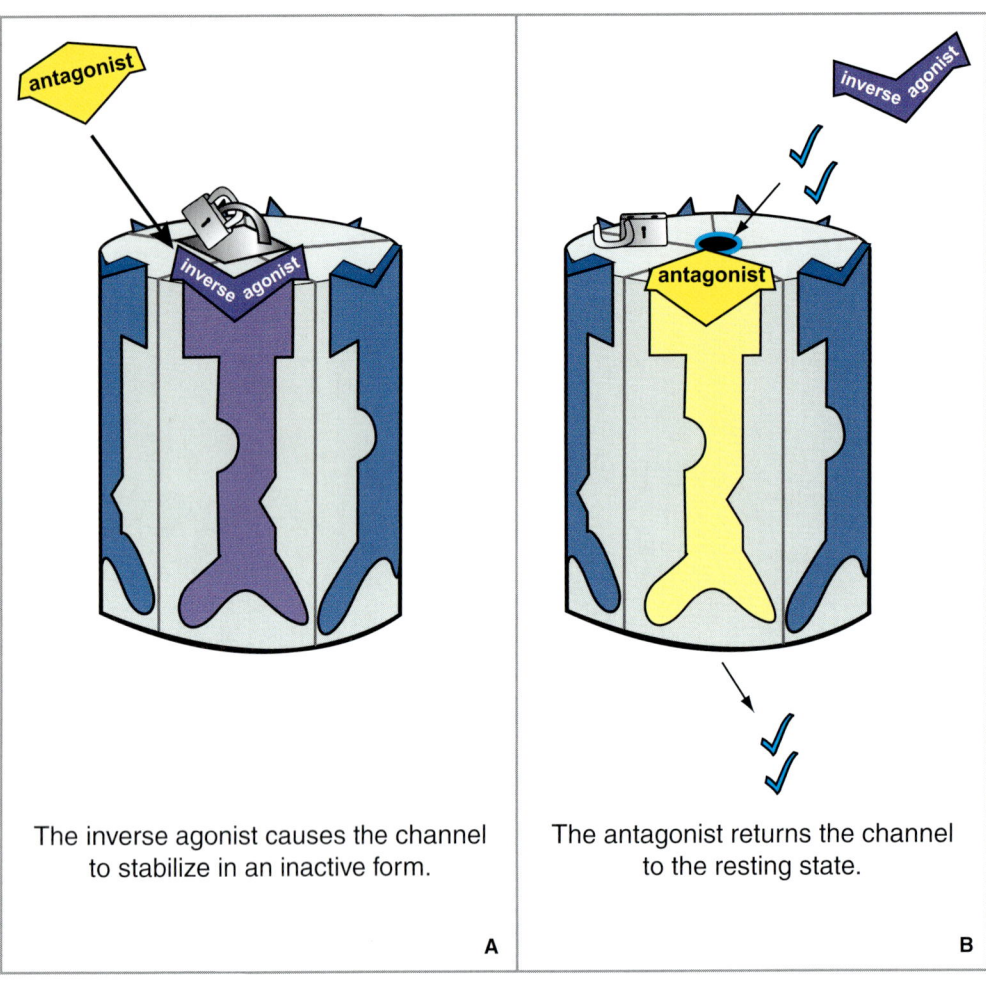

B

FIGURE 5-17 Antagonist acting in presence of inverse agonist. In panel A, the ion channel has been stabilized in an inactive form by the inverse agonist occupying its binding site on the ligand-gated ion channel. This is represented as the purple inverse agonist turning the receptor purple and closing and padlocking the ion channel. In panel B, the yellow antagonist prevails and shoves the purple inverse agonist off the binding site, returning the ion channel to its resting state. In this way, the antagonist's effects on an inverse agonist's actions are similar to its effects on an agonist's actions; namely, it returns the ion channel to its resting state. However, in the presence of an inverse agonist, the antagonist increases the frequency of channel opening, whereas in the presence of an agonist, the antagonist decreases the frequency of channel opening. Thus an antagonist can reverse the actions of either an agonist or an inverse agonist despite the fact that it does nothing on its own.

various receptor states induced by agonists are shown in Figure 5-20. Desensitization of nicotinic receptors is discussed in further detail in the chapter on substance abuse and smoking.

Allosteric modulation: PAMs and NAMs

Ligand-gated ion channels are regulated by more than the neurotransmitter(s) that bind to them. That is, there are other molecules that are not neurotransmitters but which can bind to the receptor–ion channel complex at different sites from where neurotransmitter(s) bind. These sites are called "allosteric" (literally, "at another site") and ligands that bind there are

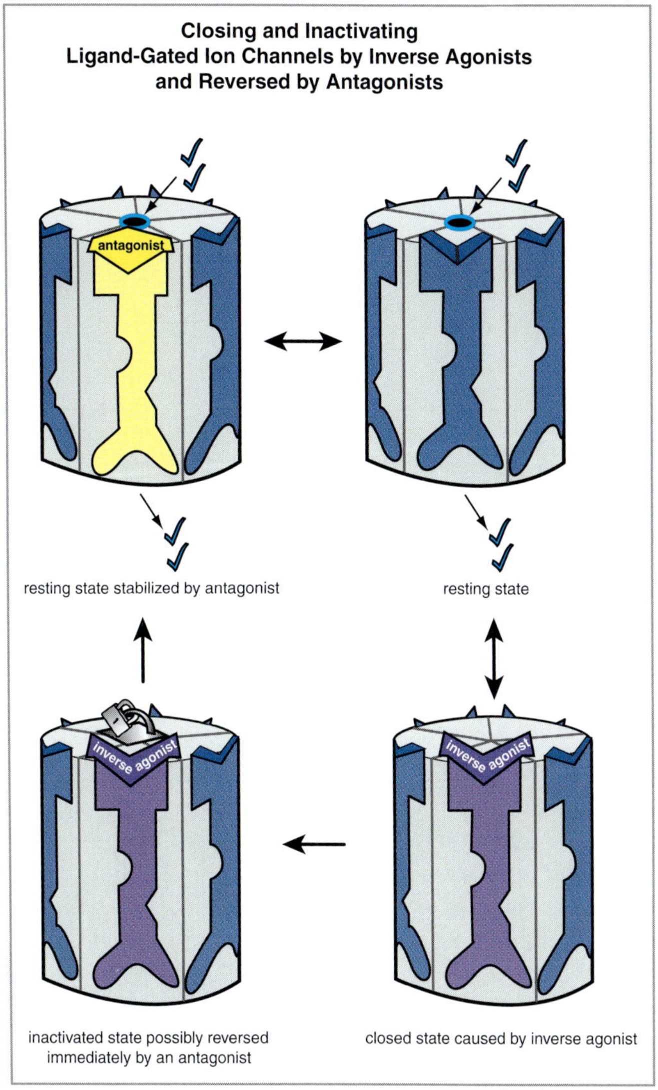

FIGURE 5-18 Inverse agonist actions reversed by antagonist. Antagonists cause conformational change in ligand-gated ion channels that stabilizes the receptors in the resting state (top left), the same state they are in when no agonist or inverse agonist is present (top right). Inverse agonists cause conformational change that closes the ion channel (bottom right). When an inverse agonist is bound over time, it may eventually stabilize the ion channel in an inactive conformation (bottom left). This stabilized conformation of an inactive ion channel can be quickly reversed by an antagonist, which restabilizes it in the resting state (top left).

called allosteric modulators. These ligands are modulators rather than neurotransmitters because they have little or no activity on their own in the absence of the neurotransmitter. Allosteric modulators thus work only in the presence of the neurotransmitter.

There are two forms of allosteric modulators: those that boost what the neurotransmitter does and are thus called positive allosteric modulators (PAMs) and those that block what the neurotransmitter does and are thus called negative allosteric modulators (NAMs).

Specifically, when PAMs or NAMs bind to their allosteric sites while the neurotransmitter is *not* binding to its site, the PAM and the NAM do nothing. However, when a PAM binds to its allosteric site while the neurotransmitter is sitting at its site, the PAM causes conformational changes in the ligand-gated ion channel that open the channel even further and more frequently than happens with a full agonist by itself (Figure 5-21). That is why the PAM is called "positive."

Ion Channels and Enzymes as Targets of Psychopharmacological Drug Action

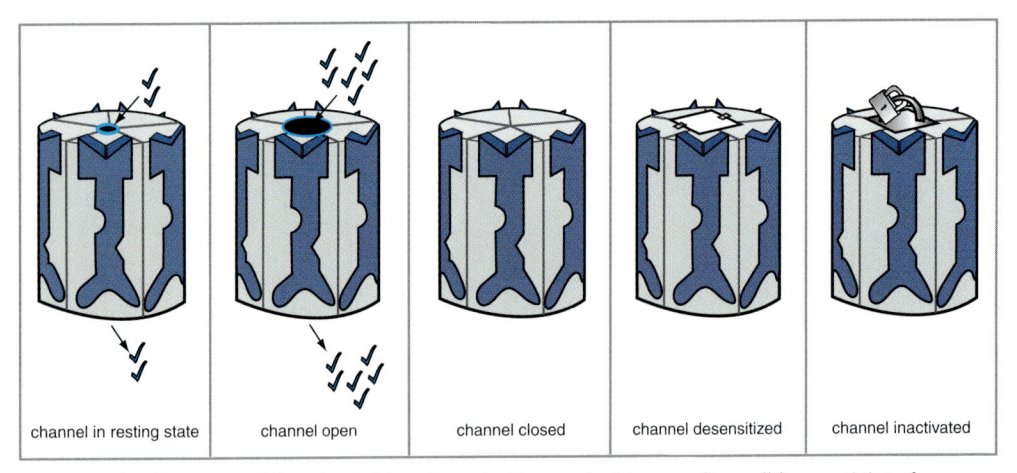

FIGURE 5-19 Five states of ligand-gated ion channels. Summarized here are five well-known states of ligand-gated ion channels. In the resting state, ligand-gated ion channels open infrequently, with consequent constitutive activity that may or may not lead to detectable signal transduction. In the open state, ligand-gated ion channels open to allow ion conductance through the channel, leading to signal transduction. In the closed state, ligand-gated ion channels are closed, allowing no ion flow to occur and thus reducing signal transduction to even less than is produced in the resting state. Channel desensitization is an adaptive state in which the receptor stops responding to agonist even if it is still bound. Channel inactivation is a state in which a closed ion channel over time becomes stabilized in an inactive conformation.

On the other hand, when a NAM binds to its allosteric site while the neurotransmitter resides at its agonist binding site, the NAM causes conformational changes in the ligand-gated ion channel that block or reduce the actions that normally occur when the neurotransmitter acts alone (Figure 5-22). That is why the NAM is called "negative."

GABA, glutamate, and regulation of ligand-gated ion channels

Good examples of PAMs are benzodiazepines. These ligands boost the action of GABA at GABA-A types of ligand-gated chloride ion channels (Figure 5-23). GABA binding to GABA-A sites increases chloride ion flux by opening the ion channel, and benzodiazepines acting as agonists at benzodiazepine receptors elsewhere on the GABA-A receptor complex cause the effect of GABA to be amplified in terms of chloride ion flux by opening the ion channel to a greater degree or more frequently (Figure 5-23). Clinically, this is exhibited as anxiolytic, hypnotic, anticonvulsant, amnestic, and muscle relaxant actions. In this example, benzodiazepines are acting as full agonists at the PAM site (Figure 5-23).

Experimentally, you can also have the opposite action. For example, NAMs acting at this same site include benzodiazepine inverse agonists. Although these are only experimental, as expected, they have the opposite actions of benzodiazepine full agonists (compare Figures 5-10 and 5-16). Specifically, inverse agonists at benzodiazepine receptors diminish chloride conductance through the ion channel so much that they cause panic attacks, seizures, and some improvement in memory – the opposite clinical effects of a benzodiazepine full agonist. Thus, the same allosteric site can have either NAM or PAM actions, depending upon whether the ligand is a full agonist or an inverse agonist.

Other examples of NAMs for ligand-gated ion channels include actions of drugs and ions at ion channels of NMDA glutamate receptors. These ionotrophic receptors can be blocked by the ion magnesium, which plugs the calcium channel associated with these types of receptors (Figure 5-24). This action of magnesium blocks the ability of the agonists

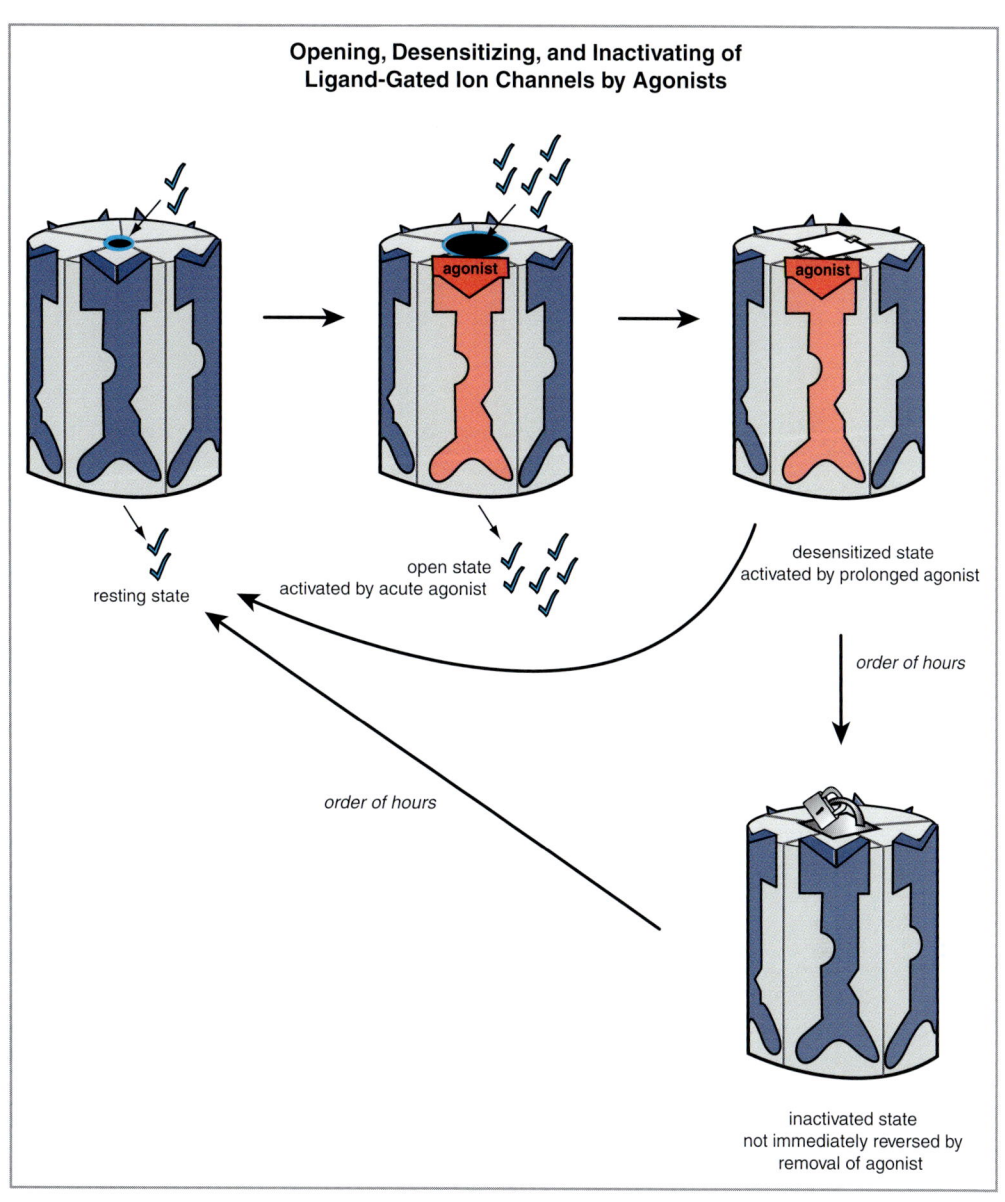

FIGURE 5-20 Opening, desensitizing, and inactivating by agonists. Agonists cause ligand-gated ion channels to open more frequently, increasing ion conductance in comparison to the resting state. Prolonged exposure to agonists can cause a ligand-gated ion channel to enter a desensitized state in which it no longer responds to the agonist even if it is still bound. Prompt removal of the agonist can reverse this state fairly quickly. However, if the agonist stays longer, it can cause a conformational change that leads to inactivation of the ion channel. This state is not immediately reversed when the agonist is removed.

glutamate and glycine to open that channel unless the nearby membrane is simultaneously depolarized (Figure 5-24). NMDA receptors are unique in that they require two agonists, called cotransmitters, to work simultaneously in order for there to be the possibility of opening the calcium channel. These coagonists or cotransmitters are glutamate and glycine, each of which binds to a different site on the NMDA complex (Figure 5-24).

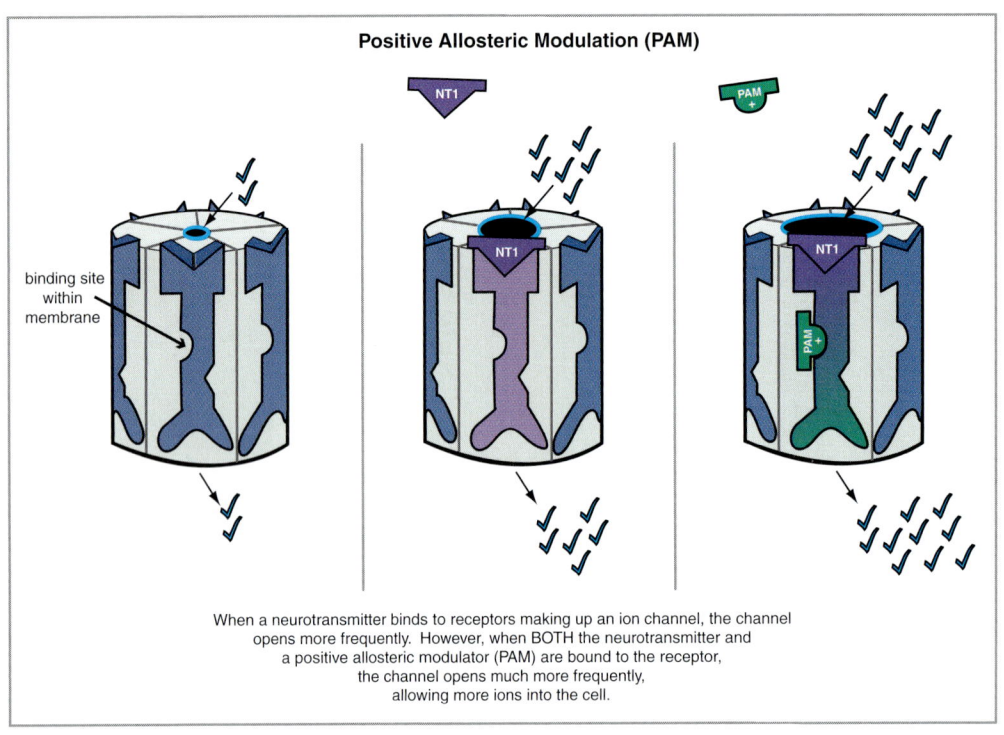

FIGURE 5-21 Positive allosteric modulators. Allosteric modulators are ligands that bind to sites other than the neurotransmitter site on an ion channel–linked receptor. Allosteric modulators have no activity of their own but rather enhance (positive allosteric modulators, or PAMs) or block (negative allosteric modulators, or NAMs) the actions of neurotransmitters. When a PAM binds to its site while an agonist is also bound, the channel opens more frequently than when only the agonist is bound, therefore allowing more ions into the cell.

Open and unblocked calcium flux through NMDA ligand-gated ion channels may be necessary for the neurophysiological phenomenon of long-term potentiation, which in turn may be necessary for long-term memory formation and may also be one mechanism that triggers synaptic plasticity (Figure 5-24). In order for this to happen, depolarization must remove the NAM magnesium while both glutamate and glycine bind to their neurotransmitter sites. Thus, these receptor systems are a form of coincidence detector – they sense the simultaneous presence of glutamate, glycine, and membrane depolarization.

Interestingly, other NAMs for NMDA receptors include PCP, or phencyclidine, also called "angel dust," and its structurally related anesthetic agent ketamine. These agents bind to a site in the calcium channel but can get into the channel to block it only when the channel is open. When either PCP or ketamine binds to its NAM site, it prevents glutamate/glycine cotransmission from opening the channel.

Other types of ionotrophic receptors for glutamate include AMPA and kainate, named for the agonists that bind to them (Figure 5-25). This ion channel–linked receptor requires only glutamate and not a cotransmitter to cause a change in its conformation in order to open it. This leads to fast excitatory neurotransmission and membrane depolarization. However, if this is sustained for too long, glutamate will desensitize this receptor via agonist-induced desensitization (Figure 5-25), which is also described above and is illustrated in Figure 5-20.

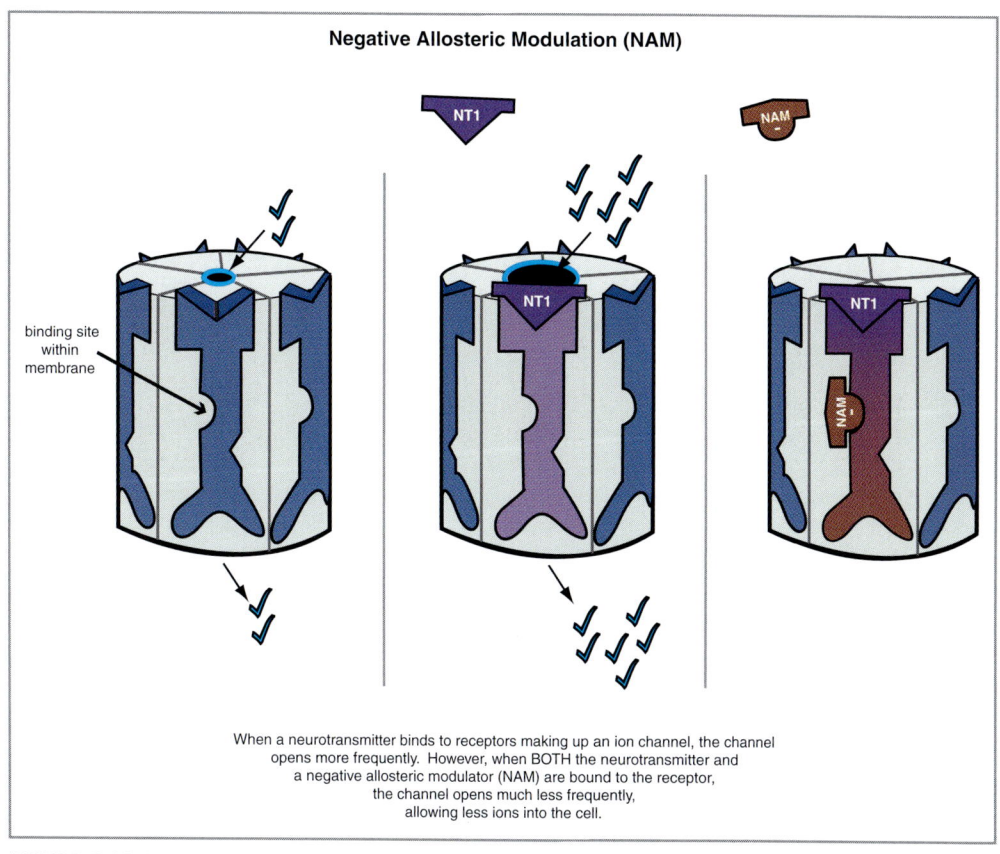

FIGURE 5-22 Negative allosteric modulators. Allosteric modulators are ligands that bind to sites other than the neurotransmitter site on an ion channel–linked receptor. Allosteric modulators have no activity of their own but rather enhance (positive allosteric modulators, or PAMs) or block (negative allosteric modulators, or NAMs) the actions of neurotransmitters. When a NAM binds to its site while an agonist is also bound, the channel opens less frequently than when only the agonist is bound, therefore allowing fewer ions into the cell.

Voltage-sensitive ion channels as targets of psychopharmacological drug action

Structure and function

Not all ion channels are regulated by neurotransmitter ligands. Indeed, critical aspects of nerve conduction, action potentials, and neurotransmitter release are all mediated by another class of ion channels, known as "voltage-sensitive" or "voltage-gated" ion channels because their opening and closing are regulated by the ionic charge or voltage potential across the membrane in which they reside. An electrical impulse in a neuron, also known as the action potential, is triggered by summation of the various neurochemical and electrical events of neurotransmission. These are discussed extensively in Chapter 2, which discusses the anatomical basis of neurotransmission, and in Chapter 3, which covers the chemical basis of neurotransmission and signal transduction.

Electrically, the action potential is shown in Figure 5-26. The first phase is sodium rushing "downhill" into the sodium-deficient, negatively charged internal milieu of the neuron (Figure 5-26A). This is made possible when voltage-gated sodium channels open the gates and let the sodium in. A few milliseconds later, the calcium channels get the same idea, with their voltage-gated ion channels opened by the change in voltage potential caused

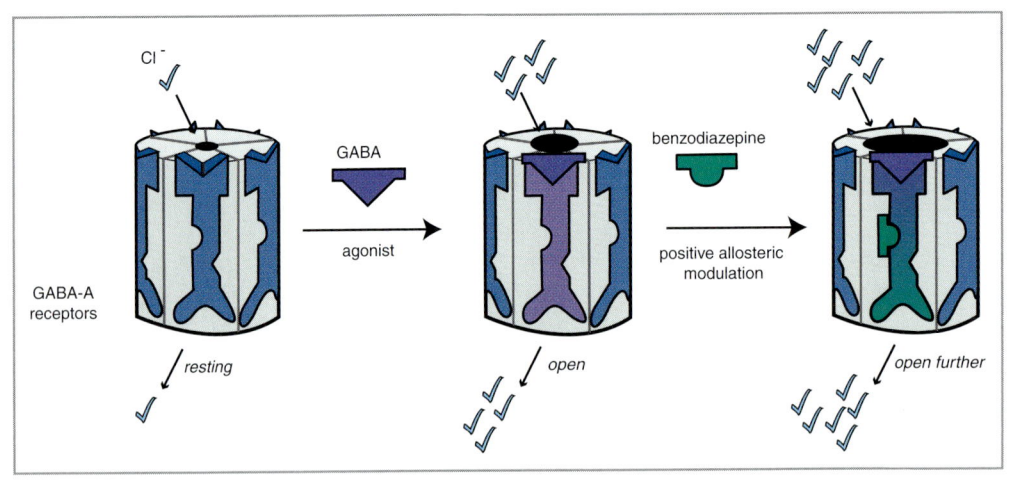

FIGURE 5-23 Benzodiazepines as positive allosteric modulators. Benzodiazepines are positive allosteric modulators (PAMs) at GABA-A receptors. When GABA binds to its site on GABA-A receptors, it causes increased chloride conductance through the ion channel. When benzodiazepines bind to GABA-A receptors in the absence of GABA, they have no effect on the ion channel. However, when benzodiazepines bind to GABA-A receptors in the presence of GABA, they enhance the effects of GABA, thus increasing chloride conductance even further.

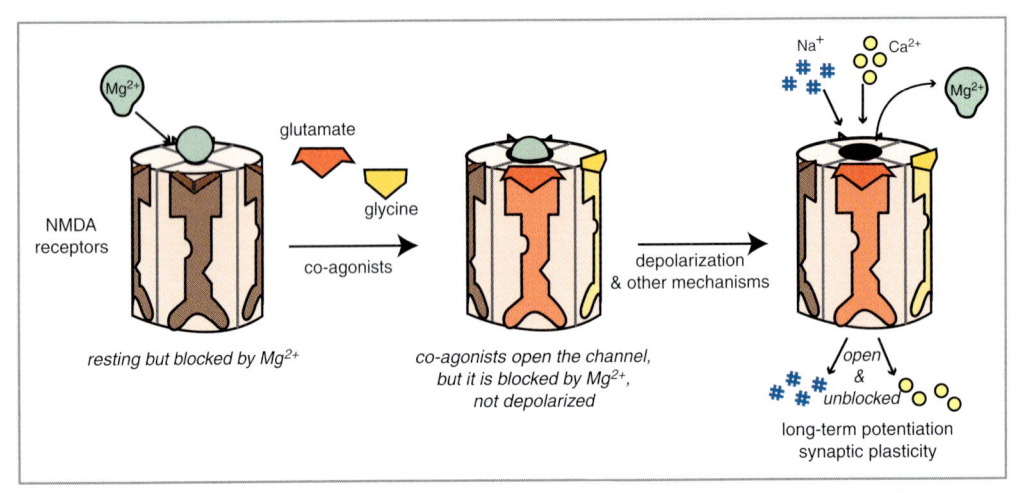

FIGURE 5-24 Magnesium as a negative allosteric modulator. Magnesium is a negative allosteric modulator (NAM) at NMDA glutamate receptors. Opening of NMDA glutamate receptors requires the presence of both glutamate and glycine, each of which bind to a different site on the receptor. When magnesium is also bound and the membrane is not depolarized, it prevents the effects of glutamate and glycine and thus does not allow the ion channel to open. In order for the channel to open, depolarization must remove magnesium while both glutamate and glycine are bound to their sites on the ligand-gated ion channel complex.

by the sodium rushing in (Figure 5-26B). Finally, after the action potential is gone, during recovery of the neuron's baseline internal electrical milieu, potassium makes its way back into the cell through potassium channels as sodium is again pumped out (Figure 5-26C). It is now known or suspected that several psychotropic drugs work on voltage-sensitive sodium channels (VSSCs) and voltage-sensitive calcium channels (VSCCs). These classes of ion channels will be discussed here. Potassium channels are less well known to be targeted by psychotropic drugs and will thus not be emphasized.

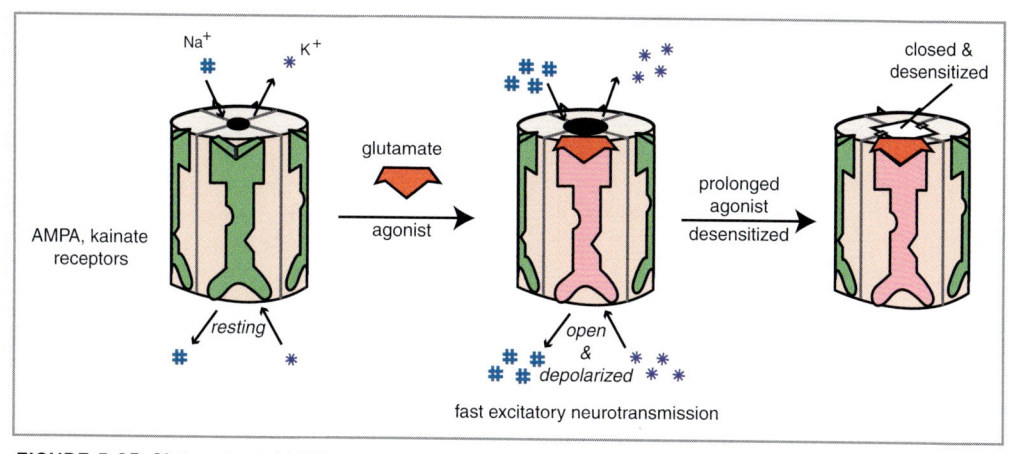

FIGURE 5-25 Glutamate at AMPA and kainate receptors. Unlike NMDA receptors, AMPA and kainate receptors require only glutamate to bind in order for the channel to open. This leads to fast excitatory neurotransmission and membrane depolarization. Sustained binding of the agonist glutamate will lead to receptor desensitization, causing the channel to close and be transiently unresponsive to agonist.

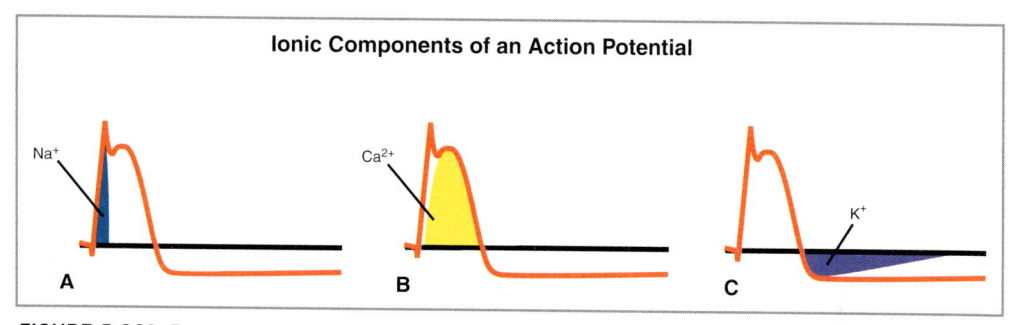

FIGURE 5-26A, B, and C Ionic components of an action potential. The ionic components of an action potential are shown graphically here. First, voltage-sensitive sodium channels open to allow an influx of "downhill" sodium into the negatively charged internal milieu of the neuron (**A**). The change of voltage potential caused by the influx of sodium triggers voltage-sensitive calcium channels to open and allow calcium influx (**B**). Finally, after the action potential is gone, potassium enters the cell while sodium is pumped out, restoring the neuron's baseline internal electrical milieu (**C**).

Voltage-sensitive sodium channels (VSSCs)

Many dimensions of ion channel structure are similar for VSSCs and VSCCs. Both have a "pore" that is the channel itself, allowing ions to travel from one side of the membrane to the other. However, voltage-gated ion channels have a more complicated structure than just a hole or pore in the membrane. These channels are long strings of amino acids, comprising subunits, and four different subunits are connected to form the critical pore, known as an alpha subunit. In addition, other proteins are associated with the four subunits, and these appear to have regulatory functions.

Let us now build a voltage-sensitive ion channel from scratch and describe the known functions for each part of the proteins that make up these channels. The subunit of an alpha pore–forming protein has six transmembrane segments (Figure 5-27). Transmembrane segment 4 can detect the difference in charge across the membrane, and is thus the most electrically sensitive part of the voltage sensitive channel. Transmembrane segment 4 thus functions like a voltmeter, and when it detects a change in ion charge across the membrane,

The Pore of a Voltage-Sensitive Ion Channel has Six Transmembrane Regions

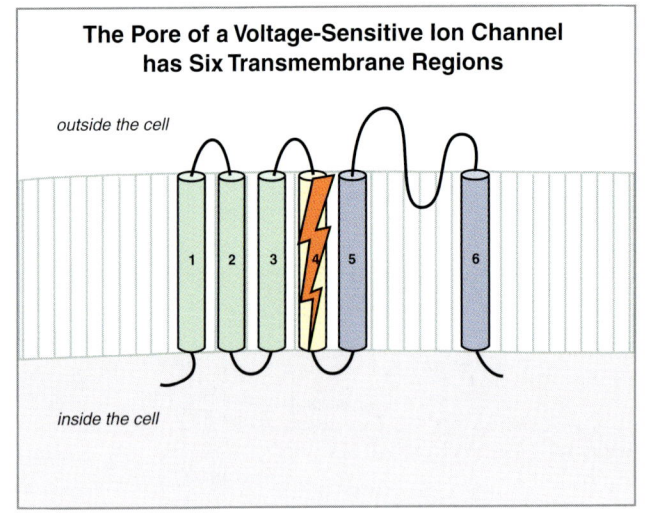

outside the cell

inside the cell

FIGURE 5-27 **Subunit of alpha pore of voltage-sensitive ion channel.** The alpha pore of a voltage-sensitive ion channel consists of four subunits, each with six transmembrane segments. A single subunit is shown here. Segment 4 is the voltage sensor, or voltmeter. It detects the difference in charge across the membrane and then alerts the rest of the protein to begin conformational changes that either open or close the ion channel. The structure of the alpha-pore unit is shared by both sodium- and calcium-sensitive ion channels, although the sequence of amino acids making up the subunit differs between the two.

it can alert the rest of the protein and begin conformational changes of the ion channel and either open it or close it (Figure 5-27). This same general structure exists for both voltage-sensitive sodium channels and voltage-sensitive calcium channels, but the exact amino acid sequence of the protein subunits is obviously different for VSSCs compared to VSCCs.

Each subunit of a voltage-sensitive ion channel has an extracellular amino acid loop between transmembrane segments 5 and 6 (see Figure 5-27). This section of amino acids serves as an "ionic filter" and is located in a position where it can cover the outside opening of the pore. This is illustrated as a colander configured molecularly to allow only sodium ions to filter through the sodium channel in Figure 5-28A and only calcium channels to filter through the calcium channel in Figure 5-28B.

Four copies of the sodium channel version of this protein are strung together to form one complete ion-channel pore of a voltage-sensitive sodium channel (Figure 5-29A). The cytoplasmic loops of amino acids that tie these four subunits together are sites that regulate various functions of the sodium channel. For example, on the connector loop between the third and fourth subunits of a VSSC, there are amino acids that act as a "plug" to close the channel. Like a ball on an amino acid chain, this "pore inactivator" stops up the channel on the inner membrane surface of the pore (Figure 5-29A). This is a physical blocking of the hole in the pore and reminiscent of an old-fashioned bathtub plug stopping up the drain in a bathtub. The alpha pore–forming unit of the voltage-sensitive sodium channel is also shown as an icon in Figure 5-29B with a hole in the middle of the pore and a pore inactivator ready to plug the hole from the inside.

Many figures in textbooks represent voltage-sensitive ion channels with the outside of the cell on the top of a figure; this is the way the ion channel is shown in Figures 5-29A and B. Here, we also show what the channel looks like when the inside of the cell is at the top of the figure, since throughout this book these channels will often be shown on presynaptic membranes where the inside of the neuron is up and the outside of the neuron, namely its synapse, is down, like the orientation represented in Figure 5-29C. In either case, the sodium is kept out of the neuron when the channel is closed or inactivated and the direction of sodium flow is into the neuron when the channel is open, activated, and the pore is not plugged up with the pore-inactivating amino acid loops.

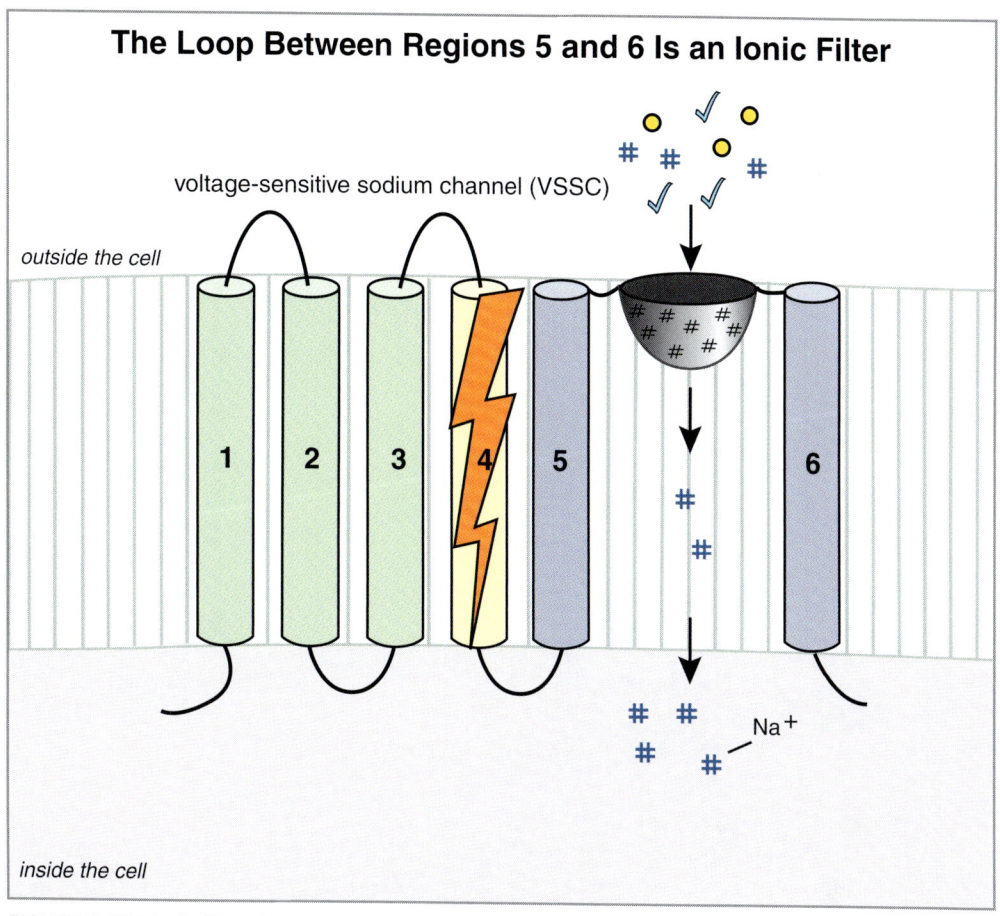

The Loop Between Regions 5 and 6 Is an Ionic Filter

FIGURE 5-28A Ionic filter of voltage-sensitive sodium channel. The extracellular loop between transmembrane segments 5 and 6 of an alpha-pore unit acts as an ionic filter (illustrated here as a colander). Shown here is an alpha-pore unit of a voltage-sensitive sodium channel, with the ionic filter allowing only sodium ions to enter the cell.

Voltage-sensitive sodium channels may have one or more regulatory proteins, some of which are called beta units, located in the transmembrane area and flanking the alpha pore–forming unit (Figure 5-30). The function of these subunits is not clearly established, but they may modify the actions of the alpha unit and thereby indirectly influence the opening and closing of the channel. It is possible that beta units may be phosphoproteins and that their state of phosphorylation or dephosphorylation could regulate how much influence they exert on ion channel regulation. Indeed, the alpha unit itself may also be a phosphoprotein, with the possibility that its own phosphorylation state could be regulated by signal transduction cascades and thus increase or decrease the sensitivity of the ion channel to changes in the ionic environment. This is discussed in Chapter 3 as part of the signal transduction cascade. Ion channels in some cases may act as third, fourth, or subsequent messengers triggered by neurotransmission (see Figures 3-19, 3-20, and 3-12). Both beta subunits and the alpha subunit itself may have various sites where psychotropic drugs act, especially anticonvulsants, some of which are also useful as mood stabilizers or as treatments for chronic pain. Specific drugs will be discussed in further detail in the chapters on mood stabilizers and pain.

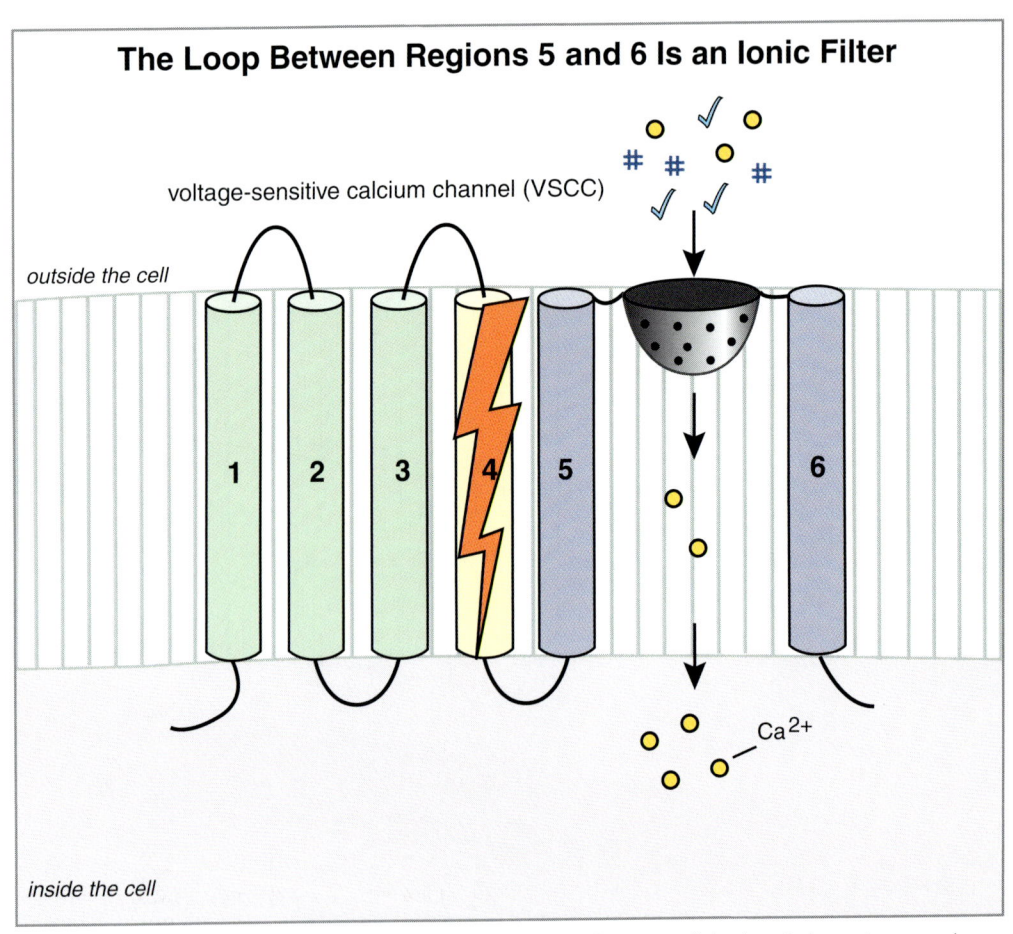

The Loop Between Regions 5 and 6 Is an Ionic Filter

FIGURE 5-28B Ionic filter of voltage-sensitive calcium channel. The extracellular loop between transmembrane segments 5 and 6 of an alpha-pore unit acts as an ionic filter (illustrated here as a colander). Shown here is an alpha-pore unit of a voltage-sensitive sodium channel, with the ionic filter allowing only sodium ions to enter the cell.

Three different states of a VSSC are shown in Figure 5-31. The channel can be open and active, a state allowing maximum ion flow through the alpha unit (Figure 5-31, left). When a sodium channel needs to stop ion flow, it has two states that can do this. One state acts very quickly to flip the pore inactivator into place, stopping ion flow so fast that the channel has not yet even closed (Figure 5-31, middle). Another state of inactivation actually closes the channel with conformational changes in the ion channel's shape (Figure 5-31, right). The pore inactivation mechanism may be for fast inactivation, and the channel closing mechanism may be for a more stable state of inactivation, but it is not entirely clear.

There are many subtypes of sodium channels, but the details of how they are differentiated from each other by differential location in the brain, by differential functions, and by differential drug actions are only beginning to be clarified. For the psychopharmacologist, what is now of interest is the fact that various sodium channels may be the sites of action of several anticonvulsants, some of which have mood-stabilizing and pain-reducing properties (Figure 5-32). Most currently available anticonvulsants probably have multiple sites of action, including multiple sites of action at multiple types of ion channels.

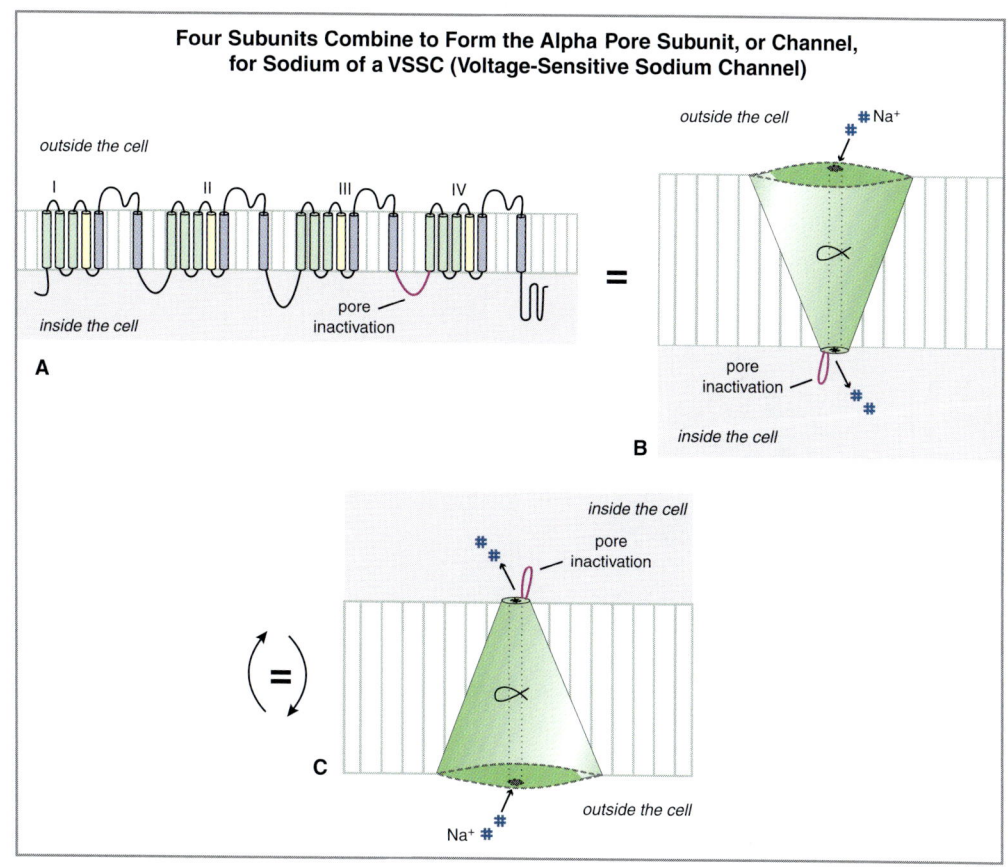

FIGURE 5-29A, B, and C Alpha pore of voltage-sensitive sodium channel. The alpha pore of a voltage-sensitive sodium channel comprises four subunits (**A**). Amino acids in the intracellular loop between the third and fourth subunits act as a pore inactivator, "plugging" the channel. An iconic version of the alpha unit is shown here, with the extracellular portion on top (**B**) and with the intracellular portion on top (**C**).

The actions of anticonvulsants at specific molecular sites on voltage-sensitive ion channels are just beginning to be clarified, especially for psychotropic drugs used currently in clinical practice. Although each of the agents shown in Figure 5-32 may bind to additional sites on various ion channels, it seems likely that there is a key site within the alpha pore, within the ion channel itself, where several anticonvulsants bind. Whether this binding site constitutes an actual receptor and whether it mediates anticonvulsant actions, mood stabilizing actions, relief from chronic pain, or side effects is not yet proven. However, a leading hypothesis suggests that agents that act at this binding site in sodium channels of epileptic neurons may reduce seizures, whereas the same agents acting at this binding site in sodium channels of neurons mediating bipolar mania may stabilize mood, and finally that the actions of these agents at sodium channels of neurons mediating chronic pain may relieve chronic pain. The specific actions of specific drugs will be discussed in the chapters that cover these specific disorders.

Voltage-sensitive calcium channels (VSCCs)

Many aspects of VSCCs and VSSCs are similar, not just their names. Like their sodium-channel cousins, the voltage-sensitive calcium channels also have subunits with six

VSSCs (Voltage-Sensitive Sodium Channels) May Have One or More Regulatory Proteins Associated (e.g., Beta Units)

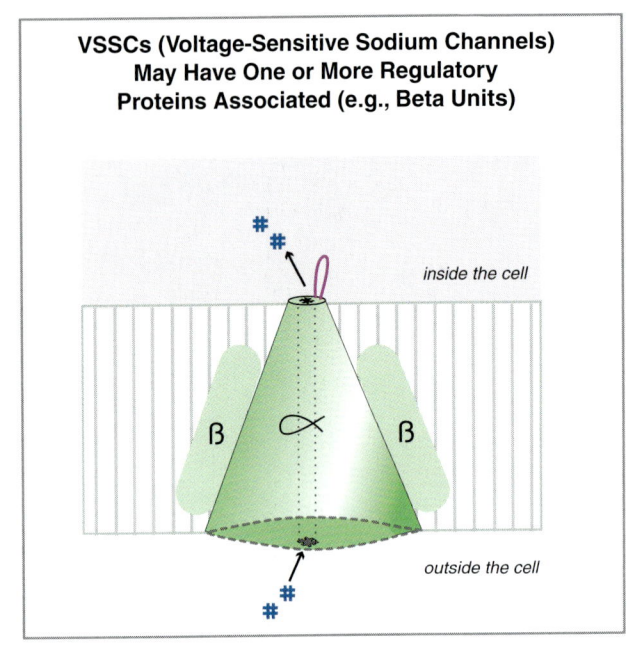

FIGURE 5-30 Structure of voltage-sensitive sodium channel. Voltage-sensitive sodium channels can have one or two regulatory proteins, called beta subunits, which flank the transmembrane portion of the alpha unit. The function of the beta subunits is not yet well understood.

Three States of a Voltage-Sensitive Sodium Channel (VSSC)

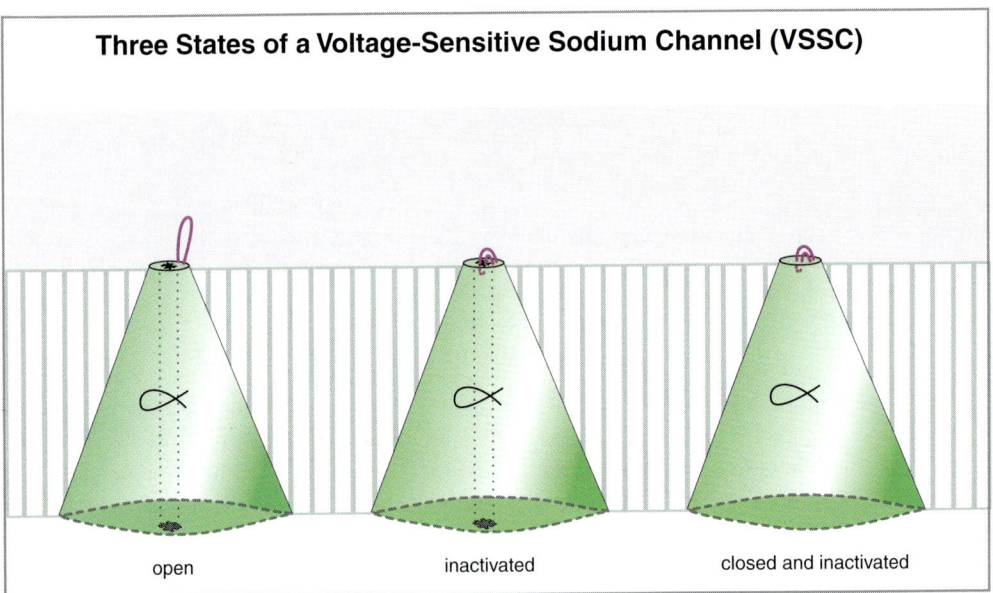

open — inactivated — closed and inactivated

FIGURE 5-31 States of voltage-sensitive sodium channel. Such channels can be in the open state, in which the ion channel is open and active and ions flow through the alpha unit (left). Voltage-sensitive sodium channels may also be in an inactivated state, in which the channel is not yet closed but has been "plugged" by the pore inactivator, preventing ion flow (middle). Finally, conformational changes in the ion channel can cause it to close, the third state (right).

transmembrane segments, with segment 4 a voltmeter, and with the extracellular amino acids connecting segments 5 and 6 acting as an ionic filter (Figure 5-27) – only this time as a colander allowing calcium, not sodium, to come into the cell (see Figure 5-28B). Obviously the exact sequence of amino acids differs between a sodium channel and a calcium channel, but they have a very similar overall organization and structure.

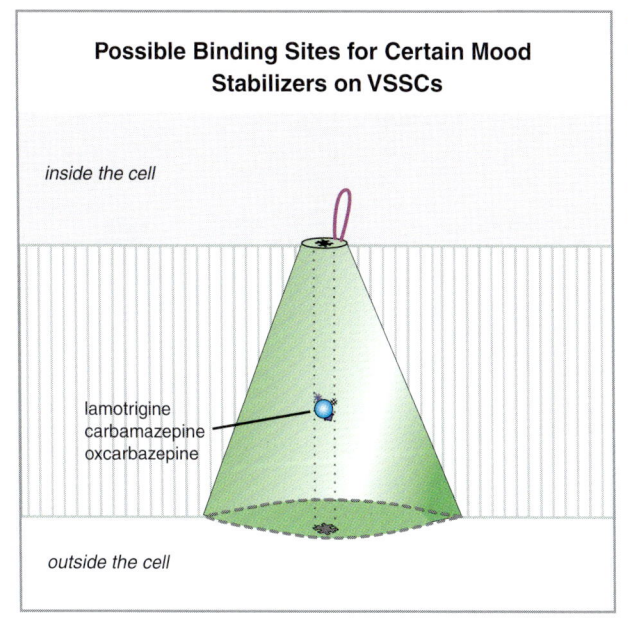

FIGURE 5-32 Binding sites for some mood stabilizers on VSSCs. Several anticonvulsant agents are believed to act at voltage-sensitive sodium channels. Lamotrigine, carbamazepine, and oxcarbazepine are believed to bind to voltage-sensitive sodium channels within the ion channel itself.

Just like voltage-gated sodium channels, VSCCs also string together four of their subunits to form a pore, called, in the case of a calcium channel, an alpha-1 unit (Figure 5-33). The connecting string of amino acids also has functional activities that can regulate the functioning of calcium channels, but in this case the functions are different from those for sodium channels. That is, there is no pore inactivator working as a plug for the VSCC, as described above for the VSSC and illustrated in Figures 5-29 and 5-31. Instead, the amino acids connecting the second and third subunits of the voltage-sensitive calcium channel work as a "snare" to hook up with synaptic vesicles and regulate the release of neurotransmitter into the synapse during synaptic neurotransmission (Figure 5-33A). The orientation of the calcium channel in Figure 5-33 is with the outside of the cell at the top of the page for Figure 5-33A and B, but with the inside of the cell at the top of the page for Figure 5-33C, so the reader can see how these channels might look in various configurations in space. In all cases, the direction of ion flow is from outside the cell to the inside when that channel opens to allow ion flow to occur.

Several proteins flank the alpha-1 pore-forming unit of a VSCC; these are called gamma, beta, and alpha-2 delta (Figure 5-34). Shown here are gamma units that span the membrane, cytoplasmic beta units, and a curious protein called alpha-2 delta, because it has two parts: a delta part that is transmembrane and an alpha-2 part that is extracellular (Figure 5-34). The functions of all these proteins associated with the alpha-1 pore-forming unit of a voltage-sensitive calcium channel are just beginning to be understood, but already it is known that the alpha-2 delta protein is the target of certain psychotropic drugs and that it may be involved in regulating conformational changes of the ion channel to change the way the ion channel opens and closes.

As would be expected, there are several subtypes of VSCCs (Table 5-5). The vast array of voltage-sensitive calcium channels indicates that the term "calcium channel" is much too general and in fact can be confusing. For example, calcium channels associated with the ligand-gated ion channels, discussed in the previous section, especially those associated

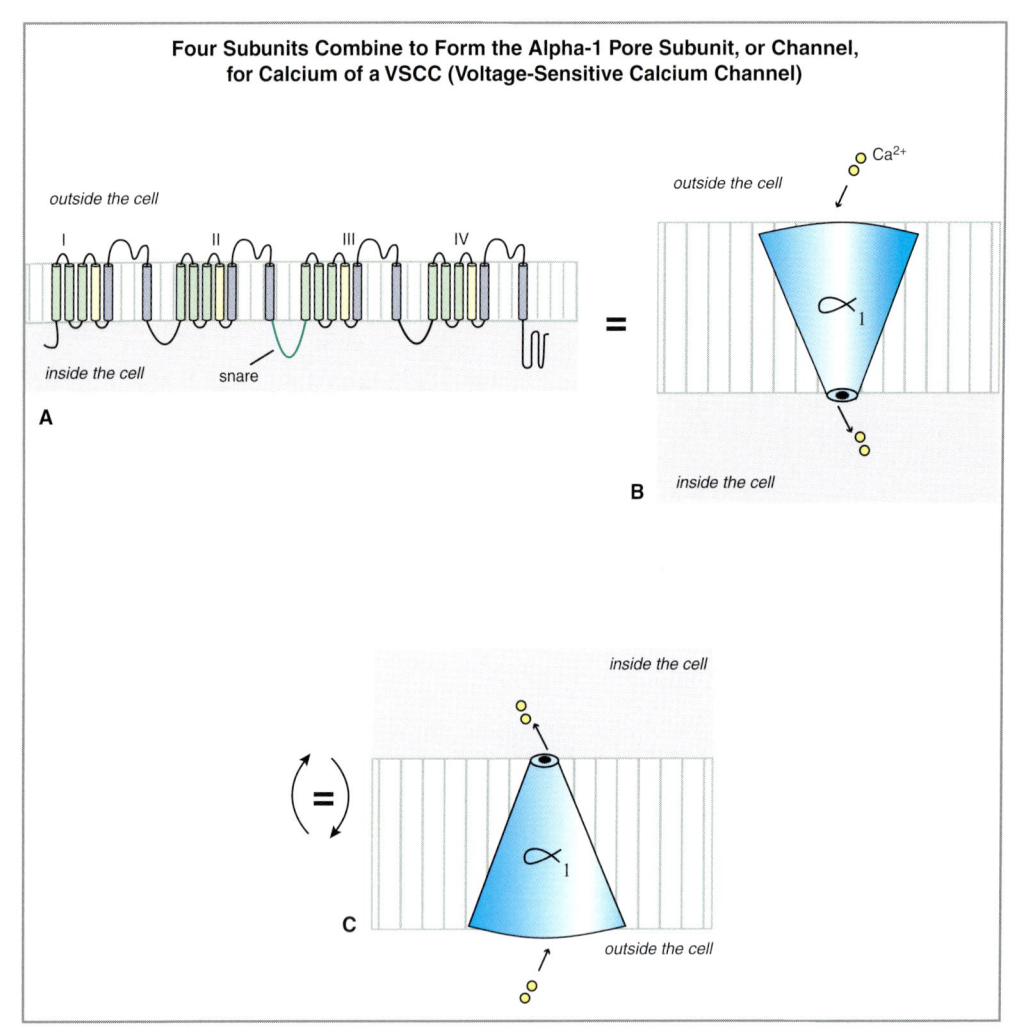

FIGURE 5-33 A, B, and C Alpha 1 pore of voltage-sensitive calcium channel. The alpha pore of a voltage-sensitive calcium channel, termed an alpha-1 unit, comprises four subunits (**A**). Amino acids in the cytoplasmic loop between the second and third subunits act as a snare to connect with synaptic vesicles, thereby controlling neurotransmitter release (**A**). An iconic version of the alpha-1 unit is shown here, with the extracellular portion on top (**B**) and with the intracellular portion on top (**C**).

with glutamate and nicotinic cholinergic ionotrophic receptors, are members of an entirely different class of ion channels from the voltage-sensitive calcium channels under discussion here. As we have mentioned, calcium channels associated with this previously discussed class of ion channels are called ligand-gated ion channels, ionotrophic receptors, or ion channel–linked receptors to distinguish them from VSCCs.

The specific subtypes of VSCCs of most interest to psychopharmacology are those that are presynaptic, that regulate neurotransmitter release, and that are targeted by certain psychotropic drugs. This subtype designation of voltage-sensitive calcium channel is shown in Table 5-5, and such channels are known as N or P/Q channels.

Another well-known subtype of VSCC is the L channel. This channel exists not only in the central nervous system, where its functions are still being clarified, but also on vascular

TABLE 5-5 Subtypes of voltage sensitive calcium channels (VSCCs)

Type	Pore-forming Subunit	Location	Function
L	Ca$_v$1.2, 1.3	Cell bodies, dendrites	Gene expression, synaptic integration
N	Ca$_v$ 2.2	*Nerve terminals* Dendrites, cell bodies	*Transmitter release* Synaptic integration
P/Q	Ca$_v$, 2.1	*Nerve terminals* Dendrites, cell bodies	*Transmitter release* Synaptic integration
R	Ca$_v$, 2.3	Cell bodies, dendrites *Nerve terminals*	Repetitive firing, synaptic integration *Transmitter release*
T	Ca$_v$, 3.1, 3.2, 3.3	Cell bodies, dendrites	Pacemaking, repetitive firing, synaptic integration

VSCCs (Voltage-Sensitive Calcium Channels) Have Multiple Associated Regulatory Proteins

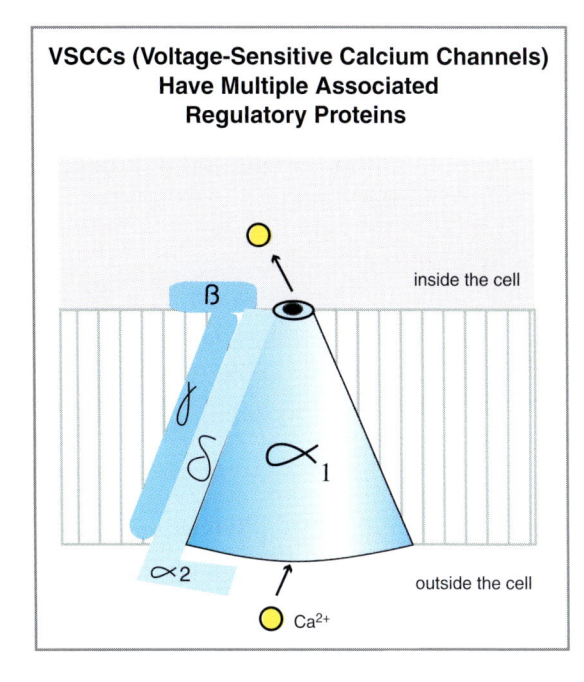

FIGURE 5-34 Structure of voltage-sensitive calcium channel. Voltage-sensitive calcium channels can have multiple regulatory proteins. Gamma units span the membrane, while beta units are intracellular. The alpha-2 delta unit consists of two parts: a delta part that spans the membrane and an alpha-2 part that is extracellular.

smooth muscle, where it regulates blood pressure and where a group of drugs known as dihydropyridine "calcium channel blockers" interact as therapeutic antihypertensives to lower blood pressure. R and T channels are also of interest, and some anticonvulsants and psychotropic drugs may also interact there, but the exact roles of these channels are still being clarified.

Presynaptic N and P/Q VSCCs have a specialized role in regulating neurotransmitter release because they are linked by molecular "snares" to synaptic vesicles (Figure 5-35). That is, these channels are hooked to synaptic vesicles. Some experts think of this as a cocked gun – loaded with neurotransmitters packed in a synaptic vesicle bullet (Figure 5-35A), ready to be fired at the postsynaptic neuron as soon as a nerve impulse arrives (Figure 5-35B). Some of the structural details of the molecular links – namely, with snare proteins – that

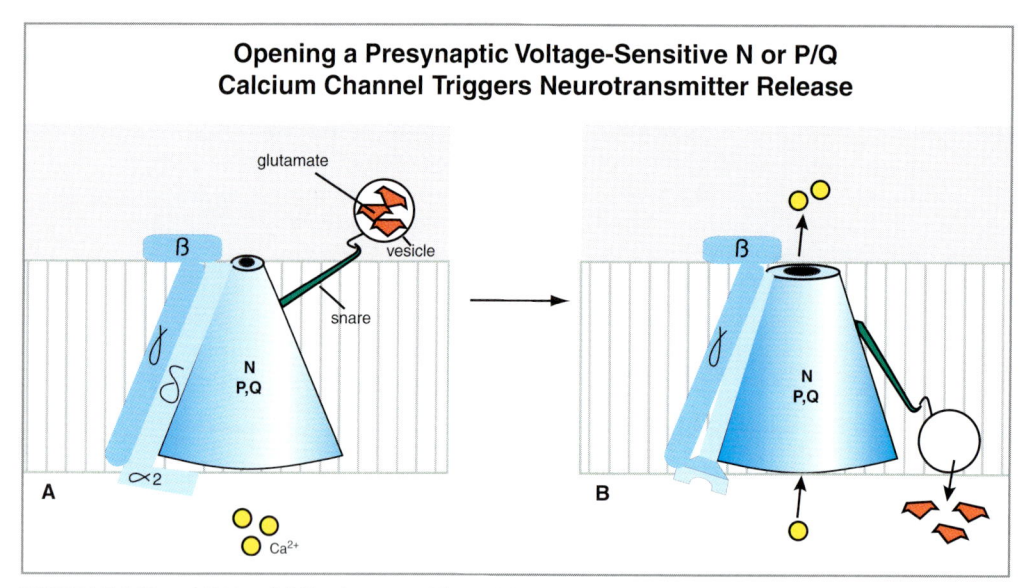

FIGURE 5-35A and B N and P/Q voltage-sensitive calcium channels. Voltage-sensitive calcium channels that are most relevant to psychopharmacology are termed N and P/Q channels. These ion channels are presynaptic and involved in the regulation of neurotransmitter release. The intracellular amino acids linking the second and third subunits of the alpha-1 unit form a snare that hooks onto synaptic vesicles (**A**). When a nerve impulse arrives, the snare "fires," leading to neurotransmitter release (**B**).

connect the N and P/Q VSCCs with the synaptic vesicle are shown in Figure 5-36. If a drug interferes with the ability of the channel to open and let in calcium, the synaptic vesicle stays tethered to the voltage-sensitive calcium channel. Neurotransmission can thus be prevented, and this may be desirable in states of excessive neurotransmission, such as pain, seizures, mania, or anxiety. This may explain the action of certain anticonvulsants (Table 5-6).

A novel transporter of uncertain mechanism is shown in Figure 5-36 on the synaptic vesicle, called SV2A. Transporters are discussed in considerable detail in Chapter 4. One of the anticonvulsants, levetiracetam, binds selectively and uniquely to this site, and by this mechanism is thought to interfere with neurotransmitter release and excitatory neurotransmission, thereby reducing seizures.

Indeed, it is neurotransmitter release that is the raison d'etre for presynaptic voltage sensitive N and P/Q channels. When a nerve impulse invades the presynaptic area, this causes the charge across the membrane to change, in turn opening the VSCC and allowing calcium to enter; this makes the synaptic vesicle dock into and merge with the presynaptic membrane, spewing its neurotransmitter contents into the synapse to effect neurotransmission (Figure 5-35). This conversion of an electrical impulse into a chemical message is triggered by calcium and sometimes called excitation-secretion coupling.

The alpha-2 delta site on N and P/Q presynaptic voltage-sensitive calcium channels is the target for a class of anticonvulsants known as alpha-2 delta ligands and comprises the drugs pregabalin and gabapentin (Figure 5-37). This is one of the best-characterized mechanisms of action of any anticonvulsant and specifically of any psychotherapeutic agent acting at a voltage-sensitive ion channel. It is known that pregabalin and gabapentin bind near the end of the alpha-2 protein, in the extracellular space, and preferentially to the

TABLE 5-6 Psychotropic drugs that hypothetically target voltage sensitive ion channels

Drug	Channel	Binding Site	Therapeutic Action
gabapentin	VSCC	alpha 2 delta ligand	anticonvulsant; neuropathic pain; anxiety; slow wave sleep
pregabalin	VSCC	alpha 2 delta ligand	anticonvulsant; neuropathic pain; anxiety; slow wave sleep
valproic acid, divalproex	? VSSC	unknown binding site	anticonvulsant; antimanic; mood stabilizer; antimigraine
lamotrigine	VSSC	channel site in alpha subunit	anticonvulsant; bipolar maintenance; bipolar depression; ? pain
carbamazepine	VSSC	channel site in alpha subunit	anticonvulsant; antimanic; neuropathic pain
oxcarbazepine	VSSC	channel site in alpha subunit	anticonvulsant; ? antimanic; ? neuropathic pain
zonisamide	? VSSC	?	anticonvulsant; ? antimanic

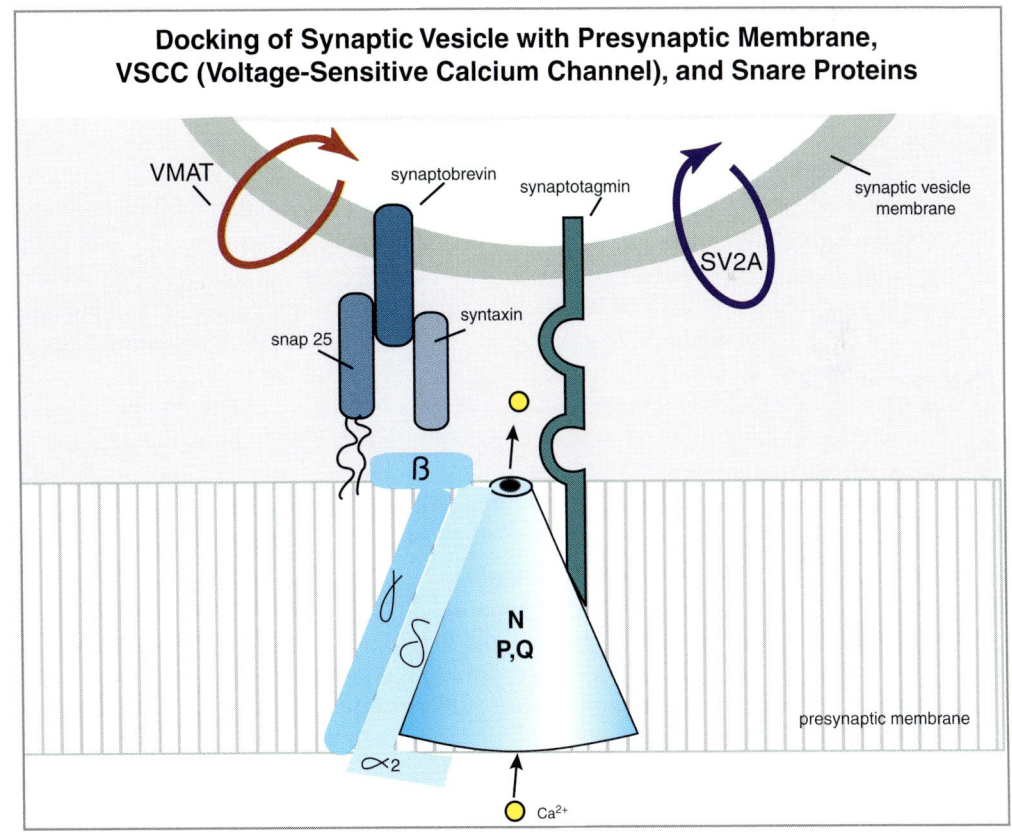

FIGURE 5-36 Snare proteins. Proteins that link the voltage-sensitive calcium channel to the synaptic vesicle, called snare proteins, are shown here; they include SNAP 25, synaptobrevin, syntaxin, and synaptotagmin. A VMAT (vesicular monoamine transporter) is shown on the left. Another transporter, SV2A, is shown on the right. The mechanism of this transporter is not yet clear, but the anticonvulsant levetiracetam is known to bind to this site.

Ion Channels and Enzymes as Targets of Psychopharmacological Drug Action | 157

Site of Action of Alpha-2 Delta Ligands as Selective Inhibitors of Presynaptic Voltage Sensitive N and P/Q Calcium Channels

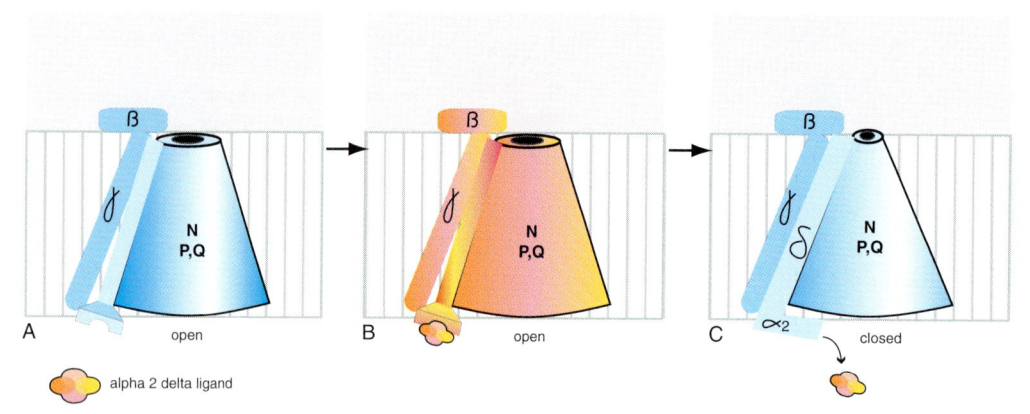

FIGURE 5-37A, B, and C Alpha-2 delta ligands. The alpha-2 delta unit is the known binding site for the alpha-2 delta ligands gabapentin and pregabalin (**A**). These agents bind to the alpha-2 delta unit at the alpha-2 protein when the channel is in the open conformation (**B**). This causes the channel to close, at which point the alpha-2 delta ligand loses its affinity for the binding site (**C**).

conformation of this protein when the ion channel is open (Figure 5-37). Thus, gabapentin and pregabalin bind to the "open channel conformation" of the alpha-2 delta protein at VSCCs (Figure 5-37B). When the drugs bind to the open VSCCs, this changes the conformation of the alpha-2 delta protein, which has the knock-on effect of closing the ion channel (Figure 5-37B). Once closed, the alpha-2 delta ligand loses its affinity for its binding site and falls off its receptor site (Figure 5-37C).

It is easy to see how this mechanism differs from the dihydropyridine antihypertensive calcium channel blockers by comparing Figure 5-37 with Figure 5-38. The antihypertensive calcium channel blockers interact with L channels, not with N or P/Q channels, and the drug binds to a very different site than does an alpha-2 delta ligand (Figure 5-38). L channel blockers bind to the channel itself, on the alpha 1 pore forming unit close to the cytoplasmic end of the channel (Figure 5-38).

Very few anticonvulsants have as well-characterized a mechanism of action as do the alpha-2 delta ligands. However, there are indications that many anticonvulsants bind to one or more voltage-sensitive ion channels, and the hypothetical sites of action of several anticonvulsants are listed in Table 5-6. Many of these anticonvulsants have several other uses in psychopharmacology, from chronic pain to migraine, from bipolar mania to bipolar depression to bipolar maintenance, and possibly as anxiolytics and sleep aids. These specific applications and more details about hypothetical mechanisms of action are explored in depth in the clinical chapters dealing with the various psychiatric disorders.

Ion channels and neurotransmission

Although the various subtypes of ligand-gated and voltage-sensitive ion channels are presented separately, the reality is that they work cooperatively during neurotransmission. When the actions of all these ion channels are well orchestrated, brain communication becomes a magical mix of electrical and chemical messages made possible by ion channels. The coordinated acts of ion channels during neurotransmission are illustrated in the next several figures (Figures 5-39 through 5-45).

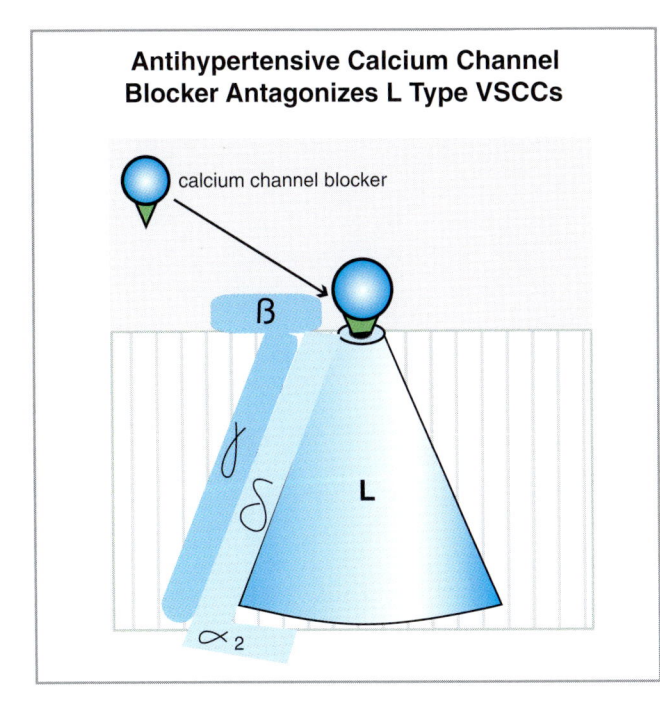

FIGURE 5-38 L voltage-sensitive calcium channels. Another type of voltage-sensitive calcium channel is the L channel, which exists both in the central nervous system and on vascular smooth muscle, where it regulates blood pressure. Dihydropyridine antihypertensive calcium channel blockers bind to this type of calcium channel by blocking the alpha-1 unit at a site near the intracellular opening.

The initiation of chemical neurotransmission by a neuron's ability to integrate all of its inputs and then translate them into an electrical impulse is presented in Chapter 3. We now show how ion channels are involved in this process (Figure 5-39). After a neuron receives and integrates its inputs from other neurons, it then encodes them into an action potential, and that nerve impulse is next sent along the axon via the voltage-sensitive sodium channels that line the axon (Figure 5-39).

The action potential may be described like lighting a fuse, with the fuse burning from the initial segment of the axon to the axon terminal. Movement of the burning edge of the fuse is carried out by a sequence of VSSCs that open one after the other, allowing sodium to pass into the neuron and then carrying the electrical impulse so generated along to the next VSSC in line (Figure 5-39). When the electrical impulse reaches the axon terminal, it meets voltage-sensitive calcium channels in the presynaptic neuronal membrane, already loaded with synaptic vesicles and ready to fire (see axon terminal of neuron A in Figure 5-39).

When the electrical impulse is detected by the voltmeter in the voltage-sensitive calcium channel, it opens the calcium channel, allows calcium to enter, and bang! the neurotransmitter is released in a cloud of synaptic chemicals from the presynaptic axon terminal via excitation-secretion coupling (see axon terminal of neuron A in Figure 5-40 and enlarged illustrations of this in Figure 5-41). Details of this process of excitation-secretion coupling are shown in Figure 5-41, beginning with the action potential about to invade the presynaptic terminal and with a closed VSSC sitting next to a closed but poised VSCC snared to its synaptic vesicle (Figure 5-41A). As the nerve impulse arrives in the axon terminal, it first hits the VSSC as a wave of positive sodium charges delivered by the openings of upstream sodium channels, which are detected by the sodium channel's voltmeter (Figure 5-41B). This opens the last sodium channel shown, allowing sodium to enter

Ion Channels and Enzymes as Targets of Psychopharmacological Drug Action

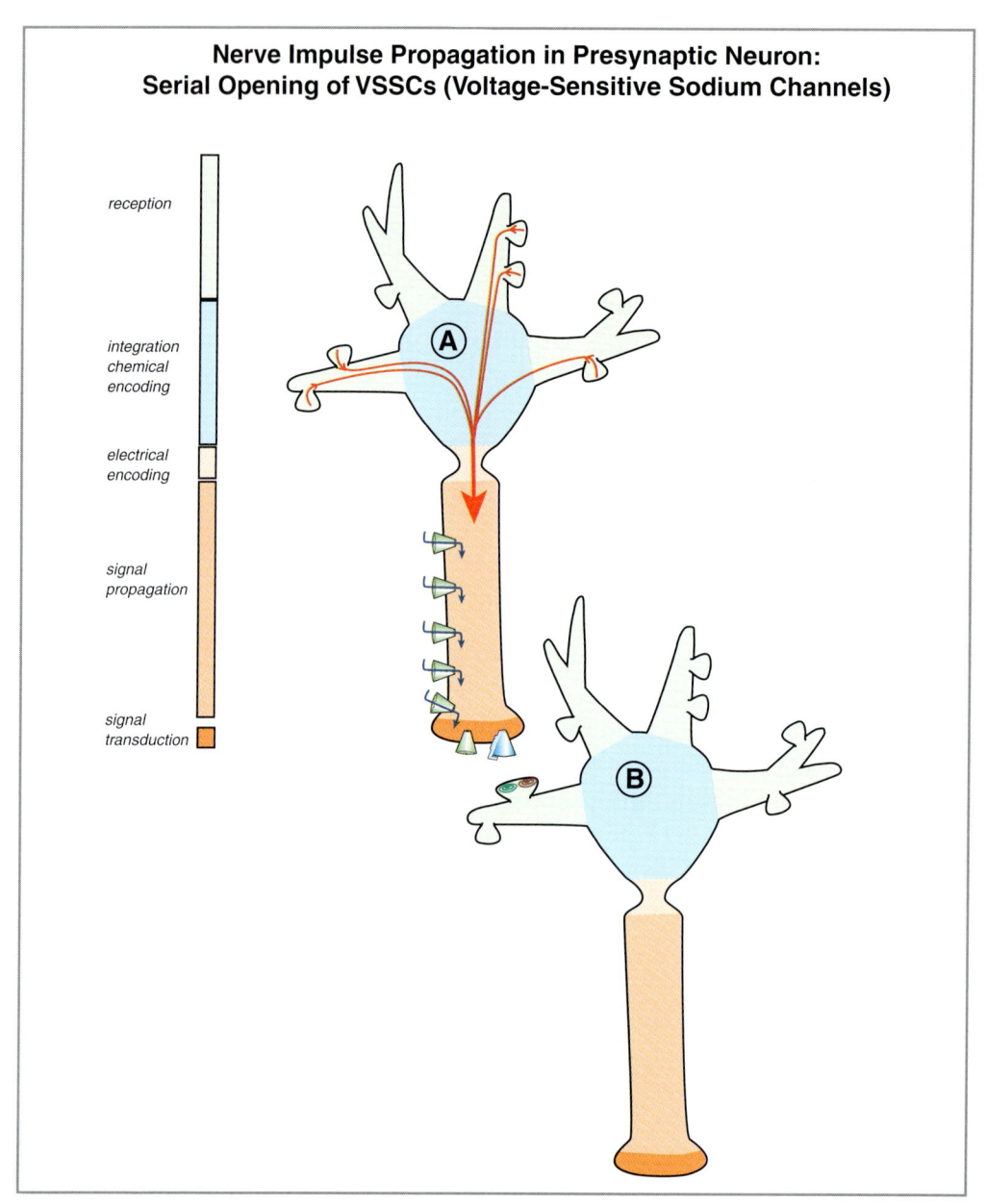

FIGURE 5-39 **Nerve impulse propagation in presynaptic neuron.** Nerve impulse propagation in the presynaptic neuron. Neuron A encodes an action potential and sends the nerve impulse along the axon via voltage-sensitive sodium channels, which open one by one to allow sodium to pass into the neuron. The electrical impulse ultimately reaches the axon terminal, where voltage-sensitive calcium channels are already primed and docked to synaptic vesicles.

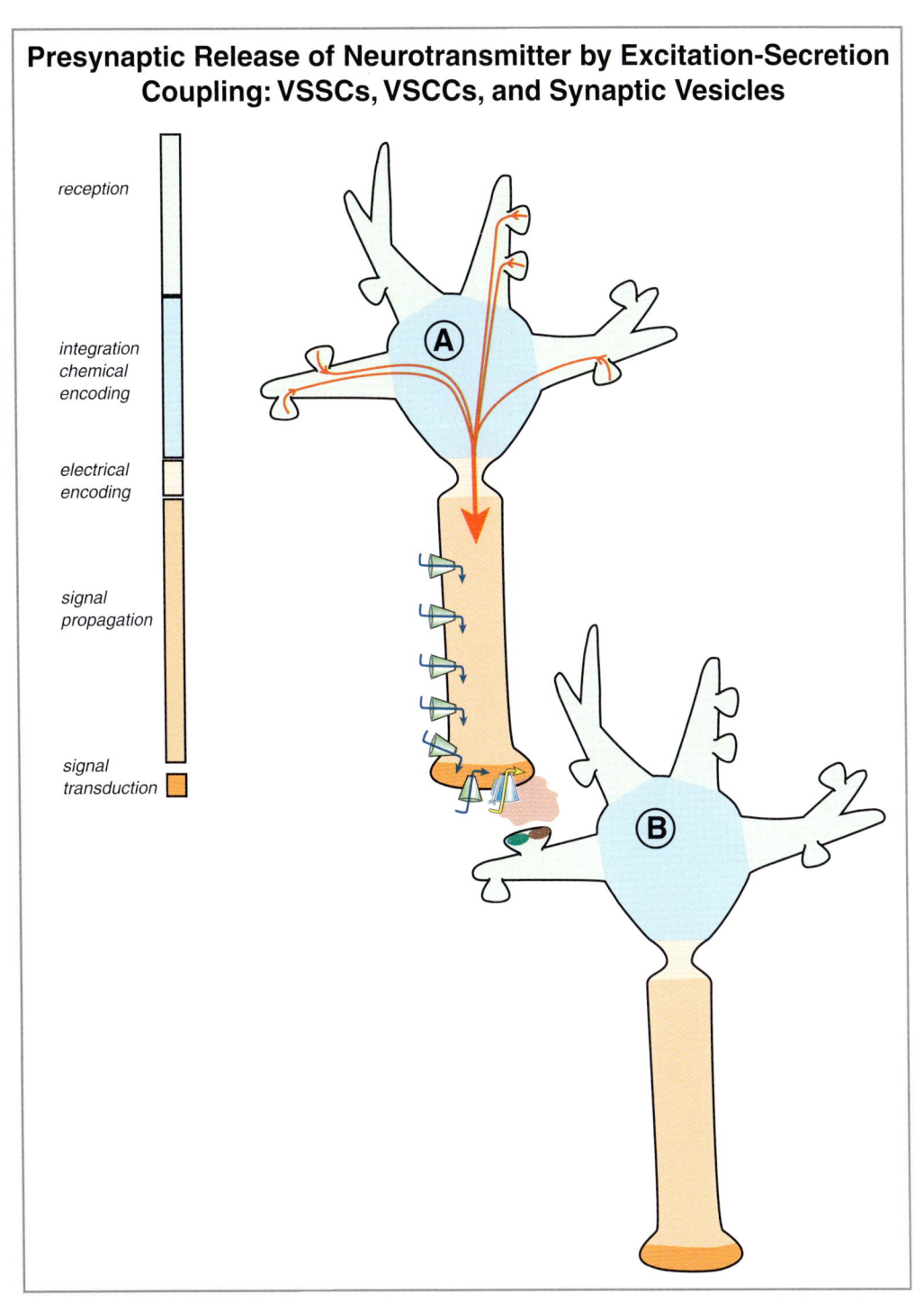

FIGURE 5-40 Presynaptic release of neurotransmitter. When voltage-sensitive calcium channels detect the electrical impulse, they open to allow calcium influx, which leads to neurotransmitter release. The conversion of the electrical impulse into a chemical message is referred to as excitation-secretion coupling and is shown here as a puff of color depicting release of the excitatory neurotransmitter glutamate.

Ion Channels and Enzymes as Targets of Psychopharmacological Drug Action | 161

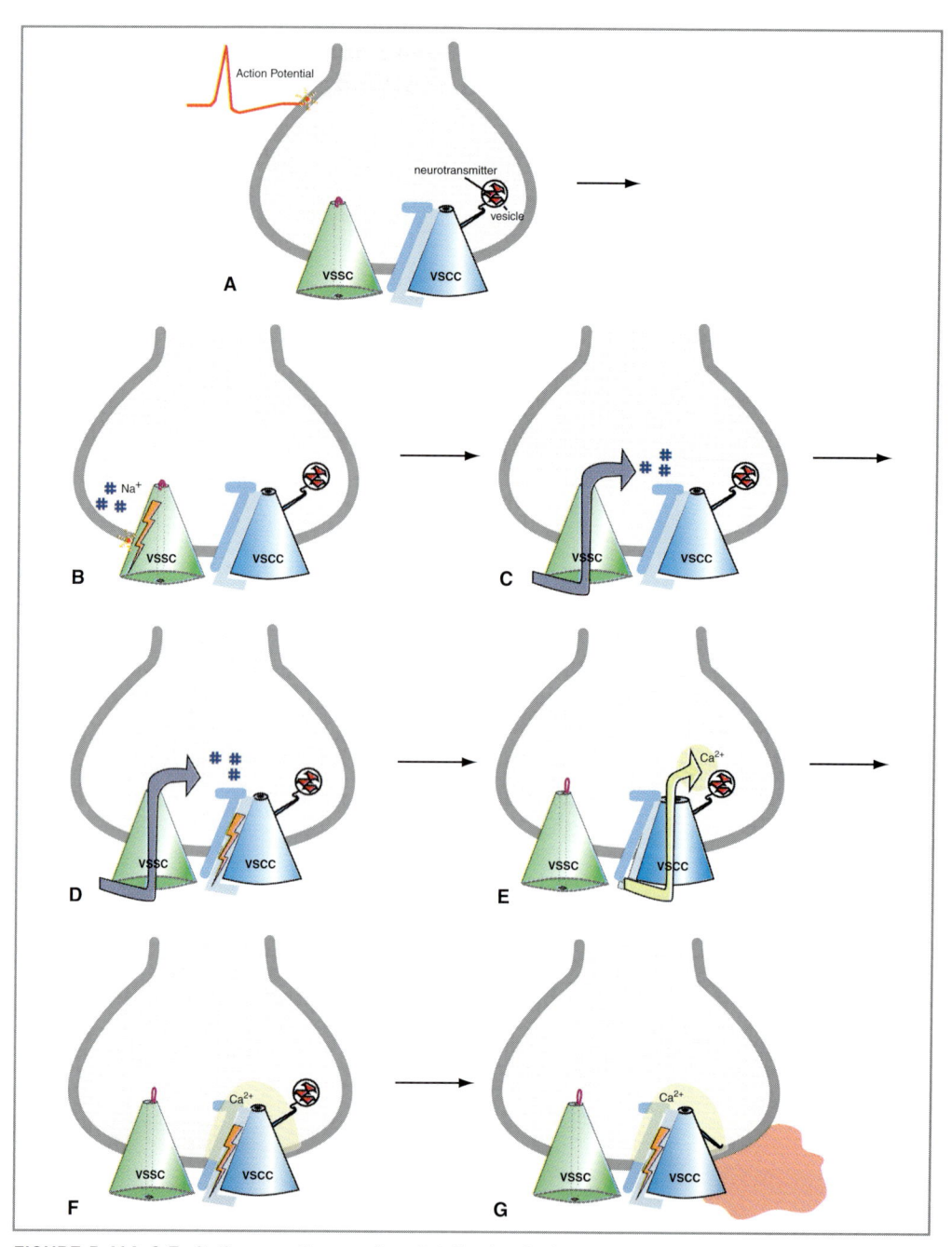

FIGURE 5-41A–G Excitation-secretion coupling. Details of excitation-secretion coupling are shown here. An action potential is encoded by the neuron and sent to the axon terminal via voltage-sensitive sodium channels along the axon (**A**). The sodium released by those channels triggers a voltage-sensitive sodium channel at the axon terminal to open (**B**), allowing sodium influx into the presynaptic neuron (**C**). Sodium influx changes the electrical charge of the voltage-sensitive calcium channel (**D**), causing it to open and allow calcium influx (**E**). As the intraneuronal concentration of calcium increases (**F**), the synaptic vesicle is caused to dock and merge with the presynaptic membrane, leading to neurotransmitter release (**G**).

162 | Essential Psychopharmacology

Signal Transduction of Glutamate into Excitatory Neurotransmission and Signal Propagation in the Postsynaptic Neuron

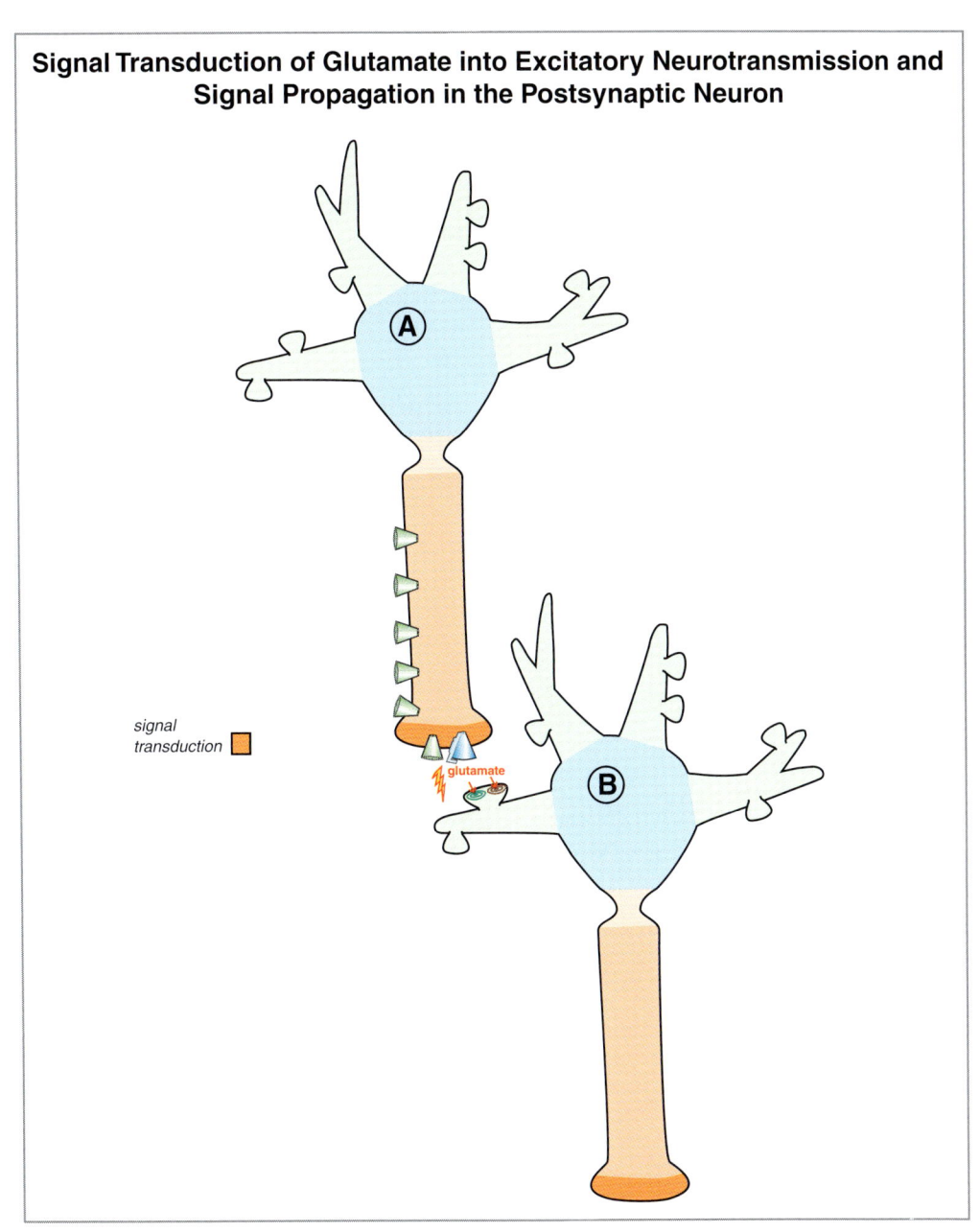

FIGURE 5-42 **Signal propagation in the postsynaptic neuron.** Signal transduction of glutamate into excitatory neurotransmission and signal propagation in the postsynaptic neuron. Neurotransmitter released presynaptically by neuron A is received at postsynaptic dendrites of neuron B.

(Figure 5-41C). The consequence of this sodium entry is to change the electrical charge near the calcium channel; this is then detected by the VSCC's voltmeter (Figure 5-41D). Next, the calcium channel opens (Figure 5-41E). At this point, chemical neurotransmission has been irreversibly triggered, and the translation of an electrical message into a chemical message has begun. Calcium entry from the VSCC now increases the local concentrations of this ion in the vicinity of the VSCC, the synaptic vesicle, and the neurotransmitter release

Ion Channels and Enzymes as Targets of Psychopharmacological Drug Action | 163

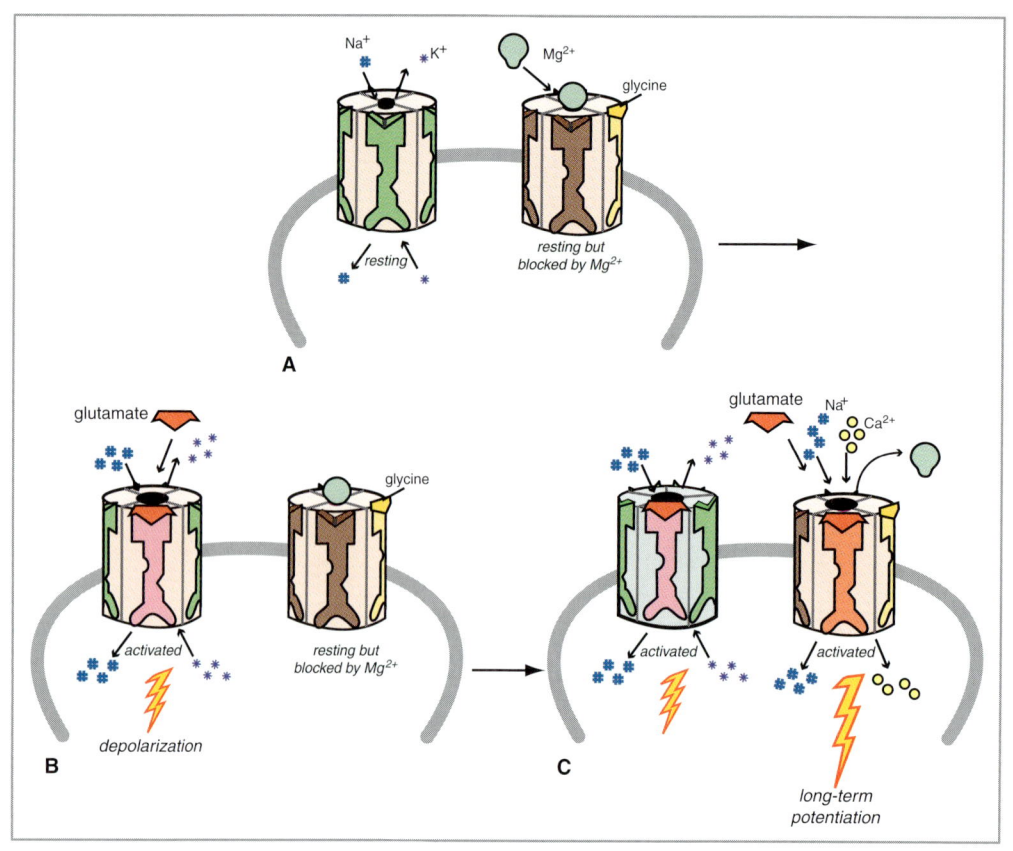

FIGURE 5-43A, B, and C Signal propagation via glutamate receptors. Enlarged view of the dendrite of neuron B from Figure 5-42. **(A)** On the left is an AMPA receptor with its sodium channel in the resting state, allowing minimal sodium to enter the cell in exchange for potassium. On the right is an NMDA receptor with magnesium blocking the calcium channel and glycine bound to its site. **(B)** When glutamate arrives, it binds to the AMPA receptor, causing the sodium channel to open, thus increasing the flow of sodium into the dendrite and of potassium out of the dendrite. This causes the membrane to depolarize and triggers a postsynaptic nerve impulse. **(C)** Depolarization of the membrane removes magnesium from the calcium channel. This, coupled with glutamate binding to the NMDA receptor in the presence of glycine, causes the NMDA receptor to open and allow calcium influx. Calcium influx through NMDA receptors contributes to long-term potentiation, a phenomenon that may be involved in long-term learning, synaptogenesis, and other neuronal functions.

machinery (Figure 5-41F). This causes the synaptic vesicle to dock into the inside of the presynaptic membrane and then merge with it, spewing its neurotransmitter contents out of the membrane and into the synapse (Figure 5-41G). This amazing process occurs almost instantaneously and simultaneously as many VSCCs release neurotransmitter from many synaptic vesicles.

By now, only about half of the sequential phenomena of chemical neurotransmission have been described. The other half occurs on the other side of the synapse. That is, reception of the released neurotransmitter now occurs in neuron B (Figure 5-42). In this example, the neurotransmitter released from the presynaptic neuron A is glutamate. Now we shall visualize how some ligand-gated ion channels can get into the act of chemical neurotransmission at the dendrite shown for neuron B in Figure 5-42 by enlarging what is happening here in Figure 5-43. Two different ionotrophic receptors for glutamate are

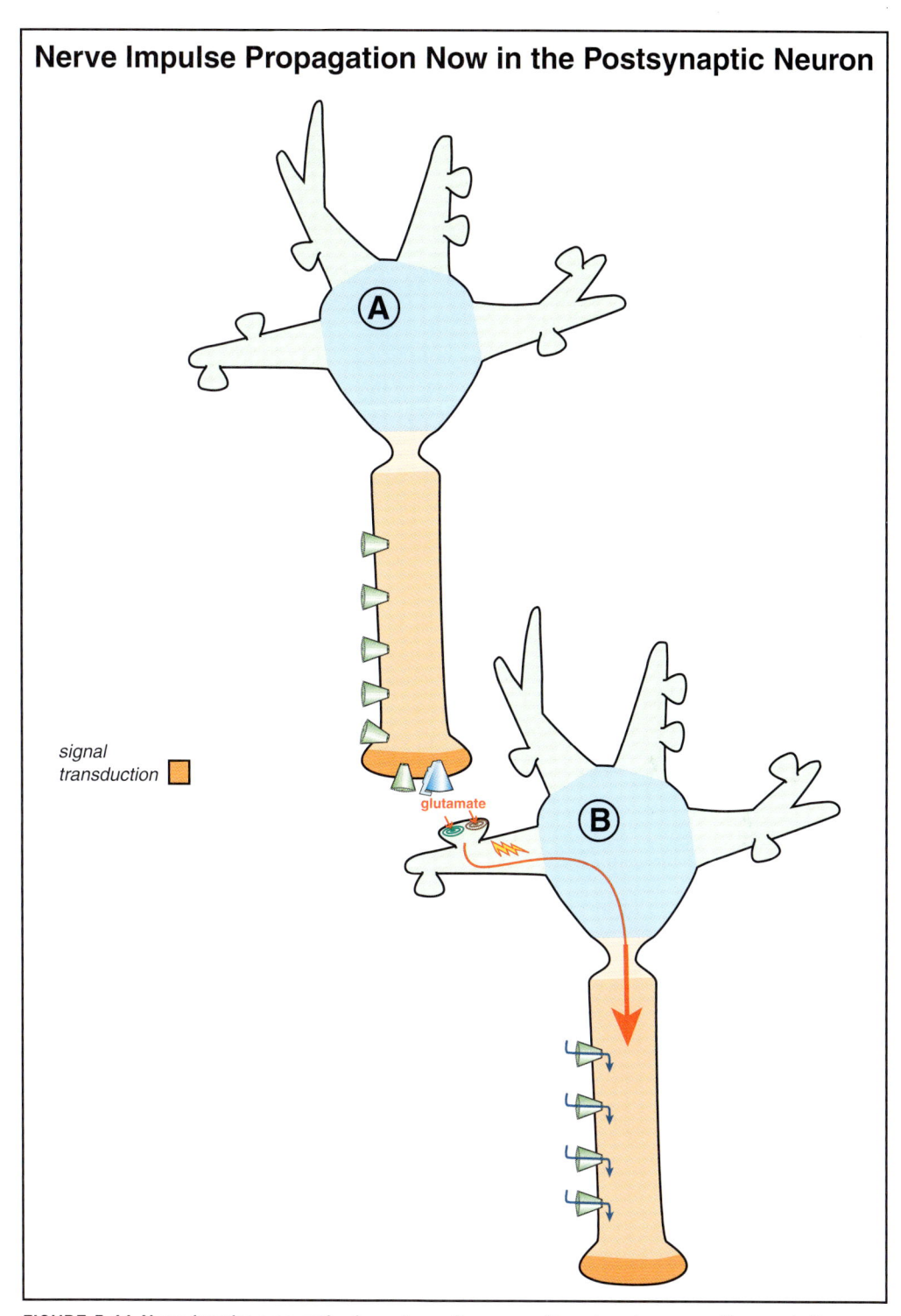

FIGURE 5-44 Nerve impulse propagation in postsynaptic neuron. Nerve impulse propagation now in the postsynaptic neuron. When glutamate binds to the AMPA receptor at the dendrite of neuron B, sodium enters the cell and causes the membrane to depolarize. This leads to encoding of an action potential, which is sent to the axon terminal via voltage-sensitive sodium channels along the axon.

Ion Channels and Enzymes as Targets of Psychopharmacological Drug Action | 165

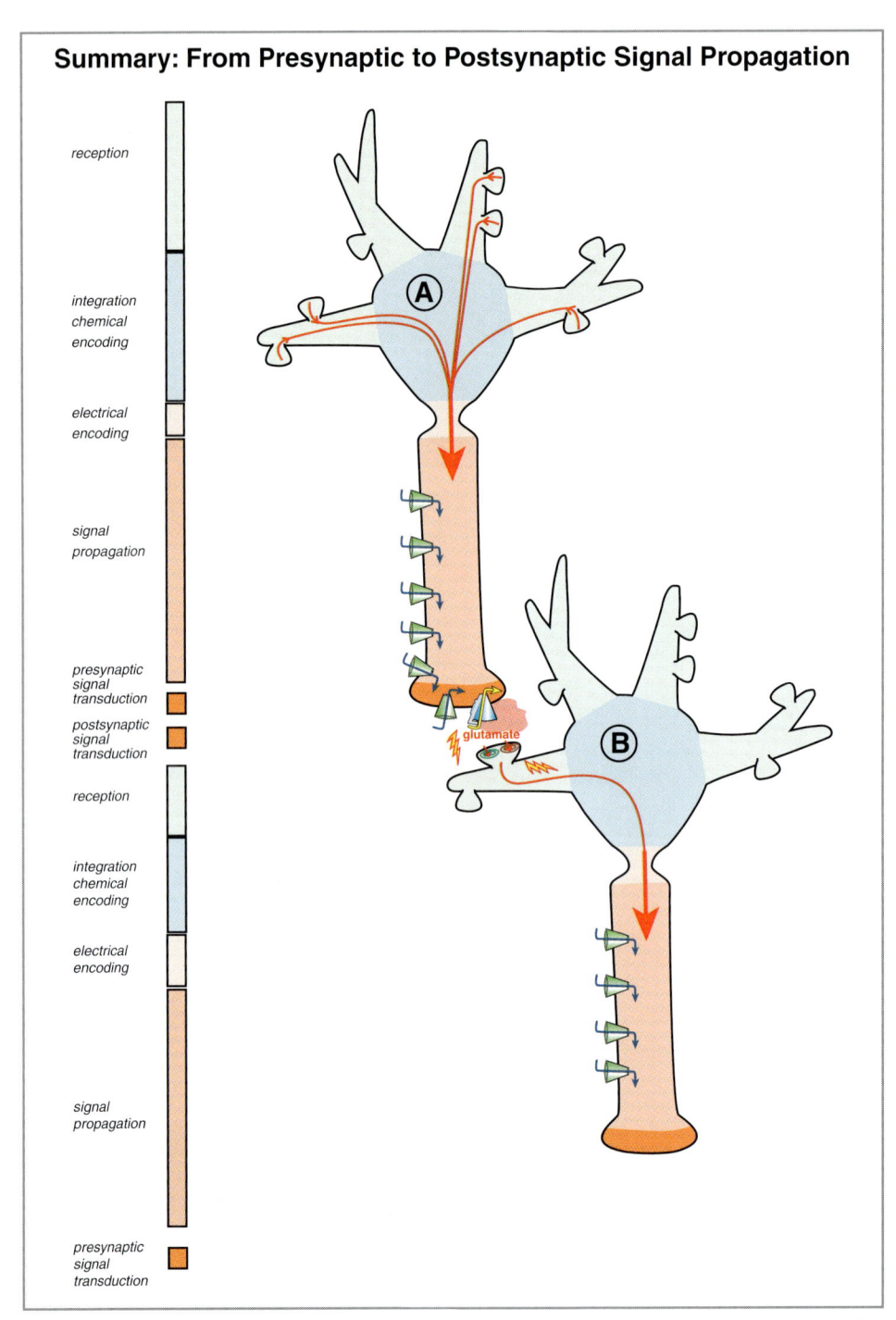

FIGURE 5-45 Signal propagation. Summary of signal propagation from presynaptic to postsynaptic neuron. A nerve impulse is generated in neuron A, and the action potential is sent along the axon via voltage-sensitive sodium channels until it reaches voltage-sensitive calcium channels linked to synaptic vesicles full of neurotransmitters in the axon terminal. Opening of the voltage-sensitive calcium channel and consequent calcium influx causes neurotransmitter release into the synapse. Arrival of neurotransmitter at postsynaptic receptors on the dendrite of neuron B triggers depolarization of the membrane in that neuron and, consequently, postsynaptic signal propagation.

Essential Psychopharmacology

awaiting the arrival of glutamate in Figure 5-43A. On the left is an AMPA receptor with its sodium channel in the resting state, allowing only a small amount of sodium to go into the cell and be exchanged with potassium. On the right is an NMDA receptor with the cotransmitter glycine already sitting in its receptor and with magnesium plugging up its calcium channel. However, this channel is still in the resting state, for two reasons. First, glutamate cotransmitter is missing from its site. Second, the membrane is not depolarized, so magnesium can block the channel.

When glutamate arrives, the first event shown is its interaction with the AMPA receptor on the left (Figure 5-43B). Glutamate is the ligand that now causes conformational changes in this ligand-gated ion channel to activate it and thus to open the associated sodium channel. Sodium entry into the dendrite causes the membrane to depolarize and send a nerve impulse along the way postsynaptically (Figure 5-43B). The view of depolarization of neuron B and propagation of this impulse along the second neuron is given in Figure 5-44.

Finally, if all the conditions are right – namely, the presence of both cotransmitters glutamate and glycine plus membrane depolarization to remove the magnesium block – a second ionotrophic channel can open on the right (Figure 5-43C). This is the NMDA receptor, and when the channel associated with it opens, calcium enters the postsynaptic dendrite and, rather than causing depolarization, contributes to a different process called long-term potentiation, a phenomenon that may be involved in long-term learning, synaptogenesis, and other neuronal functions.

This whole process – from the generation of a nerve impulse and its propagation along neuron A to its nerve terminal, then sending chemical neurotransmission to neuron B and finally propagating this second nerve impulse along neuron B – is summarized in Figure 5-45. Voltage-sensitive sodium channels in presynaptic neuron A propagate the impulse there; then voltage-sensitive calcium channels in presynaptic neuron A release the neurotransmitter glutamate. Ligand-gated ion channels on dendrites in postsynaptic neuron B next receive this chemical input and translate this chemical message back into a nerve impulse propagated in neuron B by voltage-sensitive sodium channels in that neuron. Also, ligand-gated ion channels in postsynaptic neuron B translate the glutamate chemical signal into another type of electrical phenomenon, called long-term potentiation, to cause changes in the function of neuron B.

Enzymes as sites of psychopharmacological drug action

Enzymes are involved in multiple aspects of chemical neurotransmission, as discussed extensively in Chapter 3 on signal transduction. Every enzyme is the theoretical target for a drug acting as an enzyme inhibitor. However, in practice, only a minority of currently known drugs utilized in the clinical practice of psychopharmacology are enzyme inhibitors.

Enzyme activity is the conversion of one molecule into another, namely a substrate into a product (Figure 5-46). The substrates for each enzyme are unique and selective, as are the products. A substrate (Figure 5-46A) comes to the enzyme to bind at the enzyme's active site (Figure 5-46B) and departs as a changed molecular entity called the product (Figure 5-46C). The inhibitors of an enzyme are also unique and selective for one enzyme compared to another. In the presence of an enzyme inhibitor, the enzyme cannot bind to its substrates. The binding of inhibitors can be either irreversible (Figure 5-47) or reversible (Figure 5-48).

When an irreversible inhibitor binds to the enzyme, it cannot be displaced by the substrate; thus that inhibitor binds irreversibly (Figure 5-47). This is depicted as binding

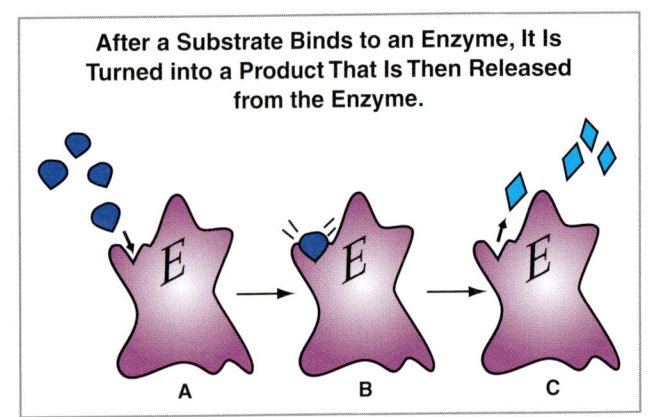

FIGURE 5-46A, B, and C Enzyme activity. Enzyme activity is conversion of one molecule into another. Thus, a substrate is said to be turned into a product by enzymatic modification of the substrate molecule. The enzyme has an active site at which the substrate can bind specifically (**A**). The substrate then finds the active site of the enzyme and binds to it (**B**) so that a molecular transformation can occur, changing the substrate into the product (**C**).

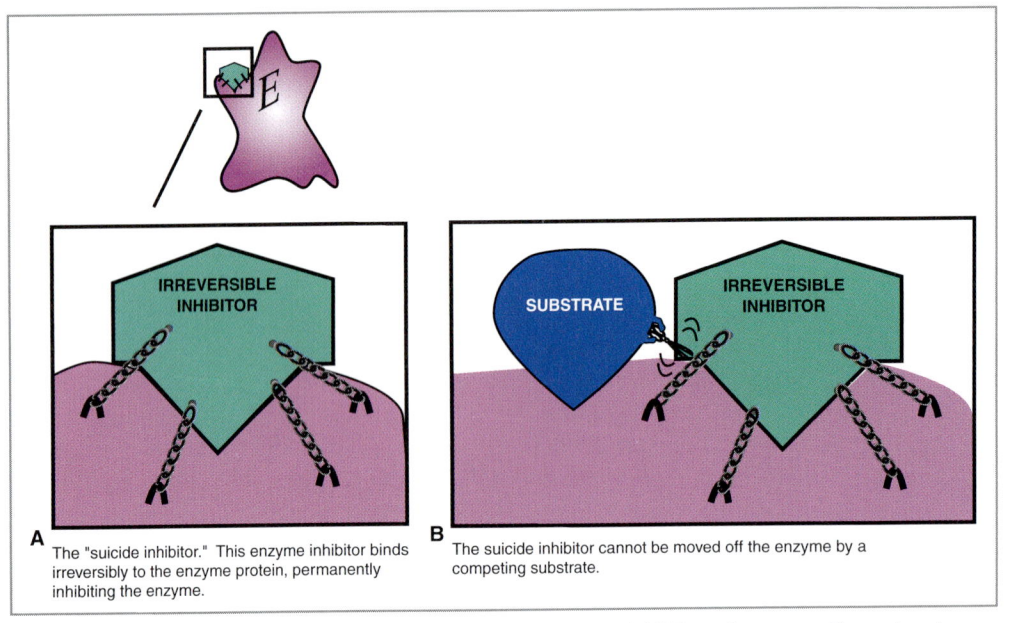

FIGURE 5-47A and B Irreversible enzyme inhibitors. Some drugs are inhibitors of enzymes. Shown here is an irreversible inhibitor of an enzyme, depicted as binding to the enzyme with chains (**A**). A competing substrate cannot remove an irreversible inhibitor from the enzyme, depicted as scissors unsuccessfully attempting to cut the chains off the inhibitor (**B**). The binding is locked so permanently that such irreversible enzyme inhibition is sometimes called the work of a "suicide inhibitor," since the enzyme essentially commits suicide by binding to the irreversible inhibitor. Enzyme activity cannot be restored unless another molecule of enzyme is synthesized by the cell's DNA.

with chains (Figure 5-47A) that cannot be cut with scissors by the substrate (Figure 5-47B). The irreversible type of enzyme inhibitor is sometimes called a "suicide inhibitor" because it covalently and irreversibly binds to the enzyme protein, permanently inhibiting it and therefore essentially "killing" it by making the enzyme nonfunctional forever (Figure 5-47). Enzyme activity in this case is restored only when new enzyme molecules are synthesized.

However, in the case of reversible enzyme inhibitors, an enzyme's substrate is able to compete with that reversible inhibitor for binding to the enzyme and can shove it off

A The reversible inhibitor. This inhibitor can come off the enzyme protein and thus can be reversed.

B

C The inhibitor can then be moved off the enzyme by a competing substrate.

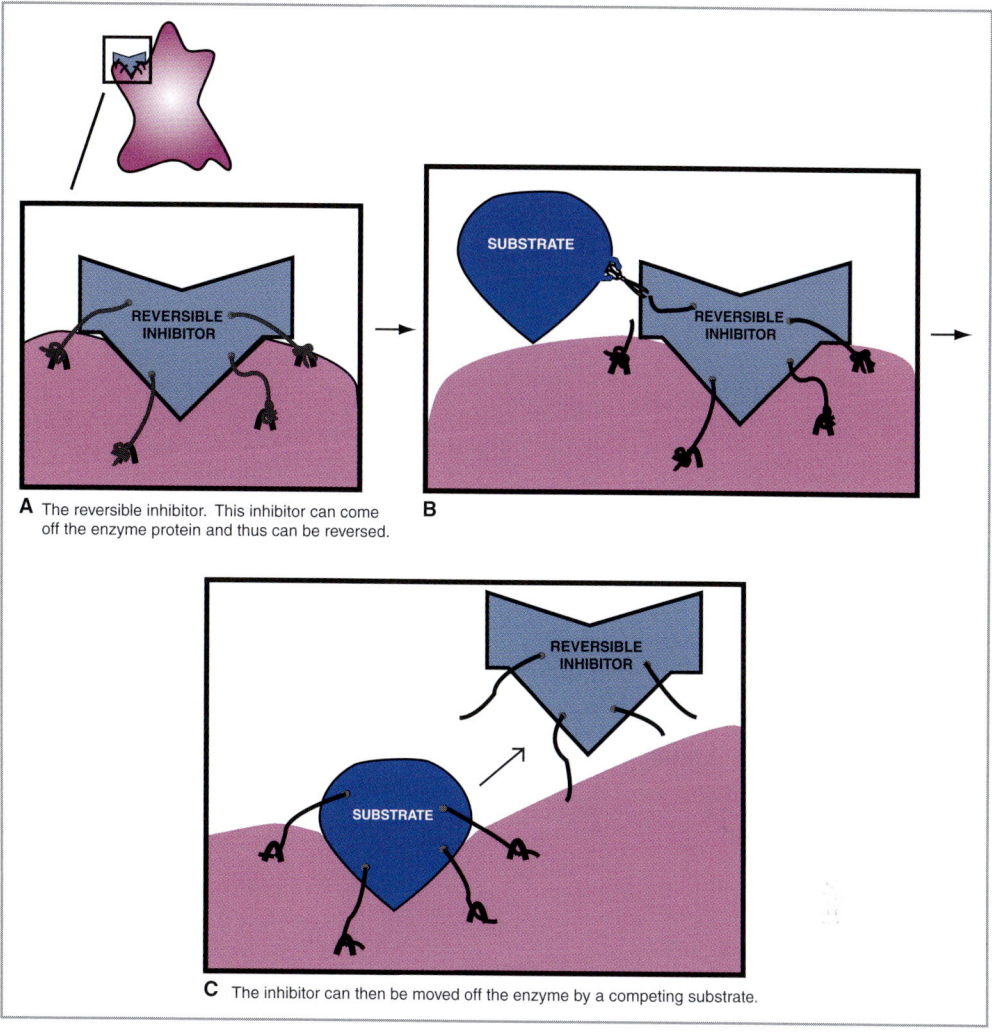

FIGURE 5-48A, B, and C Reversible enzyme inhibitors. Other drugs are reversible enzyme inhibitors, depicted as binding to the enzyme with a string (**A**). A reversible inhibitor can be challenged by a competing substrate for the same enzyme. In the case of a reversible inhibitor, the molecular properties of the substrate are such that it can get rid of the reversible inhibitor, depicted as scissors cutting the string that binds the reversible inhibitor to the enzyme (**B**). The consequence of a substrate competing successfully for reversal of enzyme inhibition is that the substrate displaces the inhibitor and shoves it off (**C**). Because the substrate has this capability, the inhibition is said to be reversible.

the enzyme (Figure 5-48). Whether the substrate or the inhibitor "wins" or predominates depends on which one has the greater affinity for the enzyme and/or is present in the greater concentration. Such binding is called "reversible." Reversible enzyme inhibition is depicted as binding with strings (Figure 5-48A), such that the substrate can cut them with scissors (Figure 5-48B), displace the enzyme inhibitor, and bind the enzyme itself with its own strings (Figure 5-48C).

These concepts can potentially be applied to any enzyme system. Several enzymes involved in neurotransmission, including in the synthesis and destruction of neurotransmitters as well as in signal transduction, are shown in Figure 5-49. Only two enzymes are

TABLE 5-7 Enzymes Directly Targeted by Psychotropic Drugs

monoamine oxidase
acetylcholine esterase

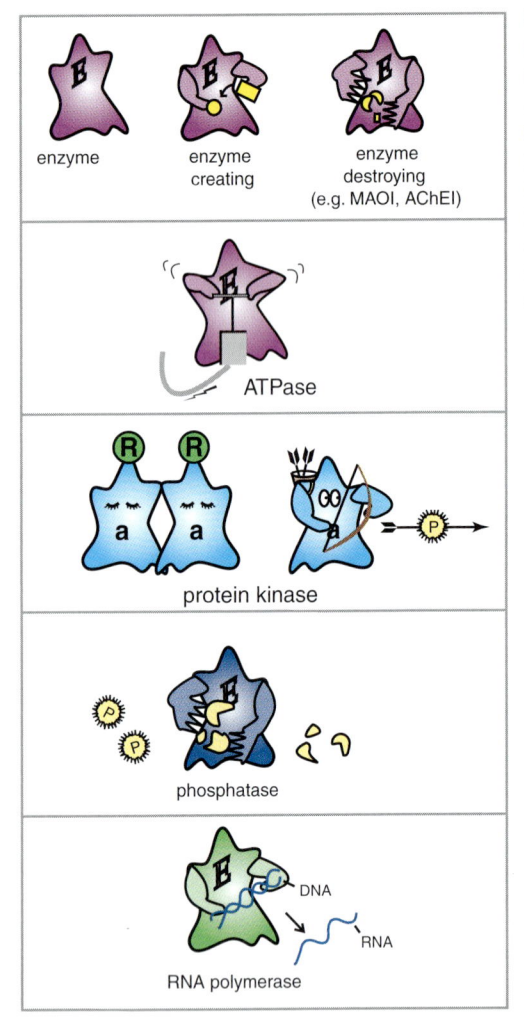

FIGURE 5-49 Enzymes. Enzymes are very important to the functioning of the cell. Some enzymes create molecules (i.e., build them up) and some enzymes destroy molecules (i.e., tear them apart). One enzyme responsible for using energy is ATPase. Three important classes of enzymes that regulate gene expression include both active and inactive forms of protein kinases; various phosphatases, which can reverse the actions of protein kinases; and finally RNA polymerase enzymes, which catalyze the transcription of DNA into RNA.

known to be targeted by psychotropic drugs currently used in clinical practice: monoamine oxidase (MAO) and acetylcholinesterase (Table 5-7). MAO inhibitors are discussed in more detail in the chapter on antidepressants, and acetylcholinesterase inhibitors are discussed in more detail in the chapter on cognition. Other enzymes may be indirectly targeted by other psychotropic drugs as a consequence of the actions of drugs on signal transduction, but the details of these actions on enzymes remain to be fully understood (Table 5-8). Given the rapid elucidation of the functions of an increasing number of enzymes, we should expect to see an ever-growing number of enzyme inhibitors entering psychopharmacology in future years.

TABLE 5-8 Enzymes possibly indirectly targeted by psychotropic drugs

Na+/K+ ATPase (sodium pump)
H+ ATPase (proton pump)
Kinases
Phosphatases
Neurotransmitter synthesizing enzymes
second messenger synthesizing enzymes
RNA polymerase

ATP = adenosine triphosphate
RNA = ribonucleic acid

TABLE 5-9 Nuclear hormone receptors as potential targets for psychotropic drugs

estrogen agonists
thyroid agonists
glucocorticoid antagonists
mineralocorticoid antagonists?

TABLE 5-10 Receptor tyrosine kinases and their signal transduction enzymes as potential targets for psychotropic drugs

Activation of BDNF cascades?
Activation of other neurotrophin cascades
Blockade of interleukins?
Blockade of cytokines?
Activation of MAP kinase cascades?
Inhibition of GSK–3? (e.g. lithium)

BDNF = brain derived neurotrophic factor
MAP = mitogen activated protein kinase
GSK = glycogen synthase kinase

Other novel or potential targets of psychopharmacological drug action

A few other novel or potential sites of drug action that may bear fruit for future psychotropic drugs are worth mentioning. Four key signal transduction pathways are described in Chapter 3, on chemical neurotransmission, and are illustrated in Figure 3-11; however, only two of these pathways are described so far in Chapters 4 and 5 as targets of psychotropic drugs. Those that are currently well-known targets of psychotropic drugs include the G protein–linked receptor systems discussed in Chapter 4 and the ligand-gated ion channels discussed in this chapter. The other two pathways include nuclear hormone receptors and receptor tyrosine kinases (Figure 3-11 and Table 3-1). Both of these are potential targets of novel psychotropics (Tables 5-9 and 5-10), but currently there are only glimpses of how this will be translated into new therapeutics (Figures 5-50 and 5-51 and Table 5-11).

Psychopharmacologists currently utilize as adjunctive treatments some hormones, such as thyroid and estrogen, that are natural agonists for nuclear hormones (Table 5-9). Another potential way to target this signal transduction system is to utilize antagonists of glucocorticoids (Table 5-9 and Figure 5-50). Excessive glucocorticoid action has long been

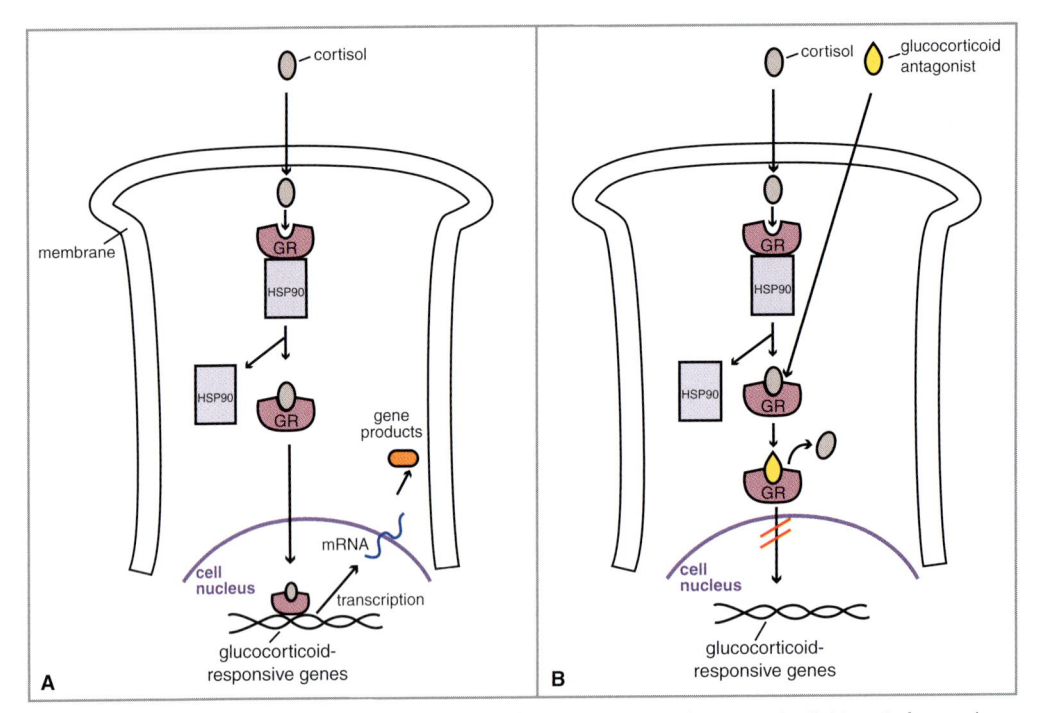

FIGURE 5-50A and B Nuclear hormone receptors. Nuclear hormone receptors are potential targets for novel psychotropic drugs. One way to target this signal transduction system is through antagonists of glucocorticoids. **(A)** Cortisol normally acts at a glucocorticoid receptor in the cell's cytoplasm that is bound to a chaperone protein called heat-shock protein 90 (HSP90). When cortisol binds to its receptor, the chaperone protein dissociates from the receptor, allowing the hormone-receptor complex to travel into the cell nucleus, where it finds glucocorticoid-responsive genes, triggering transcription into gene products. **(B)** Glucocorticoid antagonists compete with cortisol at the glucocorticoid receptor, resulting in the lack of expression of glucocorticoid genes.

hypothesized to be important in depression, anxiety, and stress, and several compounds that antagonize this system are in clinical testing. Normally, cortisol interacts with a glucocorticoid (GR) receptor in the cell's cytoplasm, not in the cell membrane (Figure 5-50A). That glucocorticoid receptor exists in the cytoplasm bound to a chaperone protein (heat-shock protein 90 or HSP 90). When cortisol binds to its glucocorticoid receptor, the chaperone protein dissociates from the receptor, allowing the hormone-receptor complex to travel into the cell nucleus, where it finds glucocorticoid-responsive genes and triggers their transcription into gene products (Figure 5-50A).

In order to interfere with excessive glucocorticoid activity in various psychiatric disorders, glucocorticoid antagonists, such as mefipristone, can be administered to compete for cortisol at the glucocorticoid receptor and inhibit glucocorticoid binding, resulting in the lack of expression of glucocorticoid genes (Figure 5-50B). The possibility that glucocorticoid antagonists will enter clinical practice for conditions such as psychotic depression or various states linked to excessive stress is a subject of current active research.

The fourth signal transduction cascade is that of receptor tyrosine kinases (Table 5-10 and Figure 5-51). Examples of the plethora of neurotrophins and growth factors that act on this system are given in Table 5-11. There are many current hypotheses concerning the therapeutic potential of targeting this pathway. For example, this signal transduction cascade has the potential to promote synaptic plasticity, neurogenesis, and neuronal survival

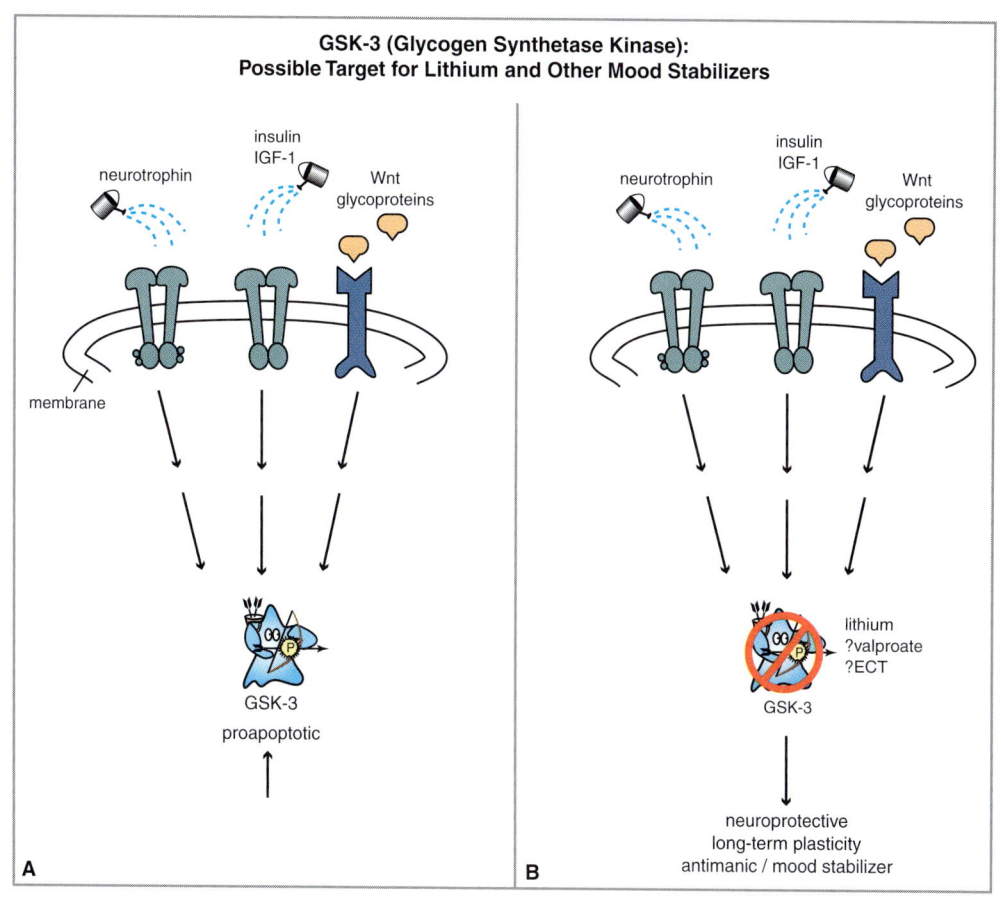

FIGURE 5-51A and B Receptor tyrosine kinases. Receptor tyrosine kinases are potential targets for novel psychotropic drugs. (**A**) Some neurotrophins, growth factors, and other signaling pathways act through a downstream phosphoprotein, an enzyme called GSK-3 (glycogen synthase kinase), to promote cell death (proapoptotic actions). (**B**) Lithium and possibly some other mood stabilizers may inhibit this enzyme, which could lead to neuroprotective actions and long-term plasticity as well as possibly contribute to mood stabilizing actions.

(described in Chapter 2). Some theoretical targets for such desirable therapeutic actions are listed in Table 5-10. Mimicking or blocking many of the neurotrophins or growth factors listed in Table 5-11 by acting on the receptor tyrosine kinase signal transduction cascade may lead to incredibly novel therapeutic agents and is the subject of intense current interest and investigation.

It is possible that one psychotropic drug, lithium, fortuitously acts somewhere in this type of a signal transduction pathway (Figure 5-51). That is, some neurotrophins, growth factors, and other signaling pathways act through a specific downstream phosphoprotein, an enzyme called GSK-3 (glycogen synthase kinase), to promote cell death (proapoptic actions). Lithium has the capacity to inhibit this enzyme (Figure 5-51B). It is possible that such inhibition may be physiologically relevant, because it could lead to neuroprotective actions and long-term plasticity and may contribute to the antimanic and mood-stabilizing actions known to be associated with lithium. Development of novel GSK-3 inhibitors is in progress.

TABLE 5-11 Examples of different neurotrophins and growth factors in the brain

Neurotrophins
- BNDF (brain derived neurotrophic factor)
- NGF (nerve growth factor)
- NT3 (neurotrophin 3)
- NT4 (neurotrophin 4)
- NT5 (neurotrophin 5)

Tissue Growth Factors
- GDNF family (glial derived neurotrophic factor)
  - GDNF
  - neurturin
  - persepkin

- TGF-β family (tumor growth factor beta)
  - TGF β1–3
  - Bone morphogenic proteins (BMB)
  - Myostatin
  - sonic hedgehog

- Insulin family
  - insulin
  - insulin like growth factor I (IGF-I)
  - insulin like growth factor II (IFG-II)

- Fibroblast growth factor family (FGF)
  - FGF (acidic)
  - FGF (basic)

- Epidermal growth factor (EGF) family
  - EGF
  - ACh–receptor inducing activity (ARIA)
  - TGF-α (tumor growth factor alpha)
  - amphiregular
  - heregulin

Cytokines
- Neuropoietic cytokines
  - CNTF (ciliary neurotrophic factor)
  - LIF (leukemia inhibitory factor)
  - cardiotrophin

- Colony stimulating factors
  - G-CSF, M-CSF, GM-CSF (granulocyte colony stimulating factor; G-CSF receptor)

- Interleukins
  - IL2
  - IL4, others (CD 132 receptor)
  - IL3, IL5, others (CD 131 receptor)
  - IL1α
  - IL2β
  - IL6 (gp 130–linked receptor)

- Leptin

Interferons
- IFN-α
- IFN-β
- IFN-γ

Tumor Necrosis Factor
- TNF-α
- TNF-β

Summary

Ion channels and enzymes are key targets of many psychotropic drugs. This is not surprising, because these targets are key regulators of chemical neurotransmission and the signal transduction cascade.

There are two major classes of ion channels: ligand-gated and voltage-sensitive ion channels. The opening of ligand-gated ion channels is regulated by neurotransmitters, whereas the opening of voltage-sensitive ion channels is regulated by the charge across the membrane in which they reside.

Ligand-gated ion channels are both ion channels and receptors. They are also commonly called ionotrophic receptors as well as ion channel–linked receptors. One subclass of ligand-gated ion channels has a pentameric structure and includes GABA-A receptors, nicotinic cholinergic receptors, serotonin-3 receptors, and glycine receptors. The other subclass of ligand-gated ion channels has a tetrameric structure and includes many glutamate receptors, including the AMPA, kainate and NMDA subtypes.

Ligands act at ligand-gated ion channels across an agonist spectrum, from full agonist, to partial agonist, to antagonist, to inverse agonist. Ligand-gated ion channels can be regulated not only by neurotransmitters acting as agonists but also by molecules interacting at other sites on the receptor, either boosting the action of neurotransmitter agonists as positive allosteric modulators (PAMs) or diminishing the action of neurotransmitter agonists as negative allosteric modulators (NAMs). In addition, these receptors exist in several states, from open, to resting, to closed, to inactivated, to desensitized.

The second major class of ion channels is called either voltage-sensitive ion channels or voltage-gated ion channels, since they are opened and closed by the voltage charge across the membrane. The major channels from this class of interest to psychopharmacologists are the voltage-sensitive sodium channels or VSSCs and the voltage-sensitive calcium channels or VSCCs. Numerous anticonvulsants bind to various sites on these channels and may exert their anticonvulsant actions by this mechanism, as well as their actions as mood stabilizers, treatments for chronic pain, anxiolytic actions, and sleep effects.

Enzymes are important regulatory elements of chemical neurotransmission but are not yet frequent targets of psychopharmacological drugs in current use. Numerous novel therapeutic agents that target enzymes are being investigated.

The signal transduction cascade for nuclear hormones is another potential site for novel therapeutics, from estrogen and thyroid agonist actions to glucocorticoid antagonist actions. Finally, the signal transduction cascade for receptor tyrosine kinases provides a rich set of new targets for novel drugs in psychopharmacology and may already include lithium, which interacts within this system.

CHAPTER 6

Psychiatric Genetics

- Genes and psychiatry: the classic theory
- Genes and psychiatry: the new paradigm
- Endophenotypes
- Traveling the hypothetical path from gene to mental illness
- Stress diathesis hypothesis
- Personality as buffer or amplifier of stress
- Degrees of genetic abnormalities and environmental stressors
- Summary

After decades of research, genetics in psychiatry may finally be coming of age. Genetic models now exist that are generating rapid and significant progress in the quest to explain the role of genes in mental illnesses. The answers are not simple and the questions remain numerous and complex, but the results are exciting and have the potential to transform the practice of psychiatry and psychopharmacology.

Here we discuss the new paradigm for genes and psychiatry that has recently emerged. That paradigm conceptualizes genes not so much as direct causes of mental illness but as direct causes of subtle molecular abnormalities that create risk for mental illness. Genes may thus act by "biasing" an individual's brain circuits toward inefficient information processing and possible breakdown into psychiatric symptoms under certain environmental circumstances.

Soon the modern psychopharmacologist in clinical practice may have tools to assess the risk of patients and their family members for various psychiatric disorders, the risk of suffering specific side effects of various drug treatments, and the likelihood that specific drugs will act effectively on their symptoms. In the future, a psychopharmacologist may even be able to investigate mental illness with information from the DNA of their patients, much as a crime scene investigator (CSI) already does for solving a mystery. Therefore, understanding the state of the art for genes and psychiatry can position psychopharmacologists to become early "CNS-Is" ("central nervous system investigators") who, as the results of research pour into clinical practice, are able to utilize data from genetic analysis of their patients' DNA.

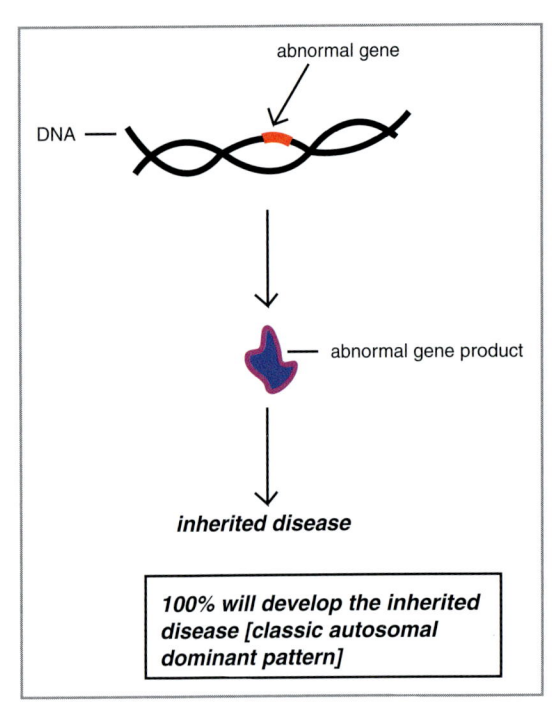

FIGURE 6-1 Classic autosomal dominant pattern. This figure depicts the classic view of an inherited disease. In this case, a single abnormal gene expresses an abnormal gene product, with the consequence of causing an inherited disease in a classic autosomal dominant pattern.

Genes and psychiatry: the classic theory

Not too many years ago, researchers were looking for the single genetic abnormality thought to cause a specific psychiatric disorder. This model has proven successful in defining other disorders, such as Huntington's disease (Figure 6-1) and cystic fibrosis. Why not, therefore, an abnormal inherited gene as the cause of schizophrenia or depression (Figure 6-2)? Decades of research and new scientific developments now make that paradigm look overly simplistic.

Why have genes for mental illnesses been so hard to find? The answer is that genes do not encode mental illnesses (Figure 6-2). This is not so hard to believe, since mental illnesses are defined as mixtures of symptoms packaged into syndromes. These syndromes are consensus statements from committees writing the nosologies of psychiatric disorders for the *Diagnostic and Statistical Manual of Mental Disorders* (DSM) of the American Psychiatric Association and the *International Classification of Diseases* (ICD). Thus, mental illnesses are not diseases.

When you think about it, the genome obviously did not evolve out of the DSM; rather, the writers of the DSM evolved out of the genome! It is no wonder that committees of experts have so far failed to define the symptoms and syndromes that have evolved out of numerous genes, since in many ways they have been working backwards – that is, from the syndrome to the gene. We are just in the earliest days of working in the other direction – namely, from the genome to the mental illness. Thus, although the DSM and ICD nosologies are useful in communicating about the symptoms of mental illness syndromes, modern genetics in many ways has freed clinicians from the tyranny of nosology in order to focus on symptoms, as we will see below in this chapter and throughout the rest of this book.

**Classic Theory:
Genes Cause Mental Illness**

hypothetical mental illness gene

abnormal gene product causes neuronal malfunction

mental illness

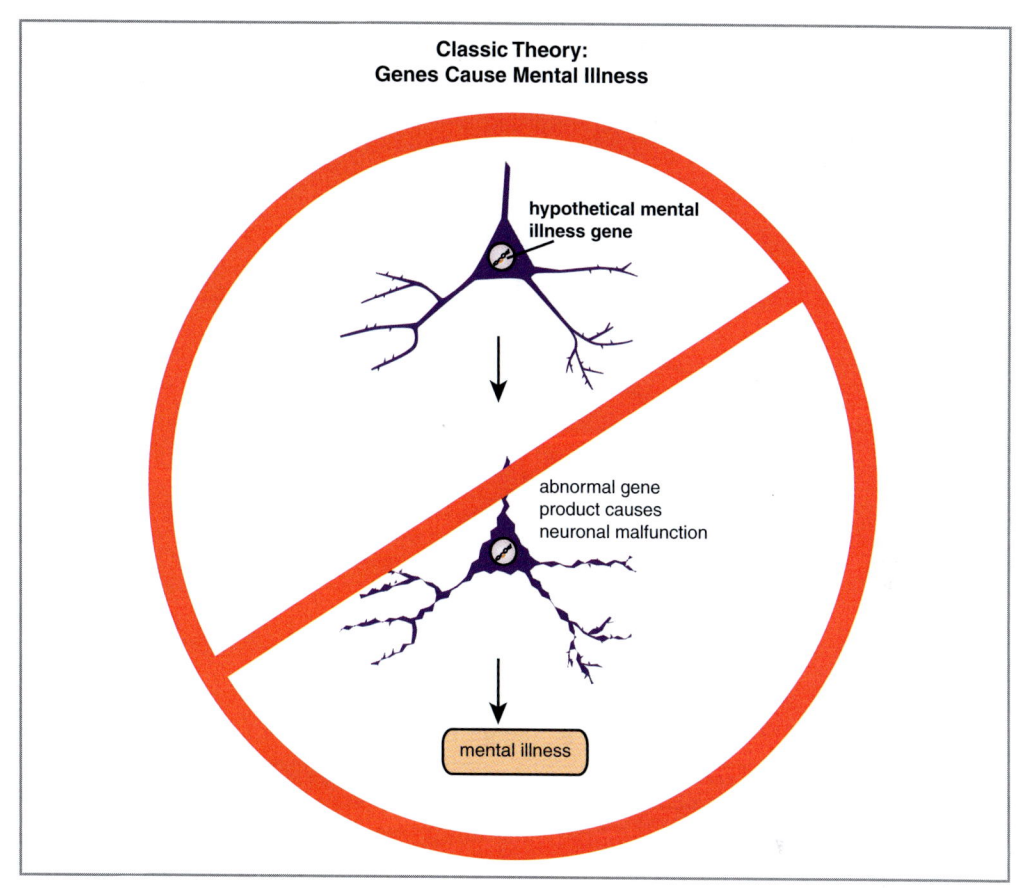

FIGURE 6-2 Classic theory of inherited disease. According to the classic theory of inherited disease, a single abnormal gene can also cause a mental illness. That is, an abnormal gene would produce an abnormal gene product, which, in turn, would lead to neuronal malfunction that directly causes a mental illness. However, no such gene has been identified, and there is no longer any expectation that such a discovery might be made. This is indicated by the red cross-out sign over this theory.

The next stage in trying to unravel the contribution of genes to mental illness was to look for genes for personality, temperament, behaviors or symptoms of a mental illness but not for a mental illness per se (Figure 6-3). However, no such genes have been found. Why have genes for personality and behaviors also been so hard to find? The answer is that genes also do not encode personality or behavior (Figure 6-3).

Genes and psychiatry: the new paradigm

Well, if genes encode neither mental illness nor behavior, what do they encode? The answer is that genes encode proteins, and that in mental illnesses, individual genes code for a subtle molecular abnormality caused by a genetically altered protein (Figure 6-4). This could include proteins that regulate neurodevelopment, such as neuronal selection, migration, differentiation, or synaptogenesis. It could also include proteins ranging from enzymes to transporters to signal transduction molecules, synaptic plasticity machinery, axonal and dendritic protein transport machinery, and many more (Figure 6-6).

It is a fact that many of the most common and puzzling illnesses of the twenty-first century are no longer thought to be caused by a huge biological contribution from

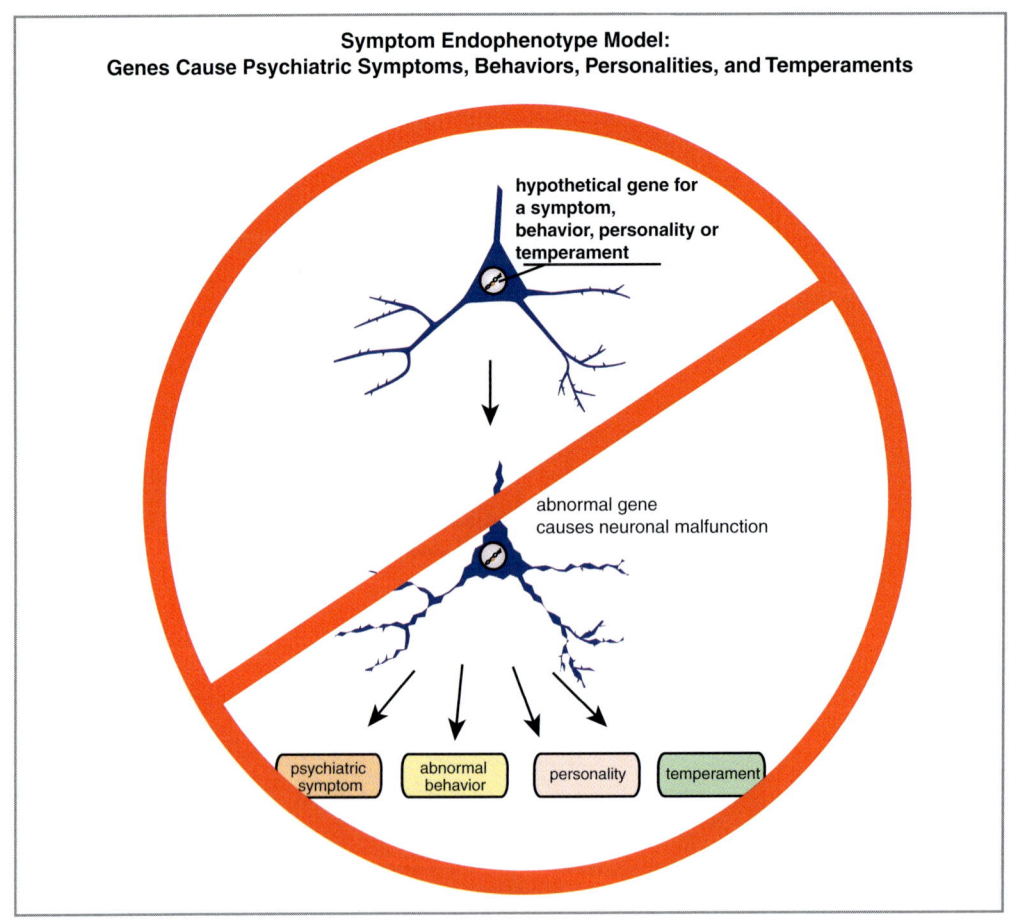

FIGURE 6-3 Symptom endophenotype model. Another theory, the symptom endophenotype model, posits that, rather than genes causing mental illness, genes instead cause individual symptoms, behaviors, personalities, or temperaments. Thus, an abnormal gene encoding for a symptom, behavior, or trait would cause neuronal malfunction leading to that symptom, behavior, or trait. However, no genes for personality or behavior have been identified, and there is no longer any expectation that such a discovery might be made – as indicated by the red cross-out sign over this theory.

a single gene (Figure 6-1). No such abnormality is sufficient to cause any known mental illness.

So what is the pathway from gene to mental illness (Figure 6-5 and 6-6)? The hypothesis is that mental illnesses are caused not by a single gene nor by a single subtle genetic abnormality but by multiple small contributions from several genes, all interacting with environmental stressors. This is sometimes called "complex genetics," for obvious reasons. It is not simple dominant or recessive genetics, but a complex set of risk factors that bias a person toward an illness but do not cause it.

This concept applies not only to mental illnesses such as schizophrenia and bipolar disorder but also to hypertension and diabetes mellitus. In this model, a person inherits risk, not illness, and there are several possible ways to combine sufficient risk with sufficient opportunity to express that risk in the environment by summing all of these factors, reaching the tipping point, and then developing the illness.

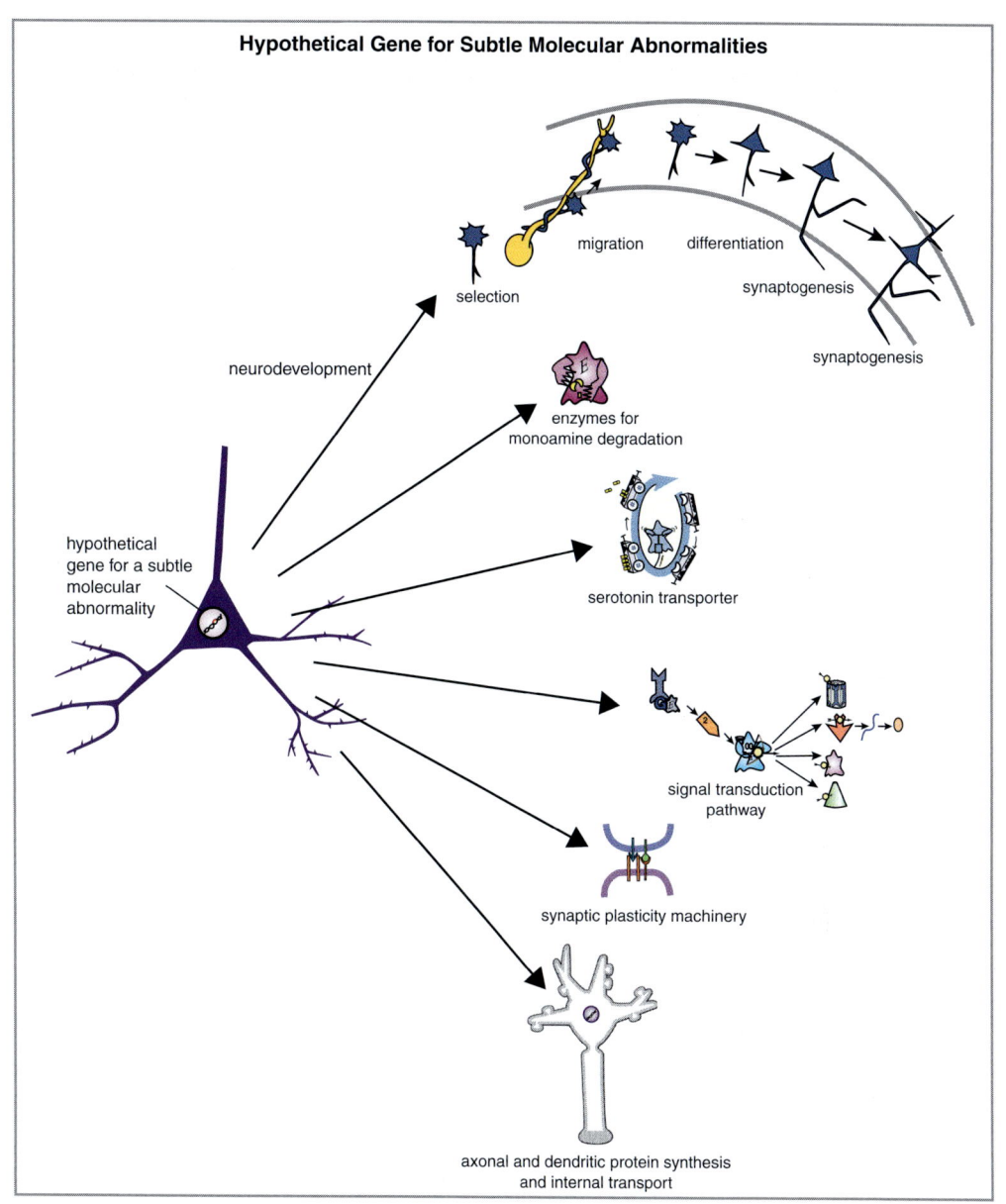

FIGURE 6-4 Subtle molecular abnormalities. Genes do not directly encode mental illnesses, behaviors, or personalities. Instead, they encode proteins. In some cases, genes may produce genetically altered proteins that code for subtle molecular abnormalities, which in turn may be linked to the development of psychiatric symptoms. Thus, a gene may code for an abnormality in the neurodevelopmental process or in the synthesis or activity of enzymes, transporters, receptors, components of signal transduction, synaptic plasticity machinery, and other neuronal components. Each subtle molecular abnormality may convey risk for the development of mental illness rather than directly causing a mental illness.

Endophenotypes

Scientists exploring along the path from gene to mental illness have discovered a few important intermediaries that assist in unraveling the contribution of genes (Figure 6-5). Lying on this pathway between the subtle molecular abnormality encoded by a gene that

Hypothetical Path from Gene to Behavior

genotype
↓
subtle molecular abnormality
↓
abnormal information processing (biological endophenotype)
↓
behavior with complex functional interactions and emergent phenomena (symptom endophenotype)

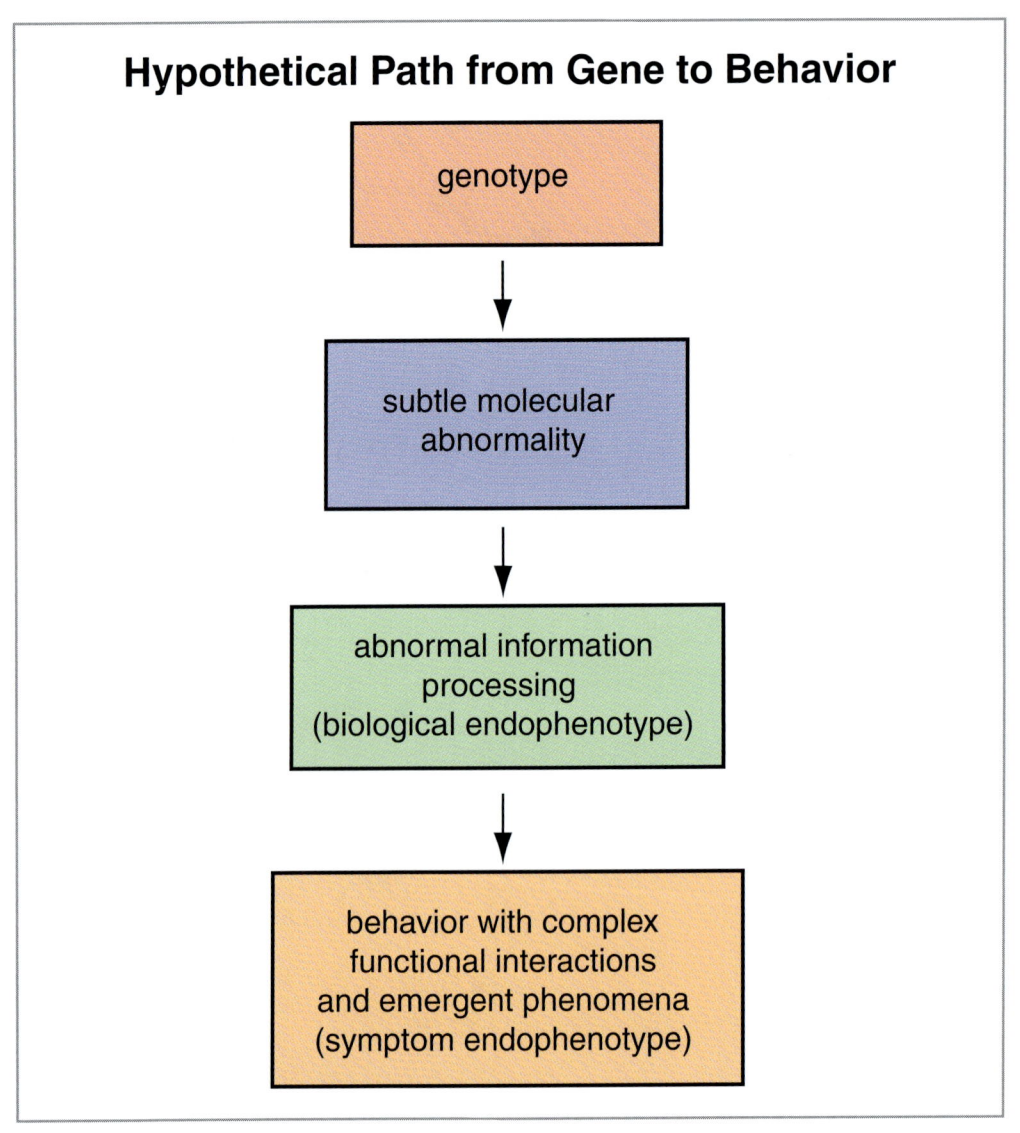

FIGURE 6-5 Hypothetical path from gene to behavior. On the hypothetical path from gene to behavior lie endophenotypes, or "intermediate phenotypes," which are measurable intermediaries more closely linked to the gene than is the disease. Abnormal cortical activity in response to stimuli (abnormal information processing) is an example of a *biological* endophenotype. A single symptom associated with a mental illness is an example of a *symptom* endophenotype. In the path from gene to mental illness, a genotype may code for a subtle molecular abnormality that is closely linked to a biological endophenotype (such as abnormal information processing in specific neuronal circuits), which, in turn, may be linked to a symptom or behavior (symptom endophenotype) associated with a mental illness.

contributes risk for a mental illness and the mental illness itself are intermediaries called "endophenotypes" (Figures 6-5 and 6-6). They are also sometimes called "intermediate phenotypes."

If the illness is the phenotype, lying at the end of the path, then there are two classes of intermediate phenotypes, called biological endophenotypes and symptom endophenotypes,

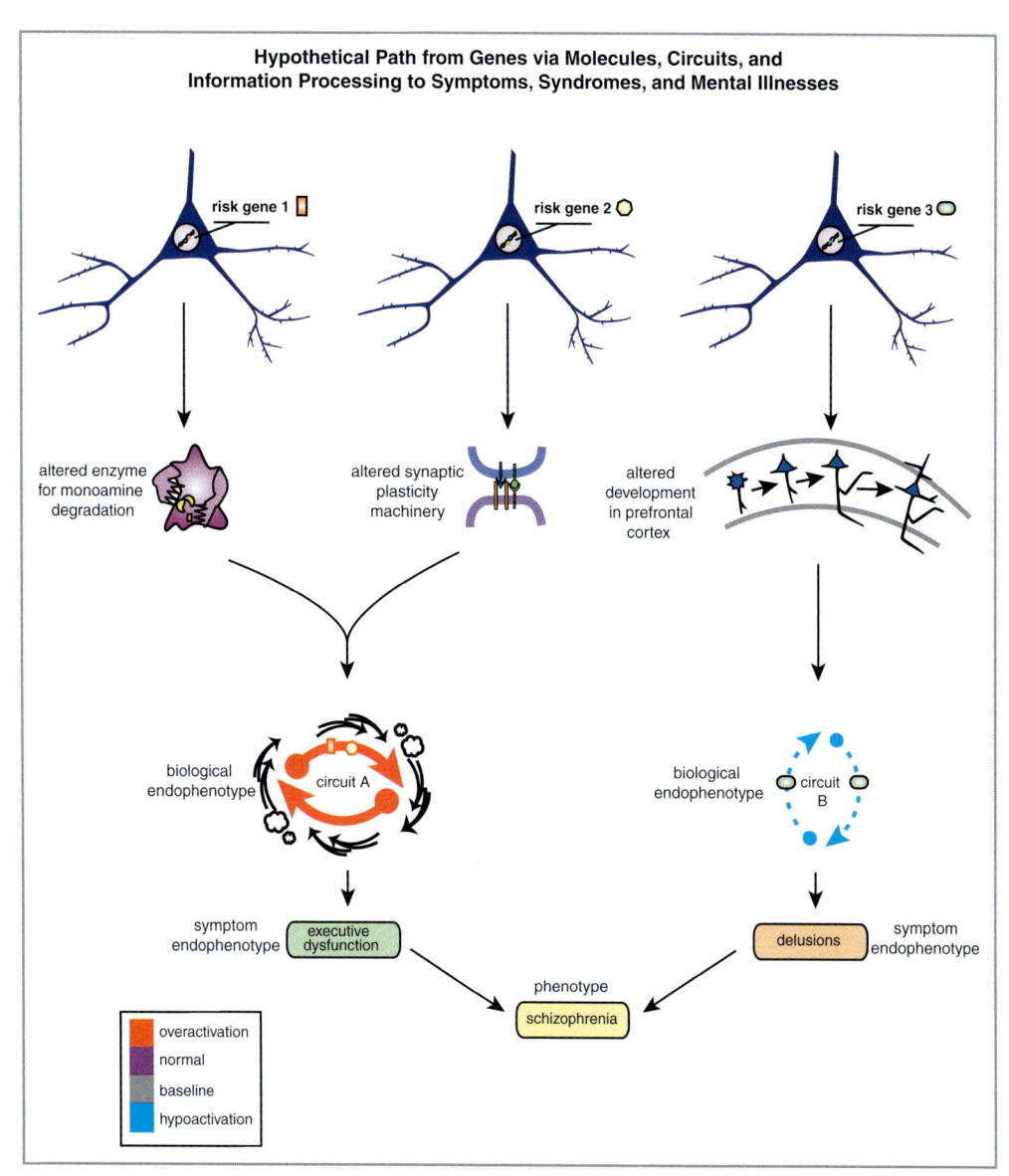

FIGURE 6-6 Hypothetical path from genes to mental illness. This figure depicts the hypothetical path from genes via molecules, circuits, and information processing to symptoms, syndromes, and mental illnesses. On the far left, the example of risk gene 1 leads to altered enzyme activity for monoamine degradation, while in the center, risk gene 2 leads to altered synaptic plasticity machinery. Both of these molecular abnormalities in this example affect the same circuit (circuit A). If only one of the genes is abnormal, the circuit may be able to compensate and prevent symptoms despite inefficient information processing. However, because both genes have caused molecular abnormalities in circuit A, this circuit can no longer compensate, and a symptom is produced (in this example, executive dysfunction). On the far right, risk gene 3 causes altered development in the prefrontal cortex, preventing adequate activation of a second circuit (circuit B) and thus producing a symptom (delusions). Multiple malfunctioning circuits expressed as multiple biological endophenotypes can cause the expression of multiple symptoms that, taken together, constitute a formally defined syndrome such as schizophrenia.

lying along the path (Figure 6-5). Both are thus intermediates between the gene and the disease and are measurable, but not always by the unaided eye of the clinician. Importantly, endophenotypes are inherited with and closely linked to the disease. They are often more precisely and reproducibly measurable than are the illnesses themselves, since each psychiatric diagnosis probably describes many different illnesses or at least many different biological routes to the same illness. Reproducibly measuring a biological endophenotype can thus reduce variability and allow scientists to link the gene to the biological endophenotype more clearly than linking the gene to the DSM illness, also known as the phenotype itself.

Biological endophenotypes are measurable biological phenomena and can range from the electrophysiological response to startle to the neuroimaging response to information processing, as well as many more. Throughout this text, we will frequently refer to the biological endophenotype of activation of brain circuits. These are now often measured by functional magnetic resonance imaging (fMRI) as a sign of information processing in specifically localized brain circuits, often in the prefrontal cortex.

Symptom endophenotypes, on the other hand, are single symptoms associated with a mental illness and usually one of the DSM criteria for that illness. Thus, guilt and insomnia are symptom endophenotypes, but the diagnosis of major depressive disorder is not; the symptoms of hallucinations and executive dysfunction are symptom endophenotypes, but the diagnosis of schizophrenia is not. Behaviors can also be more than just the symptom endophenotype of a mental illness and can range from how well you calculate something in your head, to how frightened you are of a scary face, to your temperament – that is, your heritable personality pattern present early in life and persisting throughout life, such as novelty seeking, harm avoidance, conscientiousness, etc.

Behaviors are obviously difficult to define because they have many complex functional interactions and emergent phenomena, but they are nevertheless often simpler to define than mental illnesses themselves, which include many different abnormal behaviors, and not the exact same abnormal behaviors in every patient with the same illness, but just several from a number of possibilities off the same diagnostic list. This variability makes it just too tough to link a subtle gene effect to a complex and multiply defined mental illness.

Traveling the hypothetical path from gene to mental illness

The hypothetical path from gene to mental illness goes from the gene via molecules, circuits, and information processing (a biological endophenotype), to symptom endophenotypes (a single symptom of a mental illness), to the full syndrome of symptoms of a mental illness (Figure 6-6). In the hypothetical example shown in Figure 6-6, two risk genes – one for altered enzyme activity for monoamine degradation and another for altered synaptic plasticity – conspire to bias the same circuit, "A," toward inefficient information processing. This hypothetically results in the cognitive symptom of executive dysfunction. In this case, the biological endophenotype is inefficiency of information processing in circuit A, and the symptom endophenotype is executive dysfunction. A hypothetical third risk gene – one that regulates a protein critical for prefrontal cortex neurodevelopment – acts alone to simultaneously bias circuit "B" toward breakdown of its information processing with the resulting symptom of delusions (Figure 6-6). The biological endophenotype here is loss of adequate information processing in circuit B. The symptom endophenotype is the formation of delusions. Putting these together, the patient hypothetically develops schizophrenia due to the combination of symptoms resulting from multiple abnormal circuits.

Thus, Figure 6-6 summarizes the contemporary model for how genes are hypothetically linked to mental illnesses along a pathway from gene through subtle molecular abnormalities, to biological endophenotypes, to symptom endophenotypes, and then to a set of symptoms constituting a syndrome known as a mental illness. It should be apparent from Figure 6-6 that anything on this pathway lying closer to the gene should be more readily linked to that gene. That is why genes are closely linked to the subtle molecular abnormalities they encode but only partially linked to the biological endophenotypes these genes cause and only loosely linked to symptoms and illnesses associated with these biological endophenotypes. Exact quantitative methods are emerging to measure the presence of subtle genetic abnormalities, to know what molecular abnormality they encode, and to see where they cause abnormal information processing in the brain (Figure 6-6), whereas measurement of symptoms and syndromes tends to be more qualitative and descriptive, adding to the loose nature of the linkage between genes and mental illness.

What is complicated here is that because of the loose nature of this linkage, not everyone with a subtle molecular abnormality that causes abnormal information processing in a specific circuit has a symptom, but everyone with a symptom is presumed to have, somewhere, abnormal information processing caused by a subtle molecular abnormality. Furthermore, the same inefficient information processing that causes a symptom can be caused by a whole variety of subtle molecular abnormalities working alone or along with additional subtle molecular abnormalities.

One could reasonably ask why the inherited subtle molecular abnormalities are not more "penetrant" at the behavioral level. That is, why do some people with the same subtle molecular abnormalities and the same abnormal biological endophenotypes of inefficient information processing in the same circuits have a symptom, or abnormal behavior, whereas others do not? A technical way to ask this is why, if the gene penetrates reliably to its molecular abnormality and its molecular abnormality penetrates reliably to inefficient information processing, does that gene not as reliably penetrate to abnormal behavior or a symptom?

The answers are simple. First, genes exert variable effects throughout life; second, no one has just one gene; and finally, it depends on whether you have healthy compensatory backup systems for your subtle molecular abnormality or if you have additional genetic biases, additional molecular abnormalities, and additional independent causes of inefficient information processing in that same circuit.

For example, if someone expresses an abnormal form of a gene for neurodevelopment after the brain has already developed, it might not have any clinical consequence. However, if someone else in the family expresses that same abnormal gene within a critical window of time, it could have a much more profound effect. Also, there are multiple copies of each gene and multiple genes that may have complementary or redundant effects, so that it may be possible to have an abnormal gene in the presence of other normal genes that render the abnormality clinically silent, whereas that same genetic abnormality in the presence of certain other critical abnormalities could lead to manifest malfunctioning of brain circuits.

Stress diathesis hypothesis

Adding to the complexity of "complex genetics" is the observation that genes alone are not necessarily enough to cause a mental illness. Something else generally has to occur from the environment to make the inheritance of silent risk become manifest as illness. That "something else" is often known as "stress." Environmental stressors are often life events, such as abusive childhood experiences, difficult adult experiences such as divorce or

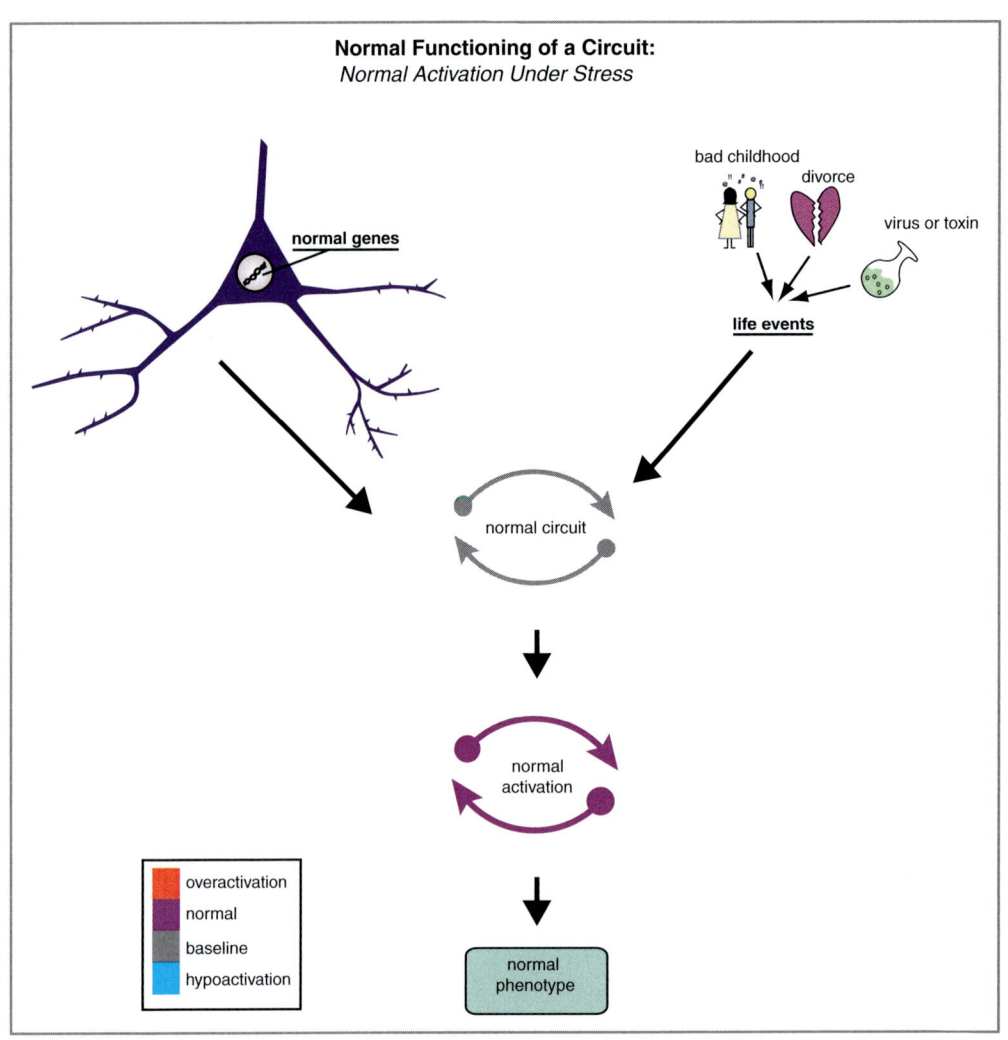

FIGURE 6-7 Normal activation after stress. Development of psychiatric symptoms is often the function of both genetic and environmental influences; this is known as the stress-diathesis model. Environmental stressors – such as childhood abuse, divorce, viruses, or toxins – can increase the risk, or diathesis, of developing a mental illness. However, individuals with a normal genome and thus normal circuits may experience only normal activation of circuits in response to stressful events; that is, they have a normal biological endophenotype. Such individuals would not express a mental illness, exhibiting instead a normal phenotype with no adverse behavioral symptoms.

financial reversals, or biological stressors such as viruses, toxins, or other illnesses (Figure 6-7). Mentally healthy individuals have a genome that is built to handle such stressors, and the normal or perhaps ideal response is hypothetically to activate neuronal circuits to process information associated with stress, to mobilize adaptive behaviors to reduce the stress, but to have no adverse behavioral symptoms and thus a "normal" phenotype (Figure 6-7).

Individuals with a risk gene for a mental illness, however, will react differently to a life stressor, but you might never know it (Figure 6-8). That is, the same stressor may cause no adverse behavioral symptoms and thus there is a "normal" phenotype (Figure 6-8) just as shown previously for the genetically and mentally healthy individual with a normal genome (Figure 6-7). However, if you had the ability to measure the effect the stressor

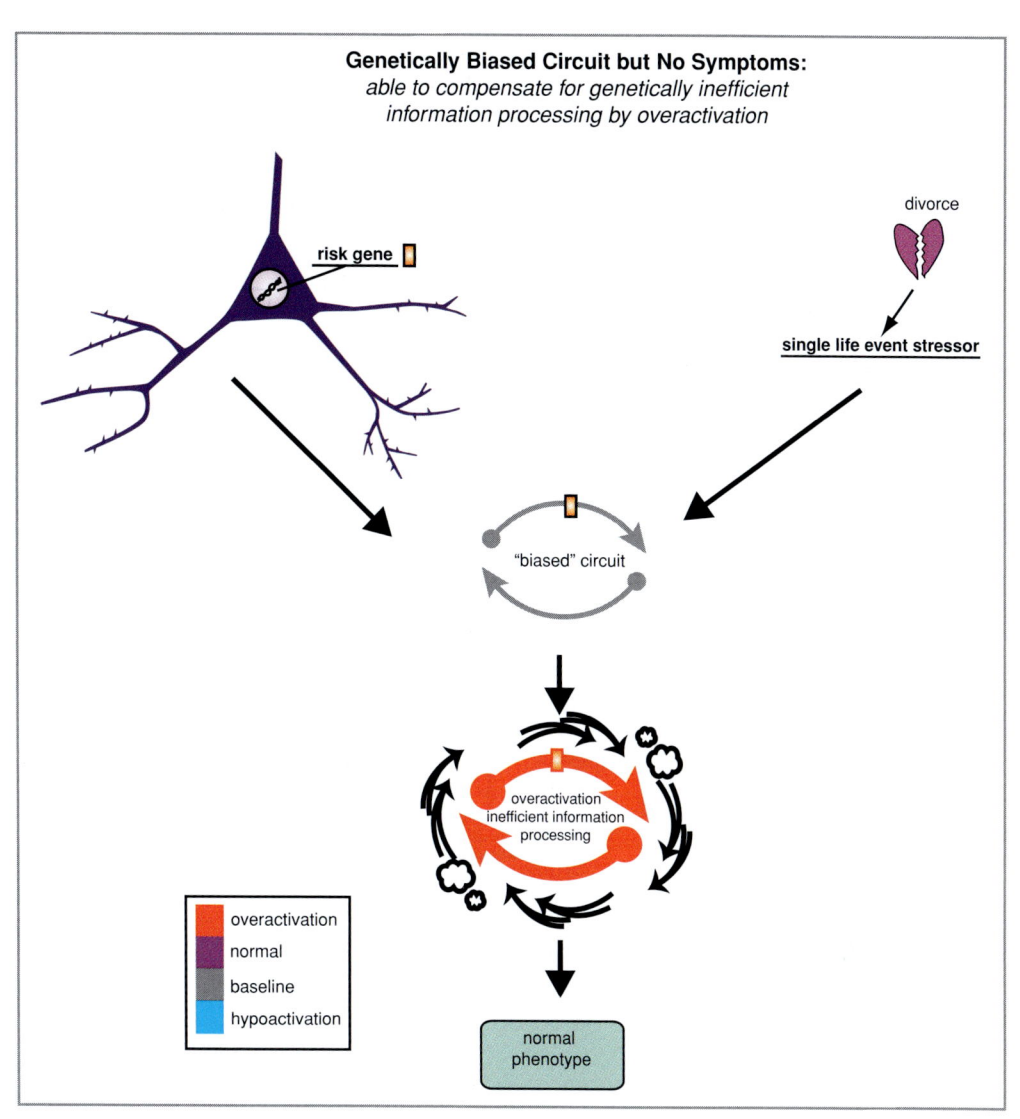

FIGURE 6-8 Genetically biased circuit but no symptoms. Environmental stress coupled with a risk gene for mental illness may lead to inefficient information processing of the "biased" circuit; however, this does not necessarily mean that behavioral symptoms will ensue. Genetically inefficient information processing may be behaviorally "silent" if it is compensated by overactivation via backup systems. In this case, the individual may still have a normal behavioral phenotype despite having an abnormal biological endophenotype. Thus, abnormal circuit activation may be detectable with functional brain scanning, but clinical interview would reveal no psychiatric symptom.

has on information processing of the circuit in the individual with the subtle molecular abnormality, you would see that there is overactivation of that circuit (Figure 6-8). Luckily in this individual, there are compensatory backup systems in place and no other critical genetic flaws, so that the circuit is behaviorally silent (Figure 6-8). Technically speaking, the abnormal biological endophenotype has a normal behavioral phenotype.

Now comes an individual with multiple genetic risk factors and with multiple life stressors who is reaching the tipping point, so that the circuit either underperforms or overactivates (Figure 6-9). The overactivation is the same biological endophenotype as that

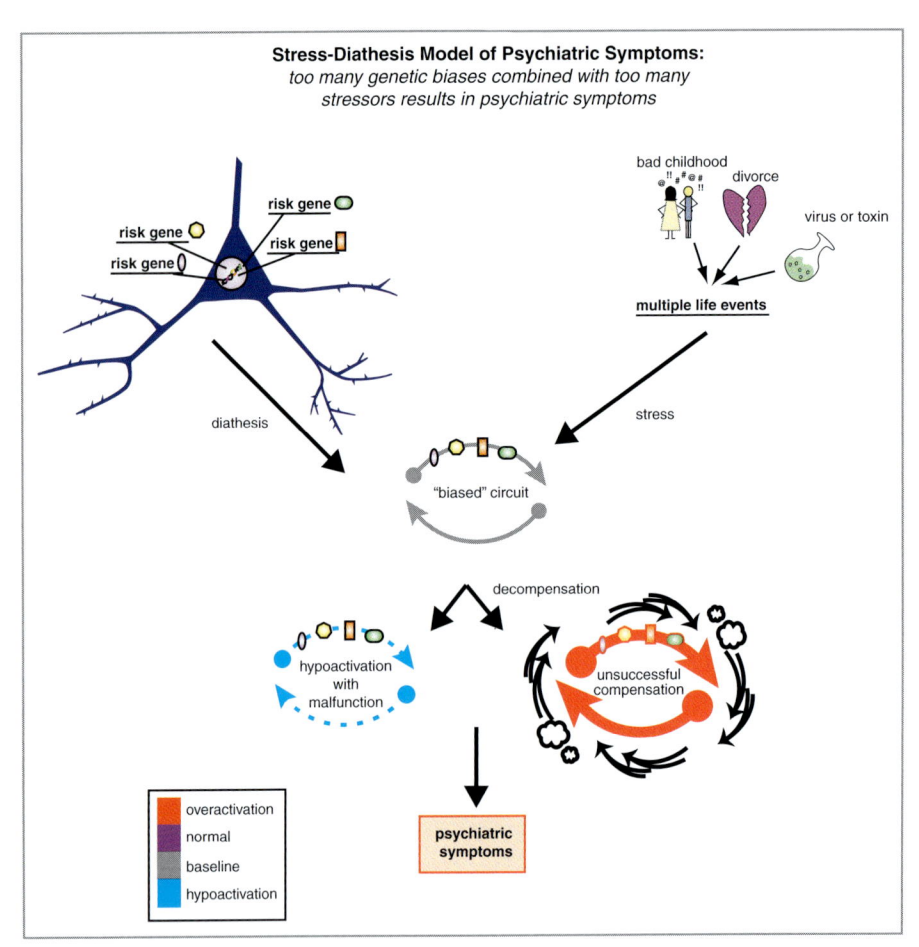

FIGURE 6-9 Stress-diathesis model of psychiatric symptoms. An individual with multiple stressors and multiple genetic risks may not have sufficient backup mechanisms to compensate for inefficient information processing within a genetically "biased" circuit. The circuit may either be unsuccessfully compensated by overactivation or it may break down and not activate at all. In either case, the abnormal biological endophenotype would be associated with an abnormal behavioral phenotype and thus a psychiatric symptom. Such abnormal circuit activation would be potentially detectable with functional brain scanning, and psychiatric symptoms would be manifest on clinical interview.

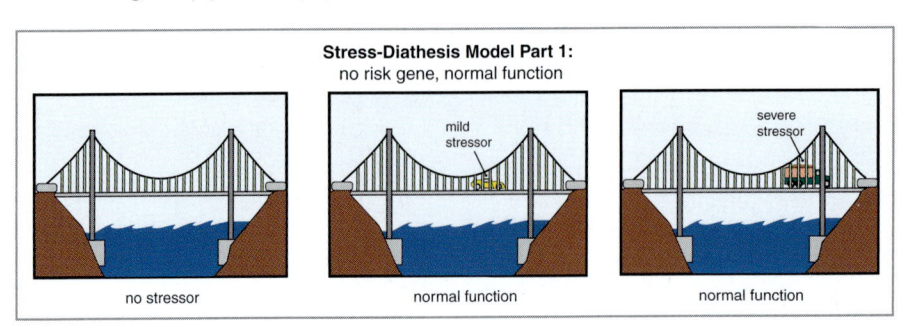

FIGURE 6-10 Stress-diathesis model. Figures 6-10 through 6-13 illustrate the stress-diathesis model using the analogy of a suspension bridge. Each suspension cable is analogous to a gene, while the vehicles that pass over the bridge represent types of environmental stressors. In this figure, there are no risk genes; thus all the suspension cables are normal and the bridge is fully intact. This allows the bridge to handle both mild stressors (small car in middle panel) and severe stressors (large truck in right panel).

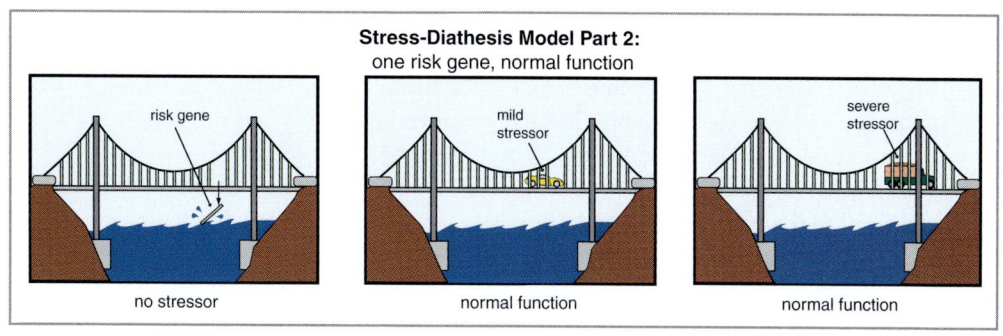

FIGURE 6-11 Stress-diathesis model. The presence of a single risk gene can lead to a subtle molecular abnormality (shown as a single cable snapping in the left panel). However, if only a single abnormality is present, the bridge remains intact and can still handle both mild (middle panel) and severe (right panel) stress loads because the other cables compensate for the broken one.

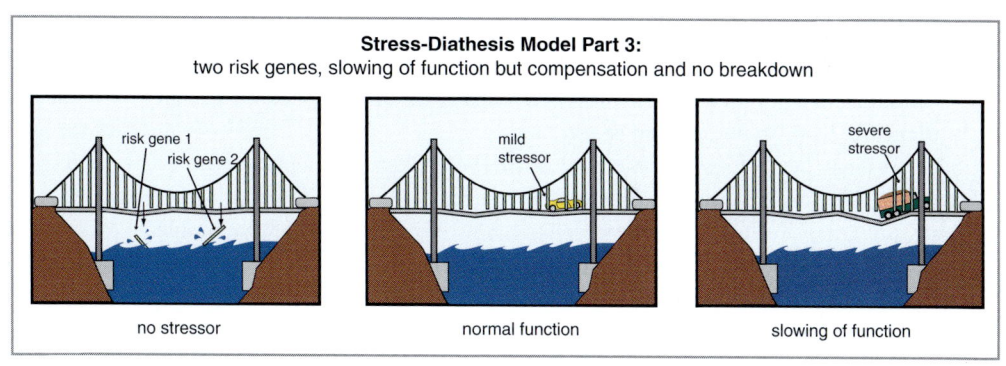

FIGURE 6-12 Stress-diathesis model. If two risk genes are present (shown as two cables snapping in the left panel), the bridge remains intact and can handle light loads (middle panel) because of compensatory actions of the other cables. The bridge can even handle heavy loads (right panel), but less efficiently and with much greater difficulty.

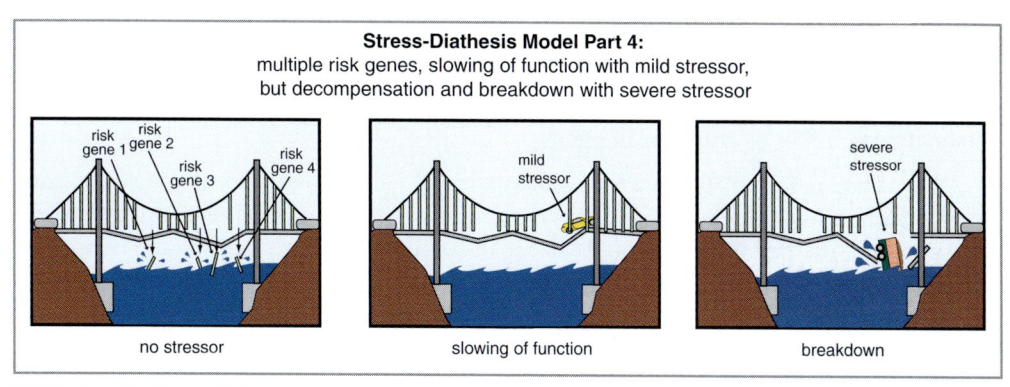

FIGURE 6-13 Stress-diathesis model. The presence of multiple risk genes and consequently multiple broken cables (left panel) puts the bridge at grave risk if any significant stressors are encountered. The bridge may remain intact in the absence of any stressors and may even accommodate light loads (middle panel), but the remaining cables may not be able to compensate for the broken ones in the event of a heavy load (left panel), causing the bridge to break and, by analogy, symptoms of a mental illness to occur.

Psychiatric Genetics | 189

of the individual with just one subtle molecular abnormality and no symptoms in Figure 6-8. An fMRI scan of both overactivated circuits would look the same. However, the patient in Figure 6-9 lacks successful compensatory mechanisms and has additional molecular flaws in backup systems; thus the abnormal biological endophenotype in this case is not silent but produces a psychiatric symptom, perhaps anxiety (Figure 6-9).

Figures 6-7 through 6-9 thus outline the idea of stress diathesis. The diathesis is the biological risk, whether one or many or none. The same stress with different diathesis can yield normal biological endophenotype and no symptoms (Figure 6-7), abnormal biological endophenotype and no symptoms (Figure 6-8), or abnormal biological endophenotype plus symptoms (Figure 6-9). It all depends on reaching the breaking point.

This idea of reaching the breaking point in the stress diathesis model of mental illnesses is illustrated in Figures 6-10 through 6-13, using the analogy of a suspension bridge holding up various loads. In the first panel of Figure 6-10, all the suspension cables, analogous to all the genes, are normal structures, and the bridge holds up not only itself but also a light stressor (small car load in the middle panel) as well as a severe stressor (big truck load in the right panel). In fact, the bridge is so well built that it has backup systems engineered into its design. If one cable snaps (analogous to one gene encoding a subtle molecular abnormality; Figure 6-11, first panel), the bridge does not fall down, and it can process any stressor loads (middle and right panels). The other cables may be working harder, but they are built for that extra load, so no problem (Figure 6-11).

Things begin to get problematic with two broken cables (analogous to two defective genes). The bridge does not fall down (Figure 6-12, left panel), and it can process a light stressor (middle panel) without problems; however, it begins to have problems processing a heavy stressor (right panel). Things therefore slow down and there is some difficulty with the speed and efficiency of processing the heavy load. Nevertheless, even the heavy stressor is successfully processed by the backup systems still in place (Figure 6-12).

However, when multiple cables are broken, as in Figure 6-13, there is too great a "diathesis" or risk if a heavy load is ever encountered. The backup systems keep the bridge up (Figure 6-13, left panel) and can even process a light load successfully if inefficiently (Figure 6-13, middle panel); but when a heavy load comes along and there are multiple broken cables, compensation is no longer possible. With functioning backup systems no longer in place, the breaking point is reached (Figure 6-13 right panel). The bridge falls down, the stressor load fails to be processed, and, by analogy, a mental illness occurs.

Personality as buffer or amplifier of stress

Even the combination of genes coding for subtle molecular abnormalities and environmental stressors is not the whole story (Figure 6-14). To add another level of complexity to the situation, the net outcome of a stressor is determined to some extent by the personality of the person experiencing that stressor, not just the genes of that person. In fact, the development of personality and temperament themselves is determined both genetically and environmentally in its own "complex genetics." Thus, if the same stressor is "filtered" through the personality of someone with good coping skills, adaptive responses to adverse circumstances, and a healthy lifestyle, the stressor is mitigated; and the effects on the genome are so subtle that there is no decompensation of information processing in the vulnerable circuit, and no symptoms appear (thus, a normal phenotype). This is shown on the left

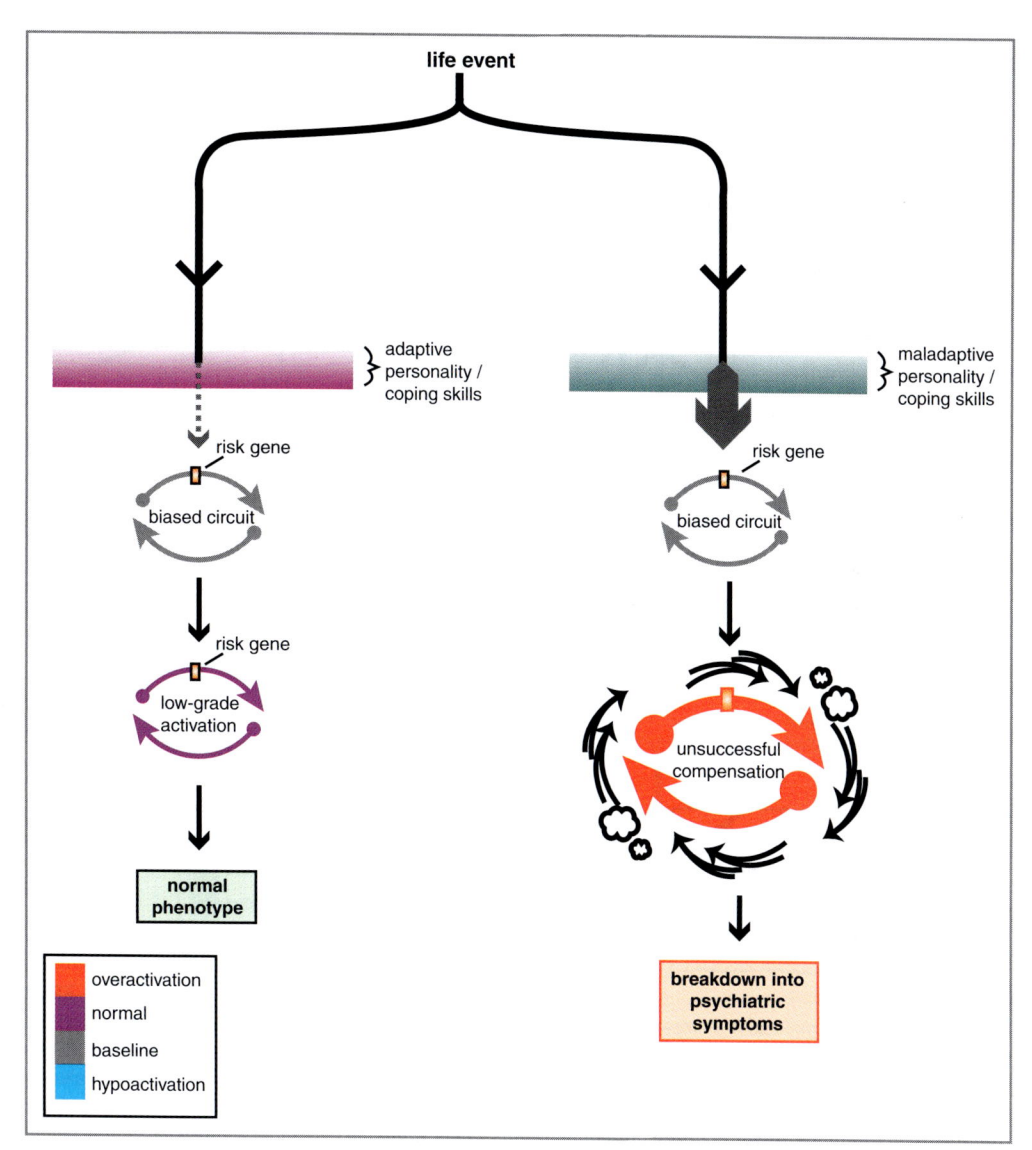

FIGURE 6-14 Stress and personality. In addition to genetically determined molecular abnormalities and environmental stressors, personality factors such as coping skills and lifestyle can also affect the impact of stressors on an individual's genome and thus his or her total risk of mental illness. As shown on the left, adaptive coping skills and healthy lifestyles may *mitigate* the effects of stressful life events on genetic risk, so that, despite a "biased" circuit, the individual still exhibits a normal phenotype (on the left). However, in an individual with poor coping skills and an unhealthy lifestyle, stressful life events may *exacerbate* the effects of genetic risk and render the "biased" circuit unable to compensate; such a person may therefore develop psychiatric symptoms (on the right).

side of Figure 6-14. Imagine, however, someone with poor coping skills, bad habits, and maladaptive responses to stress, such as arguing, drinking, or fighting, and so on. In that case, the same stressor can be amplified rather than mitigated (Figure 6-14 on the right). A stressor that would be silent in the person on the left may cause breakdown into the symptom of a mental illness on the right (Figure 6-14).

Psychiatric Genetics | 191

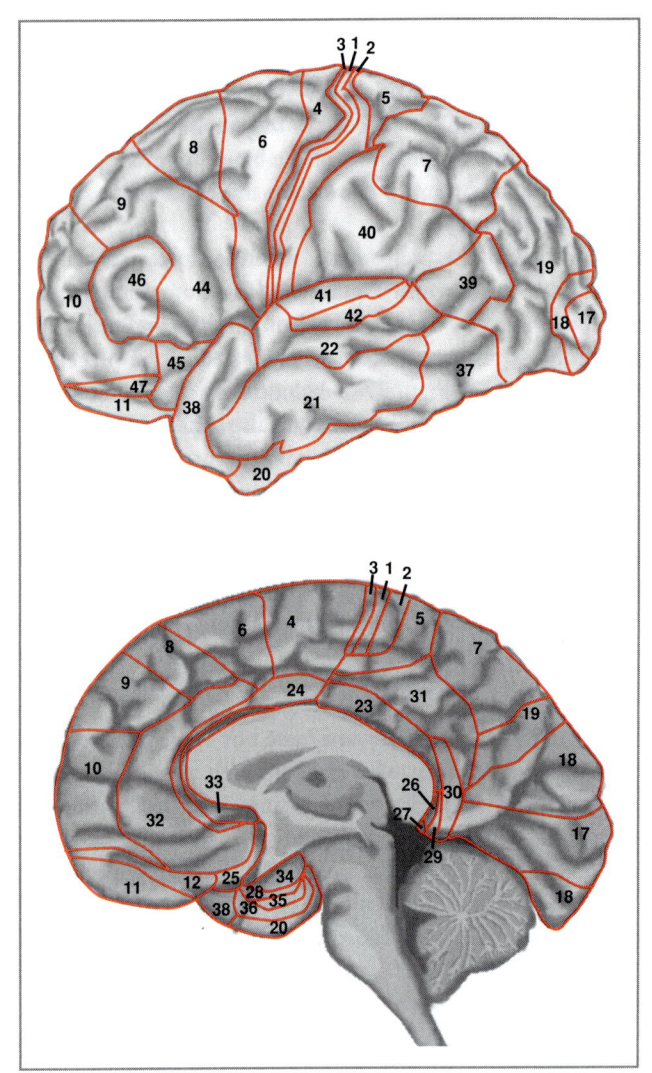

FIGURE 7-2 **Brodmann areas.** One way of identifying different brain regions is through the use of Brodmann areas. These areas are structurally though not necessarily functionally distinguishable regions of the brain, each of which is designated by a unique number. Lateral (top) and medial (bottom) views of the brain are shown here with the Brodmann areas indicated.

Dorsolateral prefrontal cortex

The dorsolateral prefrontal cortex (DLPFC) is shown in the blue-green oval and seen only on the lateral view (Figure 7-3). This is an important region of prefrontal cortex whose cortical pyramidal cells are the engines for various types of cognitive functions, such as executive functioning, problem solving, and analyzing.

Orbital frontal cortex

The orbital frontal cortex (OFC) is the part of the prefrontal cortex that sits above the eye in its orbit and is seen both on the lateral and medial views of Figure 7-3 (blue). The OFC may regulate impulses, compulsions, and drives.

Anterior cingulate cortex

The anterior cingulate cortex (ACC) is the part of prefrontal cortex shown in light pink on the medial view of Figure 7-4. The top of the ACC, also called dorsal ACC, is thought

198 | Essential Psychopharmacology

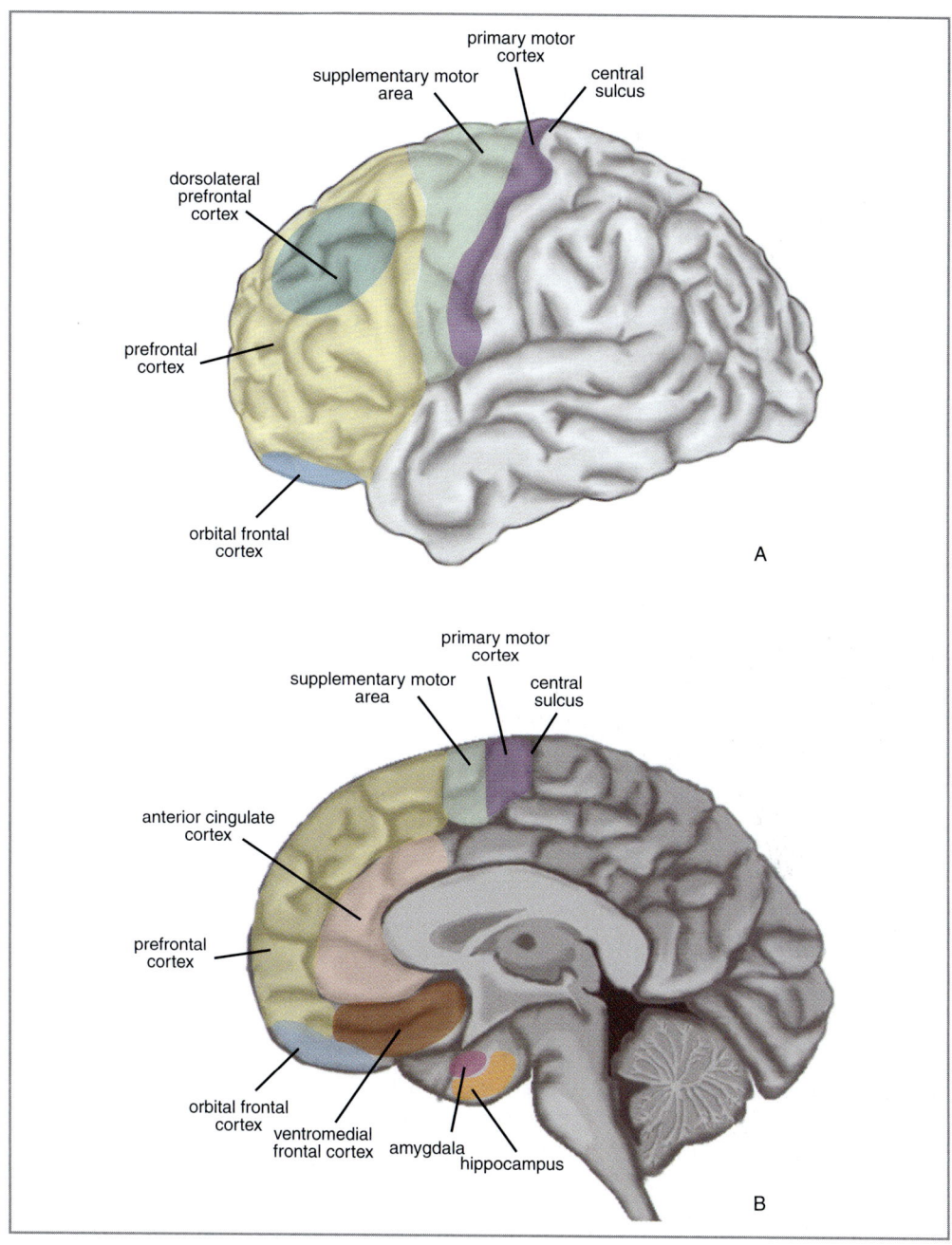

FIGURE 7-3A and B Key brain regions. Several functional anatomical divisions of the brain relevant to psychopharmacology are shown here, using both a lateral (**A**) and a medial (**B**) view. There are several subregions of the frontal cortex, including the primary motor cortex, supplementary motor area, and prefrontal cortex. The prefrontal cortex itself consists of functionally distinct subregions. These include the orbital frontal cortex (OFC), visible in both the lateral and medial views, which may regulate impulses and compulsions; the dorsolateral prefrontal cortex (DLPFC) (lateral view), which is integral to cognitive functioning; the ventromedial prefrontal cortex (medial view), which is involved in emotional processing; and the anterior cingulate cortex (ACC) (medial view), which is involved in both selective attention (dorsal ACC) and emotional regulation (ventral ACC). Two additional brain regions emphasized here are the amygdala and the hippocampus, which are important for fear processing and memory, respectively.

Planes for Visualizing the Brain

horizontal plane

coronal plane

sagittal plane

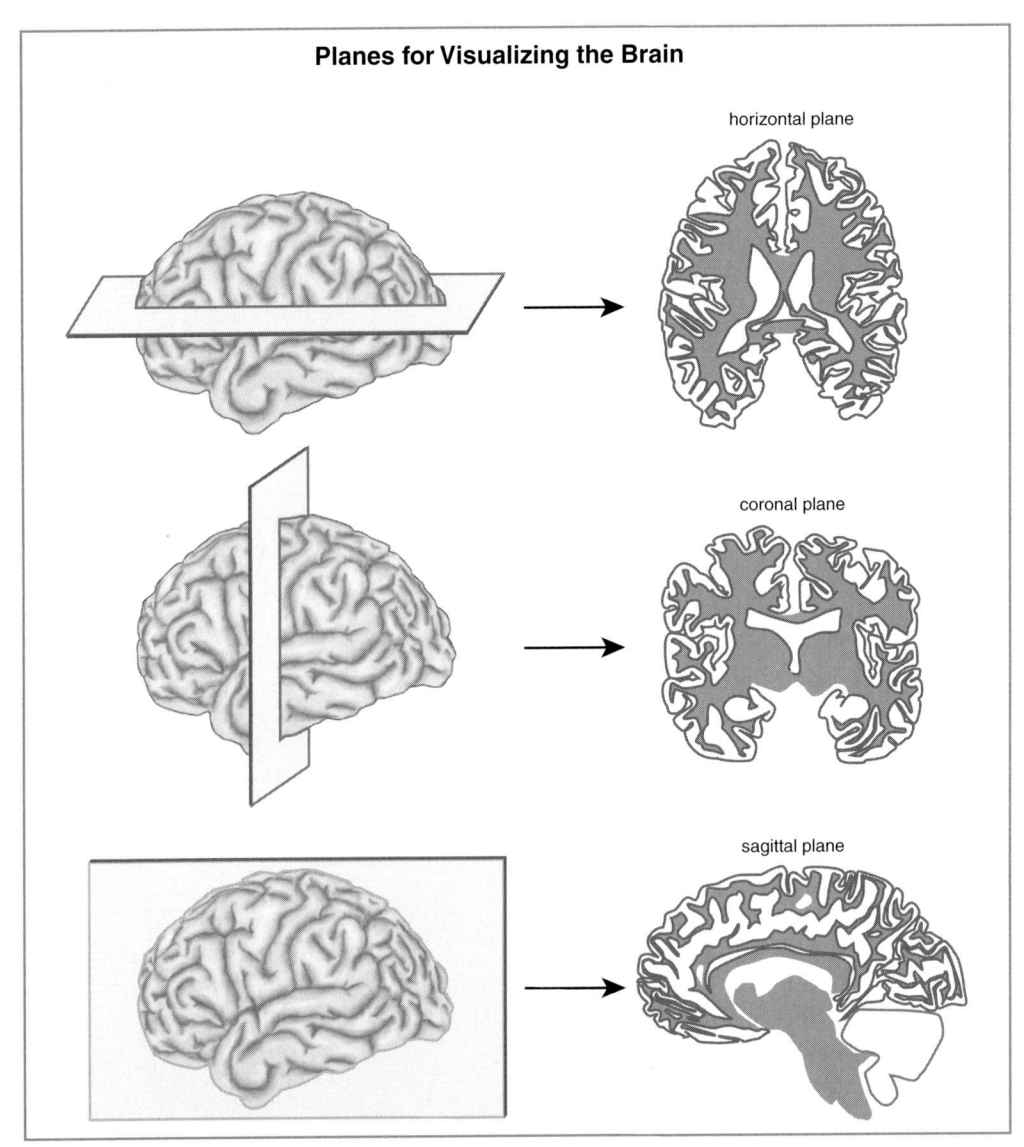

FIGURE 7-4 Horizontal, coronal, and sagittal planes. Three standard planes for visualizing the brain are shown here: horizontal, coronal, and sagittal. Each of these views may be used throughout this book to depict connectivity between different brain regions.

to play an important role in selective attention. The lower part of the ACC, called either the ventral ACC or the subgenual ACC, regulates various emotions such as depression and anxiety. The ACC is shaped like a C; some would say it bends like a knee. *Genu* is the Latin name for knee; thus the area of the C below the bend is sometimes called the subgenual area.

Ventromedial prefrontal cortex
The ventromedial prefrontal cortex, in brown, is the area between the OFC and the ventral ACC (Figure 7-3); it also plays a role in emotional processing.

Beyond prefrontal cortex to hippocampus and amygdala

Two other areas are shown on the medial view of Figure 7-3: the orange hippocampus, important for memory, and the magenta almond-shaped amygdala, buried in the temporal lobe near the hippocampus and involved very much in fear processing.

The planes of the brain

Those who are serious neuroimagers know how to slice and dice the brain, and understand the anatomical relationships of all the possible cuts that can be made through the brain by the various neuroimaging techniques available today. The modern psychopharmacologist should have some familiarity with the deeper structures of the brain so revealed by these techniques in order to interpret various brain images, especially those images showing areas that project to prefrontal cortex or receive projections from prefrontal cortex.

Thus, three standard planes for visualizing the brain are shown in Figure 7-4: the horizontal plane, the coronal plane and the sagittal plane. It may be useful to refer back to this picture when studying images throughout this book to remind yourself at times what cut of the brain you are looking at, and how the cut relates to the orientation of the whole brain.

One can also visualize the brain in some figures that attempt to show the structures underlying the cortex in a 3 dimensional perspective (Figure 7-5). The deep structures under the surface, such as the caudate, thalamus, hypothalamus, brainstem monoamine centers (VTA, ventral tegmental area; LC, locus coeruleus; raphe) can be seen here through a transparent cortex (Figure 7-5).

The brain can also be shown more as a cartoon with approximations of anatomic areas. For example, 11 key areas of the brain that will be discussed extensively in this text are shown with their rough anatomic localization and names in Figure 7-6. The hypothetical behaviors thought to be regulated by circuits running through each of these 11 nodes in various networks are indicated in Figure 7-7.

These will be important to remember, since alterations in neurotransmitters within these sites (Figure 7-6) are hypothesized to create inefficient information processing there and consequently the specific symptoms of psychiatric disorders indicated for each of these 11 areas (Figure 7-7). Also, the neurotransmitters within each of these 11 areas serve as targets for psychopharmacologic drug treatments, which are hypothesized to reduce symptoms in these specific areas by successfully altering neurotransmission and thus information processing there. Knowing where an individual patient's symptoms are hypothetically located, and the neurotransmitters that regulate them within those specific brain areas, can provide a rational basis for which drugs are chosen or combined. This theme will be emphasized repeatedly throughout the textbook and specific applications of this principle will be discussed for each of the specific psychiatric disorders in subsequent chapters.

Neurotransmitter nodes

Several different neurotransmitters have their cell bodies in the brainstem, and their axons project to prefrontal cortex and to many other areas of the brain (Figures 7-8 to 7-13). Although there is quite a bit of overlap of projection areas among the various neurotransmitters, no one neurotransmitter projects to all the same brain areas as another, and certainly not always to the same neurons in the brain areas where they project. Nevertheless, it is hypothesized that when a neurotransmitter does project to a specific area, it has the capacity to modulate the behavior or brain function thought to be associated with that area, as illustrated in Figure 7-7.

Important Functional Areas Within the Left Hemisphere

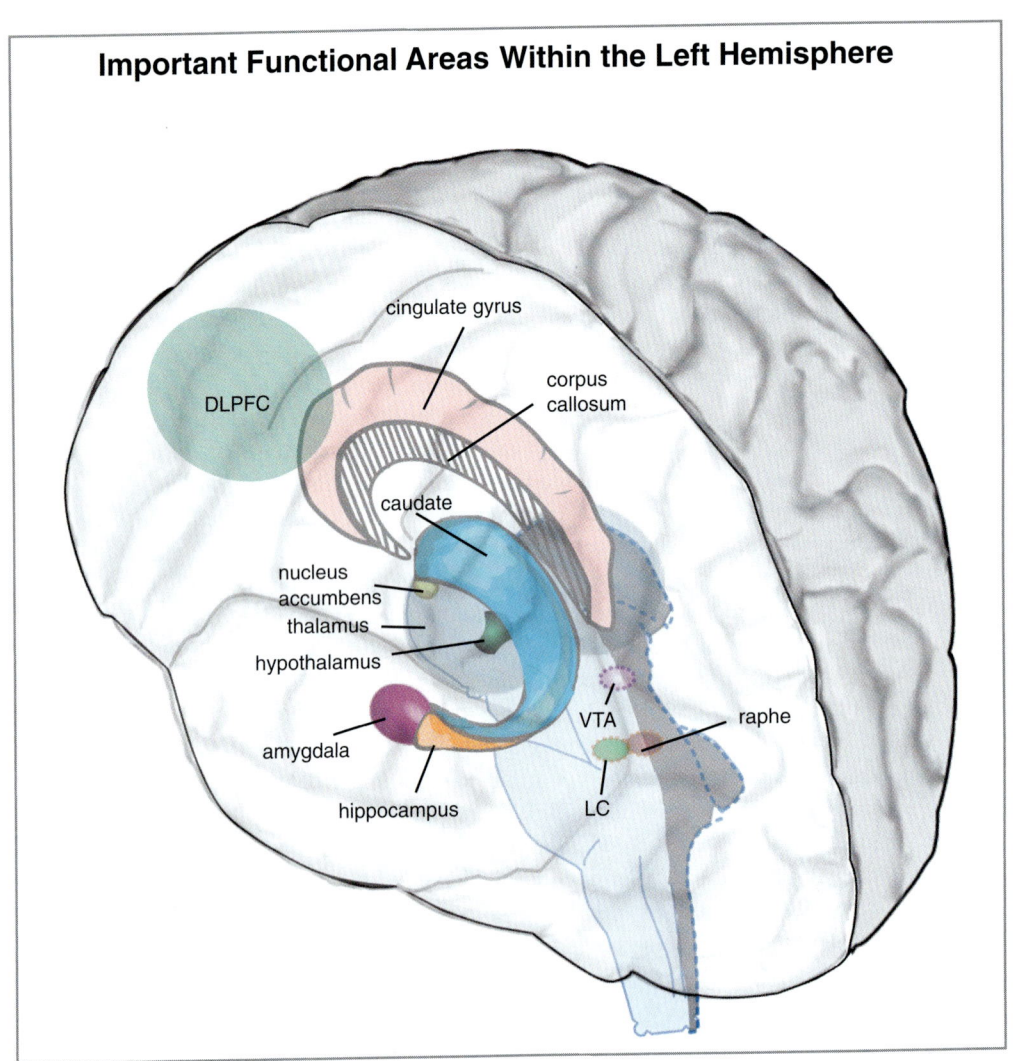

FIGURE 7-5 Key brain regions in three dimensions. This figure provides a somewhat three-dimensional depiction of the brain in which the cortex of the left hemisphere is transparent, allowing us to see the topographical relationships between structures such as the caudate, nucleus accumbens, thalamus, hypothalamus, amygdala, hippocampus, and brainstem monoamine centers. VTA, ventral tegmental area; LC, locus coeruleus; DLPFC, dorsolateral prefrontal cortex.

Neurotransmitter pathways form the molecular and anatomical substrates that "tune" neurons within circuits. This happens not only at the cortical level but at the level of all the nodes within the network of the various cortical circuits. Psychopharmacologists can rationally target these pathways and the functions they regulate by selecting and combining drugs that act on the specific neurotransmitters in the specific brain areas of interest for treatment of an individual patient. Thus, it is useful to know which neurotransmitters go where as well as the function of each brain area they innervate.

Dopamine

The major dopamine projections are shown in Figure 7-8. They arise predominantly but not exclusively from brainstem neurotransmitter centers, notably the ventral tegmental area and

202 | Essential Psychopharmacology

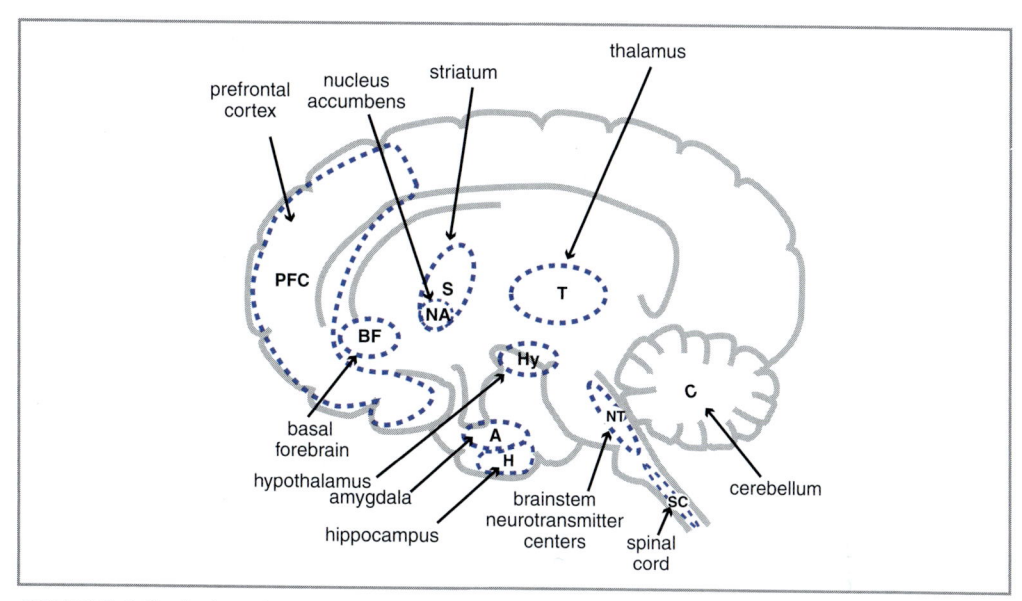

FIGURE 7-6 **Key brain regions in two dimensions.** A two-dimensional depiction of the brain (medial view) is provided here. The general locations and names of eleven brain regions are indicated. These eleven areas are connected by many different neurotransmitter circuits that are relevant to psychiatric disorders and that will be discussed in great detail throughout the rest of this book.

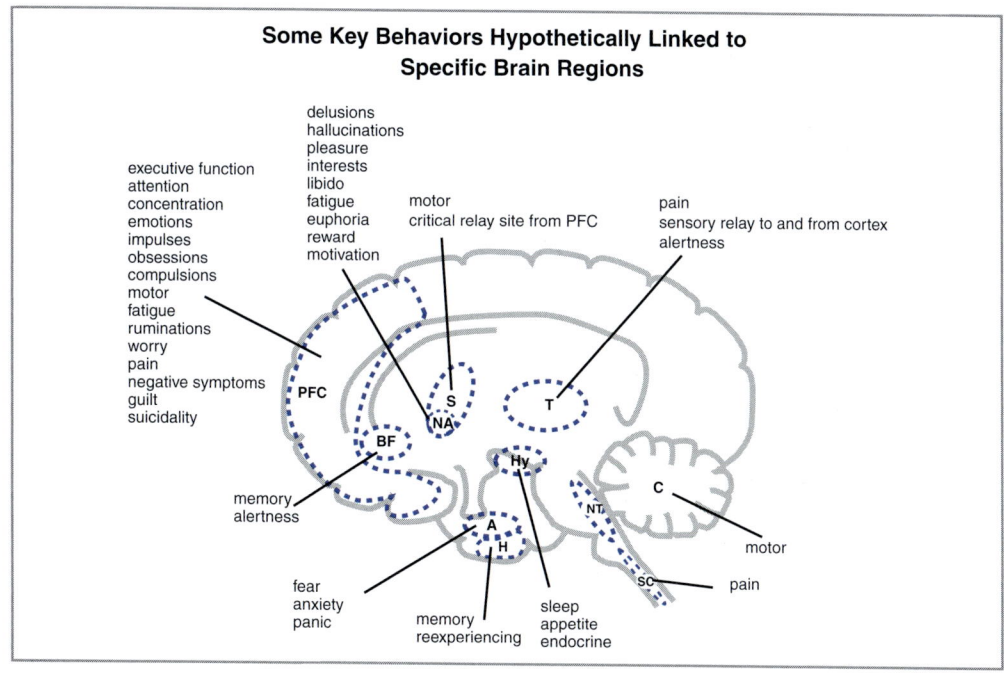

FIGURE 7-7 **Behaviors linked to key brain regions.** Alterations in neurotransmission within each of the eleven brain regions shown here and in Figure 7-6 can lead to symptoms of psychiatric disorders. Functionality in each brain region may be associated with a different constellation of symptoms. PFC, prefrontal cortex; BF, basal forebrain; S, striatum; NA, nucleus accumbens; T, thalamus; HY, hypothalamus; A, amygdala; H, hippocampus; NT, brainstem neurotransmitter centers; SC, spinal cord; C, cerebellum.

Circuits in Psychopharmacology | 203

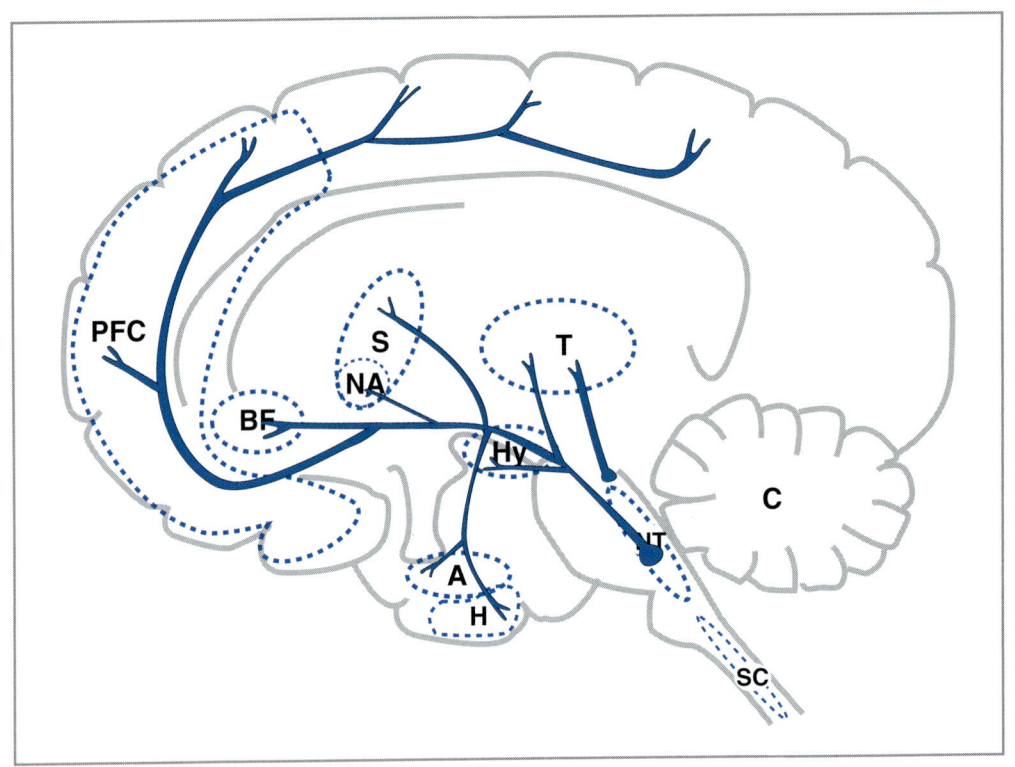

FIGURE 7-8 Major dopamine projections. Major neurotransmitter projections, part 1: dopamine. Dopamine has widespread ascending projections that originate predominantly in the brainstem (particularly the ventral tegmental area and substantia nigra) and extend via the hypothalamus to the prefrontal cortex, basal forebrain, striatum, nucleus accumbens, and other regions. Dopaminergic neurotransmission is associated with movement, pleasure and reward, cognition, psychosis, and other functions. In addition, there are direct projections from other sites to the thalamus, creating the "thalamic dopamine system," which may be involved in arousal and sleep. PFC, prefrontal cortex; BF, basal forebrain; S, striatum; NA, nucleus accumbens; T, thalamus; HY, hypothalamus; A, amygdala; H, hippocampus; NT, brainstem neurotransmitter centers; SC, spinal cord; C, cerebellum.

the substantia nigra, to project to many brain areas but not to any great extent to cerebellum or spinal cord. These neurons regulate movements, reward, cognition, psychosis, and many other functions. Recently, significant dopaminergic innervation of the thalamus has been demonstrated. Unlike the other dopaminergic pathways, this "thalamic dopamine system" arises from multiple sites, including the periaqueductal gray, the ventral mesencephalon, hypothalamic nuclei, and the lateral parabrachial nucleus. The thalamic dopamine system may contribute to the gating of information transferred through the thalamus to the neocortex, striatum, and amygdala and has recently been implicated in regulating arousal and sleep. Not shown is the small incertohypothalamic pathway, which originates from an area of the brain called the zona incerta; it innervates amygdaloid and hypothalamic nuclei involved in sexual behavior. Specific dopamine projections will be discussed in much more detail in the clinical chapters dealing with specific psychiatric disorders.

Norepinephrine

The major norepinephrine projections are shown in Figure 7-9; they arise largely from the brainstem neurotransmitter center known as the locus coeruleus, although some also

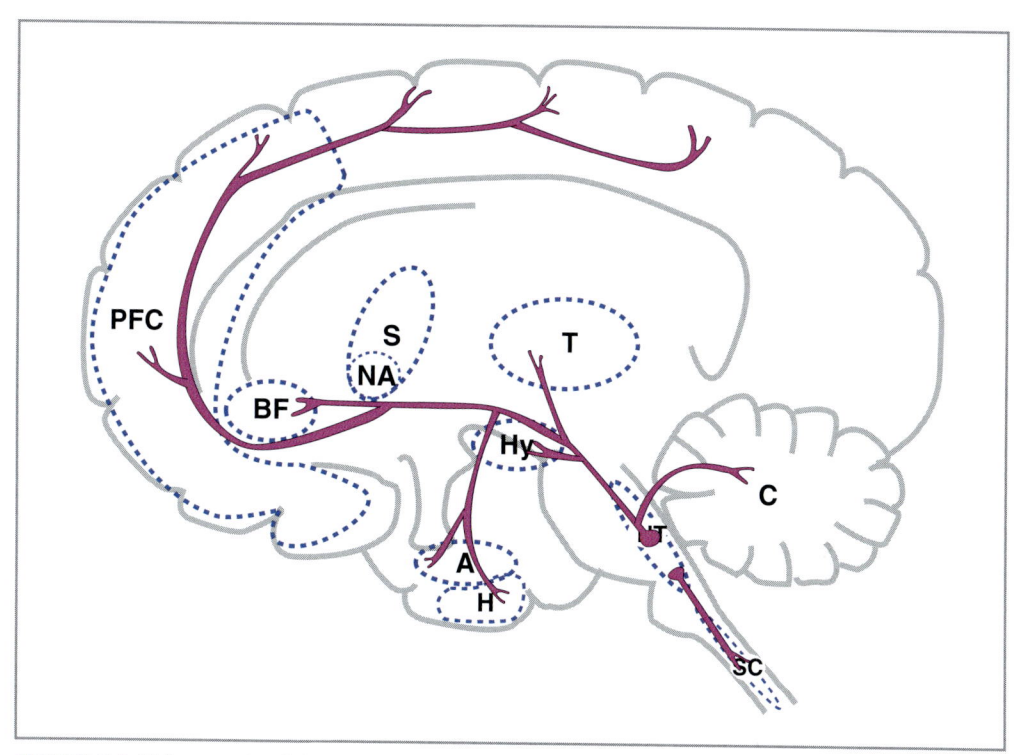

FIGURE 7-9 Major norepinephrine projections. Major neurotransmitter projections, part 2: norepinephrine. Norepinephrine has both ascending and descending projections. Ascending noradrenergic projections originate mainly in the locus coeruleus of the brainstem; they extend to multiple brain regions, as shown here, and regulate mood, arousal, cognition, and other functions. Descending noradrenergic projections extend down the spinal cord and regulate pain pathways. PFC, prefrontal cortex; BF, basal forebrain; S, striatum; NA, nucleus accumbens; T, thalamus; HY, hypothalamus; A, amygdala; H, hippocampus; NT, brainstem neurotransmitter centers; SC, spinal cord; C, cerebellum.

arise from the lateral tegmental norepinephrine cell system also in the brainstem. They regulate mood, arousal, cognition, and many other functions. Spinal projections arise from noradrenergic cell bodies in the lower (caudal) parts of the brainstem neurotransmitter center and regulate pain pathways. Ascending noradrenergic pathways arise along the middle and top (rostral) end of the brainstem centers and find their projections terminating diffusely throughout the brain, including most of the same places where serotonin pathways terminate; however, there are few noradrenergic projections to the striatum/nucleus accumbens (compare to Figure 7-10).

Serotonin

The major serotonin projections are shown in Figure 7-10; they arise from several clusters of discrete brainstem nuclei in the brainstem neurotransmitter center. The upper (rostral) nuclei include the dorsal and medial raphe as well as the nucleus linearis and the raphe pontis. These diffusely innervate most of the brain areas indicated, including the cerebellum, and regulate a wide range of functions from mood, to anxiety, to sleep, and many others. The lower (or caudal) serotonin nuclei comprise the raphe magnus, raphe pallidus, and raphe obscurus and have more limited projections to the cerebellum, brainstem, and spinal cord, where they may regulate the pain pathways.

Circuits in Psychopharmacology | 205

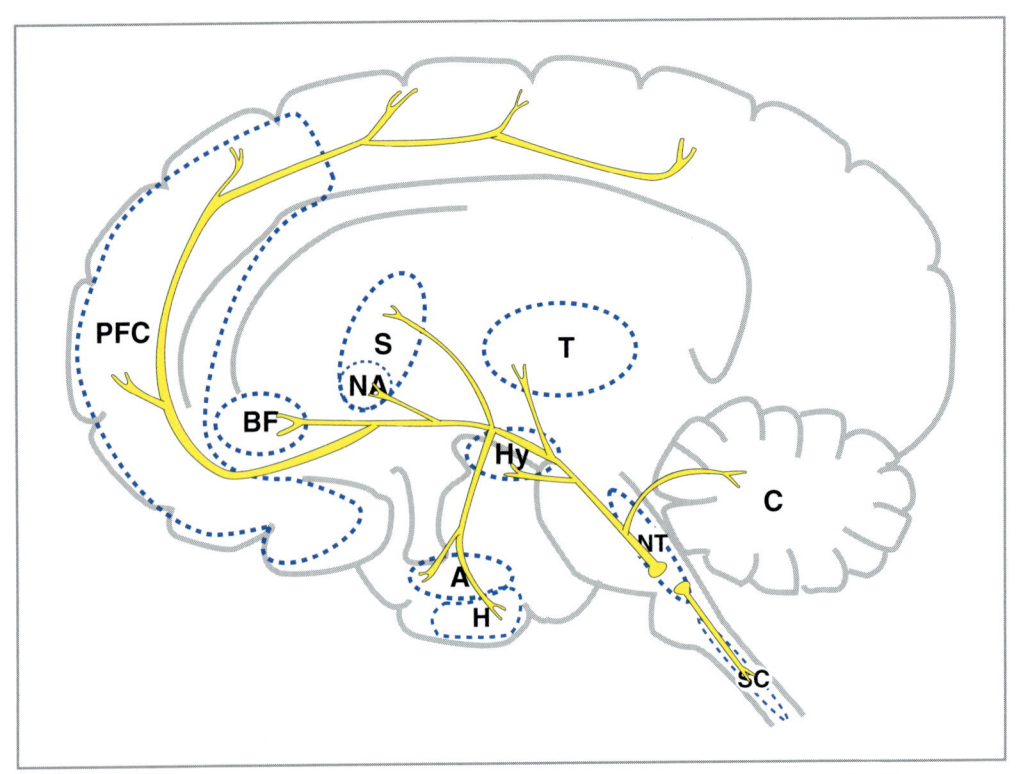

FIGURE 7-10 **Major serotonin projections.** Major neurotransmitter projections, part 3: serotonin. Like norepinephrine, serotonin has both ascending and descending projections. Ascending serotonergic projections originate in the brainstem and extend to many of the same regions as noradrenergic projections, with additional projections to the striatum and nucleus accumbens. These ascending projections may regulate mood, anxiety, sleep, and other functions. Descending serotonergic projections extend down the brainstem and through the spinal cord; they may regulate pain. PFC, prefrontal cortex; BF, basal forebrain; S, striatum; NA, nucleus accumbens; T, thalamus; HY, hypothalamus; A, amygdala; H, hippocampus; NT, brainstem neurotransmitter centers; SC, spinal cord; C, cerebellum.

Acetylcholine

Two sets of acetylcholine projections are shown in Figure 7-11, where they arise from the brainstem neurotransmitter center, and in Figure 7-12, where they arise from the basal forebrain. Some of the cell bodies for acetylcholine are not shown, including those in the striatum and some of those in the brainstem that innervate oculomotor and preganglionic autonomic neurons. Those cholinergic neurons arising from the brainstem neurotransmitter center that travel along with the monoaminergic neurons (Figures 7-8, 7-9, and 7-10) to innervate many brain areas are shown in Figure 7-11; they may regulate arousal, cognition, and many other functions. Four small nuclei in the brainstem supply this ascending cholinergic innervation.

A second and perhaps more prominent site of cholinergic cell bodies innervating the brain arise in a complex of nuclei in the basal forebrain (Figure 7-12). This includes an area called the basal nucleus, or sometimes the nucleus basalis (of Meynert), as well as the medial septal nucleus and the diagonal band (all indicated as BF, for basal forebrain, in Figure 7-12). These cholinergic fibers are thought to have a prominent role in memory.

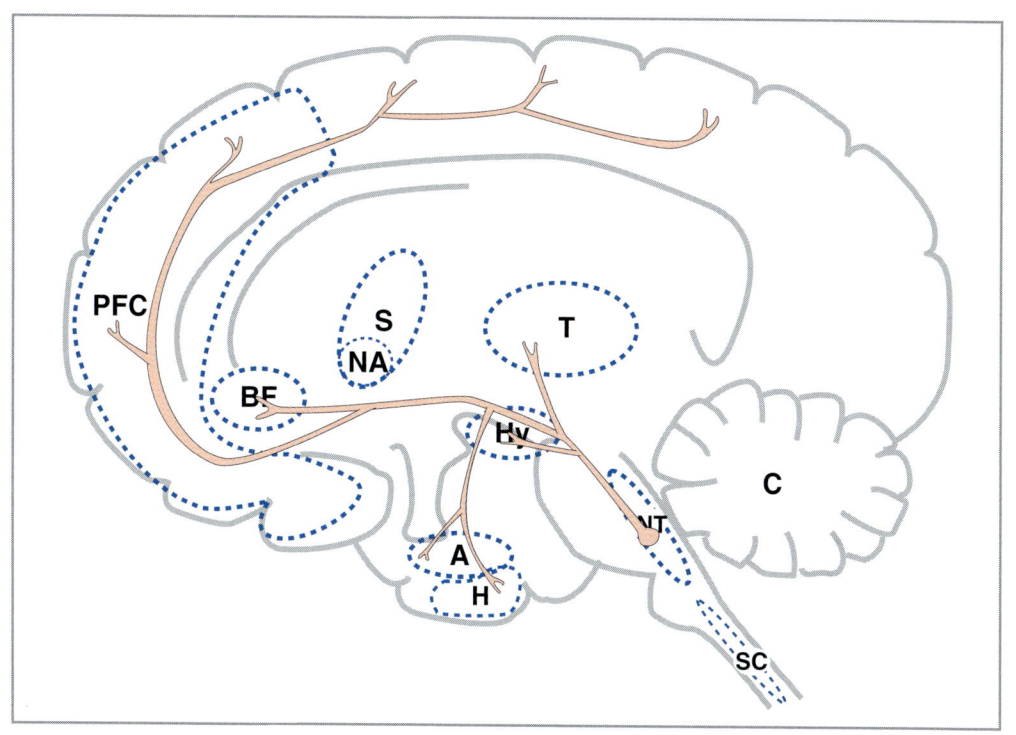

FIGURE 7-11 **Major acetylcholine projections via brainstem.** Major neurotransmitter projections, part 4: acetylcholine via brainstem. Acetylcholine projections originating in the brainstem extend to many brain regions, including the prefrontal cortex, basal forebrain, thalamus, hypothalamus, amygdala, and hippocampus. These projections may regulate arousal, cognition, and other functions. PFC, prefrontal cortex; BF, basal forebrain; S, striatum; NA, nucleus accumbens; T, thalamus; HY, hypothalamus; A, amygdala; H, hippocampus; NT, brainstem neurotransmitter centers; SC, spinal cord; C, cerebellum.

Histamine

The final set of neurotransmitter pathways illustrated here are those for histamine (Figure 7-13). This interesting neurotransmitter arises from a single small area of the hypothalamus known as the tuberomammillary nucleus (TMN), which is also part of the "sleep-wake switch" and thus plays an important part in arousal, wakefulness, and sleep. The TMN is a small bilateral nucleus that provides histaminergic input to most brain regions and to the spinal cord.

Linking it all together into functional loops

Corticocortical circuits

As we have stated above, cortical circuits provide the engine for the brain's behavioral and functional outputs. Circuits process information and then act on that information by linking neurons together into functional loops. One type of functional loop is a cortex-to-cortex circuit, where one part of the cortex talks to another, a so-called corticocortical interaction (Figure 7-14A). For example, pyramidal cells in one part of the prefrontal cortex link to pyramidal cells in another part of the prefrontal cortex. These connections utilize glutamate output from one pyramidal cell's axon directly onto the dendritic tree of another pyramidal cell.

Cholinergic Projections from Basal Forebrain

Important cholinergic neurons in the basal forebrain project to the cortex, hippocampus, and amygdala.

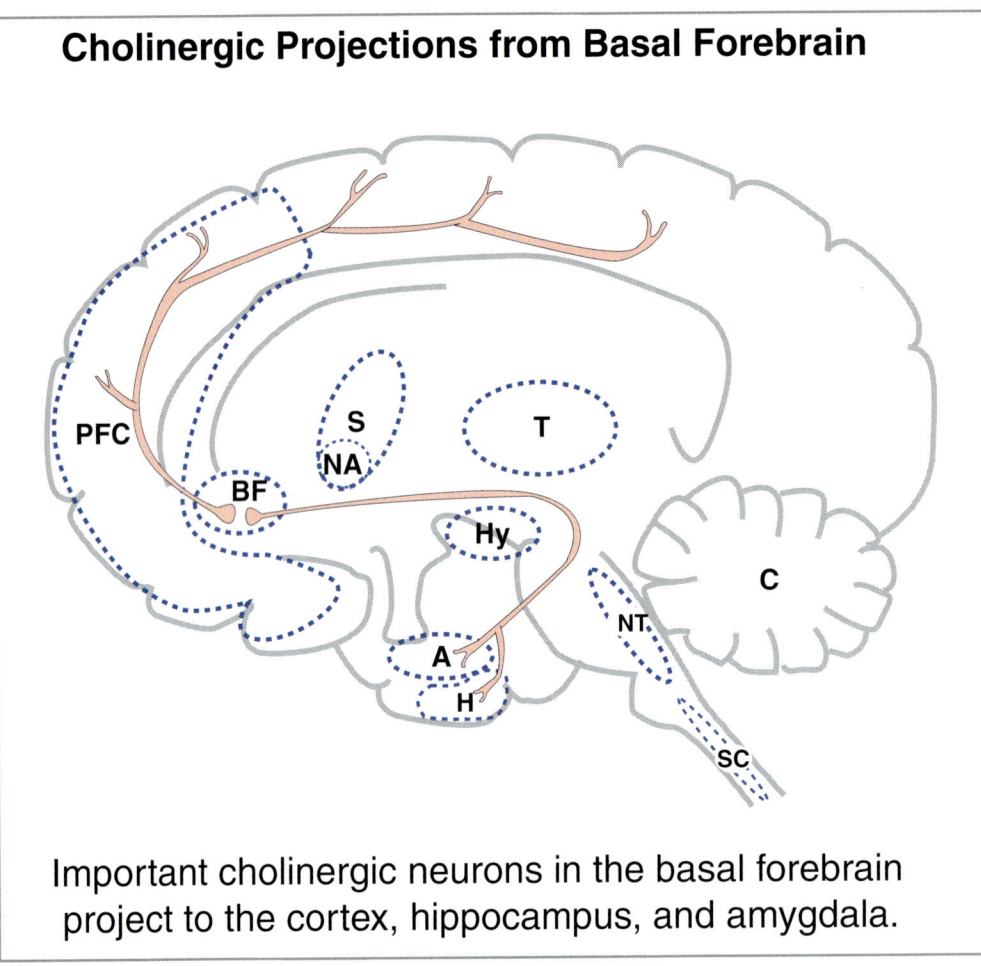

FIGURE 7-12 **Major acetylcholine projections via basal forebrain.** Major neurotransmitter projections, part 5: acetylcholine via basal forebrain. Cholinergic neurons originating in the basal forebrain project to the prefrontal cortex, hippocampus, and amygdala; they are believed to be involved in memory. PFC, prefrontal cortex; BF, basal forebrain; S, striatum; NA, nucleus accumbens; T, thalamus; HY, hypothalamus; A, amygdala; H, hippocampus; NT, brainstem neurotransmitter centers; SC, spinal cord; C, cerebellum.

Both cortical areas can be "tuned" by input from below: namely, neurotransmitter input arriving from neurotransmitter centers to innervate these very same pyramidal cells (Figure 7-14B). This is an example of how circuits allow a neurotransmitter not only to directly influence a neuron but also – by virtue of neuronal connections within a circuit – to affect a third neuron through an intermediary. That is, blue dopamine input to prefrontal cortex (PFC) area 1 in Figure 7-14B not only directly influences PFC area 1, symbolically turning it blue, but also has an indirect impact on PFC area 2 through the connections of PFC area 1 with PFC area 2. Likewise, pink acetylcholine input directly influences PFC area 2, symbolically turning it pink, yet this indirectly influences PFC area 1 as well.

Some of the more important corticocortical circuits and connections involving the prefrontal cortex are shown in Figure 7-15. Not all areas have robust, bilateral interactions with each other. For example, DLPFC has relatively sparse direct connections with limbic

Histaminergic Projections from the Hypothalamus

The histamine center is in the hypothalamus (TMN, tuberomammillary nucleus), which provides input to most brain regions and the spinal cord.

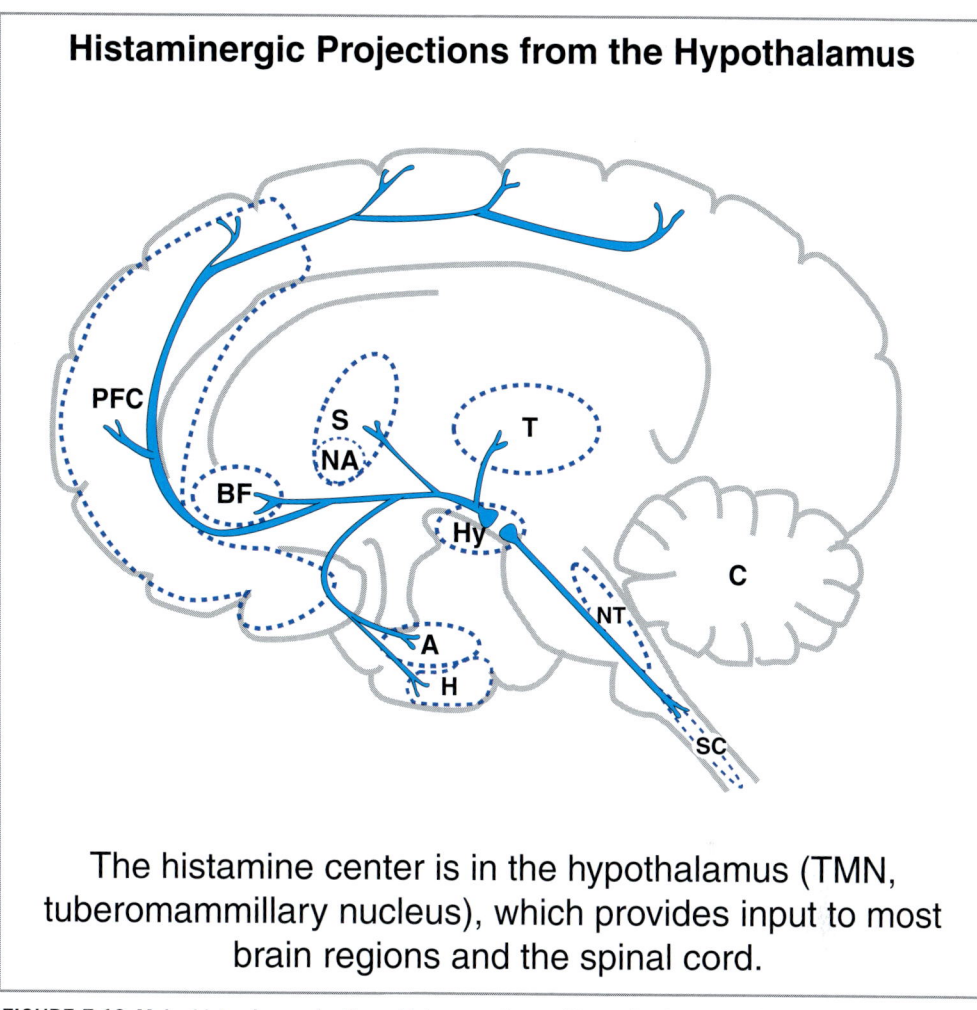

FIGURE 7-13 **Major histamine projections.** Major neurotransmitter projections, part 6: histamine. Histamine neurons arise from the tuberomammillary nucleus of the hypothalamus and project widely throughout the brain and to the spinal cord. Histamine is predominantly involved in sleep and wakefulness. PFC, prefrontal cortex; BF, basal forebrain; S, striatum; NA, nucleus accumbens; T, thalamus; HY, hypothalamus; A, amygdala; H, hippocampus; NT, brainstem neurotransmitter centers; SC, spinal cord; C, cerebellum.

structures such as amygdala and hippocampus. Thus, some brain areas must go through a second area in order to influence a third area. These corticocortical interactions are discussed in relation to specific psychiatric symptoms – ranging from fear to attention, memory, problem solving, impulses, and emotions – in chapters dealing with specific psychiatric disorders.

Cortico-striatal-thalamic-cortical circuits

Another important cortical circuit is called the "CSTC loop" – the cortico-striatal-thalamic-cortical loop. This circuit allows information to be sent "downstream" and out of the cortex, yet the cortex gets feedback on how that information was processed (Figure 7-16A). Prefrontal cortex projects to the striatal complex and then to the thalamus. Both the

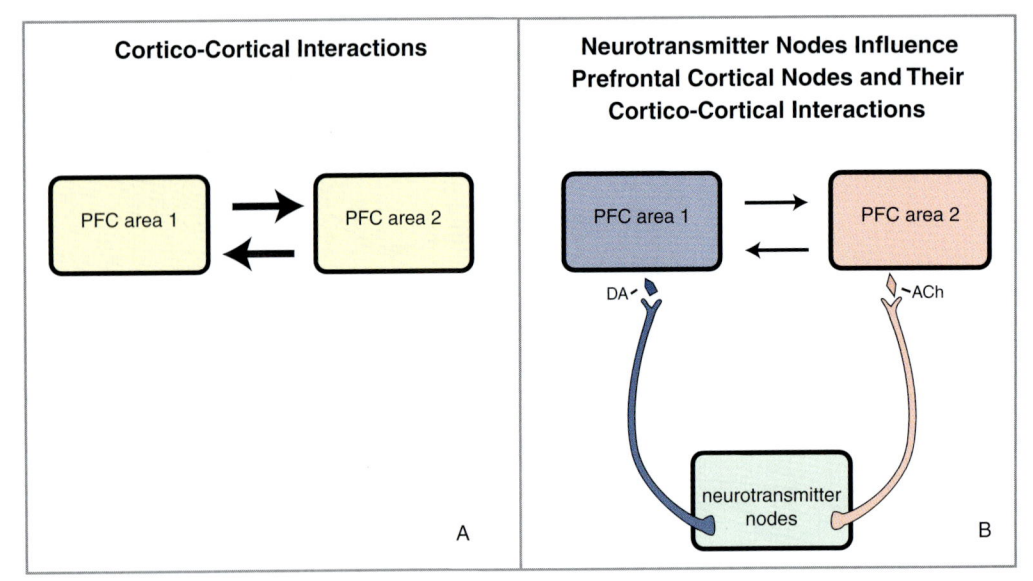

FIGURE 7-14 Cortico-cortical interactions. Information from different brain regions is processed and communicated via neuronal interconnections that form functional loops, or circuits. One type of functional loop is a cortex-to-cortex circuit, or corticocortical interaction (**A**). Corticocortical interactions can also be mediated by input from neurotransmitter nodes (**B**). As shown in panel B, dopaminergic projections directly modulate activity in prefrontal cortex (PFC) area 1 – depicted as this area turning blue – while indirectly modulating activity in PFC area 2 via its interaction with PFC area 1. Similarly, cholinergic projections directly modulate PFC area 2 – shown as this area turning pink – while indirectly modulating PFC area 1.

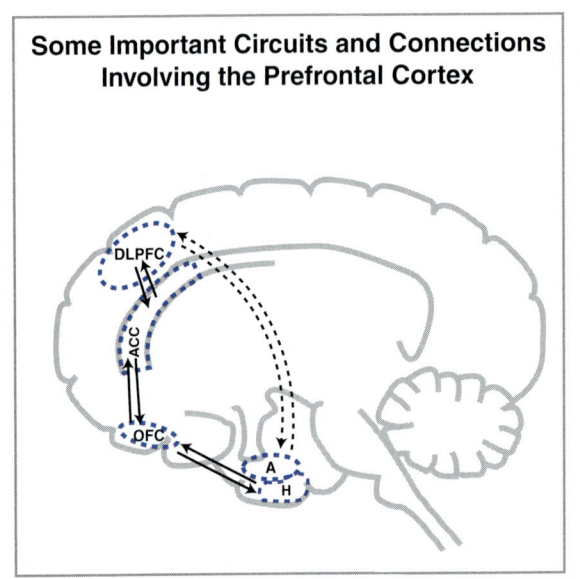

FIGURE 7-15 Key cortico-cortical circuits. Several important prefrontal corticocortical circuits are shown here. The anterior cingulate cortex (ACC) has corticocortical interactions with the dorsolateral prefrontal cortex (DLPFC) and the orbital frontal cortex (OFC). The OFC, in turn, has corticocortical interactions with the hippocampus. The DLPFC has only sparse direct connections with the amygdala and hippocampus.

striatum and the thalamus are topographically organized to interact only with specific areas of the cortex. The loop through the striatum may have a synapse through another part of the striatal complex before it leaves to go to the thalamus. The thalamus relays back to the original area of prefrontal cortex, sometimes right back to the original pyramidal cell.

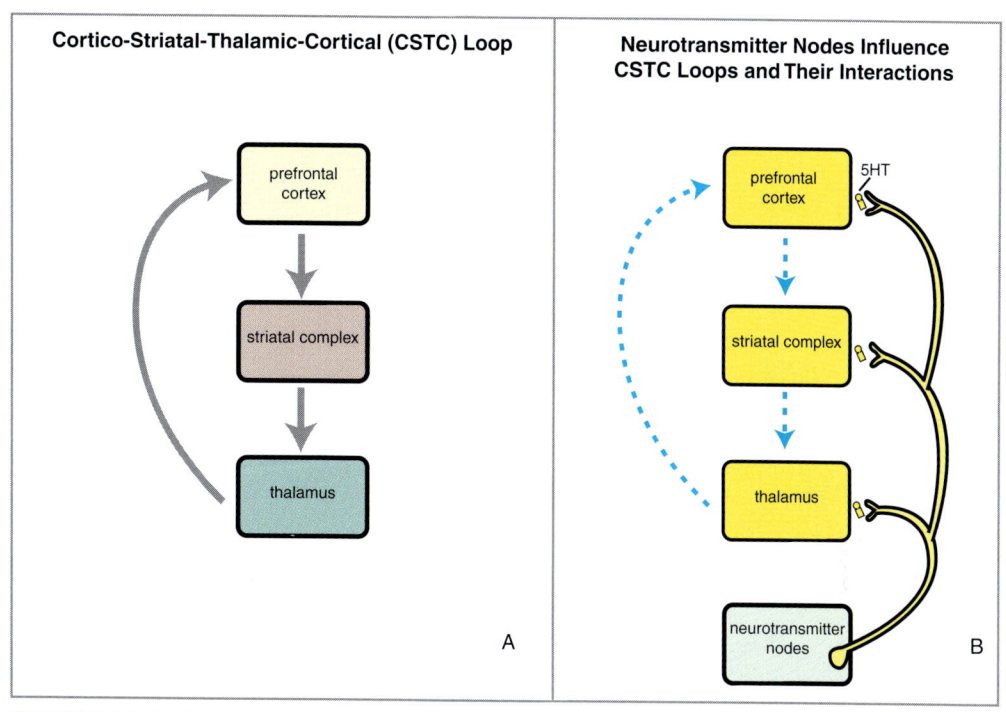

FIGURE 7-16 Cortico-striatal-thalamic-cortical loop. An important circuit is the cortico-striatal-thalamic-cortical (CSTC) loop. The prefrontal cortex projects to the striatal complex, which projects to the thalamus, which feeds back to the prefrontal cortex (**A**). The CSTC loop can be modulated by neurotransmitter nodes that project to the cortex, striatum, or thalamus (**B**). In panel B, serotonin projects to all three regions (depicted as the three regions turning yellow) and inhibits output (indicated by dotted lines connecting the regions).

Neurotransmitters have three chances to influence CSTC loops, since many neurotransmitters innervate all three levels of a CSTC loop (Figure 7-16B). Shown here is an example of serotonin projections arising from their brainstem neurotransmitter nodes and innervating the thalamus, striatal complex, and prefrontal cortex. Releasing serotonin within the CSTC loop symbolically turns all three areas yellow, with inhibition of output at all levels indicated by dotted lines connecting the CSTC loop in Figure 7-16B. This is contrasted with no yellow serotonin influence on these brain areas and fully functioning outputs within the CSTC loop in Figure 7-16A.

A look at how CSTC loops might appear in a three-dimensional brain where you can see through the cortex is shown in Figures 7-17 through 7-21. Each of these serves as an example of the principle of topographical representation of function. Thus, in Figure 7-17, the cortical engine is in the *dorsolateral prefrontal cortex* (DLPFC), projecting to the top (rostral) part of the caudate within the striatal complex, then to the thalamus, and right back to DLPFC. Loops like this are thought to regulate executive functions, problem solving, and cognitive tasks such as representing and maintaining goals and allocating attentional resources to various tasks.

However, the very same type of loop arising out of the *dorsal anterior cingulate gyrus* (ACC) modulates a very specific cognitive function – namely, selective attention. The dorsal ACC evaluates functions such as self-monitoring of performance. In this case, a pyramidal cell now in dorsal ACC projects to a different part of the striatal complex, near the bottom

Circuits in Psychopharmacology | 211

Hypothetical CSTC Loop for Executive Functions

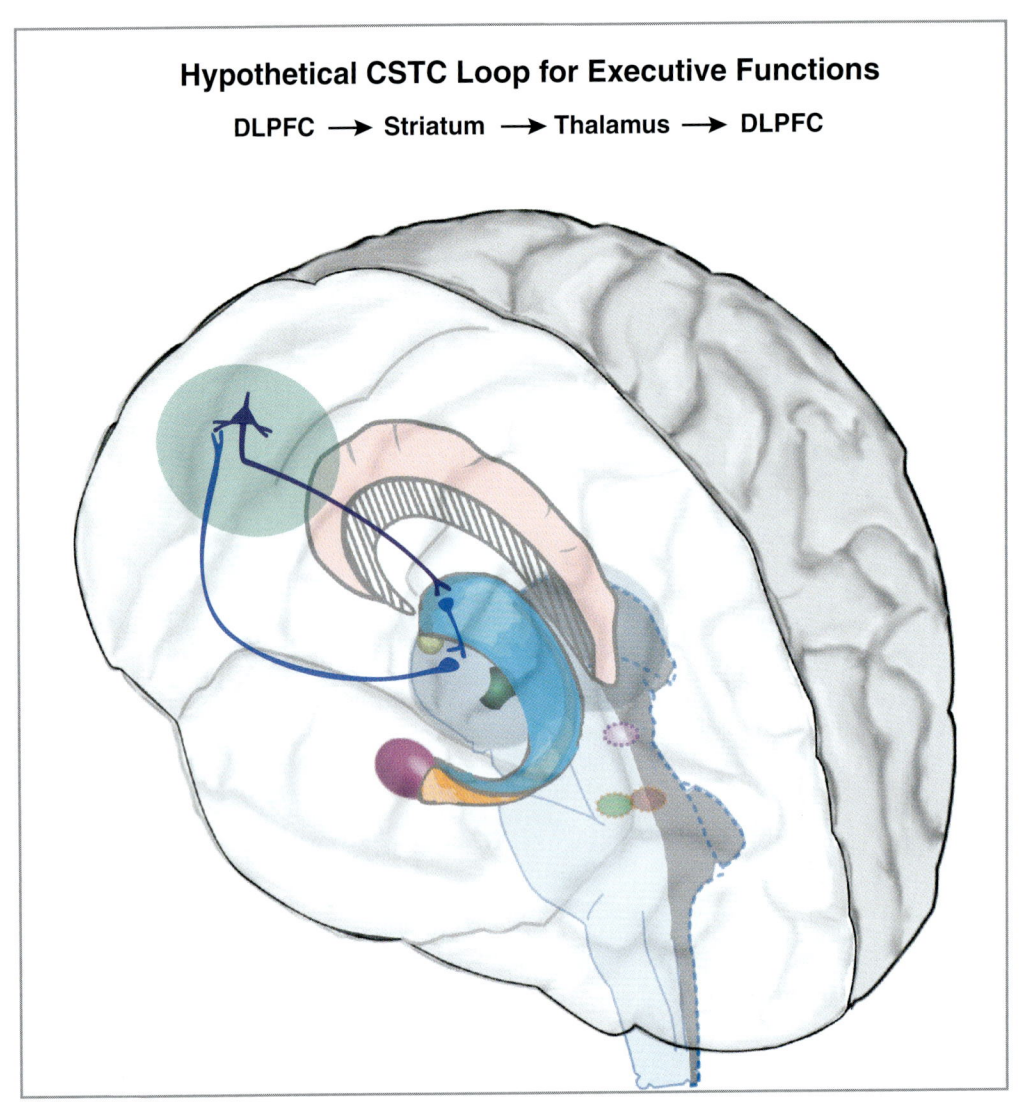

DLPFC → Striatum → Thalamus → DLPFC

FIGURE 7-17 Cortico-striatal-thalamic-cortical loop: executive function. There are many cortico-striatal-thalamic-cortical (CSTC) loops, depending on which prefrontal region is involved as well as where in the striatum and thalamus the neurons project. This figure depicts the hypothetical CSTC loop for executive functions, which involves the dorsolateral prefrontal cortex (DLPFC) and the rostral (top) part of the caudate within the striatal complex.

(or ventral) part of it, then to a different area of thalamus, and back to dorsal ACC (Figure 7-18).

Yet a third CSTC loop is shown in Figure 7-19, with the pyramidal cell engine lying in the *subgenual or ventral part of the ACC* and then projecting to a part of the striatal complex known as the nucleus accumbens; from there it extends to the thalamus and then back to subgenual ACC (Figure 7-19). This loop is thought to regulate emotions, including depression and fear.

A fourth CSTC loop is represented in Figure 7-20, starting with pyramidal output from the *orbital frontal cortex*, to the ventral part of the caudate nucleus in the striatal complex,

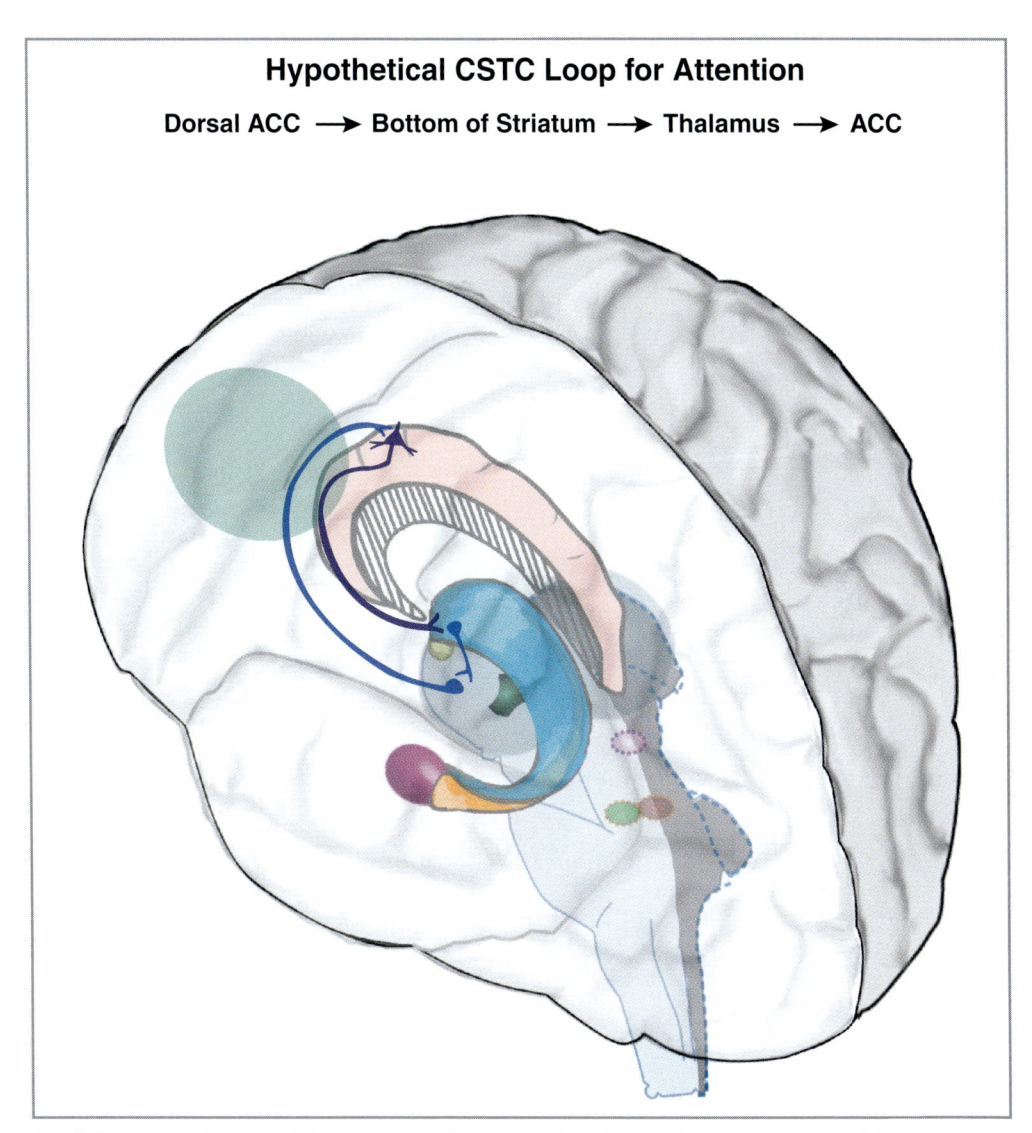

FIGURE 7-18 Cortico-striatal-thalamic-cortical loop: attention. Attention is hypothetically modulated by a cortico-striatal-thalamic-cortical (CSTC) loop arising from the dorsal anterior cingulate cortex (ACC) and projecting to the bottom of the striatum, then the thalamus, and back to the dorsal ACC.

to the thalamus, and back to OFC. Cortical loops from this brain area seem to regulate impulsivity and compulsivity.

Finally, a fifth CSTC loop starts in the *supplemental motor area of prefrontal motor cortex*, projects to the putamen in the lateral part of the striatal complex, then to the thalamus, and back to premotor cortex (Figure 7-21). These loops may modulate motor behavior such as hyperactivity, psychomotor agitation, and psychomotor retardation.

CSTC loops are a very good example of how cortical engines not only drive neuronal structures throughout the brain while receiving feedback from them, but how different functions are regulated by different topographical brain areas. One brain area does not necessarily regulate just one function, and any given function is not necessarily regulated

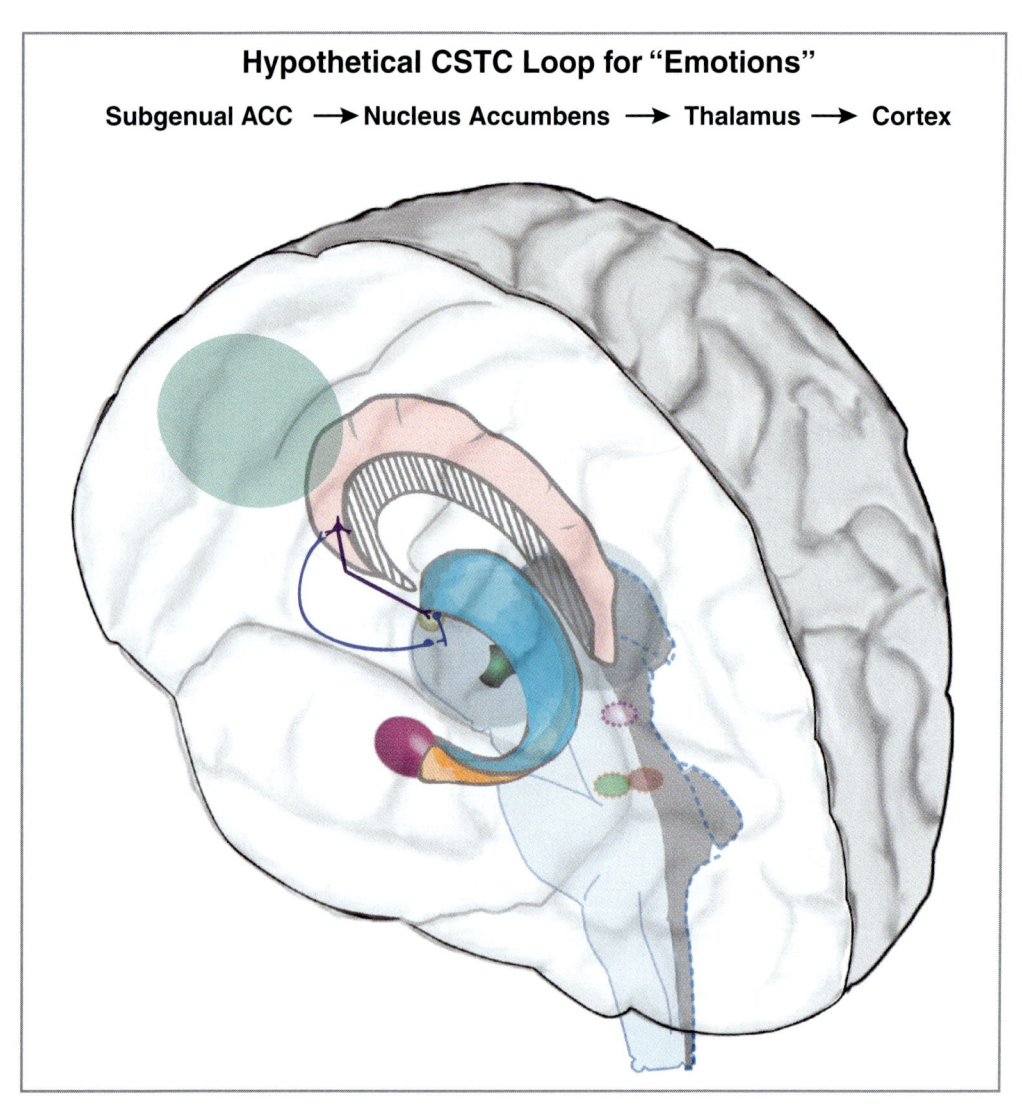

FIGURE 7-19 Cortico-striatal-thalamic-cortical loop: emotion. Emotion is hypothetically modulated by a cortico-striatal-thalamic-cortical (CSTC) loop originating in the ventral, or subgenual, anterior cingulate cortex (ACC) and projecting to the nucleus accumbens, then the thalamus, and back to the subgenual ACC.

by just one dedicated brain area. However, these notions of brain topography are useful to keep in mind when examining functional brain imaging of patients and their specific symptoms.

Pyramidal cells as drivers of cortical circuits

Each of the CSTC loops shown in Figures 7-17 through 7-21 starts and ends with a pyramidal cell in the cortex. Since pyramidal cells drive the engine of cortical circuits, influencing these neurons with drugs that alter neurotransmitter input or output from these cells has a critical role in psychopharmacology. Thus, it is useful to understand a bit about what regulates these interesting and unusual looking cortical neurons.

Hypothetical CSTC Loop for Impulsivity/Compulsivity

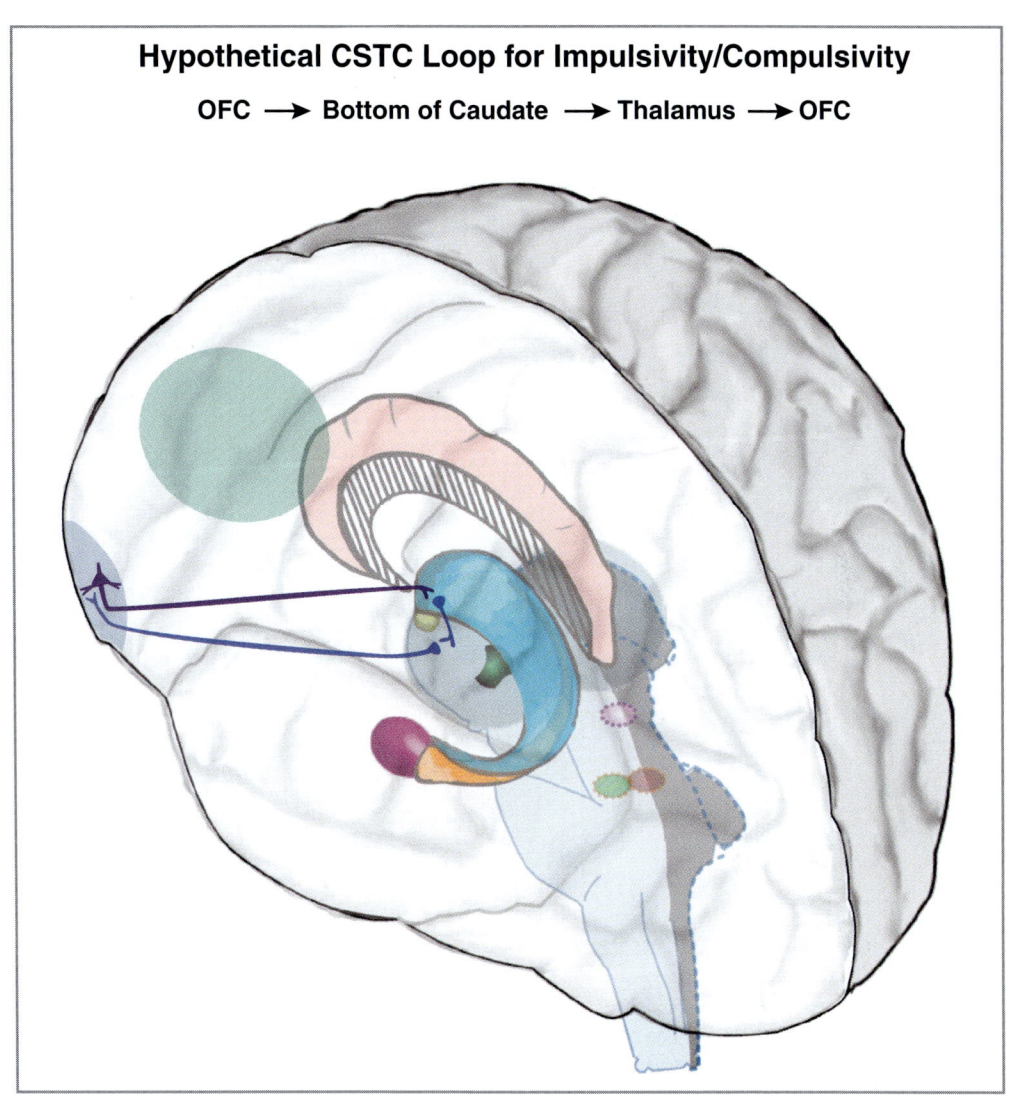

OFC → Bottom of Caudate → Thalamus → OFC

FIGURE 7-20 **Cortico-striatal-thalamic-cortical loop: impulsivity.** Impulsivity and compulsivity are associated with a cortico-striatal-thalamic-cortical (CSTC) loop that involves the orbital frontal cortex, the bottom of the caudate, and the thalamus.

Pyramidal cell excitatory outputs

Remember that pyramidal cells are discussed in Chapter 1, and are shaped like they are sitting as a triangular pyramid, each having an extensively branched spiny apical dendrite and shorter basal dendrites, as well as a single axon emerging from the basal pole of the cell body (Figure 1-2A and B).

The cortex is a series of layers or laminae, and pyramidal cells are located in four of the six cortical laminae (Figure 7-22). Where a pyramidal cell sends its output depends upon where it sits in the cortical lamina. Thus, corticocortical outputs come from pyramidal cells residing in lamina 2 or 3 (Figure 7-22). On the other hand, cortical outputs from lamina 5 drive the engine for the CSTC loops to striatum.

Hypothetical CSTC Loop for Motor Activity

Prefrontal Motor Cortex ⟶ Putamen (Lateral Striatum) ⟶ Thalamus ⟶ Cortex

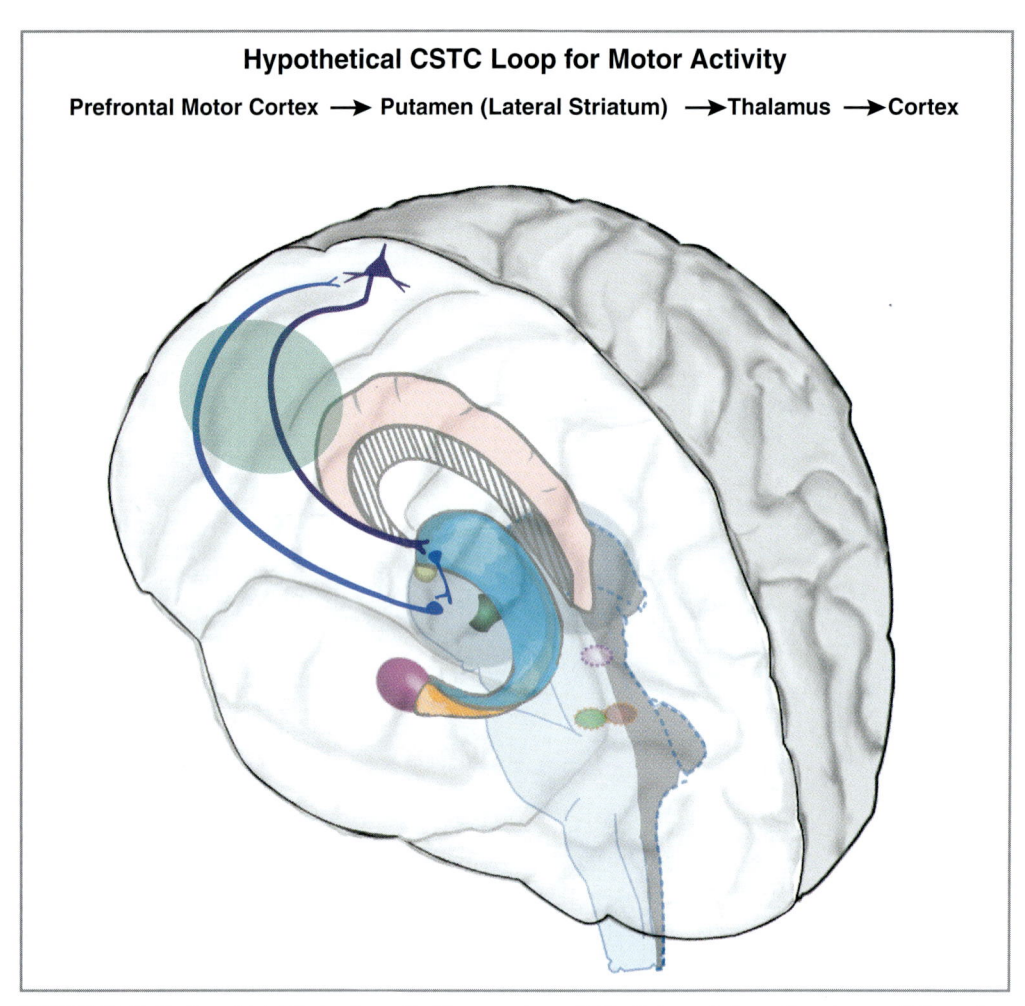

FIGURE 7-21 Cortico-striatal-thalamic-cortical loop: motor activity. Motor activity, such as hyperactivity and psychomotor agitation or retardation, can be modulated by a cortico-striatal-thalamic-cortical (CSTC) loop from the prefrontal motor cortex to the putamen (lateral striatum) to the thalamus and back to the prefrontal motor cortex.

Still other cortical circuits start from pyramidal neurons in lamina 5, which project to the brainstem, or from pyramidal neurons in lamina 6, which project to the thalamus (Figure 7-22). The neurotransmitter output of most pyramidal neurons is glutamate.

Pyramidal cell inhibitory inputs

Pyramidal neurons in the cortex also have many *inputs* from various brain areas. Those from nearby GABAergic inhibitory interneurons are shown in Figure 7-23. The structures of these neurons are also described in Chapter 1 and shown there as basket neurons in Figures 1-3A and 1-3B, as double bouquet neurons in Figures 1-4A and 1-4B, and as chandelier neurons in Figures 1-7A and 1-7B. Now we see these same neurons functioning as GABAergic interneurons in the cortex, innervating cortical pyramidal neurons with their inhibitory input (Figure 7-23). Thus, a red basket neuron is shown in Figure 7-23, on the left, with inhibitory GABA input to the pyramidal neuron's cell body, or soma. At the top of Figure 7-23, a blue double bouquet neuron is shown providing GABAergic inhibitory

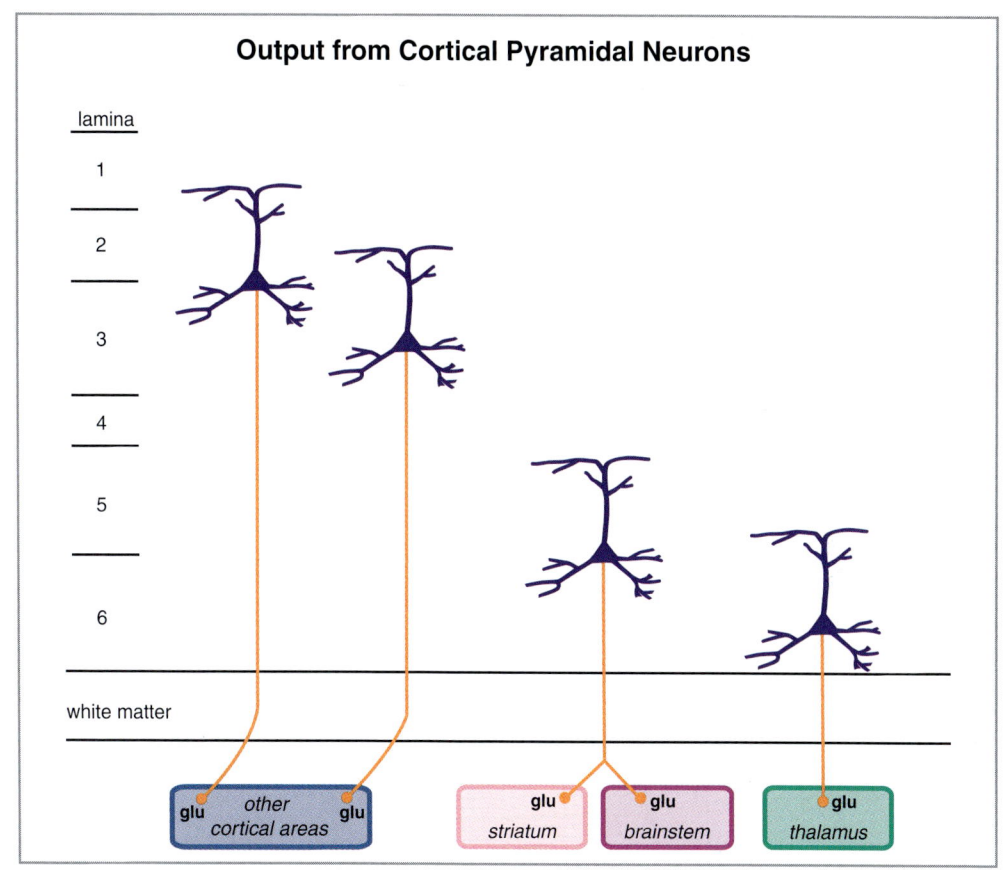

FIGURE 7-22 Output from cortical pyramidal neurons. Cortico-striatal-thalamic-cortical loops begin and end with a pyramidal neuron in the cortex. These pyramidal cells are located in various laminae, or layers, of the cortex, which influences the direction in which they send their output. Cortical pyramidal neurons located in laminae 2 and 3 send output to other cortical areas; those located in lamina 5 send output to the striatum and brainstem; and those in lamina 6 send output to the thalamus. The neurotransmitter output of all cortical pyramidal neurons is glutamate.

input to the end of an apical dendrite on the pyramidal neuron. There is even a second blue double bouquet neuron on the right, inhibiting the double bouquet neuron on the left (Figure 7-23). This arrangement has the net effect of "inhibiting the inhibition," or "disinhibiting" the pyramidal neuron, with the second double bouquet neuron thus canceling the effect of the inhibitory input of the first. Finally, a green chandelier neuron innervates the initial segment of the axon, also known as the axon hillock of the pyramidal neuron (Figure 7-23). As explained in Chapter 1, this type of inhibitory chandelier GABAergic input to the axon hillock exerts powerful control over the output of that pyramidal cell, possibly even determining whether or not that pyramidal axon will fire an action potential. One can readily see that there are many opportunities to exert inhibitory control on a pyramidal neuron as it ranges throughout the cortex, and that the presence or absence of GABA tone on the pyramidal neuron can have profound influence on the ability of that cortical pyramidal cell to serve as the driver of a cortical engine that delivers the behavioral programs of the brain.

Circuits in Psychopharmacology

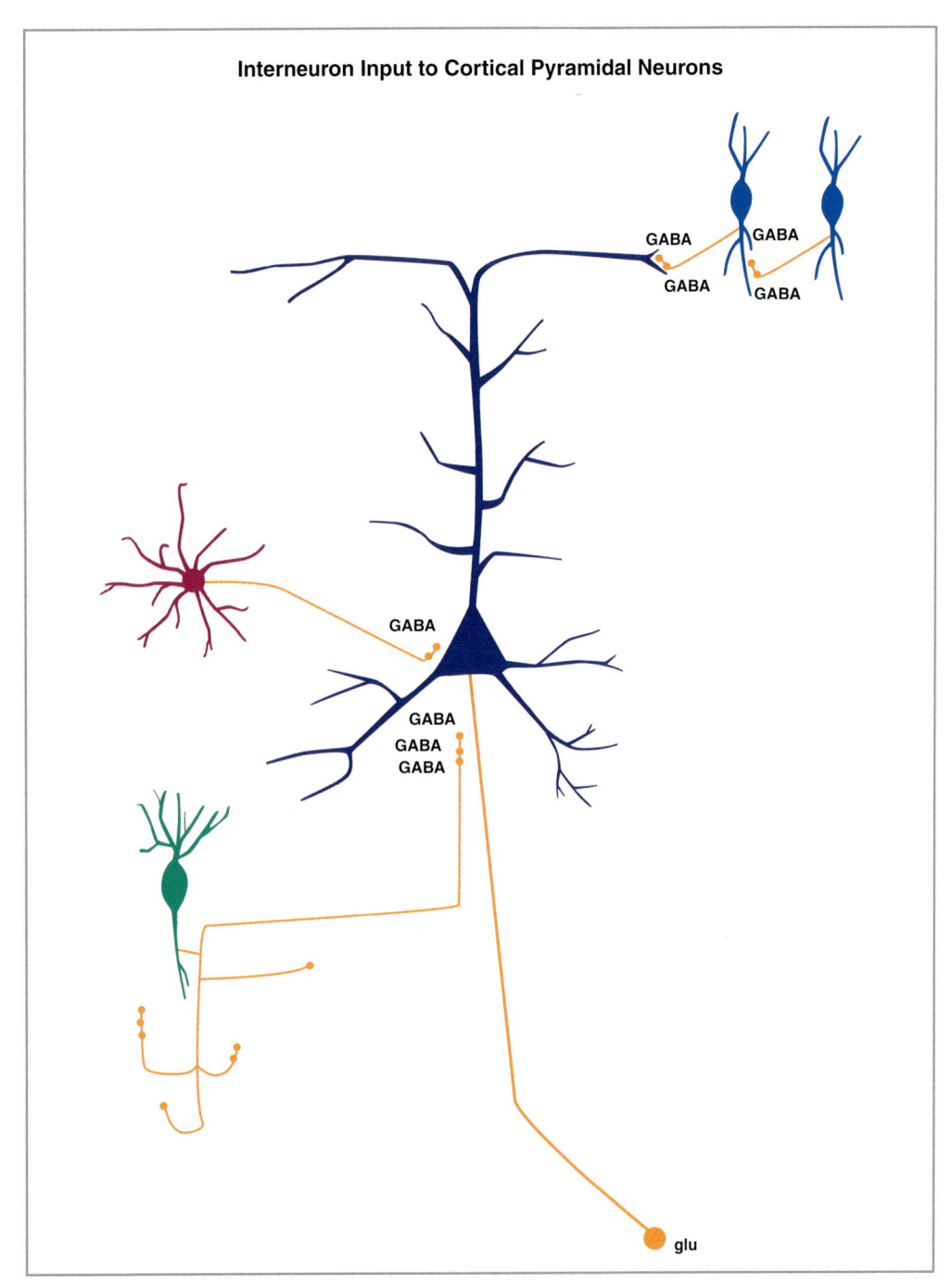

FIGURE 7-23 Interneuron input to cortical pyramidal neurons. Cortical pyramidal neurons receive inputs from many different brain areas. Shown here are different types of GABAergic inhibitory interneurons: a GABAergic basket neuron (red, left), providing inhibitory input to the pyramidal neuron's soma; a GABAergic chandelier neuron (green, bottom), providing inhibitory input to the axon hillock; and two double bouquet neurons (blue, right), providing input to a dendrite of the pyramidal neuron. The left double bouquet neuron provides direct inhibitory input to the pyramidal neuron; however, it itself is inhibited by the right double bouquet neuron, which thus inhibits the inhibition – or disinhibits – the actions of the left double bouquet neuron.

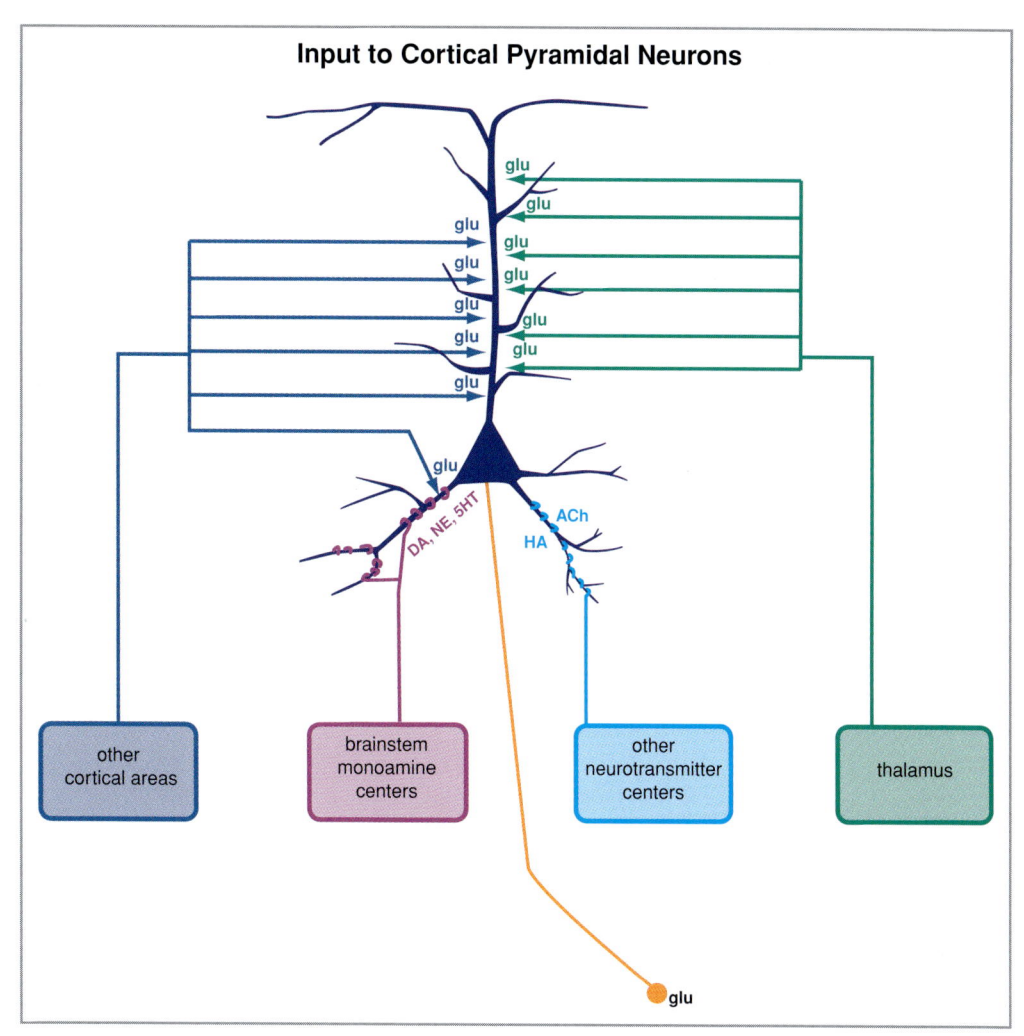

FIGURE 7-24 Input to cortical pyramidal neurons. Shown here are different inputs to cortical pyramidal neurons. Glutamatergic excitatory projections from thalamus and cortical areas synapse with apical dendrites, while monoamines and other neurotransmitters synapse with basilar dendrites (shown) as well as apical dendrites. These neurotransmitter projections can be either inhibitory or excitatory, depending on the neurotransmitter and the receptor involved; however, their actions may be more subtle than those of GABA and glutamate.

Pyramidal cell excitatory inputs

Cortical pyramidal neurons also receive many *excitatory* inputs, coming predominantly to synapse with the apical (top) dendrites and utilizing the excitatory neurontransmitter glutamate (Figure 7-24). These inputs arise from other cortical areas (corticocortical inputs) and from the thalamus (corticothalamic inputs), all utilizing glutamate as neurotransmitter. Thus it is easy to see how the cortical pyramidal neuron can either be excited by these long-distance glutamate inputs, shown in Figure 7-24, or inhibited by short-distance GABA inputs, shown in Figure 7-23.

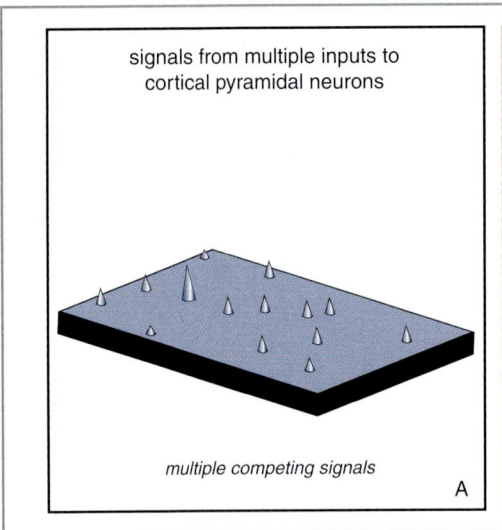

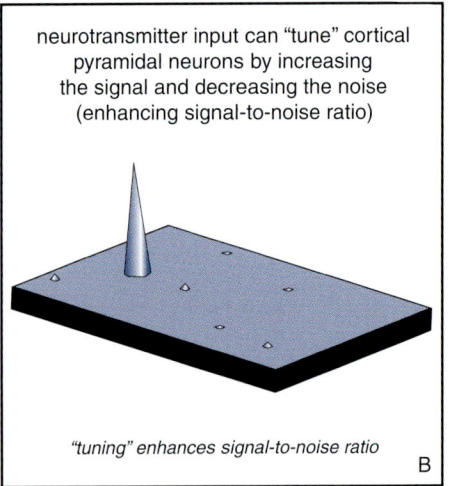

FIGURE 7-25 Signal-to-noise ratio. Cortical pyramidal neurons receive signals from multiple competing inputs, forming "noise" (**A**). Monoamine input can "tune" cortical pyramidal neurons to enhance a specific signal that should be prioritized by increasing that signal and decreasing the others (i.e., the noise) – in other words, by enhancing the signal-to-noise ratio (**B**).

Fine tuning pyramidal cells with monoamine, acetylcholine, and histamine input

If glutamate and GABA exert more of an "on-off" effect on pyramidal neurons, monoamines and other neurotransmitters may exert more of a "fine-tuning" action on pyramidal cells. Inputs from various other neurotransmitter centers – such as the monoamines dopamine, norepinephrine, and serotonin as well as other key neurotransmitters such as acetylcholine and histamine – are also shown in Figure 7-24. They synapse here on basilar dendrites, but they also have synapses on apical dendrites. These specific neurotransmitter inputs can be either excitatory or inhibitory, depending on the neurotransmitter and the specific receptor subtype expressed on the pyramidal cell at a given synapse. More often, however, their actions are more subtle than just turning a neuron on or off.

Specifically, monoamines may be particularly helpful in optimizing the output of pyramidal neurons. That is, under many circumstances, the multiple competing outputs all appear at once and can be interpreted as if they are all just "noise" (Figure 7-25A). However, graded degrees of monoamine input can "tune" a pyramidal neuron to a signal that it must prioritize while allowing it to ignore other competing signals (Figure 7-25B). This is sometimes called increasing the signal and decreasing the noise, or enhancing the signal-to-noise ratio.

Just as in tuning a guitar string, more is not always better (Figure 7-26). That is, neurotransmitter input to cause receptor stimulation may optimize pyramidal neuronal functioning, but only to a point. Too much tension on a guitar string can make it sound just as out of tune as too little. The same is apparently true for neurotransmitters such as dopamine, where finding the optimal amount of receptor stimulation is what is needed for optimal tuning of signal-to-noise ratios. Thus, for optimal tuning, some "out of tune" neurons need more neurotransmitters and others need less (Figure 7-26).

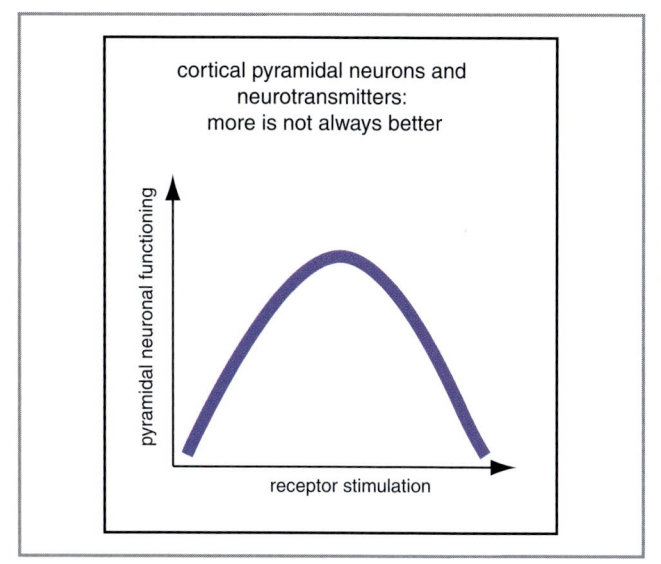

FIGURE 7-26 Pyramidal neuronal function and receptor stimulation. Receptors can be both under- and overstimulated. Finding the optimal amount of receptor stimulation is necessary for optimal tuning of signal-to-noise ratios. This means that in some cases, neurotransmission needs to be increased, but in other cases it may need to be decreased.

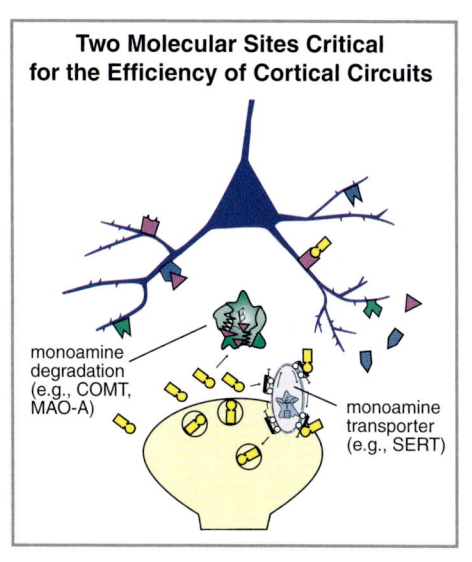

FIGURE 7-27 Molecular sites for regulating monoamines. Two molecular sites important for regulating monoamines and thus for maintaining efficiency of cortical circuits are (1) the enzymes that break down monoamines and (2) monoamine transporters. Examples of enzymes include monoamine oxidase A (MAO-A) and catechol-O-methyl transferase (COMT). Examples of monoamine transporters include the serotonin transporter (SERT).

Regulating the monoamine "tuners"

Two of the key regulators of the monoamines that help to set the tone of a pyramidal neuron are shown in Figure 7-27 – namely, the presynaptic transporters for monoamines and the catabolic enzymes for monoamine degradation. Interestingly, genetic control of these regulators of monoamines also profoundly affects the efficiency of information processing; there are two examples of this that can now be measured in living humans with psychiatric disorders. These are the neuroimaging consequences of variants of the genes for the serotonin transporter (SERT) and for the dopamine metabolizing enzyme COMT (catechol-O-methyl transferase). Both are discussed extensively in various chapters on imaging genetics and different psychiatric disorders.

Summary

Modern psychopharmacology is being transformed by the systematic mapping of psychiatric symptoms to specific brain regions and by the ability to image these regions and their functioning or malfunctioning in patients. Neurons in the cortex are connected to many other neurons, forming cortical circuits that serve as engines for brain functions. Prefrontal cortex is especially important to behaviors, with executive functioning localized to dorsolateral prefrontal cortex, selective attention to dorsal parts of the anterior cingulate, impulsivity to orbital frontal cortex, emotions to ventromedial prefrontal cortex, and motor control to supplementary motor areas. Loops of neurons out of one cortical area and into another (corticocortical circuits) as well as out of cortex to the striatum, thalamus, and back to cortex (cortico-striatal-thalamic-cortical circuits, or CSTCs) are examples of key neuronal networks that have the capacity to transform simple inputs into complex outputs which ultimately mediate brain functions and behaviors. Multiple neurotransmitters influence cortical circuits at every node in the circuit; this provides an opportunity both for genes to influence information processing in circuits by regulating neurotransmitter functioning and for psychopharmacologists to influence symptoms in circuits by administering drugs that alter neurotransmitter actions in specific brain circuits.

CHAPTER 8

From Circuits to Symptoms in Psychopharmacology

- Malfunctioning loops
  - Stress and the normal circuit
  - Stress sensitization
  - Progression from stress sensitization
  - Preemptive treatments
  - Is mental illness damaging to your brain?
  - Diabolical learning
- Imaging malfunctioning circuits
  - fMRI and PET
  - Provoking cognitive circuits
  - Imaging genetics: the role of dopamine in cognitive processing by DLPFC circuits
  - Provoking fear circuits
  - Imaging genetics: the role of serotonin in fear processing by the amygdala
  - Provoking circuits for attention
  - Seeing your grandmother in your brain
  - CNS-I (Central nervous system investigators in the psychopharmacology of tomorrow may model crime scene investigators of today)
- Symptoms and circuits for the psychopharmacologist
- Summary

Psychiatric symptoms are increasingly linked to the malfunction of specific brain circuits. Genetic and environmental influences conspire to produce inefficient information processing in these circuits, and can increasingly be detected with modern neuroimaging techniques. Brain imaging combined with genetics has thus given birth to the new discipline of "imaging genetics," which is transforming how we think about psychiatric disorders and their treatments. Therefore it is important to understand current theories about how psychiatric disorders are linked to neuronal circuitry and how this can potentially be detected in patients with modern genetic and imaging technologies. This background also provides the rationale for using and combining current treatments for the symptoms of psychiatric disorders as well as for strategies leading to new drug development in psychopharmacology.

Malfunctioning loops

When cortical circuits malfunction, the effect is felt throughout the loop it drives, and causes downstream dysfunction in other anatomical areas manifest as inefficient information processing throughout the network. In Chapter 6 we discussed how genetic abnormalities in brain molecules can bias brain circuits to break down and cause symptoms, especially when multiple risk genes combine with significant environmental stressors (Figure 6-9). Malfunction in cortical circuits can also be acquired after birth by various nongenetic factors, such as emotional and physical trauma, aberrant learning, drugs, toxins, and infection. These external factors can also act on circuits to produce inefficient information processing and psychiatric symptoms.

Stress and the normal circuit

An illustration of this concept is shown in Figure 8-1. Here a resting circuit is provoked by a single emotional trauma, causing overactivation of the circuit but no symptoms because the circuit is able to process the load. When the trauma is withdrawn, the circuit returns to baseline functioning. The whole time the circuit is overactivated, it is clinically silent. This is also the normal processing of stress, and was discussed and illustrated in Chapter 6, showing what happens whether your circuits are normal (Figure 6-7) or vulnerable (Figure 6-8).

Normally, the response to emotional trauma is to have circuits compensate, process the stressful load, and cause no symptoms. Furthermore, after the trauma is withdrawn,

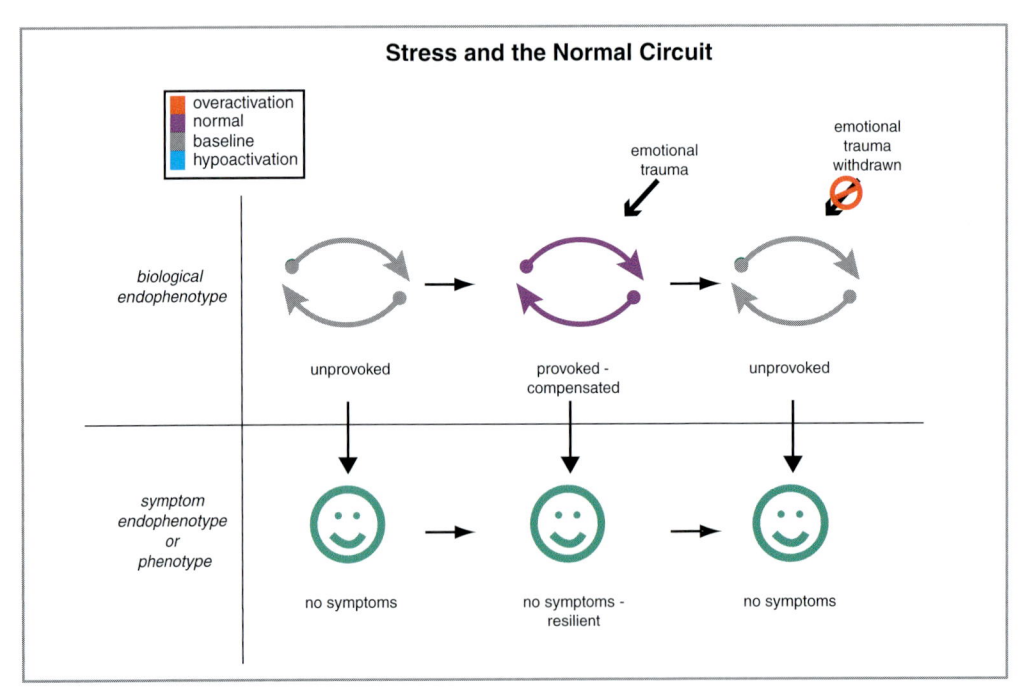

FIGURE 8-1 Stress and the normal circuit. In a healthy individual, stress can cause a temporary activation of circuits which is resolved when the stressor is removed. As shown here, when the circuit is unprovoked, no symptoms are produced. In the presence of a stressor such as emotional trauma, the circuit is provoked yet able to compensate for the effects of the stressor. By its ability to process the information load from the environment, it can avoid producing symptoms. When the stressor is withdrawn, the circuit returns to baseline functioning.

Development of Stress Sensitization in Normal Circuits

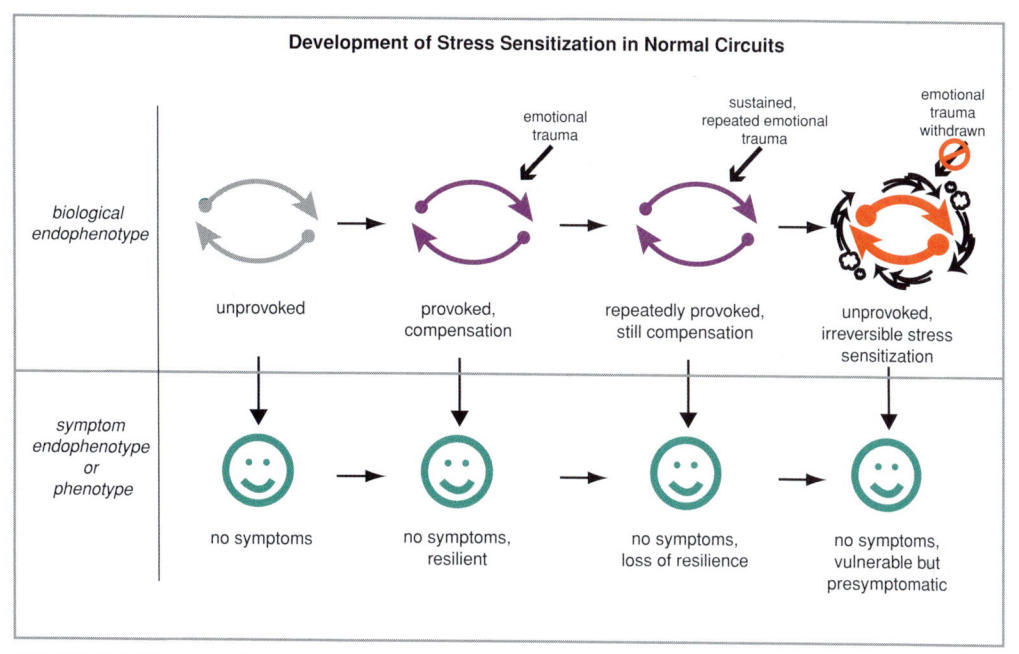

FIGURE 8-2 Stress sensitization in normal circuits. Prolonged activation of circuits due to repeated exposure to stressors can lead to a condition known as "stress sensitization," in which circuits not only become overly activated but remain overly activated even when the stressor is withdrawn. Although circuits are overly activated in this model, the individual exhibits no symptoms because these circuits can somehow still compensate for this additional load; however, the individual with "stress-sensitized" circuits is now vulnerable to the effects of future stressors, so that the risk for developing psychiatric symptoms is increased. Stress sensitization may therefore constitute a "presymptomatic" state for some psychiatric symptoms. This state might be detectable with functional brain scans of circuits but not from psychiatric interviews or patient complaints.

biological resilience is sustained. Humans are thus wired for a certain amount of stress. One might even say that some people purposely seek stress to "exercise" their circuits so that those circuits can not only handle current stress but learn to handle more. It is only when the load is mismatched with the potential of the circuit to handle the load that problems occur.

Stress sensitization

What problems can circuits develop and what symptoms can patients develop when this mismatch between the demand of a load and the capacity of a circuit occurs? Hypothetically, when circuits are repeatedly stressed, put repeatedly on overload, and not allowed to recover, as in Figure 8-2, the circuit can become "stress-sensitized," such that it starts working overtime even when the stressor is withdrawn. Despite this problem that has now developed in the circuit, there is still no symptom. However, the price paid by the circuit for compensating for this overload is loss of resilience and development of vulnerability (Figure 8-2). One might be able to detect the biological endophenotype of increased activation if the stressed circuit were measured with functional neuroimaging techniques, but there is no symptom endophenotype to observe.

This is analogous to a duck swimming quickly across a pond: the duck looks relaxed and dignified above the water, but it is paddling frantically below the surface. Stress sensitization could hypothetically happen to the circuits of children who experience early-life trauma yet do not (as children) develop psychiatric symptoms immediately following the trauma. In

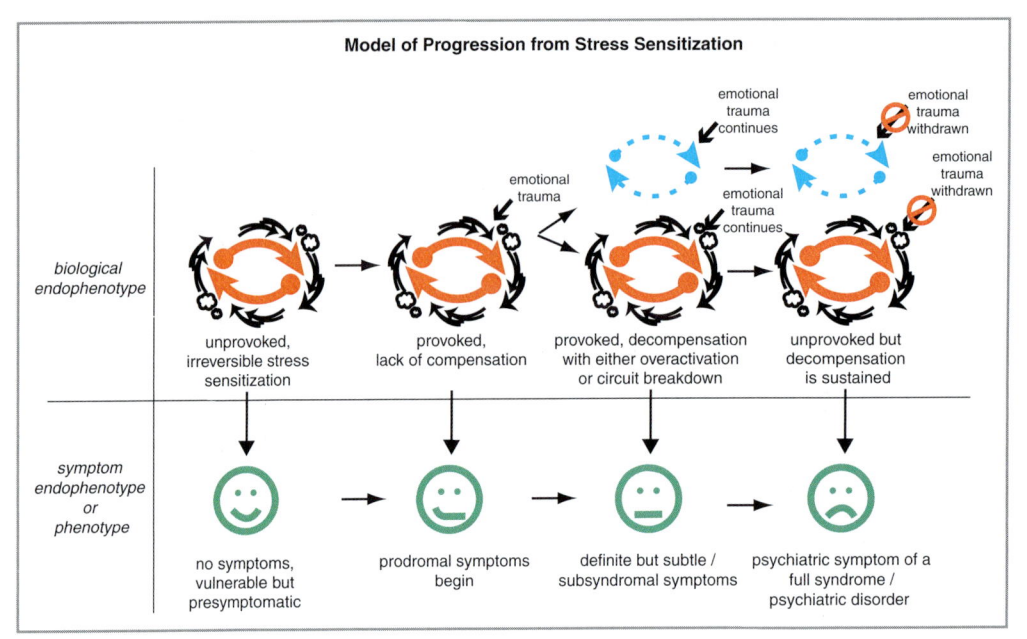

FIGURE 8-3 Progression from stress sensitization. This figure shows the progression from stress sensitization to psychiatric symptoms. That is, individuals with stress sensitization are at increased risk for developing psychiatric symptoms following exposure to subsequent stressors. Stress sensitized and overly activated circuits at rest are shown on the far left. In the absence of additional stressors, these overly activated circuits are nevertheless clinically silent, since they are able to compensate for the excessive activation. However, these overly activated circuits, in an effort to combat the effects of previous stress, are less efficient in their information processing than are normal, nonsensitized circuits. Under additional stress or emotional trauma, stress-sensitized circuits are hypothetically unable to compensate and begin to show signs of breakdown into subtle prodromal symptoms. With further emotional trauma, these failing circuits either do not compensate when they overly activate or even break down and fail to activate adequately, leading to the development of definite but subsyndromal symptoms. Finally, with continuing emotional trauma, the malfunctioning circuits break down further; thereafter psychiatric symptoms not only develop but may persist even after withdrawal of the emotional trauma (far right).

such cases, the stage is set for breakdown the next time – later in life, perhaps in adulthood – that a load is put on this circuit.

Progression from stress sensitization

Sure enough, in Figure 8-3, a stress-sensitized circuit meets a subsequent emotional trauma and the circuitry can no longer compensate. The response of this vulnerable circuit is to decompensate: either enhanced activity of the circuit is no longer able to compensate for an emotional trauma that would ordinarily be processed by a normal, nonsensitized circuit or the circuit fails and is no longer activated at all (Figure 8-3). In either case the progression of the biological endophenotype is no longer clinically silent: a vulnerable but presymptomatic state progresses to prodromal symptoms, then to definite but subtle symptoms not sufficient to qualify for a psychiatric disorder and thus subsyndromal, and finally to fully developed psychiatric symptoms as part of a full syndrome psychiatric disorder (Figure 8-3).

Preemptive treatments

The hypothesis of disease progression from stress sensitization to psychiatric disorder has raised an interesting question: what would happen if treatment were given *before* the psychiatric disorder developed? With the advent of genotyping, it may be possible to measure

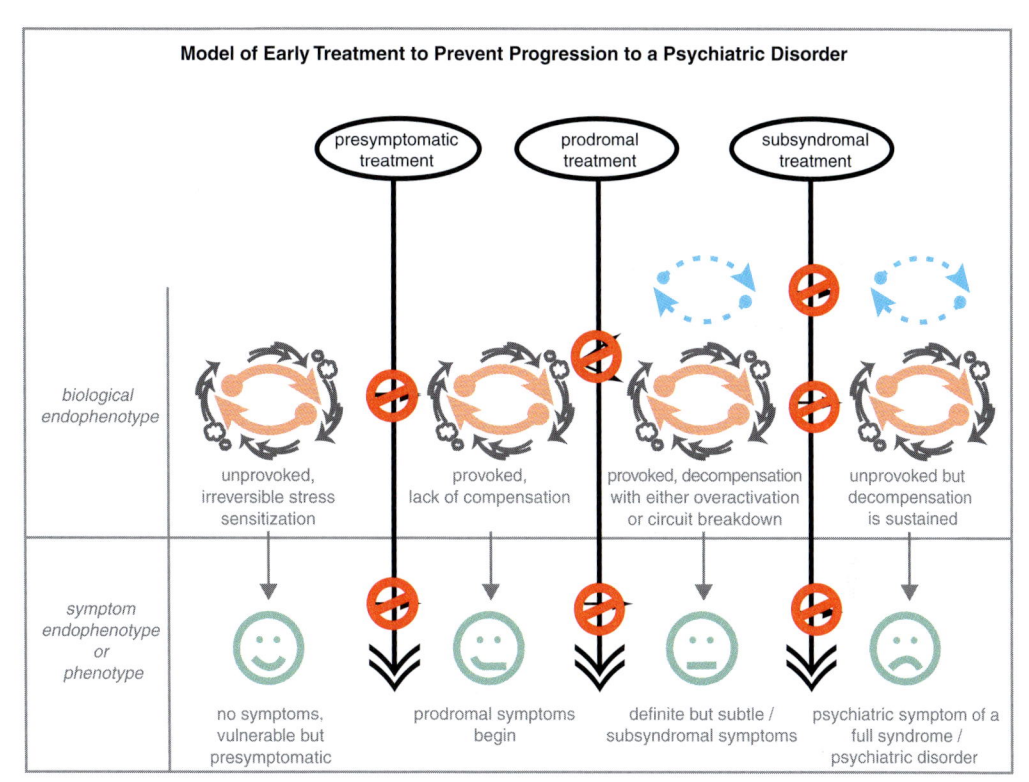

FIGURE 8-4 Presymptomatic and prodromal treatment. It is possible that individuals in presymptomatic states, recognized through the presence of biological endophenotypes identified via functional neuroimaging, could be treated in order to prevent progression to a psychiatric disorder (presymptomatic treatment). Theoretically, the treatments that would reduce the biological loads on circuits would improve the efficiency of information processing, preventing decompensation. Similarly, treatment administered during prodromal or subsyndromal states could also prevent progression to a psychiatric disorder.

preexisting genetic bias for various psychiatric disorders. With the advent of functional neuroimaging, it may be possible to uncover clinically silent but biologically distressed brain circuits laboring with inefficient information processing (that duck paddling frantically below the surface but appearing calm above it).

Specifically, could treatments that improved the efficiency of information processing in circuits buffer them by reducing their load and thus prevent the progression of disease? The concepts of preemptive and disease-modifying treatments are presented in Figure 8-4. Many ongoing studies are investigating whether the treatment of presymptomatic states (i.e., those "frantically paddling ducks" with biological vulnerability and inefficient information processing below the surface but *no symptoms* above it) could prevent progression to a prodrome (subtle premonitory symptoms predicting the development of a psychiatric disorder); whether treatments of prodromal states could prevent progression to subsyndromal states (symptoms not severe enough to qualify for a psychiatric disorder); and whether treatment of subsyndromal states could prevent progression to full-syndrome psychiatric disorders (Figure 8-4).

These are as yet futuristic concepts. The trick in proving disease prevention by future psychopharmacological interventions will be not only to find psychopharmacological treatments that reduce biological loads, but also to be able to identify reliably the biological and clinical endophenotypes along the hypothetical disease progression pathway shown in Figure 8-4. Thus, specific regions and patterns of circuit malfunction accompanying presymptomatic/stress-sensitized, prodromal, subsyndromal, and full symptom states of a psychiatric disorder must become reliably detectable – a situation that does not yet exist with sufficient clarity for clinical practice. However, current research is progressing rapidly, and there is hope that this outcome will someday be achieved. If so, it would dramatically transform the practice of psychiatry in terms of both diagnostic evaluations and of how and when treatments are prescribed.

Is mental illness damaging to your brain?

One of the ideas evolving from the association of malfunctioning circuits not only with symptoms of psychiatric disorders but also with silent risks for psychiatric disorders is that "mental illness may be damaging to your brain." That is, in addition to causing current suffering, symptoms may, if they persist over time, also alter circuits, making it easier and easier for symptoms to occur, worsen, or relapse and harder and harder for drugs to work, with resistance to treatment as a result. This concept has led to the idea that reducing symptoms is perhaps not only merciful in the short run, but good for your brain in the long run (Figure 8-5).

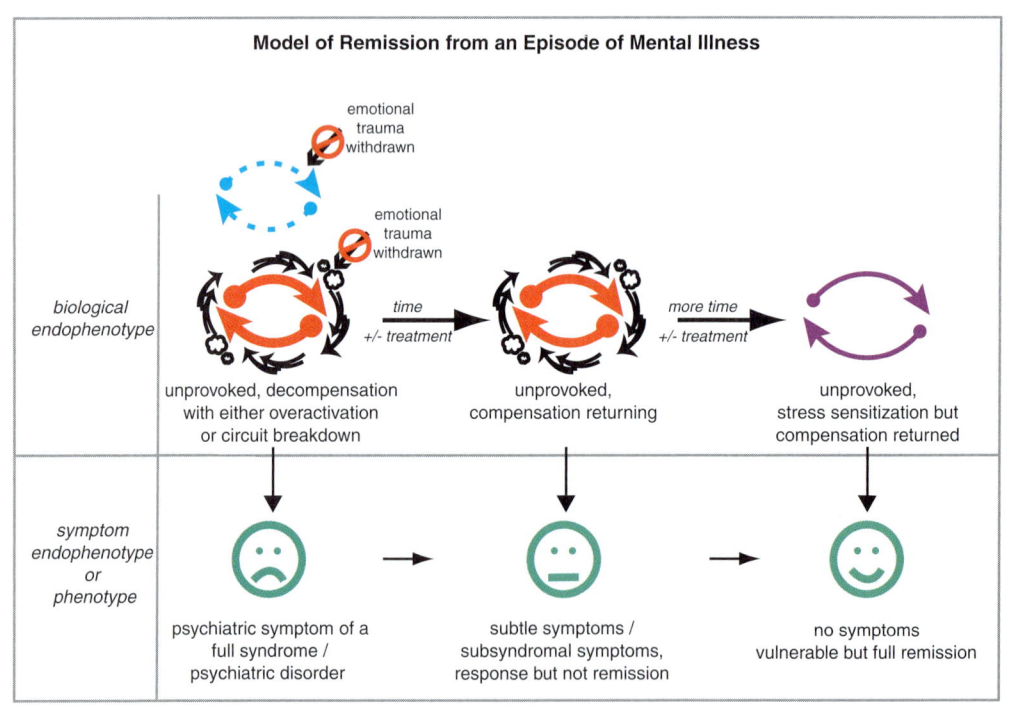

FIGURE 8-5 Remission from mental illness. Model of remission from an episode of mental illness. With treatment or, in some cases, with just the passage of time in the absence of treatment, individuals with an episode of a psychiatric disorder may experience partial or full reduction of episodic symptoms. These individuals' circuits may at first still be overactive due to prior stress sensitization, but as the load on the circuits diminishes or as compensatory mechanisms from drug treatments are instituted, these circuits begin to compensate, at first expressing fewer or less severe symptoms. With the passage of time and removal of all symptoms, the overly activated circuit may even become compensated, so that baseline overactivation is reduced, no symptoms are expressed, and full remission ensues. However, such a circuit, even if asymptomatic and in remission, would be theoretically vulnerable to the effects of future stressors.

The idea is that mental illnesses have waxing and waning symptoms over time, with episodes followed by either unremitting symptoms, partial recovery with some lower level of sustained symptoms, or full remission. Psychiatric symptoms are a proxy for malfunctioning circuits that have already decompensated, either partially or fully. With this point of view, everyone with symptoms has malfunctioning circuits, but not everyone with malfunctioning circuits has symptoms (see Figure 8-3).

A technical way of saying this is that biological endophenotype is not always matched with symptom endophenotype (Figure 8-3). Specifically, asymptomatic patients recovering from an episode of a mental illness may be vulnerable to future stressors as manifest by stress-sensitized circuits that overreact to provocation but are clinically silent in an unprovoked state once the patient has achieved remission (Figure 8-5). In such cases, the patient is not "cured"; this can be detected by neuroimaging provoked circuits (the persistently abnormal biological endophenotype) but not by observing any symptoms (the currently normal symptom endophenotype).

In order to keep the vulnerable patient with abnormal but silent circuits from having another episode of illness, it may be important to continue reducing the load on those circuits with drugs that eliminate all symptoms. Then, after remission, one could maintain these treatments while also using therapeutic and lifestyle interventions so as to buffer the circuits against future stressors.

The idea in Figure 8-5 is that circuits may potentially experience some degree of recovery from their malfunctioning when the patient goes from a state of a symptomatic psychiatric disorder to sustained remission of all symptoms, which may also require continued drug treatment and the prevention of future stress (Figure 8-5). Neuroimaging studies are now being done to prove or refute this hypothesis, but it already seems apparent that patients with full remission of some psychiatric disorders, such as major depression, have a reduced risk for relapse into another episode as compared with patients who have continuing symptoms.

Does this mean that full symptomatic recovery from an episode of mental illness could actually change asymptomatic circuits such that they once again become partially compensated? This seems to be feasible biologically and intuitively, yet it remains to be proven scientifically. In the meantime, many psychopharmacologists who are proactive with their treatment interventions would rather commit a "sin of commission" and "overtreat" symptoms rather than a "sin of omission" and "undertreat" symptoms, assuming acceptable drug risks and side effects while the proof of prevention of disease progression of continuing symptoms is being assembled.

Diabolical learning
Taking this idea in the other direction is the hypothesis of "diabolical learning" in cortical circuits. That is, symptoms allowed to run amok may be able to trigger plastic changes in circuits and synapses, recruiting additional sick circuits, eliminating healthy compensatory mechanisms, phosphorylating critical regulatory proteins, and erecting better synaptic scaffolding to make neurotransmission in sick circuits more efficient (Figures 8-6A, B, and C). A bad situation gets worse.

Some of the best examples for the model shown in Figures 8-6A, B, and C may be the symptoms of panic and chronic pain. The idea is that pain begets pain and panic begets panic; it is not a good thing to allow symptoms to persist because this can lead to continuation of these symptoms as well as their worsening, enhanced chances of relapse in the future, new symptoms, and treatment resistance. All clinicians have seen patients who

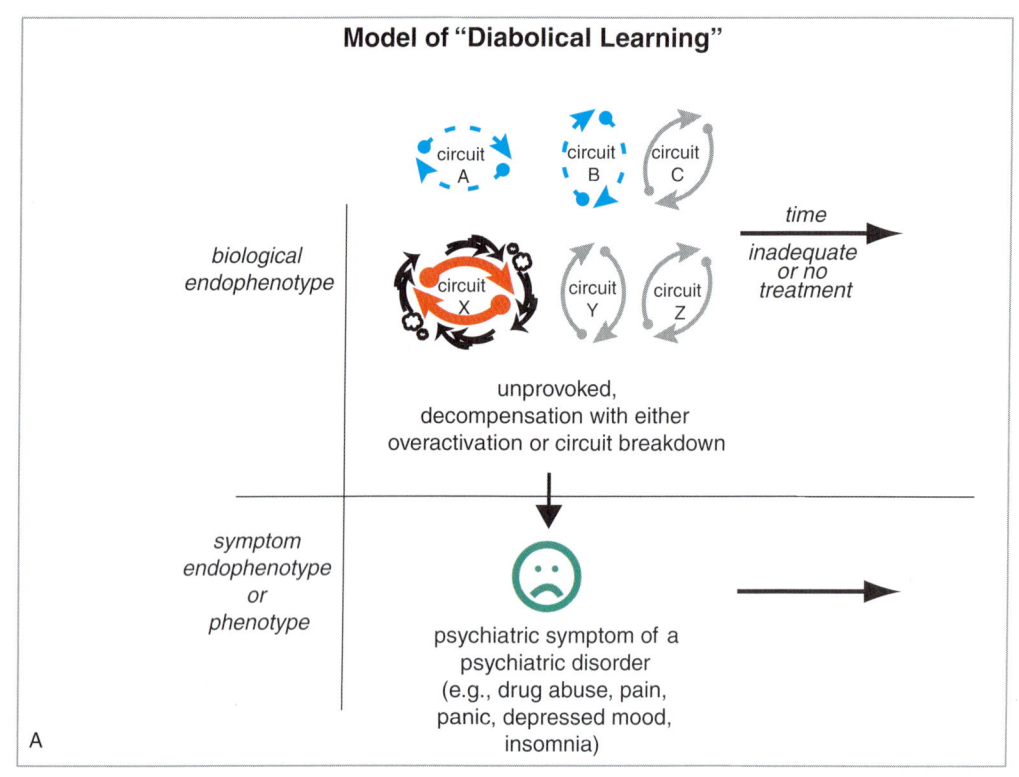

FIGURE 8-6A Diabolical learning. Model of "diabolical learning," part one. According to the model of "diabolical learning," a psychiatric symptom that persists in time may be subject to a worsening of circuit breakdown.

seem to have a progressive illness; they may then wonder whether interventions earlier in the course of that illness would have made a difference to outcome or if some patients just have bad outcomes that treatments cannot modify.

Studies of relapse prevention in a number of disorders intuitively fit with the concept that lack of treatment leads to relapse. Some institutional review boards even wonder whether it is ethical to withhold active treatment and give placebo in a number of psychiatric disorders, especially schizophrenia, due to concerns about the impact of another exacerbation of symptoms on long-term outcomes.

A wide range of psychiatric symptoms is thought to be subject to a type of "diabolical learning," including depression, anxiety, insomnia, worry, obsessions, delusions, impulsivity, and many more. The relevant circuit first experiences the state of inefficient information processing with decompensation into such symptoms; then many of the same changes hypothesized to occur with long-term memory, such as the phenomenon of long-term potentiation, may occur in the relevant circuit and at its synapses to perpetuate the circuit's inefficiencies and thus the symptoms. A learning model has been a key research perspective for both pain and addiction and can usefully be applied to our thinking about symptoms in numerous other psychiatric disorders (Figure 8-6). The circuit literally "learns" to panic, get addicted, have pain, experience anxiety, etc.

If diabolical learning were not bad enough, it is also hypothesized that sustained symptoms over time may lead to synaptic, dendritic, and neuronal loss (Figure 8-7). Thus, glutamate-mediated excitotoxicity or signal transduction that turns on apoptosis may be

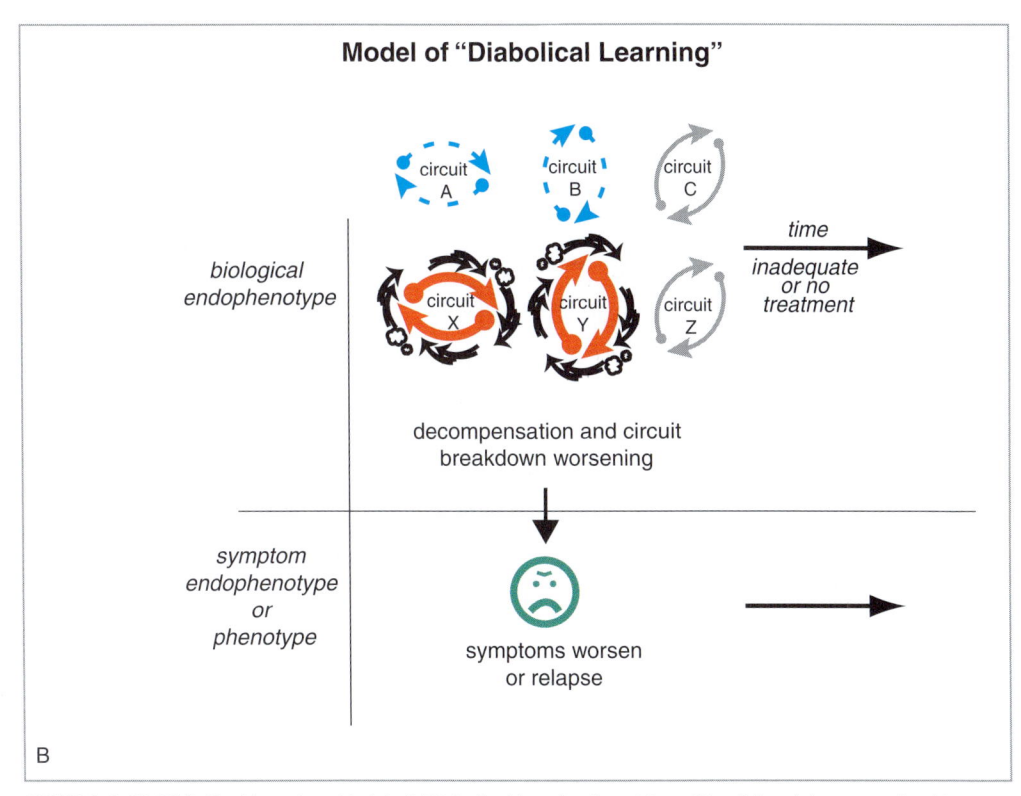

FIGURE 8-6B Diabolical learning. Model of "diabolical learning," part two. Circuit breakdown may lead to a worsening of symptoms or relapse. In this model, "symptoms beget symptoms" and circuits literally "learn" to become inefficient and overly activated.

triggered when circuits are overly active, breaking down, unable to process biological or emotional loads, and running unremittingly in a state of overload from inefficient information processing. The good news here is that these ideas are consistent with the notion that a clinician may not only be merciful in reducing symptoms for here-and-now relief but – in doing so aggressively, completely, and persistently over time – also "save" the patient's brain and prevent the development of very difficult symptoms, where the learning in the circuit may be difficult to reverse, or where loss of neurons may be impossible to reverse.

Imaging malfunctioning circuits

fMRI and PET

There are a number of neuroimaging techniques, some better for imaging of structures [such as standard magnetic resonance imaging (MRI) and computed tomography (CT)] and others better for imaging function [such as functional magnetic resonance imaging (fMRI) and positron emission tomography (PET)]. In this book, we show cartoons and visual concepts of brain functioning with fMRI and PET. Specific neuroimaging findings in particular psychiatric disorders are discussed in the clinical chapters. Here we will present some of the general ways in which functional neuroimaging is beginning to affect the field of psychopharmacology.

As goes neuronal firing, so goes blood flow and glucose utilization by the brain. This fact is exploited by several functioning neuroimaging techniques. Simply put, when fMRI scans

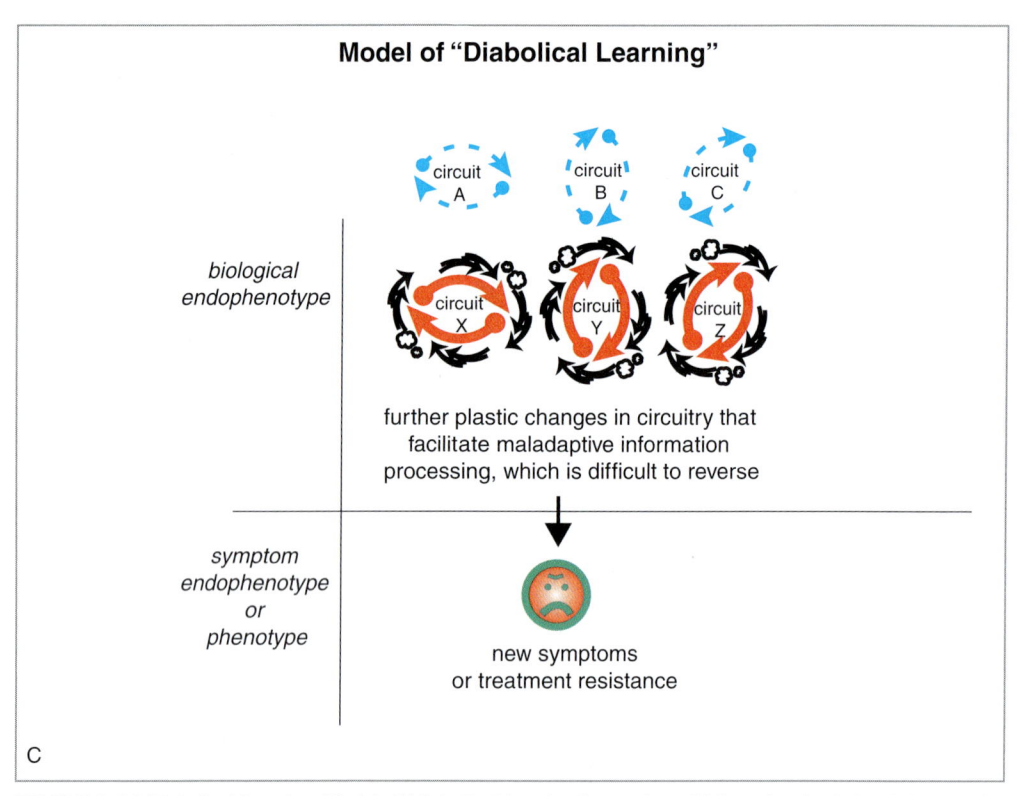

FIGURE 8-6C Diabolical learning. Model of "diabolical learning," part three. Ultimately, circuit breakdown and worsening of symptoms may cause further plastic changes in circuitry which facilitate maladaptive information processing, leading to new symptoms and even treatment resistance.

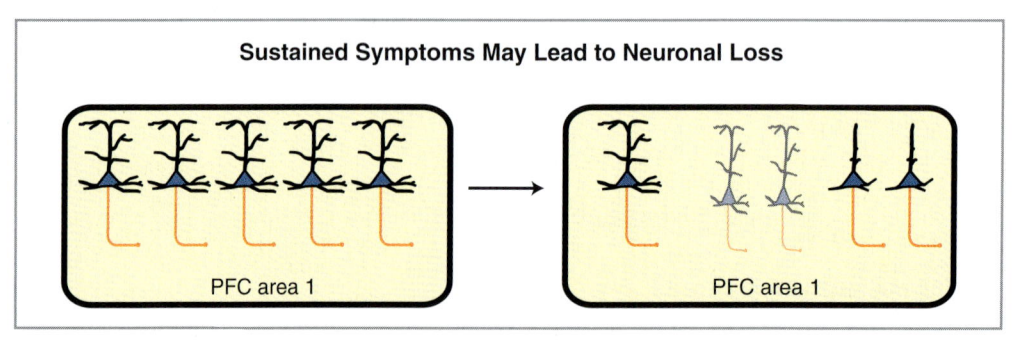

FIGURE 8-7 Sustained symptoms and neuron loss. Overactivation of circuits, expressed phenotypically as sustained psychiatric symptoms, may over time lead to the loss of dendrites and neurons.

are performed, blood oxygenation is being measured. The scan can detect the difference between oxygenated and deoxygenated blood; the implication is that if more oxygen is extracted from the blood, the neurons in that area of the image are firing more rapidly. When PET scans with a derivative of glucose are performed, glucose uptake is being measured. If more glucose is taken up by neurons, the neurons in that area of the brain are firing more rapidly. Other techniques based upon MRI and PET are reviewed in connection with specific psychiatric disorders discussed elsewhere in this book.

N-Back Test

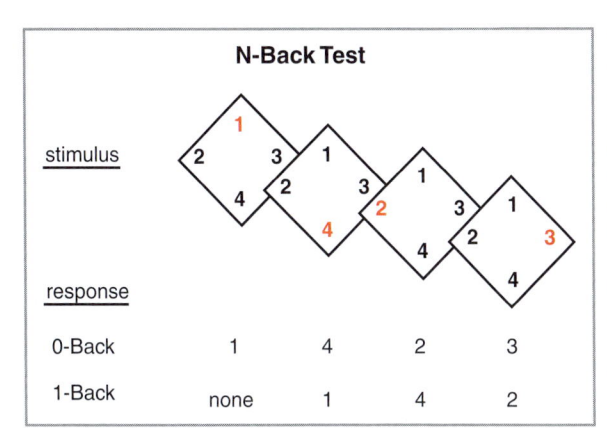

response				
0-Back	1	4	2	3
1-Back	none	1	4	2

FIGURE 8-8 N-back test. Biological endophenotypes for executive dysfunction can be identified using functional neuroimaging during mental tasks such as the n-back test. In the 0-back variant of the test, participants view a number on a screen and then indicate what that number was. In the 1-back test, the participant is shown a stimulus but does not respond; after viewing the second stimulus, the participant pushes a button corresponding to the first stimulus. The "N" can be any number, higher numbers being associated with greater difficulty.

Provoking cognitive circuits

It has been difficult to show reproducible differences in functional brain imaging when the brain is at rest or in a baseline condition without performing a conscious task. Thus, a number of provocative stimuli have been developed that activate specific parts of the brain. The n-back test is a type of mental task done while viewing a sequence of numbers (Figure 8-8). In the 0-back variant of the n-back test, the subject indicates the number that was just shown. In the 1-back test, the subject must indicate, upon presentation of a new number, what was shown one number back, thus the 1-back test. The 2-back test is harder, because the subject has to remember, in a sequence of numbers, what number was shown two numbers back; then the 3-back test, and so on.

When a patient performs this test in an fMRI scanner, his or her dorsolateral prefrontal cortex will become activated and "light up" (Figures 8-9 and 8-10). How much this lights up tells how efficient the information processing is: little or moderate activation indicates efficiency. However, a lot of activation means that information processing is inefficient and that the neurons in this area are working very hard to process the stress of the cognitive load being placed on them.

Imaging genetics: the role of dopamine in cognitive processing by DLPFC circuits

A major advance in understanding the pathway from genes to circuits is shown when imaging the amount of activation of the dorsolateral prefrontal cortex (DLPFC) in people who have variants of the gene for the dopamine metabolizing enzyme COMT (or catechol-O-methyl transferase).

The COMT gene comes in two forms, and everybody has two copies of it. One form of the gene changes a single amino acid from valine to methionine and by doing so lowers enzymatic activity by 75 percent. Subjects with two copies of the methionine version of the gene are called met-met carriers, and those with one or two copies of the valine version (met-val or val-val) are called val carriers. When performing the n-back test in an fMRI scanner, the DLPFC circuits of met-met subjects are significantly more efficient in processing this information (Figure 8-10A) than are those of val carriers (Figure 8-10B). Those met-met subjects with more efficient information processing may also make fewer mistakes.

This may reflect the impact of dopamine on information processing in DLPFC. Met-met subjects have the lowest activity of COMT. Since COMT metabolizes dopamine, this means that low COMT activity yields high dopamine. If dopamine enhances information processing in the prefrontal cortex for cognitive tasks, people with met-met genes

Provoking DLPFC with the N-Back Test

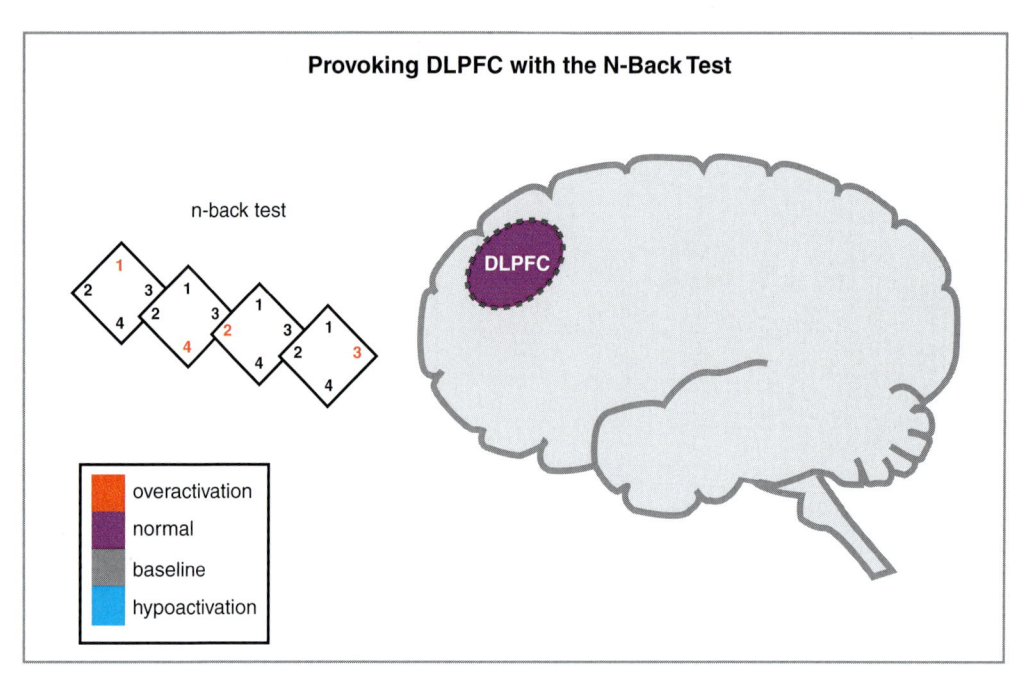

FIGURE 8-9 N-back test and dorsolateral prefrontal cortex. Performing the n-back test results in activation of the dorsolateral prefrontal cortex (DLPFC), shown here by the DLPFC turning from gray (baseline) to purple (normal activation). The degree of activation indicates how efficient the information processing in the DLPFC is – both overactivation and hypoactivation being associated with inefficient information processing.

for COMT should have more efficient information processing than people with one or two copies of the val gene for COMT. Those with the val gene for COMT should have higher COMT activity, lower DLPFC dopamine levels, and thus less efficient information processing. That is exactly what the fMRI scans in Figure 8-10A and B show. It is possible that val carriers, who have less efficient information processing when doing cognitive tasks, have more risk for psychiatric disorders characterized by executive dysfunction, particularly schizophrenia.

Provoking fear circuits
A second provocative test is to evaluate fearful faces during fMRI scanning (Figure 8-11). This provocation causes activation of the amygdala (Figure 8-12). The degree to which fearful faces light up the amygdala can suggest how reactive this part of the fear-processing circuit is to the provocation of fear.

Imaging genetics: the role of serotonin in fear processing by the amygdala
A second major advance in understanding the pathway from genes to circuits is demonstrated in imaging the degree of activation of the amygdala in people who have variants of the gene for the serotonin transporter, or SERT. The SERT gene comes in a longer (l) and a shorter (s) form; those subjects with two copies of the l form of the gene make more copies of SERT, have higher amounts of SERT reuptake activity at serotonin synapses, and have lower amounts of synaptic serotonin.

When processing fearful faces in an fMRI scanner, l/l subjects have circuits in the amygdala that are significantly more efficient in processing this information than are s

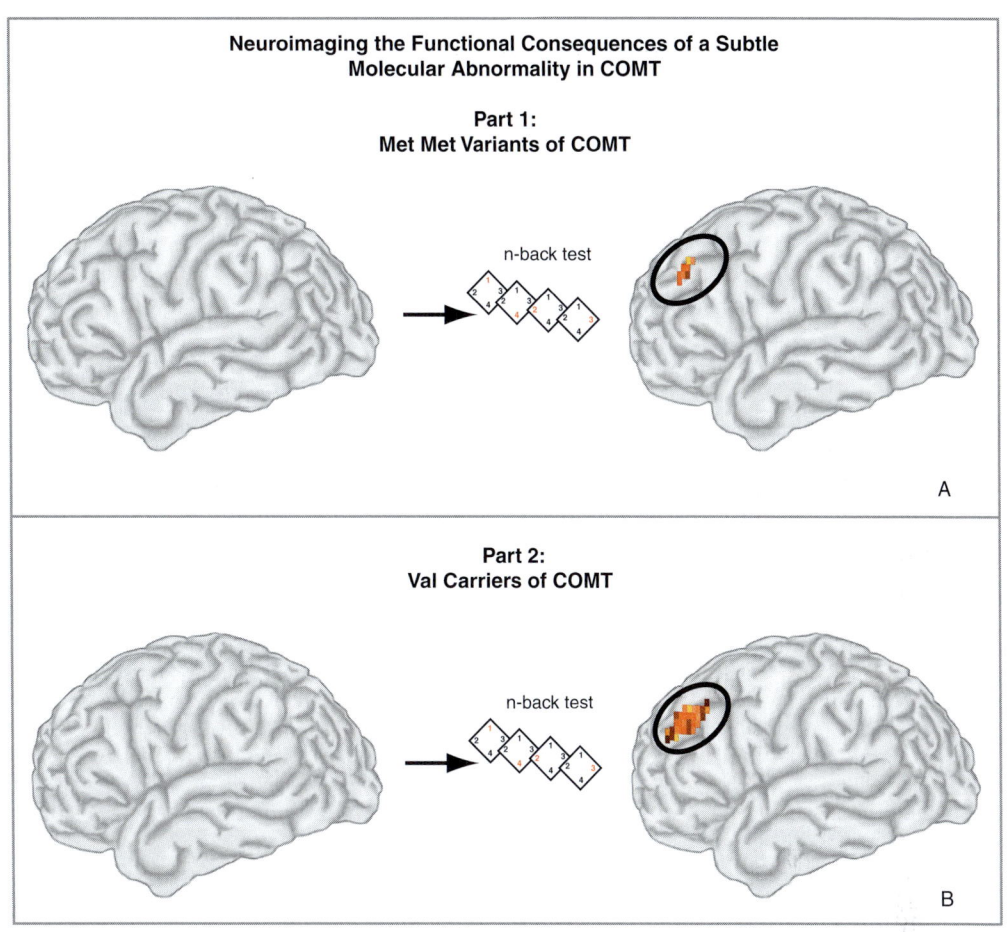

FIGURE 8-10A and B Subtle molecular abnormality in COMT. Genetic influence on circuits regulating executive functioning can be demonstrated by comparing functional neuroimaging data from individuals with different variants of the catechol-O-methyl transferase (COMT) gene while they are performing the n-back test. COMT is an enzyme that breaks down dopamine. Every individual carries two copies of the gene for COMT, which can be the valine (val) variant or the methionine (met) variant. The met variant leads to reduced enzymatic activity, reduced degradation of dopamine, and thus higher levels of dopamine. Because dopamine is important for efficient information processing in the DLPFC, carriers of two copies of the met variant – who thus have higher cortical dopamine levels – have significantly more efficient information processing in the DLPFC during cognitive provocation with the n-back test (**A**) than do individuals with either one or two copies of the val variant (**B**).

carriers (compare parts A and B of Figure 8-13). This could reflect the impact of serotonin on information processing in the amygdala.

Provoking circuits for attention

A third provocative test for fMRI scanning is the Stroop task (Figure 8-14). In this test, the subject is asked to respond to the color and suppress reading the word, which is generally mismatched with the color of the letters. This task activates the dorsal part of the anterior cingulate cortex (Figure 8-15) and is utilized in testing of subjects with problems of selective attention, such as attention deficit hyperactivity disorder.

FIGURE 8-11 Processing fearful faces. Biological endophenotypes for anxiety and fearful symptoms can be identified using functional neuroimaging while individuals view fear-related stimuli, such as the fearful faces shown here.

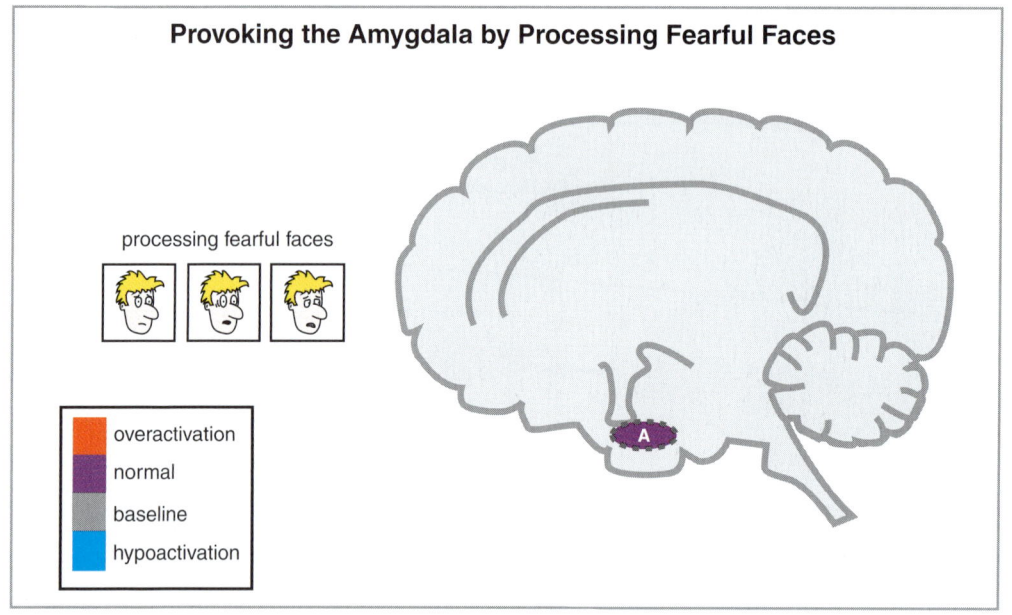

FIGURE 8-12 Processing fearful faces and amygdala. Exposure to fearful faces generally causes amygdalar activation, shown here by the amygdala turning from gray (baseline) to purple (normal activation). The degree of activation can indicate how reactive this part of the fear-processing circuit is to fear-related stimuli.

Seeing your grandmother in your brain

To explore the path between gene and mental illness, many other provocative tests are being standardized for research testing and potential correlation with genetic variants, symptoms, and psychiatric disorders.

Currently available results from imaging genetics already show that you can "see" your ancestors in your brain! That is, looking at the effects of certain variants of the genes your ancestors gave you on the images your brain makes today, in different regions and under different conditions, can already provide some idea of your inherited efficiency of information processing.

CNS-I (Central nervous system investigators in the psychopharmacology of tomorrow may model crime scene investigators of today)

The birth of this new field of imaging genetics suggests that the diagnosis and treatment of psychiatric disorders may soon be much different than it is today. Perhaps DNA analysis

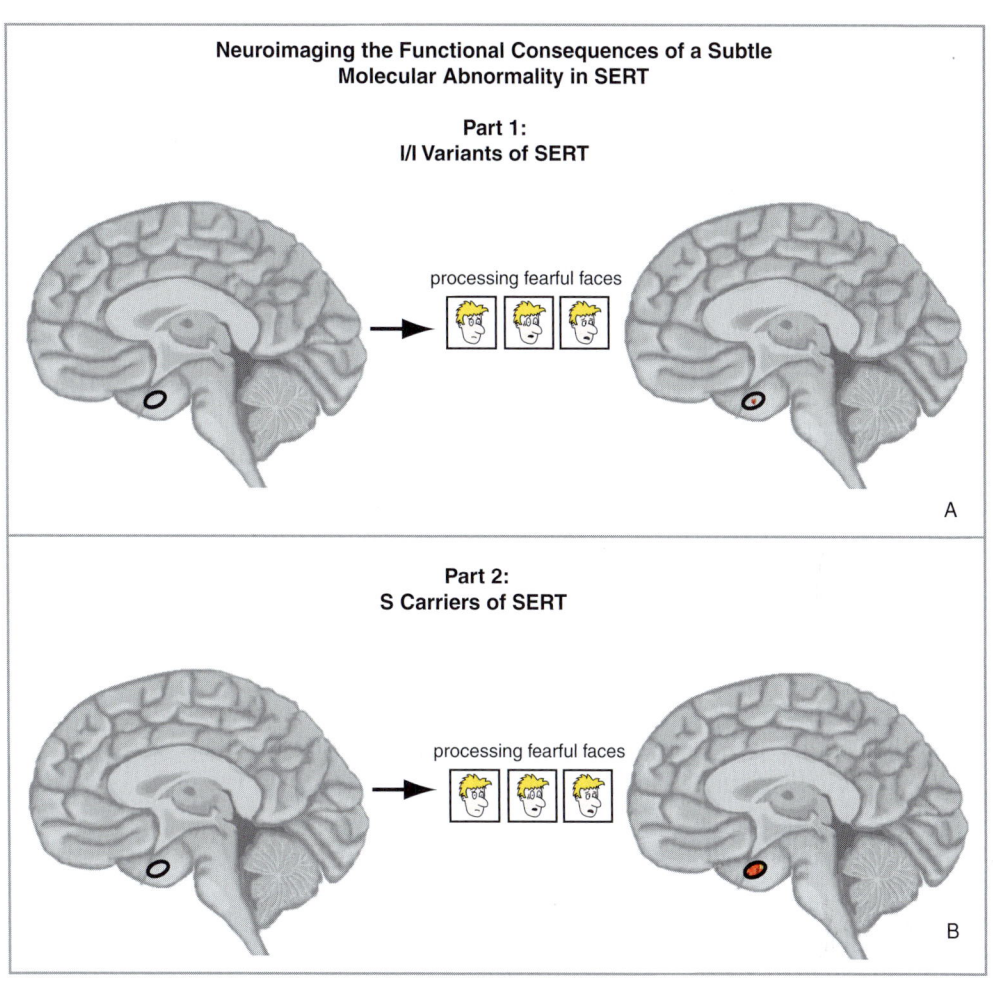

FIGURE 8-13A and B Subtle molecular abnormality and SERT. Genetic influence on circuits regulating emotions can be demonstrated by comparing functional neuroimaging data from individuals with different variants of the serotonin transporter (SERT) gene while they are viewing fearful faces. The SERT gene has two variants, a long (l) and a short (s) form. Individuals with two copies of the long form have more copies of the transporter as well as higher amounts of reuptake activity and consequently lower amounts of synaptic serotonin. When individuals view fearful faces, those with two copies of the l form of the SERT gene exhibit more efficient information processing (**A**) than those with either one or two copies of the s form of the gene (**B**).

by a psychiatric diagnostician or CNS investigator (CNS-I) will someday be part of the investigation of psychiatric illnesses in much the same way as DNA analysis is now part of crime scene investigation (CSI). Just as treadmill "stress tests" for the heart are part of cardiology assessment today, obtaining functional brain images to determine the efficiency of information processing in various parts of the provoked brain will likely someday be part of the evaluation of treatment effects on circuits and symptoms in psychiatry. Such "psychiatric treadmills" and genotyping may also become useful to assess clinically silent risk in patients without psychiatric disorders, such as first-degree relatives. Functional neuroimaging has the potential to allow clinicians to "see" more than malfunctioning circuits in a psychiatric disorder – possibly even see the linkage of genes, symptoms, stress, and treatments with the function of numerous circuits.

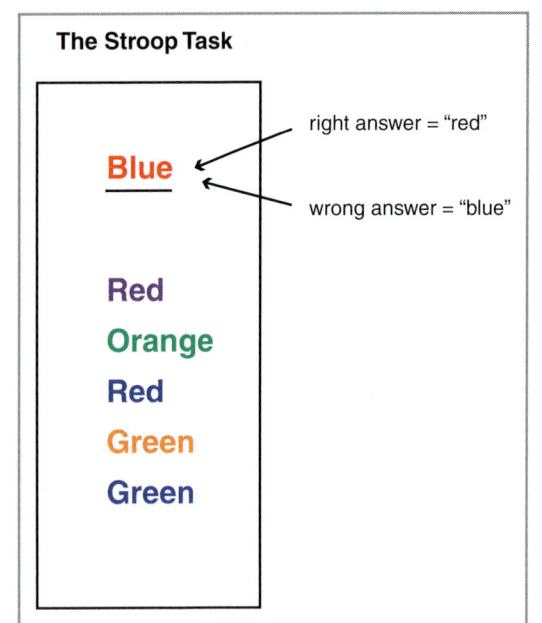

FIGURE 8-14 Stroop task. Biological endophenotypes for attention can be identified using functional neuroimaging during mental tasks such as the Stroop task. In this task, the names of colors are written in different colors, often with the color of the word not matching what it says. Individuals are not supposed to read the words but rather to indicate the color in which each word is written. For example, in this figure, the word "blue" is written in red ink. The correct answer would be "red," while an answer of "blue" would be incorrect.

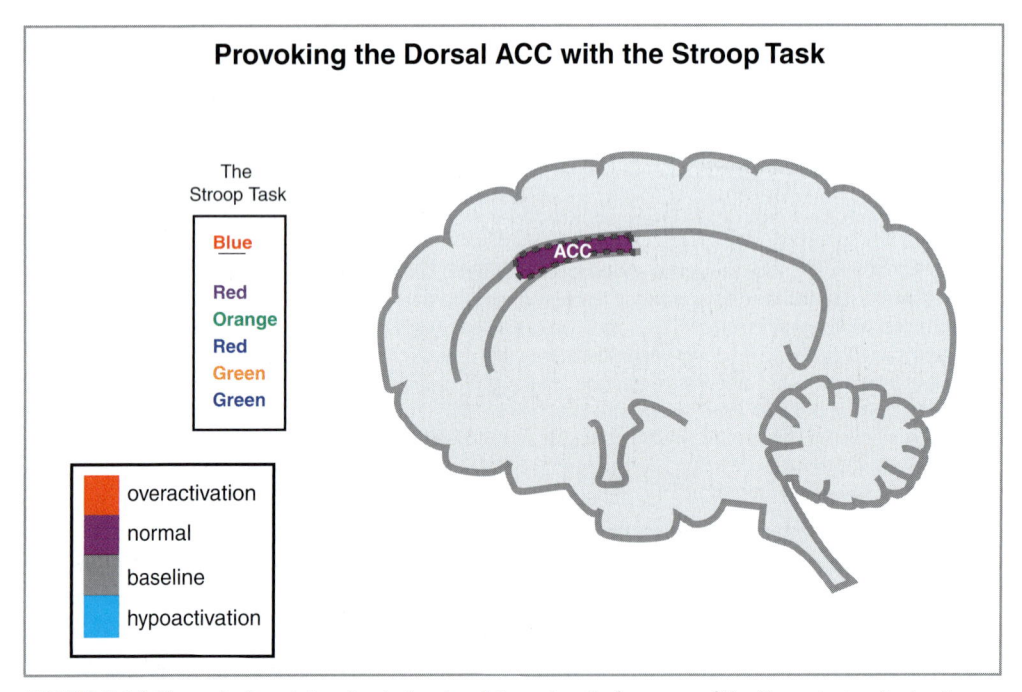

FIGURE 8-15 Stroop task and dorsal anterior cingulate cortex. Performance of the Stroop task activates the dorsal anterior cingulate cortex (ACC), demonstrated here by the ACC changing from gray (baseline) to purple (normal activation). The degree of activation indicates how efficient the information processing is – both overactivation and hypoactivation being associated with inefficient information processing.

TABLE 8-1 Symptoms and circuits can provide a rational approach to selecting and combining treatments

	Step 1	Construct a diagnosis
	Step 2	Deconstruct the diagnosis into its component symptoms
	Step 3	Match each symptom to its hypothetically malfunctioning circuit
Each circuit repeats until symptoms are gone	Step 4	Consider the portfolio of neurotransmitters that theoretically regulate each circuit
	Step 5	Select a treatment that targets the neurotransmitter regulating the hypothetically malfunctioning circuit
	Step 6	Add or switch to another treatment if the symptom is not relieved
	Step 7	Repeat for each symptom until the patient is asymptomatic or in remission whenever possible

Symptoms and circuits for the psychopharmacologist

We have presented here a discussion on the hypothetical role of genes and stressors on neuronal circuitry and, ultimately, on psychiatric symptoms. It should now be clear that genes that are robustly linked to subtle molecular abnormalities are only poorly linked to psychiatric disorders (defined as syndromes in the DSM and ICD). However, a few genes now known to be weakly related to psychiatric symptom endophenotypes are relatively strongly related to the development and function of cortical circuits involved in processing cognitive and emotional information in the brain.

Prior to the era of futuristic gene testing and provocative functional neuroimaging in standard clinical practice, is there anything the modern psychopharmacologist can do today with this information about genes, circuits, topographical localization of symptoms, and regional neurotransmitter control of information processing? The answer may be that the neurobiologically informed psychopharmacologist can already use this information to establish the strategies and tactics for current clinical practice. That is, the concepts developed in this chapter strongly suggest that the clinical strategy should be to reduce or eliminate as many symptoms as possible and that the clinical tactics are to prioritize, among all the evidence-based treatments available, those that target neurotransmission in malfunctioning brain circuits. By treating each patient – with his or her unique portfolio of symptoms – in this way, it may be possible to improve information processing and thereby reduce symptoms. This tactic would enable the rational selection and combination of treatments for each individual patient as well as the restructuring of treatment on the basis of the patient's response to prior treatment. Such an approach is outlined in Table 8-1.

Many examples of this approach will be developed for specific treatment selections in the various chapters of this book dealing with specific psychiatric disorders. In general, the approach is to first utilize a categorical approach, listing symptoms and constructing a psychiatric diagnosis according to accepted criteria, such as those DSM criteria for major depression listed in Figure 8-16 (see also Table 8-1). At this point, one could go to a list of evidence-based approved treatments for major depression and choose any one. Prior experience, side effect profile, and clinician preference may guide that choice. However, it is also possible to choose a treatment based upon the patient's symptom profile. In this case, the approach is to deconstruct a patient's psychiatric syndrome into the specific symptoms that the patient is experiencing. This is the dimensional approach, and is shown in Figure 8-17 (see also Table 8-1).

Constructing a Diagnosis: the Categorical Approach

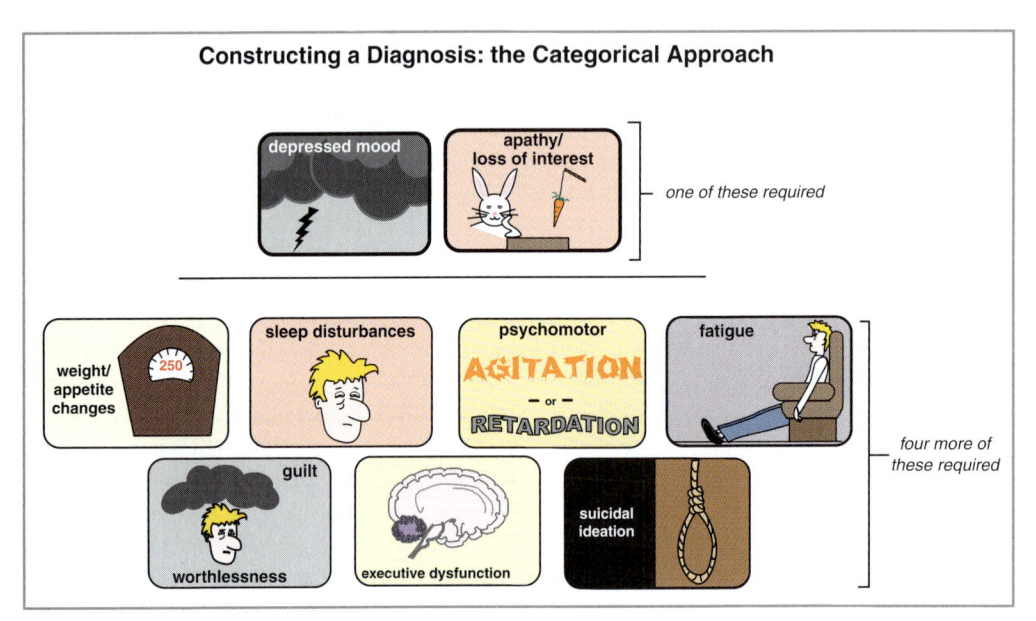

depressed mood | apathy/loss of interest — one of these required

weight/appetite changes | sleep disturbances | psychomotor AGITATION — or — RETARDATION | fatigue
guilt / worthlessness | executive dysfunction | suicidal ideation
— four more of these required

FIGURE 8-16 **Constructing a categorical diagnosis.** Constructing a diagnosis: the categorical approach. Symptoms can be constructed into a psychiatric diagnosis according to accepted criteria, such as those for a major depressive episode as defined in the *Diagnostic and Statistical Manual of Mental Disorders*. Treatment can then be based on the syndrome.

Deconstructing Psychiatric Syndromes into Symptoms: the Dimensional Approach

symptom	psychiatric syndromes with the same overlapping symptoms		
problems concentrating	major depression	ADHD	narcolepsy
anxiety	generalized anxiety disorder	social anxiety disorder	panic disorder

FIGURE 8-17 **Deconstructing syndromes into symptoms.** Deconstructing psychiatric syndromes into symptoms: the dimensional approach. Psychiatric syndromes can be deconstructed into the specific presenting symptoms of an individual patient, with treatment selected based on those symptoms rather than on a syndromic diagnosis. In this case, any given symptom may cut across several different diagnoses, involve the same circuit, and respond to the same treatment.

Essential Psychopharmacology

Many psychiatric symptoms cut across several psychiatric disorders, and the genetics, functional imaging and localization of circuits involved in these symptoms may be similar across many psychiatric disorders. For example, if a patient with major depression is experiencing both problems concentrating (as shown in Figure 8-18A) and anxiety (as shown in Figure 8-18B), these dimensions of ongoing symptomatology may share inclusion in numerous other psychiatric disorders (Figure 8-17). Furthermore, a symptom shared by different psychiatric disorders may actually share the same localization in the brain (Figure 8-18A and B).

The brain has a limited number of neuronal highways by which it can express its symptoms, so executive dysfunction or anxiety may share the same circuits in several different psychiatric disorders characterized by either of these symptoms (Figure 8-18A and B). Following the strategy set forth in Table 8-1, once the diagnosis has been made (as in Figure 8-16), and then deconstructed into its symptom components (Figure 8-17) and, furthermore, matched to a hypothetically malfunctioning circuit (Figure 8-18A and B), the next step is to consider the portfolio of neurotransmitters known to regulate each circuit. For example, dopamine and histamine may be key neurotransmitters regulating cognition in DLPFC (Figure 8-19A) whereas serotonin and GABA may be key neurotransmitters regulating anxiety in the amygdala (Figure 8-19A). This provides the rationale for specific neurochemical targeting and for priorities for treatment selection and combination (Table 8-1).

As soon as this strategy provides treatments that lead to remission of all symptoms, the job is done. However, in the frequent situation where treatments either do not work, or only work on some symptoms and leave other residual symptoms, the tactics change now to either adding or switching to another treatment that targets a different neurotransmitter in that pathway (Figure 8-19 and Table 8-1). This can be repeated for each symptom in each pathway until the patient is asymptomatic or in remission whenever possible (Table 8-1).

An example of this approach is shown in Figures 8-19 and 8-20. Perhaps an agent that boosts serotonin was chosen first-line for major depressive disorder, with improvement of sadness and depressed mood but residual symptoms of executive dysfunction and anxiety. The symptoms of executive dysfunction can be localized hypothetically to inefficient information processing in the DLPFC (Figure 8-18A), with regulation of this circuit by several neurotransmitters, including histamine and dopamine (Figure 8-19A). This could lead to additional dopamine targeting with a booster of dopamine such as bupropion and/or additional targeting of histamine with modafinil (Figure 8-20A).

On the other hand, residual symptoms of anxiety can be localized hypothetically to inefficient information processing in the amygdala (Figure 8-18B), with regulation of this circuit by several neurotransmitters, including serotonin and GABA (Figure 8-19B). Since this patient is already receiving a serotonergic treatment, this could be continued or switched to another selective serotonin reuptake inhibitor (SSRI) or serotonin-norepinephrine reuptake inhibitor (SNRI); additional GABA targeting can be done with a benzodiazepine or even cognitive behavioral therapy (Figure 8-20B).

The strategy outlined in Table 8-1 depends on the tactics of selecting and combining specific drugs on the basis of the topographical location of functions, topographical location of neurotransmitters, and mechanisms of action of psychotropic drugs. This approach is already routine practice for many clinicians on the basis of their clinical experience, but now there is an emerging science that supports this clinical approach.

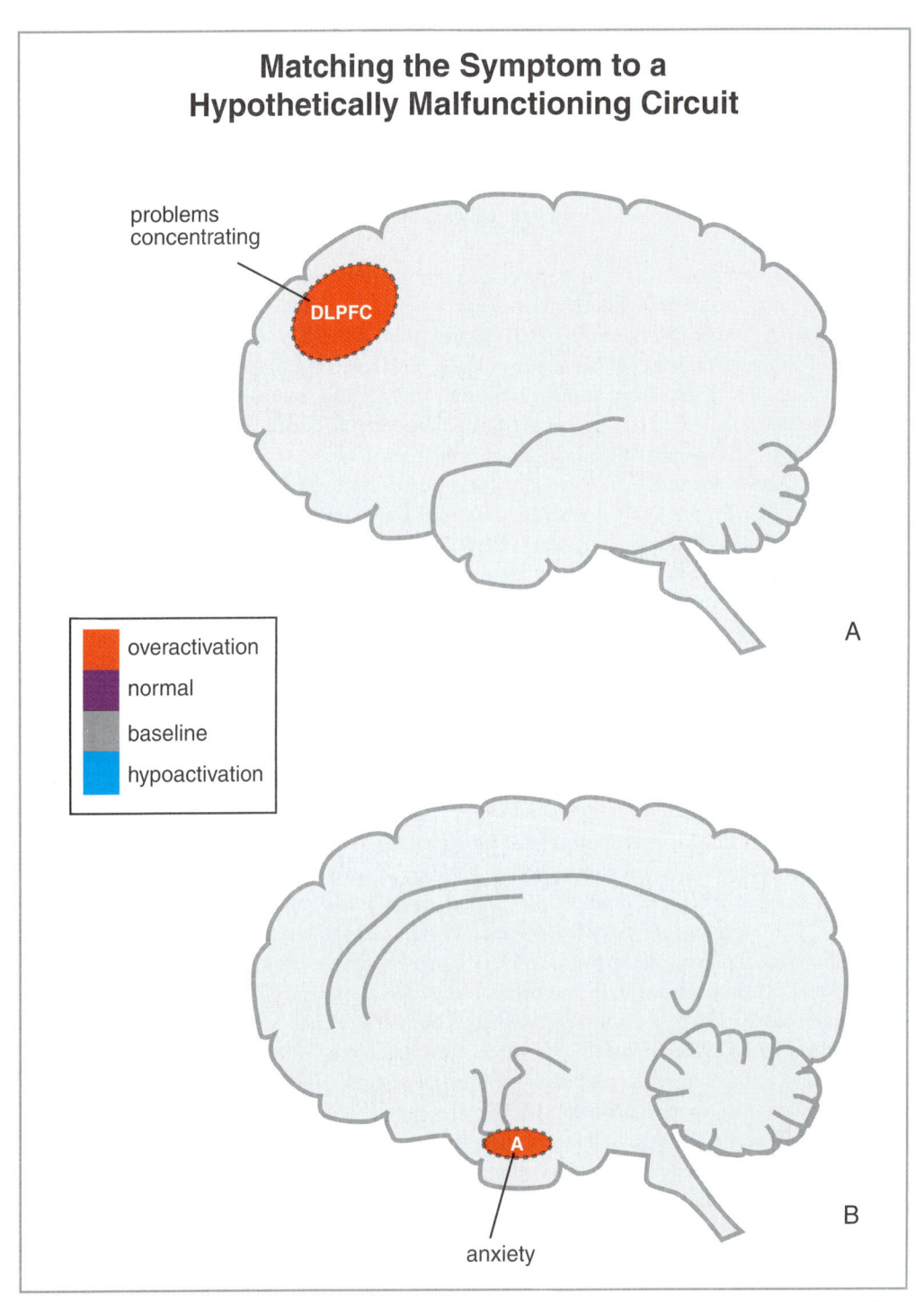

FIGURE 8-18A and B Matching symptoms to circuits. Once a patient's symptoms have been identified, each one may be matched to a hypothetically malfunctioning circuit. For example, difficulty concentrating may be associated with abnormal activity in the dorsolateral prefrontal cortex (**A**), while anxiety may be associated with abnormal amygdalar activation (**B**).

Essential Psychopharmacology

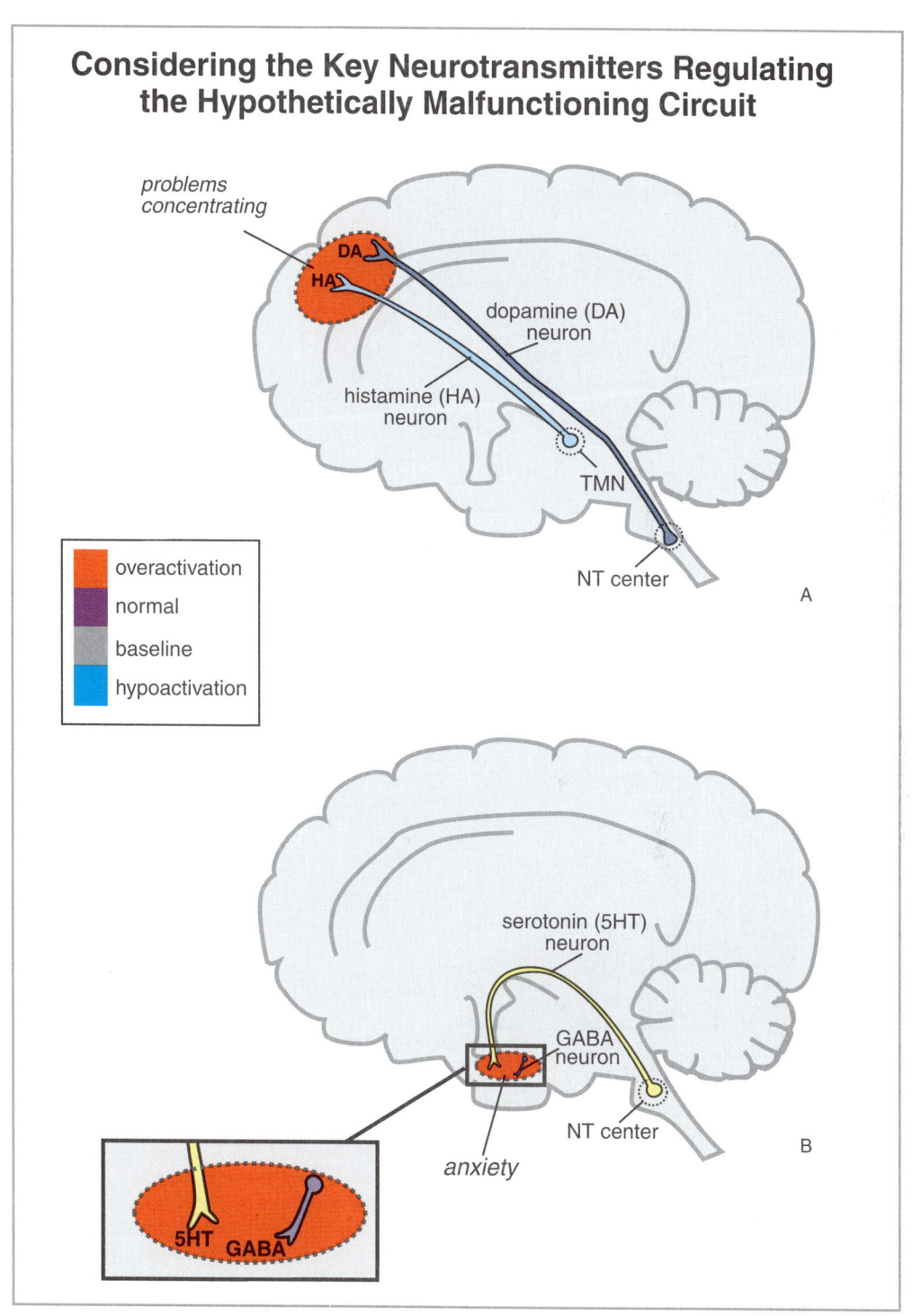

FIGURE 8-19A and B Matching neurotransmitters to circuits. In order to select treatment for a patient's symptoms, it is necessary to determine which neurotransmitters may affect information processing in the area of the brain associated with each symptom. For example, dopamine and histamine are both regulatory neurotransmitters in the dorsolateral prefrontal cortex (**A**), while serotonergic and GABAergic projections are important for amygdalar functioning (**B**).

From Circuits to Symptoms in Psychopharmacology | 243

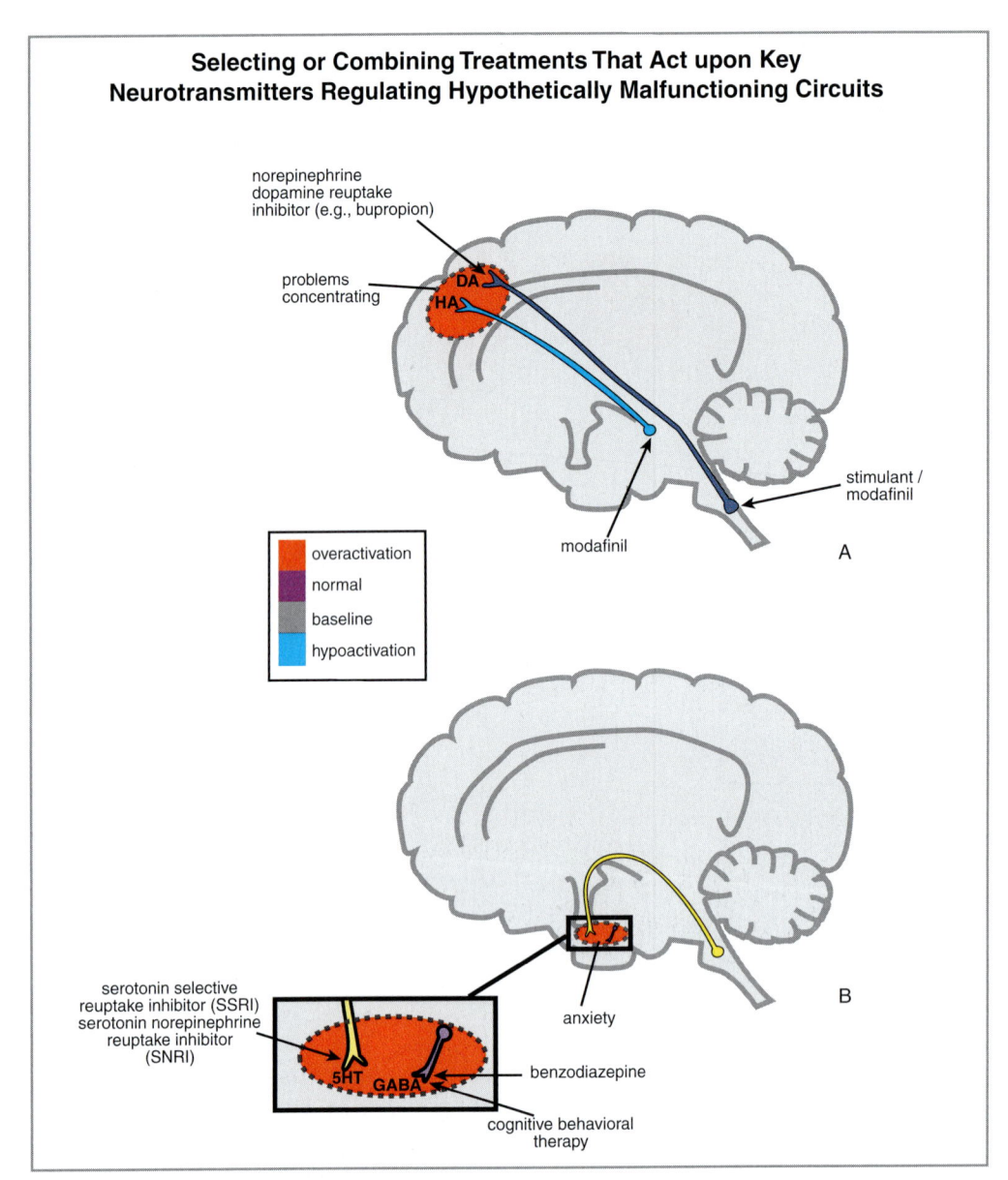

FIGURE 8-20A and B Treatment based on symptoms and circuits. Because most available psychopharmacological treatments target neurotransmitter systems, treatments for psychiatric symptoms can be selected or combined by identifying key neurotransmitters that regulate hypothetically malfunctioning circuits associated with specific symptoms. For example, bupropion, modafinil, or stimulants may modulate dopaminergic neurotransmission in the dorsolateral prefrontal cortex (DLPFC), while modafinil may modulate histaminergic neurotransmission in the DLPFC, making any of these viable options for the treatment of concentration difficulties (**A**). Selective serotonin reuptake inhibitors or dual serotonin and norepinephrine reuptake inhibitors may modulate serotonergic neurotransmission in the amygdala, while benzodiazepines may modulate GABA neurotransmission in the amygdala, making any of these viable options for the treatment of anxiety (**B**).

Table 8-1 makes a great deal of sense to many clinicians and scientists because there does not appear to be a single drug mechanism for any psychiatric disorder (such as major depressive disorder) any more than there appears to be a single gene for any psychiatric disorder (such as major depressive disorder). However, there may be one drug that acts on mechanisms that could improve information processing in one part of the brain, thus improving depressed mood, and another drug that acts on different mechanisms that could improve information processing in another part of the brain to improve insomnia, anxiety, or problems concentrating no matter what the psychiatric diagnosis. Many clinicians already follow these strategies and tactics intuitively, and now major developments in the neurosciences reinforce these actions, inform them, and allow us to anticipate more powerful strategies and tactics for psychopharmacology in the not too distant future.

Summary

Malfunctioning brain circuits may mediate specific psychiatric symptoms. A new discipline of imaging genetics now reveals how genes affect the efficiency of information processing in specific brain circuits, which can be visualized by modern brain imaging techniques. Malfunctioning circuits can be caused by genetic risk factors and/or by environmental stressors such as emotional and physical trauma, aberrant learning, drugs, toxins, and infection. Thus, stress may sensitize a circuit without necessarily causing a psychiatric disorder until a subsequent stressor is experienced. By identifying genetic risk and neuroimaging abnormalities in brain circuits and intervening early with treatment, it may be possible to interrupt the progression of psychiatric disorders from presymptomatic but malfunctioning circuits, to prodromal symptoms, to subsyndromal symptoms to full syndrome psychiatric disorders.

It may also be possible to prevent disease recurrence and progression to treatment resistance by treating not only symptoms but also inefficient brain circuits that are asymptomatic. Failing to do so may allow "diabolical learning," where circuits run amok, become more efficient in learning how to mediate symptoms, and are therefore more difficult to treat.

Malfunctioning circuits can be imaged by provoking them with cognitive and affective tasks. This approach allows visualization of the effects of risk genes on the efficiency of information processing in specific neuronal circuits. Modern psychopharmacologists can currently exploit the findings from imaging genetics to develop a rationale for selecting and combining drugs for their patients. That strategy is first to construct a categorical diagnosis and then to deconstruct it into its component symptoms. Next, one can match each symptom to a hypothetically malfunctioning circuit and – with knowledge of the neurotransmitters regulating that circuit and drugs acting on those neurotransmitters – choose a therapeutic agent to reduce that symptom. If such a strategy proves unsuccessful, it is possible that adding or switching to another agent acting on another neurotransmitter in that circuit can be effective. Repeating this strategy for each symptom can result in remission of all symptoms in many patients.

CHAPTER 9

Psychosis and Schizophrenia

- Symptom dimensions in schizophrenia
  - Clinical description of psychosis
  - Schizophrenia is more than a psychosis
  - Beyond positive and negative symptoms of schizophrenia
  - Symptoms of schizophrenia are not necessarily unique to schizophrenia
  - Brain circuits and symptom dimensions in schizophrenia
- Neurotransmitters and circuits in schizophrenia
  - Dopamine
  - Dopaminergic neurons
  - Key dopamine pathways in the brain
  - The integrated dopamine hypothesis of schizophrenia
  - Glutamate
  - Glutamate synthesis
  - Synthesis of glutamate cotransmitters glycine and d-serine
  - Glutamate receptors
  - Key glutamate pathways in the brain and the NMDA receptor hypofunction hypothesis of schizophrenia
- Neurodegenerative hypothesis of schizophrenia
  - Excitotoxicity and the glutamate system in neurodegenerative disorders such as schizophrenia
- Neurodevelopmental hypothesis and genetics of schizophrenia
  - Is schizophrenia acquired or inherited?
  - Genes that affect connectivity, synaptogenesis and NMDA receptors
  - Dysconnectivity
  - Abnormal synaptogenesis
  - NMDA receptors, AMPA receptors, and synaptogenesis
  - Convergence of susceptibility genes for schizophrenia upon glutamate synapses
  - The bottom line
- Neuroimaging circuits in schizophrenia
- Summary

Psychosis is a difficult term to define and is frequently misused, not only in the newspapers, in movies, and on television but unfortunately among mental health professionals as well. Stigma and fear surround the concept of psychosis, and the average citizen worries about long-standing myths of "mental illness," including "psychotic killers," "psychotic rage," and the equivalence of "psychosis" with the pejorative term "crazy."

There is perhaps no area of psychiatry where misconceptions are greater than in that of psychotic illnesses. The reader is well served to develop an expertise on the facts about the diagnosis and treatment of psychotic illnesses in order to dispel unwarranted beliefs and to help destigmatize this devastating group of illnesses. This chapter is not intended to list the diagnostic criteria for all the different mental disorders of which psychosis is either a defining or associated feature. The reader is referred to standard reference sources (DSM-IV and ICD-10) for that information. Although schizophrenia is emphasized here, we will approach psychosis as a syndrome associated with a variety of illnesses that are all targets for antipsychotic drug treatment.

Symptom dimensions in schizophrenia

Clinical description of psychosis

Psychosis is a syndrome – a mixture of symptoms – that can be associated with many different psychiatric disorders, but it is not a specific disorder itself in diagnostic schemes such as DSM-IV or ICD-10. At a minimum, psychosis means delusions and hallucinations. It generally also includes symptoms such as disorganized speech, disorganized behavior, and gross distortions of reality testing.

Therefore psychosis can be considered to be a set of symptoms in which a person's mental capacity, affective response, and capacity to recognize reality, communicate, and relate to others is impaired. Psychotic disorders have psychotic symptoms as their defining features; there are, however, other disorders in which psychotic symptoms may be present but are not necessary for the diagnosis.

Those **disorders that require the presence of psychosis** as a *defining* feature of the diagnosis include schizophrenia, substance-induced (i.e., drug-induced) psychotic disorder, schizophreniform disorder, schizoaffective disorder, delusional disorder, brief psychotic disorder, shared psychotic disorder, and psychotic disorder due to a general medical condition (Table 9-1). **Disorders that may or may not have psychotic symptoms** as an *associated* feature include mania and depression as well as several cognitive disorders such as Alzheimer's dementia (Table 9-2).

Psychosis itself can be paranoid, disorganized/excited, or depressive. Perceptual distortions and motor disturbances can be associated with any type of psychosis. **Perceptual distortions** include being distressed by hallucinatory voices; hearing voices that accuse, blame, or threaten punishment; seeing visions; reporting hallucinations of touch, taste, or odor; or reporting that familiar things and people seem changed. **Motor disturbances** are peculiar, rigid postures; overt signs of tension; inappropriate grins or giggles; peculiar

TABLE 9-1 Disorders in which psychosis is a defining feature

Schizophrenia
Substance-induced (i.e., drug-induced) psychotic disorders
Schizophreniform disorder
Schizoaffective disorder
Delusional disorder
Brief psychotic disorder
Shared psychotic disorder
Psychotic disorder due to a general medical condition

TABLE 9-2 Disorders in which psychosis is an associated feature

Mania
Depression
Cognitive disorders
Alzheimer's dementia

repetitive gestures; talking, muttering, or mumbling to oneself; or glancing around as if hearing voices.

In **paranoid psychosis**, the patient has paranoid projections, hostile belligerence, and grandiose expansiveness. **Paranoid projection** includes preoccupation with delusional beliefs; believing that people are talking about oneself; believing one is being persecuted or being conspired against; and believing that people or external forces control one's actions. **Hostile belligerence** is a verbal expression of feelings of hostility; expressing an attitude of disdain; manifesting a hostile, sullen attitude; manifesting irritability and grouchiness; tending to blame others for problems; expressing feelings of resentment; complaining and finding fault; as well as expressing suspicion of people. **Grandiose expansiveness** is exhibiting an attitude of superiority; hearing voices that praise and extol; and believing one has unusual powers, is a well known personality, or has a divine mission.

In a **disorganized/excited psychosis**, there is conceptual disorganization, disorientation, and excitement. **Conceptual disorganization** can be characterized by giving answers that are irrelevant or incoherent, drifting off the subject, using neologisms, or repeating certain words or phrases. **Disorientation** is not knowing where one is, the season of the year, the calendar year, or one's own age. **Excitement** is expressing feelings without restraint, manifesting speech that is hurried, exhibiting an elevated mood, showing an attitude of superiority, dramatizing oneself or one's symptoms, manifesting loud and boisterous speech, exhibiting overactivity or restlessness, and exhibiting excess of speech.

Depressive psychosis is characterized by retardation, apathy, and anxious self-punishment and blame. **Retardation and apathy** are manifesting slowed speech, indifference to one's future, fixed facial expression, slowed movements, deficiencies in recent memory, blocking in speech, apathy toward oneself or one's problems, slovenly appearance, low or whispered speech, and failure to answer questions. **Anxious self-punishment and blame** is the tendency to blame or condemn oneself; anxiety about specific matters; apprehensiveness regarding vague future events; an attitude of self-deprecation; manifesting a depressed mood; expressing feelings of guilt and remorse; preoccupation with suicidal thoughts, unwanted ideas, and specific fears; and feeling unworthy or sinful.

This discussion of clusters of psychotic symptoms does not constitute diagnostic criteria for any psychotic disorder. It is given merely as a description of several types of symptoms in psychosis to give the reader an overview of the nature of behavioral disturbances associated with the various psychotic illnesses.

Schizophrenia is more than a psychosis

Although schizophrenia is the commonest and best known psychotic illness, it is not synonymous with psychosis but is just one of many causes of psychosis. Schizophrenia affects 1 percent of the population, and in the United States there are over 300,000 acute schizophrenic episodes annually. Between 25 and 50 percent of schizophrenia patients

Schizophrenia: The Phenotype

schizophrenia

deconstruct the syndrome...

...into symptoms

positive symptoms
-delusions
-hallucinations

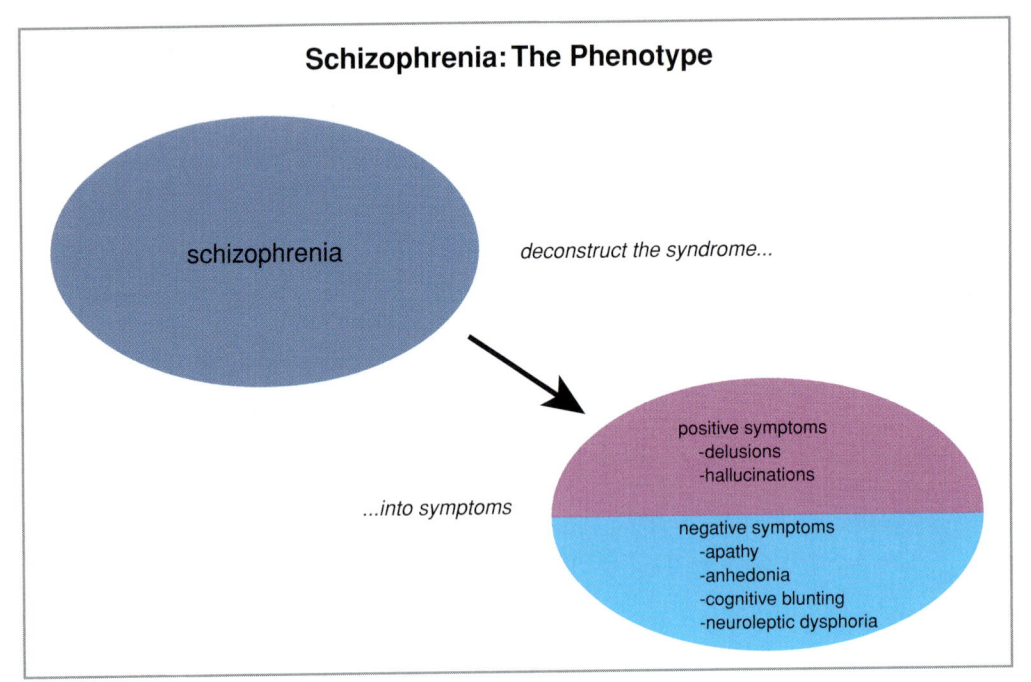

negative symptoms
-apathy
-anhedonia
-cognitive blunting
-neuroleptic dysphoria

FIGURE 9-1 Positive and negative symptoms. The syndrome of schizophrenia consists of a mixture of symptoms that are commonly divided into two major categories, positive and negative. Positive symptoms, such as delusions and hallucinations, reflect the development of the symptoms of psychosis; they can be dramatic and may reflect loss of touch with reality. Negative symptoms reflect the loss of normal functions and feelings, such as losing interest in things and not being able to experience pleasure.

attempt suicide, and 10 percent eventually succeed, contributing to a mortality rate eight times greater than that of the general population. The life expectancy of a schizophrenic patient may be 20 to 30 years shorter than that of the general population, not only due to suicide but in particular due to premature cardiovascular disease. Accelerated mortality from premature cardiovascular disease in schizophrenic patients is caused not only by genetic factors and lifestyle choices – such as smoking, unhealthy diet, and lack of exercise leading to obesity and diabetes – but also, unfortunately, by treatment with some antipsychotic drugs, which themselves cause an increased incidence of obesity and diabetes and thus increased cardiac risk. In the United States, over 20 percent of all social security benefit days are used for the care of schizophrenic patients. The direct and indirect costs of schizophrenia in the United States alone are estimated to be in the tens of billions of dollars every year.

Schizophrenia by definition is a disturbance that must last for 6 months or longer, including at least 1 month of delusions, hallucinations, disorganized speech, grossly disorganized or catatonic behavior, or negative symptoms. Thus, symptoms of schizophrenia are often divided into positive and negative symptoms (Figure 9-1).

Positive symptoms are listed in Table 9-3. These symptoms of schizophrenia are often emphasized, since they can be dramatic, can erupt suddenly when a patient decompensates into a psychotic episode (often called a psychotic "break," as in break from reality), and are the symptoms most effectively treated by antipsychotic medications. **Delusions** are one type of positive symptom; these usually involve a misinterpretation of perceptions or experiences. The most common content of a delusion in schizophrenia is persecutory, but

TABLE 9-3 Positive symptoms of psychosis and schizophrenia

Delusions
Hallucinations
Distortions or exaggerations in language and communication
Disorganized speech
Disorganized behavior
Catatonic behavior
Agitation

TABLE 9-4 Negative symptoms of schizophrenia

Blunted affect
Emotional withdrawal
Poor rapport
Passivity
Apathetic social withdrawal
Difficulty in abstract thinking
Lack of spontaneity
Stereotyped thinking
Alogia: restrictions in fluency and productivity of thought and speech
Avolition: restrictions in initiation of goal-directed behavior
Anhedonia: lack of pleasure
Attentional impairment

may comprise a variety of other themes including referential (i.e., erroneously thinking that something refers to oneself), somatic, religious, or grandiose. **Hallucinations** are also a type of positive symptom (Table 9-3) and may occur in any sensory modality (e.g., auditory, visual, olfactory, gustatory and tactile), but auditory hallucinations are by far the most common and characteristic hallucinations in schizophrenia. Positive symptoms generally reflect an **excess** of normal functions and, in addition to delusions and hallucinations, may also include distortions or exaggerations in language and communication (disorganized speech) as well as in behavioral monitoring (grossly disorganized or catatonic or agitated behavior).

Negative symptoms are listed in Tables 9-4 and 9-5. Classically, there are at least five types of negative symptoms, all starting with the letter "A" (Table 9-5):

alogia – dysfunction of communication; restrictions in the fluency and productivity of thought and speech

affective blunting or flattening – restrictions in the range and intensity of emotional expression

asociality – reduced social drive and interaction

anhedonia – reduced ability to experience pleasure

avolition – reduced desire, motivation, or persistence; restrictions in the initiation of goal-directed behavior

Psychosis and Schizophrenia | 251

TABLE 9-5 What are negative symptoms?

Domain	Descriptive Term	Translation
Dysfunction of communication	Alogia	Poverty of speech; e.g., talks little, uses few words
Dysfunction of affect	Blunted affect	Reduced range of emotions (perception, experience and expression); e.g., feels numb or empty inside, recalls few emotional experiences good or bad
Dysfunction of socialization	Asociality	Reduced social drive and interaction; e.g., little sexual interest, few friends, little interest in spending time with (or little time spent with) friends
Dysfunction of capacity for pleasure	Anhedonia	Reduced ability to experience pleasure; e.g., finds previous hobbies or interests unpleasurable
Dysfunction of motivation	Avolition	Reduced desire or motivation persistence; e.g., reduced ability to undertake and complete everyday tasks; may have poor personal hygiene

Negative symptoms in schizophrenia are commonly considered a reduction in normal functions, such as blunted affect, emotional withdrawal, poor rapport, passivity and apathetic social withdrawal, difficulty in abstract thinking, stereotyped thinking and lack of spontaneity. These symptoms are associated with long periods of hospitalization and poor social functioning. Although this reduction in normal functioning may not be as dramatic as positive symptoms, it is interesting to note that negative symptoms of schizophrenia determine whether a patient ultimately functions well or has a poor outcome. Certainly patients will have disruptions in their ability to interact with others when their positive symptoms are out of control, but their degree of negative symptoms will largely determine whether they can live independently, maintain stable social relationships, or reenter the workplace.

Negative symptoms in schizophrenia can be either primary or secondary (Table 9-6). Primary negative symptoms are considered to be those that are core features of the primary deficits of schizophrenia itself. Other deficits of schizophrenia that may manifest themselves as negative symptoms are thought to be secondary to the positive symptoms of psychosis or secondary to EPS (extrapyramidal symptoms) caused by antipsychotic medications. Negative symptoms can also be secondary to depressive symptoms or environmental deprivation. As shown in Table 9-6, there is debate as to whether this distinction of primary from secondary negative symptoms is important.

Since negative symptoms are so important to the outcome of schizophrenia, it is important to measure them in clinical practice (Table 9-7). Although formal rating scales such as those listed in Table 9-8 can be used to measure negative symptoms in research studies, in clinical practice it may be more practical to identify and monitor negative symptoms quickly by observation alone (Figure 9-2) or by some simple questioning (Figure 9-3). A more quantitative assessment for clinical practice can be rapidly made by rating just four items taken from formal rating scales and shown in Table 9-9; namely, reduced range of emotions, reduced interests, reduced social drive, and restricted speech quantity.

Negative symptoms are not just part of the syndrome of schizophrenia – they can also be part of a "prodrome" that begins with subsyndromal symptoms which do not meet the diagnostic criteria of schizophrenia and occur before the onset of the full syndrome (Figure 9-4). Prodromal negative symptoms are important to detect and monitor over time in

TABLE 9-6 Primary and secondary negative symptoms

Primary: Inherent to the disease process itself

Secondary: Result from other factors, such as depression, extrapyramidal symptoms (EPS), suspicious withdrawal

Deficit syndrome: Enduring primary negative symptoms

Is the distinction important?

YES

Secondary can mimic primary negative symptoms

e.g., unresponsive facial expression:
- Sign of reduced emotional responsiveness and experience, anhedonia?
- Result of EPS?

NO

Negative symptoms, whether primary or secondary, still impair outcomes and should be avoided

---

TABLE 9-7 Why measure negative symptoms?

1. In clinical trials
    - To measure efficacy of interventions in treating negative symptoms
      - pharmacological interventions
      - psychosocial, cognitive, and behavioral interventions
2. In clinical practice
    - To identify patients in your practice who have negative symptoms and the severity of these symptoms
    - To monitor response of your patients to pharmacological and nonpharmacological interventions

---

TABLE 9-8 Scales used to assess negative symptoms

BPRS	Brief Psychiatric Rating Scale (retardation factor)
PANSS	Positive and Negative Syndrome Scale (negative symptom subscale; negative factor)
SANS	Scale for Assessment of Negative Symptoms
NSA-16	Negative Symptom Assessment
SDS	Schedule for the Deficit Syndrome

---

high-risk patients so that treatment can be initiated at the first signs of psychosis (Figure 9-4). Negative symptoms can also persist between psychotic episodes once schizophrenia has begun and reduce social and occupational functioning in the absence of positive symptoms.

Because of the increasing recognition of the importance of negative symptoms, their detection and treatment are now being emphasized. Despite the fact that our current antipsychotic drug treatments are limited in their ability to treat negative symptoms, psychosocial interventions along with antipsychotics can be helpful in reducing negative symptoms. There is even the possibility that instituting treatment for negative symptoms during the prodromal phase of schizophrenia may delay or prevent the onset of the illness, but this is still a matter of current research.

Beyond positive and negative symptoms of schizophrenia

Although not recognized formally as part of the diagnostic criteria for schizophrenia, numerous studies subcategorize the symptoms of this illness into five dimensions: not

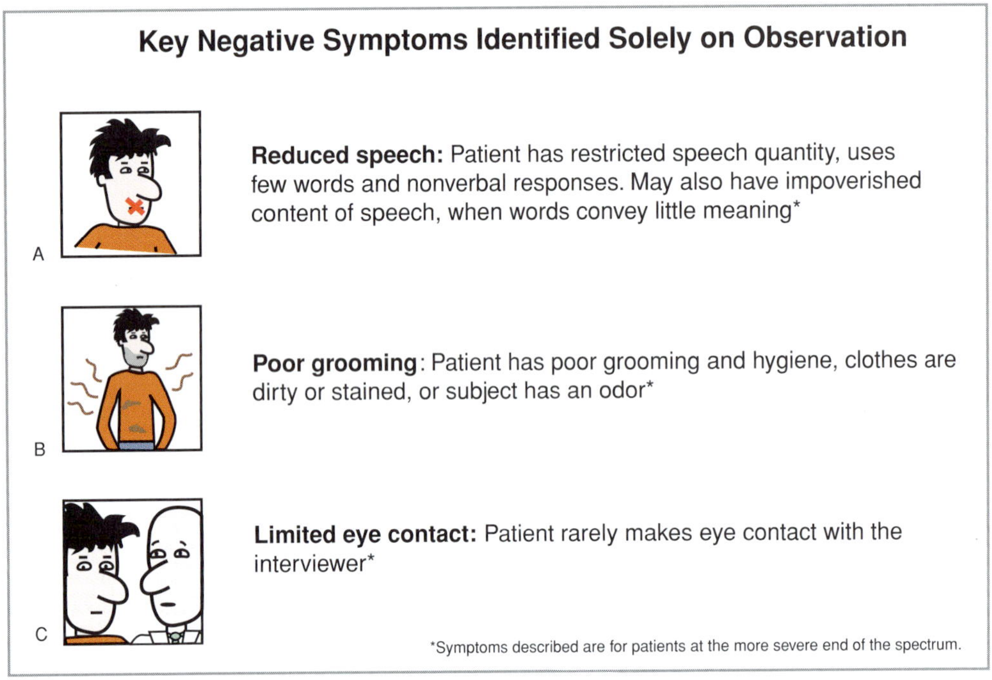

Key Negative Symptoms Identified Solely on Observation

Reduced speech: Patient has restricted speech quantity, uses few words and nonverbal responses. May also have impoverished content of speech, when words convey little meaning*

Poor grooming: Patient has poor grooming and hygiene, clothes are dirty or stained, or subject has an odor*

Limited eye contact: Patient rarely makes eye contact with the interviewer*

*Symptoms described are for patients at the more severe end of the spectrum.

FIGURE 9-2 **Negative symptoms identified by observation.** Some negative symptoms of schizophrenia – such as reduced speech, poor grooming, and limited eye contact – can be identified solely by observing the patient.

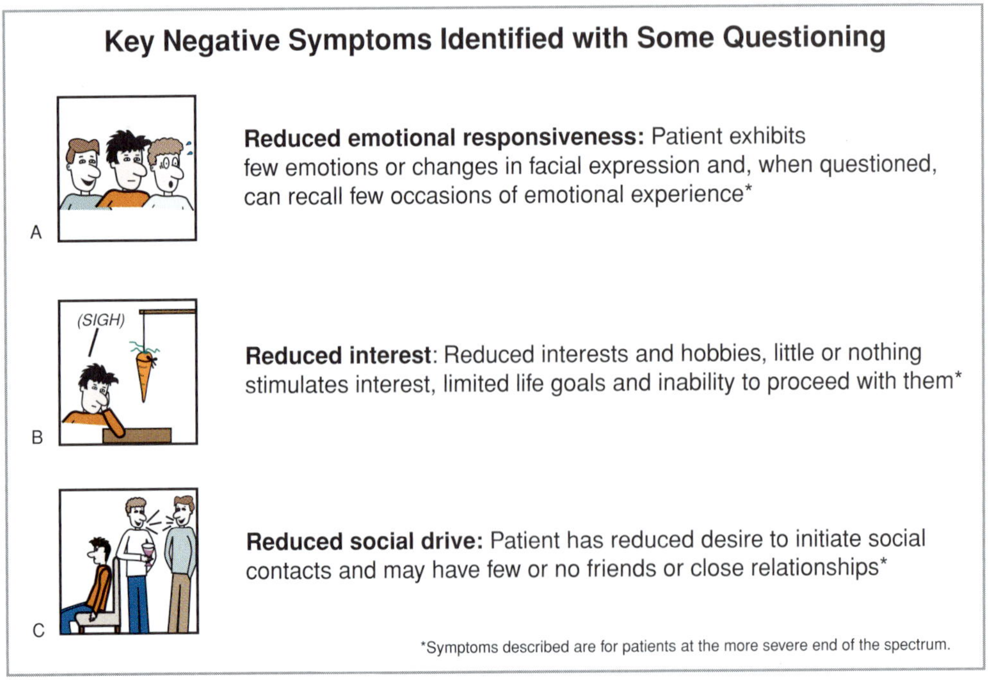

Key Negative Symptoms Identified with Some Questioning

Reduced emotional responsiveness: Patient exhibits few emotions or changes in facial expression and, when questioned, can recall few occasions of emotional experience*

Reduced interest: Reduced interests and hobbies, little or nothing stimulates interest, limited life goals and inability to proceed with them*

Reduced social drive: Patient has reduced desire to initiate social contacts and may have few or no friends or close relationships*

*Symptoms described are for patients at the more severe end of the spectrum.

FIGURE 9-3 **Negative symptoms identified by questioning.** Other negative symptoms of schizophrenia can be identified by simple questioning. For example, brief questioning can reveal the degree of emotional responsiveness, interest level in hobbies or pursuing life goals, and desire to initiate and maintain social contacts.

TABLE 9-9 Selected items for rapid clinical assessment

1. **Reduced range of emotions**

Base rating on the subject's answers to the following queries:

Have you felt anxious, nervous, or worried during the past week? What has that been like for you? What makes you feel this way? (Repeat for sad, happy, proud, scared, surprised, and angry)

During the last week, were there times when you felt numb or empty inside?

1. Normal range of emotion
2. Minimal reduction in range, may be extreme of normal
3. Range seems restricted relative to a normal person but subject convincingly reports at least four emotions
4. Subject convincingly identifies two or three emotional experiences
5. Subject can convincingly identify only one emotional experience
6. Subject reports little or no emotional range

Reduced range of emotion: Ask the patient whether he or she has experienced a range of emotions in the past week and rate according to the number of emotions described (Note that the ability to experience emotion is different from the ability to display affect)

2. **Reduced interests**

Base rating on assessment of range and intensity of subject's interests

What do you enjoy doing? What else do you enjoy? Have you done these things in past week? Are you interested in what is going on in the world? Do you read the newspapers? Do you watch the news on TV? Can you tell me about some of the important news stories of the past week? Do you like sports? What is your favorite sport? Which is your favorite team? Who are the top players in this sport? Have you played in any sport during the past week?

1. Normal sense of purpose
2. Minimal reduction in purpose, may be extreme of normal
3. Life goals somewhat vague but current activities suggest purpose
4. Subject has difficulty coming up with life goals but activities are directed toward limited goal or goals
5. Goals are very limited or have to be suggested and activities are not focused toward achieving any of them
6. No identifiable life goals

Reduced Interests: Assess whether the patient has a normal range and intensity of interests

3. **Reduced social drive**

Rate based on patient responses to queries:

Do you live alone or with someone else?

Do you like to be around other people? Do you spend much time with others?

Do you have difficulty feeling close to them?

How are your friends? How often do you see them? Did you see them this past week? Have you called them on the phone? When you got together this past week, who decided what to do and where to go?

Is anyone concerned about your happiness and well-being?

1. Normal social drive
2. Minimal reduction in social drive, may be extreme of normal
3. Desire for social interactions seems somewhat reduced
4. Obvious reduction in desire to initiate social contacts, but a number of contacts are initiated each week
5. Marked reduction in the subject's desire to initiate social contacts, but a few contacts are maintained at subject's initiation (as with family)
6. No desire to initiate any social interactions

Reduced social drive: Assess the level of social drive by probing the type of social interactions and their frequency. Remember to rate in reference to an age-matched normal.

(Cont.)

TABLE 9-9 *(Cont.)*

2. **Restricted speech quantity**
No specific question; rate based on observations during the interview.
1. Normal speech quantity
2. Minimal reduction in quantity, may be extreme of normal
3. Speech quantity is reduced, but more obtained with minimal prodding
4. Flow of speech is maintained only by regularly prodding
5. Responses usually limited to a few words and/or detail is only obtained by prodding or bribing
6. Responses usually nonverbal or limited to one or two words despite efforts to elicit more

Restricted speech quantity: This item requires no specific questions and is rated based on observing the patient's speech during the interview.

All ratings should assess the function/behavior of the patient in reference to a normal age-matched person.

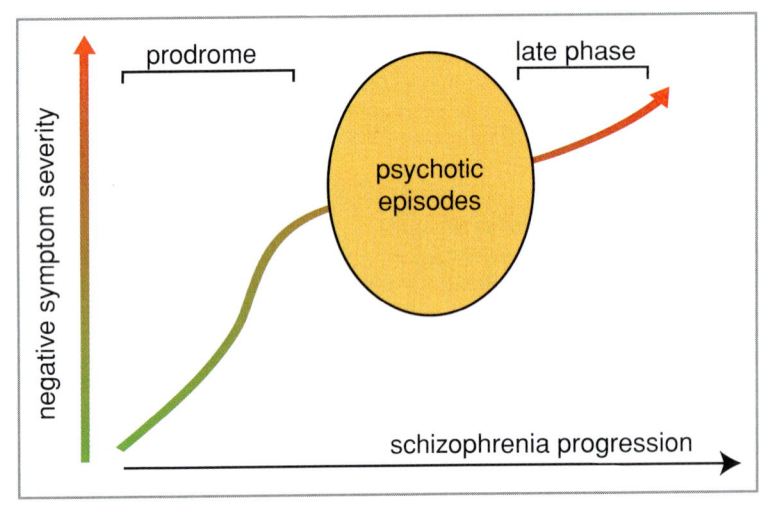

FIGURE 9-4 Negative symptoms in the prodromal phase. Negative symptoms of schizophrenia may occur during the prodromal phase, prior to developing the full syndrome of schizophrenia with both positive and negative symptoms. Theoretically, if such prodromal negative symptoms could be identified early and treated with psychosocial or pharmacological interventions prior to the onset of a psychotic break, it might be possible to delay or even prevent the onset of full-syndrome schizophrenia.

just positive and negative symptoms but also cognitive symptoms, aggressive symptoms, and affective symptoms (Figure 9-5). This is perhaps a more sophisticated if complicated manner of describing the symptoms of schizophrenia.

The overlaps among these five symptom dimensions are shown in Figure 9-6A, and some potentially overlapping symptoms are shown in Figure 9-6B. That is, aggressive symptoms such as assaultiveness, verbally abusive behaviors, and frank violence can occur with positive symptoms such as delusions and hallucinations, yet this is not always the case. It can be difficult to separate the symptoms of formal cognitive dysfunction and those of affective dysfunction from negative symptoms, as shown in Figure 9-6B. Since research is attempting to localize the specific areas of brain dysfunction for each of these

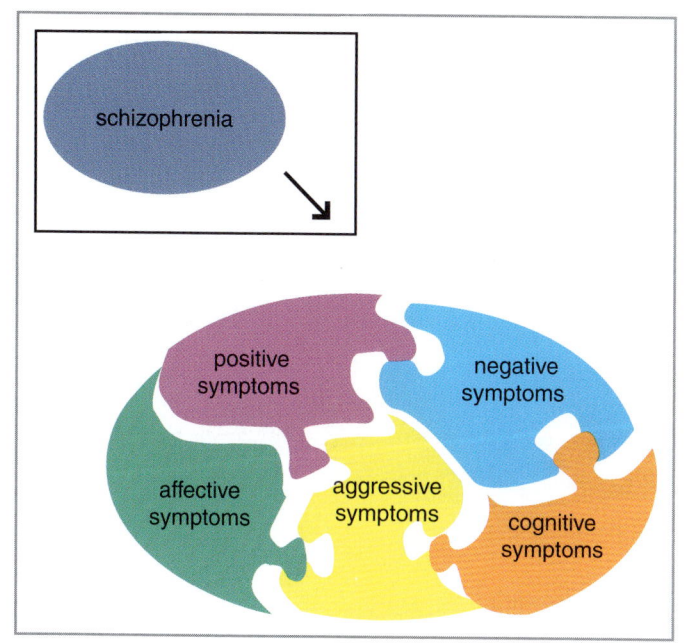

FIGURE 9-5 **Five symptom dimensions of schizophrenia.** The syndrome of schizophrenia can be conceptualized as consisting of five symptom dimensions rather than just the two dimensions of positive and negative symptoms shown in Figure 9-1. This deconstruction of the schizophrenia syndrome thus includes not only positive symptoms and negative symptoms but also cognitive, affective, and aggressive symptoms.

symptom domains and scientists are also attempting to develop better treatments for the often neglected negative, cognitive, and affective symptoms of schizophrenia, there are ongoing attempts to try to quantify and measure such symptoms independently.

In particular, neuropsychological assessment batteries are being developed to quantitate cognitive symptoms, to show how they are independent of the other symptoms of schizophrenia, and to detect cognitive improvement after treatment with a number of novel psychotropic drugs currently being tested. Cognitive symptoms of schizophrenia and other illnesses where psychosis may be an associated feature can overlap with negative symptoms, so test batteries attempt to parse cognitive symptoms from negative symptoms. Overlapping symptoms can include the thought disorder of schizophrenia and the sometimes odd use of language, including incoherence, loose associations, and neologisms. Impaired attention and impaired information processing are other specific cognitive impairments associated with schizophrenia. In fact, the most common and severe of the cognitive impairments in schizophrenia can include impaired verbal fluency (ability to produce spontaneous speech), problems with serial learning (of a list of items or a sequence of events), and impairment in vigilance for executive functioning (problems with sustaining and focusing attention, concentrating, prioritizing, and modulating behavior based on social cues).

Important cognitive symptoms of schizophrenia are listed in Table 9-10. These do not include symptoms of dementia and memory disturbance more characteristic of Alzheimer's disease, but cognitive symptoms of schizophrenia emphasize "executive dysfunction," which includes problems in representing and maintaining goals, allocating attentional resources, evaluating and monitoring performance, and utilizing these skills to solve problems. It is important to recognize and monitor cognitive symptoms of schizophrenia because they are the single strongest correlate of real-world functioning – even stronger than negative symptoms.

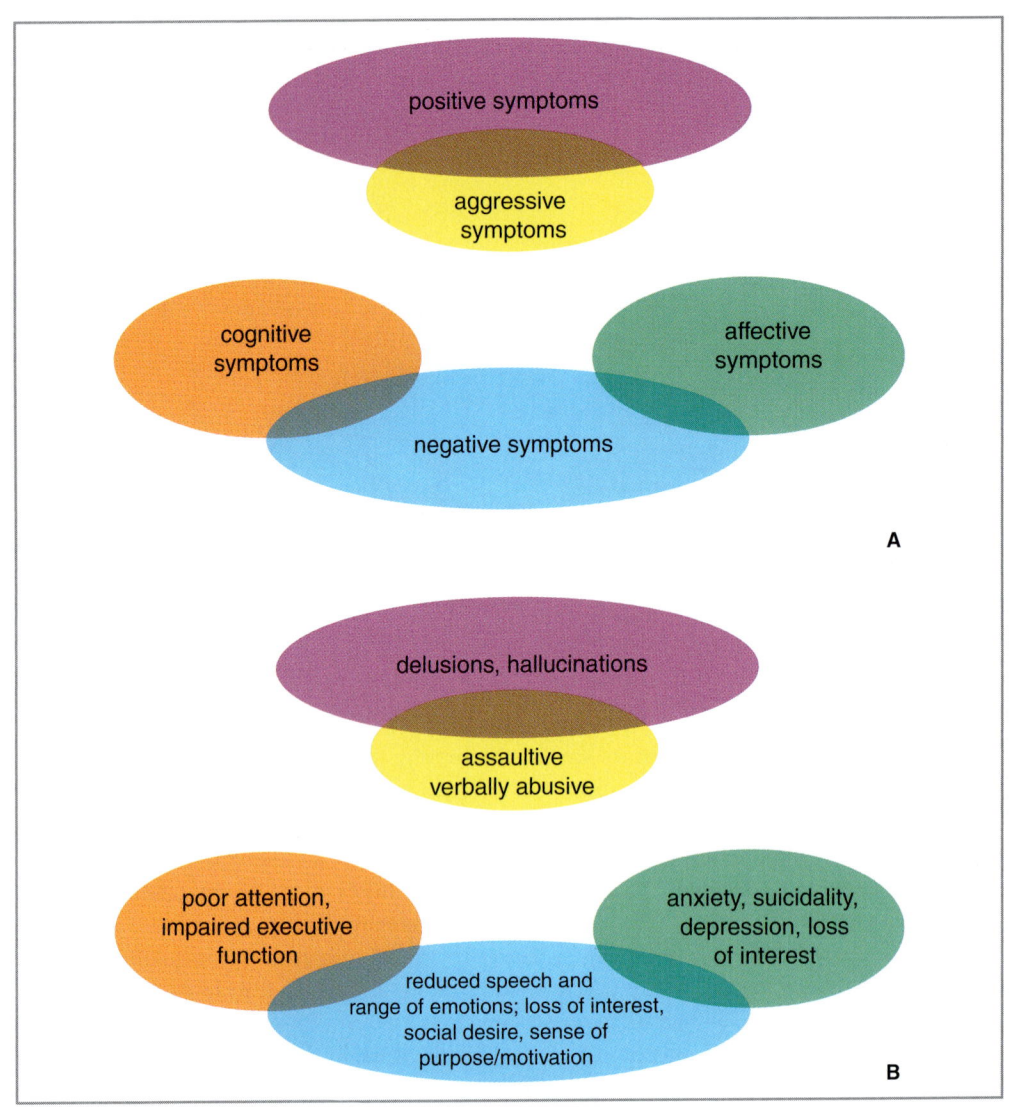

FIGURE 9-6A and B Symptom overlap. Although schizophrenia may be conceptually divided into five symptom dimensions, as shown in Figure 9-5, in reality there is a good deal of overlap among these separate symptom dimensions (**A**). In particular, aggressive symptoms such as assaultiveness and verbal abuse frequently occur in association with positive symptoms (**B**). Impairment in attention and executive functioning as well as affective symptoms such as loss of interest may be difficult to distinguish from negative symptoms (**B**).

Symptoms of schizophrenia are not necessarily unique to schizophrenia

It is important to recognize that several illnesses other than schizophrenia can share some of the same five symptom dimensions described here for schizophrenia and shown in Figure 9-5. Thus, disorders in addition to schizophrenia that can have **positive symptoms** include bipolar disorder, schizoaffective disorder, psychotic depression, Alzheimer's disease and other organic dementias, childhood psychotic illnesses, drug-induced psychoses, and others (Figure 9-7).

Negative symptoms can also occur in other disorders and can also overlap with cognitive and affective symptoms occurring in these disorders. However, as a primary deficit

TABLE 9-10 Cognitive symptoms of schizophrenia

Problems representing and maintaining goals
Problems allocating attentional resources
Problems focusing attention
Problems sustaining attention
Problems evaluating functions
Problems monitoring performance
Problems prioritizing
Problems modulating behavior based upon social cues
Problems with serial learning
Impaired verbal fluency
Difficulty with problem solving

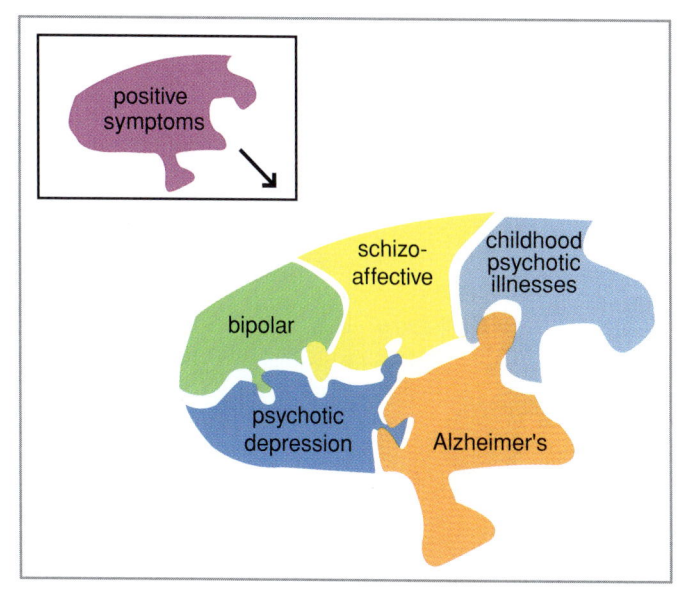

FIGURE 9-7 Positive symptoms across disorders. Positive symptoms are not associated only with schizophrenia but can also occur in several other disorders that may be associated with psychotic symptoms, including bipolar disorder, schizoaffective disorder, childhood psychotic illnesses, Alzheimer's disease and other organic dementias, psychotic depression, and others.

state (Figure 9-8), negative symptoms are unique to schizophrenia. On the other hand, negative symptoms that are secondary to other causes are common in schizophrenia but not necessarily unique to this disorder (Figure 9-8).

Schizophrenia is certainly not the only disorder with **cognitive symptoms**. Autism, poststroke (vascular or multi-infarct) dementia, Alzheimer's disease, and many other organic dementias (parkinsonian/Lewy-body dementia; Pick's disease or frontotemporal lobar degeneration, etc.) can also be associated with cognitive dysfunctions similar to those seen in schizophrenia (Figure 9-9).

Finally, **aggressive and hostile symptoms** occur in numerous other disorders, especially those with problems of impulse control. Symptoms include overt hostility, such as verbal or physical abusiveness or even assault; self-injurious behaviors including suicide; and arson or other property damage. Other types of impulsiveness, such as sexual acting out, are also in this category of aggressive and hostile symptoms. These same symptoms are frequently associated with bipolar disorder, childhood psychosis, borderline personality disorder, antisocial

Psychosis and Schizophrenia | 259

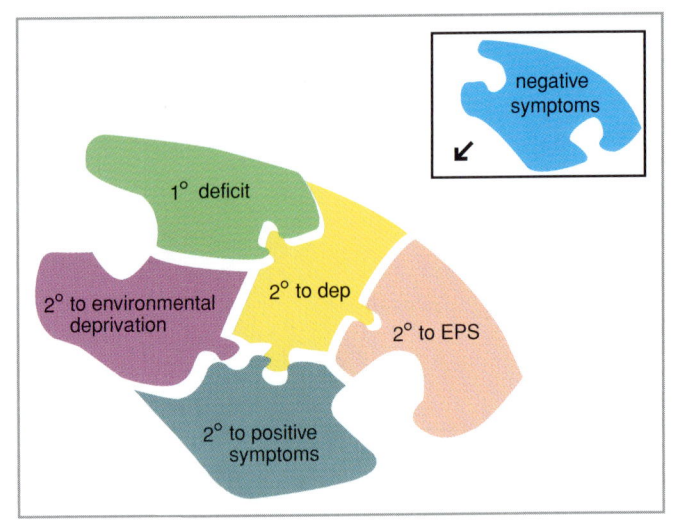

FIGURE 9-8 Causes of negative symptoms. Negative symptoms in schizophrenia can either be a primary core deficit of the illness (1° deficit), or secondary to depression (2° to dep), secondary to extrapyramidal symptoms (2° to EPS), secondary to environmental deprivation, or even secondary to positive symptoms in schizophrenia.

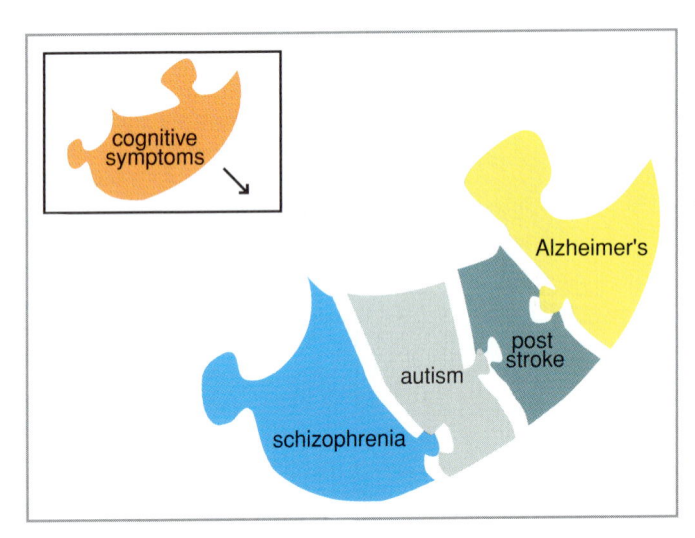

FIGURE 9-9 Cognitive symptoms across disorders. Cognitive symptoms are not associated only with schizophrenia but also with several other disorders including autism, Alzheimer's disease, following cerebrovascular accidents (poststroke) and many others.

personality disorder, drug abuse, Alzheimer's and other dementias, attention deficit hyperactivity disorder, conduct disorders in children, and many others (Figure 9-10).

Affective symptoms are frequently associated with schizophrenia, but this does not necessarily mean that they fulfill the diagnostic criteria for a comorbid anxiety or affective disorder. Nevertheless, depressed mood, anxious mood, guilt, tension, irritability, and worry frequently accompany schizophrenia. These various symptoms are also prominent features of major depressive disorder, psychotic depression, bipolar disorder, schizoaffective disorder, organic dementias, childhood psychotic disorders, and treatment-resistant cases of depression, bipolar disorder, and schizophrenia, among others (Figure 9-11).

Brain circuits and symptom dimensions in schizophrenia

Just as is the case for other psychiatric disorders, the various symptoms of schizophrenia are hypothesized to be localized in unique brain regions (Figure 9-12). Specifically, the positive

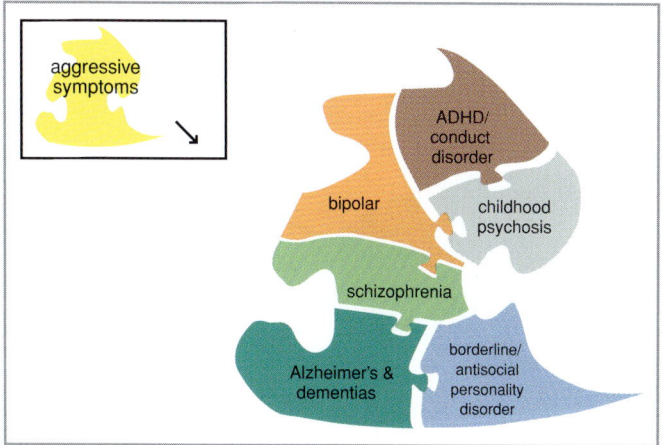

FIGURE 9-10 Aggressive symptoms across disorders. Aggressive symptoms and hostility are associated with several conditions in addition to schizophrenia, including bipolar disorder, attention deficit hyperactivity disorder (ADHD), conduct disorder, childhood psychosis, borderline personality disorder and antisocial personality disorder, Alzheimer's disease, and other dementias.

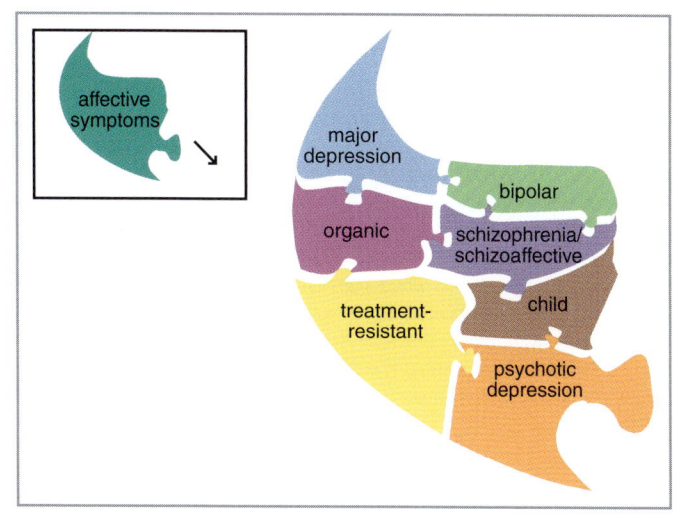

FIGURE 9-11 Affective symptoms across disorders. Affective symptoms are a hallmark not only of major depressive disorder but are also frequently associated with other psychiatric disorders, including bipolar disorder, schizophrenia and schizoaffective disorder, childhood mood disorders, psychotic forms of depression, treatment-resistant mood and psychotic disorders, and organic causes of depression such as substance abuse.

symptoms of schizophrenia have long been hypothesized to be localized to malfunctioning mesolimbic circuits, especially involving the nucleus accumbens. The nucleus accumbens is considered to be part of the brain's reward circuitry, so it is not surprising that problems with reward and motivation in schizophrenia – symptoms that can overlap with negative symptoms and lead to smoking, drug and alcohol abuse – may be linked to this brain area as well.

The prefrontal cortex is considered to be a key node in the nexus of malfunctioning cerebral circuitry responsible for each of the remaining symptoms of schizophrenia: specifically, the mesocortical and ventromedial prefrontal cortex with negative symptoms and affective symptoms, the dorsolateral prefrontal cortex with cognitive symptoms, and the orbitofrontal cortex and its connections to the amygdala with aggressive, impulsive symptoms (Figure 9-12).

This model is obviously oversimplified and reductionistic, because every brain area has several functions and every function is certainly distributed to more than more brain area.

Match Each Symptom to Hypothetically Malfunctioning Brain Circuits

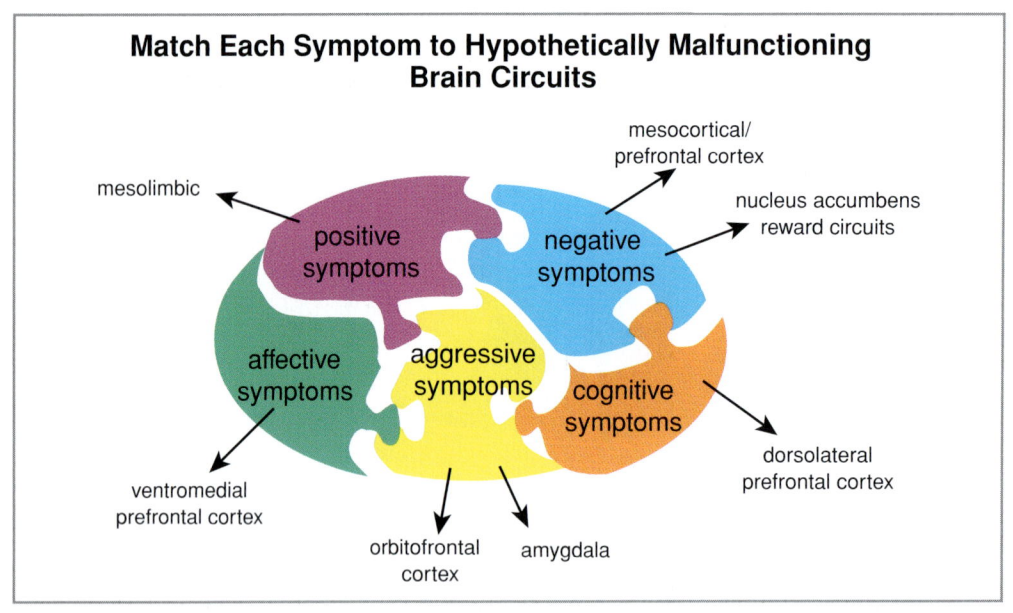

FIGURE 9-12 Localization of symptom domains. The different symptom domains of schizophrenia are hypothesized to be regulated by unique brain regions. **Positive symptoms** of schizophrenia are hypothetically modulated by malfunctioning mesolimbic circuits, while **negative symptoms** are hypothetically linked to malfunctioning mesocortical circuits and may also involve mesolimbic regions such as the nucleus accumbens, which is part of the brain's reward circuitry and thus plays a role in motivation. The nucleus accumbens may also be involved in the increased rate of substance use and abuse seen in patients with schizophrenia. **Affective symptoms** are associated with the ventromedial prefrontal cortex, while **aggressive symptoms** (related to impulse control) are associated with abnormal information processing in orbitofrontal cortex and amygdala, whereas **cognitive symptoms** are associated with problematic information processing in dorsolateral prefrontal cortex. Although there is overlap in function among different brain regions, understanding which brain regions may be predominantly involved in specific symptoms can aid in customization of treatment to the particular symptom profile of each individual patient with schizophrenia.

Nevertheless, allocating specific symptom dimensions to unique brain areas not only assists research studies but has both heuristic and clinical value. Specifically, every patient has unique symptoms and unique responses to medication. In order to optimize and individualize treatment, it can be useful to consider which specific symptoms any given patient is expressing and therefore which areas of that particular patient's brain are hypothetically malfunctioning (Figure 9-12). Each brain area has unique neurotransmitters, receptors, enzymes, and genes that regulate it, with some overlap but also with some unique regional differences; knowing this can help the clinician in choosing medications and monitoring the effectiveness of treatment.

For example, positive symptoms of schizophrenia are theoretically most robustly linked to the mesolimbic/nucleus accumbens brain area and to the neurotransmitter dopamine, with perhaps secondary involvement of the neurotransmitters serotonin, glutamate, gamma-aminobutyric acid (GABA), and others (Figure 9-13). On the other hand, emotional symptoms such as affective and social symptoms are more robustly linked to orbital, medial, and ventral areas of the prefrontal cortex, with executive cognitive symptoms related to the dorsolateral prefrontal cortex (Figure 9-14). Neurotransmitters and key regulatory molecules for the dorsolateral prefrontal cortex include not only dopamine but also several others (Figure 9-15).

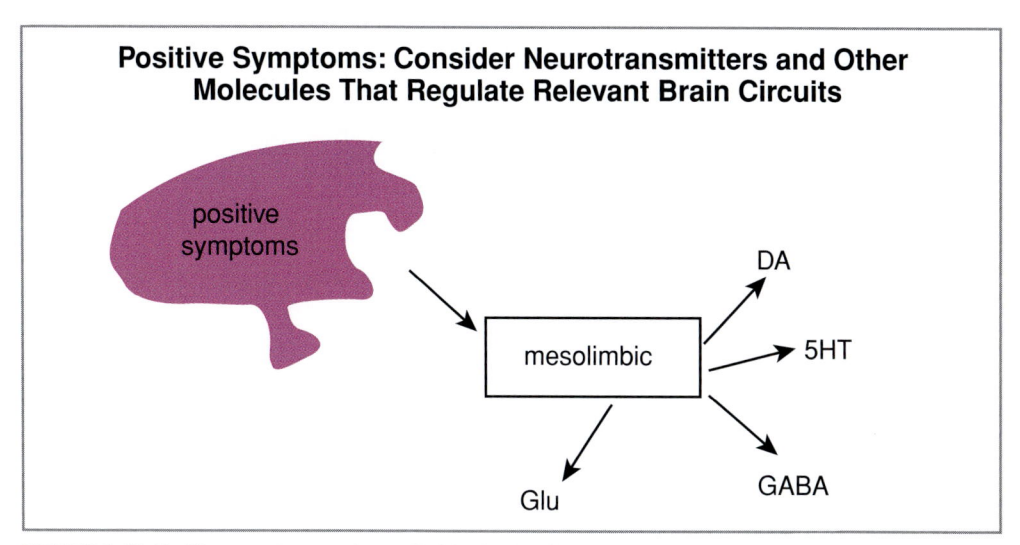

FIGURE 9-13 Positive symptoms and mesolimbic circuits. Positive symptoms of schizophrenia are associated with malfunctioning mesolimbic circuits; the neurotransmitters that regulate mesolimbic neuronal functioning include dopamine (DA), which plays a predominant regulatory role, as well as several other neurotransmitters that play important but perhaps lesser regulatory roles, such as serotonin (5HT), gamma-aminobutyric acid (GABA), and glutamate (glu).

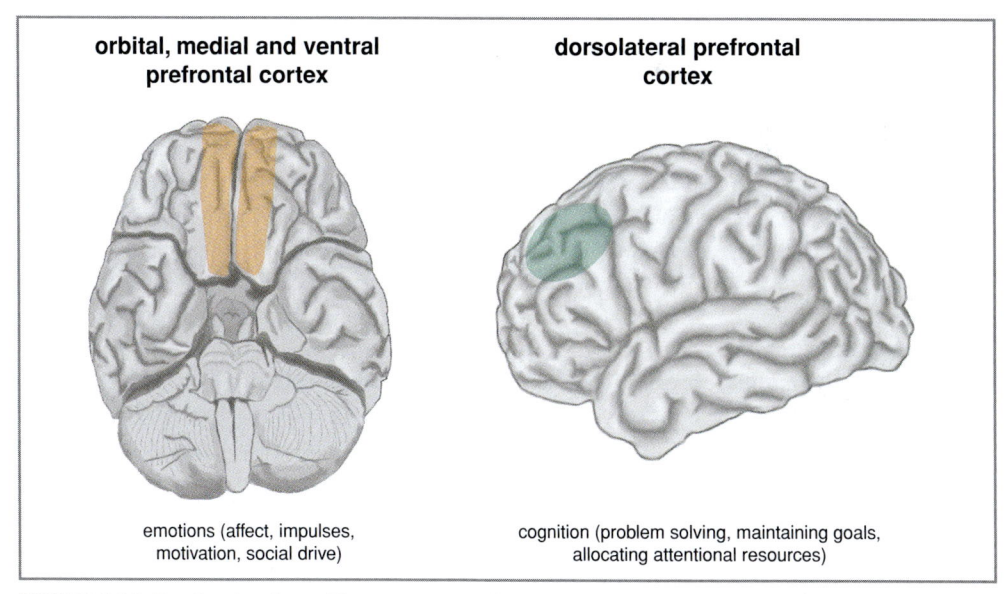

FIGURE 9-14 Emotional and cognitive symptoms and mesocortical circuits. Emotional symptoms of schizophrenia (such as affective symptoms, impulsive symptoms, absence of motivation, absence of social drive) are theoretically mediated by different regions of the prefrontal cortex than are cognitive symptoms. Specifically, emotional symptoms of schizophrenia are hypothetically associated with abnormal information processing in the orbital, medial, and ventral prefrontal cortex (left), while cognitive symptoms of schizophrenia are hypothetically associated with abnormal information processing in the dorsolateral prefrontal cortex (right).

Cognitive Symptoms: Consider Neurotransmitters and Other Molecules That Regulate Relevant Brain Circuits

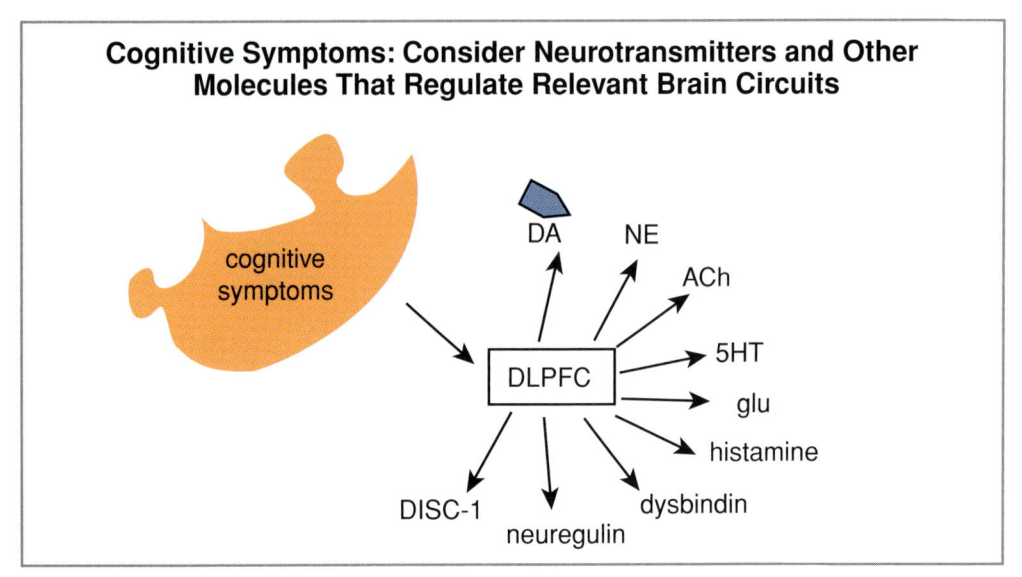

FIGURE 9-15 Cognitive symptoms and dorsolateral prefrontal cortex. The dorsolateral prefrontal cortex, which is linked to cognitive symptoms of schizophrenia, is modulated by the neurotransmitter dopamine (DA) as well as by several other neurotransmitters, including norepinephrine (NE), acetylcholine (ACh), serotonin (5HT), glutamate (glu), and histamine (HA). Circuits in prefrontal cortex are also modulated by numerous molecules important in synapse formation such as dysbindin, neuregulin, and DISC-1 (disrupted in schizophrenia-1).

What is the point of deconstructing the diagnosis of schizophrenia into its symptom domains and then matching each symptom to a hypothetically malfunctioning brain circuit and the neurotransmitters that regulate that brain area? This strategy not only helps the clinician to develop a unique profile of symptoms to target in each individual patient but also provides a specifically tailored set of psychopharmacological treatment tactics for each individual. That is, each neurotransmitter regulating a given circuit is associated with unique pharmacological agents that either boost or block it, depending on the outcome desired (Figure 9-16). When one agent for a given neurotransmitter is ineffective, this approach suggests not only another agent for that same neurotransmitter but also agents for other neurotransmitters that may work together to form a logical set of cotherapies to relieve symptoms. An additional bonus to this approach is that it also suggests which specific genes may be involved in any given symptom in any given brain area (Figure 9-17). This latter information will be critical for developing rational genetic approaches to risk assessment for individual patients and their families and will help in interpreting the results of functional neuroimaging tests to assess these patients' biological endophenotypes, indicating how efficient their information processing is in specific brain regions and whether they are enhancing their chances of symptom relief and reducing their chances of relapse.

Neurotransmitters and circuits in schizophrenia

Dopamine
The biological basis of schizophrenia remains unknown. However, the monoamine neurotransmitter dopamine (DA) has long played a prominent role in the hypotheses of

Identify Pharmacologic Mechanisms That Influence Those Regulators to Select or Combine Treatments

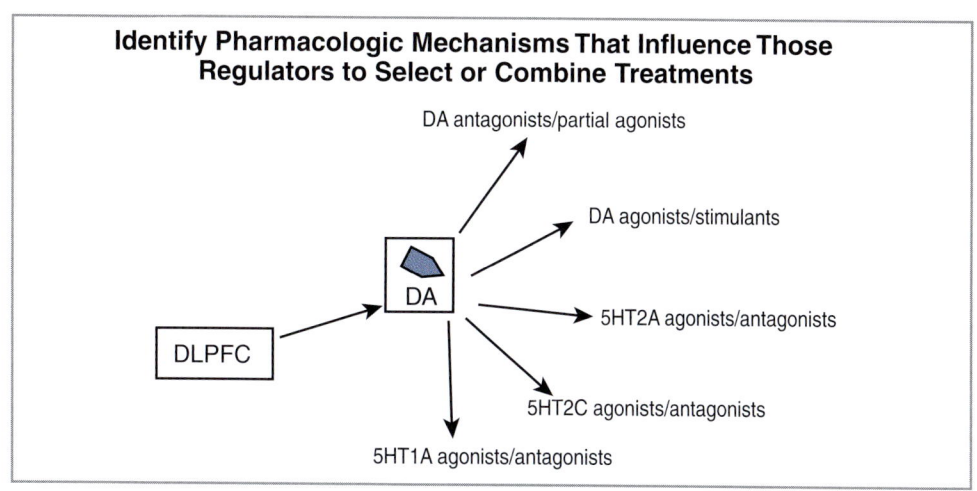

- DA antagonists/partial agonists
- DA agonists/stimulants
- 5HT2A agonists/antagonists
- 5HT2C agonists/antagonists
- 5HT1A agonists/antagonists

DLPFC → DA

FIGURE 9-16 Pharmacological mechanisms influencing dopamine. By matching individual symptoms to a particular brain region and the neurotransmitters that regulate it, clinicians can identify pharmacological mechanisms that influence those regulators. This information can then be utilized to select specific drugs acting on desired pharmacological mechanisms to target the relief of specific symptoms. Theoretically, this occurs by drugs acting on neurotransmitters to change the efficiency of information processing in specific brain areas with hypothetically malfunctioning circuitry. For example, as shown in Figure 9-15, the dorsolateral prefrontal cortex (DLPFC) is regulated by dopamine (DA) and serotonin (5HT). Thus, agents that act on DA and/or serotonin, such as agonists or antagonists of dopamine at D1 and D2 receptors, as well as agonists and antagonists of serotonin at 5HT2A, 5HT2C, and 5HT1A receptors, may all affect information processing in this brain area and thus, cognitive function.

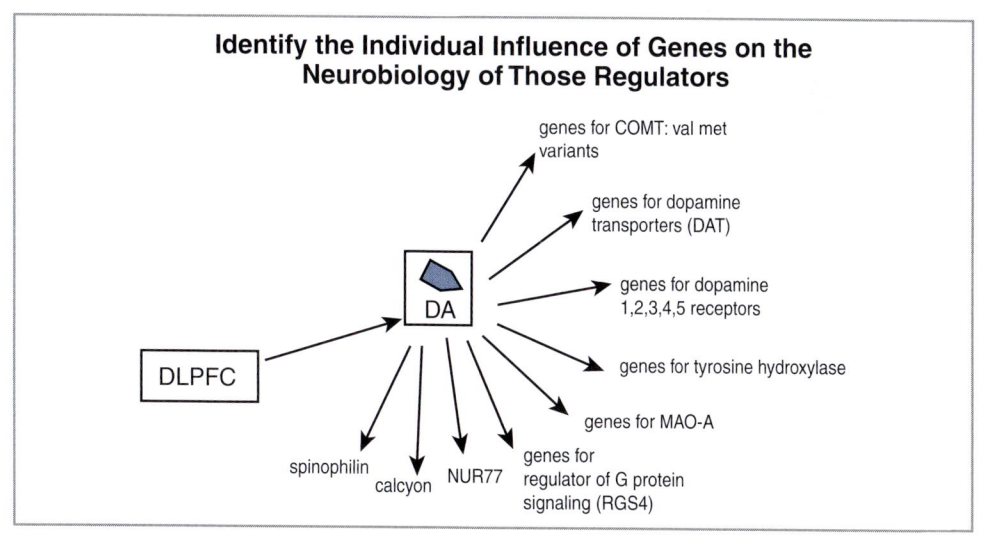

Identify the Individual Influence of Genes on the Neurobiology of Those Regulators

- genes for COMT: val met variants
- genes for dopamine transporters (DAT)
- genes for dopamine 1,2,3,4,5 receptors
- genes for tyrosine hydroxylase
- genes for MAO-A
- genes for regulator of G protein signaling (RGS4)
- spinophilin
- calcyon
- NUR77

DLPFC → DA

FIGURE 9-17 Genes influencing dopamine. Determining the brain regions and regulatory neurotransmitters involved in specific symptoms of schizophrenia aids in the identification of genes that may be involved in the manifestation of those symptoms. For example, dopamine (DA) neurotransmission, which modulates activity in the dorsolateral prefrontal cortex (DLPFC), is influenced by several genes including genes for catechol-O-methyl-transferase (COMT), genes for the dopamine transporter (DAT), genes for various dopamine receptors, and many other genes, several of which are shown here. Identifying genetic contributions to symptoms of schizophrenia may ultimately allow for genetic approaches to risk assessment for patients and their families as well as assist in the design of more effective psychopharmacological agents for treating the symptoms of schizophrenia.

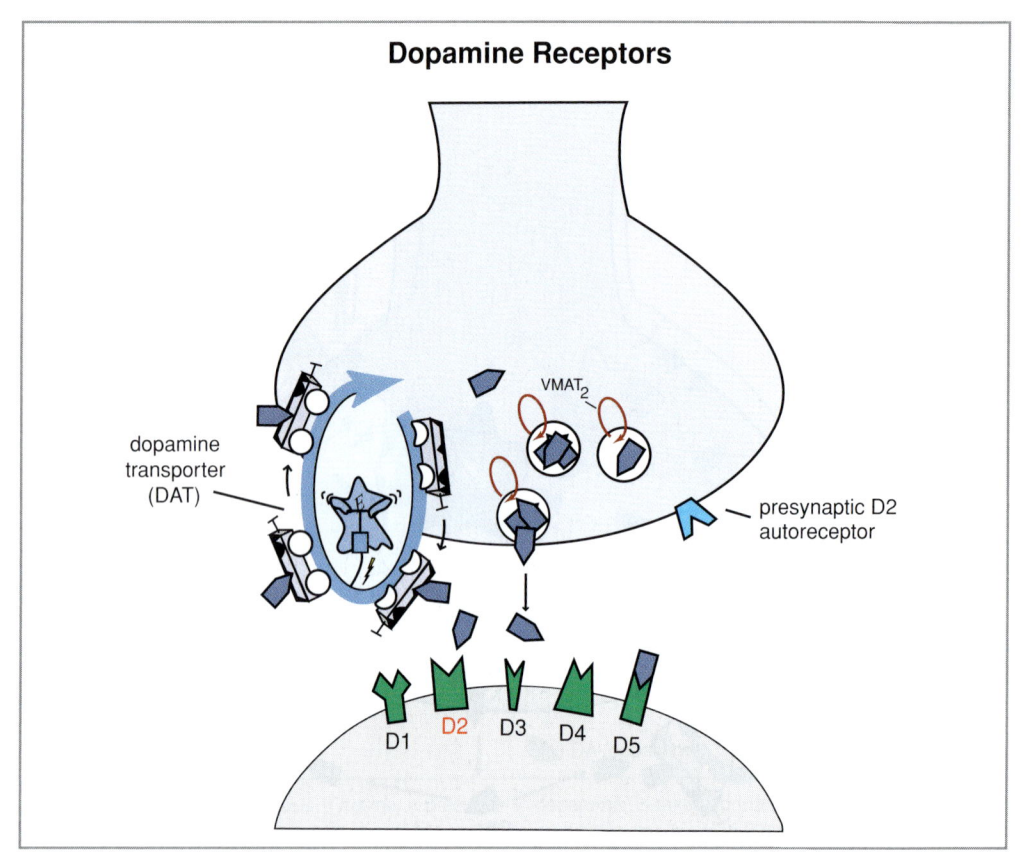

FIGURE 9-20 Dopamine receptors. Shown here are receptors for dopamine that regulate its neurotransmission. The dopamine transporter (DAT) exists presynaptically and is responsible for clearing excess dopamine out of the synapse. The vesicular monoamine transporter (VMAT2) takes dopamine up into synaptic vesicles for future neurotransmission. There is also a presynaptic dopamine-2 autoreceptor, which regulates release of dopamine from the presynaptic neuron. In addition, there are several postsynaptic receptors. These include dopamine-1, dopamine-2, dopamine-3, dopamine-4, and dopamine-5 receptors. The functions of the dopamine-2 receptors are best understood, because this is the primary binding site for virtually all antipsychotic agents as well as for dopamine agonists used to treat Parkinson's disease.

Dopamine D2 receptors can be presynaptic, where they function as autoreceptors (Figure 9-20). Presynaptic D2 receptors thus act as "gatekeepers," either allowing DA release when they are not occupied by DA (Figure 9-21A) or inhibiting DA release when DA builds up in the synapse and occupies the gatekeeping presynaptic autoreceptor (Figure 9-21B). Such receptors are located either on the axon terminal (Figure 9-22) or on the other end of the neuron in the somatodendritic area (Figure 9-23). In both cases, occupancy of these D2 receptors provides negative feedback input, or a braking action on the release of dopamine from the presynaptic neuron.

Key dopamine pathways in the brain

Four well-defined dopamine pathways in the brain plus a newly discovered fifth pathway for dopamine are shown in Figure 9-24. They include the mesolimbic, mesocortical, nigrostriatal, and tuberoinfundibular dopamine DA pathways. The new pathway innervates the thalamus.

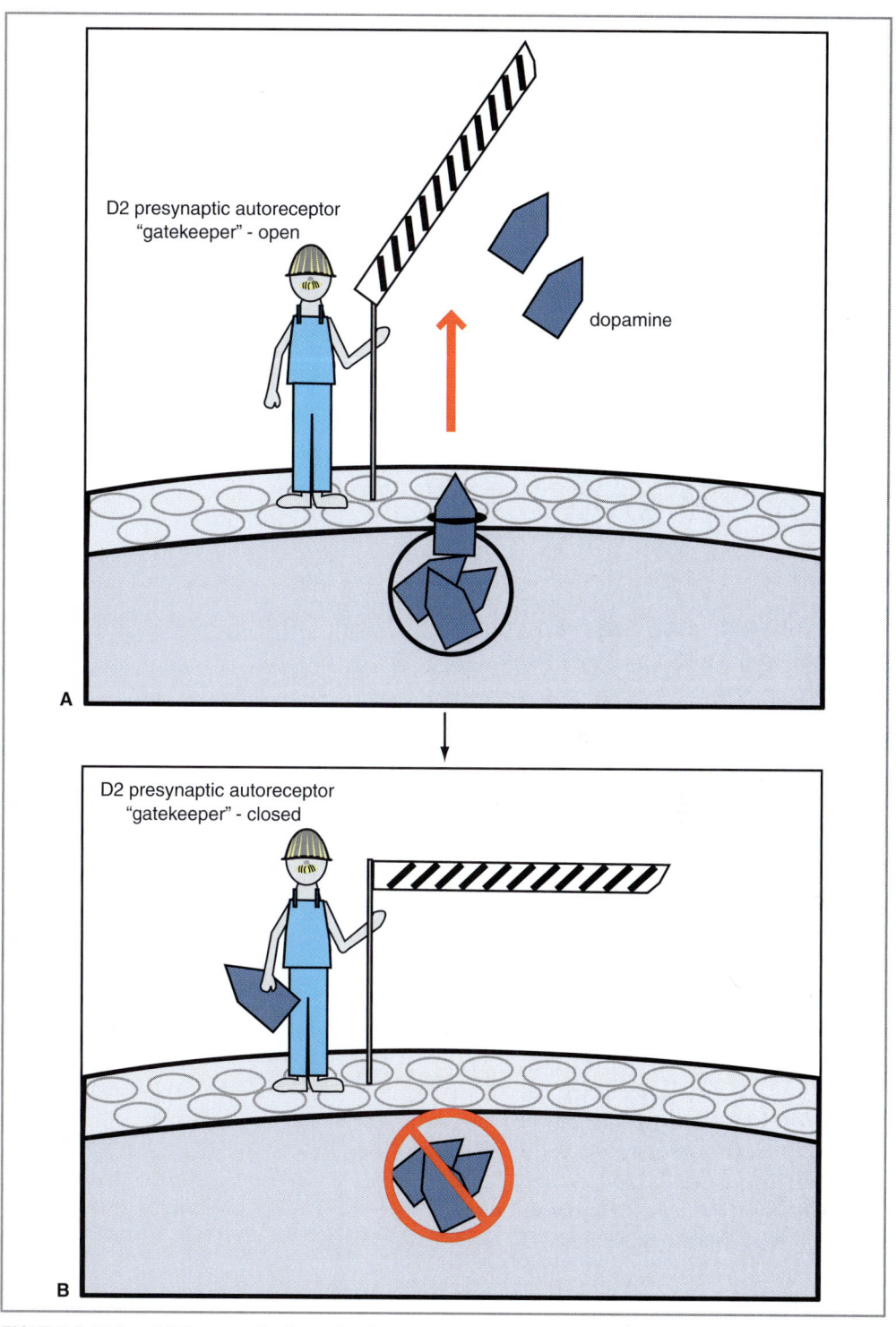

FIGURE 9-21A and B Presynaptic dopamine-2 autoreceptors. Presynaptic dopamine-2 autoreceptors are "gatekeepers" for dopamine. That is, when these gatekeeping receptors are not bound by dopamine (no dopamine in the gatekeeper's hand), they open a molecular gate, allowing dopamine release (**A**). However, when dopamine binds to the gatekeeping receptors (now the gatekeeper has dopamine in his hand), they close the molecular gate and prevent dopamine from being released (**B**).

Psychosis and Schizophrenia | 269

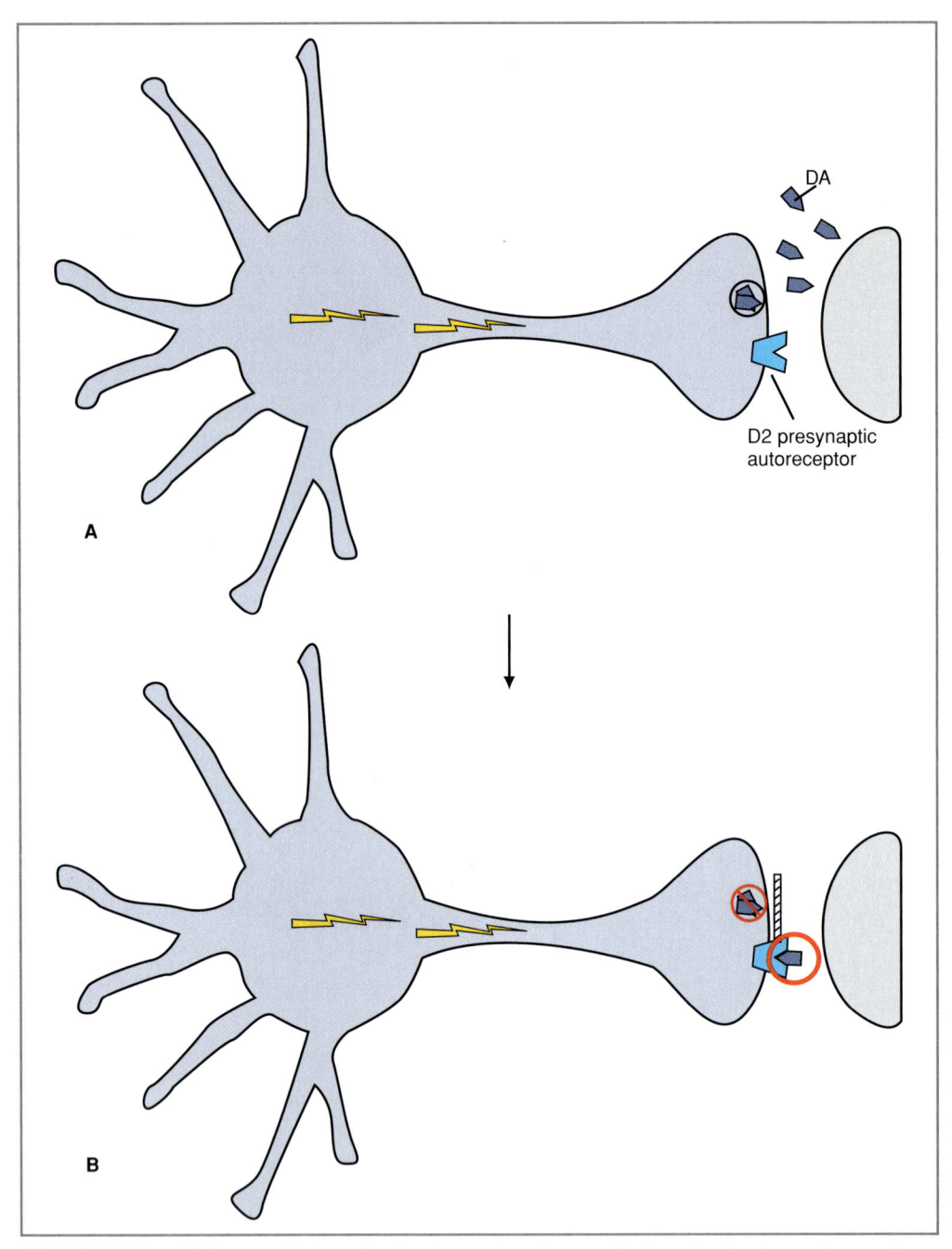

FIGURE 9-22A and B Presynaptic dopamine-2 autoreceptors. Presynaptic dopamine-2 autoreceptors can be located on the axon terminal, as shown here. When dopamine builds up in the synapse (**A**), it is available to bind to the autoreceptor, which then inhibits dopamine release (**B**).

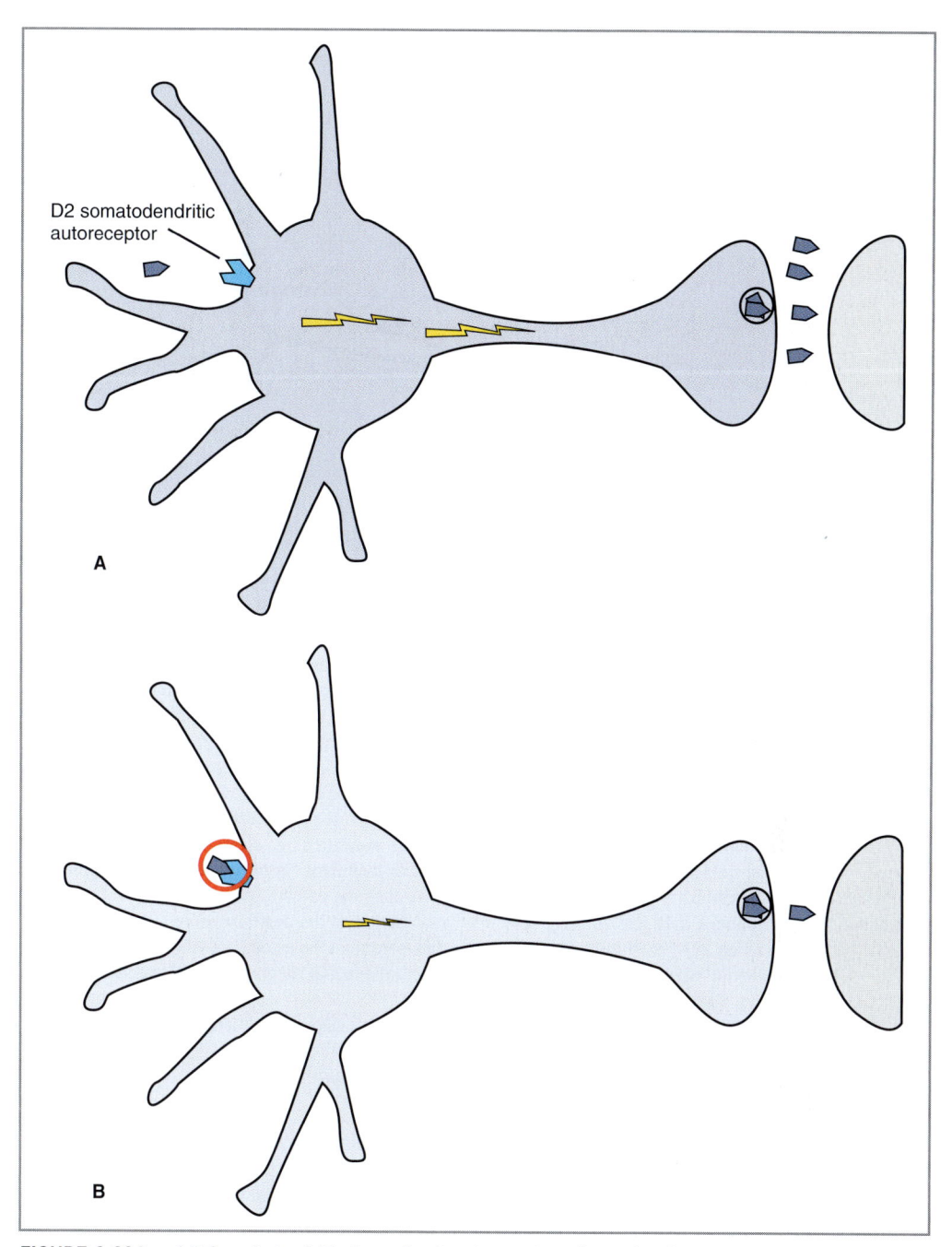

FIGURE 9-23A and B Somatodendritic dopamine-2 autoreceptors. Dopamine-2 autoreceptors can also be located in the somatodendritic area, as shown here (**A**). When dopamine binds to the receptor here, it shuts off neuronal impulse flow in the dopamine neuron (see loss of lightning bolts in the neuron in **B**), and this stops further dopamine release.

Psychosis and Schizophrenia | 271

Dopamine Pathways and Key Brain Regions

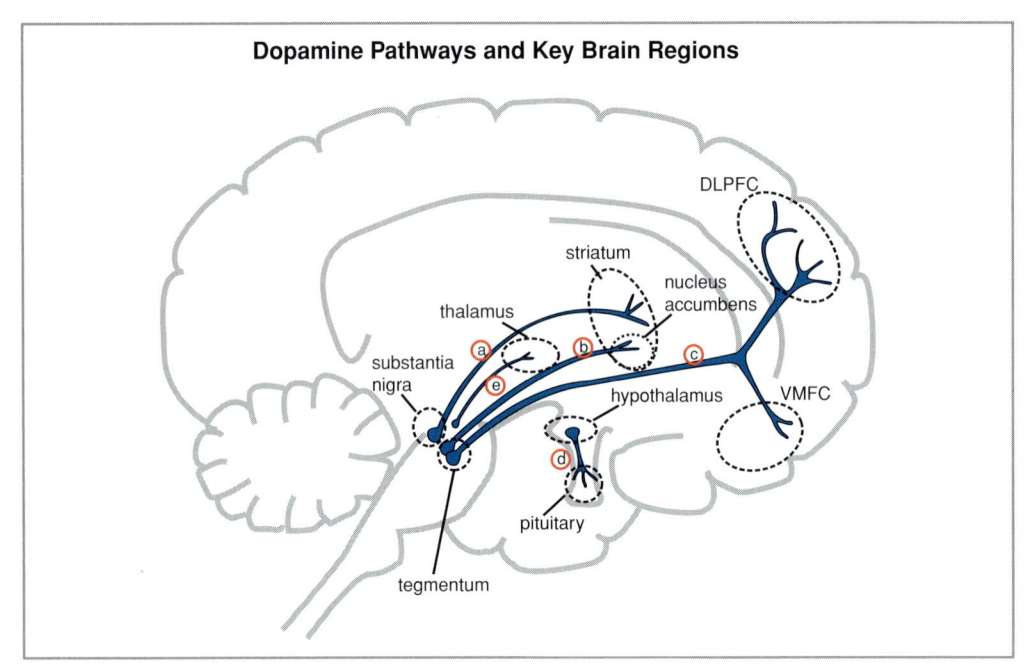

FIGURE 9-24 **Five dopamine pathways in the brain.** The neuroanatomy of dopamine neuronal pathways in the brain can explain the symptoms of schizophrenia as well as the therapeutic effects and side effects of antipsychotic drugs. (a) The **nigrostriatal dopamine pathway**, which projects from the substantia nigra to the basal ganglia or striatum, is part of the extrapyramidal nervous system and controls motor function and movement. (b) The **mesolimbic dopamine pathway** projects from the midbrain ventral tegmental area to the nucleus accumbens, a part of the limbic system of the brain thought to be involved in many behaviors such as pleasurable sensations, the powerful euphoria of drugs of abuse, as well as delusions and hallucinations of psychosis. (c) A pathway related to the mesolimbic dopamine pathway is the **mesocortical dopamine pathway**. It also projects from the midbrain ventral tegmental area but sends its axons to areas of the prefrontal cortex, where they may have a role in mediating cognitive symptoms (dorsolateral prefrontal cortex) and affective symptoms (ventromedial prefrontal cortex) of schizophrenia. (d) The fourth dopamine pathway of interest, the **tuberoinfundibular dopamine pathway**, projects from the hypothalamus to the anterior pituitary gland and controls prolactin secretion. (e) The fifth dopamine pathway arises from multiple sites, including the periaqueductal gray, ventral mesencephalon, hypothalamic nuclei, and lateral parabrachial nucleus, and it projects to the thalamus. Its function is not currently well known.

Mesolimbic dopamine pathway and the mesolimbic dopamine hypothesis of positive symptoms of schizophrenia

The **mesolimbic dopamine pathway** projects from dopaminergic cell bodies in the ventral tegmental area of the brainstem to axon terminals in one of the limbic areas of the brain, namely the nucleus accumbens in the ventral striatum (Figure 9-24). This pathway is thought to have an important role in several emotional behaviors, including the positive symptoms of psychosis, such as delusions and hallucinations (Figure 9-25). The mesolimbic dopamine pathway is also important for motivation, pleasure, and reward.

For more than 30 years, it has been observed that diseases or drugs that increase dopamine will enhance or produce positive psychotic symptoms, whereas drugs that decrease dopamine will decrease or stop positive symptoms. For example, stimulant drugs such as amphetamine and cocaine release dopamine and, if given repetitively, can cause a paranoid psychosis virtually indistinguishable from the positive symptoms of schizophrenia. Stimulant drugs are discussed in detail in subsequent chapters on the treatment of attention

Mesolimbic Pathway

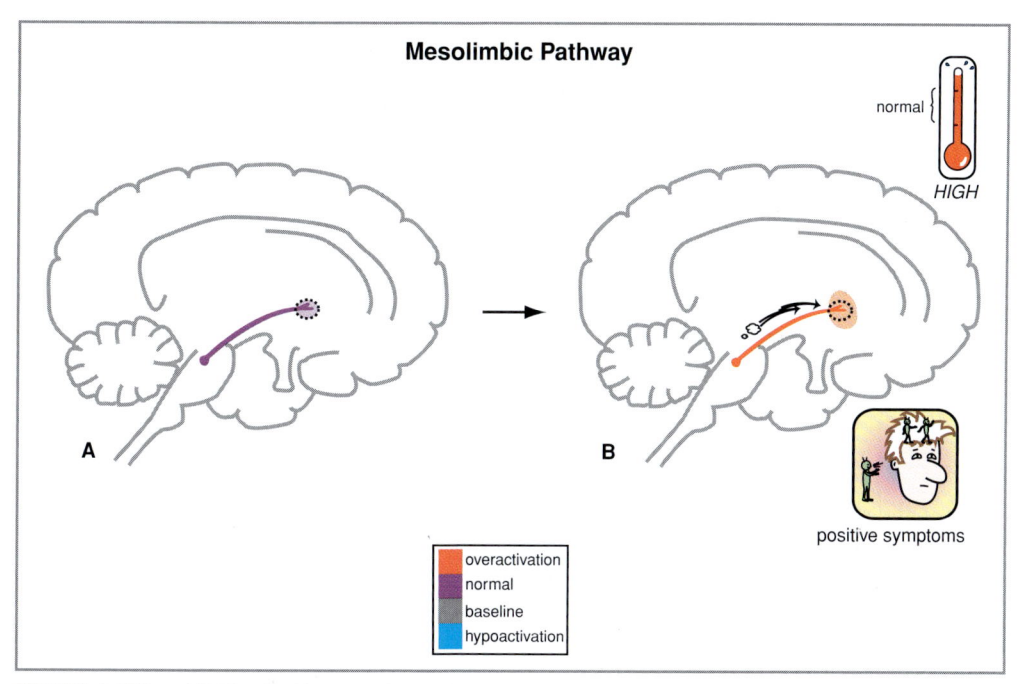

FIGURE 9-25A and B Mesolimbic dopamine pathway. The mesolimbic dopamine pathway, which projects from the ventral tegmental area in the brainstem to the nucleus accumbens in the ventral striatum (**A**), is involved in regulation of emotional behaviors and is believed to be the predominant pathway regulating positive symptoms of psychosis. Specifically, hyperactivity of this pathway is believed to account for delusions and hallucinations (**B**).

deficit hyperactivity disorder and on drug abuse. Their mechanism of action is also discussed in Chapter 4 and illustrated in Figures 4-14 and 4-15.

All known antipsychotic drugs capable of treating positive psychotic symptoms are blockers of the D2 dopamine receptor. Antipsychotic drugs are discussed in Chapter 10. These observations have been formulated into a theory of psychosis sometimes referred to as the "dopamine hypothesis of schizophrenia." Perhaps a more precise modern designation is the "mesolimbic dopamine hypothesis of positive symptoms of schizophrenia," since it is believed that it is hyperactivity specifically in this particular dopamine pathway that mediates the positive symptoms of psychosis (Figure 9-25 and 9-26). Hyperactivity of the mesolimbic dopamine pathway hypothetically accounts for positive psychotic symptoms, whether those symptoms are part of the illness of schizophrenia or of drug-induced psychosis or whether positive psychotic symptoms accompany mania, depression, or dementia. Hyperactivity of mesolimbic dopamine neurons may also play a role in aggressive and hostile symptoms in schizophrenia and related illnesses, especially if serotonergic control of dopamine is aberrant in patients who lack impulse control.

Mesocortical dopamine pathways and the mesocortical dopamine hypothesis of cognitive, negative, and affective symptoms of schizophrenia

Another pathway also arising from cell bodies in the ventral tegmental area but projecting to areas of the prefrontal cortex is known as the **mesocortical dopamine pathway** (Figures 9-27 and 9-28). Branches of this pathway into the dorsolateral prefrontal cortex are hypothesized to regulate cognition and executive functions (Figure 9-27), whereas its branches into the

The Mesolimbic Dopamine Hypothesis of Positive Symptoms of Schizophrenia

mesolimbic overactivity =
positive symptoms of schizophrenia

positive symptoms

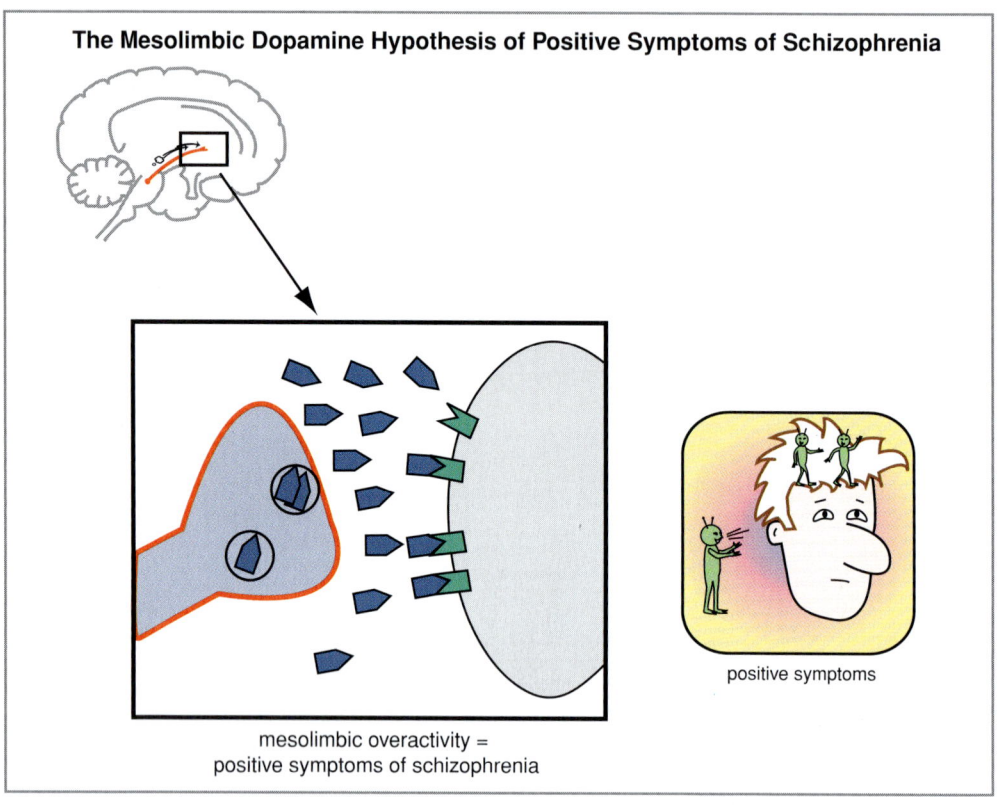

FIGURE 9-26 Mesolimbic dopamine hypothesis. Hyperactivity of dopamine neurons in the mesolimbic dopamine pathway theoretically mediates the positive symptoms of psychosis such as delusions and hallucinations. This pathway is also involved in pleasure, reward, and reinforcing behavior, and many drugs of abuse interact here.

ventromedial parts of prefrontal cortex are hypothesized to regulate emotions and affect (Figure 9-28). The exact role of the mesocortical dopamine pathway in mediating symptoms of schizophrenia is still a matter of debate, but many researchers believe that cognitive and some negative symptoms of schizophrenia may be due to a **deficit** of dopamine activity in mesocortical projections to dorsolateral prefrontal cortex (Figure 9-27), whereas affective and other negative symptoms of schizophrenia may be due to a **deficit** of dopamine activity in mesocortical projections to ventromedial prefrontal cortex (Figure 9-28).

The behavioral deficit state suggested by negative symptoms certainly implies underactivity or even "burnout" of neuronal systems. This may be related to the consequences of prior excitotoxic overactivity of **glutamate systems** (discussed below). An ongoing degenerative process in the mesocortical dopamine pathway could explain a progressive worsening of symptoms and an ever-increasing deficit state in some schizophrenic patients. This deficit of dopamine in mesocortical projections could also be the consequences of neurodevelopmental abnormalities in the N-methyl-d-aspartate (NMDA) glutamate system, described in the next section. Whatever the cause, a corollary to the original DA hypothesis of schizophrenia now incorporates theories for the cognitive, negative, and affective symptoms and might be more precisely designated as the "mesocortical dopamine hypothesis of cognitive, negative, and affective symptoms of schizophrenia" since it is believed that underactivity specifically in

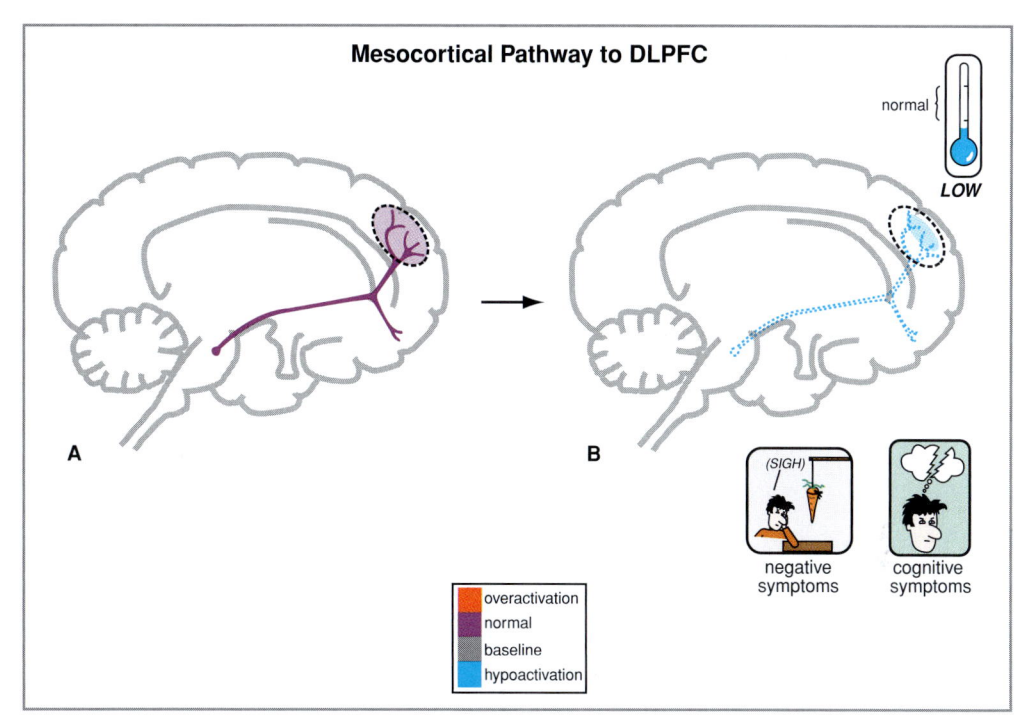

FIGURE 9-27A and B Mesocortical pathway to dorsolateral prefrontal cortex. Another major dopaminergic pathway is the mesocortical dopamine pathway, which projects from the ventral tegmental area to the prefrontal cortex (**A**). Projections specifically to the dorsolateral prefrontal cortex (DLPFC) are believed to be involved in the negative and cognitive symptoms of schizophrenia. In this case, expression of these symptoms is thought to be associated with *hypo*activity of this pathway (**B**).

mesocortical projections to prefrontal cortex mediates the cognitive, negative, and affective symptoms of schizophrenia (Figure 9-29).

Theoretically, increasing dopamine in the mesocortical dopamine pathway might improve the negative, cognitive, and affective symptoms of schizophrenia. However, since there is hypothetically an excess of dopamine elsewhere in the brain within the mesolimbic dopamine pathway, any further increase of dopamine in that pathway would actually worsen positive symptoms. Thus, this state of affairs for dopamine activity in the brain of schizophrenic patients poses a therapeutic dilemma: how do you increase dopamine in the mesocortical pathway while, at the same time, also decreasing dopamine activity in the mesolimbic dopamine pathway? The extent to which atypical antipsychotic medications have provided a solution to this therapeutic dilemma will be discussed in Chapter 10.

Mesolimbic dopamine pathway, reward, and negative symptoms
Dopamine function in schizophrenia may be more complicated than just "too high" in mesolimbic areas and "too low" in mesocortical areas. Instead, it may be that dopamine neurons are better characterized as "out of tune" or "chaotic." This idea of neuronal "tuning" is discussed in Chapter 7 and illustrated in Figures 7-25 and 7-26. A similar phenomenon may be occurring in the mesolimbic dopamine system, with one subset of mesolimbic dopamine neurons out of tune and hyperactive, mediating positive symptoms, and another set of mesolimbic dopamine neurons out of tune but hypoactive, mediating some negative symptoms and malfunctioning reward mechanisms.

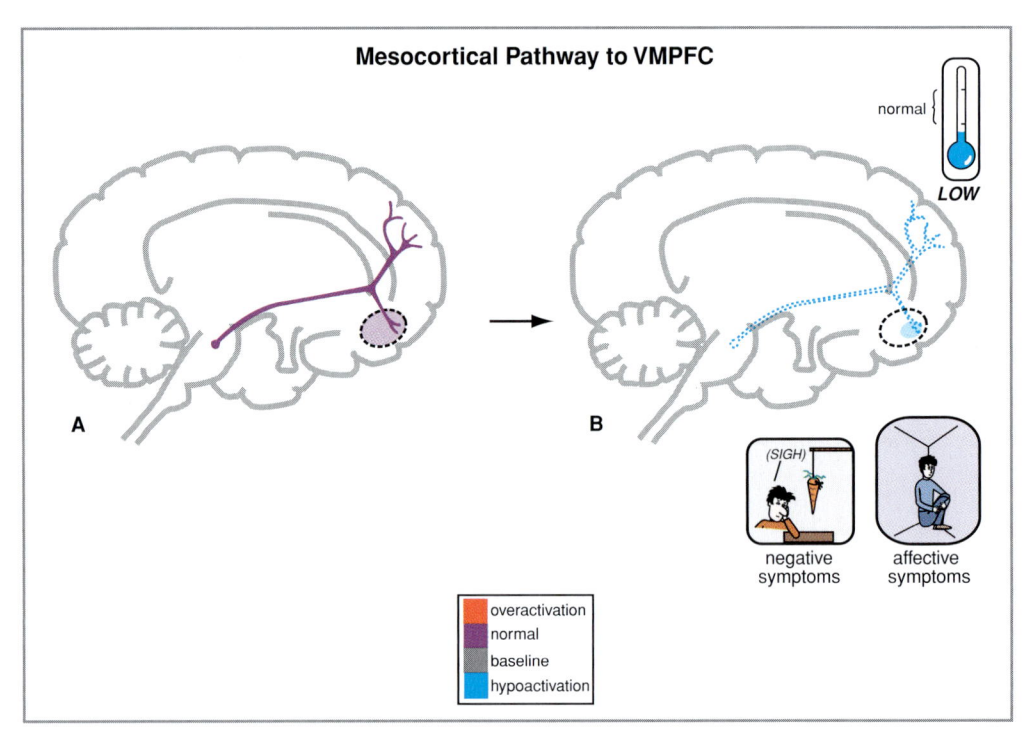

FIGURE 9-28A and B Mesocortical pathway to ventromedial prefrontal cortex. Mesocortical dopamine projections specifically to the ventromedial prefrontal cortex (VMPFC) are believed to mediate negative and affective symptoms associated with schizophrenia (**A**). These symptoms are believed to arise from hypoactivity in this pathway (**B**).

The mesolimbic dopamine pathway is not only the postulated site for the positive symptoms of psychosis but is also thought to be the site of the brain's reward system or pleasure center. This aspect of the mesolimbic dopamine pathway is discussed in later chapters on substance abuse. When a patient with schizophrenia loses motivation and interest and has anhedonia and lack of pleasure, such symptoms could also implicate a deficient functioning of the mesolimbic dopamine pathway, not just deficient functioning in the mesocortical dopamine pathway.

This idea is further supported by observations that patients treated with antipsychotics, particularly the conventional antipsychotics, can produce a worsening of negative symptoms and a state of "neurolepsis" that looks very much like negative symptoms of schizophrenia. Since the prefrontal cortex does not have a high density of D2 receptors, this implicates possible deficient functioning within the mesolimbic dopamine system, causing inadequate reward mechanisms exhibited as behaviors such as anhedonia and drug abuse as well as negative symptoms exhibited as lack of rewarding social interactions and lack of general motivation and interest. Perhaps the much higher incidence of substance abuse in schizophrenia than in normal adults, especially of nicotine but also of stimulants and other substances of abuse, could be partially explained as an attempt to boost the function of defective mesolimbic dopaminergic pleasure centers, possibly at the cost of activating positive symptoms.

The Mesocortical Dopamine Hypothesis of Cognitive, Negative, and Affective Symptoms of Schizophrenia

cognitive symptoms

negative symptoms

affective symptoms

mesocortical underactivity = negative, cognitive and affective symptoms of schizophrenia

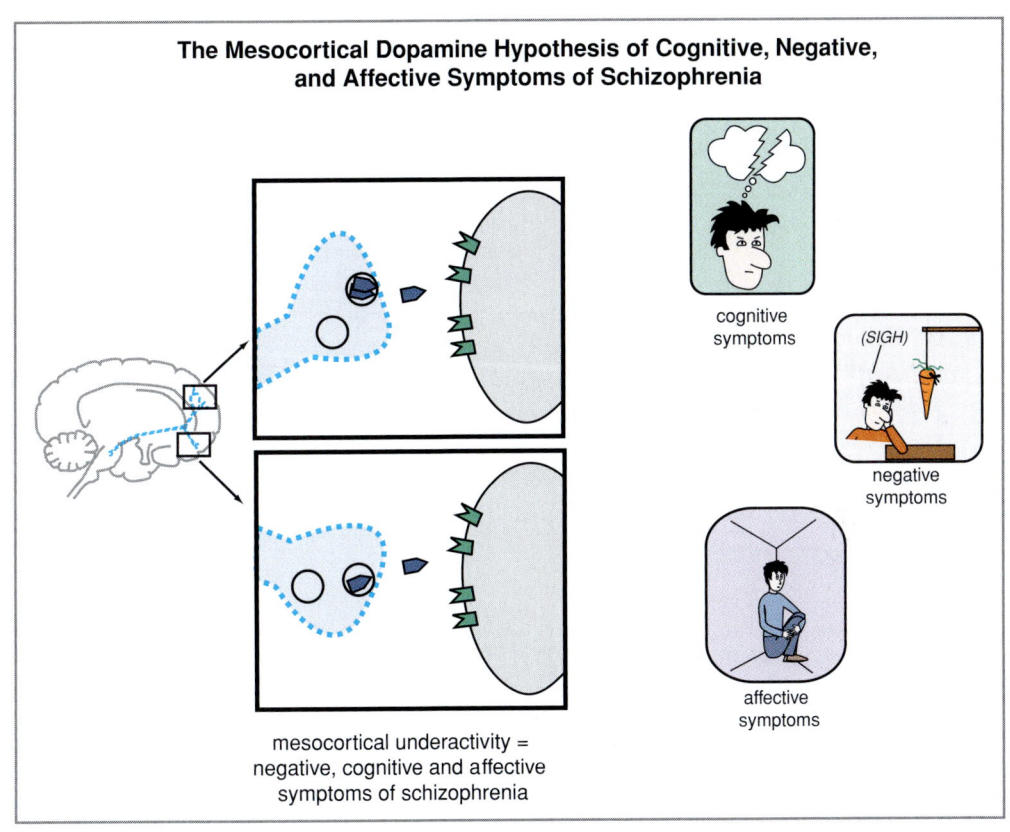

FIGURE 9-29 **Mesocortical dopamine hypothesis of negative, cognitive, and affective symptoms of schizophrenia.** Hypoactivity of dopamine neurons in the mesocortical dopamine pathway theoretically mediates the cognitive, negative, and affective symptoms of schizophrenia.

Nigrostriatal dopamine pathway

Another key dopamine pathway in the brain is the **nigrostriatal dopamine pathway**, which projects from dopaminergic cell bodies in the brainstem substantia nigra via axons terminating in the basal ganglia or striatum (Figure 9-30). The nigrostriatal dopamine pathway is a part of the extrapyramidal nervous system, and controls motor movements. Deficiencies in dopamine in this pathway cause movement disorders, including Parkinson's disease, characterized by rigidity, akinesia/bradykinesia (i.e., lack of movement or slowing of movement), and tremor. Dopamine deficiency in the basal ganglia can also produce akathisia (a type of restlessness) and dystonia (twisting movements, especially of the face and neck). These movement disorders can be replicated by drugs that block dopamine-2 receptors in this pathway and will be discussed briefly in Chapter 10.

Hyperactivity of dopamine in the nigrostriatal pathway is thought to underlie various hyperkinetic movement disorders such as chorea, dyskinesias, and tics. Chronic blockade of dopamine-2 receptors in this pathway may result in a hyperkinetic movement disorder known as neuroleptic-induced tardive dyskinesia. This will also be discussed briefly in Chapter 10. In schizophrenia, the nigrostriatal pathway in untreated patients may be relatively preserved (Figure 9-30).

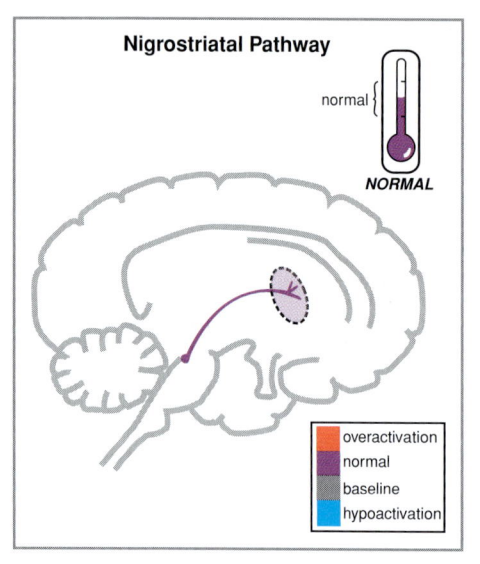

FIGURE 9-30 Nigrostriatal dopamine pathway. The nigrostriatal dopamine pathway projects from the substantia nigra to the basal ganglia or striatum. It is part of the extrapyramidal nervous system and plays a key role in regulating movements. When dopamine is deficient, it can cause parkinsonism with tremor, rigidity, and akinesia/bradykinesia. When DA is in excess, it can cause hyperkinetic movements like tics and dyskinesias. In untreated schizophrenia, activation of this pathway is believed to be "normal."

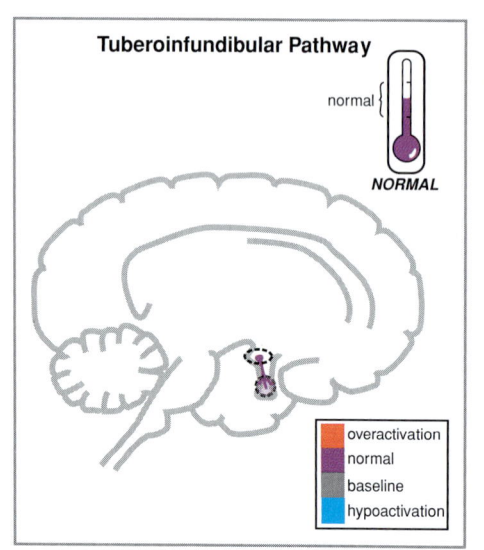

FIGURE 9-31 Tuberoinfundibular dopamine pathway. The tuberoinfundibular dopamine pathway from hypothalamus to anterior pituitary regulates prolactin secretion into the circulation. Dopamine inhibits prolactin secretion. In untreated schizophrenia, activation of this pathway is believed to be "normal."

Tuberoinfundibular dopamine pathway

The dopamine neurons that project from the hypothalamus to the anterior pituitary are known as the tuberoinfundibular dopamine pathway (Figure 9-31). Normally, these neurons are active and **inhibit** prolactin release. In the postpartum state, however, the activity of these dopamine neurons is decreased. Prolactin levels can therefore rise during breast-feeding so that lactation will occur. If the functioning of tuberoinfundibular dopamine neurons is disrupted by lesions or drugs, prolactin levels can also rise. Elevated prolactin levels are associated with galactorrhea (breast secretions), amenorrhea (loss of ovulation and menstrual periods), and possibly other problems such as sexual dysfunction. Such problems can occur after treatment with many antipsychotic drugs that block dopamine-2 receptors and will be discussed further in Chapter 10. In untreated schizophrenia, the function of the tuberoinfundibular pathway may be relatively preserved (Figure 9-31).

Thalamic dopamine pathway

A dopamine pathway that innervates the thalamus in primates has recently been described. It arises from multiple sites, including the periaqueductal gray matter, ventral mesencephalon, various hypothalamic nuclei, and lateral parabrachial nucleus (Figure 9-24). Its function is still under investigation but may be involved in sleep and arousal mechanisms by gating information passing through the thalamus to the cortex and other brain areas. There is no evidence at this point for abnormal functioning of this dopamine pathway in schizophrenia.

The integrated dopamine hypothesis of schizophrenia

Putting all this information together, the integrated dopamine hypothesis of schizophrenia attempts to explain all of the major symptoms of this disorder by dysregulation of either the mesolimbic dopamine pathway or the mesocortical dopamine pathway, with relative preservation of functioning of the nigrostriatal, tuberoinfundibular, and thalamic dopamine pathways (Figure 9-32). Specifically, positive symptoms of psychosis are hypothesized to be due to hyperactive mesolimbic dopamine neurons and negative, cognitive, and affective symptoms of schizophrenia are hypothesized to be due to underactivity of mesocortical dopamine neurons and their projections to prefrontal cortex (Figure 9-32). Underactive mesolimbic dopamine neurons may also contribute to reward-related negative symptoms in schizophrenia.

Glutamate

In recent years, the neurotransmitter glutamate has attained a key theoretical role in the pathophysiology of schizophrenia. It is also now a key target of novel psychopharmacological agents for future treatments of schizophrenia. In order to understand theories about glutamate in schizophrenia, how the malfunctioning of glutamate systems impacts dopamine systems in schizophrenia, and how glutamate systems might become important targets of new therapeutic drugs for schizophrenia, it is necessary to review the regulation of glutamate neurotransmission. Glutamate is the major excitatory neurotransmitter in the central nervous system and sometimes considered to be the "master switch" of the brain, since it can excite and turn on virtually all CNS neurons. The synthesis, metabolism, receptor regulation and key pathways of glutamate are therefore critical to the functioning of the brain and will be reviewed here.

Glutamate synthesis

Glutamate or glutamic acid is a neurotransmitter that is an amino acid. Its predominant use is not as a neurotransmitter but as an amino acid building block for protein biosynthesis. When used as a neurotransmitter, it is synthesized from glutamine in glial cells, which also assist in the recycling and regeneration of more glutamate following glutamate release during neurotransmission. Thus, glutamate is first released from synaptic vesicles that store this neurotransmitter in glutamate neurons and secondly taken up into neighboring glial cells by a reuptake pump known as an excitatory amino acid transporter (EAAT) (Figure 9-33A). The presynaptic glutamate neuron and the postsynaptic site of glutamate neurotransmission may also have EAATs (not shown in the figures), but these EAATs do not appear to play as important a role in glutamate recycling and regeneration as the EAATs in glial cells

The Integrated Dopamine Hypothesis of Schizophrenia

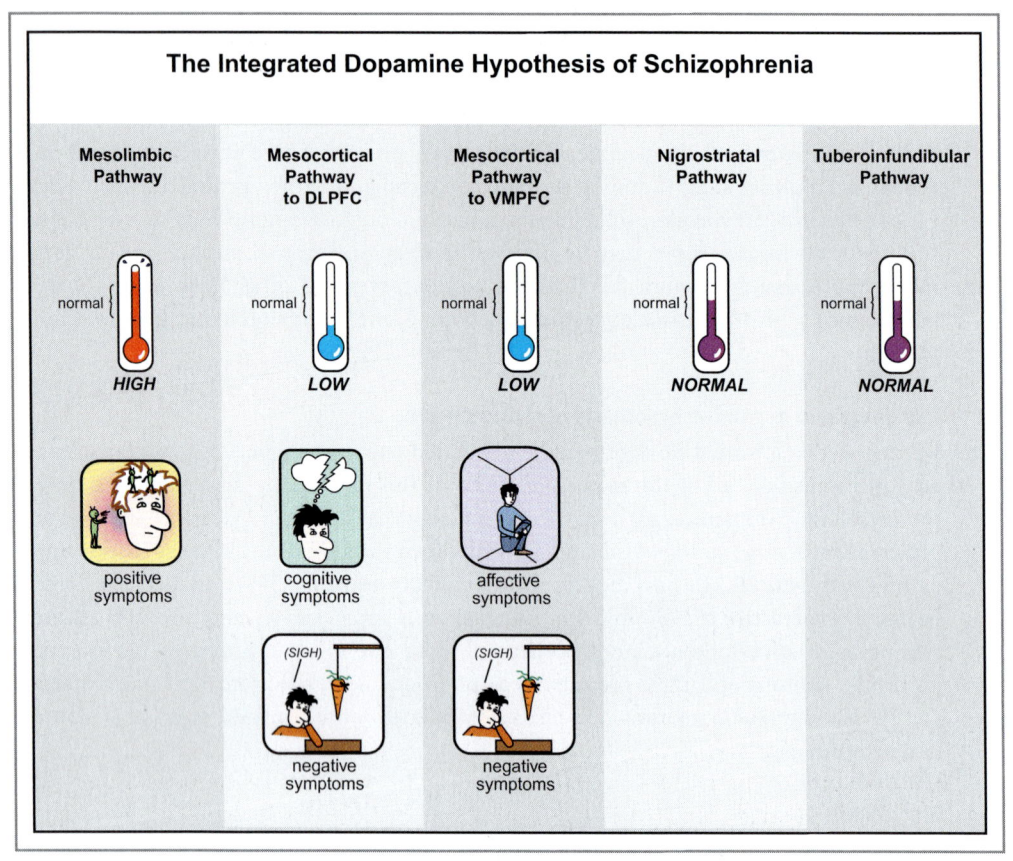

Mesolimbic Pathway	Mesocortical Pathway to DLPFC	Mesocortical Pathway to VMPFC	Nigrostriatal Pathway	Tuberoinfundibular Pathway
HIGH	LOW	LOW	NORMAL	NORMAL
positive symptoms	cognitive symptoms	affective symptoms		
	negative symptoms	negative symptoms		

FIGURE 9-32 Integrated dopamine hypothesis of schizophrenia. The majority of symptoms associated with schizophrenia may be explained by dysregulation of dopaminergic pathways; specifically by hyperactivity of the mesolimbic dopamine pathway (positive symptoms), hypoactivity of the mesocortical dopamine pathway to dorsolateral prefrontal cortex (DLPFC) (cognitive and negative symptoms), and hypoactivity of the mesocortical dopamine pathway to ventromedial prefrontal cortex (VMPFC) (affective and negative symptoms). The nigrostriatal and tuberoinfundibular dopamine pathways, though affected by antipsychotics used to treat schizophrenia, are believed to be "normal" in untreated schizophrenia.

(Figure 9-33A). EAATs are discussed in Chapter 4 and illustrated in Figure 4-11 and EAATs subtypes 1 through 5 listed in Table 4-2.

Next, glutamate is converted into glutamine inside of glial cells by an enzyme known as glutamine synthetase (arrow 3 in Figure 9-33B). Glutamine is released from glial cells via reverse transport by a pump or transporter known as a specific neutral amino acid transporter (glial SNAT and arrow 4 in Figure 9-33C). Glutamine may also be transported out of glial cells by a second transporter known as a glial alanine-serine-cysteine transporter or ASC-T (not shown). When glial SNATs and ASC-Ts operate in the inward direction, they transport glutamine and other amino acids into the glial cell. Here, they are reversed, so that glutamine can get out of the glial cell and hop a ride into a neuron via a different type of neuronal SNAT operating inwardly in a reuptake manner (arrow 5 in Figure 9-33C).

Once inside the neuron, glutamine is converted into glutamate by an enzyme in mitochondria called glutaminase (arrow 6 in Figure 9-33D). Glutamate is then transported into synaptic vesicles via a vesicular glutamate transporter (vGluT, arrow 7 in Figure 9-33D),

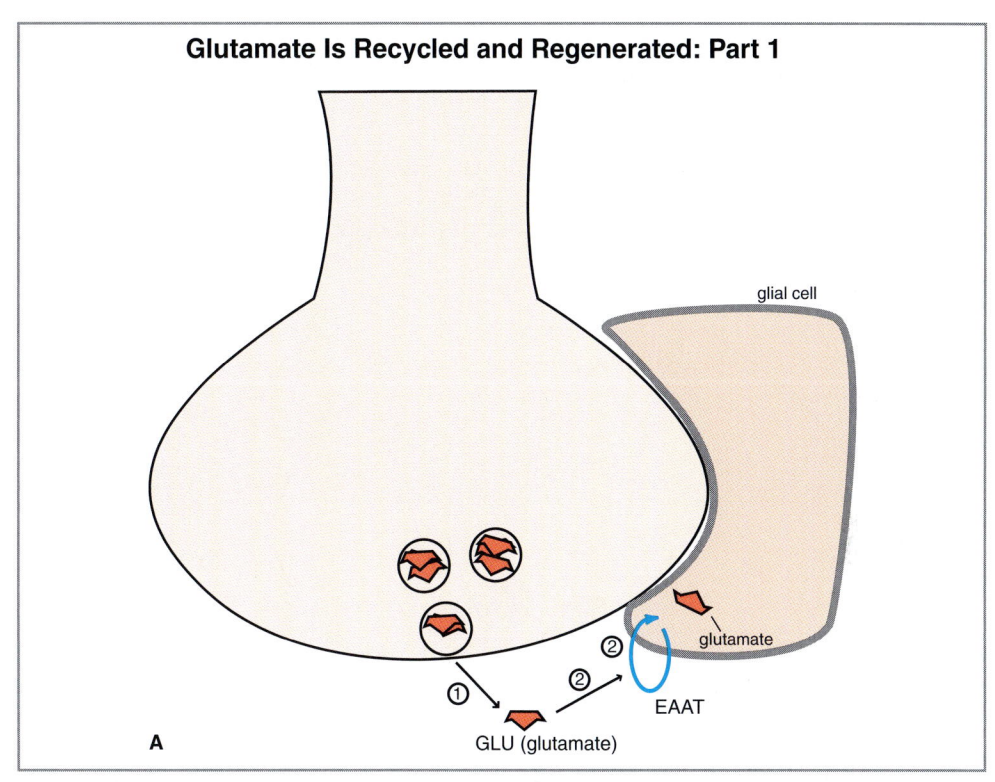

FIGURE 9-33A Glutamate is recycled and regenerated, part 1. After release of glutamate from the presynaptic neuron (1), it is taken up into glial cells via the EAAT, or excitatory amino acid transporter (2).

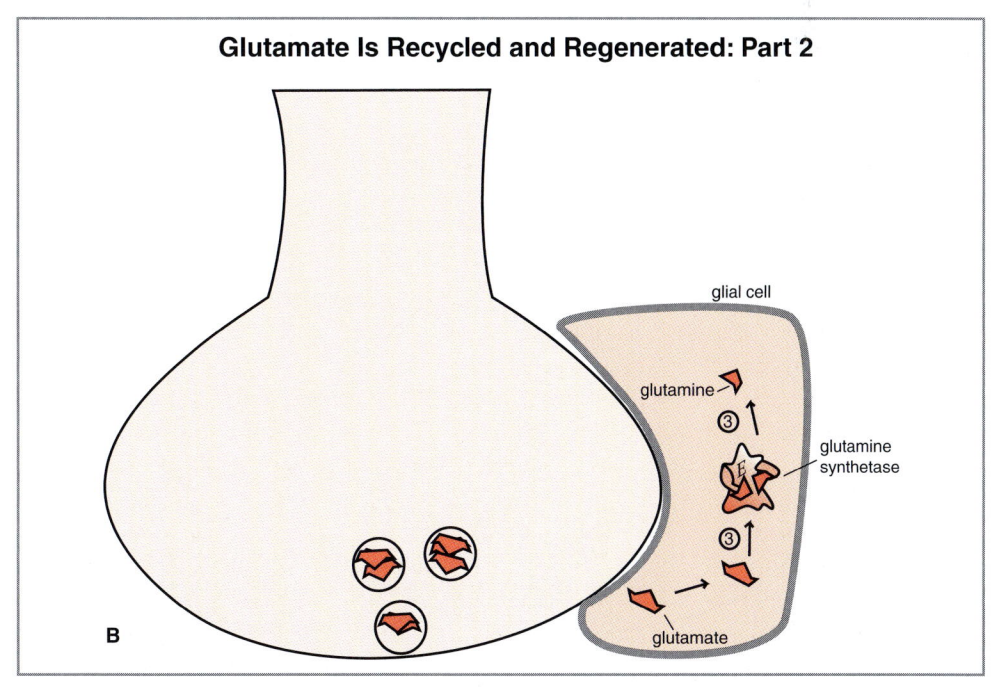

FIGURE 9-33B Glutamate is recycled and regenerated, part 2. Once inside the glial cell, glutamate is converted into glutamine by the enzyme glutamine synthetase (3).

Psychosis and Schizophrenia | 281

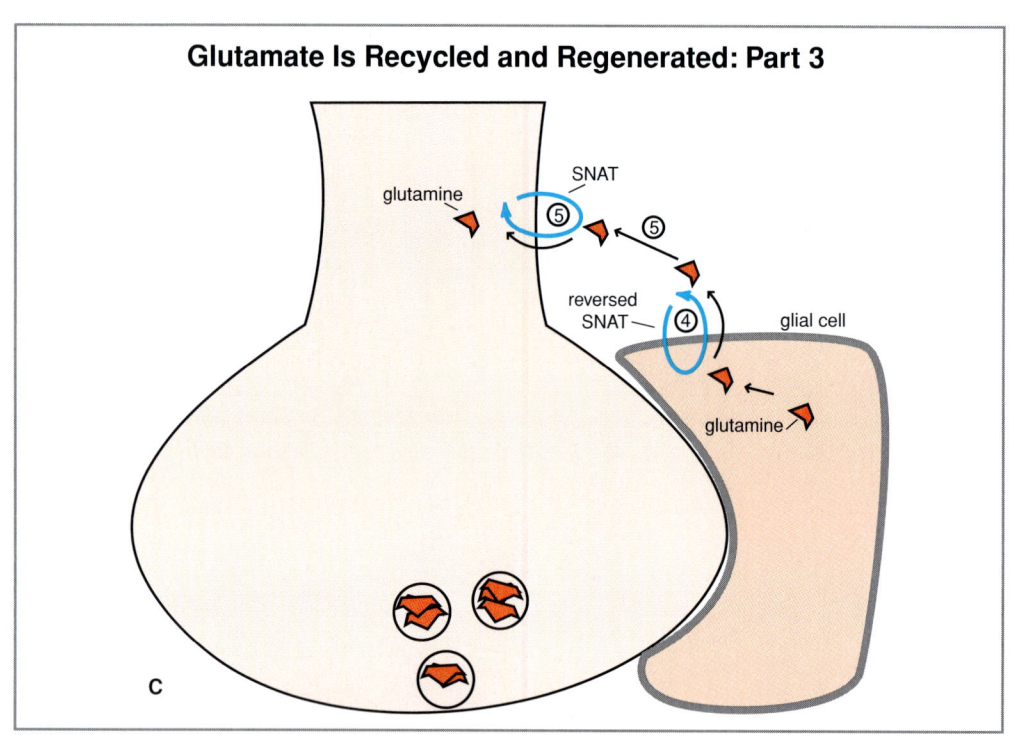

FIGURE 9-33C Glutamate is recycled and regenerated, part 3. Glutamine is released from glial cells by a specific neutral amino acid transporter (glial SNAT) through the process of reverse transport (4), and then taken up by SNATs on glutamate neurons (5).

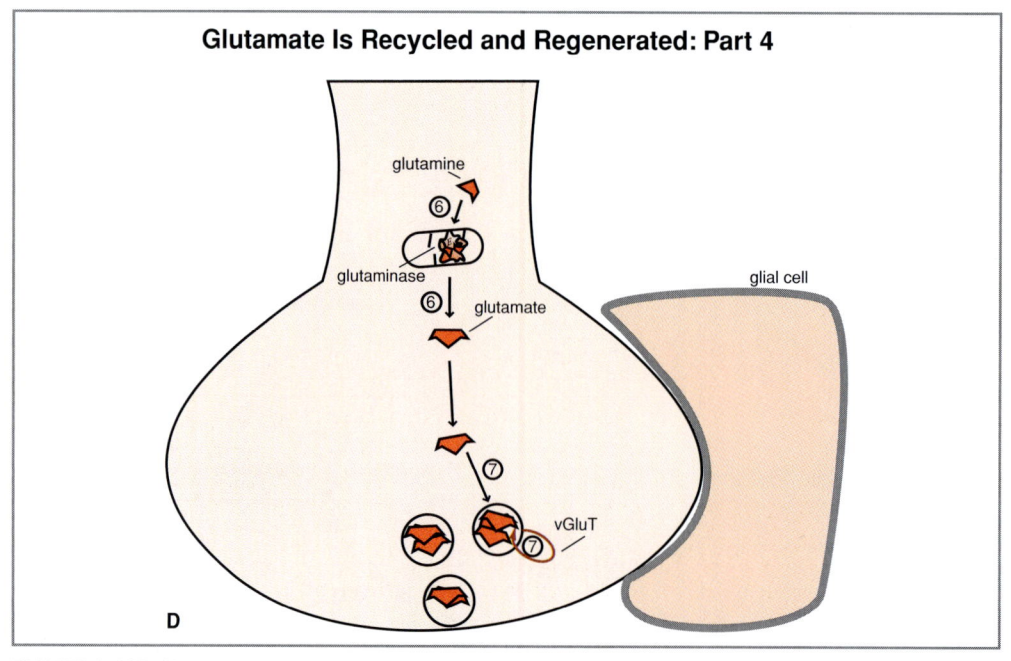

FIGURE 9-33D Glutamate is recycled and regenerated, part 4. Glutamine is converted into glutamate within the presynaptic glutamate neuron by the enzyme glutaminase (6) and taken up into synaptic vesicles by the vesicular glutamate transporter (vGluT), where it is stored for future release.

where it is stored for subsequent release during neurotransmission. vGluTs are discussed in Chapter 4 and illustrated in Figure 4-11; subtypes are listed in Table 4-3. Once released, glutamate's actions are stopped not by enzymatic breakdown, like in other neurotransmitter systems, but by removal by EAATs on neurons or glia, and the whole cycle is started again (Figure 9-33A through D).

Synthesis of glutamate cotransmitters glycine and d-serine

Glutamate systems are curious in that one of the key receptors for glutamate requires a cotransmitter in addition to glutamate in order to function. That receptor is the NMDA receptor, described below, and the cotransmitter is either the amino acid glycine (Figure 9-34), or another amino acid closely related to glycine, known as d-serine (Figure 9-35).

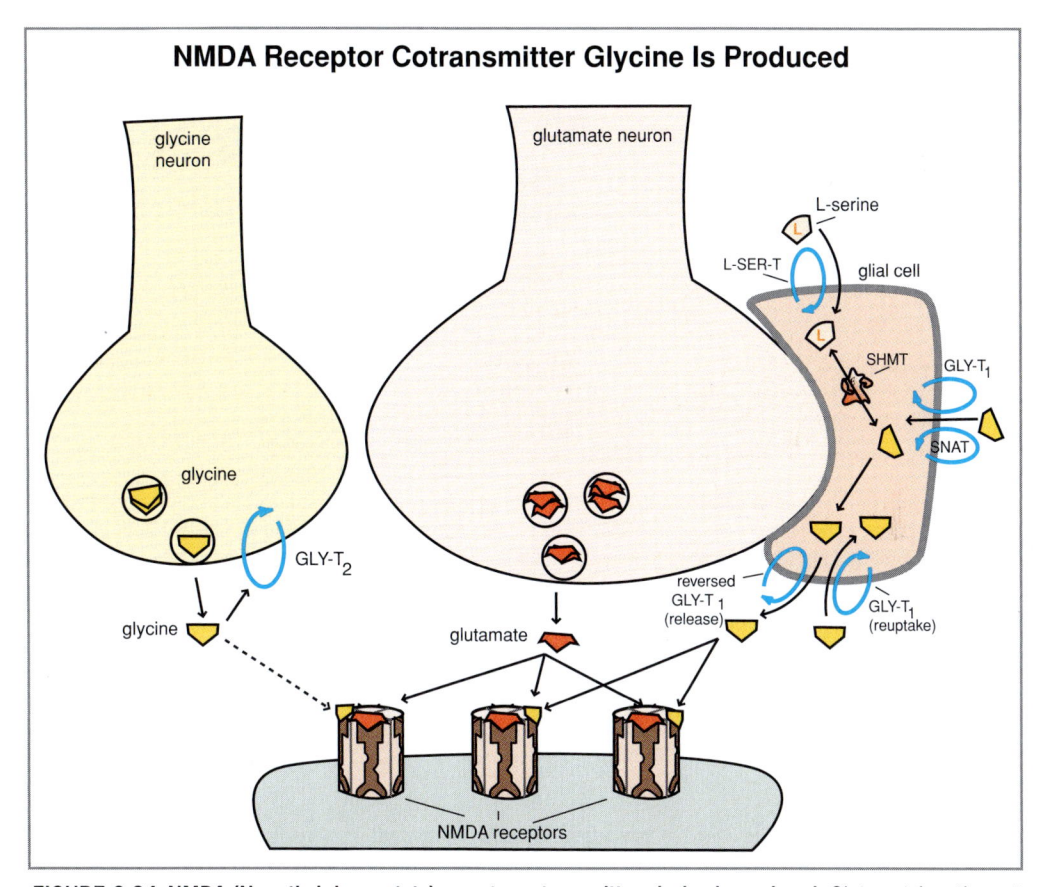

FIGURE 9-34 NMDA (N-methyl-d-aspartate) receptor cotransmitter glycine is produced. Glutamate's actions at NMDA receptors are dependent in part upon the presence of a cotransmitter, either glycine or d-serine. Glycine can be derived directly from dietary amino acids and transported into glial cells either by a glycine transporter (GlyT1) or by a specific neutral amino acid transporter (SNAT). Glycine can also be produced both in glycine neurons and in glial cells. Glycine neurons provide only a small amount of the glycine at glutamate synapses, because most of the glycine released by glycine neurons is used only at glycine synapses and then taken back up into presynaptic glycine neuron via the glycine 2 transporter (GLY-T2) before much glycine can diffuse to glutamate synapses. Glycine produced by glial cells plays a larger role at glutamate synapses. Glycine is produced in glial cells when the amino acid l-serine is taken up into glial cells via the l-serine transporter (l-SER-T), and then converted into glycine by the enzyme serine hydroxy methyl transferase (SHMT). Glycine from glial cells is released into the glutamate synapse through reverse transport by the glycine 1 transporter (GLY-T1). Extracellular glycine is then transported back into glial cells via a reuptake pump, namely GLY-T1.

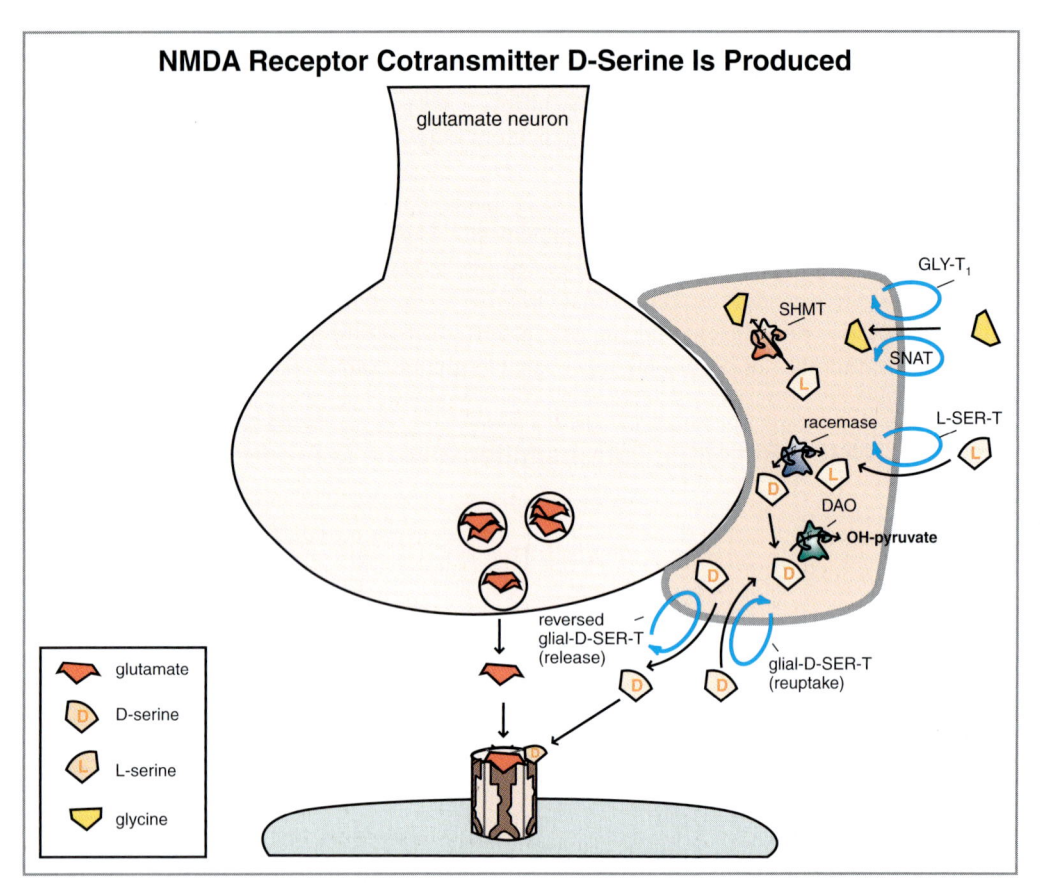

FIGURE 9-35 NMDA receptor cotransmitter d-serine is produced. Glutamate requires the presence of either glycine or d-serine at N-methyl-d-aspartate (NMDA) receptors in order to exert some of its effects there. In glial cells, the enzyme serine racemase converts l-serine into d-serine, which is then released into the glutamate synapse via reverse transport on the glial d-serine transporter (glial d-SER-T). l-serine's presence in glial cells is a result either of its transport there via the l-serine transporter (l-SER-T) or its conversion into l-serine from glycine via the enzyme serine hydroxy methyl transferase (SHMT). Once d-serine is released into the synapse, it is taken back up into the glial cell by a reuptake pump, namely d-SER-T. Excess d-serine within the glial cell can be destroyed by the enzyme d-amino acid oxidase (DAO), which converts d-serine into hydroxy-pyruvate (OH-pyruvate).

Glycine is not known to be synthesized by glutamate neurons, so glutamate neurons must get the glycine they need for their NMDA receptors either from glycine neurons or from glial cells (Figure 9-34). Glycine neurons release glycine, but they contribute only a small amount of glycine to glutamate synapses, since glycine is unable to diffuse very far from neighboring glycine neurons because the glycine they release is taken back up into those neurons by a type of glycine reuptake pump known as the type 2 glycine transporter, or Gly-T2 (Figure 9-34).

Thus, neighboring glial cells are thought to be the source of most of the glycine available for glutamate synapses. Glycine itself can be taken up into glial cells from the extracellular space or bloodstream by a type 1 glycine transporter, or Gly-T1 (Figure 9-34). Glycine can also be taken up into glial cells by a glial SNAT. Glycine is not known to be stored within synaptic vesicles of glial cells, but as we will learn below, the companion neurotransmitter d-serine is thought to be stored within some type of synaptic vesicle in glial cells. Glycine in the cytoplasm of glial cells is nevertheless somehow available for release into synapses, and it escapes from glial cells by riding outside them and into the glutamate synapse on a reversed Gly-T1 transporter (Figure 9-34). Once outside, glycine can get right back into the glial cell by an inwardly directed Gly-T1, which functions as a reuptake pump and is the main mechanism responsible for terminating the action of synaptic glycine (Figure 9-34). Later, in Chapter 10, we will discuss novel treatments for schizophrenia that boost glycine action and thus glutamate action at NMDA receptors; these are in testing and include inhibitors of the key glycine transporter Gly-T1.

Glycine can also be synthesized from the amino acid l-serine, derived from the extracellular space, bloodstream, and diet; transported into the glial cell by an l-serine transporter (SER-T); and converted from l-serine into glycine by the glial enzyme serine hydroxy methyl transferase (SHMT) (Figure 9-34). This enzyme works in both directions, either converting l-serine into glycine or glycine into l-serine.

How is the cotransmitter d-serine produced? D-serine is unusual in that it is a d-amino acid, whereas the twenty known essential amino acids are all l-amino acids, including d-serine's mirror image amino acid l-serine. It just so happens that d-serine has high affinity for the glycine site on NMDA receptors and that glial cells are equipped with an enzyme that can convert regular l-serine into the neurotransmitting amino acid d-serine by means of an enzyme that can go back and forth between d and l serine known as d-serine racemase (Figure 9-35). Thus, d-serine can be derived either from glycine or from l-serine, both of which can be transported into glial cells by their own transporters. Glycine is converted to l-serine by the enzyme SHMT and l-serine is converted into d-serine by the enzyme d-serine racemase (Figure 9-35). Interestingly, the d-serine so produced may be stored in some sort of vesicle in the glial cell for subsequent release on a reversed glial d-serine transporter (or d-SER-T) for neurotransmitting purposes at glutamate synapses containing NMDA receptors. D-serine's actions are terminated not only by synaptic reuptake via the inwardly acting glial d-SER-T but also by the enzyme d-amino acid oxidase (DAO), which converts d-serine into hydroxypyruvate (Figure 9-35). Below, an activator of DAO made by the brain, known not surprisingly as d-amino acid oxidase activator (DAOA), is discussed. The gene that makes DAOA may be one of the important regulatory genes that contribute to the genetic basis of schizophrenia, as explained below in the section on the neurodevelopmental hypothesis of schizophrenia.

Glutamate receptors

There are several types of glutamate receptors (Figure 9-36 and Table 9-11), including the neuronal presynaptic reuptake pump (excitatory amino acid transporter, or EAAT) and the vesicular transporter for glutamate into synaptic vesicles (vGluT). Shown also on the presynaptic neuron as well as the postsynaptic neuron are metabotropic glutamate receptors (Figure 9-36). Metabotropic glutamate receptors are linked to G proteins. G protein–linked receptors are discussed in Chapter 4.

There are at least eight subtypes of metabotropic glutamate receptors, which are organized into three separate groups (Table 9-11). Research suggests that the metabotropic receptors of groups II and III can occur presynaptically, where they function as autoreceptors to block glutamate release (Figure 9-37). Drugs that stimulate these presynaptic autoreceptors as agonists may therefore reduce glutamate release and be potentially useful as anticonvulsants and mood stabilizers and also in protecting against glutamate excitotoxicity, as explained below. Group I metabotropic glutamate receptors may be located

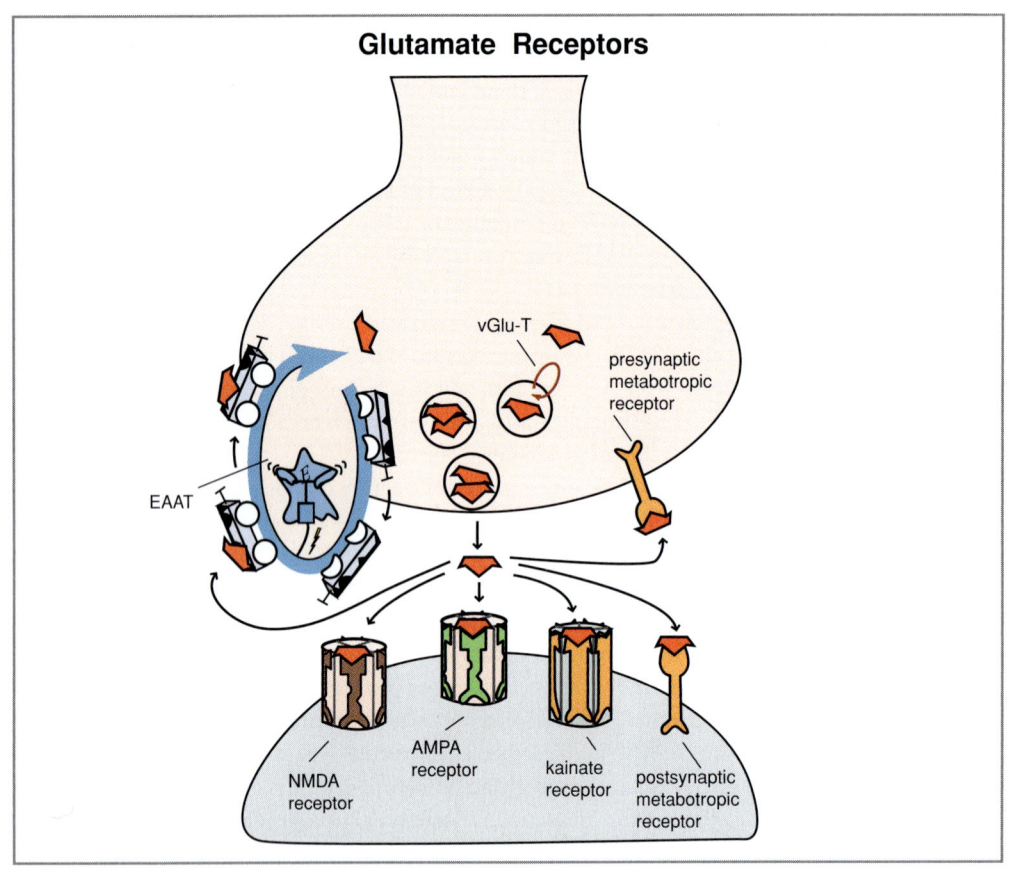

FIGURE 9-36 Glutamate receptors. Shown here are receptors for glutamate that regulate its neurotransmission. The excitatory amino acid transporter (EAAT) exists presynaptically and is responsible for clearing excess glutamate out of the synapse. The vesicular transporter for glutamate (v-Glu-T) transports glutamate into synaptic vesicles, where it is stored until used in a future neurotransmission. Metabotropic glutamate receptors (linked to G-proteins) can occur either pre- or postsynaptically. Three types of postsynaptic glutamate receptors are linked to ion channels, and are known as ligand-gated ion channels: N-methyl-d-aspartate (NMDA) receptors, alpha-amino-3-hydroxy-5-methyl-4-isoxazolepropionic acid (AMPA) receptors, and kainate receptors, all named for the agonists that bind to them.

predominantly postsynaptically, where they hypothetically interact with other postsynaptic glutamate receptors to facilitate and strengthen responses mediated by ligand-gated ion channel receptors for glutamate during excitatory glutamatergic neurotransmission (Figure 9-36; see also Figure 5-43A, B, and C).

NMDA, AMPA (alpha-amino-3-hydroxy-5-methyl-4-isoxazole-propionic acid), and kainate receptors for glutamate, named after the agonists that selectively bind to them, are all members of the ligand-gated ion channel family of receptors (Figure 9-36 and Table 9-11). These ligand-gated ion channels are also known as ionotropic receptors or ion channel–linked receptors (discussed in Chapter 5 and shown in Figures 5-24, 5-25, and 5-43A, B, and C). They all tend to be postsynaptic and work together to modulate excitatory postsynaptic neurotransmission triggered by glutamate. Specifically, AMPA and kainate receptors may mediate fast, excitatory neurotransmission, allowing sodium to enter

TABLE 9-11 Types of glutamate receptors

Metabotropic

Group I	mGluR1
	mGluR5
Group II	mGluR2
	mGluR3
Group III	mGluR4
	mGluR6
	mGluR7
	mGluR8

Ionotropic (ligand-gated ion channels; ion channel–linked receptors)

Functional class	gene family	agonists	antagonists
AMPA	GluR1	glutamate	
	GluR2	AMPA	
	GluR3	kainate	
	GluR4		
Kainate	GluR5	glutamate	
	GluR6	kainate	
	GluR7		
	KA1		
	KA2		
NMDA	NR1	glutamate	
	NR2A	aspartate	
	NR2B	NMDA	MK801
	NR2C		ketamine
	NR2D		PCP (phencyclidine)

the neuron to depolarize it (see Figures 5-25 and 5-43). NMDA receptors in the resting state are normally blocked by magnesium, which plugs its calcium channel (Figures 5-24 and 5-43). NMDA receptors are an interesting type of "coincidence detector" that can open to let calcium into the neuron to trigger postsynaptic actions from glutamate neurotransmission only when three things occur at the same time: glutamate occupies its binding site on the NMDA receptor, glycine or d-serine binds to its site on the NMDA receptor, and depolarization occurs, allowing the magnesium plug to be removed (Figures 5-25 and 5-43). Some of the many important signals by NMDA receptors that are activated when NMDA calcium channels are opened include not only long-term potentiation and synaptic plasticity but also excitotoxicity, as explained later in this chapter.

Key glutamate pathways in the brain and the NMDA receptor hypofunction hypothesis of schizophrenia

Glutamate is an ubiquitous excitatory neurotransmitter that seems to be able to excite nearly any neuron in the brain; that is why it is sometimes called the "master switch." Nevertheless, there are several specific glutamatergic pathways that are of particular relevance to psychopharmacology and especially to the pathophysiology of schizophrenia (Figure 9-38). These five pathways all relate to glutamatergic pyramidal neurons in the prefrontal cortex.

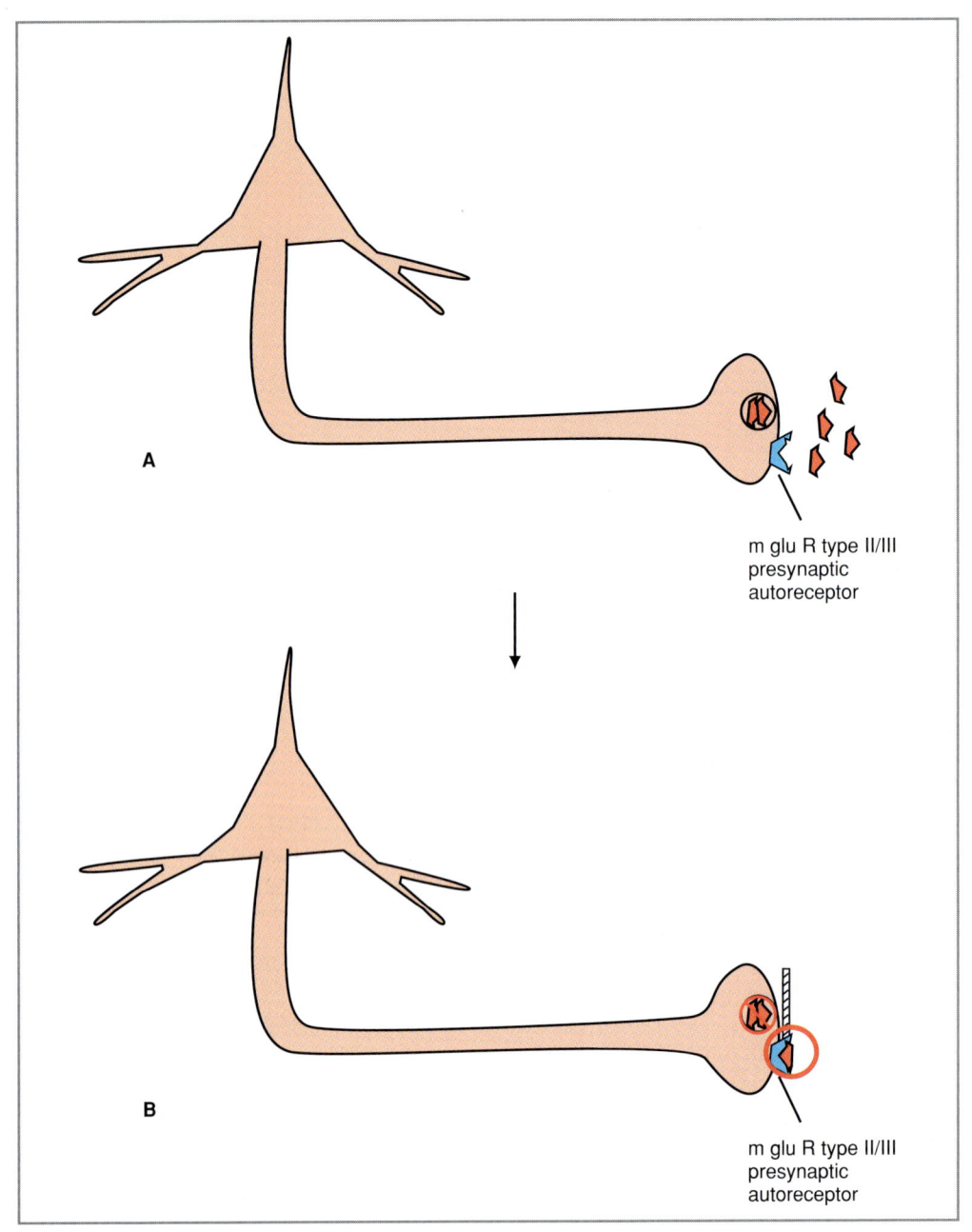

FIGURE 9-37A and B Metabotropic glutamate autoreceptors. Groups II and III metabotropic glutamate receptors can exist presynaptically as autoreceptors to regulate the release of glutamate. When glutamate builds up in the synapse (**A**), it is available to bind to the autoreceptor, which then inhibits glutamate release (**B**).

Corticobrainstem glutamate pathways and the NMDA receptor hypofunction hypothesis of schizophrenia

A very important descending glutamatergic pathway projects from cortical pyramidal neurons mostly in lamina 5 (see Figure 7-22) to brainstem neurotransmitter centers, including the raphe for serotonin, the ventral tegmental area (VTA) and substantia nigra for dopamine,

Key Glutamate Pathways

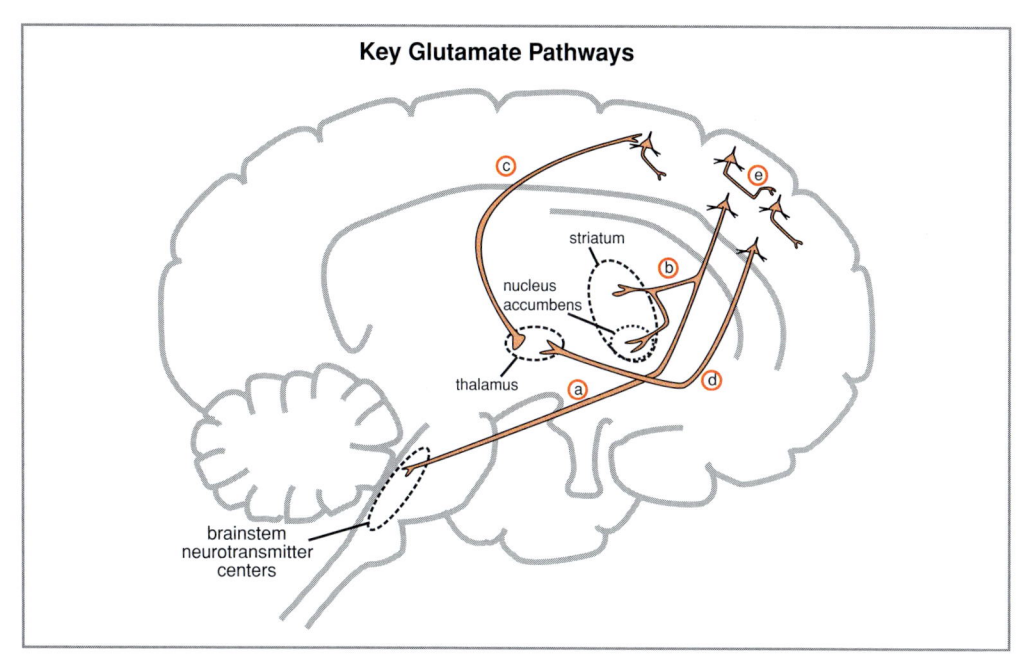

FIGURE 9-38 Five glutamate pathways in the brain. Although glutamate can have actions at virtually all neurons in the brain, there are five glutamate pathways particularly relevant to schizophrenia. (a) The **cortical brainstem glutamate projection** is a descending pathway that projects from cortical pyramidal neurons in the prefrontal cortex to brainstorm neurotransmitter centers (raphe, locus coeruleus, ventral tegmental area, substantia nigra) and regulates neurotransmitter release. (b) Another descending glutamatergic pathway projects from the prefrontal cortex to the striatum (**corticostriatal glutamate pathway**) and to the nucleus accumbens (corticoaccumbens glutamate pathway), and constitutes the "corticostriatal" portion of cortico-striatal-thalamic loops. (c) **Thalamocortical glutamate pathways** are pathways that ascend from the thalamus and innervate pyramidal neurons in the cortex. (d) **Corticothalamic glutamate pathways** descend from the prefrontal cortex to the thalamus. (e) Intracortical pyramidal neurons can communicate with each other via the neurotransmitter glutamate. These pathways are known as **corticocortical glutamatergic pathways**.

and the locus coeruleus for norepinephrine (pathway a in Figure 9-38). This pathway is the cortical brainstem glutamate projection and is a key regulator of neurotransmitter release. Specifically, this descending corticobrainstem glutamate pathway normally acts as a brake on the mesolimbic dopamine pathway. It does this by communicating with these dopamine neurons through an inhibitory GABA interneuron in the VTA (Figure 9-39A). This normally results in tonic inhibition of dopamine release from the mesolimbic pathway (Figure 9-39A).

A major current hypothesis for schizophrenia involves NMDA receptors in this pathway. The NMDA receptor hypofunction hypothesis of schizophrenia arises from observations that when NMDA receptors are made hypofunctional by means of the NMDA receptor antagonist phencyclidine (PCP), this produces a psychotic condition in normal humans very similar to the positive symptoms of schizophrenia, including hallucinations and delusions. To a lesser extent, the NMDA receptor antagonist ketamine can also produce a schizophrenia-like psychosis in normals.

Such observations have led to the hypothesis that NMDA receptors specifically in the corticobrainstem glutamate projection might be hypoactive in untreated schizophrenia and thus cannot do their job of tonically inhibiting mesolimbic dopamine neurons. When this happens, mesolimbic dopamine hyperactivity is the result. This is theoretically

Psychosis and Schizophrenia

NMDA Receptor Regulation of Mesolimbic Dopamine Pathway: Tonic Inhibition

NMDA Receptor Hypofunction in Cortico-Brainstem Projections: Hyperactivity of Mesolimbic Dopamine Pathway

- overactivation
- normal
- baseline
- hypoactivation

positive symptoms

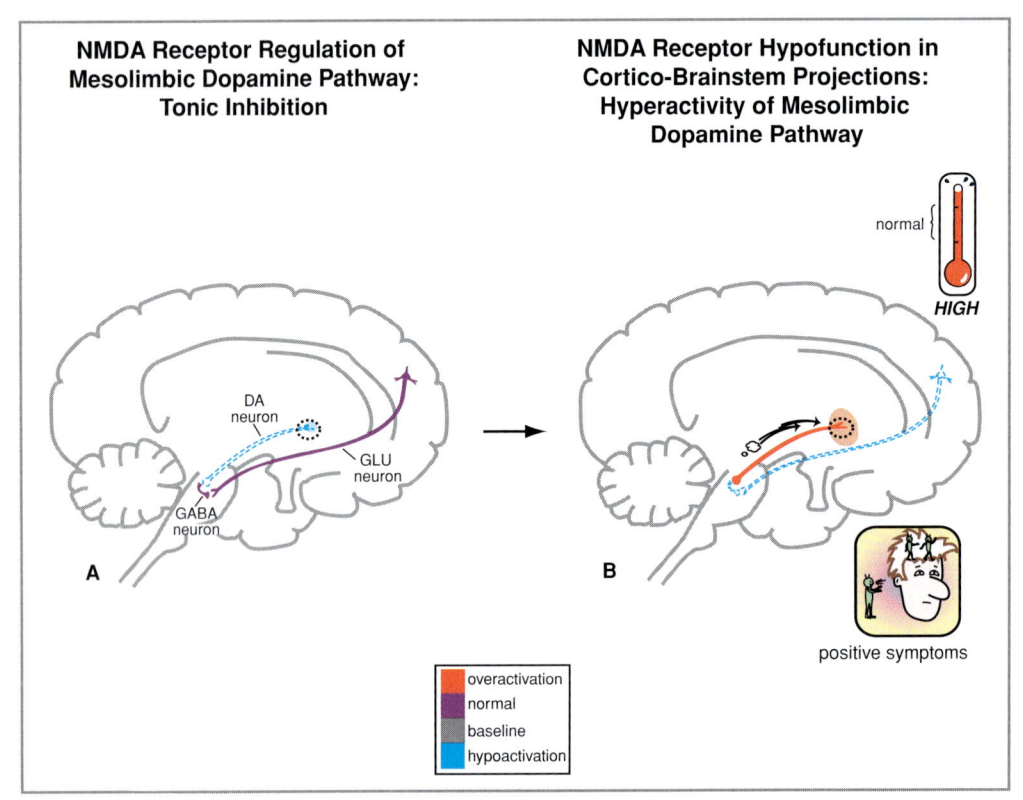

FIGURE 9-39A and B NMDA receptor hypofunction hypothesis and positive symptoms of schizophrenia. (A) The cortical brainstem glutamate projection communicates with the mesolimbic dopamine pathway via a gamma aminobutyric acid (GABA) interneuron in the ventral tegmental area. Excitatory glutamate stimulates N-methyl-d-aspartate (NMDA) receptors on the interneuron, causing GABA release, and GABA, in turn, inhibits release of dopamine from the mesolimbic dopamine pathway; thus the descending glutamatergic pathway normally acts as a brake on the mesolimbic dopamine pathway. (B) If NMDA receptors in the cortical brainstem glutamate projection are *hypo*active, then the downstream effect of tonic inhibition of the mesolimbic dopamine pathway will not occur, leading to *hyper*activity in this pathway. This is the theoretical biological basis for the mesolimbic dopamine hyperactivity thought to be associated with the positive symptoms of psychosis.

the consequence of corticobrainstem glutamate hypoactivity at NMDA receptors (Figure 9-39B).

Thus the mesolimbic dopamine hypothesis of positive symptoms of schizophrenia shown in Figures 9-25B and 9-26 may be explained by the NMDA receptor hypofunction hypothesis of schizophrenia shown in Figure 9-39B. That is, mesolimbic dopamine hyperactivity that produces positive symptoms of schizophrenia may actually be the consequence of NMDA receptor hypoactivation in corticobrainstem glutamate projections, as shown in Figure 9-39B.

What is so attractive about the NMDA receptor hypofunction hypothesis of schizophrenia is that unlike amphetamine which activates only positive symptoms, PCP also mimics the cognitive, negative and affective symptoms of schizophrenia. That is, normal humans who take PCP and render their NMDA receptors hypofunctional not only experience positive symptoms such as delusions and hallucinations, but also affective symptoms such as blunted affect, negative symptoms such as social withdrawal, and cognitive

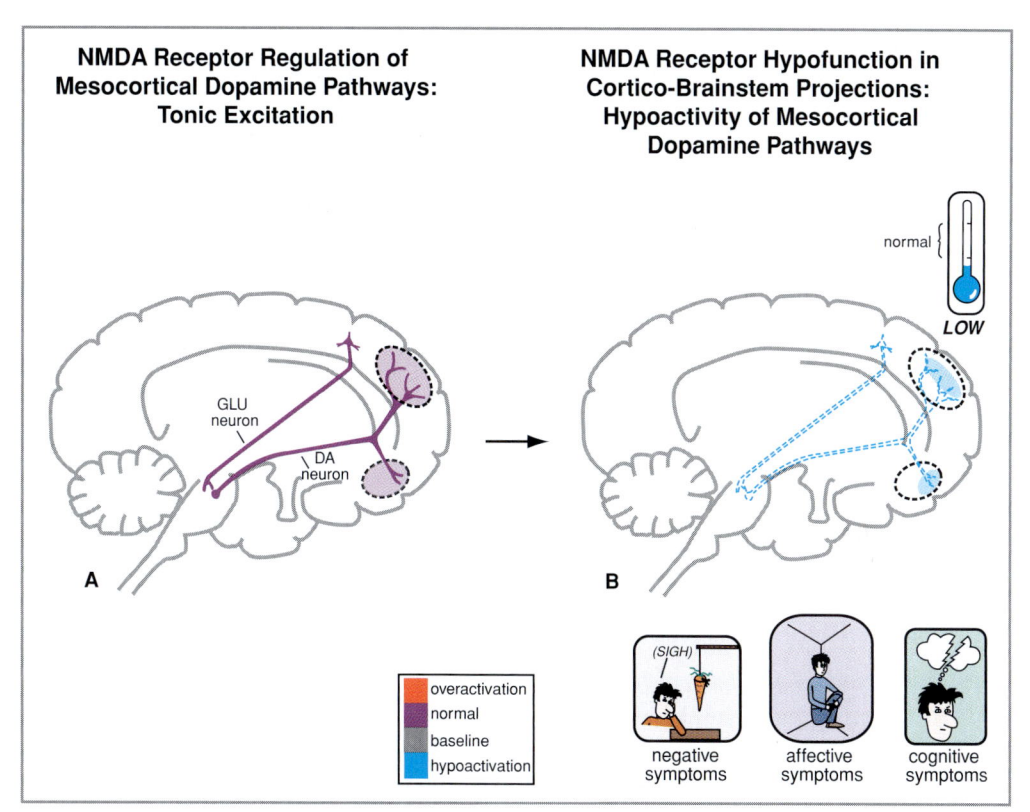

FIGURE 9-40A and B NMDA receptor hypofunction hypothesis and negative, cognitive, and affective symptoms of schizophrenia. (A) The cortical brainstem glutamate projection communicates directly with the mesocortical dopamine pathway in the ventral tegmental area, normally causing tonic excitation. (B) If N-methyl-d-aspartate (NMDA) receptors in cortical brainstem glutamate projections are hypoactive, tonic excitation here is lost and mesocortical dopamine pathways become hypoactive, potentially explaining the cognitive, negative, and affective symptoms of schizophrenia.

symptoms such as executive dysfunction. These additional clinical observations have led to the idea that NMDA receptors in corticobrainstem glutamate projections that regulate mesocortical dopamine pathways may also be hypoactive in schizophrenia.

How can this be explained? Normally, these descending corticobrainstem glutamate neurons act as accelerators to mesocortical dopamine neurons. Unlike the actions of corticobrainstem glutamate neurons on mesolimbic dopamine neurons shown in Figure 9-39A, where they act via an intermediary GABA interneuron, corticobrainstem glutamate neurons synapse directly on those dopamine neurons in the ventral tegmental area that project to the cortex, those so-called mesocortical dopamine neurons (Figure 9-40A). This means that corticobrainstem glutamate neurons normally function as accelerators of these mesocortical dopamine neurons; therefore they excite them tonically (Figure 9-40A).

The consequence of this neuronal circuitry is that when corticobrainstem projections to mesocortical dopamine neurons have NMDA receptor hypoactivity, they lose their excitatory drive and become hypoactive, as shown in Figure 9-40B. This could hypothetically explain why mesocortical dopamine neurons are hypoactive and thus their link to the cognitive, negative, and affective symptoms of schizophrenia, as shown in Figures 9-27B, 9-28B, and 9-29.

Corticostriatal glutamate pathways

A second descending glutamatergic output from pyramidal neurons projecting to the striatum is shown as pathway b in Figure 9-38. This pathway is known as the corticostriatal glutamate pathway when it projects to the striatum itself or the corticoaccumbens glutamate pathway when it projects to a specific area of the ventral striatum known as the nucleus accumbens. In either case, it originates from pyramidal neurons in lamina 5 of the cortex (Figure 7-22). This corticostriatal pathway is the first leg of cortico-striatal-thalamic-cortical (CSTC) loops, which are the brain's engines for behavioral and functional outputs; they are discussed in Chapter 7 and illustrated in Figures 7-16 through 7-21.

Normally, this corticostriatal glutamate projection to the striatum terminates on GABA neurons in the striatum (number 1 in Figure 9-41A), which in turn project to the thalamus (number 2 in Figure 9-41A). In the thalamus, these GABA neurons create a "sensory filter" to prevent too much of the sensory traffic coming into the thalamus from escaping to the cortex, where it may confuse or overwhelm cortical information processing (arrow 3 in Figure 9-41A).

Dopamine functions in this CSTC loop to inhibit the GABA neurons projecting to the thalamus, thus reducing the effectiveness of the thalamic filter (Figure 9-41B). This opposes the excitatory input of glutamate from corticostriatal glutamate projections to the striatum (Figures 9-41A and B).

Thalamocortical glutamate pathways

An ascending glutamate pathway starts from the thalamus and innervates pyramidal neurons and is known as the thalamocortical pathway (pathway c in Figure 9-38). This is the return leg of the CSTC loop (see Figures 7-16 to 7-21), namely from thalamus to cortex, and provides not only feedback to the original pyramidal cell "cortical engine" from information processing that occurs in the CSTC loop (see number 3 in Figure 9-41A), but also input diffusely throughout the cortex to numerous other pyramidal neurons and their CSTC loops (see arrow 3 in Figure 9-41C). A properly functioning thalamic filter prevents too much sensory input from penetrating the thalamus into the cortex, so that information processing can occur in an orderly manner (Figure 9-41C).

How does NMDA receptor hypofunction affect information processing in CSTC loops? First, when descending corticobrainstem glutamate pathways have hypofunctioning NMDA receptors in the ventral tegmental area, this creates mesolimbic dopamine hyperactivity and positive symptoms of psychosis, as already explained above and illustrated in Figure 9-39B. The effects of this on CSTC loops are shown in Figure 9-41D, where dopamine hyperactivity reduces the thalamic filter and permits the escape of excessive sensory information coming into the thalamus, thus allowing it to get into the cortex by means of ascending thalamocortical neurons.

If this were not bad enough, there is hypothetical NMDA receptor hypofunction in the descending corticostriatal glutamate pathway as well (Figure 9-41E). This reduces the excitatory drive on the GABA neurons that create the thalamic filter. Coupled with the excessive dopamine drive from mesolimbic neurons, the thalamic filter fails, and too much information escapes diffusely into the cortex, where it can cause cortical manifestations of hallucinations or may also create other cortical symptoms such as cognitive, affective, and negative symptoms of schizophrenia (Figure 9-41E).

Corticothalamic glutamate pathways

A third descending glutamatergic pathway, mostly from lamina 6 in the cortex (Figure 7-22), projects directly to the thalamus, where it may provide sensory and other types

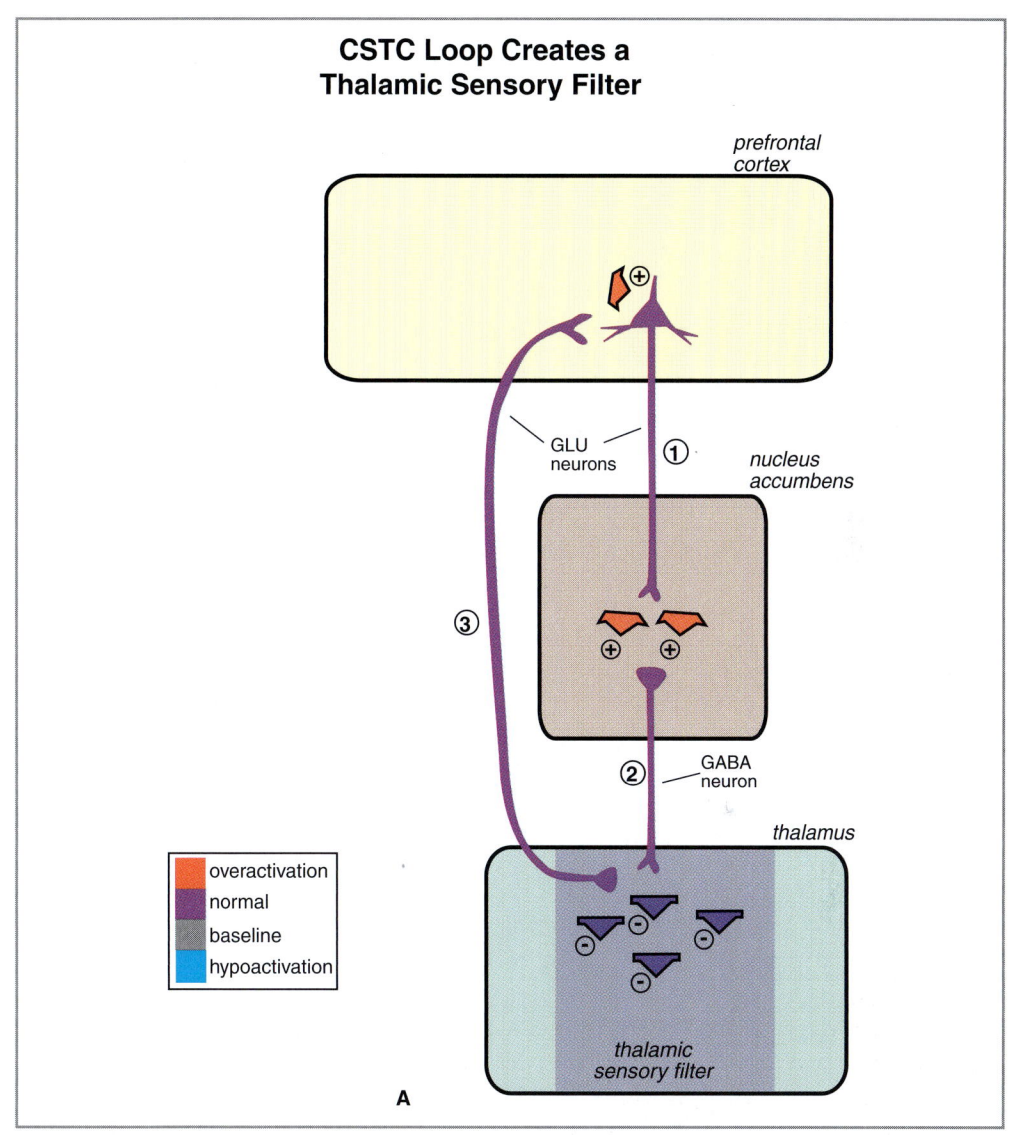

FIGURE 9-41A The cortico-striatal-thalamic-cortical loop creates a thalamic sensory filter. Pyramidal glutamatergic neurons descend from the prefrontal cortex to the striatum (1), where they terminate on gamma aminobutyric acid (GABA) neurons (2) that project to the thalamus. The release of GABA in the thalamus creates a sensory filter that prevents too much sensory information traveling through the thalamus from reaching the cortex, including the feedback thalamocortical glutamate neurons that project back to the original cortical pyramidal neuron (3).

of input (pathway d in Figure 9-38). This is known as the corticothalamic pathway. This may represent some of the sensory input that arrives via glutamate neurons to the thalamus in Figure 9-41C, D, and E. Hypofunction of NMDA receptors at this level may also cause dysregulation of the information that arrives in the cortex due to sensory overload and a malfunctioning of cortical glutamate input directly to the thalamic filter (Figure 9-41E).

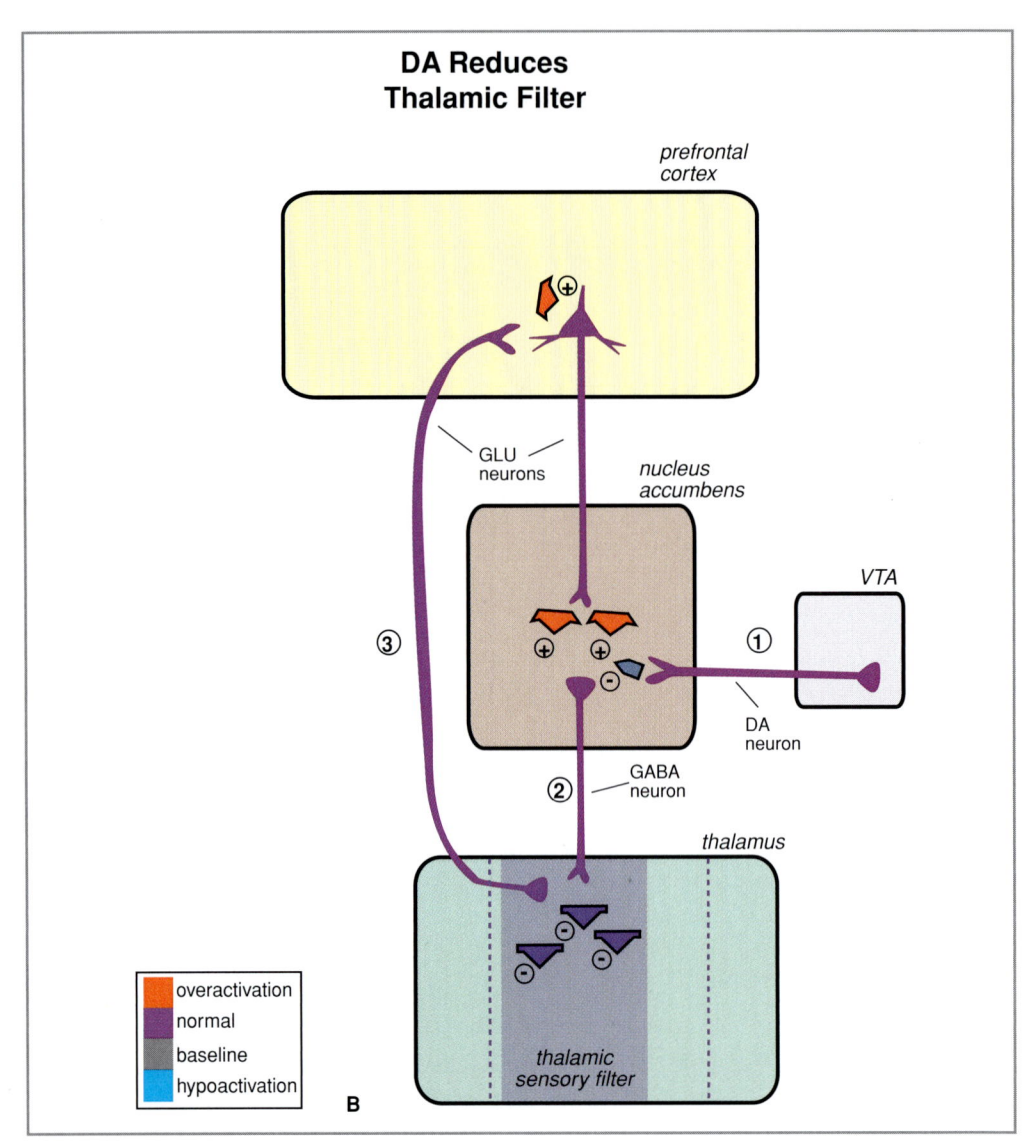

FIGURE 9-41B Dopamine reduces the thalamic filter. Dopaminergic input to the nucleus accumbens via the mesolimbic dopamine pathway (1) has an inhibitory effect on gamma aminobutyric acid (GABA) neurons (2). Thus, dopamine input (1) reduces the stimulatory glutamatergic input to these neurons from the prefrontal cortex, and thereby reduces the effectiveness of the thalamic sensory filter since less GABA is released by GABA neurons projecting from the nucleus accumbens to the thalamus (2). This means that more sensory input can escape from the thalamus to the cortex (3).

Corticocortical glutamate pathways

One pyramidal neuron communicates with another via the neurotransmitter glutamate (Figure 9-38, pathway e). These pathways are known as corticocortical glutamatergic pathways. Glutamatergic output from cortical pyramidal neurons is also discussed in Chapter 7; specific glutamatergic output from pyramidal neurons in laminas 2 and 3 of prefrontal cortex is illustrated in Figure 7-22. Corticocortical glutamatergic interactions are also illustrated in Figures 7-14 and 7-15.

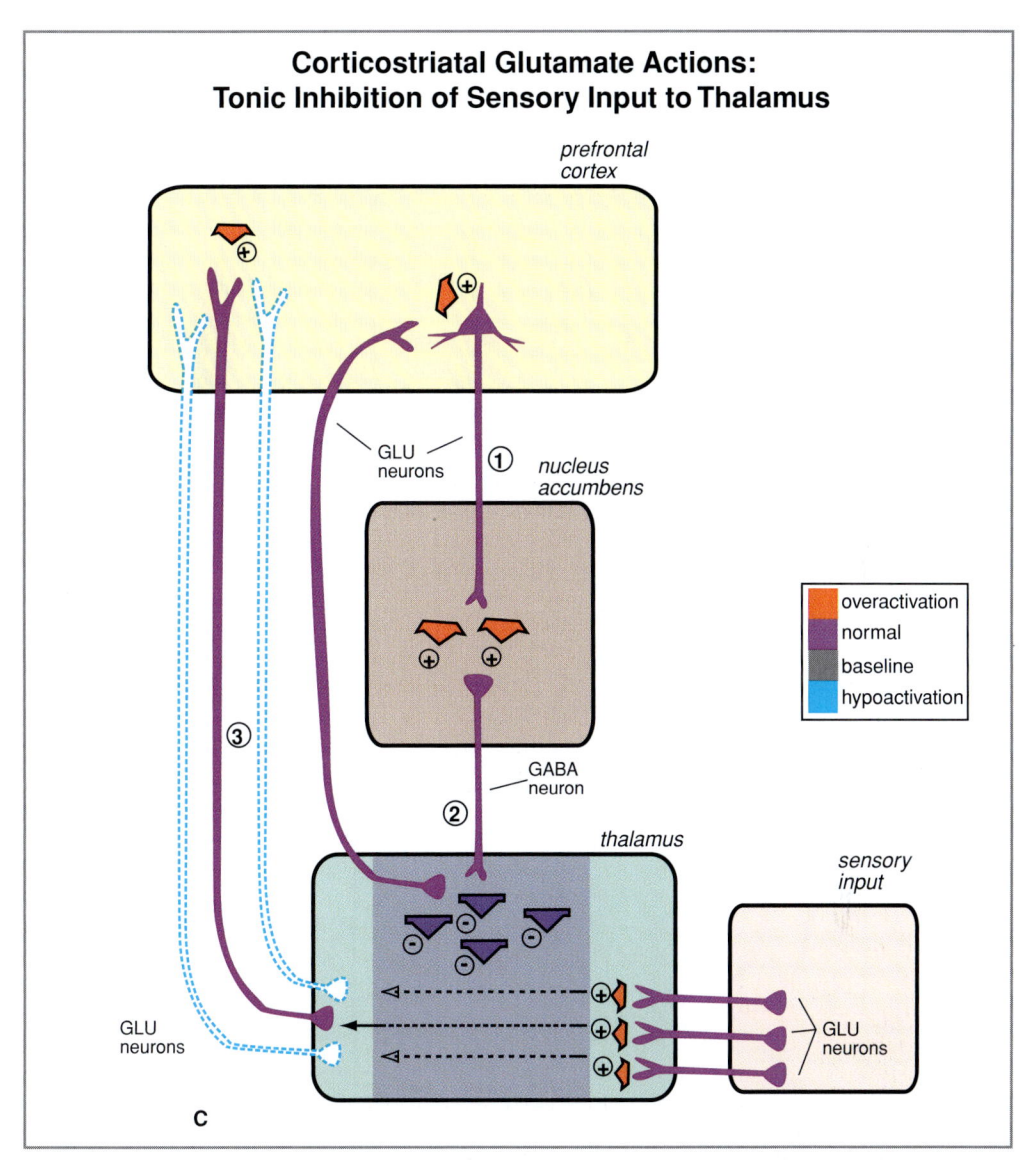

FIGURE 9-41C Tonic inhibition of sensory input from thalamus. A thalamic filter for sensory input to the cortex is set up by glutamate neurons projecting to nucleus accumbens (1), stimulating GABA release in the thalamus (2). When effective, this inhibitory GABA filters out most sensory input arriving in the thalamus, so that only selected types of sensory input are relayed to the cortex (3).

Cortical pyramidal neurons thus utilize glutamate to communicate back and forth: they not only send information to other pyramidal neurons with glutamate but also receive information from other neurons via glutamate (Figure 9-38). Glutamate is the main neurotransmitter utilized to send information as output from pyramidal neurons, but these neurons can receive a whole host of chemical neurotransmitting messages as input from other neurons, as discussed in Chapter 7 and illustrated for GABAergic interneuron input to pyramidal neurons in Figure 7-23 and for numerous other neurotransmitter inputs to pyramidal neurons in Figure 7-24.

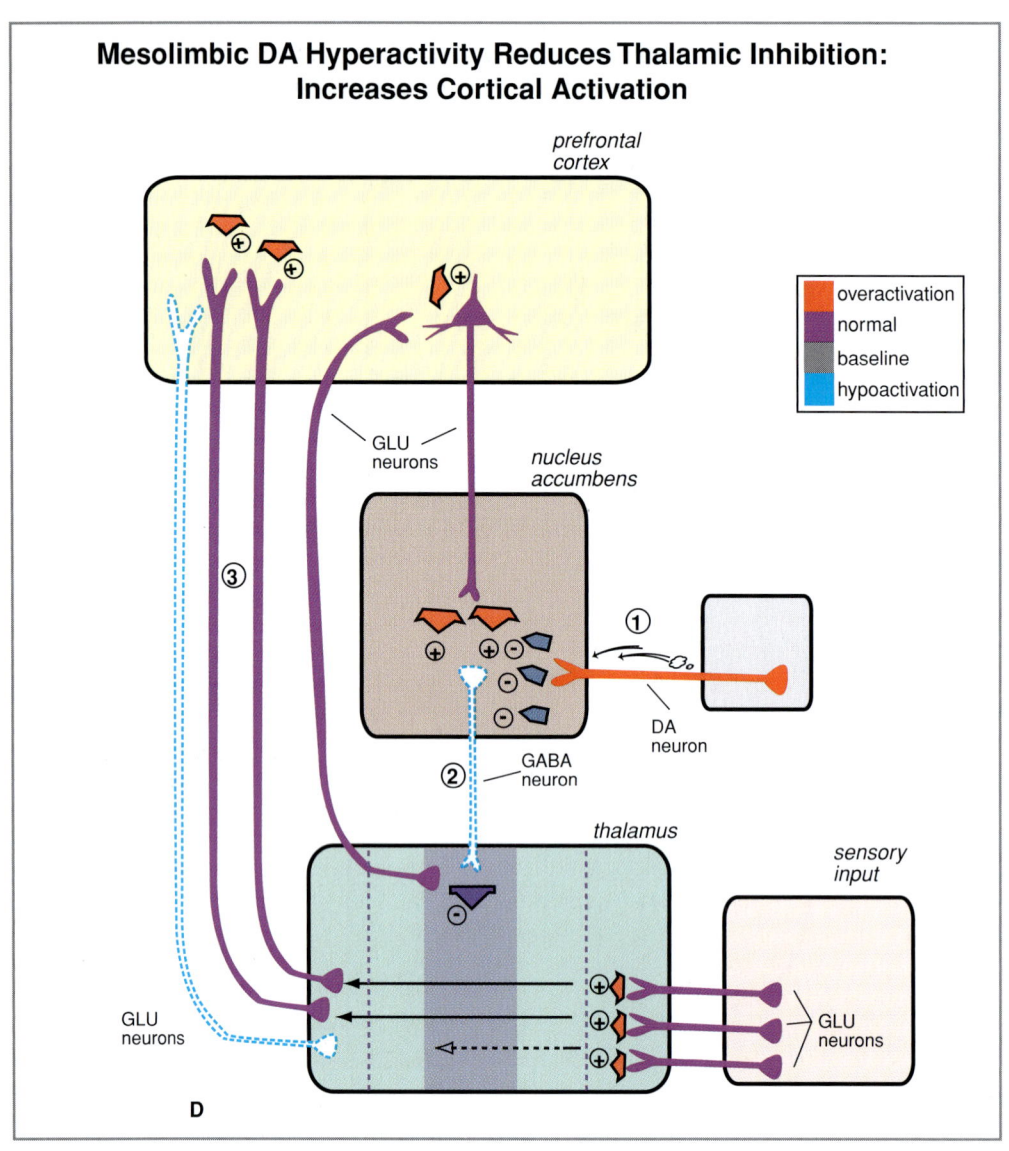

FIGURE 9-41D Mesolimbic dopamine hyperactivity reduces thalamic inhibition and increases cortical activation. The inhibitory effect of dopamine represented in Figure 9-41B is shown here as being much enhanced when this mesolimbic dopamine pathway is hyperactive (1). Too much dopamine activity in the nucleus accumbens (1), reduces GABA output to the thalamus (2), thus greatly reducing the effectiveness of the thalamic filter. When this occurs, more sensory input gets through the thalamic filter and increases the amount of cortical activation by ascending thalamocortical glutamate neurons (3). This definitely causes increased cortical activation and could potentially even cause overload in the prefrontal cortex, and positive symptoms of schizophrenia. See also Figure 9-41E.

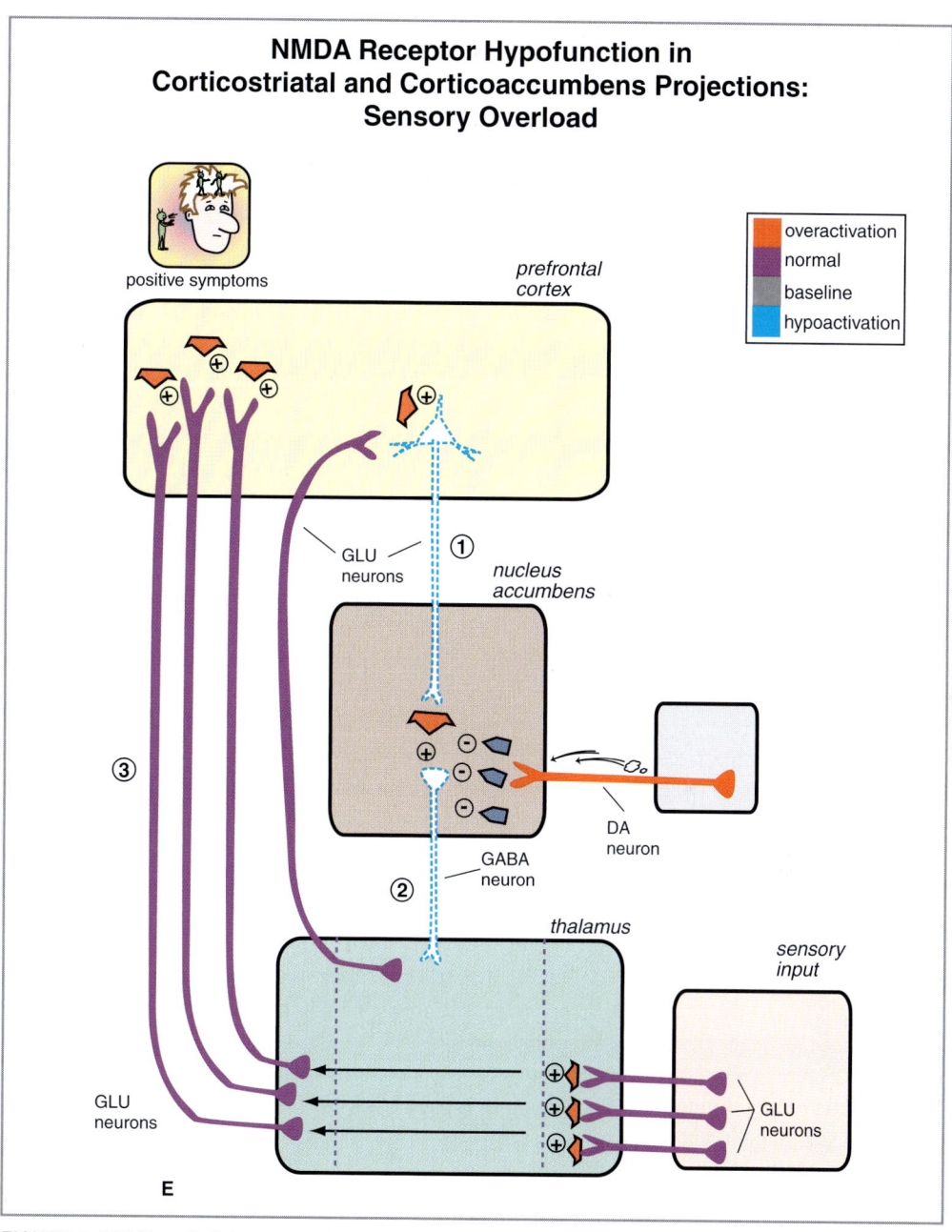

FIGURE 9-41E N-methyl-d-aspartate (NMDA) receptor hypofunction in corticostriatal and corticoaccumbens projections: sensory overload. NMDA receptor hypofunction in glutamatergic corticostriatal and corticoaccumbens projections (1) reduces the excitatory drive on gamma aminobutyric acid (GABA) neurons that create the thalamic filter (2), which can lead to excess sensory information escaping to the cortex (3). When this NMDA receptor hypofunction (1) is coupled with hyperactivity of mesolimbic dopamine neurons (shown here on the right and also in Figure 9-41D), this can cause the thalamic filter (2) to fail to the point where so much sensory information reaches the cortex that positive symptoms of psychosis occur (3) (see positive symptom icon in the cortex).

Psychosis and Schizophrenia | 297

In terms of the NMDA receptor hypofunction hypothesis of schizophrenia, it is not difficult to see how malfunctioning of glutamate input into cortical pyramidal neurons, not just from thalamocortical neurons (shown in Figure 9-41) but also from corticocortical neurons communicating within the cortex (shown in Figure 9-38 as well as in Figures 7-14 and 7-15) could contribute to symptoms of schizophrenia that theoretically reside in prefrontal cortex, such as cognitive, affective, and negative symptoms.

That is, normally corticocortical projections and loops between key areas of prefrontal cortex communicate effectively and process information efficiently (Figure 9-42A). When NMDA receptors are hypofunctional, this changes the nature of information processing such that corticocortical communication of one glutamatergic pyramidal cell to another becomes dysfunctional (Figure 9-42B). Theoretically, this can range from hypoactivation of the entire loop, as shown for the corticocortical loop between dorsolateral prefrontal cortex (DLPFC) and ventromedial prefrontal cortex (VMPFC) in Figure 9-42B, to overactivation of the entire loop as shown from VMPFC to orbitofrontal cortex (OFC) to partial overactivation with partial hypoactivation as shown for OFC to DLPFC in Figure 9-42B. Whatever the actual activation pattern, communication when NMDA receptors are hypofunctional can be faulty if not chaotic, thus, according to the NMDA receptor hypofunction hypothesis, leading to the symptoms of schizophrenia.

In summary, NMDA receptor hypofunction within the five major glutamate pathways described in Figure 9-38 can potentially explain not only the positive, negative, affective, and cognitive symptoms of schizophrenia but also how dopamine becomes dysregulated as a consequence of NMDA receptor hypofunction, and thus too active in the mesolimbic dopamine pathway for positive symptoms and too hypoactive in the mesocortical dopamine pathway for cognitive, affective, and negative symptoms of schizophrenia. Many contemporary theories on the genetic basis of schizophrenia now focus on the NMDA receptor, as discussed below, as do new drug development efforts for novel treatments of schizophrenia, discussed in Chapter 10.

Neurodegenerative hypothesis of schizophrenia

The presence of both functional and structural abnormalities demonstrated in neuroimaging studies of the brain of schizophrenics suggests that a neurodegenerative process with progressive loss of neuronal function may be ongoing during the course of schizophrenia (Figure 9-43). Numerous neurodegenerative processes are hypothesized, ranging from genetic programming of abnormal apoptosis and subsequent degeneration of critical neurons, to prenatal exposure to anoxia, toxins, infection, or malnutrition, to a process of neuronal loss known as excitotoxicity (Figure 9-43). If neurons are excited while mediating positive symptoms and then die off from a toxic process caused by excessive excitatory neurotransmission, this may lead to a residual burnout state and thus negative symptoms (Figure 9-43).

A neurodegenerative condition in schizophrenia is also suggested by the progressive nature of the course of this illness (Figure 9-44). Such a course is not consistent with simply being the result of a static and previously completed pathologic process. Thus, schizophrenia progresses from a largely asymptomatic stage prior to the teen years (phase I in Figure 9-44), to a prodromal stage of "oddness" and the onset of subtle negative symptoms in the late teens to early twenties (phase II in Figure 9-44). The active phase of the illness begins and continues throughout the twenties and thirties, with destructive positive symptoms characterized by an up-and-down course with treatment and relapse, never quite returning

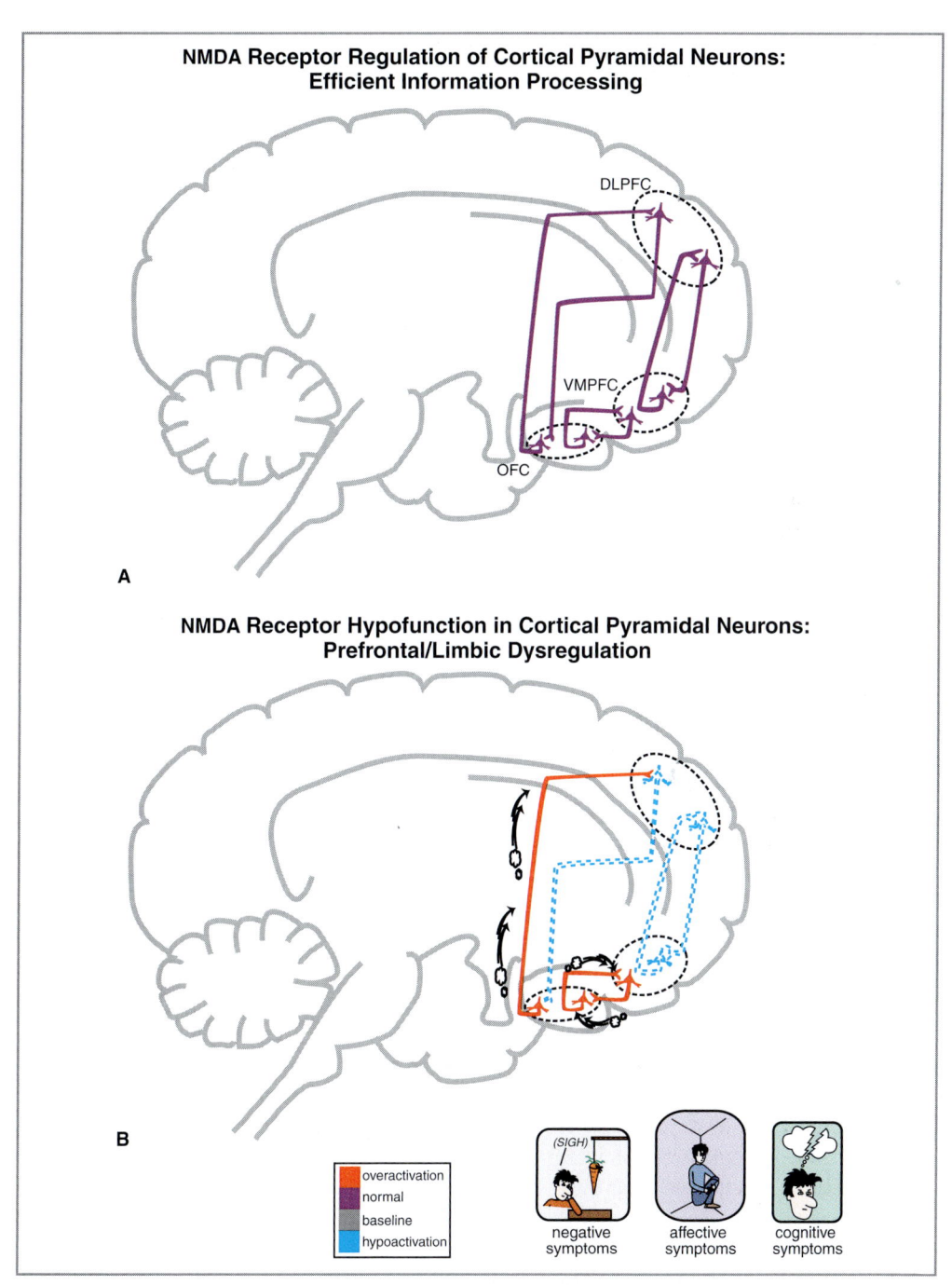

FIGURE 9-42A and B N-methyl-d-aspartate (NMDA) receptor regulation of corticocortical glutamate pathways. (**A**) When NMDA receptors function normally, corticocortical glutamate loops communicate effectively and process information efficiently. (**B**) NMDA receptor hypofunction in cortical pyramidal neurons can impair communication between neurons by causing hypoactivation of loops [shown here, for example, between dorsolateral prefrontal cortex (DLPFC) and ventral medial prefrontal cortex (VMPFC)], hyperactivation of loops [shown here, for example, between orbitofrontal cortex (OFC) and VMPFC], and even partial hyperactivation with partial hypoactivation (shown here, for example, between OFC and DLPFC). Dysfunction of corticocortical glutamate pathways due to NMDA receptor hypofunction could be an underlying cause of schizophrenia symptoms.

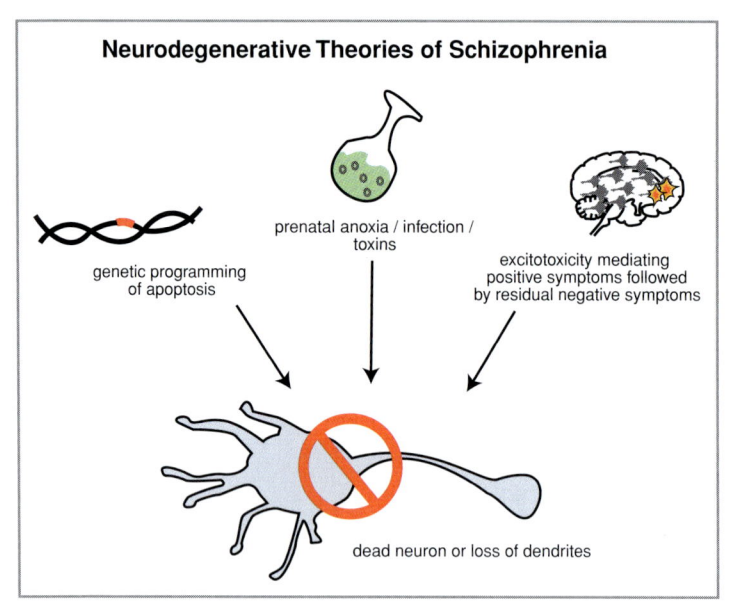

FIGURE 9-43 **Neurodegenerative theories of schizophrenia.** Neurodegenerative theories of schizophrenia posit that progressive loss of neuronal function – whether through loss of dendrites, destruction of synapses, or neuronal death – may underlie symptoms and progression of schizophrenia. Causes of neurodegeneration can range from predetermined genetic programming of neuronal or synaptic destruction; to fetal insults such as anoxia, infection, toxins, or maternal starvation; to glutamate-mediated excitotoxicity that initially can cause positive symptoms, and, as neurons die, lead to residual negative symptoms.

to the same level of functioning following acute relapses or exacerbations (phase III in Figure 9-44). Finally, the disease can go into a largely stable stage of poor social functioning and prominent negative and cognitive symptoms, with some ups and downs but at a considerable decline from baseline functioning, suggesting a more static phase of illness, sometimes called burnout, in the forties or later in life (phase IV in Figure 9-44).

The fact that a schizophrenic patient's responsiveness to antipsychotic treatment can change (and lessen) over the course of illness also suggests an ongoing neurodegenerative process of some kind. For example, the time it takes for a schizophrenic patient to go into remission increases with each successive psychotic relapse. Patients may be less responsive to antipsychotic treatment during successive episodes or exacerbations, such that residual symptoms remain as well as decrements in the patients' functional capacities. This development of treatment resistance during successive episodes of the illness suggests that "psychosis is hazardous to the brain." It thus seems possible that patients who receive early and effective continuous treatment may avoid disease progression or at least the development of treatment resistance.

One major idea that proposes to explain the downhill course of schizophrenia and the development of treatment resistance is that neurodegenerative events in schizophrenia may be mediated by a type of excessive action of the neurotransmitter glutamate that has come to be known as "excitotoxicity." The "excitotoxic hypothesis of schizophrenia" proposes that neurons degenerate because of excessive excitatory neurotransmission at glutamate neurons. This process of excitotoxicity is not only a hypothesis to explain neurodegeneration in schizophrenia; it has also been invoked as an explanation for neurodegeneration in any number of neurologic and psychiatric conditions, including Alzheimer's disease and other

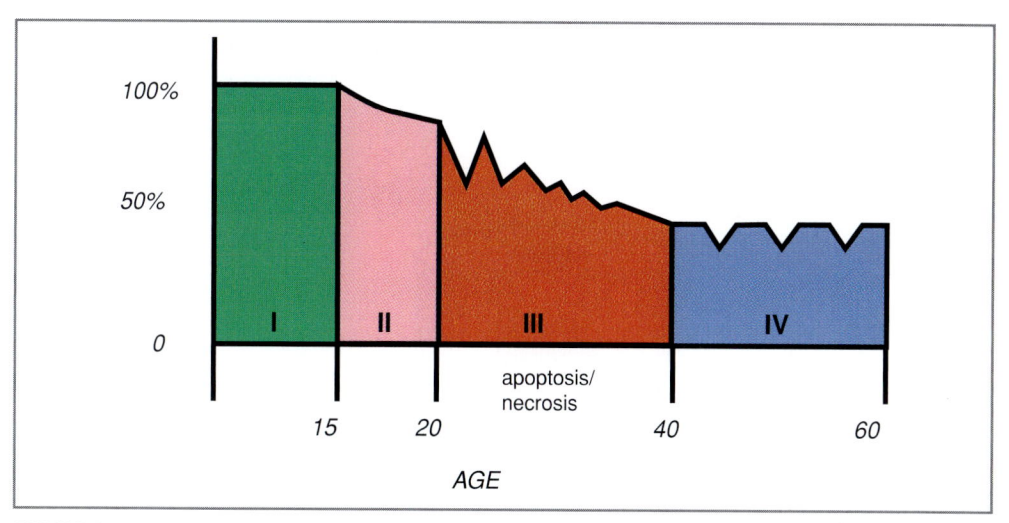

FIGURE 9-44 **Stages of schizophrenia.** The stages of schizophrenia are shown here over a lifetime. The progressive nature of schizophrenia, illustrated here, supports a neurodegenerative basis for the disorder. The patient has full functioning (100 percent) early in life, and is virtually asymptomatic (Stage I). However, during a prodromal phase (Stage II) starting in the teens, there may be odd behaviors and subtle negative symptoms. The acute phase of the illness usually announces itself fairly dramatically in the twenties (Stage III) with positive symptoms, remissions, and relapses but never quite getting back to previous levels of functioning. This is often a chaotic stage of illness with a progressive downhill course. The final phase of the illness may begin in the forties or later, with prominent negative and cognitive symptoms and some waxing and waning, but often more of a "burnout" stage of continuing disability. There may not necessarily be a continuing and relentless downhill course, but the patient may become progressively resistant to treatment with antipsychotic medications during this stage (Stage IV).

degenerative dementias, Parkinson's disease, amytrophic lateral sclerosis (ALS, or Lou Gehrig's disease), and even stroke.

Excitotoxicity and the glutamate system in neurodegenerative disorders such as schizophrenia

The NMDA subtype of glutamate receptor is thought to mediate both normal excitatory neurotransmission, leading to vital functions such as neuronal plasticity and long-term potentiation (Figure 9-45), as well as neurodegenerative excitotoxicity along the glutamate excitation spectrum shown in Figure 9-46. Excitotoxicity could be the final common pathway that leads to progressive worsening in any number of neurologic and psychiatric disorders characterized by a neurodegenerative course. The basic idea is that the normal process of excitatory neurotransmission runs amok, and instead of normal excitatory neurotransmission, things get out of hand and the neuron is literally excited to death (Figures 9-46 and 9-47). The excitotoxic mechanism is thought to begin with a pathologic process of overexcitation that may accompany symptoms such as psychosis, mania, or even panic (Figures 9-46 and 9-48). The storm of excitatory symptoms could be the trigger for reckless glutamate activity leading ultimately to neuronal death (Figure 9-47). The sequence of ever more dangerous excitatory neurotransmission could begin with potentially reversible excess calcium entering neurons during excitatory neurotransmission with glutamate, mediating positive symptoms of psychosis, and possibly allowing full recovery of the neuron (left-hand part of the spectrum in Figures 9-46 and 9-48). However, such a state of overexcitation could also lead to dangerous opening of the calcium channel, because if too much calcium

Normal Excitatory Neurotransmission at NMDA Receptors

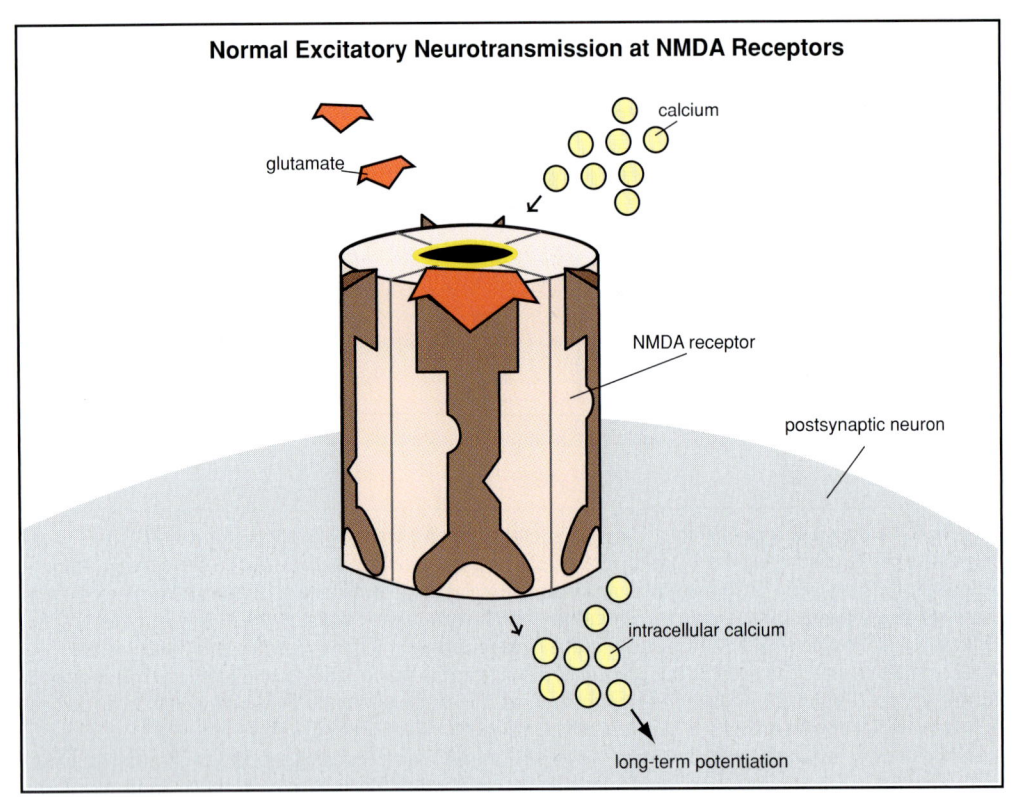

FIGURE 9-45 Normal excitatory neurotransmission at NMDA receptors. Shown here is normal excitatory neurotransmission at the N-methyl-d-aspartate (NMDA) type of glutamate receptor. The NMDA receptor is a ligand-gated ion channel. This fast transmitting ion channel is an excitatory calcium channel. Occupancy of NMDA glutamate receptors by glutamate causes calcium channels to open and the neuron to be excited for neurotransmission.

enters the cell through open channels, it would poison the cell due to calcium activation of intracellular enzymes (Figure 9-48) that form pesky free radicals (Figure 9-49). Initially, free radicals begin destroying just the dendrites that serve as postsynaptic targets of glutamate (Figure 9-50). However, too many free radicals would eventually overwhelm the cell with toxic actions on cellular membranes and organelles (Figure 9-51), ultimately killing the neuron.

A limited form of excitotoxicity may be useful as a "pruning" mechanism for normal maintenance of the dendritic tree (see Figure 2-32), getting rid of cerebral "deadwood" like a good gardener; excitotoxicity to excess, however, is hypothesized to be a form of pruning out of control (Figure 2-33). This hypothetically results in various forms of neurodegeneration, ranging from slow, relentless neurodegenerative conditions such as schizophrenia and Alzheimer's disease to sudden, catastrophic neuronal death such as stroke (Figure 9-46).

Neurodevelopmental hypothesis and genetics of schizophrenia

Is schizophrenia acquired or inherited?

Many contemporary theories for the etiology of schizophrenia propose that this illness originates from abnormalities in brain development. Some suggest that the problem is acquired

Spectrum of Excitation by Glutamate at NMDA Receptors

- normal excitation and long-term potentiation
- excess excitation
  - psychosis
  - mania
  - panic
- excitotoxicity - damage to neurons
- excitotoxicity - slow neurodegeneration
- excitotoxicity - catastrophic neurodegeneration

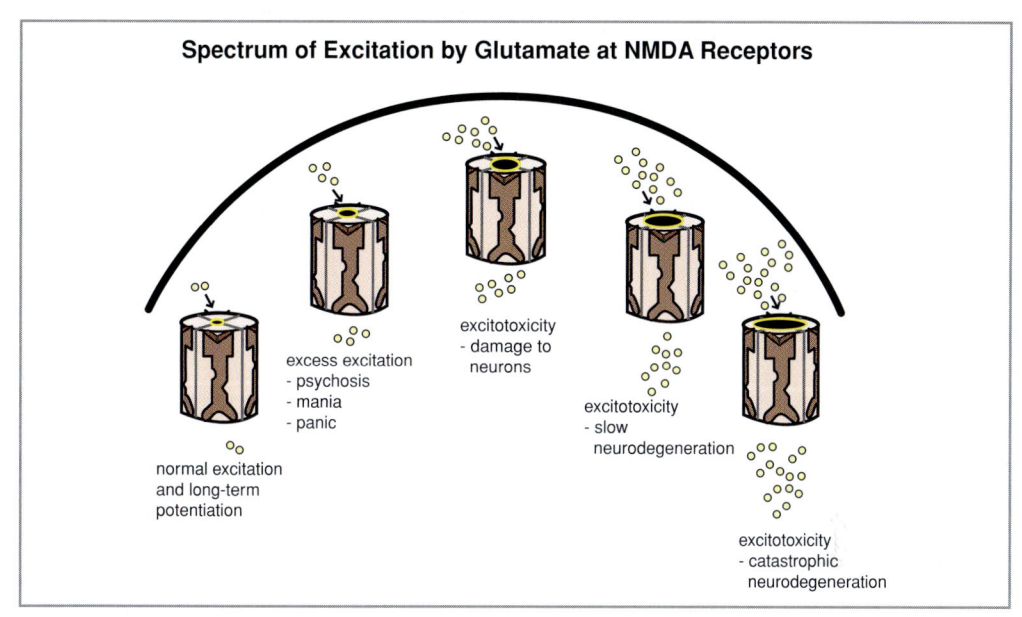

FIGURE 9-46 **Spectrum of excitation by glutamate at N-methyl-d-aspartate (NMDA) receptors.** A major hypothesis for the pathophysiology of neurologic and psychiatric disorders that run a neurodegenerative course is that glutamate may cause neuronal damage or death by a process of normal excitatory neurotransmission run amok, called excitotoxicity. The spectrum of excitation by glutamate ranges from normal neurotransmission, which is necessary for such neuronal activities as long-term potentiation, memory formation, and synaptogenesis; to an excessive amount of excitatory neurotransmission that may occur while a patient is experiencing pathologic symptoms such as psychosis, mania, or panic; to excitotoxicity that results in damage to dendrites but not neuronal death; to slow progressive excitotoxicity resulting in neuronal degeneration of many neurons over an extended period of time, as occurs in Alzheimer's disease or possibly schizophrenia; to sudden and catastrophic excitotoxicity causing neurodegeneration leading to loss of a large number of neurons at once, as in stroke.

from the fetal brain's environment, as shown in Figure 9-43. Schizophrenia may thus start with an acquired neurodegenerative process that interferes with neurodevelopment. For example, schizophrenia is increased in those with a fetal history of obstetric complications in the pregnant mother – ranging from viral infections to starvation to autoimmune processes and other such problems – suggesting that an insult to the brain early in fetal development could contribute to the cause of schizophrenia. These risk factors may all have the final common pathway of reducing nerve growth factors (see Figure 2-17) and also stimulating certain noxious processes that kill off critical neurons, such as cytokines, viral infection, hypoxia, trauma, starvation, or stress. This may be mediated by either apoptosis or necrosis (Figure 2-10).

Neuronal insult could also be mediated by excitotoxicity, as discussed earlier (Figures 9-46 through 9-51). In particular, if excitotoxicity occurred specifically in the ventral hippocampus before the completion of connections in the developing brain, some neurodevelopmental theories suggest that this could impact the development of the prefrontal cortex and result in dysconnectivity with the prefrontal cortex (Figure 9-52). Such an abnormal set of neuronal connections could be the biological substrate for symptoms in schizophrenia (Figure 9-52). The excitotoxicity that causes such dysconnectivity could be genetically programmed or environmentally triggered.

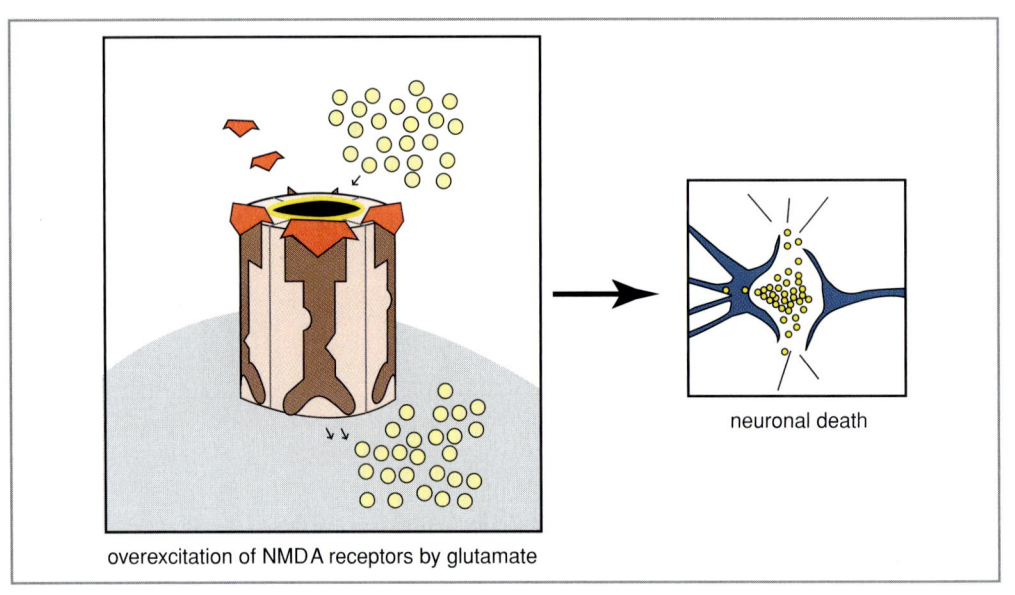

FIGURE 9-47 Cellular events occurring during excitotoxicity, part 1. Excitotoxicity is a major current hypothesis for explaining a neuropathologic mechanism that could mediate the final common pathway of any number of neurologic and psychiatric disorders characterized by a neurodegenerative course. The basic idea is that the normal process of excitatory neurotransmission runs amok, and instead of normal excitatory neurotransmission, things get out of hand and the neuron is literally excited to death. The excitotoxic mechanism is thought to begin with a pathologic process that triggers excessive glutamate activity. This causes excessive opening of the calcium channel, shown here, beginning the process of poisoning of the cell by allowing too much calcium to enter it.

Genes that affect connectivity, synaptogenesis and NMDA receptors

Although abnormal neuronal connectivity can be triggered in many ways by the environment (Figure 9-43), it is increasingly believed that the neurodevelopmental processes underlying schizophrenia are mostly influenced by genes. Strong evidence for a genetic basis of schizophrenia comes from the classic schizophrenia twin studies showing that monozygotic twins are much more frequently concordant for schizophrenia than are dizygotic twins. For many years, scientists have therefore been trying to identify abnormal genes in schizophrenia. Once it was recognized that single genes do not directly cause schizophrenia (Figure 6-2) or the behavioral symptoms of schizophrenia (Figure 6-3), attention turned to the discovery of "susceptibility" genes that code for subtle molecular abnormalities that could provide a genetic bias toward inefficient information processing in brain circuits mediating the symptoms of schizophrenia (Figures 6-4, 6-5, and 6-6). A sufficient combination of such genetic bias (Figure 6-6), particularly when coupled with stressful input from the environment (Figure 6-15), is the modern formulation for how genes and the environment conspire to produce schizophrenia.

More than a dozen susceptibility genes have been identified, several of which have been reproducibly linked to schizophrenia (Table 9-12). The pathogenic mechanisms of the most prominent genes described by current genetic research in schizophrenia include abnormal neuronal connectivity, defective synaptogenesis, and dysregulation of the NMDA glutamate receptor (Figures 9-53 through 9-58). Four key genes that regulate neuronal connectivity and synaptogenesis in schizophrenia are shown in Figure 9-53. These are the genes for four key proteins: **BDNF** (brain-derived neurotrophic factor), a known trophic factor

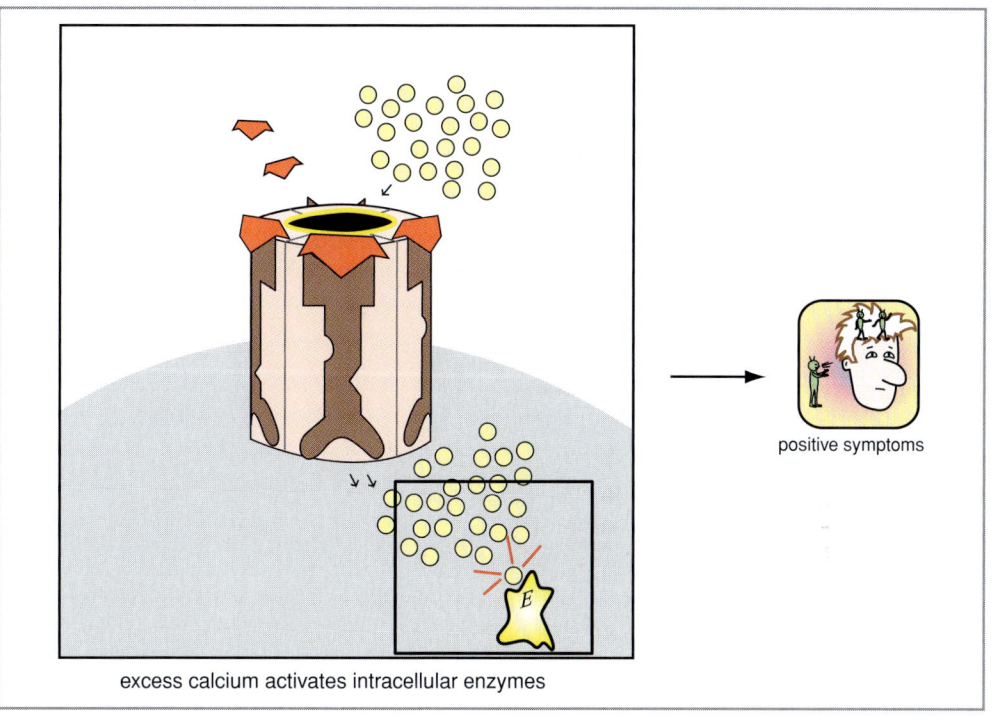

FIGURE 9-48 Cellular events occurring during excitotoxicity, part 2. The internal milieu of a neuron is very sensitive to calcium, as a small increase in calcium concentration will alter the activities of various enzymes as well as cause alterations in neuronal membrane excitability. If calcium levels rise too much, then they will begin to activate enzymes that can be dangerous for the cell owing to their ability to trigger a destructive chemical cascade. The beginning of this process may be an underlying cause of pathologic symptoms of schizophrenia such as delusions and hallucinations.

discussed in Chapter 2, listed in Table 2-1, and illustrated in Figures 2-7 and 2-17; **dysbindin**, also known as dystrobrevin-binding protein 1, involved in the formation of synaptic structures (Figures 9-53 and 9-55A and B); **neuregulin**, involved in neuronal migration (Figures 9-53 and 9-54B) and in the genesis of glial cells and subsequent myelination of neurons by these cells (Figure 9-54D); and **DISC-1** (disrupted in schizophrenia-1), aptly named for a disrupted gene linked to schizophrenia that makes a protein involved in neurogenesis (Figure 9-54A), neuronal migration (Figure 9-54B), and dendritic organization (Figures 9-53 and 9-54C).

It is not known exactly how these genes cause the hypothesized subtle molecular abnormalities that are thought to bias neuronal circuits towards schizophrenia or whether these genes make abnormal proteins or just do not turn on and off synthesis of their gene product protein when they should during neurodevelopment. The specific combinations of abnormal genes that are either necessary or sufficient for the development of schizophrenia are also not known. Nevertheless, the fact that several genes linked to schizophrenia are all involved in neurodevelopment strongly indicates that in schizophrenia, something has gone wrong with the connections between neurons.

Dysconnectivity
The results of abnormal genetic programming during critical periods of neurodevelopment could include selecting the wrong neurons to survive in the fetal brain (Figures 2-9 and

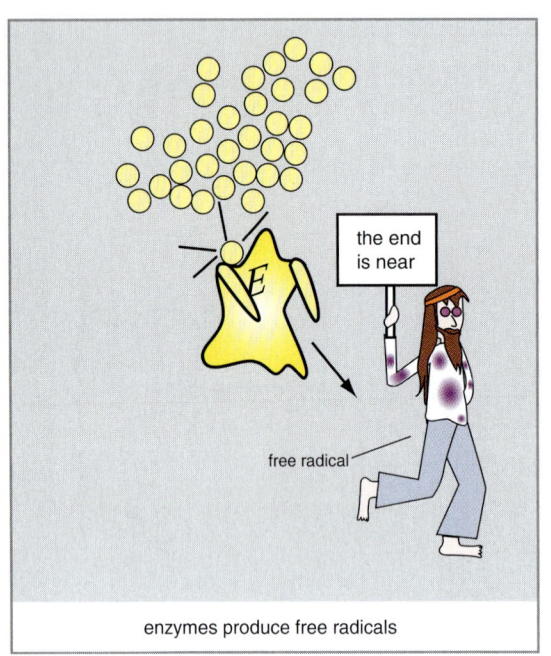

FIGURE 9-49 Cellular events occurring during excitotoxicity, part 3. Once excessive glutamate causes too much calcium to enter the neuron and calcium activates dangerous enzymes, these enzymes go on to produce troublesome free radicals. Free radicals are chemicals that are capable of destroying other cellular components, such as organelles and membranes, by destructive chemical reactions.

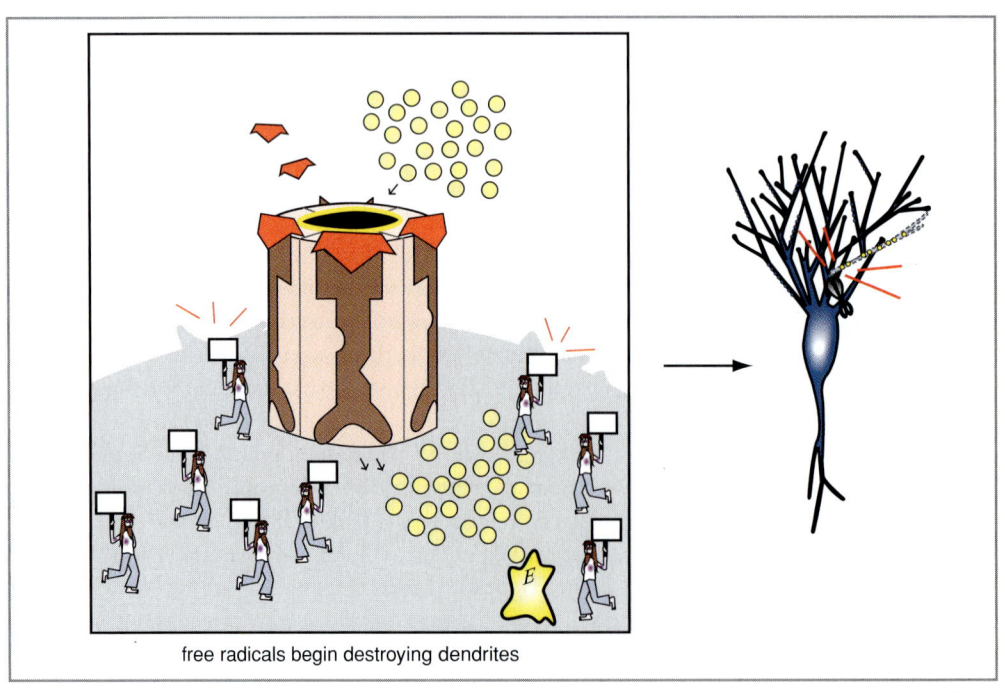

FIGURE 9-50 Cellular events occurring during excitotoxicity, part 4. As the calcium accumulates in the cell, and the enzymes produce more and more free radicals, they begin to destroy the dendrites that serve as postsynaptic targets of glutamate.

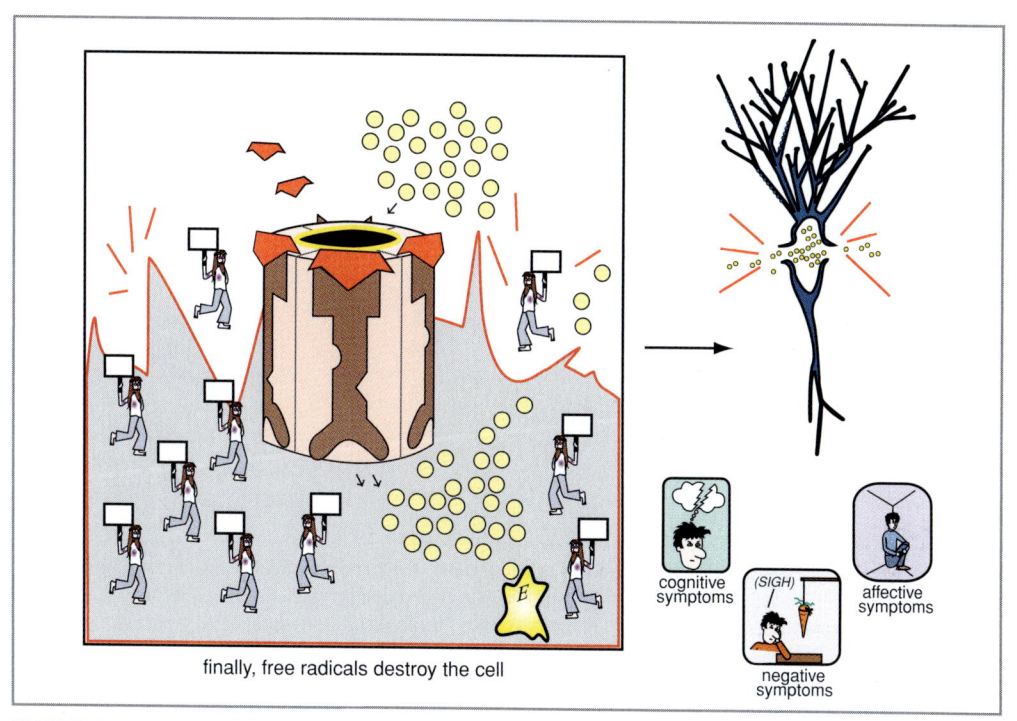

FIGURE 9-51 Cellular events occurring during excitotoxicity, part 5. Eventually, too many free radicals lead to indiscriminate destruction of various parts of the neuron, especially its neuronal and nuclear membranes and critical organelles such as energy-producing mitochondria. The damage can be so great that the free radicals essentially destroy the whole neuron. This level of destruction may be related to deficit states in schizophrenia and be associated with cognitive, negative, and affective symptoms.

9-54A), having neurons migrate to the wrong places (Figures 2-11, 2-12, and 9-54B), having neurons innervate the wrong targets, perhaps from getting the nurturing signals mixed up so that what innervates these neurons is also mixed up (Figures 2-13 through 2-16, 2-19, 9-53, and 9-54C), or having abnormal development of the glial cells so that they are unable to myelinate neurons properly (Figure 9-54D).

To the extent that something is wrong with major susceptibility genes for schizophrenia during the formation of the brain before birth, DISC-1 could affect early neurogenesis (Figure 9-54A), neuronal migration (Figure 9-54B) and dendritic organization (Figure 9-54C), whereas neuregulin could affect neuronal migration, especially of GABA-ergic interneurons (Figure 9-54B) as well as myelination of neurons once they have migrated into place in the forming brain (Figure 9-54D). These neurodevelopmental processes are absolutely critical for normal brain development, occur over large distances, and impact the functioning of the brain for an entire lifetime.

Abnormal synaptogenesis

Although it is possible that schizophrenia susceptibility genes may impact brain development once and forever in a type of fetal "hit and run" damage that is complete by the time the brain is formed, it is also possible that an abnormal neurodevelopmental process continues in the schizophrenic brain throughout a lifetime. Most neurons form, are selected, migrate, differentiate, and myelinate before birth, but the process of neurogenesis continues for a

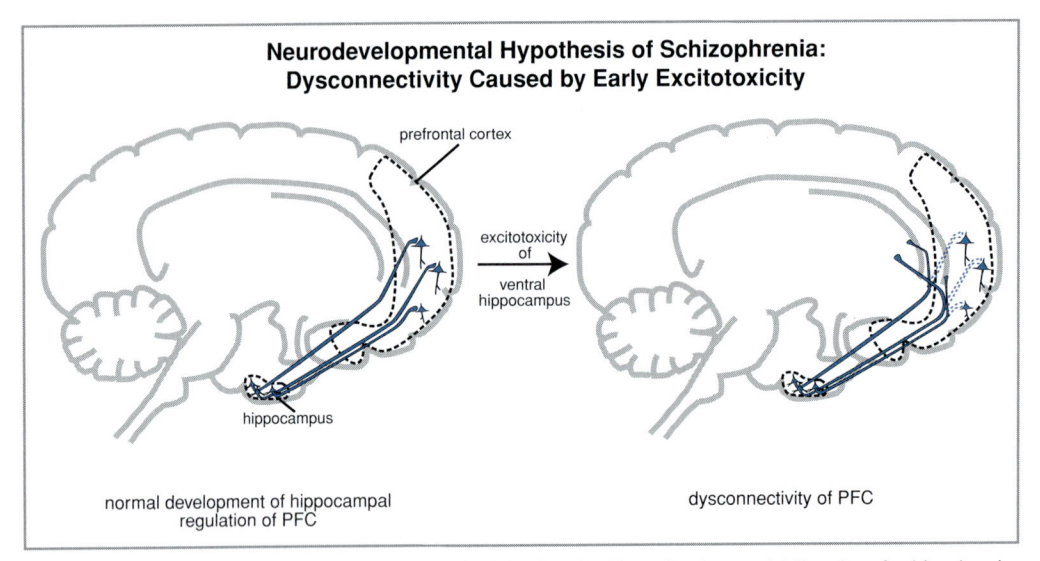

FIGURE 9-52 Neurodevelopmental hypothesis of schizophrenia. Neurodevelopmental theories of schizophrenia suggest that the disorder occurs as a result of abnormalities in brain development. Excitotoxicity that occurs early in development, before the completion of synaptic connections, could result in dysconnectivity between brain regions and consequently symptoms of mental illness. For example, with normal development the ventral hippocampus forms connections with cortical pyramidal neurons to regulate activity in the prefrontal cortex (left). Excitotoxicity in the ventral hippocampus prior to completion of these connections could impact development of the prefrontal cortex, causing abnormal neuronal connections that may lead to symptoms of schizophrenia (right).

lifetime in selected brain areas (discussed in Chapter 2 and illustrated in Figures 2-3 and 2-4). Perhaps more importantly, synaptogenesis, synaptic strengthening, elimination, and reorganization continue over a lifetime (Figures 2-1 and 2-22 through 2-32). Thus, to the extent that schizophrenia susceptibility genes affect synapse formation (Figure 9-53), they have the potential to affect ongoing brain function for a lifetime.

Many of the known susceptibility genes for schizophrenia have a profound impact on synaptogenesis (Figures 9-53 and 9-55A and B). Dysbindin, BDNF, DISC-1, and neuregulin all affect normal synapse formation; thus some combination of abnormalities in these molecules could lead to abnormal synapse formation in schizophrenia (Figure 9-55A). For example, abnormal genetic programming of dysbindin could affect synaptic cytoarchitecture and scaffolding in schizophrenia, whereas abnormal programming of DISC-1 and neuregulin could affect dendritic morphology and together lead to structurally abnormal synapses in schizophrenia (Figure 9-55B).

NMDA receptors, AMPA receptors, and synaptogenesis

Earlier in this chapter we reviewed the NMDA receptor hypofunction hypothesis of schizophrenia (illustrated in Figures 9-39 through 9-42). Supporting this hypothesis are observations that several of the known susceptibility genes for schizophrenia impact the NMDA receptor (Figures 9-55C and D and 9-56 through 9-58). Dysbindin, DISC-1, and neuregulin are all involved in the normal "strengthening" of glutamate synapses (Figure 9-55C). Normally, when glutamate synapses are active, their NMDA receptors trigger an electrical phenomenon known as long-term potentiation (LTP). With the help of dysbindin, DISC-1, and neuregulin, LTP leads to structural and functional changes of the

TABLE 9-12 Susceptibility genes for schizophrenia

Genes for:
Dysbindin (dystrobrevin binding protein 1 or DTNBP1)
Neuregulin (NRG1)
DISC1 (disrupted in schizophrenia 1)
DAOA (d-amino acid oxidase activator; G72/G30)
DAO (d-amino acid oxidase)
RGS4 (regulator of G protein signaling 4)
COMT (Catechol-O-methyl transferase)
CHRNA7 (alpha-7 nicotinic cholinergic receptor)
GAD1 (glutamic acid decarboxylase 1)
GRM3 (mGluR3)
PPP3CC
PRODH2
AKT1
ERBB4
FEZ1
MUTED
MRDS1 (OFCC1)
BDNF (brain-derived neurotrophic factor)
Nur77
MAO-A (monoamine oxidase A)
Spinophylin
Calcyon
Tyrosine hydroxylase
Dopamine-D2 receptor (D2R)
Dopamine-D3 receptor (D3R)

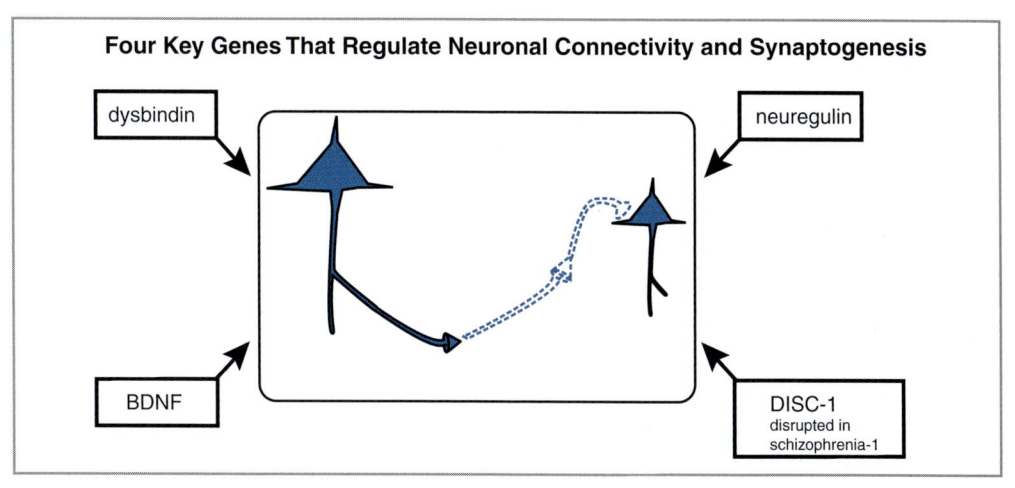

FIGURE 9-53 BDNF, dysbindin, neuregulin, and DISC-1. Four key genes that regulate neuronal connectivity and synaptogenesis in schizophrenia are the genes that code for the proteins brain derived neurotrophic factor (BDNF), dysbindin, neuregulin, and DISC-1 (disrupted in schizophrenia-1).

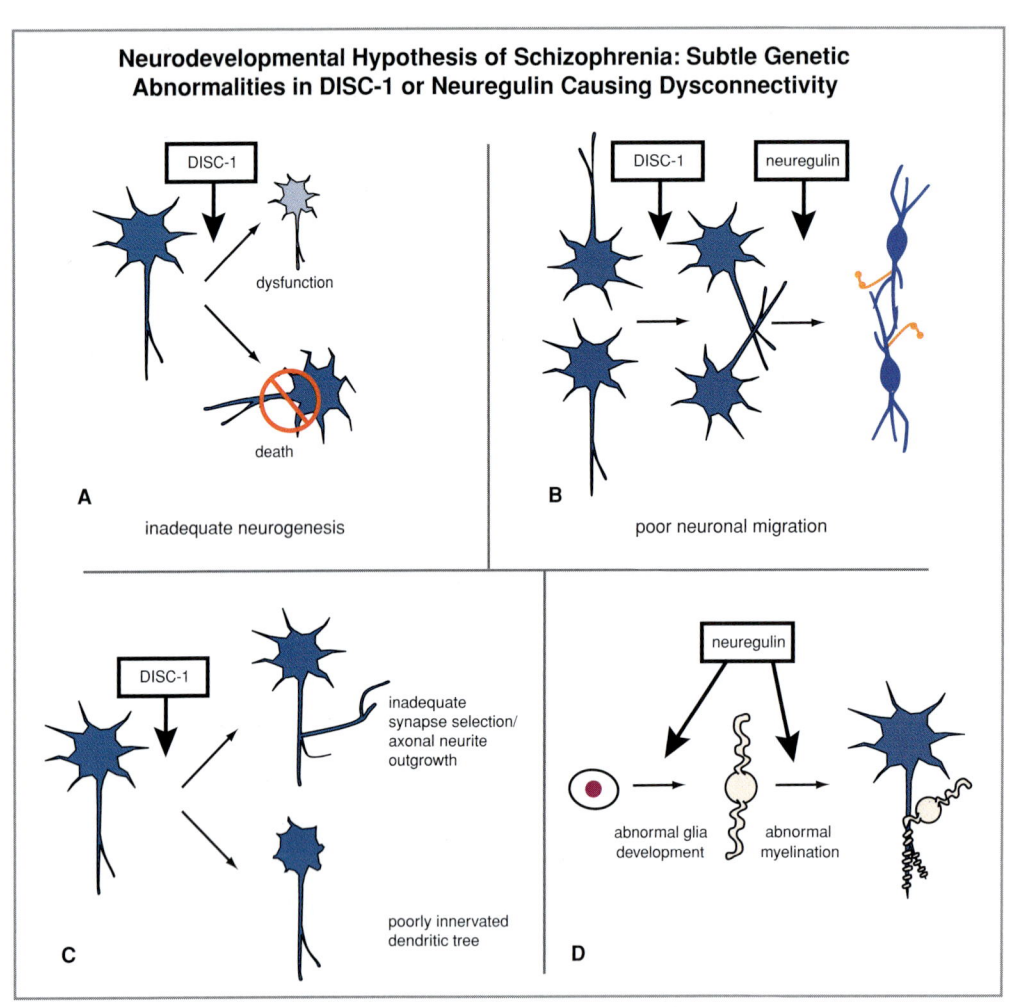

FIGURE 9-54A, B, C, and D Neurodevelopmental hypothesis of schizophrenia: subtle genetic abnormalities in DISC-1 or neuregulin causing dysconnectivity. DISC-1 (disrupted in schizophrenia-1) is a protein that is involved in neurogenesis (**A**), neuronal migration (**B**), and dendritic organization (**C**). Neuregulin is involved in neuronal migration (**B**), genesis of glial cells (**D**), and myelination of neurons by glial cells (**D**). Thus, subtle genetic abnormalities in the genes for DISC-1 or neuregulin can disrupt these processes, causing dysconnectivity among neurons, abnormal functioning of neuronal circuits among neurons linked together, increased risk of schizophrenia, and ultimately the symptoms of schizophrenia.

synapse that make neurotransmission more efficient. This includes increasing the number of AMPA receptors (Figure 9-55C).

AMPA receptors are important for mediating excitatory neurotransmission and depolarization at glutamate synapses (discussed in Chapter 5 and illustrated in Figures 5-25 and 5-43). Thus, more AMPA receptors can mean a "strengthened" synapse (Figure 9-55C). If something is wrong with the genes that regulate synaptic strengthening, it is possible that this causes NMDA receptors to be hypoactive, leading to ineffective LTP and fewer AMPA receptors trafficking into the postsynaptic neuron. Such a synapse would be "weak," theoretically causing inefficient information processing in its circuit and thus symptoms of schizophrenia (Figure 9-55C).

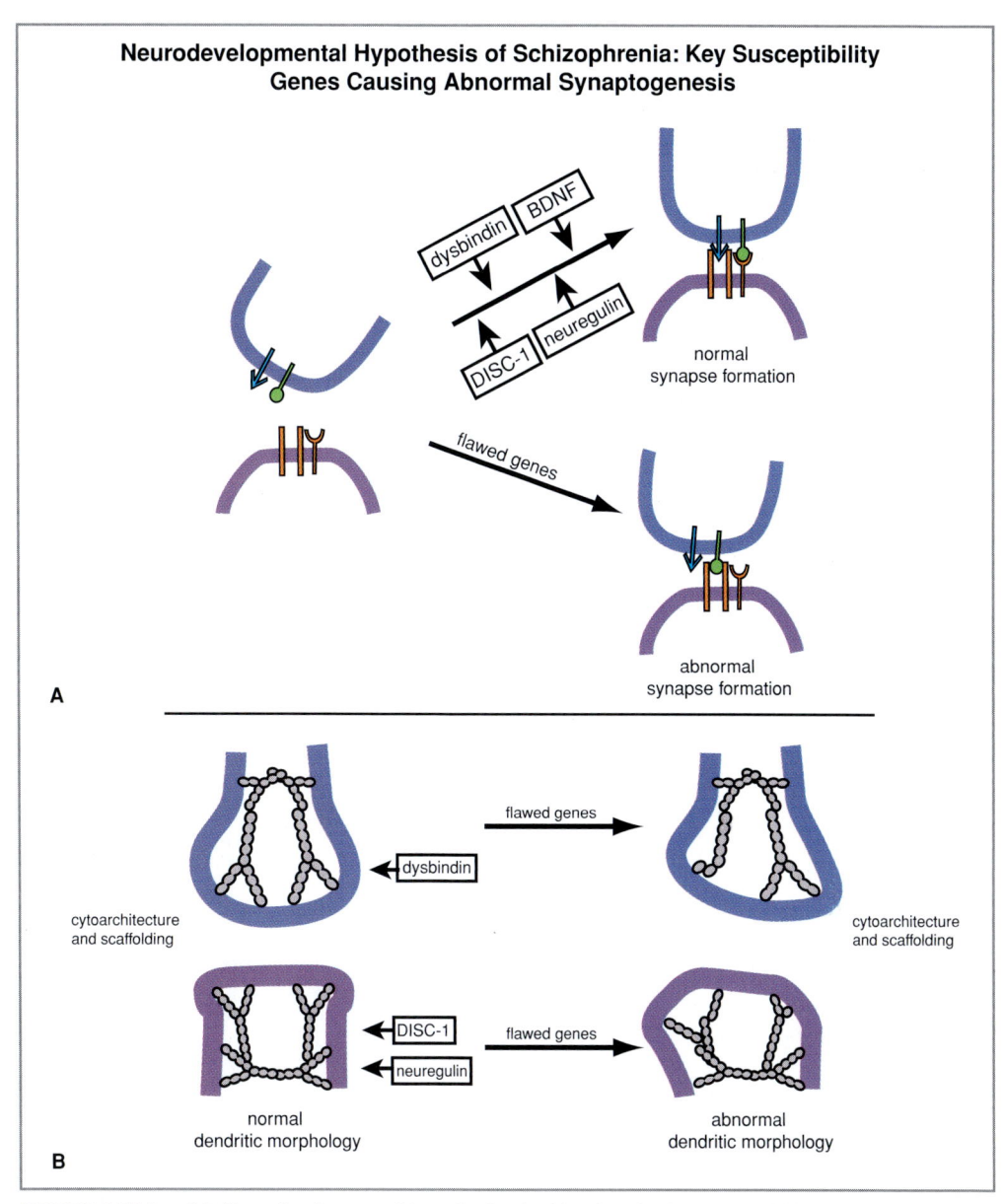

FIGURE 9-55A and B Neurodevelopmental hypothesis of schizophrenia: key susceptibility genes causing abnormal synaptogenesis, part 1. Dysbindin, brain-derived neurotrophic factor (BDNF), DISC-1 (disrupted in schizophrenia-1), and neuregulin are all involved in synapse formation. Any subtle molecular abnormalities in these genes could therefore lead to abnormal synapse formation (**A**). Specifically, abnormal genetic programming of dysbindin could affect synaptic cytoarchitecture and scaffolding, while abnormal genetic programming of DISC-1 and neuregulin could affect dendritic morphology; any of these could contribute to abnormal synapse formation and increased risk for schizophrenia (**B**).

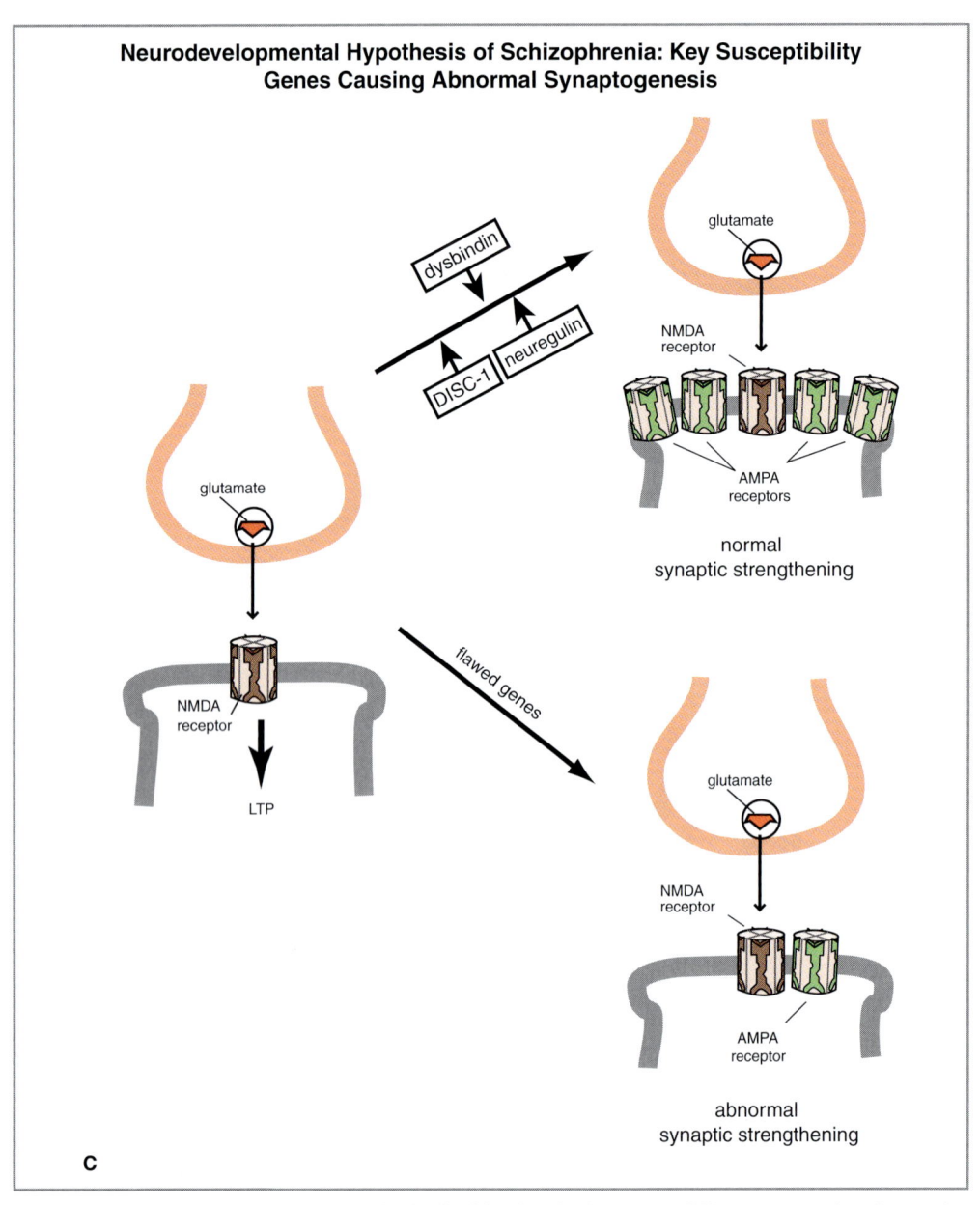

FIGURE 9-55C Neurodevelopmental hypothesis of schizophrenia: key susceptibility genes causing abnormal synaptogenesis, part 2. Dysbindin, DISC-1 (disrupted in schizophrenia-1), and neuregulin are all involved in "strengthening" of glutamate synapses. Under normal circumstances, N-methyl-d-aspartate (NMDA) receptors in active glutamate synapses trigger long-term potentiation (LTP), which leads to structural and functional changes of the synapse to make it more efficient, or "strengthened." In particular, this process leads to an increased number of alpha-amino-3-hydroxy-5-methyl-4-isoxazolepropionic acid (AMPA) receptors, which are important for mediating glutamatergic neurotransmission. If the genes that regulate strengthening of glutamate synapses are abnormal, then this could cause hypofunctioning of NMDA receptors, with a resultant decrease in LTP and fewer AMPA receptors. This would theoretically lead to increased risk of developing schizophrenia, and these abnormal synapses could mediate the symptoms of schizophrenia.

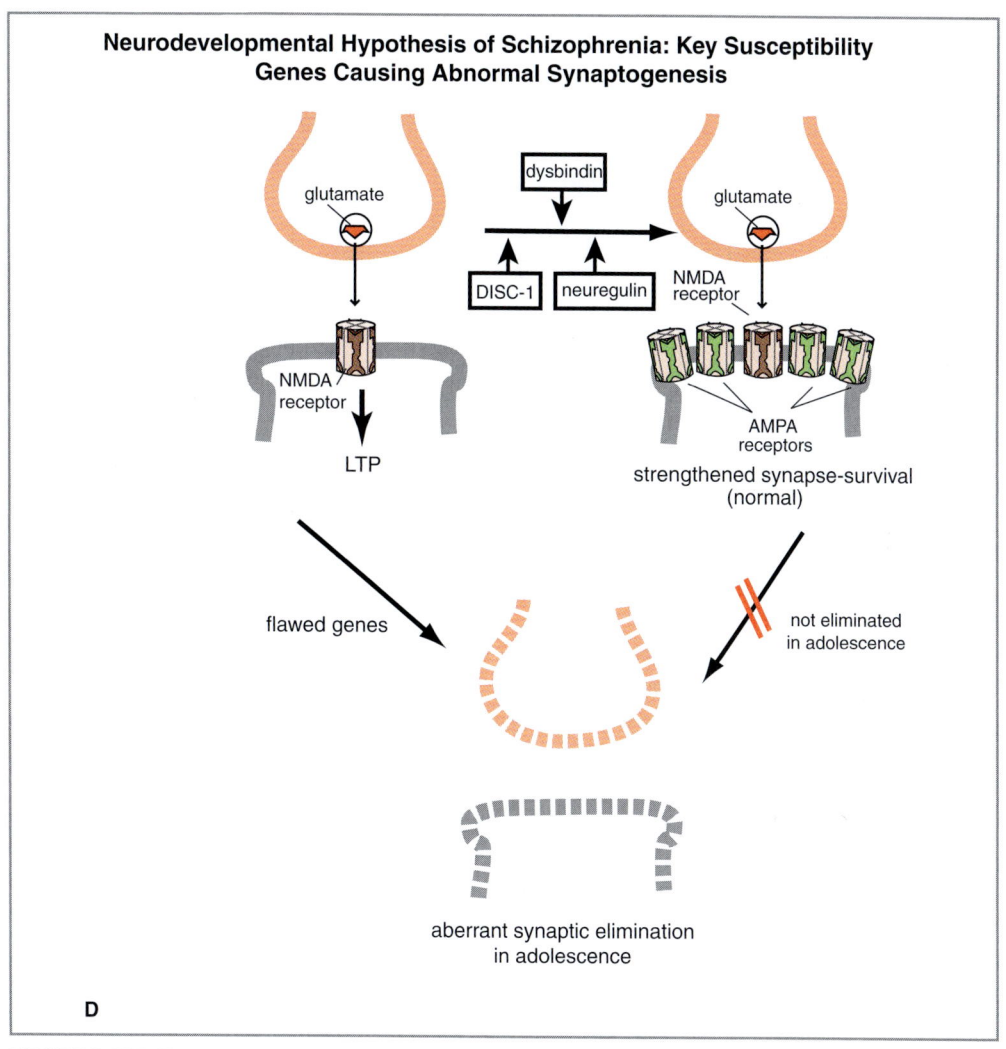

FIGURE 9-55D Neurodevelopmental hypothesis of schizophrenia: key susceptibility genes causing abnormal synaptogenesis, part 3. Strengthened synapses [for glutamate, synapses with efficient N-methyl-d-aspartate (NMDA) neurotransmission and multiple alpha-amino-3-hydroxy-5-methyl-4-isoxazolepropionic acid (AMPA) receptors] are more likely to survive than weak synapses. If the genes that regulate strengthening of glutamate synapses are abnormal, then not only might these synapses be weak but they also may be at increased risk for elimination, especially during adolescence, when there is massive restructuring of the synapses in the brain.

Furthermore, the "strength" of a synapse is likely to determine whether it is eliminated or maintained (Figure 9-55D). Specifically, "strong" synapses with efficient NMDA neurotransmission and many AMPA receptors survive, whereas "weak" synapses with few AMPA receptors may be targets for elimination (Figure 9-55D). This normally shapes the brain's circuits so that the most critical synapses are not only strengthened but also enabled to survive the selection process, keeping the most efficient and most frequently utilized synapses while eliminating those that are inefficient and rarely utilized. However, if critical synapses are not adequately strengthened in schizophrenia, it could lead to their

Four Key Genes That Regulate NMDA Receptors

dysbindin

neuregulin

DAOA
D-amino acid
oxidase activator

DISC-1
disrupted in
schizophrenia-1

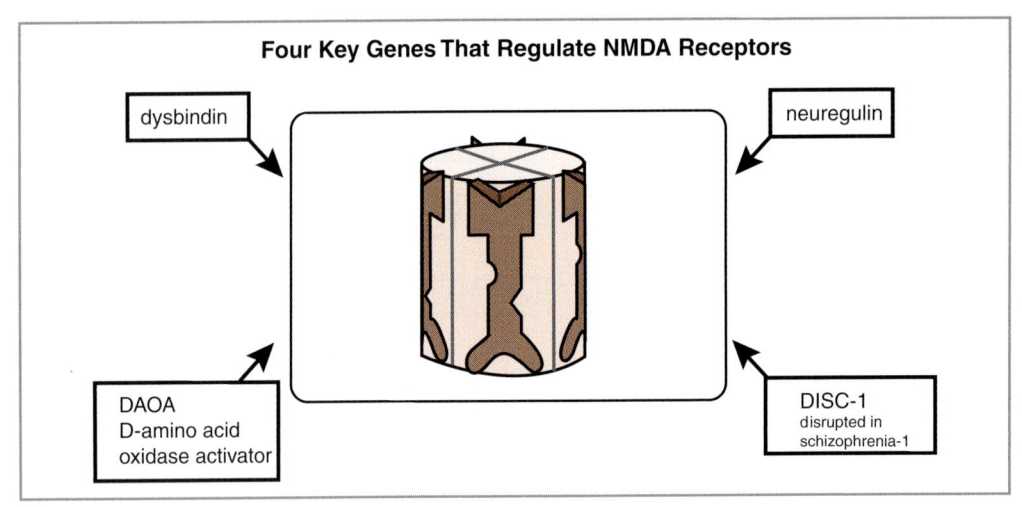

FIGURE 9-56 **Dysbindin, neuregulin, DISC-1 and DAOA.** Four key genes that regulate N-methyl-d-aspartate (NMDA) receptors are dysbindin, neuregulin, DISC-1 (disrupted in schizophrenia-1), and d-amino acid oxidase activator (DAOA).

elimination, disrupting information flow from circuits now deprived of synaptic connections where communication needs to be efficient (Figure 9-55D).

Competitive elimination of "weak" but critical synapses during adolescence could even explain why schizophrenia has onset at this time. Normally, almost half of the brain's synapses are eliminated in adolescence (discussed in Chapter 2 and illustrated in Figure 2-38). If abnormalities in genes for dysbindin, neuregulin, and/or DISC-1 lead to the failure of critical synapses to be strengthened, these critical synapses may be mistakenly eliminated during adolescence, with disastrous consequences – namely, the onset of symptoms of schizophrenia.

It is possible that "the die is cast" much earlier, due to aberrant neuronal selection, migration, and connections that remain silent until adolescence. However, in the late teens to twenties, abnormal synaptic restructuring due to elimination of necessary synapses that are not adequately strengthened could unmask neurodevelopmental problems that were previously hidden. To add insult to injury, ongoing problems in synaptic strengthening throughout adulthood in a schizophrenic patient may lead to perpetual elimination of critical synapses, causing the formation of new symptoms or exacerbation of ongoing symptoms due to circuits with progressively and unremittingly aberrant synaptogenesis.

Convergence of susceptibility genes for schizophrenia upon glutamate synapses
Many of the known susceptibility genes for schizophrenia (Table 9-12) regulate not only synaptogenesis at glutamate synapses (Figure 9-53), but also many other functions linked to glutamate neurotransmission, such as the NMDA receptor (Figure 9-56).

For example, the gene for DAOA (d-amino acid oxidase activator) codes for a protein that activates the enzyme DAO (d-amino acid oxidase) (Figures 9-56 and 9-57). We have previously discussed how DAO degrades the cotransmitter d-serine, which acts at glutamate synapses and at NMDA receptors (Figure 9-35). DAOA activates this enzyme (Figure 9-57A); therefore abnormalities in the gene for DAOA would be expected to alter the metabolism of d-serine. This, in turn, would alter glutamate neurotransmission at NMDA receptors (Figure 9-57A).

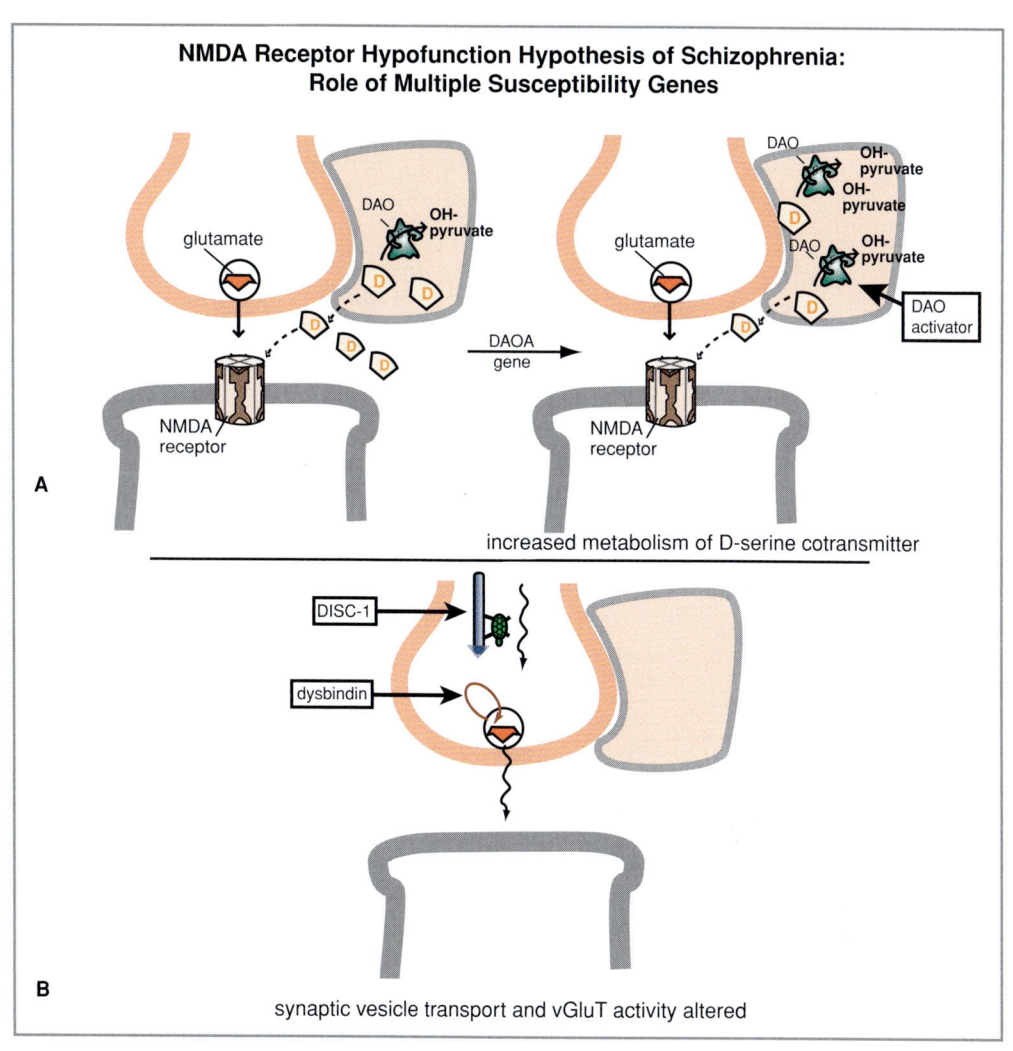

FIGURE 9-57A and B NMDA receptor hypofunction hypothesis of schizophrenia: role of multiple susceptibility genes, part 1. (**A**) d-amino acid oxidase activator (DAOA) is a protein that activates the enzyme d-amino acid oxidase (DAO). DAO converts d-serine into OH-pyruvate (on the left). Thus, abnormalities in the gene for DAOA could lead to abnormal functioning of the enzyme DAO, and this would change the metabolism of d-serine. Changes in the availability of d-serine would affect glutamate neurotransmission at N-methyl-d-aspartate (NMDA) receptors. If DAO activity were increased and d-serine levels thus decreased, this would lead to hypofunctioning of NMDA receptors (on the right). Thus, an abnormality in the gene for DAOA could increase risk for schizophrenia by altering the function of NMDA receptors. (**B**) Abnormalities in dysbindin and DISC-1 (disrupted in schizophrenia-1) could lead to alterations in the transport of synaptic vesicles into the presynaptic nerve terminal and could also lead to changes in the vesicular transport of glutamate by the glutamate transporter (vGluT). Both would be predicted to cause changes in the presynaptic storage of glutamate, and these could alter the function of NMDA receptors during glutamate neurotransmission. Thus, abnormalities in dysbindin and/or DISC-1 could lead to hypofunctioning of NMDA receptors and increase the risk for schizophrenia.

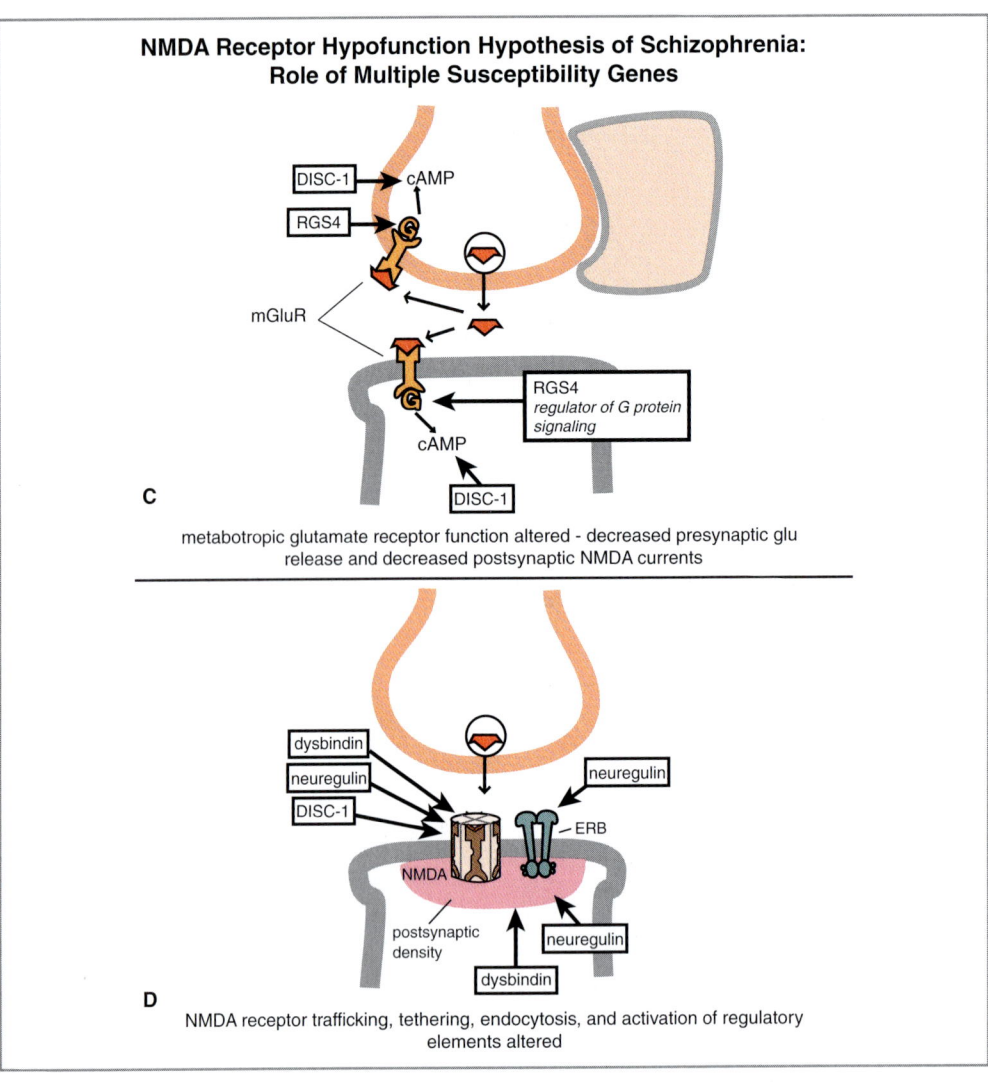

FIGURE 9-57C and D NMDA receptor hypofunction hypothesis of schizophrenia: role of multiple susceptibility genes, part 2. (**C**) Abnormalities in the genes for DISC-1 (disrupted in schizophrenia-1) could lead to disruptions of cyclic adenosine monophosphate (cAMP) signaling and consequently to alterations in the functioning of metabotropic glutamate receptors. Abnormalities in the gene that codes for the regulator of G protein signaling (RGS4) could also alter metabotropic glutamate receptor signaling. These changes would alter glutamate neurotransmission by decreasing the release of presynaptic glutamate, thus leading to a decrease in postsynaptic N-methyl-d-aspartate (NMDA) currents. Together, this would cause NMDA receptor hypofunctioning, which could increase the risk for schizophrenia. (**D**) Abnormalities in dysbindin, neuregulin, and/or DISC-1 could lead to alterations in NMDA receptor trafficking, tethering, endocytosis, and activation of postsynaptic regulatory elements. That would cause NMDA receptor hypofunctioning and could increase the risk for developing schizophrenia.

Dysbindin regulates the activity of vGluT, the vesicular transporter for glutamate (Figure 9-57B). DISC-1 affects the transport of synaptic vesicles into presynaptic glutamate nerve terminals (Figure 9-57B) and also regulates cAMP signaling, which would affect the functions of glutamate neurotransmission mediated by metabotropic glutamate receptors (Figure 9-57C). Another schizophrenia susceptibility gene is RGS4 (regulator of G protein signaling) (Table 9-12), and this gene product also impacts metabotropic glutamate receptor signaling through the G protein – coupled signal transduction system (Figure 9-57C).

Finally, numerous susceptibility genes regulate various elements of NMDA receptor – mediated signaling (Figure 9-57D). Dysbindin, neuregulin, and DISC-1 all affect NMDA receptor number by altering NMDA receptor trafficking to the postsynaptic membrane, NMDA receptor tethering within that membrane, and NMDA receptor endocytosis, which cycles receptors out of the postsynaptic membrane to remove them (Figure 9-57D). Both dysbindin and neuregulin affect the formation and function of the postsynaptic density, a set of proteins that interact with the postsynaptic membrane to provide both structural and functional regulatory elements for neurotransmission and for NMDA receptors (Figure 9-57D). Neuregulin also activates an ERB signaling system that is colocalized with NMDA receptors (Figure 9-57D). This signaling system is a member of the receptor tyrosine kinase and neurotrophin signal transduction system discussed in Chapter 3 and illustrated in Figure 3-11. These ERB receptors also interact with the postsynaptic density and may be involved in mediating the neuroplasticity triggered by NMDA receptors (Figure 9-57D).

Thus, there is a powerful convergence of the known susceptibility genes for schizophrenia upon connectivity, synaptogenesis, and neurotransmission at glutamate synapses and specifically at NMDA receptors (Figures 9-55C and D, 9-56, 9-57, and 9-58). These observations strongly support the hypothesis of NMDA receptor hypofunction as a plausible theory for schizophrenia. Genes that code for any number of subtle molecular abnormalities linked to NMDA receptor function in specific brain circuits theoretically create inefficient information processing at glutamate synapses, which can produce the symptoms of schizophrenia. If enough of these genetically mediated abnormalities occur simultaneously in a permissive environment, the syndrome of schizophrenia could be the result.

What are the candidate susceptibility genes for schizophrenia and how do they affect the NMDA receptor? Several of these are listed in Table 9-12 and many are shown in Figure 9-58. Clearly, numerous susceptibility genes can affect glutamate and its cotransmitter d-serine directly (e.g., DISC-1, neuregulin, dysbindin, DAOA, RGS4); their hypothesized actions on the glutamate system are illustrated in Figures 9-53 through 9-58. In addition, a number of other neurotransmitters such as dopamine, serotonin, GABA, and acetylcholine also affect the NMDA receptor, not only by direct interaction with glutamate neurons via brain circuits that utilize these other neurotransmitters but also by virtue of the fact that several of the genes that affect glutamate (e.g., neuregulin, RGS4) also affect these other neurotransmitters (Figure 9-58). Additional susceptibility genes may modulate these other neurotransmitter systems, leading to their aberrant modulation of NMDA plasticity and thus contributing to the genetic risk for schizophrenia. Some of these other genes regulate the receptors, enzymes, signaling molecules, and synapses for serotonin, dopamine, and acetylcholine (Table 9-12 and Figure 9-58). With sufficient combinations of directly and indirectly acting genetic influences, the NMDA receptor may not function properly, become hypofunctional, and – in addition to causing the changes in neuronal activity within brain circuits already described (see Figures 9-39 through 9-42) – also cause abnormal

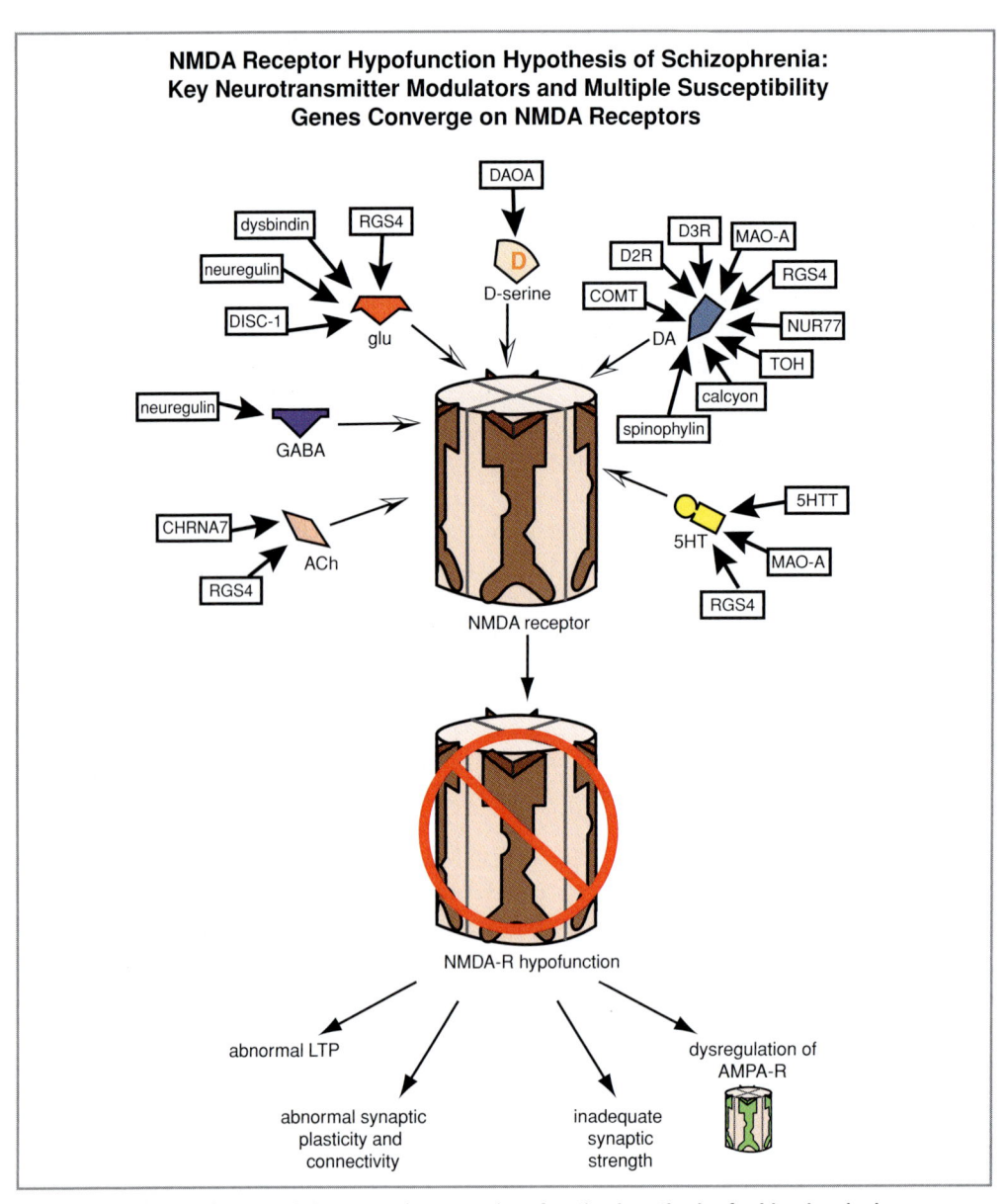

FIGURE 9-58 NMDA (N-methyl-d-aspartate) receptor hypofunction hypothesis of schizophrenia: key neurotransmitter modulators and multiple susceptibility genes converge on NMDA receptors. There is a powerful convergence of susceptibility genes for schizophrenia upon the connectivity, synaptogenesis, and neurotransmission at glutamate synapses and specifically at NMDA receptors, supporting the NMDA receptor hypofunction hypothesis of schizophrenia. The specific hypothesized actions of four key genes shown here are illustrated in detail in Figure 9-57 [i.e., the susceptibility genes DAOA (d-amino acid oxidase activator), dysbindin, neuregulin, and DISC-1 (disrupted in schizophrenia-1)]. Additional susceptibility genes are also shown here, including those that affect various neurotransmitters involved in modulating glutamate and NMDA receptors, namely gamma-aminobutyric acid (GABA), acetylcholine (ACh), dopamine (DA) and serotonin (5HT). That is, abnormalities in genes for various neurotransmitters that regulate NMDA receptors could have additional downstream actions on glutamate functioning at NMDA receptors. Thus, genes that regulate these other neurotransmitters may also constitute susceptibility genes for schizophrenia. This includes genes that affect ACh, such as the genes for RGS4 (regulator of G protein signaling 4) and for CHRNA7 (the alpha-7 nicotinic cholinergic receptor subtype); genes that affect 5HT (RGS4 as well as the genes for the monoamine oxidase A,

long-term potentiation, abnormal synaptic plasticity and connectivity, dysregulation of AMPA receptors, and inadequate synaptic strength with those circuits (Figure 9-58).

The bottom line

Genetics studies in schizophrenia have identified a number of susceptibility genes that increase risk for schizophrenia but do not cause schizophrenia. Since the best-understood and most replicated of these genes are involved in neurodevelopment, neuronal connectivity, and synaptogenesis, most scientists now believe that schizophrenia is caused by various possible combinations of many different genes plus stressors from the environment conspiring to cause abnormal neurodevelopment. Genetic and pharmacological evidence in schizophrenia also points to abnormal neurotransmission at glutamate synapses, possibly involving hypofunctional NMDA receptors. Several new therapies that target NMDA receptors are being tested, and new treatments for schizophrenia are discussed in Chapter 10.

Neuroimaging circuits in schizophrenia

Functional imaging of circuits in patients with schizophrenia suggests that information processing is abnormal in key brain areas linked to specific symptoms of this disorder. For example, schizophrenia is characterized by cognitive symptoms that are theoretically linked to information processing by circuits that involve the dorsolateral prefrontal cortex (DLPFC). The n-back test can be used to activate the DLPFC (Figure 9-59). This is also discussed in Chapter 8 and illustrated in Figures 8-8 through 8-10.

Some studies show that activation of the prefrontal cortex is low in schizophrenia, but other studies show that it is high (Figure 9-60). The best explanation for this may be that prefrontal cortical dysfunction in schizophrenia is likely to be more complicated than just "up" (hyperactivation) or "down" (hypoactivation) but might be better characterized as "out of tune." Tuning of prefrontal pyramidal neurons is discussed in Chapter 7 and illustrated in Figures 7-25 and 7-26. According to this concept, either too much or too little activation of neuronal activity in the prefrontal cortex is suboptimal and can potentially be symptomatic.

How can circuits in schizophrenia be both hyper- and hypoactive? Schizophrenic patients appear to utilize greater prefrontal resources in performing cognitive tasks and yet achieve lower accuracy because they have cognitive impairment despite their best efforts. To perform near normally, schizophrenic patients engage the DLPFC, but they do so inefficiently, recruiting greater neural resources and hyperactivating the DLPFC (Figure 9-60). When they are performing poorly, schizophrenic patients do not appropriately engage and sustain the DLPFC and thus show hypoactivation (Figure 9-60). Thus, DLPFC circuits in schizophrenic patients can either be underactive and hypofrontal or overactive and inefficient.

FIGURE 9-58 (Cont.) or MAO-A); and the genes for the serotonin transporter (5HTT); finally, multiple genes that affect DA (RGS4, MAO-A), and also genes for the enzymes catechol-O-methyl-transferase (COMT) and tyrosine hydroxylase (TOH); genes for the D2- and D3-dopamine receptors (D2R and D3R), and finally genes for the regulatory proteins spinophylin and calcyon. The idea is that any of these susceptibility genes could conspire to cause NMDA receptor hypofunction, which would lead to abnormal long-term potentiation (LTP), abnormal synaptic plasticity and connectivity, inadequate synaptic strength, and/or dysregulation of alpha-amino-3-hydroxy-5-methyl-4-isoxazolepropionic acid (AMPA) receptors. Any combination of sufficient genetic risk factors with sufficient stress or environmental risk will result in the susceptibility for schizophrenia to become manifest as the disease of schizophrenia with the presence of full syndrome symptoms.

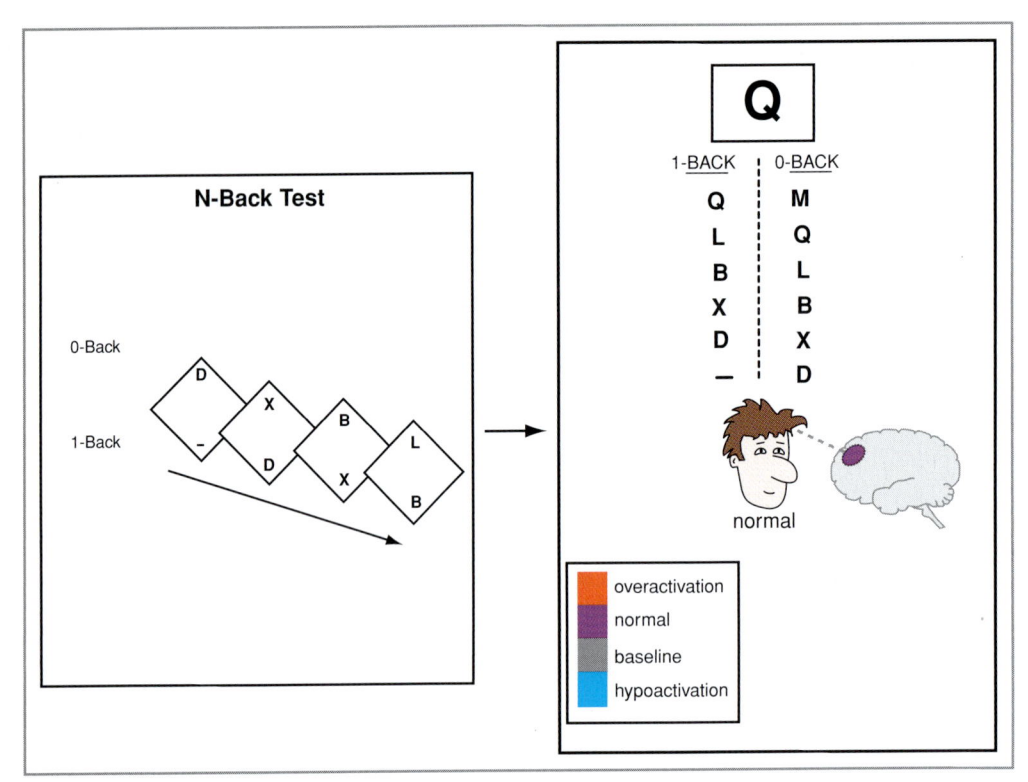

FIGURE 9-59 n-back test. Functional neuroimaging studies have suggested that information processing in schizophrenia is abnormal in certain brain regions. Information processing during cognitive tasks has been evaluated using the n-back test. In the 0-back variant of the test, participants view a number on a screen and then indicate what the number was. In the 1-back test, participants are shown a stimulus but do not respond; after viewing the second stimulus, the participant then pushes a button corresponding to the first stimulus. The "n" can be any number, with higher numbers associated with greater difficulty. Performing the n-back test results in activation of the dorsolateral prefrontal cortex (DLPFC), shown here by the DLPFC lit up as purple (normal activation). The degree of activation indicates how efficient the information processing is in DLPFC, with both overactivation and hypoactivation associated with inefficient information processing.

It is interesting to note that unaffected siblings of patients with schizophrenia may have the very same inefficient information processing in DLPFC that schizophrenic patients have (Figure 9-61). Although such unaffected siblings might have a mild degree of cognitive impairment, they do not share the full clinical phenotype of the syndrome of schizophrenia; however, neuroimaging reveals that they may share the same biological endophenotype of inefficient DLPFC functioning while performing cognitive tasks that characterizes their schizophrenic siblings (Figure 9-61). The unaffected siblings of a schizophrenic patient may thus share some of the susceptibility genes for schizophrenia with their affected sibling but not enough of these risk genes to have the full syndrome of schizophrenia itself. Functional neuroimaging has the potential of unmasking clinically silent biological endophenotypes in the unaffected siblings of schizophrenic patients who share some of the same risk genes, but do not have sufficient combinations of risk genes to develop the illness of schizophrenia. Functional neuroimaging also has the potential of unmasking clinically silent biological endophenotypes in presymptomatic patients destined to progress to the full schizophrenia syndrome. However, much further research is required to see if this will become clinically useful.

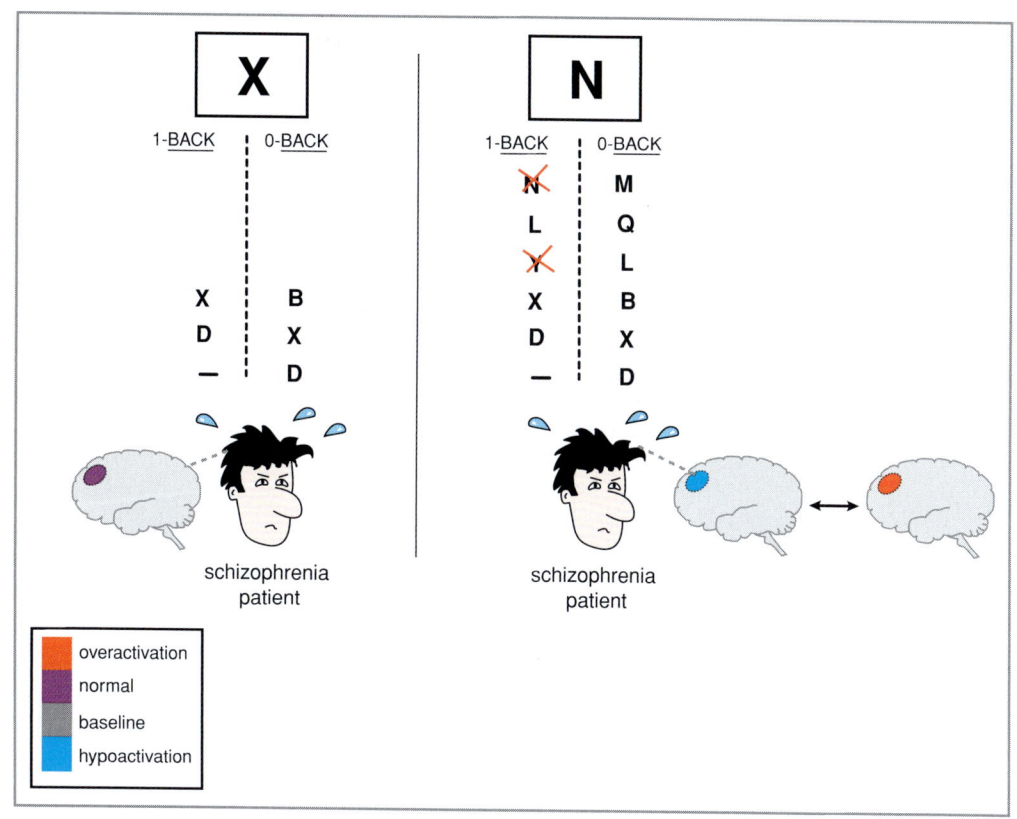

FIGURE 9-60 n-back test in schizophrenia. Patients with schizophrenia exhibit inefficient information processing during cognitive challenges such as the n-back test. To perform near normal, these individuals must recruit greater neuronal resources, resulting in hyperactivation of the dorsolateral prefrontal cortex (DLPFC). Under increased cognitive load, however, schizophrenic patients do not appropriately engage and sustain the DLPFC, with resultant hypoactivation.

Affective and negative symptoms of schizophrenia may involve other areas of the prefrontal cortex, such as orbital, medial, and ventral areas (see Figure 9-14). These brain areas, along with the amygdala, nucleus accumbens, and other regions, comprise a "ventral" system involved in emotional processing. This ventral system interacts with a "dorsal" system that includes the DLPFC and modulates the output from the ventral system (Figure 9-62).

The ventral system (Figure 9-62) includes orbital, ventral, and medial areas of prefrontal cortex (shown in Figure 9-14), amygdala (shown in Figure 9-63), and nucleus accumbens (shown in Figure 9-62) – brain regions that are all important for the identification and appraisal of emotional stimuli and for generating an appropriate emotional response. The dorsal system includes not just the DLPFC but also the hippocampus. This system marshals the cognitive resources necessary either to maintain the emotional response from the ventral system or to modulate it. The dorsal system selects an appropriate behavioral output in response not only to emotions but also to demands from the environment and from the individual's internal goals.

Schizophrenia has long been recognized as having impairments in the ability to identify and accurately interpret emotions from overt sources, including facial expressions. This may

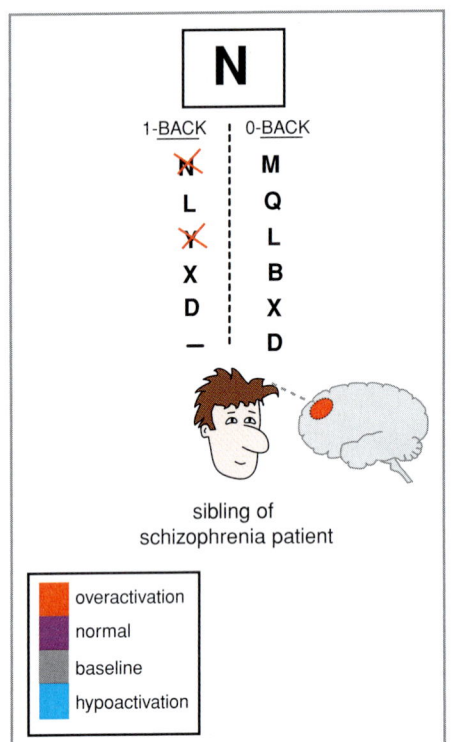

FIGURE 9-61 n-back test in sibling of schizophrenic. Because siblings share some of the same genes, the siblings of schizophrenic patients could inherit the genes that compromise the ability to process information without inheriting all the genes necessary for schizophrenia. Thus their cortical activation and cognitive performance may be abnormal, but they may not have any of the other features of schizophrenia.

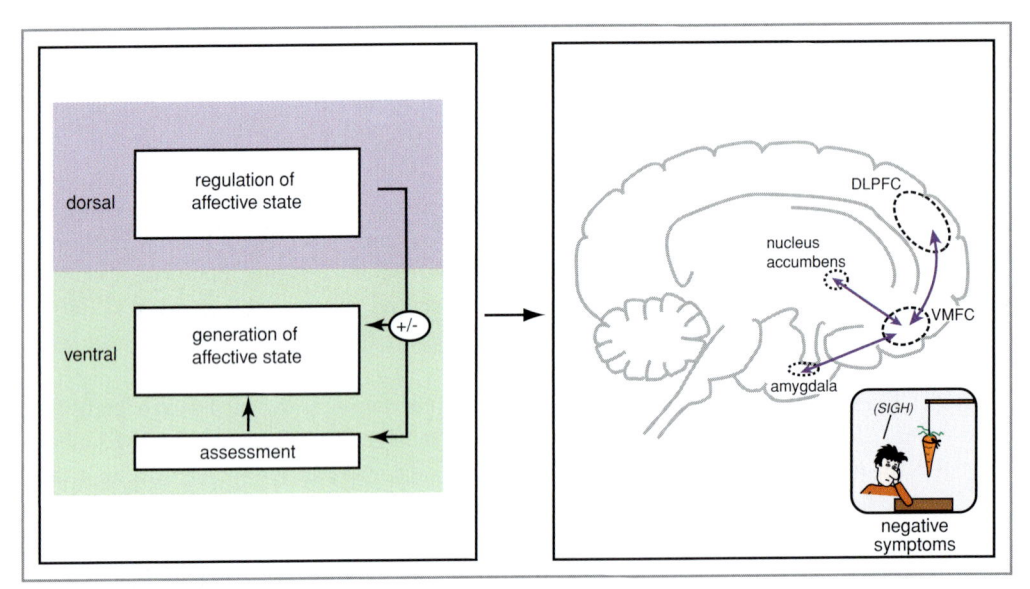

FIGURE 9-62 Dorsal versus ventral regulation of affect. Affective and negative symptoms of schizophrenia may be generated by a ventral system that includes the ventromedial prefrontal cortex (VMFC), nucleus accumbens, and amygdala and regulated by a dorsal system that includes the dorsolateral prefrontal cortex (DLPFC).

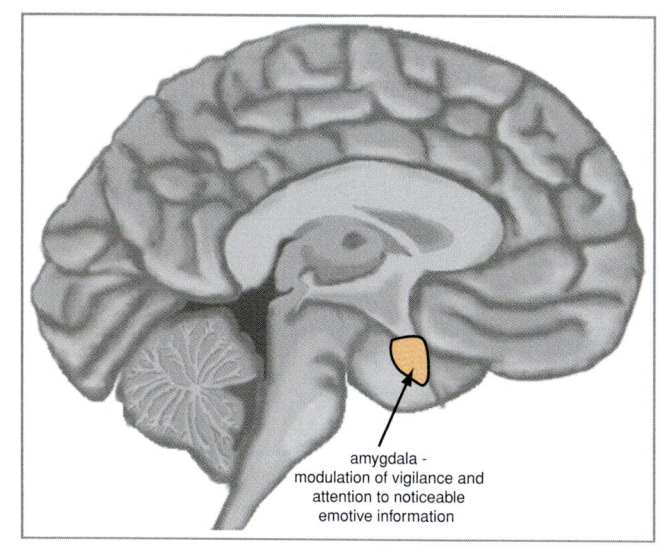

FIGURE 9-63 Amygdala. The amygdala is involved in modulation of vigilance, attention, and reactions to noticeable emotive information. Functional neuroimaging studies have examined activity in the amygdala to determine the efficiency of information processing in schizophrenic patients during exposure to emotional stimuli.

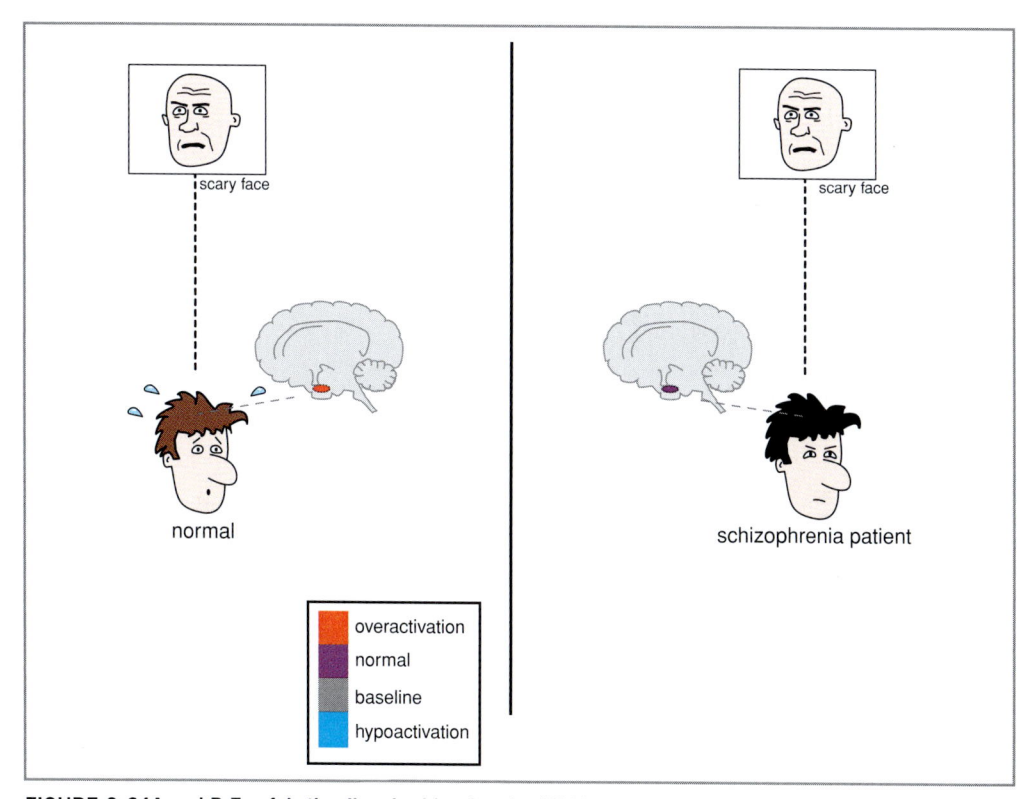

FIGURE 9-64A and B Fearful stimuli and schizophrenia. (**A**) Normally, exposure to an emotional stimulus, such as a scary face, causes hyperactivation in the amygdala. (**B**) Schizophrenic patients often have impairments in the ability to identify and interpret emotional stimuli. The underlying neurobiological explanation for this may be inefficient information processing within the ventral system. In this example, the amygdala is not appropriately engaged during exposure to an emotional stimulus.

Psychosis and Schizophrenia | 323

be due to inefficient information processing within the ventral system and can be measured by imaging the response of the amygdala (Figure 9-63) to emotional input, especially from facial expressions. The amygdala is normally activated by looking at scary, threatening faces or by assessing how happy or sad a face may be and while attempting to match the emotions of one face to another (Figure 9-64A). This is discussed in Chapter 8 and illustrated in Figures 8-11 through 8-13.

Whereas normals may activate the amygdala in response to scary or fearful or emotionally charged faces (Figure 9-64A), patients with schizophrenia may not (Figure 9-64B). This may represent distortion of reality as well as an impairment in recognizing negative emotions and in decoding negative emotions in schizophrenia. Failure to mount the "normal" emotional response to a scary face can also represent an inability to interpret social cues and may lead to distortions in judgment and reasoning in schizophrenia. Thus, these negative and affective symptoms of schizophrenia may be due in part to lack of emotional processing under circumstances when this should be occurring.

On the other hand, a neutral face or neutral stimulus may provoke little activation of the amygdala in a normal person (Figure 9-65A), yet an overreaction in a schizophrenic patient, who may mistakenly judge people negatively or conclude wrongly that another holds strong unfavorable impressions of him or her or may even be threatening (Figure 9-65B). The activation of emotional processing in the amygdala when it is inappropriate may accompany the symptom of paranoia and lead to impaired interpersonal functioning, including problems

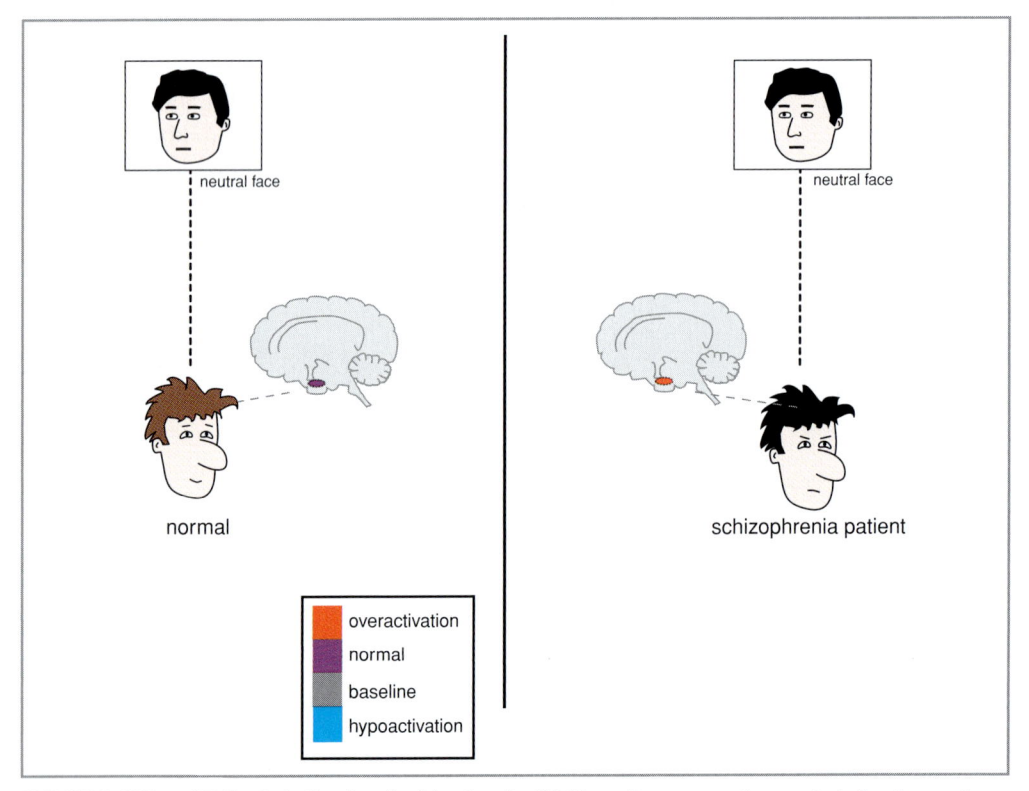

FIGURE 9-65A and B Neutral stimuli and schizophrenia. (**A**) Normally, exposure to a neutral stimulus, such as a neutral face, causes little activation of the amygdala. (**B**) Schizophrenic patients may mistakenly judge others as threatening, with associated inappropriate hyperactivation of the amygdala.

in social communication. Thus, schizophrenic patients may exhibit deficits in recognizing emotions, which may become manifest as either positive or negative symptoms of this disorder. The underlying biological endophenotype of amygdala activation (or lack of it) in the ventral emotional processing circuitry can be assessed with neuroimaging, whether the patient is experiencing these symptoms or not. Looking at the efficiency of emotional information processing may help clinicians identify and understand emotional symptoms that are difficult for schizophrenic patients to express.

Summary

This chapter has provided a clinical description of psychosis, with special emphasis on the psychotic illness schizophrenia. We have explained the dopamine hypothesis of schizophrenia, and the related NMDA receptor hypofunction hypothesis of schizophrenia, which are the major hypotheses for explaining the mechanism underlying positive, negative, cognitive, and affective symptoms of schizophrenia.

The major dopamine and glutamate pathways in the brain have been described. Overactivity of the mesolimbic dopamine system may mediate the positive symptoms of psychosis and may be linked to hypofunctioning NMDA glutamate receptors in the descending corticobrainstem glutamate pathway. Underactivity of the mesocortical dopamine system may mediate the negative, cognitive, and affective symptoms of schizophrenia and could also be linked to hypofunctioning NMDA receptors.

The synthesis, metabolism, reuptake, and receptors for both dopamine and glutamate have been described above. Dopamine-2 receptors are targets of all known antipsychotic drugs. NMDA glutamate receptors require interaction not only with the neurotransmitter glutamate but also with the cotransmitters glycine or d-serine.

Both the neurodegenerative hypothesis and the neurodevelopmental hypothesis of schizophrenia have been discussed. Although neurodegenerative events such as fetal brain insults or excitotoxicity may contribute to schizophrenia, current research points most strongly to a neurodevelopmental basis, mediated by a whole host of susceptibility genes that regulate neuronal connectivity and synapse formation. A great deal of genetic research converges on the possibility that abnormal formation of synapses – particularly those that utilize glutamate as neurotransmitter and those that function with NMDA receptors – is a central biological flaw in schizophrenia.

Malfunctioning neural circuits can be imaged in schizophrenic patients, including those in the dorsolateral prefrontal cortex linked to cognitive symptoms and those in the amygdala linked to symptoms of emotional dysregulation.

CHAPTER 10

Antipsychotic Agents

- What makes an antipsychotic conventional?
  - D2 receptor antagonism makes an antipsychotic conventional
  - Neurolepsis
  - Extrapyramidal symptoms (EPS) and tardive dyskinesia
  - Prolactin elevation
  - The dilemma of blocking D2 dopamine receptors in all dopamine pathways
  - Muscarinic cholinergic blocking properties of conventional antipsychotics
  - Other pharmacological properties of conventional antipsychotic drugs
  - Risks and benefits of long-term treatment with conventional antipsychotics
- What makes an antipsychotic atypical?
  - Serotonergic neurotransmission and serotonin dopamine antagonism
  - Serotonin synthesis and termination of action
  - Serotonin receptors
  - 5HT1A and 5HT2A receptors have opposite actions in regulating dopamine release
  - 5HT2A antagonism makes an antipsychotic atypical
  - Rapid dissociation of D2 antagonism makes an antipsychotic atypical
  - D2 partial agonism (DPA) makes an antipsychotic atypical
  - 5HT1A partial agonism (SPA) actions make an antipsychotic atypical
- Receptor binding properties and pharmacokinetics of antipsychotics
  - Links between antipsychotic binding properties and clinical actions
  - Cardiometabolic risk and antipsychotics
  - Sedation and antipsychotics
  - Antipsychotic pharmacokinetics
  - Pharmacological properties of individual antipsychotics
- Antipsychotics in clinical practice
  - Schizophrenia symptom pharmacies
  - The art of switching antipsychotics
  - Combos and polypharmacy
- Future treatments for schizophrenia
  - Presymptomatic and prodromal treatments for schizophrenia: putting the cart before the horse or preventing disease progression?
  - Glutamate-linked mechanisms and new treatments for schizophrenia
  - Glutamate agonists or antagonists for schizophrenia?
  - Novel serotonin- and dopamine-linked mechanisms
  - Acetylcholine-linked mechanisms
  - Peptide-linked mechanisms
  - Future combination chemotherapies for schizophrenia and other psychotic disorders
- Summary

This chapter explores antipsychotic drugs with an emphasis on treatments for schizophrenia. These treatments include not only conventional antipsychotic drugs but also the newer atypical antipsychotic drugs, which have largely replaced the older conventional agents in many countries. Atypical antipsychotics are also used as mood stabilizers for the manic, depressed, and maintenance phases of bipolar disorder in both adults and in children, but this is discussed in Chapter 13 on mood stabilizers. Atypical antipsychotics have many other "off-label" uses, from augmentation of antidepressants in treatment-resistant depression and of anxiolytics in treatment-resistant anxiety disorders to treatment of psychosis and behavioral disturbances in Alzheimer's disease and other dementias. The use of atypical antipsychotics for indications other than the treatment of psychosis and schizophrenia is discussed in chapters dealing with those other disorders. Here we will discuss the use of conventional and atypical antipsychotics for the treatment of schizophrenia and also take a look into the future by discussing numerous new drugs under development for schizophrenia.

Antipsychotic drugs exhibit possibly the most complex pharmacological mechanisms of any drug class in the field of clinical psychopharmacology. To assist the reader in mastering this critical area of therapeutics in psychopharmacology, we have organized this chapter into five sections: first, the classic conventional antipsychotics; second, the contrasting pharmacological properties that make an antipsychotic atypical; third, a discussion of the multiple receptor actions of antipsychotics as well as their pharmacokinetics, comparing and contrasting the properties of the various individual atypical antipsychotics; fourth, a practical analysis of how these agents are put to use in clinical practice; and fifth, a discussion of new therapeutics for schizophrenia currently in development.

The reader is referred to standard reference manuals and textbooks for practical prescribing information, such as drug doses, because this chapter emphasizes basic pharmacological concepts regarding mechanisms of action and not practical issues such as how to prescribe these drugs (for that information, see, for example, S. M. Stahl, *Essential Psychopharmacology: The Prescriber's Guide*, which is a companion to this book). The pharmacological concepts developed here should, however, help the reader understand the rationale for how to use antipsychotic agents based on their interactions with different neurotransmitter systems. Such interactions can often explain both the therapeutic actions and the side effects of antipsychotic medications and thus can provide very helpful background information for prescribers of these therapeutic agents.

What makes an antipsychotic conventional?

In this section we will discuss the pharmacological properties of the first drugs that were proven to treat schizophrenia effectively. These drugs are usually called conventional antipsychotics, but they are sometimes also called classic or "typical" antipsychotics. The earliest effective treatments for schizophrenia and other psychotic illnesses arose from serendipitous clinical observations more than 50 years ago, rather than from scientific knowledge of the neurobiologic basis of psychosis or of the mechanism of action of effective antipsychotic agents. Thus, the first antipsychotic drugs were discovered by accident in the 1950s, when a drug with antihistamine properties (chlorpromazine) was observed to have antipsychotic effects when tested in schizophrenic patients. Chlorpromazine indeed has antihistaminic activity, but its therapeutic actions in schizophrenia are not mediated by this property. Once chlorpromazine was observed to be an effective antipsychotic agent, it was tested experimentally to uncover its mechanism of antipsychotic action.

What Makes an Antipsychotic Conventional?
D2 Antagonist Actions

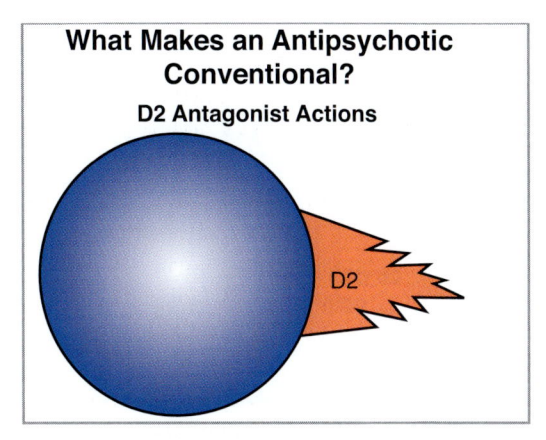

FIGURE 10-1 D2 antagonist. Conventional antipsychotics, also called first-generation antipsychotics or typical antipsychotics, share the primary pharmacological property of D2 antagonism, which is responsible not only for their antipsychotic efficacy but also for many of their side effects. Shown here is an icon representing this single pharmacological action.

Early in the testing process, chlorpromazine and other antipsychotic agents were all found to cause "neurolepsis," an extreme form of slowness or absence of motor movements as well as behavioral indifference in experimental animals. The original antipsychotics were first discovered largely by their ability to produce this effect in experimental animals and are thus sometimes called "neuroleptics." A human counterpart of neurolepsis is also caused by these original (i.e., conventional) antipsychotic drugs and is characterized by psychomotor slowing, emotional quieting, and affective indifference.

D2-receptor antagonism makes an antipsychotic conventional

By the 1970s, it was widely recognized that the key pharmacological property of all neuroleptics with antipsychotic properties was their ability to block dopamine-2 (D2) receptors (Figure 10-1). This action has proven to be responsible not only for the antipsychotic efficacy of conventional antipsychotic drugs but also for most of their undesirable side effects, including neurolepsis.

The therapeutic actions of conventional antipsychotic drugs are due to blockade of D2 receptors, specifically in the mesolimbic dopamine pathway (Figure 10-2). This has the effect of reducing the hyperactivity in this pathway, which is postulated to cause the positive symptoms of psychosis, as discussed in Chapter 9 (see Figures 9-25 and 9-26). All conventional antipsychotics reduce positive psychotic symptoms about equally in schizophrenic patients studied in large multicenter trials. That is not to say that one individual patient might not occasionally respond better to one conventional antipsychotic agent than another, but there is no consistent difference in antipsychotic efficacy among the conventional antipsychotic agents. A list of many conventional antipsychotic drugs is given in Table 10-1.

Unfortunately it is not possible to block just these D2 receptors in the mesolimbic DA pathway with conventional antipsychotics because antipsychotic drugs are delivered throughout the entire brain after oral ingestion. Thus, conventional antipsychotics will seek out every D2 receptor throughout the brain and block them all (see Figures 10-3 through 10-7). This leads to a high "cost of doing business" in order to get the mesolimbic D2 receptors blocked for the treatment of positive symptoms.

Neurolepsis

D2 receptors in the mesolimbic dopamine system are postulated to mediate not only the positive symptoms of psychosis but also the normal reward system of the brain, and the nucleus accumbens is widely considered to be the "pleasure center" of the brain. It may be the final common pathway of all reward and reinforcement, including not only normal

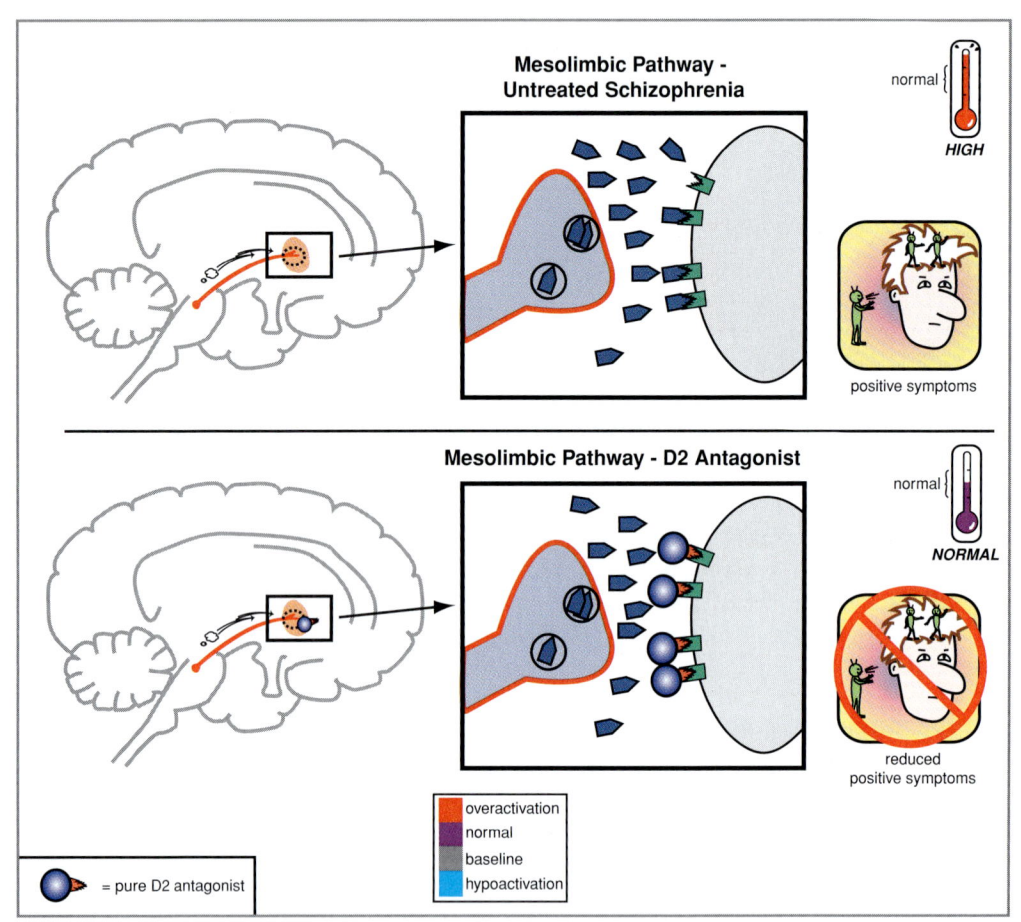

FIGURE 10-2 Mesolimbic dopamine pathway and D2 antagonists. In untreated schizophrenia, the mesolimbic dopamine pathway is hypothesized to be hyperactive, indicated here by the pathway appearing red as well as by the excess dopamine in the synapse. This leads to positive symptoms such as delusions and hallucinations. Administration of a D2 antagonist, such as a conventional antipsychotic, blocks dopamine from binding to the D2 receptor, which reduces hyperactivity in this pathway and thereby reduces positive symptoms as well.

reward (such as the pleasure of eating good food, orgasm, listening to music) but also the artificial reward of substance abuse. If D2 receptors are stimulated in some parts of the mesolimbic pathway, this can lead to the experience of pleasure. Thus if D2 receptors in the mesolimbic system are blocked, this may not only reduce positive symptoms but also block reward mechanisms, leaving patients apathetic, anhedonic, lacking motivation, and with reduced interest and joy from social interactions – a state very similar to that due to the negative symptoms of psychosis and sometimes called secondary negative symptoms.

Antipsychotics also block D2 receptors in the mesocortical DA pathway (Figure 10-3), where DA may already be deficient in schizophrenia (see Figures 9-27 through 9-29). This can cause or worsen negative and cognitive symptoms. However, since the density of D2 receptors in the cortex is much lower than in other brain areas, the lack of pleasure and negative symptoms produced by antipsychotic drugs may be more closely linked to profound blockade of D2 receptors in the mesolimbic dopamine system than to blockade of D2 receptors in the mesocortical dopamine system. An adverse behavioral state can be produced by conventional antipsychotics and is sometimes called the "neuroleptic-induced deficit

TABLE 10-1 Some conventional antipsychotics still in use

Generic Name	Trade Name
chlorpromazine	Thorazine
cyamemazine	Tercian
flupenthixol	Depixol
fluphenazine	Prolixin
haloperidol	Haldol
loxapine	Loxitane
mesoridazine	Serentil
molindone	Moban
perphenazine	Trilafon
pimozide	Orap
pipothiazine	Piportil
sulpiride	Dolmatil
thioridazine	Mellaril
thiothixene	Navane
trifluoperazine	Stelazine
zuclopenthixol	Clopixol

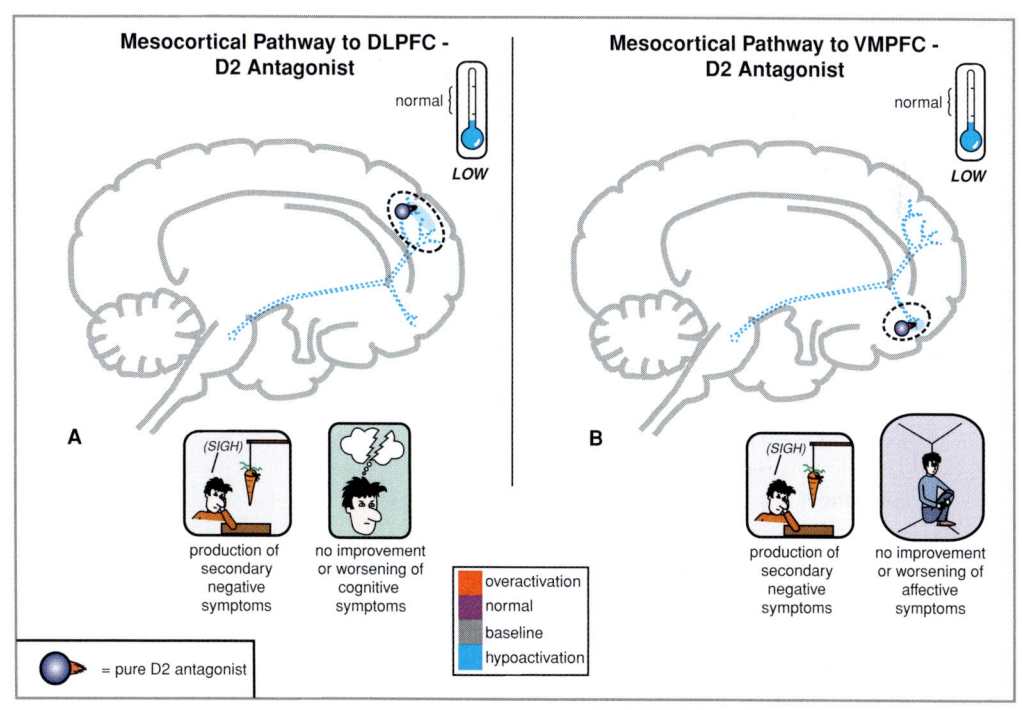

FIGURE 10-3 Mesocortical dopamine pathway and D2 antagonists. In untreated schizophrenia, the mesocortical dopamine pathways to dorsolateral prefrontal cortex (DLPFC) and to ventromedial prefrontal cortex (VMPFC) are hypothesized to be hypoactive, indicated here by the pathways appearing blue. This hypoactivity is related to cognitive symptoms (in the DLPFC), negative symptoms (in the DLPFC and VMPFC), and affective symptoms of schizophrenia (in the VMPFC). Administration of a D2 antagonist could further reduce activity in this pathway and thus not only not improve such symptoms but actually potentially worsen them.

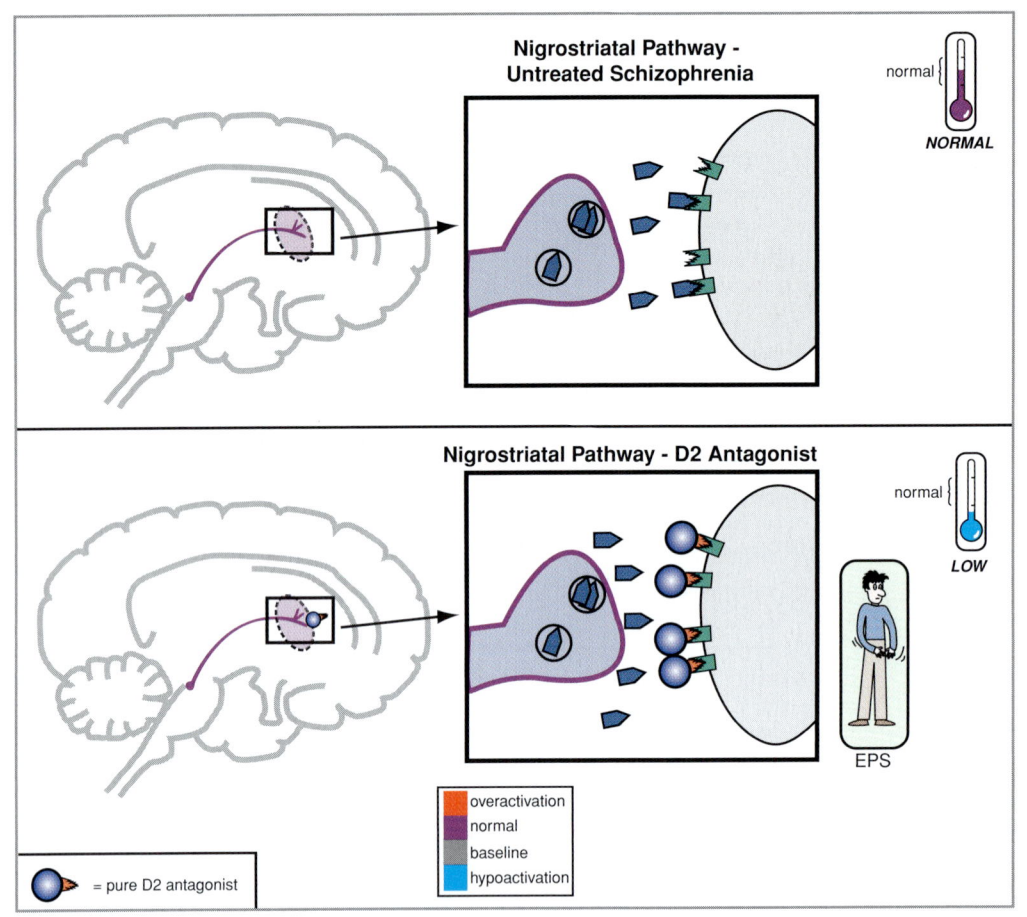

FIGURE 10-4 **Nigrostriatal dopamine pathway and D2 antagonists.** The nigrostriatal dopamine pathway is theoretically unaffected in untreated schizophrenia, illustrated here by the purple hue of the pathway. However, blockade of D2 receptors, as with a conventional antipsychotic, prevents dopamine from binding there and can cause motor side effects that are often collectively termed extrapyramidal symptoms (EPS).

syndrome" because it looks so much like the negative symptoms produced by schizophrenia itself and is reminiscent of neurolepsis in animals.

Extrapyramidal symptoms (EPS) and tardive dyskinesia

When D2 receptors are blocked in the nigrostriatal DA pathway, it produces disorders of movement that can appear very much like those of Parkinson's disease; that is why this is sometimes called drug-induced parkinsonism (Figure 10-4). Since the nigrostriatal pathway is part of the extrapyramidal nervous system, these motor side effects associated with blocking D2 receptors in this part of the brain are sometimes also called extrapyramidal symptoms, or EPS.

Worse yet, if these D2 receptors in the nigrostriatal DA pathway are blocked chronically (Figure 10-5), they can produce a hyperkinetic movement disorder known as tardive dyskinesia. This causes facial and tongue movements, like constant chewing, tongue protrusions, and facial grimacing as well as limb movements that can be quick, jerky, or choreiform ("dancing"). Tardive dyskinesia is thus caused by long-term administration of conventional

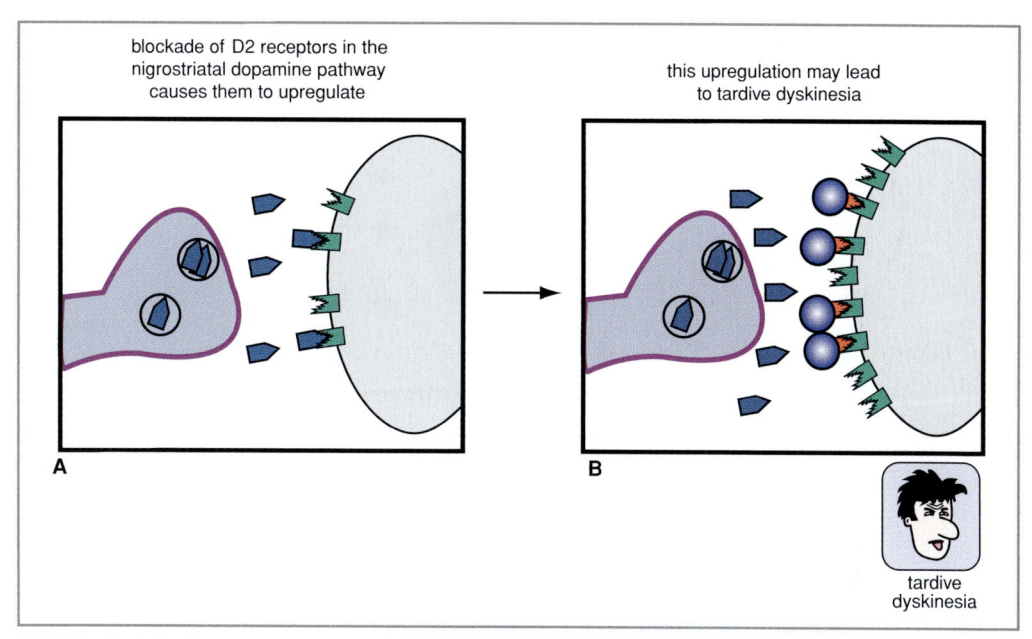

FIGURE 10-5 Tardive dyskinesia. Long-term blockade of D2 receptors in the nigrostriatal dopamine pathway can cause upregulation of those receptors, which may lead to a hyperkinetic motor condition known as tardive dyskinesia, characterized by facial and tongue movements (e.g., tongue protrusions, facial grimaces, chewing) as well as quick, jerky limb movements. This upregulation may be the consequence of the neuron's futile attempt to overcome drug-induced blockade of its dopamine receptors.

antipsychotics and is thought to be mediated by changes, sometimes irreversible, in the D2 receptors of the nigrostriatal DA pathway. Specifically, these receptors are hypothesized to become supersensitive or to "upregulate" (i.e., increase in number), perhaps in a futile attempt to overcome drug-induced blockade of these receptors (Figure 10-5).

About 5 percent of patients maintained on conventional antipsychotics will develop tardive dyskinesia every year (i.e., about 25 percent of patients by 5 years) – not a very encouraging prospect for a lifelong illness starting in the early twenties. The risk of developing tardive dyskinesia in elderly subjects may be as high as 25 percent within the first year of exposure to conventional antipsychotics. Thus, the number of patients that a psychopharmacologist needs to treat in order to harm 1 patient with tardive dyskinesia may be only 4 young patients over 5 years of conventional antipsychotic treatment or only 4 elderly patients over 1 year of conventional antipsychotic treatment. Statisticians sometimes call this the "number needed to harm."

If the D2 receptor blockade is removed early enough, tardive dyskinesia may reverse. This reversal is theoretically due to a "resetting" of these receptors by an appropriate decrease in the number or sensitivity of D2 receptors in the nigrostriatal pathway once the drug that had been blocking these receptors is removed. However, after long-term treatment, the D2 receptors apparently cannot or do not reset back to normal, even when conventional antipsychotic drugs are discontinued. This leads to irreversible tardive dyskinesia, which continues whether conventional antipsychotic drugs are administered or not.

Is there any way to predict those who will be harmed with the development of tardive dyskinesia after chronic treatment with conventional antipsychotics? Patients who develop

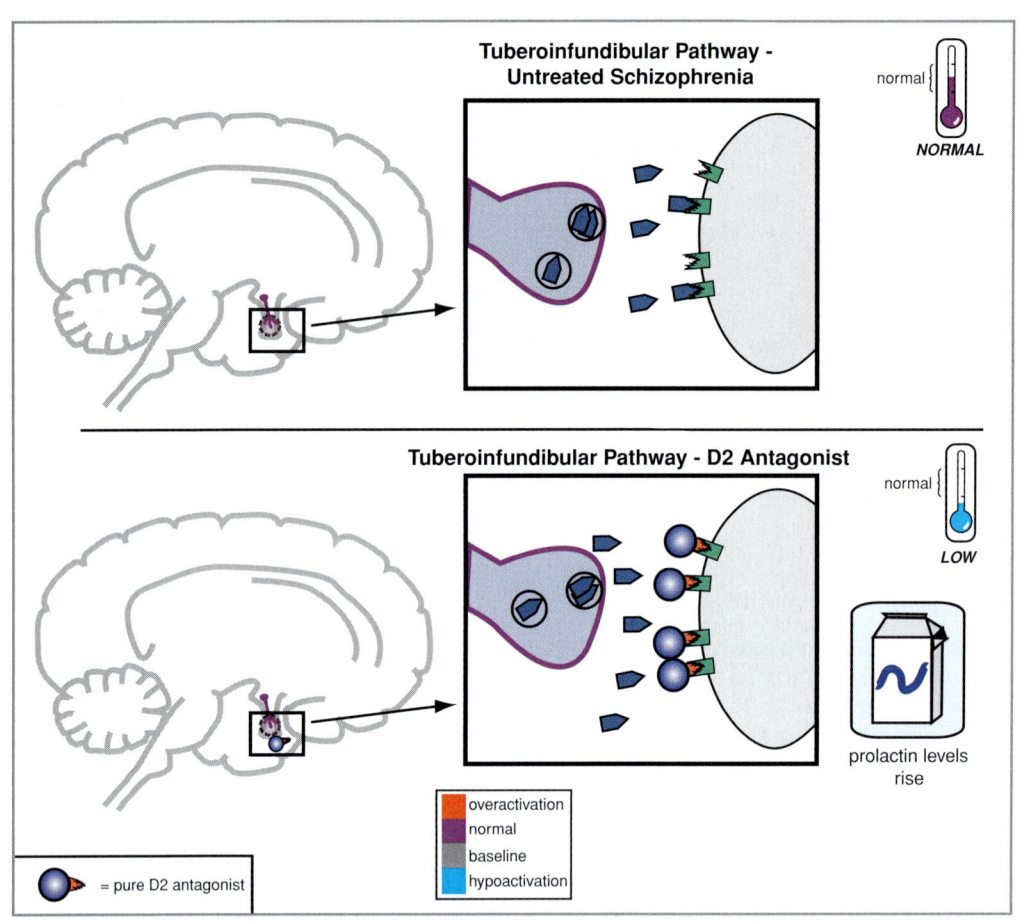

FIGURE 10-6 Tuberoinfundibular dopamine pathway and D2 antagonists. The tuberoinfundibular dopamine pathway, which projects from the hypothalamus to the pituitary gland, is theoretically "normal" in untreated schizophrenia. D2 antagonists reduce activity in this pathway by preventing dopamine from binding to D2 receptors. This causes prolactin levels to rise, which is associated with side effects such as galactorrhea (breast secretions) and amenorrhea (irregular menstrual periods).

FIGURE 10-7 Integrated theory of schizophrenia and D2 antagonists. In untreated schizophrenia, dopamine output is high in the mesolimbic pathway, causing positive symptoms; it is low in the mesocortical pathway to the dorsolateral prefrontal cortex (DLPFC), causing cognitive and negative symptoms; it is low in the mesocortical pathway to ventromedial prefrontal cortex (VMPFC), causing affective and negative symptoms; and it is normal in the nigrostriatal and tuberoinfundibular pathways (upper panel). With administration of a D2 antagonist, dopamine output is reduced throughout the brain (lower panel). This can reduce the positive symptoms of psychosis, although it may also reduce the experience of pleasure or reward, since these emotions are also mediated by the mesolimbic pathway. Reduction of dopamine output in mesocortical pathways would not improve cognitive, negative, or affective symptoms and might even worsen them. In the nigrostriatal and tuberoinfundibular pathways, reduction of dopamine output could lead to extrapyramidal symptoms (EPS) and prolactin elevation, respectively.

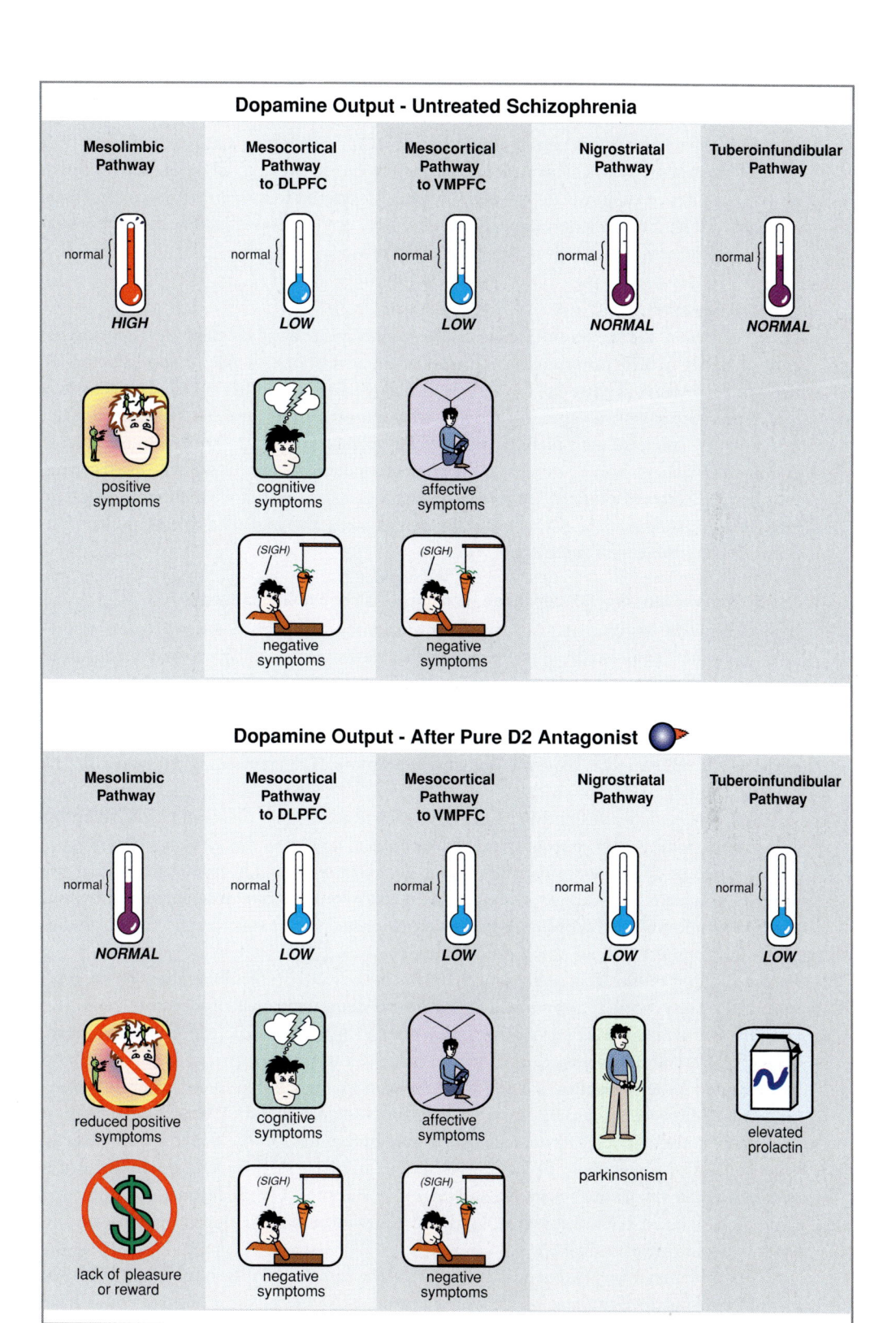

Dopamine Output - Untreated Schizophrenia

Mesolimbic Pathway	Mesocortical Pathway to DLPFC	Mesocortical Pathway to VMPFC	Nigrostriatal Pathway	Tuberoinfundibular Pathway
HIGH	LOW	LOW	NORMAL	NORMAL
positive symptoms	cognitive symptoms	affective symptoms		
	negative symptoms (SIGH)	negative symptoms (SIGH)		

Dopamine Output - After Pure D2 Antagonist

Mesolimbic Pathway	Mesocortical Pathway to DLPFC	Mesocortical Pathway to VMPFC	Nigrostriatal Pathway	Tuberoinfundibular Pathway
NORMAL	LOW	LOW	LOW	LOW
reduced positive symptoms	cognitive symptoms	affective symptoms	parkinsonism	elevated prolactin
lack of pleasure or reward	negative symptoms (SIGH)	negative symptoms (SIGH)		

Antipsychotic Agents

EPS early in treatment may be twice as likely to develop tardive dyskinesia if treatment with a conventional antipsychotic is continued chronically. Also, specific genotypes of dopamine receptors may confer important genetic risk factors for developing tardive dyskinesia with chronic treatment with a conventional antipsychotic. However, risk of a new onset of tardive dyskinesia can diminish considerably after 15 years of treatment with a conventional antipsychotic, presumably because patients who have not developed tardive dyskinesia over this treatment period have lower genetic risk factors.

Prolactin elevation

D2 receptors in the tuberoinfundibular DA pathway are also blocked by conventional antipsychotics, which causes plasma prolactin concentrations to rise, a condition called hyperprolactinemia (Figure 10-6). This is associated with a condition called galactorrhea (i.e., breast secretions) and amenorrhea (i.e., irregular menstrual periods). Hyperprolactinemia may thus interfere with fertility, especially in women. It might also lead to more rapid demineralization of bones, especially in postmenopausal women who are not receiving estrogen replacement therapy. Other possible problems associated with elevated prolactin levels may include sexual dysfunction and weight gain, although the role of prolactin in causing such problems is not clear.

The dilemma of blocking D2 dopamine receptors in all dopamine pathways

It should now be obvious that the use of conventional antipsychotic drugs presents a powerful dilemma. That is, there is no doubt that conventional antipsychotic medications have dramatic therapeutic effects on positive symptoms of psychosis by blocking hyperactive dopamine neurons in the mesolimbic dopamine pathway. However, there are **several** dopamine pathways in the brain. It appears that blocking dopamine receptors in **only one** of them is useful, whereas blocking dopamine receptors in the remaining pathways may be harmful (Figure 10-7).

Specifically, delusions and hallucinations are reduced when mesolimbic D2 receptors are blocked, but this may come at the expense of loss of reward in this same pathway (Figure 10-7). The near shutdown of the mesolimbic dopamine pathway necessary to improve the positive symptoms of psychosis in some patients may contribute to anhedonia, apathy, and negative symptoms of schizophrenia; this may be a partial explanation for the high incidence of smoking and drug abuse among such patients.

In addition to blocking reward mechanisms in the mesolimbic dopamine system, conventional antipsychotic actions in other dopamine systems may cause the negative, cognitive, and affective symptoms of psychosis to be worsened when mesocortical D2 receptors are blocked; EPS and tardive dyskinesia may be produced when nigrostriatal D2 receptors are blocked; and hyperprolactinemia and its complications may be produced when tuberoinfundibular D2 receptors are blocked. The pharmacological quandary here is what to do if one wishes simultaneously to **decrease** dopamine in the mesolimbic dopamine pathway in order to treat positive psychotic symptoms and yet **increase** dopamine in the mesocortical dopamine pathway to treat negative and cognitive symptoms while leaving dopaminergic tone unchanged in both the nigrostriatal and tuberoinfundibular dopamine pathways in order to avoid side effects.

This dilemma may have been solved in part by the atypical antipsychotic drugs described in the following sections and is one of the reasons why the atypical antipsychotics have largely replaced conventional antipsychotic agents in the treatment of schizophrenia and other psychotic disorders throughout the world.

Which Antipsychotics Are Conventional?

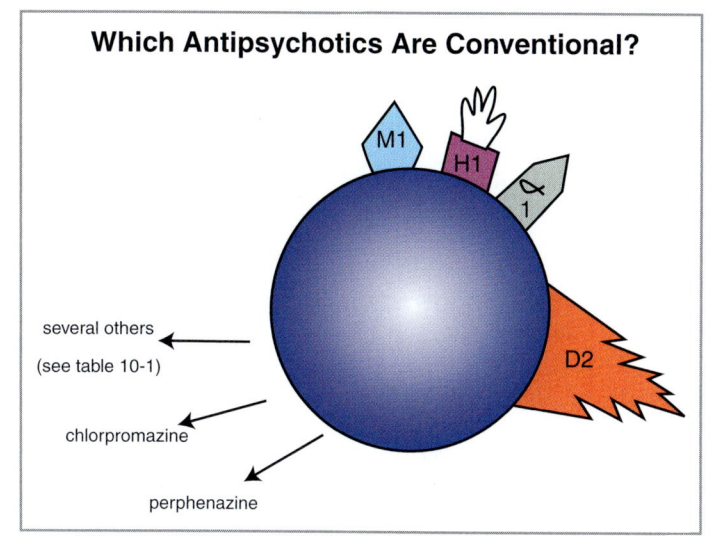

several others (see table 10-1)

chlorpromazine

perphenazine

FIGURE 10-8 Conventional antipsychotic. Shown here is an icon representing a conventional antipsychotic drug. Conventional antipsychotics have pharmacological properties in addition to dopamine D2 antagonism. The receptor profiles differ for each agent, contributing to divergent side-effect profiles. However, some important characteristics that multiple agents share are the ability to block muscarinic cholinergic receptors, histamine-1 receptors, and/or alpha-1 adrenergic receptors.

Haloperidol: Selective Conventional

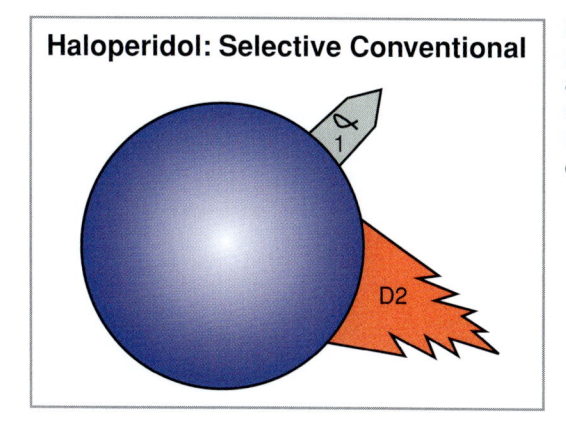

FIGURE 10-9 Haloperidol. Haloperidol pharmacological icon. Haloperidol is a conventional antipsychotic that, in addition to blocking D2 receptors, also inhibits alpha-1 adrenergic receptors. Haloperidol has little or no affinity for muscarinic cholinergic or histaminergic receptors.

Muscarinic cholinergic blocking properties of conventional antipsychotics

In addition to blocking D2 receptors in all dopamine pathways (Figure 10-7), conventional antipsychotics have other important pharmacological properties (Figures 10-8 through 10-13). One particularly important pharmacological action of some conventional antipsychotics is their ability to block muscarinic cholinergic receptors (Figures 10-8, 10-10, and 10-11). This can cause undesirable side effects such as dry mouth, blurred vision, constipation, and cognitive blunting (Figure 10-10). Differing degrees of muscarinic cholinergic blockade may also explain why some conventional antipsychotics have a greater propensity to produce extrapyramidal side effects (EPS) than others. That is, those conventional antipsychotics that cause more EPS are the agents that have only **weak** anticholinergic properties, whereas those conventional antipsychotics that cause fewer EPS are the agents that have **stronger** anticholinergic properties.

How does muscarinic cholinergic receptor blockade reduce the EPS caused by dopamine D2 receptor blockade in the nigrostriatal pathway? This effect seems to be

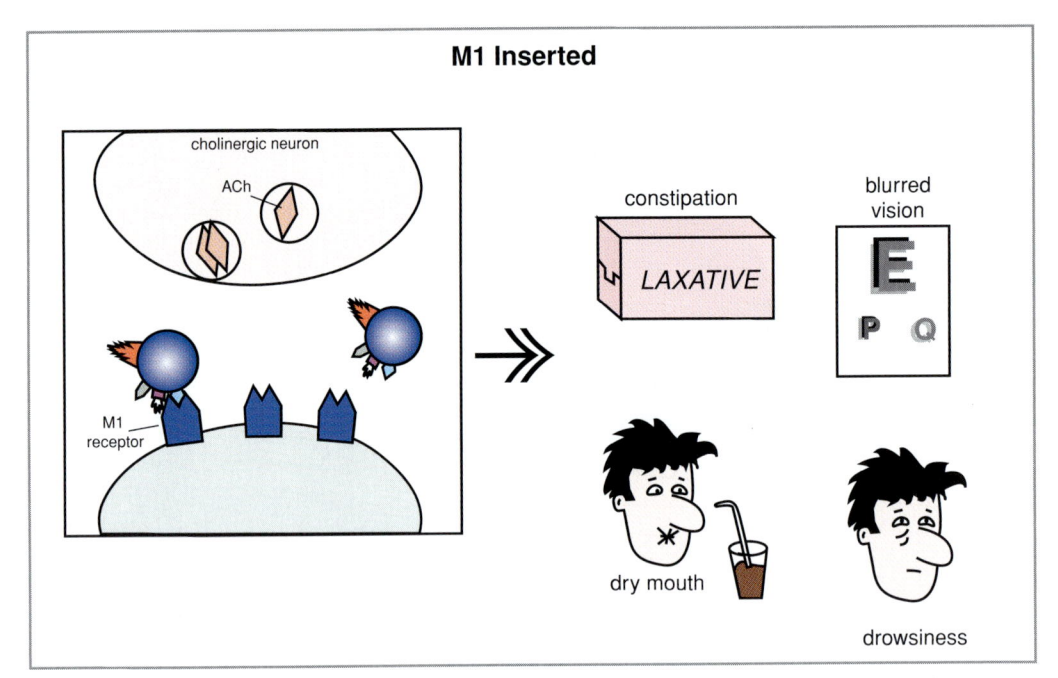

FIGURE 10-10 Side effects of muscarinic cholinergic receptor blockade. In this diagram, the icon of a conventional antipsychotic drug is shown with its M1-anticholinergic/antimuscarinic portion inserted into acetylcholine receptors, causing the side effects of constipation, blurred vision, dry mouth, and drowsiness.

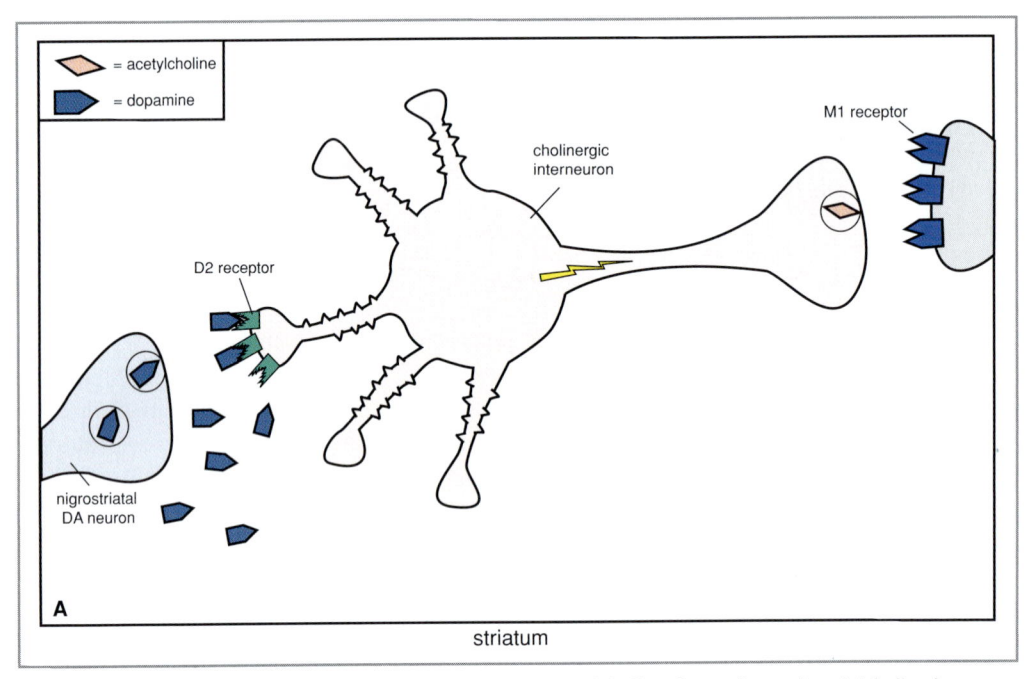

FIGURE 10-11A Reciprocal relationship of dopamine and acetylcholine. Dopamine and acetylcholine have a reciprocal relationship in the nigrostriatal dopamine pathway. Dopamine neurons here make postsynaptic connections with the dendrite of a cholinergic neuron. Normally, dopamine suppresses acetylcholine activity (no acetylcholine being released from the cholinergic axon on the right).

338 | Essential Psychopharmacology

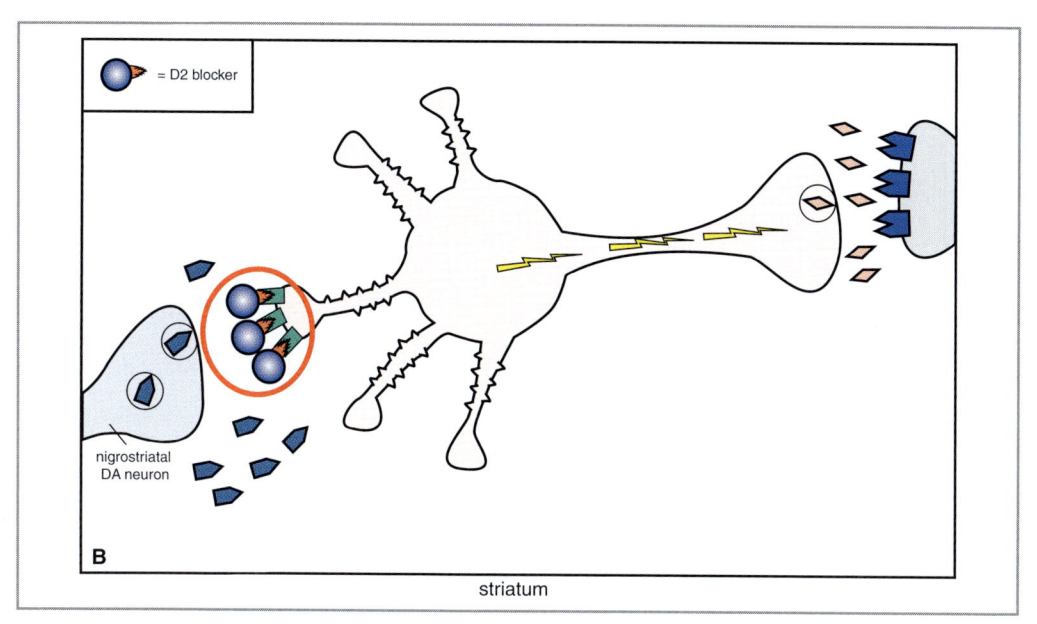

FIGURE 10-11B Dopamine, acetylcholine, and D2 antagonism. This figure shows what happens to acetylcholine activity when dopamine receptors are blocked. As dopamine normally suppresses acetylcholine activity, removal of dopamine inhibition causes an increase in acetylcholine activity. Thus if dopamine receptors are blocked at the D2 receptors on the cholinergic dendrite on the left, then acetylcholine becomes overly active, with enhanced release of acetylcholine from the cholinergic axon on the right. This is associated with the production of extrapyramidal symptoms (EPS). The pharmacological mechanism of EPS therefore seems to be a relative dopamine deficiency and a relative acetylcholine excess.

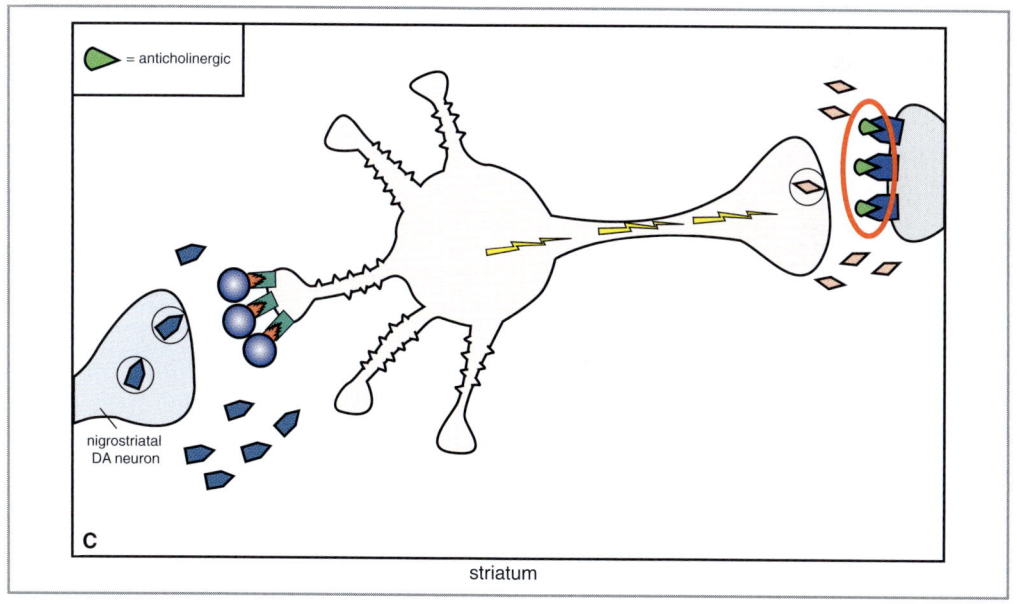

FIGURE 10-11C D2 antagonism and anticholinergic agents. One compensation for the overactivity that occurs when dopamine receptors are blocked is to block the acetylcholine receptors with an anticholinergic agent (M1 receptors being blocked by an anticholinergic on the far right). Thus, anticholinergics overcome excess acetylcholine activity caused by removal of dopamine inhibition when dopamine receptors are blocked by conventional antipsychotics. This also means that extrapyramidal symptoms (EPS) are reduced.

Antipsychotic Agents | 339

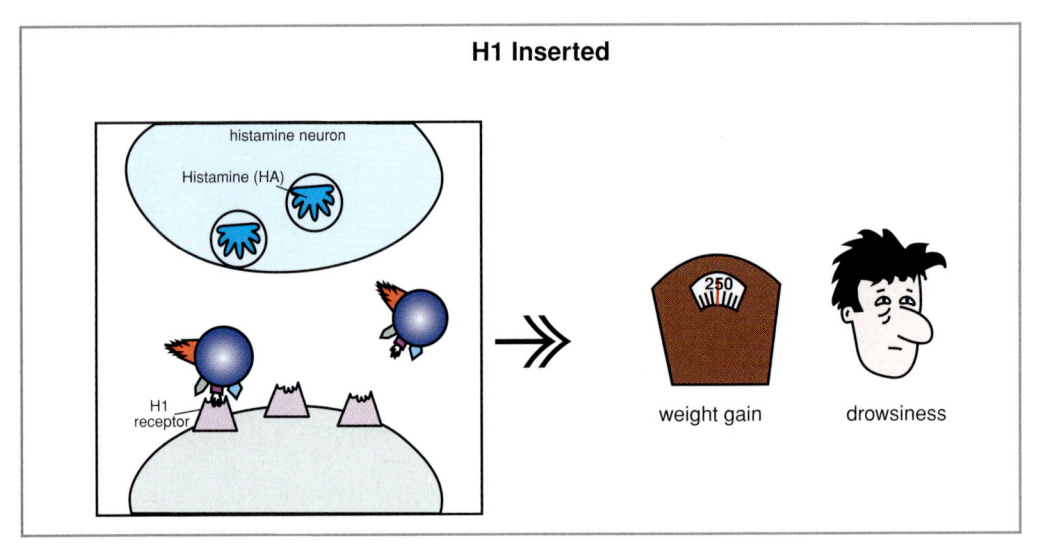

FIGURE 10-12 Histamine 1 receptor antagonism. In this diagram, the icon of a conventional antipsychotic drug is shown with its H1 (antihistamine) portion inserted into histamine receptors, causing the side effects of weight gain and drowsiness.

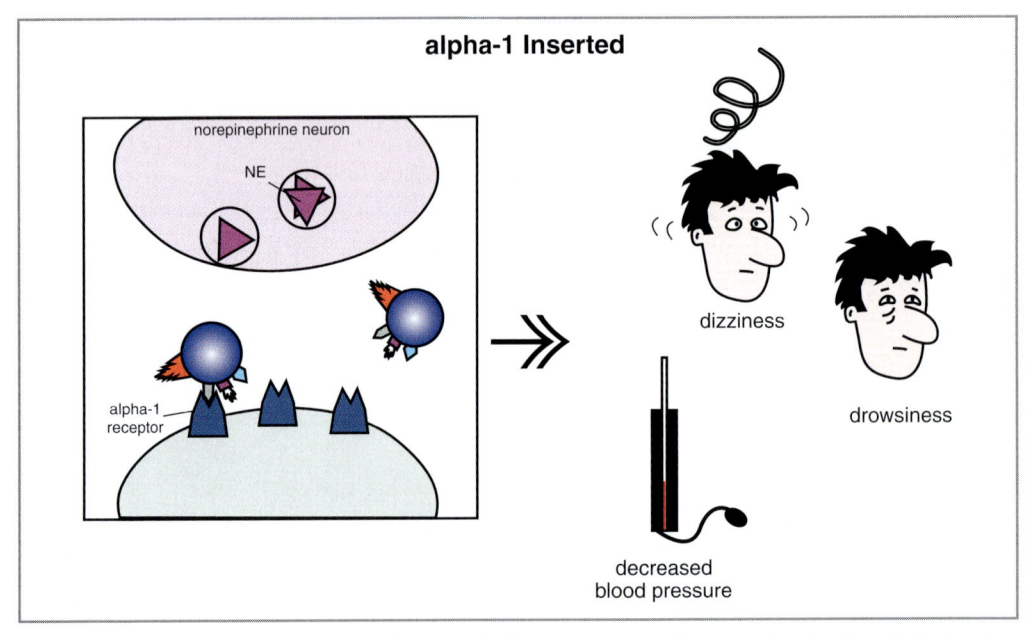

FIGURE 10-13 Alpha-1 receptor antagonism. In this diagram, the icon of a conventional antipsychotic drug is shown with its alpha-1 (alpha-1 antagonist) portion inserted into alpha-1 adrenergic receptors, causing the side effects of dizziness, decreased blood pressure, and drowsiness.

based on the fact that dopamine and acetylcholine have a reciprocal relationship with each other in the nigrostriatal pathway (see Figure 10-11). Dopamine neurons in the nigrostriatal dopamine pathway make postsynaptic connections with cholinergic neurons (Figure 10-11A). Dopamine normally **inhibits** acetylcholine release from postsynaptic nigrostriatal cholinergic neurons, thus suppressing acetylcholine activity there (Figure 10-11A).

340 | Essential Psychopharmacology

If dopamine can no longer suppress acetylcholine release because dopamine receptors are being blocked by a conventional antipsychotic drug, then acetylcholine becomes overly active (Figure 10-11B).

One compensation for this overactivity of acetylcholine is to block it with an anticholinergic agent (Figure 10-11C). Thus drugs with anticholinergic actions will diminish the excess acetylcholine activity caused by removal of dopamine inhibition when dopamine receptors are blocked (Figure 10-8 and Figure 10-11C). If anticholinergic properties are present in the same drug with D2-blocking properties, they will tend to mitigate the effects of D2 blockade in the nigrostriatal dopamine pathway. Thus, conventional antipsychotics with potent anticholinergic properties (for example, Figure 10-8) have a lower tendency to cause EPS than conventional antipsychotics with weak anticholinergic properties (Figure 10-9). Furthermore, the effects of D2 blockade in the nigrostriatal system can be mitigated by coadministering an agent with anticholinergic properties. This has led to the common strategy of giving anticholinergic agents along with conventional antipsychotics in order to reduce EPS. Unfortunately, this concomitant use of anticholinergic agents does not lessen the ability of the conventional antipsychotics to cause tardive dyskinesia. It also causes the well-known side effects associated with anticholinergic agents, such as dry mouth, blurred vision, constipation, urinary retention, and cognitive dysfunction (Figure 10-10).

Other pharmacological properties of conventional antipsychotic drugs

Still other pharmacologic actions are associated with the conventional antipsychotic drugs. These include generally undesired blockade of histamine-1 receptors (Figures 10-8 and 10-12), causing weight gain and drowsiness, as well as blockade of alpha-1 adrenergic receptors (Figures 10-8, 10-9, and 10-13), causing cardiovascular side effects such as orthostatic hypotension and drowsiness. Conventional antipsychotic agents differ in terms of their ability to block the various receptors represented in Figures 10-8 and 10-9. [For example, haloperidol, a popular conventional antipsychotic (Figure 10-9), has relatively little anticholinergic or antihistaminic binding activity.] Because of this, conventional antipsychotics differ somewhat in their side-effect profiles even if they do not differ overall in their therapeutic profiles. That is, some conventional antipsychotics are more sedating than others, some have more ability to cause cardiovascular side effects than others, and some have more ability to cause EPS than others.

Risks and benefits of long-term treatment with conventional antipsychotics

Although the conventional antipsychotics reduce positive psychotic symptoms in most patients after several weeks of treatment, discontinuing these drugs causes relapse of psychosis in patients with schizophrenia at the rate of approximately 10 percent per month, so that 50 percent or more have relapsed by 6 months after medication discontinuation. Despite this powerful incentive for patients to continue long-term treatment with conventional antipsychotics to prevent relapse, the unfortunate fact that all dopamine pathways are blocked by these drugs means that many patients do not consider the benefits of long-term treatment worth the resultant problems they cause. This leads many to discontinue treatment, become noncompliant, and relapse with a "revolving door" lifestyle in and out of the hospital. Patients too commonly select the risk of relapse over the subjectively unacceptable side effects of the conventional antipsychotics. Especially unacceptable to patients are motor restlessness and EPS such as akathisia, ridigity, and tremor as well as cognitive blunting and social withdrawal, anhedonia, and apathy. There is even the possibility of a rare but potentially fatal complication called the "neuroleptic malignant syndrome," which is associated with extreme muscular rigidity, high fevers, coma, and even death.

Given these problems with conventional antipsychotics, when are these agents worthwhile to administer? Recently, long-term cardiometabolic risks for some of the atypical antipsychotics have been uncovered (discussed later in this chapter), and this, combined with their higher cost, is leading to a resurgence of interest among some psychopharmacologists in going back to conventional antipsychotic treatment, where the cardiometabolic risks (and costs) may be lower. This may be prudent for some patients who experience a robust therapeutic effect at low doses of a conventional antipsychotic and thus show improvement in positive symptoms without worsening of negative symptoms and without "neurolepsis." Furthermore, if such patients have had 15 years of treatment with a conventional antipsychotic without developing tardive dyskinesia, there may be little additional risk that this will occur with continued treatment with a conventional antipsychotic. It is interesting to note that some so-called first generation conventional antipsychotics (such as loxapine, cyamemazine, and sulpiride) may have the pharmacological properties of an atypical antipsychotic, particularly at low doses (discussed later in this chapter). Administering one of these agents may be a way to treat with a less expensive agent that could potentially have atypical antipsychotic properties.

On the other hand, psychopharmacologists who no longer see tardive dyskinesia in their patients (owing to the conversion of most of their patients to an atypical antipsychotic) must not forget that most patients remain at much higher risk for developing tardive dyskinesia on a conventional antipsychotic than for developing cardiometabolic risks on an atypical antipsychotic, particularly on certain atypical antipsychotics that pose little cardiometabolic risk.

Selecting which antipsychotic to administer to an individual patient thus requires weighing tardive dyskinesia, neurolepsis, EPS, and cardiometabolic risks for that individual against the particular clinical benefits for that same patient in terms of improvement in negative, cognitive, and affective symptoms as well as positive symptoms. In order to make prudent antipsychotic choices for each individual patient, it is necessary to understand the differentiating properties not only of conventional antipsychotics compared to atypical antipsychotics but of each individual antipsychotic drug. These issues are developed in detail throughout this chapter.

What makes an antipsychotic atypical?

What is an "atypical" antipsychotic? From a clinical perspective, it is defined in part by the "atypical" clinical properties that distinguish such drugs from conventional antipsychotics, namely "low EPS" and "good for negative symptoms." From a pharmacological perspective, the atypical antipsychotics as a class may be defined in at least four ways: as "serotonin dopamine antagonists" (Figure 10-14), as "D2 antagonists with rapid dissociation" (Figure 10-39), as "D2 partial agonists (DPA)" (Figure 10-45) or as "serotonin partial agonists (SPA)" at 5HT1A receptors (Figure 10-55). In the following section, we will discuss all four of these proposed pharmacological mechanisms of action of atypical antipsychotics.

Serotonergic neurotransmission and serotonin dopamine antagonism

Here, we will first discuss how some atypical antipsychotics obtain their atypical clinical properties by exploiting the different ways that serotonin and dopamine interact within the key dopamine pathways in the brain. In order to understand the powerful consequences of adding 5HT2A receptor antagonism to D2 antagonism, it is very important to grasp the

What Makes an Antipsychotic Atypical?
Adding 5HT2A Antagonist / Inverse Agonist Actions

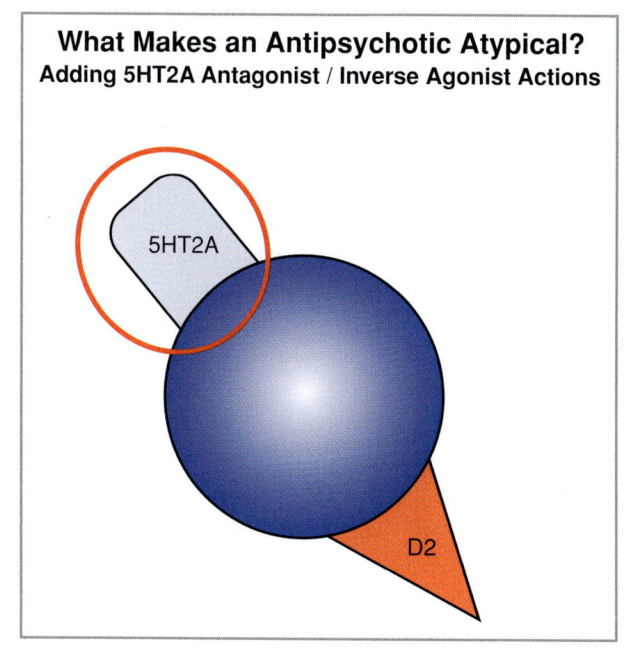

FIGURE 10-14 **Serotonin-dopamine antagonist.** The "atypicality" of atypical antipsychotics has often been attributed to the coupling of D2 antagonism with serotonin-2A antagonism. Shown here is an icon representing this dual pharmacological action.

principles of serotonin receptor pharmacology and also the nature of serotonin-dopamine interactions in each of the dopamine pathways.

Serotonin synthesis and termination of action

Serotonin is also known as 5-hydroxytryptamine and abbreviated as 5HT. Synthesis of 5HT begins with the amino acid tryptophan, which is transported into the brain from the plasma to serve as the 5HT precursor (Figure 10-15). Two synthetic enzymes then convert tryptophan into serotonin: first tryptophan hydroxylase (TRY-OH) converts tryptophan into 5-hydroxy-tryptophan and then aromatic amino acid decarboxylase (AAADC) converts 5HTP into 5HT (Figure 10-15). After synthesis, 5HT is taken up into synaptic vesicles by a vesicular monoamine transporter (VMAT2) and stored there until it is used during neurotransmission.

The action of 5HT is terminated when it is enzymatically destroyed by MAO and converted into an inactive metabolite (Figure 10-16). Serotonergic neurons themselves contain MAO B, which has low affinity for 5HT; therefore much of 5HT is thought to be enzymatically degraded by MAO A outside of the neuron once 5HT is released. The 5HT neuron also has a presynaptic transport pump for serotonin called the serotonin transporter (SERT), which is unique for 5HT and terminates serotonin's actions by pumping it out of the synapse and back into the presynaptic nerve terminal, where it can be re-stored in synaptic vesicles for subsequent use in another neurotransmission (Figure 10-15).

Serotonin receptors

Serotonin has many different receptor subtypes (Figures 10-17 through 10-20). For a general understanding of 5HT receptors, the reader can begin with the two key receptors that are presynaptic (5HT1A and 5HT1B/D) (Figures 10-17 through 10-19) and several that are postsynaptic (5HT1A, 5HT1B/D as well as 5HT2A, 5HT2C, 5HT3, 5HT4, 5HT5, 5HT6, and 5HT7) (Figure 10-17).

Serotonin Is Produced

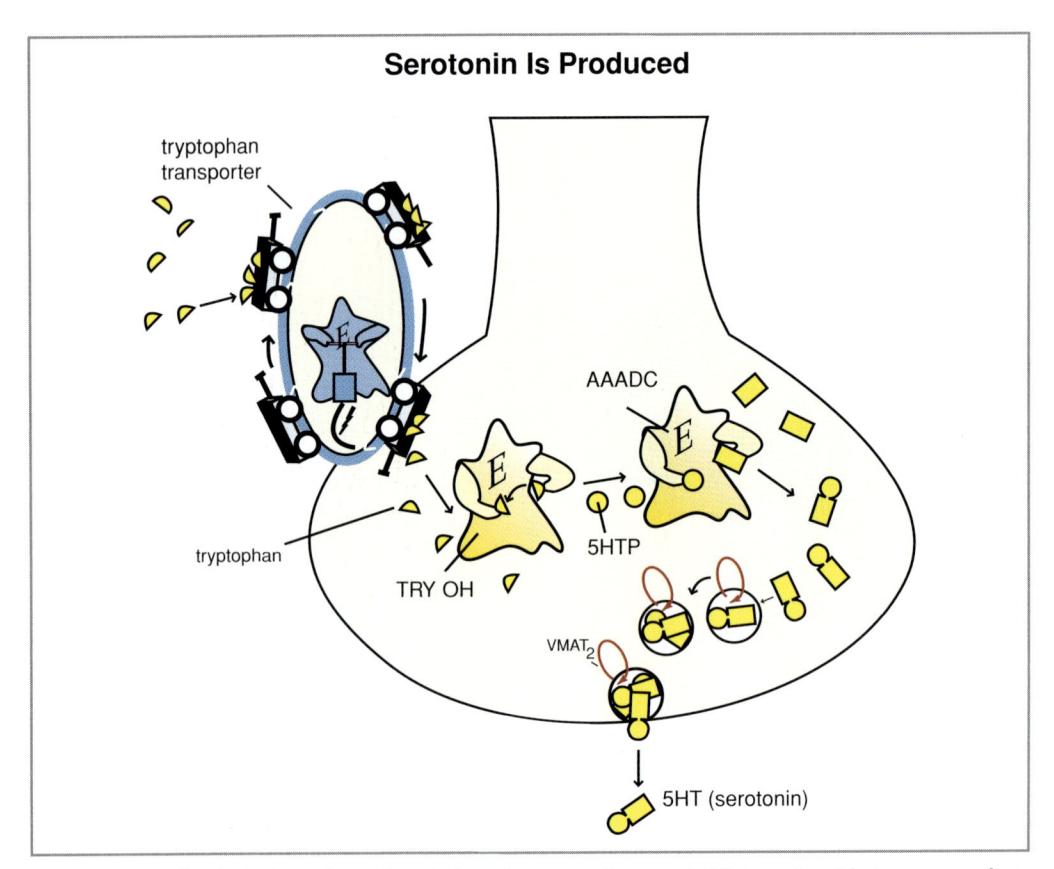

FIGURE 10-15 Serotonin is produced. Serotonin (5-hydroxytryptamine [5HT]) is produced from enzymes after the amino acid precursor tryptophan is transported into the serotonin neuron. The tryptophan transport pump is distinct from the serotonin transporter. Once transported into the serotonin neuron, tryptophan is converted by the enzyme tryptophan hydroxylase (TRY-OH) into 5-hydroxytryptophan (5HTP), which is then converted into 5HT by the enzyme aromatic amino acid decarboxylase (AAADC). Serotonin is then taken up into synaptic vesicles via the vesicular monoamine transporter (VMAT2), where it stays until released by a neuronal impulse.

Presynaptic 5HT receptors are autoreceptors and detect the presence of 5HT, causing a shutdown of further 5HT release and 5HT neuronal impulse flow. When 5HT is detected in the synapse by presynaptic 5HT receptors on axon terminals, it occurs via a 5HT1B/D receptor, which is also called a **terminal autoreceptor** (Figure 10-18A). In the case of the 5HT1B/D terminal autoreceptor, 5HT occupancy of this receptor causes a blockade of 5HT release (Figure 10-18B). On the other hand, drugs that block the 5HT1B/D autoreceptor can promote 5HT release. When 5HT is detected in the cell dendrites and cell body, it occurs via a 5HT1A receptor, which is also called a **somatodendritic** autoreceptor (Figure 10-19). This causes a slowing of neuronal impulse flow through the serotonin neuron (Figure 10-19B).

Postsynaptic 5HT receptors translate the chemical signal from serotonin into a signal within the postsynaptic neuron (Figures 10-17 and 10-20). All of these receptors in one way or another regulate various neuronal circuits. More specifically, postsynaptic 5HT1A receptors inhibit cortical pyramidal neurons and are thought to regulate hormones, cognition, anxiety, and depression (Figure 10-20). 5HT2A receptors, on the other hand, excite cortical pyramidal neurons, enhance glutamate release, and inhibit dopamine release while

Serotonin Action Is Terminated

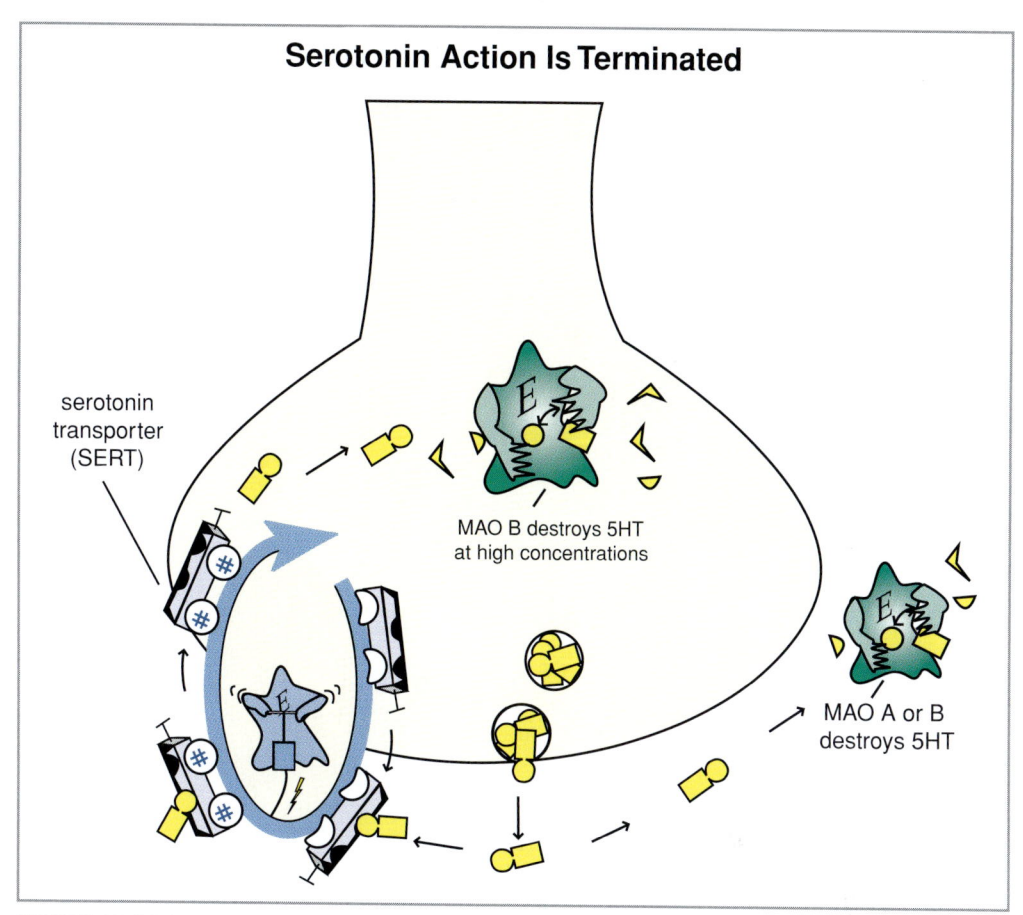

FIGURE 10-16 Serotonin's action is terminated. Serotonin's (5HT) action is terminated by the enzymes monoamine oxidase A (MAO-A) and MAO-B outside the neuron, and by MAO-B within the neuron when it is present in high concentrations. These enzymes convert serotonin into an inactive metabolite. There is also a presynaptic transport pump selective for serotonin, called the serotonin transporter or SERT, that clears serotonin out of the synapse and back into the presynaptic neuron.

playing a role in both sleep and hallucinations (Figure 10-20). 5HT2C receptors regulate both dopamine and norepinephrine release and may play a role in obesity, mood, and cognition (Figure 10-20). 5HT3 receptors regulate inhibitory interneurons in the cortex and mediate vomiting via the vagal nerve (Figure 10-20). 5HT6 receptors are under intense investigation, as they may be key in regulating the release of neurotrophic factors such as brain derived neurotrophic factor (BDNF), which in turn regulates the formation of long-term memory. Finally, the role of 5HT7 receptors is being clarified; these seem to be linked to circadian rhythms, sleep, and mood (Figure 10-20).

5HT1A and 5HT2A receptors have opposite actions in regulating dopamine release

Some serotonin receptors have a major influence on dopamine release; when serotonin acts on them, they can determine whether dopamine release is stimulated or inhibited. Specifically, 5HT1A receptors act as an accelerator for dopamine release, whereas 5HT2A receptors act as a brake on dopamine release (Figure 10-21). How does this happen?

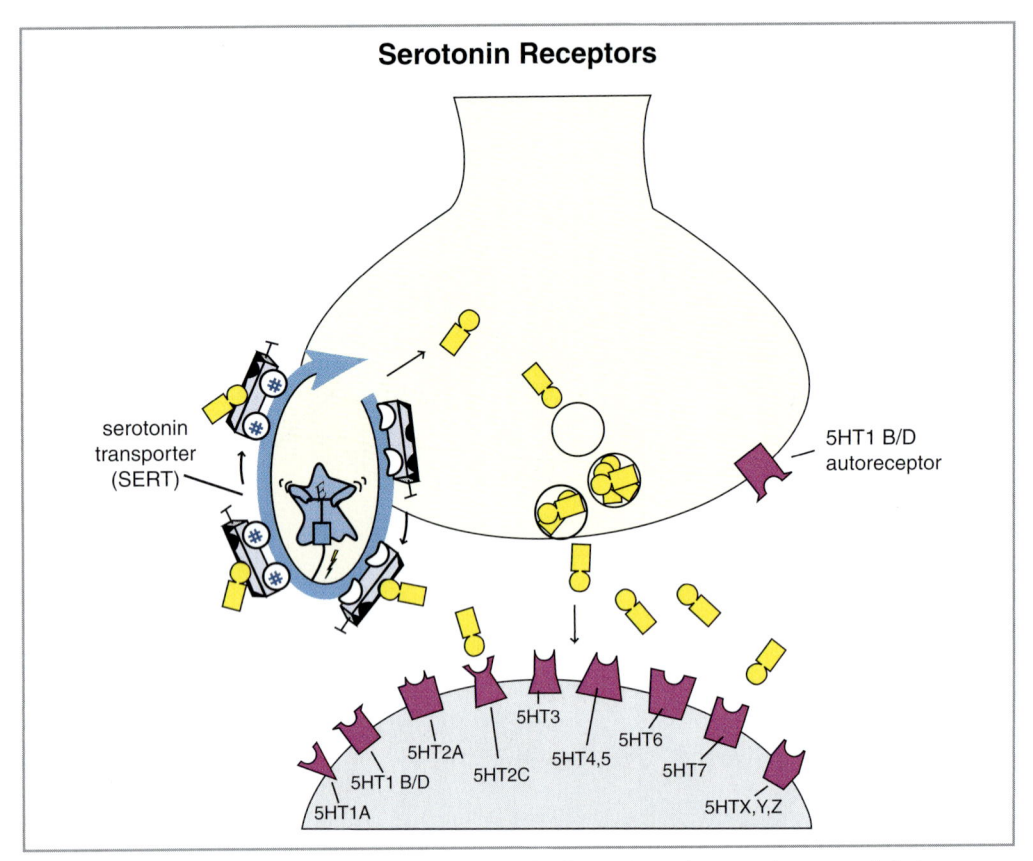

FIGURE 10-17 Serotonin receptors. Receptor subtyping for the serotonergic neuron has proceeded at a very rapid pace. On the presynaptic side, in addition to the well-known serotonin (5HT) transporter, there is a key presynaptic 5HT receptor (5HT1B/D) that functions as an autoreceptor. Several postsynaptic 5HT receptors (5HT1A, 5HT1B/D, 5HT2A, 5HT2C, 5HT3, 5HT4, 5HT6, 5HT7, and many others denoted by 5HTX,Y,Z) are shown here as well.

The 5HT2A receptor is a dopamine brake

Serotonin neurons innervate dopamine neurons either directly via postsynaptic 5HT2A receptors on the dopamine neuron, or indirectly via 5HT2A receptors on GABA interneurons (Figure 10-21). When serotonin is released onto these postsynaptic 5HT2A receptors, the dopamine neuron is inhibited, providing a braking action on dopamine release (lower left of Figure 10-21).

The 5HT1A receptor is a dopamine accelerator

How does serotonin also act as an accelerator to stimulate dopamine release via 5HT1A receptors? Recall that 5HT1A receptors in the somatodendritic region of serotonin neurons are autoreceptors that act to inhibit serotonin release (Figure 10-19). When 5HT1A receptors inhibit serotonin release (Figure 10-19B), the 5HT2A postsynaptic receptors on dopamine neurons cannot be activated (lower right of Figure 10-21). In other words, the 5HT2A dopamine brake is not applied and dopamine neurons will lose the inhibitory action of serotonin via 5HT2A receptors. This lack of 5HT2A inhibition is also known as "disinhibition," which is just a fancy way of saying "turned on." Technically speaking,

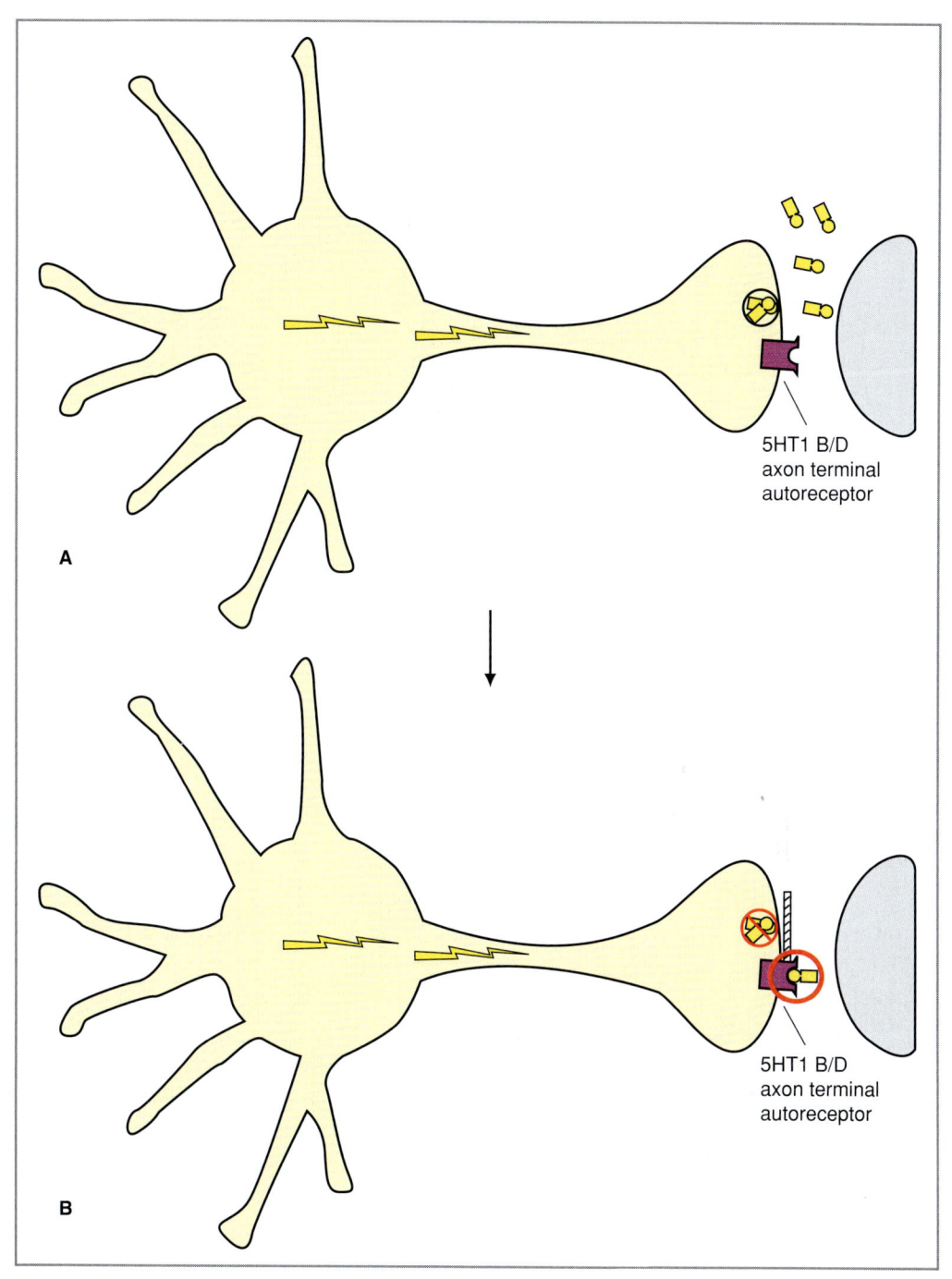

FIGURE 10-18A and B 5HT1B/D autoreceptors. Presynaptic 5HT1B/D receptors are autoreceptors located on the presynaptic axon terminal. They act by detecting the presence of serotonin (5HT) in the synapse and causing a shutdown of further 5HT release. When 5HT builds up in the synapse (**A**), it is available to bind to the autoreceptor, which then inhibits serotonin release (**B**).

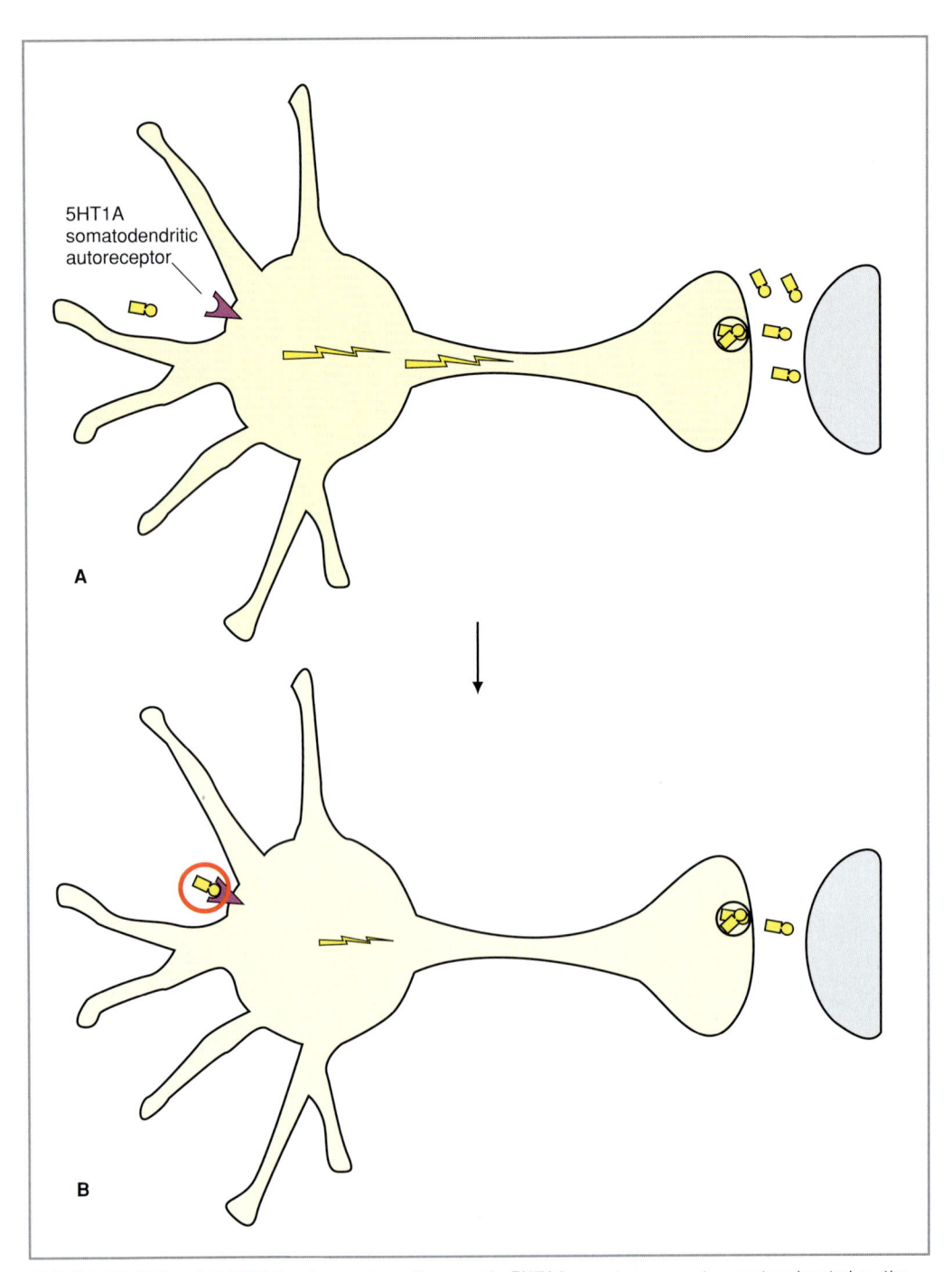

FIGURE 10-19A and B 5HT1A autoreceptors. Presynaptic 5HT1A receptors are autoreceptors located on the cell body and dendrites, and are therefore called somatodendritic autoreceptors (**A**). When serotonin (5HT) binds to these 5HT1A receptors, it causes a shutdown of 5HT neuronal impulse flow, depicted here as decreased electrical activity and a reduction in the release of 5HT from the synapse on the right (**B**).

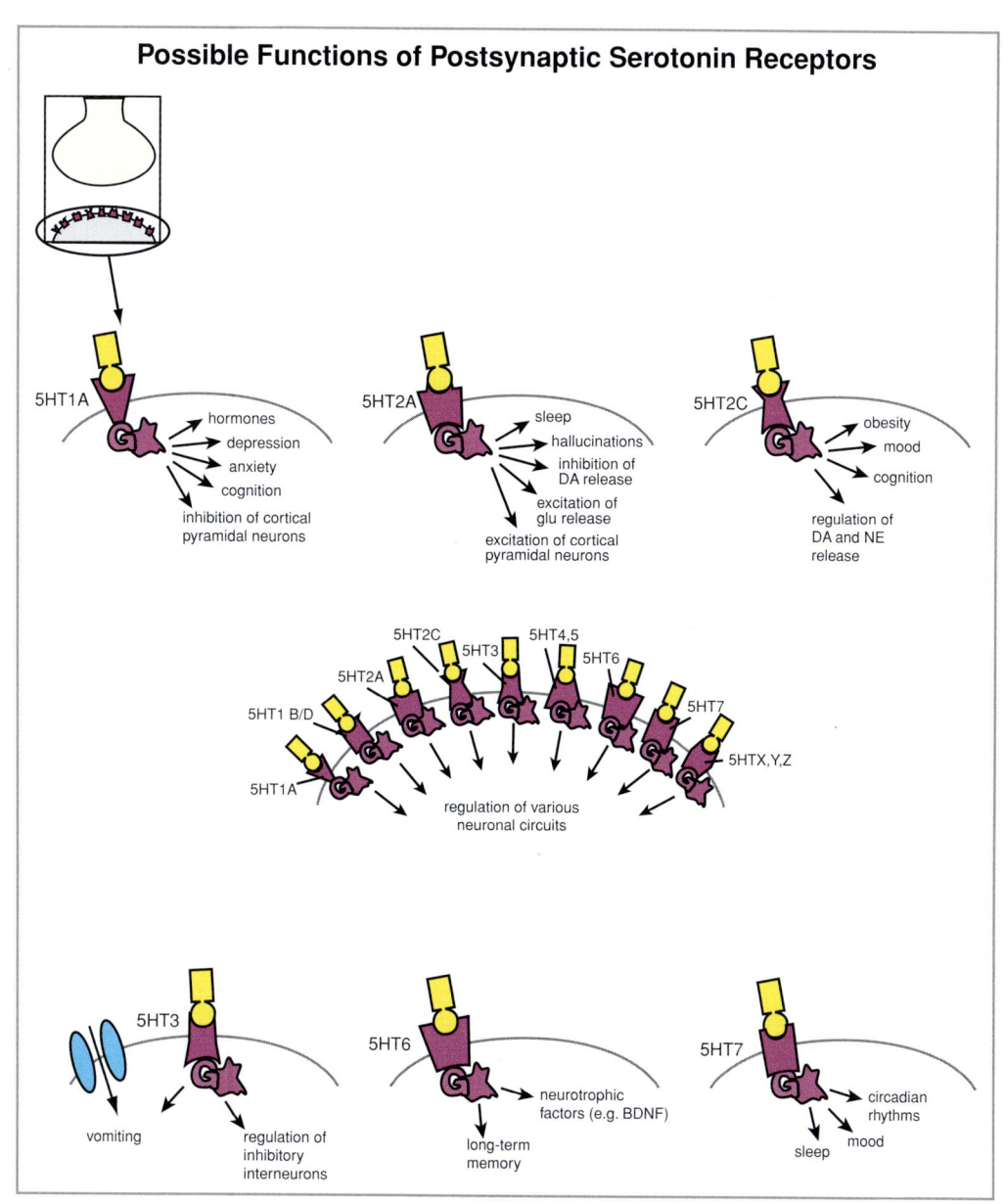

FIGURE 10-20 **Possible functions of postsynaptic serotonin receptors.** Postsynaptic serotonin (5HT) receptors are G protein–linked receptors. 5HT binding to these receptors causes signal transduction and downstream events that regulate various neuronal circuits. In particular, postsynaptic 5HT1A receptors inhibit cortical pyramidal neurons, regulate hormones, and play a role in depression, anxiety, and cognition. 5HT2A receptors excite cortical pyramidal neurons, increase glutamate release, decrease dopamine release, and are involved in sleep and hallucinations. 5HT2C receptors regulate dopamine and norepinephrine release and play a role in obesity, mood and cognition. 5HT3 receptors regulate inhibitory interneurons in the brain and also mediate vomiting via the vagal nerve. 5HT6 receptors may regulate release of neurotrophic factors (e.g., brain-derived neurotrophic factor, or BDNF), which could affect long-term memory. 5HT7 receptors may be involved in circadian rhythms, mood, and sleep.

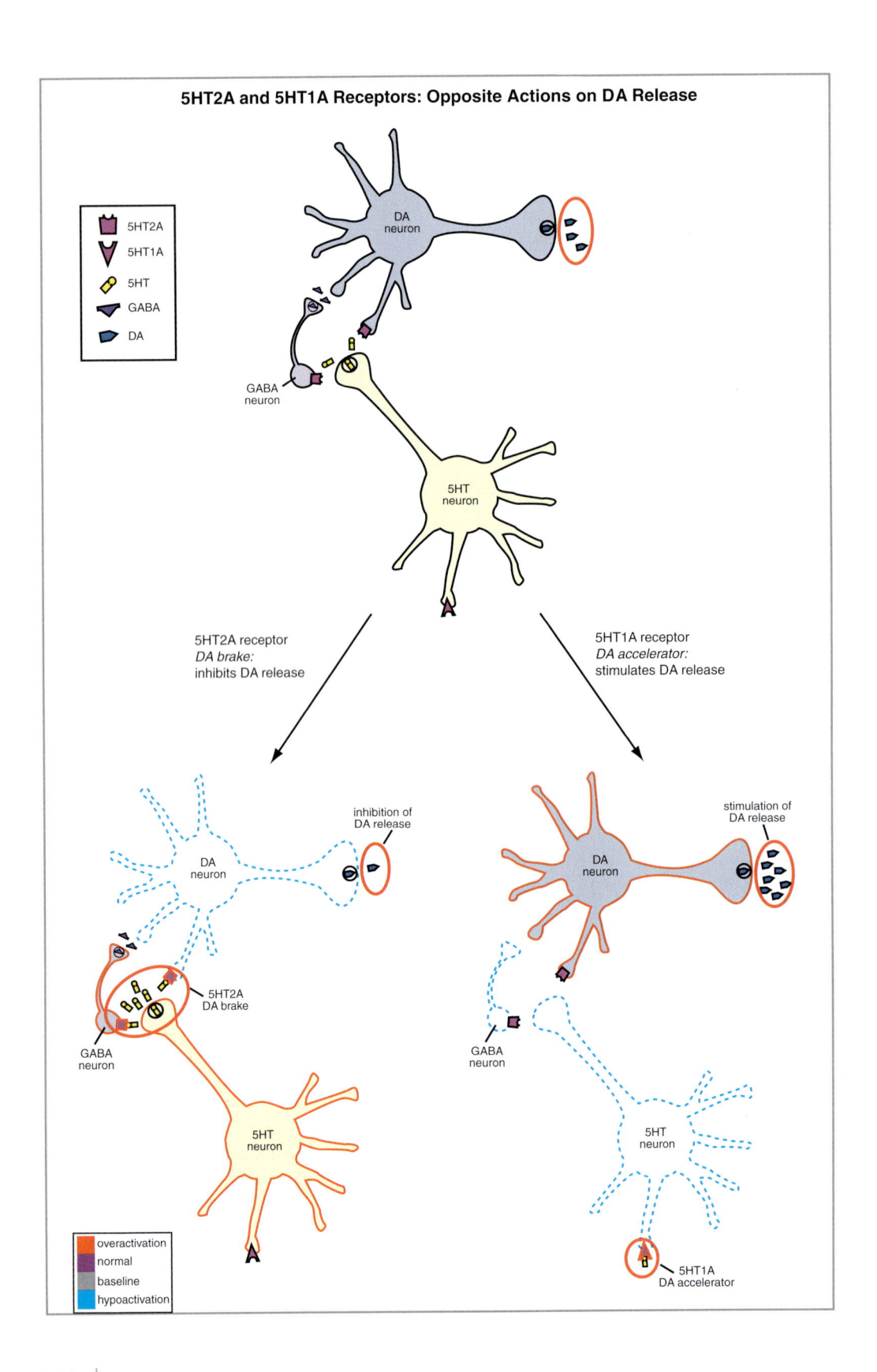

5HT2A and 5HT1A Receptors: Opposite Actions on DA Release

350 | Essential Psychopharmacology

activation of 5HT1A autoreceptors disinhibits the dopamine neuron, and thus dopamine release is enhanced (Figure 10-21, lower right). Thus, the presynaptic somatodendritic 5HT1A autoreceptor is a DA accelerator.

5HT2A antagonism makes an antipsychotic atypical
5HT2A antagonists stimulate dopamine release

Many atypical antipsychotics are antagonists at the 5HT2A receptor as well as at the D2 receptor (Figure 10-14). Some research suggests that this antagonist action is actually more precisely described as inverse agonist action at 5HT2A receptors, but the clinical differences between antagonists and inverse agonists are not yet clear. The pharmacological distinctions between so-called "silent" antagonists and inverse agonists are discussed in Chapters 4 and 5 and illustrated in Figures 4-21 through 4-28 and in Figures 5-9 through 5-18. Here we will continue to refer to the actions of atypical antipsychotics at 5HT2A receptors as antagonist actions.

What is so important about 5HT2A antagonist actions of atypical antipsychotics? 5HT2A antagonism can cause dopamine release in certain brain areas (Figure 10-22), and this pharmacological action hypothetically explains the atypical clinical properties of these agents that distinguish them from conventional antipsychotics, namely "low EPS" and "good for negative symptoms." Thus, the 5HT2A receptor "brake" on dopamine release shown in Figure 10-21 and on the left in Figure 10-22 is disrupted by a 5HT2A antagonist, essentially cutting the brake cable, disinhibiting the dopamine neuron, and stimulating dopamine release (Figure 10-22, the right).

5HT2A antagonism reduces EPS

So far, we have shown how serotonin neurons act on the somatodendritic regions of dopamine neurons (Figures 10-21 and 10-22). However, serotonin neurons may also act on the axon terminals of dopamine neurons (Figures 10-23 through 10-26). For example, serotonin actions on nigrostriatal dopamine neurons may occur both at the level of the brainstem in the substantia nigra, where the somatodendritic regions of these dopamine neurons are located, and also in the striatum, where the axon terminals of these dopamine neurons are located (Figure 10-23). In both cases, a 5HT2A receptor mediates the action of serotonin at the dopamine neuron, via either a direct connection between the serotonin neuron and the dopamine neuron or an indirect connection with a GABA interneuron (Figure 10-24A). Specifically, Figure 10-24B shows actions of 5HT2A receptors in the somatodendritic region of the dopamine neuron in the substantia nigra, inhibiting dopamine release in the striatum, as in Figure 10-21, lower left. In addition, the actions of 5HT2A receptors on dopamine axon terminals in the striatum are shown in Figure 10-24C, also inhibiting the release of dopamine in the striatum. A closeup depiction of these actions of 5HT at axon terminal 5HT2A receptors in the striatum is shown in Figure 10-25, where striatal

---

FIGURE 10-21 5HT2A and 5HT1A receptors: opposite actions on DA release. Serotonin (5HT) 1A and 2A receptors influence dopamine (DA) release, either directly or via gamma aminobutyric acid (GABA) neurons. However, these receptors actually have opposite effects on DA release. Specifically, 5HT2A receptors act as a DA brake. When 5HT binds to 5HT2A receptors on postsynaptic DA neurons, this inhibits DA release (bottom left). Similarly, 5HT binding to 5HT2A receptors on GABA interneurons causes GABA release, which in turn inhibits DA release (also bottom left). 5HT1A somatodendritic autoreceptors, on the other hand, act as DA accelerators. That is, when 5HT binds to these receptors, it inhibits 5HT release; thus, 5HT is unable to inhibit DA release, and dopamine release is thus disinhibited, and therefore increased (bottom right).

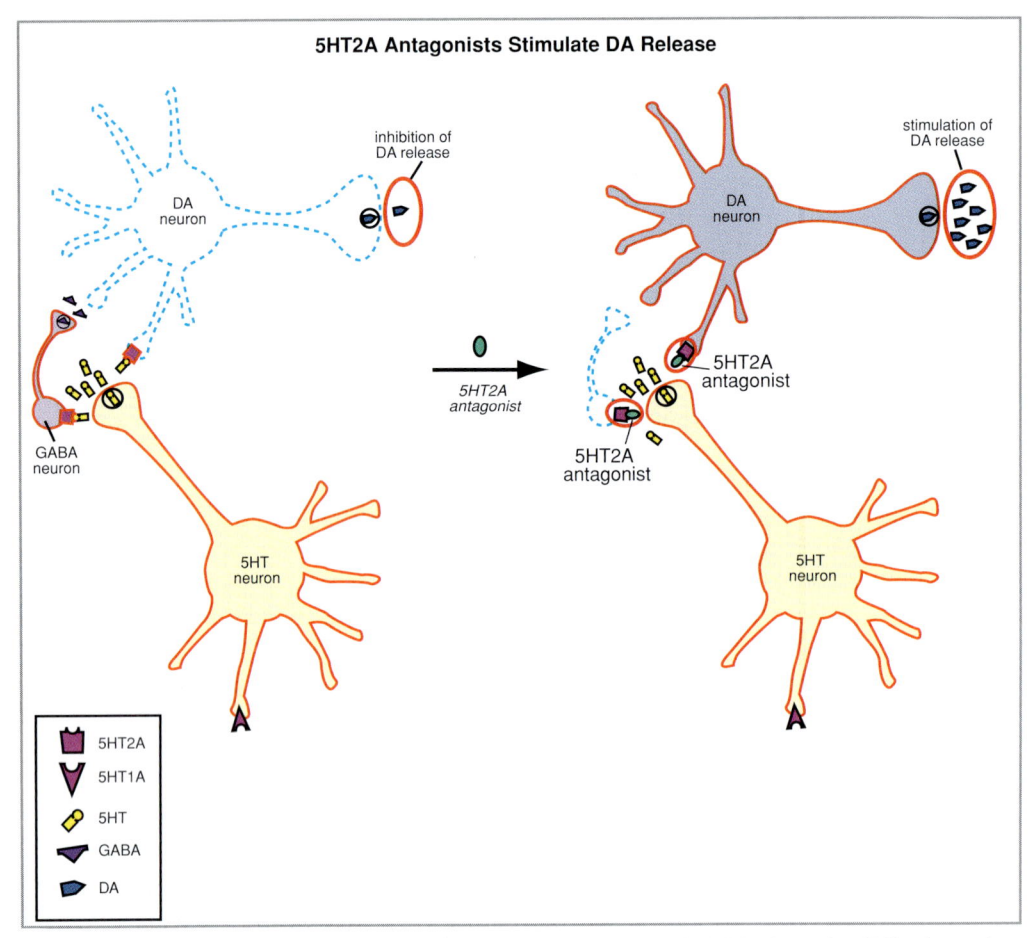

FIGURE 10-22 5HT2A antagonists stimulate DA release. Serotonin (5HT) inhibits dopamine (DA) release via stimulation of 5HT2A receptors (left); when this action is blocked by a 5HT2A antagonist, this leads to an increase in DA release, either by blocking 5HT2A receptors on postsynaptic DA neurons or by blocking 5HT2A receptors on gamma aminobutyric acid (GABA) interneurons (on the right).

dopamine release (Figure 10-25A) is inhibited by serotonin actions at postsynaptic 5HT2A receptors located at an axoaxonic synapse of a serotonin neuron on a striatal dopamine nerve terminal (Figure 10-25B).

How does 5HT2A antagonist action reduce EPS? The answer to this is shown in Figure 10-26, where both the D2 and 5HT2A antagonist actions of an atypical antipsychotic are illustrated in the striatum. First, the D2 actions of an atypical antipsychotic are shown in Figure 10-26A. In this case, most of the D2 receptors in the striatum are occupied, and if this persisted, it would cause EPS, as this would be no different than the actions of a conventional antipsychotic with pure D2 antagonist actions (Figure 10-1). However, in Figure 10-26B, the additional action of the 5HT2A antagonist is shown. Adding this second action results in disinhibition of the dopamine neuron, which causes stimulation of dopamine release, just as has already been explained and illustrated in Figure 10-22. The result of this increased dopamine release is that dopamine competes with drug at D2 receptors and reduces binding there enough to eliminate EPS (Figure 10-26B).

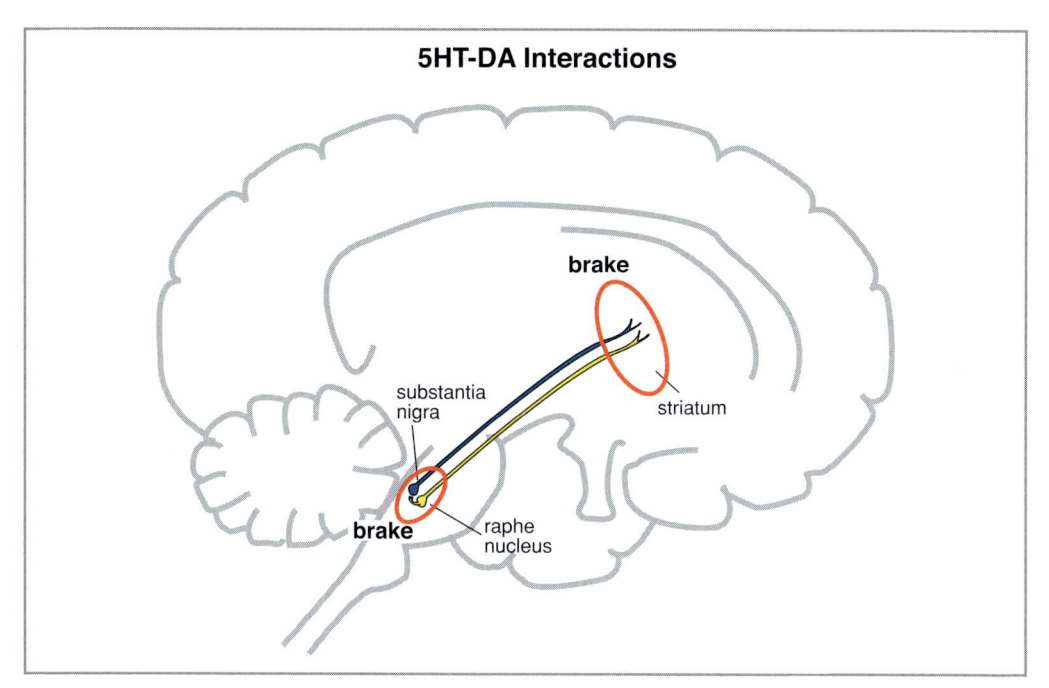

FIGURE 10-23 5HT-DA interactions. Serotonin-dopamine interactions in the nigrostriatal dopamine pathway. Serotonin inhibits dopamine release, both at the level of the dopamine cell bodies in the brainstem substantia nigra and at the level of the axon terminals in the basal ganglia-neostriatum. In both cases, the release of serotonin acts as a brake on dopamine release.

These actions of an atypical antipsychotic with both D2 antagonist actions and 5HT2A antagonist actions are confirmed when imaging D2 receptors in the striatum of patients receiving antipsychotic drugs (Figure 10-27). In the case of a conventional antipsychotic given at clinically effective doses, it is estimated that up to 90 percent of D2 receptors are blocked in every dopamine pathway in the brain. This degree of blockade of D2 receptors in the nucleus accumbens of the mesolimbic dopamine pathway is presumably necessary to reduce positive symptoms of psychosis, but this degree of simultaneous blockade of D2 receptors in the striatum causes EPS and eventually, tardive dyskinesia. An artist's conception of occupancy of 90 percent of D2 receptors by a conventional antipsychotic drug is shown in Figure 10-27A. Real neuroimaging scans with positron emission tomography (PET) ligands are much more complicated, but we know that if we could selectively label the D2 receptors in the striatum after a clinically effective dose of a conventional antipsychotic, a high proportion of D2 receptors in the striatum would be occupied (Figure 10-27A).

However, in the case of an atypical antipsychotic, the number of D2 receptors that are occupied in the striatum is notably less at clinically effective doses (Figure 10-27B). How can this be? Presumably it is due to the actions of drug blocking 5HT2A receptors and leading to increased striatal dopamine release (as shown in Figure 10-26B), which in turn causes dopamine to knock enough drug off D2 receptors that the occupancy drops below the threshold for producing EPS (i.e., presumably less than 70 to 80 percent of D2 receptor occupancy).

Antipsychotic Agents | 353

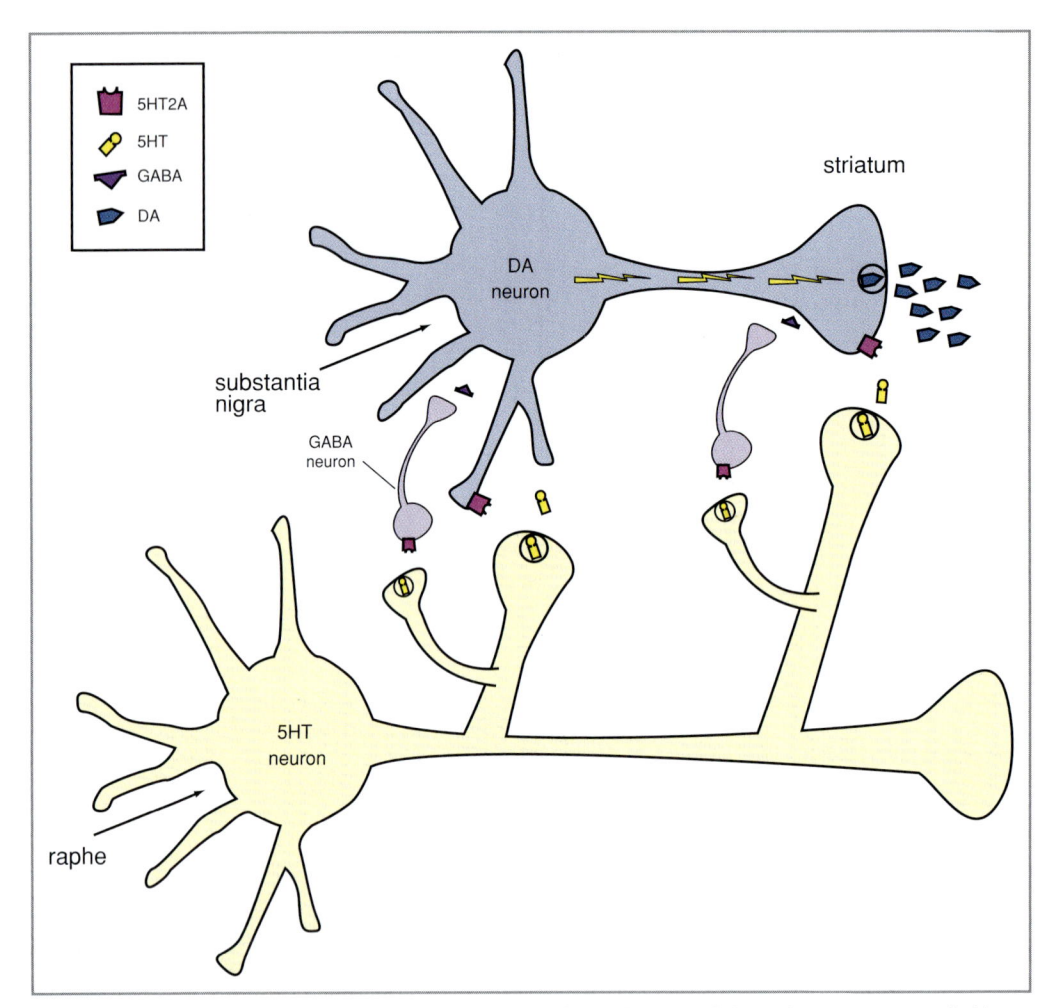

FIGURE 10-24A Serotonin regulation of dopamine release from nigrostriatal dopamine neurons, part 1. Here, dopamine is being freely released from its axon terminal in the striatum because there is no serotonin causing direct or indirect inhibition of dopamine release.

5HT2A antagonism reduces negative symptoms

There is a debate as to how robustly atypical antipsychotics compared to conventional antipsychotics reduce negative symptoms. Some experts believe that atypical antipsychotics do not really reduce negative symptoms but that conventional antipsychotics increase them, presumably due to the induction of secondary negative symptoms related to EPS. If conventional antipsychotics cause EPS and thus secondary negative symptoms but atypical antipsychotics do not (as explained in the section above and illustrated in Figures 10-26 and 10-27), this could explain some of the apparent differences in the severity of negative symptoms in patients taking conventional antipsychotics versus atypical antipsychotics.

However, the lack of production of secondary negative symptoms does not appear to be an adequate explanation for all the reduction in severity of negative symptoms by atypical antipsychotics compared to conventional antipsychotics. Another mechanism that could explain this apparent reduction is that atypical antipsychotics, working through their 5HT2A antagonist properties, may increase dopamine release in hypoactive mesolimbic

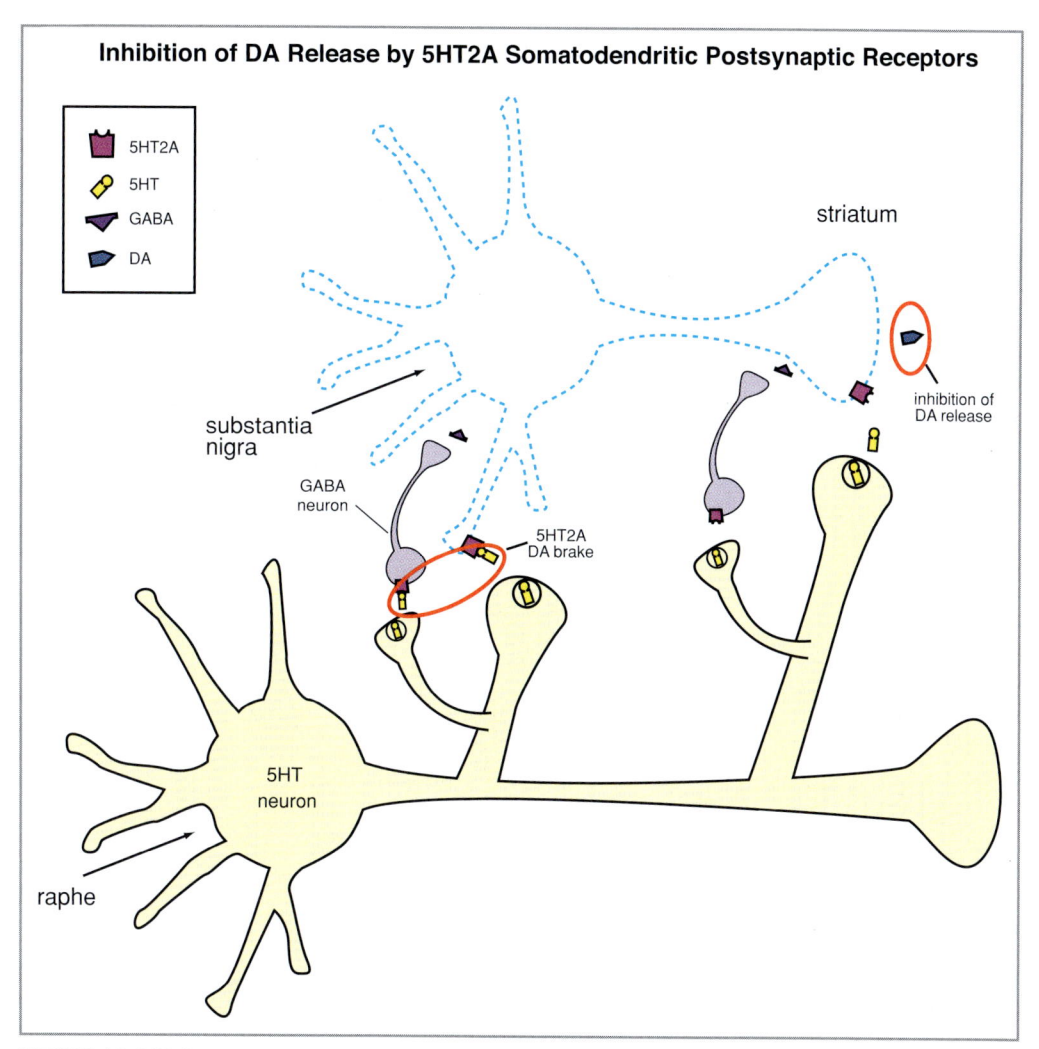

FIGURE 10-24B Serotonin regulation of dopamine release from nigrostriatal dopamine neurons, part 2. Now, serotonin is being released from a synaptic connection projecting from the raphe to the substantia nigra and terminating on somatodendritic postsynaptic serotonin 2A (5HT2A) receptors on dopamine and gamma aminobutyric acid (GABA) neurons (bottom red circle). Because of this, dopamine release from its axonal terminal is now inhibited (top red circle).

pleasure centers. If this were the case to any great extent, one might expect to see an activation of positive symptoms by atypical antipsychotics as well, but this is not observed. Apparently, dopamine release by 5HT2A receptor antagonism in the nucleus accumbens is not as robust as in other brain areas.

What, then, is the mechanism whereby atypical antipsychotics improve the negative, cognitive, and affective symptoms of schizophrenia in those patients in whom these actions are observed? The answer is illustrated in Figure 10-28 where the 5HT2A antagonist actions of atypical antipsychotics are shown to be increasing DA release in prefrontal cortex. Note that no blockade of D2 receptors in the prefrontal cortex is shown, since D2 receptors are not very dense in this part of the brain. Note also that dopamine deficiency can be primary, due to hypoactive mesocortical dopamine neurons (Figure 10-28A), or secondary, due to

Inhibition of DA Release by 5HT2A Axon Terminal Postsynaptic Receptors

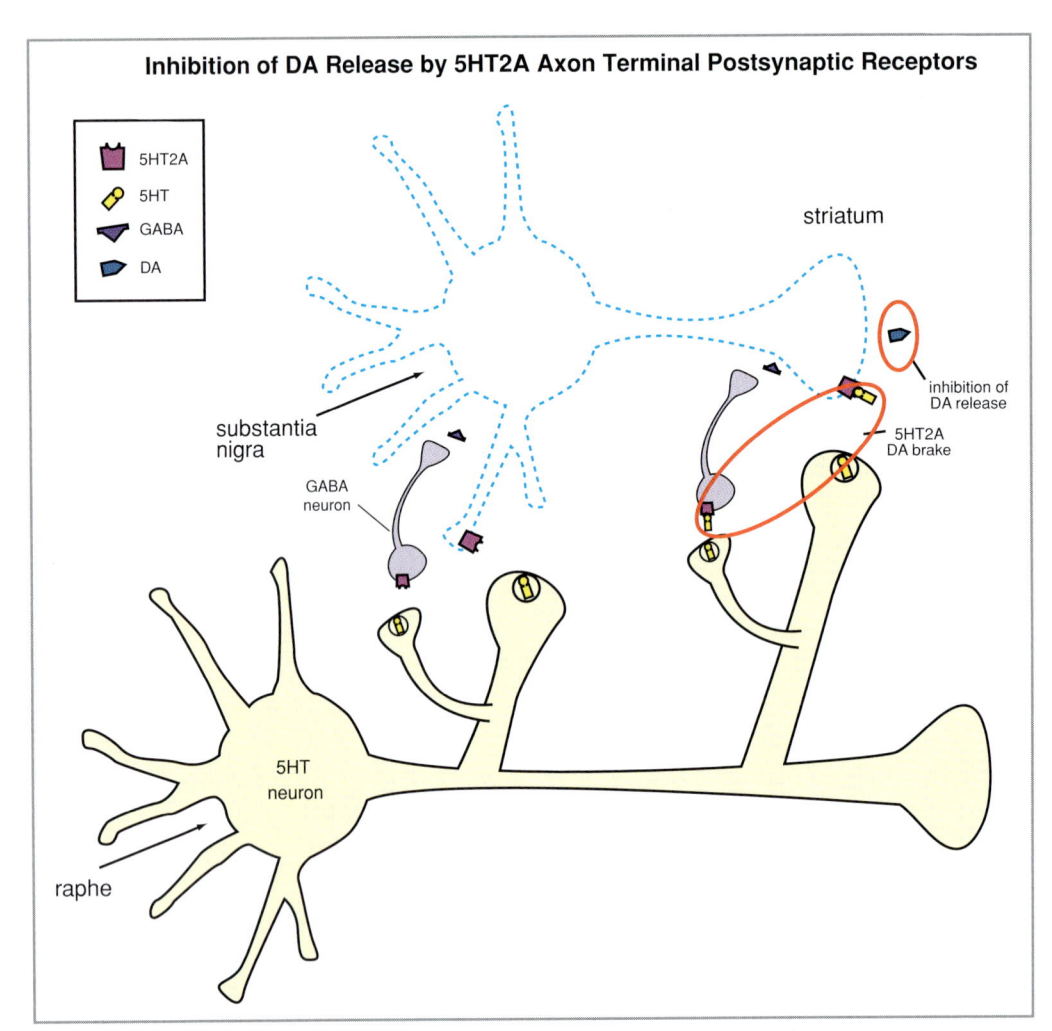

FIGURE 10-24C Serotonin regulation of dopamine release from nigrostriatal dopamine neurons, part 3. Here, serotonin is being released from a synaptic connection projecting from axoaxonal contacts or by volume neurotransmission between serotonergic axon terminals and dopamine axon terminals, resulting in serotonin occupying postsynaptic serotonin 2A (5HT2A) receptors on dopamine and gamma aminobutyric acid (GABA) neurons (bottom red circle). Because of this, dopamine release from its axonal terminal is inhibited (top red circle).

high levels of serotonin acting at 5HT2A receptors, causing inhibition of dopamine release (Figure 10-28B). Secondary dopamine deficiency in mesocortical dopamine pathways is sometimes seen in patients taking serotonin selective reuptake inhibitors (SSRIs), which boost the action of serotonin at 5HT2A receptors on mesocortical dopamine neurons, thus producing the side effect of cognitive dulling and affective flattening. Figure 10-28C shows what happens when a 5HT2A antagonist occupies 5HT2A receptors on mesolimbic dopamine neurons: namely, dopamine release is increased. Thus, affective, cognitive, and negative symptoms in schizophrenia may be reduced (Figure 10-28C).

These actions of atypical antipsychotics are confirmed when 5HT2A receptors in the cortex of a patient receiving antipsychotic drugs are imaged (Figure 10-29). In the case of a conventional antipsychotic given at clinically effective doses, essentially no 5HT2A

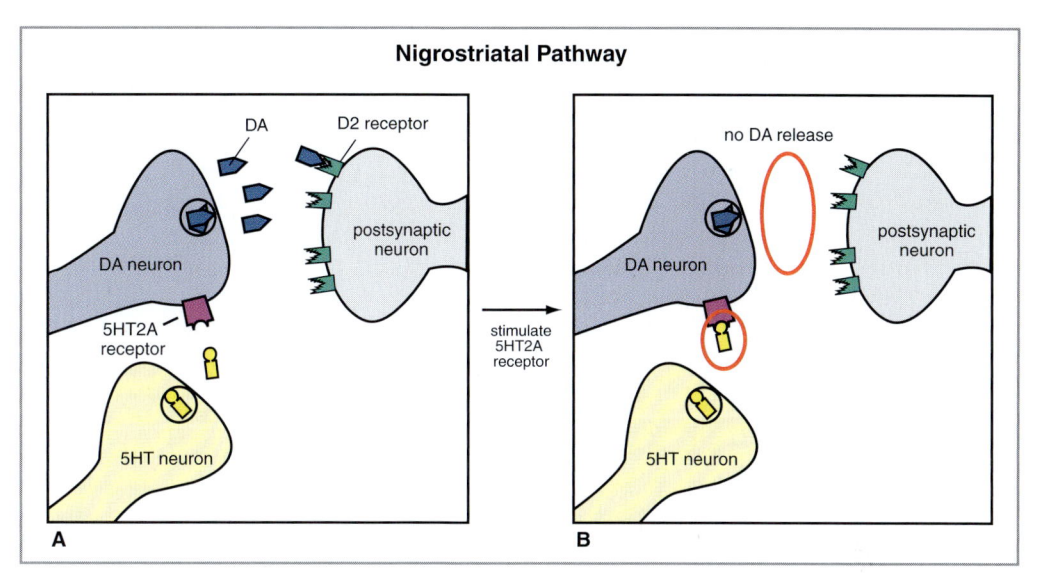

FIGURE 10-25A and B Enlarged view of serotonin (5HT) and dopamine (DA) interactions in the nigrostriatal DA pathway at axon terminals in the striatum. Normally, 5HT inhibits DA release. **(A)** DA is being released because no 5HT is stopping it. Specifically, no 5HT is present at its 5HT2A receptor on the nigrostriatal DA neuron. **(B)** Now DA release is being inhibited by 5HT in the nigrostriatal dopamine pathway. When 5HT occupies its 5HT2A receptor on the DA neuron (lower red circle), this inhibits DA release, so there is no DA in the synapse (upper red circle).

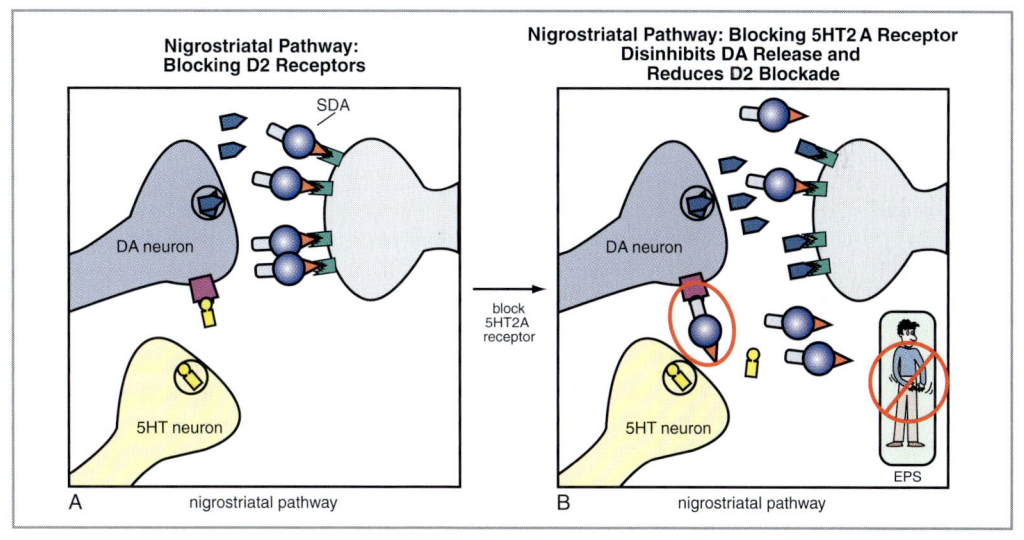

FIGURE 10-26A and B Serotonin 2A antagonists in nigrostriatal pathway. In panel **A** postsynaptic dopamine 2 (D2) receptors are being blocked by a serotonin-dopamine antagonist (SDA) in the nigrostriatal dopamine pathway. This shows what would happen if only the D2 blocking action of an atypical antipsychotic were active – namely, the drug would only bind to postsynaptic D2 receptors and block them. In contrast, panel **B** shows the dual action of the SDAs, in which both D2 and serotonin 2A (5HT2A) receptors are blocked. The interesting thing is that the second action of 5HT2A antagonism actually reverses the first action of D2 antagonism. This happens because dopamine is released when serotonin can no longer inhibit its release. Another term for this is disinhibition. Thus, blocking a 5HT2A receptor disinhibits the dopamine neuron, causing dopamine to pour out of it. The consequence of this is that dopamine can then compete with the SDA for the D2 receptor and reverse the inhibition there. As D2 blockade is thereby reversed, SDAs cause little or no extrapyramidal symptoms (EPS) or tardive dyskinesia.

A   conventional antipsychotic:
90% of striatal D2 receptors occupied

B   serotonin-dopamine antagonist:
70% to 80% of striatal D2 receptors occupied

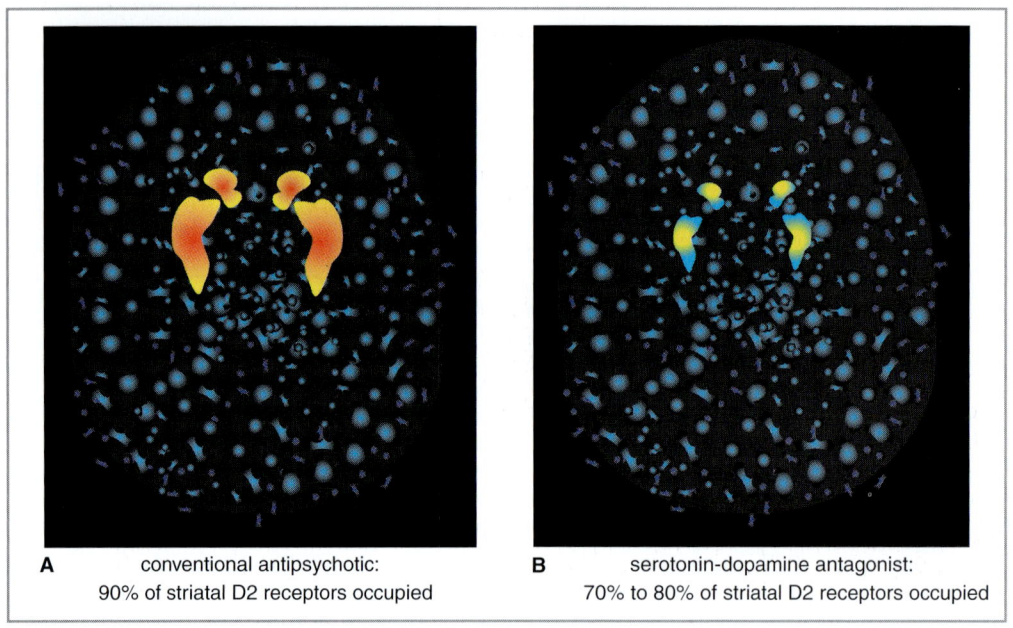

FIGURE 10-27A and B Artist's conception of a conventional antipsychotic drug vs. an atypical antipsychotic drug binding to postsynaptic D2 receptors in the nigrostriatal pathway. (**A**) Autoradiographic and radioreceptor labeling studies in experimental animals as well as positron emission tomography (PET) scans in schizophrenic patients have established that antipsychotic doses of conventional antipsychotic drugs saturate a substantial proportion of the binding capacity of these receptors. Here, bright colors indicate binding to D2 receptors and show that about 90 percent of D2 receptors are being blocked at an antipsychotic dose of a conventional antipsychotic in a schizophrenic patient, which explains why such doses also cause extrapyramidal symptoms (EPS). (**B**) Although this patient is receiving an antipsychotic dose of an atypical antipsychotic, the binding of drug to D2 receptors in the striatum is less intense in color than the scan in panel A, indicating only about 70 to 80 percent blockade of receptors. This reduction is sufficient to put the patient below the threshold for EPS. Thus, this patient has the benefit of the drug's antipsychotic actions without having EPS. Presumably blockade of D2 receptors in the mesolimbic dopamine pathway (not shown), which is the target for reducing positive symptoms of psychosis, is matched for patients in both panels, which is why they both have relief of psychosis.

receptors are occupied in the cortex because conventional antipsychotic drugs do not have high affinity for 5HT2A receptors (Figure 10-29A). However, at clinically effective doses of an atypical antipsychotic, a very high proportion of 5HT2A receptors are occupied (Figure 10-29B). Areas where a 5HT2A antagonist is binding to 5HT2A receptors on mesolimbic dopamine neurons represent areas where dopamine release is presumably enhanced as well. The increased availability of dopamine to areas with hypoactive dopamine release in schizophrenia may lead to improvement in the negative, cognitive, and affective symptoms thought to be mediated by these areas of the brain.

Theoretically, the ideal treatment of schizophrenia would be a drug with actions at clinical doses that fully saturate 5HT2A receptors in the prefrontal cortex (Figure 10-29B) while blocking enough D2 receptors in the mesolimbic area to reduce positive symptoms but not abolish reward; also, the drug would block too few D2 receptors in the nigrostriatal pathway to cause EPS (Figure 10-27B). The atypical antipsychotics with 5HT2A antagonist properties at least as potent as their D2 antagonist properties seem to fulfill that role (see Figures 10-27B and 10-29B).

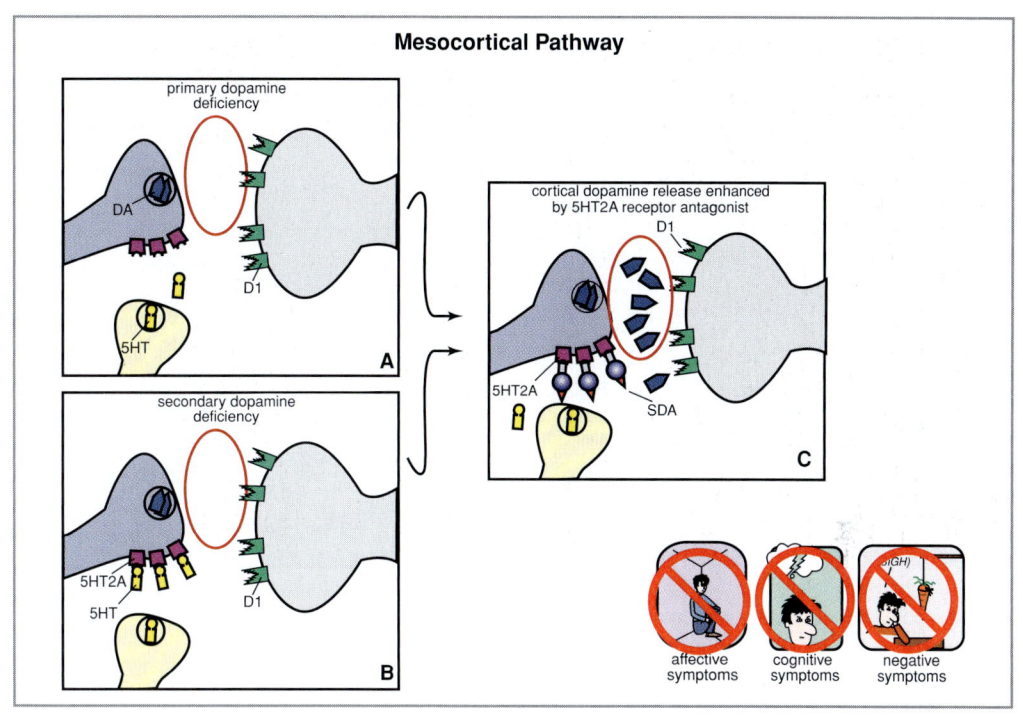

FIGURE 10-28A, B and C Mesocortical pathway and serotonin-dopamine antagonism. The mesocortical dopamine (DA) pathway may mediate affective, cognitive, and negative symptoms in schizophrenia because of a relative deficiency in DA, due either to a primary deficiency (**A**) or to various secondary causes, such as serotonin (5HT) excess (**B**). In either case, blockade of 5HT2A receptors with an atypical antipsychotic should lead to DA release (**C**), which could compensate for the DA deficiency and improve affective, cognitive, and negative symptoms.

5HT2A antagonism may improve positive symptoms

We have already discussed how 5HT1A receptors and 5HT2A receptors regulate dopamine release (Figure 10-21). These same receptors also regulate glutamate release, with 5HT1A receptors acting as brakes to inhibit glutamate release and 5HT2A receptors acting as accelerators to stimulate glutamate release (Figure 10-30). This is the opposite of their regulatory actions on dopamine release (illustrated in Figures 10-21 and 10-22).

The regulatory effects of serotonin on glutamate may play a role in schizophrenia, since it is possible that the stimulatory effects of 5HT2A receptors on glutamate release may be linked to the causation of hallucinations. That is, most hallucinogens are partial agonists at 5HT2A receptors, implicating possible abnormal activation of 5HT2A receptors on cortical glutamate neurons not only in hallucinogen abuse but also in schizophrenia. The role of 5HT2A receptors in the mechanism of action of drugs of abuse is discussed in the chapter on substance abuse.

Furthermore, in schizophrenia, the action of 5HT2A receptors in enhancing cortical glutamate output (Figure 10-30) can be linked to the pathophysiology of positive symptoms such as hallucinations within a three-neuron circuit: one utilizing serotonin, one utilizing dopamine, and one utilizing glutamate (Figure 10-31). That is, glutamate input via projections to mesolimbic dopaminergic neurons in the VTA can be direct (as shown in Figure 10-31) or indirect (the predominant circuit already shown in Figure 9-39). The direct excitatory input of glutamate descending to the VTA shown in Figure 10-31 is hypothetically

A conventional antipsychotic:
no cortical 5HT2A receptors occupied

B serotonin-dopamine antagonist:
90% of cortical 5HT2A receptors occupied

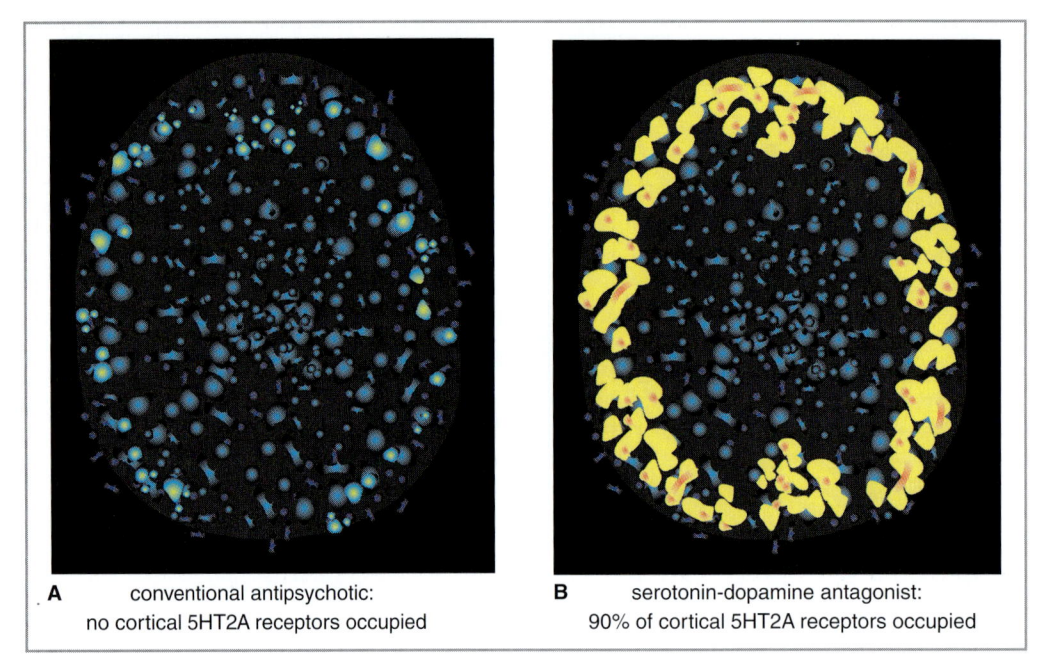

FIGURE 10-29A and B Artist's conception of a conventional antipsychotic drug vs. an atypical antipsychotic drug binding to postsynaptic serotonin 2A (5HT2A) receptors in the cerebral cortex. (**A**) Autoradiographic and radioreceptor labeling studies in experimental animals as well as positron emission tomography (PET) scans in schizophrenic patients have established that antipsychotic doses of conventional antipsychotic drugs essentially bind to none of these receptors. Bright colors indicate binding to 5HT2A receptors, and the lack of any receptors lighting up here confirms the lack of binding to cortical 5HT2A receptors. (**B**) Autoradiographic and radioreceptor labeling studies in experimental animals as well as PET scans in schizophrenic patients have established that 5HT2A receptors in the cortex are essentially saturated by antipsychotic doses of atypical antipsychotic drugs. Presumably dopamine release occurs at the sites where there is 5HT2A binding, which could lead to improvement in cognitive functioning and negative symptoms by a mechanism not possible for conventional antipsychotic agents.

controlled by serotonin projections ascending to glutamatergic cortical pyramidal neurons (as shown in Figure 10-31).

In schizophrenia, activation of 5HT2A receptors in the prefrontal cortex may contribute to positive symptoms of hallucinations by enhancing the excitation of this descending glutamate neuron, which in turn further excites the mesolimbic dopamine neuron it innervates downstream (Figure 10-31A). The take-away message here is that understanding the pharmacology of this three-neuron circuit shows why 5HT2A antagonist actions could reduce positive symptoms such as hallucinations (Figure 10-31B). That is, when 5HT2A antagonists block the serotonergic excitation of cortical pyramidal cells, their glutamate release is reduced, and this lowers the hyperactive drive on the mesolimbic dopamine pathway downstream, thus reducing hallucinations and other positive symptoms.

This idea suggests that the ideal atypical antipsychotic would have not only 5HT2A antagonist actions but also more potent such actions than D2 antagonist actions in order to optimize antipsychotic therapeutic efficacy and reduce the risk of D2-mediated side effects. In fact, this idea has led to proposals that adding a pure 5HT2A antagonist to either a conventional or atypical antipsychotic drug could result in better control of positive symptoms without producing unwanted side effects. The goal would be to achieve perhaps

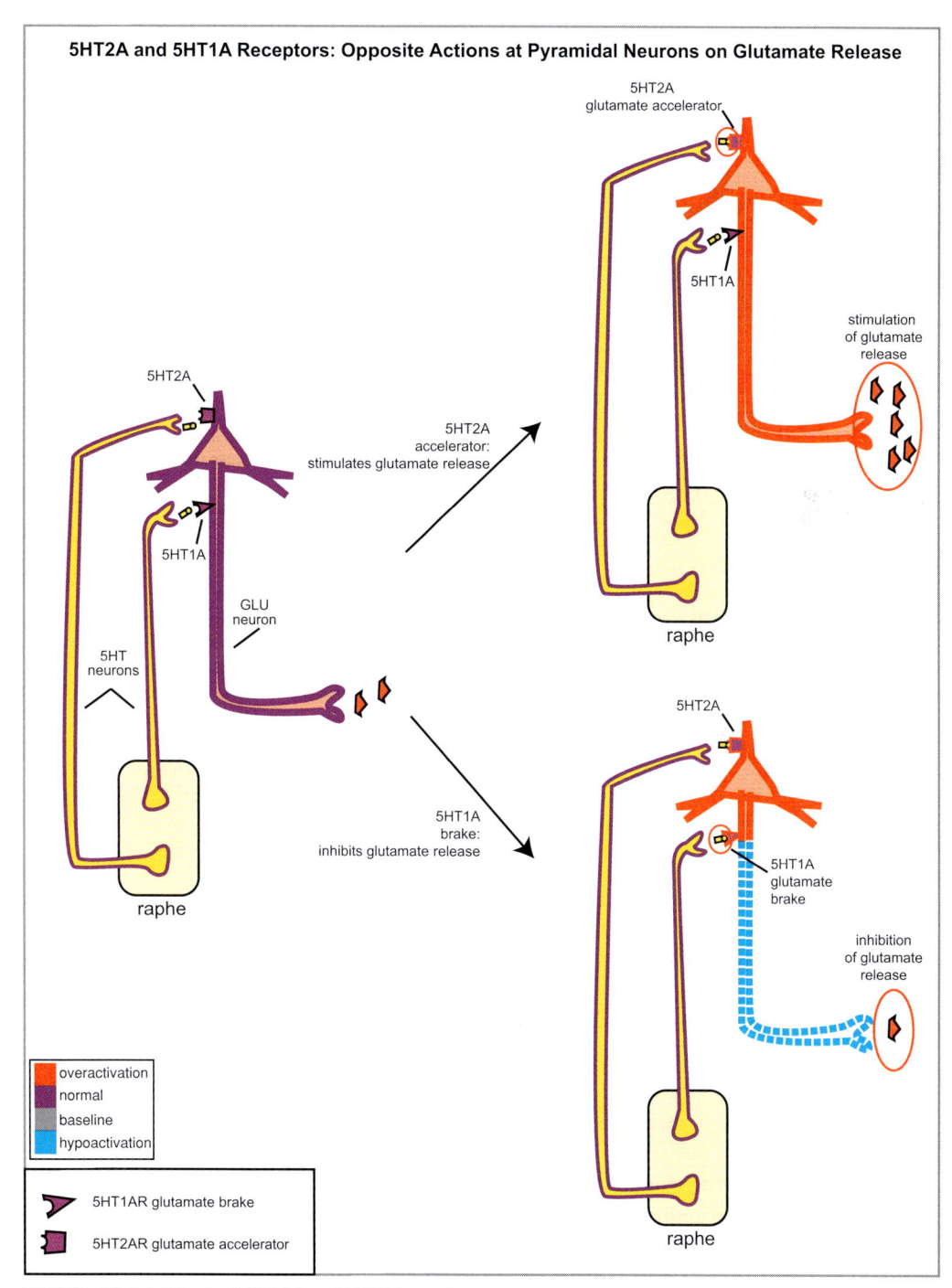

FIGURE 10-30 Effects of 5HT1A and 5HT2A on glutamate release. Serotonin (5HT) 2A and 5HT1A receptors have opposing actions on glutamate release from cortical pyramidal neurons. Specifically, 5HT2A receptors act as glutamate accelerators, stimulating glutamate release when 5HT binds to them (top right). 5HT1A receptors, on the other hand, act as glutamate brakes. That is, when 5HT binds to cortical 5HT1A receptors, this inhibits glutamate release (bottom right). Thus, the regulatory actions of 5HT2A and 5HT1A on glutamate release are the opposite of their actions on dopamine release, where 5HT2A acts as a brake and 5HT1A acts as an accelerator.

Antipsychotic Agents | 361

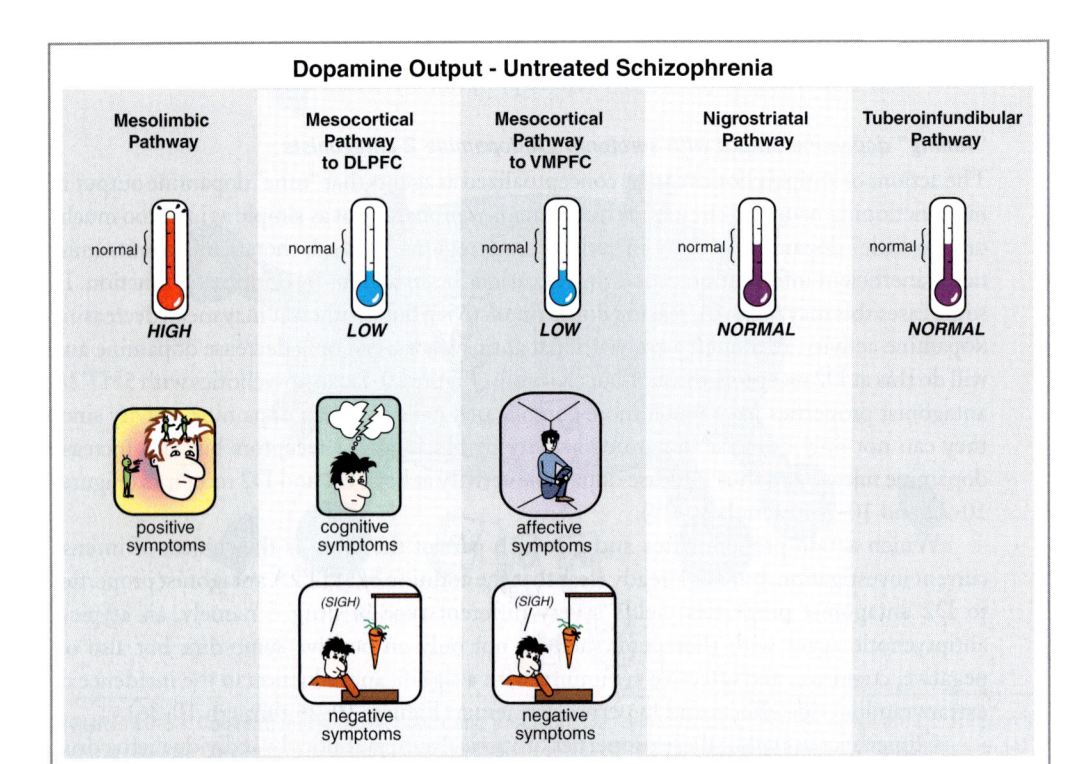

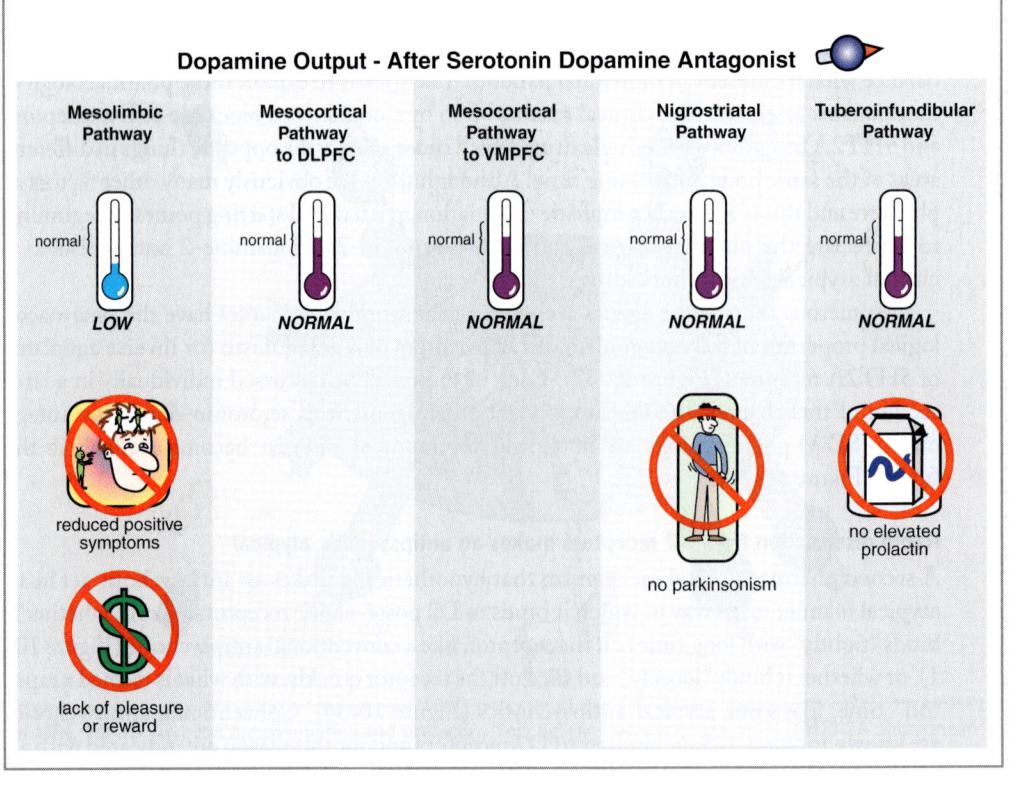

Dopamine Output - Untreated Schizophrenia

Mesolimbic Pathway	Mesocortical Pathway to DLPFC	Mesocortical Pathway to VMPFC	Nigrostriatal Pathway	Tuberoinfundibular Pathway
HIGH	LOW	LOW	NORMAL	NORMAL
positive symptoms	cognitive symptoms	affective symptoms		
	negative symptoms (SIGH)	negative symptoms (SIGH)		

Dopamine Output - After Serotonin Dopamine Antagonist

Mesolimbic Pathway	Mesocortical Pathway to DLPFC	Mesocortical Pathway to VMPFC	Nigrostriatal Pathway	Tuberoinfundibular Pathway
LOW	NORMAL	NORMAL	NORMAL	NORMAL
reduced positive symptoms; lack of pleasure or reward			no parkinsonism	no elevated prolactin

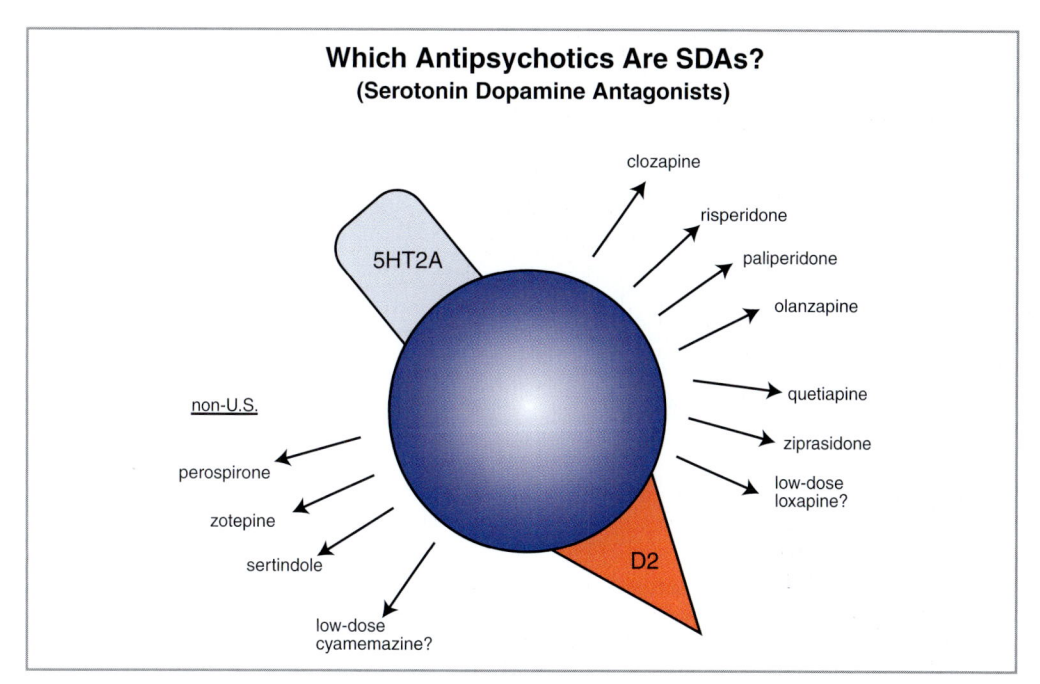

FIGURE 10-37 Serotonin-dopamine antagonists on the market. Which antipsychotics are SDAs (serotonin 2A/dopamine 2 antagonists)? There are several pharmacological agents available with the dual properties of D2 antagonism and serotonin (5HT) 2A antagonism. These include clozapine, risperidone, paliperidone, olanzapine, quetiapine, and ziprasidone in the United States as well as perospirone, zotepine, and sertindole outside of the United States. In addition, at low doses the conventional antipsychotics loxapine and cyamemazine may be serotonin-dopamine antagonists.

is that conventional antipsychotics outlive their welcome: that is, they don't just stay on the D2 receptor long enough to relieve the positive symptoms of psychosis but instead actually stay too long and thus cause extrapyramidal side effects (Figure 10-41).

By contrast, atypical antipsychotics, even if they also have the 5HT2A antagonist properties discussed above, also have the ability to rapidly dissociate from D2 receptors. This is indicated by a smooth icon for the binding property of an atypical antipsychotic at D2 receptors (Figures 10-14, 10-39, and 10-42). Rapid dissociation from the D2 receptor, or "hit and run" binding, is indicated in Figure 10-42, with the smooth D2 binding surface of the atypical antipsychotic fitting into the D2 receptor (the "hit") but not getting caught in the grooves and thus slipping off (the "run"). Theoretically, such an agent is able to stay at D2 receptors long enough to exert an antipsychotic action but then

FIGURE 10-36 Integrated theory of schizophrenia and serotonin-dopamine antagonists. In untreated schizophrenia, dopamine output is high in the mesolimbic pathway, causing positive symptoms; it is low in the mesocortical pathway to dorsolateral prefrontal cortex (DLPFC), causing cognitive and negative symptoms; it is low in the mesocortical pathway to ventromedial prefrontal cortex (VMPFC), causing affective and negative symptoms; and it is normal in the nigrostriatal and tuberoinfundibular pathways (top panel). With administration of a D2/serotonin 2A antagonist, dopamine output is decreased in the mesolimbic pathway, which can reduce the positive symptoms of psychosis, although it may also reduce the experience of pleasure or reward, since these are mediated by the mesolimbic pathway (bottom panel). Any potential decrease in mesocortical dopamine with D2 antagonism may be offset by serotonin 2A antagonism; in fact, the net effect may actually be that dopamine in the cortex is increased, which could reduce cognitive, negative, or affective symptoms. In the nigrostriatal and tuberoinfundibular pathways, the net effect of serotonin-dopamine antagonism may be that dopamine output is unchanged, thus reducing the risk of extrapyramidal symptoms (EPS) or prolactin elevation (bottom panel).

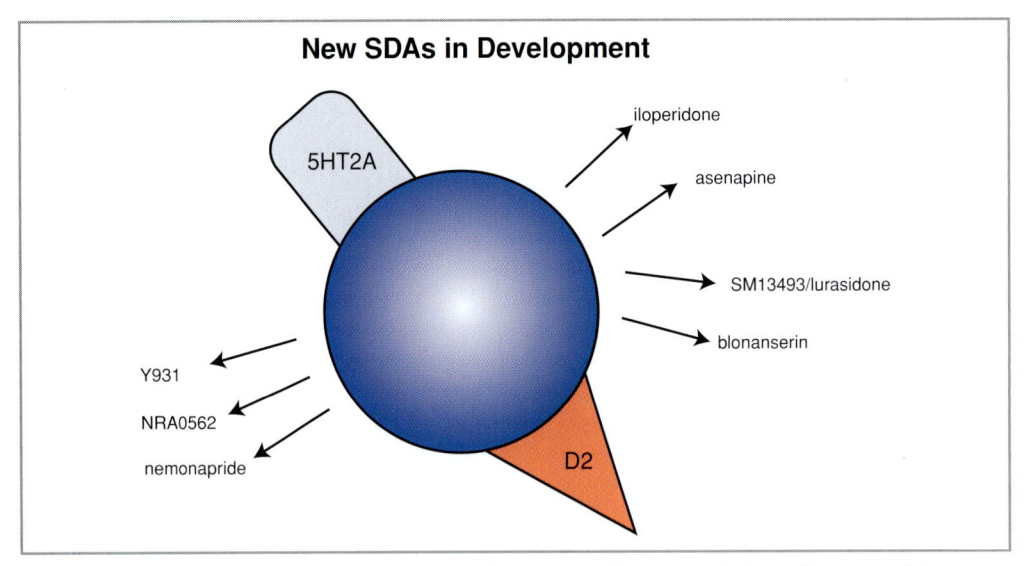

FIGURE 10-38 Serotonin-dopamine antagonists in development. New serotonin-dopamine antagonists currently in development include iloperidone, asenapine, SM13493/lurasidone, blonanserin, nemonapride, NRA0562, and Y931.

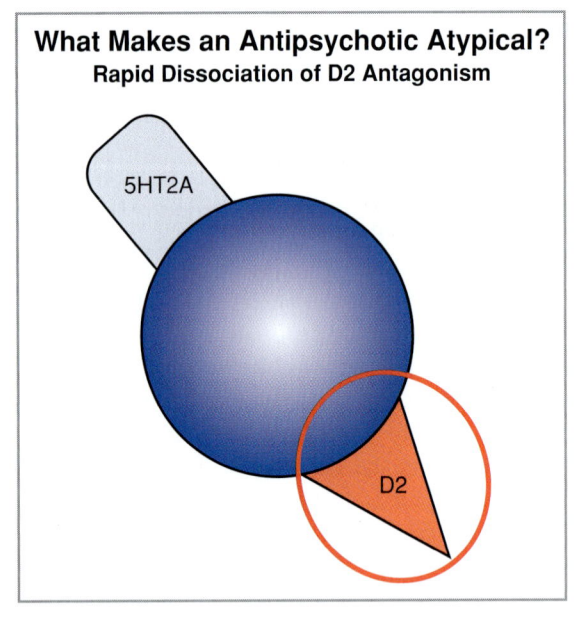

FIGURE 10-39 Rapid dissociation of D2 antagonism. In addition to serotonin 2A antagonism, the "atypicality" of an antipsychotic may be related to how quickly it dissociates from the D2 receptor, such that long-lasting binding is a feature of conventional antipsychotics and rapid dissociation is a feature of atypical antipsychotics.

leaves prior to producing an extrapyramidal side effect, elevation of prolactin, or worsening of negative symptoms (Figure 10-43). The hit-and-run theory is summarized in Figure 10-44.

One of the interesting clinical aspects of atypical antipsychotics is the observation that they need to be administered less frequently than would be required to keep D2 receptors occupied 24 hours a day. Drugs with short half-lives therefore often need to be administered only once a day. Why is this? It seems possible that continuous receptor occupancy is not

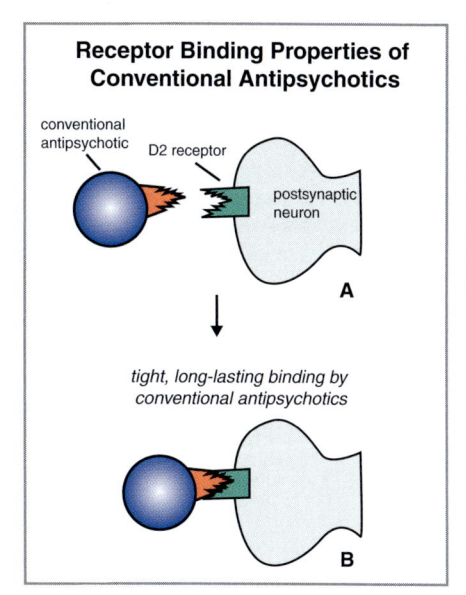

FIGURE 10-40A and B D2 binding of conventional antipsychotics. (**A**) Shown here is an icon for conventional antipsychotic drugs. Because of the biochemical properties of these drugs, their binding to postsynaptic D2 receptors is tight and long-lasting, as shown by the teeth on the binding site of the conventional antipsychotic. The D2 receptor has grooves at which the teeth of the drug can bind tightly. (**B**) Here, the conventional antipsychotic is binding to the postsynaptic D2 receptor, with its teeth locking the drug into the receptor binding site to block it in a long-lasting manner.

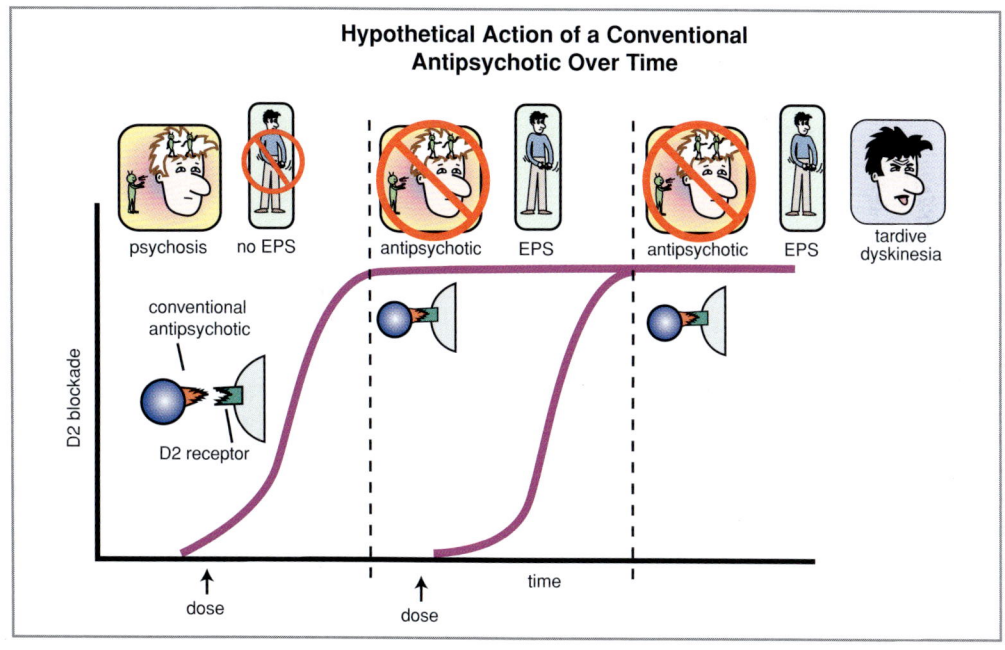

FIGURE 10-41 Hypothetical action of a conventional antipsychotic over time. This figure shows a curve of D2 receptor blockade after two doses of a conventional antipsychotic as well as the concomitant clinical effects. Prior to dosing a schizophrenic patient with a conventional antipsychotic (far left), there is no D2 receptor blockade, and the schizophrenic patient has positive symptoms of psychosis such as delusions and hallucinations. Also, since there is no drug present, there will be no EPS. Following a dose of a conventional antipsychotic (middle), D2 receptors are blocked so tightly that they both cause antipsychotic actions and induce EPS. Following another dose of a conventional antipsychotic (far right), the D2 receptors stay persistently blocked, so that antipsychotic actions are always associated with EPS and eventually tardive dyskinesia may even occur.

Antipsychotic Agents | 369

Receptor Binding Properties of Atypical Antipsychotics

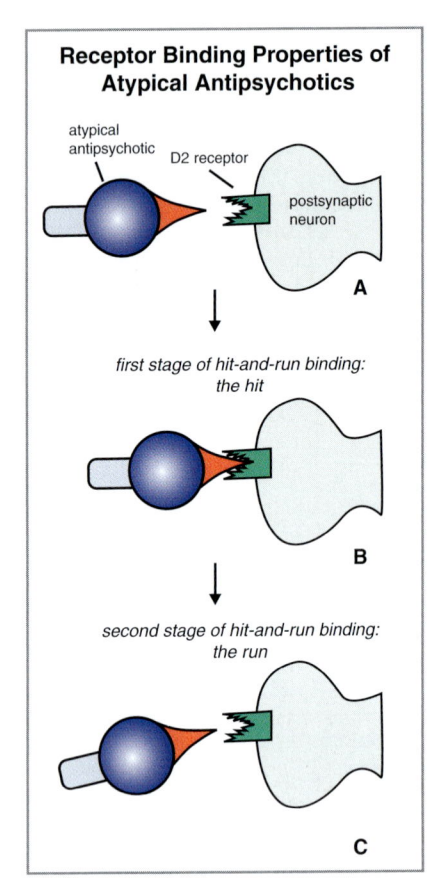

FIGURE 10-42A, B and C Hit-and-run receptor binding properties of atypical antipsychotics. (**A**) Shown here is the icon for atypical antipsychotic drugs. Because of their biochemical nature, the binding of atypical antipsychotics to postsynaptic D2 receptors (shown on the right) is loose, as shown by a smooth binding site for the atypical antipsychotic that does not fit into the teeth of the receptor. (**B**) First stage of hit-and-run binding: the hit. Here the atypical antipsychotic is binding to the D2 receptor. Note that it fits loosely into the D2 receptor without getting locked into the grooves of the receptor as do the conventional antipsychotics. (**C**) Second stage of hit-and-run binding: the run. Since an atypical antipsychotic fits loosely into the D2 receptors, it slips off easily after binding only briefly and then runs away. This is also called rapid dissociation.

required for the desired antipsychotic actions but may in fact contribute to the undesired side effects. Indeed, what may be required for antipsychotic efficacy may be akin to "ringing a bell" by clanging the D2 receptor just once a day. The D2 receptor continues to resonate with antipsychotic actions long after the atypical antipsychotic hits it.

These observations suggest that antipsychotics are atypical because they stay around D2 receptors long enough to cause an antipsychotic action but not long enough to cause side effects. One of the consequences of fast dissociation is that the drug is gone from the receptor until the next dose arrives (Figure 10-43). This means that natural dopamine can bathe the receptor for a while before the next pulse of drug. Perhaps a bit of real dopamine in the nigrostriatal dopamine system is all that is needed to prevent motor side effects. If this happens while there is yet insufficient dopamine in the mesolimbic dopamine system to reactivate psychosis between doses, the drug has atypical antipsychotic clinical properties (Figures 10-42 through 10-44).

The idea of rapid D2 receptor dissociation as a pharmacological property that can explain atypical clinical actions of some antipsychotic drugs is supported by the observation that rapid dissociation from the D2 receptor in vitro is a good predictor of low extrapyramidal side-effect potential in patients. Since rapid dissociation generally also means low potency, this also means that low-potency agents (i.e., those requiring higher milligram doses, such as clozapine and quetiapine) have faster dissociation from the D2 receptor than high-potency agents (i.e., those requiring lower milligram doses, such as risperidone), with

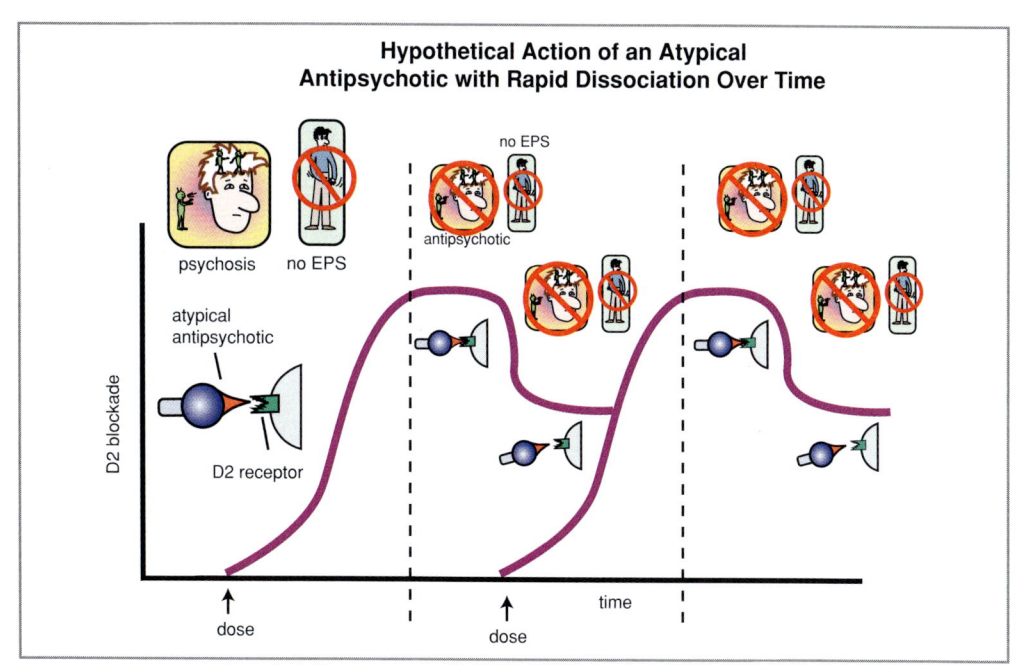

FIGURE 10-43 Hypothetical action of atypical antipsychotic over time. This figure shows a curve of D2 receptor blockade after two doses of an atypical antipsychotic as well as the concomitant clinical effects. Prior to dosing a schizophrenic patient with an atypical antipsychotic (far left), there is no D2 receptor blockade, and the schizophrenic patient has positive symptoms of psychosis, just as in Figure 10-41. Also, since there is no drug present, there will be no extrapyramidal symptoms (EPS). Following a dose of an atypical antipsychotic (middle), D2 receptors are blocked initially, but then the drug slides off the receptor and they are no longer blocked. Theoretically, antipsychotic actions require only initial blockade of D2 receptors, whereas EPS require persistent blockade of D2 receptors. Since the nature of atypical antipsychotic binding is such that the drugs rapidly dissociate from D2 receptors after binding to them, these drugs can have antipsychotic actions without inducing EPS by hitting the D2 receptor hard enough to cause antipsychotic effects and then running before they cause EPS. Since this happens dose after dose (far right), there are persistent and long-lasting antipsychotic actions, but EPS do not develop over time.

intermediate-potency agents such as olanzapine in the middle. This roughly correlates with the abilities of these drugs to cause motor side effects within the group of atypical antipsychotics and also sets them all apart from the conventional antipsychotics. It may also help explain some of the atypical clinical actions of benzamide antipsychotics, such as sulpiride and amisulpride, discussed in the following section, which have low potency at D2 receptors and lack serotonin 2A-antagonist properties yet have some atypical clinical properties.

D2 partial agonism (DPA) makes an antipsychotic atypical

A new class of antipsychotics is emerging that stabilizes dopamine neurotransmission in a state between silent antagonism and full stimulation. This is due to partial agonist actions at the D2 receptor (Figure 10-45). Partial agonist actions are explained in Chapters 4 and 5 and illustrated in Figures 4-21 through 4-28 and Figures 5-9 through 5-18. Dopamine partial agonists (DPAs) theoretically bind to the D2 receptor in a manner that is neither too antagonizing, like a conventional antipsychotic ("too cold," with antipsychotic actions but also EPS, as in Figure 10-46A), nor too stimulating, like a stimulant or dopamine itself ("too hot," with positive symptoms of psychosis, as in Figure 10-46B). Instead, a partial

Dopamine Output - Untreated Schizophrenia

Mesolimbic Pathway	Mesocortical Pathway to DLPFC	Mesocortical Pathway to VMPFC	Nigrostriatal Pathway	Tuberoinfundibular Pathway
HIGH	LOW	LOW	NORMAL	NORMAL
positive symptoms	cognitive symptoms	affective symptoms		
	negative symptoms	negative symptoms		

Hit-and-Run Theory

Mesolimbic Pathway	Mesocortical Pathway to DLPFC	Mesocortical Pathway to VMPFC	Nigrostriatal Pathway	Tuberoinfundibular Pathway
LOW	NORMAL	NORMAL	NORMAL	NORMAL
reduced positive symptoms			no parkinsonism	no elevated prolactin
lack of pleasure or reward				

Essential Psychopharmacology

What Makes an Antipsychotic Atypical?
D2 Partial Agonist Actions (DPA)

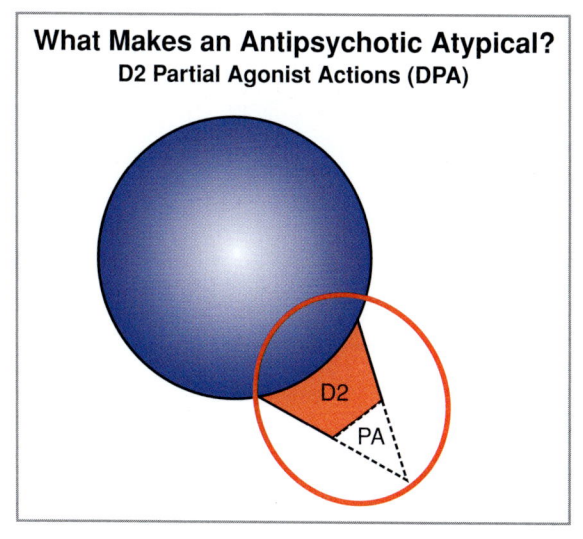

FIGURE 10-45 **D2 partial agonism.** What makes an antipsychotic atypical? D2 partial agonist actions (DPA). A third property that may render an antipsychotic atypical is that of partial dopamine 2 antagonism. These agents may stabilize dopamine neurotransmission in a state between silent antagonism and full stimulation.

agonist binds in an intermediary manner ("just right," with antipsychotic actions but no EPS, as in Figure 10-46C). For this reason, partial agonists that get the balance "just right" between full agonism and complete antagonism are sometimes called "Goldilocks" drugs. However, as we will see, this explanation is an oversimplification.

Partial agonists have the intrinsic ability to bind receptors in a manner that causes signal transduction from the receptor to be intermediate between full output and no output (Figure 10-47). The naturally occurring neurotransmitter generally functions as a full agonist and causes maximum signal transduction from the receptor it occupies (Figure 10-47, top), whereas antagonists essentially shut down all output from the receptor they occupy and make them "silent" in terms of communicating with downstream signal transduction cascades (Figure 10-47, middle). Partial agonists cause receptor output that is more than the silent antagonist but less than the full agonist (Figure 10-47, bottom). Thus many degrees of partial agonism between these two extremes are possible.

Partial agonist actions have unique functional and clinical consequences. Dopamine partial agonists (DPAs) used to treat schizophrenia reduce D2 hyperactivity in mesolimbic dopamine neurons to a degree that is sufficient to exert an antipsychotic action on positive symptoms, even though they do not completely shut down the D2 receptor, as a conventional

FIGURE 10-44 **Integrated theory of schizophrenia and hit-and-run actions.** In untreated schizophrenia, dopamine output is high in the mesolimbic pathway, causing positive symptoms; is low in the mesocortical pathway to dorsolateral prefrontal cortex (DLPFC), causing cognitive and negative symptoms; is low in the mesocortical pathway to ventromedial prefrontal cortex (VMPFC), causing affective and negative symptoms, and is normal in the nigrostriatal and tuberoinfundibular pathways (upper panel). With administration of an agent that rapidly dissociates from D2 receptors, dopamine output is decreased in the mesolimbic pathway, which can reduce the positive symptoms of psychosis, although it may also reduce the experience of pleasure or reward since these are mediated by the mesolimbic pathway (lower panel). Theoretically, decreased dopamine in mesocortical pathways may require persistent blockade of D2 receptors, and thus worsening of affective, cognitive, or negative symptoms may not occur with agents that dissociate rapidly. Similarly, decreased dopamine in the nigrostriatal and tuberoinfundibular pathways may require persistent blockade of D2 receptors; thus, agents that dissociate rapidly may have reduced risk for extrapyramidal symptoms (EPS) and prolactin elevation, respectively (lower panel).

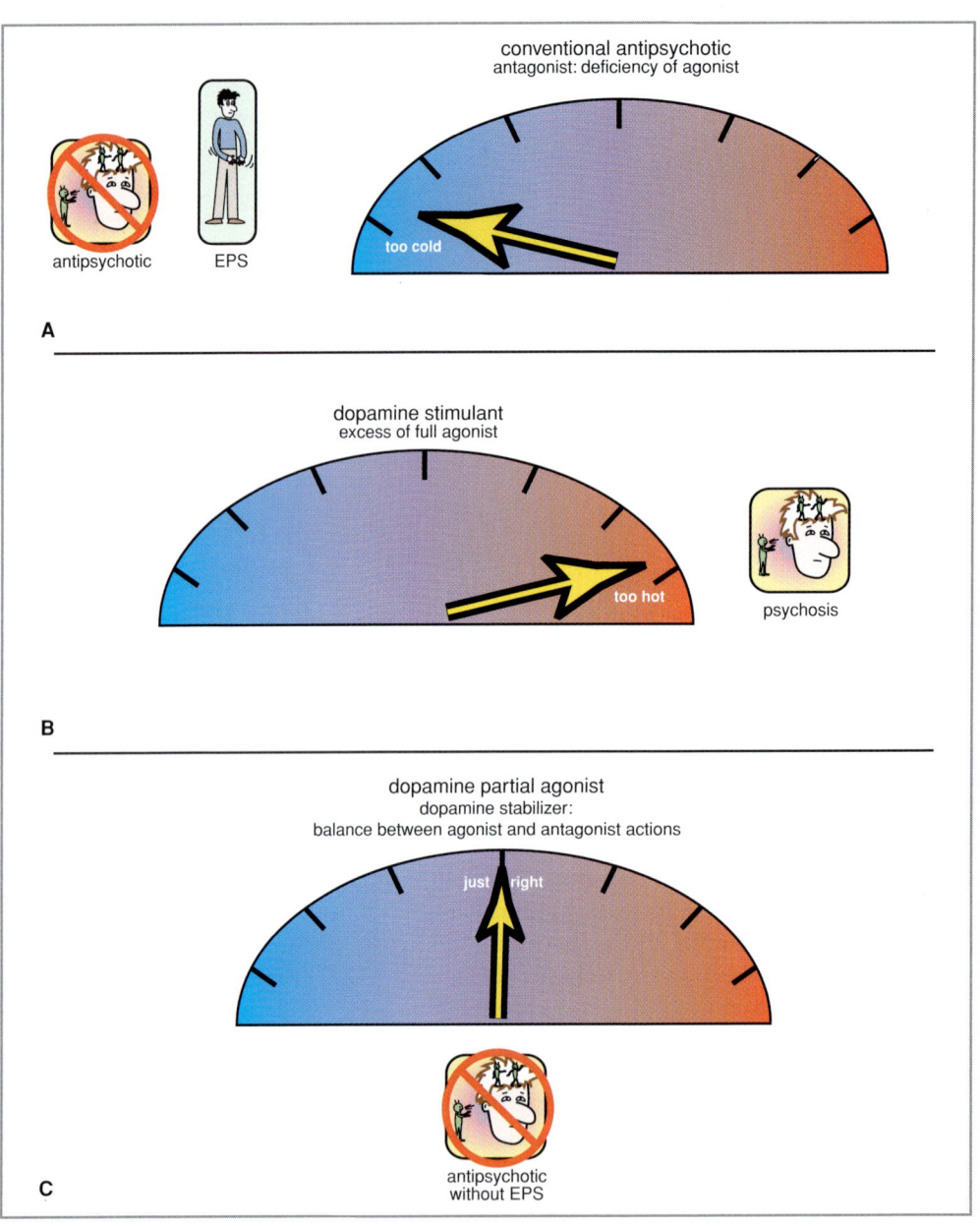

FIGURE 10-46A, B and C Spectrum of dopamine neurotransmission. Simplified explanation of actions on dopamine. (**A**) Conventional antipsychotics bind to the D2 receptor in a manner that is "too cold"; that is, they have powerful antagonist actions while preventing agonist actions and thus can reduce positive symptoms of psychosis but also cause extrapyramidal symptoms (EPS). (**B**) D2 receptor agonists, such as dopamine itself, are "too hot" and can therefore lead to positive symptoms. (**C**) D2 partial agonists bind in an intermediary manner to the D2 receptor and are therefore "just right" with antipsychotic actions but no EPS.

antipsychotic does (Figure 10-48). At the same time, DPAs reduce dopamine activity in the nigrostriatal system to a degree that is insufficient to cause EPS (Figure 10-49). Only a small amount of signal transduction through D2 receptors in the striatum seems to be necessary for a DPA to avoid EPS, and this seems to be the property of DPAs used to treat

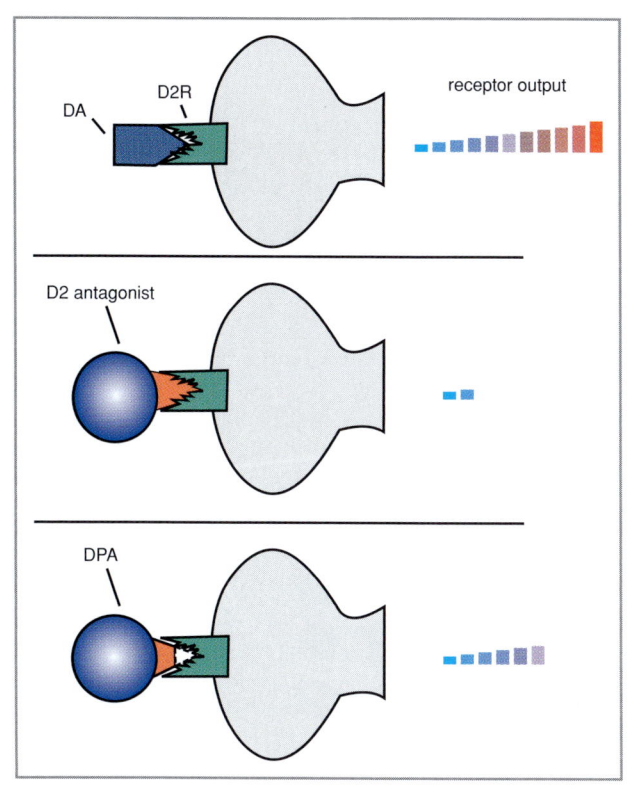

FIGURE 10-47 Dopamine receptor output. Dopamine itself is a full agonist and causes full receptor output (top). Conventional antipsychotics are full antagonists and allow little if any receptor output (middle). The same is true for atypical antipsychotics that are serotonin dopamine antagonists. However, D2 partial agonists can partially activate dopamine receptor output and cause a stabilizing balance between stimulation and blockade of dopamine receptors (bottom).

schizophrenia (Figure 10-49). Full agonists, antagonists, and partial agonists may cause different changes in receptor conformation, which lead to a corresponding range of signal transduction output from the receptor (Figure 10-50). The effects of DPAs on dopamine output are summarized in Figure 10-51.

Antipsychotics that act as DPAs include not only aripiprazole but also a new agent called bifeprunox (Figure 10-52). Older agents that may have DPA actions include amisulpride and possibly even low doses of sulpiride, but the partial agonist properties of amisulpride or sulpiride are not well characterized with modern techniques. Many new DPAs are in development (Figure 10-53), and several others have been tested and dropped from further development (Figure 10-54). Bifeprunox is in late stage development in several countries, and related compounds SLV313 and SLV314 are early in clinical testing (Figure 10-53). ACP-104 is a clozapine metabolite that may have DPA actions, but it is still in early testing, and many other compounds shown in Figure 10-53 are also in early testing.

The plethora of new DPAs establishes the point that there is a spectrum of partial agonist action, and clinical testing has shown that too much agonism is not acceptable for a DPA in the treatment of schizophrenia (Figure 10-54). This is perhaps best demonstrated by the successful development of aripiprazole, compared to the failure of a related compound from the same laboratory, OPC 4293. That is, OPC 4293 is a partial agonist that is closer to a full agonist on the DPA spectrum than is aripiprazole (Figure 10-54). This compound did show the ability to improve negative symptoms of schizophrenia, but it caused worsening of positive symptoms, similar to the psychotomimetic actions of a stimulant. Aripiprazole was then developed with a DPA profile closer to the antagonist part of the spectrum and

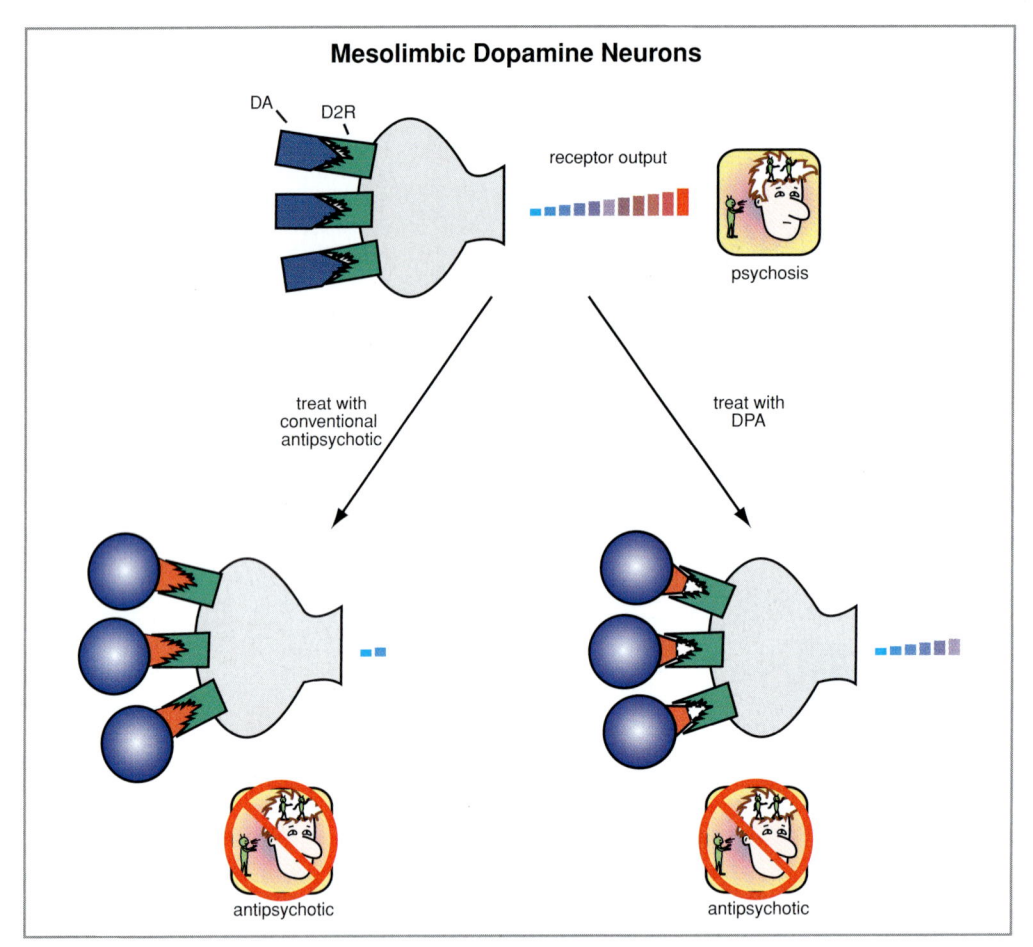

FIGURE 10-48 **Dopamine partial agonist in mesolimbic pathway.** Excessive dopamine output from mesolimbic dopamine neurons causes psychosis. Both conventional antipsychotics and dopamine partial agonists (DPAs) reduce this output. Although the reduction in dopamine output is not as robust for DPAs (lower right) as it is for the conventional antipsychotics (lower left), dopamine output is reduced sufficiently by a DPA yet with enough stabilization to produce a comparable degree of antipsychotic action to conventional antipsychotics.

has proven to be an atypical antipsychotic without psychotomimetic actions and without significant EPS in most patients.

Several other DPAs that are "too hot" on the spectrum are shown in Figure 10-54. Although there has not been sufficient head-to-head testing of the agents listed as DPAs in Figure 10-52 to determine how they may be distinguishable from each other or exactly where they should be placed along the partial agonist spectrum, hints from both preclinical and clinical investigations suggest that bifeprunox may be closer to the full agonist part of the spectrum than aripiprazole, whereas amisulpride and sulpiride may be closer to the silent antagonist part of the spectrum than aripiprazole. Although it does appear that sulpiride is too close to a silent antagonist to have an ideal clinical profile, it is not clear what the clinical differences are for agents within the effective portion of the DPA spectrum. Perhaps different patients will have better responses to one of these agents versus another, but establishing where different agents may lie on the DPA spectrum and what clinical significance this may have will require much further testing.

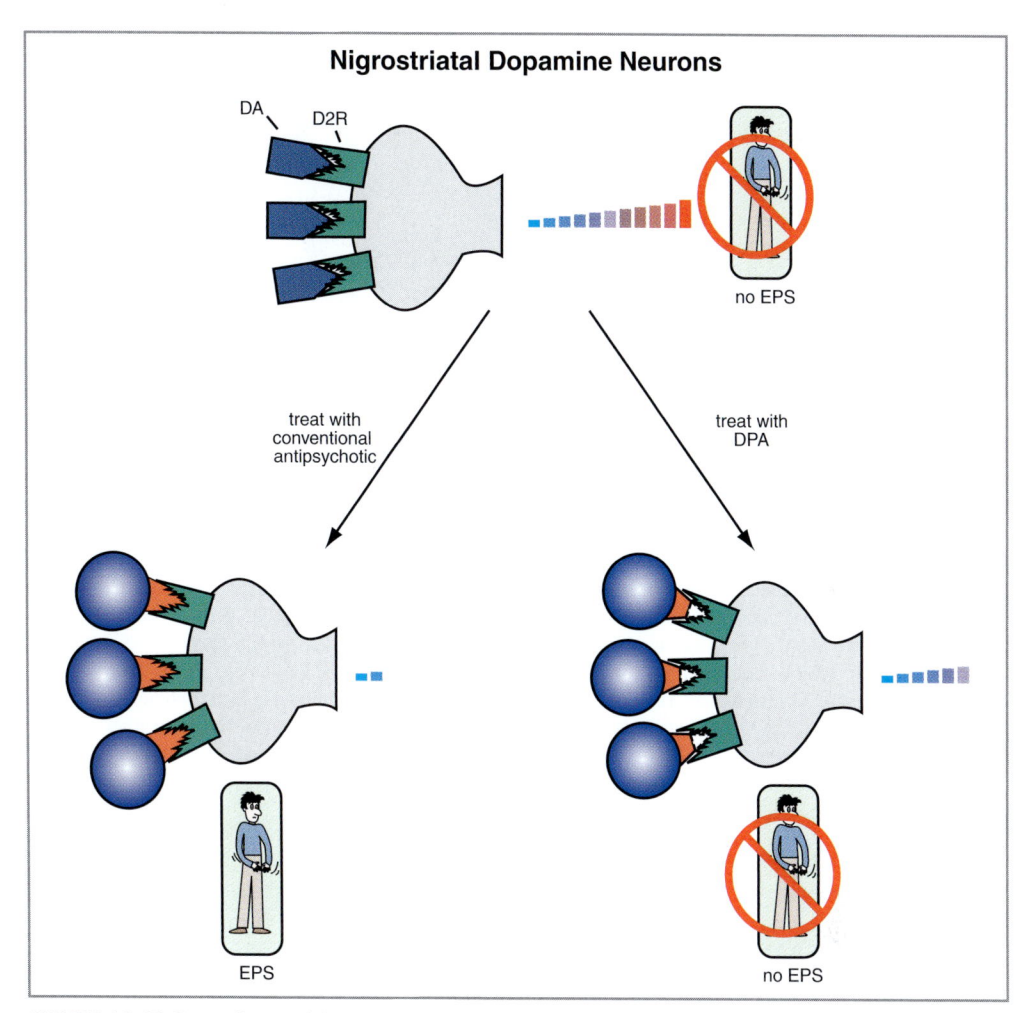

FIGURE 10-49 Dopamine partial agonist and nigrostriatal pathway. Dopaminergic tone in nigrostriatal neurons must be maintained for optimal motor functioning. Conventional antipsychotics reduce this tone so much that extrapyramidal symptoms (EPS) are produced (lower left). On the other hand, dopamine partial agonists allow continuing dopaminergic tone in these neurons, so that EPS are not present (lower right).

5HT1A partial agonist (SPA) actions make an antipsychotic atypical

The fourth pharmacological mechanism that may contribute to the atypical clinical properties of an antipsychotic is the ability of some of these agents to act at 5HT1A receptors either as full agonists or partial agonists (serotonin partial agonist, or SPA) (Figure 10-55). We have already discussed the 5HT2A antagonist actions of some atypical antipsychotics, and have also contrasted the regulatory influence of 5HT1A receptors with 5HT2A receptors on dopamine release (Figure 10-21) and on glutamate release (Figure 10-30). Thus, agonist actions at 5HT1A receptors would be expected to increase dopamine release (Figure 10-21) and reduce glutamate release (Figure 10-30). Enhanced dopamine release by SPA action in the striatum would theoretically improve extrapyramidal actions; enhanced dopamine release by SPA action in the pituitary would theoretically reduce the risk of hyperprolactinemia; and enhanced dopamine release by SPA action in the prefrontal cortex would theoretically improve negative, cognitive, and affective symptoms of schizophrenia.

Antipsychotic Agents | 377

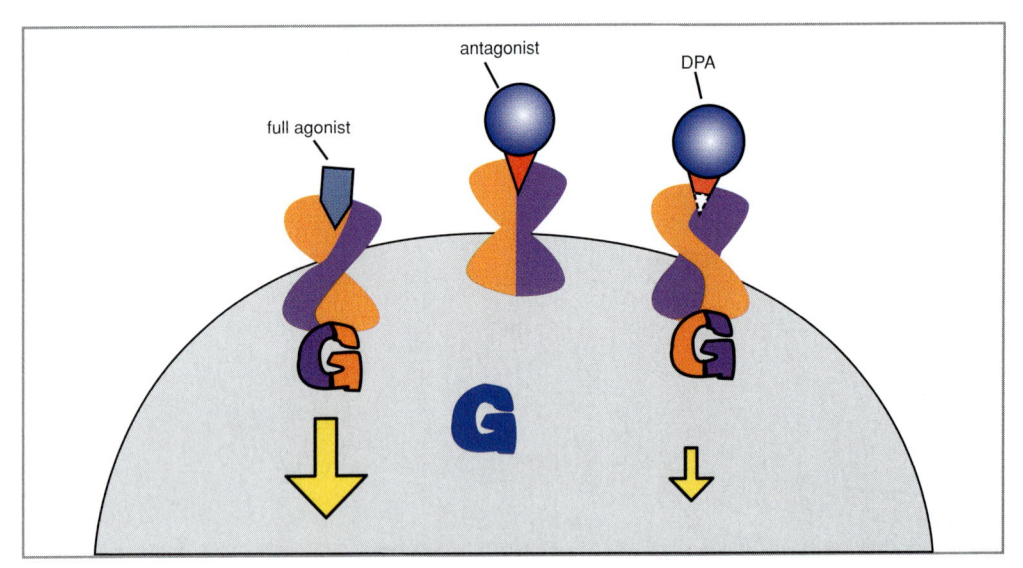

FIGURE 10-50 Agonist spectrum and receptor conformation. This figure shows an artist's depiction of changes in receptor conformation in response to full agonists versus antagonists versus partial agonists. With full agonists, the receptor conformation is such that there is robust signal transduction through the G protein–linked second messenger system of D2 receptors (on the left). Antagonists, on the other hand, bind to the D2 receptor in a manner that produces a receptor conformation that is not capable of any signal transduction (middle). Partial agonists, such as a dopamine partial agonist (DPA), cause a receptor conformation such that there is an intermediate amount of signal transduction (on the right). However, the partial agonist does not induce as much signal transduction (on the right) as a full agonist (on the left).

Reduced glutamate release by SPA action in prefrontal cortex could theoretically reduce positive symptoms. Thus, 5HT1A agonist action has similar net effects to 5HT2A antagonism. Some drugs have both 5HT1A agonist actions and 5HT2A antagonist actions, an action that could be additive or synergistic (Figure 10-56). Other drugs have SPA actions without 5HT2A antagonist actions; furthermore SPA actions can be combined either with D2 antagonism or with DPA to create an atypical antipsychotic drug (Figure 10-56).

Receptor binding properties and pharmacokinetics of antipsychotics

Over two dozen antipsychotic drugs are in clinical use; and so far in this chapter we have discussed pharmacological properties that are shared among some drugs in this class and how those actions are linked to therapeutic efficacy and certain side effects. Many

FIGURE 10-51 Integrated theory of schizophrenia and dopamine partial agonists. In untreated schizophrenia, dopamine output is high in the mesolimbic pathway, causing positive symptoms; it is low in the mesocortical pathway to dorsolateral prefrontal cortex (DLPFC), causing cognitive and negative symptoms; it is low in the mesocortical pathway to ventromedial prefrontal cortex (VMPFC), causing affective and negative symptoms; and it is normal in the nigrostriatal and tuberoinfundibular pathways (upper panel). Dopamine partial agonists decrease dopamine output in comparison to dopamine but allow more dopamine output than a dopamine antagonist (bottom panel). Thus, dopamine output is decreased in the mesolimbic pathway, which can reduce the positive symptoms of psychosis, but the decrease may not be sufficient to affect the experience of pleasure or reward (bottom panel). Because dopamine output in mesocortical pathways is likely already too low, dopamine partial agonists may actually increase dopamine output there and thus potentially improve cognitive, negative, or affective symptoms (bottom panel). In the nigrostriatal and tuberoinfundibular pathways, theoretically, dopamine partial agonism would not reduce dopamine output sufficiently to cause extrapyramidal symptoms (EPS) or prolactin elevation (bottom panel).

Dopamine Output - Untreated Schizophrenia

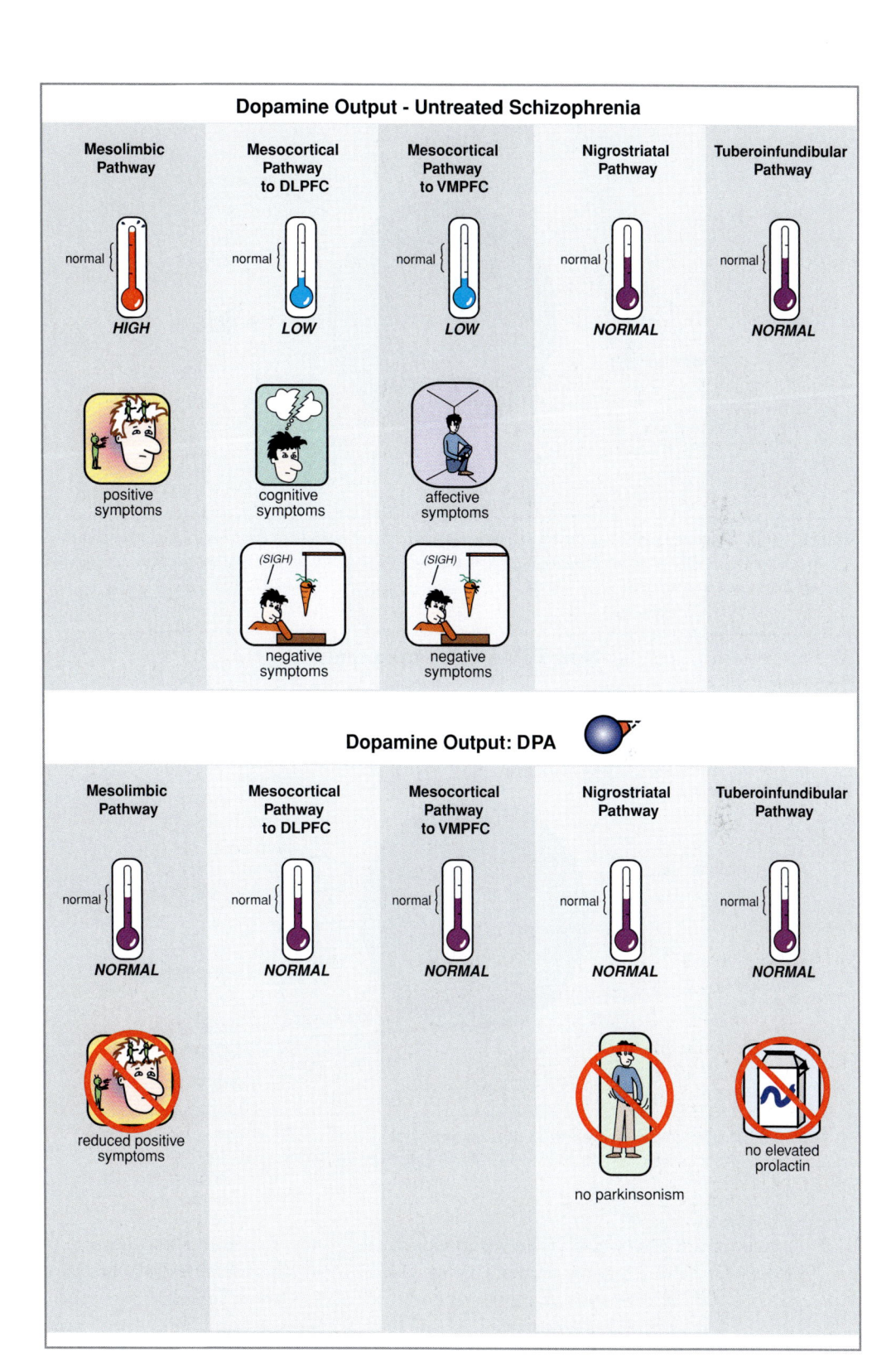

Mesolimbic Pathway	Mesocortical Pathway to DLPFC	Mesocortical Pathway to VMPFC	Nigrostriatal Pathway	Tuberoinfundibular Pathway
HIGH	LOW	LOW	NORMAL	NORMAL
positive symptoms	cognitive symptoms	affective symptoms		
	negative symptoms	negative symptoms		

Dopamine Output: DPA

Mesolimbic Pathway	Mesocortical Pathway to DLPFC	Mesocortical Pathway to VMPFC	Nigrostriatal Pathway	Tuberoinfundibular Pathway
NORMAL	NORMAL	NORMAL	NORMAL	NORMAL
reduced positive symptoms			no parkinsonism	no elevated prolactin

Antipsychotic Agents

Which Antipsychotics Are DPAs?

amisulpride?
aripiprazole
bifeprunox
low-dose sulpiride?
D2
PA

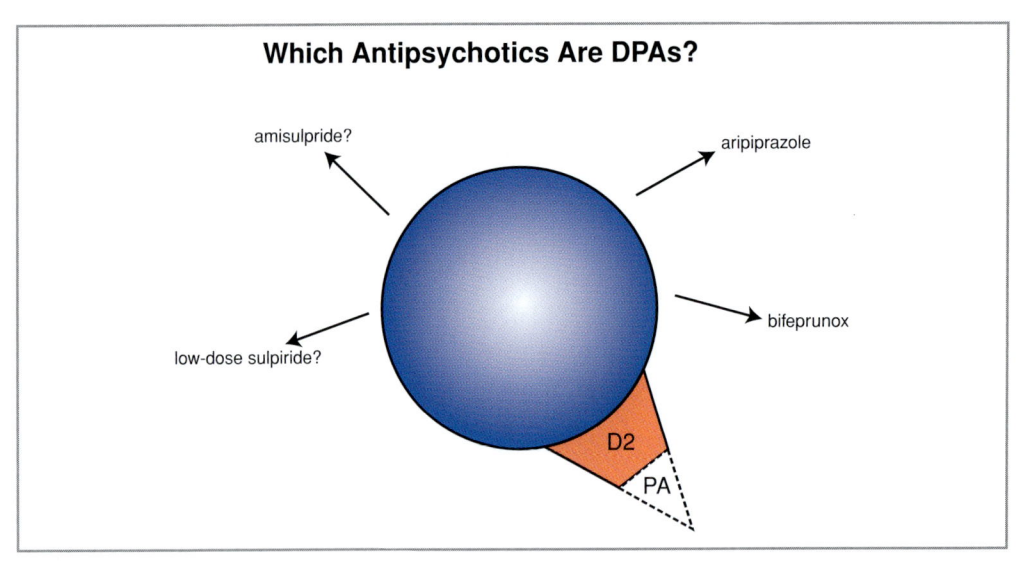

FIGURE 10-52 **Dopamine partial agonists on the market.** Which antipsychotics are DPAs? Dopamine partial agonists that are currently available or soon to be available include aripiprazole, bifeprunox, possibly amisulpride, and perhaps sulpiride when used at low doses.

New DPAs in Development

RGH188
3PPP
sarizotan
bifeprunox
SSR-181507
SLV313
SLV314
ACR16
ACP-104
PNU 9639/OSU 6162
CI1007
D2
PA

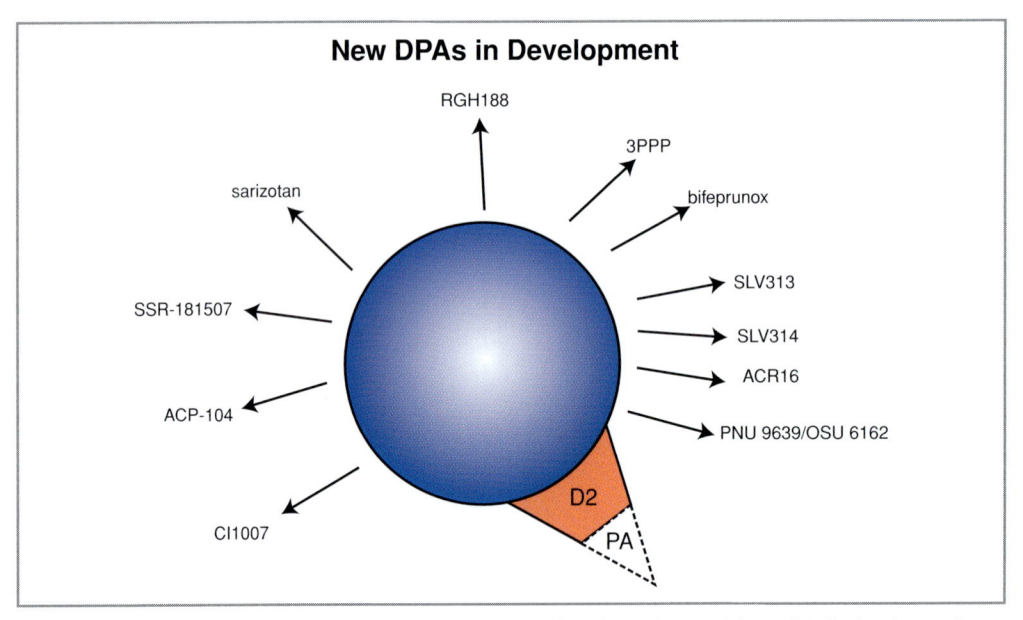

FIGURE 10-53 **Dopamine partial agonists in development.** New dopamine partial agonists in development include RGH188, 3PPP, bifeprunox, SLV313, SLV314, ACR16, PNU 9639/OSU 6162, CI1007, ACP-104, SSR181507, and sarizotan.

drugs in the antipsychotic class have additional binding properties at receptors other than the dopamine and serotonin receptors discussed above, and many of these drugs also have additional side effects, such as cardiometabolic risk and sedation. In many cases, there is good evidence to link pharmacological actions with clinical actions, but in other cases these links are only hypothetical or even tenuous. In the following section, we will review a number of receptor interactions for antipsychotic drugs and show where there may be

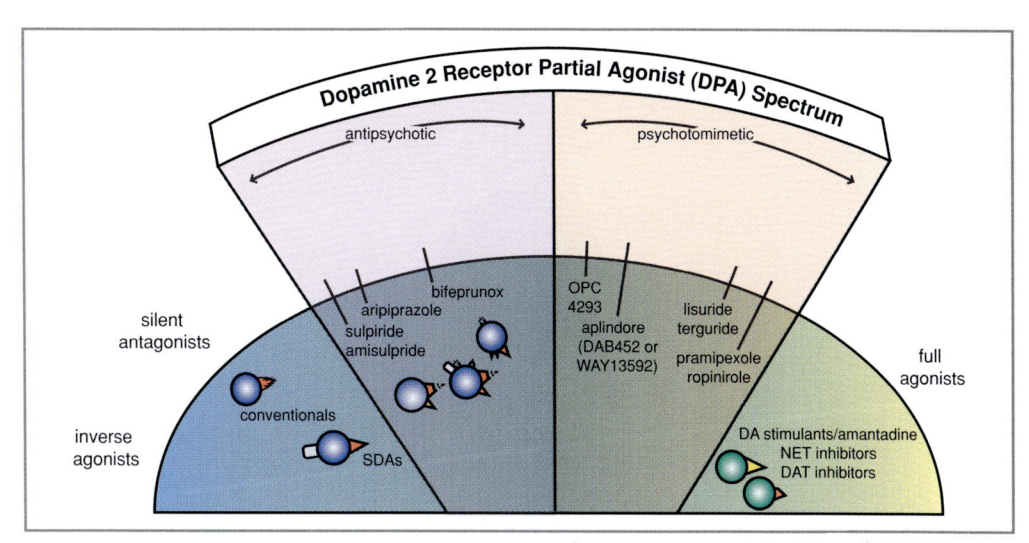

FIGURE 10-54 Spectrum of dopamine partial agonists. Dopamine partial agonists may themselves fall along a spectrum, with some having actions closer to a silent antagonist and others having actions closer to a full agonist. Agents with too much agonism (such as failed agent OPC 4293) may be psychotomimetic and thus not effective antipsychotics. Instead, partial agonists that are closer to the antagonist end of the spectrum (such as aripiprazole or bifeprunox) seem to have favorable profiles. Amisulpride and sulpiride may be very partial agonists, with their partial agonist clinical properties more evident at lower doses.

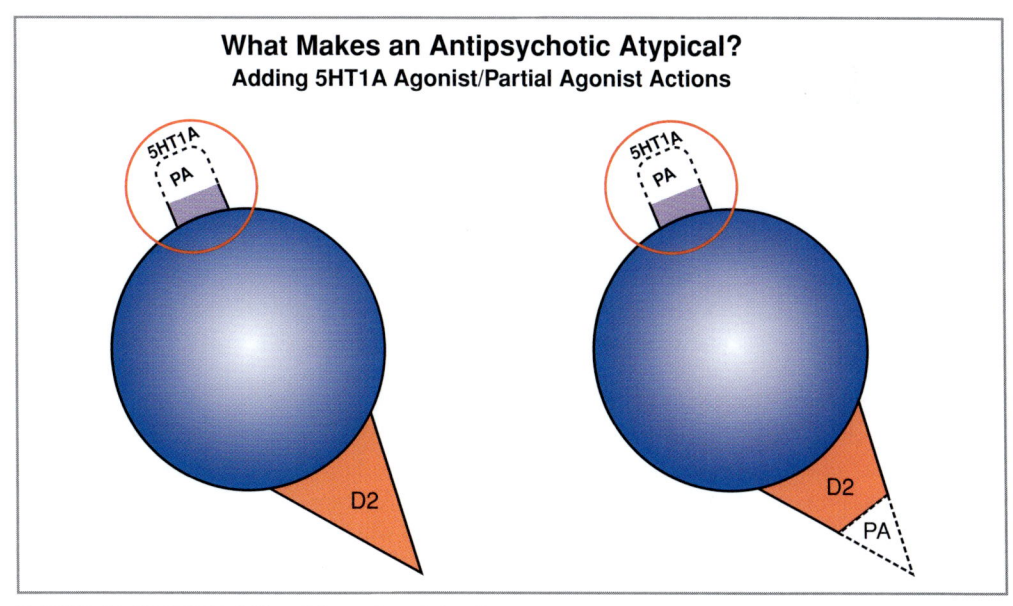

FIGURE 10-55 5HT1A full/partial agonism. A fourth property that may contribute to the atypicality of an antipsychotic is full or partial agonism of serotonin 1A receptors. Agonism of serotonin 1A receptors can increase dopamine release, which could improve affective, cognitive, and negative symptoms while also reducing the risk of extrapyramidal symptoms (EPS) and prolactin elevation. Serotonin 1A agonism can also decrease glutamate release, which could indirectly reduce positive symptoms of psychosis.

Antipsychotic Agents | 381

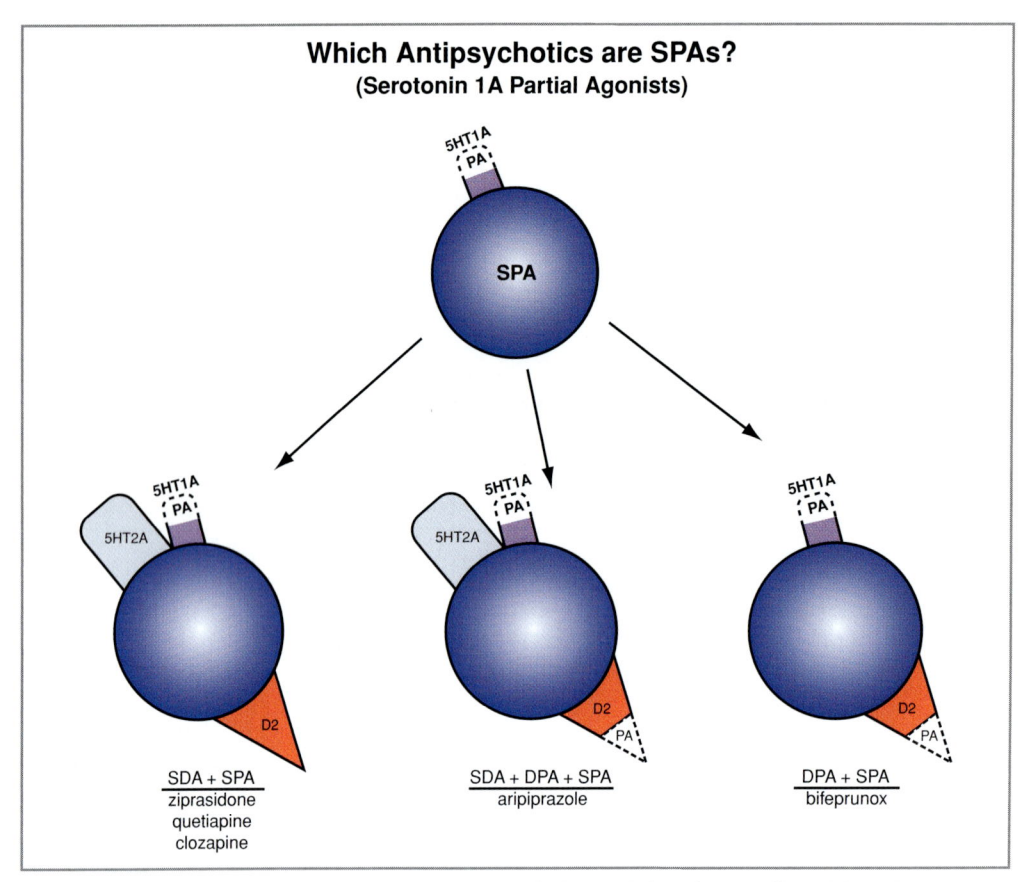

FIGURE 10-56 5HT1A partial agonists. Ziprasidone, quetiapine, and clozapine are all partial agonists at serotonin (5HT) 1A receptors, in addition to being antagonists at 5HT1A receptors. Aripiprazole is not only a partial agonist at D2 receptors but also an antagonist at 5HT2A receptors and a partial agonist at 5HT1A receptors. Bifeprunox is partial agonist at both D2 and 5HT1A receptors.

potential links between pharmacology and clinical actions. Wherever there is evidence of differentiation among the many members of the antipsychotic class, we will emphasize potential pharmacological explanations for clinical distinctions. Pharmacokinetic properties as well as neurotransmitter receptor binding actions and clinical effects are discussed for antipsychotics in general and for fifteen important antipsychotics in particular.

Links between antipsychotic binding properties and clinical actions

Antipsychotics have perhaps the most complicated pattern of binding to neurotransmitter receptors of any drug class in psychopharmacology. So far, we have concentrated on just three receptors: the D2 dopamine receptor, the 5HT2A receptor, and the 5HT1A receptor. In reality, there are at least a dozen more receptors to which one or another of the antipsychotic drugs also bind (Figure 10-57A). Scientists are just beginning to unravel the clinical significance of these receptor actions, but it is clear that many of them are clinically relevant, contributing to therapeutic actions (Figure 10-57B), side effects (Figure 10-57C), and the clinical differentiation between one agent in this class and another (discussed later in this section and illustrated in Figures 10-90 through 10-104).

Although the actions of these drugs on the various receptors are fairly well established, the link of this receptor binding to clinical actions remains hypothetical, with some links better established than others. We have already discussed the side effects mediated by unwanted D2 receptor blockade, namely extrapyramidal side effects, tardive dyskinesia, hyperprolactinemia, and worsening of negative, cognitive, and affective symptoms in schizophrenia. Here we tackle the possible pharmacological mechanisms involved in mediating two other important side effects: cardiometabolic risk and sedation (Figures 10-57A, 10-58, and 10-66). Later, we will attempt to link other pharmacological properties to both the efficacy and differential side effects of individual atypical antipsychotics (Figures 10-90 through 10-104).

Cardiometabolic risk and antipsychotics

Atypical antipsychotics have been on the market for over a decade, and only now is it becoming clear that some of these agents are associated with significant cardiometabolic risk (Tables 10-2 through 10-4) and with pharmacological actions that may mediate this cardiometabolic risk (Figure 10-58). At first, weight gain and obesity were clearly linked to atypical antipsychotics (Table 10-2 and Figure 10-59), but more recently, increased risk for dyslipidemia, diabetes, accelerated cardiovascular disease, and premature death have been linked to certain drugs in this class as well (Tables 10-3 and 10-4; Figures 10-60 through 10-65).

All of us in western civilization and particularly in the United States, live in a society experiencing an epidemic of obesity and diabetes. The "metabolic highway" begins with increased appetite and weight gain and progresses to obesity, insulin resistance, and dyslipidemia with increases in fasting triglyceride levels (Figure 10-60). Ultimately, hyperinsulinemia advances to pancreatic beta cell failure, prediabetes, and then diabetes. Once diabetes is established, risk for cardiovascular events is further increased, as is the risk of premature death (Figure 10-60).

Cardiovascular disease and diabetes are illnesses determined by both the environment and genetics. Lifestyle factors such as poor diet, lack of exercise, stress, and smoking interact with genetic risk factors such as family history of cardiovascular disease and diabetes associated with genes coding for subtle molecular abnormalities that appear to "bias" the body towards developing cardiovascular disease and diabetes. In the twenty-first century, the schizophrenic patient thus comes to treatment with the same environmental cardiometabolic risk factors that affect all of us. In addition, there is some indication that whatever genes add risk for serious mental illness may also add incremental risk for cardiometabolic disorders. For these reasons, it was not recognized early following the introduction of atypical antipsychotics that some of these agents enhanced cardiometabolic risk beyond these background factors of genes and environment (see Tables 10-2 through 10-4 and Figures 10-58 through 10-65).

As already mentioned, the first indication that certain atypical antipsychotics are associated with increased cardiometabolic risk was the recognition that weight gain, sometimes profound, is associated with some antipsychotics (Table 10-2). Receptors associated with increased weight gain are the H1 histamine receptor and the 5HT2C serotonin receptor; when these receptors are blocked, particularly at the same time, patients can experience weight gain (Table 10-2 and Figures 10-58 and 10-59). Such weight gain is at least in part due to enhanced appetite in hypothalamic eating centers (Figure 10-59), although peripheral factors unrelated to appetite may also be involved in antipsychotic-induced weight gain. Antipsychotics associated with the greatest degree of weight gain are those that have the most potent antagonist actions simultaneously at H1 and 5HT2C receptors (Table 10-2 and Figures 10-58 and 10-59; see also Figures 10-90 through 10-104). Since weight gain

384 | Essential Psychopharmacology

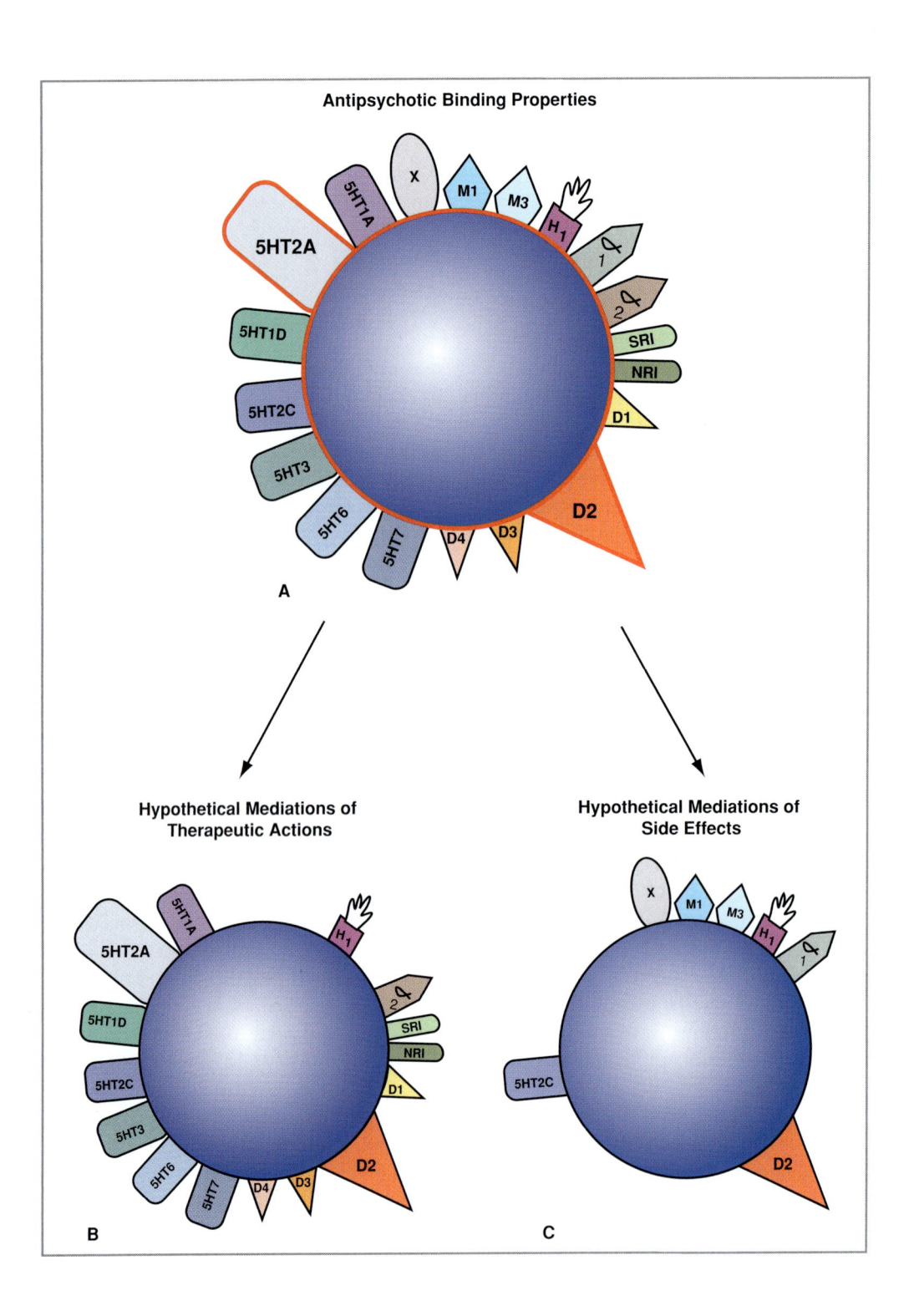

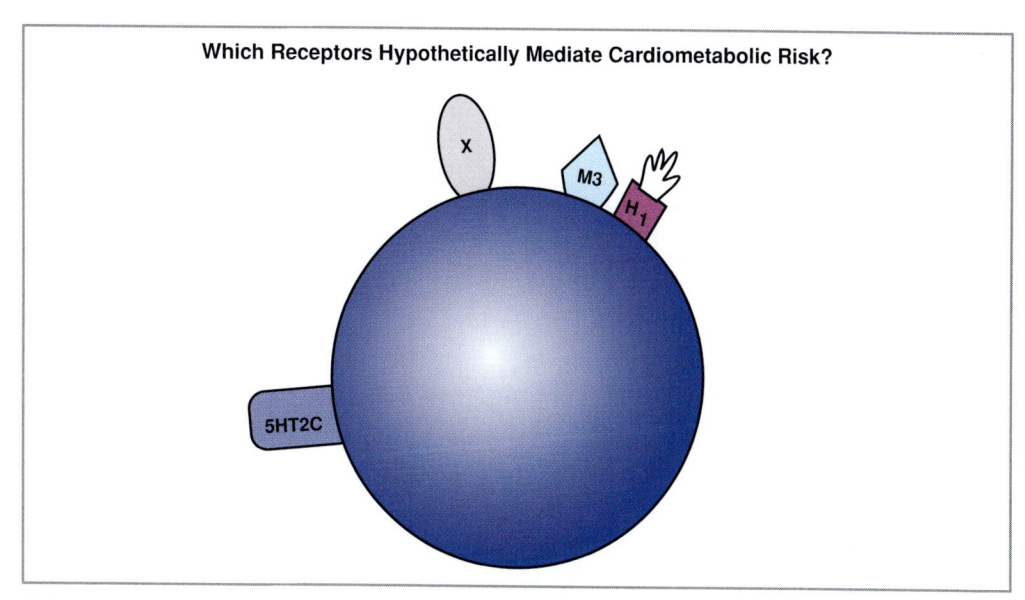

FIGURE 10-58 Receptors mediating cardiometabolic risk. Which receptors hypothetically mediate cardiometabolic risk? Serotonin-2C, muscarinic-3, and histamine-1 receptors as well as receptors yet to be identified (signified here as receptor X), are all hypothetically linked to cardiometabolic risk. In particular, antagonism of serotonin-2C and histamine-1 receptors is associated with weight gain, while antagonism at muscarinic-3 receptors can impair insulin regulation. An unknown receptor X may be involved in the rapid production of insulin resistance and may also rapidly cause elevated fasting plasma triglyceride levels in some patients who experience increased cardiometabolic risk on certain atypical antipsychotics.

can lead to obesity, obesity to diabetes, and diabetes to cardiac disease along the metabolic highway (Figure 10-60), it seemed feasible at first that weight gain might explain all the other cardiometabolic complications linked to treatment with those atypical antipsychotics that cause weight gain (Table 10-2).

However, it now appears that the cardiometabolic risk of certain atypical antipsychotics cannot simply be explained by increased appetite and weight gain, even though they certainly do represent the first steps down the slippery slope toward cardiometabolic complications (Figure 10-61). That is, some atypical antipsychotics can elevate fasting triglyceride levels and cause increased insulin resistance in a manner that cannot be explained by weight gain alone (Tables 10-3 and 10-4; Figures 10-62 and 10-63; see also Figures 10-90 through 10-104). When dyslipidemia and insulin resistance occur, this moves a patient along the

---

FIGURE 10-57A, B and C Pharmacological properties of atypical antipsychotics. Atypical antipsychotics have some of the most complex mixtures of pharmacological properties in psychopharmacology. (**A**) Beyond antagonism of serotonin (5HT) 2A and D2 receptors, agents in this class interact with multiple other receptor subtypes for both dopamine and serotonin, including 5HT1A, 5HT1D, 5HT2C, 5HT3, 5HT6, 5HT7, the 5HT transporter, and D1, D3, and D4. Atypical antipsychotics may have effects on other neurotransmitter systems as well, with inhibition of the norepinephrine transporter as well as muscarinic-1, muscarinic-3, histamine-1, alpha-1 adrenergic, and alpha-2 adrenergic receptors. In addition, some atypical antipsychotics may have actions that alter cellular insulin resistance and increase fasting plasma triglyceride levels, hypothetically due to action at receptors that are not yet well understood, signified by receptor X in this picture. Some of these multiple pharmacological properties can contribute to the therapeutic effects of atypical antipsychotics (**B**), whereas others can contribute to their side effects (**C**). No two atypical antipsychotics have identical binding properties, which probably helps to explain why they all have distinctive clinical properties.

Antipsychotic Agents | 385

TABLE 10-2 Atypical antipsychotics and risk of weight gain: FDA and experts agree on three tiers of risk

Antipsychotic	Risk for Weight Gain
Clozapine	+++
Olanzapine	+++
Risperidone*	++
Quetiapine	++
Ziprasidone	+/−
Aripiprazole	+/−

*Risperidone's active metabolite paliperidone likely poses the same risk of weight gain as risperidone itself.
FDA, US Food and Drug Administration.

TABLE 10-3 Atypical antipsychotics and cardiometabolic risk: FDA and experts disagree on one versus three tiers of risk

| Antipsychotic | Cardiometabolic/Dyslipidemia/Diabetes Risk |||
	Expert consensus	CATIE	FDA
Clozapine	Definite risk	ND	Diabetes warning
Olanzapine	Definite risk	Definite risk	Diabetes warning
Risperidone*	Inconclusive	Intermediate	Diabetes warning
Quetiapine	Inconclusive	Definite risk	Diabetes warning
Ziprasidone	+/− limited data	Low-risk	Diabetes warning
Aripiprazole	+/− limited data	ND	Diabetes warning

*Risperidone's active metabolite paliperidone likely poses the same cardiometabolic risk as risperidone itself.
ND, not done (clozapine and aripiprazole not studied in early phases of this trial).
CATIE, Clinical Antipsychotic Trials of Intervention Effectiveness.
FDA, US Food and Drug Administration.

TABLE 10-4 Are there "metabolically friendly" atypical antipsychotics? Low-risk agents for weight gain and cardiometabolic illness

Antipsychotic	Cardiometabolic Risk
Ziprasidone	Low
Aripiprazole	Low
Amisulpride	Possibly low but not well studied
Bifeprunox	Possibly low, studies in progress

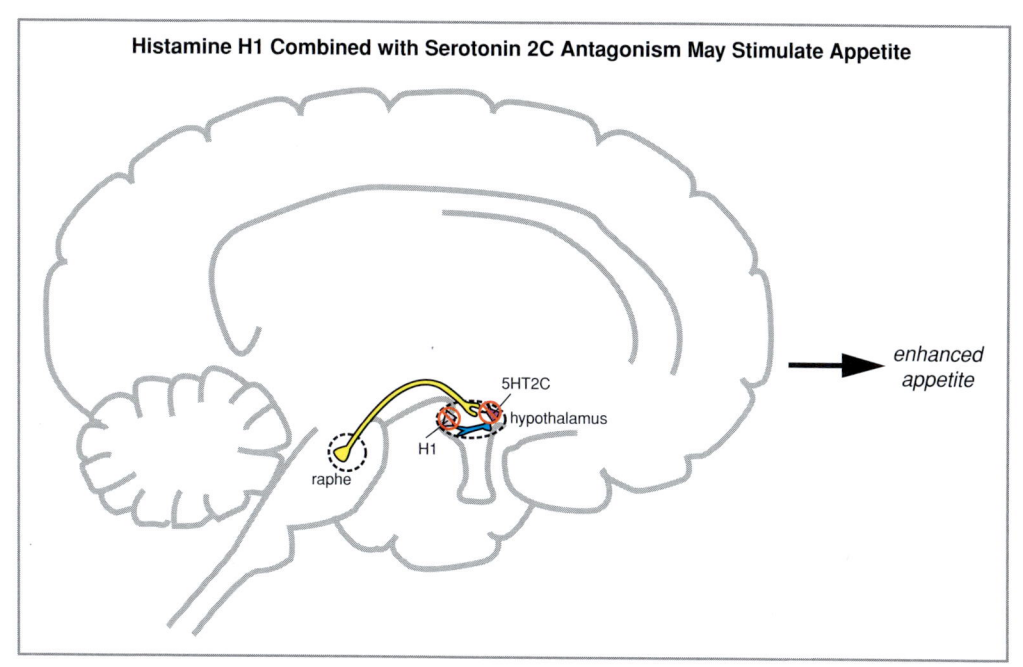

FIGURE 10-59 H1 combined with 5HT2C antagonism. Histamine 1 (H1) combined with serotonin-2C antagonism may stimulate appetite. Antagonism of serotonin-2C and/or H1 receptors can lead to weight gain, perhaps at least in part due to stimulation of appetite regulated by the hypothalamus.

metabolic highway toward diabetes and cardiovascular disease (Figure 10-60). Although this happens in many patients with weight gain alone, it also occurs in some patients who take atypical antipsychotics prior to gaining weight, as though there were an acute receptor-mediated action of these drugs on insulin regulation.

This hypothesized mechanism is indicated as receptor X on the drug icon in Figures 10-57 and 10-58 and on the icons for those agents hypothesized to have this action on insulin resistance and fasting triglycerides (see Tables 10-3 and 10-4 and Figures 10-90 through 10-104). To date, the mechanism of this increased insulin resistance and elevation of fasting triglycerides has been vigorously pursued but has not yet been identified. The rapid elevation of fasting triglycerides on initiation of some antipsychotics and the rapid fall of fasting triglycerides on discontinuation of such drugs (Table 10-3) is highly suggestive that an unknown pharmacological mechanism causes these changes, although this remains speculative. The hypothetical actions of atypical antipsychotics with this postulated receptor action are shown in Figure 10-62, where adipose tissue, liver, and skeletal muscle all develop insulin resistance in response to administration of certain antipsychotic drugs (e.g., high-risk drugs listed in Table 10-3 but not metabolically friendly drugs listed in Table 10-4), at least in certain patients.

Whatever the mechanism of this effect, it is clear that fasting plasma triglycerides and insulin resistance can be elevated significantly in some patients taking certain antipsychotics (Tables 10-3 and 10-4) and that this enhances cardiometabolic risk, moves such patients along the metabolic highway (Figure 10-60), and functions as a second step down the slippery slope toward the diabolical destination of cardiovascular events and premature death (Figure 10-63). This does not happen in all patients taking an antipsychotic (Tables 10-3 and 10-4), but the development of this problem can be detected by monitoring

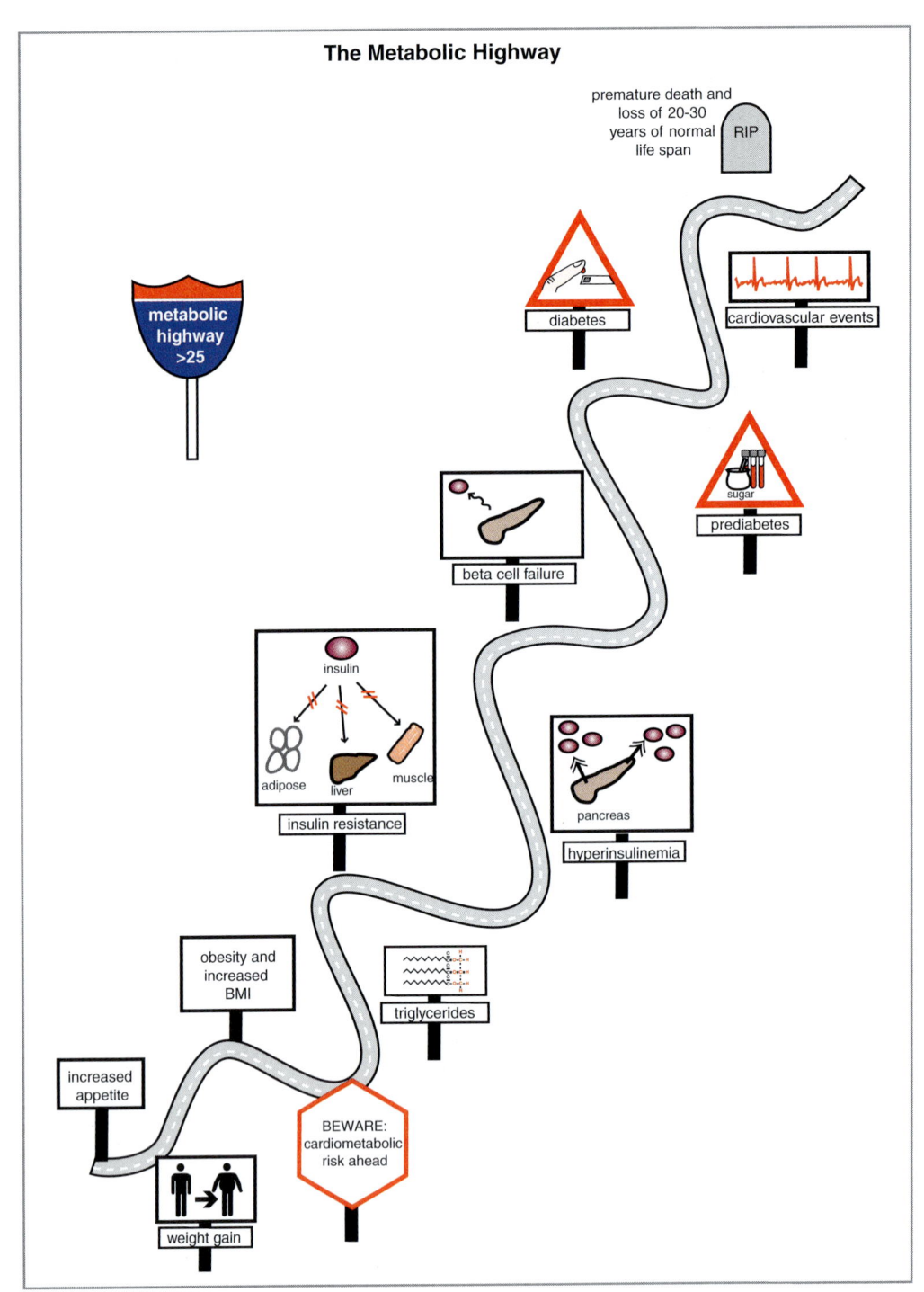

FIGURE 10-60 Metabolic highway. The metabolic highway depicts stages of metabolic changes and illnesses that progressively increase risk of cardiovascular disease and premature death. The "entrance ramp" for the metabolic highway may be increased appetite and weight gain that leads to a body mass index (BMI) greater than 25. This can progress to obesity, insulin resistance, and dyslipidemia, with increases in fasting triglyceride levels. Ultimately, hyperinsulinemia advances to pancreatic beta cell failure, prediabetes, and then diabetes. Diabetes in turn increases risk for cardiovascular events as well as premature death.

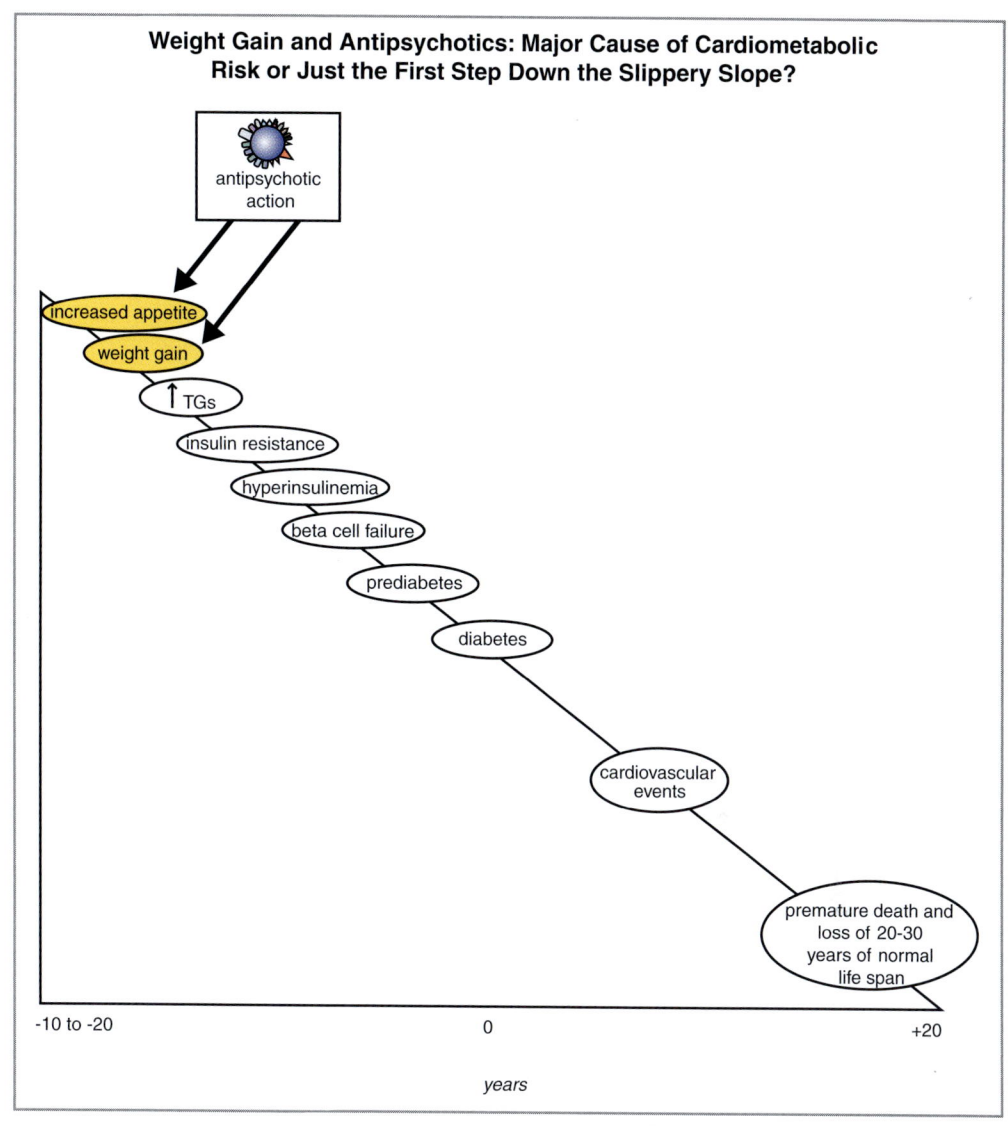

FIGURE 10-61 Weight gain and slippery slope. Weight gain and antipsychotics: major cause of cardiometabolic risk or just the first step down the slippery slope? Rather than being the only risk or even the single major cardiometabolic risk caused by atypical antipsychotics, weight gain associated with increased appetite and that leads ultimately to obesity, appears to be just the first step down the slippery slope of cardiometabolic risk factors leading to premature death. Other cardiometabolic risks caused by atypical antipsychotics are shown in subsequent figures.

(Figures 10-66 through 10-68), and it can be managed easily when it does occur (Figures 10-67 and 10-69).

Another rare but life-threatening cardiometabolic problem is known to be associated with atypical antipsychotics: namely, an association with the sudden occurrence of diabetic ketoacidosis (DKA) or the related condition hyperglycemic hyperosmolar syndrome (HHS) (Figures 10-64 and 10-65). The mechanism of this complication is under intense investigation and is probably complex and multifactorial. In some cases, it may be that patients

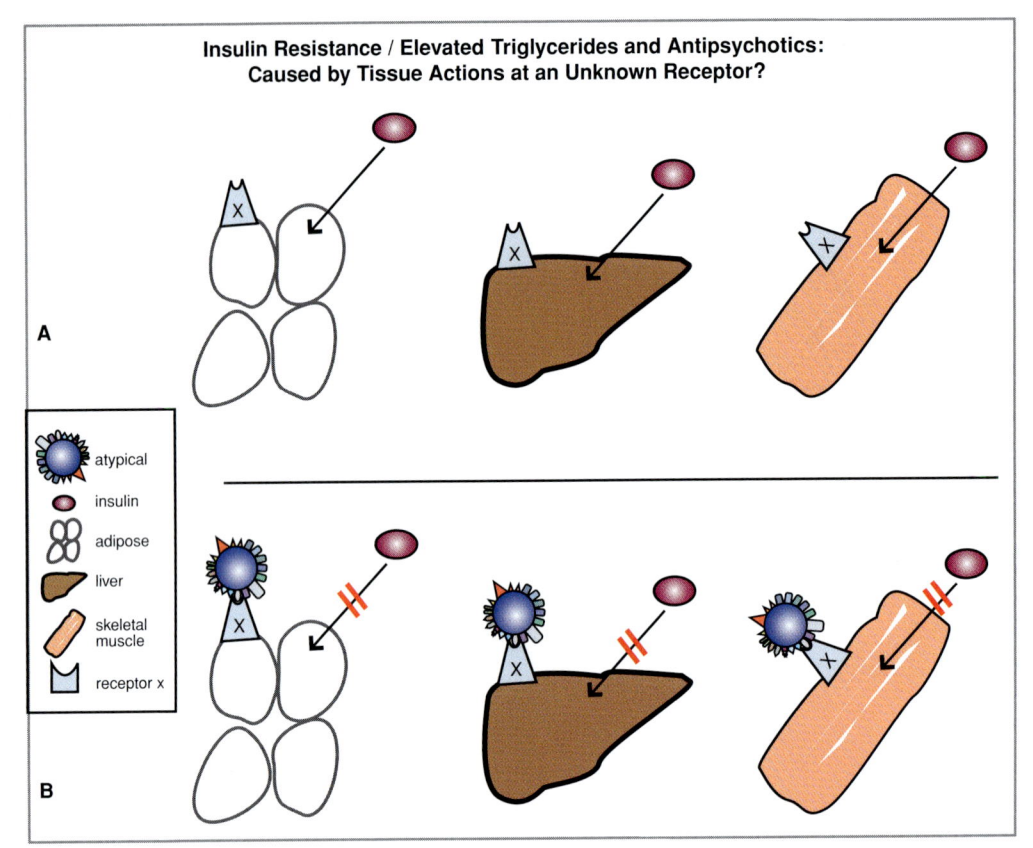

FIGURE 10-62 Insulin resistance, elevated triglycerides, and antipsychotics: caused by tissue actions at an unknown receptor? Some atypical antipsychotics may lead to insulin resistance and elevated triglycerides independently of weight gain, although the mechanism is not yet established. This figure depicts a hypothesized mechanism in which antipsychotic binds to receptor X at adipose tissue, liver, and skeletal muscle to cause insulin resistance.

with undiagnosed insulin resistance, prediabetes, or diabetes who are in a state of compensated hyperinsulinemia on the metabolic highway (Figure 10-60) become decompensated when given an atypical antipsychotic agent because of some pharmacological mechanism associated with these drugs.

One hint for the cause in some patients taking agents such as olanzapine and clozapine is antagonism of the M3 muscarinic cholinergic receptor (Figures 10-57, 10-58, 10-64 and 10-65; see also Figures 10-90 and 10-91). That is, it is known that insulin secretion is regulated in part by parasympathetic cholinergic neurons that innervate the pancreas and act on postsynaptic M3 receptors localized on pancreatic beta cells, the cells that secrete insulin (Figure 10-64A and B). Preclinical research suggests that agents that can block the M3 cholinergic receptor in the pancreatic beta cell may reduce insulin release (Figure 10-64C). If this occurs in a patient dependent on cholinergic regulation of insulin release, it could be a factor in causing insulin deficiency and lead to DKA/HHS. This remains speculative, and many patients have no problem with insulin secretion when M3 receptors are blocked, so this may be just one of several possible mechanisms that could explain the induction of DKA/HHS only in vulnerable patients taking atypical antipsychotics. Because of the risk of DKA/HHS, it is important to know the patient's location along the metabolic

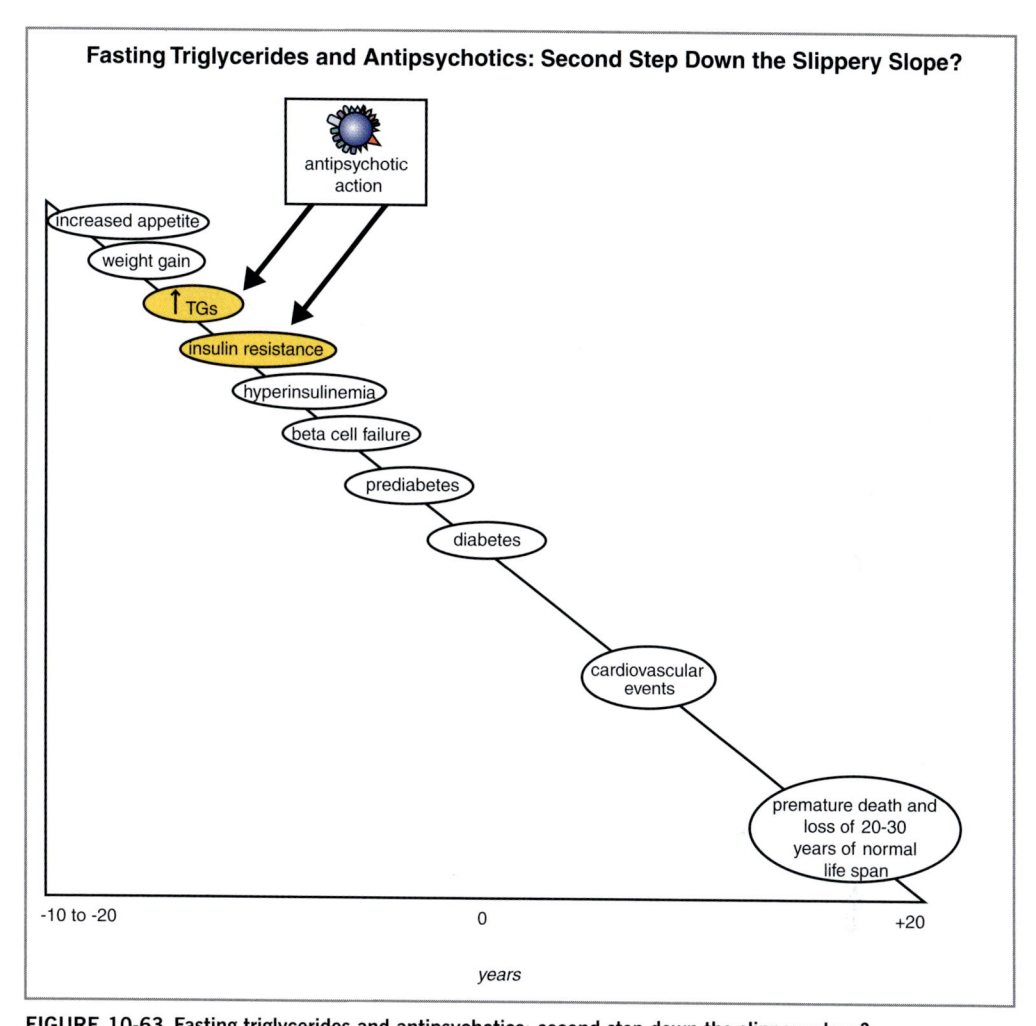

FIGURE 10-63 Fasting triglycerides and antipsychotics: second step down the slippery slope? Antipsychotic-induced elevation of triglycerides (TGs) and insulin resistance may be the second step down the slippery slope of increased cardiometabolic risk. These actions can be independent of weight gain and occur prior to significant weight gain, which suggests that they are mediated by an unknown receptor where certain atypical antipsychotics may interact to cause this risk.

highway (Figure 10-60) prior to prescribing an antipsychotic, particularly if the patient has hyperinsulinemia, prediabetes, or diabetes. It is also important to monitor (Figures 10-66 through 10-68) and manage the metabolic response of the patient to administration of an antipsychotic (Figures 10-67 through 10-69).

There are at least three stops along the metabolic highway where a psychopharmacologist should monitor a patient taking an atypical antipsychotic (Figure 10-66) and manage the cardiometabolic risks of atypical antipsychotics (Tables 10-2, 10-3 and 10-4; Figure 10-67). This starts with monitoring weight and body mass index to detect weight gain and the development of diabetes (Figure 10-66). It also means getting a baseline of fasting triglyceride levels and determining whether there is a family history of diabetes. The second thing to determine, by measuring fasting triglyceride levels before and after starting an atypical antipsychotic, is whether atypical antipsychotics are causing dyslipidemia and increased

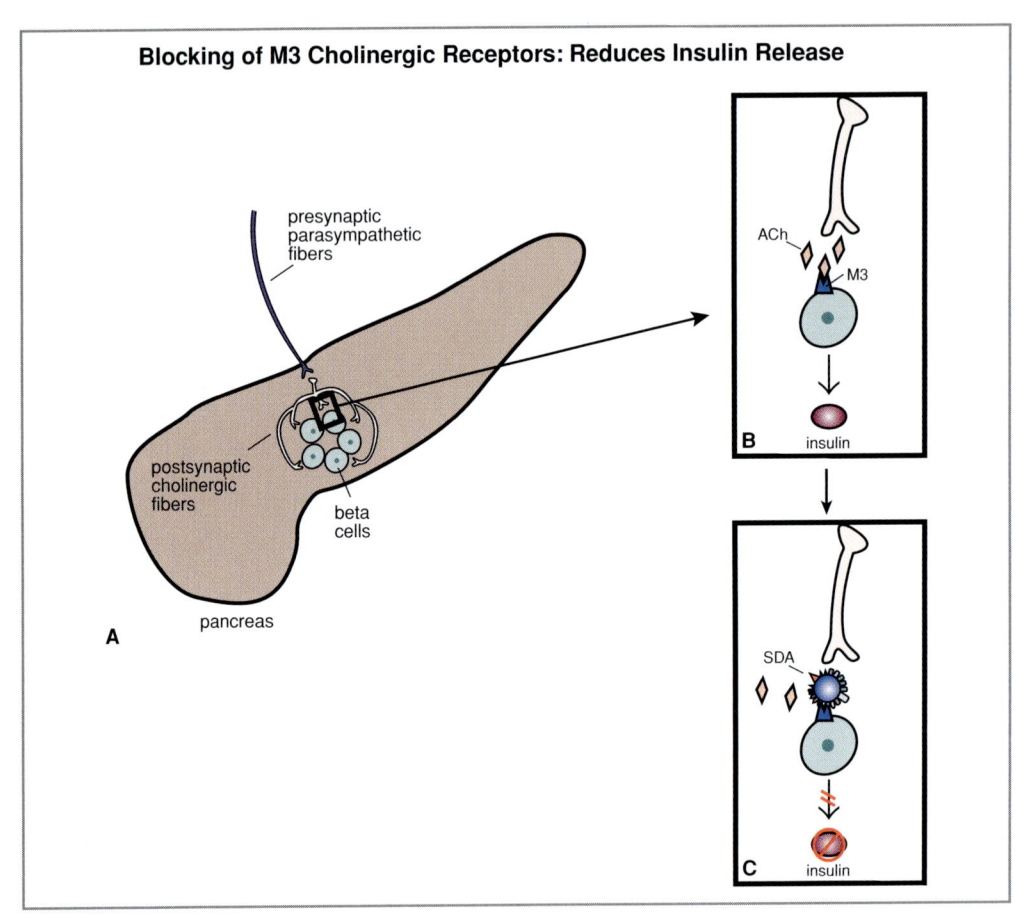

FIGURE 10-64A, B and C Blocking M3-cholinergic receptors reduces insulin release. (**A**) Insulin secretion is regulated in part by parasympathetic cholinergic neurons that synapse with pancreatic beta cells. (**B**) When acetylcholine (ACh) binds to muscarinic-3 (M3) receptors on pancreatic beta cells, this causes insulin secretion. (**C**) Thus, agents that block M3 receptors – such as certain atypical antipsychotics like olanzapine and clozapine – may reduce insulin release.

insulin resistance (Figure 10-66). If body mass index or fasting triglycerides increase significantly, a switch to a different antipsychotic that does not cause these problems should be considered (Figure 10-67). In patients who are obese, have dyslipidemia, and are in either a prediabetic or diabetic state, it is especially important to monitor blood pressure, fasting glucose, and waist circumference before and after initiating an atypical antipsychotic. Best practices are to monitor these parameters in anyone taking any atypical antipsychotic (Figure 10-67). In high-risk patients, it is especially important to be vigilant for DKA/HHS, and possibly to reduce that risk by maintaining such patients on an antipsychotic with lower cardiometabolic risk (Tables 10-3 and 10-4; Figure 10-67). In high-risk patients, especially those with pending or actual pancreatic beta cell failure as manifested by hyperinsulinemia, prediabetes, or diabetes, fasting glucose and other chemical and clinical parameters can be monitored to detect early signs of rare but potentially fatal DKA/HHS (Figure 10-66).

So, does a psychopharmacologist have to become an endocrinologist? The answer is no. The psychopharmacologist's metabolic tool kit is quite simple (Figure 10-68). It involves a flowchart that tracks perhaps as few as four parameters over time, with documentation

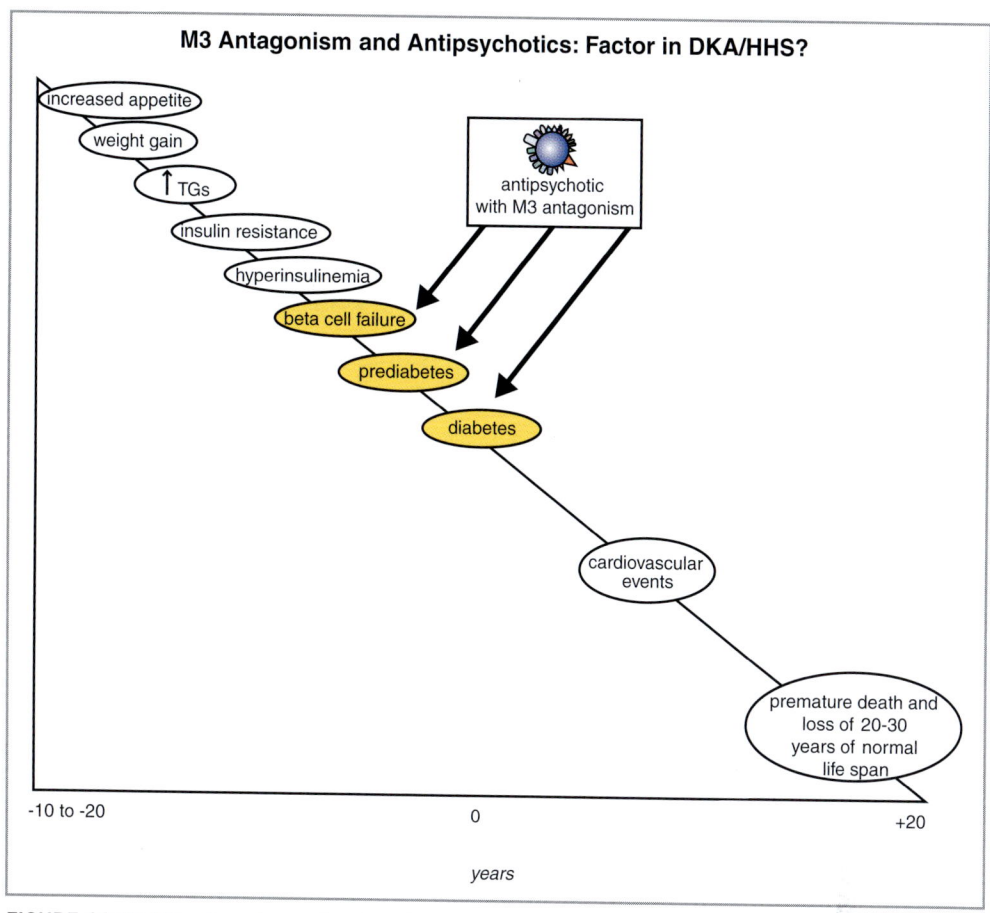

FIGURE 10-65 **M3 antagonism and antipsychotics: factor in DKA/HHS?** An atypical antipsychotic with muscarinic 3 (M3) antagonism could reduce insulin release by binding to M3 receptors on pancreatic beta cells. In patients with undiagnosed insulin resistance, prediabetes, or diabetes, this could potentially lead to diabetic ketoacidosis (DKA) or hyperglycemic hyperosmolar syndrome (HHS). However, not all patients have problems with insulin secretion when M3 receptors are blocked; additional mechanisms are likely to be important in the production of DKA/HHS by atypical antipsychotics.

being especially important before and after switches from one antipsychotic to another or as new risk factors evolve. These four parameters are weight (as body mass index), fasting triglycerides, fasting glucose, and blood pressure.

The management of patients at risk for cardiometabolic disease can be quite simple as well, although patients who have already developed dyslipidemia, hypertension, diabetes, and heart disease will likely require management of these problems by a medical specialist. However, the psychopharmacologist is left with a very simple set of options for managing patients with cardiometabolic risk who are taking an atypical antipsychotic (Figure 10-69). The major factors that determine whether such a patient progresses along the metabolic highway to premature death include those that are unmanageable (e.g., the patient's genetic makeup and age), those that are modestly manageable (e.g., change in lifestyle, such as diet, exercise, and stopping smoking), and those that are most manageable, namely the selection of antipsychotic and perhaps switching from one that is causing increased risk in a particular

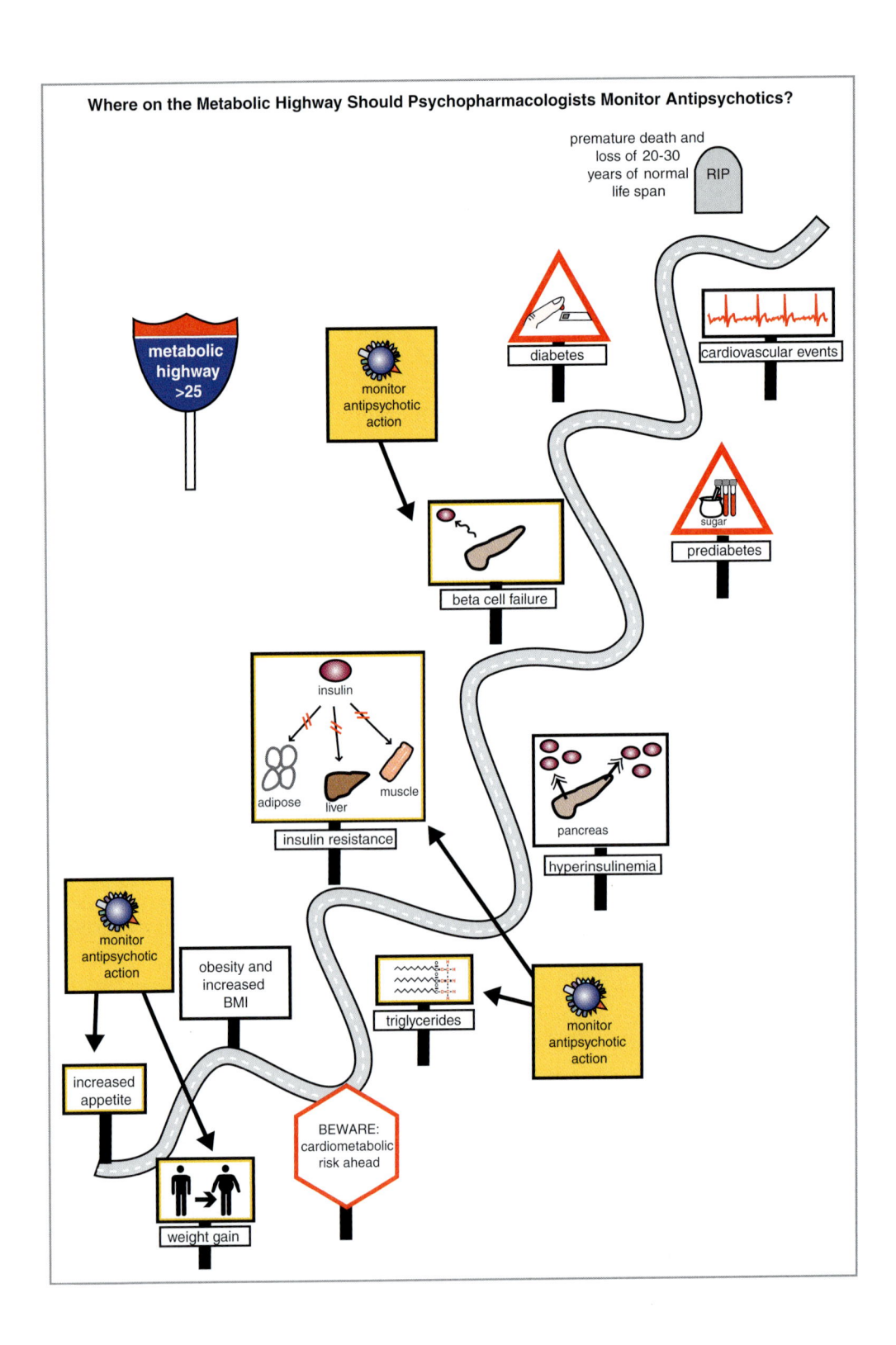

Where on the Metabolic Highway Should Psychopharmacologists Monitor Antipsychotics?

premature death and loss of 20-30 years of normal life span — RIP

metabolic highway >25

monitor antipsychotic action

diabetes

cardiovascular events

beta cell failure

sugar

prediabetes

insulin

adipose liver muscle

insulin resistance

pancreas

hyperinsulinemia

monitor antipsychotic action

increased appetite

obesity and increased BMI

triglycerides

monitor antipsychotic action

BEWARE: cardiometabolic risk ahead

weight gain

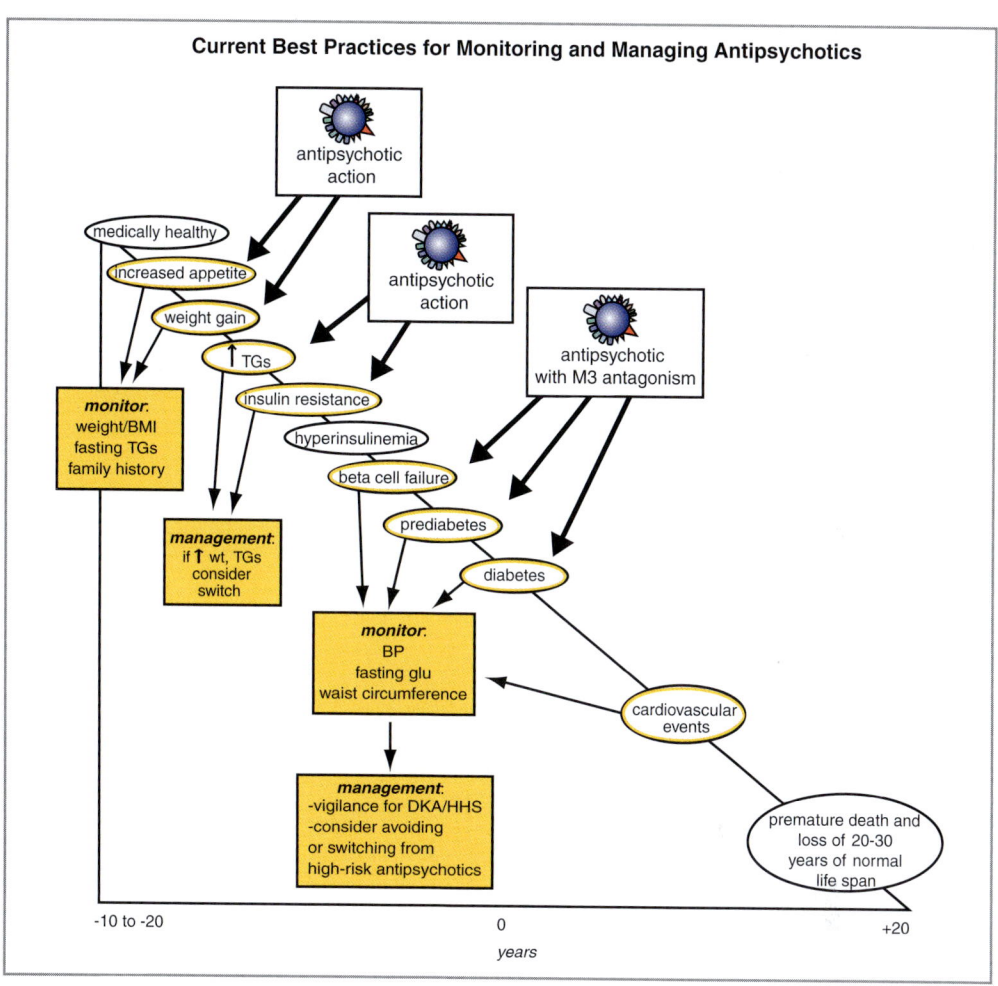

FIGURE 10-67 **Current best practices for monitoring and managing antipsychotics.** Monitoring should occur prior to the initiation of an antipsychotic, with baseline measurements including weight, body mass index (BMI), fasting triglyceride levels (TGs), and family history of diabetes. Weight, BMI, and fasting triglycerides should continue to be monitored throughout treatment. If patients do show an increase in weight or triglyceride levels, they may need to be switched to a different antipsychotic, adopt lifestyle changes, or both. For patients who are obese, have dyslipidemia, or are prediabetic or diabetic, it is important to monitor blood pressure, fasting glucose, and waist circumference both before and after starting an antipsychotic as well as to be vigilant for diabetic ketoacidosis (DKA) and hyperglycemic hyperosmolar syndrome (HHS). One may choose to avoid or switch from antipsychotics with higher risk of cardiometabolic effects.

FIGURE 10-66 **Monitoring on the metabolic highway.** Where on the metabolic highway should psychopharmacologists monitor antipsychotics? Key stages along the metabolic highway where antipsychotics can produce cardiometabolic risks are the places where the actions of these drugs should be monitored. Thus, there are at least three "on" ramps where the cardiometabolic risk of some atypical antipsychotics can enter the metabolic highway, and they are all shown here. First, increased appetite and weight gain can lead to elevated body mass index (BMI) and ultimately obesity. Thus, weight and BMI should be monitored here. Second, atypical antipsychotics can cause insulin resistance by an unknown mechanism; this can be detected by measuring fasting plasma triglyceride levels. Finally, atypical antipsychotics can cause sudden onset of diabetic ketoacidosis (DKA) or hyperglycemic hyperosmolar syndrome (HHS) by unknown mechanisms, possibly including blockade of M3-cholinergic receptors. This can be detected by informing patients of the symptoms of DKA/HHS and by measuring fasting glucose levels.

Psychopharmacologist's Metabolic Monitoring Tool Kit

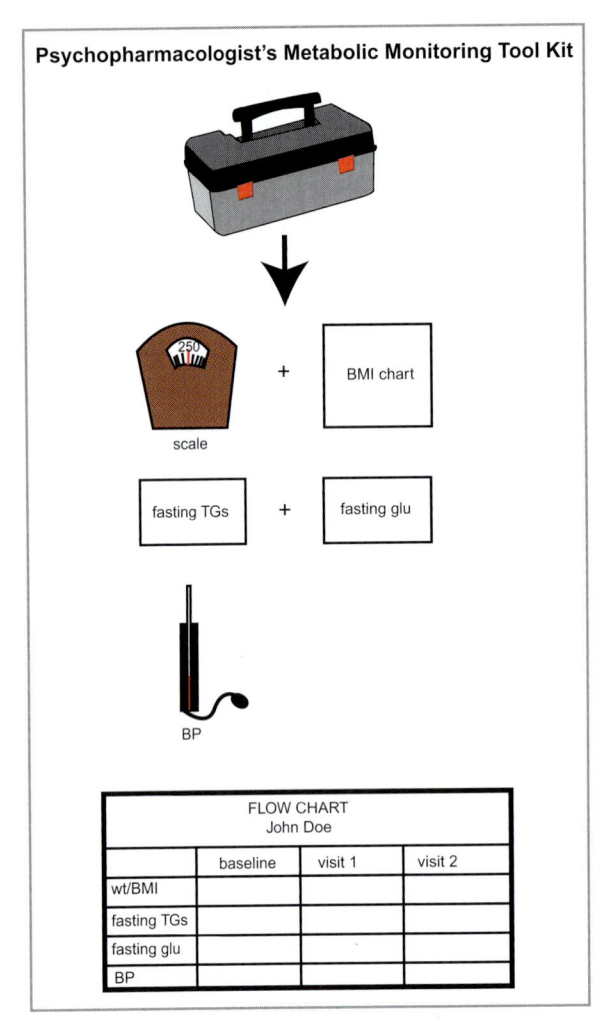

FIGURE 10-68 Metabolic monitoring tool kit. The psychopharmacologist's metabolic monitoring tool kit includes items for tracking four major parameters: weight/body mass index, fasting triglycerides (TGs), fasting glucose, and blood pressure. These items are simply a flowchart that can appear at the beginning of a patient's chart with entries for each visit, a scale, a BMI chart to convert weight into BMI, a blood pressure cuff, and laboratory results for fasting triglycerides and fasting glucose.

patient to one that, on monitoring, demonstrates a reduced risk (Tables 10-2 through 10-4; Figure 10-69).

Sedation and antipsychotics

Antipsychotics are associated with sedation, and sedation has several potential mechanisms (Figures 10-70 and 10-71). Not only can blocking D2 receptors cause sedation, particularly at high doses that cause neurolepsis, but so can blocking M1-muscarinic cholinergic receptors, H1-histamine receptors, and alpha-1 adrenergic receptors (Figures 10-70 and 10-71). Dopamine, acetylcholine, histamine, and norepinephrine are all involved in arousal pathways (Figure 10-71), so it is not surprising that the blocking of one or more of these systems can lead to sedation. Arousal pathways are discussed in detail in the chapters on sleep and cognition, respectively. For our purposes, it is useful to point out that one can produce or avoid sedation by understanding the pharmacology of this clinical effect (Figures 10-70 and 10-71) and by knowing which drugs have such pharmacological properties and which do not (see later discussion of individual drugs and Figures 10-90 through 10-104).

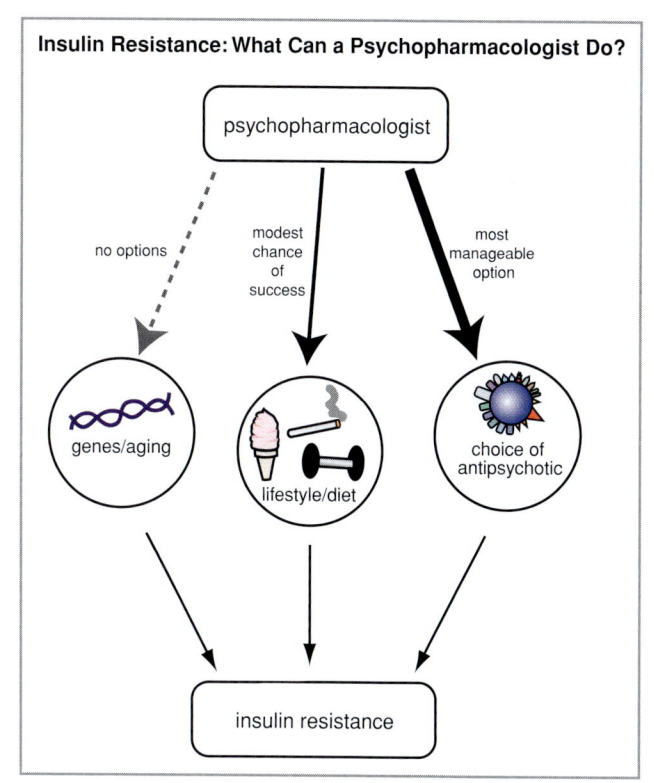

FIGURE 10-69 Insulin resistance: what can a psychopharmacologist do? Several factors influence whether or not an individual develops insulin resistance, some of which are manageable by a psychopharmacologist and some of which are not. Unmanageable factors include genetic makeup and age, while items that are modestly manageable include lifestyle (e.g., diet, exercise, smoking). Psychopharmacologists exert their greatest influence on managing insulin resistance through selection of antipsychotics that either do or do not cause insulin resistance.

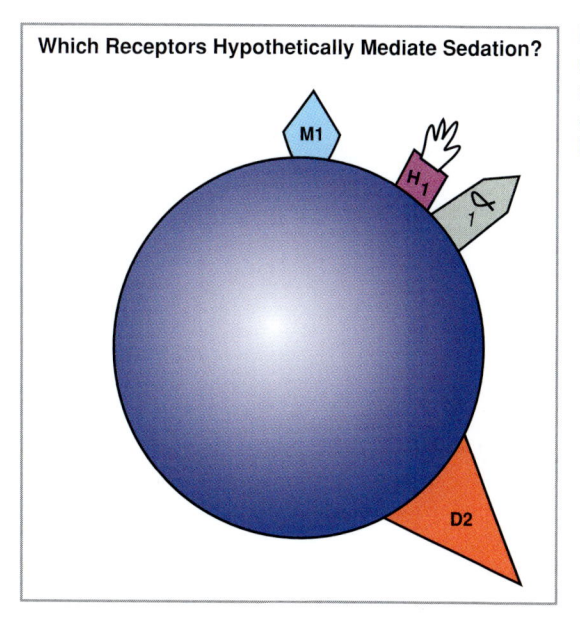

FIGURE 10-70 Which receptors hypothetically mediate sedation? Antagonism of D2 receptors, as well as of muscarinic-1, histamine-1, and alpha-1 adrenergic receptors, could hypothetically mediate sedation.

Antipsychotic Agents | 397

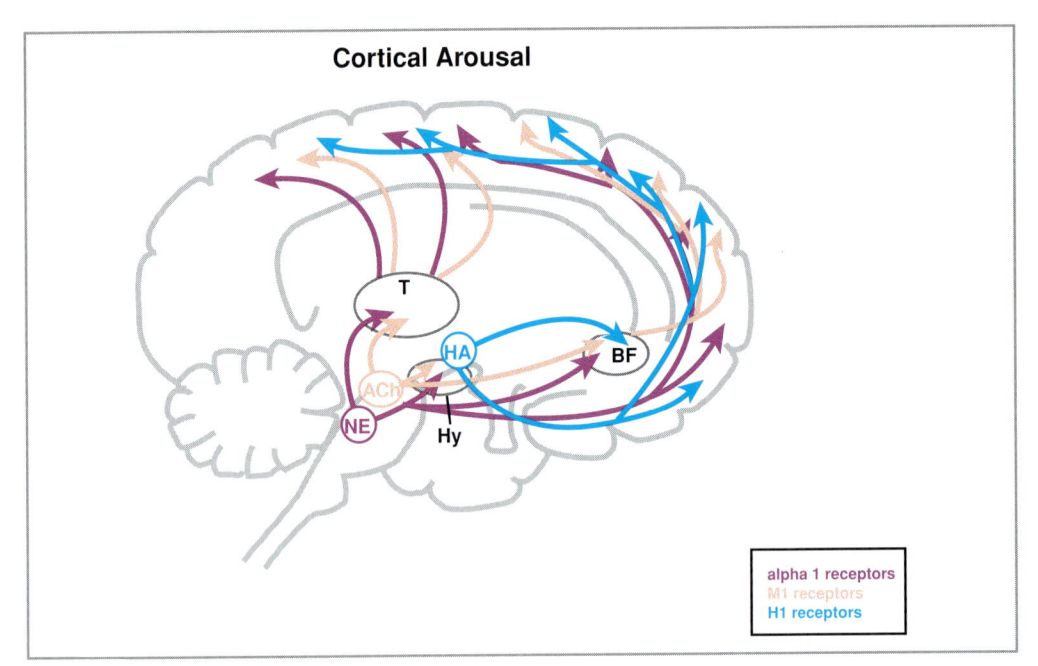

FIGURE 10-71 Neurotransmitters of cortical arousal. The neurotransmitters acetylcholine (ACh), histamine (HA), and norepinephrine (NE) are all involved in arousal pathways connecting neurotransmitter centers with the thalamus (T), hypothalamus (Hy), basal forebrain (BF), and cortex. Thus, pharmacological actions at their receptors could influence arousal. In particular, antagonism of muscarinic M1, histamine H1, and alpha-1 adrenergic receptors are all associated with sedating effects.

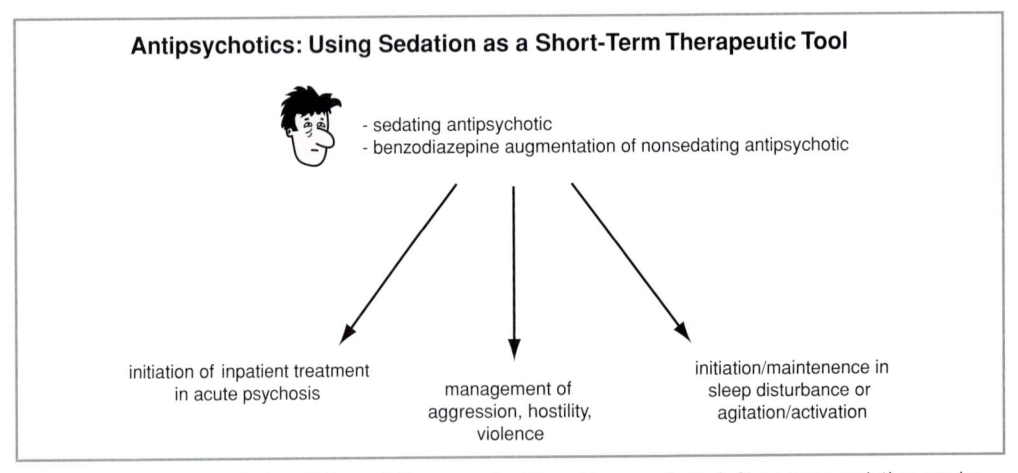

FIGURE 10-72 Antipsychotics: Using sedation as a short term therapeutic tool. Short-term, sedation can be beneficial for management of acute psychosis; aggression, hostility, or violence; sleep disturbances; or agitation/activation. This can be achieved with sedating antipsychotics or by augmentation with a benzodiazepine.

In some cases, sedation is a desired therapeutic effect, particularly early in treatment, during hospitalization, and when patients are aggressive, agitated, or needing sleep induction (Figure 10-72). This can be accomplished either with a sedating antipsychotic that has muscarinic, histaminic, and adrenergic blocking properties or by adding a sedating

Antipsychotics: Side Effects and Compliance

A

most common side effect
4 out of 5 antipsychotics in CATIE
olanzapine, risperidone, quetiapine,
perphenazine, but not ziprasidone

→ hypersomnia/sedation

---

most common reasons to
discontinue due to intolerability

→

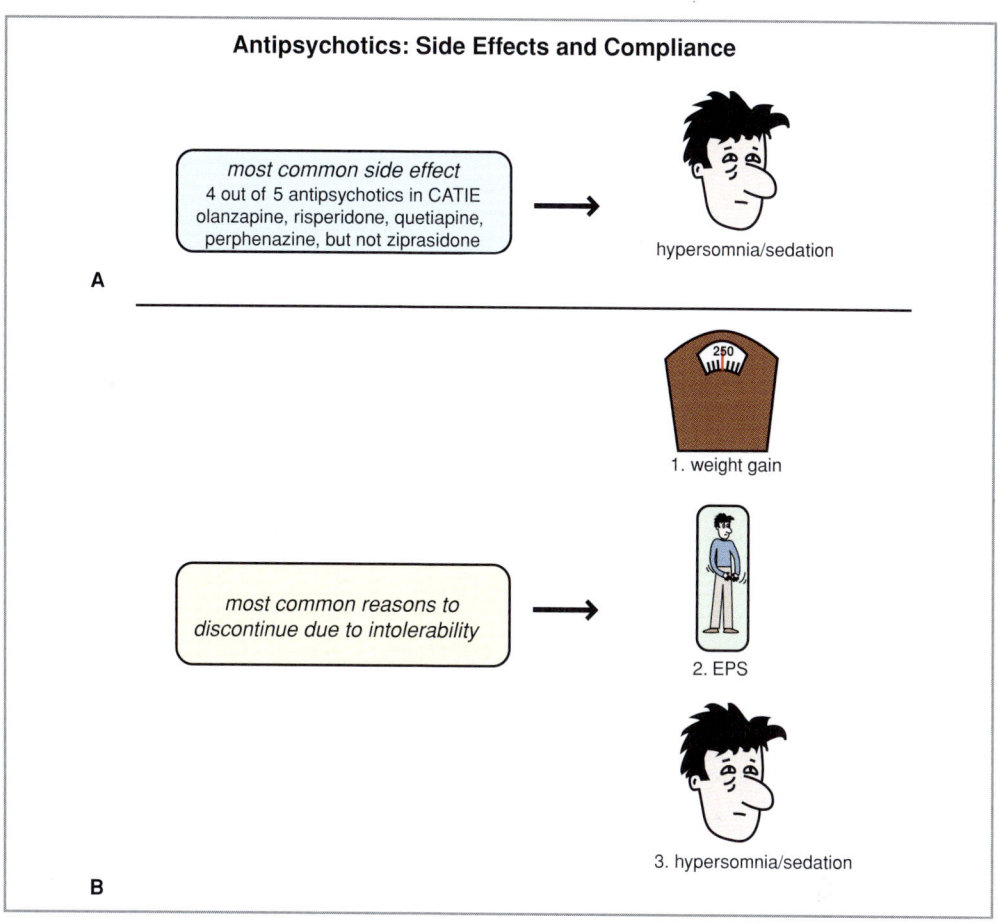

1. weight gain

2. EPS

3. hypersomnia/sedation

B

FIGURE 10-73A and B Antipsychotics, side effects and compliance. (**A**) Sedation is a common side effect of several antipsychotics, including many of the atypical antipsychotics, as shown in studies such as CATIE (Clinical Antipsychotic Trials of Intervention Effectiveness). (**B**) Long-term sedation may need to be avoided, as it is among the top three reasons for discontinuation due to intolerability, falling just behind weight gain and extrapyramidal symptoms (EPS).

benzodiazepine to any antipsychotic, especially those that are not sedating and lack these pharmacological properties (Figure 10-72).

In other cases, particularly for long-term treatment, sedation is generally a side effect to be avoided. Sedation is the most common side effect reported for many antipsychotics, especially those with a mixture of muscarinic, histaminic, and adrenergic blocking properties. Along with weight gain and EPS, sedation is one of the most common reasons for a patient to discontinue treatment with an antipsychotic drug (Figure 10-73). Furthermore, diminished arousal, sedation, and somnolence can lead to cognitive impairment, since cognitive functioning is mediated by these same pathways (Figure 10-71). When cognition is impaired, functional outcomes are compromised (Figures 10-74 through 10-77).

Pharmacological evidence suggests that the best long-term outcomes in schizophrenia result from adequate D2/5HT2A/5HT1A receptor occupancy, improving positive and especially negative and cognitive symptoms, rather than from nonspecific sedation resulting from muscarinic, histaminic, and adrenergic receptor blockade (Figures 10-74 through

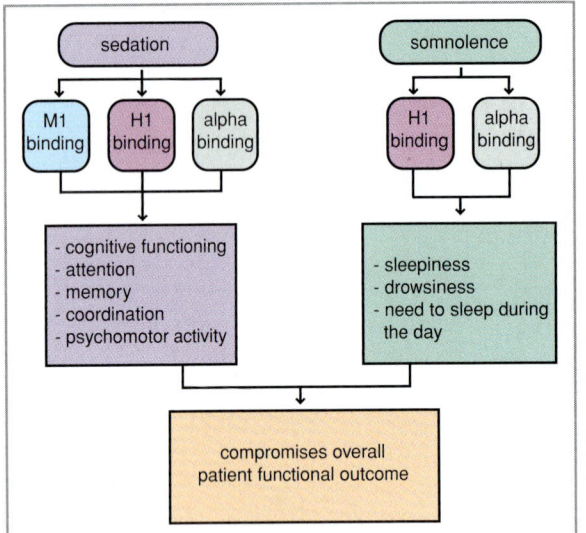

FIGURE 10-74 Sedation vs. somnolence. Sedation may be caused by antagonism of muscarinic M1, histamine H1, and/or alpha-1 adrenergic receptors. Sedation as a result of blocking these receptors may contribute to impaired cognitive functioning, attention, memory, and coordination, which in turn could affect overall patient functioning. Somnolence may be distinct from sedation and become manifest more as sleepiness, drowsiness, and the need to sleep during the day. These symptoms may be regulated by H1 and alpha 1 adrenergic receptors and can also affect overall patient functioning.

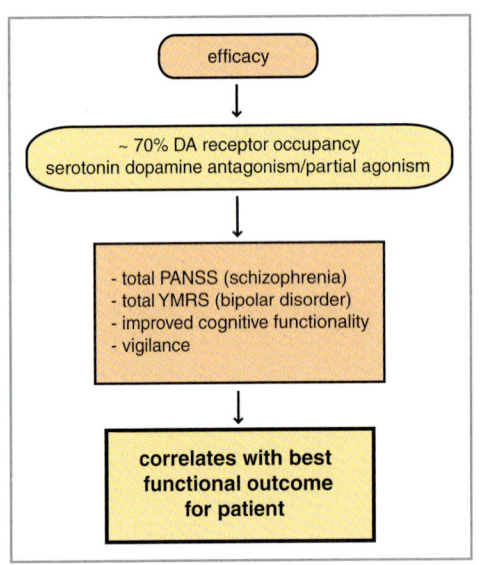

FIGURE 10-75 Efficacy profile. The best long-term outcomes in schizophrenia occur when patients experience relief not only from positive symptoms but also from affective, cognitive, and negative symptoms. From a pharmacological perspective, this can be achieved through blocking approximately 70 percent of D2 receptors in the nucleus accumbens plus antagonism/partial agonism of D2, serotonin-2A, and serotonin-1A receptors in other key brain regions and not from interaction with histamine H1, muscarinic M1, or alpha-1 adrenergic receptors. PANSS, Positive and Negative Symptom Scale; YMRS, Young Mania Rating Scale.

10-76). Thus, if sedation and somnolence cause cognitive impairment and cognitive impairment is linked to poor patient outcomes, sedation and somnolence may also be linked to poor patient outcomes (Figure 10-76). On the other hand, if optimum D2/5HT2A/5HT1A receptor actions are combined with levels of muscarinic, histaminic, and adrenergic receptor blockade that do not cause sedation, perhaps the best patient outcomes will be achieved (Figure 10-75 through 10-77). Sometimes this is easier said than done, but drug selection based on desired pharmacological profile can result in managing sedation in a clinically useful manner while obtaining the best patient outcomes (Figure 10-77).

The Path to Efficacy

if

| A sedation and somnolence (M1 + H1 + alpha 1 actions) | = | B cognitive impairment |

and

| B cognitive impairment | = | C poor patient outcomes |

then

| A sedation and somnolence (M1 + H1 + alpha 1 actions) | = | C poor patient outcomes |

therefore

if

| A more 5HT/D2 actions + less M1, H1, alpha 1 actions | = | B antipsychotic/antimanic efficacy |

and

| B antipsychotic/antimanic efficacy | = | C best patient outcomes |

then

| A more 5HT/D2 actions + less M1, H1, alpha 1 actions | = | C best patient outcomes |

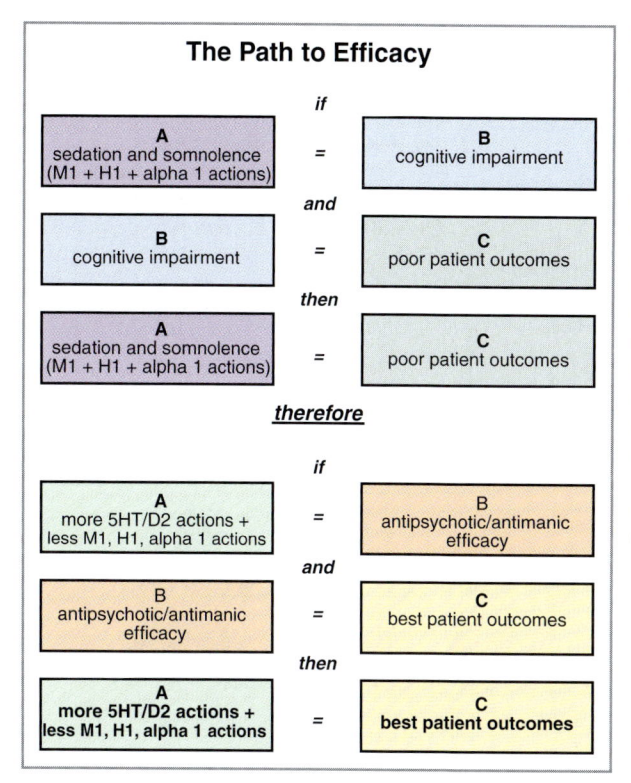

FIGURE 10-76 The path to efficacy. If sedation and somnolence (mediated by M1, H1, and alpha-1 actions) lead to cognitive impairment and cognitive impairment is associated with poor patient outcomes, sedation and somnolence (mediated by M1, H1, and alpha-1) would therefore be related to poor patient outcomes. On the other hand, if serotonergic and dopaminergic actions with minimal effects on M1, H1, and alpha-1 receptors are related to antipsychotic and antimanic efficacy and if antipsychotic/antimanic efficacy is associated with good patient outcomes, an antipsychotic with a serotonergic and dopaminergic profile but without actions at M1, H1, or alpha-1 receptors should lead to good patient outcomes.

Antipsychotics: Strategies to Avoid Sedation and Enhance Long-Term Outcome

- tolerance to sedating antipsychotic
- d/c benzodiazepines
- nonsedating antipsychotic

↓ ↓ ↓

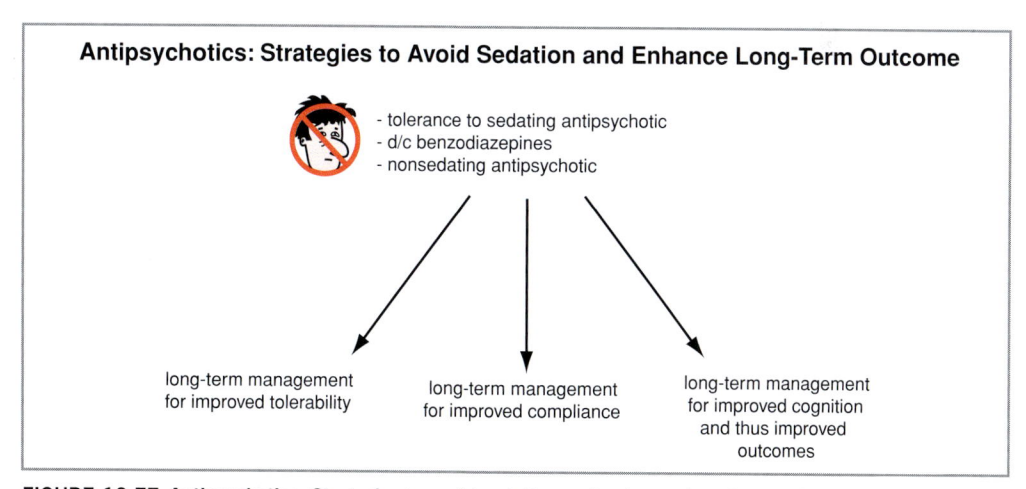

long-term management for improved tolerability

long-term management for improved compliance

long-term management for improved cognition and thus improved outcomes

FIGURE 10-77 Antipsychotics: Strategies to avoid sedation and enhance long-term outcome. Achieving the best long-term outcomes in schizophrenia may require avoiding long-term sedation. For patients whose treatment was initiated with a nonsedating antipsychotic but who received an adjunct benzodiazepine, this may mean discontinuing the benzodiazepine. Some patients initiated on a sedating antipsychotic may develop tolerance to the sedating side effects and not require treatment adjustment; however, others may need to be switched to a nonsedating agent.

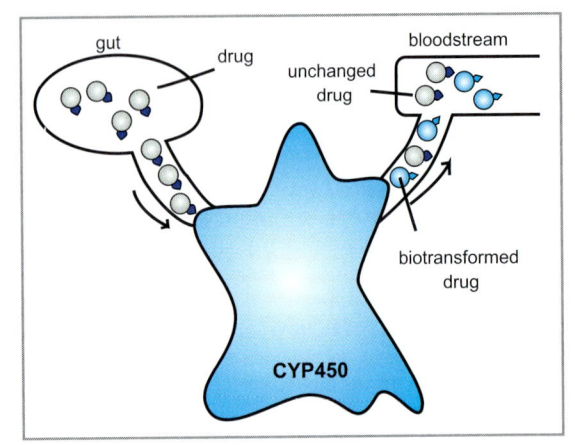

FIGURE 10-78 CYP450. The cytochrome P450 (CYP450) enzyme system mediates how the body metabolizes many drugs, including antipsychotics. The CYP450 enzyme in the gut wall or liver converts the drug into a biotransformed product in the bloodstream. After passing through the gut wall and liver (left), the drug will exist partly as unchanged drug and partly as biotransformed drug (right).

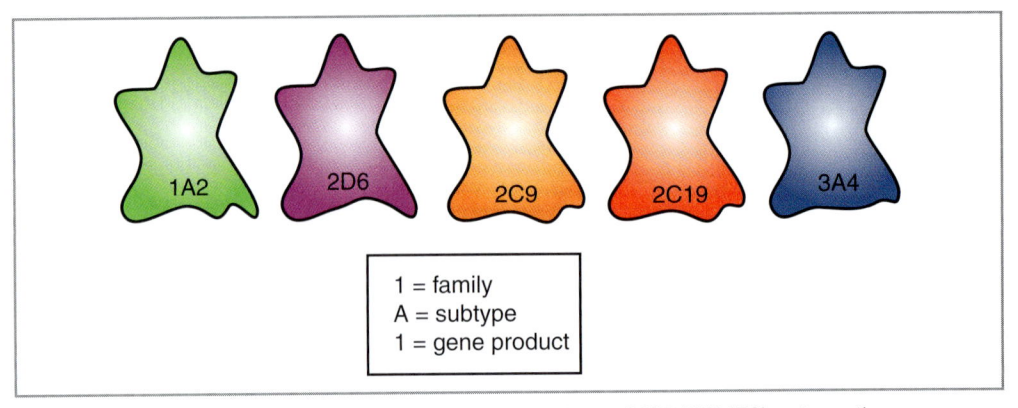

FIGURE 10-79 Five CYP450 enzymes. There are many cytochrome P450 (CYP450) systems; these are classified according to family, subtype, and gene product. Five of the most important are shown here, and include CYP450 1A2, 2D6, 2C9, 2C19, and 3A4.

Antipsychotic pharmacokinetics

Pharmacokinetics is the study of how the body acts on drugs, especially to absorb, distribute, metabolize, and excrete them. These pharmacokinetic actions are mediated through the hepatic and gut drug metabolizing system known as the cytochrome P450 (CYP450) enzyme system. The CYP450 enzymes and the **pharmacokinetic** actions they represent must be contrasted with the **pharmacodynamic** actions of the antipsychotics discussed extensively so far in this chapter. Although most of this book deals with the **pharmacodynamics** of psychopharmacological agents, especially how drugs act on the brain, the following section will discuss the **pharmacokinetics** of antipsychotics, or how the body acts on these drugs.

CYP450 enzymes follow the same principles of enzymes transforming substrates into products as discussed in Chapter 5 and illustrated in Figures 5-46 through 5-48. Figure 10-78 shows how an antipsychotic is absorbed and delivered through the gut wall to the liver to be biotransformed so that it can be excreted from the body. Specifically, CYP450 enzymes in the gut wall or liver convert the drug substrate into a biotransformed product in the bloodstream. After passing through the gut wall and liver, the drug exists partially as unchanged drug and partially as biotransformed product (Figure 10-78).

There are several known CYP450 systems. Five of the most important enzymes for antidepressant drug metabolism are shown in Figure 10-79. There are over thirty known

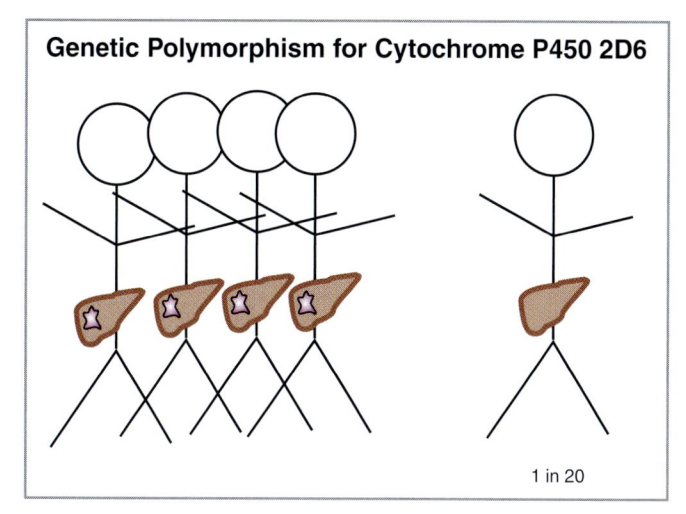

FIGURE 10-80 Genetic polymorphism for CYP450 2D6. Not all individuals have the same CYP450 enzymes. For example, about 1 in 20 Caucasians is a poor metabolizer via 2D6 and must metabolize drugs by an alternative route, which may not be as efficient.

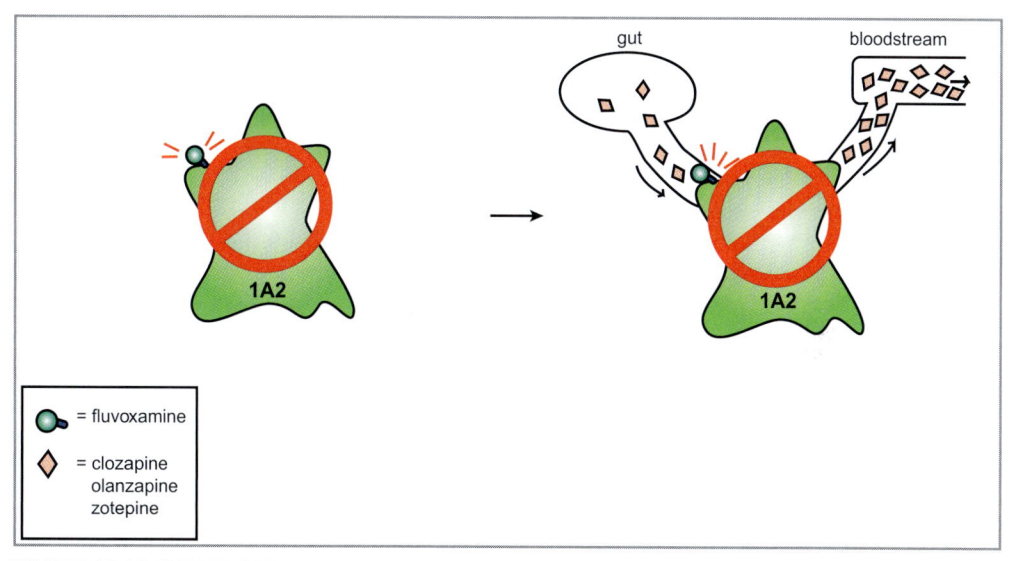

FIGURE 10-81 CYP450 1A2 substrates. Clozapine, olanzapine, and zotepine are substrates for CYP450 1A2. When these antipsychotics are given with an inhibitor of this enzyme, such as the antidepressant fluvoxamine, their plasma levels can rise.

CYP450 enzymes and probably many more awaiting discovery and classification. Not all individuals have all the same CYP450 enzymes. In such cases, the enzyme is said to be polymorphic. For example, about 5 to 10 percent of Caucasians are poor metabolizers via the enzyme CYP450 2D6 (Figure 10-80). They must metabolize drugs by alternative routes, which may not be as efficient as the CYP450 2D6 route. Another CYP450 enzyme, 2C19, has reduced activity in approximately 20 percent of Japanese and Chinese individuals and in 3 to 5 percent of Caucasians.

CYP450 1A2. One CYP450 enzyme of relevance to antipsychotics is 1A2 (Figures 10-81 and 10-82). Three atypical antipsychotics are substrates for 1A2, namely olanzapine, clozapine, and zotepine. This means that when they are given concomitantly with

Antipsychotic Agents | 403

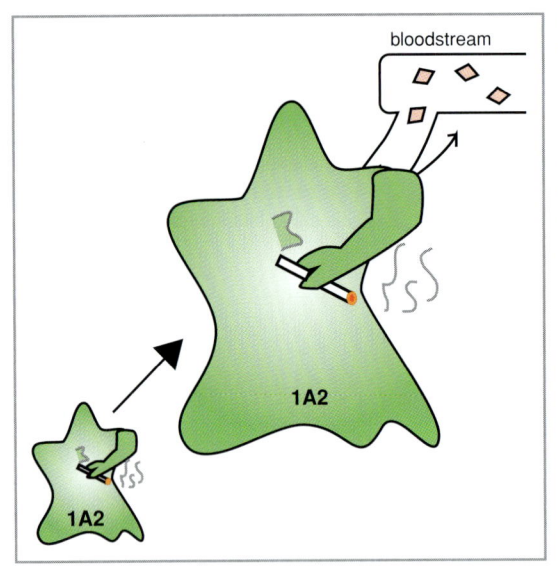

FIGURE 10-82 CYP450 1A2 and smoking. Cigarette smoking, quite common among schizophrenic patients, can induce the enzyme CYP450 1A2 and lower the concentration of drugs metabolized by this enzyme, such as olanzapine, clozapine, and zotepine. Smokers may also require higher doses of these drugs than nonsmokers.

an inhibitor of this enzyme, such as the antidepressant fluvoxamine, their levels may rise (Figure 10-81). Although this may not be particularly important clinically for olanzapine (possibly causing slightly increased sedation), it could potentially raise plasma levels sufficiently in the case of clozapine or zotepine to increase the risk of seizures. Thus, the dose of clozapine or zotepine may need to be lowered when it is administered with fluvoxamine, or another antidepressant may need to be chosen.

On the other hand, when an inducer of 1A2 is given concomitantly with any of the three antipsychotic substrates for 1A2, their levels may fall. This happens when a patient begins to smoke, because smoking induces 1A2, and this would cause levels of olanzapine and clozapine to fall (Figure 10-82). Theoretically this might cause patients stabilized on an antipsychotic dose to relapse if the drug levels fell too low. Also, cigarette smokers may require higher doses of these atypical antipsychotics than nonsmokers.

CYP 2C9. The new DPA (dopamine partial agonist) bifeprunox is a substrate of 2C9, and its levels are increased by coadministration of a 2C9 inhibitor such as fluconazole.

CYP 2D6. Another CYP450 enzyme of importance to atypical antipsychotic drugs is the enzyme 2D6. Risperidone, clozapine, olanzapine, and aripiprazole are all substrates for this enzyme (Figure 10-83). Risperidone's metabolite is paliperidone, itself recently approved as a new atypical antipsychotic (Figure 10-84). Paliperidone itself thus bypasses the 2D6 enzyme, is not a substrate for 2D6, and is therefore not affected by alterations in the activity of the 2D6 enzyme, unlike its precursor risperidone (Figures 10-83 and 10-84).

Several antidepressants are inhibitors of 2D6 and thus can raise the levels of the atypical antipsychotics that are substrates of 2D6 (Figure 10-85). For risperidone, this shifts the balance away from formation of the active metabolite paliperidone, which could potentially increase EPS. Theoretically, the dose of olanzapine, clozapine, or aripiprazole may have to be lowered when given with an antidepressant that blocks 2D6, although this is not often necessary in practice.

CYP 3A4. This enzyme metabolizes several atypical antipsychotics including clozapine, quetiapine, ziprasidone, sertindole, aripiprazole, zotepine, and bifeprunox (Figure 10-86). Several psychotropic drugs are weak inhibitors of this enzyme, including the

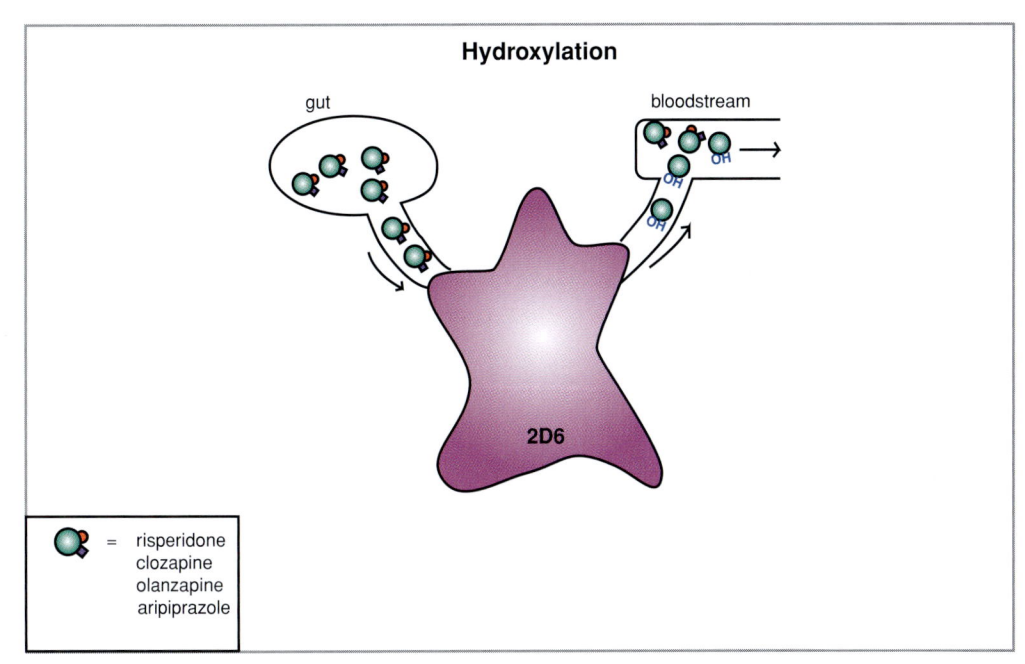

FIGURE 10-83 CYP450 2D6 substrates. Several atypical antipsychotics are substrates for CYP450 2D6, including risperidone, clozapine, olanzapine, and aripiprazole. 2D6 often hydroxylates drug substrates.

FIGURE 10-84 Paliperidone. Conversion of risperidone to paliperidone by CYP450 2D6. Risperidone is converted to the active metabolite paliperidone by the enzyme CYP450 2D6. Paliperidone is now available as an antipsychotic.

antidepressants fluvoxamine, nefazodone, and the active metabolite of fluoxetine, norfluoxetine. Several nonpsychotropic drugs are powerful inhibitors of 3A4, including ketoconazole (antifungal), protease inhibitors (for AIDS/HIV) and erythromycin (antibiotic). For atypical antipsychotics that are substrates of 3A4, the clinical implication is that concomitant administration with a 3A4 inhibitor may require dosage reduction of the atypical antipsychotic (Figure 10-87).

Antipsychotic Agents | 405

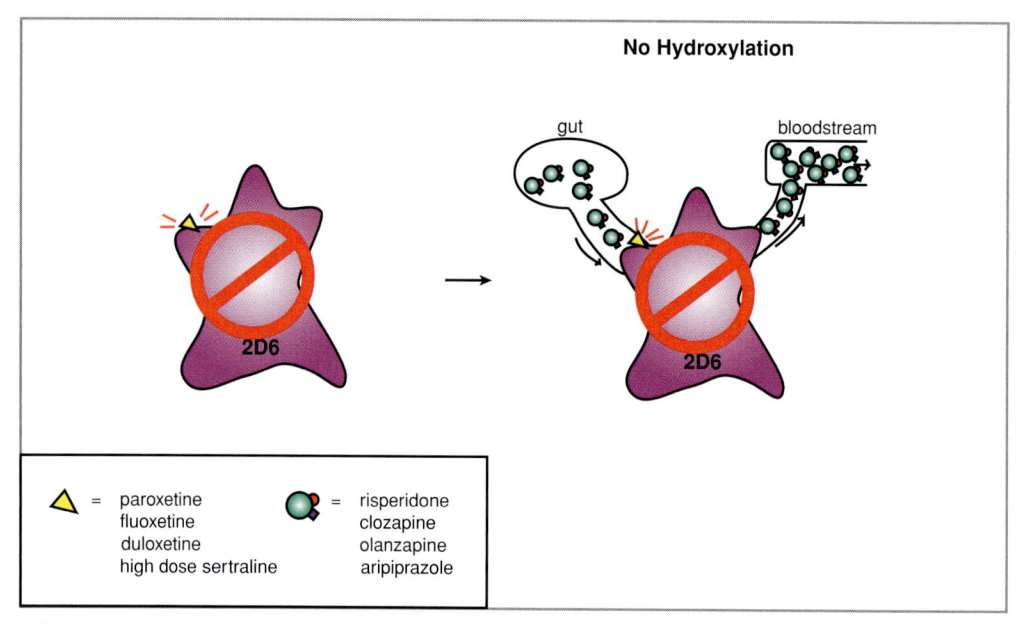

FIGURE 10-85 CYP450 2D6 inhibitors. Several antidepressants are inhibitors of CYP450 2D6 and could theoretically raise the levels of 2D6 substrates such as risperidone, clozapine, olanzapine, and aripiprazole. However, this is not usually clinically significant.

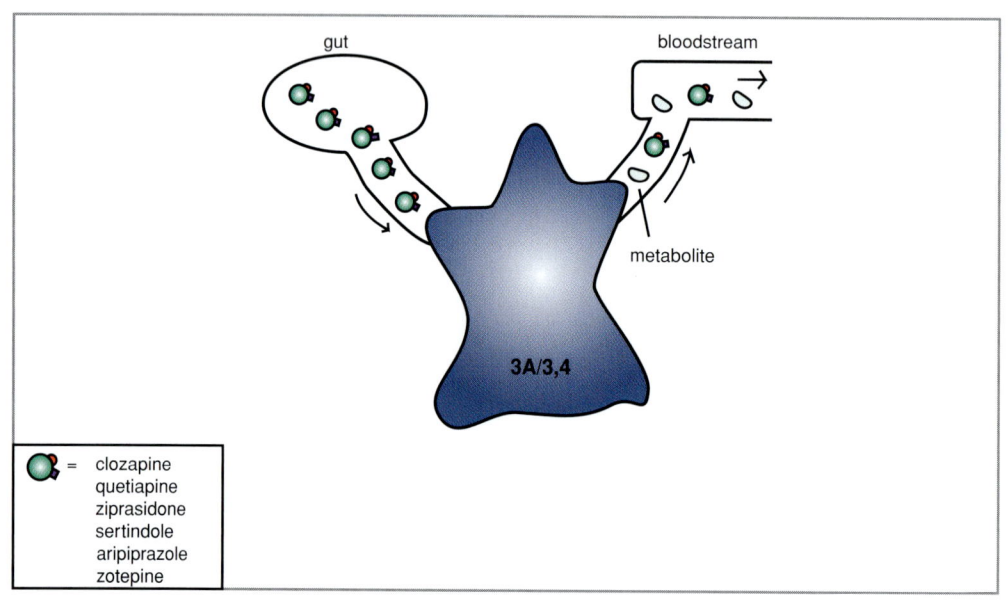

FIGURE 10-86 CYP450 3 A/3,4 substrates. Several atypical antipsychotics are substrates for CYP450 3A4, including clozapine, quetiapine, ziprasidone, sertindole, aripiprazole, and zotepine.

Drugs can not only be substrates for a CYP450 enzyme or inhibitors of a P450 enzyme but also inducers of a CYP450 enzyme, thereby increasing the activity of that enzyme. An example of this is the anticonvulsant and mood stabilizer carbamazepine, which induces the activity of 3A4 (Figure 10-88). Since mood stabilizers may frequently be mixed with atypical antipsychotics, it is possible that carbamazepine may be added to the regimen of a

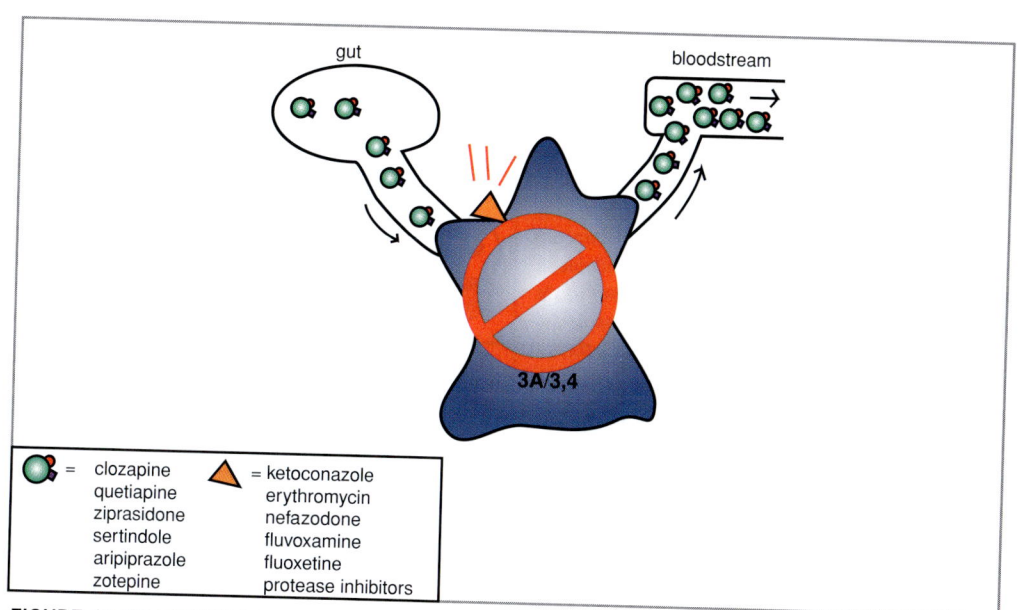

FIGURE 10-87 CYP450 3 A/3,4 inhibitors. There are several inhibitors of CYP450 3A4 that may increase levels of those atypical antipsychotics that are substrates for 3A4. The inhibitors for 3A4 are shown here, as are the atypical antipsychotics that are substrates for 3A4.

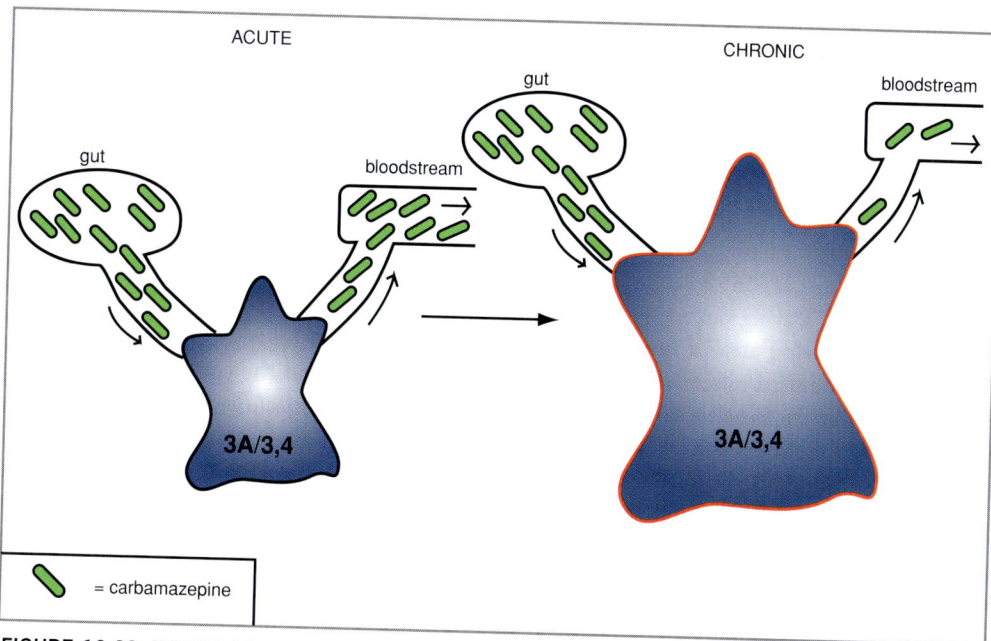

FIGURE 10-88 CYP450 3A4 induced by carbamazepine. The enzyme CYP450 3A4 can be induced by the anticonvulsant and mood stabilizer carbamazepine. This would lead to increased metabolism of substrates for 3A4 (e.g., clozapine, quetiapine, ziprasidone, sertindole, aripiprazole, and zotepine) and may therefore require higher doses of these agents when given concomitantly with carbamazepine.

Antipsychotic Agents | 407

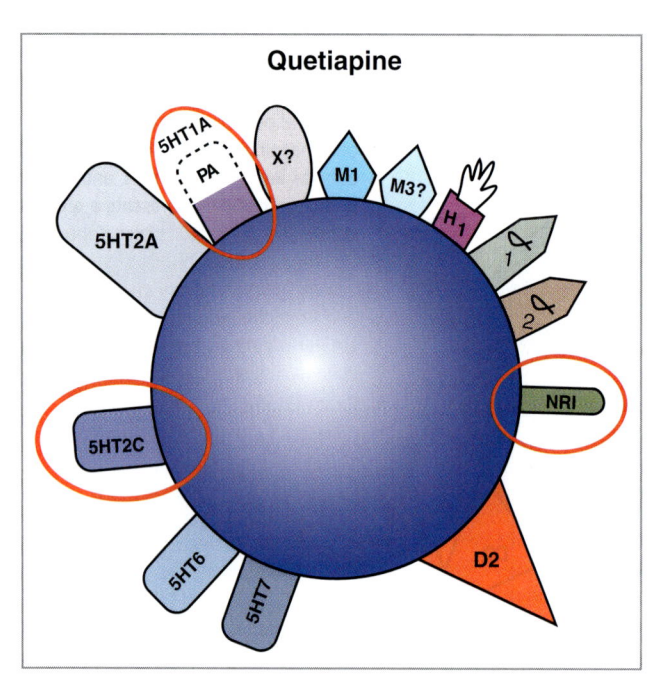

FIGURE 10-94 Quetiapine. Quetiapine's pharmacological icon, portraying a qualitative consensus of current thinking about the binding properties of this drug. It has a unique pharmacological profile, different from those of all other atypical antipsychotics. As with all atypical antipsychotics discussed in this chapter, binding properties vary greatly with technique and from one laboratory to another; they are constantly being revised and updated. Quetiapine's prominent H1-antagonist properties probably contribute to its ability to enhance sleep, and this may contribute as well to its ability to improve sleep disturbances in bipolar and unipolar depression as well as in anxiety disorders. However, this property can also contribute to daytime sedation, especially combined with M1-antimuscarinic and alpha-1 adrenergic antagonist properties. Recently, a potentially important active metabolite of quetiapine, norquetiapine, has been identified; in addition to some of the pharmacological properties noted here for the parent compound, norquetiapine may contribute additional actions at 5HT1A receptors and unique actions as a norepinephrine (NE) reuptake inhibitor (NRI) or NE transport inhibitor (NET) as well as antagonist actions at 5HT2C receptors (see red circles for unique actions contributed by the active metabolite norquetiapine). 5HT1A partial agonist actions, NET inhibition, and 5HT2C antagonist actions may all contribute to mood-improving properties as well as to cognitive enhancement by quetiapine. However, 5HT2C antagonist actions combined with H1 antagonist actions may contribute to weight gain.

Paliperidone's efficacy may be linked in part to alpha-2 antagonist properties, specifically for improving depression (Figure 10-93), especially since it may have less potent alpha-1 than alpha-2 antagonist potency. Alpha-2 antagonism as a mechanism of antidepressant action is discussed in Chapter 12, on antidepressants. Risperidone also has alpha-2 antagonist properties, but its somewhat more potent alpha-1 antagonist properties can not only potentially mitigate antidepressant actions but also cause more orthostatic hypotension, particularly on dose initiation, compared to paliperidone.

Weight gain, insulin resistance, and diabetes may be associated with the use of paliperidone, as may elevations of plasma prolactin, with much the same risk as that of risperidone. Paliperidone has not been shown to bind to M3 cholinergic receptors.

Quetiapine. Quetiapine also has a chemical structure related to clozapine and is an SDA, but it has several differentiating pharmacological properties (Figure 10-94). In addition, norquetiapine – an active metabolite that has unique pharmacological properties which may contribute to quetiapine's overall pharmacological profile – has recently been characterized (Figure 10-94).

Quetiapine is "very atypical" in that it causes virtually no EPS at any dose; neither does it cause elevations in prolactin, perhaps related to its particularly rapid dissociation from D2 receptors (discussed above and illustrated in Figures 10-39 through 10-44). Thus, quetiapine tends to be the preferred atypical antipsychotic for patients with Parkinson's disease and psychosis. When dosed adequately, quetiapine is also highly effective in the treatment of schizophrenia and bipolar mania, and is the first atypical antipsychotic proven effective as a monotherapy for the treatment of the depressed phase of bipolar disorder. Quetiapine's 5HT1A partial agonist properties and those of its active metabolite norquetiapine may contribute to the overall efficacy of this agent for treating disorders of mood and cognition (Figure 10-94). In addition, norquetiapine can block the norepinephrine transporter (NET) (Figure 10-94), which would theoretically enhance norepinephrine (and dopamine) levels as do other known antidepressants and cognitive enhancers with this mechanism (explained in detail in the chapters on antidepressants and attention deficit hyperactivity disorder). Furthermore, norquetiapine can block 5HT2C receptors (Figure 10-94), which should enhance the release of both norepinephrine and dopamine and contribute to antidepressant action and cognitive improvement (explained in detail in Chapter 12). An oral controlled-release formulation is now available that may not only enhance the duration of action of quetiapine and reduce its peak-dose actions, such as sedation, but also enhance the formation of the active metabolite norquetiapine and its contributions to the overall actions of this agent.

Although an agent with a short half-life that was originally studied with thrice-daily administration, quetiapine is clearly effective with once-daily administration for many patients, particularly at night, so that the sedating H1-antihistamine actions treat insomnia and wear off by morning, thus preventing daytime sedation. Quetiapine proves the point discussed earlier in this chapter that antipsychotics may not need to be administered often enough to keep D2 receptors occupied by drug for 24 hours a day. As mentioned earlier, this may be due to the possibility that continuous receptor occupancy may not be required for therapeutic actions but may in fact contribute to the undesired side effects. Indeed, what may be required for therapeutic efficacy may be akin to "ringing a bell" by clanging the receptor just once a day. The receptor continues to resonate long after the atypical antipsychotic hits it. That clearly is the case for the use of quetiapine in general and for its particular use as an agent to treat the depressed phase of bipolar disorder.

Quetiapine can cause weight gain (Table 10-2), particularly when given in moderate to high doses, as it blocks histamine-1 receptors (Figures 10-59 and 10-94). The 5HT2C actions of its active metabolite norquetiapine may contribute to weight gain at moderate to high doses of quetiapine (Figure 10-94). Quetiapine can also cause significant sedation because of its binding of histamine-1 receptors as well as to alpha-1 adrenergic receptors and M1-cholinergic receptors (Figures 10-70, 10-71, and 10-94). However, the binding of H1 receptors may also enhance its ability to treat insomnia, which can be beneficial in treating not only psychosis and mania but also the depressed phase of bipolar disorder and for off-label uses such as difficult-to-treat cases of unipolar depression, various anxiety disorders, and sleep disorders.

Quetiapine can increase fasting triglyceride levels and insulin resistance, particularly at moderate to high doses, and with intermediate to high risk compared to other atypical antipsychotics (Table 10-3), possibly via the same unknown pharmacological mechanism postulated to be active for some other atypical antipsychotics (receptor X in

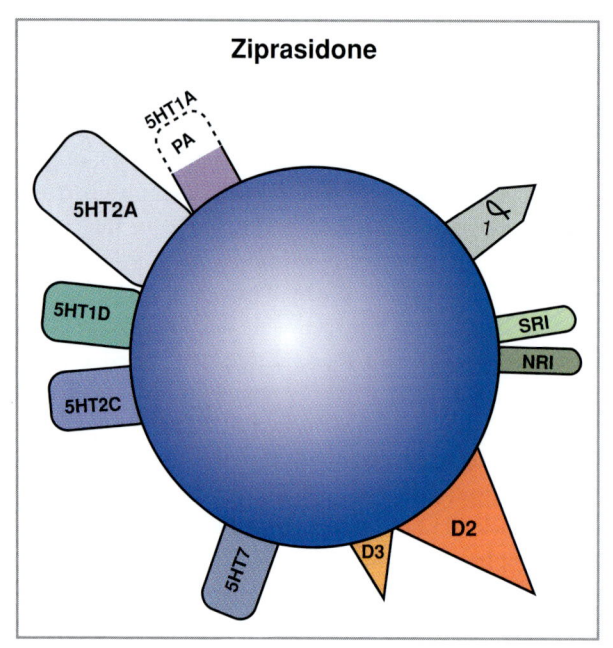

FIGURE 10-95 Ziprasidone. Ziprasidone's pharmacological icon, portraying a qualitative consensus of current thinking about the binding properties of this drug. It is the only atypical antipsychotic with serotonin (5HT) 1D antagonist and both serotonin and norepinephrine reuptake blocking properties. As with all atypical antipsychotics discussed in this chapter, binding properties vary greatly with technique and from one laboratory to another; they are constantly being revised and updated. The 5HT1A partial agonist actions as well as the 5HT2C antagonist actions may contribute to the mood-improving properties and to the cognitive enhancement observed with ziprasidone. This compound seems to lack the pharmacological actions associated with weight gain and increased cardiometabolic risk such as increasing fasting plasma triglyceride levels or increasing insulin resistance. Ziprasidone also lacks many of the pharmacological properties associated with significant sedation.

Figures 10-58, 10-62, 10-63, 10-66, 10-67, and 10-94). Like all atypical antipsychotics, quetiapine can be associated rarely with sudden and life-threatening hyperglycemic hyperosmolar syndrome/diabetic ketoacidosis; M3-cholinergic antagonism might be a factor in this, but the importance of this mechanism is still unproven (Figures 10-58, 10-64, 10-65, 10-66, 10-67, and 10-94). Actual risks versus benefits for quetiapine must be determined — as for all atypical antipsychotics — patient by patient while monitoring both efficacy and side effects, including cardiometabolic risks.

Ziprasidone. Ziprasidone has a novel chemical structure and a quite novel pharmacological profile compared to the other atypical antipsychotics (Figure 10-95). It is an SDA and is atypical in that it is associated with a low incidence of EPS and prolactin elevation. Numerous studies demonstrate that ziprasidone is highly effective for positive symptoms of schizophrenia and also improves negative symptoms of schizophrenia and the symptoms of mania in bipolar disorder. It has an intramuscular dosage formulation for rapid use in urgent circumstances that is robustly and predictably effective in acute psychosis. This is interesting, since it proves the point that ziprasidone has robust and consistent efficacy when dosed correctly, something that is not always done when ziprasidone is administered orally. When underdosed, ziprasidone, like all antipsychotics, may not exhibit full efficacy. It is now appreciated that rapid oral dose escalation to the middle or top of the dose range, while being administered twice daily with food to assure its absorption, is what provides predictability to ziprasidone's efficacy in psychosis and mania. Low doses, particularly when they are not administered with food, probably occupy too few D2 receptors for consistent efficacy. As discussed above for quetiapine, it is possible that once-daily administration of ziprasidone could be appropriate for some patients, especially if ziprasidone is taken reliably with a small (500-calorie) meal, but this has not been adequately studied.

Earlier concerns about dangerous QTc prolongation by ziprasidone now appear to be unjustified. Unlike zotepine, sertindole, and amisulpride, ziprasidone does not cause dose-dependent QTc prolongation, and few drugs have the potential to increase ziprasidone's plasma levels. Paliperidone (and by association, risperidone) also have warnings of a modest increase in QTc interval. All of these agents should be given cautiously if at all to patients receiving other drugs known to prolong QTc interval, but routine EKGs are generally not recommended. It is obviously prudent to be cautious when using any atypical antipsychotic or psychotropic drug in patients with cardiac problems or in patients taking other drugs that affect cardiac function; this is part of the routine risk-benefit calculation made for each individual patient prior to prescribing any of the atypical antipsychotic drugs.

The major differentiating feature of ziprasidone is that it has little or no propensity to promote weight gain (Table 10-2), perhaps because it has no antihistamine properties, although it does have 5HT2C-antagonist actions (Figures 10-59 and 10-95). Furthermore, there seems to be little association of ziprasidone with dyslipidemia, elevation of fasting triglycerides, or insulin resistance (Tables 10-3 and 10-4). In fact, when patients who have developed weight gain and dyslipidemia from high-risk antipsychotics (Table 10-3) are switched from those antipsychotics to ziprasidone, there can be weight loss and often lowering of fasting triglycerides while continuing to receive treatment with ziprasidone.

Is it clinically meaningful when one antipsychotic elevates cardiometabolic risk (Table 10-3) and another does not (Table 10-4)? An answer to this question can be found by considering how many patients a psychopharmacologist would have to treat with an agent that elevates cardiometabolic risk to cause one of them to get diabetes or have a heart attack (myocardial infarction), known as the number needed to harm. Progress along the metabolic highway from no disease to diabetes or myocardial infarction takes about 10 years (Figure 10-60), with loss of about 25 years of life expectancy in patients with serious mental illnesses. Statistics from clinical trials suggest that psychopharmacologists who treat patients with antipsychotics for 10 years would need to treat only about 25 male patients with olanzapine or 100 male patients with either risperidone or quetiapine to cause one of them to become diabetic in that period of time due to use of the atypical antipsychotic drug, whereas this might be predicted not to happen in anyone treated with ziprasidone (Table 10-3). Aripiprazole may also not cause increased risk of diabetes; this may also prove to be true for bifeprunox and for amisulpride, but further investigation of the latter drugs is needed (Table 10-4).

Similarly, over a 10-year period of treatment, it might require that olanzapine be administered to about 200 patients, quetiapine to 300 patients, and risperidone to 1500 patients to cause one patient to have a myocardial infarction due to the antipsychotic drug treatment, with relatively no additional risk with agents such as ziprasidone or aripiprazole. Thus, over a career of several decades, choice of atypical antipsychotic drug can make a big difference to many patients in each psychopharmacologist's practice. Sometimes incremental risks are justified by the severity of the psychotic illness, but only with metabolic monitoring can a psychopharmacologist be in a position to weigh that risk against the benefit of clinical efficacy.

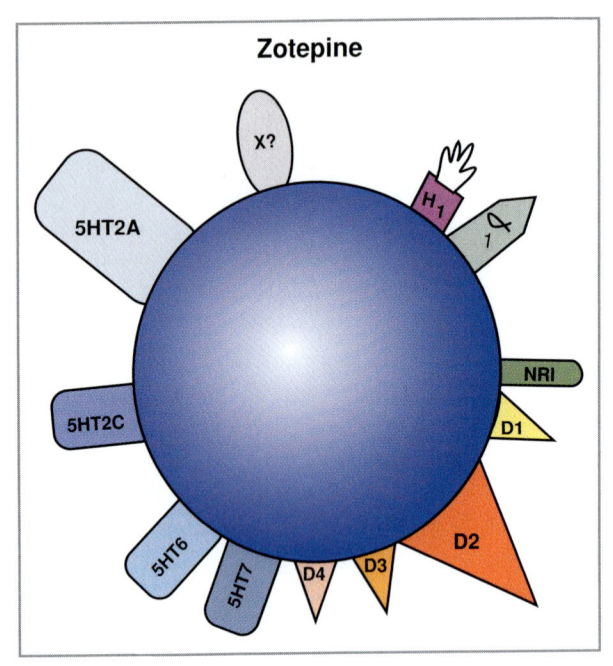

FIGURE 10-96 Zotepine. Zotepine's pharmacological icon, portraying a qualitative consensus of current thinking about the binding properties of this drug. As with all atypical antipsychotics discussed in this chapter, binding properties vary greatly with technique and from one laboratory to another; they are constantly being revised and updated. 5HT2C and histamine H1-antagonist properties can contribute to weight gain, H1 and alpha-1 adrenergic antagonist properties can contribute to sedation, and 5HT2C and norepinephrine reuptake inhibition (NRI) suggest possible efficacy for mood symptoms.

The pharmacological properties that make ziprasidone different in terms of its lower cardiometabolic risk are unknown but could be explained if ziprasidone lacks the ability to bind to receptors postulated to mediate insulin resistance and hypertriglyceridemia. Furthermore, ziprasidone does not bind to M3-cholinergic receptors.

Ziprasidone is the only atypical antipsychotic with 5HT1D antagonist actions as well as moderate inhibition of both 5HT reuptake and NE reuptake (Figure 10-95). These latter pharmacological actions would be expected to be both proserotonergic and pronoradrenergic, which might contribute to ziprasidone's favorable actions with regard to weight but would also predict antidepressant and anxiolytic actions. In addition, potent 5HT1A partial agonist and 5HT2C antagonist actions (Figure 10-95) may explain not only potential cognitive and affective actions of ziprasidone – due to theoretical increases in dopamine and norepinephrine in prefrontal cortex – but also the activating actions of this agent when given in subtherapeutic doses. Paradoxically, ziprasidone's activating actions may be diminished by increasing its dose. Antidepressant actions of ziprasidone are being actively tested and are discussed further in Chapter 12, on antidepressants.

Zotepine. Zotepine is an SDA available in several countries, including Japan and in Europe, has a chemical structure related to that of clozapine, but with distinguishing pharmacological (Figure 10-96) and clinical properties. Although zotepine is an SDA, some EPS have nevertheless been observed, as have prolactin elevations. Like clozapine, there is an increased risk of seizures, especially at high doses, as well as weight gain and sedation. Zotepine probably increases risk for insulin resistance, dyslipidemia, and diabetes, but it has not been extensively studied for these side effects. Unlike the case for clozapine, however, there is no clear evidence yet that zotepine is as effective for patients who fail to respond to conventional antipsychotics. Zotepine dose-dependently prolongs the QTc interval. It is generally administered three times daily. Zotepine inhibits norepinephrine reuptake

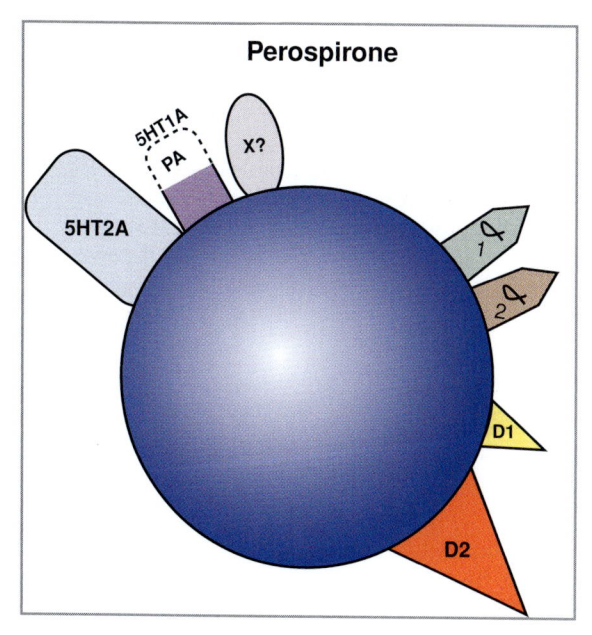

FIGURE 10-97 Perospirone. Perospirone's pharmacological icon, portraying a qualitative consensus of current thinking about the binding properties of this drug. As with all atypical antipsychotics discussed in this chapter, binding properties vary greatly with technique and from one laboratory to another; they are constantly being revised and updated. 5HT1A partial agonist actions may contribute to efficacy for mood and cognitive symptoms.

(Figure 10-96), suggesting potential antidepressant actions. Because of its side effects, zotepine is generally considered a second-line agent.

Perospirone. Perospirone is an SDA available in Japan. Its 5HT1A partial agonist actions may contribute to its efficacy (Figure 10-97). Its ability to cause weight gain, dyslipidemia, insulin resistance, and diabetes has not been well investigated. It is generally administered three times a day, and there is more experience with its use in the treatment of schizophrenia than in that of mania.

Sertindole. Sertindole is an atypical antipsychotic with SDA properties (Figure 10-98). It was originally approved in some European countries, then withdrawn for further testing of its cardiac safety and QTc-prolonging potential, and finally reintroduced into certain countries as a second-line agent. It may be useful for some patients in whom other antipsychotics have failed and who can have close monitoring of their cardiac status and drug interactions.

Loxapine. Loxapine is another SDA with a structural formula related to that of clozapine but generally classified as a conventional antipsychotic (Figure 10-99). As usually dosed, it indeed has the clinical profile of a conventional antipsychotic, causing EPS and prolactin elevation. There are hints, however, that it may be somewhat atypical at doses lower than those usually administered, and this is confirmed by human PET scans confirming its ability to block serotonin 2A receptors (see red circle in Figure 10-99) as well as D2 receptors. It is possible that loxapine's atypical properties were masked because it was used in high doses, just as high-dose use can convert other atypical antipsychotics into drugs with EPS and prolactin elevation. Testing at low doses (perhaps one-tenth of those usually administered) could confirm whether loxapine has atypical clinical properties.

Loxapine is available for intramuscular administration and usually causes no weight gain, but its cardiometabolic risk is not well characterized. A principal metabolite is N-methyl loxapine, a tricyclic antidepressant better known as amoxapine. Amoxapine has noradrenergic reuptake blocking properties, suggesting possible antidepressant actions for loxapine as well.

Antipsychotic Agents | 419

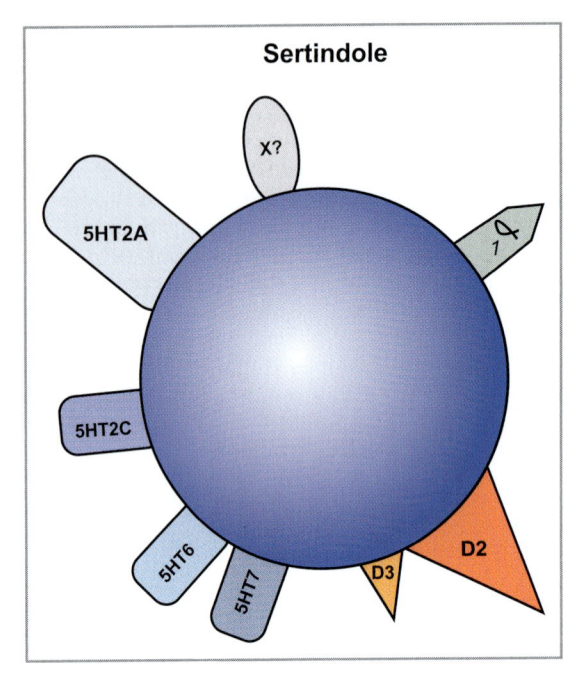

FIGURE 10-98 Sertindole. Sertindole's pharmacological icon, portraying a qualitative consensus of current thinking about the binding properties of this drug. As with all atypical antipsychotics discussed in this chapter, binding properties vary greatly with technique and from one laboratory to another; they are constantly being revised and updated. Potent antagonist actions at alpha-1 receptors may account for some of sertindole's side effects.

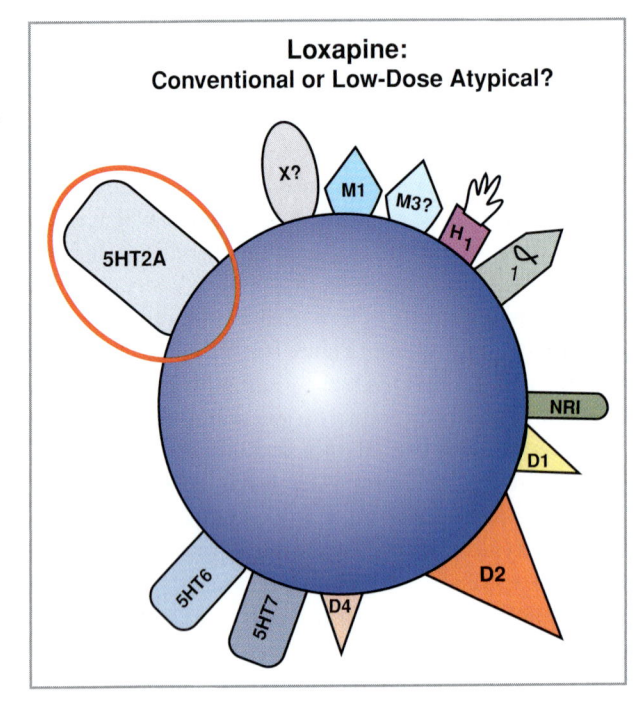

FIGURE 10-99 Loxapine. Loxapine's pharmacological icon, portraying a qualitative consensus of current thinking about the binding properties of this drug. As usually dosed, loxapine has a profile more consistent with a conventional antipsychotic than an atypical antipsychotic. However, it may be somewhat atypical at lower doses. As with all atypical antipsychotics discussed in this chapter, binding properties vary greatly with technique and from one laboratory to another; they are constantly being revised and updated. This so-called conventional antipsychotic nevertheless has antagonist actions at 5HT2A receptors (red circle), just like atypical antipsychotics, and may thus have some atypical antipsychotic properties, particularly at low doses. It also has norepinephrine reuptake inhibition (NRI) properties and has amoxapine, a known antidepressant, as one of its active metabolites; it may therefore have additional actions for mood symptoms.

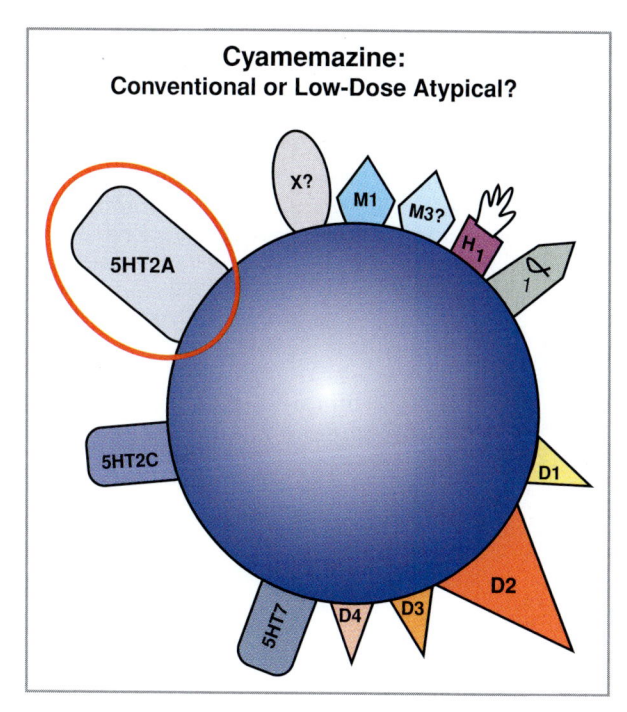

FIGURE 10-100 Cyamemazine. Cyamemazine's pharmacological icon, portraying a qualitative consensus of current thinking about the binding properties of this drug. Like loxapine, cyemamazine's profile may be more that of a conventional antipsychotic when used at higher doses. As with all atypical antipsychotics discussed in this chapter, binding properties vary greatly with technique and from one laboratory to another; they are constantly being revised and updated. This so-called conventional antipsychotic nevertheless has antagonist actions at 5HT2A receptors (red circle) and may thus have some atypical antipsychotic properties, particularly at low doses.

Cyamemazine. Cyamemazine is another antipsychotic originally developed at high doses as a conventional antipsychotic agent with EPS and prolactin elevations, but it was subsequently found to have 5HT2A antagonist properties (see red circle in Figure 10-100). This agent is available in some European countries and has long been popular in France at low doses, especially for treating anxiety associated with psychosis. Its ability to cause weight gain and to increase cardiometabolic risk has not been extensively investigated.

Aripiprazole. This agent is the first antipsychotic developed as a D2-receptor partial agonist (DPA), a major differentiating feature from serotonin dopamine antagonists or SDAs that are silent antagonists at D2 receptors (see Figures 10-45 and 10-101). Aripiprazole does have the 5HT2A antagonist properties associated with SDAs but not the full antagonist actions at D2 receptors associated with SDAs (Figure 10-101). Aripiprazole also has 5HT1A partial agonist properties which, together with its 5HT2A antagonist properties, may contribute to its tolerability profile and efficacy (Figure 10-101). As for all antipsychotics, the actions of aripiprazole at D3 receptors remains unclear. Aripiprazole is highly effective in treating the positive symptoms of schizophrenia and manic symptoms in mania and has shown promising results as an augmenting agent in major depressive disorder. Early clinical results in bipolar depression have been disappointing. An intramuscular dosage formulation is now available. An orally disintegrating tablet and a liquid formulation are available.

Aripiprazole lacks the pharmacological properties normally associated with sedation, namely, robust alpha-1 adrenergic, M1-muscarinic cholinergic, and H1-histamine antagonist properties and thus is not generally sedating (Figure 10-101). In fact, aripiprazole can be activating in some patients, causing mild agitation or akathisia, which diminishes over time or is often decreased by dose reduction or by administering an anticholinergic agent or a benzodiazepine. In some people, therefore, the partial agonist properties might be too

Antipsychotic Agents | 421

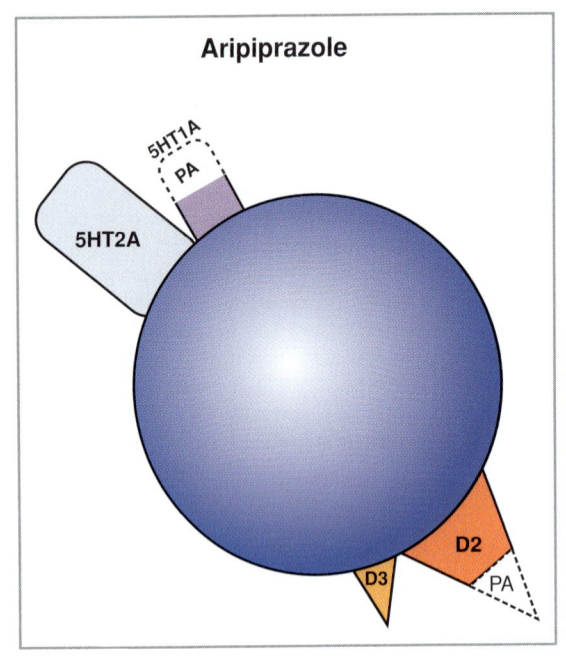

FIGURE 10-101 Aripiprazole. Aripiprazole's pharmacological icon, portraying a qualitative consensus of current thinking about the binding properties of this drug. Aripiprazole differs from most other antipsychotics in that it is a partial agonist at D2 receptors rather than an antagonist. As with all atypical antipsychotics discussed in this chapter, binding properties vary greatly with technique and from one laboratory to another; they are constantly being revised and updated. Additional important pharmacological properties that may contribute to its clinical profile include 5HT2A antagonist actions and 5HT1A partial agonist actions. Aripiprazole lacks the pharmacological actions usually associated with significant sedation and also seems to lack the pharmacologic actions associated with weight gain and increased cardiometabolic risk, such as increasing fasting plasma triglyceride levels or increasing insulin resistance.

close to full antagonism, with mild EPS such as akathisia (Figure 10-54), at least on dosage initiation and in patients without prior exposure to D2 full antagonists.

In other patients, the partial agonist properties might be too close to those of a dopamine agonist (Figure 10-54), with activation, nausea, and occasionally vomiting. In these cases, the use of time, dose adjustment, and short-term concomitant benzodiazepines can smooth the transition to a DPA and optimize tolerability.

A major differentiating feature of aripiprazole is that it has, like ziprasidone, little or no propensity to promote weight gain (Table 10-2), perhaps because it has no antihistamine properties or 5HT2C antagonist actions (Figures 10-59 and 10-101). Furthermore, there seems to be little association of aripiprazole with dyslipidemia, elevation of fasting triglycerides, or insulin resistance (Tables 10-3 and 10-4). In fact, as in the case of ziprasidone, when patients with weight gain and dyslipidemia caused by other antipsychotics switch to aripiprazole, there can be weight loss and a lowering of fasting triglyceride levels. The pharmacological properties that make aripiprazole different in terms of its lower metabolic risk are unknown but could be explained if aripiprazole lacks the ability to bind to postulated receptors that mediate insulin resistance and hypertriglyceridemia.

Amisulpride. Amisulpride was developed in Europe and other countries prior to full appreciation of the concept of dopamine partial agonism (DPA) (Figure 10-102). Thus it has not been tested in the same systems as newer agents, but there are some clinical hints that amisulpride is not only an atypical antipsychotic but that it has these clinical properties because it is a DPA at D2 receptors. Amisulpride has no appreciable affinity for 5HT2A or 5HT1A receptors to explain its low propensity for EPS and the observation of improvement of negative symptoms in schizophrenia, particularly at low doses. As in the case of all antipsychotics, it is not known how amisulpride's actions at D3 receptors may contribute to its clinical profile.

Amisulpride's ability to cause weight gain, dyslipidemia, and diabetes has not been extensively investigated. It may cause dose-dependent QTc prolongation. Since amisulpride

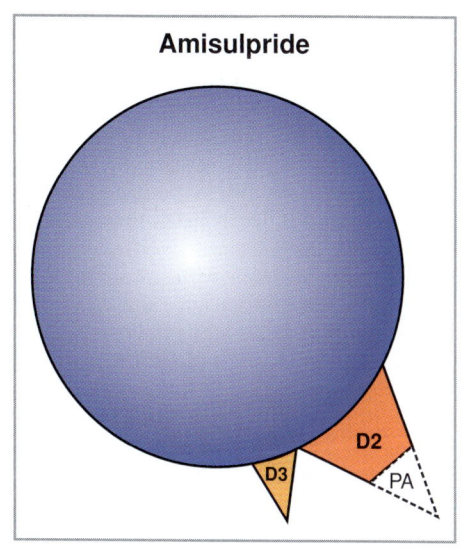

FIGURE 10-102 Amisulpride. Amisulpride's pharmacological icon, portraying a qualitative consensus of current thinking about the binding properties of this drug. Amisulpride does not have affinity for serotonin 2A or 1A receptors, but it may be a partial agonist at D2 receptors rather than an antagonist. As with all atypical antipsychotics discussed in this chapter, binding properties vary greatly with technique and from one laboratory to another; they are constantly being revised and updated.

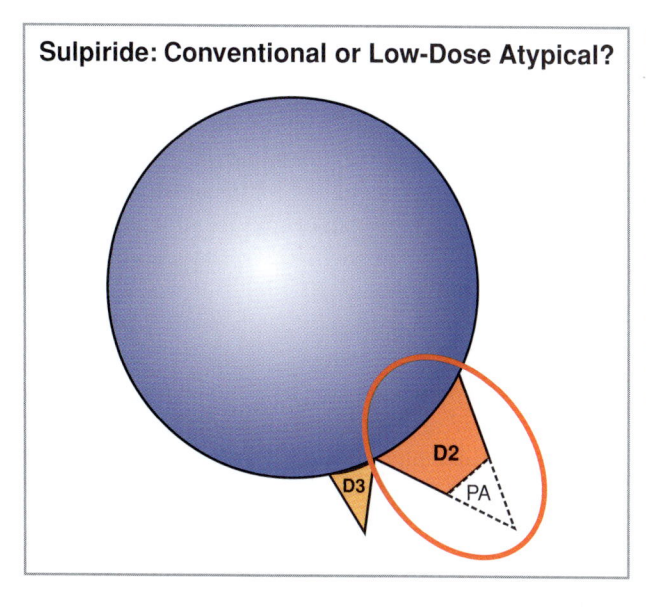

FIGURE 10-103 Sulpiride. Sulpiride's pharmacological icon, portraying a qualitative consensus of current thinking about the binding properties of this drug. At usual doses, sulpiride has the profile of a conventional antipsychotic, but at low doses it may be a partial agonist at D2 receptors, though likely still closer to the antagonist end of the spectrum. As with all atypical antipsychotics discussed in this chapter, binding properties vary greatly with technique and from one laboratory to another; they are constantly being revised and updated.

can cause prolactin elevation, if it is appropriately classifiable as a DPA, it is likely closer to a silent antagonist than is aripiprazole on the DPA spectrum and may only function as a DPA at low doses and as a more conventional D2 antagonist at high doses (see Figure 10-54).

Sulpiride. Sulpiride is an earlier compound structurally related to amisulpride that was developed as a conventional antipsychotic (Figure 10-103). Although it generally causes EPS and prolactin elevation at usual antipsychotic doses, it may be activating and have efficacy for negative symptoms of schizophrenia as well as for depression at low doses. This agent, if a DPA, is likely to have pharmacological properties very close to those of a silent antagonist and may function as a DPA only at low doses and as a more conventional D2 antagonist at high doses (Figure 10-54).

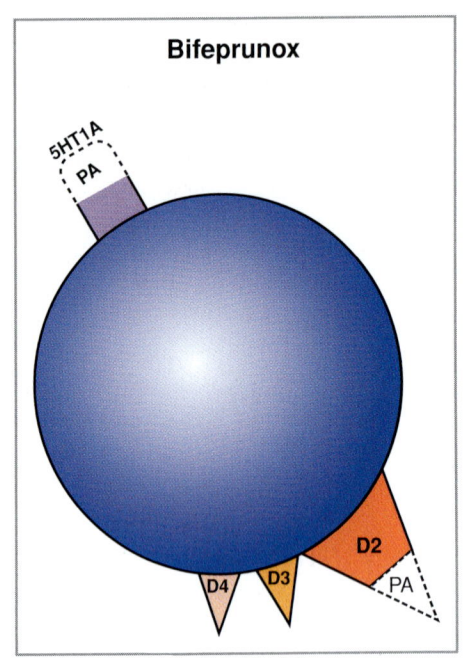

FIGURE 10-104 Bifeprunox. Bifeprunox's pharmacological icon, portraying a qualitative consensus of current thinking about the binding properties of this drug. Bifeprunox does not have appreciable affinity for serotonin 2A receptors, but instead seems to be a partial agonist at both D2 receptors and serotonin 1A receptors. As with all atypical antipsychotics discussed in this chapter, binding properties vary greatly with technique and from one laboratory to another; they are constantly being revised and updated. Bifeprunox seems to lack the pharmacological properties associated with sedation and may lack the actions that cause weight gain, or increases in fasting plasma triglycerides, or insulin resistance.

Bifeprunox. A new DPA with efficacy for positive symptoms in schizophrenia and for manic symptoms in bipolar disorder is bifeprunox (Figure 10-104). This agent is interesting in that it has no significant 5HT2A antagonist properties but couples its DPA actions with potent 5HT1A serotonin partial agonist (SPA) actions to attain its atypical clinical profile of low EPS and a low incidence of hyperprolactinemia (Figure 10-104). Bifeprunox lacks the pharmacological properties normally associated with sedation, namely, alpha-1 adrenergic, M1-muscarinic cholinergic and H1-histamine antagonist properties; thus it is not sedating (Figure 10-104). In fact, bifeprunox can be a bit more activating than the DPA aripiprazole, thus moving it along the spectrum closer to a full agonist than aripiprazole (Figure 10-54). As a partial agonist closer to agonist actions than aripiprazole, it may cause more nausea and vomiting than aripiprazole. This can slow down the ideal rate of dose titration and thus delay onset of action in situations of acute psychosis or acute mania. On the other hand, its partial agonist actions may lead to enhanced long term tolerability during long term maintenance by having a lack of sedating side effects plus the theoretical potential to brighten patients by improving both cognitive and affective symptoms, clinical possibilities that are currently under investigation. Bifeprunox does not appear to pose a great risk of weight gain or of increasing cardiometabolic risk such as dyslipidemia, increased insulin resistance, or elevated fasting plasma triglycerides, but it is still under investigation for these properties (Table 10-4). Bifeprunox is also under study as an antidepressant for the depressed phase of bipolar disorder. The emerging clinical profile of bifeprunox is one that may be advantageous for long-term use as a maintenance agent in schizophrenia and bipolar disorder.

Antipsychotics in clinical practice

The prescription of antipsychotics in clinical practice can be very different from studying them in clinical trials. Real patients are often more complicated, may have diagnoses that do not meet diagnostic criteria for the formally studied indications, and generally have much more comorbidity than patients studied in clinical trials. Thus, it is important for the practicing psychopharmacologist to appreciate that different atypical antipsychotics can have clinically distinctive effects in different patients in clinical practice. What this also means is that median clinical effects in clinical trials may not be the best indicator of the range of clinical responses possible for individual patients. Furthermore, optimal doses suggested from clinical trials often do not match optimal doses used in clinical practice (too high for some drugs; too low for others). Finally, although virtually all studies are head-to-head comparisons of monotherapies and/or placebo, many patients receive two antipsychotics or antipsychotics plus other psychotropic drugs in clinical practice settings. Sometimes this is rational and justified, but sometimes it is not. Here we will briefly discuss some of the issues that arise in trying to apply knowledge about the pharmacological mechanisms of action discussed so far in this chapter to the utilization of atypical antipsychotics in clinical practice.

Schizophrenia symptom pharmacies
Although it is important to make accurate psychiatric diagnoses, throughout this book it has been emphasized that in reality, clinicians treat symptoms, not diseases. Psychiatric disorders are clusters of symptoms for which the underlying disease is not known, but psychopharmacological agents can be powerful agents to relieve suffering by reducing symptoms. Here we break down the syndrome of schizophrenia and psychotic illnesses into symptom dimensions in order to customize the application of treatments to specific symptoms.

Positive symptom pharmacy (Figure 10-105). The most robust action of any antipsychotic is generally its ability to reduce the positive symptoms of psychosis, such as delusions and hallucinations, and these are the symptoms often targeted first in the treatment of schizophrenia. It is very difficult to consider treatment for other symptoms until the positive symptoms are somewhat under control. When the situation is urgent, rapid delivery with a short-acting intramuscular injection may be required, and this formulation is available for several atypical and conventional antipsychotics (Figure 10-105, in case of emergency). Positive symptoms can also be treated in urgent situations for the short term with an injectable benzodiazepine.

First-line treatment of positive symptoms includes any atypical antipsychotic, either a serotonin dopamine antagonist (SDA) or a dopamine partial agonist (DPA). For noncompliant patients, positive symptoms can be managed with a depot, for which one atypical antipsychotic (the SDA risperidone) as well as several conventional antipsychotics are available. Second-line treatment of positive symptoms that have not been controlled with adequate trials of a first-line SDA or DPA would include either clozapine or a conventional antipsychotic. If all else fails, either heroic doses of one of the first- or second-line agents might be considered, a combination (combo) such as augmentation of a first-line treatment with a mood stabilizer, or polypharmacy of two antipsychotics, particularly one atypical antipsychotic with one conventional antipsychotic.

Aggressive symptom pharmacy (Figure 10-106). Patients with schizophrenia can be hostile and aggressive, toward self, staff, family, and property. This may take the form of suicide attempts, self-mutilation, poor impulse control, drug abuse, verbal abuse, physical abuse, or threatening behavior and may not directly correlate with positive symptoms. It can be a particularly difficult problem among patients in a forensic setting. Such problems are also common symptom dimensions in many psychiatric disorders other than schizophrenia, including many childhood and adolescent disorders such as conduct disorder, oppositional

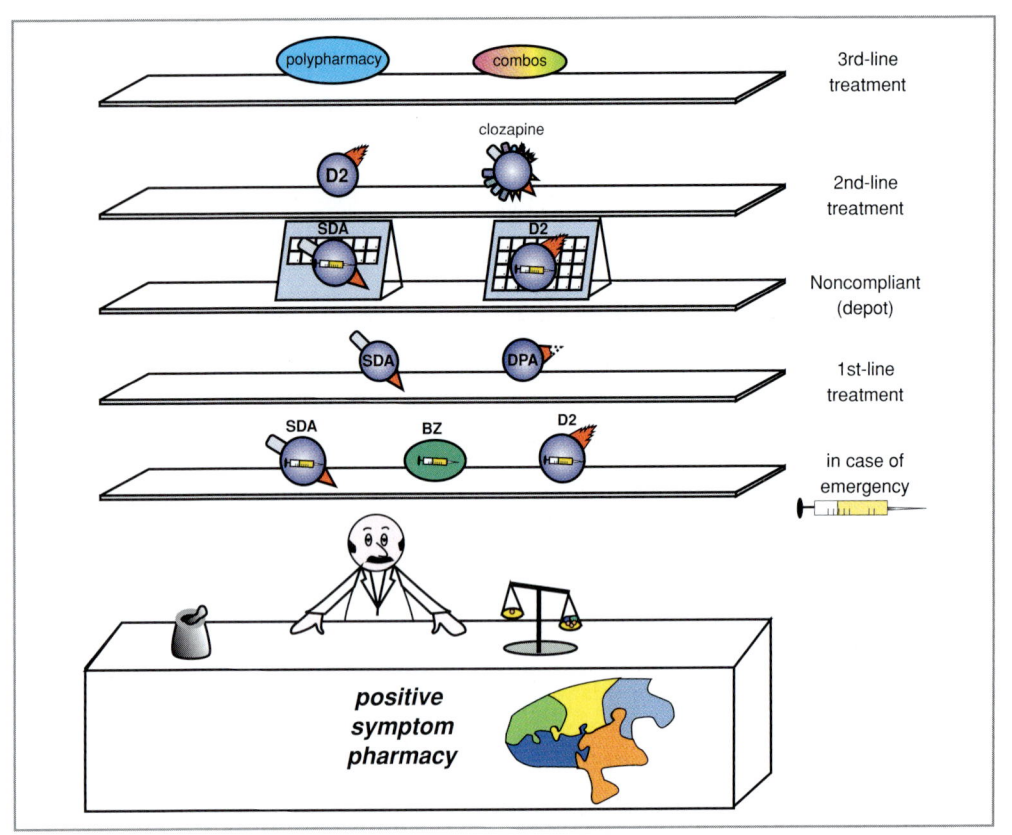

FIGURE 10-105 Positive symptom pharmacy. First-line treatment of positive symptoms is now atypical antipsychotics [serotonin-dopamine antagonists (SDAs) or dopamine partial agonists (DPAs)], not only for schizophrenia but also for positive symptoms associated with bipolar disorder, Alzheimer's disease, childhood psychoses, and other psychotic disorders. Several atypical antipsychotics are available in intramuscular formulations, which can be used acutely (in case of emergency). Conventional antipsychotics (D2) and benzodiazepines (BZ) can also be useful for acute intramuscular administration (in case of emergency). Depot injections are available for one atypical antipsychotic, risperidone (every 2 weeks) or for several conventional antipsychotics (monthly). This can be especially useful for noncompliant patients as well as for second-line use after several atypical agents fail. Clozapine, conventional antipsychotics, polypharmacy, and combinations (combos) are relegated to second- and third-line treatment for positive symptoms of psychosis.

defiant disorder, autism, mental retardation, attention deficit hyperactivity disorder, as well as borderline personality disorder, bipolar disorders, and various types of organic disorders and brain damage including head injury, traumatic brain injury, stroke, and Alzheimer's disease. This dimension of psychopathology obviously cuts a wide swath across psychiatric disorders and is not necessarily associated with psychosis.

Both conventional and atypical antipsychotics may reduce such symptoms, but there are far more studies of hostility and aggression in psychotic illnesses than in nonpsychotic illnesses. The treatment of aggressive symptoms in schizophrenia can be much like the treatment of positive symptoms with injectable antipsychotics and benzodiazepines for urgent situations, with SDA or DPA atypical antipsychotics preferred for first-line treatment (Figure 10-106). Not only clozapine or conventional antipsychotics can be helpful for aggressive symptoms in some patients when first-line treatments are not satisfactory but also oral benzodiazepines or mood stabilizers (Figure 10-106). The treatment of

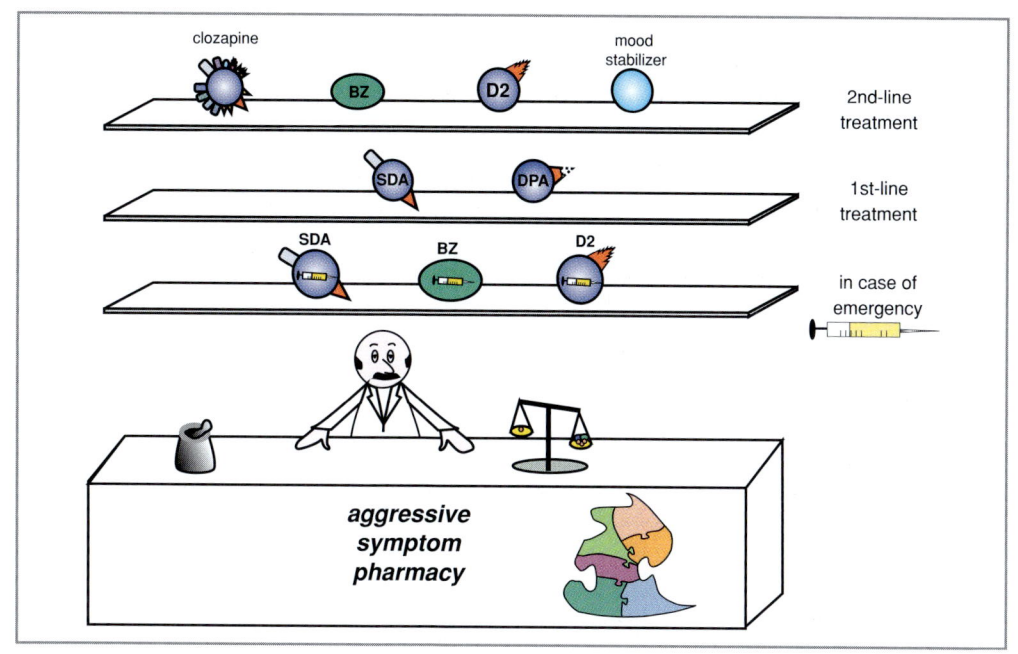

FIGURE 10-106 Aggressive symptom pharmacy. Atypical antipsychotics [serotonin-dopamine antagonists (SDAs) or dopamine partial agonists (DPAs)] are preferable (first-line) to conventional antipsychotics (D2) for the management of aggression, hostility, and impulse control because of their more favorable side effect profiles. In an acute situation, intramuscular atypical (SDA) or conventional (D2) antipsychotics as well as intramuscular benzodiazepines (BZ) may be useful. Conventional antipsychotics, clozapine, benzodiazepines, or mood stabilizers may be required when atypical antipsychotics are not effective (second-line).

hostility, aggression, and poor impulse control is always controversial; it requires good clinical judgment and consideration of other interventions such as seclusion, restraint, and environmental and milieu techniques, with prevention of utilizing drugs as punishment or excessive behavioral control vehicles ("chemical straight jackets").

The treatment of aggressive symptoms is particularly controversial when the patient does not have schizophrenia, and antipsychotics are not approved for such uses, although it may be necessary to use antipsychotics off-label for these symptoms in some cases. As mentioned earlier in this chapter, one antipsychotic, risperidone, has proven to be effective for irritability associated with autistic disorder in children and adolescents (ages 5 to 16), including symptoms of aggression toward others, deliberate self-injury, tantrums, and quickly changing moods. Although frequently used to help reduce aggression and related behavioral disturbances in dementia as well, this use must be carefully weighed against the other available options and against the risks of treatment versus the risks of nontreatment.

Negative symptom pharmacy (Figure 10-107). This symptom dimension is thought to be a particularly unique feature of schizophrenia, although certain aspects of these symptoms can overlap with symptoms that are not unique to schizophrenia itself, such as cognitive and affective symptoms. Any improvement in negative symptoms that can be gained from treatment with atypical antipsychotics is very important, because the long-term outcome of schizophrenia is more closely correlated with severity of negative symptoms than it is with that of positive symptoms. However, it is already clear that significantly more robust treatment effects will be necessary than those offered by any currently available

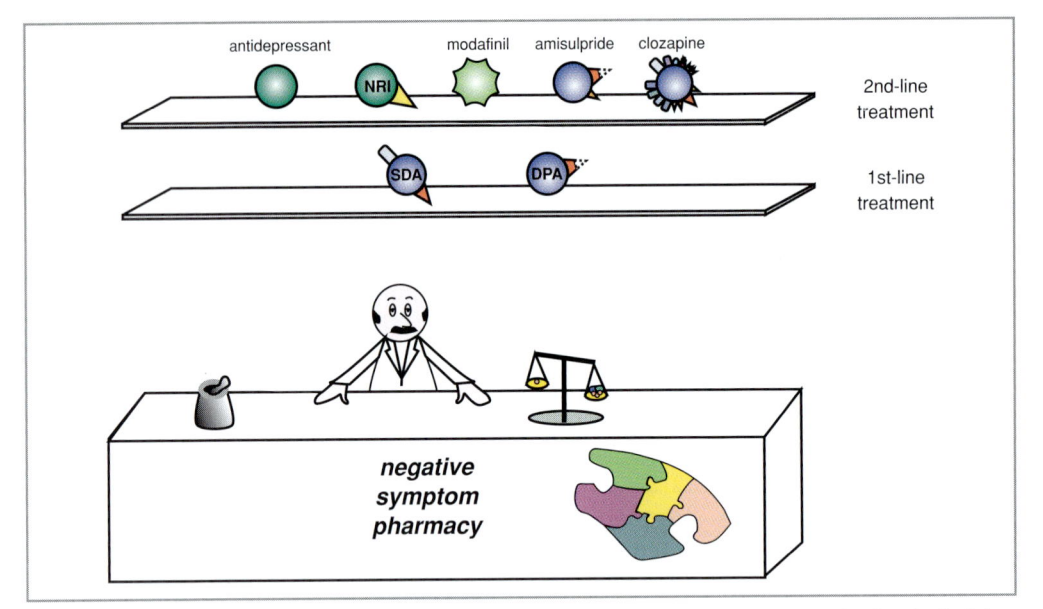

FIGURE 10-107 **Negative symptom pharmacy.** Negative symptoms can be improved in schizophrenia, both by switching from conventional antipsychotics (which can make these symptoms worse) to atypical antipsychotics [serotonin-dopamine antagonists (SDAs) or dopamine partial agonists (DPAs)] that do not generally worsen negative symptoms and may even improve negative symptoms. As second-line options, amisulpride or clozapine may be beneficial, as may augmentation with antidepressants, norepinephrine reuptake inhibitors (NRIs), or modafinil.

antipsychotic if such symptoms are to improve enough to transform the poor outcomes of many schizophrenic patients.

In the meantime, there are some approaches which are currently available for improving negative symptoms in the short run. First, negative symptoms secondary to antipsychotics can be readily reduced by avoiding conventional antipsychotics and by avoiding high doses of atypical antipsychotics whenever possible. Second, atypical antipsychotics actually improve negative symptoms in some patients, so first-line treatment is with either an SDA or a DPA (Figure 10-107). Finally, off-label use of certain antidepressants or cognitive enhancers can be considered as augmentation to an atypical antipsychotic. This may be helpful in selected cases.

Cognitive symptom pharmacy (Figure 10-108). Severity of cognitive symptoms correlates with the long-term prognosis of schizophrenia, so reduction of these symptoms is a vital treatment goal. The pharmacy for cognitive treatment of schizophrenia includes atypical but not conventional antipsychotics. Otherwise the cupboard is relatively bare. Augmentation with antidepressants or cognitive enhancers may be helpful in selected cases, just as these agents are occasionally helpful for negative symptoms. Discontinuing drugs with sedating or anticholinergic properties may also be useful in improving cognition in some cases. However, it is hoped that the multiple experimental interventions currently under study will be able to treat the cognitive symptoms of schizophrenia much more effectively than any of the interventions currently available, probably by adding treatments with new mechanisms to atypical antipsychotics. Many therapeutics in testing as future cognitive treatments for schizophrenia are discussed next in the final section of this chapter.

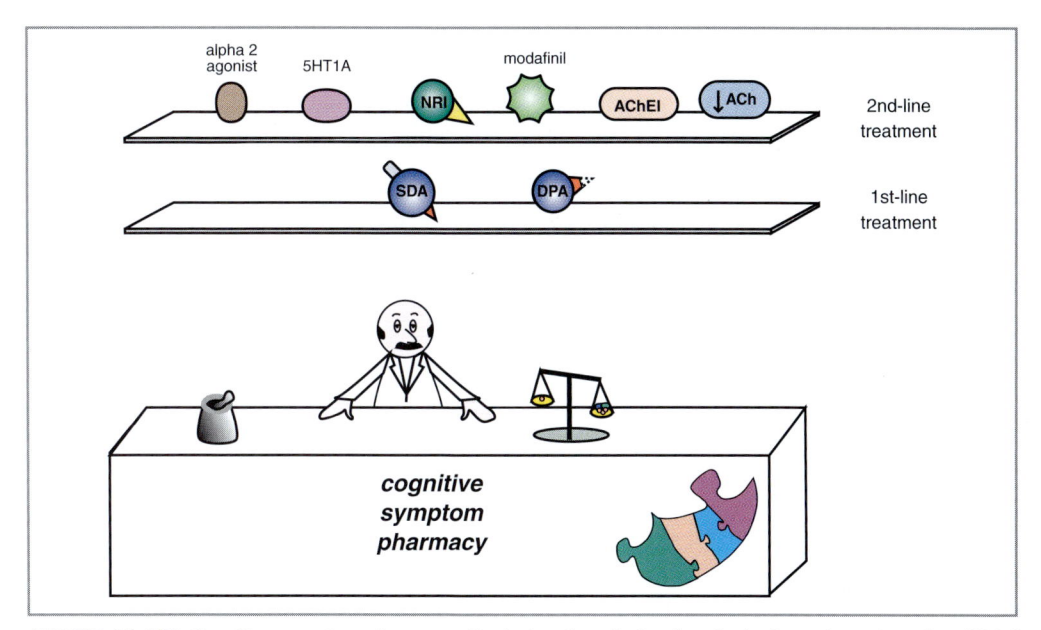

FIGURE 10-108 **Cognitive symptom pharmacy.** Atypical antipsychotics [serotonin-dopamine antagonists (SDAs) or dopamine partial agonists (DPAs)] may improve cognitive functions in schizophrenic patients (first-line). It may also be useful to discontinue any anticholinergic medications that you can, a welcome bonus when switching from conventional antipsychotics to atypical antipsychotics (decreased ACh). Augmentation with alpha-2 agonists, 5HT1A agonists, norepinephrine reuptake inhibitors (NRIs), modafinil, or acetylcholinesterase inhibitors (AChEIs) may all be second-line options for treating cognitive symptoms of psychosis.

Affective symptom pharmacy (Figure 10-109). Affective symptoms are a dimension of schizophrenia and are a major feature of bipolar disorder, schizoaffective disorder, and of course major depressive disorder. Further, patients with schizophrenia can even have a major depressive episode that is comorbid with their schizophrenia. Thus, it is important to treat affective symptoms in schizophrenia and bipolar disorder not only first-line with an atypical antipsychotic but also, if remission is not fully achieved with this approach, to consider augmentation with lithium, a mood stabilizer, or an antidepressant to relieve all affective symptoms and stabilize mood. Antidepressants and mood stabilizers are discussed in much further detail in Chapters 12 and 13. Clozapine is the only atypical antipsychotic proven to reduce suicide in schizophrenia, although other antipsychotics may also be useful for this symptom. Lithium is the only mood stabilizer proven to reduce suicide in bipolar disorder, but it could possibly have a similar effect in schizophrenia, even though this has not yet been proven.

Metabolic pharmacy (Figure 10-110). Although all atypical antipsychotics approved for use in the United States are associated with metabolic warnings, experts generally believe that there are tiers of risk for weight gain (Table 10-2) as well as cardiometabolic risk among these agents (Tables 10-3 and 10-4). Thus, to avoid weight gain and cardiometabolic risk, first line treatment is either ziprasidone or aripiprazole. Monitoring is still necessary with these agents, as some patients nevertheless may exhibit weight gain or elevations in fasting triglycerides. Second-tier risk may apply to risperidone, paliperidone, and quetiapine, but monitoring is even more important among all these second tier agents (Table 10-3). Other agents that may eventually prove to belong in either the first or the second tier include bifeprunox (in testing) and amisulpride (needs further testing and available only outside the

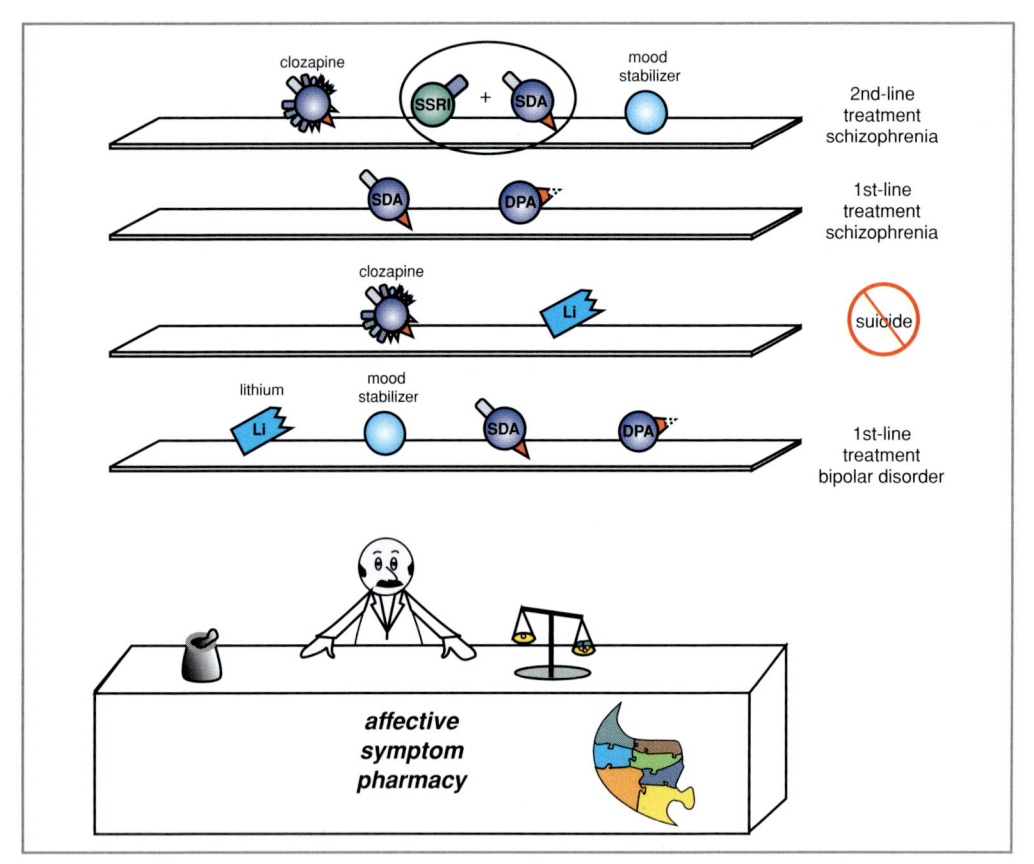

FIGURE 10-109 Affective symptom pharmacy. Atypical antipsychotics [serotonin-dopamine antagonists (SDAs) or dopamine partial agonists (DPAs)] are surprisingly effective in stabilizing mood in a number of disorders and are now becoming treatments for affective symptoms of schizophrenia (first-line), and also for stabilizing mood, mixed, rapid cycling, and treatment-resistant mood states in bipolar patients along with lithium and various anticonvulsant mood stabilizers (first-line treatment). Suicide may be reduced by clozapine (in schizophrenia) and by lithium (Li) (in bipolar disorder). Atypical antipsychotics are also combined with antidepressants such as serotonin selective reuptake inhibitors (SSRIs) or serotonin norepinephrine reuptake inhibitors (SNRIs) for affective symptoms, with clozapine or with various anticonvulsant mood stabilizers as other second-line options.

United States) (Table 10-3). The highest risk is posed by clozapine and olanzapine (Table 10-3). The actual risks of conventional antipsychotics and certain atypical antipsychotics that are available only outside the United States are not well characterized.

Sedation pharmacy (Figure 10-111). Not all antipsychotics are sedating. However, this is a side effect that can be quite variable and difficult to predict in individual patients. Those agents with the lowest risk of sedation might be aripiprazole and ziprasidone, although both can be sedating in some individuals and especially at higher doses. Bifeprunox is not often sedating. Many patients may not experience sedation with either risperidone or paliperidone, but individual experience is necessary to determine what the exact effects will be. When sedation is present with either risperidone or paliperidone, it often comes at the beginning of dosing, can return with dose escalation, and can wear off with time or be managed with once-daily nighttime administration.

In some cases, sedation may be desired. For intermittent sedation, at night or during the day, benzodiazepines are a good choice to "top up" one of the agents with a lower incidence of

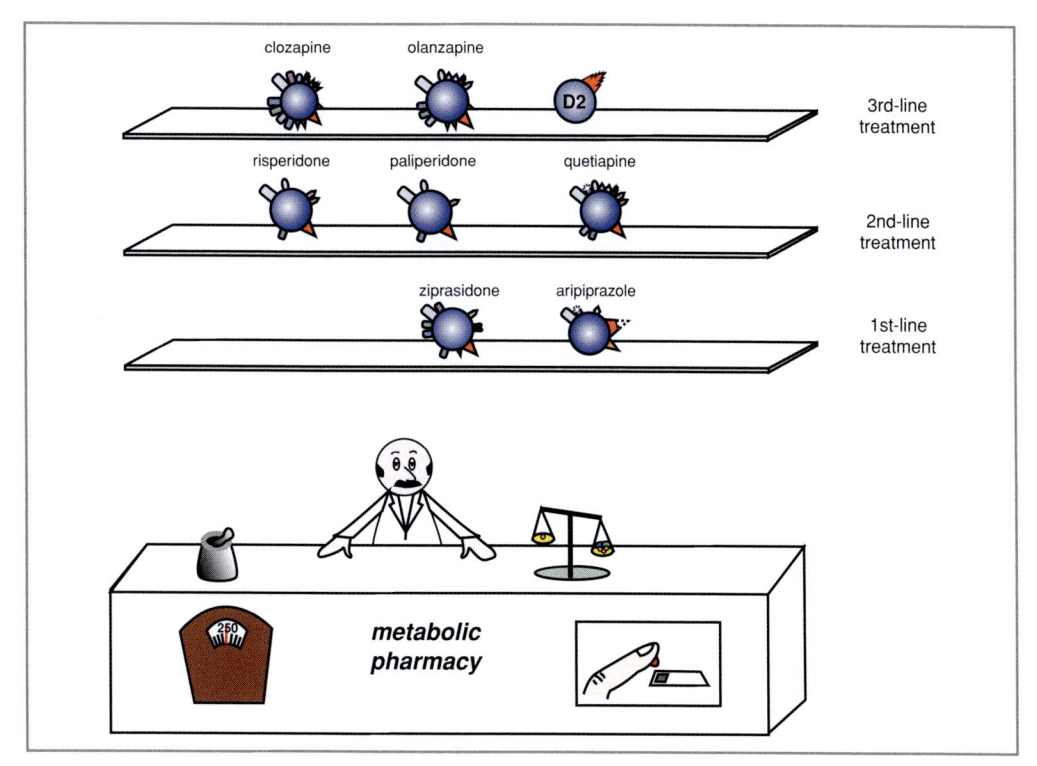

FIGURE 10-110 Metabolic pharmacy. Agents that seem to have the lowest risk of weight gain and cardiometabolic problems include ziprasidone and aripiprazole (first-line). Second-line treatment options include risperidone, paliperidone and quetiapine, while olanzapine and clozapine carry the greatest risk of weight gain and cardiometabolic effects. The risks associated with the various conventional antipsychotics (D2) are not well characterized but may be lower than the highest risk atypical antipsychotics.

sedation. However, if sedation is necessary because of incessant daytime agitation, persistent insomnia, or lack of control, patients may benefit from the artful production of sedation with appropriate doses of either quetiapine, clozapine, or olanzapine, including either daytime administration in some cases or split doses with some medication given during the day and some at night.

The art of switching antipsychotics

It might seem that it would be easy to switch from one antipsychotic to another, but this has proven to be problematic for many patients. Switching actually requires skill to convert patients from one agent to another. Otherwise, they can develop agitation, activation, insomnia, rebound psychosis, and withdrawal effects, especially anticholinergic rebound if done too quickly or without finesse (Figure 10-112).

The sophisticated clinician realizes that the way to switch patients depends on the specific antipsychotics involved and the urgency of the clinical situation. For example, clozapine might be most likely to cause rebound psychosis if rapidly discontinued. Another observation is that switching from a sedating antipsychotic to a nonsedating antipsychotic is different than switching between two sedating antipsychotics. Furthermore, switching between two agents that block D2 receptors as antagonists can be much different than switching between a D2 receptor antagonist and a DPA. These concepts are shown in the next few figures.

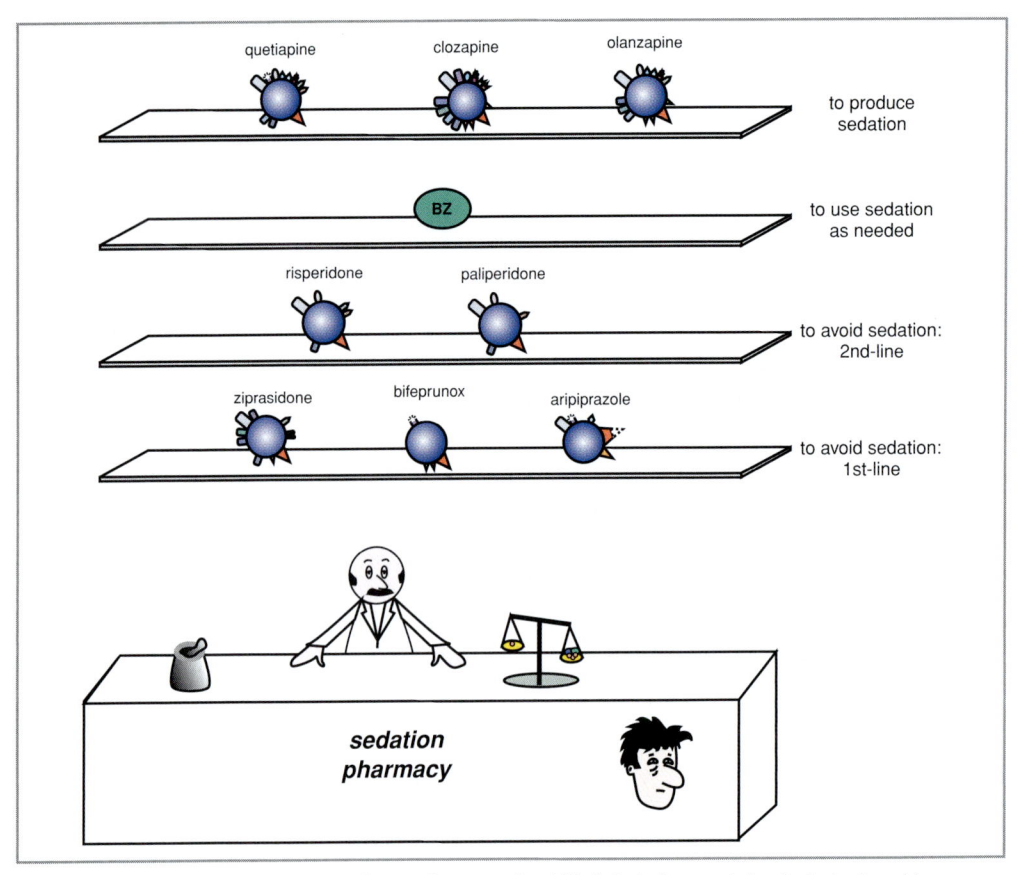

FIGURE 10-111 **Sedation pharmacy.** Agents that seem least likely to induce sedation include ziprasidone, aripiprazole, and bifeprunox. Risperidone and paliperidone may also not cause sedation in many patients but may cause sedation in others. In cases where sedation would be beneficial, options include quetiapine, clozapine, or olanzapine as well as augmentation with a benzodiazepine.

In general, it is rarely a good idea to precipitously stop one antipsychotic and start the other at full dose. Full doses, of course, can be given to patients who are not taking any antipsychotic at the time when one is started. However, in a switch scenario, some form of transition is usually necessary if the clinical situation is to stay stable or improve. For example, switching between two similar agents might be the easiest, such as two agents with D2 antagonist properties that are both somewhat sedating (Figure 10-113). In this case, the best results are usually obtained by cross titration over several days (Figure 10-113). This creates concomitant administration of two antipsychotics for a while as one goes up and the other goes down in dose, and this is acceptable and in fact desirable polypharmacy until the transition is complete.

Sometimes the transition between two similar agents can take up to a few weeks rather than a few days. Nevertheless, it is important to complete the transition and not get caught in cross titration, as shown in Figure 10-114. Sometimes, as the dose of the second drug goes up and the dose of the first drug comes down, the patient begins to do better, and the clinician just stops without completing the transition to a full dose of the second agent and complete discontinuation of the first. That is not generally recommended, since a full trial on the second agent is the goal, and long-term polypharmacy of two agents is not well

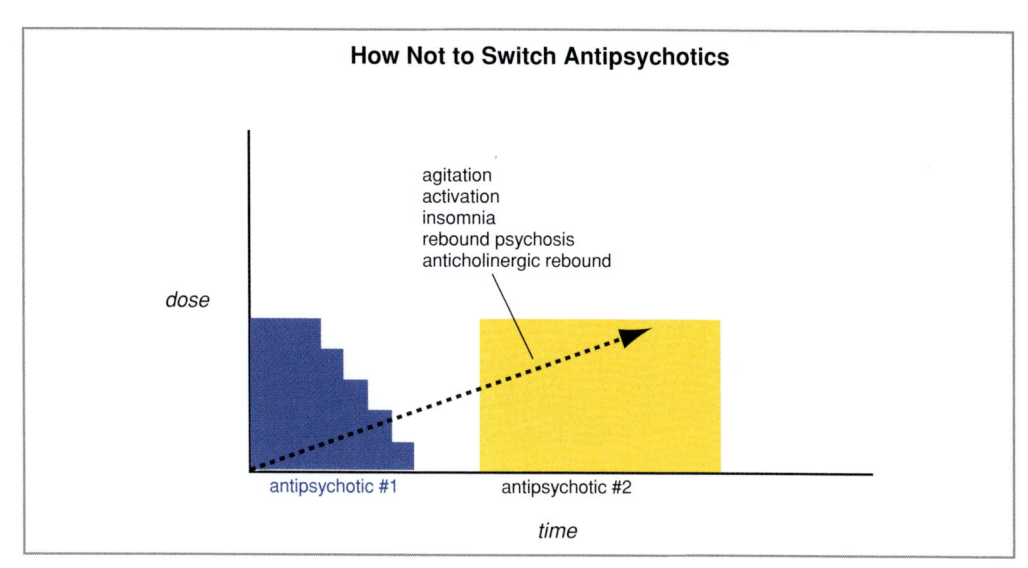

FIGURE 10-112 How not to switch antipsychotics. Converting patients from one antipsychotic to another requires great care in order to ensure that they do not develop withdrawal symptoms, rebound psychosis, or aggravation of side effects. Generally, as shown here, this means not precipitously discontinuing the first antipsychotic, allowing gaps between the administration of the two antipsychotics, or starting the second antipsychotic at full dose.

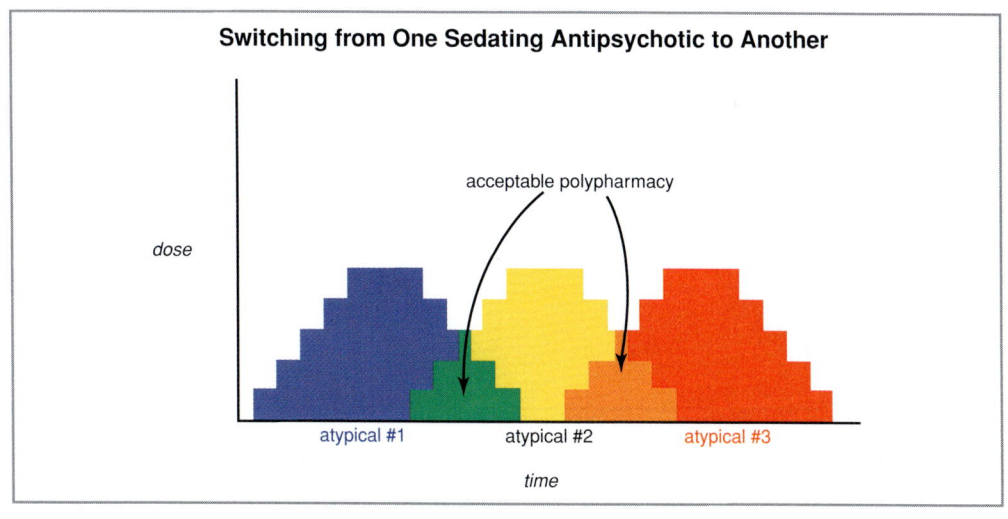

FIGURE 10-113 Switching from one sedating antipsychotic to another. When switching from one sedating antipsychotic to another, it is frequently prudent to "cross-titrate"; that is, to build down the dose of the first drug while building up the dose of the other over a few days to a few weeks. This leads to transient administration of two drugs but is justified in order to reduce side effects and the risk of rebound symptoms and to accelerate the successful transition to the second drug.

studied and can be quite expensive. If the second agent is not satisfactory, it is generally preferable to try a third rather than backtrack to the use of two agents together indefinitely (Figure 10-114).

Since the first atypical antipsychotics were all characterized as having some degree of sedation, especially at higher doses (e.g., risperidone, olanzapine, and quetiapine), it was

Antipsychotic Agents | 433

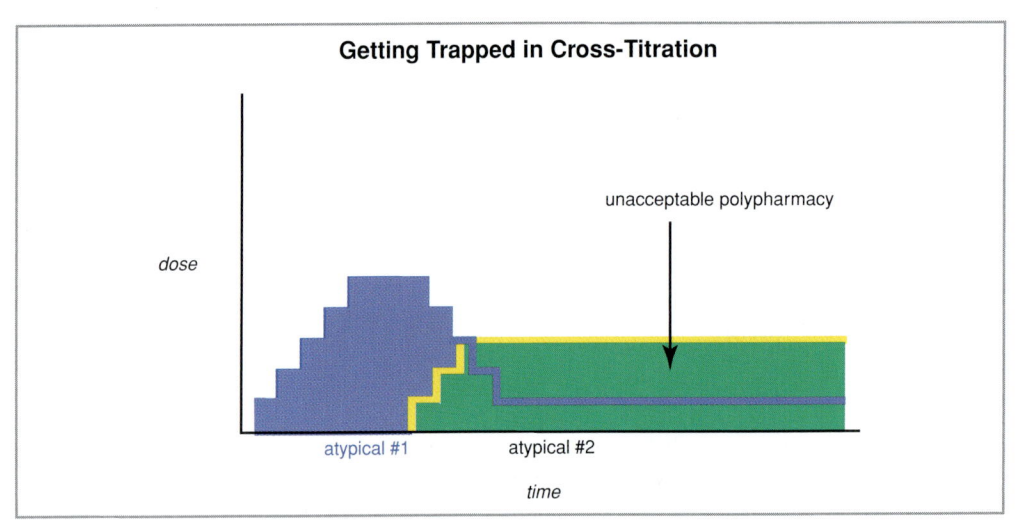

FIGURE 10-114 Getting caught in cross-titration. When switching from one atypical antipsychotic to another, the patient may improve in the middle of cross-titration. Polypharmacy results if cross-titration is stopped at this point and the patient continues both drugs indefinitely. It is generally better to complete the cross titration as shown in Figure 10-113, with discontinuation of the first agent and an adequate monotherapy trial of the second drug before trying long-term polypharmacy.

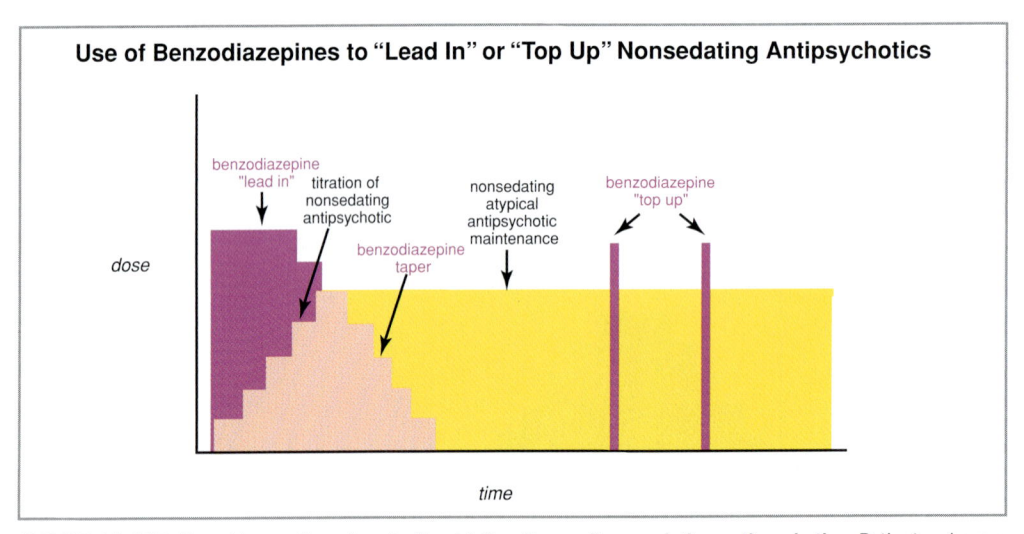

FIGURE 10-115 Use of benzodiazepines to "lead in" or "top up" nonsedating antipsychotics. Patients who are agitated and cannot sleep may need short-term augmentation with a benzodiazepine when initiating a nonsedating antipsychotic. The benzodiazepine can be discontinued once the patient is stabilized, with the potential to occasionally top up as needed.

not appreciated early that initiating treatment with a nonsedating antipsychotic (such as ziprasidone or aripiprazole, introduced later to the market) and switching from a sedating to a nonsedating antipsychotic can be different. Experience now tells us that patients who are agitated and cannot sleep might need short-term supplementation with a benzodiazepine when treatment with a nonsedating agent such as aripiprazole, ziprasidone, or bifeprunox is being initiated (Figure 10-115). The disadvantage of this approach is the need to use a second drug, especially when the antipsychotic is initiated or given as a "top up" during dose

Switching from a Sedating Antipsychotic to a Nonsedating Antipsychotic

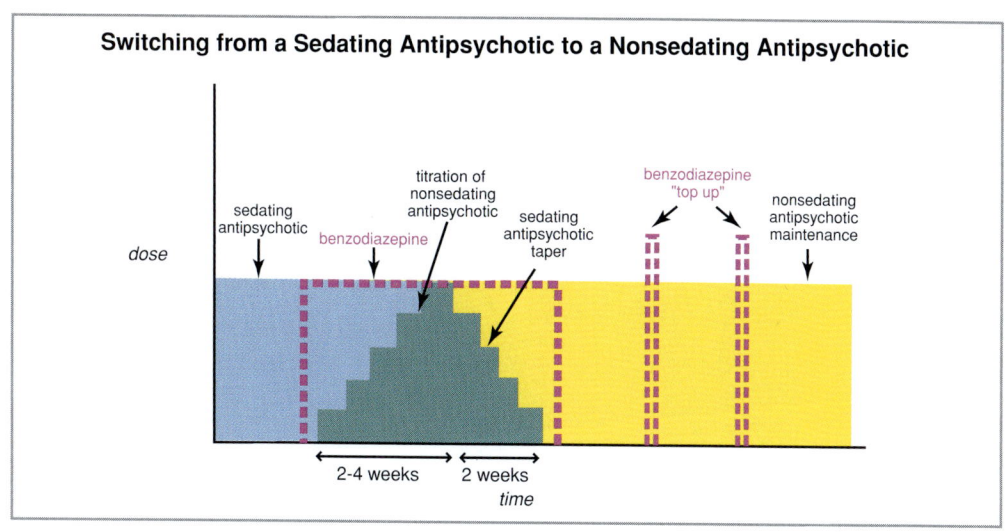

FIGURE 10-116 Switching from a sedating antipsychotic to a nonsedating antipsychotic. One method for switching from a sedating antipsychotic to a nonsedating antipsychotic shown here is to add a benzodiazepine first, and then start the up-titration of the nonsedating agent while maintaining the full dose of the sedating agent. Once the nonsedating agent is at a therapeutic dose, the sedating agent can be tapered while maintaining the benzodiazepine. Once the sedating antipsychotic is fully tapered and the patient is stable, the benzodiazepine can be tapered or stopped. In addition, once the benzodiazepine has been discontinued, it can be used as needed occasionally to top up the patient for treatment of any breakthrough agitation or insomnia. This switching method may be best for patients who are switching due to lack of adequate control of symptoms on their sedating antipsychotic rather than for those who are switching due to intolerability, as the temporary use of three agents concomitantly may cause side effects.

stabilization. The advantage of this approach is the ability to control sedation and use it as a therapeutic tool, discontinuing the benzodiazepine to remove unwanted sedation when it is no longer needed or desired for maintenance as well as to prevent cognitive problems and unacceptable daytime sedation once psychosis has stabilized.

Benzodiazepines can not only be useful in "leading in" and "topping up" antipsychotics when a nonsedating agent is initiated (Figure 10-115); they can also be very helpful in easing the transition from a sedating to a nonsedating antipsychotic (Figure 10-116). Thus, in preparing for a switch from a sedating agent such as quetiapine to a nonsedating agent such as aripiprazole, the switch can be anticipated by initiating a benzodiazepine before doing anything and then starting the uptitration of the nonsedating agent while maintaining the full dose of the sedating agent. This can mean the short-term use of three drugs, which can cause side effects and may not be desirable in mildly ill patients whose symptoms are under control or who are very sensitive to side effects; however, in a schizophrenic patient who is switching because of inadequate symptom control by the sedating agent, this approach, shown in Figure 10-116, should be considered, since behavioral control can be attained with the three drugs for a few days to a few weeks prior to beginning slow downtitration of the sedating antipsychotic over a few more weeks. Once the second antipsychotic has full-dose buildup and the first is completely tapered, the benzodiazepine can then be tapered and also used to top up later if necessary (Figure 10-116). This may seem complicated, but it is actually quite intuitive and allows for a successful slow transition to a nonsedating agent over several weeks without the risk of rebound psychosis or emergence of agitation and insomnia prior to giving the new agent a chance to work.

Switching from an SDA to a DPA: Not Too Fast

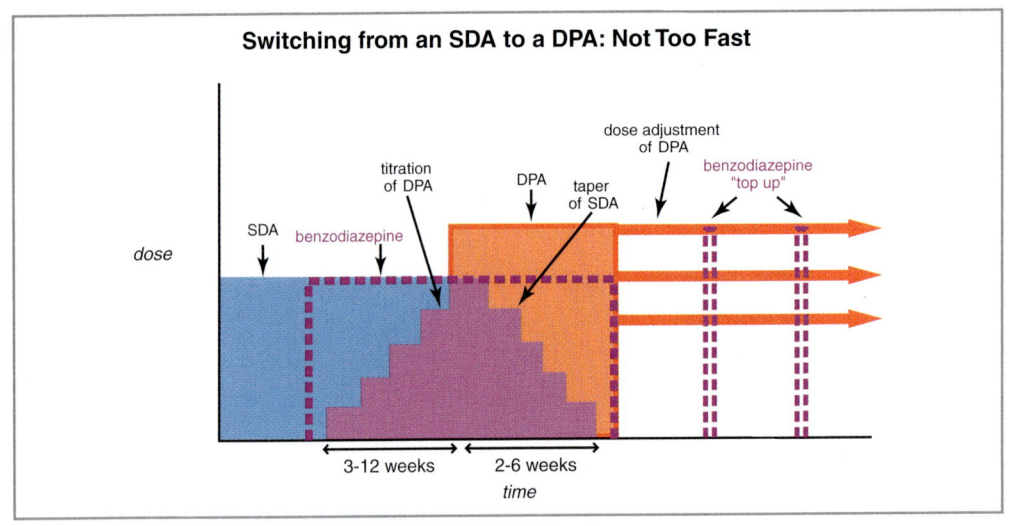

FIGURE 10-117 Switching from SDA to DPA. When switching from an agent with full D2 antagonist properties (e.g., from a serotonin-dopamine antagonist, or SDA) to a partial dopamine agonist (DPA), patients could potentially experience emergence of psychosis, agitation, or insomnia. Thus, a gradual switch may be best, with patients continuing to receive a full dose of the first antipsychotic both during uptitration of the second and perhaps for a few weeks afterward. Adding a benzodiazepine short-term may also be beneficial. Once the second antipsychotic has attained a full therapeutic dose, the first antipsychotic can be tapered while the benzodiazepine is maintained for a short time. When the patient is stable, the benzodiazepine can be discontinued, and possibly utilized again as needed occasionally to top up the patient for treatment of any breakthrough agitation or insomnia. This switch method allows the dose of the DPA to be optimized and for the dopamine receptors to potentially "reset" their sensitivity so that partial agonist actions can be optimally therapeutic.

Similar principles are at play when switching a patient from a D2 antagonist, such as an SDA, to a D2 partial agonist (DPA) (Figure 10-117). Patients accustomed to full D2 antagonism may experience less than full blockade of D2 receptors at first as they transition to a partial agonist. This can be experienced as emergence of psychosis, agitation, or insomnia but can be anticipated both by the prior initiation of a benzodiazepine and the maintenance of a full dose of the first antipsychotic for a while (Figure 10-117). It can take from a few weeks to a few months for the dopamine receptors to reset and become adequately blocked as the patient accommodates to the partial agonist and stabilizes clinically. Then, the first antipsychotic can be fully tapered, and soon thereafter the benzodiazepine as well. Dose adjustment of the DPA can be optimized once the first antipsychotic and the benzodiazepine have both been discontinued. Observing patients, anticipating and responding to their changing symptoms of psychosis and side effects during the transition, is the way to apply these tools, often utilizing time as an agent to ease the switch.

Combos and polypharmacy
Mood stabilizers can sometimes be helpful in augmenting incomplete or unsatisfactory responses of schizophrenic patients to antipsychotic monotherapy, including unsatisfactory responses to high-dose monotherapy (Figure 10-118). Lithium may not be particularly helpful in schizophrenia, but divalproex and lamotrigine or even an antidepressant can sometimes be useful as an augmenting agent to atypical antipsychotics in the treatment of schizophrenia inadequately responsive to monotherapy. Mood stabilizers are discussed in further detail in Chapter 13.

When Several Antipsychotic Monotherapies Fail

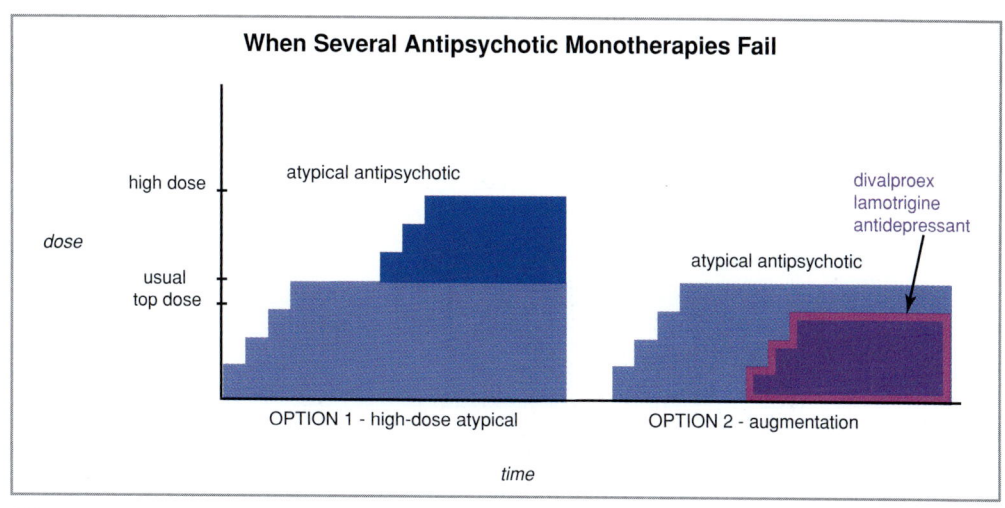

FIGURE 10-118 High dose and augmentation. When several atypical antipsychotic monotherapies fail, it may be necessary to use high doses of an antipsychotic (on the left). Although this can sometimes lead to improved efficacy, this is also quite costly and can lead to loss of the atypical therapeutic advantages of some atypical antipsychotics as well as other side effects. Another option is to add a mood stabilizer such as divalproex or lamotrigine, or an antidepressant to augment an inadequately efficacious atypical antipsychotic (on the right).

Schizophrenic patients usually respond to treatment with any single antipsychotic drug, whether conventional or atypical, by improving their positive symptoms and their total symptoms by at least 20 to 30 percent on standardized rating scales after a month or two of treatment. However, if a treatment effect of this order of magnitude is not observed after an adequate trial with the first antipsychotic agent, clinicians usually try a second, third, and fourth agent until a satisfactory response is achieved. If no satisfactory response exists to a series of monotherapies, including high doses, clozapine, and augmentation with mood stabilizers, then administration of two antipsychotics may be considered (Figure 10-119, when all else fails).

Some clinicians prefer augmenting clozapine for treatment-resistant cases, and this form of antipsychotic polypharmacy has been studied the most. Others try augmenting an atypical antipsychotic with a conventional antipsychotic or giving two atypical antipsychotics together – a very expensive proposition (Figure 10-119). Audits of antipsychotic use in clinical practice suggest that up to one-fourth of outpatients and up to half of inpatients take two antipsychotic drugs for long-term maintenance treatment. Is this a viable therapeutic option for treatment-resistant patients or a dirty little secret of irrational drug use? Whatever it is, the use of two antipsychotics seems to be one of the most practiced and least investigated phenomena in clinical psychopharmacology. It may occasionally be useful to combine two agents when no single agent is effective. On the other hand, it has not proven useful to combine two antipsychotics to get supra-additive antipsychotic effects, such as "wellness" or "awakenings." Although **depressed** patients frequently recover (see Chapter 11), **schizophrenic** patients rarely achieve wellness, no matter what drug or drug combination is given. Thus, current treatment guidelines suggest that maintenance of patients on two antipsychotics or even very high doses of atypical antipsychotics should be done sparingly and perhaps only "when all else fails" (Figure 10-119), and even in such cases only when clearly demonstrated to be beneficial.

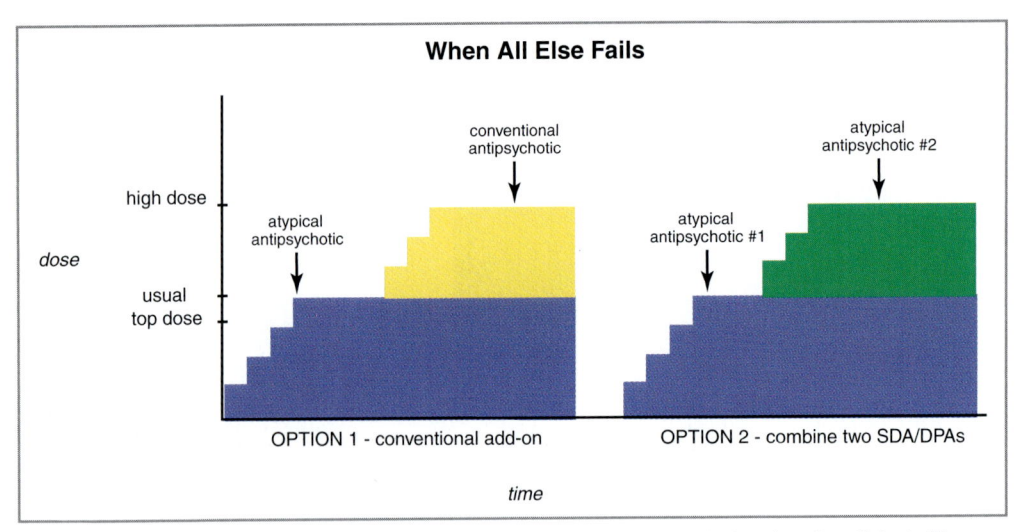

FIGURE 10-119 Polypharmacy: when all else fails. If many atypical antipsychotics show insufficient efficacy even at high doses and when augmenting agents also do not help, then a final option is to add a second antipsychotic to the first. This can be done by adding an agent from the conventional class to an atypical antipsychotic or by combining two atypical antipsychotics, whether serotonin-dopamine antagonists (SDAs) or dopamine partial agonists (DPAs). Antipsychotic polypharmacy is not well studied though frequently practiced and should truly be reserved for cases in which "all else fails."

Future treatments for schizophrenia

Innovation in the area of schizophrenia is among the most actively researched areas in psychopharmacology. New concepts of prodromal and presymptomatic treatments to prevent disease progression as well as new mechanisms aimed primarily at the devastating negative and cognitive symptoms of schizophrenia have captured the imagination of new drug discovery efforts and will be briefly reviewed here.

Presymptomatic and prodromal treatments for schizophrenia: putting the cart before the horse or preventing disease progression?

An emerging concept in psychopharmacology is the possibility that treatments that reduce symptoms could also be disease-modifying (Figure 10-120). In this chapter we have discussed how atypical antipsychotics treat symptoms of schizophrenia (first- and second-episode treatment in Figure 10-120). These same agents are also proven to prevent the reemergence of symptoms and thus relapse (maintenance treatment in Figure 10-120). It now is being debated whether these agents given to high-risk individuals either in a presymptomatic state or with only mild prodromal symptoms could prevent or delay progression to schizophrenia.

Current concepts about the natural history of schizophrenia hypothesize that this illness progresses from a state of high risk without symptoms (presymptomatic) to a prodrome with cognitive and negative but not psychotic symptoms and ultimately to a first episode with psychotic symptoms (Figure 10-120). Throughout the field of psychiatry, it is being debated whether remission of symptoms of any psychiatric disorder with psychopharmacological treatments can prevent disease progression, possibly by preventing the plastic changes in brain circuits that fully establish and worsen psychiatric disorders. In schizophrenia, therefore, the question is whether "prophylactic" antipsychotics can keep an individual from "catching" schizophrenia.

Presymptomatic/Prodromal Treatment of Schizophrenia

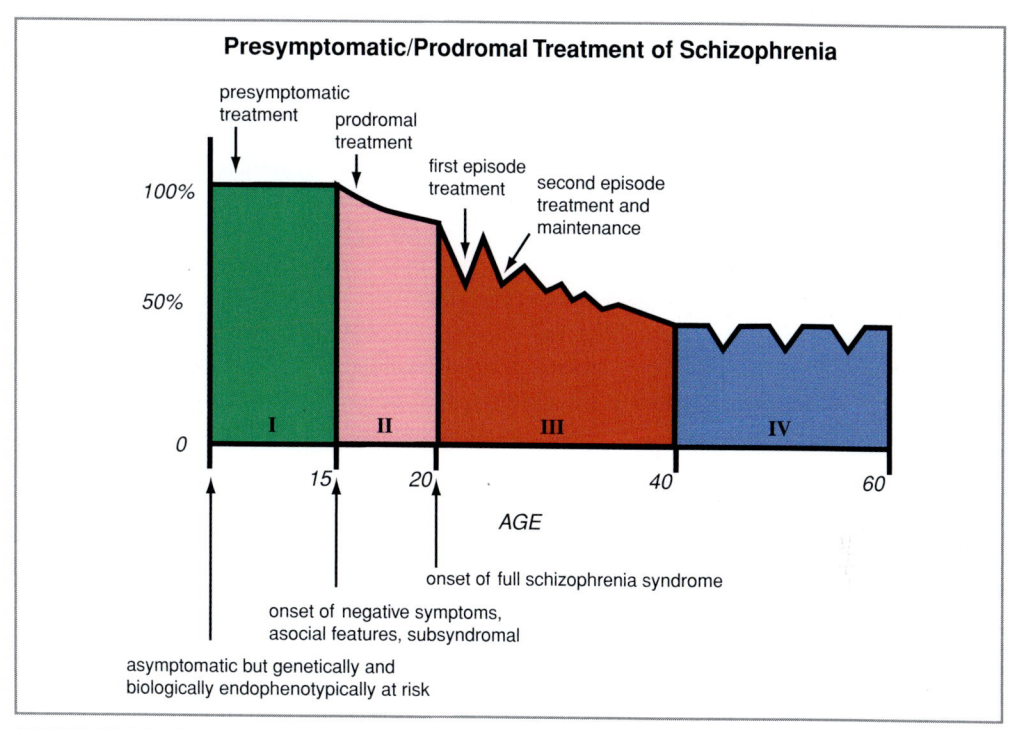

FIGURE 10-120 Presymptomatic/prodromal treatment of schizophrenia. The stages of schizophrenia are shown here over a lifetime. The patient often has full functioning (100 percent) early in life and is virtually asymptomatic (stage I). However, during a prodromal phase (stage II) starting in the teens, there may be odd behaviors and subtle negative symptoms. The acute phase of the illness usually announces itself fairly dramatically in the twenties (stage III), with positive symptoms, remissions, and relapses but never a complete return to previous levels of functioning. This is often a chaotic stage of the illness, with a progressive downhill course. The final phase of the illness (stage IV) may begin in the forties or later, with prominent negative and cognitive symptoms and some waxing and waning during its course, but often more of a burnout stage of continuing disability. There may not necessarily be a continuing and relentless downhill course, but the patient may become progressively resistant to treatment with antipsychotic medications during this stage. An emerging concept in psychopharmacology is that the treatments that reduce symptoms could also be disease modifying. That is, perhaps these agents given to high risk individuals either in a presymptomatic (stage I) or prodromal (stage 2) state could prevent or delay progression through the subsequent stages of schizophrenia.

Pilot results from early intervention studies in first-episode cases of schizophrenia already suggest that treatment with atypical antipsychotics as soon as possible after onset of the first psychotic symptoms can improve outcomes (first-episode treatment in Figure 10-120). What if high-risk patients without symptoms could be identified from genetic or neuroimaging techniques? How about patients with the prodromal cognitive and negative symptoms that frequently precede the onset of psychotic symptoms? Could treatment of patients at these points prevent the long-term course of schizophrenia – for many patients one of waxing and waning positive symptoms with ever-worsening cognitive and negative symptoms (Figure 10-120)?

Early results with atypical antipsychotics are indeed promising. Treating prodromal symptoms with antidepressants and anxiolytics may also delay the onset of schizophrenia. At this point, much more research will be required before presymptomatic or prodromal treatment can be recommended for schizophrenia, but the promise of disease-modifying treatments for psychiatric disorders in general and schizophrenia in particular is leading to studies to fully investigate this exciting possibility.

Glutamate-linked mechanisms and new treatments for schizophrenia

Much of the discussion of treatments for schizophrenia in this chapter has revolved around modifying the neurotransmitters dopamine and serotonin. A major new area of research is to investigate whether modifications of glutamate pharmacology will lead to new psychopharmacological therapeutics for schizophrenia. Targeting of the glutamate system is a logical extension of the NMDA receptor hypofunction hypothesis of schizophrenia discussed in detail in Chapter 9 and illustrated in Figures 9-39 through 9-42.

Glutamate agonists or antagonists for schizophrenia?

NMDA antagonists. Throughout this chapter, we have discussed the idea that the dopamine system should be optimized or even "stabilized" in schizophrenia, with neither too much nor too little dopamine activity in various pathways throughout the brain. A very similar concept could be applied to the glutamate system. That is, one hypothesis of schizophrenia suggests that early in the illness, excessive glutamate activity could lead to excitotoxicity (discussed in Chapter 9 and illustrated in Figures 9-45 through 9-52) and thus interfere with normal neurodevelopment (Figure 9-52). Excitotoxicity could also continue during the course of the illness and be linked to disease progression in schizophrenia (Figures 9-44 and 10-120). However, it is now also widely hypothesized that once the illness of schizophrenia has developed, NMDA glutamate receptors are actually hypofunctional (discussed in Chapter 9 and illustrated in Figures 9-39 through 9-41). So what is the best approach to treatment for schizophrenia, glutamate agonists or glutamate antagonists? The answer may be that it depends on what stage of the illness is being treated, what specific symptoms are being targeted, and whether either the agonist or antagonist action modulates the glutamate system by tuning it, stabilizing it, and optimizing it, or is too powerful and either shuts it down or overly stimulates it.

Thus, the idea has arisen that blocking excessive and excitotoxic glutamate neurotransmission (Figures 9-45 through 9-52) with NMDA antagonists might prevent damage or death to neurons in schizophrenia (Figure 10-121). It may also be possible to prevent neuronal death or damage after excessive glutamate neurotransmission by administering free radical scavengers (Figure 10-122), which destroy free radicals generated during glutamate-mediated excitotoxicity (Figures 9-49 through 9-51). Although this idea of blocking NMDA neurotransmission and its consequences has a certain theoretical appeal for the treatment of schizophrenia, especially for preventing possible neuronal damage at critical points during neurodevelopment (Figure 9-52), it may be more applicable to other conditions where excitotoxic neurodegenerative activity remains an active component of the disease mechanism, such as Alzheimer's disease and other neurodegenerative conditions. In schizophrenia, there may be a combination both of excitotoxicity, particularly early in the disease process (Figure 9-52), and NMDA receptor hypoactivation during the later course of the disease (Figures 9-39 to 9-42), making the use of agents that block NMDA receptors potentially quite complicated.

Thus potent NMDA antagonists might block excitotoxicity, but at a price: they would also cause or worsen positive, cognitive, and negative symptoms of schizophrenia (Figure 10-121). In fact, we have already discussed how the observations that NMDA antagonists such as phencyclidine (PCP) or ketamine can produce the symptoms of schizophrenia in normal volunteers is consistent with the NMDA receptor hypofunction hypothesis of schizophrenia. This seems to be too dear a price to pay for neuroprotection in schizophrenia.

One response to this quandary is to consider whether less robust NMDA antagonists such as memantine or even amantadine (discussed later, in the chapter on Alzheimer's

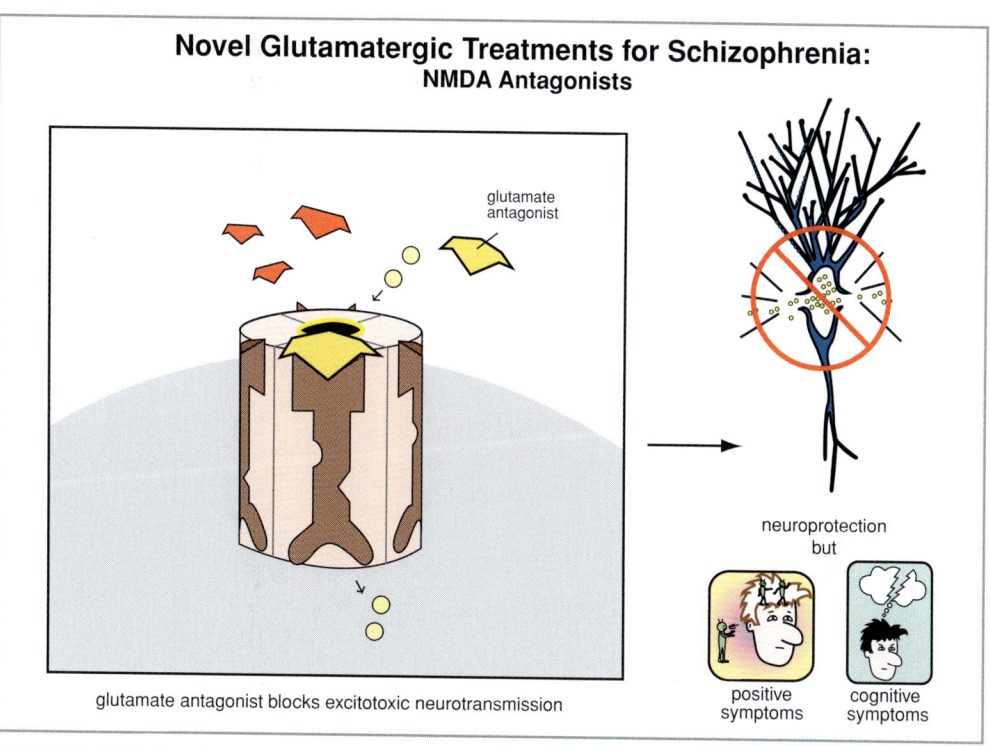

FIGURE 10-121 Novel glutamatergic treatments for schizophrenia: NMDA antagonists? Antagonists of glutamate either at the N-methyl-d-aspartate (NMDA) agonist site as shown here, or at any number of allosteric sites around this receptor complex, could potentially block excitotoxic neurotransmission and exert neuroprotective actions. Such agents would potentially be treatments for conditions characterized by ongoing excitotoxic neurodegeneration such as schizophrenia, Alzheimer's disease, or other neurodegenerative conditions. Theoretically, they could also be useful for preventing early excitotoxic neuronal damage in schizophrenia. However, later in the course of schizophrenia there seems to be NMDA receptor hypoactivation that contributes to the pathophysiology of positive and cognitive symptoms. Thus, NMDA antagonists could actually worsen those symptoms.

disease), that only partially block NMDA neurotransmission, might be better options. Another possibility is to block the presynaptic release of glutamate, which is the hypothesized mechanism of certain anticonvulsants that also act as mood stabilizers, like lamotrigine and riluzole. Mood stabilizers are discussed in detail in Chapter 13. Blockade of presynaptic release of glutamate by agonists acting at presynaptic metabotropic glutamate receptors (mGluR2/3) is discussed below and illustrated in Figure 10-125. Much of the current targeting of the glutamate system in schizophrenia, however, is now aiming at psychopharmacological mechanisms whereby glutamate neurotransmission can actually be **increased** to compensate for NMDA receptor **hypoactivity**, but without increasing it so much as to become neurotoxic.

Glycine agonists. In Chapter 9 we discussed the actions of coagonists at the glycine site of NMDA receptors (Figures 9-34 and 9-35). Agonists at the glycine site of NMDA receptors include the naturally occurring amino acids glycine (Figure 9-34) and d-serine (Figure 9-35). An analogue of d-serine called d-cycloserine is also active at the glycine coagonist site of NMDA receptors. All of these agents have been tested in schizophrenia, with evidence that they can reduce negative and/or cognitive symptoms (Figure 10-123). Further testing is in progress, and synthetic agonists with greater potency are in

Antipsychotic Agents | 441

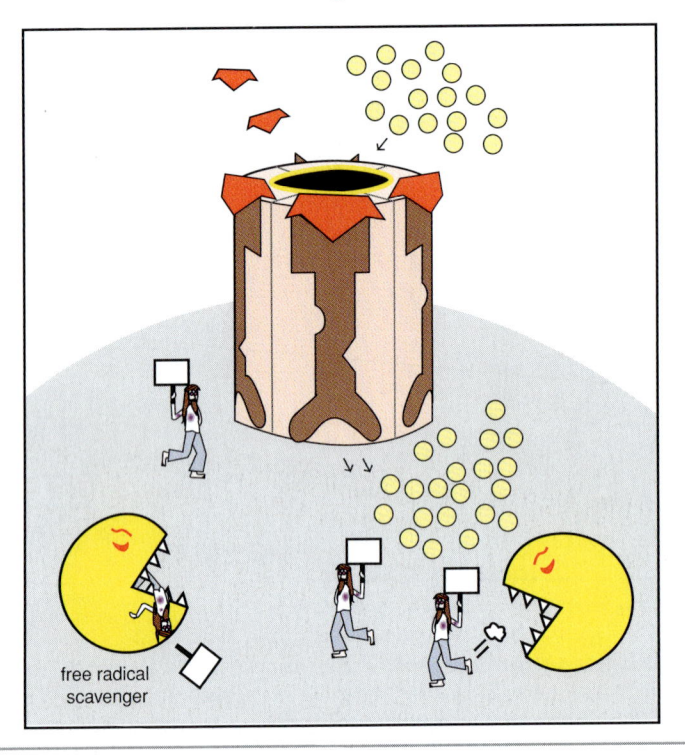

FIGURE 10-122 Novel glutamatergic treatments for schizophrenia: free radical scavengers for excitotoxicity. Free radicals are generated in the neurodegenerative process of excitotoxicity. A drug acting as a free radical scavenger, which works as a "chemical sponge," soaking up toxic free radicals and removing them, would be theoretically neuroprotective. Vitamin E is one such weak scavenger. Other free radical scavengers, such as the lazaroids (so named because of their putative properties of raising degenerating neurons, like Lazarus, from the dead) are also being tested.

discovery. Perhaps stimulation of the glycine site will boost NMDA receptor activity enough to overcome its hypothetical hypofunction (Figures 9-39 to 9-42) and thereby reduce not only negative and cognitive symptoms, but possibly even affective symptoms in schizophrenia (Figure 10-123) without worsening positive symptoms or becoming neurotoxic.

GlyT1 inhibitors. Earlier, in Chapter 9, we also discussed how glycine transporters on glial cells, known as GlyT1, terminate the action of glycine released by glial cells into the synapses to act at the glycine site of NMDA receptors (Figure 9-34). Several GlyT1 inhibitors are now in testing, including the natural agent N-methyl-glycine, also known as sarcosine, as well as drugs in preclinical testing, such as SSR 504734, SSR 241586, JNJ17305600, and Org 25935. GlyT1 inhibitors are analogous to drugs that inhibit reuptake of other neurotransmitters, such as the serotonin selective reuptake inhibitors (SSRIs) and their actions at the serotonin transporter, or SERT. When GlyT1 pumps are blocked by a GlyT1 inhibitor, this increases the synaptic availability of glycine and thus enhances NMDA neurotransmission (Figure 10-124). Sarcosine has been shown to improve negative, cognitive, and depressive symptoms, including symptoms such as alogia and blunted affect in schizophrenia. The hope is that GlyT1 inhibitors with greater potency, such as those in preclinical testing mentioned above, will be able to reduce the hypofunctioning of NMDA potentially convert conventional antipsychotics into atypical antipsychotics or allow dose sparing of atypical antipsychotics, or it could optimize the efficacy and safety profile of various antipsychotics; however, further testing will be required. Earlier testing of MDL 100907 was discontinued. Another compound with this mechanism at 5HT2A receptors is eplivanserin (SR 46349).

Serotonin 1A agonists or antagonists. Theoretically, the 5HT1A actions of some atypical antipsychotics may contribute to their clinical properties, from procognitive actions to antidepressant actions to anxiolytic actions. There is debate as to whether the ideal 5HT1A actions are agonist, partial agonist, or antagonist actions, although in many cases the net long-term consequences are similar since antagonists block and chronic agonists down regulate 5HT1A receptors. Early studies with 5HT1A partial agonists such as buspirone and tandospirone added on to antipsychotics suggest possible improvement in cognition in schizophrenia. Other agents in this class include the 5HT1A partial agonist gepirone ER, the 5HT1A partial agonist/serotonin reuptake inhibitors vilazodone and Lu AA21004, and the selective 5HT1A antagonists lecozotan (SRA133) and AV965.

Serotonin 2C agonists or antagonists. Theoretically, the 5HT2C actions of some atypical antipsychotics may also contribute to their clinical actions, including procognitive and antidepressant actions. A 5HT2C agonist may be expected to reduce positive symptoms by reducing dopamine release in the mesolimbic dopamine pathway. Vabicaserin (SCA-136) is a 5HT2C agonist that has shown promise in preliminary testing in schizophrenia.

On the other hand, 5HT2C antagonists may be expected to reduce depression and improve cognition by enhancing dopamine release in the mesocortical dopamine pathway and also to release norepinephrine in the same brain areas. Several atypical antipsychotics have 5HT2C antagonist actions (see Figures 10-90 through 10-104), as does the SSRI antidepressant fluoxetine and the novel antidepressant agomelatine. The mechanism of 5HT2C actions on dopamine and norepinephrine release as well as the link of these actions to possible antidepressant effects is discussed in Chapter 12. The debate on whether the desired 5HT2C actions are agonist, partial agonist, or antagonist actions continues, as it does for 5HT1A receptors, although long-term actions may be similar for agents across the agonist spectrum, since antagonists block and chronic agonists may downregulate 5HT2C receptors.

5HT6 antagonists. The physiological role of 5HT6 receptors is still being clarified, but it does appear that these receptors may be linked to the production and/or release of neurotrophic factors such as brain derived neurotrophic factor (BDNF). Some atypical antipsychotics do have 5HT6-antagonist properties (clozapine, Figure 10-90; olanzapine, Figure 10-91; quetiapine, Figure 10-94; zotepine, Figure 10-96; sertindole, Figure 10-98; loxapine, Figure 10-99; and perhaps others), which might increase the release of BDNF, although it is not known whether this contributes to any of the possible protrophic effects seen with antipsychotics. Selective 5HT6-receptor antagonists such as GW742457 are in development for testing in both schizophrenia and depression and other disorders where protrophic actions on BDNF could exert a therapeutic action.

5HT7 antagonists. The physiological role of 5HT7 receptors is also being clarified, and some atypical antipsychotics do have 5HT7 actions (clozapine, Figure 10-90; risperidone, Figure 10-91; paliperidone, Figure 10-92; quetiapine, Figure 10-94; ziprasidone, Figure 10-95; zotepine, Figure 10-96; sertindole, Figure 10-98; loxapine, Figure 10-99; cyamemazine, Figure 10-100; and possibly others), even though it is not known whether this contributes to their therapeutic effects. 5HT7 receptors may be linked to circadian rhythms, sleep, anxiety and depression; selective 5HT7 antagonists are being developed and tested not only in schizophrenia but also in other psychiatric disorders such as sleep, mood, and anxiety disorders.

New DPAs. Several new dopamine partial agonists (DPAs) are in development, including bifeprunox (DU 127090), a DPA with 5HT1A partial agonist properties that is pending marketing and in late clinical development in many countries (Figure 10-53). Several compounds mix DPA actions (dopamine 2-receptor partial agonist) with SPA actions (serotonin 1A partial agonist), including sarizotan (EMD128130), SSR181507, SLV313, and SLV314. Two of these compounds are related to bifeprunox, including SLV313, which appears to balance relatively selective D2 and 5HT1A partial agonist activities, and SLV314, which is a potent DPA with serotonin reuptake inhibition properties but less potent actions at 5HT1A receptors.

Selective D3 antagonists. The function of D3 receptors remains unknown, and until recently was difficult to study since it was not possible to separate D2-antagonist properties from D3-antagonist properties of antipsychotics. Now that D3-selective agents are available, preclinical testing suggests that these agents may be useful for both negative symptoms and cognitive symptoms and might reduce stimulant abuse both in schizophrenia and in patients with substance abuse disorders who do not have schizophrenia. One example of this is RGH 188, with D3 and D2 partial agonist actions.

Other dopamine mechanisms. D1-selective agonists may be useful as procognitive agents. This may be helpful in other cognitive disorders as well. Since some atypical antipsychotics are D1 antagonists, D1-agonist action may help reverse the undesirable actions of D1 antagonism.

Many atypical antipsychotics are also D4 antagonists, and selective D4 antagonists (such as YM-43611, nemonapride, fananserin, L-745870, PNU-101387G, NGD-94–4, LU-111995, and LU35138) have been synthesized and several tested in schizophrenia, but they have not been found to be helpful.

Modafinil is an agent approved for sleepiness and may improve attention in several sleep disorders. It has also been shown to improve cognitive functioning in attention deficit hyperactivity disorder (discussed in detail in chapters on sleep disorders and cognitive disorders). Modafinil may act in part as a dopamine transport (DAT) inhibitor, and it as well as other DAT inhibitors could potentially improve cognition in schizophrenia and other disorders but might also activate psychosis.

Centrally acting COMT inhibitors. Catechol-O-methyl transferase inhibitors can boost the actions of dopamine, and those that act peripherally can be given with levodopa to reduce the peripheral metabolism of levodopa and enhance the central actions of dopamine. Centrally acting COMT inhibitors have the potential of increasing dopamine neurotransmission directly in the brain, especially in prefrontal cortex, where COMT is the key metabolic pathway for dopamine degradation.

Norepinephrine-linked mechanisms. Norepinephrine-selective reuptake inhibitors have been tested in depression and in attention deficit hyperactivity disorder; they are discussed in later chapters on these topics. Norepinephrine reuptake inhibitors enhance the release not just of norepinephrine but also of dopamine in prefrontal cortex and thus may enhance executive functioning. Some preliminary investigation of this mechanism for cognitive dysfunction in schizophrenia is in progress.

Acetylcholine-linked mechanisms

Alpha-7-nicotinic cholinergic agonists. The alpha-7-nicotinic cholinergic receptor has been implicated in the familial transmission of sensory gating deficits in families with schizophrenia. Deficits in activity at this receptor could theoretically predispose patients to problems with learning efficiency and accuracy and underlie delusional thinking and social dysfunction. In addition, heavy smoking in many schizophrenics (about two-thirds of a North American population of schizophrenics are smokers; in comparison, about one-fourth of nonschizophrenics are smokers) is consistent with the high concentration of nicotine necessary to activate the receptor and with the receptor's rapid desensitization. Thus there are numerous theoretically appealing hypotheses to targeting this receptor to improve particularly cognitive functioning in schizophrenia and other cognitive disorders. Preliminary testing of DMXB-A {3-[(2,4-dimethoxy) benzylidene] anabaseine}, a natural alkaloid derivative and partial agonist at alpha-7-nicotinic cholinergic receptors, appears to have some positive effects on cognition in schizophrenia. Other alpha-7-nicotinic cholinergic agonists in testing include ABT089, MEM3454, and SSR180711.

Alpha-4 Beta-2 partial agonists (nicotinic partial agonists, or NPAs). A second subtype of nicotinic receptor may be involved in mediating the reward mechanisms of smoking – namely the alpha-4 beta-2 nicotinic acetylcholine receptor located in the mesolimbic reward pathway. Recently a number of partial agonists for this receptor have been identified, namely selective alpha-4 beta-2 nicotinic acetylcholine partial agonists, or NPAs. One of these, varenicline, has been approved for smoking cessation, and other compounds such as SSR591813 and TC1827 are in testing. Since a great number of schizophrenic patients smoke, which enhances their cardiometabolic risk and can reduce their life expectancy, already abnormal due to factors linked to their psychiatric illness, lifestyle, and some of their treatments, it seems important to investigate treatments that could reduce smoking. Most studies of varenicline have involved patients without psychiatric disorders and who do not take psychotropic drugs; testing is now needed to determine to what extent NPAs are effective in reducing smoking specifically in schizophrenic patients who take antipsychotics.

Muscarinic-1 agonists. Muscarinic-1 (M1) antagonist properties of antipsychotics contribute to sedation and cognitive dysfunction, so it seems logical to determine whether an M1 agonist would be procognitive in schizophrenia or other cognitive disorders. ACP104, a metabolite of clozapine (which is a muscarinic antagonist), is itself actually an M1 agonist, and possibly a dopamine partial agonist. This compound is currently in testing in schizophrenia.

Cannabinoid antagonists. Cannabinoid receptors, linked to reward mechanisms in the mesolimbic system, are discussed in further detail in the chapter on drug abuse. An antagonist to cannabinoid 1 (CB1) receptors known as rimonabant, or SR141716 A, has been tested in schizophrenia, but without clearly improving psychosis. However, rimonabant is approved in some countries for obesity, as it may lead to weight loss; it is in testing also for smoking cessation and alcohol abuse. A related compound is SR 147778 (AVE 1625). Testing of rimonabant as a weight-loss agent in obesity has not yet been extensively completed for schizophrenic patients taking antipsychotics, but it could be an important intervention in reducing obesity and cardiometabolic risk in these patients.

Peptide-linked mechanisms

Neurokinin antagonists (NK1, NK2, and NK3). The three principal neurokinin neurotransmitters and their receptors are discussed in detail in Chapter 12, on antidepressants. Testing with NK1 antagonists (also known as substance P antagonists) has generally been disappointing for all psychiatric indications, from schizophrenia to depression to pain. Testing with an NK2 antagonist for depression is promising and is discussed in Chapter 12, on antidepressants. Finally, testing of various NK3 antagonists is in progress but without as yet any clear results of efficacy in schizophrenia. These drugs include talnetant (SB223412), osanetant (SR142801), SSR 146977, and the NK3/NK2 antagonist SR 241586.

Neurotensin antagonists. Neurotensin is a peptide neurotransmitter that is colocalized with dopamine in the mesolimbic dopamine pathway, but is much lower in concentration in nigrostriatal and mesocortical dopaminergic pathways. A nonpeptide antagonist SR-142948 is in clinical testing in schizophrenia as a theoretical agent that could reduce positive symptoms without producing EPS by exploiting differential actions on the mesolimbic rather than nigrostriatal dopamine systems; it has thus far not yielded definitive results.

Cholecystokinin. Cholecystokinin (CCK) is also colocalized with dopaminergic neurons and has two receptor subtypes, with CCK-A being predominantly outside the CNS and CCK-B within the CNS. Studies of CCK agonists and antagonists to date have not given clear clues as to their potential for therapeutic actions in schizophrenia.

Peptide treatments for obesity
Pramlintide. Pramlintide (Symlin) is a synthetic analog of the human peptide hormone amylin, a naturally occurring neuroendocrine hormone synthesized by pancreatic beta cells that contributes to glucose control during the postprandial period. Pramlintide is given at mealtimes as an adjunctive treatment to diabetics who fail to achieve desired glucose control despite adequate insulin (and oral hypoglycemic) therapy. It works by modulating gastric emptying, preventing the postprandial rise in plasma glucagon, and causing satiety, probably by a central mechanism leading to decreased caloric intake and potential weight loss. Thus it is being tested for obesity in general and – given the high incidence of obesity, cardiometabolic risk, and complications in schizophrenia – should be tested in schizophrenic patients taking atypical antipsychotic drugs.

Future combination chemotherapies for schizophrenia and other psychotic disorders
Given the economic incentives for providing the "cure" and treatment of choice for psychotic disorders, it is not difficult to understand why most drug development activities for the psychoses target a single disease mechanism with the goal of being the only therapy for a given disorder. In reality, it is overly simplistic to conceptualize disorders with psychotic features as the product of a single disease mechanism. Schizophrenia has not only psychotic features but also negative symptoms, affective symptoms, cognitive symptoms, and probably neurodevelopmental and neurodegenerative dimensions. It is difficult to conceptualize how such a complex disorder could ever be satisfactorily treated with a single entity acting by a single pharmacological mechanism.

Psychopharmacological treatments for schizophrenia in the future will need to borrow a chapter out of the book of cancer chemotherapy and HIV/AIDS therapy, where the standard of treatment is to use multiple drugs simultaneously to attain therapeutic synergy. "Combination chemotherapy" for malignancy utilizes the approach of combining several independent therapeutic mechanisms. When successful, this results in a total therapeutic response that is greater than the sum of its parts. This approach often has the favorable consequence of simultaneously diminishing total side effects, since adverse experiences of multiple drugs are mediated by different pharmacological mechanisms and therefore should not be additive. Clinical trials with multiple therapeutic agents working by several mechanisms can be quite difficult to undertake; but as there is a clinical trials methodology that exists in the cancer chemotherapy and HIV/AIDS literature, it is an approach that should be applied for complex disorders with multiple underlying disease mechanisms, such as schizophrenia. Thus, schizophrenia treatments of the near future will almost certainly combine new agents with one of the known atypical antipsychotics. Thus a platform of at least partial control of positive and negative symptoms, mood, cognition, and hostility will be provided with the known atypical antipsychotic, hopefully without causing EPS, tardive dyskinesia, hyperprolactinemia, or metabolic disturbances. New agents with new mechanisms can then "top up" the atypical antipsychotic, particularly in the hope of boosting the relief of negative and cognitive symptoms. In the long run, some sort of molecularly based therapy to prevent genetically programmed disease onset or progression or to reverse the consequences of aberrant neurodevelopment may also form part of the portfolio of treatments for schizophrenia.

Summary

This chapter has reviewed the pharmacology of conventional D2 antagonist antipsychotic drugs as well as the new atypical antipsychotic agents that are largely replacing them in clinical practice. The features of serotonin-2A/D2 antagonism (or SDA) of the atypical antipsychotic are discussed, as are several other pharmacological mechanisms that may contribute to atypical antipsychotic clinical actions, including D2 partial agonism (or DPA), rapid dissociation from D2 receptors, and serotonin-1A partial agonism (or SPA). Multiple receptor binding properties hypothesized to be linked to cardiometabolic risk and sedation of antipsychotics are explored. Pharmacokinetics of antipsychotics are briefly reviewed, as are the unique pharmacological and clinical properties of 15 specific antipsychotic agents. Use of these agents in a clinical practice setting, including considerations of how to treat individual symptoms of schizophrenia and how to dose, switch, and combine these agents for difficult patients are all reviewed. Finally, many new treatments under development for schizophrenia are presented.

CHAPTER 11

Mood Disorders

- Description of mood disorders
- The bipolar spectrum
- Can unipolar depression be distinguished from bipolar depression?
- Are mood disorders progressive?
- Neurotransmitters and circuits in mood disorders
  - Noradrenergic neurons
  - Monoamine interactions: NE regulation of 5HT release
  - Monoamine interactions: 5HT regulation of NE and DA release
- The monoamine hypothesis of depression
- The monoamine hypothesis, monoamine receptors, and gene expression
- Symptoms and circuits in depression
- Symptoms and circuits in mania
- Genes and neuroimaging in mood disorders
- Summary

This chapter discusses disorders characterized by abnormalities of mood: namely, depression, mania, or both. Included are descriptions of a wide variety of mood disorders that occur over a broad clinical spectrum. Also included is an analysis of how abnormalities in regulation of the trimonoaminergic neurotransmitter system – comprising the three monoamine neurotransmitters norepinephrine (NE; also called noradrenaline, or NA), dopamine (DA), and serotonin (also called 5-hydroxytryptamine, or 5HT) – are hypothesized to explain the biological basis of mood disorders. The approach taken here is to deconstruct each mood disorder into its component symptoms, followed by matching each symptom to hypothetically malfunctioning brain circuits, each regulated by one or more of the neurotransmitters within the trimonoaminergic neurotransmitter system. The genetic regulation and neuroimaging of these hypothetically malfunctioning brain circuits are also briefly mentioned. The discussion of symptoms and circuits in this chapter is intended to set the stage for understanding the pharmacological concepts underlying the mechanisms of action and use of antidepressants and mood-stabilizing drugs reviewed in the following two chapters (Chapters 12 and 13).

Mood Chart

mania

– – – – – – – – – – HYPOMANIA – – – – – – – – – – –

euthymia
(normal mood)

– – – – – – – – – – DYSTHYMIA – – – – – – – – – – –

depression

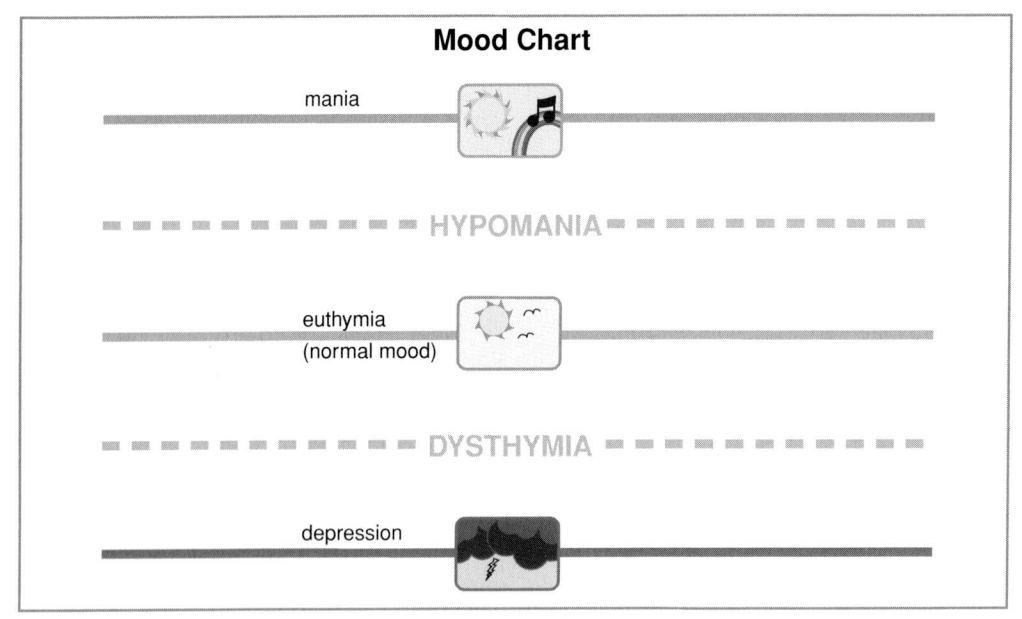

FIGURE 11-1 Mood chart. Disorders of mood can be mapped on a mood chart to track the course of illness, identify phase of illness, and aid in differential diagnosis. As shown in this chart, mood can range from mania at the top, to hypomania, to euthymia (normal mood) in the middle, and to dysthymia and depression at the bottom.

Clinical descriptions and criteria for the diagnosis of disorders of mood are mentioned only in passing. The reader should consult standard reference sources for this material. Here we discuss how the discovery of various neurotransmitters and brain circuits has influenced the understanding of symptoms in mood disorders. The goal of this chapter is to outline current ideas about the clinical and biological aspects of mood disorders in order to prepare the reader to understand the various treatments for these disorders discussed in later chapters.

Description of mood disorders

Disorders of mood are often called affective disorders, since affect is the external display of mood or emotion which is, however, felt internally. Depression and mania are often seen as opposite ends of an affective or mood spectrum. Classically, mania and depression are "poles" apart, thus generating the terms "unipolar" depression (i.e., as in patients who just experience the *down* or depressed pole) and "bipolar" [i.e., as in patients who at different times experience either the *up* (manic) pole or the *down* (depressed) pole]. In practice, however, depression and mania may occur simultaneously, in which case a "mixed" mood state exists. Mania may also occur in lesser degrees, known as "hypomania"; or a patient may switch so quickly between mania and depression that it is called "rapid cycling."

Mood disorders can be usefully visualized not only to distinguish different mood disorders from one another but also to summarize the course of illness for individual patients by showing them their disorders mapped onto a mood chart. Thus, mood ranges from hypomania to mania at the top, to euthymia (or normal mood) in the middle, to dysthymia and depression at the bottom (Figure 11-1). Mood abnormalities for the major diagnostic entities are summarized in Figure 11-2 and shown in more detail in Figures 11-3 through 11-29.

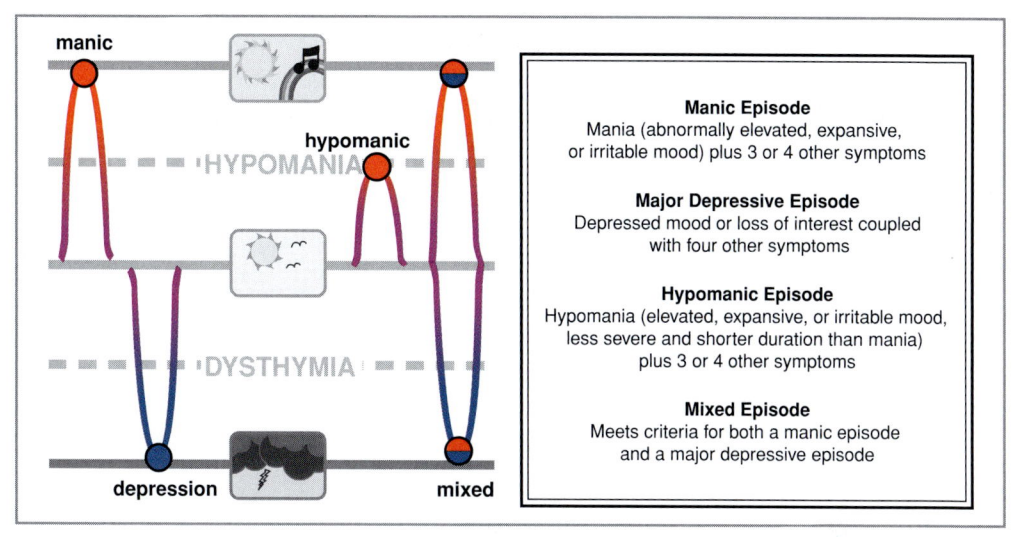

FIGURE 11-2 Mood episodes. Bipolar disorder is generally characterized by four types of illness episodes: manic, major depressive, hypomanic, and mixed. A patient may have any combination of these episodes over the course of illness; subsyndromal manic or depressive episodes also occur during the course of illness, in which case there are not enough symptoms or the symptoms are not severe enough to meet the diagnostic criteria for one of these episodes. Thus the presentation of mood disorders can vary widely.

Manic Episode
Mania (abnormally elevated, expansive, or irritable mood) plus 3 or 4 other symptoms

Major Depressive Episode
Depressed mood or loss of interest coupled with four other symptoms

Hypomanic Episode
Hypomania (elevated, expansive, or irritable mood, less severe and shorter duration than mania) plus 3 or 4 other symptoms

Mixed Episode
Meets criteria for both a manic episode and a major depressive episode

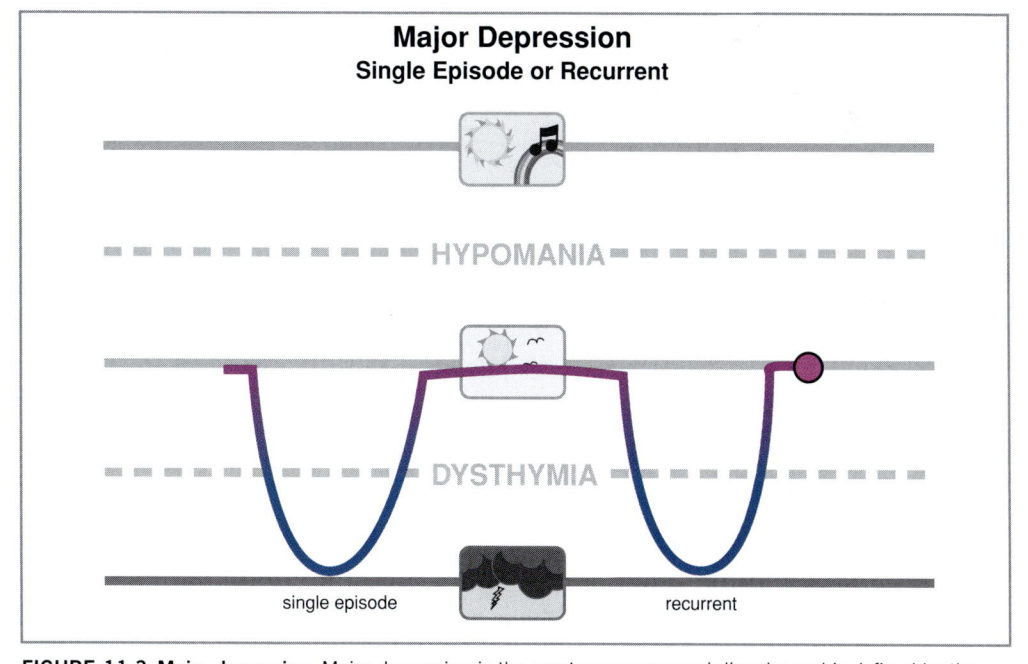

FIGURE 11-3 Major depression. Major depression is the most common mood disorder and is defined by the occurrence of at least a single major depressive episode, although most patients will experience recurrent episodes.

Mood Disorders | 455

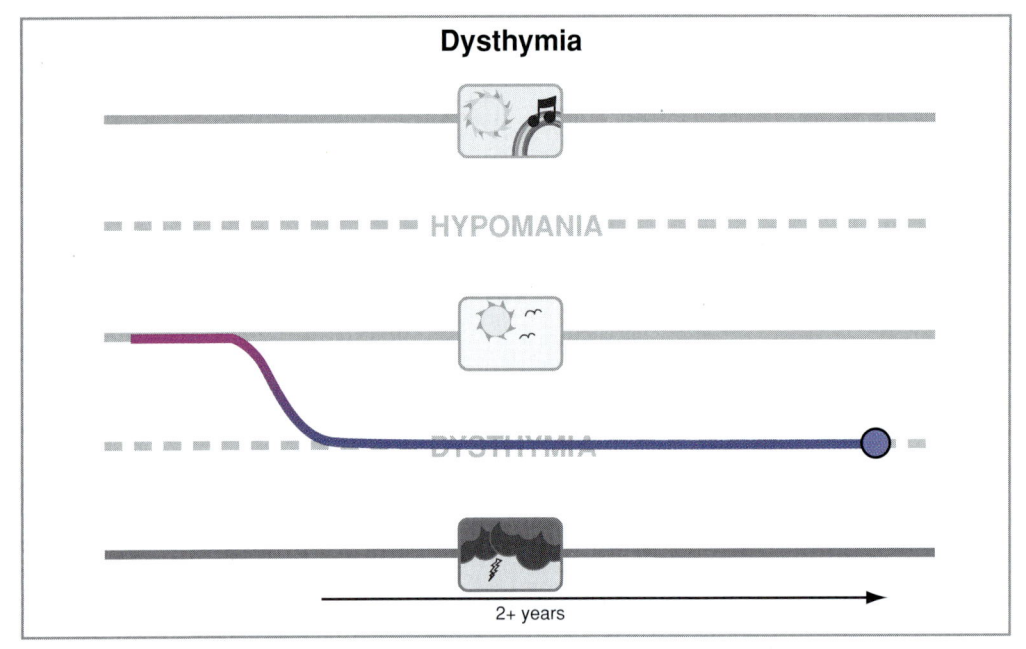

FIGURE 11-4 Dysthymia. Dysthymia is a less severe form of depression than major depression but long-lasting (over two years in duration) and is often unremitting.

The most common and readily recognized mood disorder is major depression (Figure 11-3) as a single episode or recurrent episodes. Dysthymia is a less severe but often longer-lasting form of depression (Figure 11-4). Patients with a major depressive episode who have poor inter-episode recovery, only to the level of dysthymia, which is then followed by another episode of major depression, are sometimes said to have "double depression," alternating between major depression and dysthymia but not remitting (Figure 11-5).

Bipolar I patients have full-blown manic episodes and/or mixed episodes of full mania plus simultaneous full depression, often followed by a full depressive episode (Figure 11-6). When mania recurs at least four times a year, it is called rapid cycling (Figure 11-17A). Bipolar I patients can also have rapid switches from mania to depression and back (Figure 11-17B). By definition, this occurs at least four times a year, but it can happen much more frequently than that.

Bipolar II disorder is characterized by at least one hypomanic episode and one full depressive episode (Figure 11-8). Cyclothymic disorder is characterized by mood swings less severe than full mania and full depression but still waxing and waning above and below the boundaries of normal mood (Figure 11-9). There may be lesser degrees of variation from normal mood that are stable and persistent, including both depressive temperament (below normal mood but not a mood disorder) (Figure 11-10) and hyperthymic temperament (above normal mood but also not a mood disorder) (Figure 11-11). Temperaments are lifelong personality styles of responding to environmental stimuli; they can be heritable patterns present early in life and persisting thereafter and include such independent personality dimensions as novelty seeking, harm avoidance, and conscientiousness. Some patients may have mood-related temperaments that may render them vulnerable to mood disorders, especially bipolar spectrum disorders, later in life.

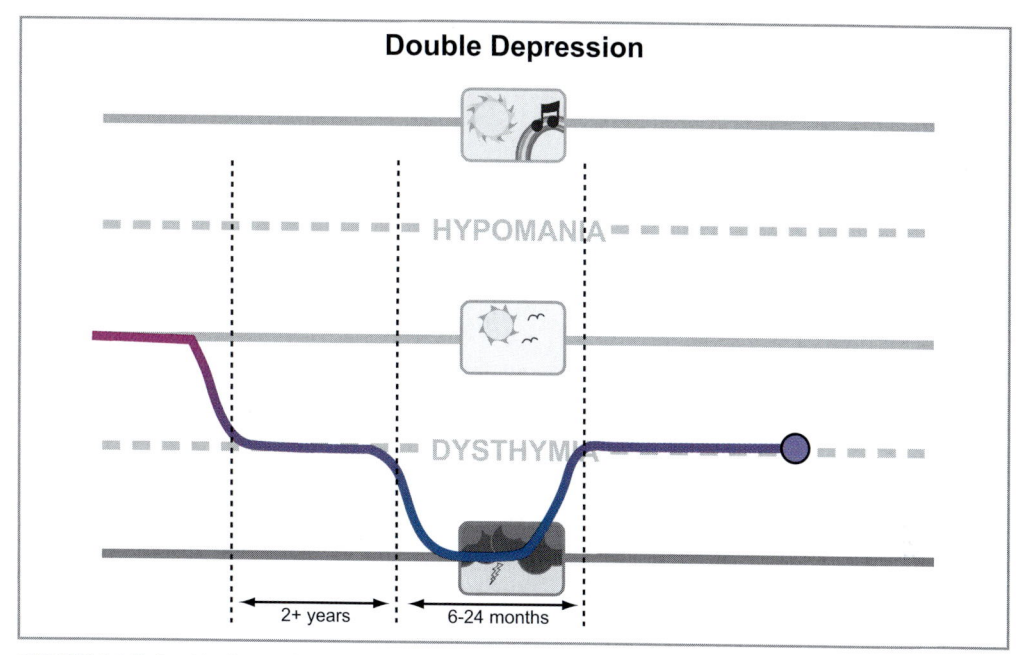

FIGURE 11-5 Double depression. Patients with unremitting dysthymia who also experience the superimposition of one or more major depressive episodes are described as having double depression. This is also a form of recurrent major depressive episodes with poor inter-episode recovery.

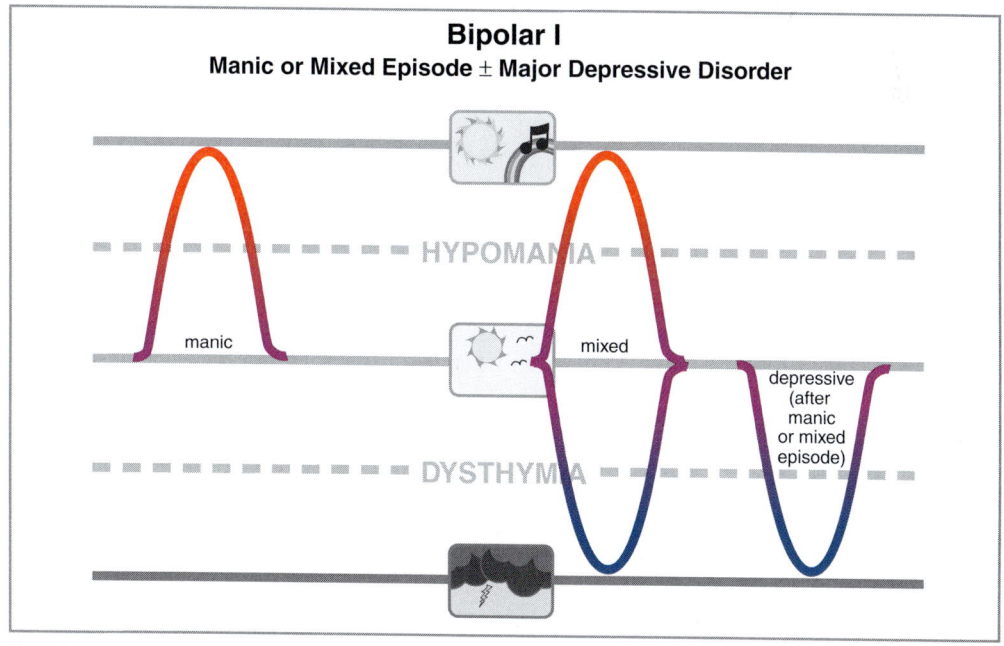

FIGURE 11-6 Bipolar I disorder. Bipolar I disorder is defined as the occurrence of at least one manic or mixed (full mania and full depression simultaneously) episode. Patients with bipolar I disorder typically experience major depressive episodes as well, although this is not necessary for the bipolar I diagnosis.

Mood Disorders | 457

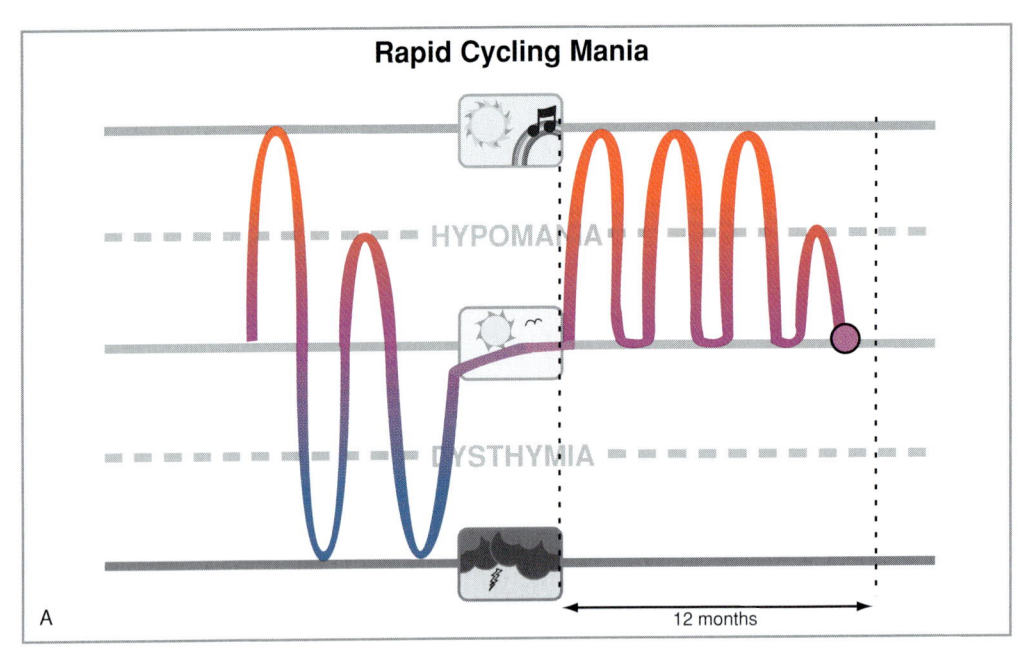

FIGURE 11-7A Rapid cycling mania. The course of bipolar disorder can be rapid cycling, which means that at least four episodes occur within a one-year period. This can manifest itself as four distinct manic episodes, as shown here. Many patients with this form of mood disorder experience switches much more frequently than four times a year.

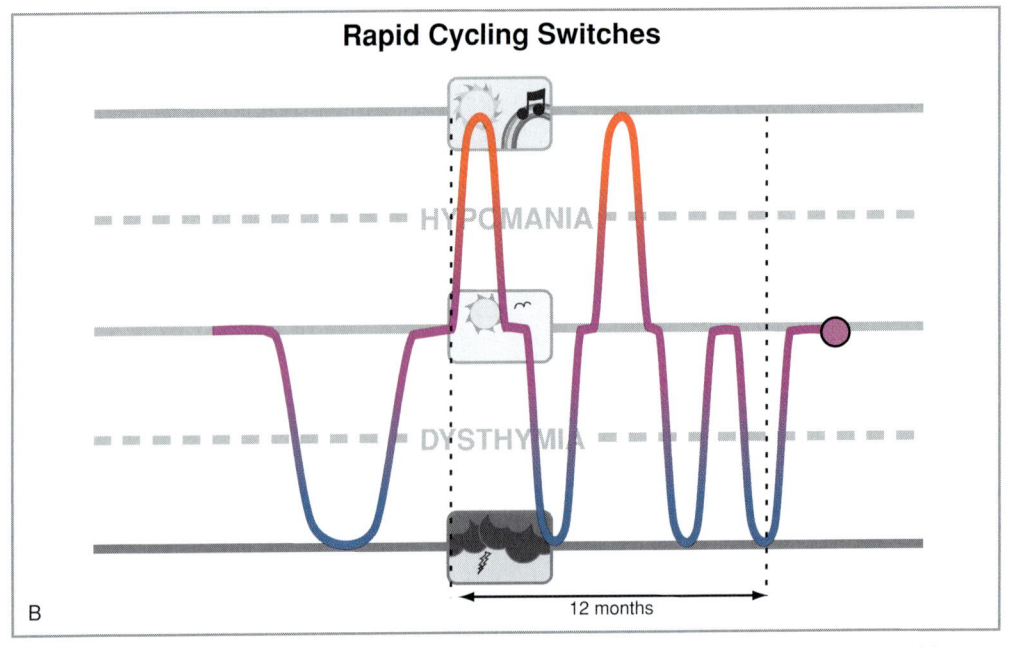

FIGURE 11-7B Rapid cycling switches. A rapid cycling course (at least four distinct mood episodes within one year) can also manifest as rapid switches between manic and depressive episodes.

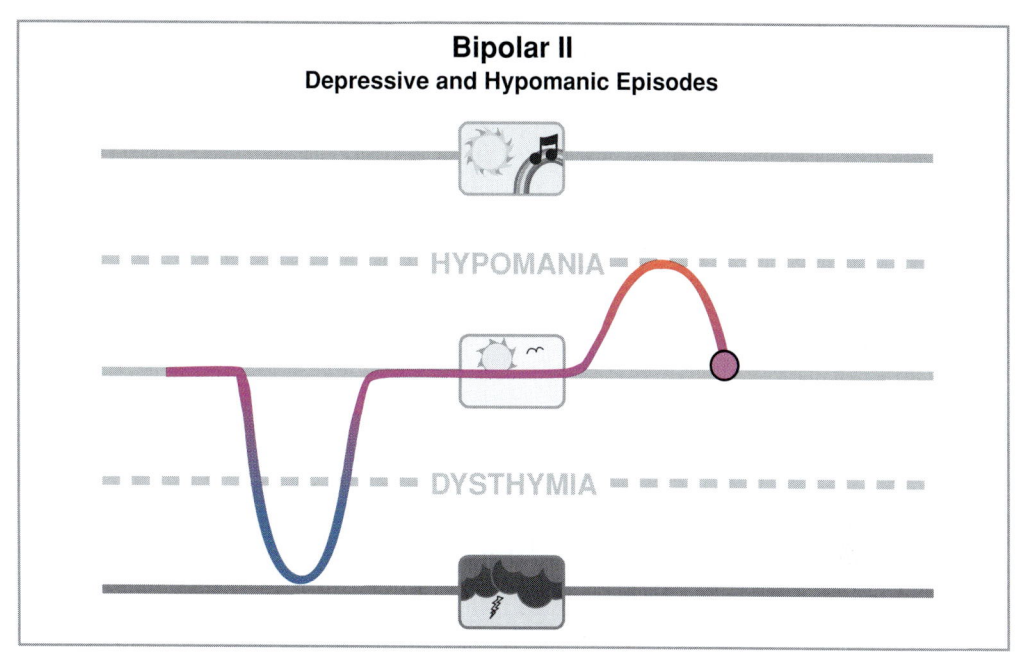

FIGURE 11-8 Bipolar II disorder. Bipolar II disorder is defined as an illness course consisting of one or more major depressive episodes and at least one hypomanic episode.

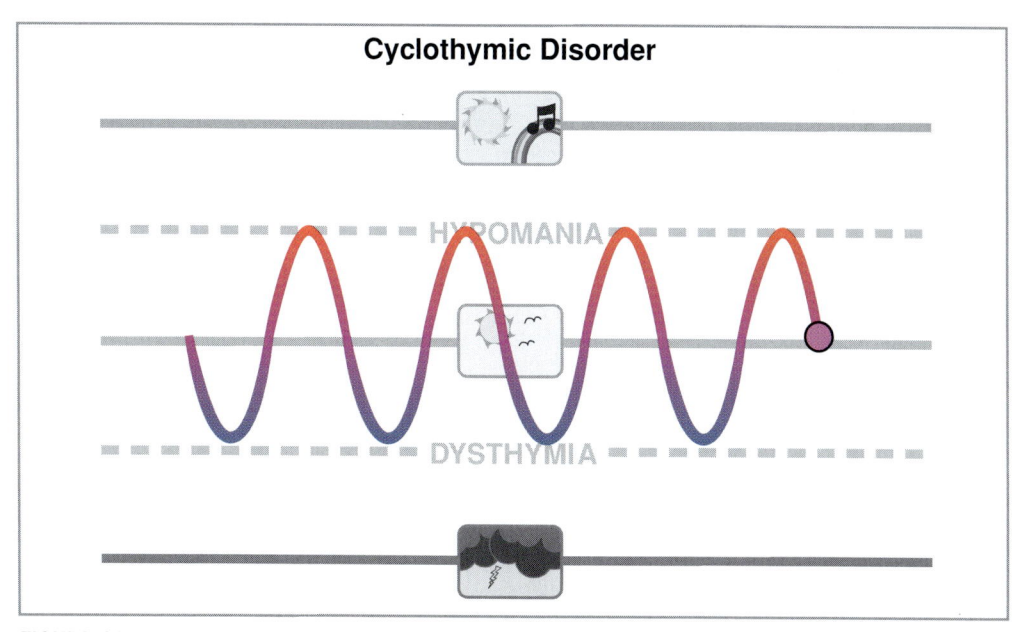

FIGURE 11-9 Cyclothymic disorder. Cyclothymic disorder is characterized by mood swings between hypomania and dysthymia but without any full manic or major depressive episodes.

Mood Disorders | 459

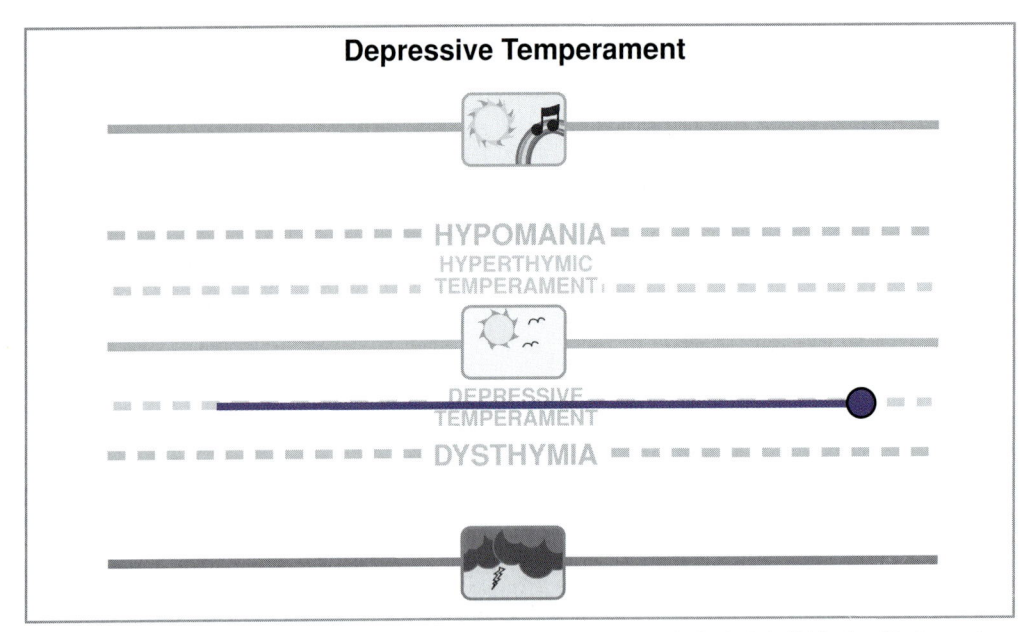

FIGURE 11-10 Depressive temperament. Not all mood variations are pathological. Individuals with depressive temperament may be consistently sad or apathetic but do not meet the criteria for dysthymia and do not necessarily experience any functional impairment. However, individuals with depressive temperament may be at greater risk for the development of a mood disorder later in life.

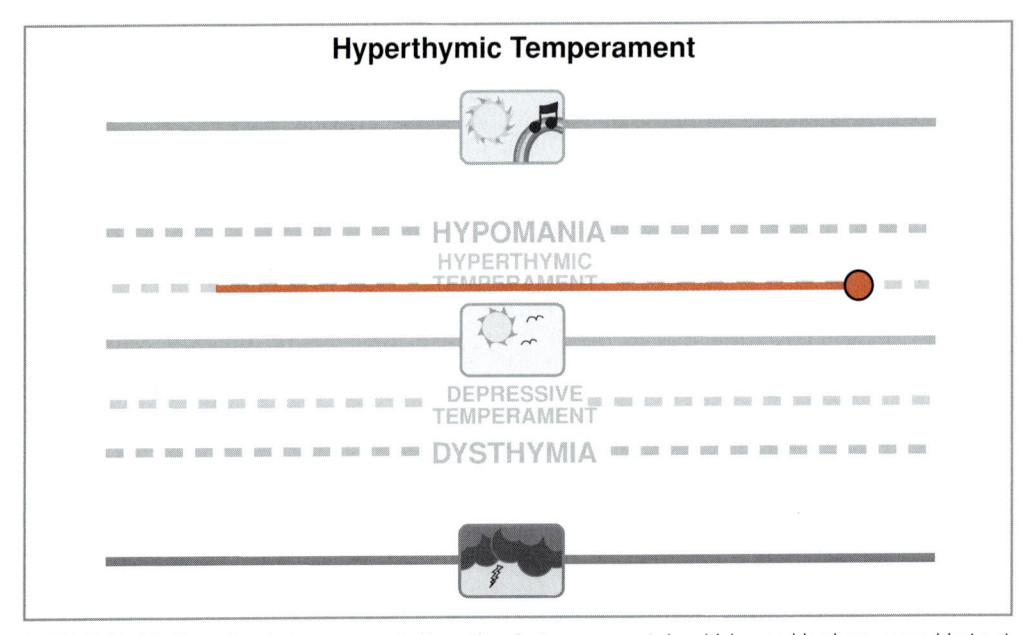

FIGURE 11-11 Hyperthymic temperament. Hyperthymic temperament, in which mood is above normal but not pathological, includes stable characteristics such as extroversion, optimism, exuberance, impulsiveness, overconfidence, grandiosity, and lack of inhibition. Individuals with hyperthymic temperament may be at greater risk for the development of a mood disorder later in life.

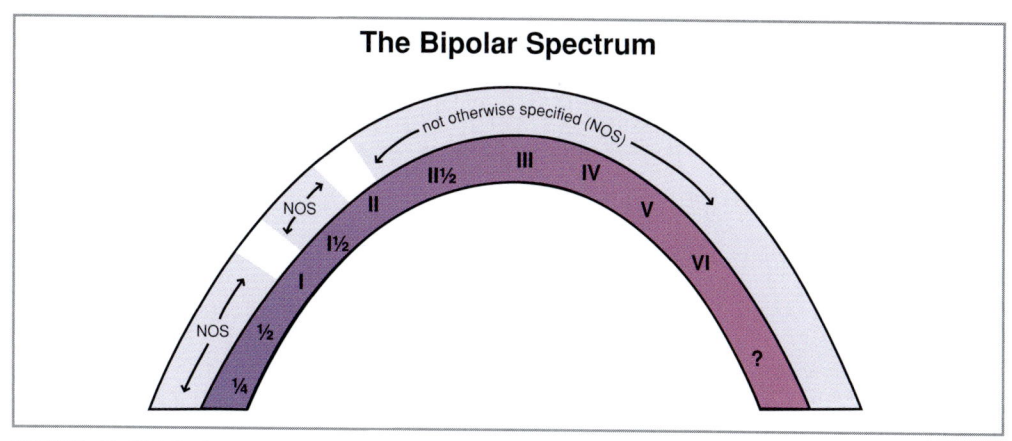

FIGURE 11-12 Bipolar spectrum. The only formal unique bipolar diagnoses identified in the *Diagnostic and Statistical Manual of Mental Disorders*, fourth edition (DSM-IV), are bipolar I, bipolar II, and cyclothymic disorder, with all other presentations that include mood symptoms above the normal range lumped together in a single category called "not otherwise specified (NOS)." However, there is a huge variation in the presentation of patients within this bipolar NOS category. It may be more useful, instead, to think of these patients as belonging to a bipolar spectrum and to identify subcategories of presentations, as has been done by Akiskal and other experts and as illustrated in the next several figures.

The bipolar spectrum

From a strict diagnostic point of view, our discussion of mood disorders might now be complete. However, there is growing recognition that many or even most patients seen in clinical practice may have a mood disorder that is not well described by the categories outlined above. Formally, they would be called "not otherwise specified" or "NOS," but this creates a huge single category for many patients that belies the richness and complexity of their symptoms. Increasingly, such patients are seen as belonging in general to the "bipolar spectrum" (Figure 11-12) and, in particular, to one of several additional descriptive categories proposed by experts such as Akiskal (Figures 11-12 through 11-21).

Two forms of mood disorder often considered to be "not quite bipolar" may include bipolar ¼ and bipolar ½ (Figures 11-13 and 11-14). Bipolar ¼ (or 0.25) could designate an unstable form of unipolar depression that responds sometimes rapidly but in an unsustained manner to antidepressants. Such an uneven response is sometimes called antidepressant "poop out" (Figure 11-13). These patients have unstable mood but not a formal bipolar disorder, yet they can sometimes benefit from mood-stabilizing treatments added to robust antidepressant treatments. Bipolar ½ (or 0.5) may indicate a type of "schizobipolar" disorder, also sometimes called schizoaffective disorder, combining positive symptoms of psychosis with manic, hypomanic, and depressive episodes (Figure 11-14). The placement of these patients within the bipolar spectrum can provide a rationale for treating them with mood stabilizers and atypical antipsychotics as well as antidepressants.

Although patients with protracted or recurrent hypomania without depression are not formally diagnosed as having bipolar II disorder, they are definitely part of the bipolar spectrum and may benefit from the mood stabilizers studied mostly in bipolar I disorder (Figure 11-15). Eventually such patients often develop a major depressive episode, and their diagnosis then changes to bipolar II disorder. In the meantime, they can be treated for hypomania while being vigilantly watched for the onset of a major depressive episode.

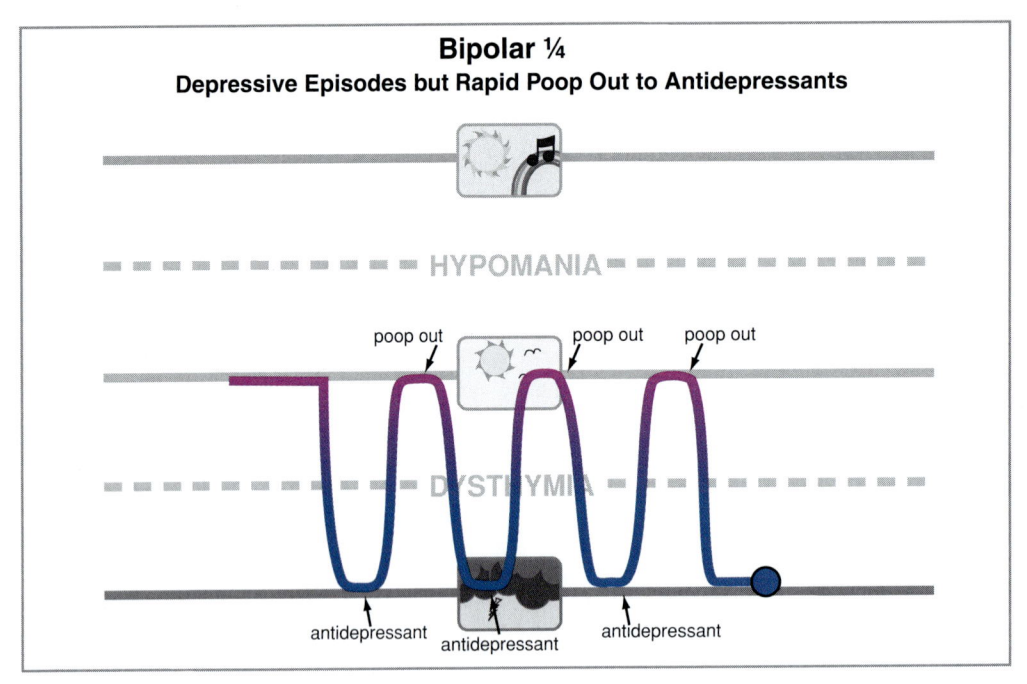

FIGURE 11-13 Bipolar ¼. Some patients may present only with depressive symptoms yet exhibit rapid but unsustained response to antidepressant treatment (sometimes called rapid "poop out"). Although such patients may have no spontaneous mood symptoms above normal, they potentially could benefit from mood-stabilizing treatment. This presentation may be termed bipolar 0.25 (or bipolar 1/4).

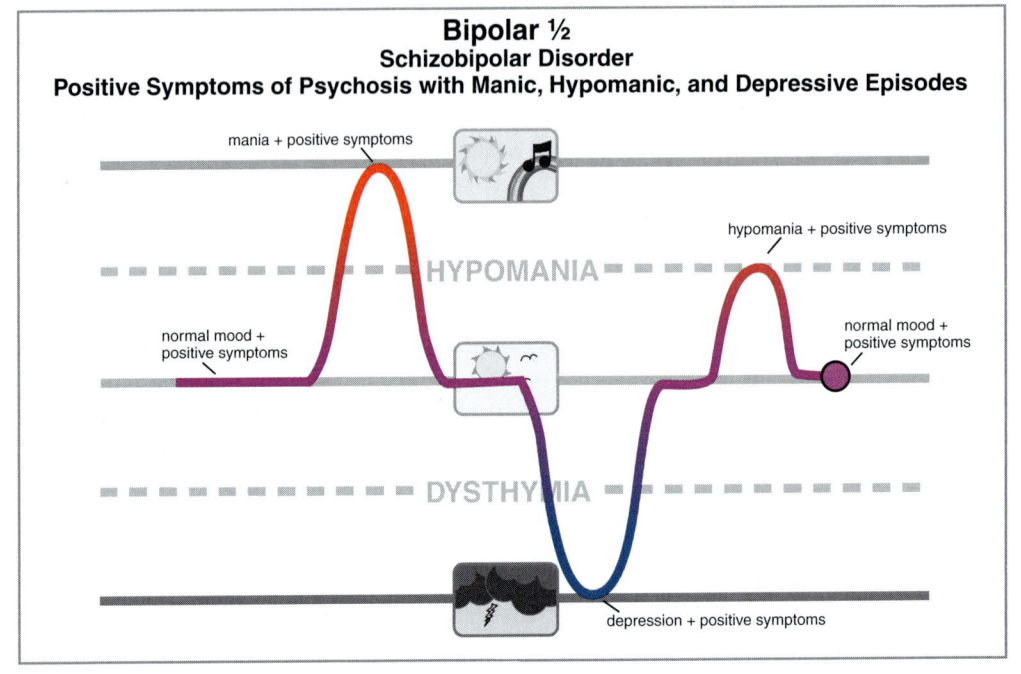

FIGURE 11-14 Bipolar 1/2. Bipolar 1/2 has been described as schizobipolar disorder, which combines positive symptoms of psychosis with manic, hypomanic, and depressive episodes.

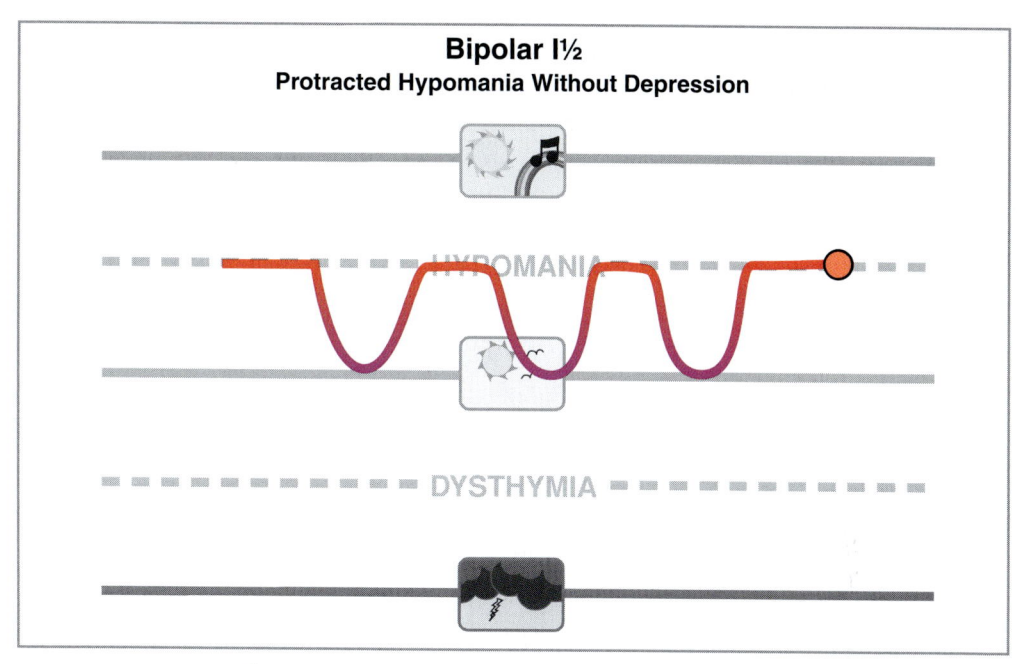

FIGURE 11-15 Bipolar I ½. A formal diagnosis of bipolar II disorder requires the occurrence of not only hypomanic episodes but also depressive episodes. However, some patients may experience recurrent hypomania without having experienced a depressive episode – a presentation that may be termed bipolar I ½. These patients may be at risk of eventually developing a depressive episode and are candidates for mood stabilizing treatment, although no treatment is formally approved for this condition.

Bipolar II ½ is the designation for patients with cyclothymic temperament who develop major depressive episodes (Figure 11-16). Many patients with cyclothymic temperament are just considered "moody" and do not consult professionals until they experience a full depressive episode. It is important to recognize patients in this part of the bipolar spectrum because treatment of their major depressive episodes with antidepressant monotherapy may actually cause increased mood cycling or even induce a full manic episode, just as can happen in patients with bipolar I or II depressive episodes.

In fact, patients who develop a manic or hypomanic episode on an antidepressant are sometimes called bipolar III (Figure 11-17). According to formal diagnostic criteria, however, when an antidepressant causes mania or hypomania, the diagnosis is not bipolar disorder but rather "substance-induced mood disorder." Many experts disagree with this designation and feel that patients who have a hypomanic or manic response to an antidepressant do so because they have a bipolar spectrum disorder and can be more appropriately diagnosed as bipolar III disorder (Figure 11-17) until they experience a spontaneous manic or hypomanic episode while taking no drugs, at which point their diagnosis would be bipolar I or II, respectively. The bipolar III designation is helpful in the meantime, reminding clinicians that such patients are not good candidates for antidepressant monotherapy.

A variant of bipolar III disorder has been called bipolar III ½ to designate a type of bipolar disorder associated with substance abuse (Figure 11-18). Although some of these patients can utilize substances of abuse to treat depressive episodes, others have previously experienced natural or drug-induced mania and take substances of abuse to induce mania. This combination of a bipolar disorder with substance abuse is a formula for chaos and can often be the story of a patient prior to seeking treatment from a mental health professional.

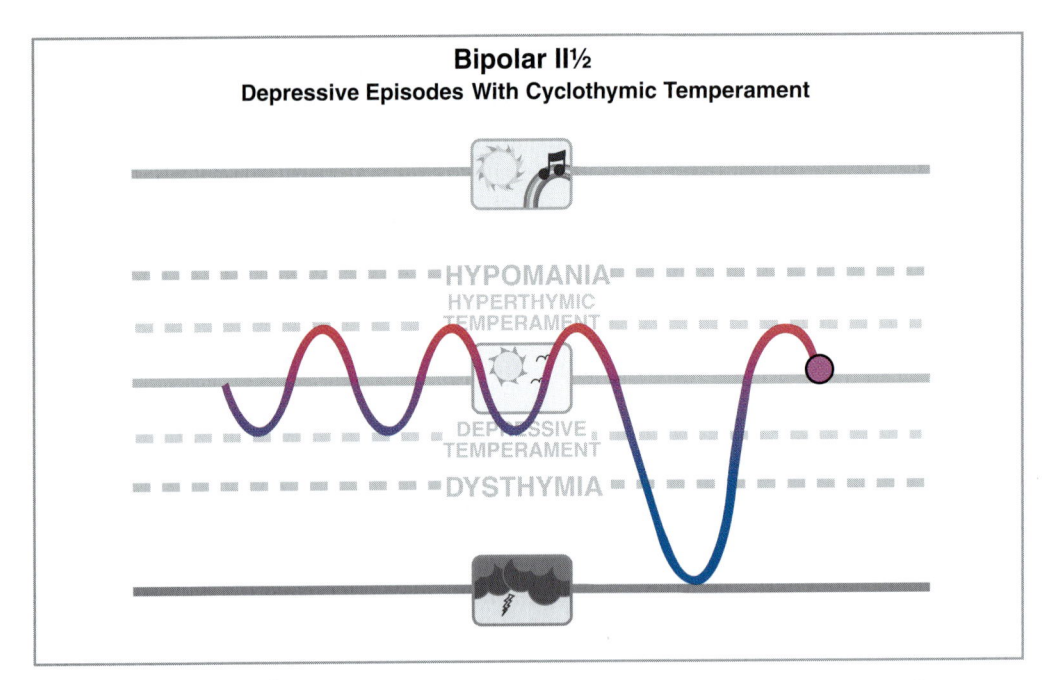

FIGURE 11-16 Bipolar II ½. Patients may present with a major depressive episode in the context of cyclothymic temperament, which is characterized by oscillations between hyperthymic or hypomanic states (above normal) and depressive or dysthymic states (below normal) upon which a major depressive episode intrudes (bipolar II ½). Individuals with cyclothymic temperament who are treated for the major depressive episodes may be at increased risk for antidepressant-induced mood cycling.

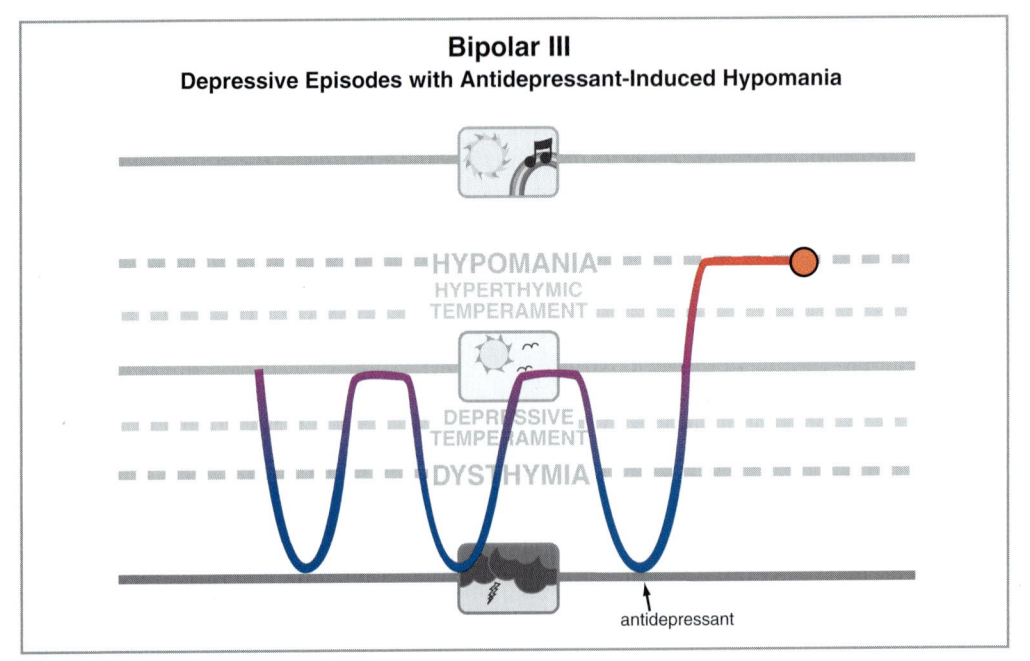

FIGURE 11-17 Bipolar III. Although the *Diagnostic and Statistical Manual of Mental Disorders*, fourth edition (DSM-IV), defines antidepressant-induced (hypo)mania as a substance-induced mood disorder, some experts believe that individuals who experience substance-induced (hypo)mania are actually predisposed to these mood states and thus belong to the bipolar spectrum (bipolar III).

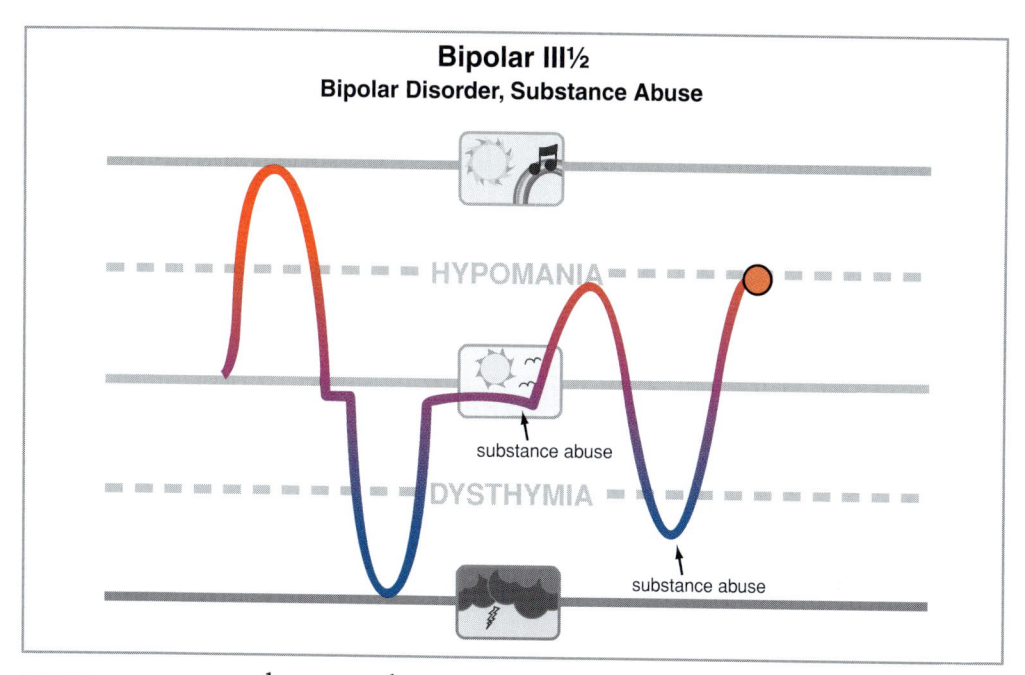

FIGURE 11-18 Bipolar III ½. Bipolar III ½ is bipolar disorder with substance abuse, in which the substance abuse is associated with efforts to achieve hypomania. Such patients should be evaluated closely to determine if (hypo)mania has ever occurred in the absence of substance abuse.

Bipolar IV disorder is the association of depressive episodes with a preexisting hyperthymic temperament (Figure 11-19). Patients with hyperthymia are often sunny, optimistic, high-output, successful individuals whose temperaments have been stable for years but who then suddenly collapse into a severe depression. In such cases, it may be useful to be vigilant to the need for more than antidepressant monotherapy if the patient is unresponsive to such treatment or develops rapid cycling, hypomanic, or mixed states in response to antidepressants. Despite not having a formal bipolar disorder, such patients may respond best to mood stabilizers.

Bipolar V disorder is depression with mixed hypomania (Figure 11-20). Formal diagnostic criteria for mixed states require full expression of both depression and mania simultaneously. In the real world, however, many depressed patients can have additional symptoms that qualify as only hypomania or even just a few or mild manic symptoms. Depression coexisting with full hypomania is represented in Figure 11-20 and requires mood stabilizer treatment, not antidepressant monotherapy.

Related states include mood states where full diagnostic criteria are not reached; these can range from full mixed states [both full mania diagnostic criteria (M) and full depression diagnostic criteria (D)] to depression with hypomania or only a few hypomanic symptoms (mD), as already discussed. In addition, other combinations of mania and depression range from full mania with only a few depressive symptoms (Md, sometimes also called "dysphoric" mania), to subsyndromal but unstable states characterized by some symptoms of both mania and depression but not diagnostic of either (md) (Table 11-1). All of these states differ from unipolar depression and belong in the bipolar spectrum; they may require treatment with the same agents used to treat bipolar I or II disorder, with appropriate caution for antidepressant monotherapy. The fact that a patient is depressed does not mean that he or she should start

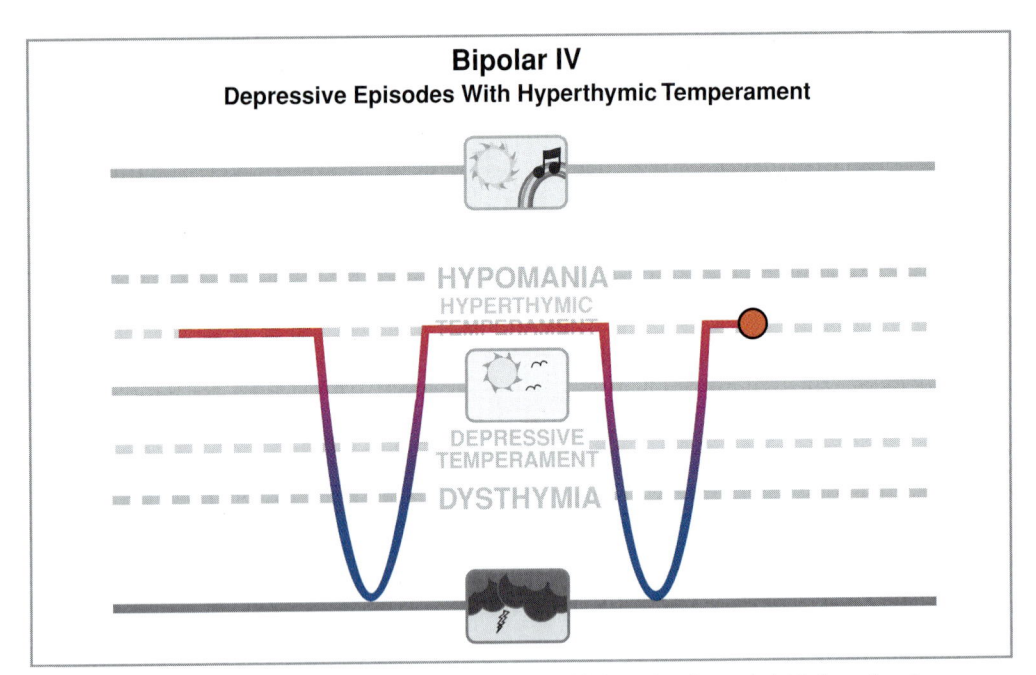

FIGURE 11-19 Bipolar IV. Bipolar IV is seen in individuals with long-standing and stable hyperthymic temperament into which a major depressive episode intrudes. Individuals with hyperthymic temperament who are treated for depressive episodes may be at increased risk for antidepressant-induced mood cycling and may instead respond better to mood stabilizers.

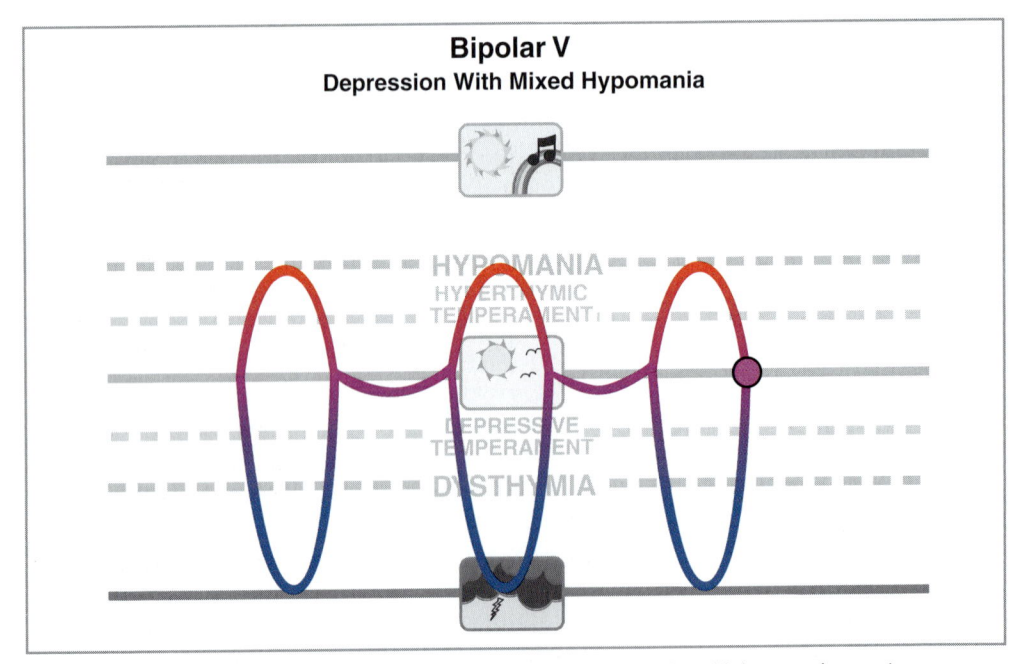

FIGURE 11-20 Bipolar V. Bipolar V is defined as major depressive episodes with hypomanic symptoms occurring during the major depressive episode but without the presence of discrete hypomanic episodes. Because the symptoms do not meet the full criteria for mania, these patients would not be considered to have a full mixed episode, but they nonetheless exhibit a mixed presentation and may require mood stabilizer treatment as opposed to antidepressant monotherapy.

TABLE 11-1 Mixed States of Mania and Depression

Description	Designation	Comment/Other Names
DSM-IV mixed	MD	Full diagnostic criteria for both mania and depression
Depression with hypomania	mD	Bipolar V
Depression with some manic symptoms	mD	Bipolar NOS
Mania with some depressive symptoms	Md	Dysphoric mania
Subsyndromal mania with subsyndromal depression	md	Prodrome or presymptomatic or state of incomplete remission

Bipolar VI
Bipolarity in the Setting of Dementia

irritability, agitation

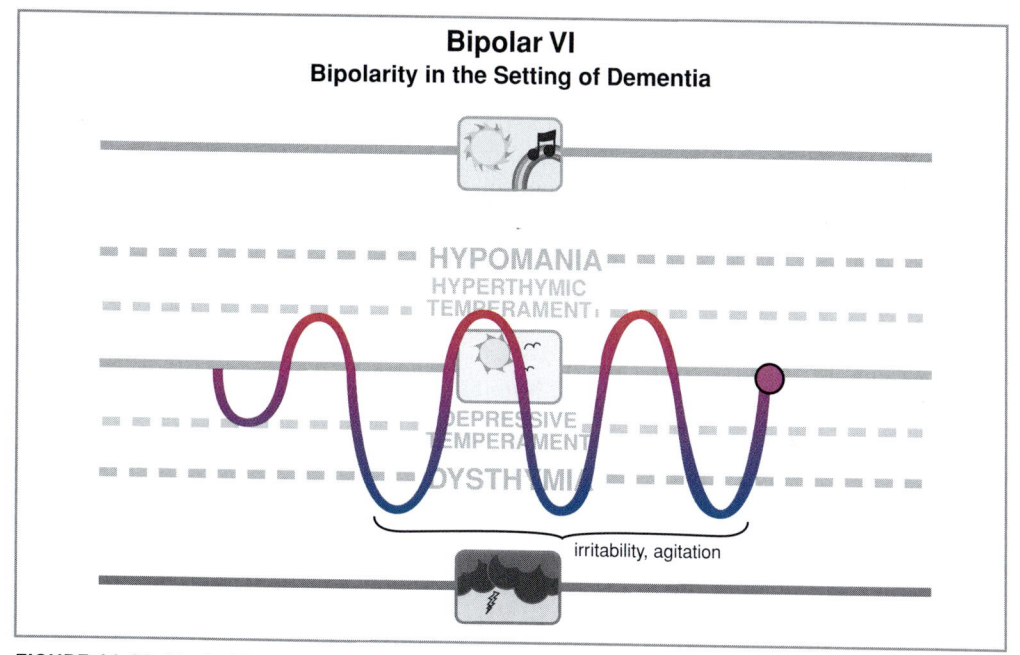

FIGURE 11-21 Bipolar VI. Another subcategory within the bipolar spectrum may be "bipolarity in the setting of dementia," termed bipolar VI. Mood instability here begins late in life, followed by impaired attention, irritability, reduced drive, and disrupted sleep. The presentation may initially appear to be attributable to dementia or be considered unipolar depression, but it is likely to be exacerbated by antidepressants and may respond to mood stabilizers.

treatment with an antidepressant. Patients with mixed states of depression and mania may be particularly vulnerable to the induction of activation, agitation, rapid cycling, dysphoria, hypomania, mania, or suicidality when treated with antidepressants, particularly without the concomitant use of a mood stabilizer or an atypical antipsychotic.

Finally, bipolar VI disorder (Figure 11-21) represents bipolarity in the setting of dementia, where it can be incorrectly attributed to the behavioral symptoms of dementia rather than recognized as a comorbid mood state and treated with mood stabilizers and even with atypical antipsychotics. Many more subtypes of mood disorders can be described within the bipolar spectrum. The important thing to take away from this discussion is that not all patients with depression have major depressive disorder requiring treatment with antidepressant monotherapy and that there are many states of mood disorder within the bipolar spectrum beyond just bipolar I and II disorders.

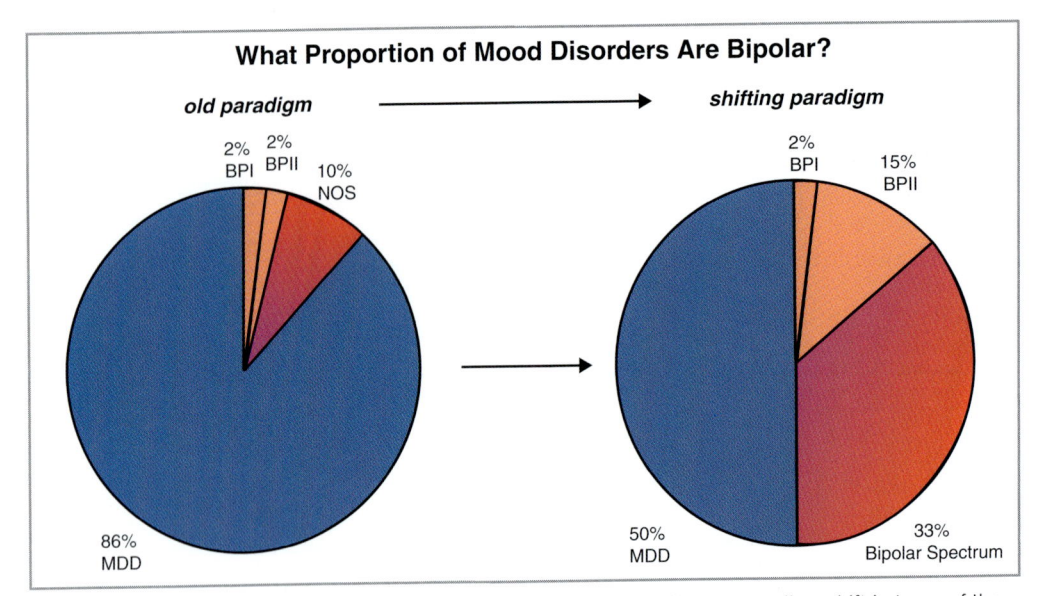

FIGURE 11-22 Prevalence of mood disorders. In recent years there has been a paradigm shift in terms of the recognition and diagnosis of patients with mood disorders. That is, many patients once considered to have major depressive disorder (old paradigm, left) are now recognized as having bipolar II disorder or another form of bipolar illness within the bipolar spectrum (shifting paradigm, right).

Can unipolar depression be distinguished from bipolar depression?

One of the important developments in the field of mood disorder in recent years, in fact, is the recognition that many patients once considered to have major depressive disorder actually have a form of bipolar disorder, especially bipolar II disorder or one of the conditions within the bipolar spectrum (Figure 11-22). Since symptomatic patients with bipolar disorder spend much more of their time in the depressed state than in the manic, hypomanic, or mixed state, this means that many depressed patients in the past were incorrectly diagnosed with unipolar major depression and treated with antidepressant monotherapy instead of being diagnosed as having a bipolar spectrum disorder and treated first with lithium, anticonvulsant mood stabilizers, and/or atypical antipsychotics prior to being given an antidepressant.

Up to half of patients once considered to have a unipolar depression are now considered to have a bipolar spectrum disorder (Figure 11-22), and although they would not necessarily be good candidates for antidepressant monotherapy, this is often the treatment that they receive when the bipolar nature of their condition is not recognized. Antidepressant treatment of unrecognized bipolar disorder may not only increase mood cycling, mixed states, and conversion to hypomania and mania, as mentioned above, but also contribute to the increase in suicidality of patients treated with antidepressants, with adults below twenty-five years of age being at greater risk for antidepressant-induced suicidality than older adults, adolescents more at risk than younger adults, and children more at risk than adolescents.

Thus it becomes important to recognize whether a depressed patient has a bipolar spectrum disorder or a unipolar major depressive disorder. How can this be done? In reality, these patients can have identical current symptoms (Figure 11-23), so obtaining the profile of current symptomatology is obviously not sufficient to distinguish unipolar from bipolar

TABLE 11-2 Is it unipolar or bipolar depression? Questions to ask

Who's your daddy?
- What is your family history of:
  – Mood disorder
  – Psychiatric hospitalizations
  – Suicide
  – Anyone who took lithium, mood stabilizers, antipsychotics, antidepressants
  – Anyone who received ECT

These can be indications of a unipolar or bipolar spectrum disorder in relatives.

Where's your mama?
- Additional history is needed about you from someone close to you, such as your mother or spouse. Patients may especially lack insight about their manic symptoms and underreport them.

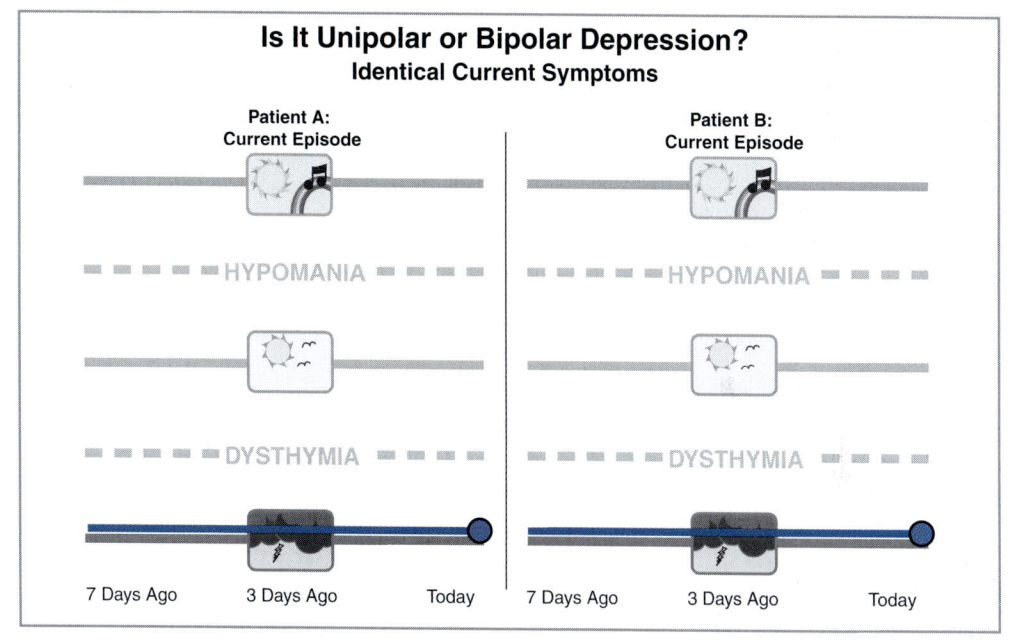

FIGURE 11-23 Unipolar versus bipolar depression presentation. The presenting symptoms of a major depressive episode in bipolar illness (Patient B) may be indistinguishable from those of a major depressive episode in unipolar depression (Patient A). Thus, the current presentation is not sufficient for making the differential diagnosis. The additional information needed includes family history, symptom and treatment-response history, and feedback from a friend or relative.

depression. The answer may be to ask the two questions shown in Table 11-2, namely, "Who's your daddy?" and "Where's your mama?"

What this means is "What is your family history?" since the existence of a first-degree relative with a bipolar spectrum disorder can strongly suggest that the patient also has a bipolar spectrum disorder rather than unipolar depression. This also means, "I need to get additional history from someone else close to you," since patients tend to underreport their manic symptoms, and the insight and observations of an outside informant such as a mother or spouse can give a past history quite different from the one the patient is reporting and thus help establish a bipolar spectrum diagnosis that patients themselves do not perceive or may deny.

Mood Disorders | 469

Is It Unipolar or Bipolar Depression?
Different Past Symptoms Make the Diagnosis

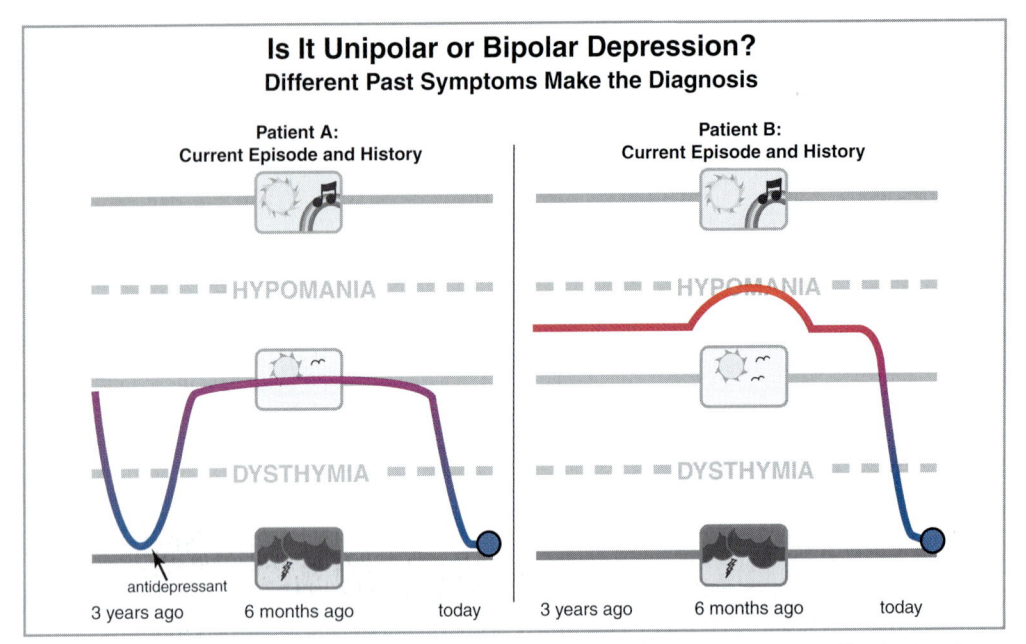

FIGURE 11-24 Unipolar versus bipolar depression history. Patterns of past symptoms as well as treatment-response history may aid in distinguishing between unipolar and bipolar illness. As shown here, although Patients A and B both present with major depressive episodes, they have divergent histories that suggest a unipolar illness for Patient A and a bipolar illness for Patient B.

Pattern of past symptoms can also give a hint as to whether a patient has a bipolar spectrum depression rather than a unipolar depression, as discussed above and as shown in Figure 11-24. Thus, prior response to antidepressants, prior hyperthymia or hypomania, can be hints from past symptoms to help distinguish unipolar from bipolar spectrum depression. Some hints, but not sufficient for diagnostic certainty, can even come from current symptoms to suggest a bipolar spectrum depression, such as more time sleeping, overeating, comorbid anxiety, motor retardation, mood lability, or psychotic or suicidal thoughts (Figure 11-25). Hints that the depression may be in the bipolar spectrum can come from the course of the untreated illness prior to the current symptoms, such as early age of onset, high frequency of depressive symptoms, high proportion of time spent ill, and acute abatement or onset of symptoms (Figure 11-26). Prior responses to antidepressants that suggest bipolar depression can be multiple antidepressant failures, rapid recovery, and the activation of side effects such as insomnia, agitation, and anxiety (Figure 11-27).

Although none of these features can discriminate bipolar depression from unipolar depression with certainty, the point is to be vigilant to the possibility that what looks like a unipolar depression might actually be a bipolar spectrum depression when investigated more carefully, and when response to treatment is monitored.

Are mood disorders progressive?

One of the major unanswered questions about the natural history of depressive illnesses is whether they are progressive (Figures 11-28 and 11-29). Specifically, it appears that many more patients in mental health practices have bipolar spectrum illnesses than unipolar illnesses, especially compared to a few decades ago. Is this merely the product of

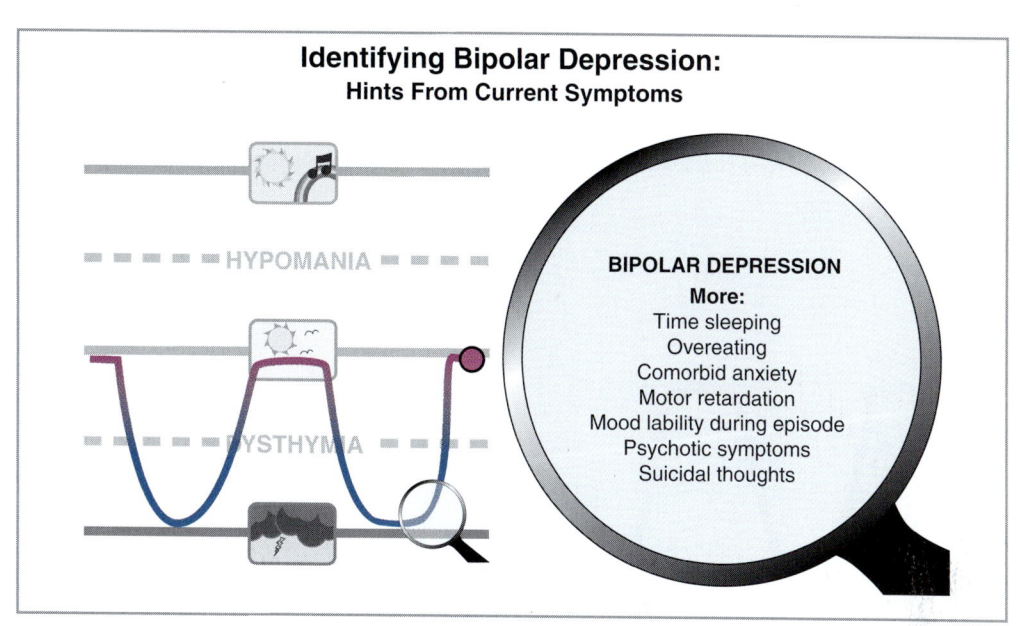

FIGURE 11-25 Bipolar depression symptoms. Although all symptoms of a major depressive episode can occur in either unipolar or bipolar depression, some symptoms may present more often in bipolar versus unipolar depression, providing hints if not diagnostic certainty that the patient has a bipolar spectrum disorder. These symptoms include increased time sleeping, overeating, comorbid anxiety, psychomotor retardation, mood lability during episodes, psychotic symptoms, and suicidal thoughts.

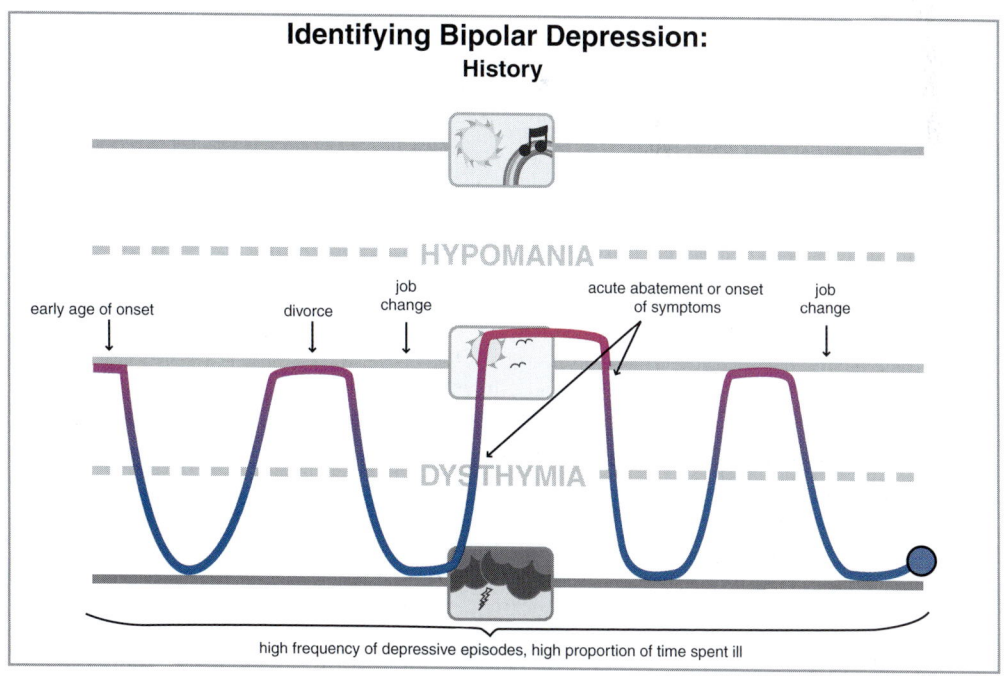

FIGURE 11-26 Identifying bipolar depression: history. Even in the absence of any previous (hypo)manic episodes, there are often specific hints in the untreated course of illness that suggest depression as part of the bipolar spectrum. These include early age of onset, high frequency of depressive episodes, high proportion of time spent ill, acute onset or abatement of symptoms, and behavioral symptoms such as frequent job or relationship changes.

Mood Disorders | 471

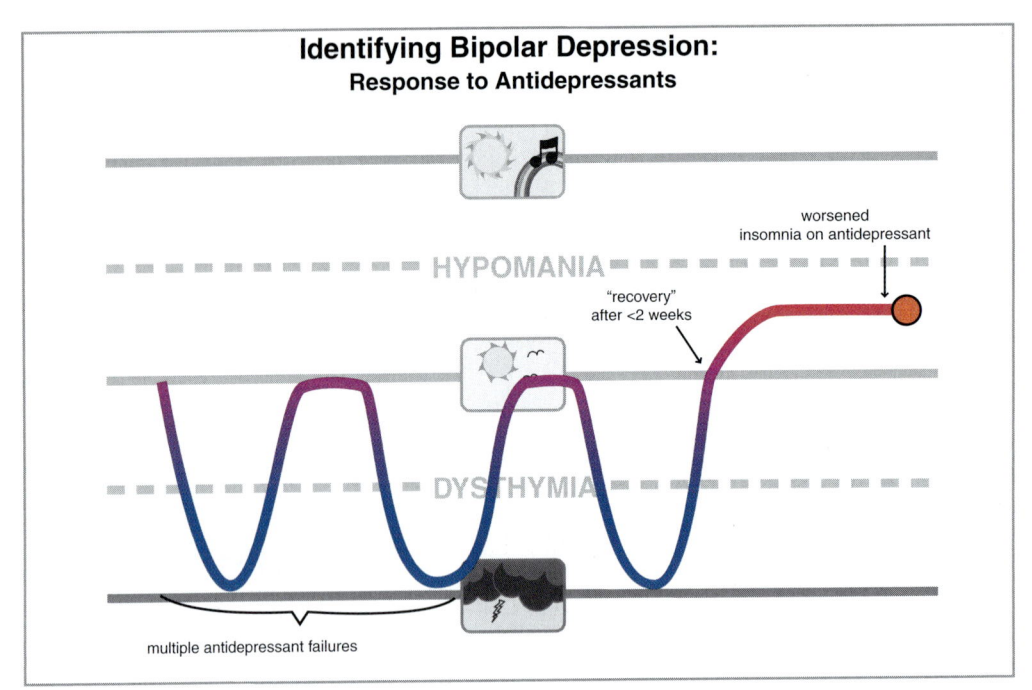

FIGURE 11-27 **Identifying bipolar depression: response to antidepressants.** Treatment-response history, particularly prior response to antidepressants, may provide insight into whether depression is unipolar or bipolar. Prior responses that suggest bipolar depression may include multiple antidepressant failures, rapid response to an antidepressant, and activating side effects such as insomnia, agitation, and anxiety.

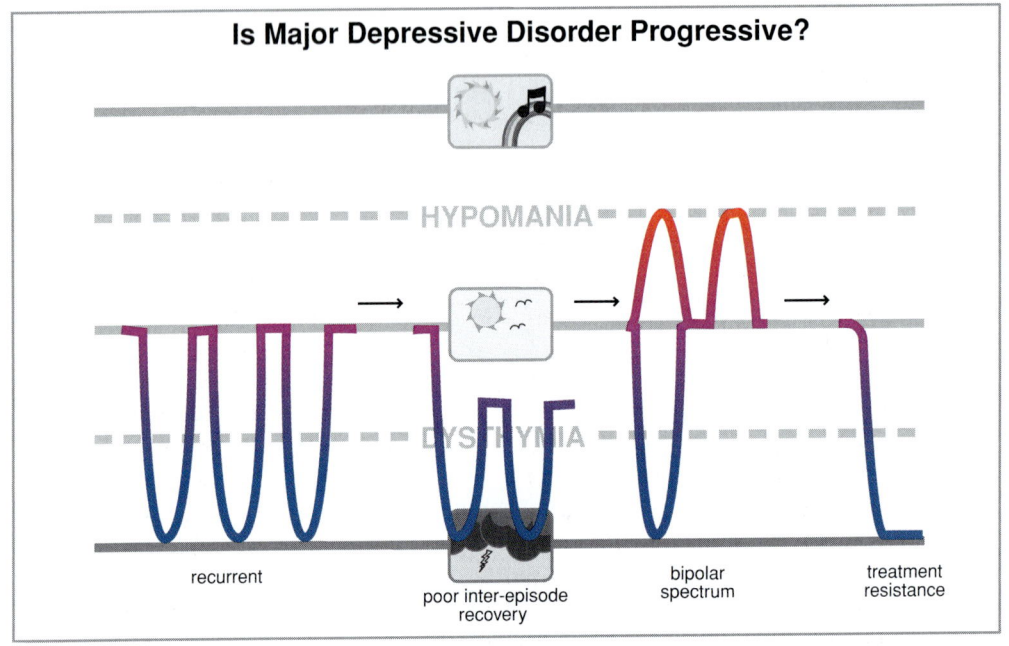

FIGURE 11-28 **Is major depressive disorder progressive?** A currently unanswered question is whether mood disorders are progressive. Does undertreatment of unipolar depression, in which residual symptoms persist and relapses occur, lead to progressive worsening of illness, such as more frequent recurrences and poor inter-episode recovery? And can this ultimately progress to a bipolar spectrum condition and finally treatment resistance?

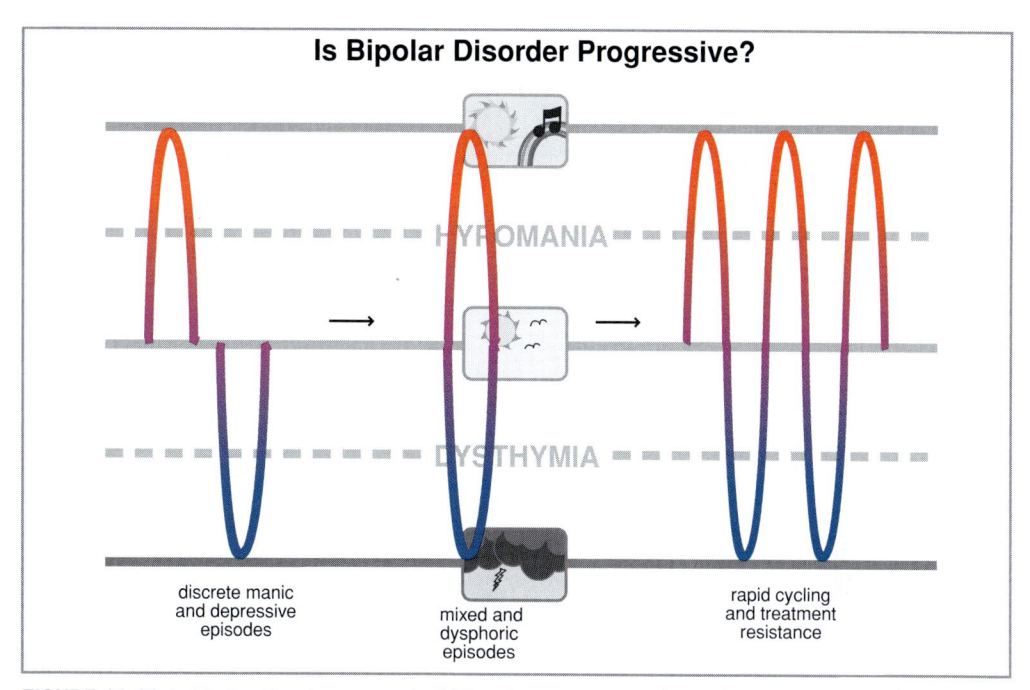

FIGURE 11-29 Is bipolar disorder progressive? There is some concern that undertreatment of discrete manic and depressive episodes may progress to mixed and dysphoric episodes and finally to rapid cycling and treatment resistance.

changing diagnostic criteria, or does unipolar depression progress to bipolar depression (Figure 11-28)?

A corollary of this question is whether chronic and widespread undertreatment of unipolar depression, allowing residual symptoms to persist and relapses and recurrences to occur, results first in more rapidly recurring episodes of major depression, then in poor interepisode recovery, then progression to a bipolar spectrum condition, and finally to treatment resistance (Figure 11-28). Many treatment-resistant mood disorders in psychiatric practices have elements of bipolar spectrum disorder that can be identified, and many of these patients require treatment with more than antidepressants or with mood stabilizers and atypical antipsychotics instead of antidepressants. This is discussed in detail in Chapter 12, which covers antidepressants, and in Chapter 13, which covers mood stabilizers.

For patients already diagnosed with bipolar disorder, there is similar concern that the disorder may be progressive, especially without adequate treatment. Thus, discrete manic and depressive episodes may progress to mixed and dysphoric episodes and finally to rapid-cycling instability and treatment resistance (Figure 11-29). The hope is that recognition and treatment of both unipolar and bipolar depressions, causing all symptoms to remit for long periods of time, might prevent progression to more difficult states. This is not proved but is a major hypothesis in the field at present.

In the meantime, practitioners must decide whether to commit "sins of omission" and be conservative with the diagnosis of bipolar spectrum disorder, thus erring on the side of undertreatment, or "sins of commission," thus overdiagnosing and overtreating symptoms in the hope that this will prevent disease progression and "diabolical learning" in brain circuits, as discussed in Chapter 8 and illustrated in Figures 8-4 through 8-7.

Mood Disorders | 473

Neurotransmitters and circuits in mood disorders

Three principle neurotransmitters have long been implicated in both the pathophysiology and treatment of mood disorders. They are norepinephrine, dopamine, and serotonin and comprise what is sometimes called the "trimonoaminergic" neurotransmitter system. These three monoamines often work in concert. Many of the symptoms of mood disorders are hypothesized to involve dysfunction of various combinations of these three systems. Essentially all known treatments for mood disorders act on one or more of these three systems.

We have extensively discussed the dopamine system in Chapter 9 and illustrated it in Figures 9-18 to 9-24. We have extensively discussed the serotonin system in Chapter 10 and illustrated it in Figures 10-15 to 10-20. Here we introduce both the norepinephrine system and also some interactions among these three monoaminergic neurotransmitter systems, showing how they interregulate one another. Although other neurotransmitter systems are undoubtedly involved in mood disorders, most is known about the links between trimonoaminergic neurotransmitters and mood disorders, so these neurotransmitters are emphasized here. New therapeutics based on glutamate and neurokinins are discussed briefly in Chapters 12 and 13. Neurotransmitters and hormones of the hypothalamic-pituitary-adrenal (HPA) axis are discussed briefly in Chapter 14, on anxiety and stress.

Noradrenergic neurons

The noradrenergic neuron utilizes norepinephrine (noradrenaline) as its neurotransmitter. Norepinephrine is synthesized, or produced, from the precursor amino acid tyrosine, which is transported into the nervous system from the blood by means of an active transport pump (Figure 11-30). Once inside the neuron, the tyrosine is acted on by three enzymes in sequence: first, tyrosine hydroxylase (TOH), the rate-limiting and most important enzyme in the regulation of NE synthesis. Tyrosine hydroxylase converts the amino acid tyrosine into dopa. The second enzyme then acts, namely, dopa decarboxylase (DDC), which converts dopa into dopamine (DA). DA itself is a neurotransmitter in dopamine neurons, as discussed in Chapter 9 and illustrated in Figure 9-18. However, for NE neurons, DA is just a precursor of NE. In fact the third and final NE synthetic enzyme, dopamine beta hydroxylase (DBH), converts DA into NE. NE is then stored in synaptic packages called vesicles until it is released by a nerve impulse (Figure 11-30).

NE action is terminated by two principal destructive or catabolic enzymes that turn NE into inactive metabolites. The first is monoamine oxidase (MAO) A or B, which is located in mitochondria in the presynaptic neuron and elsewhere (Figure 11-31). The second is catechol-O-methyl-transferase (COMT), which is thought to be located largely outside of the presynaptic nerve terminal (Figure 11-31).

The action of NE can be terminated not only by enzymes that destroy NE but also by a transport pump for NE that prevents NE from acting in the synapse without destroying it (Figure 11-31). In fact, such inactivated NE can be restored for reuse in a later neurotransmitting nerve impulse. The transport pump that terminates synaptic action of NE is sometimes called the "NE transporter" or "NET" and sometimes the "NE reuptake pump." This NE reuptake pump is located on the presynaptic noradrenergic nerve terminal as part of the presynaptic machinery of the neuron, where it acts like a vacuum cleaner, whisking NE out of the synapse, off the synaptic receptors, and stopping its synaptic actions. Once inside the presynaptic nerve terminal, NE can either be stored again for subsequent reuse when another nerve impulse arrives or it can be destroyed by NE-destroying enzymes (Figure 11-31).

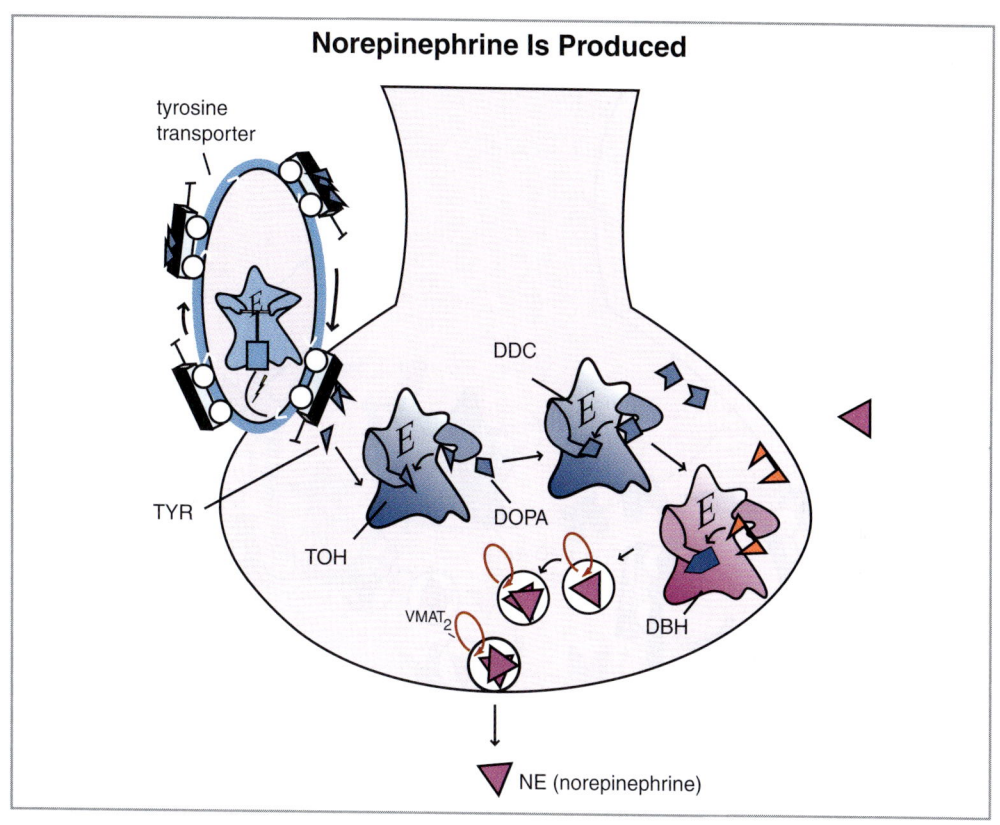

FIGURE 11-30 Norepinephrine is produced. Tyrosine, a precursor to norepinephrine (NE), is taken up into NE nerve terminals via a tyrosine transporter and converted into dopa by the enzyme tyrosine hydroxylase (TOH). Dopa is then converted into dopamine (DA) by the enzyme dopa decarboxylase (DDC). Finally, DA is converted into NE by dopamine beta hydroxylase (DBH). After synthesis, NE is packaged into synaptic vesicles via the vesicular monoamine transporter (VMAT2) and stored there until its release into the synapse during neurotransmission.

The noradrenergic neuron is regulated by a multiplicity of receptors for NE (Figure 11-32). The norepinephrine transporter or NET is one type of receptor, as is the vesicular monoamine transporter (VMAT2), which transports NE in the cytoplasm of the presynaptic neuron into storage vesicles (Figure 11-32). NE receptors are classified as alpha 1A, 1B, 1C or alpha 2A, 2B, or 2C, or as beta 1, beta 2, or beta 3. All can be postsynaptic, but only alpha 2 receptors can act as presynaptic autoreceptors (Figures 11-32 through 11-34). Postsynaptic receptors convert their occupancy by norepinephrine at alpha 1A, B, or C; alpha 2A, B, or C; or beta 1, 2, or 3 receptors into physiological functions and ultimately into changes in signal transduction and gene expression in the postsynaptic neuron (Figure 11-32).

Presynaptic alpha 2 receptors regulate norepinephrine release, so they are called "autoreceptors" (Figures 11-32 and 11-33). Presynaptic alpha 2 autoreceptors are located both on the axon terminal (i.e., terminal alpha 2 receptors; Figures 11-32 and 11-33) and at the cell body (soma) and nearby dendrites; thus, these latter alpha 2 presynaptic receptors are called somatodendritic alpha 2 receptors (Figure 11-34). Presynaptic alpha 2 receptors are important because both the terminal and somatodendritic alpha 2 receptors are autoreceptors. That is, when presynaptic alpha 2 receptors recognize NE, they turn off further release

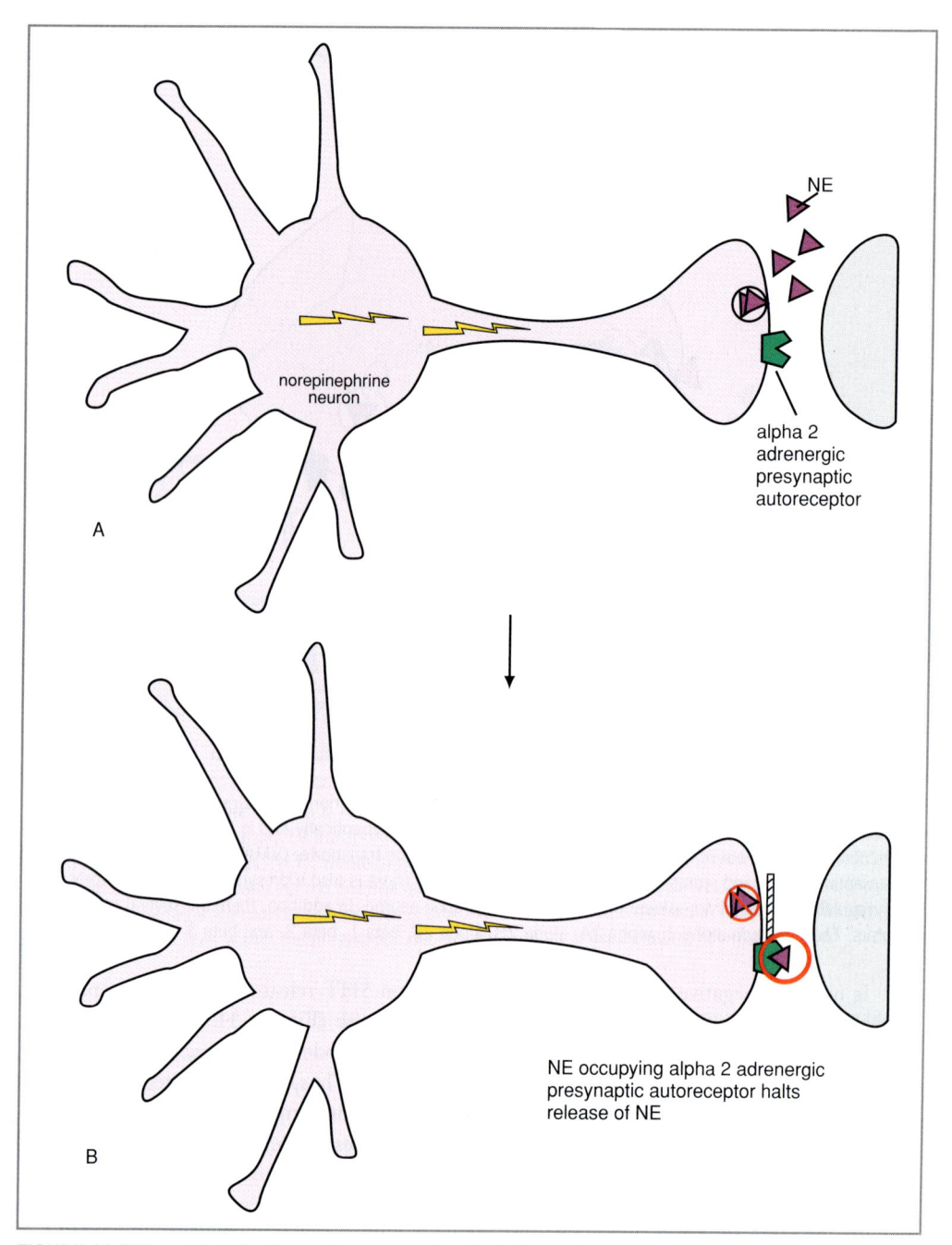

FIGURE 11-33A and B Alpha 2 receptors on axon terminal. Shown here are presynaptic alpha 2 adrenergic autoreceptors located on the axon terminal of the norepinephrine neuron. These autoreceptors are "gatekeepers" for norepinephrine. That is, when they are not bound by norepinephrine, they are open, allowing norepinephrine release (**A**). However, when norepinephrine binds to the gatekeeping receptors, they close the molecular gate and prevent norepinephrine from being released (**B**).

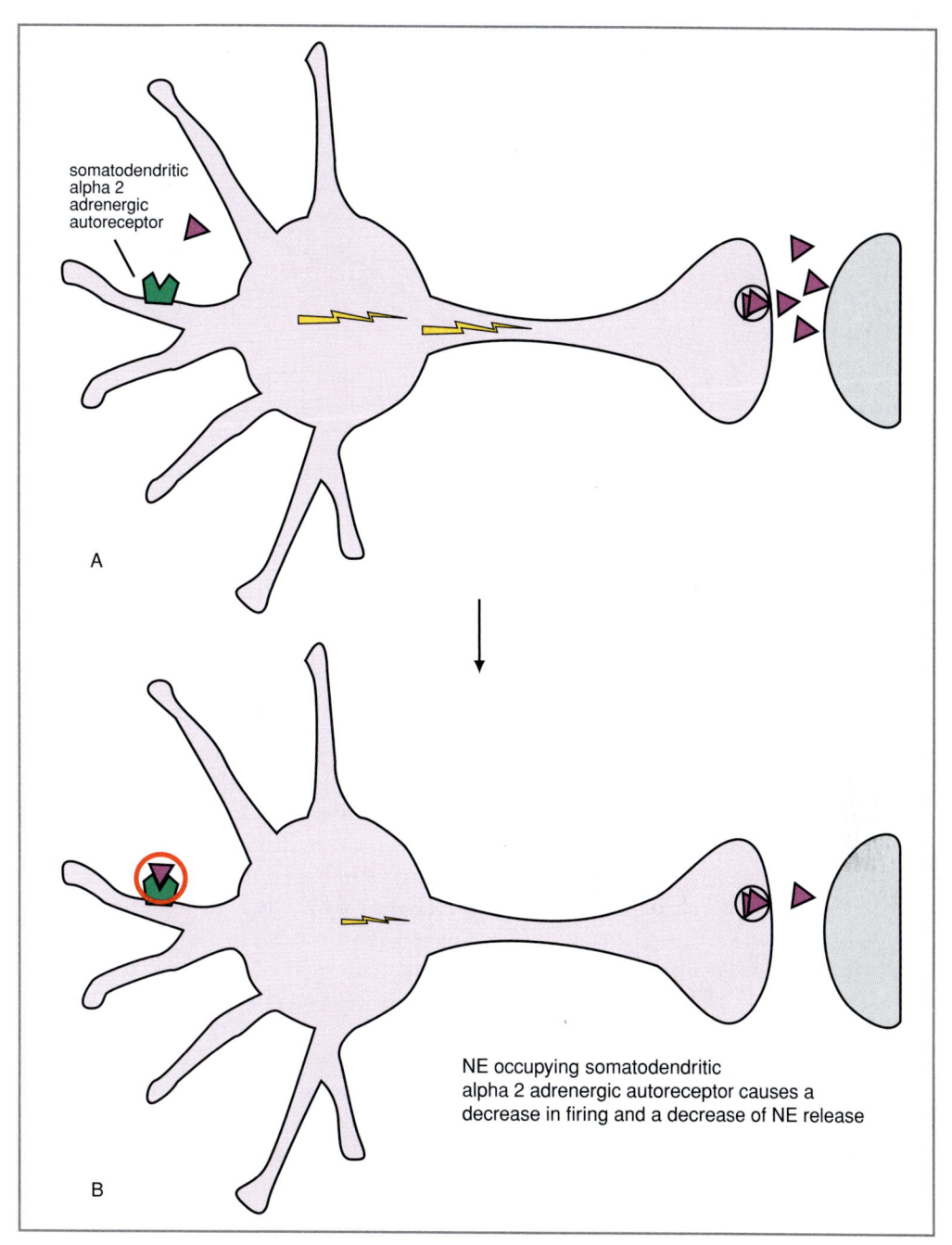

FIGURE 11-34 Somatodendritic alpha 2 receptors. Presynaptic alpha 2 adrenergic autoreceptors are also located in the somatodendritic area of the norepinephrine neuron, as shown here. When norepinephrine binds to these alpha 2 receptors, it shuts off neuronal impulse flow in the norepinephrine neuron (see loss of lightning bolts in the neuron in the lower figure), and this stops further norepinephrine release.

Mood Disorders | 479

NE-5HT Interactions: NE Regulation of 5HT

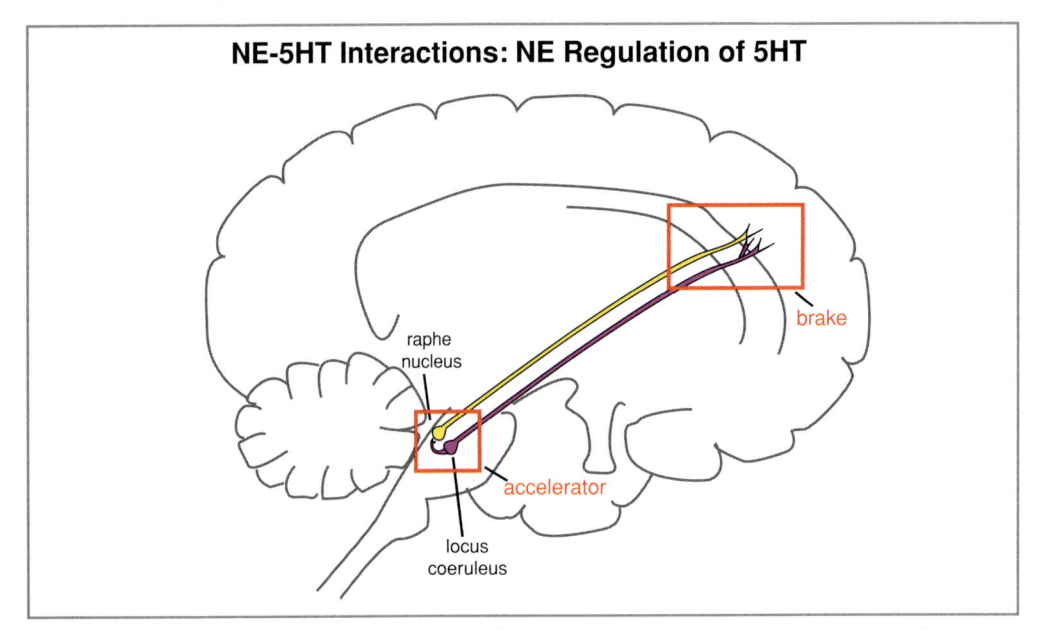

FIGURE 11-35 **Norepinephrine regulation of serotonin.** Norepinephrine regulates serotonin release. It does this by acting as a brake on serotonin release at alpha 2 receptors on axon terminals and as an accelerator of serotonin release at alpha 1 receptors at the somatodendritic area.

our discussion here is aimed at providing a background for understanding the actions of atypical antipsychotics in mood disorders; this is not meant to be a comprehensive review of all aspects of 5HT2A receptor regulation of DA release. Other evidence suggests that some 5HT2A receptors in some brain areas under certain circumstances can actually facilitate DA release (as discussed in Chapter 10 and illustrated in Figure 10-31).

A separate circuit also regulates 5HT2C inhibition of DA release in the nucleus accumbens (Figure 11-41). In this case, 5HT acts upon GABA neurons in the brainstem, one of which inhibits the mesolimbic dopamine projection when 5HT2C receptors are occupied (Figure 11-41). 5HT actions on a second GABA neuron that projects to prefrontal cortex result in inhibition of a descending excitatory glutamate projection to the dopamine neuron, further inhibiting dopamine release in the nucleus accumbens (Figure 11-41).

In summary, there are numerous known interregulatory pathways and receptor interactions among the trimonoaminergic neurontransmitter systems so that they can influence each other and change the release not only of their own neurotransmitters but also of others within this system.

The monoamine hypothesis of depression

The classic theory about the biological etiology of depression hypothesizes that depression is due to a deficiency of monoamine neurotransmitters. At first, there was a great argument about whether norepinephrine (NE) or serotonin (5-hydroxytryptamine; 5HT) was the more important deficiency, and dopamine was relatively neglected. Now the monoamine theory suggests that the entire trimonoaminergic neurotransmitter system may be malfunctioning in various brain circuits, with different neurotransmitters involved depending on the patient's symptom profile.

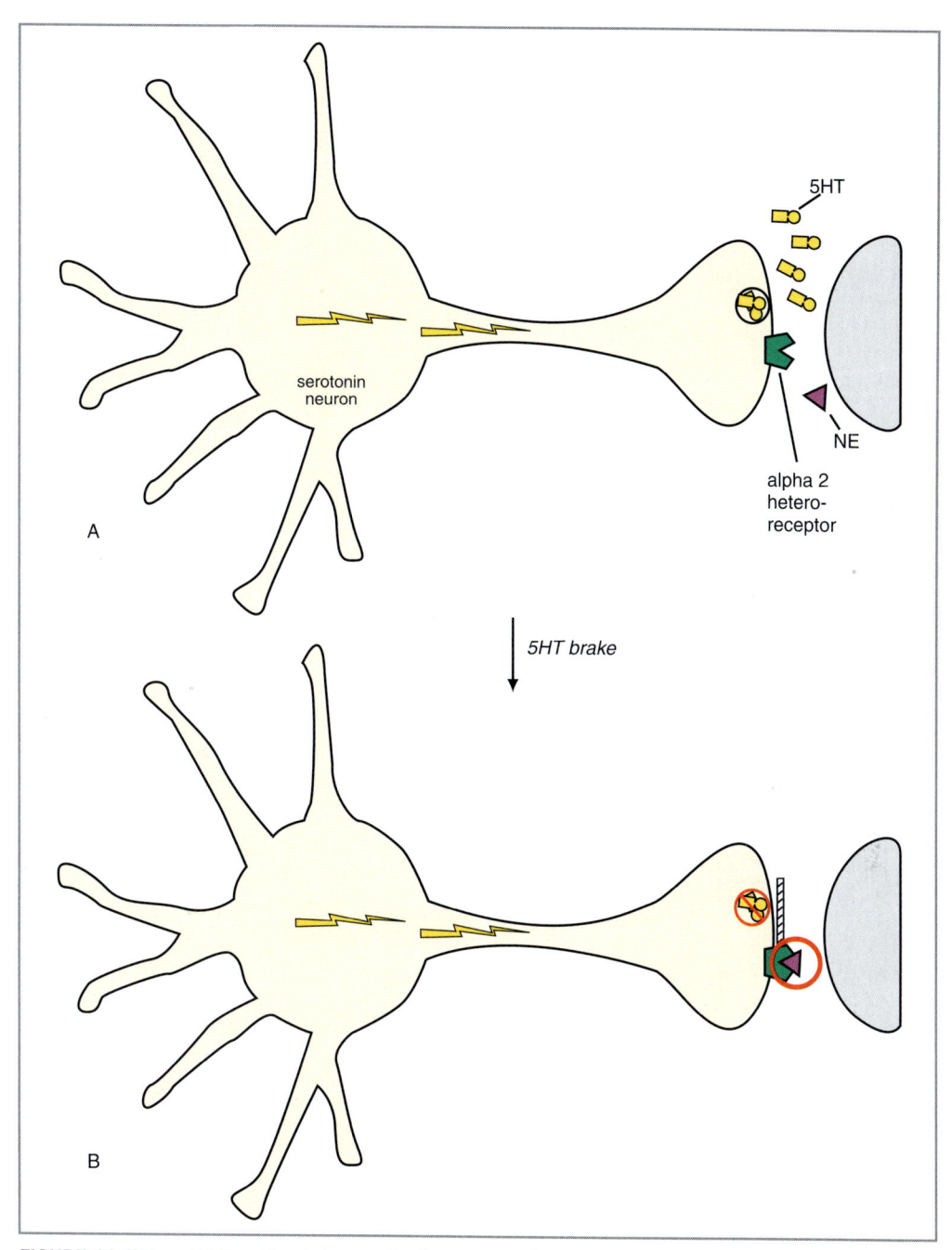

FIGURE 11-36A and B Norepinephrine as a brake on serotonin release. Alpha 2 adrenergic heteroreceptors are located on the axon terminals of serotonin neurons. When these receptors are unoccupied by norepinephrine, serotonin is released from the serotonin neuron (**A**). However, when norepinephrine binds to the alpha 2 receptor this closes the molecular gate and prevents serotonin from being released (**B**).

Mood Disorders

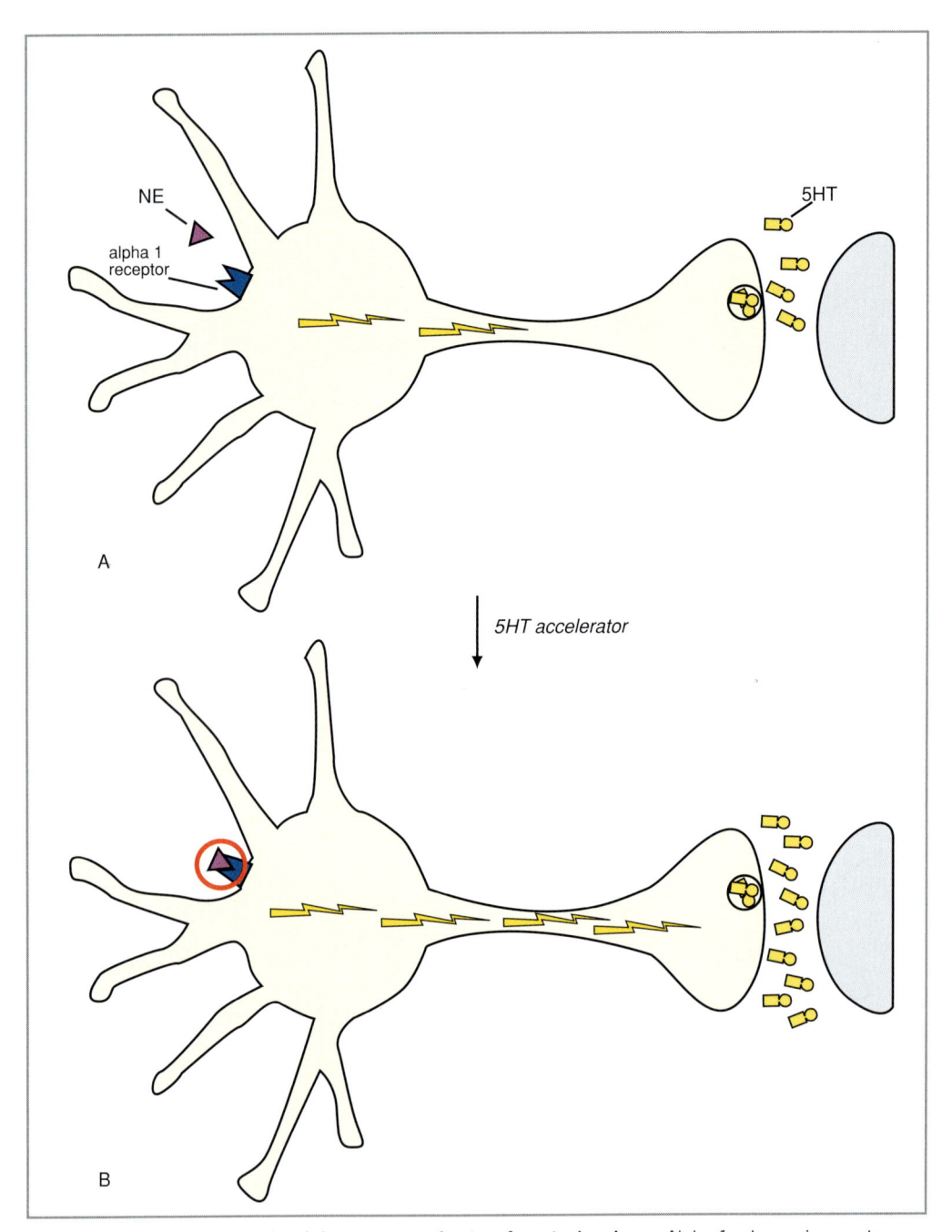

FIGURE 11-37A and B Norepinephrine as an accelerator of serotonin release. Alpha 1 adrenergic receptors are located in the somatodendritic regions of serotonin neurons. When these receptors are unoccupied by norepinephrine, some serotonin is released from the serotonin neuron (**A**). However, when norepinephrine binds to the alpha 1 receptor this stimulates the serotonin neuron, accelerating release of serotonin (**B**).

482 | Essential Psychopharmacology

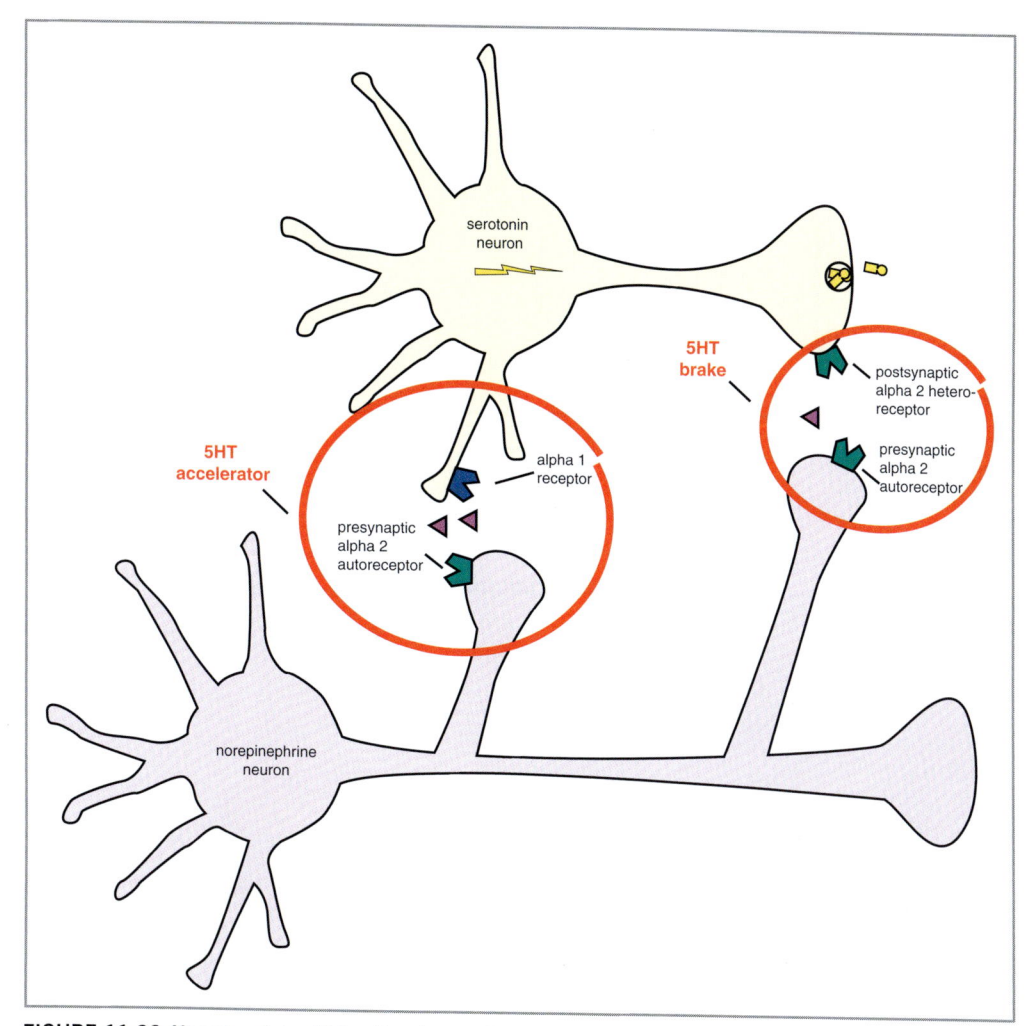

FIGURE 11-38 Norepinephrine bidirectional control of serotonin. Norepinephrine can act as a brake on serotonin release when it binds to alpha 2 receptors at the axon terminal and as an accelerator of serotonin release when it binds to alpha 1 receptors at somatodendritic regions. Thus norepinephrine has bidirectional control of serotonin release.

The original conceptualization was rather simplistic and based on observations that certain drugs which depleted these neurotransmitters could induce depression, and, further, that all effective antidepressants act by boosting one or more of these three monoamine neurotransmitters. Thus the idea was that the "normal" quantity of monoamine neurotransmitters (Figure 11-42A) somehow became depleted – perhaps by an unknown disease process, stress, or drugs (Figure 11-42B) – leading to the symptoms of depression.

Direct evidence for the monoamine hypothesis is still largely lacking. A good deal of effort was expended, especially in the 1960s and 1970s, to identify the theoretically predicted deficiencies of the monoamine neurotransmitters. This effort to date has unfortunately yielded mixed and sometimes confusing results. Some studies suggest that NE metabolites are deficient in some patients with depression, but this has not been uniformly observed. Other studies suggest that the 5HT metabolite 5HIAA (5-hydroxy-indole acetic acid) is

Mood Disorders | 483

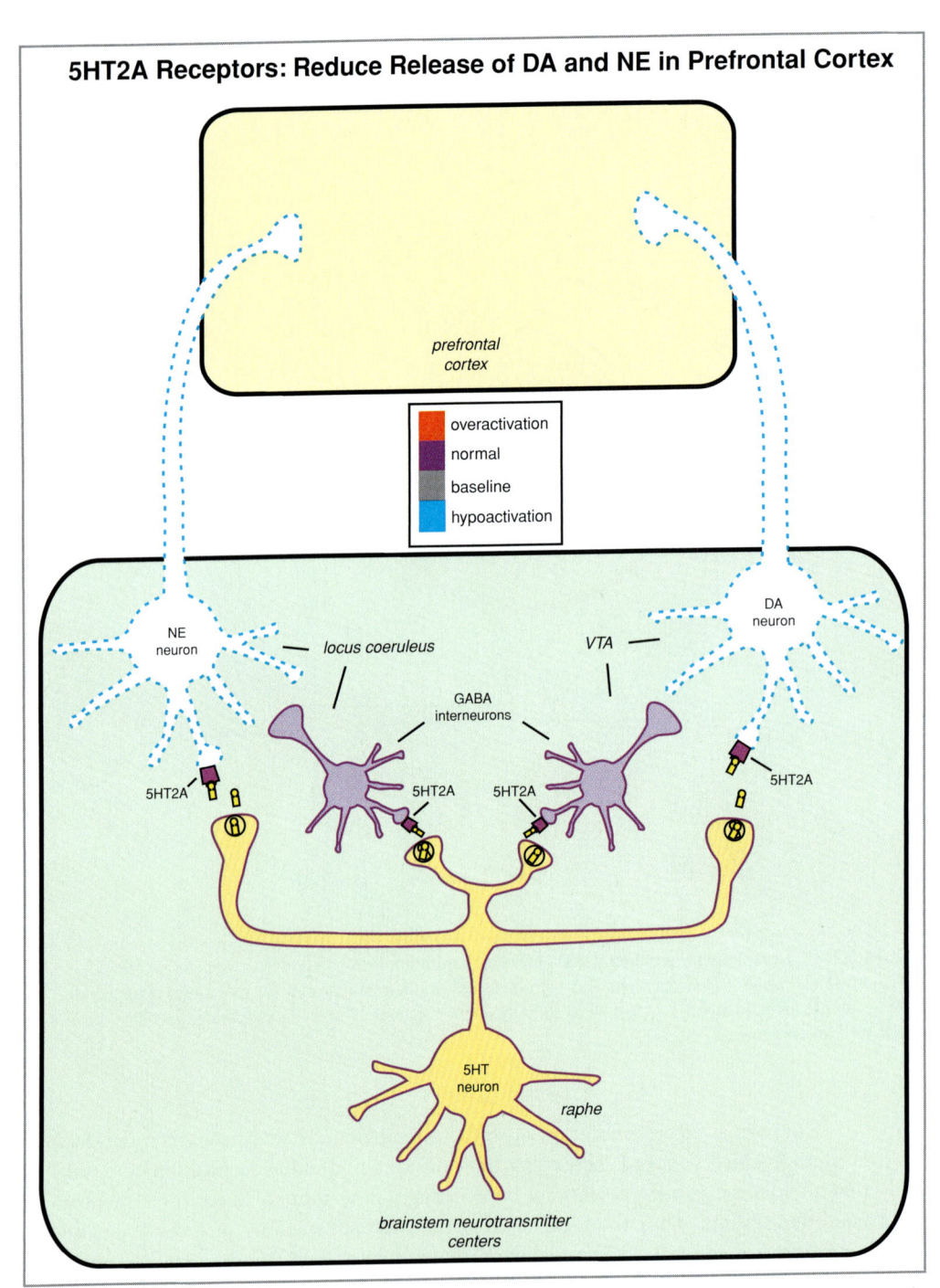

FIGURE 11-39 5HT2A receptors regulate norepinephrine and dopamine. Serotonin (5HT) regulates release of norepinephrine (NE) and dopamine (DA) in the prefrontal cortex via 5HT2A receptors located at the somatodendritic ends of NE, DA, and gamma-aminobutyric acid (GABA) neurons. Binding of 5HT at 5HT2A receptors on some NE and DA neurons in the brainstem directly inhibits release of these neurotransmitters into the prefrontal cortex. In addition, binding of 5HT at 5HT2A receptors on some GABA interneurons in the brainstem *increases* GABA release, which then inhibits NE and DA release.

484 | Essential Psychopharmacology

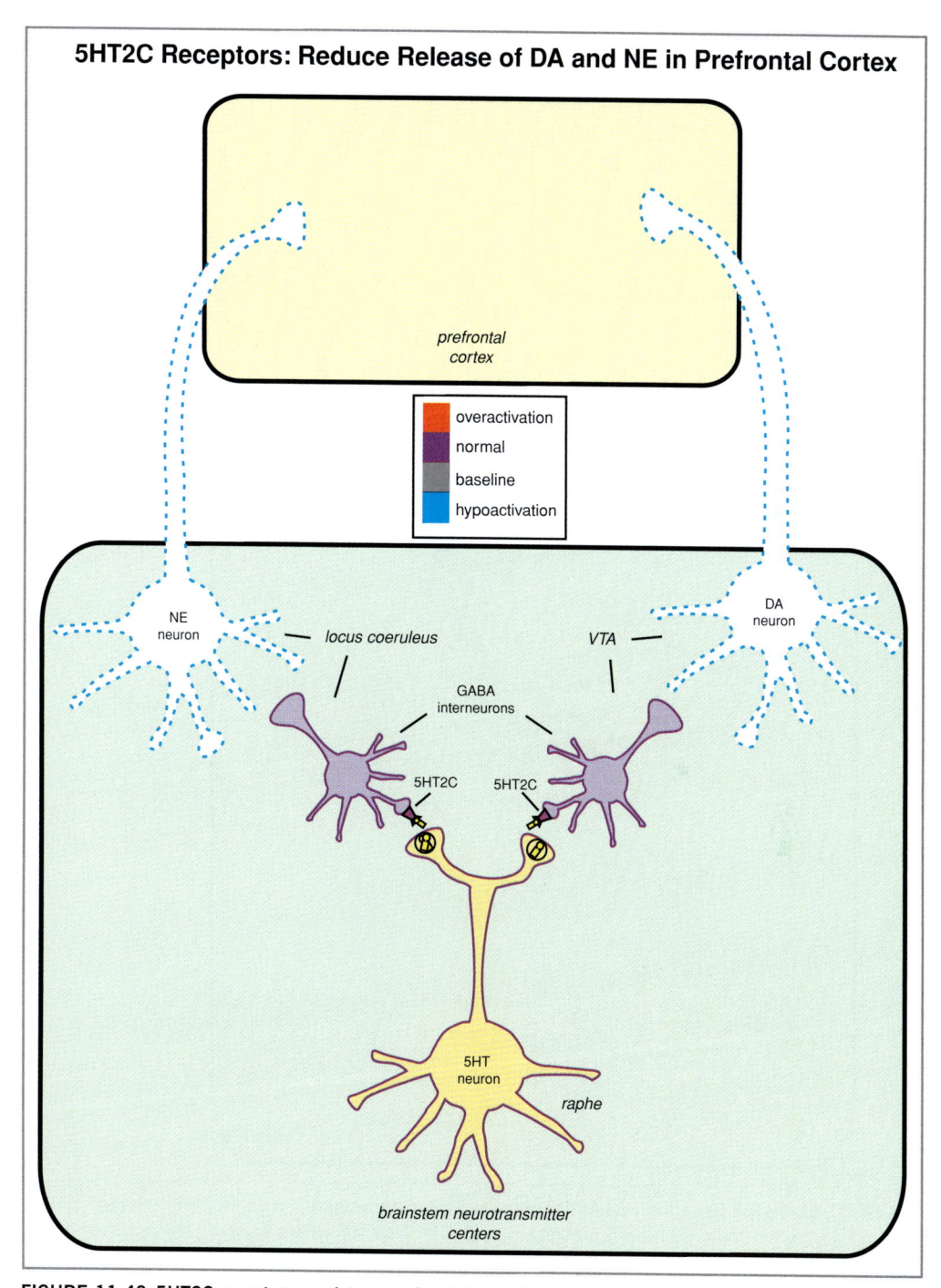

FIGURE 11-40 5HT2C receptors regulate norepinephrine and dopamine. Serotonin (5HT) also regulates release of norepinephrine (NE) and dopamine (DA) in the prefrontal cortex via 5HT2C receptors located on gamma-aminobutyric acid (GABA) interneurons in the brainstem. Binding of 5HT at 5HT2C receptors on these GABA interneurons *increases* GABA release, which then inhibits NE and DA release from their respective neurons.

Mood Disorders | 485

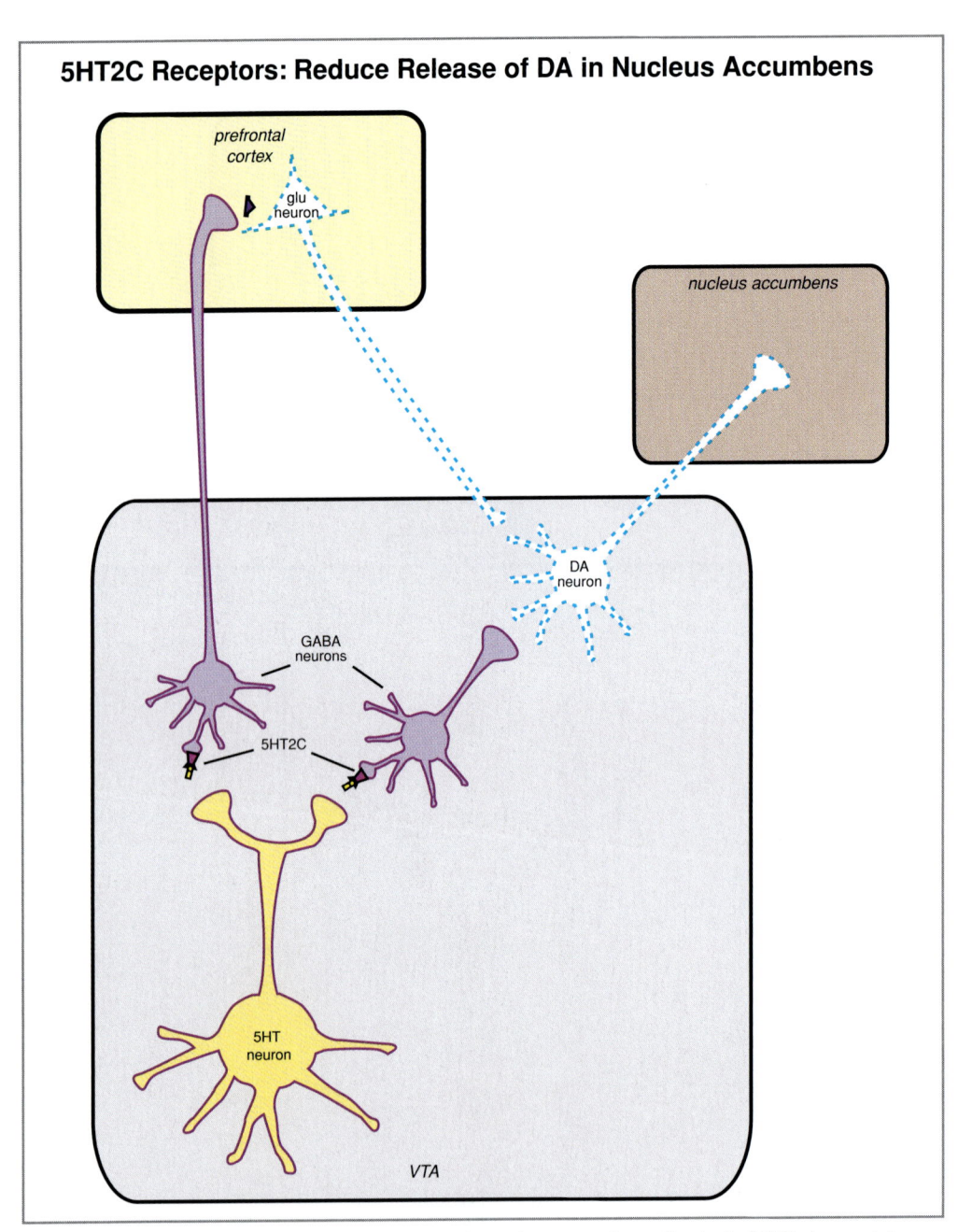

FIGURE 11-41 5HT2C receptors regulate dopamine in nucleus accumbens. Serotonin (5HT) also regulates release of dopamine (DA) in the nucleus accumbens via 5HT2C receptors on two types of gamma-aminobutyric acid (GABA) neurons. First, stimulation of 5HT2C receptors on GABA interneurons within the brainstem (on the right) causes release of GABA there, which in turn inhibits activity of ascending mesolimbic dopamine projections. This results in reduced DA release in the nucleus accumbens. Second, stimulation of 5HT2C receptors on GABA neurons that project out of the brainstem and into the prefrontal cortex (on the left) leads to inhibition of descending glutamate projections to brainstem dopamine neurons. This, in turn, also leads to reduced DA in the nucleus accumbens.

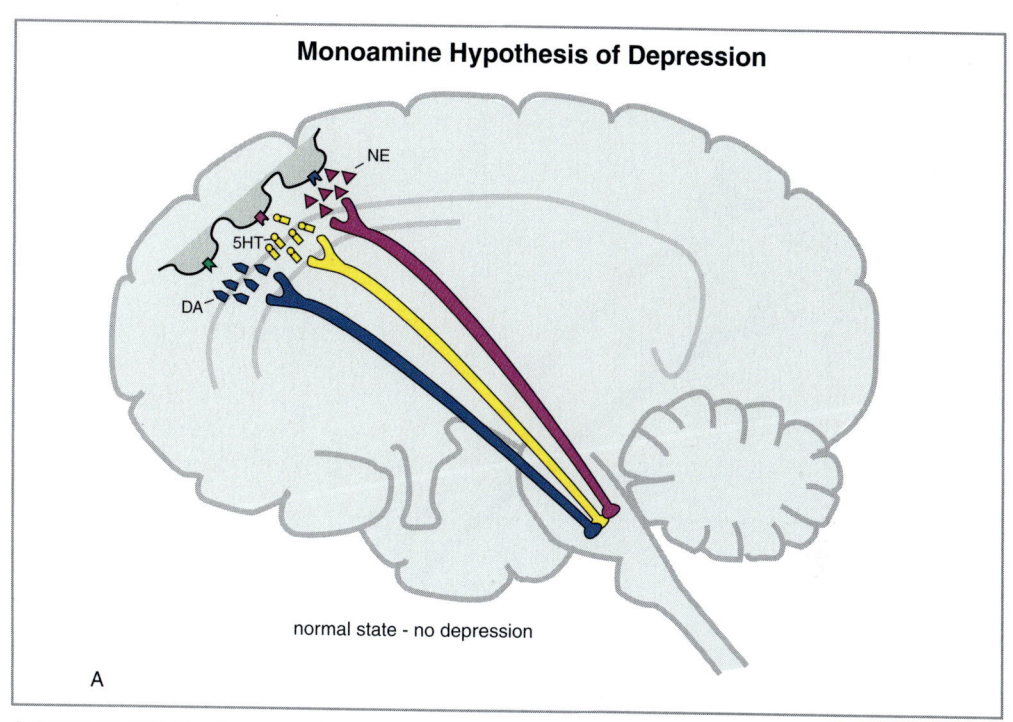

FIGURE 11-42A Classic monoamine hypothesis of depression, part 1. According to the classic monoamine hypothesis of depression, when there is a "normal" amount of monoamine neurotransmitter activity, there is no depression present.

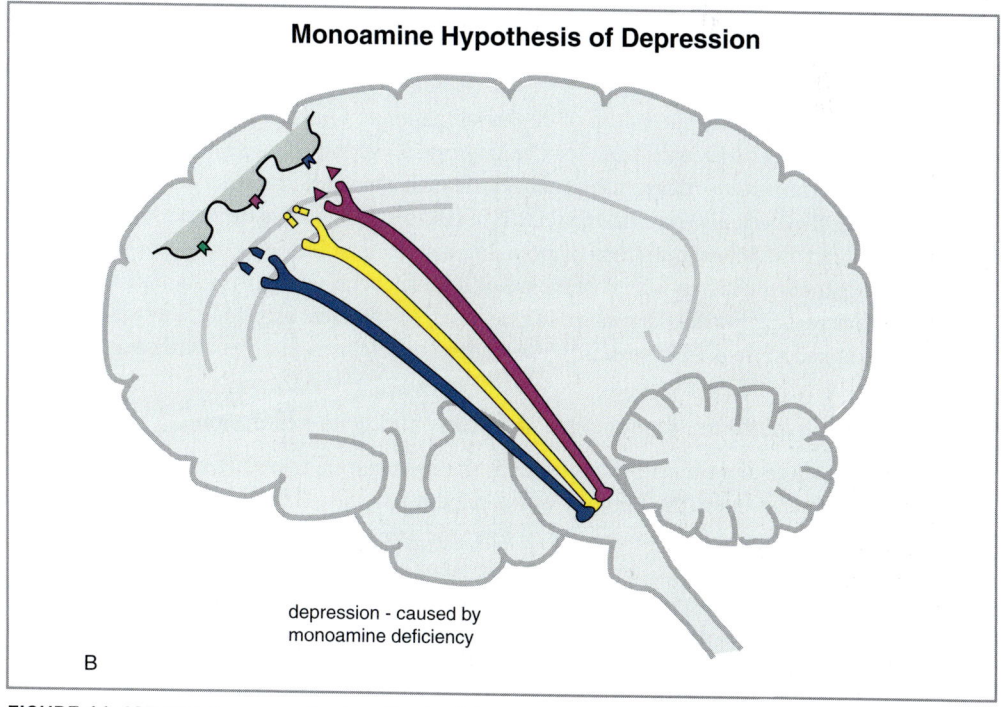

FIGURE 11-42B Classic monoamine hypothesis of depression, part 2. The monoamine hypothesis of depression posits that if the "normal" amount of monoamine neurotransmitter activity becomes reduced, depleted, or dysfunctional for some reason, depression may ensue.

Mood Disorders | 487

Monoamine Receptor Hypothesis of Depression

receptors upregulate
due to lack of monoamines

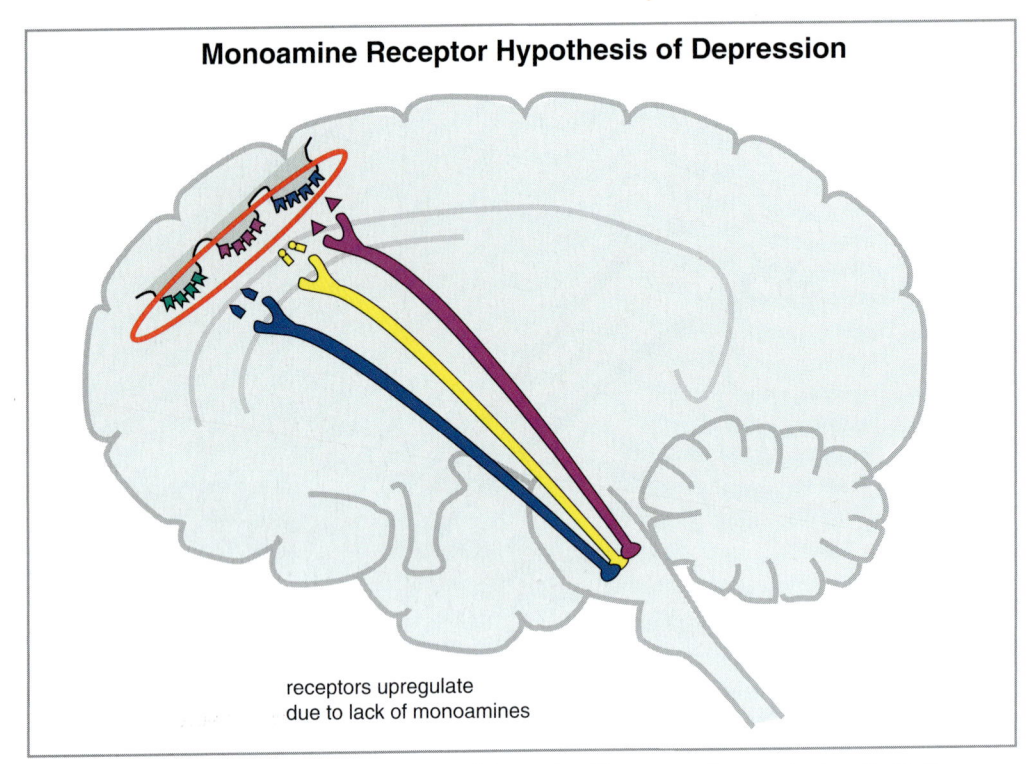

FIGURE 11-43 Monoamine receptor hypothesis of depression. The monoamine receptor hypothesis of depression extends the classic monoamine hypothesis of depression, positing that deficient activity of monoamine neurotransmitters causes upregulation of postsynaptic monoamine neurotransmitter receptors, and that this leads to depression.

reduced in the cerebrospinal fluid of depressed patients. On closer examination, however, it has been found that only some of the depressed patients have low CSF 5HIAA, and they tend to be those with impulsive behaviors, such as suicide attempts of a violent nature. Subsequently, it was also reported that CSF 5HIAA is decreased in other populations noted to be subject to violent outbursts or poor impulse control but who were not depressed – namely, patients with antisocial personality disorder who were arsonists and those with borderline personality disorder who engaged in self-destructive acts. Thus, low CSF 5HIAA may be linked more closely with impulse-control problems rather than with depression.

The monoamine hypothesis, monoamine receptors, and gene expression

Because of these and other difficulties with the monoamine hypothesis of depression, the focus of hypotheses for the etiology of depression has shifted from the monoamine neurotransmitters themselves to their receptors and the downstream molecular events that these receptors trigger, including the regulation of gene expression. For example, the neurotransmitter receptor hypothesis of depression posits that an abnormality in the receptors for monoamine neurotransmitters leads to depression (Figure 11-43). Thus, if depletion of monoamine neurotransmitters is the central theme of the monoamine hypothesis of depression (Figure 11-42B), the neurotransmitter receptor hypothesis of depression takes this theme one step further: namely, that the depletion of neurotransmitter causes compensatory upregulation of postsynaptic neurotransmitter receptors (Figure 11-43).

Essential Psychopharmacology

Direct evidence for this is also generally lacking. Postmortem studies do consistently show increased numbers of serotonin 2 receptors in the frontal cortex of patients who commit suicide. Also, some neuroimaging studies have identified abnormalities in serotonin receptors of depressed patients, but this approach has not yet been successful in identifying consistent and replicable molecular lesions in receptors for monoamines in depression.

Thus, there is no clear and convincing evidence that monoamine deficiency accounts for depression; that is, there is no "real" monoamine deficit. Likewise, there is no clear and convincing evidence that abnormalities in monoamine receptors account for depression. Emphasis is now turning to the possibility that in depression there may be a deficiency in downstream signal transduction of the monoamine neurotransmitter and its postsynaptic neuron that is occurring in the presence of normal amounts of neurotransmitter and receptor. Thus the hypothesized molecular problem in depression could lie within the molecular events distal to the receptor, in the signal transduction cascade system and in appropriate gene expression. This is the subject of much current research into the potential molecular basis of affective disorders.

One candidate mechanism that has been proposed as the site of a possible flaw in signal transduction from monoamine receptors is the target gene for brain-derived neurotrophic factor (BDNF) (see discussion in Chapter 2 and illustrations in Figures 2-5 through 2-7 and Figure 2-10). Normally, BDNF sustains the viability of brain neurons; but under stress, the gene for BDNF may be repressed, leading to the atrophy and possible apoptosis of vulnerable neurons in the hippocampus when their neurotrophic factor BDNF is cut off. The idea is that this, in turn, leads to depression and to the consequences of repeated depressive episodes; namely, more and more episodes and less and less responsiveness to treatment. This possibility that hippocampal neurons are decreased in size and impaired in function during depression and anxiety disorders is supported by recent clinical imaging studies showing decreased brain volume of related structures.

This provides a molecular and cellular hypothesis of depression consistent with a mechanism distal to the neurotransmitter receptor and involving an abnormality in gene expression. Thus, stress-induced vulnerability decreases the expression of genes that make neurotrophic factors such as BDNF, which are critical to the survival and function of key neurons. A corollary to this hypothesis is that antidepressants act by reversing this by causing the genes for neurotrophic factors to be activated. The biological consequences of stress are discussed further in Chapter 14, on anxiety disorders.

Although the monoamine hypothesis is obviously an overly simplified notion about depression, it has been very valuable in focusing attention on the three monoamine neurotransmitter systems: norepinephrine, dopamine, and serotonin. This has led to a much better understanding of the physiological functioning of these three neurotransmitters and especially the various mechanisms by which all known antidepressants act to boost neurotransmission at one or more of these three monoamine neurotransmitter systems.

Symptoms and circuits in depression

The monoamine hypothesis of depression is now being applied to elucidating how the trimonoaminergic neurotransmitter system regulates the efficiency of information processing in a wide variety of neuronal circuits that may be responsible for mediating the various symptoms of depression. Obviously numerous symptoms are required for the diagnosis of a major depressive episode (Figure 11-44). Each symptom is hypothetically associated

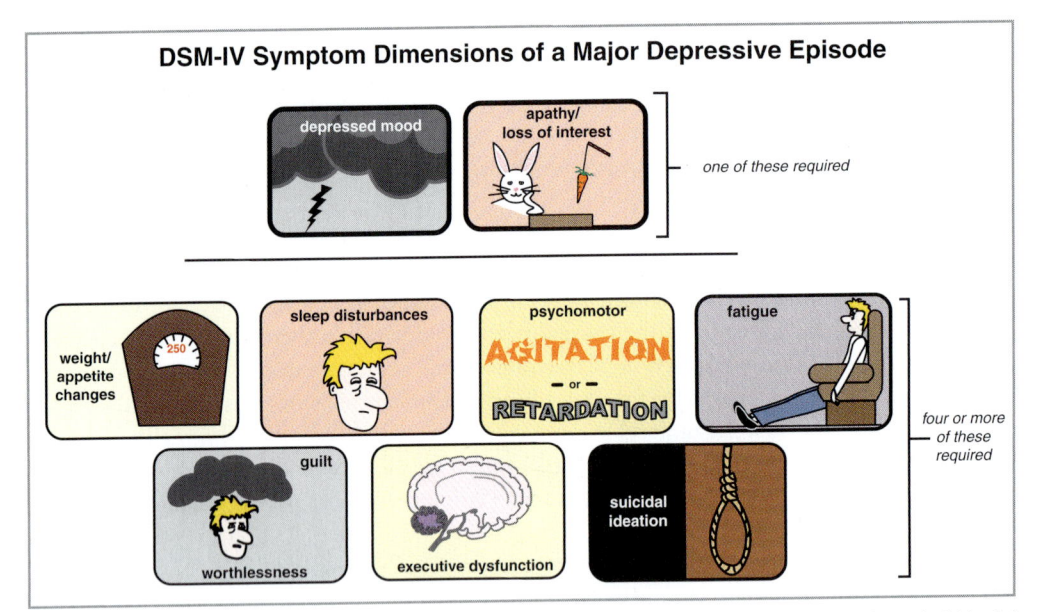

FIGURE 11-44 DSM-IV symptoms of depression. According to the *Diagnostic and Statistical Manual of Mental Disorders*, fourth edition (DSM-IV), a major depressive episode consists of either depressed mood or loss of interest and at least four of the following: weight/appetite changes, insomnia or hypersomnia, psychomotor agitation or retardation, fatigue, feelings of guilt or worthlessness, executive dysfunction, and suicidal ideation.

with inefficient information processing in various brain circuits, with different symptoms topographically localized to specific brain regions (Figure 11-45).

Not only can each of the nine symptoms listed for the diagnosis of a major depressive episode be mapped onto brain circuits that theoretically mediate these symptoms (Figure 11-45), but the hypothetical trimonoaminergic regulation of each of these brain areas can also be mapped onto each brain region they innervate (Figures 11-46 to 11-54). This creates a set of monoamine neurotransmitters that regulate each specific hypothetically malfunctioning brain region. Targeting each region with drugs that act on the relevant neurotransmitters within the trimonoaminergic neurotransmitter system could potentially lead to reduction of each individual symptom experienced by a specific patient by enhancing the efficiency of information processing in malfunctioning circuits for each specific symptom. If successful, this targeting of monoamines in specific brain areas could eliminate symptoms and cause a major depressive episode to go into remission (Figures 11-46 through 11-54).

Generally, the monoaminergic functioning in these circuits in major depressive disorder are represented as being blue, or reduced, consistent with the monoamine hypothesis. However, the more accurate portrayal may be "out of tune" rather than simply deficient. Some brain regions in depression, in fact, have enhanced neuronal activation, and others have reduced neuronal activation. Nevertheless, trimonoaminergic treatments available today for depression all generally boost one or more of the monoamines.

For example, the core symptom of a major depressive episode is depressed mood, thought to be linked to inefficient information processing in the amygdala and in "emotional" areas of the prefrontal cortex, especially the ventromedial prefrontal cortex (VMPFC) and the nearby subgenual area of the anterior cingulate cortex (Figure 11-46). Each of the three monoamine neurotransmitters of the trimonoaminergic neurotransmitter system

490 | Essential Psychopharmacology

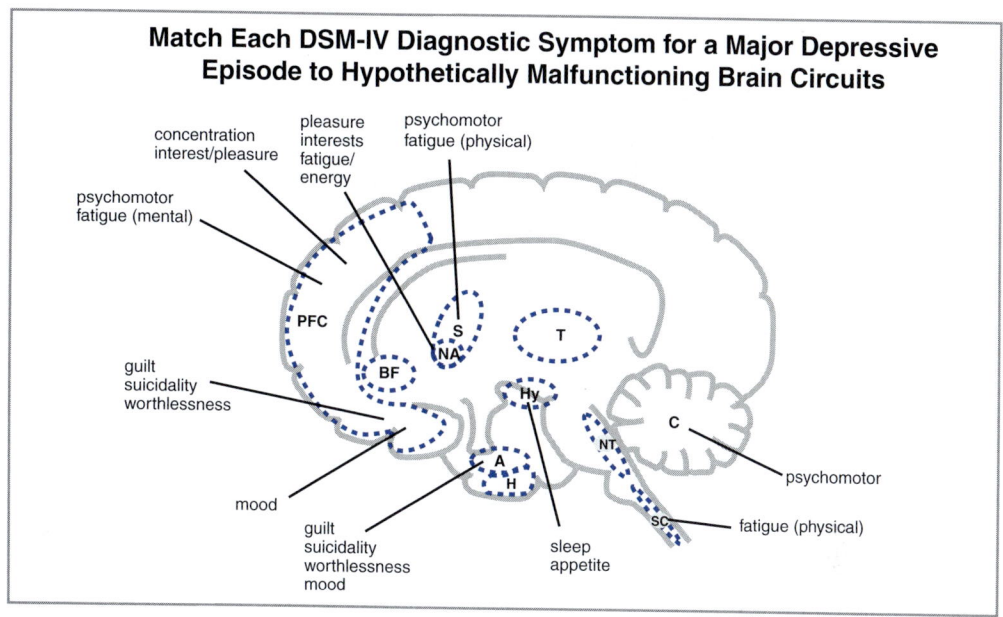

FIGURE 11-45 Matching depression symptoms to circuits. Alterations in neuronal activity and in the efficiency of information processing within each of the eleven brain regions shown here can lead to symptoms of a major depressive episode. Functionality in each brain region is hypothetically associated with a different constellation of symptoms. PFC, prefrontal cortex; BF, basal forebrain; S, striatum; NA, nucleus accumbens; T, thalamus; HY, hypothalamus; A, amygdala; H, hippocampus; NT, brainstem neurotransmitter centers; SC, spinal cord; C, cerebellum.

innervates these areas; it is therefore not surprising that antidepressants that boost any of these neurotransmitters can improve mood in depression (Figure 11-46).

Apathy or loss of interest is another key symptom of depression and may be more common in elderly patients with depression, even in the absence of depressed mood. How can someone have apathy without depressed mood? The answer is because these symptoms may involve different brain circuits and different neurotransmitters. That is, apathy may involve the prefrontal cortex diffusely, including not only VMPFC but also especially dorsolateral prefrontal cortex as well as the hypothalamic "drive" centers and the nucleus accumbens "pleasure" or interest center (Figure 11-47). Furthermore, whereas deficient dopamine and norepinephrine may regulate these areas and boosting them with antidepressants may help relieve such symptoms associated with these areas, boosting serotonin may actually act to reduce both of these neurotransmitters and make symptoms worse. The mechanisms by which serotonin reduces them are discussed earlier in this chapter and illustrated in Figures 11-39 to 11-41. Thus only NE and DA are shown in Figure 11-47.

Sleep disturbances may be diffusely represented in several brain areas, especially hypothalamus, thalamus, basal forebrain, and diffusely throughout prefrontal cortex, with regulatory input by all three monoamines (Figure 11-48). Fatigue or loss of energy is linked to deficient functioning of NE and DA in prefrontal cortex, especially for mental fatigue, as well as in striatum and nucleus accumbens, especially for physical fatigue (Figure 11-49). Executive dysfunction is fairly well characterized as having localization in the dorsolateral prefrontal cortex (DLPFC) and being regulated mostly by DA and NE (Figure 11-50). Psychomotor symptoms, either agitation or retardation, are linked to motor circuits, especially in the striatum but also in the prefrontal cortex and secondarily perhaps in the cerebellum

Mood Disorders | 491

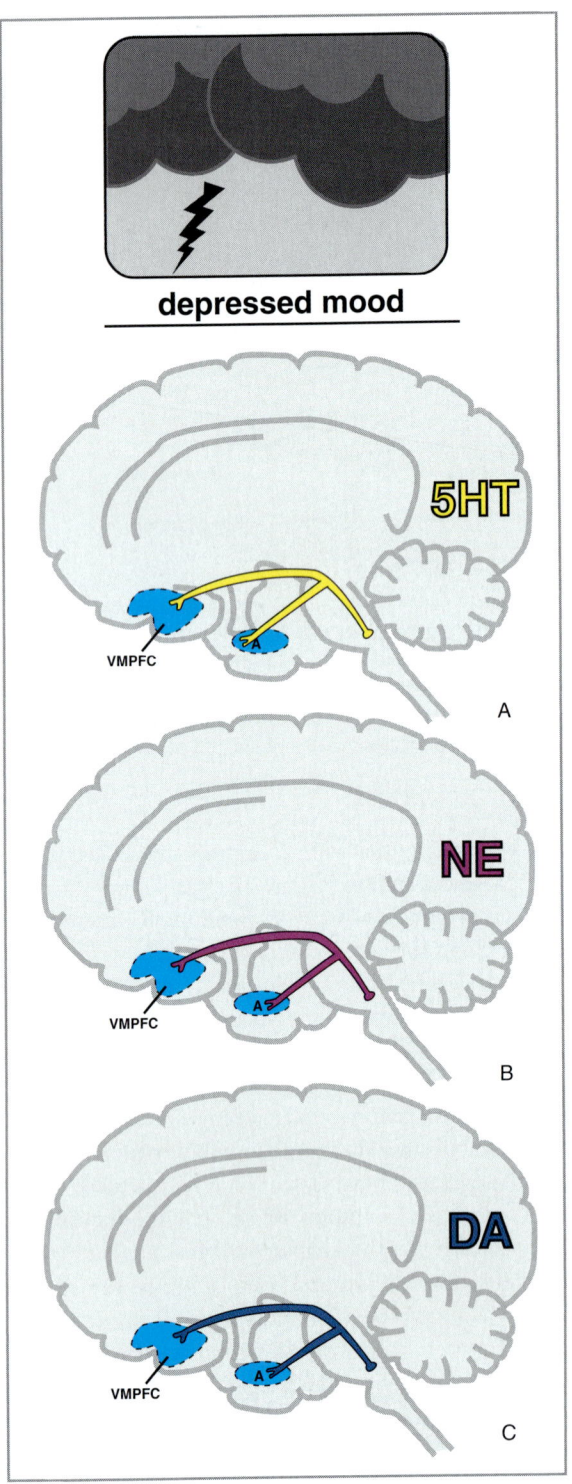

FIGURE 11-46A, B, and C Depressed mood circuits. Depressed mood is believed to be linked to inefficient information processing in the amygdala (A) and the ventromedial prefrontal cortex (VMPFC), both of which are innervated by serotonergic (**A**), noradrenergic (**B**), and dopaminergic (**C**) projections from brainstem nuclei. Reduced, dysfunctional, and inefficient monoaminergic functioning in these regions is depicted here as hypoactive (blue color).

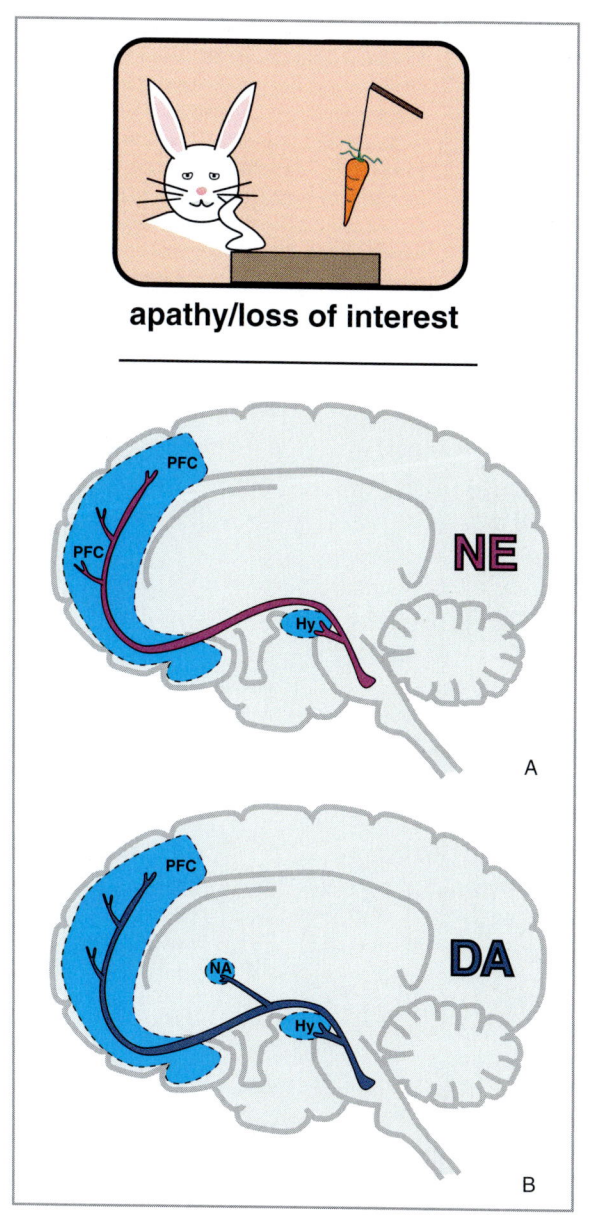

FIGURE 11-47A and B Apathy circuits. Although apathy and depressed mood are often considered similar symptoms, they are hypothetically regulated by different brain circuits. Apathy is believed to be related to inefficient information processing (depicted here as blue or hypoactive) diffusely through the prefrontal cortex (PFC) as well as in hypothalamic centers (Hy) and the nucleus accumbens (NA). These functions within the prefrontal cortex and hypothalamus are thought to be regulated in part by noradrenergic neurons that project there (**A**), while within prefrontal cortex, hypothalamus, and nucleus accumbens these functions are also thought to be regulated by dopaminergic projections (**B**).

as well (Figure 11-51). Changes in weight and appetite, either increased or decreased, have important hypothalamic and serotonergic components to their regulation (Figure 11-52). Suicidal ideation (Figure 11-53) as well as feelings of guilt and worthlessness (Figure 11-54) all have profound connections to serotonin and to circuits connecting to amygdala and emotional regulatory areas of the prefrontal cortex, including the ventromedial prefrontal cortex and perhaps the orbitofrontal cortex.

Many of the mood-related symptoms of depression can be categorized as having either too little positive affect or too much negative affect (Figure 11-55). This idea is linked to the fact that there are diffuse anatomic connections of the trimonoaminergic neurotransmitter system throughout the brain, with diffuse dopamine dysfunction in this system

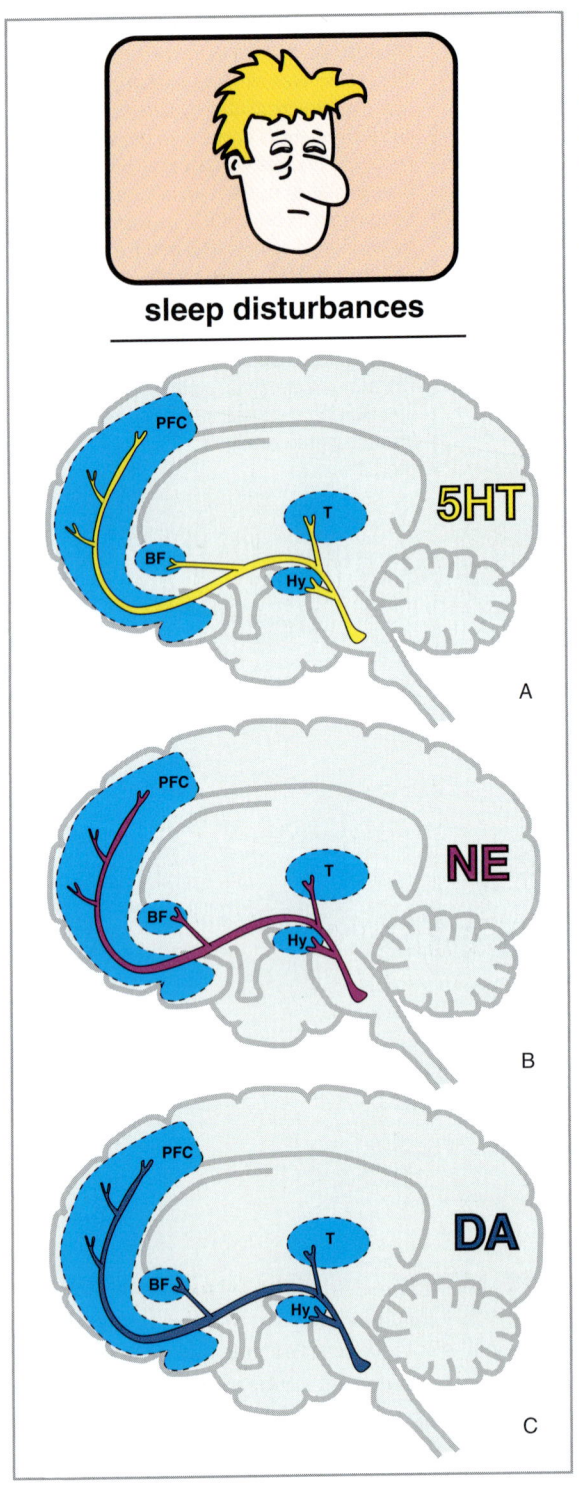

FIGURE 11-48A, B, and C Sleep circuits. Sleep disturbances are believed to be linked to inefficient information processing in the hypothalamus (Hy), thalamus (T), basal forebrain (BF), and diffusely in the prefrontal cortex (PFC), depicted here by the blue color representing hypoactivity. All of these brain regions are regulated by serotonergic (**A**), noradrenergic (**B**), and dopaminergic (**C**) projections from brainstem nuclei.

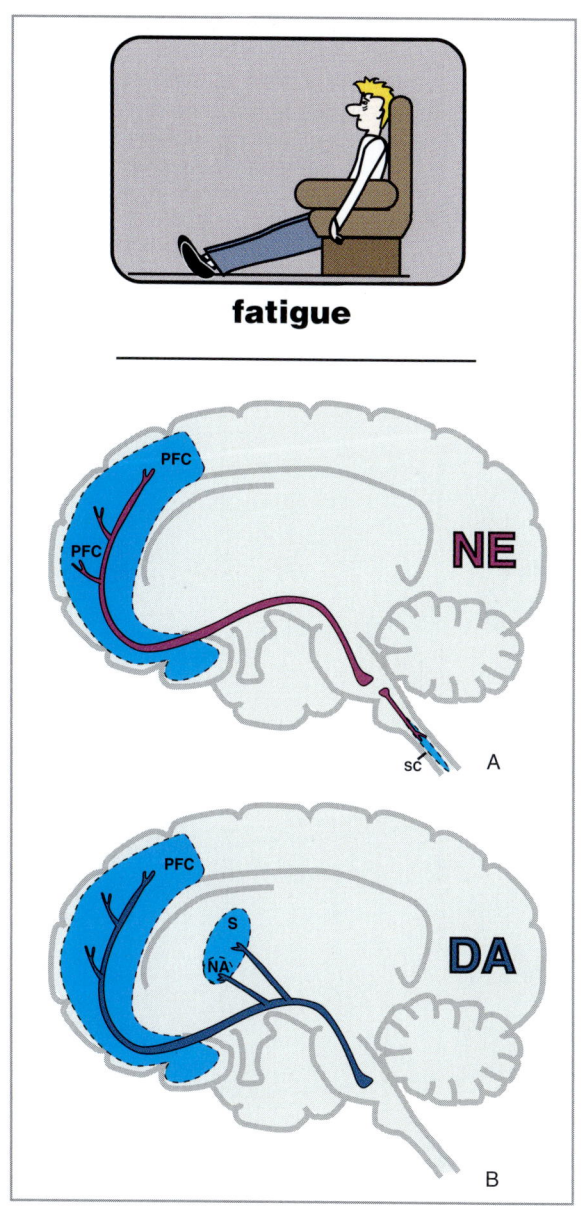

FIGURE 11-49A and B Fatigue circuits. Fatigue or loss of energy is linked to inefficient information processing in several brain regions as well as in the spinal cord, shown here as hypoactivity (blue color). Specifically, mental fatigue is related to deficient noradrenergic functioning in the prefrontal cortex (PFC), while physical fatigue is related to deficient noradrenergic functioning in descending spinal cord (SC) projections (**A**). Dopamine also plays a role in fatigue, with deficient dopaminergic functioning in the PFC related to mental fatigue and deficient dopaminergic functioning in the striatum (S), nucleus accumbens (NA), hypothalamus (Hy), and SC related to physical fatigue (**B**).

driving predominantly the reduction of positive affect, with diffuse serotonin dysfunction driving predominantly the increase in negative affect, and with norepinephrine dysfunction being involved in both. Thus reduced positive affect includes such symptoms as depressed mood but also loss of happiness, joy, interest, pleasure, alertness, energy, enthusiasm, and self-confidence (Figure 11-55, on the left). Enhancing dopamine function and possibly also norepinephrine function may improve information processing in the circuits mediating this cluster of symptoms. On the other hand, increased negative affect includes not only depressed mood but also guilt, disgust, fear, anxiety, hostility, irritability, and loneliness (Figure 11-55, on the right). The enhancement of serotonin function and possibly also norepinephrine function may improve information processing in the circuits that

Mood Disorders | 495

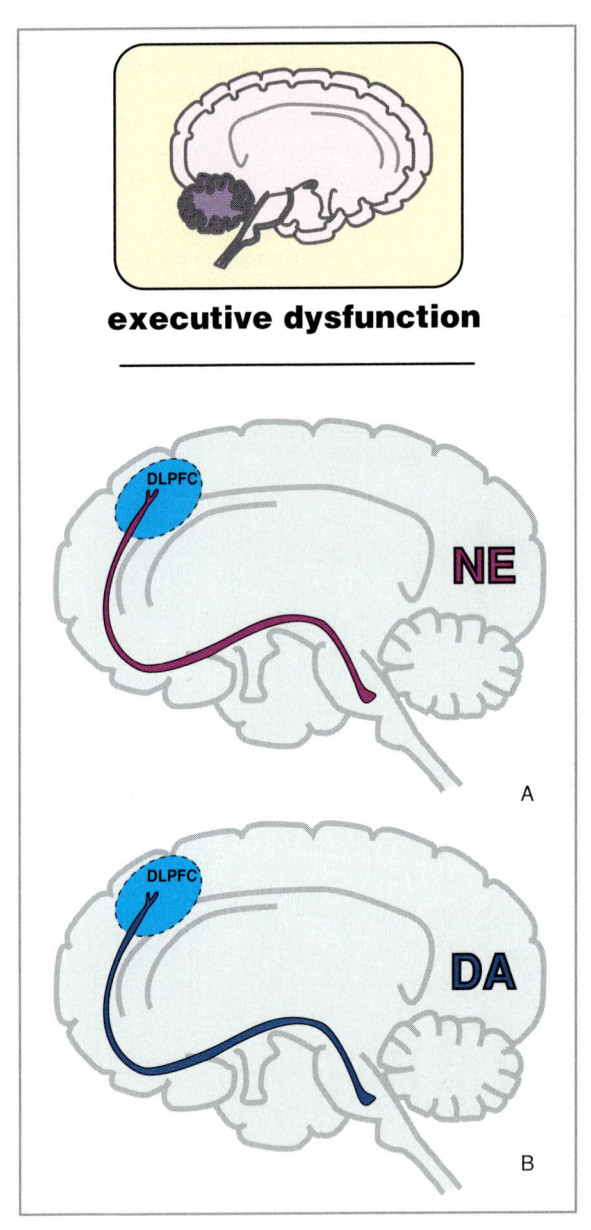

FIGURE 11-50A and B Executive dysfunction circuits. Executive dysfunction is associated with inefficient information processing (depicted here as blue or hypoactive), specifically in the dorsolateral prefrontal cortex (DLPFC), which receives important regulatory projections from both noradrenergic (**A**) and dopaminergic (**B**) neurons.

hypothetically mediate this cluster of symptoms. Patients with symptoms of both clusters may require triple-action treatments that boost all three of the trimonoamine neurotransmitters.

Symptoms and circuits in mania

The same general paradigm of trimonoaminergic neurotransmitter system regulation of the efficiency of information processing in specific brain circuits can be applied to mania as well as depression, although this is frequently thought to be in the opposite direction and in some overlapping but some different brain regions compared to depression. The numerous

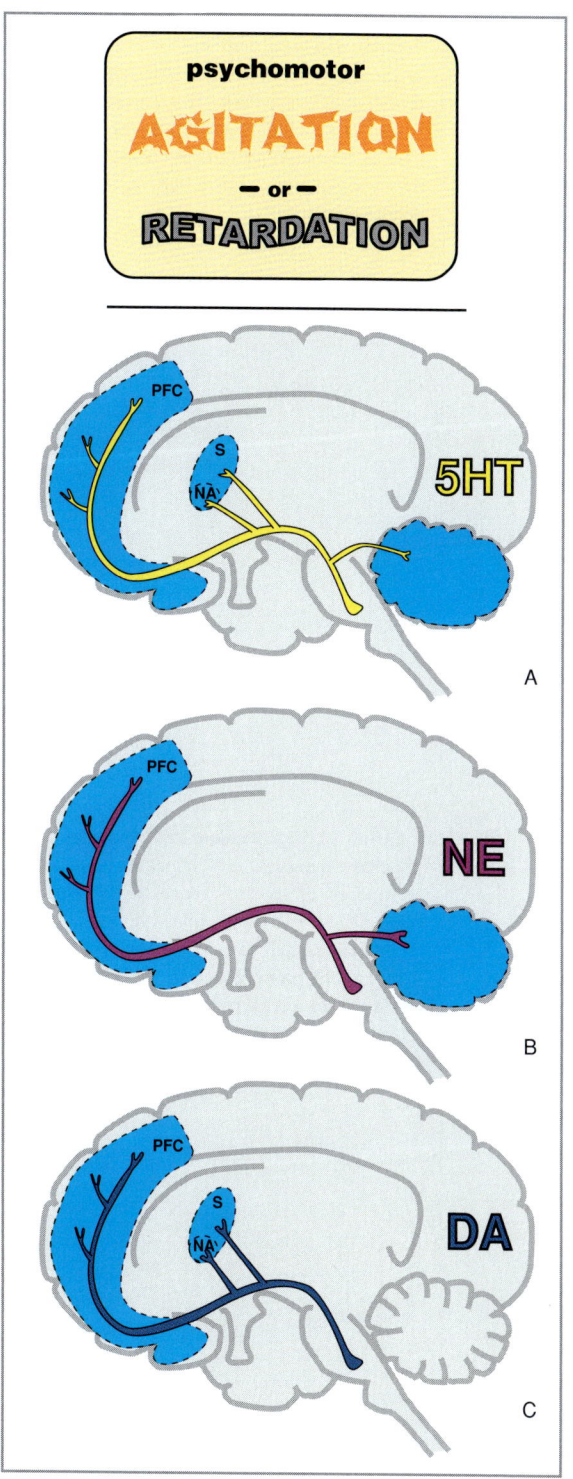

FIGURE 11-51A, B, and C Psychomotor symptom circuits. Psychomotor agitation or retardation may be related to inefficient information processing in multiple brain regions innervated by serotonergic (**A**), noradrenergic (**B**), and/or dopaminergic (**C**) projections. These regions include the cerebellum, which receives serotonergic and noradrenergic projections, the striatum and nucleus accumbens, which receive serotonergic and dopaminergic projections, and the prefrontal cortex (PFC), which receives projections from all three monoamines. In this figure, the monoaminergic functioning is depicted as hypoactive (blue color).

Mood Disorders | 497

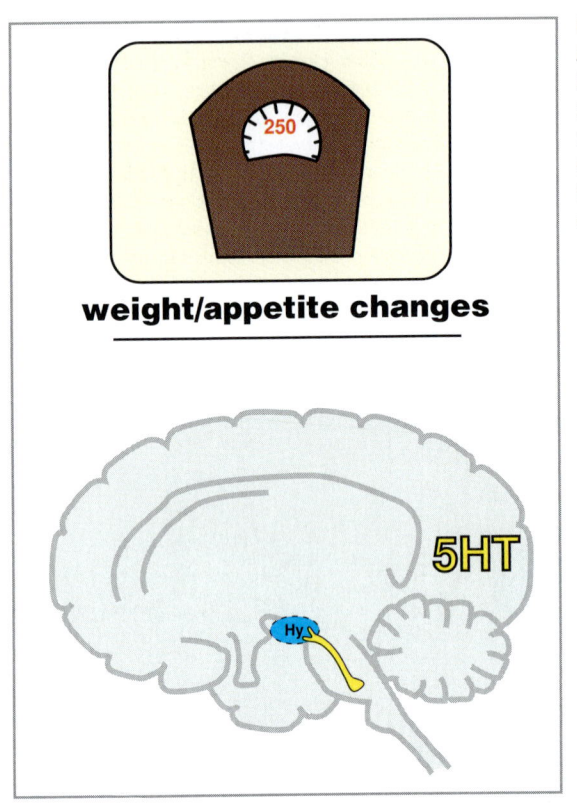

FIGURE 11-52 Weight and appetite circuit. Appetite and weight are mediated in large part by the hypothalamus (Hy), which receives serotonergic projections. Thus, any changes in weight or appetite as a symptom of depression may be related in part to serotonergic control of the hypothalamus (shown here as blue to denote hypoactivity).

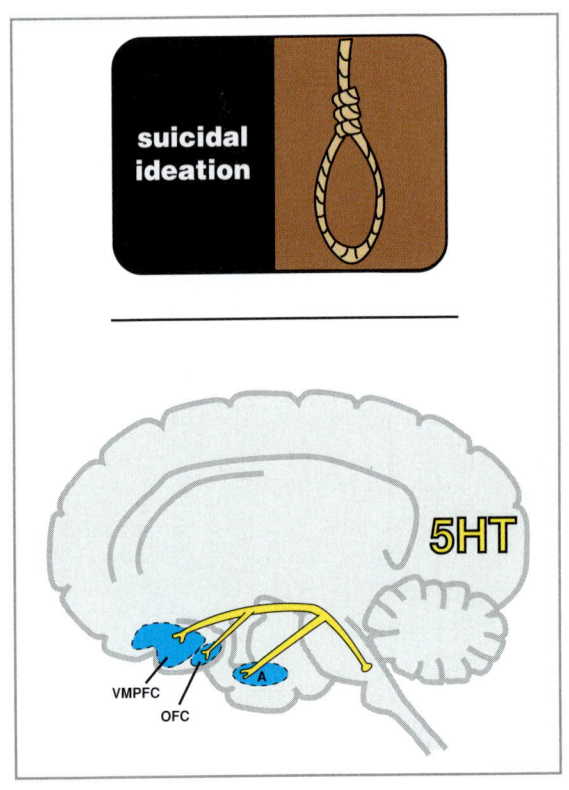

FIGURE 11-53 Suicide circuit. Suicidal ideation is believed to be regulated by inefficient information processing (shown here in blue for hypoactivity) in brain regions associated with emotionality, such as the amygdala (A), ventromedial prefrontal cortex (VMPFC), and orbital frontal cortex (OFC). These brain regions receive important regulatory control for suicidality from serotonergic projections.

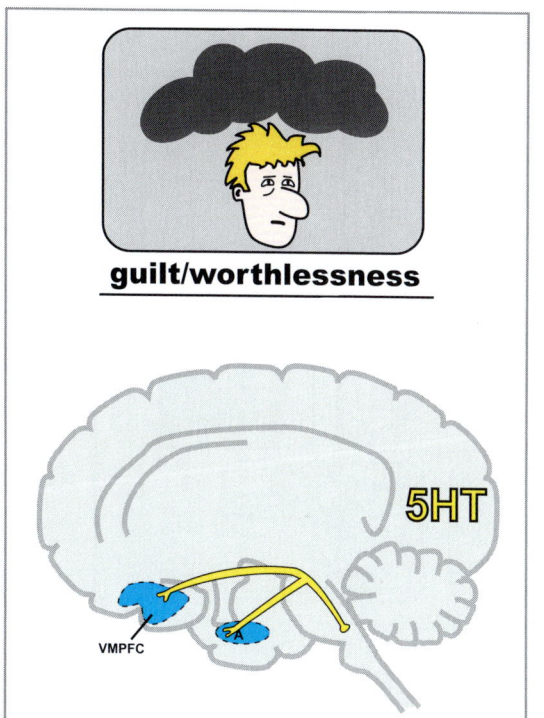

FIGURE 11-54 **Guilt/worthlessness circuit.** As with suicidal ideation, feelings of guilt or worthlessness are regulated by "emotional" brain regions such as the amygdala (A) and ventromedial prefrontal cortex (VMPFC), which are innervated by important serotonergic regulatory projections. Inefficient information processing in these regions (depicted here as blue or hypoactive) may cause these symptoms to occur.

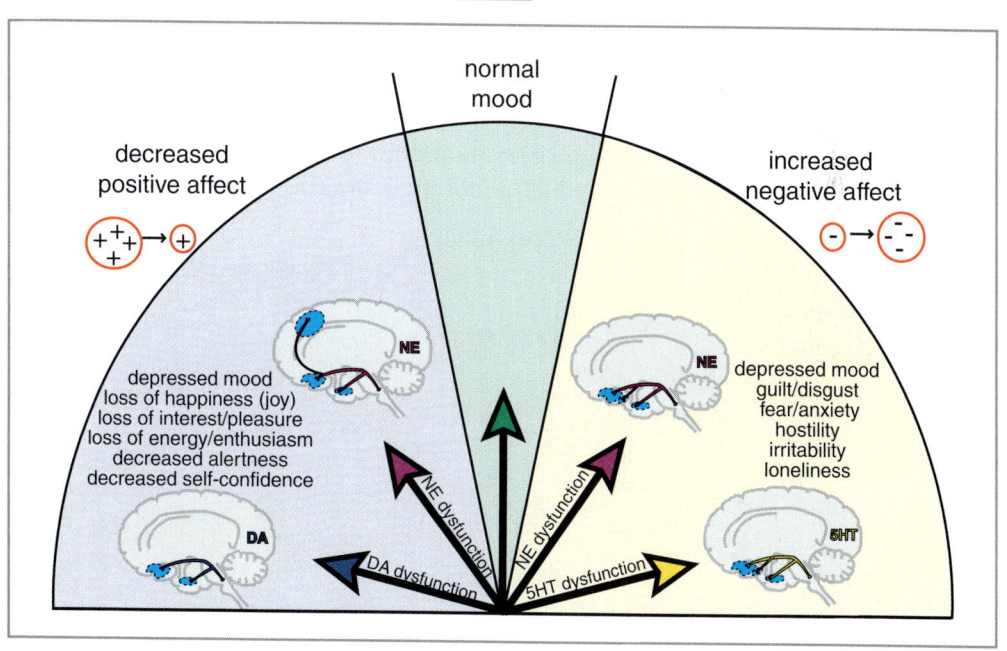

FIGURE 11-55 **Positive and negative affect.** Mood-related symptoms of depression can be characterized by their affective expression – that is, whether they cause a reduction in positive affect or an increase in negative affect. Symptoms related to reduced positive affect include depressed mood; loss of happiness, interest, or pleasure; loss of energy or enthusiasm; decreased alertness; and decreased self-confidence. Reduced positive affect may be hypothetically related to dopaminergic dysfunction, with a possible role of noradrenergic dysfunction as well. Symptoms associated with increased negative affect include depressed mood, guilt, disgust, fear, anxiety, hostility, irritability, and loneliness. Increased negative affect may be linked hypothetically to serotonergic dysfunction and perhaps also noradrenergic dysfunction.

Mood Disorders | 499

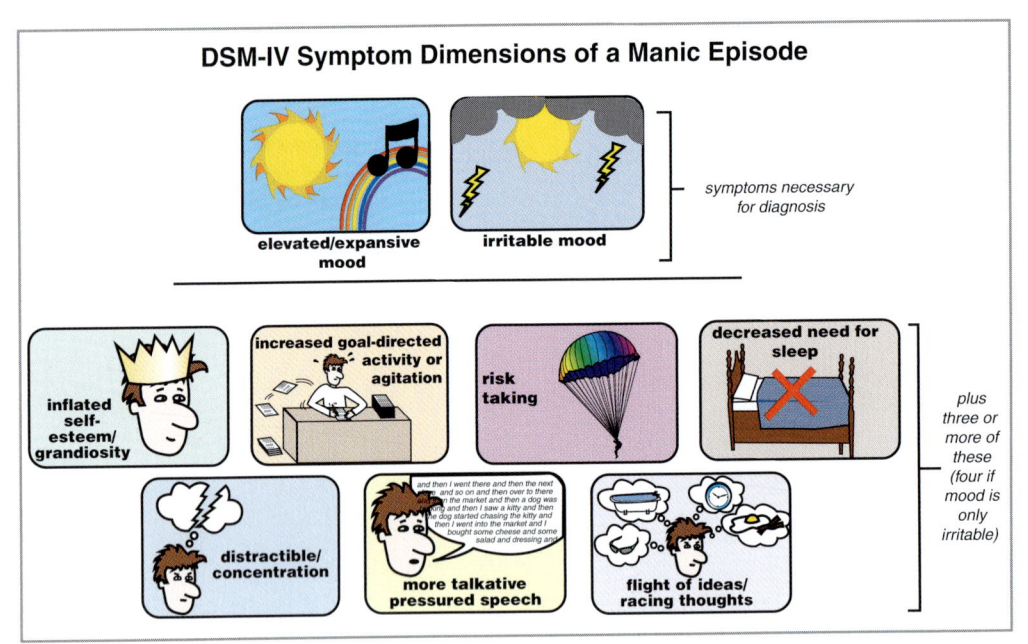

FIGURE 11-56 DSM-IV symptoms of mania. According to the *Diagnostic and Statistical Manual of Mental Disorders*, fourth edition (DSM-IV), a manic episode consists of either elevated/expansive mood or irritable mood. In addition, at least three of the following must be present (four if mood is irritable): inflated self-esteem/grandiosity, increased goal-directed activity or agitation, risk taking, decreased need for sleep, distractibility, pressured speech, and racing thoughts.

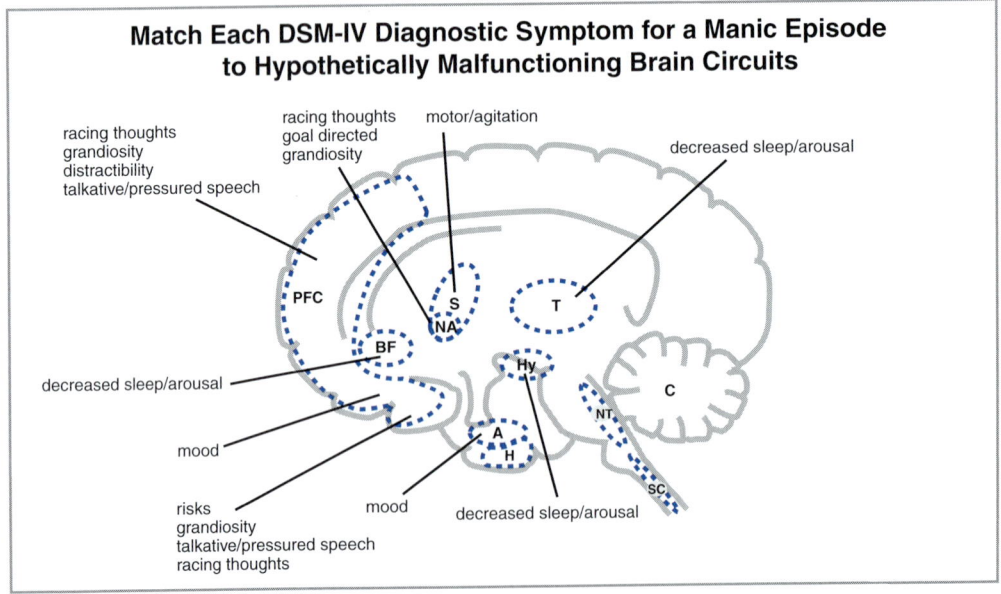

FIGURE 11-57 Matching mania symptoms to circuits. Alterations in neurotransmission within each of the eleven brain regions shown here can be hypothetically linked to the various symptoms of a manic episode. Functionality in each brain region may be associated with a different constellation of symptoms. PFC, prefrontal cortex; BF, basal forebrain; S, striatum; NA, nucleus accumbens; T, thalamus; HY, hypothalamus; A, amygdala; H, hippocampus; NT, brainstem neurotransmitter centers; SC, spinal cord; C, cerebellum.

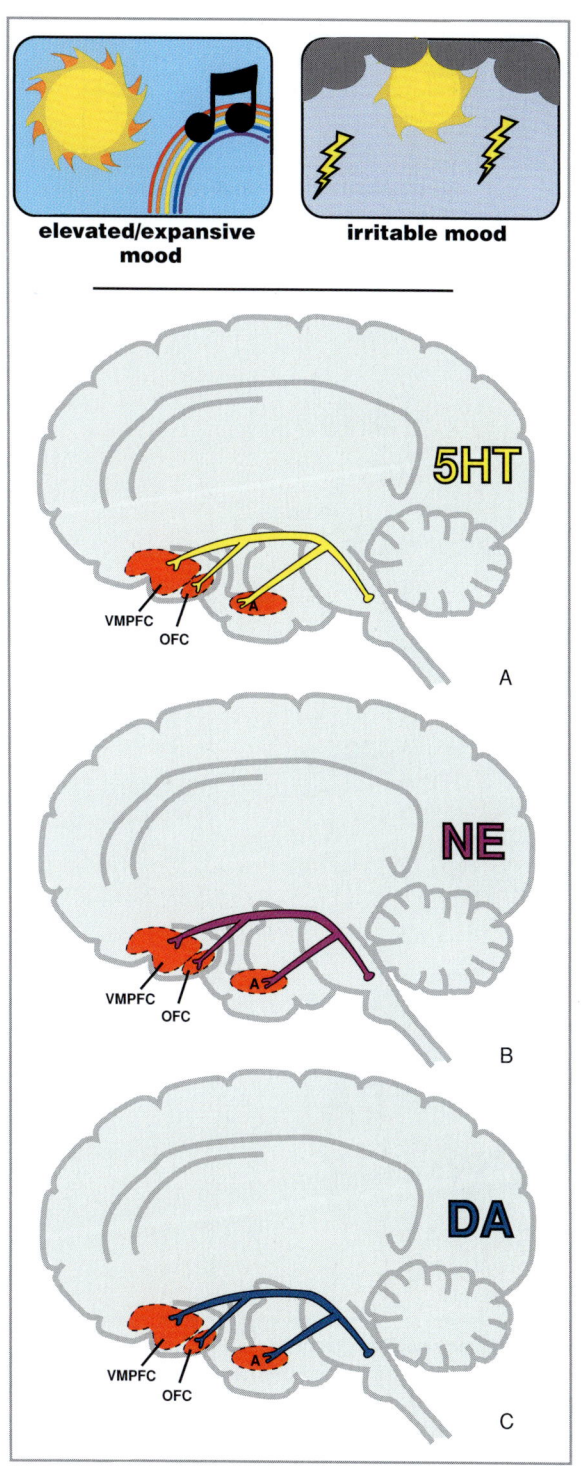

FIGURE 11-58A, B, and C Elevated/irritable mood circuits. Elevated/expansive or irritable mood may be hypothetically linked to inefficient information processing (depicted here in red to denote hyperactivity) in the amygdala (A), ventromedial prefrontal cortex (VMPFC), and orbital frontal cortex (OFC), all of which are innervated by serotonergic (**A**), noradrenergic (**B**), and dopaminergic (**C**) projections from brainstem nuclei.

Mood Disorders | 501

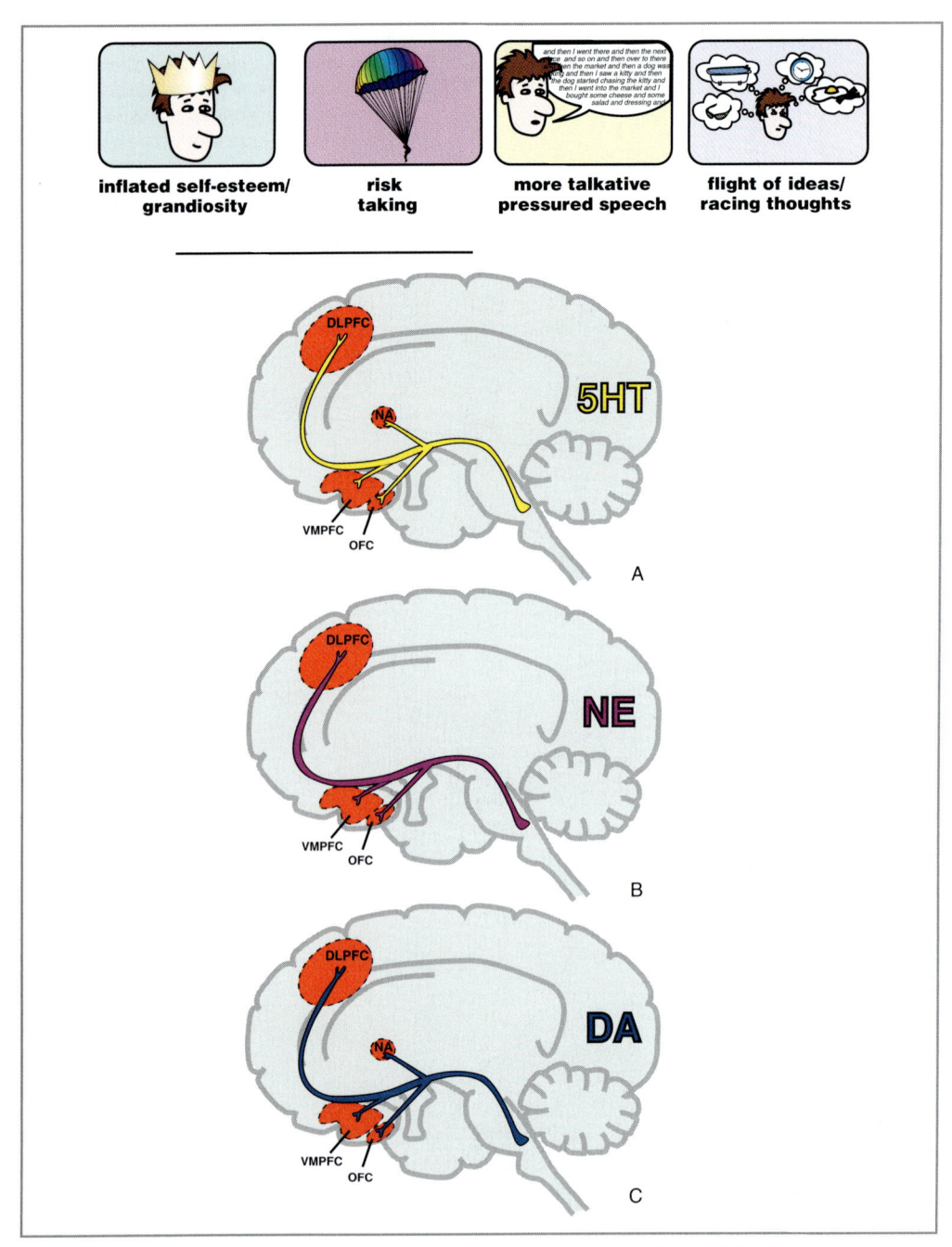

FIGURE 11-59A, B, and C Mania symptom circuits. Symptoms such as grandiosity, flight of ideas, and racing thoughts may be hypothetically linked to inefficient information processing (depicted here in red as hyperactivity) in the same brain regions associated with positive symptoms of psychosis [i.e., nucleus accumbens (NA)]. Other manic symptoms, such as risk taking and pressured speech, may be manifestations of poor impulse control and thus regulated by the orbital frontal cortex (OFC). Other areas of the prefrontal cortex, such as the dorsolateral prefrontal cortex (DLPFC) and ventromedial prefrontal cortex (VMPFC), may also be involved in these symptoms. Regulation of these areas of presumed inefficient information processing in prefrontal cortex include serotonergic (**A**), noradrenergic (**B**), and dopaminergic (**C**) projections, while the nucleus accumbens is innervated by serotonergic (**A**) and dopaminergic (**C**) projections.

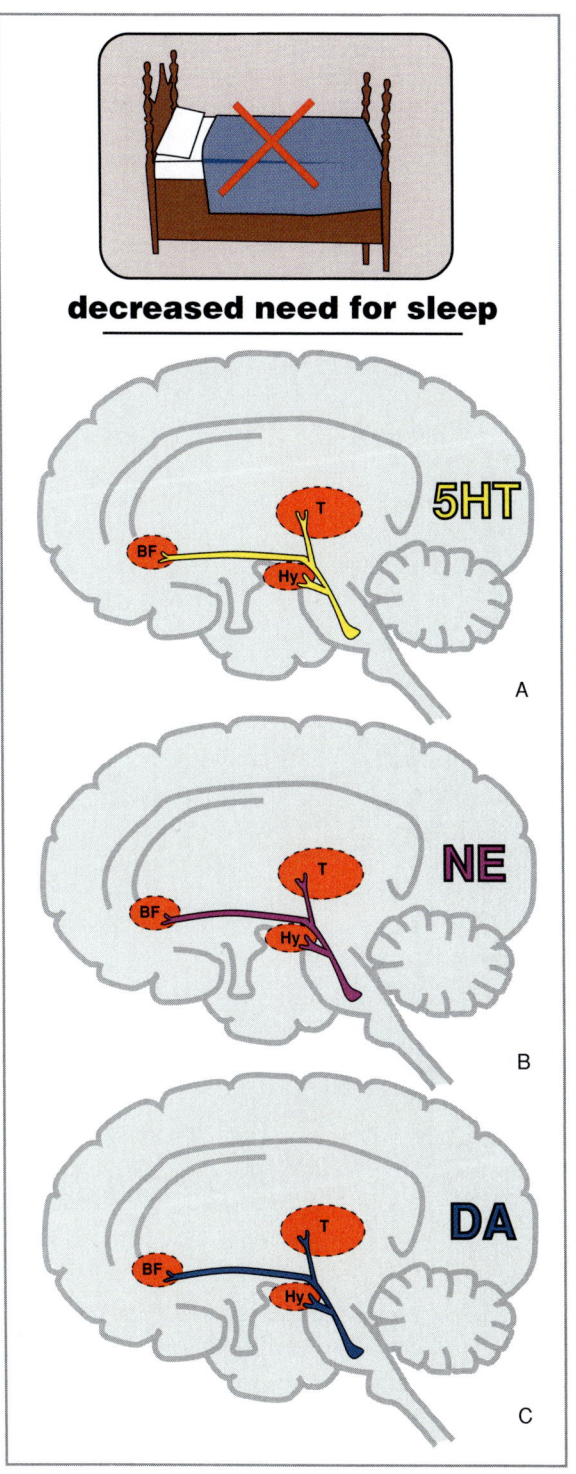

FIGURE 11-60A, B, and C Sleep circuits. Although sleep disturbances manifest themselves differently in a major depressive versus a manic episode (i.e., insomnia or hypersomnia versus decreased subjective need for sleep), they may still be regulated by many of the same brain regions. Thus decreased need for sleep may be linked to inefficient information processing in the hypothalamus (Hy), thalamus (T), and basal forebrain (BF), depicted here by the red color representing hyperactivity. All of these brain regions are innervated by serotonergic (**A**), noradrenergic (**B**), and dopaminergic (**C**) projections from brainstem nuclei.

Mood Disorders | 503

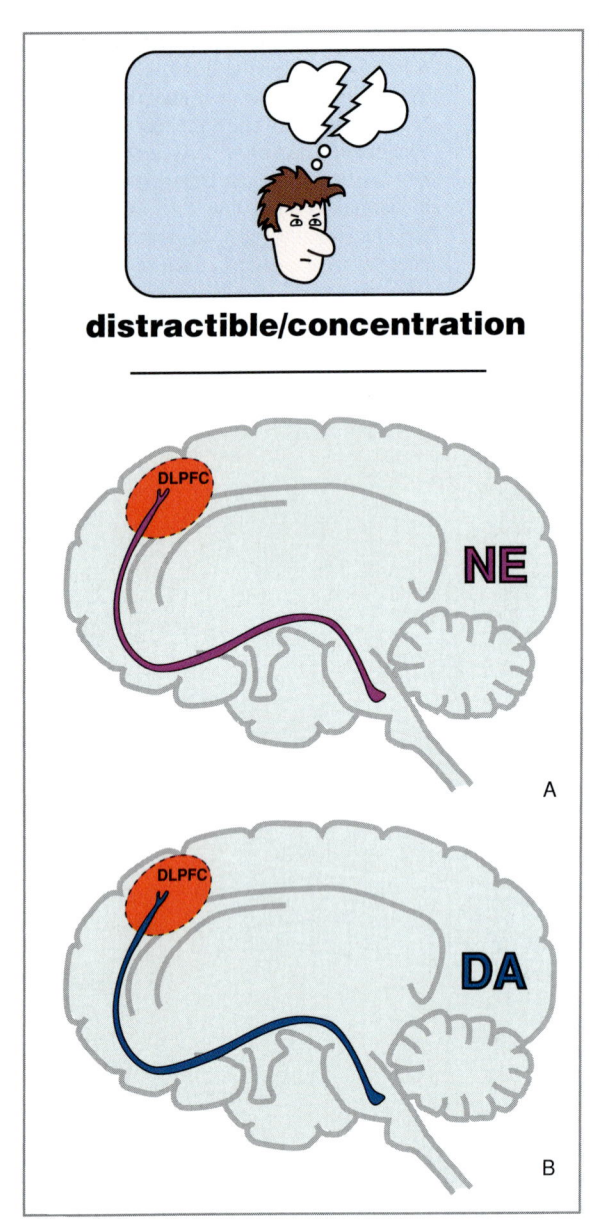

FIGURE 11-61A and B Distractibility circuit. Cognitive problems in mania, such as distractibility or poor concentration, may be associated with aberrant information processing (depicted here as red or hyperactive) specifically in the dorsolateral prefrontal cortex (DLPFC), which receives important regulatory projections from both noradrenergic (**A**) and dopaminergic (**B**) neurons.

symptoms required for the diagnosis of a manic episode are shown in Figure 11-56. As in the case of major depression, each symptom of mania is also hypothetically associated with inefficient information processing in various brain circuits, with different symptoms topographically localized to specific brain regions (Figure 11-57).

Generally, the monoaminergic functioning in these circuits in mania is represented as being red, or hyperactive, and thus essentially the opposite of the malfunctioning hypothesized for depression (see Figures 11-46 through 11-54). As for depression, however, the more accurate portrayal may be "out of tune" rather than simply excessive, especially since some patients can simultaneously have both manic and depressed symptoms. Generally,

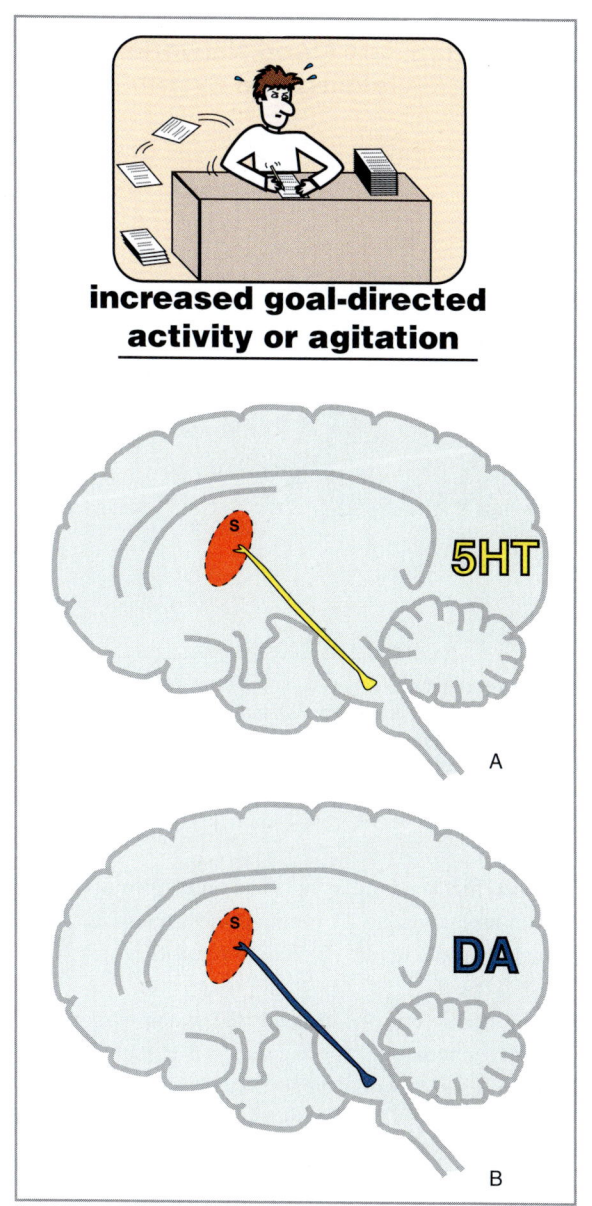

FIGURE 11-62A and B Goal-directed activity circuit. Increased goal-directed activity or agitation in mania may be associated with inefficient information processing in the striatum, perhaps related to hyperactivity of serotonergic (**A**) and dopaminergic (**B**) projections (depicted as red).

however, treatments of mania either reduce or stabilize trimonoaminergic regulation of circuits associated with symptoms of mania.

Just as shown for depression, each of the nine symptoms listed for the diagnosis of mania (Figure 11-56) can also be mapped onto brain circuits that theoretically mediate these symptoms (Figure 11-57), and the hypothetical trimonoaminergic regulation of each of these brain areas can be mapped onto each of the brain regions they innervate as well (Figures 11-58 through 11-62). Targeting each affected region with drugs that act on the relevant neurotransmitters within the trimonoaminergic neurotransmitter system could potentially lead to reduction of each individual manic symptom experienced by a specific

Mood Disorders | 505

**Key Genes That Hypothetically Regulate Mood Networks:
Convergence Upon Trimonoamine Neurotransmitter System**

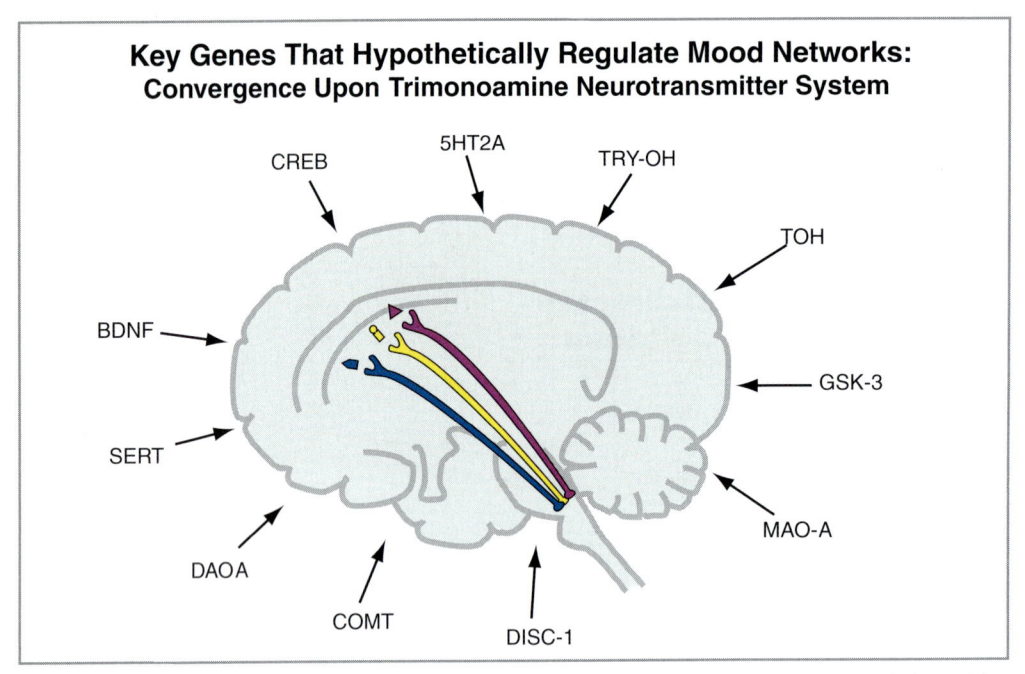

Labels: CREB, 5HT2A, TRY-OH, TOH, BDNF, GSK-3, SERT, MAO-A, DAOA, COMT, DISC-1

FIGURE 11-63 Key genes that hypothetically regulate mood networks. Several key genes that code for proteins that regulate mood networks are shown here. Many of these genes converge on the trimonoaminergic neurotransmitter system, supporting the role of these three neurotransmitters – serotonin, norepinephrine, and dopamine – in both the symptoms and treatments of mood disorders.

patient by enhancing the efficiency of information processing in malfunctioning circuits for each specific symptom. If successful, this targeting of monoamines in specific brain areas could eliminate manic symptoms and cause a manic episode to remit (Figures 11-58 through 11-62).

For example, the core symptoms of a manic episode are elevated, expansive, or irritable mood (Figure 11-58). Thus, patients may have some elements of enhanced negative affect, such as irritability and dysphoria, as experienced by some depressed patients (Figure 11-55). As is the case for depressed mood, these other moods are hypothetically linked to the amygdala, ventromedial prefrontal cortex, and orbitofrontal cortex, with regulation by all three monoamine neurotransmitters (Figure 11-58).

On the other hand, symptoms of inflated self-esteem, grandiosity, flight of ideas, and racing thoughts may be linked to the psychotic symptoms discussed in Chapter 10 and thus to limbic areas such as nucleus accumbens, with risk taking and pressured speech linked to poor impulse control and perhaps therefore to orbitofrontal cortex (Figure 11-59). Sleep disturbance as a symptom of a manic episode (Figure 11-60) may be linked to many of the same areas as sleep disturbance as a symptom of depression (Figure 11-48), although the symptom in mania is not really insomnia but rather a decreased subjective need for sleep. Similarly, distractibility and problems concentrating as symptoms of a manic episode (Figure 11-61) are likely associated with the same brain area as that associated with executive dysfunction such as problems concentrating in a major depressive episode (Figure 11-50) – namely, the dorsolateral prefrontal cortex. Increased goal-directed activity or agitation may be linked to the striatum in mania (Figure 11-62).

**Brain Activation in Depression:
Resting Activity Is Low in DLPFC and High in VMPFC/Amygdala**

normal - resting   normal - resting

depressed - resting   depressed - resting

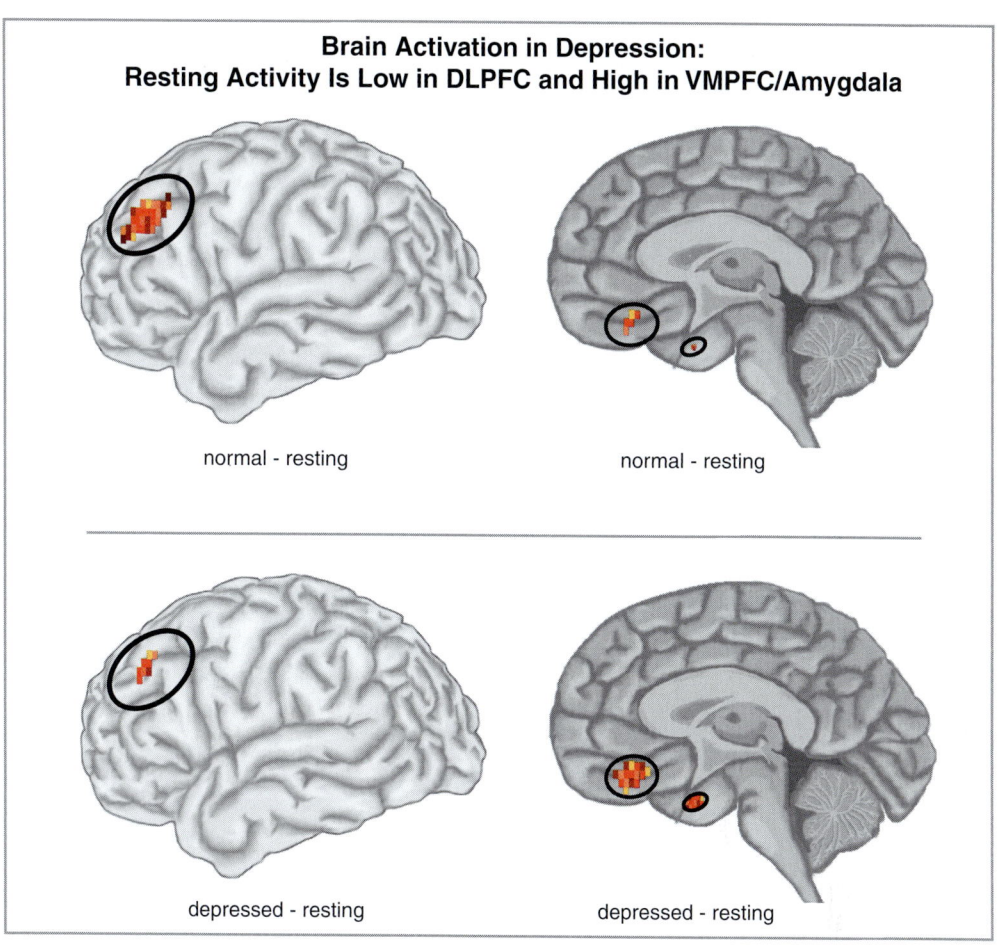

FIGURE 11-64 **Neuroimaging of brain activation in depression.** Neuroimaging studies of brain activation suggest that resting activity in the dorsolateral prefrontal cortex (DLPFC) of depressed patients is low compared to that in nondepressed individuals (left, top and bottom), whereas resting activity in the amygdala and ventromedial prefrontal cortex (VMPFC) of depressed patients is high compared to that in nondepressed individuals (right, top and bottom).

As the reader can see, there is considerable overlap between mania and depression, and common symptoms are hypothetically mediated by the same circuits. Obviously this is a simplistic and reductionistic approach to mapping symptoms of mania and depression; many brain areas are involved, since each brain area is linked to many others. Nevertheless, this idea of constructing a diagnosis, then deconstructing it into its symptom components, and then matching each symptom to a hypothetically malfunctioning brain circuit can be useful in choosing treatments for individual patients. This approach is sometimes called symptom-based treatment selection and combination and is discussed in much further detail in Chapter 12, on antidepressants, and in Chapter 13, on mood stabilizers.

Genes and neuroimaging in mood disorders

Many of the issues in identifying gene abnormalities in mood disorders are the same as those discussed in Chapter 9 for identifying gene abnormalities in schizophrenia. In fact, many of the same genetic abnormalities associated with schizophrenia may apply in part to mood

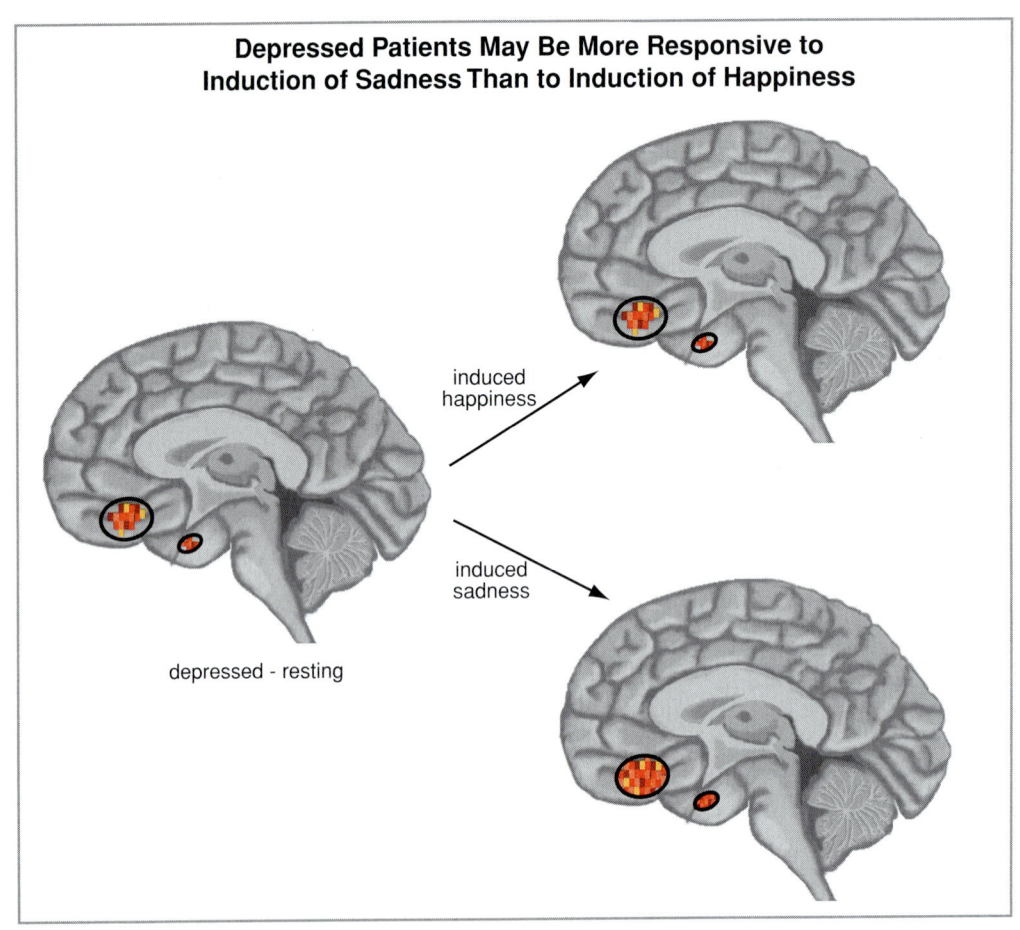

FIGURE 11-65 Depressed patient's neuronal response to induced sadness versus happiness. Emotional symptoms such as sadness or happiness are regulated by the ventromedial prefrontal cortex (VMPFC) and the amygdala, two regions in which activity is high in the resting state of depressed patients (left). Interestingly, provocative tests in which these emotions are induced show that neuronal activity in the amygdala is overreactive to induced sadness (bottom right) but underreactive to induced happiness (top right).

disorders, especially bipolar disorder (see Figures 9-53 through 9-58). The confluence of genetic risk plus environmental stressors is thought to be the same general paradigm for mood disorders, as previously discussed for schizophrenia. The role of stress and genes is also discussed in Chapter 14, on anxiety. Several of the key genes that hypothetically regulate mood networks not surprisingly all converge on the trimonoamine neurotransmitter system (Figure 11-63). How these genes influence neurodevelopment, synaptic plasticity, neuronal connectivity, and the efficiency of neuronal information processing in mood disorders is currently under intense investigation.

In terms of neuroimaging mood disorders, there is general agreement that in depression, the dorsolateral prefrontal cortex, associated with cognitive symptoms, may have reduced activity, and the amygdala and ventromedial prefrontal cortex, associated with various emotional symptoms including depressed mood, may have increased activity (Figure 11-64). Furthermore, provocative testing of patients with mood disorders may provide some insight into the malfunctioning of brain circuits that are exposed to environmental input and required to process it. For example, some studies of depressed patients show that their

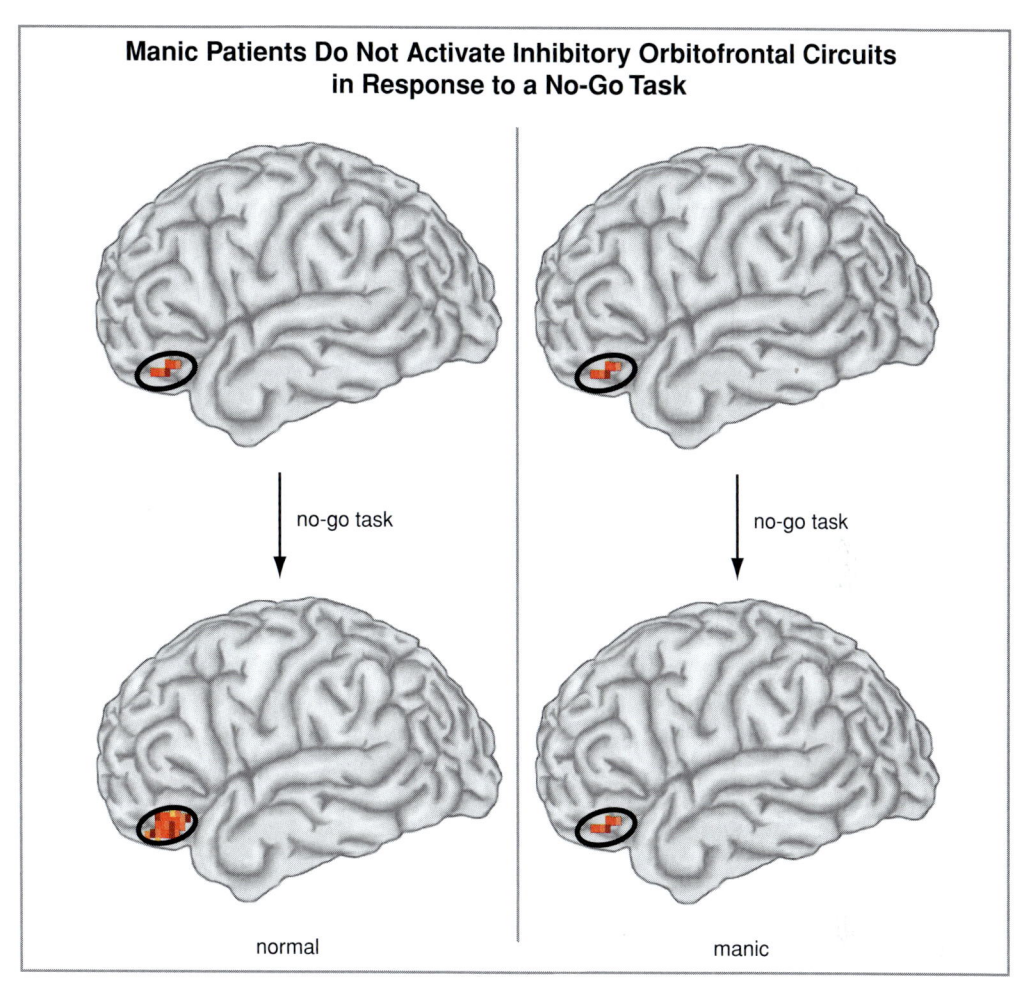

Manic Patients Do Not Activate Inhibitory Orbitofrontal Circuits in Response to a No-Go Task

FIGURE 11-66 Manic patient's neuronal response to no-go task. Impulsive symptoms of mania, such as risk taking and pressured speech, are related to activity in the orbital frontal cortex (OFC). Neuroimaging data show that this brain region is hypoactive in manic (bottom right) versus normal (bottom left) individuals during the no-go task, which is designed to test response inhibition.

neuronal circuits at the level of the amygdala and ventromedial prefrontal cortex are overly reactive to induced sadness but underreactive to induced happiness (Figure 11-65). On the other hand, imaging the orbitofrontal cortex of manic patients shows that they fail to appropriately activate this brain region in a test that requires them to suppress a response, suggesting problems with impulsivity associated with mania and with this specific brain region (Figure 11-66). In general, these neuroimaging findings support the mapping of symptoms to brain regions discussed earlier in this chapter, but much further work is currently in progress and must be completed before the results of neuroimaging can be applied to diagnostic or therapeutic decision making in clinical practice.

Summary

This chapter has described the mood disorders, including those across the bipolar spectrum. For prognostic and treatment purposes, it is increasingly important to be able to distinguish unipolar depression from bipolar spectrum depression. Although mood disorders are indeed disorders of mood, they are much more, and several different symptoms in addition to a mood symptom are required to make a diagnosis of a major depressive episode or a manic episode. Each symptom can be matched to a hypothetically malfunctioning neuronal circuit. The monoamine hypothesis of depression suggests that dysfunction – generally due to underactivity – of one or more of the three monoamines DA, NE, or 5HT of the trimonoaminergic neurotransmitter system may be linked to symptoms in major depression. Boosting one or more of the monoamines in specific brain regions may improve the efficiency of information processing there and reduce the symptom caused by that area's malfunctioning. Other brain areas associated with the symptoms of a manic episode can similarly be mapped to various hypothetically malfunctioning brain circuits. Understanding the localization of symptoms in circuits – as well as the neurotransmitters that regulate these circuits in different brain regions – can set the stage for choosing and combining treatments for each individual symptom of a mood disorder, with the goal being to reduce all symptoms and bring about remission.

CHAPTER 12

Antidepressants

- General principles of antidepressant action
- Antidepressant classes
  - Serotonin selective reuptake inhibitors (SSRIs)
  - Serotonin norepinephrine reuptake inhibitors (SNRIs)
  - Norepinephrine and dopamine reuptake inhibitors (NDRIs)
  - Selective norepinephrine reuptake inhibitors (NRIs)
  - Alpha 2 antagonists as serotonin and norepinephrine disinhibitors (SNDIs)
  - Serotonin antagonist/reuptake inhibitors (SARIs)
  - Classic antidepressants: monoamine oxidase inhibitors
  - Classic antidepressants: tricyclic antidepressants
- Antidepressant pharmacokinetics
- Trimonoaminergic modulators (triple monoamine modulators, or TMMs)
  - Estrogen as a trimonoaminergic, GABA, and glutamate modulator
  - L-methylfolate (6-(S)-5-methyltetrahydrofolate, or MTHF) as a trimonoamine modulator (TMM)
  - S-adenosyl-methionine (SAMe), MTHF, and methylation
  - Thyroid
  - Lithium
  - Brain stimulation: creating a "perfect storm" in brain circuits of depressed patients
  - Psychotherapy
- Antidepressants in clinical practice
- Future treatments for mood disorders
- Summary

This chapter reviews the pharmacological concepts underlying the use of antidepressant drugs. There are many different classes of antidepressants and dozens of individual drugs. The goal of this chapter is to acquaint the reader with current ideas about how the various antidepressants work. It explains the mechanisms of action of these drugs by building upon general pharmacological concepts introduced in earlier chapters. It also discusses concepts about how to use these drugs in clinical practice, including strategies for what to do if initial treatments fail and how to rationally combine one antidepressant with another or with a modulating agent. Finally, the reader is introduced to several new antidepressants in clinical development.

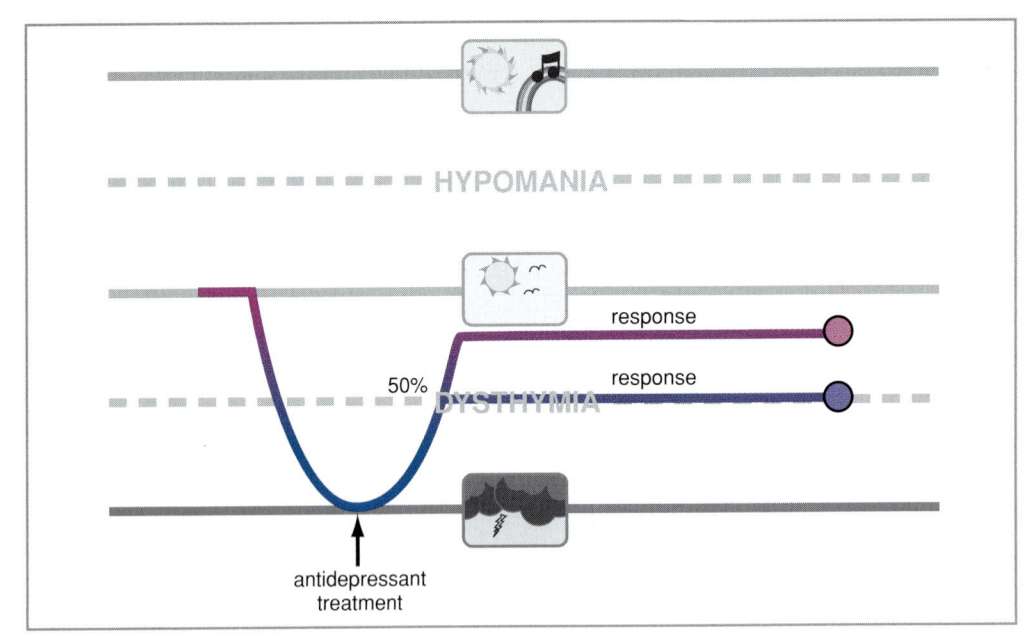

FIGURE 12-1 Response. When treatment of depression results in at least 50% improvement in symptoms, it is called a response. Such patients are better but not well. Previously, this was considered the goal of depression treatment.

The treatment of antidepressants in this chapter is at the conceptual level, not at the pragmatic level. The reader should consult standard drug handbooks (such as the companion *Essential Psychopharmacology: Prescriber's Guide*) for details of doses, side effects, drug interactions, and other issues relevant to the prescribing of these drugs in clinical practice.

General principles of antidepressant action

Patients undergoing a major depressive episode who receive treatment with any antidepressant often experience improvement in their symptoms; when this improvement reaches the level of reducing symptoms by 50% or more, it is called a response (Figure 12-1). This used to be the goal of treatment with antidepressants: namely, to reduce symptoms substantially, at least by 50%. However, the paradigm for antidepressant treatment has shifted dramatically in recent years, so that now the goal of treatment is complete remission of symptoms (Figure 12-2) and maintaining that level of improvement, so that the patient's major depressive episode does not relapse shortly after remission and the patient will not have a recurrent episode in the future (Figure 12-3). Given the known limits to the efficacy of available antidepressants, especially when multiple antidepressant treatment options are not deployed aggressively, this goal of treatment can be difficult to reach. In fact, the goal of remission (Figure 12-3) is not usually reached with the first antidepressant treatment administered.

There are various strategies for putting together an antidepressant treatment portfolio for each patient. This is often accomplished by utilizing multiple pharmacological mechanisms and that increasingly requires treatment with more than one drug in order to generate numerous therapeutic options for reaching the important if sometimes difficult goal of remission. This treatment strategy for depression is very different from that for schizophrenia, where the expected improvement in symptomatology may be only a

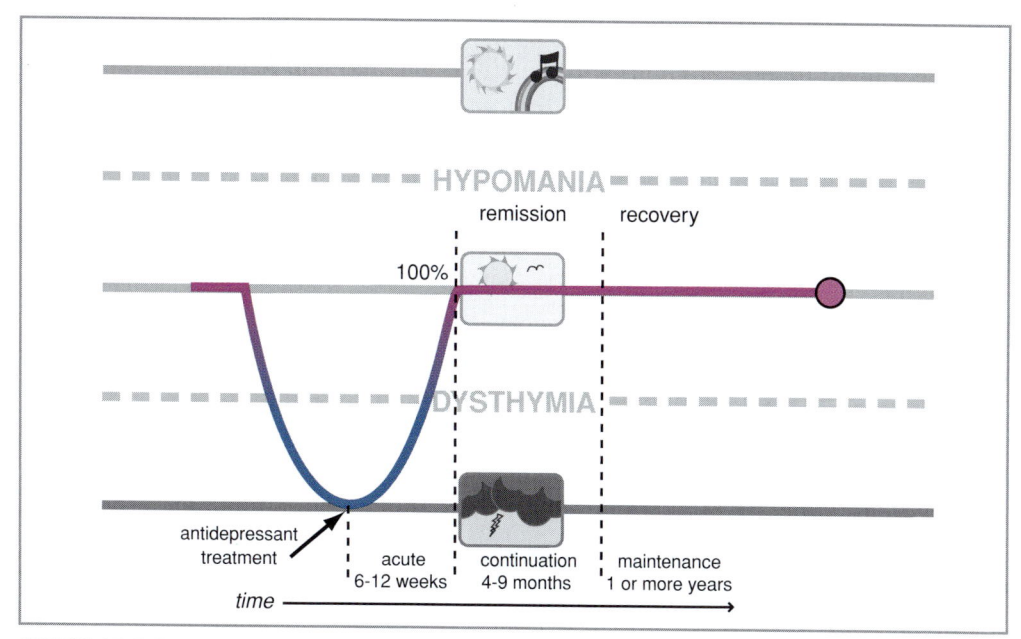

FIGURE 12-2 Remission. When treatment of depression results in removal of essentially all symptoms, it is called remission for the first several months and then recovery if it is sustained for longer than six to twelve months. Such patients are not just better – they are well. However, they are not cured, since depression can still recur. Remission and recovery are now the goals when treating patients with depression.

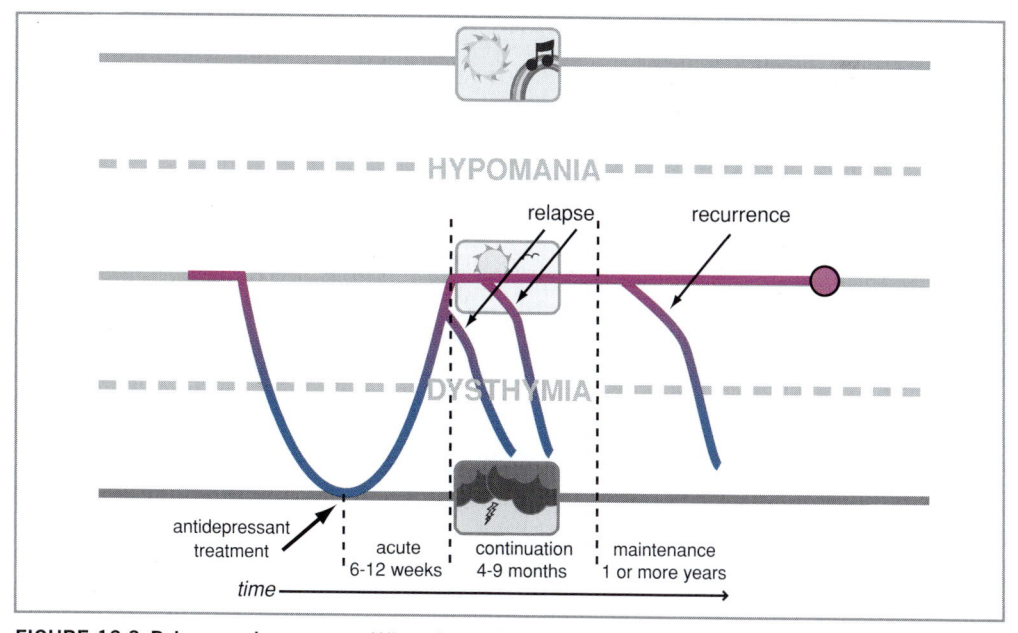

FIGURE 12-3 Relapse and recurrence. When depression returns before there is a full remission of symptoms or within the first several months following remission of symptoms, it is called a relapse. When depression returns after a patient has recovered, it is called a recurrence.

Antidepressants | 513

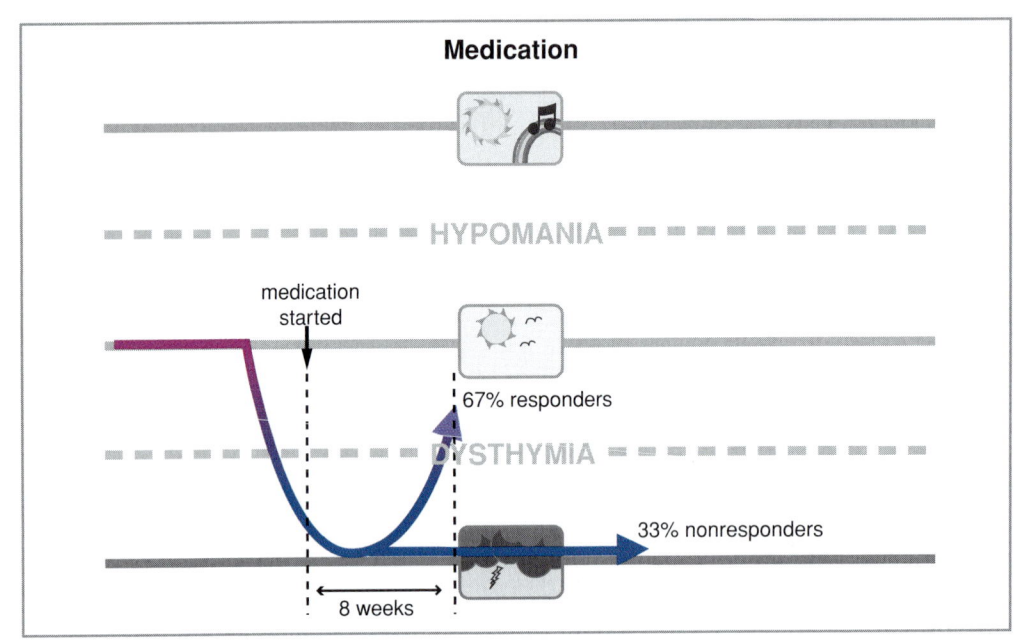

FIGURE 12-4 Antidepressant response rates. Virtually every known antidepressant has the same response rate: 67% of depressed patients respond to any given medication and 33% fail to respond.

20% to 30% reduction of symptoms, and few if any patients become truly asymptomatic or go into remission. Thus the attainment of a genuine state of asymptomatic remission in major depression is the current challenge for those who treat this disorder; this is the reason for learning the mechanisms of action of so many drugs, the complex biological rationale for combining specific sets of drugs, and the practical tactics for tailoring a unique drug treatment portfolio to fit the needs of an individual patient.

All known antidepressants studied in clinical trials designed for marketing approval cause about two-thirds of patients to respond within 8 weeks of initiating treatment (Figure 12-4), whereas placebo causes only about one-third of patients to respond within 8 weeks (Figure 12-5). In addition, patients who respond to an antidepressant and continue it (Figure 12-6) have a much lower relapse rate than those who are switched to placebo (Figure 12-7). These are classic statements but belie the fact that it is becoming more and more difficult to prove that antidepressants – even well-established antidepressants – actually work any better than placebo in clinical trials. This problem of translating results from clinical trials into clinical practice may be due to fluctuating placebo response rates, which occasionally are as high as drug response rates in clinical trial settings, as well as to many other complex factors, such as the highly structured treatment environment of the clinical trial setting, where some are receiving placebo, payments are being made to investigators and sometimes to patients, and patients with comorbid conditions as well as those who are severely ill, suicidal, or treatment-resistant are excluded from trials.

Further complicating the translation of clinical trial findings to the clinical practice setting is the fact that up to one-third of patients in clinical practice never fill their first antidepressant prescription; of those who do, perhaps less than half get a second month of treatment and maybe less than one-fourth get an adequate trial of 3 months or longer. One thing is for sure about antidepressants, and that is that they don't work if you don't take them. Thus, the effectiveness of antidepressants in clinical practice settings is reduced by

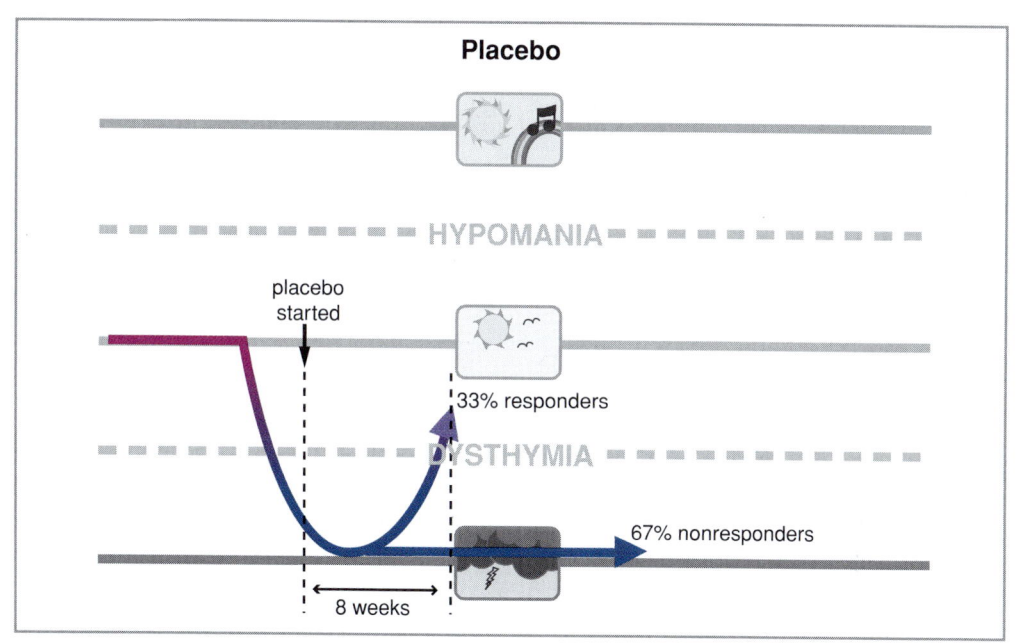

FIGURE 12-5 **Placebo response rates.** In controlled clinical trials, 33% of patients respond to placebo treatment and 67% fail to respond.

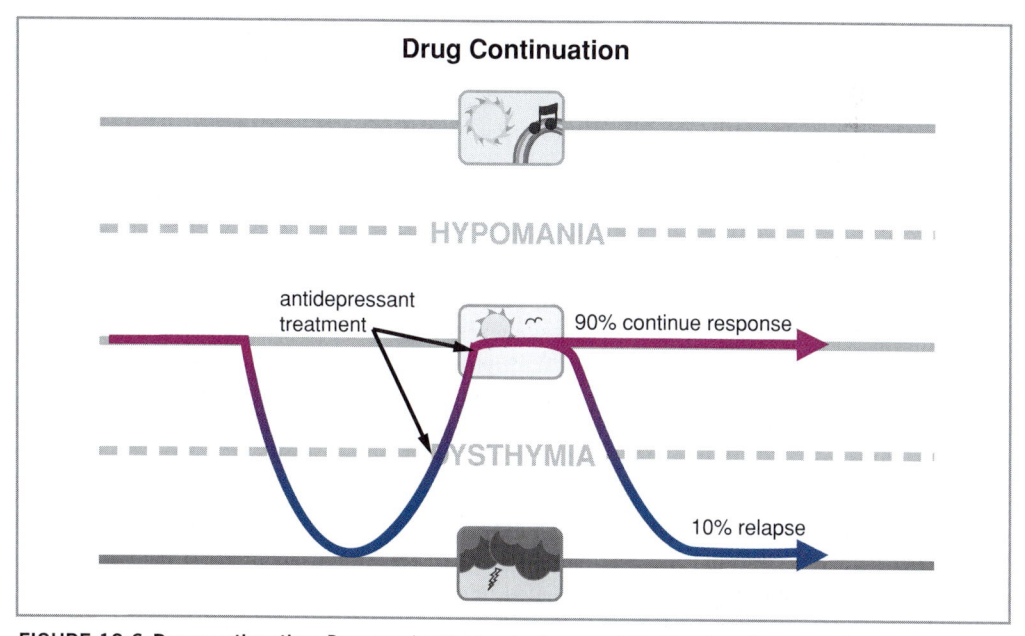

FIGURE 12-6 **Drug continuation.** Depressed patients who have an initial treatment response to an antidepressant will relapse at a rate only of about 10% to 20% if their medication is continued for six months to a year following recovery.

Antidepressants | 515

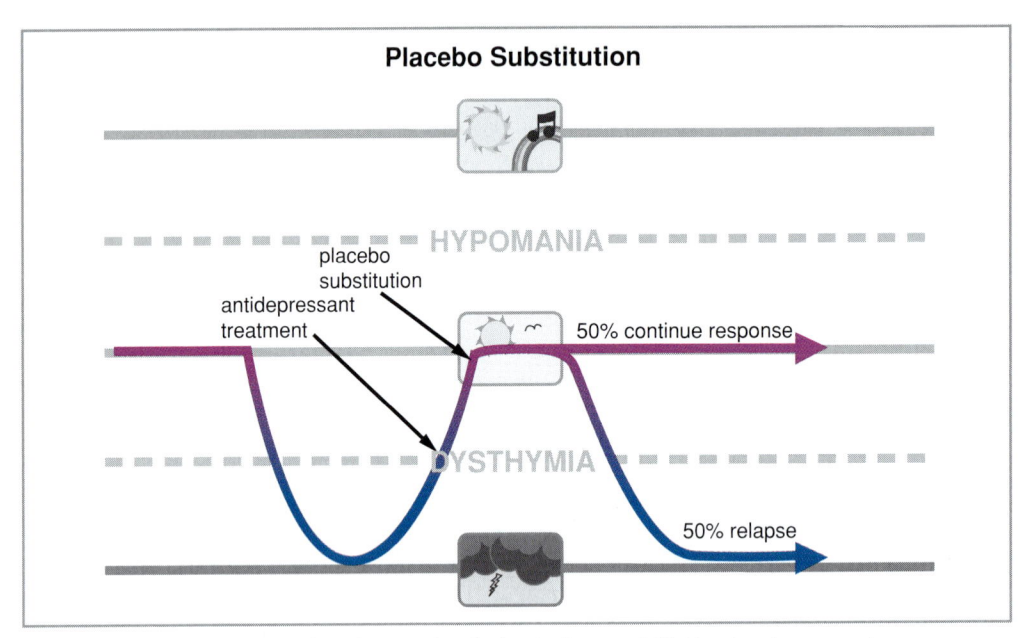

FIGURE 12-7 Placebo substitution. Depressed patients who have an initial treatment response to an antidepressant will relapse at the rate of 50% within six to twelve months if their medication is withdrawn and a placebo is substituted.

this failure of "persistency" of treatment for a long enough period of time to give the drug a chance to work.

"Real world" trials of antidepressants test them in clinical practice settings that include patients normally excluded from marketing trials, such as the STAR-D (Sequenced Treatment Alternatives to Relieve Depression) trial of antidepressants. These trials have recently provided sobering results. Only one-third of such patients remit on their first antidepressant treatment; even after a year of treatment with a sequence of four different antidepressants given for twelve weeks each, only about two-thirds of depressed patients achieve remission (Figure 12-8).

What are the most common symptoms that persist after antidepressant treatment, causing this disorder not to go into remission? The answer is shown in Figure 12-9, and the symptoms include insomnia, fatigue, multiple painful physical complaints (even though these are not part of the formal diagnostic criteria for depression), as well as problems concentrating and lack of interest or motivation. Antidepressants appear to work fairly well in improving depressed mood, suicidal ideation, and psychomotor retardation (Figure 12-9).

Why should we care whether a patient is in remission from major depression or has just a few persistent symptoms? The answer can be found in Figure 12-10, which shows both good news and bad news about antidepressant treatment over the long run. The good news is that if an antidepressant gets your patient into remission, that patient has a significantly lower relapse rate. The bad news is that there are still very frequent relapses in the remitters, and these relapse rates get worse the more treatments the patient needs to take in order to get into remission (Figure 12-10).

Data like these have galvanized researchers and clinicians alike to treat patients to the point of remission of all symptoms whenever possible and to try to intervene as early as

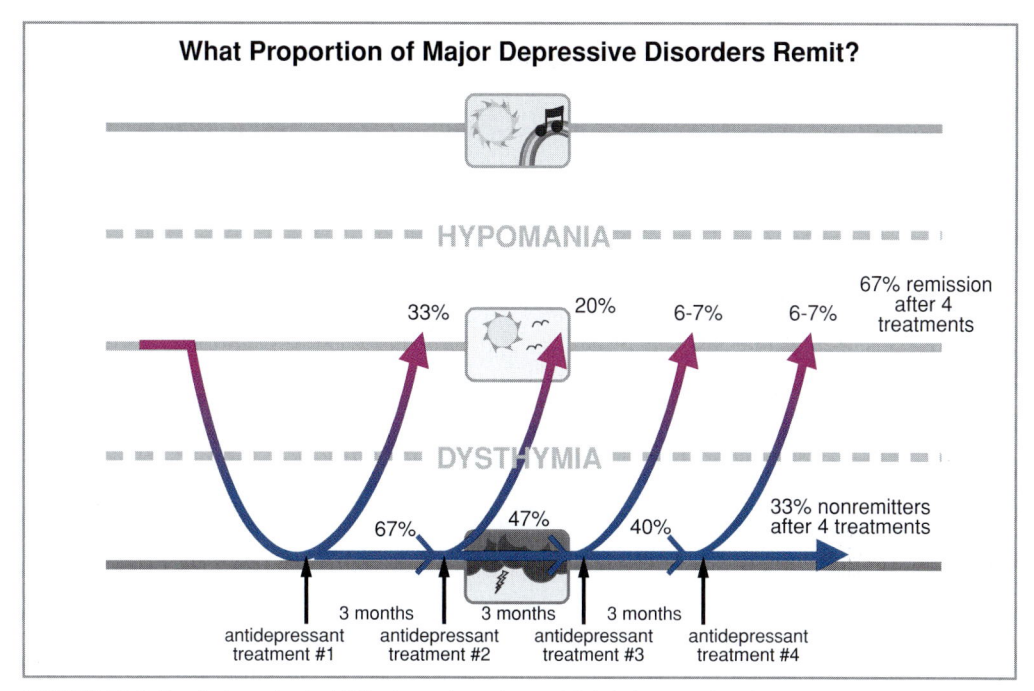

FIGURE 12-8 Remission rates in MDD. Approximately one-third of depressed patients will remit during treatment with any antidepressant initially. Unfortunately, for those who fail to remit, the likelihood of remission with another antidepressant monotherapy goes down with each successive trial. Thus, after a year of treatment with four sequential antidepressants taken for twelve weeks each, only two-thirds of patients will have achieved remission.

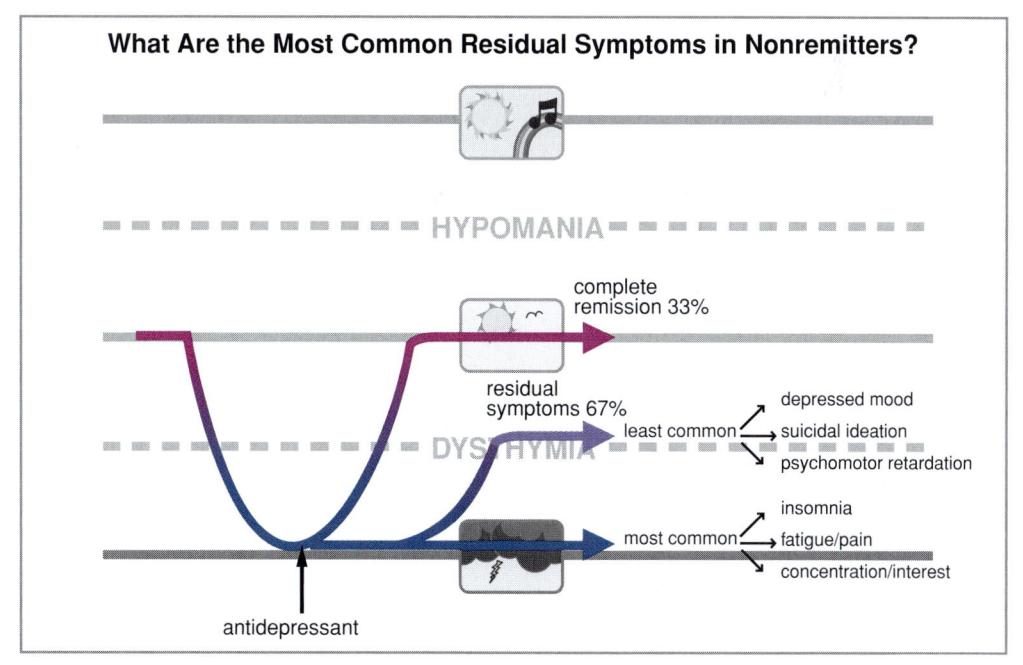

FIGURE 12-9 Common residual symptoms. In patients who do not achieve remission, the most common residual symptoms are insomnia, fatigue, painful physical complaints, problems concentrating, and lack of interest. The least common residual symptoms are depressed mood, suicidal ideation, and psychomotor retardation.

Antidepressants | 517

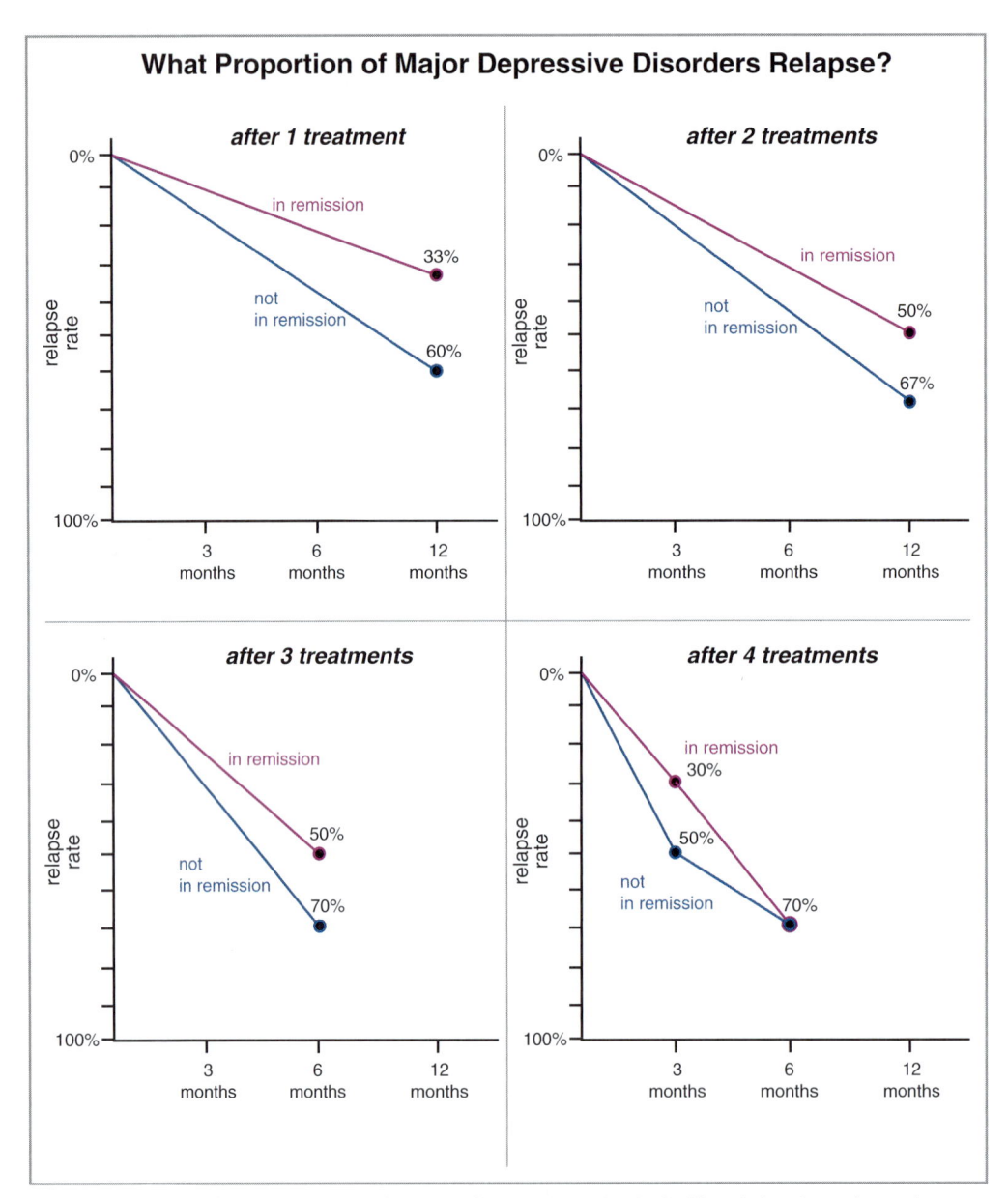

FIGURE 12-10 Relapse rates. The rate of relapse of major depression is significantly less for patients who achieve remission. However, there is still risk of relapse even in remitters, and the likelihood increases with the number of treatments it takes to get the patient to remit. Thus the relapse rate for patients who do not remit ranges from 60% at twelve months after one treatment to 70% at six months after four treatments; but for those who do remit, it ranges from only 33% at twelve months after one treatment all the way to 70% at six months after four treatments. In other words, the protective nature of remission virtually disappears once it takes four treatments to achieve remission.

When Do Antidepressants Start and Stop Working Over the Life Cycle for Major Depressive Disorder?

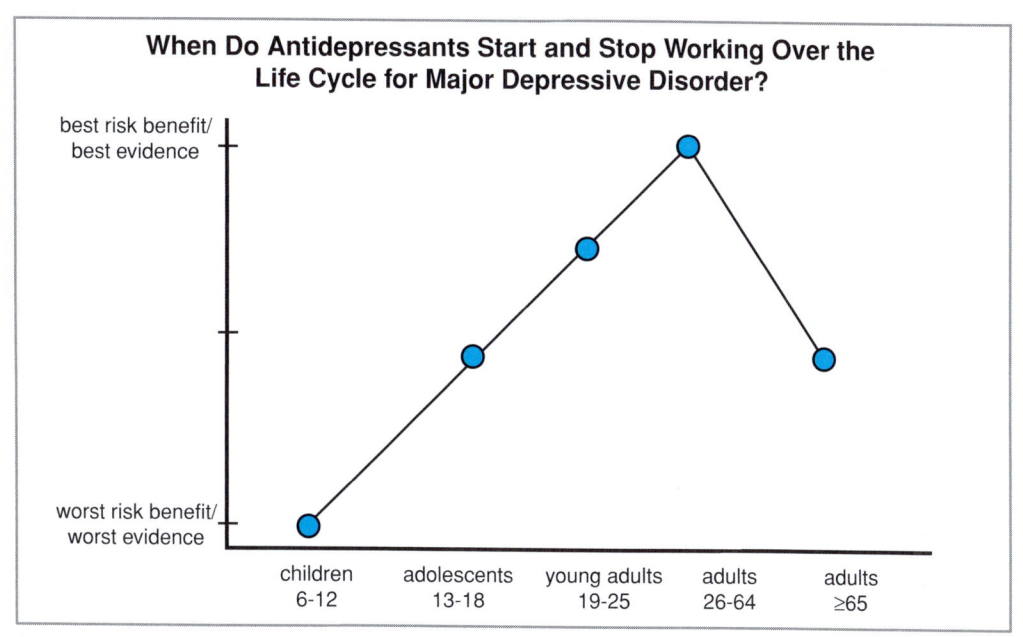

FIGURE 12-11 Antidepressants over the life cycle. The efficacy, tolerability, and safety of antidepressants have been studied mostly in individuals between the ages of 25 to 64. Existing data across all age groups suggest that the risk/benefit ratio is most favorable for adults between the ages of 25 to 64 and somewhat less so for adults between the ages of 19 to 25 due to a possibly increased risk of suicidality in younger adults. Limited data in children and adolescents also suggest increased risk of suicidality; this, coupled with a lack of data demonstrating clear antidepressant efficacy, gives children between the ages of 6 to 12 the worst risk/benefit ratio, with adolescents intermediate between young adults and children. Elderly patients 65 years of age and older may not respond as well or as quickly to antidepressants as other adults and may also experience more side effects than younger adults.

possible in major depression, not only to be merciful in trying to relieve current suffering from depressive symptoms but also because of the possibility that aggressive treatment may prevent disease progression. The concept of disease progression in major depression is controversial, unproven, and provocative, but it makes a good deal of sense intuitively for many clinicians and investigators. It is being vigorously researched at the present time. This concept of disease progression is also discussed in Chapter 8 and illustrated in Figures 8-1 through 8-7 and in Chapter 11 and illustrated in Figures 11-28 and 11-29. The idea is that chronicity of major depression, development of treatment resistance, and likelihood of relapse could all be reduced with aggressive treatment of major depressive episodes that leads to remission of all symptoms, thus potentially modifying the course of illness. This may pose an especially difficult challenge for the treatment of younger patients, where antidepressant efficacy and safety are currently being debated.

Do antidepressants work in the same way over the entire life cycle? The answer seems to be no. Adults between the ages of 25 and 65 might have the best chance of getting a good response and having good tolerability to an antidepressant (Figure 12-11). However, adults above age 65 may not respond as quickly or as robustly to antidepressants, especially if their first episode starts at this age and their presenting symptoms are lack of interest and cognitive dysfunction rather than depressed mood. Depression in elderly patients is discussed in Chapter 18, on dementia and its treatments.

Monoamine Hypothesis of Depression: Antidepressants Increase Monoamines

reuptake pump blocked by antidepressant

increase in neurotransmitters causes return to normal state

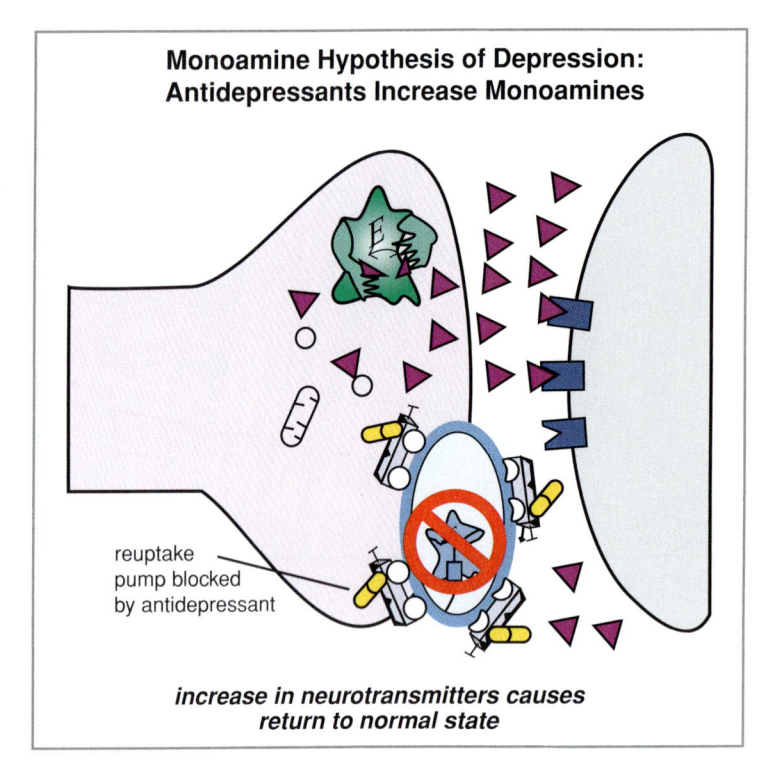

FIGURE 12-12 Antidepressants increase monoamines. According to the monoamine hypothesis of depression, a deficiency in serotonin, norepinephrine, and/or dopamine leads to depression. Thus an increase in these neurotransmitters should cause a return to a normal state. In general, all antidepressants boost the synaptic action of one or more of the monoamines, in most cases by blocking presynaptic transporters. In this figure, an antidepressant is blocking the norepinephrine transporter (NET), thus increasing synaptic availability of norepinephrine and theoretically reducing symptoms of depression.

At the other end of the adult age range, those between the ages of 18 and 24 may benefit from antidepressant efficacy. However, there is now concern that the risk of antidepressants inducing suicidality may be greater in these young adults than in adults above age 25 (Figure 12-11). Thus there is possibly more risk in treating these patients with antidepressants. Finally, the younger the patient, the less evidence there is for antidepressant efficacy and the more evidence for the induction of suicidality. That is, children show the highest risk and least proven benefit from antidepressants, whereas adolescents rank intermediate in benefit and risk of suicidality between children and young adults (Figure 12-11). These findings are an important part of the consideration of whether, when, and how to treat a patient with antidepressants throughout the life cycle.

Antidepressant classes

Although the details of individual antidepressants' mechanisms of action are complex and are described in detail throughout the rest of this chapter, the general principle is actually quite simple: namely, all effective antidepressants boost the synaptic action of one or more of the three monoamines – dopamine, norepinephrine, and serotonin (Figure 12-12). This is often but not exclusively done by acutely blocking one or more of the presynaptic transporters for these monoamines, namely the dopamine transporter (DAT) (see Figures 4-14 and 9-10), the norepinephrine transporter (NET) (see Figure 11-31), and/or the serotonin transporter (SERT) (see Figures 4-7, 4-8, and 10-17).

This pharmacological action at monoamine transporters is entirely consistent with the monoamine hypothesis of depression, which states that monoamines are somehow depleted (Figure 11-42) and, when boosted with effective antidepressants (Figure 12-12), relieve depression. One problem for the monoamine hypothesis, however, is that the action

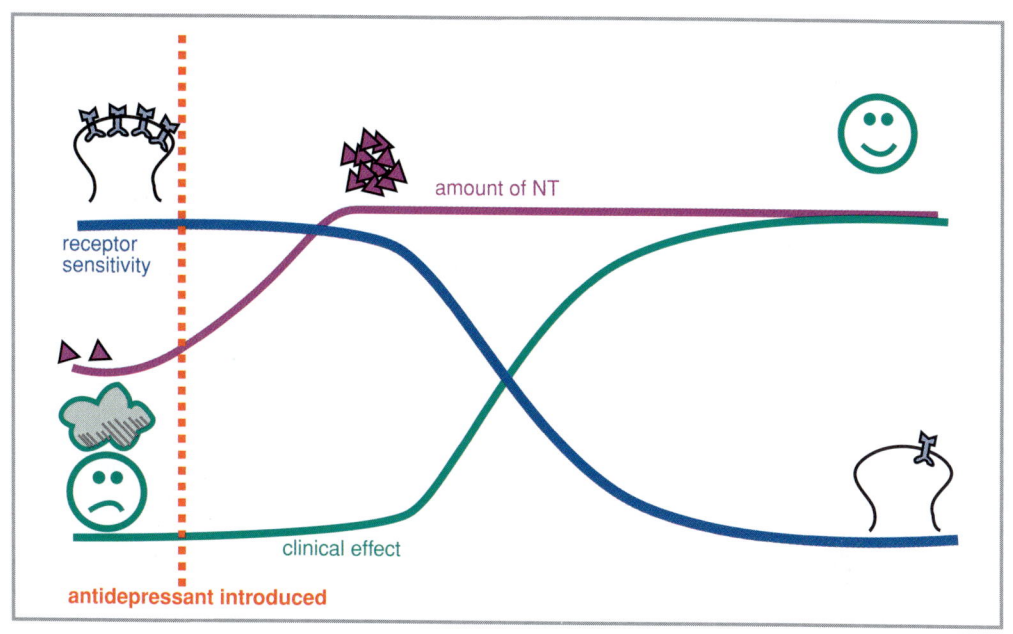

FIGURE 12-13 Time course of antidepressant effects. This figure depicts the different time courses for three effects of antidepressant drugs – namely, clinical changes, neurotransmitter (NT) changes, and receptor sensitivity changes. Specifically, the amount of NT changes relatively rapidly after an antidepressant is introduced. However, the clinical effect is delayed, as is the desensitization, or downregulation, of neurotransmitter receptors. This temporal correlation of clinical effects with changes in receptor sensitivity has given rise to the hypothesis that changes in neurotransmitter receptor sensitivity may actually mediate the clinical effects of antidepressant drugs. These clinical effects include not only antidepressant and anxiolytic actions but also the development of tolerance to the acute side effects of antidepressant drugs.

of antidepressants at monoamine transporters can raise monoamine levels quite rapidly in some brain areas, and certainly sooner than the antidepressant clinical effects occur in patients weeks later (Figure 12-13). How could immediate changes in neurotransmitter levels caused by antidepressants be linked to clinical actions seen much later in time? The answer may be that the acute increases in neurotransmitter levels cause adaptive changes in neurotransmitter **receptor sensitivity** in a delayed time course consistent with the onset of clinical antidepressant actions (Figure 12-13). Specifically, acutely enhanced synaptic levels of neurotransmitter (Figure 12-14A) could lead to adaptive downregulation and desensitization of postsynaptic neurotransmitter receptors over time (Figure 12-14B).

This concept of antidepressants causing changes in neurotransmitter receptor sensitivity is also consistent with the neurotransmitter receptor hypothesis of depression causing upregulation of neurotransmitter receptors in the first place (Figures 11-43 and 12-14A). Thus antidepressants theoretically reverse this pathological upregulation of receptors over time (Figure 12-14B). Furthermore, the time course of receptor adaptation fits both with the onset of therapeutic effects and with the onset of tolerance to many side effects. Different receptors likely mediate these different actions, but both the onset of therapeutic action and the onset of tolerance to side effects may occur with the same delayed time course.

Adaptive changes in receptor number or sensitivity are likely the result of alterations in gene expression (Figure 12-15). This may include not only turning off the synthesis of neurotransmitter receptors but also increasing the synthesis of various neurotrophic factors

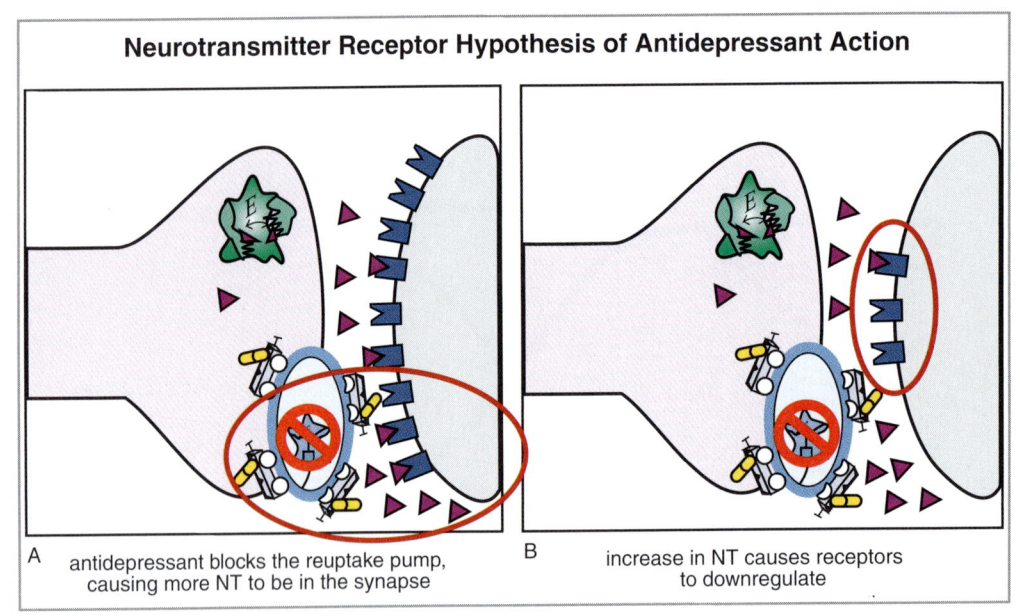

FIGURE 12-14A and B Neurotransmitter receptor hypothesis of antidepressant action. Although antidepressants cause an immediate increase in monoamines, they do not have immediate therapeutic effects. This may be explained by the monoamine receptor hypothesis of depression, which states that depression is caused by upregulation of monoamine receptors; thus antidepressant efficacy would be related to downregulation of those receptors, as shown here. (**A**) When an antidepressant blocks a monoamine reuptake pump, this causes more neurotransmitter (NT) (in this case, norepinephrine) to accumulate in the synapse. (**B**) The increased availability of NT ultimately causes receptors to downregulate. The time course of receptor adaptation is consistent both with the delayed clinical effects of antidepressants and with development of tolerance to antidepressant side effects.

such as brain-derived neurotrophic factor (BDNF) (Figure 12-15). Such mechanisms may apply broadly to all effective antidepressants and may provide a final common pathway for the action of antidepressants.

Serotonin selective reuptake inhibitors (SSRIs)

Rarely has a class of drugs transformed a field as dramatically as the SSRIs have transformed clinical psychopharmacology (Table 12-1). Introduced in the late 1980s, most are now off patent, but not before becoming so widely prescribed within psychiatry, mental health, and primary care that up to six prescriptions per second, around the clock and around the year, are said to be written for these agents. Clinical indications for the use of SSRIs range far beyond major depressive disorder to premenstrual dysphoric disorder, many different anxiety disorders (discussed in Chapter 14, on anxiety), eating disorders (discussed in Chapter 19, on disorders of reward), and beyond. There are six principal agents in this group (Table 12-1). All six of these drugs share the common property of serotonin reuptake inhibition; thus they all belong to the same drug class, known as SSRIs (Figure 12-16). However, each of these six drugs also has unique pharmacological properties that allow it to be distinguished from the others. First, what these six drugs share in common is discussed, and then their distinctive individual properties are explored – properties that allow sophisticated prescribers to match specific drug profiles to individual patient symptom profiles.

TABLE 12-1 Serotonin selective reuptake inhibitors

fluoxetine (Prozac)
sertraline (Zoloft)
paroxetine (Paxil, Aropax, Seroxat)
fluvoxamine (Luvox, Faverin)
citalopram (Celexa, Cipramil)
escitalopram (Lexapro, Cipralex)

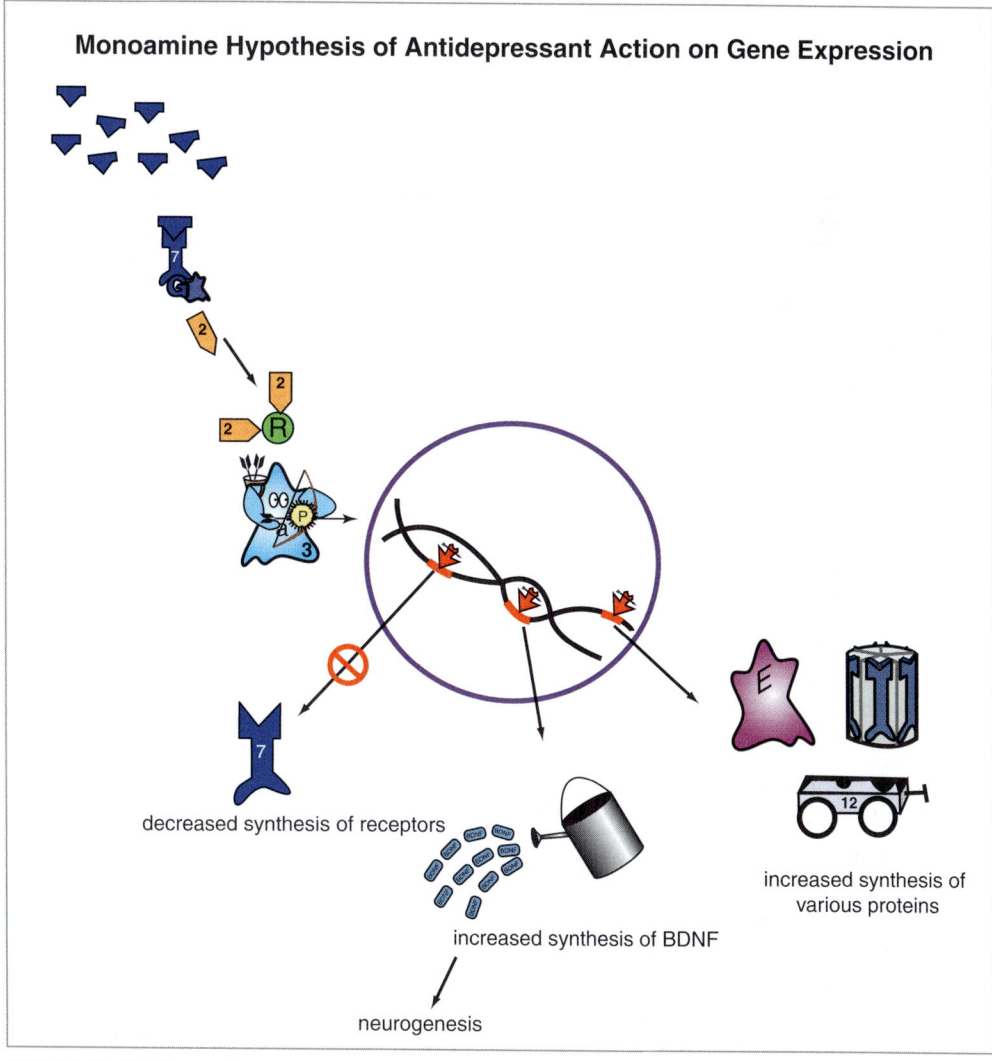

FIGURE 12-15 Monoamine hypothesis of antidepressant action on gene expression. Adaptations in receptor number or sensitivity are likely due to alterations in gene expression, as shown here. The neurotransmitter at the top is presumably increased by an antidepressant. The cascading consequence of this is ultimately to change the expression of critical genes in order to effect an antidepressant response. This includes downregulating some genes so that there is decreased synthesis of receptors as well as upregulating other genes so that there is increased synthesis of critical proteins, such as brain-derived neurotrophic factor (BDNF).

Antidepressants | 523

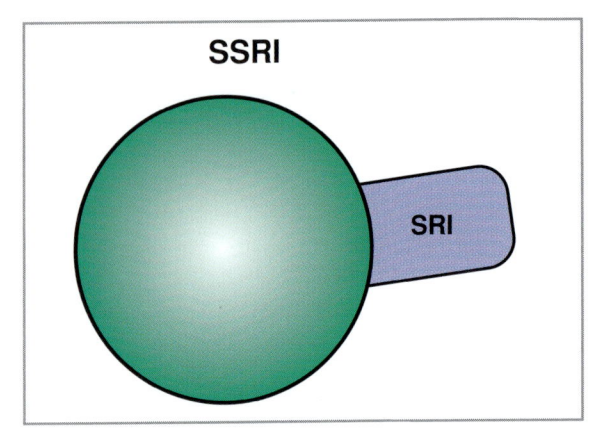

FIGURE 12-16 Serotonin selective reuptake inhibitors. Shown here is an icon depicting the core feature of serotonin selective reuptake inhibitors (SSRIs), namely serotonin reuptake inhibition. Although the six agents in this class have unique pharmacological profiles, they all share the common property of serotonin transporter (SERT) inhibition.

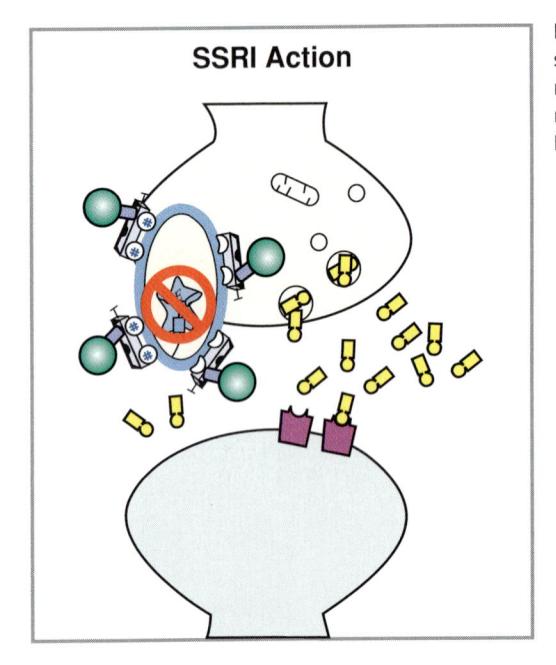

FIGURE 12-17 SSRI action. In this figure, the serotonin reuptake inhibitor (SRI) portion of the SSRI molecule is shown inserted into the serotonin reuptake pump (the serotonin transporter, or SERT), blocking it and causing an antidepressant effect.

What the six SSRIs have in common

These drugs include fluoxetine, sertraline, paroxetine, fluvoxamine, citalopram, and escitalopram (Table 12-1). All share a single major pharmacological feature: selective and potent inhibition of serotonin reuptake, also known as inhibition of the serotonin transporter, or SERT. This simple concept was introduced in Chapter 4 and illustrated in Figures 4-7 and 4-8; it is shown here in Figure 12-17.

Pharmacological and molecular mechanism of action of the SSRIs

Although the action of SSRIs at the **presynaptic axon terminal** has classically been emphasized (Figure 12-17), it now appears that events occurring at the **somatodendritic end** of the serotonin neuron (near the cell body) may be more important in explaining the therapeutic actions of the SSRIs (Figures 12-18 through 12-22). That is, in the depressed state, the monoamine hypothesis of depression states that serotonin may be deficient, both at

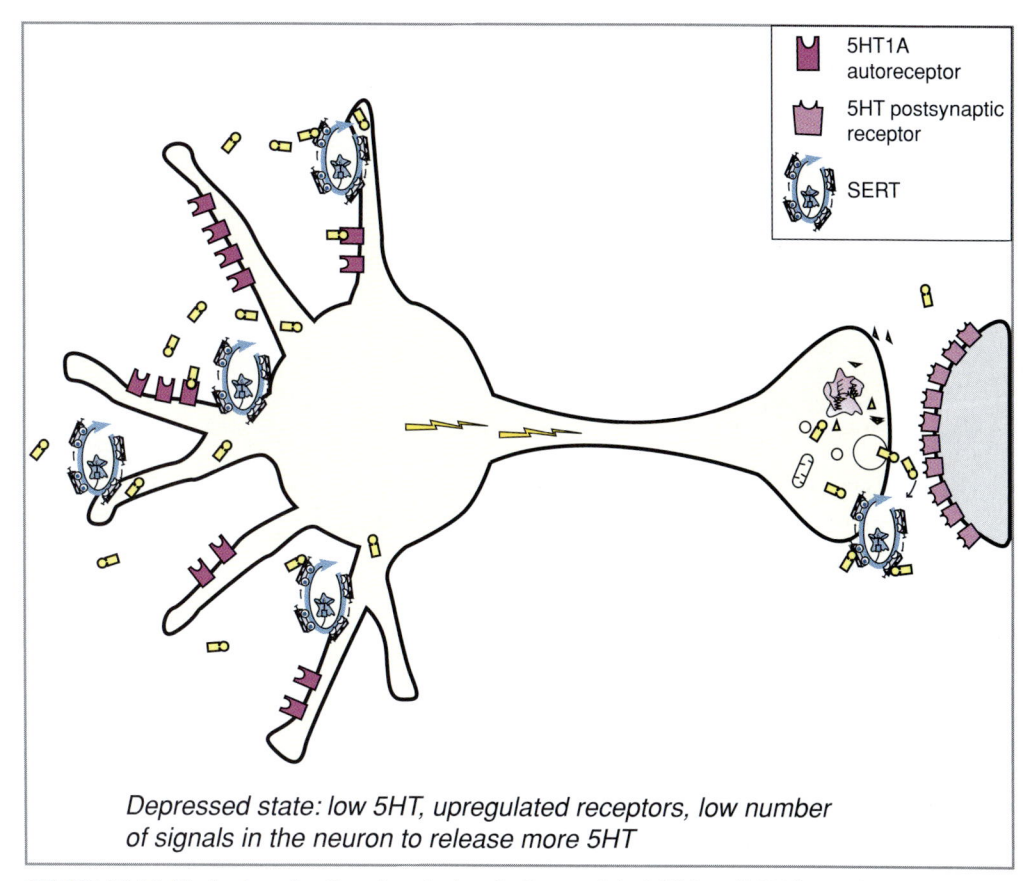

FIGURE 12-18 Mechanism of action of serotonin selective reuptake inhibitors (SSRIs), part 1. Depicted here is a serotonin (5HT) neuron in a depressed patient. In depression, the 5HT neuron is conceptualized as having a relative deficiency of the neurotransmitter 5HT. Also, the number of 5HT receptors is upregulated, including presynaptic 5HT1A autoreceptors as well as postsynaptic 5HT receptors.

presynaptic somatodendritic areas near the cell body (on the left in Figure 12-18) and in the synapse itself near the axon terminal (on the right in Figure 12-18). This is discussed in Chapter 11 and illustrated in Figure 11-42.

Furthermore, the neurotransmitter receptor hypothesis states that pre- and postsynaptic receptors may be upregulated; this is also discussed in Chapter 11 and illustrated in Figure 11-43. Both of these elements are shown for the serotonin neuron in Figure 12-18, which represents the depressed state before treatment. Neuronal firing rates for this neuron may also be dysregulated in depression, contributing to regional abnormalities in information processing and the development of specific symptoms, depending on the region affected, as discussed in Chapter 11 and shown in Figures 11-45 to 11-55.

When an SSRI is given acutely, it is well known that 5HT rises due to blockade of SERT. What is somewhat surprising, however, is that blocking the presynaptic SERT does *not* immediately lead to a great deal of serotonin in many synapses. In fact, when SSRI treatment is initiated, 5HT rises much more at the somatodendritic area located in the midbrain raphe (on the left in Figure 12-19), due to blockade of SERTs there, rather than in the areas of the brain where the axons terminate (on the right in Figure 12-19).

Antidepressants | 525

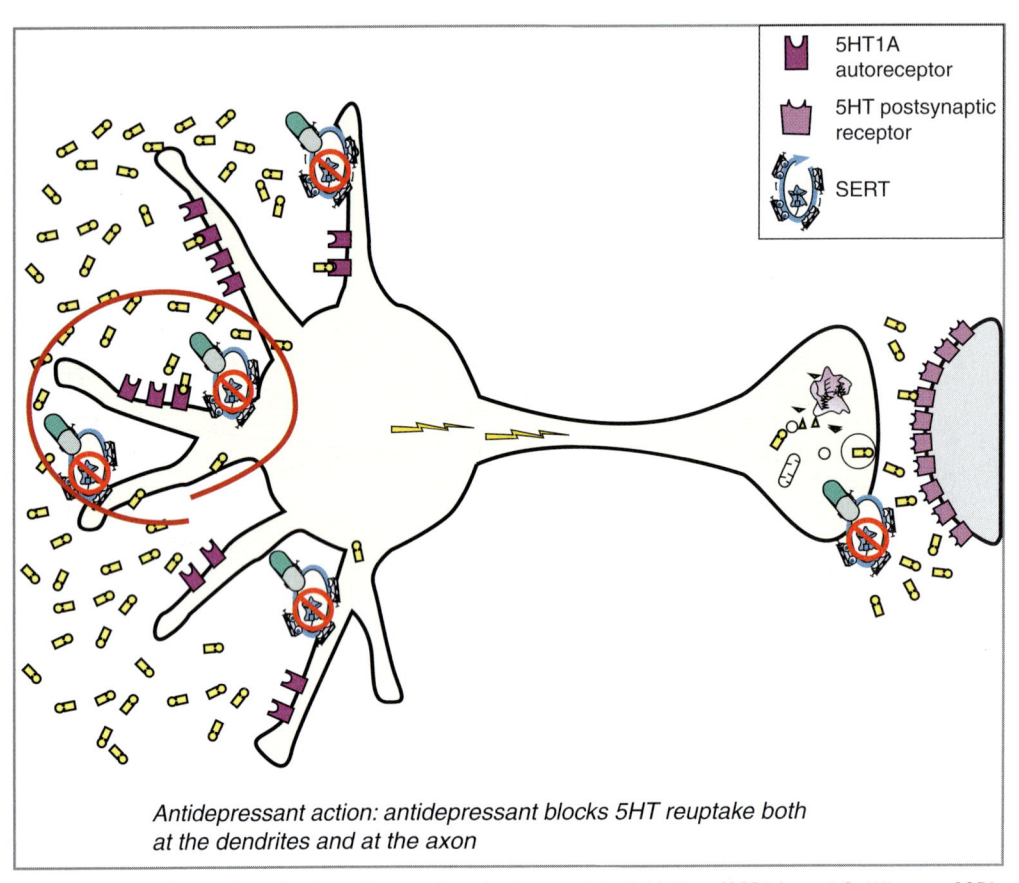

Antidepressant action: antidepressant blocks 5HT reuptake both at the dendrites and at the axon

FIGURE 12-19 Mechanism of action of serotonin selective reuptake inhibitors (SSRIs), part 2. When an SSRI is administered, it immediately blocks the serotonin reuptake pump [see icon of an SSRI drug capsule blocking the reuptake pump, or serotonin transporter (SERT)]. However, this causes serotonin to increase initially only in the somatodendritic area of the serotonin neuron (left) and not very much in the axon terminals (right).

The somatodendritic area of the serotonin neuron is therefore where 5HT increases first (on the left in Figure 12-19). Serotonin receptors in this brain area have 5HT1A pharmacology, as discussed in Chapter 10 and illustrated in Figure 10-19. When serotonin levels rise in the somatodendritic area, they stimulate nearby 5HT1A autoreceptors (also on the left in Figure 12-19). These immediate pharmacological actions obviously cannot explain the delayed therapeutic actions of the SSRIs. However, they may explain the side effects caused by the SSRIs when treatment is initiated.

Over time, the increased 5HT levels acting at the somatodendritic 5HT1A autoreceptors cause them to downregulate and become desensitized (on the left in Figure 12-20). This desensitization occurs because the increase in serotonin is recognized by these presynaptic 5HT1A receptors, and this information is sent to the cell nucleus of the serotonin neuron. The genome's reaction to this information is to issue instructions that cause these same receptors to become desensitized over time. The time course of this desensitization correlates with the onset of therapeutic actions of the SSRIs.

Once the 5HT1A somatodendritic autoreceptors are desensitized, 5HT can no longer effectively turn off its own release. Since 5HT is no longer inhibiting its own release, the serotonin neuron is therefore disinhibited (Figure 12-21). This results in a flurry of 5HT

The increase in 5HT causes the autoreceptors to desensitize / downregulate

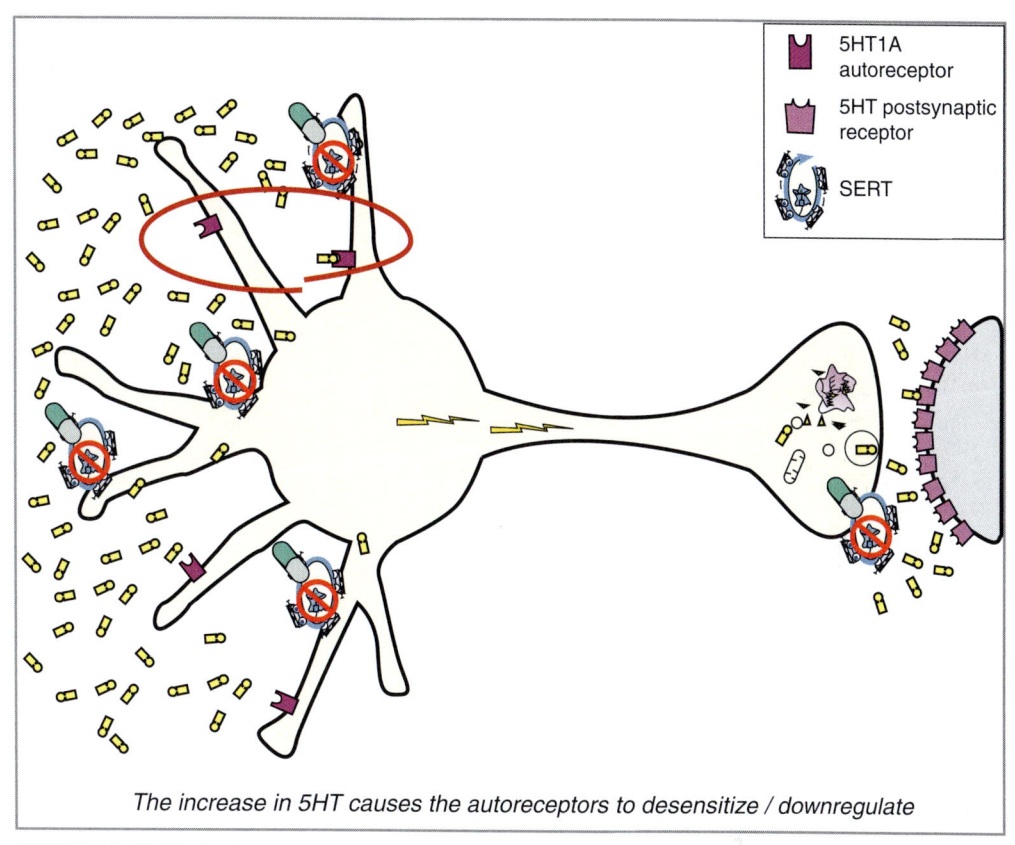

FIGURE 12-20 Mechanism of action of serotonin selective reuptake inhibitors (SSRIs), part 3. The consequence of serotonin increasing in the somatodendritic area of the serotonin (5HT) neuron, as depicted in Figure 12-19, is that the somatodendritic 5HT1A autoreceptors desensitize or downregulate (red circle).

release from axons and an increase in neuronal impulse flow (shown as lightning in Figure 12-21 and release of serotonin from the axon terminal on the right). This is just another way of saying that the serotonin release is "turned on" at the axon terminals. The serotonin that now pours out of the various projections of serotonin pathways in the brain is what theoretically mediates the various therapeutic actions of the SSRIs.

While the presynaptic somatodendritic 5HT1A autoreceptors are desensitizing (Figure 12-20), serotonin builds up in synapses (Figure 12-21) and causes the postsynaptic serotonin receptors to desensitize as well (on the right in Figure 12-22). This happens because the increase in synaptic serotonin is recognized by postsynaptic serotonin 2A, 2C, 3, and many other serotonin receptors there (see Figure 10-20). These various postsynaptic serotonin receptors, in turn, send information to the cell nucleus of the **postsynaptic** neuron that serotonin is targeting (on the far right of Figure 12-22). The reaction of the genome in the postsynaptic neuron is also to issue instructions to downregulate or desensitize these receptors as well. The time course of this desensitization correlates with the onset of tolerance to the side effects of the SSRIs (Figure 12-22).

This theory suggests a pharmacological cascading mechanism whereby the SSRIs exert their therapeutic actions: namely, powerful but delayed disinhibition of serotonin release in key pathways throughout the brain. Furthermore, side effects are hypothetically caused

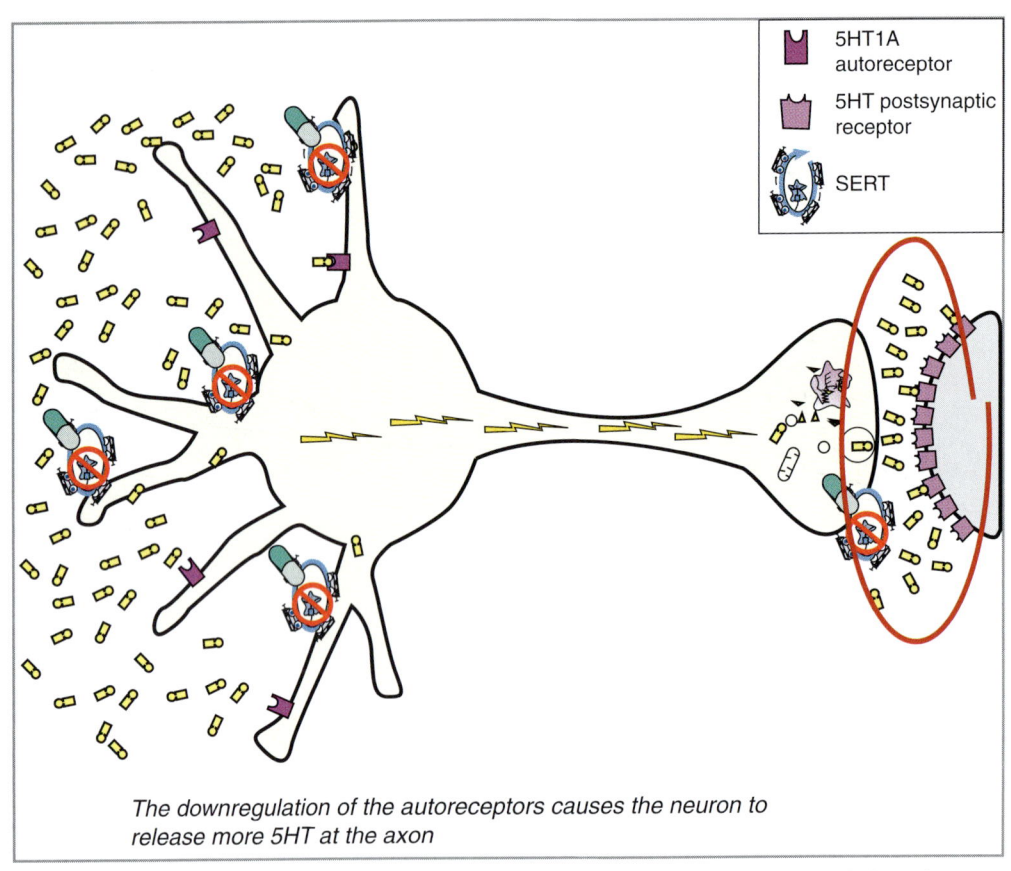

The downregulation of the autoreceptors causes the neuron to release more 5HT at the axon

FIGURE 12-21 **Mechanism of action of serotonin selective reuptake inhibitors (SSRIs), part 4.** Once the somatodendritic receptors downregulate, as depicted in Figure 12-21, there is no longer inhibition of impulse flow in the serotonin (5HT) neuron. Thus, neuronal impulse flow is turned on. The consequence of this is release of 5HT in the axon terminal (red circle). However, this increase is delayed as compared with the increase of 5HT in the somatodendritic areas of the 5HT neuron, depicted in Figure 12-20. This delay is the result of the time it takes for somatodendritic 5HT to downregulate the 5HT1A autoreceptors and turn on neuronal impulse flow in the 5HT neuron. This delay may explain why antidepressants do not relieve depression immediately. It is also the reason why the mechanism of action of antidepressants may be linked to increasing neuronal impulse flow in 5HT neurons, with 5HT levels increasing at axon terminals before an SSRI can exert its antidepressant effects.

by the acute actions of serotonin at undesirable receptors in undesirable pathways. Finally, side effects may attenuate over time by desensitization of the very receptors that mediate them.

There are potentially exciting corollaries to this hypothesis. First, if the ultimate increase in 5HT at critical synapses is required for therapeutic actions, then its failure to occur may explain why some patients respond to an SSRI and some do not. Also, if new drugs could be designed to increase 5HT at the right places at a faster rate or to a greater degree, it could result in a much needed rapid-acting antidepressant, an antidepressant with greater efficacy than an SSRI, or one that could be used to augment an SSRI. Such ideas are active research hypotheses at this time and are leading to many new approaches to modulating the serotonin system with new drugs, which are discussed in the final section of this chapter on future antidepressants.

The increase of 5HT at the axon causes the postsynaptic receptors to desensitize / downregulate, reducing side effects

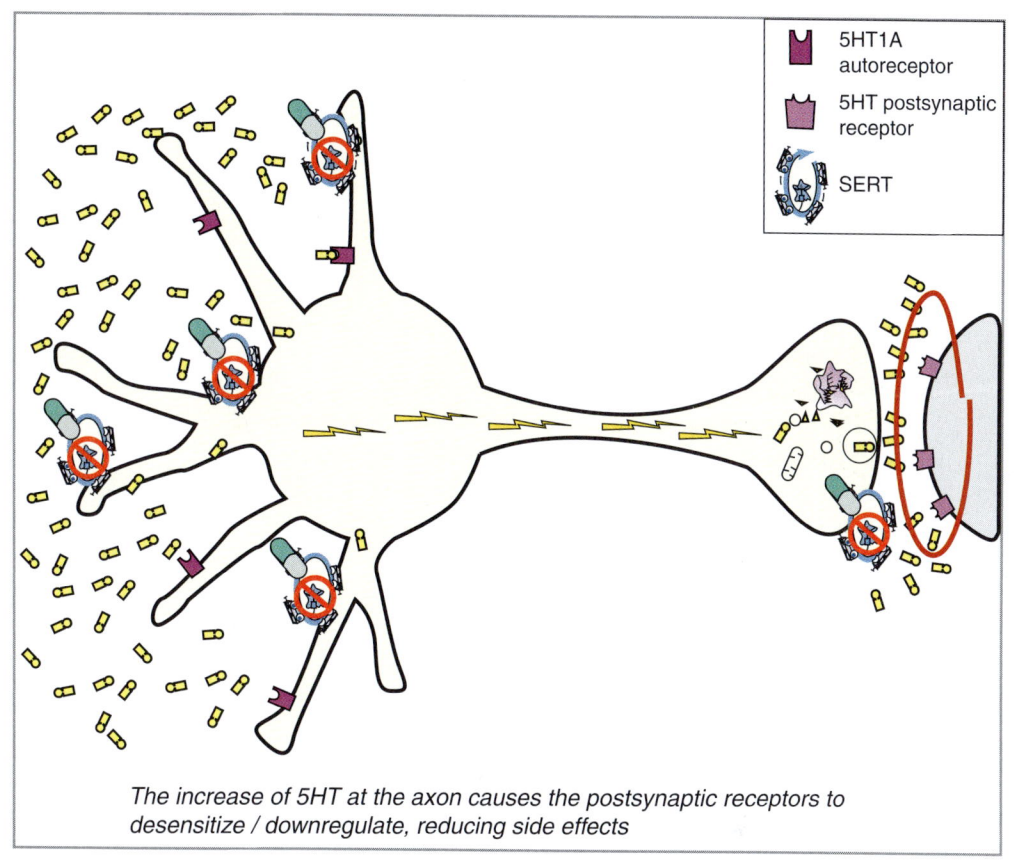

FIGURE 12-22 Mechanism of action of serotonin selective reuptake inhibitors (SSRIs), part 5. Finally, once the SSRIs have blocked the reuptake pump [or serotonin transporter (SERT) in Figure 12-19], increased somatodendritic serotonin (5HT) (Figure 12-19), desensitized somatodendritic 5HT1A autoreceptors (Figure 12-20), turned on neuronal impulse flow (Figure 12-21), and increased release of 5HT from axon terminals (Figure 12-21), the final step (shown here) may be the desensitization of postsynaptic 5HT receptors. This desensitization may mediate the reduction of side effects of SSRIs as tolerance develops.

Serotonin pathways and receptors that hypothetically mediate therapeutic actions and side effects of SSRIs

As mentioned above, the SSRIs cause both their therapeutic actions and their side effects by increasing serotonin at synapses where reuptake is blocked and serotonin release is disinhibited. In general, increasing serotonin in desirable pathways and at targeted receptor subtypes leads to the well-known therapeutic actions of these drugs. However, SSRIs increase serotonin in virtually every serotonin pathway and at virtually every serotonin receptor, and some of these actions are undesirable; these therefore account for the side effects. By understanding the functions of the various serotonin pathways and the distribution of the various serotonin receptor subtypes, it is possible to gain insight into both the therapeutic actions and the side effects that the SSRIs share as a class.

In terms of the potential therapeutic actions of boosting serotonin for the many symptoms of depression, Chapter 11 extensively discusses the various specific projections of serotonin neurons from the midbrain raphe as hypothetical regulators of various specific symptoms of depression (Figures 11-44 through 11-55). Pathways hypothesized to mediate the therapeutic effects of SSRIs in anxiety disorders are discussed in Chapter 14, on anxiety. Pathways hypothesized to mediate the therapeutic effects of SSRIs in eating disorders are discussed in Chapter 19, on reward.

Since serotonin does not influence all brain areas equally, it does not necessarily influence all the symptoms of depression equally. Furthermore, the therapeutic effects from boosting serotonin in the brain will not have the same clinical profile as the therapeutic effects that result from boosting other neurotransmitters, such as NE or DA, since there is not an identical overlap of all three monoamine inputs to all brain circuits. Specifically, a "serotonin deficiency syndrome" in major depression is linked to the concept of "increased negative affect" discussed in Chapter 11 and illustrated in Figure 11-55. SSRIs are often considered to have an excellent profile in such patients, who not only have depressed mood but also guilt, disgust, fear, anxiety, hostility, irritability, and loneliness (Figure 11-55).

On the other hand, because of the distribution of serotonin pathways in the brain, SSRIs often fail to target the other symptoms of major depression as robustly as they target the symptoms of increased negative affect. That is, SSRIs often fail to relieve symptoms of "reduced positive affect" or can even produce some of these symptoms as side effects, including loss of happiness, joy, interest, pleasure, energy, enthusiasm, alertness, and self-confidence (Figure 11-55). When symptoms of increased negative affect improve but symptoms of reduced positive affect persist or are induced by SSRI treatment, this can sometimes be called an "apathetic" recovery. For these latter symptoms to improve, it may require adding or switching to agents that act on NE and/or DA, as discussed below.

In terms of the potential side effects of SSRIs, acute stimulation of any of the plethora of serotonin receptor subtypes (Figure 10-20) may be responsible for mediating these undesirable actions. This includes at least 5HT2A, 5HT2C, 5HT3, and 5HT4 postsynaptic receptors. Since many SSRI side effects are acute, starting from the first dose, and attenuate over time, it may be that a small but acute increase in synaptic serotonin is sufficient to mediate these side effects (Figure 12-19) but insufficient to mediate therapeutic effects until the much more robust disinhibition of the neuron "kicks in" once autoreceptors are downregulated (Figure 12-22). If the postsynaptic serotonin receptors that theoretically mediate side effects downregulate or desensitize, the side effects attenuate or go away (Figure 12-23). Presumably the signal of receptor occupancy of serotonin to the postsynaptic receptor is detected by the genome of the target neuron, and by changing the genetic expression of those receptors that mediate specific side effects, those side effects will go away.

The undesirable side effects of SSRIs seem not only to involve specific serotonin receptor subtypes but also the action of serotonin at these receptors in specific areas of the body, including brain, spinal cord, and gut. The topography of serotonin receptor subtypes in different serotonin pathways may thus help to explain how side effects are mediated. In fact, the same pathways that appear to mediate the delayed therapeutic effects of SSRIs may also mediate the acute side effects of SSRIs, acting at different receptors and in a different time course. Thus, acute stimulation of serotonin 2A and 2C receptors in the serotonin projection from raphe to amygdala and limbic cortex, such as ventromedial prefrontal cortex, may cause acute mental agitation, anxiety, or panic attacks, which can be observed with early dosing of an SSRI prior to anxiolytic actions kicking in (Figure 11-46). Acute stimulation of 5HT2A receptors in the basal ganglia may lead to acute changes in motor movements due to serotonin's inhibition of dopamine neurotransmission there (Figure 10-24,

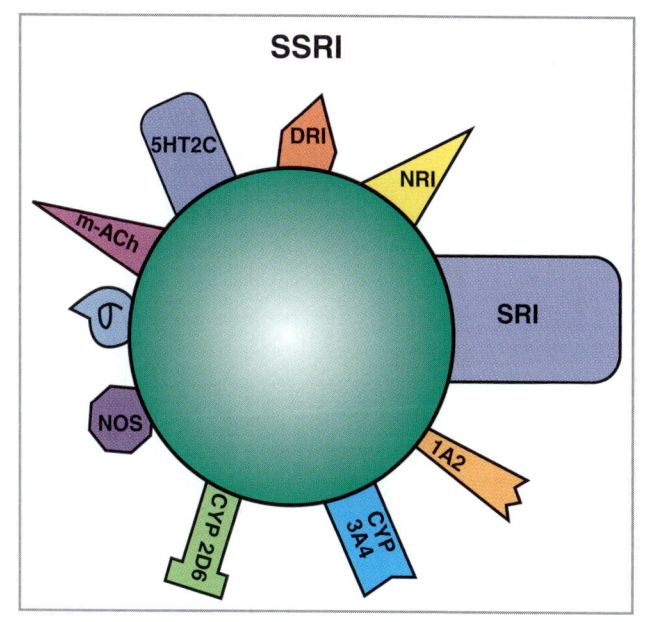

FIGURE 12-23 Secondary pharmacological properties of SSRIs. This icon depicts the various secondary pharmacological properties that may be associated with one or more of the six different serotonin selective reuptake inhibitors (SSRIs). These include not only serotonin reuptake inhibition (SRI) but also lesser degrees of actions at other neurotransmitters and enzymes, including norepinephrine reuptake inhibition (NRI), dopamine reuptake inhibition (DRI), serotonin 2C antagonist actions (5HT2C), muscarinic/cholinergic antagonist actions (M1), sigma 1 receptor actions (σ), inhibition of nitric oxide synthetase (NOS), and inhibition of CYP450 2D6, 3A4, and 1A2.

Figure 10-25, and Figure 11-51). Thus, akathisia (restlessness), psychomotor retardation, or even mild parkinsonism and dystonic movements can result from acute SSRI administration. Stimulation of serotonin 2A receptors in the brainstem sleep centers may contribute to the induction of rapid muscle movements, called myoclonus, during the night; it may also disrupt slow-wave sleep and cause nocturnal awakenings (Figure 11-48). Stimulation of serotonin 2A and 2C receptors in the spinal cord may inhibit the spinal reflexes of orgasm and ejaculation and cause sexual dysfunction. Pathways related to sexual dysfunction are discussed in Chapter 19, on reward. Stimulation of serotonin 2A receptors in mesocortical pleasure centers may reduce dopamine activity there and cause apathy or decreased libido (Figure 11-47). Thus, in a patient treated with an SSRI who has agitation, anxiety, sexual dysfunction, and apathy, it can be difficult to know whether this represents incomplete recovery from depression or drug-induced side effects! In either case, persistence of these symptoms will likely require adding or switching to a different pharmacological mechanism that boosts DA, NE, and/or GABA (gamma-aminobutyric acid). This strategy is discussed below, in the section on antidepressants in clinical practice.

Stimulation of serotonin 3 receptors in the hypothalamus or brainstem may cause nausea or vomiting after SSRI administration (Figure 11-52). Stimulation of serotonin 3 and/or serotonin 4 receptors in the GI tract may cause increased bowel motility, GI cramps, and diarrhea. Tolerance to these side effects usually develops rapidly.

Thus, virtually all side effects of the SSRIs can be understood as undesirable actions of serotonin in undesirable pathways at undesirable receptor subtypes. This appears to be the "cost of doing business," as it is not possible for a systemically administered SSRI to act only at the desirable receptors in the desirable places; it must act everywhere it is distributed, which means all over the brain and all over the body. Fortunately SSRI side effects are more of a nuisance than a danger, and they generally attenuate over time, although they can cause an important subset of patients to discontinue an SSRI prematurely due to intolerance or to lack of remission of all symptoms of depression.

The not-so-selective serotonin reuptake inhibitors: six unique drugs or one class of six drugs?

Although the SSRIs clearly share the same mechanism of action, therapeutic profiles, and side effect profiles, individual patients often react very differently to one SSRI versus another. This is not generally observed in large clinical trials, where group differences between two SSRIs either in efficacy or side effects are very difficult to document. Rather, such differences are seen by prescribers treating patients one at a time, with some patients experiencing a therapeutic response to one SSRI and not another and other patients tolerating one SSRI and not another.

If blockade of SERT explains the shared clinical and pharmacological actions of SSRIs, what explains their differences? Although there is no generally accepted explanation that accounts for the commonly observed clinical phenomena of different efficacy and tolerability of various SSRIs in individual patients, it makes sense to consider those unique pharmacological characteristics of the six SSRIs that are not shared among them as candidates to explain the broad range of individual patient reactions to different SSRIs (Figure 12-23 and Table 12-1). Each SSRI has secondary pharmacological actions other than SERT blockade, and no two SSRIs have identical secondary pharmacological characteristics. These are depicted in Figure 12-23 for the class of SSRIs and include actions such as norepinephrine reuptake blockade, dopamine reuptake blockade, serotonin 2C antagonism, muscarinic cholinergic antagonism, sigma 1 receptor actions, inhibition of the enzyme nitric oxide synthetase, and inhibition of the various cytochrome P450 enzymes 1A2, 2D6, and 3A4. Whether these secondary binding profiles can account for the differences in efficacy and tolerability in individual patients remains to be proven. However, it does lead to provocative hypothesis generation and gives a rational basis for physicians not to be denied access to one or another of the SSRIs by payors claiming that "they are all the same." Sometimes only an empirical trial of different SSRIs will lead to the best match of drug to an individual patient.

Fluoxetine: an SSRI with 5HT2C antagonist and thus norepinephrine and dopamine disinhibiting (NDDI) properties

This SSRI has 5HT2C antagonist actions, which may explain many of its unique clinical properties (Figure 12-24). This is a novel concept for antidepressant action (Table 12-2) and is now a recognized property of several known antidepressants (discussed in the sections on various antidepressants below) and atypical antipsychotics (discussed in Chapter 10) and is an important action of some novel antidepressants still in testing (discussed below in the section on future antidepressants).

Serotonin action at 5HT2C receptors normally *inhibits* both NE and DA release, as discussed in Chapter 11 and as illustrated in Figures 11-40 through 11-42. Drugs that *block* 5HT2C receptors have the opposite action and thus *disinhibit* both NE and DA release (Figure 12-25). Therefore fluoxetine, as a 5HT2C antagonist, is not only an SSRI but also a norepinephrine and dopamine disinhibitor, or NDDI. NDDI actions may lead to increases in DA and NE release in prefrontal cortex (Figure 12-25) and contribute to therapeutic actions in major depression.

The good news about this action is that it is generally activating and may be why many patients, even from the first dose, detect an energizing and fatigue-reducing effect of fluoxetine, with improvement in concentration and attention as well. This mechanism is perhaps best matched to depressed patients with reduced positive affect, hypersomnia, psychomotor retardation, apathy, and fatigue but perhaps least well matched to patients

TABLE 12-2 Putative antidepressant mechanisms

SSRI	Serotonin selective reuptake inhibitor
SNRI	Serotonin norepinephrine reuptake inhibitor
NDRI	Norepinephrine dopamine reuptake inhibitor
selective NRI	Selective norepinephrine reuptake inhibitor
A2A	Alpha 2 antagonist
SARI	Serotonin antagonist/reuptake inhibitor
MAOI	Monoamine oxidase inhibitor
TCA	Tricyclic antidepressant
5HT2C antagonist*	Serotonin 2C antagonist
SNDI*	Serotonin norepinephrine disinhibitor
NDDI*	Norepinephrine dopamine disinhibitor
TMM*	Trimonoamine modulator

*New concepts/mechanisms

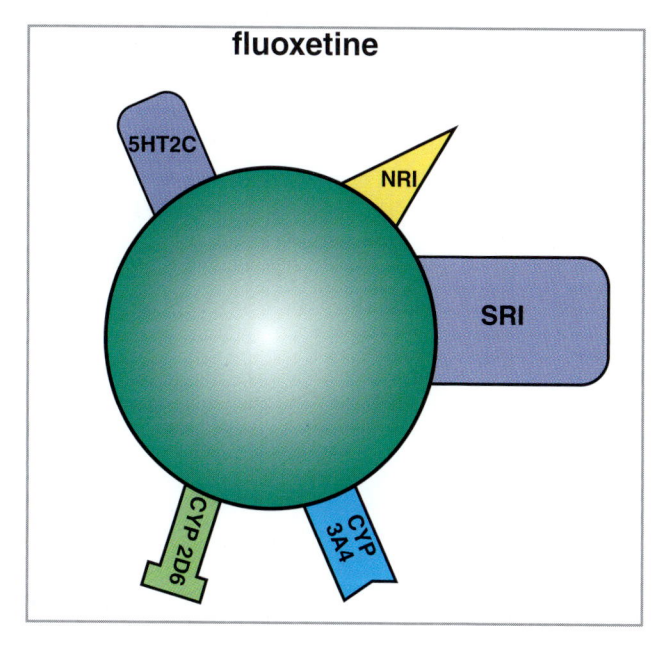

FIGURE 12-24 Icon of fluoxetine. In addition to serotonin reuptake inhibition, fluoxetine has norepinephrine reuptake inhibition (NRI), CYP450 2D6 and 3A4 inhibition, and serotonin 2C antagonist actions (5HT2C). Fluoxetine's activating effects may be due to its actions at serotonin 2C receptors. Norepinephrine reuptake inhibition may be clinically relevant only at very high doses.

with agitation, insomnia, and anxiety who may experience unwanted activation and even a panic attack if given an agent that further activates them.

5HT2C antagonism may also contribute to the anorexia and antibulimia therapeutic actions approved only for this SSRI and only at high doses. Finally, 5HT2C antagonism may explain fluoxetine's ability to boost the antidepressant actions of olanzapine in bipolar depression. Olanzapine also has 5HT2C antagonist actions (discussed in Chapter 10 and illustrated in Figure 10-91). Adding together the 5HT2C antagonist actions of both drugs could theoretically lead to enhanced DA and NE release in cortex to mediate antidepressant actions in bipolar depression, since the combination of both drugs is approved for the treatment of bipolar depression, whereas neither of the individual drugs is approved as monotherapy for this indication.

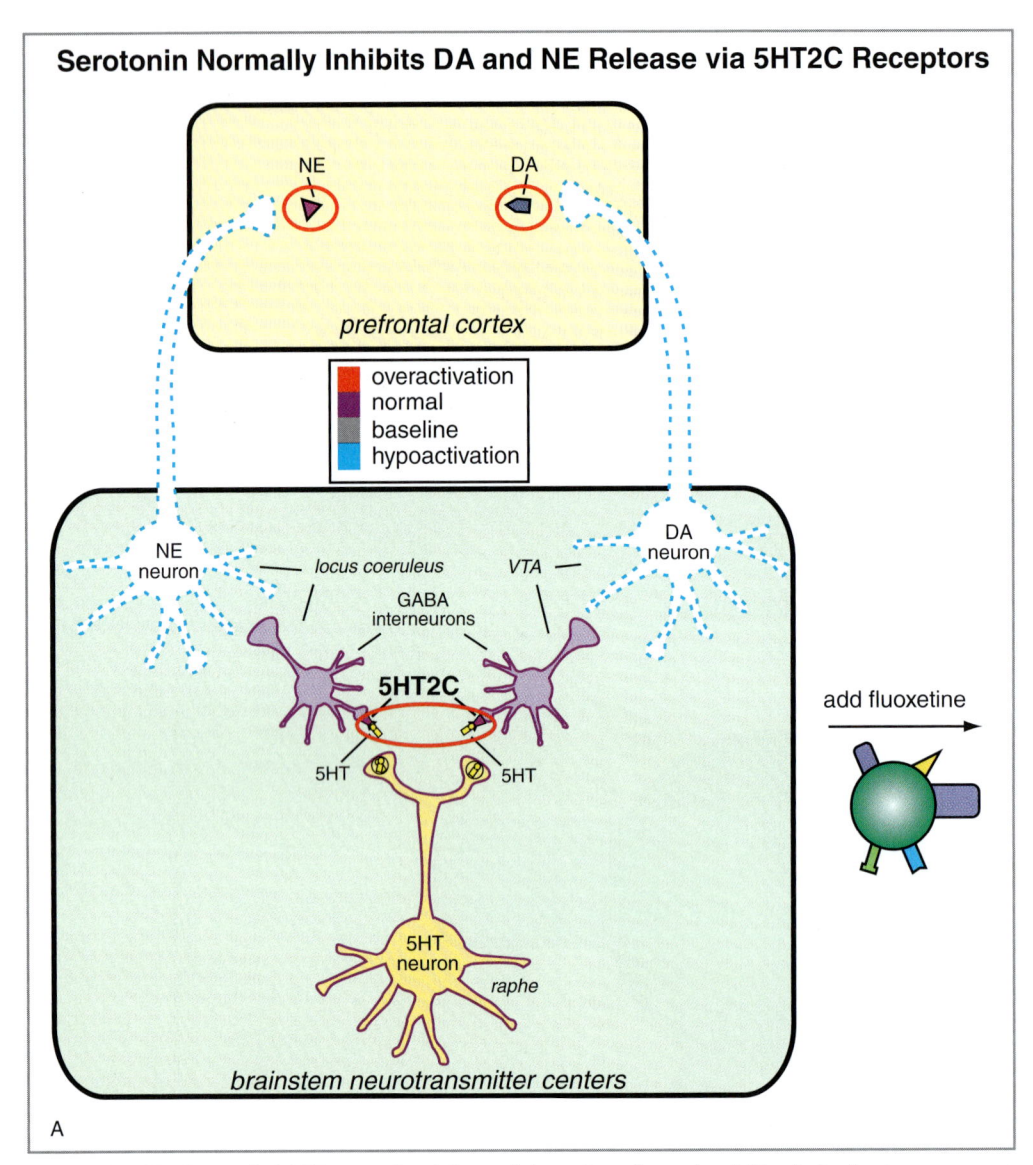

FIGURE 12-25A Serotonin inhibits norepinephrine and dopamine release. In addition to its direct pharmacological effects, fluoxetine can also indirectly increase norepinephrine and dopamine release via blockade of 5HT2C receptors. Normally, serotonin binding at 5HT2C receptors on gamma-aminobutyric acid (GABA) interneurons (bottom red circle) inhibits norepinephrine and dopamine release in the prefrontal cortex (top red circles).

Other unique properties of fluoxetine (Figure 12-24) are weak NE reuptake blocking properties, which may become clinically relevant at very high doses, and inhibition of CYP 2D6 and 3A4 by the parent compound and its active metabolite. Also, fluoxetine has a very long half-life (two to three days); its active metabolite has an even longer half-life (two weeks). This long half-life is advantageous in that it seems to reduce the withdrawal reactions characteristic of sudden discontinuation of some SSRIs, but it also means that it takes a long time to clear the drug and its active metabolite after discontinuing fluoxetine and prior to starting other agents, such as an MAO inhibitor. Fluoxetine is available not

Mechanism of Fluoxetine as a 5HT2C Antagonist and Norepinephrine and Dopamine Disinhibitor in Prefrontal Cortex

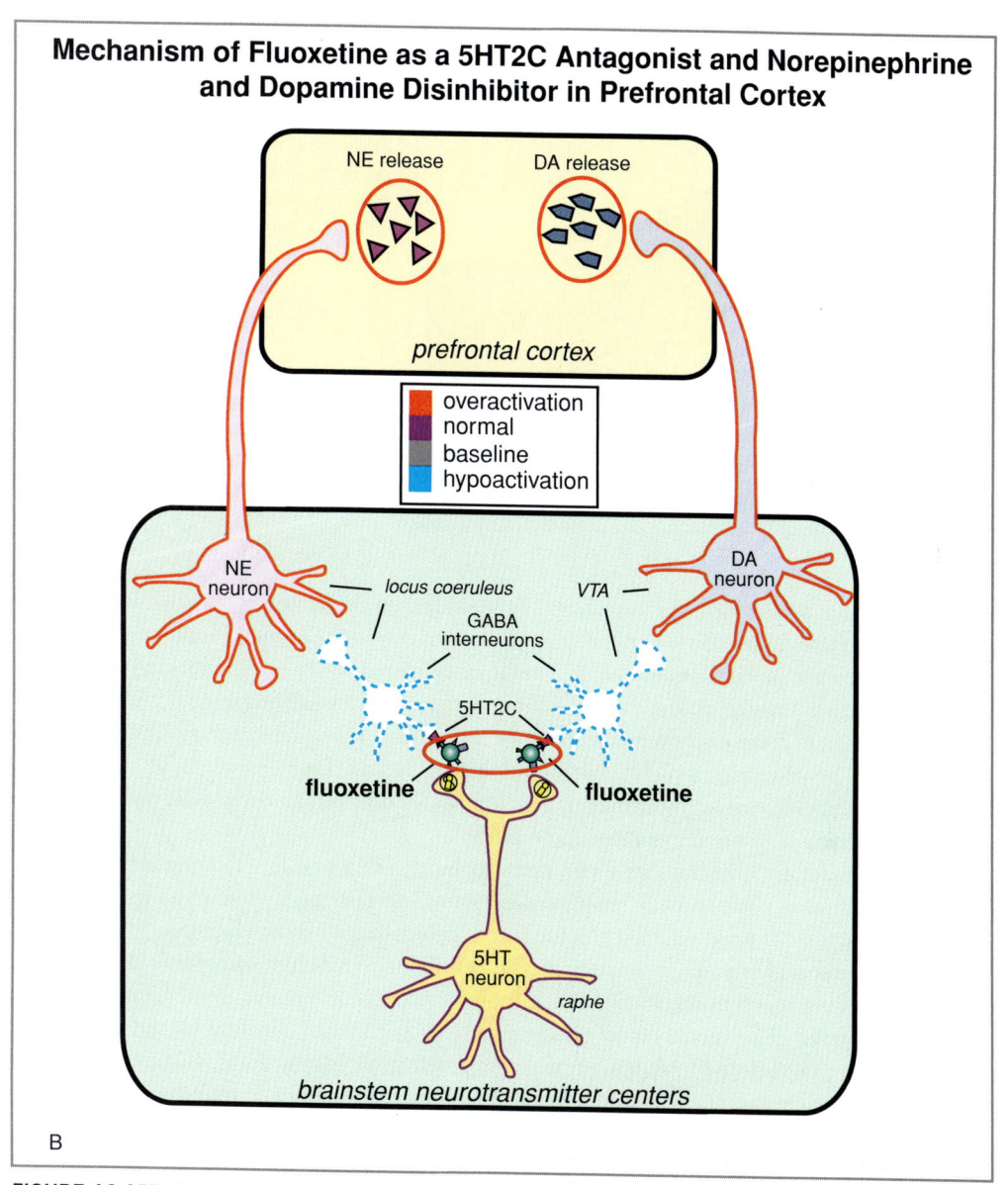

FIGURE 12-25B Fluoxetine disinhibits norepinephrine and dopamine release. When fluoxetine binds to 5HT2C receptors on gamma-aminobutyric acid (GABA) interneurons (bottom red circle), it prevents serotonin from binding there and thus prevents inhibition of norepinephrine and dopamine release in the prefrontal cortex; in other words, it disinhibits their release (top red circles).

only as a once-daily formulation but also as a once-weekly oral dosage formulation; however, the weekly formulation has never become popular.

Sertraline: an SSRI with dopamine transporter (DAT) inhibition

This SSRI has two candidate mechanisms that distinguish it: dopamine transporter (DAT) inhibition and sigma 1 receptor binding (Figure 12-26). It may also have some weak CYP 2D6 inhibitory properties at high doses. The DAT inhibitory actions are controversial since they are weaker than the SERT inhibitory actions, thus leading some experts to suggest that

Antidepressants | 535

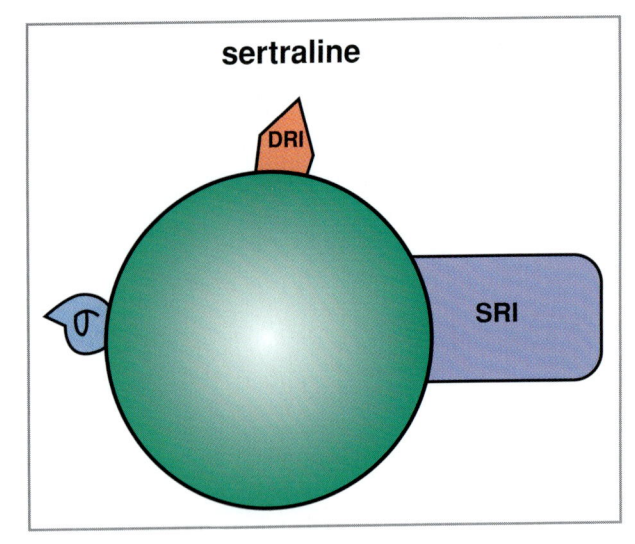

FIGURE 12-26 Icon of sertraline. Sertraline has dopamine reuptake inhibition (DRI) and sigma 1 receptor binding in addition to serotonin reuptake inhibition (SRI). The clinical relevance of sertraline's DRI is unknown, although it may improve energy, motivation, and concentration. Its sigma properties may contribute to anxiolytic actions and may also be helpful in patients with psychotic depression.

there is not sufficient DAT occupancy by sertraline to be clinically relevant. However, as discussed later in the section on norepinephrine and dopamine reuptake inhibitors (NDRIs), it is not clear that high degrees of DAT occupancy are necessary or even desirable in order to contribute to antidepressant actions. That is, perhaps only a small amount of DAT inhibition is sufficient to cause improvement in energy, motivation, and concentration, especially when added to another action such as SERT inhibition. In fact, high-impact DAT inhibition is the property of reinforcing stimulants, including cocaine and methylphenidate, and would not generally be desired in an antidepressant.

Anecdotally, clinicians have observed the mild and desirable activating actions of sertraline in some patients with "atypical depression," improving symptoms of hypersomnia, low energy, and mood reactivity. A favorite combination of some clinicians for depressed patients is to add bupropion to sertraline (i.e., Wellbutrin to Zoloft, sometimes called "Welloft"), adding together the weak DAT inhibitory properties of each agent. Clinicians have also observed the overactivation of some patients with panic disorder by sertraline, thus requiring slower dose titration in some patients with anxiety symptoms. All of these actions of sertraline are consistent with the weak DAT inhibitory actions of sertraline contributing to its clinical portfolio of actions. Combination of the NDRI bupropion with SSRIs is discussed below in the section on NDRIs.

The sigma 1 actions of sertraline are not well understood but might contribute to its anxiolytic effects and especially to its effects in psychotic and delusional depression, where sertraline may have advantageous therapeutic effects compared to some other SSRIs. Sigma 1 actions could theoretically contribute both to anxiolytic actions and to antipsychotic actions as will be discussed further in the section on fluvoxamine below.

Paroxetine: an SSRI with muscarinic anticholinergic and norepinephrine transporter (NET) inhibitory actions

This SSRI is preferred by many clinicians for patients with anxiety symptoms. It tends to be more calming, even sedating, early in treatment compared to the more activating actions of both fluoxetine and sertraline discussed above. Perhaps the mild anticholinergic actions of paroxetine contribute to this clinical profile (Figure 12-27). Paroxetine also has weak NET inhibitory properties, which could contribute to efficacy in depression, especially at high

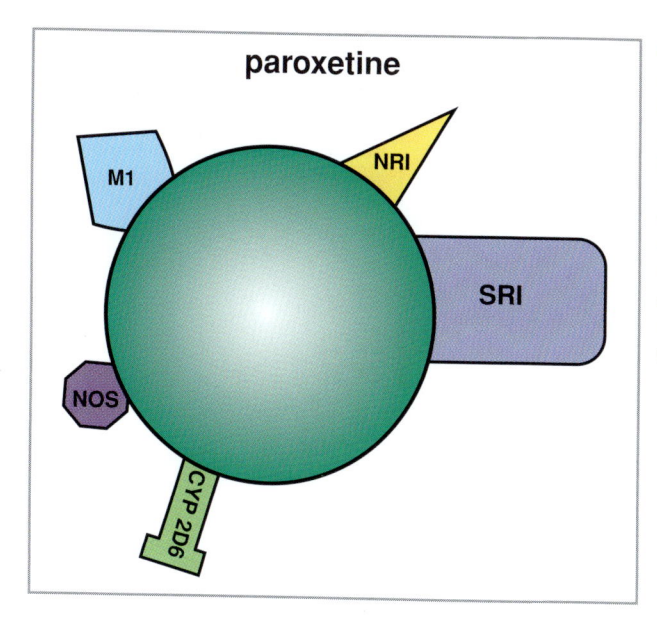

FIGURE 12-27 Icon of paroxetine. In addition to serotonin reuptake inhibition (SRI), paroxetine has mild anticholinergic actions (M1), which can be calming or possibly sedating, weak norepinephrine reuptake inhibition (NRI), which may contribute to further antidepressant actions, and inhibition of the enzyme nitric oxide synthetase (NOS), which may contribute to sexual dysfunction. Paroxetine is also a potent inhibitor of CYP450 2D6.

doses. The advantages of dual serotonin plus norepinephrine reuptake–inhibiting properties, or SNRI actions, are discussed below in the section on SNRIs. The possibility that weak to moderate NET inhibition may nevertheless contribute importantly to antidepressant actions is discussed below not only in the section on SNRIs but also in the section on NDRIs.

Paroxetine is a potent 2D6 inhibitor and also may inhibit the enzyme nitric oxide synthetase, which could theoretically contribute to sexual dysfunction, especially in men. Paroxetine is also notorious for causing withdrawal reactions upon sudden discontinuation, with symptoms such as akathisia, restlessness, gastrointestinal upset, dizziness, and tingling, especially when suddenly discontinued from long-term high-dose treatment. This is possibly due not only to SERT inhibition properties, since all SSRIs can cause discontinuation reactions, but with additional contributions from anticholinergic rebound when paroxetine is rapidly discontinued. Furthermore, paroxetine is both a substrate and an inhibitor for CYP 2D6, which leads to a very rapid decline in plasma drug levels when paroxetine is discontinued, possibly contributing to withdrawal symptoms. Paroxetine is available in a controlled-release formulation, which may mitigate some of its side effects, including discontinuation reactions, but this form of the drug is not widely used in clinical practice.

Fluvoxamine: an SSRI with sigma 1 receptor binding properties

This SSRI was among the first to be launched for the treatment of depression worldwide but was never officially approved for depression in the United States, where it has been considered more of an agent for the treatment of obsessive compulsive disorder and anxiety. Use of SSRIs for treatment of anxiety is discussed in Chapter 14, on anxiety. A secondary binding property of fluvoxamine, like sertraline, is its interaction at sigma 1 sites, but this action is more potent for fluvoxamine than for sertraline (Figure 12-28). The physiological function of sigma 1 sites is still a mystery, sometimes called the "sigma enigma," but has been linked both to anxiety and psychosis. Although it is not entirely clear how to define an agonist or antagonist at sigma 1 sites, recent studies suggest that fluvoxamine may be an agonist at sigma 1 receptors and that this property may contribute an additional pharmacological

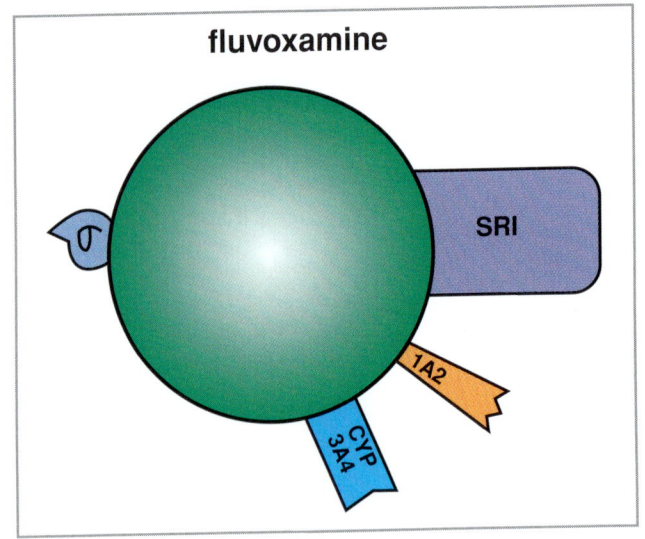

FIGURE 12-28 Icon of fluvoxamine. Fluvoxamine's secondary properties include actions at sigma 1 receptors, which may be anxiolytic as well as beneficial for psychotic depression, and inhibition of CYP450 1A2 and 3A4.

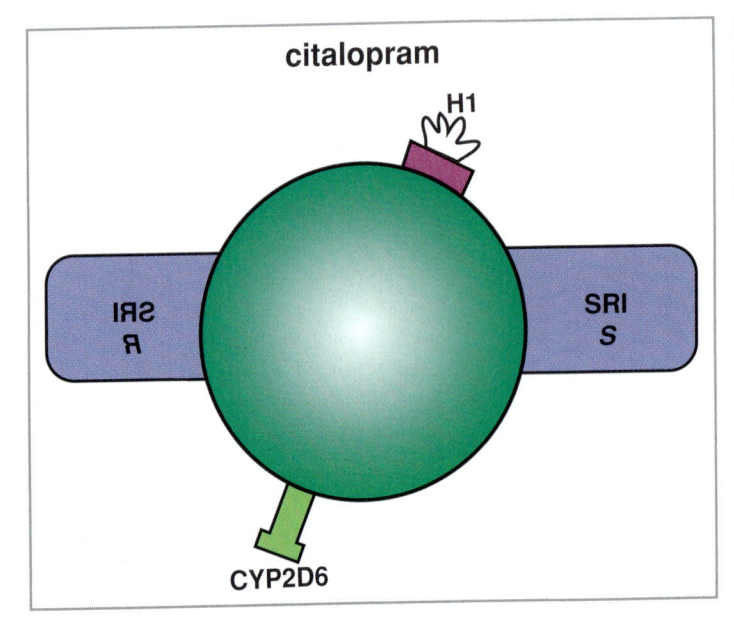

FIGURE 12-29 Icon of citalopram. Citalopram consists of two enantiomers, R and S. The R enantiomer has weak antihistamine properties and is a weak inhibitor of CYP450 2D6.

action to help explain fluvoxamine's well-known anxiolytic properties. Fluvoxamine has also shown therapeutic activity in both psychotic and delusional depression, where it, like sertraline, may have advantages over other SSRIs.

Fluvoxamine is now available as a controlled-release formulation, which makes once-a-day administration possible, unlike immediate-release fluvoxamine, whose shorter half-life often requires twice-daily administration. In addition, recent trials of controlled-release fluvoxamine show impressive remission rates in both obsessive compulsive disorder and social anxiety disorder as well as possibly less peak-dose sedation.

Citalopram: an SSRI with a "good" and a "bad" enantiomer

This SSRI (Figure 12-29) comprises two enantiomers, R and S, one of which is the mirror image of the other (Figure 12-30). The mixture of these enantiomers is known as racemic

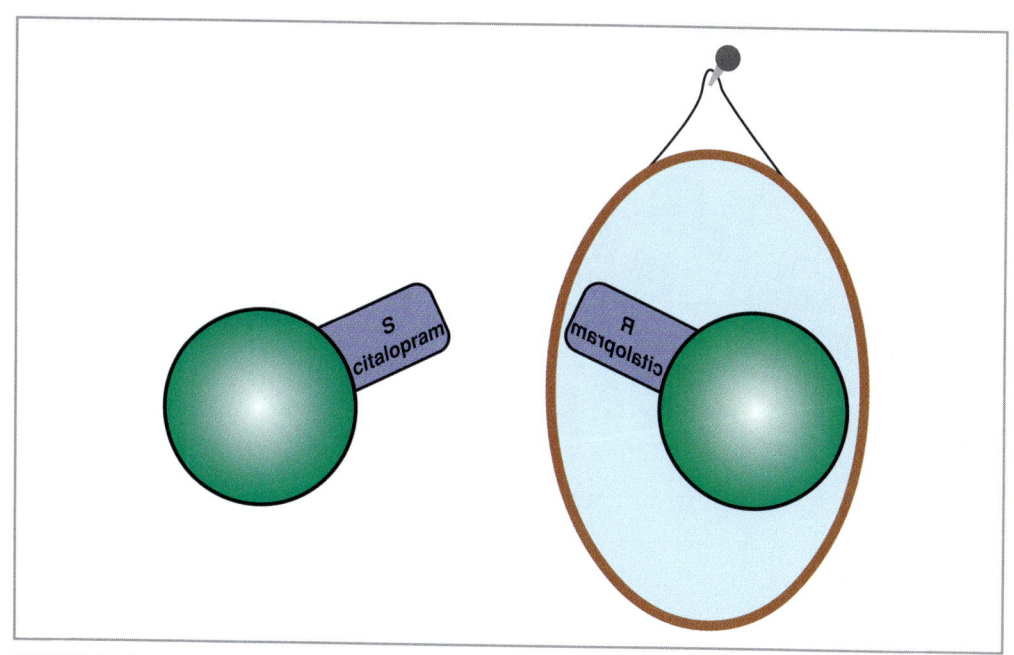

FIGURE 12-30 R and S enantiomers of citalopram. The R and S enantiomers of citalopram are mirror images of each other but have slightly different clinical properties. The R enantiomer is the one with weak antihistamine properties and weak inhibition of CYP450 2D6, while the S enantiomer does not have these properties. The R and S enantiomers may also differ in their effects at the serotonin transporter, as shown in Figure 12-31.

citalopram, or commonly just as citalopram, and has mild antihistamine properties and mild inhibition of CYP450 2D6, with both of these properties residing in the R enantiomer (Figure 12-29). Racemic citalopram is generally one of the better tolerated SSRIs and has favorable findings in the treatment of depression in the elderly. However, it has a somewhat inconsistent therapeutic action at the lowest dose, often requiring dose increases to optimize treatment. This may be due to a recent finding suggesting that the R enantiomer may be pharmacologically active at SERT in a manner that does not inhibit SERT but actually interferes with the ability of the active S enantiomer to inhibit SERT. This could lead to reduced inhibition of SERT, reduced synaptic 5HT, and possibly reduced net therapeutic actions, especially at low doses (Figure 12-31).

Escitalopram: the quintessential SSRI

The solution to improving the properties of racemic citalopram (which is still a very safe and effective SSRI) is to remove the unwanted R enantiomer. The resulting drug is known as escitalopram, as it is made up of only the pure active S enantiomer (Figure 12-32). This maneuver appears to remove the antihistaminic and CYP450 2D6 inhibitory properties (compare Figures 12-29 and 12-32). In addition, removal of the potentially interfering R isomer makes the lowest dose of escitalopram more predictably efficacious (Figure 12-31). Escitalopram is therefore the SSRI for which pure SERT inhibition is most likely to explain almost all of its pharmacological actions. Escitalopram is considered perhaps the best-tolerated SSRI, with the fewest CYP450-mediated drug interactions, although it is still an expensive agent in many countries, since it is not yet available as a generic.

Antidepressants | 539

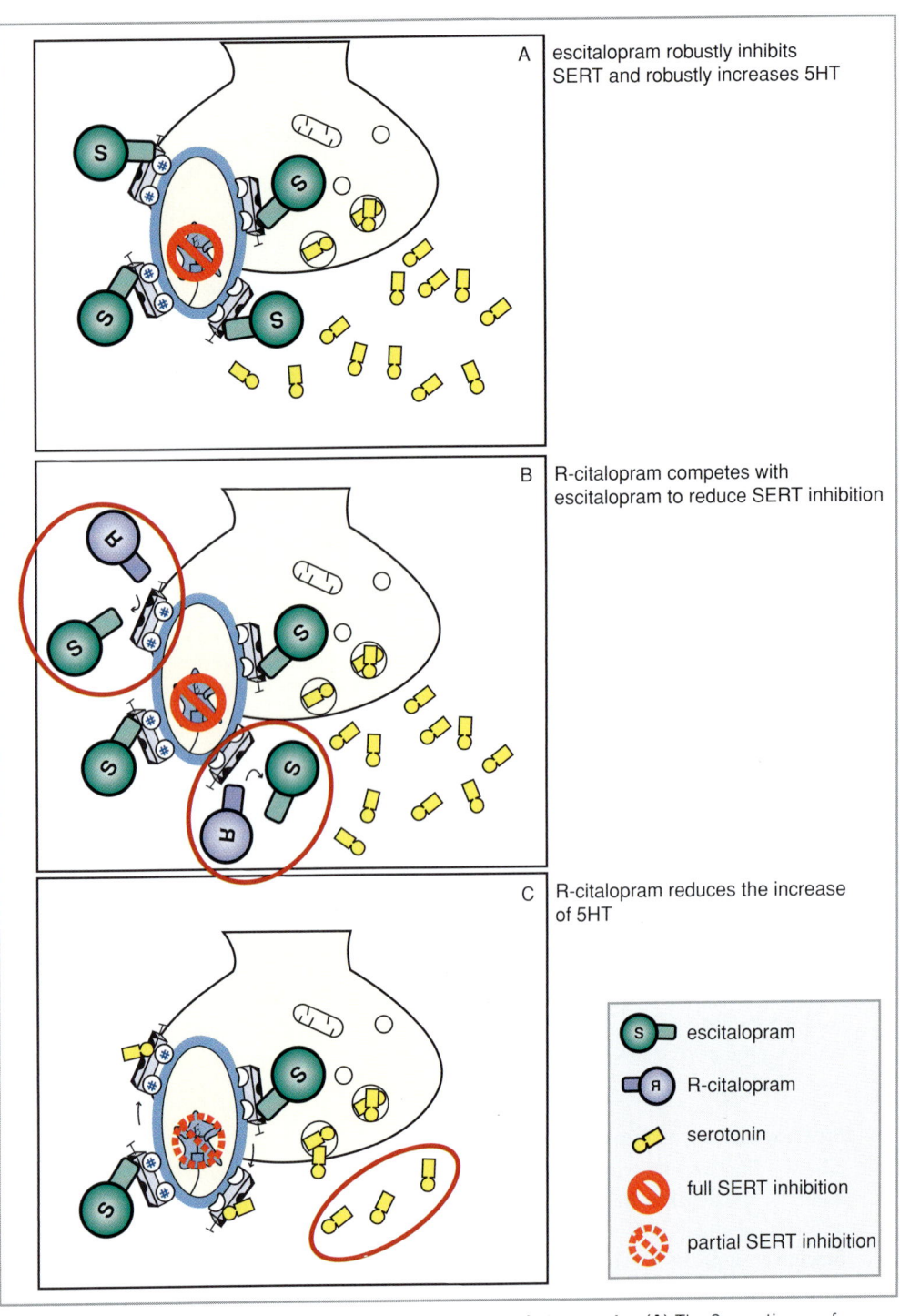

FIGURE 12-31A, B, and C R versus S enantiomer at the serotonin transporter. (**A**) The S enantiomer of citalopram (escitalopram) robustly inhibits the serotonin transporter (SERT) and robustly increases serotonin (5HT) (**A**). The R enantiomer of citalopram (R-citalopram) binds to SERT but does not inhibit it (**B**). Thus it competes with escitalopram to reduce SERT inhibition (**B**), which reduces the ability of the S enantiomer to increase 5HT (**C**).

540 | Essential Psychopharmacology

TABLE 12-3 Serotonin norepinephrine reuptake inhibitors

venlafaxine XR (Effexor XR; Efexor XR)
desvenlafaxine XR (Pristiq)
duloxetine (Cymbalta, Xeristar)
milnacipran (Ixel, Toledomin)

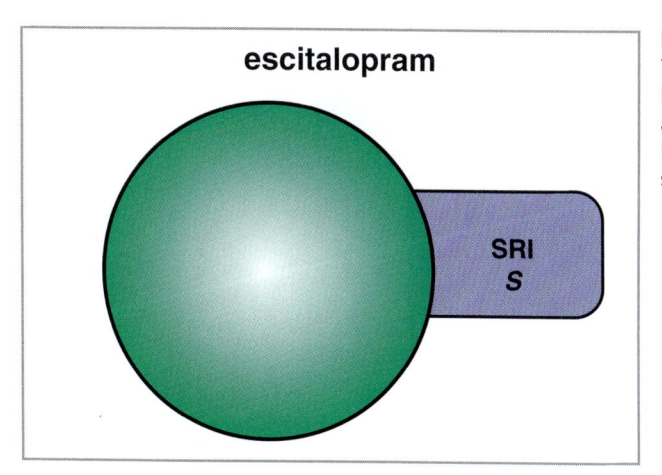

FIGURE 12-32 Icon of escitalopram. The S enantiomer of citalopram has been developed and marketed as the antidepressant escitalopram. This agent is the most selective of the serotonin selective reuptake inhibitors (SSRIs).

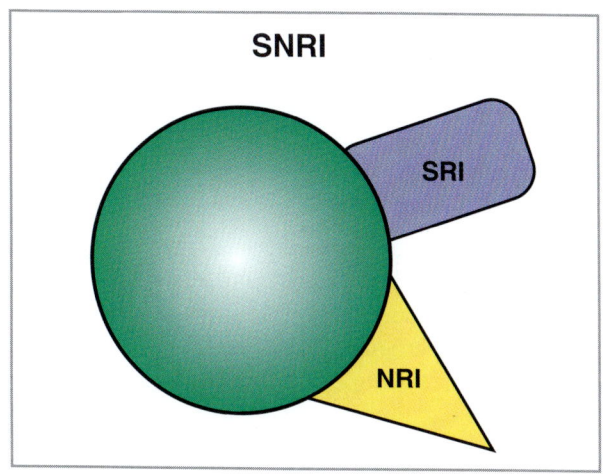

FIGURE 12-33 Icon of a serotonin norepinephrine reuptake inhibitor (SNRI). Dual reuptake inhibitors of serotonin and norepinephrine by definition combine the actions of both a serotonin reuptake inhibitor (SRI) and a norepinephrine reuptake inhibitor (NRI).

Serotonin norepinephrine reuptake inhibitors (SNRIs)

Antidepressants that block the reuptake of both serotonin and norepinephrine – known as SNRIs – have rapidly become among the most frequently prescribed classes of antidepressants, particularly in mental health practices (Table 12-3). These agents combine the robust SERT inhibition of the SSRIs with various degrees of inhibition of the norepinephrine transporter (or NET) (Figure 12-33). This has led to this highly debated question: Are two mechanisms better than one (Figure 12-34)?

Antidepressants | 541

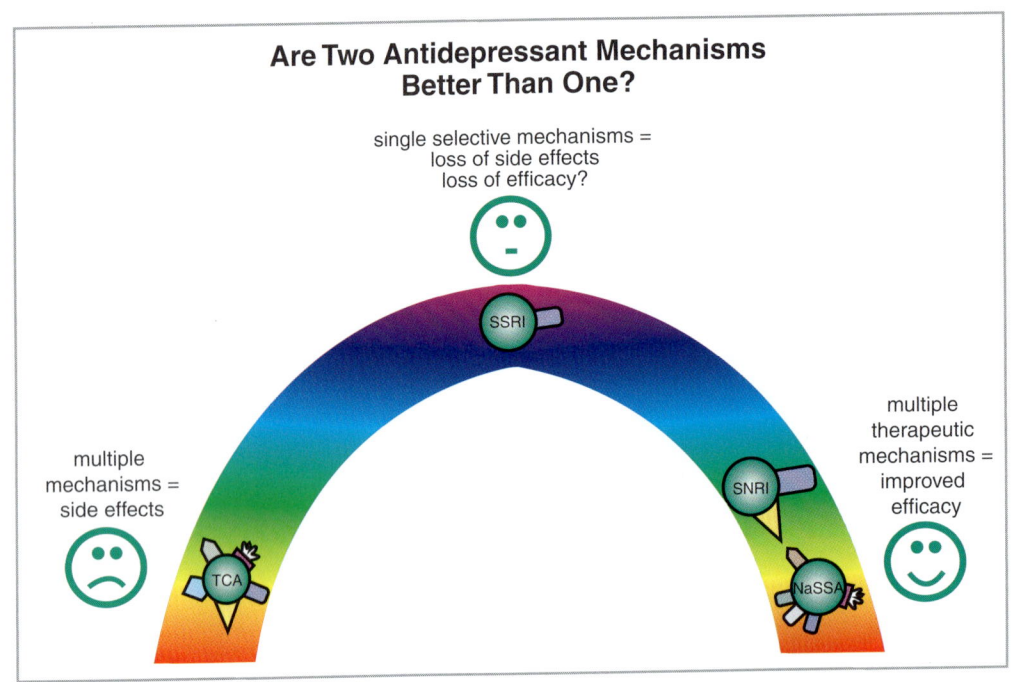

FIGURE 12-34 Are two antidepressant mechanisms better than one? Originally, multiple pharmacological mechanisms were synonymous with "dirty drugs," because they implied unwanted side effects. This is shown as tricyclic antidepressants on the left, with serotonin and norepinephrine reuptake inhibition but also anticholinergic, antihistaminic, and antiadrenergic actions. The trend to develop selective drugs (center) led to the removal of unwanted side effects and to the inclusion of only a single therapeutic action. More recently, the trend has again been to add multiple therapeutic actions together so as to improve tolerability and enhance efficacy. Enhanced efficacy from synergistic pharmacological mechanisms may increase response in some patients, especially those resistant to single-mechanism agents.

Are two antidepressant mechanisms better than one?

The original tricyclic antidepressants (TCAs) had multiple pharmacological mechanisms and were termed "dirty drugs" because many of these mechanisms were undesirable, as they caused side effects (Figure 12-34). The idea was then to "clean up" these agents by making them selective; thus, the SSRI era was born. Indeed, the development of such selective agents made them devoid of pharmacological properties mediating the *side effects* of the first generation tricyclic antidepressants, such as anticholinergic, antihistaminic, and antiadrenergic side effects (tricyclic antidepressants are discussed below). However, selectivity may be less desired when that means loss of multiple *therapeutic* mechanisms (Figure 12-34). In practice, many difficult, severe, or treatment-resistant cases require multiple therapeutic mechanisms before an adequate therapeutic effect is attained, and serotonergic action alone is frequently not enough for such patients.

Thus psychotropic drug development is trending back to incorporating multiple pharmacological mechanisms in the hope that this will exploit potential synergies among two or more independent therapeutic mechanisms. For antidepressants, this has led to the development of drugs that exhibit "intramolecular polypharmacy," such as the dual action of the SNRIs discussed here (Figure 12-35). It has also led to the increasing use of two antidepressants together for treatment-resistant cases, combining two or more synergistic therapeutic mechanisms, as discussed below in the section on antidepressants in clinical practice.

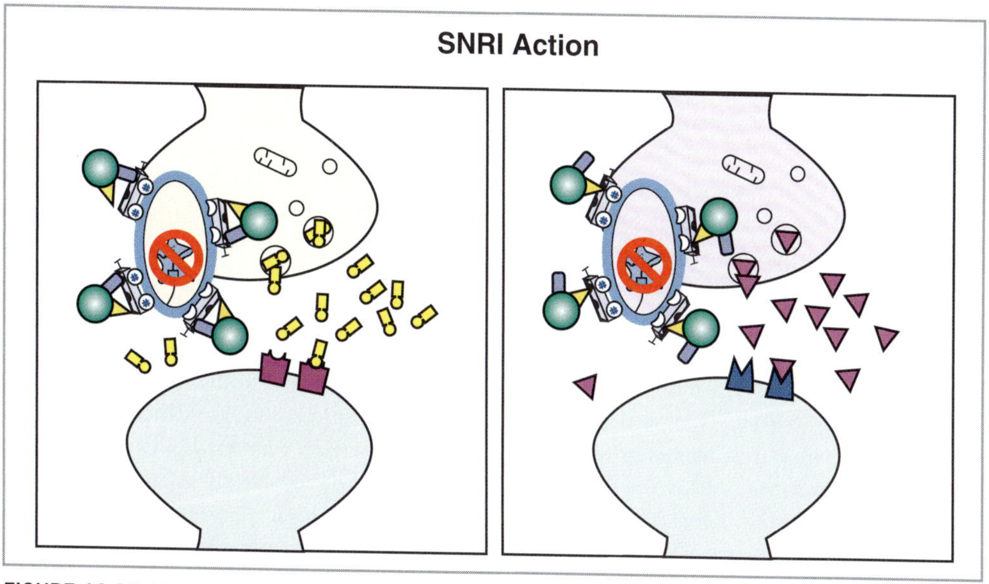

FIGURE 12-35 SNRI actions. In this figure, the dual actions of the serotonin norepinephrine reuptake inhibitors (SNRIs) are shown. Both the serotonin reuptake inhibitor (SRI) portion of the SNRI molecule (left panel) and the norepinephrine reuptake inhibitor (NRI) portion of the SNRI molecule (right panel) are inserted into their respective reuptake pumps. Consequently, both pumps are blocked, and the drug mediates an antidepressant effect.

Of course there is "no free lunch," meaning that adding more mechanisms almost always means adding more mechanism-related side effects. Nevertheless, the hallmark of the current era of antidepressant treatment is to aim for sustained remission of all symptoms, and it frequently takes more than one mechanism to get this degree of therapeutic efficacy. In fact, the field is now moving to the use of as many mechanisms as necessary to gain remission, whether that means utilizing one drug with several different mechanisms or utilizing several drugs, each with a different mechanism.

Clinicians and experts currently debate whether remission rates are higher with SNRIs compared to SSRIs or whether SNRIs are more helpful in patients who fail to respond to SSRIs than are other options. The data may lean in favor of higher remission rates for SNRIs compared to SSRIs, but that is not really the point. The important thing to keep in mind is the need to attain remission in any patient, and to do this in any way that works. SSRI treatment frequently results in remission. When it does not, certainly a dual-action SNRI could be considered. However, when treatment with any antidepressant does not result in remission, the point is to do something else, generally substituting or adding an additional pharmacological mechanism until remission is achieved. This is discussed in detail in the section below on antidepressants in clinical practice.

Theoretically, there should be some therapeutic advantage of adding NET inhibition to SERT inhibition, since one mechanism may add efficacy to the other by widening the reach of the trimonoamine neurotransmitter system throughout more brain regions (Figures 11-46 through 11-55). A practical indication that dual monoamine mechanisms may lead to more efficacy is the finding that the SNRI venlafaxine frequently seems to have greater efficacy as the dose increases, theoretically due to the recruitment of more and more NET inhibition as the dose is raised (i.e., the noradrenergic "boost").

Antidepressants | 543

NET inhibition increases DA in prefrontal cortex

Although SNRIs are commonly called "dual action" serotonin-norepinephrine agents, they actually have a third action on dopamine in the prefrontal cortex but not elsewhere in the brain. Thus they are not "full" triple-action agents, since they do not inhibit the dopamine transporter (DAT); but SNRIs can perhaps be considered to have "two and a half actions" (Figure 12-36) and not just two (Figure 12-35). That is, SNRIs boost not only serotonin and norepinephrine throughout the brain (Figure 12-35) but also dopamine specifically in prefrontal cortex (Figure 12-36). This third mechanism of boosting dopamine in an important area of the brain associated with several symptoms of depression should add another theoretical advantage to the pharmacology of SNRIs and to their efficacy in the treatment of major depression.

How does NET inhibition boost DA in prefrontal cortex? The answer is illustrated in Figure 12-36. In prefrontal cortex, SERTs and NETs are present in abundance on serotonin and norepinephrine nerve terminals, respectively, but there are very few DATs on dopamine nerve terminals in this part of the brain (Figure 12-36). The consequence of this is that once DA is released, it is free to cruise away from the synapse (Figure 12-36A). The diffusion radius of DA is thus wider (Figure 12-36A) than that of NE in prefrontal cortex (Figure 12-36B), since there is NET at the NE synapse (Figure 12-36B) but no DAT at the DA synapse (Figure 12-36A). This arrangement may enhance the regulatory importance of dopamine in prefrontal cortex functioning, since DA in this part of the brain can interact with DA receptors not only at its own synapse but also at a distance, perhaps enhancing the ability of DA to regulate cognition in an entire area within its diffusion radius, not just at a single synapse.

Dopamine action is therefore not terminated by DAT in prefrontal cortex but by two other mechanisms. That is, DA diffuses away from the DA synapse until it either encounters the enzyme COMT (catechol-O-methyl transferase), which degrades it (see Figure 9-19), or it encounters a norepinephrine reuptake pump or NET that transports it into the NE neuron (Figure 12-36A). NETs, in fact, have a greater affinity for DA than they do for NE, so they will pump DA as well as NE into NE nerve terminals, halting the action of either.

It is interesting what happens when NET is inhibited in prefrontal cortex. As expected, NET inhibition enhances synaptic NE levels and increases the diffusion radius of NE (Figure 12-36B). Somewhat surprising may be the fact that NET inhibition also enhances DA levels and increases DA's diffusion radius (Figure 12-36C). The bottom line is that NET inhibition increases both NE and DA in prefrontal cortex. Thus, SNRIs have "two and a half" mechanisms: boosting serotonin throughout the brain, boosting norepinephrine throughout the brain, and boosting dopamine in prefrontal cortex (but not in other DA projection areas).

Serotonergic, noradrenergic, and dopaminergic pathways and receptors as mediators of therapeutic actions and side effects of SNRIs

The role of serotonin receptors and pathways in the therapeutic actions and side effects of SSRIs is discussed above, and this discussion applies to the serotonergic aspect of SNRI actions as well. In addition, SNRIs have additional considerations due to their NET inhibitory actions. For a full understanding of the mechanism of therapeutic actions and side effects of SNRIs, we must therefore add a discussion of the role of norepinephrine pathways and receptors and, in prefrontal cortex, the role of dopamine pathways and receptors.

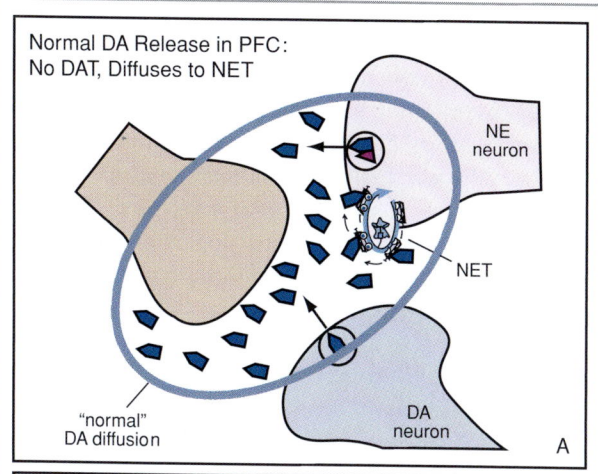

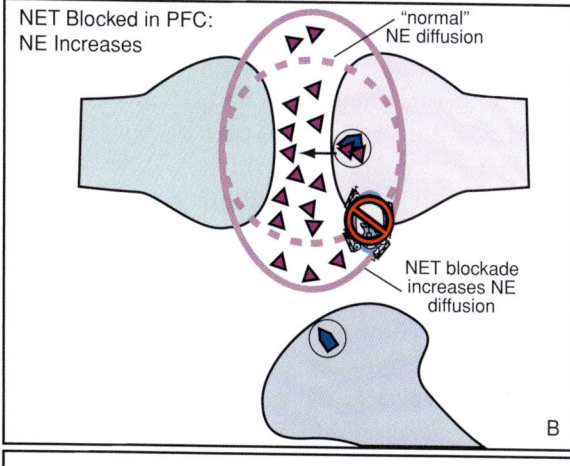

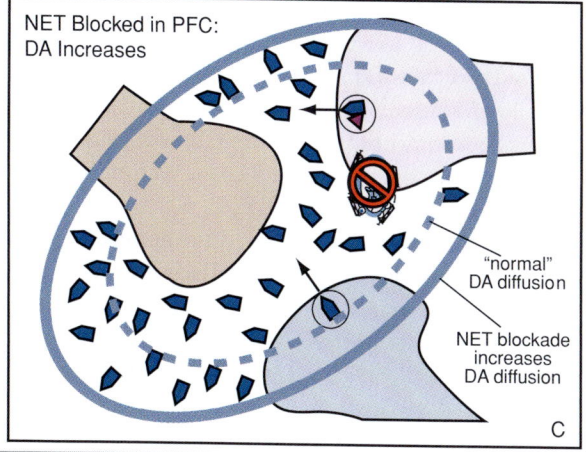

FIGURE 12-36A, B, and C Norepinephrine transporter blockade and dopamine in the prefrontal cortex. (**A**) Although there are abundant serotonin transporters (SERTs) and norepinephrine transporters (NETs) in the prefrontal cortex, there are very few dopamine transporters (DATs). This means that dopamine can diffuse away from the synapse and therefore exert its actions within a larger radius. Dopamine's actions are terminated at norepinephrine axon terminals, because DA is taken up by NET. (**B**) NET blockade in the prefrontal cortex leads to an increase in synaptic norepinephrine, thus increasing norepinephrine's diffusion radius. (**C**) Because NET takes up dopamine as well as norepinephrine, NET blockade also leads to an increase in synaptic dopamine, further increasing its diffusion radius. Thus, agents that block NET increase norepinephrine throughout the brain and both norepinephrine and dopamine in the prefrontal cortex.

Antidepressants | 545

That is, increasing norepinephrine and/or dopamine at desirable synapses and desirable noradrenergic or dopaminergic receptors would theoretically lead to the therapeutic properties of SNRIs. However, increasing norepinephrine or dopamine at undesirable places would theoretically lead to side effects as the "cost of doing business" owing to NET inhibition, thus increasing norepinephrine in virtually every noradrenergic pathway and at virtually every noradrenergic receptor. As has been discussed, NET inhibition also increases DA in some dopamine pathways and at some dopamine receptors in prefrontal cortex. By understanding the functions of the various norepinephrine and prefrontal dopamine pathways and the distribution of the various noradrenergic and dopamine receptor subtypes, it is possible to gain insight into both the therapeutic actions and side effects that can be attributed to the NET inhibitory actions of SNRIs.

In terms of therapeutic actions of NET inhibition, Chapter 11 extensively discusses the various specific projections of noradrenergic neurons from the midbrain locus coeruleus and of dopamine neurons from midbrain dopamine centers as hypothetical regulators of various specific symptoms of depression (Figures 11-44 through 11-55). Pathways hypothesized to mediate the therapeutic effects of NET inhibition in ADHD (attention deficit hyperactivity disorder) are discussed in Chapter 17 on ADHD. Pathways hypothesized to mediate the therapeutic effects of NET inhibition (along with SERT inhibition) in chronic painful conditions such as fibromyalgia and neuropathic pain are discussed in Chapter 15, on pain.

Since norepinephrine does not influence all brain areas equally, it does not necessarily influence all the symptoms of depression equally. Furthermore, the therapeutic effects from boosting norepinephrine or dopamine in the brain will not have the same clinical profile as the therapeutic effects that result from boosting other neurotransmitters such as 5HT, since there is not an identical overlap of all three monoamine inputs to all brain circuits. Specifically, a "norepinephrine deficiency syndrome" in major depression is linked to the concept of "reduced positive affect" (Figure 11-55), although this concept may fit even better with the idea of a "dopamine deficiency syndrome" (discussed below in the section on NDRIs and MAO inhibitors). Norepinephrine, in fact, may be linked across the affective spectrum, including both "reduced positive affect" as well as "increased negative affect," and it certainly has a wider theoretical clinical spectrum than serotonin (see Figure 11-55). This may be the reason why a larger portfolio of symptoms is relieved by SNRIs than by SSRIs in some patients. Add to this the regional boosting of DA in prefrontal cortex, and there is a broad set of pharmacological targets within the trimonoaminergic neurotransmitter system that are linked to the therapeutic mechanism of action of SNRIs.

Nevertheless, like SSRIs, SNRIs not infrequently fail to relieve all symptoms of reduced positive affect or may even produce some of these symptoms as side effects, including loss of happiness, joy, interest, pleasure, energy, enthusiasm, alertness, and self-confidence (Figure 11-55). It has already been mentioned that when symptoms of increased negative affect improve but symptoms of reduced positive affect persist or are induced by either SSRI or SNRI treatment, this can sometimes be called an "apathetic" recovery. For such symptoms to improve, it may be necessary to raise the dose of the SNRI or to add or switch to agents that act more robustly on DA, particularly in brain regions outside of the prefrontal cortex, as discussed below.

In terms of potential side effects of NET inhibition by SNRIs, these can hypothetically be linked to acute stimulation of several clinically important noradrenergic receptor subtypes in various parts of the brain and body: alpha 1, alpha 2, and/or beta 1 adrenergic receptors. The undesirable side effects linked to NET inhibition seem to involve not only specific norepinephrine receptor subtypes but also the action of NE at receptors in specific areas of the body, including the brain, spinal cord, peripheral autonomic nervous system, heart, and bladder. The topography of NE receptor subtypes in different NE pathways and peripheral tissues may thus help to explain how side effects are mediated.

Thus, acute stimulation of beta 1 and/or beta 2 receptors in the cerebellum or peripheral sympathetic nervous system may cause motor activation or tremor (Figure 11-51). Acute stimulation of noradrenergic receptors in the amygdala or limbic cortex, such as ventromedial prefrontal cortex, may cause agitation (Figure 11-46). Acute stimulation of noradrenergic receptors in the brainstem cardiovascular centers and descending into the spinal cord may alter blood pressure. This can be a particularly troubling side effect in some patients taking SNRIs, especially at high doses. Stimulation of beta 1 receptors in the heart may cause changes in heart rate.

Stimulation of noradrenergic receptors in the sympathetic nervous system may also cause a net reduction of parasympathetic cholinergic tone, since these systems often have reciprocal roles in peripheral organs and tissues. Thus increased norepinephrine activity at alpha 1 receptors may produce symptoms reminiscent of "anticholinergic" side effects. This is not due to direct blockade of muscarinic cholinergic receptors but to indirect reduction of net parasympathetic tone due to increased sympathetic tone. Thus, a "pseudo-anticholinergic" syndrome of dry mouth, constipation, and urinary retention may be caused by high degrees of NET inhibition, even though SNRIs have no direct actions on muscarinic cholinergic receptors. Usually, however, the indirect reduction of cholinergic tone yields milder symptoms than does direct blockade of muscarinic cholinergic receptors.

Thus, virtually all side effects of the selective NET inhibition can be understood as undesirable actions of norepinephrine in undesirable pathways at undesirable receptor subtypes. Just as for the SSRIs, this occurs because it is not possible for a systemically administered drug to act only at the desirable receptors in the desirable places; it must act everywhere it is distributed, which means all over the brain and all over the body. Fortunately, side effects from NET inhibition are more of a nuisance than a danger and they generally attenuate over time, although they can cause an important subset of patients to discontinue treatment.

Venlafaxine

Venlafaxine is the first SNRI marketed in the United States (Figure 12-37 and Table 12-3). It has now become generally the most frequently prescribed individual antidepressant by most mental health professionals and by many primary care physicians in many countries. Depending on the dose, venlafaxine has different degrees of inhibition of 5HT reuptake (most potent and present even at low doses) versus NE reuptake (moderate potency and present at higher doses) (Figure 12-37). However, there are no significant actions on other receptors.

Venlafaxine has pioneered the concept that multiple pharmacological mechanisms in a single agent may be linked to greater efficacy than single pharmacological mechanisms, either in terms of enhanced remission rates, more robust sustained remission over long-term treatment, or greater efficacy for treatment-resistant depression. Recent long-term recurrence prevention studies with venlafaxine show very low recurrence rates not only over the first year but surprisingly over the second year of maintenance treatment. It is not clear whether these recurrence rates are lower than for single mechanism SSRIs, but they do appear to be lower than those reported in the STAR-D study with a variety of antidepressants (Figure 12-10). However, the study populations in these different studies may not be comparable. Although this concept of greater efficacy with multiple mechanisms

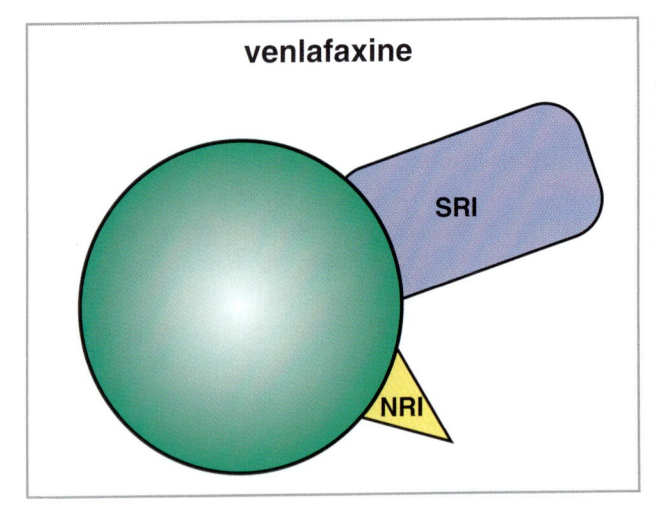

FIGURE 12-37 Icon of venlafaxine. Venlafaxine inhibits reuptake of both serotonin (SRI) and norepinephrine (NRI), thus combining two therapeutic mechanisms in one agent. Venlafaxine's serotonergic actions are present at low doses, while its noradrenergic actions are progressively enhanced as dose increases.

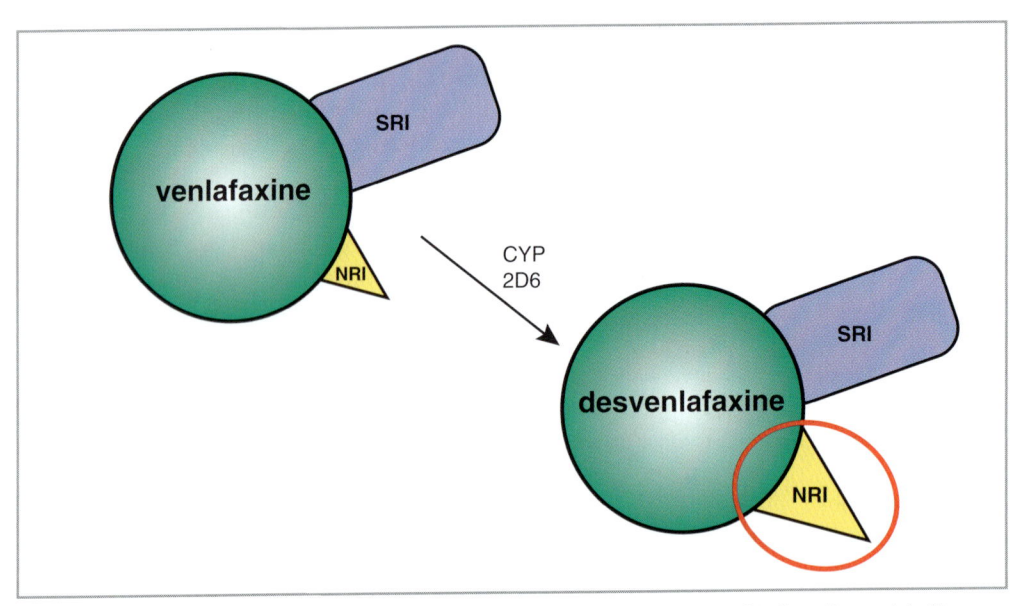

FIGURE 12-38 Venlafaxine conversion to desvenlafaxine. Venlafaxine is converted to its active metabolite desvenlafaxine by CYP450 2D6. Like venlafaxine, desvenlafaxine inhibits reuptake of serotonin (SRI) and norepinephrine (NRI), but its NRI actions are greater relative to its SRI actions compared to venlafaxine. Venlafaxine administration usually results in plasma levels of venlafaxine that are about half those of desvenlafaxine; however, this can vary depending on genetic polymorphisms of CYP450 2D6 and if patients are taking drugs that are inhibitors or inducers of CYP450 2D6. Thus the degree of NET inhibition with venlafaxine administration may be unpredictable.

is widely embraced as a strategy for achieving and maintaining remission in depression, it remains controversial whether the specific mixing of SERT and NET inhibition by venlafaxine itself is consistently and robustly more efficacious than SERT inhibition by SSRIs alone for the treatment of depression.

Venlafaxine is a substrate for CYP450 2D6, which converts it to the active metabolite desvenlafaxine (Figure 12-38). Desvenlafaxine has greater NET inhibition relative to SERT inhibition compared to venlafaxine (Figures 12-37 to 12-39). After venlafaxine

548 | Essential Psychopharmacology

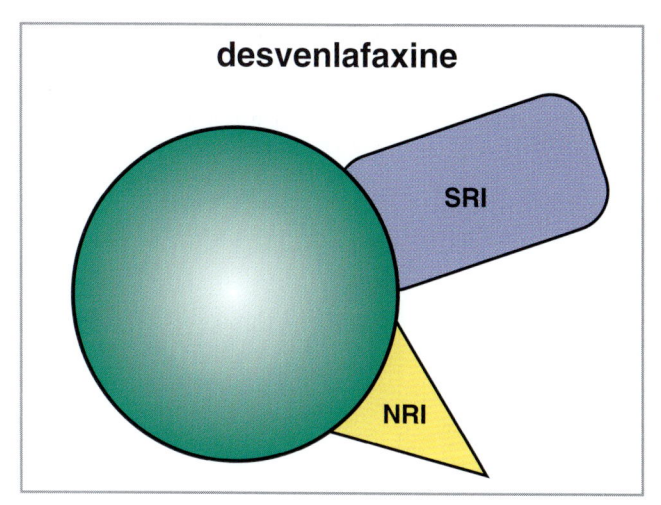

FIGURE 12-39 Icon of desvenlafaxine. Desvenlafaxine, the active metabolite of venlafaxine, has now been developed as a separate drug. It has relatively greater norepinephrine reuptake inhibition (NRI) than venlafaxine but is still more potent at the serotonin transporter.

administration, the plasma levels of venlafaxine are normally about half of those for desvenlafaxine. However, this is highly variable, depending on whether the patient is taking another drug that is a CYP450 2D6 inhibitor, which shifts the plasma levels toward more venlafaxine and less desvenlafaxine, also reducing the relative amount of NET inhibition. Variability in plasma levels of venlafaxine versus desvenlafaxine is also due to genetic polymorphisms for CYP450 2D6, such that poor metabolizers will shift the ratio of these two drugs toward more parent venlafaxine and away from the active metabolite desvenlafaxine and thus reduce the relative amount of NET inhibition. As a result of these considerations, how much NET inhibition a given dose of venlafaxine will have in a given patient at a given time can be somewhat unpredictable. Expert clinicians have learned to solve this problem with skilled dose titration, but the recent development of desvenlafaxine as a separate drug may also solve this problem with less need for dose titration and more consistent NET inhibition at a given dose across all patients.

Venlafaxine is available as an extended-release formulation (venlafaxine XR), which not only allows for once daily administration but also significantly reduces side effects, especially nausea. In contrast to several other psychotropic drugs available in controlled-release formulations, venlafaxine XR is a considerable improvement over the immediate-release formulation, which has fallen into little or no use because of unacceptable nausea and other side effects associated with the immediate-release formulation, especially when started or stopped. However, venlafaxine even in controlled-release formulation can cause withdrawal reactions, sometimes quite bothersome, especially after sudden discontinuation from high-dose long-term treatment. Nevertheless, the controlled-release formulation is highly preferred because of enhanced tolerability.

Use of SNRIs such as venlafaxine for the treatment of various anxiety disorders is discussed in Chapter 14, on anxiety. Venlafaxine is approved and widely used for several anxiety disorders.

Desvenlafaxine

This is the active metabolite of venlafaxine (Figure 12-38); it has relatively greater NET inhibition than venlafaxine but still has less potent actions on NET than on SERT (Figure 12-39). It is not a substrate of CYP450 enzymes, including 2D6, so its plasma drug concentrations are not influenced by 2D6 inhibitors or by genetic polymorphisms in 2D6, as

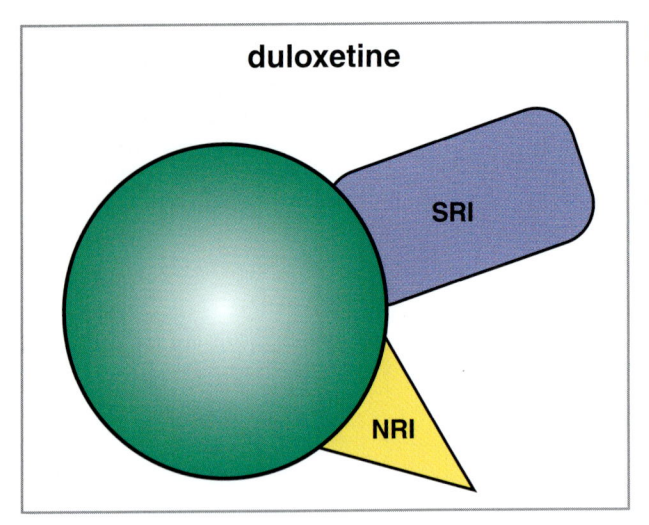

FIGURE 12-40 Icon of duloxetine. Duloxetine inhibits reuptake of both serotonin (SRI) and norepinephrine (NRI). Its noradrenergic actions may contribute to efficacy for painful physical symptoms. Duloxetine is also an inhibitor of CYP450 2D6.

those of venlafaxine are. The bottom line is that the plasma levels of desvenlafaxine should be more consistent than those of venlafaxine and that the relative amount of NET versus SERT should generally be more consistent and greater at comparable doses.

Whether this will lead to any advantages in the treatment of depression remains to be seen, although it might prove to be easier to dose and be more predictable than venlafaxine. What is perhaps more interesting is that owing to its relatively more robust and predictable NET inhibition, desvenlafaxine has been tested in two novel indications: vasomotor symptoms and fibromyalgia, both theoretically thought to require robust NET inhibition as well as SERT inhibition. Many perimenopausal women develop hot flushes and other vasomotor symptoms, including night sweats, insomnia, and even depression, but do not wish to take estrogen replacement therapy. Desvenlafaxine appears to have robust efficacy in reducing vasomotor symptoms in such women and provides an alternative to estrogen replacement therapy. Other considerations, such as the treatment of perimenopausal women who have both vasomotor symptoms and either depression or risk of depression are discussed later in this chapter in the section on trimonoamine modulators and estrogen.

Desvenlafaxine, like the other SNRIs milnacipran and duloxetine, is also being tested with promising results for the treatment of fibromyalgia. Fibromyalgia and other chronic painful conditions are discussed in Chapter 15, on pain.

Duloxetine

This is an SNRI (Figure 12-40 and Table 12-3) that not only is indicated for the treatment of depression and for anxiety disorders but is also the first SNRI approved as a treatment for painful neuropathy associated with diabetes. Use of SNRIs for the treatment of chronic painful conditions is discussed in Chapter 15, on pain, and for the treatment of anxiety disorders in Chapter 14. It is worth noting that duloxetine has established efficacy not only in depression and chronic pain but also in patients with chronic painful physical symptoms of depression. These symptoms are frequently ignored or missed by patients and clinicians alike. Until recently, the link of these symptoms to major depression was not well appreciated, in part because painful physical symptoms are not included in the list of symptoms for the formal diagnostic criteria for depression. Nevertheless, it is now widely appreciated that painful physical symptoms are frequently associated with a major

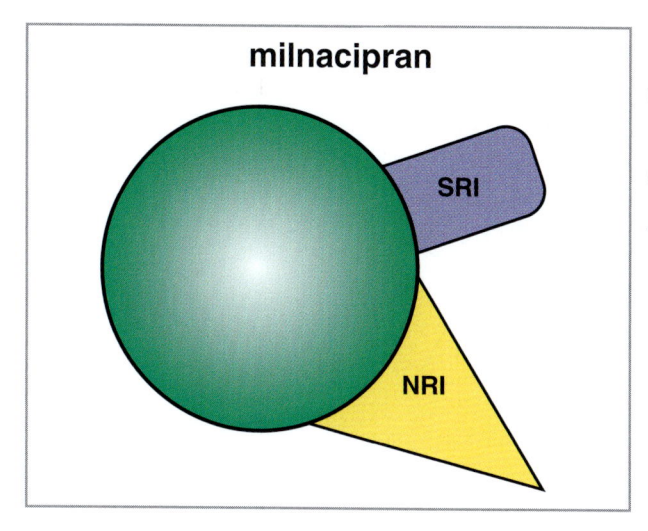

FIGURE 12-41 Icon of milnacipran. Milnacipran inhibits reuptake of both serotonin (SRI) and norepinephrine (NRI) but is a more potent inhibitor of the norepinephrine transporter (NET) than the serotonin transporter (SERT). Its robust NET inhibition may contribute to efficacy for painful physical symptoms.

depressive episode and are also among the leading residual symptoms after treatment with an antidepressant (Figure 12-9). It appears that the dual SNRI actions of duloxetine and other SNRIs may be superior to the selective serotonergic actions of SSRIs for treating conditions such as the neuropathic pain of diabetes and chronic painful physical symptoms associated with depression. Duloxetine also appears to be effective in the treatment of fibromyalgia.

Duloxetine has shown efficacy in the treatment of the cognitive symptoms of depression prominent in geriatric depression, possibly exploiting the NET inhibition of the SNRI mechanism in the prefrontal cortex (see Figure 12-36). Cognitive symptoms are discussed in further detail in Chapter 18, on dementia and its treatments.

Duloxetine can supposedly be given once a day, but this is usually a good idea only after the patient has had a chance to become tolerant to it after initiating it at twice-daily dosing, especially during titration to the higher doses often used in psychiatry and in the treatment of painful conditions. Duloxetine may need to be given in some difficult-to-treat patients at doses higher than the normal prescribing range; in this case, twice-daily dosing may be preferred. Duloxetine may be associated with a lower incidence of hypertension and milder withdrawal reactions than venlafaxine. Duloxetine is a CYP450 2D6 inhibitor, which may cause some drug interactions (see section on antidepressant pharmacokinetics, below).

Milnacipran

Milnacipran is the first SNRI marketed in Japan and many European countries such as France, where it is currently marketed as an antidepressant. As of this writing, milnacipran is not yet marketed in the United States (Table 12-3).

Milnacipran is a somewhat atypical SNRI in that it is a more potent NET than SERT inhibitor (Figure 12-41) whereas the others are more potent SERT than NET inhibitors (Figures 12-37 to 12-40). This unique pharmacological profile may explain milnacipran's somewhat different clinical profile compared to other SNRIs. Since noradrenergic actions may be equally or more important for the treatment of pain-related conditions compared to serotonergic actions, the robust NET inhibition of milnacipran suggests that it may be particularly useful in conditions ranging from the painful physical symptoms associated with depression to chronic neuropathic pain to fibromyalgia. Among these conditions, milnacipran is probably best studied in fibromyalgia, where it shows positive evidence of efficacy and is in the late stages of testing in the United States and other countries.

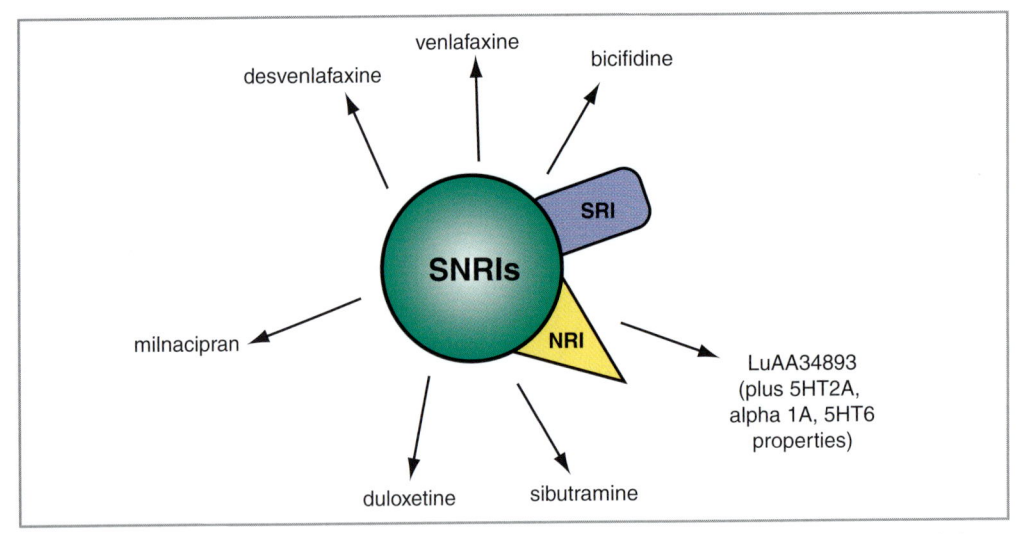

FIGURE 12-42 Other serotonin norepinephrine reuptake inhibitors (SNRIs). SNRIs in addition to venlafaxine, desvenlafaxine, duloxetine, and milnacipran include sibutramine, which is marketed as an appetite suppressant; bicifidine, which is in testing for painful conditions and depression; and LuAA34893, which, in addition to SNRI actions, is an antagonist at serotonin 2A, alpha 1A, and serotonin 6 receptors.

Milnacipran's potent NET inhibition also suggests a potentially favorable pharmacological profile for the treatment of cognitive symptoms, including cognitive symptoms of depression as well as those frequently associated with fibromyalgia, sometimes called "fibrofog." Fibromyalgia is discussed in more detail in Chapter 15, on pain.

Other clinical observations possibly linked to milnacipran's robust NET inhibition are that it can be more energizing and activating than other SNRIs while perhaps also causing more sweating and urinary hesitancy. For patients with urinary hesitancy, generally due theoretically to robust pro-noradrenergic actions at bladder alpha 1 receptors, an alpha 1 antagonist can be helpful. Milnacipran must generally be given twice daily due to its relatively short half-life.

Other SNRIs (Figure 12-42)

Sibutramine is marketed as an appetite suppressant but also has SNRI pharmacological properties, yet it is not approved for the treatment of depression. Bicifidine is an agent in clinical testing for back pain, other painful conditions, and depression. LuAA34893 is an early-stage compound with "SNRI plus" properties, namely SNRI actions plus 5HT2A, alpha 1A, and 5HT6 antagonist actions.

Norepinephrine and dopamine reuptake inhibitors (NDRIs)

Bupropion is the prototypical agent of this group (Figure 12-43 and Table 12-2). For many years, the mechanism of action of bupropion has been unclear, and it still remains somewhat controversial. Bupropion itself has only weak reuptake blocking properties for dopamine (DAT inhibition) and for norepinephrine (NET inhibition) (Figure 12-44). No other specific or potent pharmacologic actions have been consistently identified for this agent. Bupropion's actions both as an antidepressant and upon norepinephrine and dopamine neurotransmission, however, have always appeared to be more powerful than

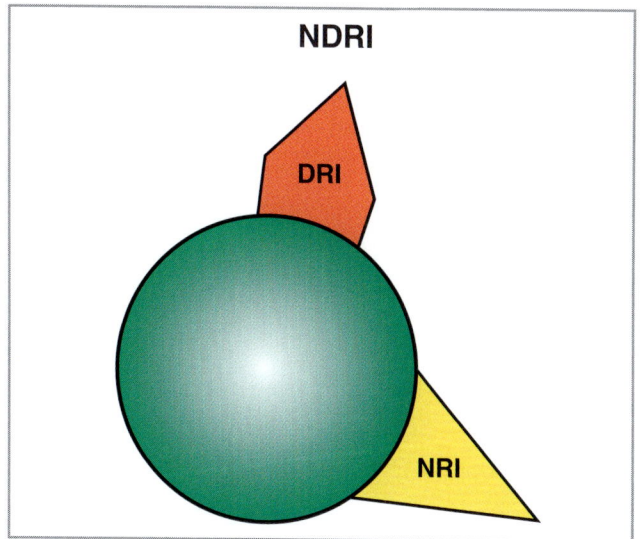

FIGURE 12-43 Icon of a norepinephrine and dopamine reuptake inhibitor (NDRI). Another class of antidepressant consists of norepinephrine and dopamine reuptake inhibitors (NDRIs), for which the prototypical agent is bupropion. Bupropion has weak reuptake blocking properties for dopamine (DRI) and norepinephrine (NRI) but is an efficacious antidepressant, which may be explained in part by the more potent inhibitory properties of its metabolites.

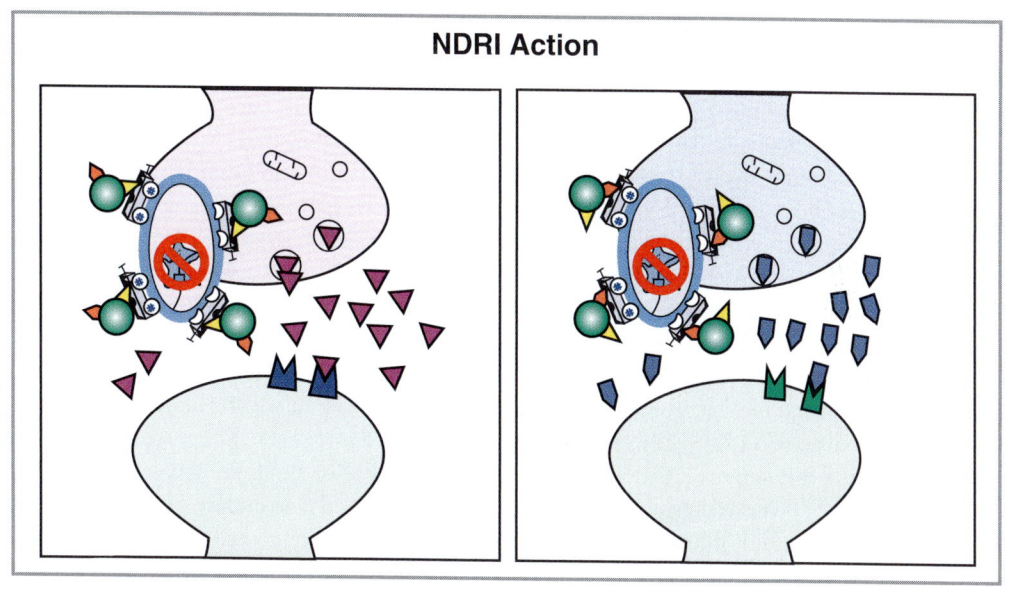

FIGURE 12-44 NDRI actions. In this figure the norepinephrine reuptake inhibitor (NRI) portion of the NDRI molecule (left panel) and the dopamine reuptake inhibitor (DRI) portion of the NDRI molecule (right panel) are inserted into their respective reuptake pumps. Consequently both pumps are blocked, and the drug mediates an antidepressant effect.

these weak properties could explain, leading to the proposal that bupropion acts rather vaguely as an adrenergic modulator of some type.

More recently, it has been found that bupropion is metabolized to a number of active metabolites, some of which are not only more potent NET inhibitors than bupropion itself (and equally potent DAT inhibitors) but are also concentrated in the brain. In some ways, therefore, bupropion is both an active drug and a precursor for other active drugs (i.e., a

Antidepressants | 553

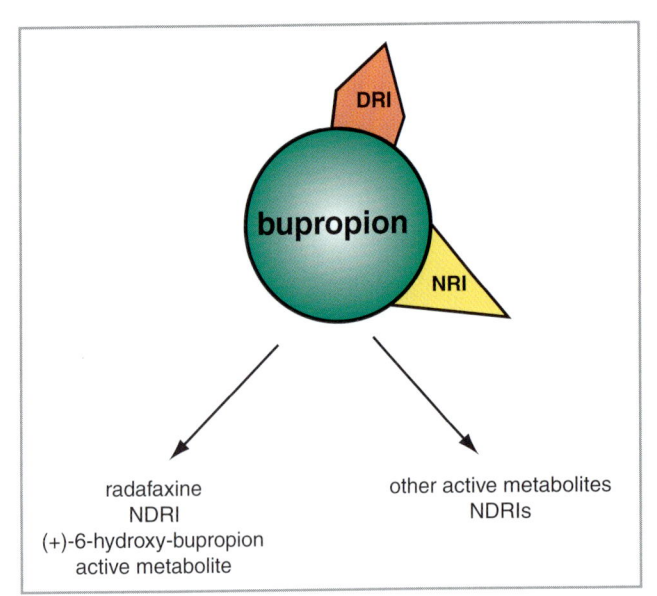

FIGURE 12-45 Bupropion conversion to its metabolites. Bupropion is converted to multiple active metabolites, the most potent of which is (+)-6-hydroxy-bupropion, also called radafaxine.

prodrug for multiple active metabolites) (Figure 12-45). The most potent of these is the + enantiomer of the 6-hydroxy metabolite of bupropion, also known as radafaxine (Figure 12-45). Radafaxine is also a weak NDRI (Figure 12-44).

Can the net effects of bupropion on NET (Figure 12-46A and 12-46B) and DAT (Figure 12-46C) account for its clinical actions in depressed patients at therapeutic doses? If one believes that 90% transporter occupancy of DAT and NET are required for antidepressant actions, the answer would be no. Human positron emission tomography (PET) scans suggest that as little as 10% to 15% and perhaps no more than 20% to 30% of striatal DATs may be occupied at therapeutic doses of bupropion. NET occupancy would be expected to be in this same range. Is this enough to explain bupropion's antidepressant actions?

Whereas it is clear from many research studies that SSRIs must be dosed to occupy a substantial fraction of SERT, perhaps up to 80% or 90% of these transporters in order to be effective antidepressants, this is far less clear for NET or DAT occupancy, particularly in the case of drugs with an additional pharmacological mechanism that may be synergistic with NET or DAT inhibition. That is, when most SNRIs are given in doses that occupy 80% to 90% of SERT, substantially fewer NETs are occupied, yet there is evidence of both additional therapeutic actions and NE-mediated side effects of these agents with perhaps as little as 50% NET occupancy.

Furthermore, there appears to be such a thing as "too much DAT occupancy." That is, when 50% or more of DATs are occupied rapidly and briefly, this can lead to unwanted clinical actions, such as euphoria and reinforcement. In fact, a rapid, short-lasting, high degree of DAT occupancy is the pharmacological characteristic of abusable stimulants such as cocaine and is discussed in Chapter 19, on drug abuse and reward. When 50% or more of DATs are occupied more slowly and in a more lasting manner, especially with controlled-release formulations, stimulants are less abusable and more useful for attention deficit hyperactivity disorder (ADHD), discussed in more detail in Chapter 17, on ADHD. The issue to be considered here is whether a low level of slow-onset and long-lasting DAT

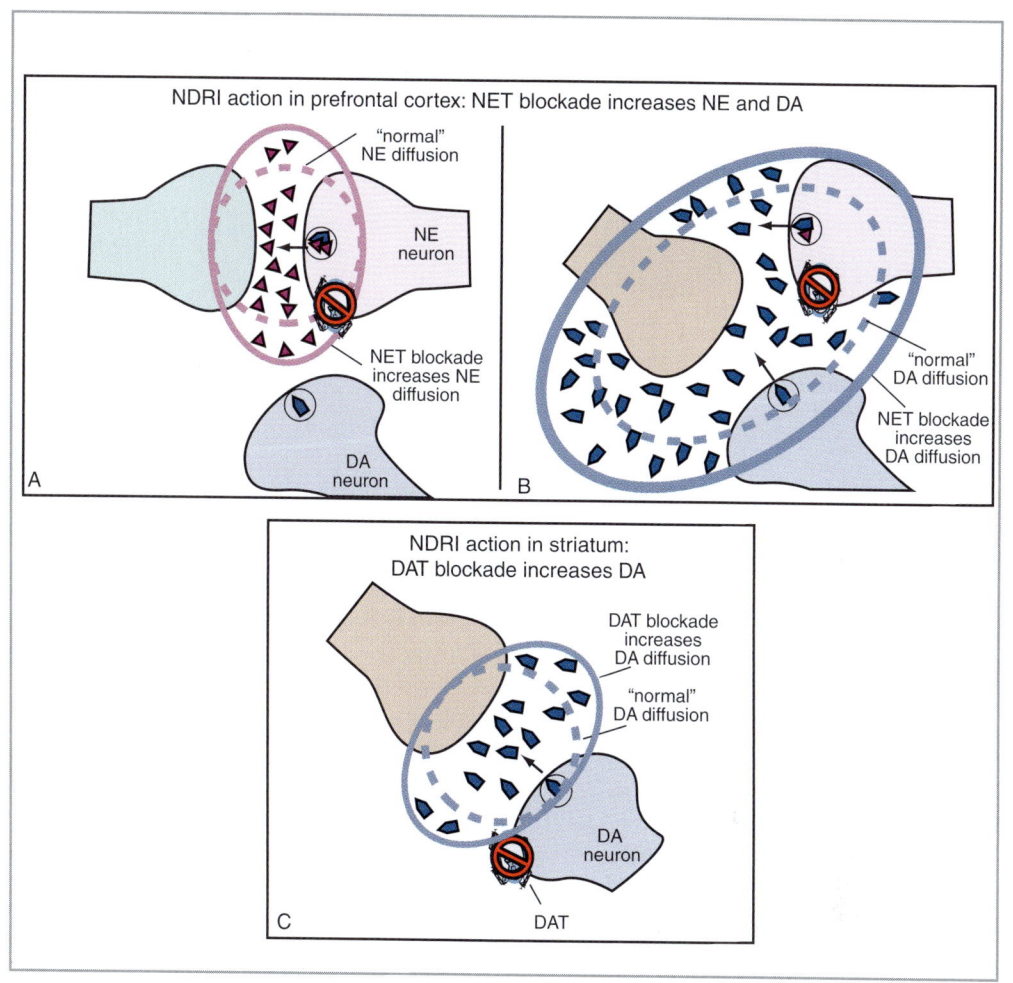

FIGURE 12-46A, B and C NDRI actions in prefrontal cortex and striatum. Norepinephrine and dopamine reuptake inhibitors (NDRIs) block the transporters for both norepinephrine (NET) and dopamine (DAT). (**A**) NET blockade in the prefrontal cortex leads to an increase in synaptic norepinephrine, thus increasing norepinephrine's diffusion radius. (**B**) Because the prefrontal cortex lacks DATs, and NETs transport dopamine as well as norepinephrine, NET blockade also leads to an increase in synaptic dopamine as well as NE in the prefrontal cortex, further increasing DA's diffusion radius. Thus, despite the absence of DAT in the prefrontal cortex, NDRIs still increase dopamine in the prefrontal cortex. (**C**) DAT is present in the striatum, and thus DAT inhibition increases dopamine diffusion there.

occupancy is the "goldilocks" solution for this mechanism to be useful as an antidepressant: thus, not "too hot" and therefore abusable; not "too cold" and therefore ineffective; but "just right" – namely an antidepressant? This issue is also mentioned below in the section on future antidepressants in relation to the new triple reuptake inhibitors in clinical development, which are currently determining the optimal amount of DAT inhibition to add to SERT and NET inhibition.

The fact that bupropion is not known to be particularly abusable, is not a scheduled substance, yet is proven effective for treating nicotine addiction is consistent with the possibility that it is occupying DATs in the striatum and nucleus accumbens in a manner sufficient

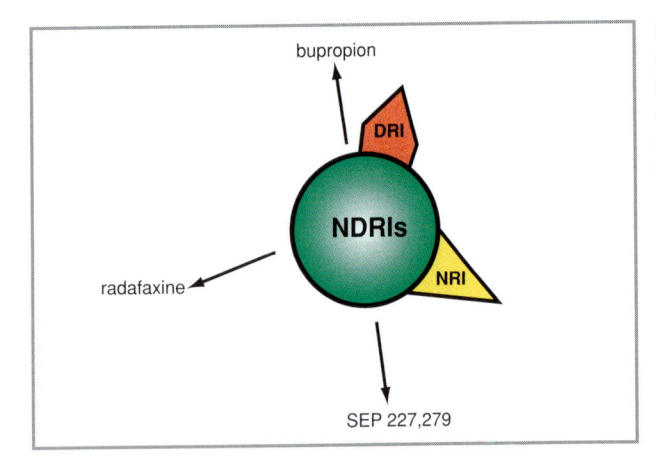

FIGURE 12-47 Other norepinephrine and dopamine reuptake inhibitors (NDRIs). There are at least two NDRIs in clinical testing: radafaxine (the active metabolite of bupropion) and SEP 227,279.

to mitigate craving but not sufficient to cause abuse (Figure 12-46C). This is discussed further in Chapter 19, on drug abuse and reward. Perhaps this is also how bupropion works in depression, combined with an equal action on NETs (Figure 12-46A and 12-46B). Clinical observations of depressed patients are also consistent with DAT and NET inhibition as bupropion's mechanism of action (Figure 12-46A, B, and C), since this agent appears especially useful in targeting the symptoms of "reduced positive affect" within the affective spectrum (see Figure 11-55), including improvement in the symptoms of loss of happiness, joy, interest, pleasure, energy, enthusiasm, alertness, and self-confidence.

Bupropion was originally marketed only in the United States as an immediate-release dosage formulation for thrice-daily administration as an antidepressant. Development of a twice-daily formulation (bupropion SR) and more recently a once-daily formulation (bupropion XL) has not only reduced the frequency of seizures at peak plasma drug levels, which are reduced with these formulations, but also increased convenience and enhanced compliance. Thus, the use of immediate-release bupropion has been all but abandoned in favor of once- or twice-daily administration.

Bupropion is generally activating or even stimulating. Interestingly, bupropion does not appear to cause the bothersome sexual dysfunction that frequently occurs with antidepressants acting by SERT inhibition, probably because bupropion lacks a significant serotonergic component to its mechanism of action. Thus, bupropion has proven to be a useful antidepressant not only for patients who cannot tolerate the serotonergic side effects of SSRIs but also for those whose depression does not respond to serotonergic boosting by SSRIs. As discussed above, given its pharmacological profile, bupropion is especially targeted at the symptoms of the "dopamine-deficiency syndrome" and "reduced positive affect" (Figure 11-55). Almost every active clinician knows that patients who have residual symptoms of reduced positive affect following treatment with an SSRI or an SNRI or who develop these symptoms as a side effect of an SSRI or SNRI frequently benefit from switching to bupropion or from augmenting their SSRI or SNRI treatment with bupropion. The combination of bupropion with an SSRI or an SNRI has a theoretical rationale as a strategy for covering the entire symptom portfolio from symptoms of reduced positive affect to symptoms of increased negative affect (Figure 11-55).

Other NDRIs

At least two other NDRIs have entered clinical testing, including not only the active metabolite of bupropion, radafaxine, but also SEP 227,279 (Figure 12-47).

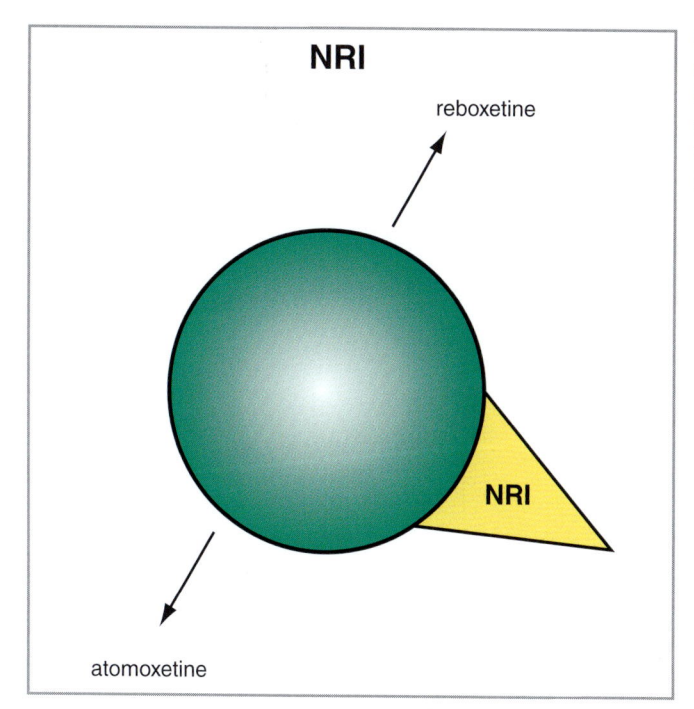

FIGURE 12-48 Icon of a selective norepinephrine reuptake inhibitor. Reboxetine and atomoxetine are two antidepressants that have selective actions at the norepinephrine reuptake inhibitor (NRI).

Selective norepinephrine reuptake inhibitors (NRIs)

Although some tricyclic antidepressants (e.g., desipramine, maprotilene) block norepinephrine reuptake more potently than serotonin reuptake, even these tricyclics are not really selective, since they still block many other receptors such as alpha 1, histamine 1, and muscarinic cholinergic receptors, as all tricyclics do. Tricyclic antidepressants are discussed later in this chapter.

The first truly selective noradrenergic reuptake inhibitor marketed in Europe and other countries is reboxetine; the first in the United States is atomoxetine (Figure 12-48 and Table 12-2). Both of these compounds are selective NRIs (Figure 12-49) and lack the additional undesirable binding properties of tricyclic antidepressants. Reboxetine is approved as an antidepressant in Europe but not in the United States. Extensive testing in the United States suggested inconsistent efficacy in major depression with the possibility of less effectiveness than the SSRIs, so reboxetine was dropped from further development as an antidepressant. Atomoxetine was never developed as an antidepressant but is marketed for the treatment of attention deficit hyperactivity disorder in the United States and other countries. ADHD treatments are discussed in Chapter 17, on ADHD.

Many of the important concepts about NET inhibition have already been covered in the section on SNRIs above. This includes the observations that NET inhibition raises not only NE diffusely throughout all NE neuronal projections but also DA levels in the prefrontal cortex (Figure 12-36). It also includes both the therapeutic and side effect profile of NET inhibition. There is some question about whether NET inhibition by itself has any different clinical profile than when NET inhibition occurs simultaneously with SERT inhibition, as when administering an SNRI or giving a selective NRI with an SSRI. One thing that may be different is that NET inhibitors that are selective tend to be dosed so that there is a greater proportion of NET occupancy, close to saturation, compared to NET

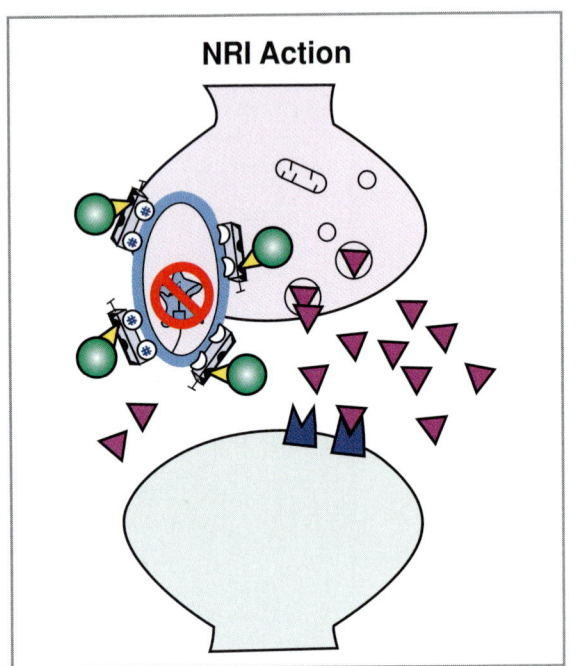

FIGURE 12-49 NRI actions. In this figure, the norepinephrine reuptake inhibitor (NRI) is inserted into the norepinephrine reuptake pump, thus blocking it and mediating the drug's effects.

occupancy when dosed as an SNRI or as an NDRI, which, as mentioned above, may occupy substantially fewer NETs at clinically effective antidepressant doses. This higher degree of NET occupancy of selective NET inhibitors may be necessary for optimal efficacy for either depression or ADHD if there is no simultaneous SERT or DAT inhibition with which to add or synergize. One of the interesting observations is that high degrees of selective NET inhibition, although often activating, can also be sedating in some patients. Perhaps this is due to "over-tuning" noradrenergic input to cortical pyramidal neurons, which is discussed in Chapter 7 and illustrated in Figures 7-24 and 7-25; it is also discussed in Chapter 17, on ADHD.

There is less documentation that NET inhibition is as helpful for anxiety disorders as SERT inhibition, and neither of the selective NRIs shown here (Figure 12-48) is approved for anxiety disorders, although atomoxetine is approved for adult ADHD, which is frequently comorbid with anxiety disorders.

Alpha 2 antagonists as serotonin norepinephrine disinhibitors (SNDIs)

Blocking the reuptake pumps for monoamines is not the only way to increase their levels or their release. Another way to raise both serotonin and norepinephrine levels is to block alpha 2 receptors (Figure 12-50 and Table 12-2). This results in disinhibition of both serotonin and norepinephrine release by a mechanism to be explained below and is why this mechanism is sometimes also called SNDI action (Table 12-2).

Recall that norepinephrine turns off its own release by interacting with presynaptic alpha 2 autoreceptors on noradrenergic neurons (Figures 11-33 and 11-34); norepinephrine also turns off serotonin release by interacting with presynaptic alpha 2 heteroreceptors on serotonergic neurons (Figure 11-36). If an alpha 2 antagonist is administered,

Alpha 2 Antagonists

- mirtazapine
- mianserin
- risperidone
- paliperidone
- quetiapine
- perospirone
- clozapine
- asenapine

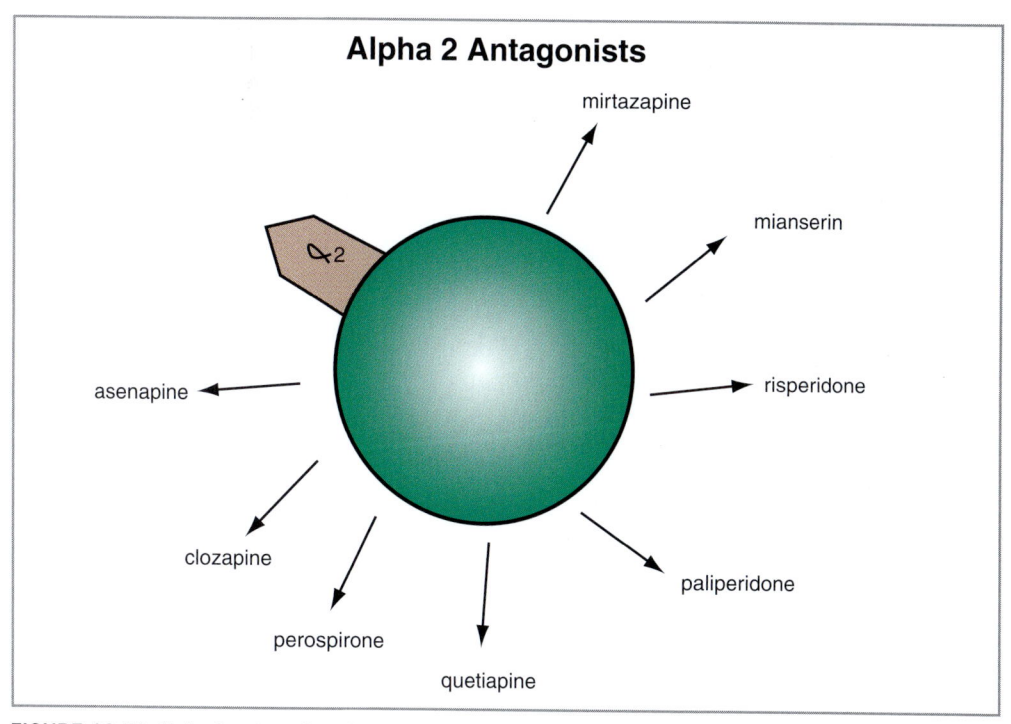

FIGURE 12-50 Alpha 2 antagonists. Blockade of alpha 2 receptors by alpha 2 antagonists can increase both serotonergic and noradrenergic neurotransmission, since alpha 2 antagonism causes serotonin and norepinephrine disinhibition. Dual enhancement of both serotonin and norepinephrine release by alpha 2 antagonism thus generates an antidepressant effect. Alpha 2 antagonists include mirtazapine, mianserin, risperidone, paliperidone, quetiapine, perospirone, clozapine, and asenapine.

norepinephrine can no longer turn off its own release and noradrenergic neurons are thus disinhibited (Figure 12-51). That is, the alpha 2 antagonist "cuts the brake cable" of the noradrenergic neuron and norepinephrine release is therefore increased.

Similarly, alpha 2 antagonists do not allow norepinephrine to turn off serotonin release. Therefore serotonergic neurons become disinhibited (Figure 12-52). Like their actions at noradrenergic neurons, alpha 2 antagonists act at serotonergic neurons to "cut the brake cable" of noradrenergic inhibition (NE brake on 5HT shown in Figures 11-36 and 11-38). Serotonin release is therefore increased (Figure 12-52).

A second mechanism to increase serotonin release after an alpha 2 antagonist is administered may be even more important. Recall that norepinephrine neurons from the locus coeruleus innervate the cell bodies of serotonergic neurons in the midbrain raphe (Figures 11-35 and 11-38). This noradrenergic input enhances serotonin release via a postsynaptic alpha 1 receptor. Thus, when norepinephrine is disinhibited in the noradrenergic pathway to the raphe, it will increase norepinephrine release there, stimulating alpha 1 receptors and thereby provoking more serotonin release (Figure 12-53). This is like stepping on the serotonin accelerator. Thus alpha 2 antagonists both "cut the brake cable" and "step on the accelerator" for serotonin release (Figure 12-54). The bottom line is that an alpha 2 antagonist is a serotonin and norepinephrine disinhibitor (SNDI) (Table 12-2).

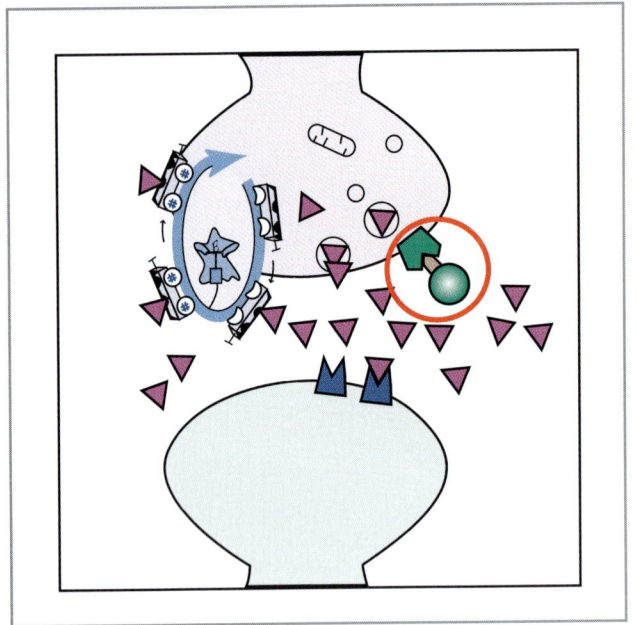

FIGURE 12-51 Alpha 2 antagonists and norepinephrine. Alpha 2 antagonists can increase noradrenergic neurotransmission by "cutting the brake cable" for noradrenergic neurons. That is, alpha 2 antagonists block presynaptic alpha 2 autoreceptors (red circle), which are the "brakes" on noradrenergic neurons. This causes noradrenergic neurons to become disinhibited, since norepinephrine can no longer block its own release. Thus noradrenergic neurotransmission is enhanced.

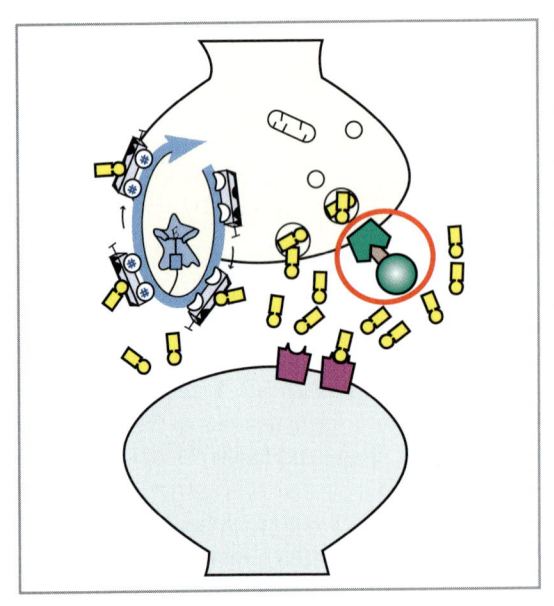

FIGURE 12-52 Alpha 2 antagonists and serotonin. Alpha 2 antagonists can also increase serotonergic neurotransmission by "cutting the brake cable" for serotonergic neurons (compare with Figure 12-51). That is, alpha 2 antagonists block presynaptic alpha 2 heteroreceptors (red circle), the "brakes" on serotonergic neurons. This causes serotonergic neurons to become disinhibited, since norepinephrine can no longer block serotonin release. Thus serotonergic neurotransmission is enhanced.

Alpha 2 antagonist actions therefore yield dual enhancement of both 5HT and NE release (see Figures 12-51 through 12-54) but, unlike SNRIs, they have this effect by a mechanism independent of blockade of monoamine transporters. These two mechanisms, monoamine transport blockade and alpha 2 antagonism, are synergistic, so that blocking them simultaneously gives a much more powerful disinhibitory signal to these two neurotransmitters than if only one mechanism were blocked. For this reason, the alpha 2 antagonist mirtazapine is often combined with an SNRI to treat patients who do not

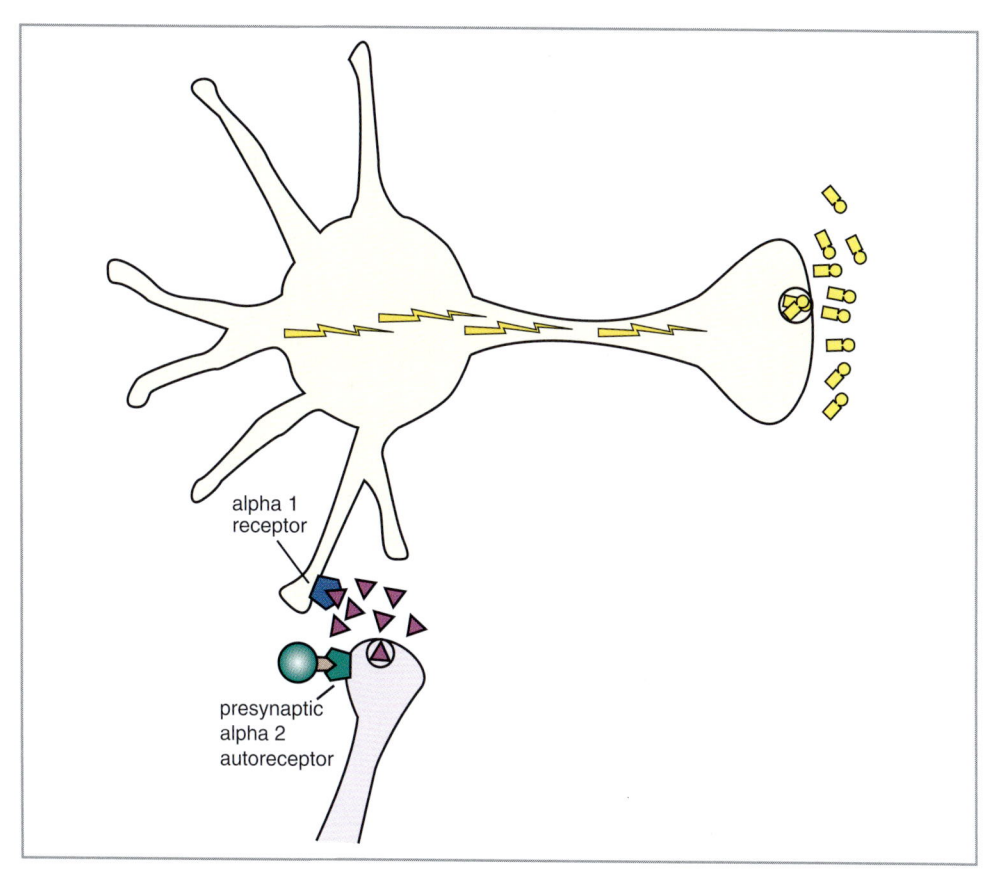

FIGURE 12-53 Alpha 2 antagonists and serotonin. Alpha 2 antagonists can also increase serotonergic neurotransmission by "stepping on the serotonin accelerator." First, antagonism of alpha 2 autoreceptors increases norepinephrine output from noradrenergic neurons in the locus coeruleus (bottom). Norepinephrine then stimulates postsynaptic excitatory alpha 1 receptors on the cell bodies of serotonergic neurons in the midbrain raphe. This increases serotonergic neuronal firing and serotonin release from the serotonin nerve terminal (right).

respond to an SNRI alone. This is discussed further in the section on antidepressants in clinical practice later in this chapter (i.e., "California rocket fuel").

Although no selective alpha 2 antagonist is available for use as an antidepressant, there are several drugs with prominent alpha 2 properties (Figure 12-50), including some atypical antipsychotics, discussed in Chapter 10, and at least one antidepressant, mirtazapine (Figure 12-55). Although mirtazapine does not block any monoamine transporter, it has additional potent antagonist actions upon 5HT2A receptors, 5HT2C receptors, 5HT3 receptors, and histamine 1 receptors (Figure 12-55).

A summary of the serotonergic actions of mirtazapine is shown in Figure 12-56. When mirtazapine disinhibits serotonin release by the alpha 2 antagonist mechanism, it causes serotonin to be released onto all serotonin receptors; however, mirtazapine simultaneously blocks the actions of serotonin at 5HT2A, 5HT2C, and 5HT3 receptors, leaving net stimulation of only 5HT1A receptors (Figure 12-56).

Net 5HT1A agonist action of mirtazapine due to serotonin itself stimulating 5HT1A receptors results in release of dopamine (discussed in Chapter 10 and illustrated in Figure 10-21). This would theoretically be helpful for depression and cognition (Figure 12-56).

Antidepressants | 561

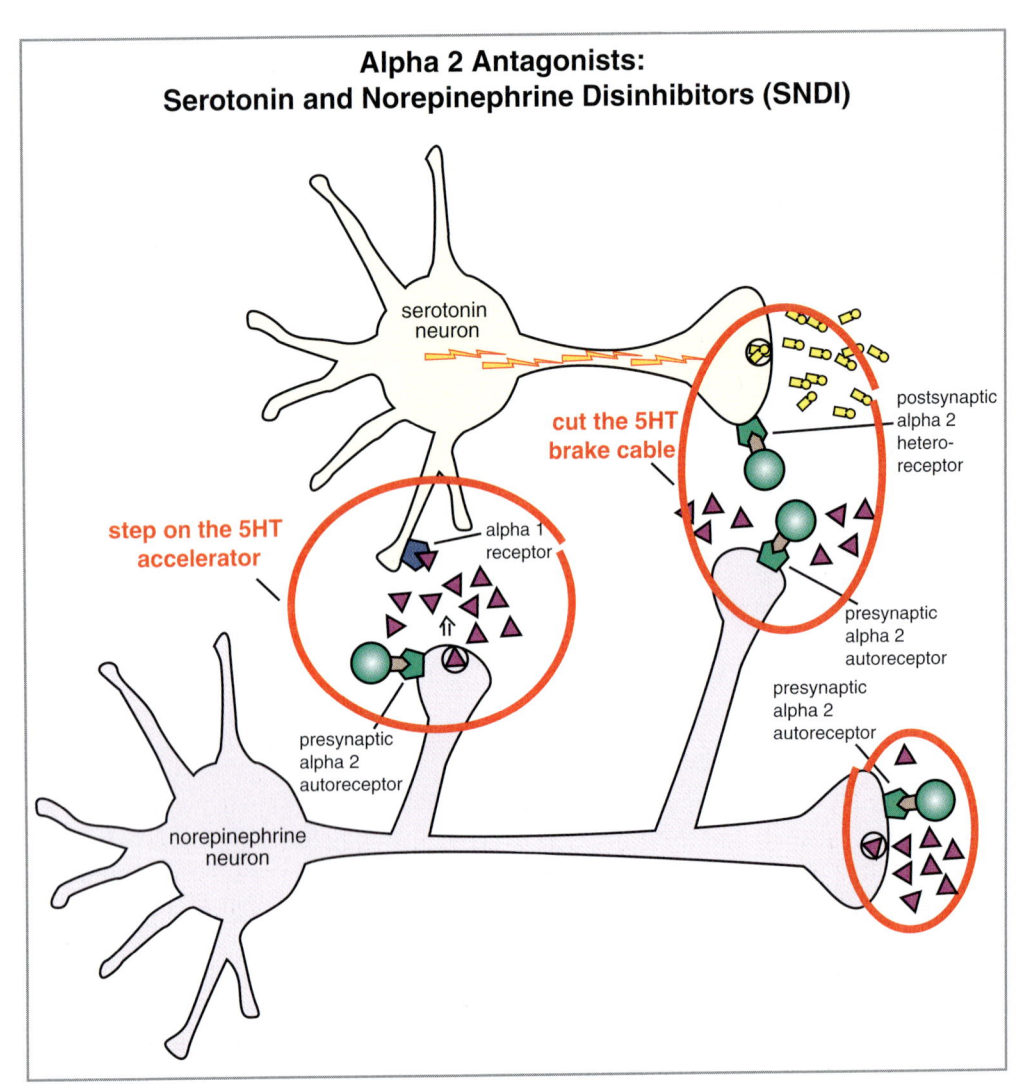

FIGURE 12-54 Alpha 2 antagonists: serotonin and norepinephrine disinhibitors (SNDI). This figure shows how both noradrenergic and serotonergic neurotransmission are enhanced by alpha 2 antagonists. The noradrenergic neuron at the bottom is interacting with the serotonergic neuron at the top. The noradrenergic neuron is disinhibited at all of its axon terminals because an alpha 2 antagonist is blocking all of its presynaptic alpha 2 autoreceptors. This has the effect of "cutting the brake cables" for norepinephrine (NE) release at all of its noradrenergic nerve terminals (NE released in all three red circles). Serotonin (5HT) release is enhanced by NE via two distinct mechanisms. First, alpha 2 antagonists "step on the 5HT accelerator" when NE stimulates alpha 1 receptors on the 5HT cell body and dendrites (left red circle). Second, alpha 2 antagonists "cut the 5HT brake cable" when alpha 2 presynaptic heteroreceptors are blocked on the 5HT axon terminal (middle red circle).

5HT1A agonist actions linked to anxiolytic effects are discussed later, in Chapter 14, on anxiety disorders. Mirtazapine is anecdotally useful in many anxiety disorders but is not approved for this use.

5HT2A/5HT2C antagonist actions of mirtazapine should theoretically contribute to anxiolytic, sleep-restoring, and antidepressant effects while not causing sexual dysfunction (Figure 12-56). In fact, mirtazapine is one of the few antidepressants that can increase serotonin release and not cause significant sexual dysfunction. The therapeutic benefits of

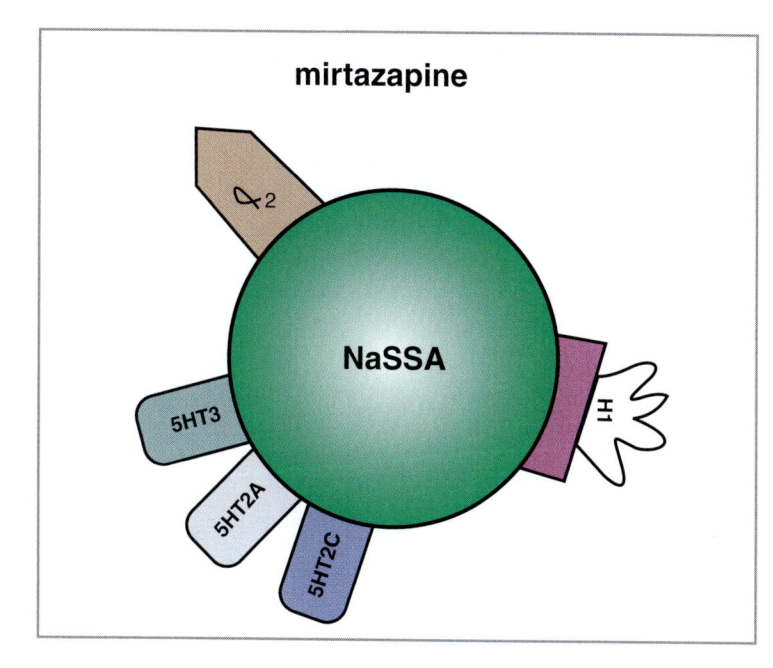

FIGURE 12-55 Icon of mirtazapine. Mirtazapine is sometimes called a noradrenergic and specific serotonergic antidepressant (NaSSA). Its primary therapeutic action is alpha 2 antagonism, as shown in Figures 12-51 through 12-54. It also blocks three serotonin (5HT) receptors: 5HT2A, 5HT2C, and 5HT3. Finally, it blocks histamine 1 (H1) receptors.

5HT2A/5HT2C antagonism for anxiety are discussed later, in Chapter 14, on anxiety; the therapeutic benefits of 5HT2A/5HT2C antagonism for sleep are also discussed later, in Chapter 16, on sleep. In terms of antidepressant effects, 5HT2A antagonist action can be difficult to separate from 5HT2C antagonist actions. Both may contribute to increasing dopamine and norepinephrine release, as discussed extensively in Chapter 10 for atypical antipsychotics and illustrated in Figures 10-22, 10-26, and 10-28; also discussed in Chapter 11 for antidepressants and illustrated in Figure 11-40.

5HT2C antagonist action as a mechanism for increasing both NE and DA release in prefrontal cortex may be more important than 5HT2A antagonist actions for a drug such as mirtazapine, which lacks the D2 antagonism of an atypical antipsychotic. It turns out that 5HT2A regulation of dopamine release is quite complex and depends on the specific circuit, the area of the brain where 5HT2A receptors are located, and the baseline amount of dopamine and serotonin release as well as the presence of other simultaneous pharmacological mechanisms, such as D2 antagonism. However, 5HT2C antagonism may be more consistently linked to norepinephrine and dopamine disinhibition in the prefrontal cortex regardless of these various factors. The bottom line is that in addition to being an SNDI (serotonin norepinephrine disinhibitor; Table 12-2) due to alpha 2 antagonist properties, mirtazapine is also an NDDI (norepinephrine and dopamine disinhibitor; Table 12-2) due to 5HT2C (and possibly 5HT2A) antagonist properties. Both of these concepts of SNDI and NDDI are novel explanations for the pharmacological actions of this established antidepressant (Table 12-2). These novel concepts may also help to explain the antidepressant actions not only of some atypical antipsychotics but also of several new drugs in development (discussed in the section on future antidepressants, below).

Although it is not clear that 5HT2C antagonist properties alone can cause weight gain, when combined with mirtazapine's simultaneous H1 antihistamine properties (Figure 12-55), weight gain appears more likely (see discussion in Chapter 10 and Figure 10-59).

Antidepressants | 563

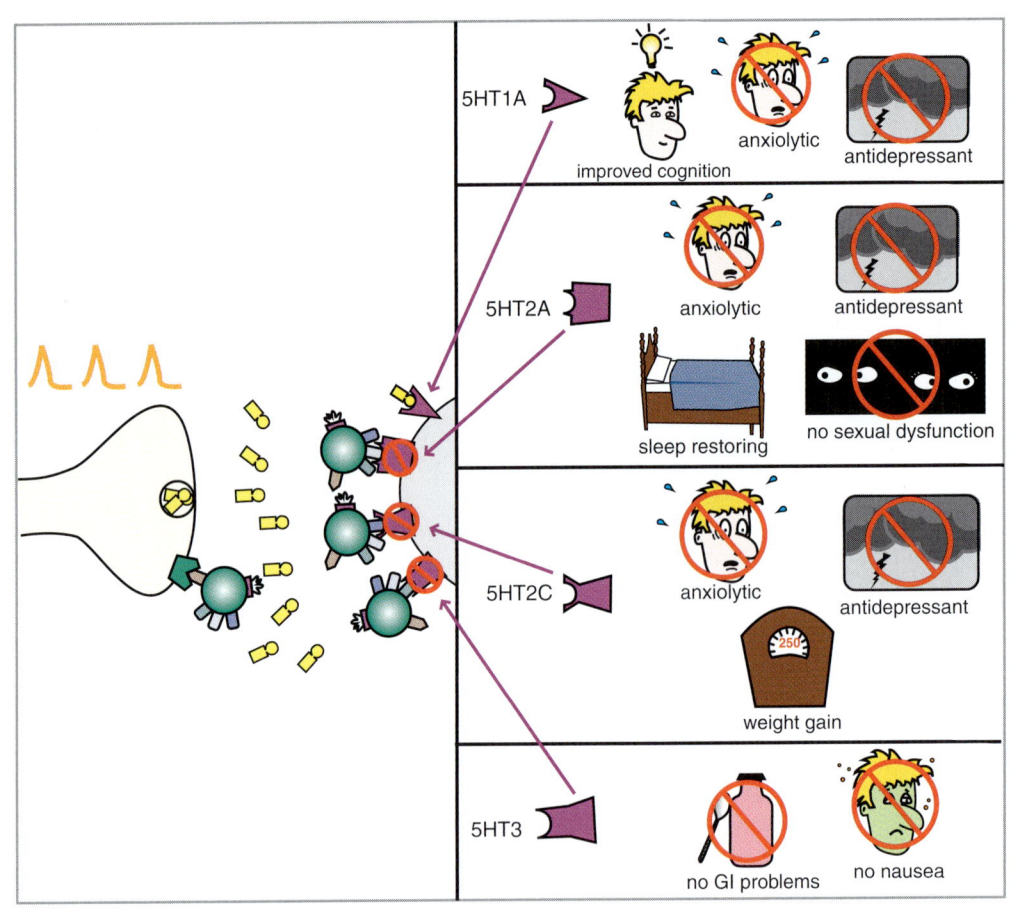

FIGURE 12-56 Mirtazapine actions at serotonin (5HT) synapses. When presynaptic alpha 2 heteroreceptors are blocked by mirtazapine, 5HT is released with the potential to activate any 5HT receptors. However, because mirtazapine blocks 5HT2C, 5HT2A, and 5HT3 receptors, the increased serotonin release is directed largely to the 5HT1A receptor. The result is that antidepressant and anxiolytic actions are preserved but the side effects associated with stimulating 5HT2A, 5HT2C, and 5HT3 are blocked. Mirtazapine's antagonism of 5HT2C receptors could contribute to weight gain.

5HT3 antagonist action should theoretically reduce any nausea or gastrointestinal problems caused by mirtazapine's ability to increase serotonin release (Figure 12-56).

H1 antihistamine actions of mirtazapine (Figure 12-57) should theoretically relieve insomnia at night and improve anxiety during the day, but they could also cause drowsiness during the day. Combined with the 5HT2C antagonist properties described above, the H1 antihistamine actions of mirtazapine could also cause weight gain (Figure 12-57). Interestingly, the histamine 1 antagonist properties of mirtazapine are so potent that both mirtazapine and its active enantiomer esmirtazapine can be given in such low doses that they are essentially selective histamine 1 antagonists. The active enantiomer at very low doses is under investigation as a novel hypnotic and is discussed in Chapter 16, on sleep.

So, there you have it. Mirtazapine is a molecule with very complex pharmacology that does not block any monoamine transporter yet is a very effective antidepressant. In summary, the therapeutic actions of mirtazapine are thought to be mainly mediated through its alpha 2 antagonist and 5HT2C antagonist properties. The other properties add to

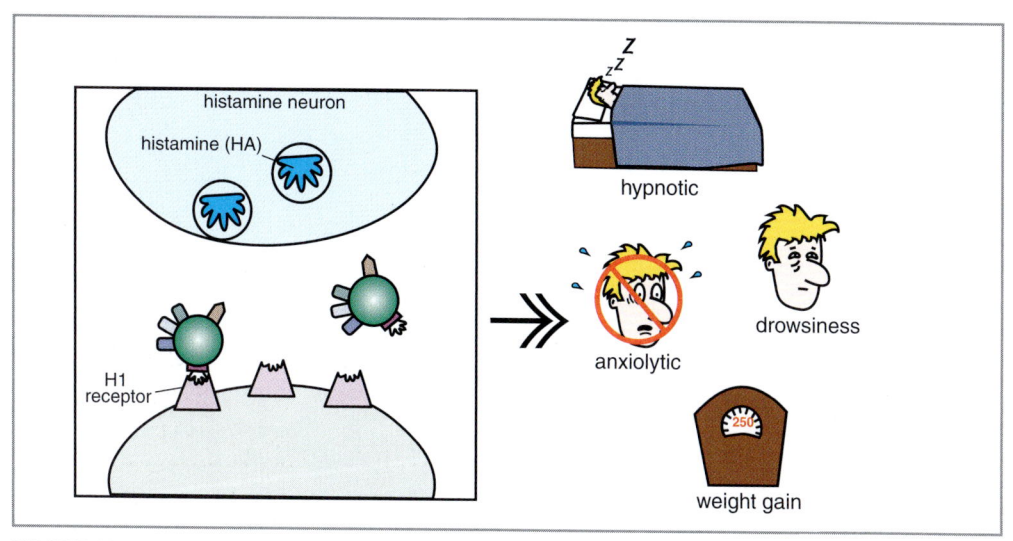

FIGURE 12-57 Mirtazapine at histamine 1 receptors. When mirtazapine blocks histamine 1 receptors, it can cause anxiolytic actions and possibly reduce nighttime insomnia, but it may also contribute to weight gain and daytime drowsiness.

therapeutic actions, cause some side effects, but probably allow patients to tolerate the powerful alpha 2 and 5HT2C antagonist actions that boost serotonin, norepinephrine, and possibly dopamine. An integrated view of mirtazapine's pharmacological actions is shown in Figure 12-58. Because of these unique pharmacological properties, it is worthwhile to understand this molecule and add it to the therapeutic armamentarium for depression, especially as an augmenting agent for difficult cases.

Two other alpha 2 antagonists are marketed as antidepressants in some countries (but not the United States), namely mianserin (worldwide except in the United States) and setiptilene (Japan). Unlike mirtazapine, mianserin has potent alpha 1 antagonist properties that tend to mitigate its ability to enhance serotonergic neurotransmission, so that this drug enhances predominantly noradrenergic neurotransmission yet with associated 5HT2A, 5HT2C, 5HT3, and histamine 1 antagonist properties. Yohimbine is also an alpha 2 antagonist, but its alpha 1 antagonist properties similarly mitigate its pro-serotonergic actions. Several selective alpha 2 antagonists, including idazoxan and fluparoxan, have been tested, but they have not demonstrated sufficiently robust antidepressant efficacy with sufficient tolerability, as they may provoke panic, anxiety, and prolonged erections in men, side effects that are not generally observed with alpha 2 antagonists such as mirtazapine, which have additional pharmacological properties that tend to block these side effects.

Serotonin antagonist/reuptake inhibitors (SARIs)

Several antidepressants share the ability to block serotonin 2A and 2C receptors as well as serotonin reuptake. The prototype drug with this antidepressant mechanism is trazodone (Figure 12-59), which is classified as a serotonin antagonist/reuptake inhibitor (SARI) (Table 12-2) or, more fully, as a serotonin 2A/2C antagonist and serotonin reuptake inhibitor (Figure 12-60). However, moderate to high doses of trazodone are required to inhibit SERT and 5HT2C receptors as well as 5HT2A receptors sufficiently for trazodone to be an effective antidepressant.

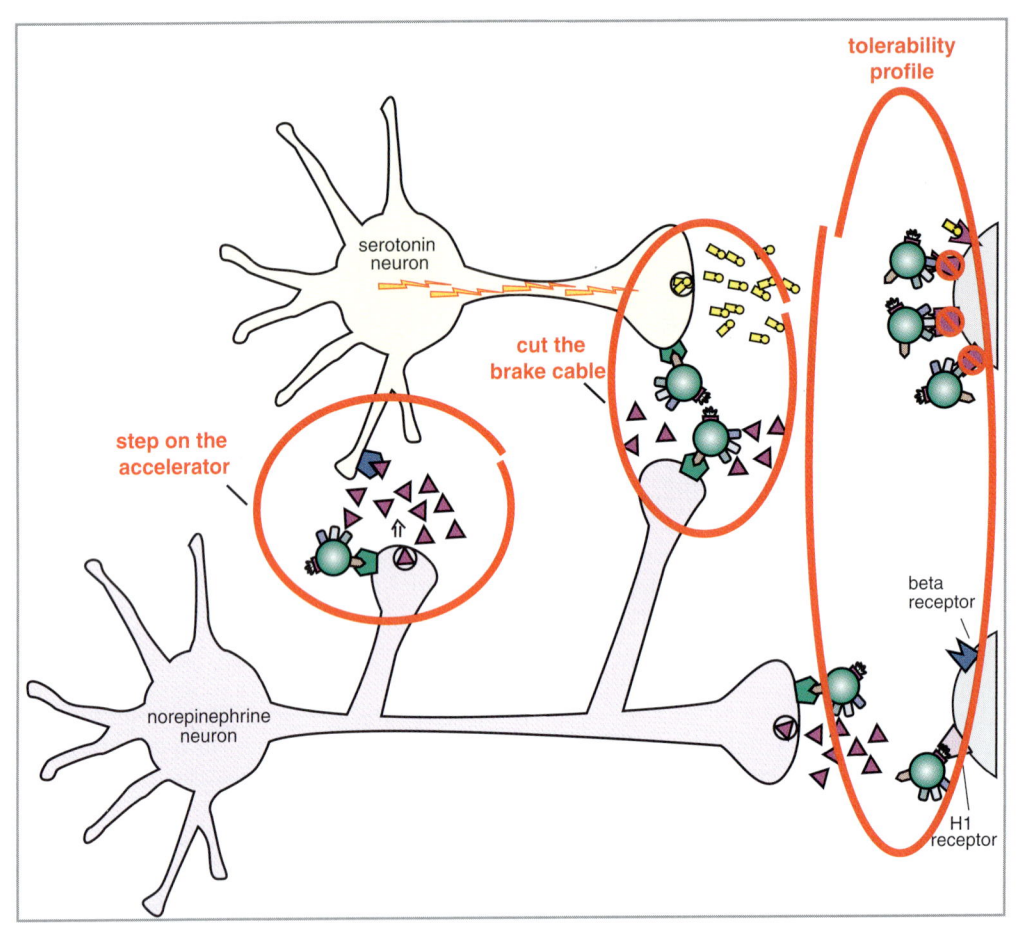

FIGURE 12-58 Overview of mirtazapine's actions. Mirtazapine's actions include those of alpha 2 antagonism, already shown in Figure 12-54: therapeutic actions of cutting the norepinephrine (NE) brake cable while stepping on the serotonin (5HT) accelerator (left circle) as well as cutting the 5HT brake cable (middle circle). This increases both 5HT and NE neurotransmission. On the right are the additional actions of mirtazapine beyond alpha 2 antagonism. These postsynaptic actions mainly account for the tolerability profile of mirtazapine.

Doses of trazodone lower than those effective for antidepressant action are frequently used for the effective treatment of insomnia. Low doses exploit trazodone's potent actions as a 5HT2A antagonist and also its properties as an antagonist of histamine 1 and alpha 1 adrenergic receptors, but they do not adequately exploit its SERT or 5HT2C inhibition properties, which are weaker (Figure 12-59). As discussed in Chapter 10 and illustrated in Figure 10-71, blocking the brain's arousal system with histamine 1 and alpha 1 antagonism can cause sedation or sleep; along with 5HT2A antagonist properties, this may explain the mechanism of how a low dose of trazodone works as a hypnotic. Since insomnia is one of the most frequent residual symptoms of depression after treatment with an SSRI (discussed earlier in this chapter and illustrated in Figure 12-9), a hypnotic is often necessary for patients with a major depressive episode. A hypnotic can not only potentially relieve the insomnia itself but – as recent data suggest – treating insomnia in patients with major depression also increases remission rates due to improvement of other symptoms, such as loss of energy and depressed mood. This ability of low doses of trazodone to improve sleep

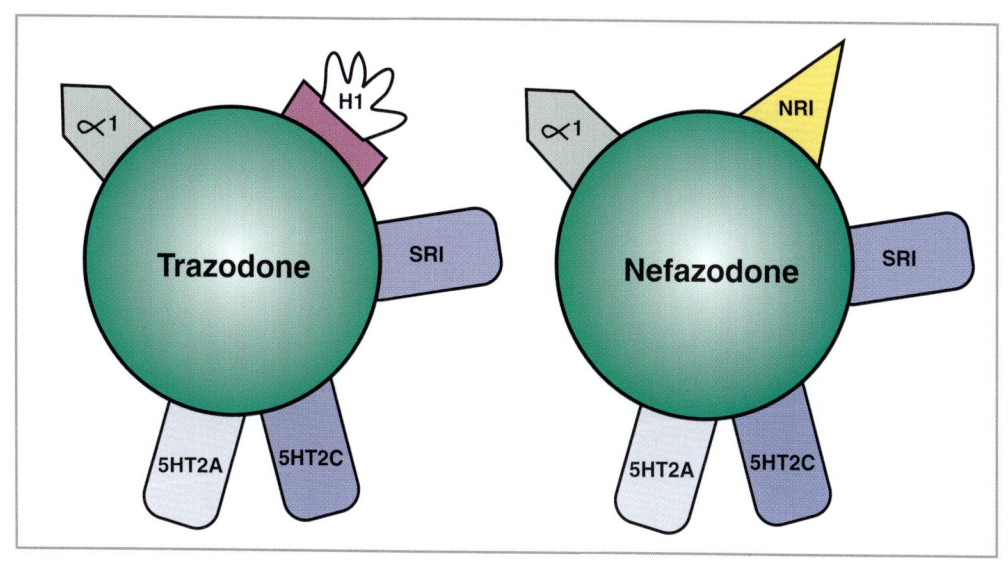

FIGURE 12-59 Serotonin antagonist/reuptake inhibitors. Shown here are icons for two serotonin 2A antagonist/reuptake inhibitors (SARIs): trazodone and nefazodone. These agents have a dual action, but the two mechanisms are different from the dual action of the serotonin norepinephrine reuptake inhibitors (SNRIs). The SARIs act by potent blockade of serotonin 2A (5HT2A) receptors as well as dose-dependent blockade of serotonin 2C (5HT2C) receptors and the serotonin transporter (SRI). SARIs also block alpha 1 adrenergic receptors. In addition, trazodone has the unique property of histamine 1 receptor antagonism and nefazodone has the unique property of norepinephrine reuptake inhibition (NRI).

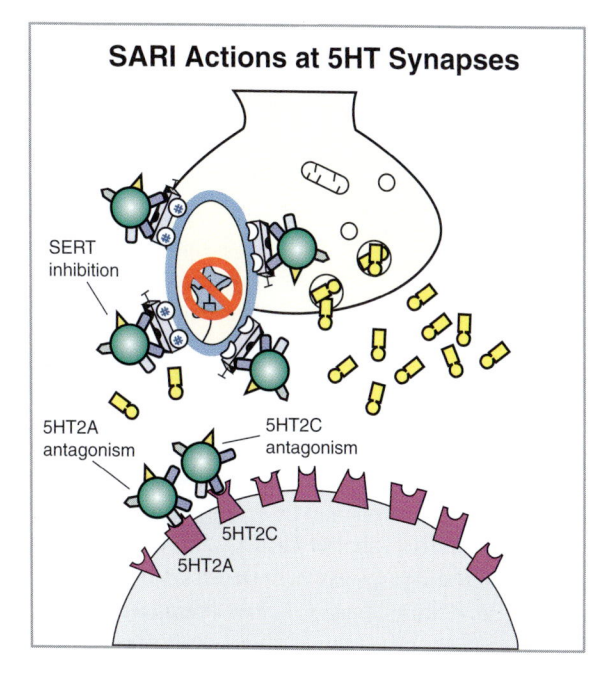

FIGURE 12-60 SARI actions at serotonin (5HT) synapses. This figure shows the dual actions of a serotonin 2A antagonist/reuptake inhibitor (SARI). This agent acts both presynaptically and postsynaptically. Presynaptic actions are indicated by the serotonin reuptake inhibitor (SRI) portion of the icon, which is inserted into the serotonin reuptake pump, blocking it. Postsynaptic actions are indicated by the serotonin 2A receptor antagonist portion of the icon (5HT2A) inserted into the 5HT2A receptor and by the serotonin 2C antagonist portion of the icon (5HT2C) inserted into the 5HT2C receptor. It is believed that all three blocking actions contribute to the antidepressant effects of SARIs. The 5HT2A antagonist actions are more potent than the serotonin reuptake properties or 5HT2C antagonism.

Antidepressants | 567

Mechanism of Action of SARIs: Baseline Postsynaptic Action

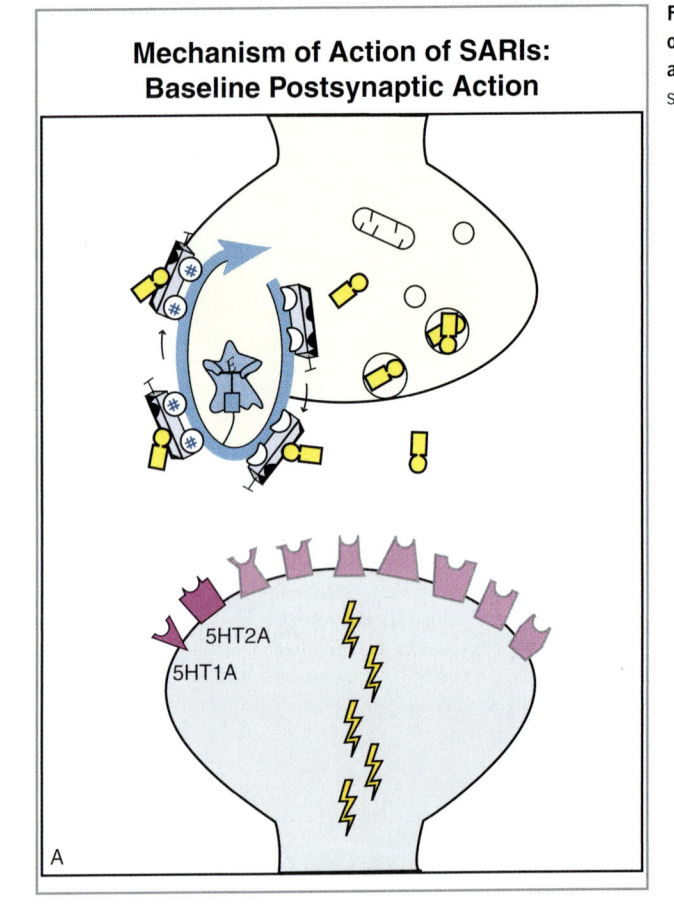

FIGURE 12-61A Mechanism of action of SARIs, part 1: baseline postsynaptic actions. Shown here is a postsynaptic serotonin neuron with baseline firing.

in depressed patients may thus be an important mechanism whereby trazodone can augment the efficacy of other antidepressants. The use of trazodone as a general hypnotic is discussed further in Chapter 16, on sleep.

Beyond the treatment of insomnia associated with depression, recruiting SERT inhibition with trazodone by increasing the dose is an important pharmacological mechanism that can be potentially synergistic with 5HT2A/5HT2C antagonism for broader antidepressant actions (Figures 12-61 through 12-64). However, in order to get this synergy of multiple mechanisms with trazodone monotherapy, a moderate to high dose must be used, which can often be attained without unacceptable daytime sedation by slow dose titration, allowing tolerance to develop, or giving the dose mostly at night to avoid unacceptable daytime sedation. Controlled-release formulations of trazodone are also in testing to reduce peak-dose sedation. Alternatively, low to moderate doses of trazodone can be added to a full dose of a known SERT inhibitor such as an SSRI or an SNRI to exploit 5HT2A/SERT synergy, as shown in Figures 12-60 through 12-63. An interesting aspect of trazodone's actions is the relative lack of sexual side effects at any dose, something it shares with mirtazapine, another 5HT2A/5HT2C antagonist.

How does 5HT2A/2C antagonism synergize with SERT inhibition to enhance the treatment of depressive symptoms other than insomnia? There are four possible ways in which this happens; these are illustrated in Figures 12-61 though 12-64.

568 | Essential Psychopharmacology

Mechanism of Action of SARIs: Serotonin Is Excitatory at 5HT2A Receptors

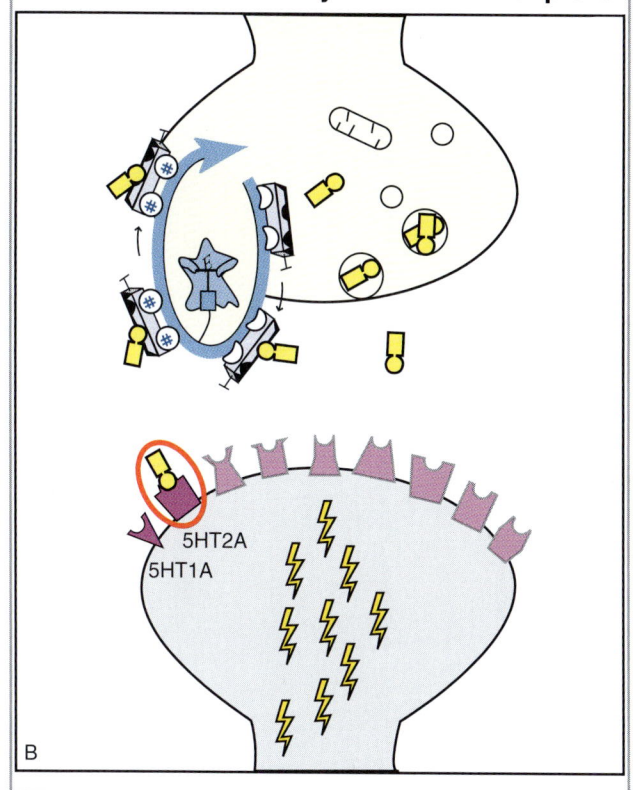

FIGURE 12-61B Mechanism of action of SARIs, part 2: serotonin (5HT) is excitatory at 5HT2A receptors. Stimulation of 5HT2A receptors by 5HT (red circle) increases firing of the postsynaptic 5HT neuron compared to baseline.

Serotonin 2A antagonism potentiates the inhibitory action of serotonin at 5HT1A receptors (Figure 12-61A)

Recall that serotonin 1A receptors in general can have the opposite actions of serotonin 2A receptors (see discussion in Chapter 10 and Figures 10-21 and 10-30). Thus, serotonin itself is excitatory at 5HT2A receptors (compare Figures 12-61A and 12-61B) and inhibitory at 5HT1A receptors (compare Figures 12-61A and 12-61C). Whether serotonin excites or inhibits the neuron depends on the density of each receptor at a given synapse and the amount of serotonin released. If the excitatory action of serotonin at 5HT2A receptors is blocked, this potentiates the inhibitory action of 5HT1A receptors (compare Figure 12-61D with Figures 12-61C and 12-61A).

Trazodone will cause 5HT2A inhibition at essentially any clinical dose, but to get the potentiation of serotonin's inhibition at 5HT1A receptors, there must be SERT inhibition that raises serotonin in the synapse and therefore increases serotonin levels so serotonin itself can interact at 5HT1A receptors at the same time that trazodone is blocking 5HT2A receptors (Figure 12-61D). This can be accomplished either by raising the trazodone dose or by adding a SERT inhibitor. The potentiation of 5HT1A inhibition of serotonin neurons may also be useful in relieving anxiety and in reducing overactivity in neuronal circuits in some brain regions associated with the various symptoms of depression (see reduction in

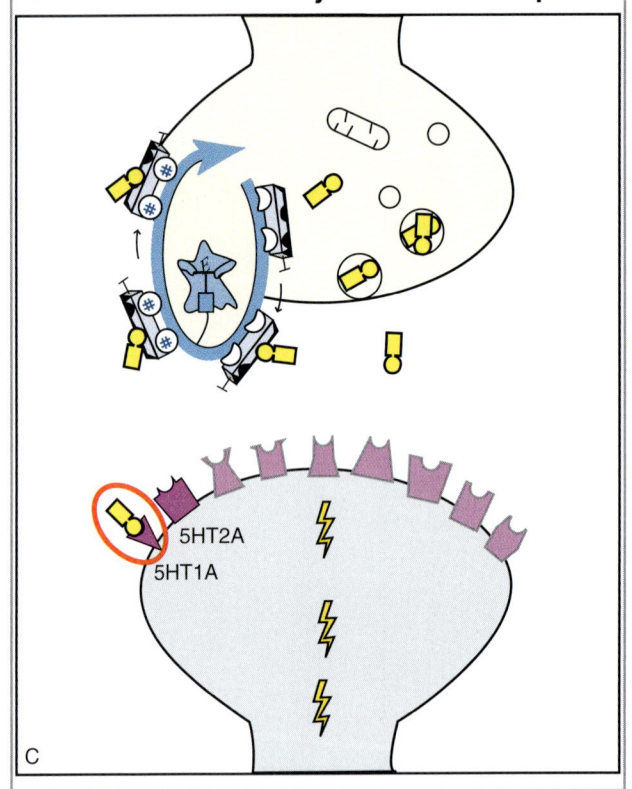

FIGURE 12-61C Mechanism of action of SARIs, part 3: serotonin (5HT) is inhibitory at 5HT1A receptors. Stimulation of 5HT1A receptors by 5HT (red circle) decreases firing of the postsynaptic 5HT neuron compared to baseline.

nerve impulse flow shown in Figure 12-61D and hypothetical areas of neuronal hyperactivity in depression in Figure 11-64).

Serotonin 2A antagonism potentiates gene expression stimulated by 5HT1A receptors (Figure 12-62)

Another action of serotonin at 5HT1A receptors that is opposed by serotonin actions at 5HT2A receptors is the stimulation of gene expression. That is, 5HT1A receptors stimulate gene expression by signal transduction through a second messenger system that utilizes cAMP (Figure 12-62A). Serotonin blocks this signal cascade system through actions downstream from 5HT2A receptors (Figure 12-62B). When this action of serotonin at 5HT2A receptors is blocked, the stimulation of gene expression by serotonin actions at 5HT1A receptors is potentiated (Figure 12-62C). Again, any clinical dose of trazodone will block 5HT2A receptors, but a higher dose of trazodone or a concomitantly administered SERT inhibitor is necessary to increase serotonin levels so that there is stimulation of 5HT1A receptors and thus 5HT2A/SERT synergy (Figure 12-62C). Potentiation of gene expression may be helpful in facilitating the regulation of neurotransmitter receptors or neurotrophic factors associated with improvement in the symptoms of depression.

**Mechanism of Action of SARIs:
Serotonin 2A Antagonism Potentiates the
Inhibitory Action of Serotonin at 5HT1A Receptors**

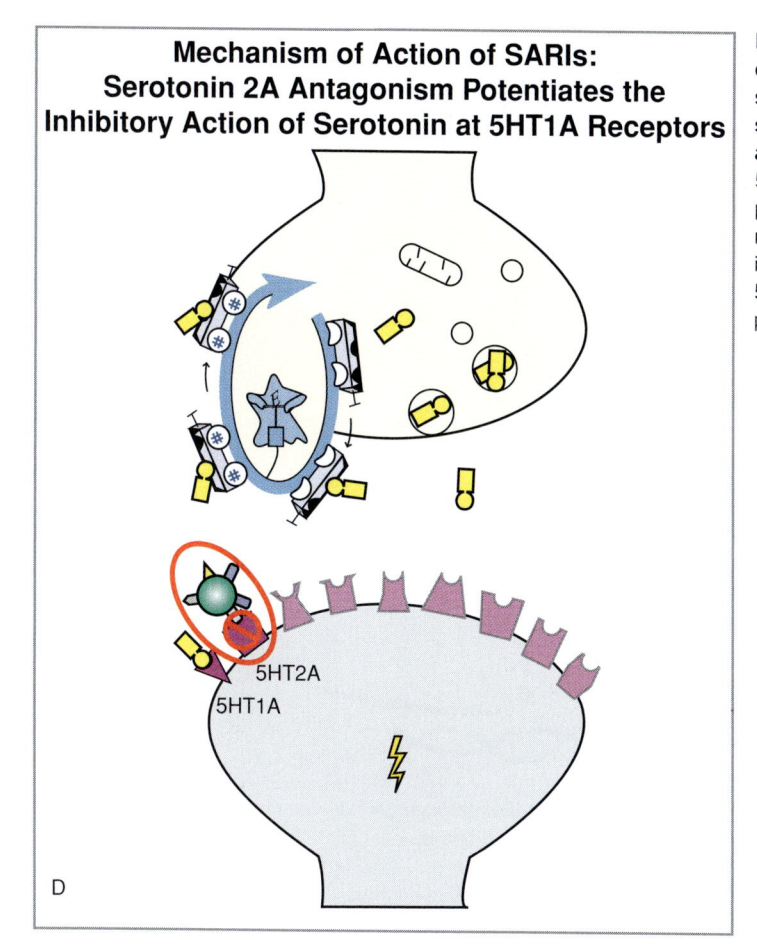

FIGURE 12-61D Mechanism of action of SARIs, part 4: synergy between 5HT1A stimulation and 5HT2A antagonism. When 5HT2A receptors are pharmacologically blocked rather than stimulated, the inhibitory actions of 5HT at 5HT1A receptors are potentiated.

Serotonin 2A antagonism potentiates the inhibitory action of serotonin 1A on glutamate release from cortical pyramidal neurons (Figure 12-63)

Serotonin stimulates glutamate release from pyramidal neurons in prefrontal cortex by its actions at 5HT2A receptors (Figure 12-63A) but inhibits glutamate release from these same neurons by its actions at 5HT1A receptors (Figure 12-63B). When 5HT2A receptors are blocked, it potentiates the inhibitory actions of serotonin at 5HT1A receptors (Figure 12-63C), but this can occur only if trazodone's potent 5HT2A antagonist properties are coupled with simultaneous SERT inhibition. Preventing the release of too much glutamate from dysfunctional pyramidal neurons that have inefficient information processing may improve information processing and reduce symptoms of depression in patients who have abnormal pyramidal cell functioning in various prefrontal cortex areas that mediate specific symptoms of depression (Figure 12-63C and Figure 11-64).

Serotonin 2A/2C potentiation of NE and DA disinhibition at serotonin 1A receptors (Figure 12-64)

Finally, as already discussed above in the sections on fluoxetine (Figure 12-25) and mirtazapine, serotonin's actions at 5HT2C receptors inhibit both DA and NE release (Figure 12-64). This same inhibition may also occur under certain circumstances at 5HT2A

Mechanism of Action of SARIs:
Serotonin Stimulates Gene Expression at 5HT1A Receptors

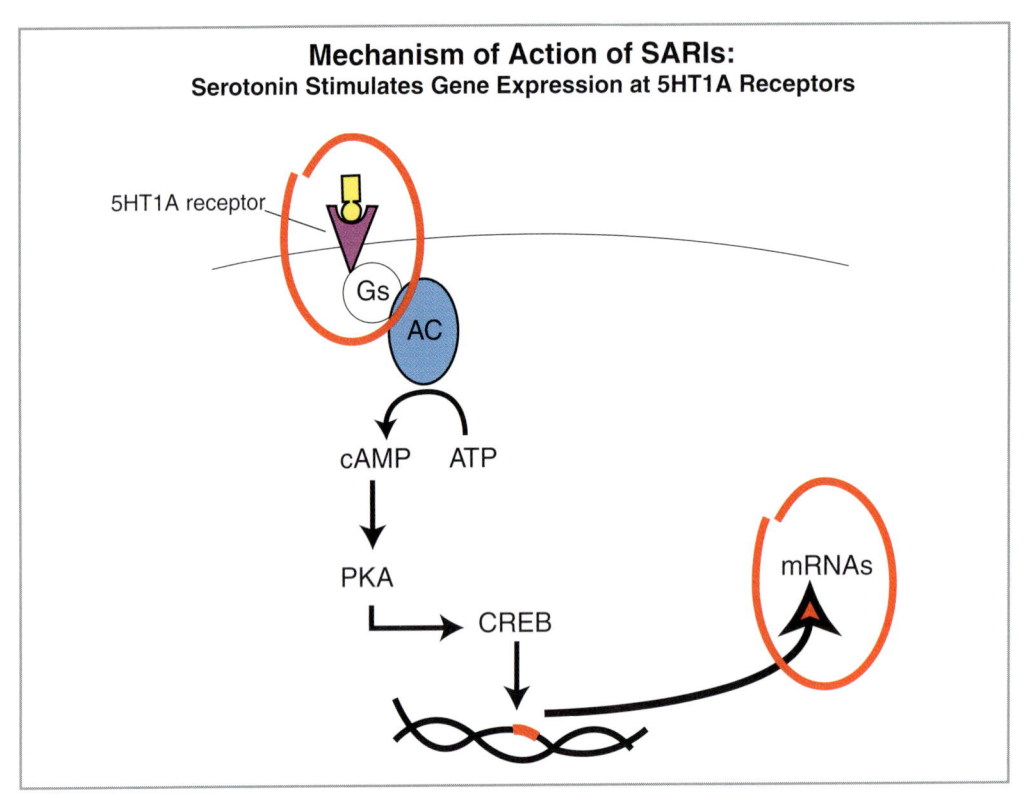

FIGURE 12-62A Serotonin (5HT) stimulates gene expression through 5HT1A receptors. The molecular consequences of 5HT1A stimulation alone, shown here, result in a certain amount of gene expression corresponding to the pharmacological actions shown in Figure 12-61C. 5HT occupancy of its 5HT1A receptor (top red circle) causes a certain amount of gene transcription (see bottom red circle on the right). The 5HT1A receptor is coupled to a stimulatory G protein (Gs) and adenylate cyclase (AC), which produces the second messenger cyclic AMP from ATP. This, in turn, activates protein kinase A (PKA), so that transcription factors such as cyclic AMP response element binding protein (CREB) can activate gene expression (mRNAs).

receptors, as discussed in Chapter 10 for atypical antipsychotics. Also already discussed is how stimulation of serotonin 1A receptors acutely reduces the serotonergic inhibition of DA and NE release at 5HT2C receptors and possibly at 5HT2A receptors, thus disinhibiting DA and NE release (Figure 12-64). Because this 5HT1A mechanism tends to desensitize, it may be important to potentiate this action of serotonin at 5HT1A receptors by simultaneously blocking 5HT2C and/or 5HT2A receptors, leading to release of both DA and NE in prefrontal cortex (Figure 12-64). The bottom line is that producing disinhibition of NE and DA in prefrontal cortex by whatever mechanism could theoretically help to enhance the efficiency of information processing there and lead to a reduction in the symptoms of depression mediated in this brain region.

Nefazodone is another SARI with robust 5HT2A antagonist actions and weaker 5HT2C antagonism and SERT inhibition, but it is no longer commonly used because of rare liver toxicity (Figure 12-59). Several tricyclic antidepressants – such as amitriptyline, nortriptyline, doxepin, and amoxapine – also have a combination of serotonin 2A and 2C antagonism with serotonin reuptake inhibition along with several other pharmacological actions; these are discussed later in this chapter in the section on tricyclic antidepressants. Since the potency of blockade of serotonin 2A and 2C receptors varies considerably among

Mechanism of Action of SARIs:
Serotonin at 5HT2A Receptors Blocks Signal Transduction
and Gene Expression From 5HT1A Receptors

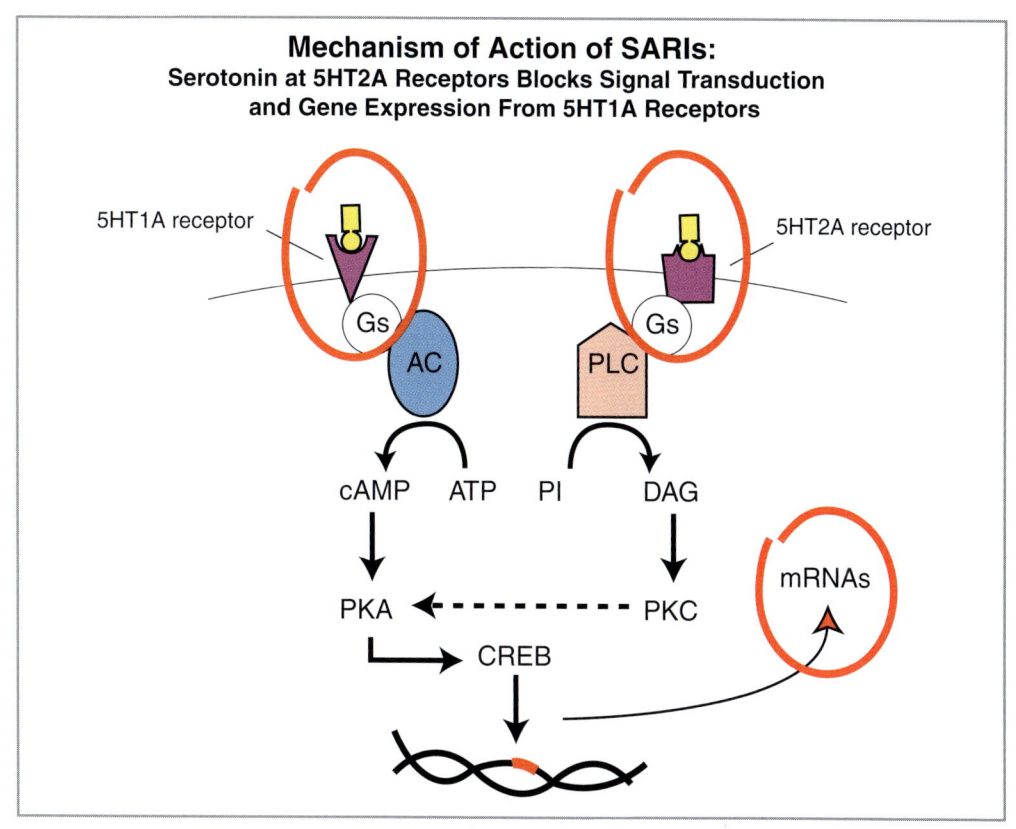

FIGURE 12-62B **Serotonin (5HT) at 5HT2A receptors blocks gene expression from 5HT1A receptors.** The molecular consequence of 5HT2A receptor stimulation concomitant with 5HT1A receptor stimulation is to reduce the gene expression of 5HT1A stimulation alone (i.e., that shown in Figure 12-62A). These molecular consequences correlate with the pharmacological actions of simultaneous 5HT1A and 5HT2A stimulation. Simultaneous activation of the 5HT2A receptor by 5HT (top right red circle) will alter the consequences of activating 5HT1A receptors (top left red circle) in a negative way and reduce the gene expression of 5HT1A receptors acting alone (Figure 12-62A). Thus, occupancy of 5HT2A receptor (top right red circle) causes coupling of a stimulatory G protein (Gs) with the enzyme phospholipase C (PLC). This, in turn, activates calcium flux and converts phosphatidylinositol (PI) into diacylglycerol (DAG). This activates the enzyme phosphokinase C (PKC), which has an inhibitory action on phosphokinase A (PKA). This reduces the activation of transcription factors such as cyclic AMP response element binding protein (CREB) and leads to a decrease in gene expression (bottom red circle).

the tricyclics, it is not clear how important this action is to the therapeutic actions of tricyclic antidepressants in general.

Many other drugs are 5HT2A/2C antagonists, including mirtazapine, just discussed in the previous section, and the atypical antipsychotics discussed in Chapter 10, all of which are potent 5HT2A antagonists and some of which are also potent 5HT2C antagonists (Figures 10-90 to 10-101). The use of atypical antipsychotics as augmenting agents for treatment-resistant depression is discussed later in this chapter in the section on antidepressants in clinical practice; their use for treatment of bipolar depression is discussed in Chapter 13, on mood stabilizers.

YM992 is another SARI (serotonin 2A/2C antagonist with moderately potent serotonin reuptake inhibition properties) that is in testing as an antidepressant. Selective 5HT2A antagonists, however, do not appear to be effective antidepressants. On the other hand, drugs

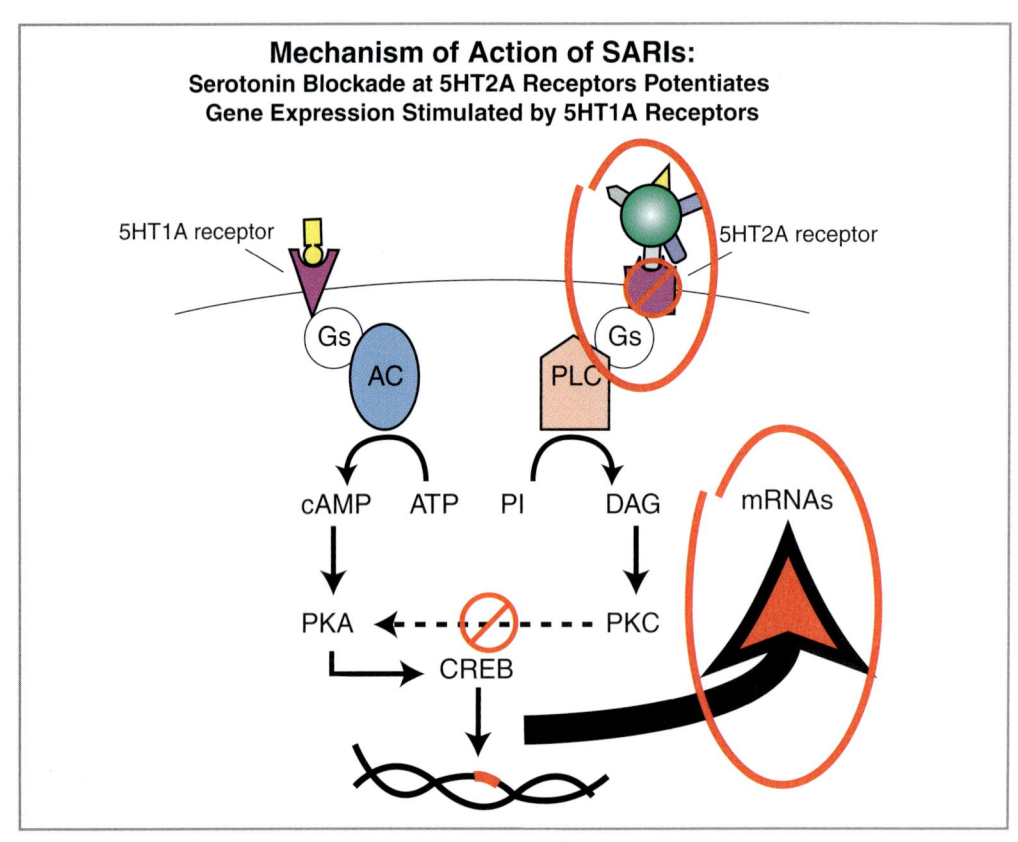

FIGURE 12-62C Serotonin (5HT) blockade at 5HT2A receptors potentiates gene expression from 5HT1A receptors. The molecular consequence of 5HT1A receptor disinhibition by 5HT2A receptor blockade is shown here – namely, enhanced gene expression. These molecular events are the consequence of the pharmacological actions shown in Figure 12-61D. Simultaneous inhibition of the 5HT2A receptor (top right circle) can stop the negative consequences that 5HT2A receptor stimulation by 5HT can have on gene expression, as shown in Figure 12-62B. Thus gene expression of the 5HT1A receptor is enhanced when 5HT2A receptors are blocked (bottom red circle) rather than diminished when they are stimulated (Figure 12-62B).

with 5HT2A/2C antagonist properties plus direct-acting 5HT1A agonist properties are in testing as potential novel antidepressants and disinhibitors of DA release for improving sexual dysfunction, including the agents flibanserin, adatanserin, BMS181,101, and others. One particularly novel agent with 5HT2C antagonist properties in testing as an antidepressant is agomelatine, discussed in the section on future antidepressants below.

Classic antidepressants: monoamine oxidase inhibitors

The first clinically effective antidepressants to be discovered were inhibitors of the enzyme monoamine oxidase (MAO). They were discovered by accident when an antituberculosis drug, iproniazid, was observed to help depression that coexisted in some of the patients who had tuberculosis. This antituberculosis drug was eventually found to work in depression by inhibiting the enzyme MAO. However, inhibition of MAO was unrelated to its antituberculosis actions.

This discovery soon led to the synthesis of more drugs in the 1950s and 1960s that inhibited MAO but lacked unwanted additional properties (such as antituberculosis properties and liver toxicity). Although best known as powerful antidepressants, the MAOIs are

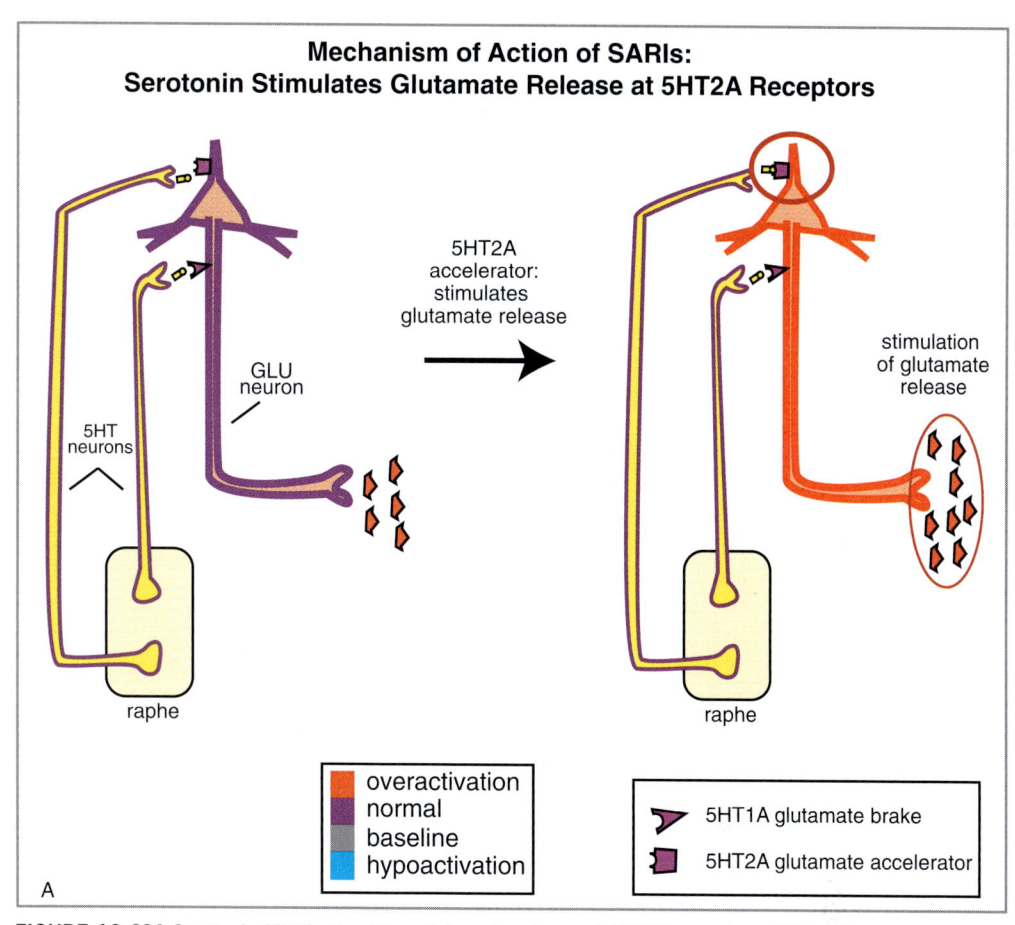

FIGURE 12-63A Serotonin (5HT) stimulates glutamate release at 5HT2A receptors. 5HT projections from the midbrain raphe synapse with pyramidal glutamate neurons in the prefrontal cortex (right). Binding of 5HT to 5HT2A receptors stimulates glutamate release from pyramidal neurons (left).

also highly effective therapeutic agents for certain anxiety disorders, such as panic disorder and social phobia (mentioned in Chapter 14, on anxiety). MAO inhibitors, however, tend to be underutilized in clinical practice. There are many reasons for this, including the fact that there are many other options for treatment today, preventing modern-day clinicians from becoming familiar with them. Since these are old drugs, and there is essentially no marketing for them, there is a good deal of misinformation and mythology about their dietary and drug interaction dangers. For these reasons, these agents are discussed in this chapter, which in this respect is uncharacteristic of modern psychopharmacology texts. Readers with no interest in MAO inhibitors can, of course, skip this section as well as the following section on tricyclic antidepressants and go on to antidepressant pharmacokinetics, but in so doing they may miss information on a few secret weapons in the therapeutic armamentarium for patients who fail to respond to the better-known agents.

Three of the original MAO inhibitors that are still available for clinical use today are phenelzine, tranylcypromine, and isocarboxazid (Table 12-4). These are all irreversible enzyme inhibitors and thus bind to MAO covalently and irreversibly and destroy its function forever. Enzyme activity returns only after new enzyme is synthesized. Sometimes such

Antidepressants | 575

Mechanism of Action of SARIs:
Serotonin Inhibits Glutamate Release at 5HT1A Receptors

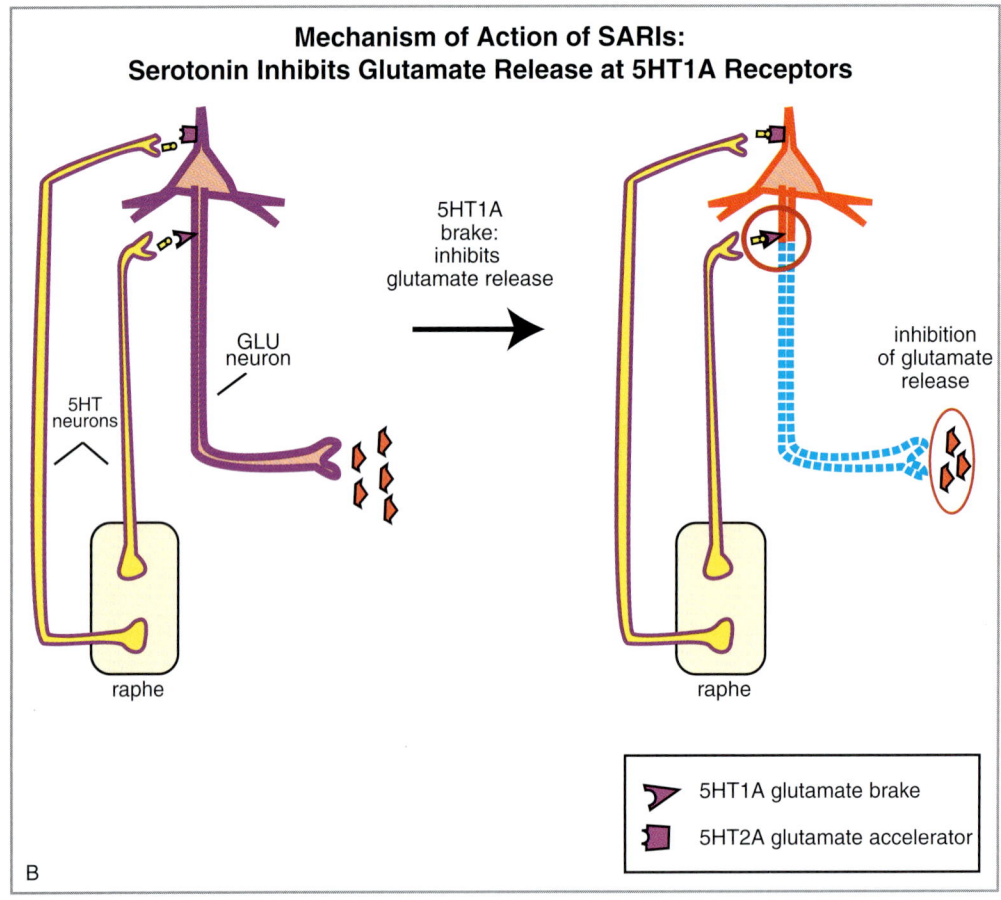

FIGURE 12-63B Serotonin (5HT) inhibits glutamate release at 5HT1A receptors. Binding of 5HT to 5HT1A receptors inhibits glutamate release from pyramidal neurons (left).

enzyme inhibitors are called "suicide inhibitors," because once this kind of inhibitor binds to the enzyme, the enzyme essentially commits suicide in that it can never function again until a new enzyme protein is synthesized by the neuron's DNA in the cell nucleus. This is an unfortunate terminology for a very effective class of antidepressants and perhaps is a concept better utilized by enzymologists, not by clinicians.

Amphetamine is itself a weak MAO inhibitor (Table 12-5). Some MAO inhibitors, such as tranylcypromine, have chemical structures modeled on amphetamine; thus, in addition to MAO inhibitor properties, they also have amphetamine-like dopamine-releasing properties (Tables 12-4 and 12-5). Amphetamine's actions on the dopamine transporter (DAT) that trigger dopamine release are discussed in Chapter 4 and illustrated in Figure 4-15. Tranylcypromine has these same actions on DAT as well. Selegiline itself does not have amphetamine-like properties but is metabolized to both l-amphetamine and l-methamphetamine, which do have inhibitory actions on DAT and dopamine-releasing properties (Tables 12-4 and 12-5). Thus there is a close mechanistic link between some MAO inhibitors and DAT inhibition as well as between the MAO-inhibiting properties and DAT-inhibiting properties of amphetamine itself (Tables 12-4 and 12-5). It is therefore not surprising that one of the augmenting agents utilized to boost MAO inhibitors

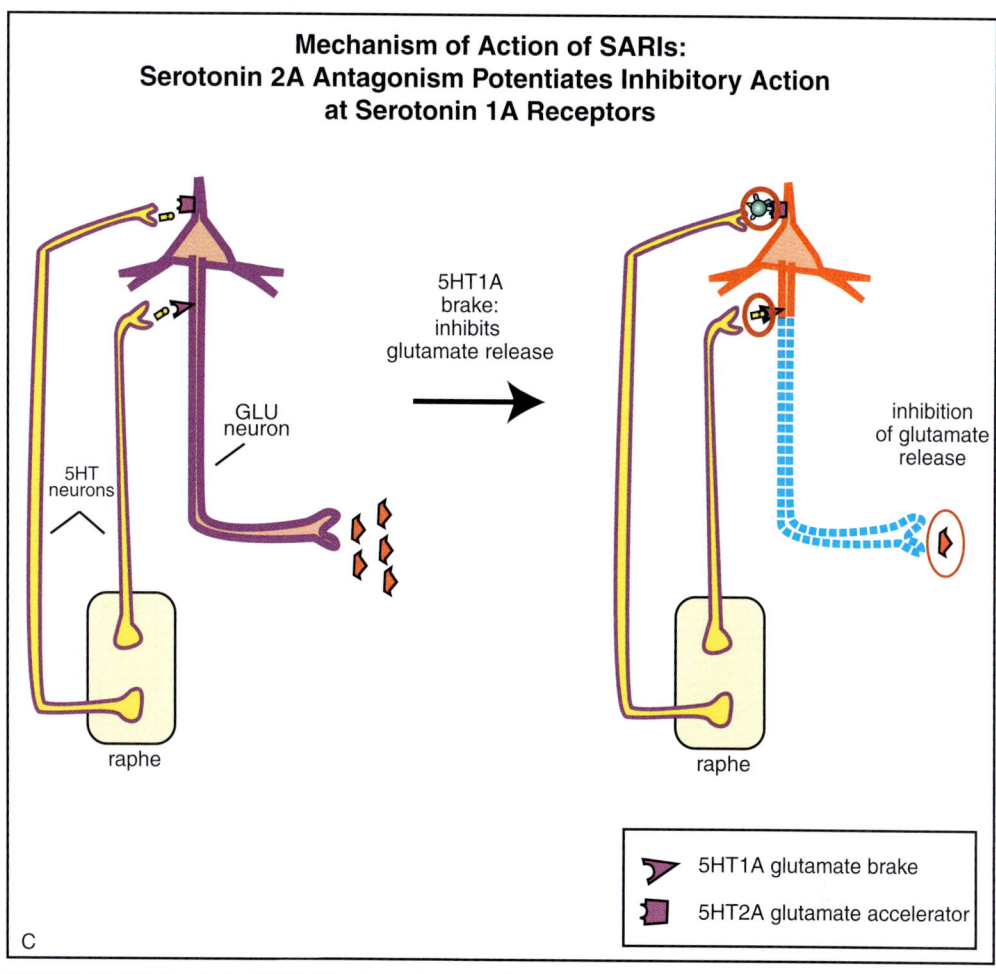

FIGURE 12-63C Serotonin (5HT) 2A antagonism potentiates inhibitory action at 5HT1A receptors. Blockade of 5HT2A receptors can potentiate the inhibitory actions of serotonin at 5HT1A receptors on glutamate release (left).

in treatment-resistant patients is amphetamine, administered by experts with great caution while monitoring blood pressure.

MAO subtypes

MAO exists in two subtypes, A and B (Table 12-6). Both forms are inhibited by the original MAO inhibitors, which are therefore nonselective (Table 12-4). The A form preferentially metabolizes the monoamines most closely linked to depression (i.e., serotonin and norepinephrine), whereas the B form preferentially metabolizes trace amines such as phenethylamine (Table 12-6). Both MAO-A and MAO-B metabolize dopamine and tyramine (Table 12-6). Both MAO-A and MAO-B are in the brain (Table 12-6). Noradrenergic neurons (Figure 11-31) and dopaminergic neurons (Figure 9-19) are thought to contain both MAO-A and MAO-B, with perhaps MAO-A activity predominant, whereas serotonergic neurons are thought to contain only MAO-B (Figure 10-16). With the exception of platelets and lymphocytes, which have MAO-B, MAO-A is the major form of this enzyme outside of the brain (Table 12-6).

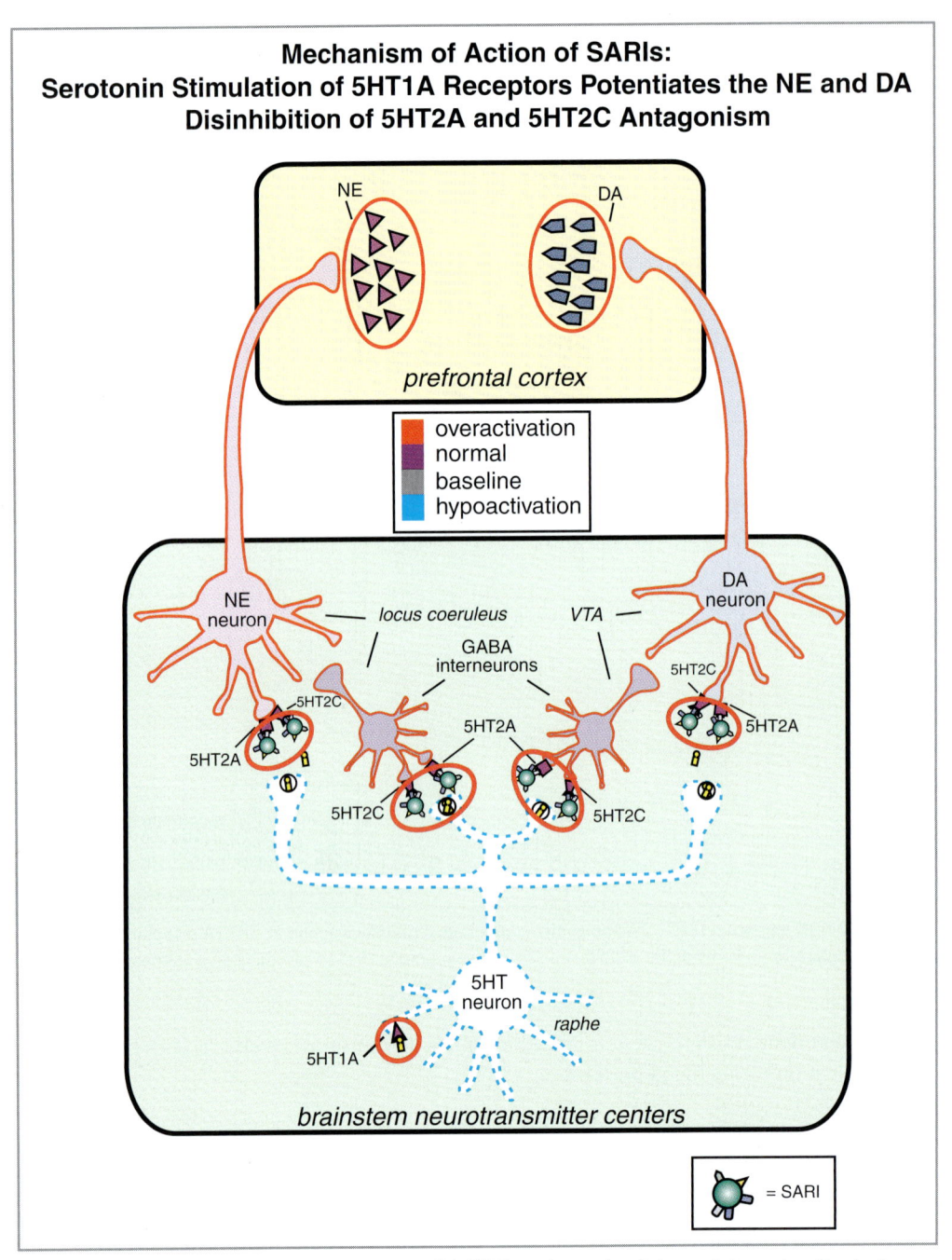

FIGURE 12-64 Stimulation of 5HT1A receptors: disinhibition of norepinephrine and dopamine. Serotonin (5HT) actions at 5HT2C and 5HT2A receptors inhibit both norepinephrine (NE) and dopamine (DA) release. Indirect stimulation of presynaptic 5HT1A receptors via SERT inhibition by high doses of trazodone can reduce this inhibition of NE and DA by 5HT via reducing the concentrations of 5HT at postsynaptic sites on NE and DA neurons. Furthermore, if 5HT2C and 5HT2A receptors are blocked, this may potentiate the disinhibiting effects of 5HT1A stimulation on NE and DA.

578 | Essential Psychopharmacology

TABLE 12-4 Currently approved MAO inhibitors

Name (trade name)	Inhibition of MAO-A	Inhibition of MAO-B	Amphetamine properties
phenelzine (Nardil)	+	+	
tranylcypromine (Parnate)	+	+	+
isocarboxazid (Marplan)	+	+	
amphetamines (at high doses)	+	+	+
selegiline transdermal system (Emsam)			
brain	+	+	+
gut	+/−	+	+
selegiline low dose oral (Deprenyl, Eldepryl)	−	+	+
rasaligine (Agilect/Azilect)	−	+	−
moclobemide (Aurorix, Manerix)	+	−	−

TABLE 12-5 MAO inhibitors with amphetamine actions or amphetamines with MAO inhibition?

Drug	Comment
amphetamine	MAOI at high doses
tranylcypromine (Parnate)	also called phenylcyclopropylamine
selegiline	metabolized to L-methamphetamine
	metabolized to L-amphetamine
	less amphetamine formed transdermally

TABLE 12-6 MAO enzymes

	MAO-A	MAO-B
Substrates	5-HT	Phenylethylamine
	NE	DA
	DA	Tyramine
	Tyramine	
Tissue distribution	Brain, gut, liver, placenta, skin	Brain, platelets, lymphocytes

Brain MAO-A must be inhibited for antidepressant efficacy to occur (Figure 12-65). This is not surprising, since this is the form of MAO that preferentially metabolizes serotonin and norepinephrine, two of the three components of the trimonoaminergic neurotransmitter system linked to depression and to antidepressant actions, both of which demonstrate increased brain levels after MAO-A inhibition (Figure 12-65). MAO-A, along with MAO-B, also metabolizes dopamine, but inhibition of MAO-A alone does not appear to lead to robust increases in brain dopamine levels, since MAO-B can still metabolize dopamine (Figure 12-65).

Inhibition of MAO-B is not effective as an antidepressant, as there is no direct effect on either serotonin or norepinephrine metabolism and little or no dopamine accumulates owing to the continued action of MAO-A (Figure 12-66). What, therefore, is the therapeutic value of MAO-B inhibition? When this enzyme is selectively inhibited, it can boost the action of concomitantly administered levodopa in Parkinson's disease. Evidently, in the presence

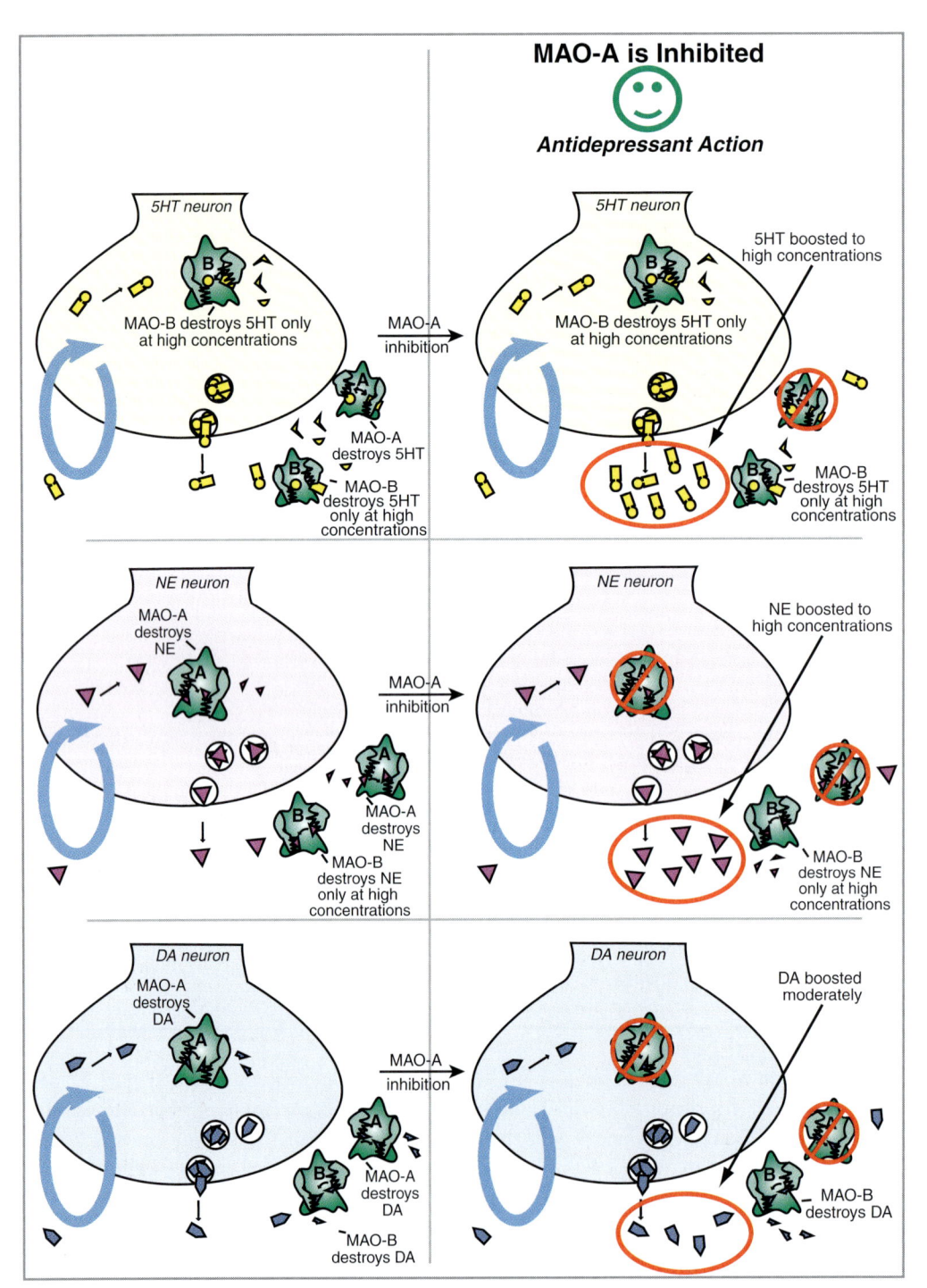

FIGURE 12-65 Monoamine oxidase A (MAO-A) inhibition. The enzyme MAO-A metabolizes serotonin (5HT) and norepinephrine (NE) as well as dopamine (DA) (left panels). Monoamine oxidase B (MAO-B) also metabolizes DA, but it metabolizes 5HT and NE only at high concentrations (left panels). This means that MAO-A inhibition increases 5HT, NE, and DA (right panels) but that the increase in DA is not as great as that of 5HT and NE because MAO-B can continue to destroy DA (bottom right panel). Inhibition of MAO-A is an efficacious antidepressant strategy.

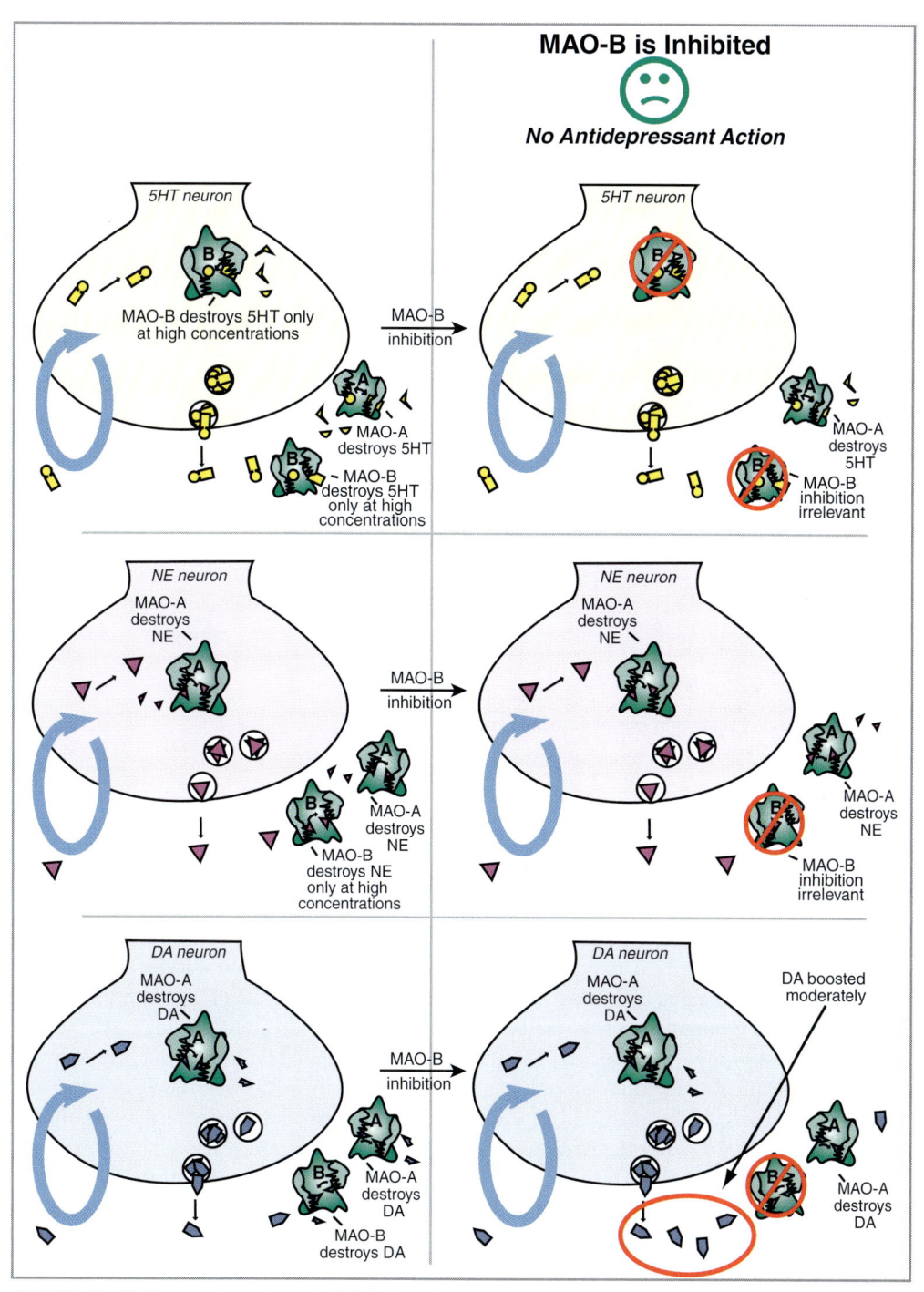

FIGURE 12-66 Monoamine oxidase B (MAO-B) inhibition. Selective inhibitors of MAO-B do not have antidepressant efficacy. This is because MAO-B metabolizes serotonin (5HT) and norepinephrine (NE) only at high concentrations (top two left panels). Since MAO-B's role in destroying 5HT and NE is small, its inhibition is not likely to be relevant to the concentrations of these neurotransmitters (top two right panels). Selective inhibition of MAO-B also has somewhat limited effects on dopamine (DA) concentrations, because MAO-A continues to destroy DA. However, inhibition of MAO-B does increase DA to some extent, which can be therapeutic in other disease states, such as Parkinson's disease.

of a large load of dopamine derived from administration of a large dose of its precursor levodopa, selective MAO-B inhibition is sufficient to boost dopamine action in the brain. MAO-B is also thought to convert some environmentally derived amine substrates, called protoxins, into toxins that may cause damage to neurons and possibly contribute to the cause or decline of function in Parkinson's disease. Inhibition of MAO-B may thus halt this process, and there is speculation that this might slow the degenerative course of various neurodegenerative disorders, including Parkinson's disease. Thus, two MAO inhibitors in Table 12-4, selegiline and rasaligine, when administered orally in doses selective for inhibition of MAO-B, are approved for use in patients with Parkinson's disease but are not effective at these selective MAO-B doses as antidepressants.

Perhaps the most important role of MAO-B in psychopharmacology is when it is inhibited simultaneously with MAO-A (Figure 12-67). In that case, there is a triple and very robust monoaminergic boost of dopamine as well as serotonin and norepinephrine (Figure 12-67). This would theoretically provide the most powerful antidepressant efficacy across the range of depressive symptoms, from diminished positive affect to increased negative affect (see Figure 11-55). Thus MAO-A plus B inhibition is one of the few therapeutic strategies available to increase dopamine in depression and therefore to treat refractory symptoms of diminished positive affect. This is a good reason for specialists in psychopharmacology to become adept at administering MAO inhibitors, so that they can have an additional strategy within their armamentarium for patients with treatment-resistant symptoms of diminished positive affect, which is a very common problem in a referral practice.

Tyramine reactions and dietary restrictions

One of the biggest barriers to utilizing MAO inhibitors has traditionally been the risk that a patient taking one of these drugs might develop a hypertensive reaction after ingesting tyramine in the diet. How does the combination of tyramine in the diet plus MAO-A inhibition in the gut lead to a dangerous elevation in blood pressure? Tyramine works to elevate blood pressure because it is a potent releaser of norepinephrine. Normally, NE is not allowed to accumulate to dangerous levels, owing in part to efficient destruction of NE by MAO-A once NE is released during neurotransmission (Figure 12-68). Thus there is no vasoconstriction and no elevated blood pressure because there is no excessive stimulation of postsynaptic alpha 1 or other adrenergic receptors (Figure 12-68). When foods high in tyramine content – such as tap beers, smoked meat or fish, fava beans, aged cheeses, sauerkraut, or soy – are ingested (Table 12-7), MAO-A in the intestinal wall goes to work, safely destroying tyramine before it is absorbed; MAO-A in the liver safely destroys any tyramine that gets absorbed; and even if any tyramine reaches the noradrenergic sympathetic neuron (Figure 12-69), the MAO-A there destroys any synaptic norepinephrine that this tyramine would release. The body thus has a huge capacity for processing tyramine, and the average person is able to handle around 400 mg of ingested tyramine before blood pressure is elevated. A high-tyramine meal, by contrast, represents only around 40 mg of tyramine.

However, when MAO-A is inhibited, this capacity to handle dietary tyramine is much reduced, and a high-tyramine meal is sufficient to raise blood pressure when a substantial amount of MAO-A is irreversibly inhibited (Figure 12-70). In fact, it may take as little as 10 mg of dietary tyramine to increase blood pressure when MAO-A is essentially knocked out by high doses of an MAO inhibitor. Some blood pressure elevations can be very large, sudden, and dramatic, causing a condition known as a hypertensive crisis (Table 12-8), which can rarely cause intracerebral hemorrhage or even death. This risk is normally controlled

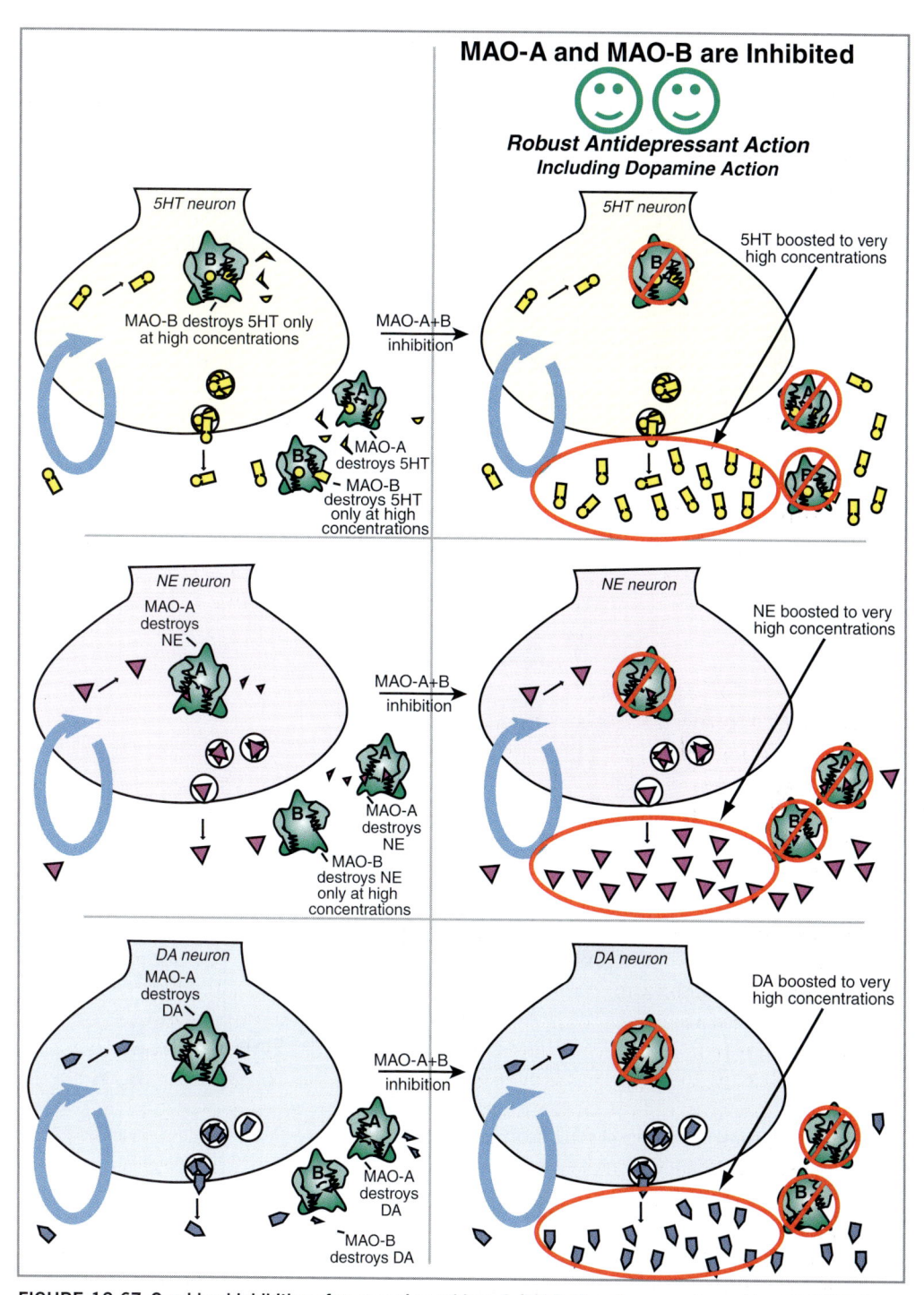

FIGURE 12-67 Combined inhibition of monoamine oxidase A (MAO-A) and monoamine oxidase B (MAO-B). Combined inhibition of MAO-A and MAO-B may have robust antidepressant actions owing to increases not only in serotonin (5HT) and norepinephrine (NE) but also dopamine (DA). Inhibition of both MAO-A, which metabolizes 5HT, NE, and DA, and MAO-B, which metabolizes primarily DA (left panels), leads to greater increases in each of these neurotransmitters than inhibition of either enzyme alone.

Antidepressants | 583

TABLE 12-7 Suggested tyramine dietary modifications for MAO inhibitors*

Food to avoid	Food allowed
Dried, aged, smoked, fermented, spoiled, or improperly stored meat, poultry, and fish	Fresh or processed meat, poultry, and fish
Broad bean pods	All other vegetables
Aged cheeses	Processed and cottage cheese, ricotta cheese, yogurt
Tap and nonpasteurized beers	Canned or bottled beers and alcohol (have little tyramine)
Marmite, sauerkraut	Brewer's and baker's yeast
Soy products/tofu	

*No dietary modifications needed for low doses of transdermal selegiline or for low oral doses of selective MAO-B inhibitors.

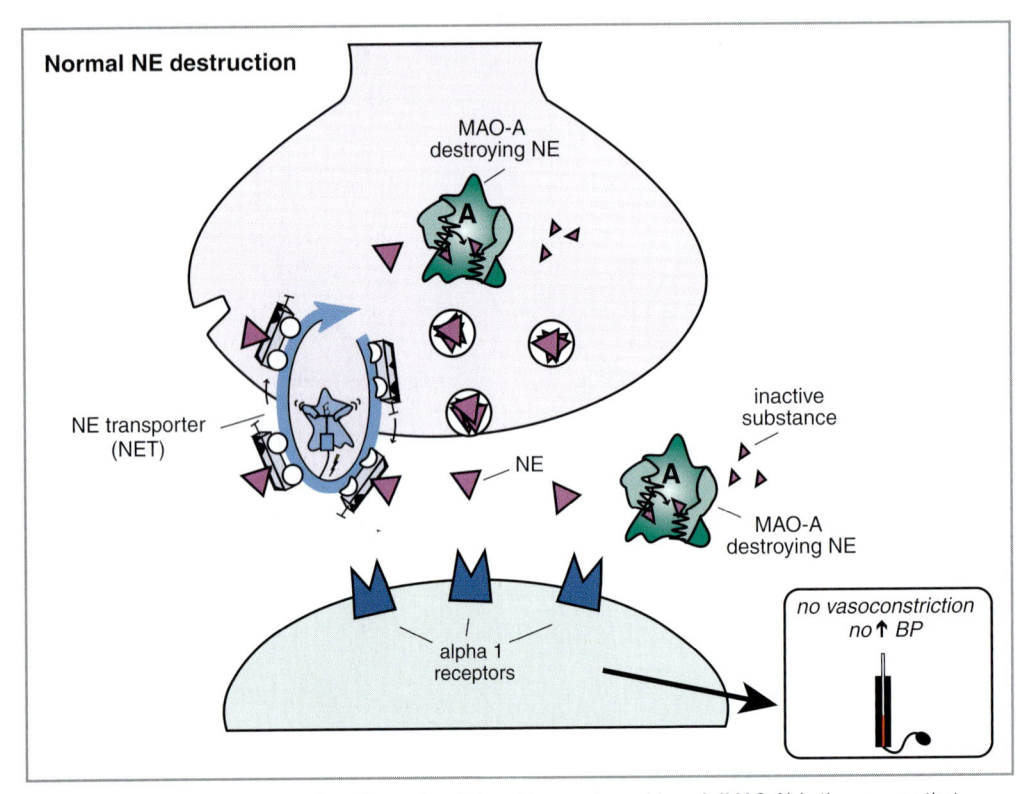

FIGURE 12-68 Normal destruction of norepinephrine. Monoamine oxidase A (MAO-A) is the enzyme that normally acts to destroy norepinephrine (NE) to keep it in balance. Since accumulated NE can cause vasoconstriction and elevated blood pressure via increased binding at alpha 1 and other adrenergic receptors, its normal destruction by MAO-A helps prevent these negative effects.

by restricting the diet so that foods dangerously high in tyramine content are eliminated (Table 12-7). Until recently, the risk of hypertensive crisis and the hassle of restricting diet have generally been the price that a patient has had to pay in order to get the therapeutic benefits of the MAO inhibitors in treating depression.

Because of the potential danger of a hypertensive crisis from a tyramine reaction in patients taking irreversible MAO inhibitors, a certain mythology has grown up around how

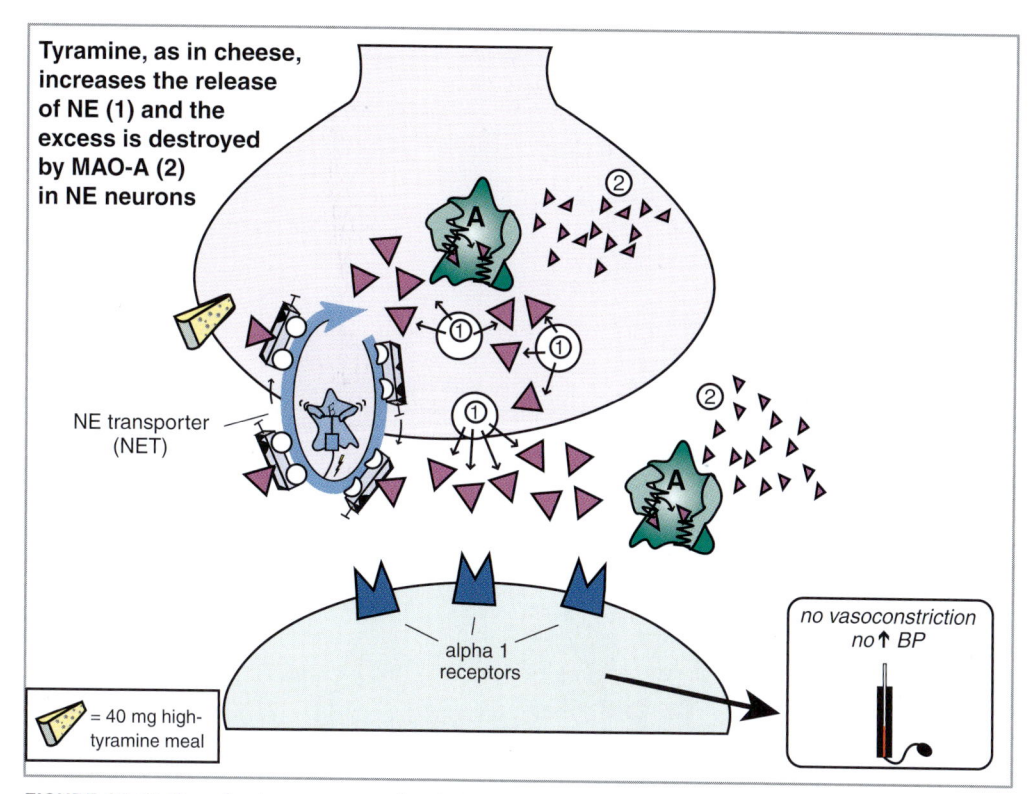

FIGURE 12-69 Tyramine increases norepinephrine release. Tyramine is an amine present in various foods, including cheese. Indicated in this figure is how a high-tyramine meal (40 mg, depicted here as cheese) acts to increase the release of norepinephrine (NE) (1). However, in normal circumstances the enzyme monoamine oxidase A (MAO-A) readily destroys the excess NE released by tyramine (2), and no harm is done (i.e., no vasoconstriction or elevation in blood pressure).

much tyramine is in various foods and therefore what dietary restrictions are necessary. Since the tyramine reaction is sometimes called a "cheese reaction," there is a myth that all cheese must be restricted. However, that is true only for aged cheeses such as English Stilton, but not for most processed cheese (Figure 12-71) or for most cheeses utilized in most commercial chain pizzas (Figure 12-72). Thus, it is not true that a patient on an MAO inhibitor must avoid all ingestion of any cheese. Also, it is not true that such patients must avoid all wine and beer. Canned and bottled beer are low in tyramine; generally only tap and nonpasteurized beers must be avoided (Table 12-8), and many wines, including Chianti, are actually quite low in tyramine (Figure 12-73). Thus, unless someone taking an irreversible inhibitor of MAO-A is going to eat 25 to 100 pieces of pizza or drink 25 to 100 glasses of wine or beer at a party, it is likely that he or she can still have a moderate amount of fun. Of course, every prescriber should counsel patients taking the classic MAO inhibitors about diet and keep up to date with the tyramine content of foods their patients wish to eat.

New developments for MAO inhibitors

Two developments have occurred with MAO inhibitors in recent years that appear to mitigate the risk of tyramine reactions. One is the production of inhibitors that are not only selective for MAO-A but also reversible. The other is the production of an MAO

TABLE 12-8 Hypertensive crisis

Defined by diastolic blood pressure >120 mm Hg
Potentially fatal reaction characterized by:
- Occipital headache which may radiate frontally
- Palpitation
- Neck stiffness or soreness
- Nausea
- Vomiting
- Sweating (sometimes with fever)
- Dilated pupils, photophobia
- Tachycardia or bradycardia, which can be associated with constricting chest pain

Here, the tyramine increases the release of NE (1) and the irreversible MAO-A inhibitor causes the MAO enzyme to stop destroying NE (2). This increase in NE (3) can lead to dangerous elevations of blood pressure.

② MAO-A inhibitor stops the enzyme from destroying NE

alpha 1 receptors

vasoconstriction and hypertension

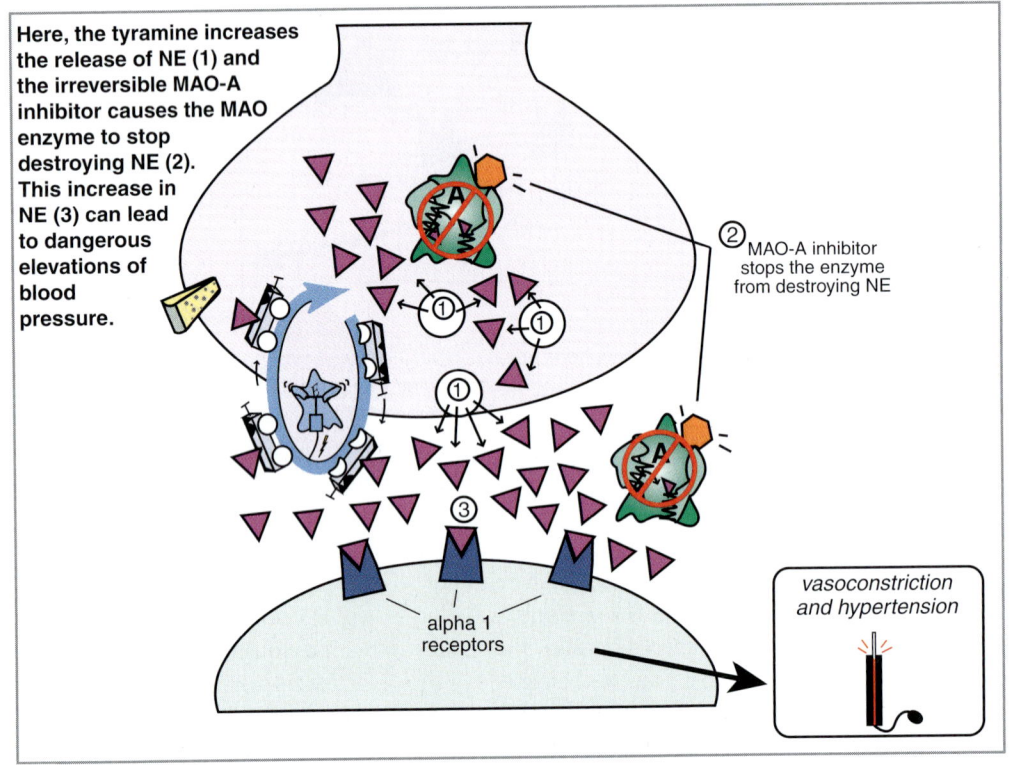

FIGURE 12-70 Inhibition of monoamine oxidase A (MAO-A) and tyramine. Here tyramine is releasing norepinephrine (NE) (1) just as shown in Figure 12-69. However, this time MAO-A is also being inhibited by an irreversible MAO-A inhibitor (2). This results in MAO-A stopping its destruction of NE (2). As indicated in Figure 12-65, such MAO-A inhibition in itself causes accumulation of NE. When MAO-A inhibition is taking place in the presence of tyramine, the combination can lead to a very large accumulation of NE (3). Such a great NE accumulation can lead to excessive stimulation of postsynaptic adrenergic receptors (3) and therefore dangerous vasoconstriction and elevation of blood pressure.

inhibitor that can be delivered through a skin patch such that both MAO-A and MAO-B are inhibited in the brain but much less MAO-A is inhibited in the gut. Neither of these innovations enhances the efficacy of MAO inhibition in depression, but both reduce the risk of hypertensive crisis, which can occur when tyramine is ingested in the diet after MAO-A is inhibited in the gut. One of these innovations is listed in Table 12-4 as moclobemide, a

Tyramine Content of Cheese		
Cheese		**mg per 15 g serving**
English STILTON	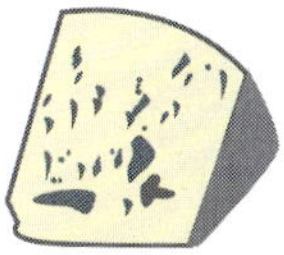	17.3
Kraft ® grated PARMESAN	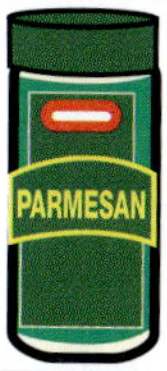	0.2
Philadelphia ® CREAM CHEESE	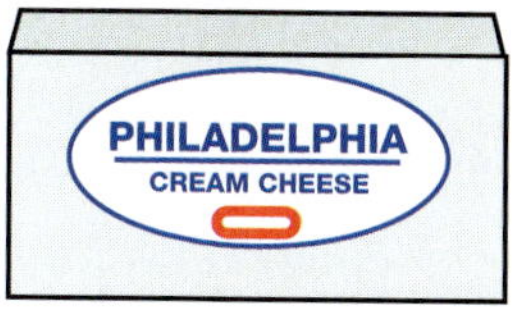	0

FIGURE 12-71 Tyramine content of cheese, part 1. The tyramine content of different types of cheeses varies. Aged cheeses such as English Stilton are high in tyramine; however, most processed cheeses are quite low in tyramine.

selective and reversible inhibitor of MAO-A, sometimes also called a RIMA (or reversible inhibitor of MAO-A). This agent is approved in Canada, Mexico, and many European and other countries but not in the United States.

The other innovation listed in Table 12-4 is the transdermal delivery system for selegiline, cleverly dosed high when delivered to the brain to inhibit both MAO-A and MAO-B there for antidepressant actions yet simultaneously dosed low when delivered to the gut to inhibit, preferentially, MAO-B so as to reduce hypertensive reactions to tyramine. Transdermal selegiline is currently available only in the United States. How it attains this clever differential inhibition of brain versus gut MAO-A is explained below.

RIMAs

The RIMAs are a nifty development in new drug therapeutics for depression because they have the potential of providing MAO-A inhibition yet with decreased risk of a tyramine reaction (Figure 12-74). How can one inhibit MAO-A to have antidepressant actions yet not inhibit MAO-A to avoid tyramine reactions? Enter the reversible inhibitors of MAO-A. If someone taking a RIMA eats aged cheese with high tyramine content in a meal, as the tyramine is absorbed it will release norepinephrine, but this will chase the reversible inhibitor off the MAO-A enzyme, reactivating MAO-A in the intestine, liver, and sympathomimetic neurons and therefore allowing the dangerous amines to be destroyed

Tyramine Content of Commercial-Chain Pizzas

Serving		mg per serving
1/2 medium double cheese, double pepperoni	Domino's Pizza	0.378
1/2 medium double cheese, double pepperoni	Pizza Hut	0.063
1/2 medium double cheese, double pepperoni	pizza pizza	0

FIGURE 12-72 Tyramine content of cheese, part 2. The tyramine content of several commercial chain pizzas is shown here. As can be seen, these types of cheese are actually quite low in tyramine content.

(Figures 12-74 and 12-75). This is sort of like having your cake – or cheese – and eating it too. The RIMAs may thus have the same therapeutic profile as the irreversible inhibitors of MAO, particularly when they are adequately dosed, but without the same likelihood of a cheese reaction if a patient inadvertently eats otherwise dangerous dietary tyramine. However, many regulators in different countries still post a warning about tyramine reactions associated with moclobemide; thus some degree of dietary caution or restriction of tyramine intake is generally still recommended with this drug.

Transdermal delivery of selective MAO-B inhibitor

In the case of selective MAO-B inhibitors administered at low doses, no significant amount of MAO-A is inhibited and there is very little risk of hypertension from dietary amines. Patients taking MAO-B inhibitors to prevent the progression of Parkinson's disease, for example, do not require any special diet. On the other hand, MAO-B inhibitors are not effective antidepressants at doses that are selective for MAO-B. Only when the MAO-B inhibitor selegiline is given orally in doses that make it lose its selectivity and inhibit MAO-A as well is this agent effective orally as an antidepressant. However, these oral doses also cause tyramine reactions.

How can selegiline be administered so that it irreversibly inhibits MAO-A and MAO-B in the brain to provide robust antidepressant actions yet inhibits MAO-B only in the gut to avoid tyramine reactions? The answer is to deliver selegiline by a transdermal patch

Tyramine Content of Wine

Wine		mg per 4 oz serving
Ruffino CHIANTI	CHIANTI RUFFINO	0.36
Blue Nun ® WHITE	BLUE NUN QUALATSWEIN	0.32
Cinzano VERMOUTH	CINZANO	0

FIGURE 12-73 Tyramine content of wine. Although patients taking a monoamine oxidase inhibitor (MAOI) have historically been told to avoid all wine and beer because of the risk of a tyramine reaction, canned and bottled beers as well as many wines are actually low in tyramine.

(Figure 12-76). That is, transdermal administration through a skin patch is like an intravenous infusion without the needle, delivering drug directly into the systemic circulation, hitting the brain in high doses, and avoiding a first pass through the liver (Figure 12-76). By the time drug recirculates to the intestine and liver, it has much decreased levels and significantly inhibits only MAO-B in these tissues. This action is sufficiently robust that, at least for low doses of transdermal selegiline, no dietary restrictions are necessary (Figure 12-77).

To show the profound reduction in risk of tyramine reactions with transdermal selegiline, it is useful to compare how much tyramine it takes to make blood pressure rise when patients take various MAO inhibitors, remembering that a high-tyramine diet is 40 mg of tyramine and that normals can handle around 400 mg of tyramine before blood pressure is increased (Figure 12-77). As stated earlier, perhaps as little as 10 mg of dietary tyramine is all that it takes for a traditional nonselective and irreversible oral MAO inhibitor to cause a tyramine reaction (Figure 12-77, first column). In that case, MAO-A and MAO-B are both inhibited in the brain for antidepressant actions, and they are also both inhibited in the gut, which increases the risk of tyramine reactions.

Contrast this with the patient taking an oral selective MAO-B inhibitor, who has only MAO-B inhibited in the brain and in the gut and can ingest as much tyramine as someone not taking any MAO inhibitor (Figure 12-77, the two far right columns). No tyramine reaction, but also no antidepressant action.

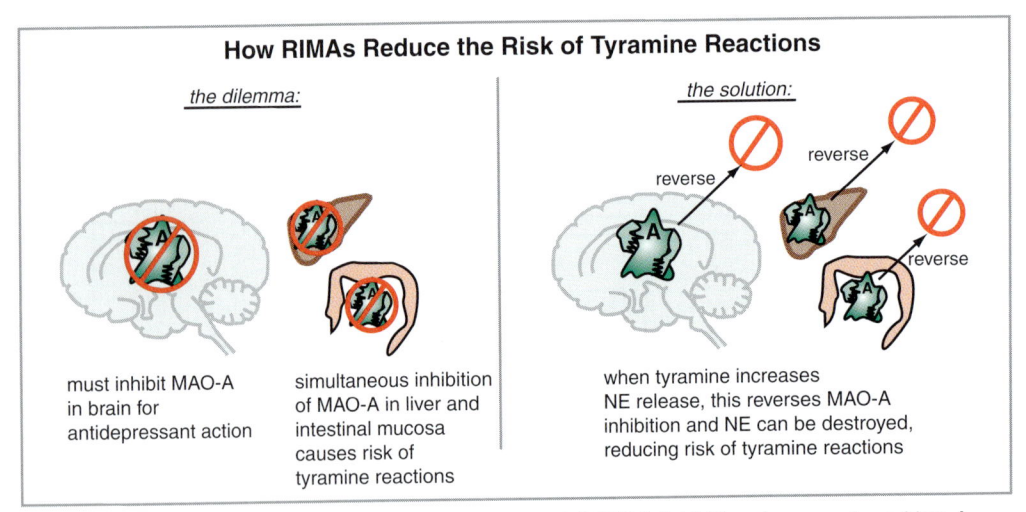

FIGURE 12-74 Reversible inhibitors of monoamine oxidase A (RIMAs). Inhibition of monoamine oxidase A (MAO-A) in the brain is necessary for an antidepressant effect. However, MAO-A is present not only in the brain but also in the gut. Inhibition of MAO-A in the liver and intestinal mucosa poses the risk of a tyramine reaction. How can the effects in the brain be preserved while those in the gut are avoided? Reversible inhibitors of monoamine oxidase A (RIMAs) can be removed from the enzyme by competitors. Thus when tyramine increases norepinephrine (NE) release, it is increasing the competition for MAO-A, which leads to the reversal of MAO-A inhibition; thus NE can be destroyed, reducing risk of a tyramine reaction.

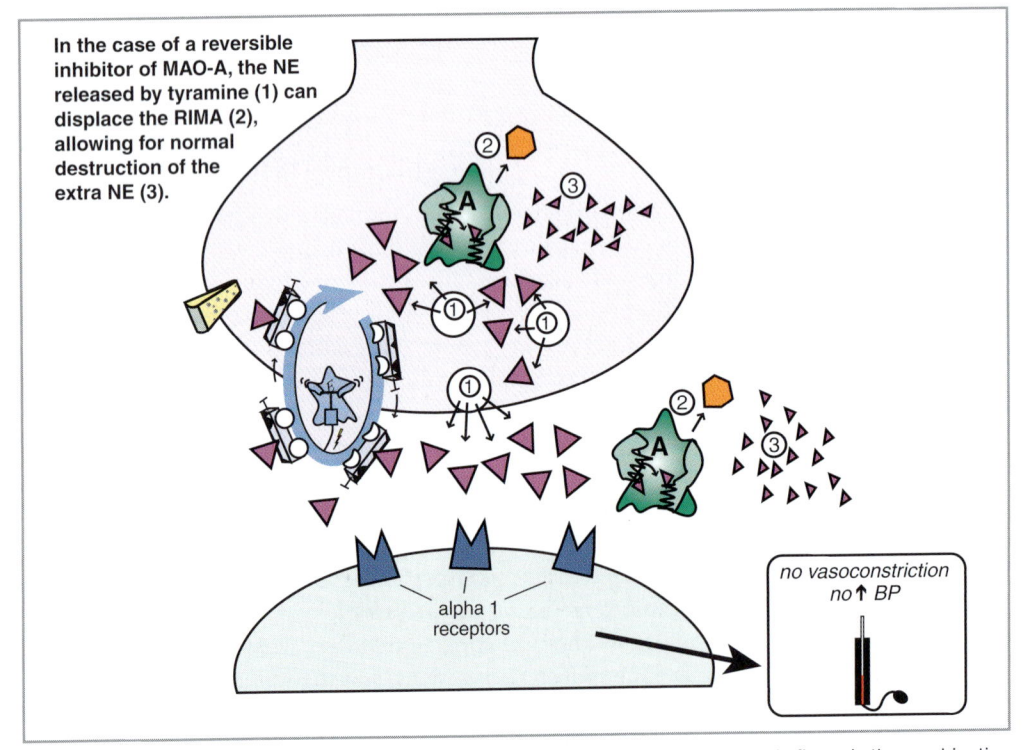

FIGURE 12-75 Reversible inhibition of monoamine oxidase A (MAO-A). Shown in this figure is the combination of an MAO-A inhibitor and tyramine. However, in this case the MAO-A inhibitor is of the reversible type (reversible inhibitor of MAO-A, or RIMA). The accumulation of norepinephrine (NE) released by tyramine (1) can displace the RIMA (2), allowing for normal destruction of the extra NE (3).

How Transdermal Selegiline Reduces the Risk of Tyramine Reactions

the dilemma:

must inhibit MAO-A and MAO-B in brain for antidepressant action

simultaneous inhibition of MAO-A in liver and intestinal mucosa causes risk of tyramine reactions

the solution:

selegiline transdermal patch

high brain delivery

bypasses gut delivery (first pass)

antidepressant actions

no risk of tyramine reactions at low dose

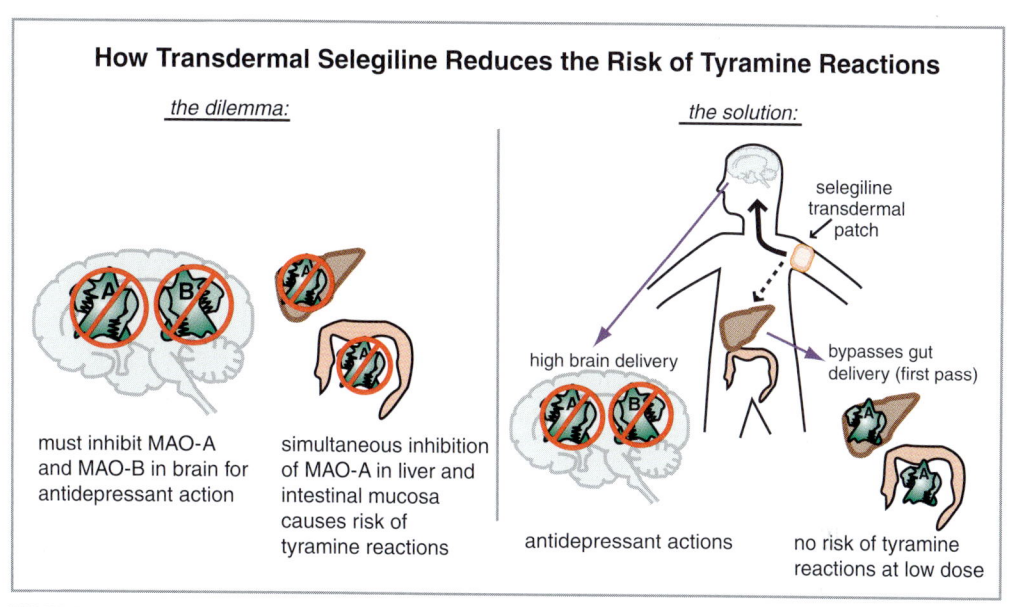

FIGURE 12-76 Transdermal selegiline. The selective monoamine oxidase B (MAO-B) inhibitor selegiline has antidepressant efficacy only when given at doses high enough also to inhibit monoamine oxidase A (MAO-A); yet when it is administered orally at these doses, it can also cause a tyramine reaction. How can selegiline inhibit both MAO-A and MAO-B in the brain to have antidepressant effects while inhibiting MAO-B only in the gut, so as to avoid a tyramine reaction? Transdermal administration of selegiline delivers the drug directly into the systemic circulation, hitting the brain in high doses and thus having antidepressant effects but avoiding a first pass through the liver and thus reducing risk of a tyramine reaction.

What is interesting are the two columns in Figure 12-77 for transdermal selegiline, showing that the average patient can take in much more than 40 mg of tyramine in a meal before showing a hypertensive reaction. At low doses of transdermal selegiline, there is substantial inhibition of both MAO-A and MAO-B in the brain but sufficiently selective inhibition of MAO-B in the gut such that no dietary restrictions are currently warranted. At high doses of transdermal selegiline, there is probably some MAO-A inhibition in the gut, with less tyramine therefore needed to raise blood pressure but still about twice as much as in a high-tyramine meal. Thus, at high doses of transdermally administered selegiline, some dietary caution against very high dietary intake of tyramine may be prudent.

Dangerous drug interactions: decongestants and drugs that boost sympathomimetic amines

Although the MAO inhibitors are famous in any pharmacology textbook for their notorious tyramine reactions, the truth is that drug–drug interactions are potentially more important clinically than dietary interactions because drug interactions are potentially more common, and some drug interactions can be much more dangerous and even lethal. Thus, when drugs that boost adrenergic stimulation by other mechanisms are added to MAO inhibitors that boost adrenergic stimulation by MAO inhibition, dangerous hypertensive reactions can ensue (Table 12-8). These interactions are generally well recognized; but, as for tyramine reactions, a certain mythology has grown up around what drugs can be given safely with MAO inhibitors.

It is true, for example, that many decongestants can adversely interact with MAO inhibitors to elevate blood pressure (Table 12-9 and Figure 12-78). However, that does

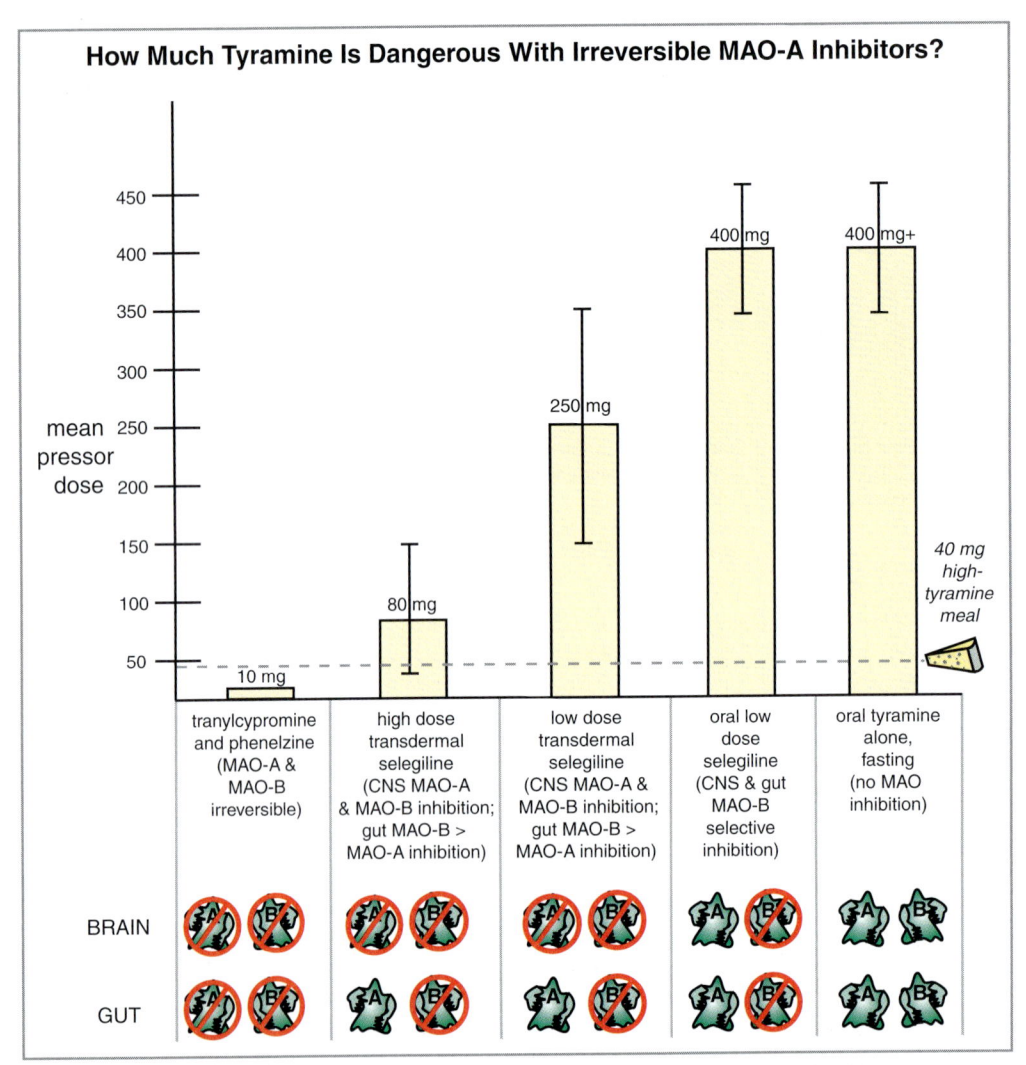

FIGURE 12-77 Dangerous tyramine levels with irreversible monoamine oxidase A (MAO-A) inhibitors. When it contains 40 mg of tyramine, a meal is considered high in this substance; however, in normal individuals (i.e., those not taking an MAO-A inhibitor) it takes as much as 400 mg of tyramine to elevate blood pressure (far right column). Patients taking low dose oral selegiline, which inhibits monoamine oxidase B (MAO-B) only, may ingest as much tyramine as someone not taking any MAO inhibitor; however, they also will not experience antidepressant effects (fourth column). In contrast, patients who take nonselective irreversible MAO inhibitors such as tranylcypromine or phenelzine may be able to ingest as little as 10 mg of tyramine before experiencing a tyramine reaction (first column). These patients experience antidepressant effects but are highly at risk for a tyramine reaction. Transdermal selegiline, on the other hand, inhibits MAO-A and MAO-B in the brain but only MAO-B in the gut; this means that it achieves antidepressant efficacy but is less likely to cause tyramine reactions. Patients taking transdermal selegiline may be able to ingest a high-tyramine meal of 40 mg or more with safety.

not mean that a patient can never take any cold preparation with an MAO inhibitor. What must be avoided are agents that add to the pro-noradrenergic actions of MAO inhibition to stimulate alpha 1 postsynaptic vascular receptors excessively (Figure 12-78). Currently, this applies mostly to phenylephrine, a relatively selective alpha 1 agonist, since three other related agents have been withdrawn from the U.S. and some other

TABLE 12-9 Potentially dangerous hypertensive combos: agents when combined with MAOIs that can cause hypertension (theoretically via adrenergic stimulation)

Decongestants
phenylephrine (alpha 1 selective agonist)
ephedrine* (ma huang, ephedra) (alpha and beta agonist; central NE and DA releaser)
pseudoephedrine* (active stereoisomer of ephedrine – same mechanism as ephedrine)
phenylpropanolamine* (alpha 1 agonist; less effective central NE/DA releaser than ephedrine)

Stimulants
amphetamines
methylphenidate

Antidepressants with NRI
TCAs
NRIs
SNRIs
NDRIs

Appetite suppressants with NRI
sibutramine
phentermine

*withdrawn from markets in the United States and some other countries.

markets – namely ephedrine, pseudoephedrine, and phenylpropanolamine (Table 12-9). Another ingredient in cold preparations that should be avoided is the cough suppressant and opiate derivate dextromethorphan, discussed in more detail in the following section.

Stimulants such as methylphenidate, which potentiate NE at adrenergic synapses by blocking NE reuptake, and amphetamines, which do not only this but also release NE and DA, can elevate blood pressure; in combination with MAO inhibitors, they should either be avoided or used with the utmost caution and monitoring in heroic cases (Table 12-10). Any drugs that block norepinephrine reuptake, from antidepressants to ADHD drugs to appetite suppressants, should also be avoided or utilized only by experts when the risks and benefits are justified in an individual patient who is given adequate monitoring.

The mechanism of excessive noradrenergic stimulation when MAO inhibitors are combined with these various agents mentioned in Table 12-9 is illustrated in Figure 12-78. Specifically, decongestants work by vasoconstricting nasal blood vessels. When topically applied or given in reasonable oral doses, however, they generally do not have sufficient systemic actions to elevate blood pressure by themselves (Figure 12-78A). Nevertheless, in some vulnerable patients, these agents can elevate blood pressure even by themselves. MAO inhibitors given by themselves do potentiate norepinephrine, but this generally is not sufficient to cause hypertension, as shown in Figure 12-78B and as already discussed above. In fact, if anything, MAO inhibitors administered by themselves may be more likely to cause hypotension, especially orthostatic hypotension. The problem comes when the two mechanisms of decongestants and MAO inhibitors are combined, especially in vulnerable patients, in whom the pro-noradrenergic actions of MAO inhibition in concert with the direct stimulation of alpha 1 receptors by an agent such as phenylephrine can result in elevated blood pressure or even a hypertensive crisis (Figure 12-78C).

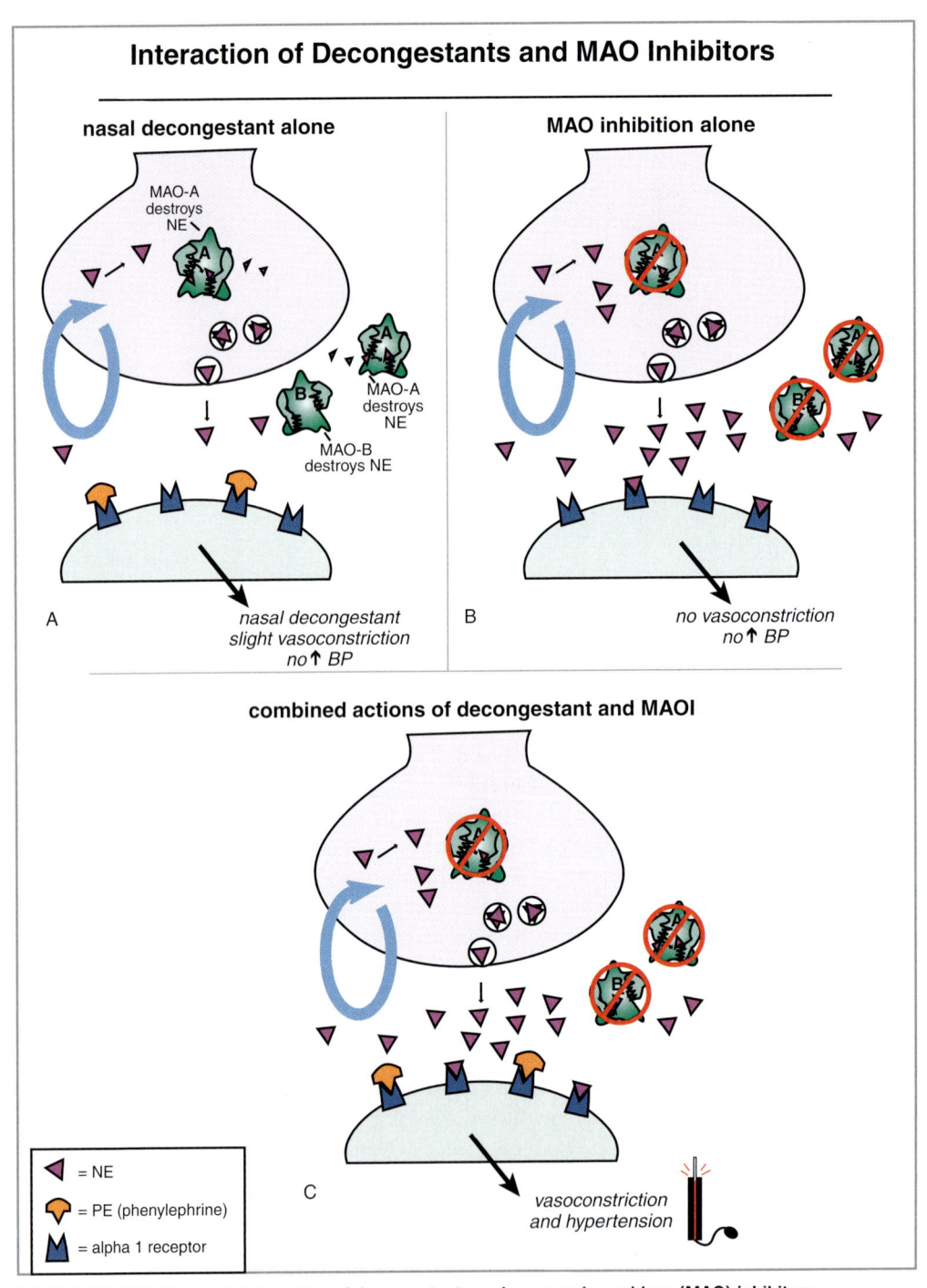

FIGURE 12-78A, B, and C Interaction of decongestants and monoamine oxidase (MAO) inhibitors. Decongestants that stimulate postsynaptic alpha 1 receptors, such as phenylephrine, may interact with MAO inhibitors to increase risk of a tyramine reaction. Decongestants work by constricting nasal blood vessels, but they do not typically elevate blood pressure at the doses used (**A**). An MAO inhibitor given alone (and without the ingestion of tyramine) increases norepinephrine but does not usually cause vasoconstriction or hypertension (**B**). However, the noradrenergic actions of an MAO inhibitor combined with the direct alpha 1 stimulation of a decongestant may be sufficient to cause hypertension or even hypertensive crisis (**C**).

TABLE 12-10 Potentially lethal combos: agents when combined with MAOIs that can cause hyperthermia/serotonin syndrome (theoretically via SERT inhibition)

Antidepressants
SSRIs
SNRIs
TCAs (especially clomipramine)

Other TCA structures
cyclobenzaprine
carbamazepine

Appetite suppressants with SRI
sibutramine

Opioids
dextromethorphan
meperidine
tramadol
methadone
propoxyphene

Dangerous drug interactions: combining MAO inhibition with serotonin reuptake blockade

More dangerous than the combination of adrenergic stimulants with MAO inhibitors may be the combination of agents that inhibit serotonin reuptake with MAO inhibitors. Although experts can sometimes cautiously administer some of the agents listed in Table 12-9 concomitantly with MAO inhibitors under heroic circumstances, one can essentially never combine agents that have potent serotonin reuptake inhibition (listed in Table 12-10) with agents given in doses that cause substantial MAO inhibition. This includes certainly any SSRI (serotonin selective reuptake inhibitor), any SNRI (serotonin norepinephrine reuptake inhibitor, including the appetite suppressant sibutramine), and the tricyclic antidepressant clomipramine (Table 12-10). Occasionally, tricyclics with weak serotonin reuptake inhibition can be combined with MAO inhibitors for heroic cases by experts, but this is rarely done any more because of the presence of many powerful and less dangerous therapeutic options. Opioids that block serotonin reuptake, especially meperidine but also methadone and even propoxyphene, dextromethorphan, and tramadol, especially at high doses, must be avoided when an MAO inhibitor is being given. Coadministration of an MAO inhibitor with an injection of mepiridine may be the drug combination from the lists in Tables 12-9 and 12-10 that most frequently causes serious complications and even death. In fact, any agent with serotonin reuptake blockade has the potential to cause a fatal "serotonin syndrome," noted by hyperthermia, coma, seizures, brain damage, and death. Theoretically, agents with a tricyclic structure such as carbamazepine and cyclobenzaprine are put on this list as a precautionary measure, but they are not known for potent serotonin reuptake blockade (Table 12-10).

The mechanism whereby serotonin reuptake inhibition combined with MAO-A inhibition causes the serotonin syndrome and its complications is illustrated in Figure 12-79. Already discussed extensively and illustrated many times is the serotonin reuptake pump, or serotonin transporter, also known as SERT, and the consequences of SERT inhibition (see Figure 12-79A as well as Figures 4-7 and 4-8, Figure 10-16, and Figure 12-17). We have also discussed the actions of irreversible MAO-A and B inhibitors in increasing synaptic

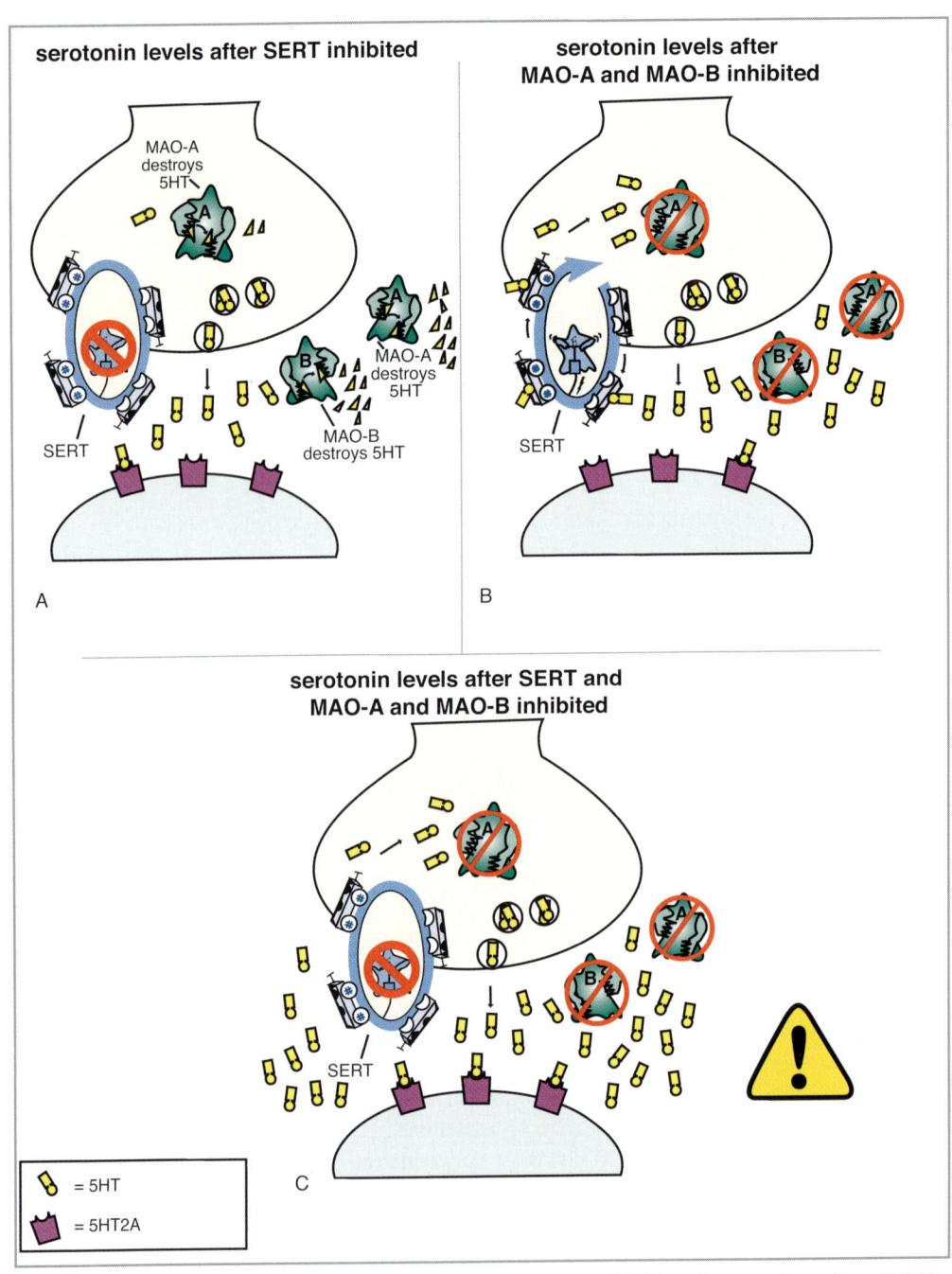

FIGURE 12-79A, B, and C Interaction of serotonin reuptake inhibitors (SRIs) and monoamine oxidase (MAO) inhibitors. Inhibition of the serotonin transporter (SERT) leads to increased synaptic availability of serotonin (**A**). Similarly, inhibition of MAO leads to increased serotonin levels (**B**). These two mechanisms in combination can cause excessive stimulation of postsynaptic serotonin receptors, which may lead to hyperthermia, seizures, coma, cardiovascular collapse, or even death.

TABLE 12-11 Some tricyclic antidepressants still in use

Generic name	Trade name
clomipramine	Anafranil
imipramine	Tofranil
amitriptyline	Elavil, Endep, Tryptizol, Loroxyl
nortriptyline	Pamelor, Endep, Aventyl
protriptyline	Vivactil
maprotiline	Ludiomil
amoxapine	Asendin
doxepin	Sinequan, Adapin
desipramine	Norpramin, Pertofran
trimipramine	Surmontil
dothiepin	Prothiaden
lofrepramine	Deprimyl, Gamanil
tianeptine	Coaxil, Stablon

concentrations of serotonin by the mechanism of MAO inhibition (see Figure 12-79B as well as Figures 12-65 to 12-67). When these two mechanisms are combined, dangerous consequences can ensue (Figure 12-79C).

Theoretically, excessive stimulation of postsynaptic serotonin receptors, possibly the most important of which is the 5HT2A receptor in the hypothalamus, causes, among other things, a disruption in thermoregulation, resulting in dangerous hyperthermia and temperatures $\geq 106°$ F or over $40°$ C. Perhaps because the serotonin neuron has MAO-B (the "wrong" form of MAO for a substrate that is metabolized preferentially by MAO-A), preventing excessive concentrations of serotonin from accumulating may be quite dependent on the serotonin reuptake pump. In contrast, norepinephrine and dopamine neurons are equipped with the "right" form of MAO (namely, MAO-A). Thus, blocking SERT alone elevates 5HT robustly at 5HT neurons, and when the extrasynaptic removal of 5HT by MAO-A is also inhibited, a potentially disastrous accumulation of 5HT can occur. The consequences can range from migraines, myoclonus, diarrhea, agitation, and even psychosis on the milder end of the spectrum of potential symptomatology to hyperthermia, seizures, coma, cardiovascular collapse, permanent hyperthermic brain damage, and even death at the severe end of the spectrum of symptoms. For this reason, it is important to monitor closely all concomitant medication for patients on MAO inhibitors, even in patients taking the new RIMAs or the selegiline patch, where these drug interactions also apply.

Classic antidepressants: tricyclic antidepressants

The tricyclic antidepressants (Table 12-11) were so named because their chemical structure contains three rings (Figure 12-80). The tricyclic antidepressants were synthesized about the same time as other three-ringed molecules that were shown to be effective tranquilizers for schizophrenia (i.e., the early antipsychotic neuroleptic drugs such as chlorpromazine) (Figure 12-80). The tricyclic antidepressants were a disappointment when tested as antipsychotics. Even though they had a three-ringed structure, they were not effective in the treatment of schizophrenia and were almost discarded. However, during testing for schizophrenia, they were discovered to be antidepressants. That is, careful clinicians detected

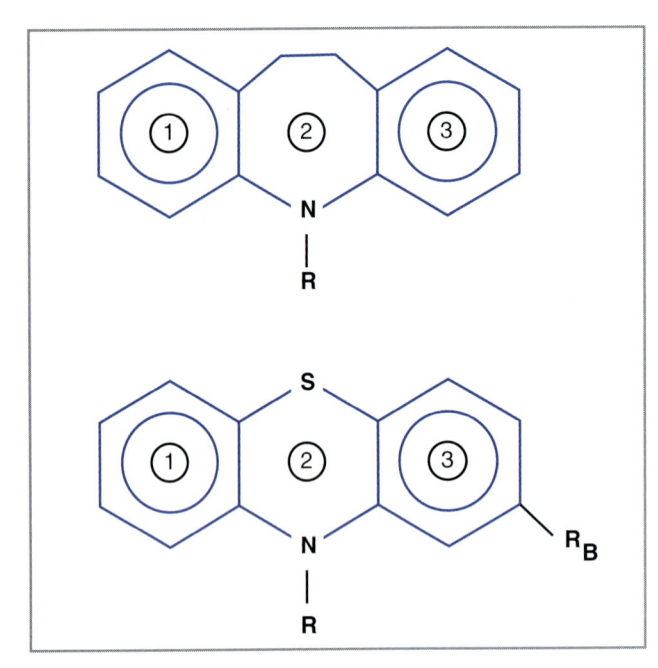

FIGURE 12-80 Tricyclic structure. At top is the chemical structure of a tricyclic antidepressant (TCA). The three rings show how this group of drugs got its name. At bottom is the general chemical formula for the phenothiazine antipsychotic drugs. These drugs also have three rings, and the first antidepressants – the TCAs – were modeled after such drugs.

antidepressant properties in schizophrenic patients, although not antipsychotic properties in these patients. Thus, the antidepressant properties of the tricyclic antidepressants were serendipitously observed in the 1950s and 1960s and eventually the TCAs were marketed for the treatment of depression.

Long after their antidepressant properties were observed, the tricyclic antidepressants were discovered to block the reuptake pumps for norepinephrine or for both norepinephrine and serotonin (Figures 5-16, 6-5, 6-6, 12-81, 12-82, and 12-83). Some tricyclics have much more potency for inhibition of the serotonin reuptake pump (e.g., clomipramine) (Figures 12-81A and 12-82); others are more selective for norepinephrine over serotonin (e.g., desipramine, maprotiline, nortriptyline, protriptyline) (Figures 12-81B and 12-83). Most, however, block both serotonin and norepinephrine reuptake to some extent. The molecular action of monoamine transporters was discussed in detail in Chapter 4 and illustrated in Figures 4-4 through 4-8.

In addition, some tricyclic antidepressants have antagonist actions at 5HT2A and 5HT2C receptors. Although these properties have not been emphasized in classic explanations of the mechanism of action of these drugs, recent developments showing the importance of blocking 5HT2A and 5HT2C receptors in mediating the mechanism of therapeutic action of other drugs strongly suggest that these properties could contribute to the therapeutic profile of those tricyclics that have such pharmacologic actions (Figures 12-84 and 12-85). Specifically, blocking 5HT2A receptors is associated with improvement of sleep and has a potential antidepressant action in its own right (Figure 12-84), possibly linked to the ability of 5HT2A/5HT2C receptor blockade to disinhibit both DA and NE release. This was discussed extensively above in relation to SARI action and trazodone and illustrated in Figure 12-64.

The major limitation to the tricyclic antidepressants has never been their efficacy: these are quite efficacious agents. The problem with drugs in this class is the fact that all of them share at least four other unwanted pharmacological actions shown in Figure 12-81, namely,

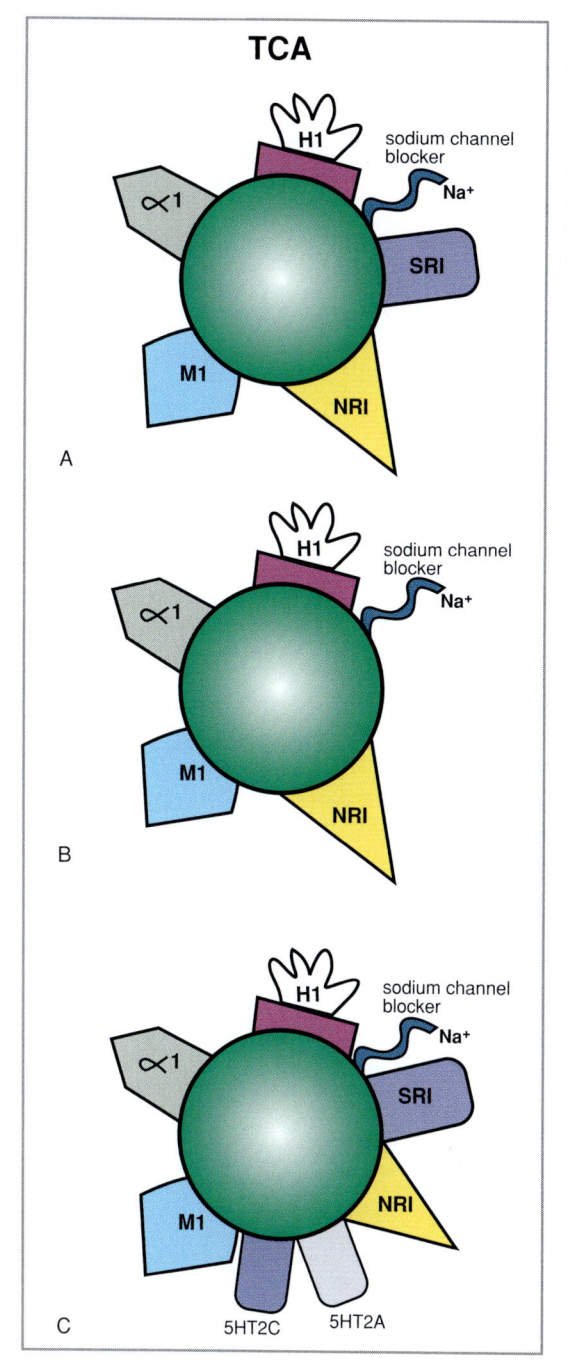

FIGURE 12-81 Icons of tricyclic antidepressants. All tricyclic antidepressants block reuptake of norepinephrine and are antagonists at histamine 1, alpha 1 adrenergic, and muscarinic cholinergic receptors; they also block voltage-sensitive sodium channels (**A, B, and C**). Some tricyclic antidepressants are also potent inhibitors of the serotonin reuptake pump (**A**), and some may additionally be antagonists at serotonin 2A and 2C receptors (**C**).

blockade of muscarinic cholinergic receptors, histamine 1 receptors, alpha 1 adrenergic receptors, and voltage-sensitive sodium channels (see Figures 12-86 through 12-88).

Blockade of histamine 1 receptors, also called antihistaminic action, causes sedation and may cause weight gain (Figure 12-86). Blockade of M1 muscarinic cholinergic receptors, also known as anticholinergic actions, causes dry mouth, blurred vision, urinary retention,

Antidepressants | 599

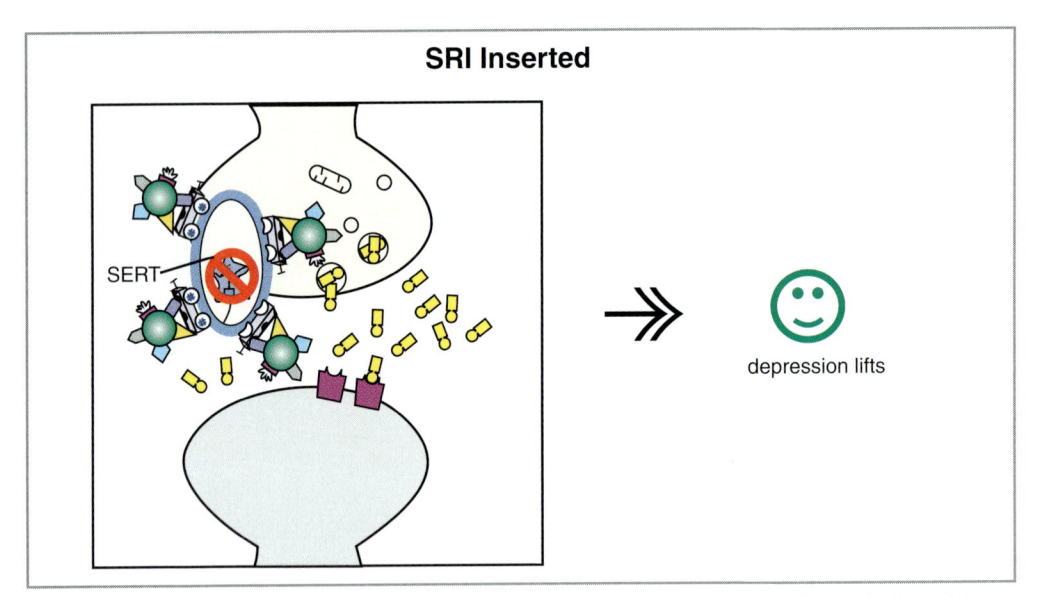

FIGURE 12-82 Therapeutic actions of tricyclic antidepressants (TCAs), part 1. In this figure, the icon of the TCA is shown with its serotonin reuptake inhibitor (SRI) portion inserted into the serotonin transporter (SERT), blocking it and causing an antidepressant effect.

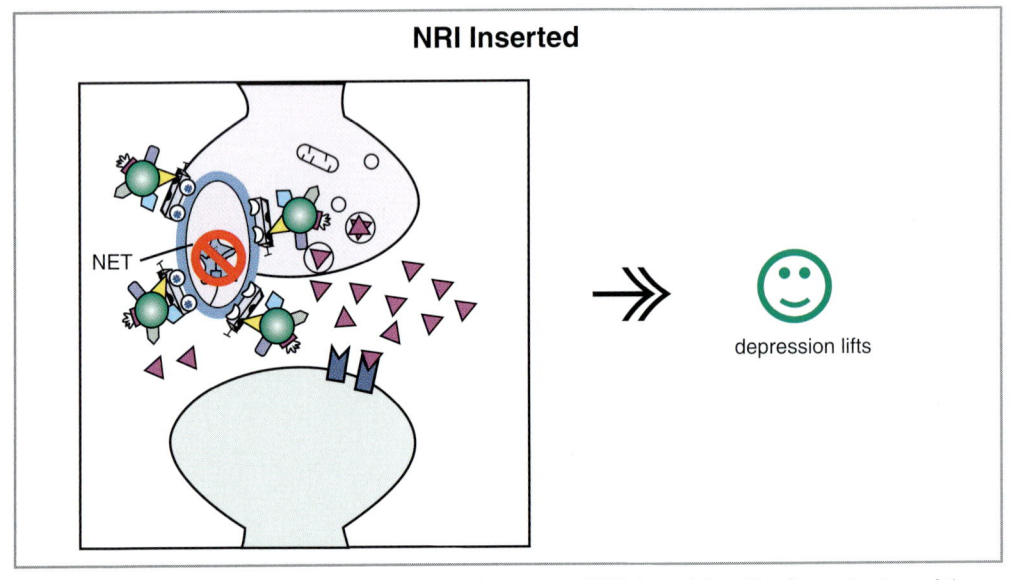

FIGURE 12-83 Therapeutic actions of tricyclic antidepressants (TCAs), part 2. In this figure, the icon of the TCA is shown with its norepinephrine reuptake inhibitor (NRI) portion inserted into the norepinephrine transporter (NET), blocking it and causing an antidepressant effect. Thus both the serotonin reuptake portion (see Figure 12-82) and the norepinephrine reuptake portion of the TCA act pharmacologically to cause an antidepressant effect.

and constipation (Figure 12-87). To the extent that these agents can block M3 cholinergic receptors, they may interfere with insulin action, as discussed in Chapter 10 and illustrated in Figure 10-64. Blockade of alpha 1 adrenergic receptors causes orthostatic hypotension and dizziness (Figure 12-88). Tricyclic antidepressants also weakly block voltage-sensitive sodium channels in the heart and brain; in overdose, this action is thought to be the cause

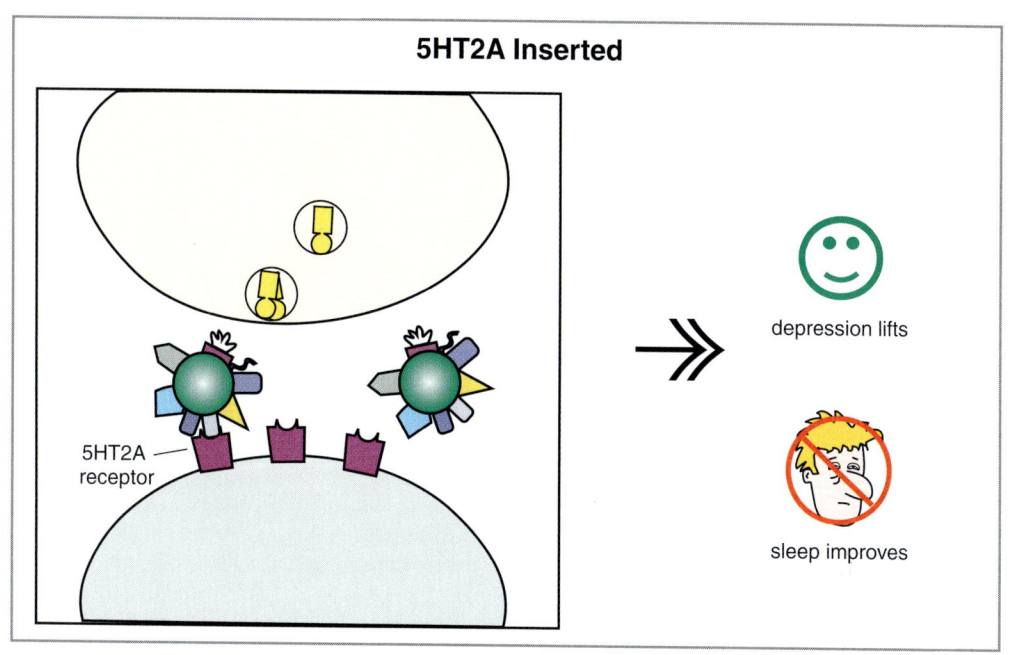

FIGURE 12-84 Therapeutic actions of tricyclic antidepressants (TCAs), part 3. In this figure, the icon of the TCA is shown with its 5HT2A portion inserted into the 5HT2A receptor, blocking it and causing an antidepressant effect as well as potentially improving sleep.

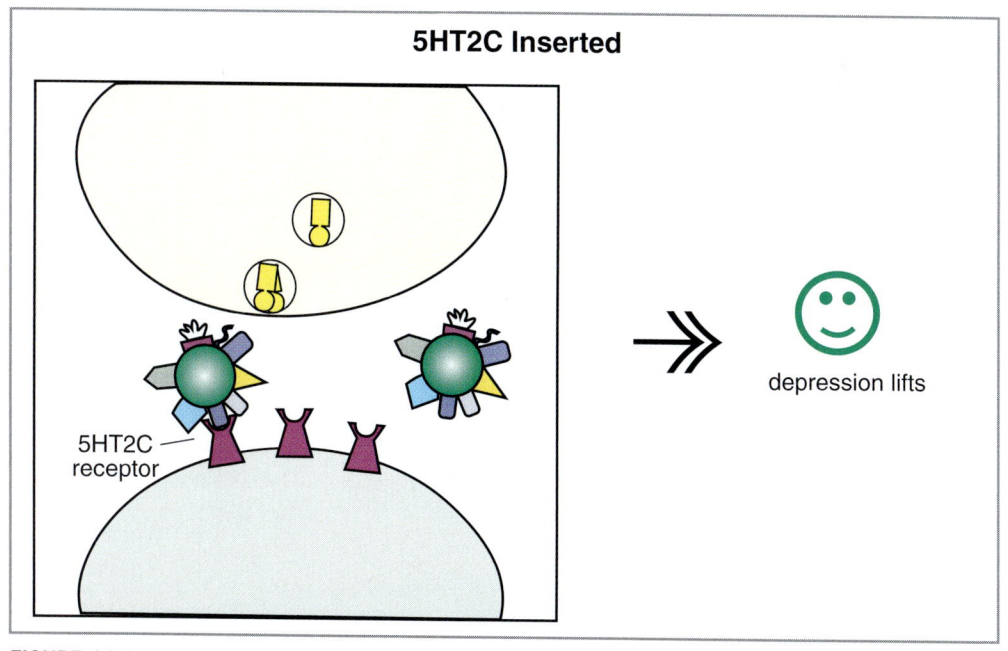

FIGURE 12-85 Therapeutic actions of tricyclic antidepressants (TCAs), part 4. In this figure, the icon of the TCA is shown with its 5HT2C portion inserted into the 5HT2C receptor, blocking it and causing an antidepressant effect.

Antidepressants | 601

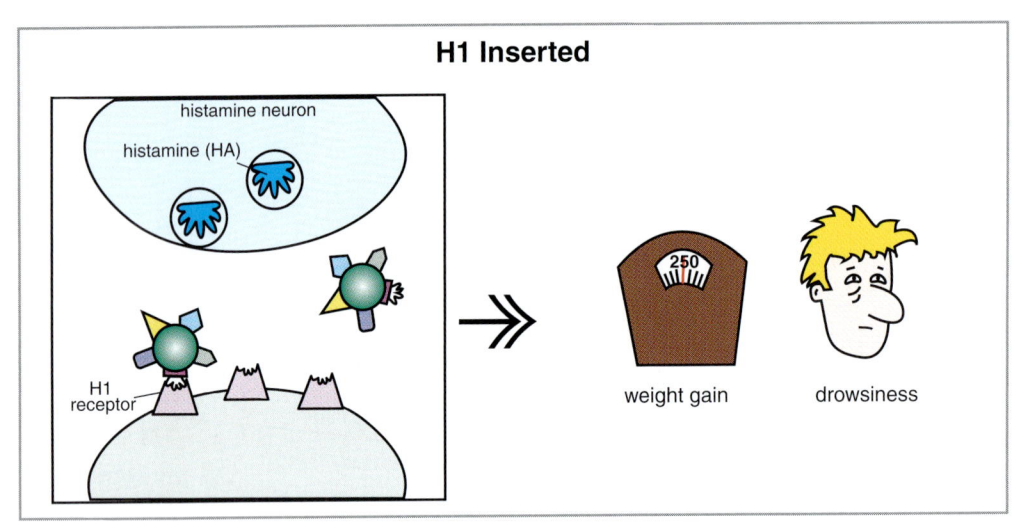

FIGURE 12-86 Side effects of tricyclic antidepressants (TCAs), part 1. In this figure, the icon of the TCA is shown with its antihistamine (H1) portion inserted into histamine receptors, causing the side effects of weight gain and drowsiness.

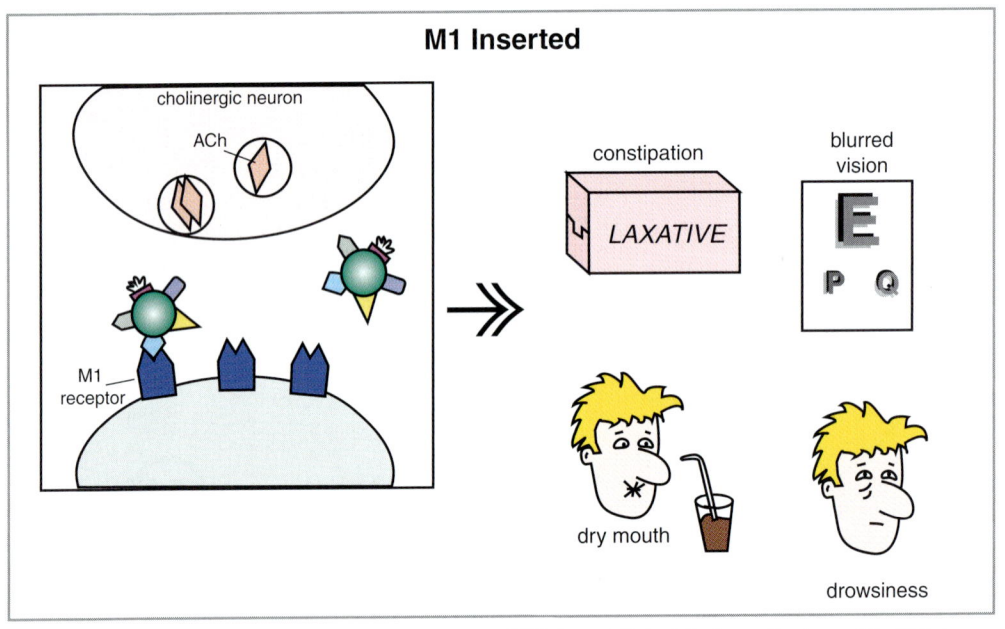

FIGURE 12-87 Side effects of tricyclic antidepressants (TCAs), part 2. In this figure, the icon of the TCA is shown with its anticholinergic/antimuscarinic (M1) portion inserted into acetylcholine receptors, causing the side effects of constipation, blurred vision, dry mouth, and drowsiness.

of coma and seizures due to central nervous system (CNS) actions as well as cardiac arrhythmias and cardiac arrest and death due to peripheral cardiac actions (Figure 12-89).

The term "tricyclic antidepressant" is archaic in today's pharmacology. First, the antidepressants that block monoamine transporters are not all tricyclic anymore: the new agents can have one, two, three, or four rings in their structures. Second, the tricyclic antidepressants are not merely antidepressants, since some of them have anti–obsessive compulsive

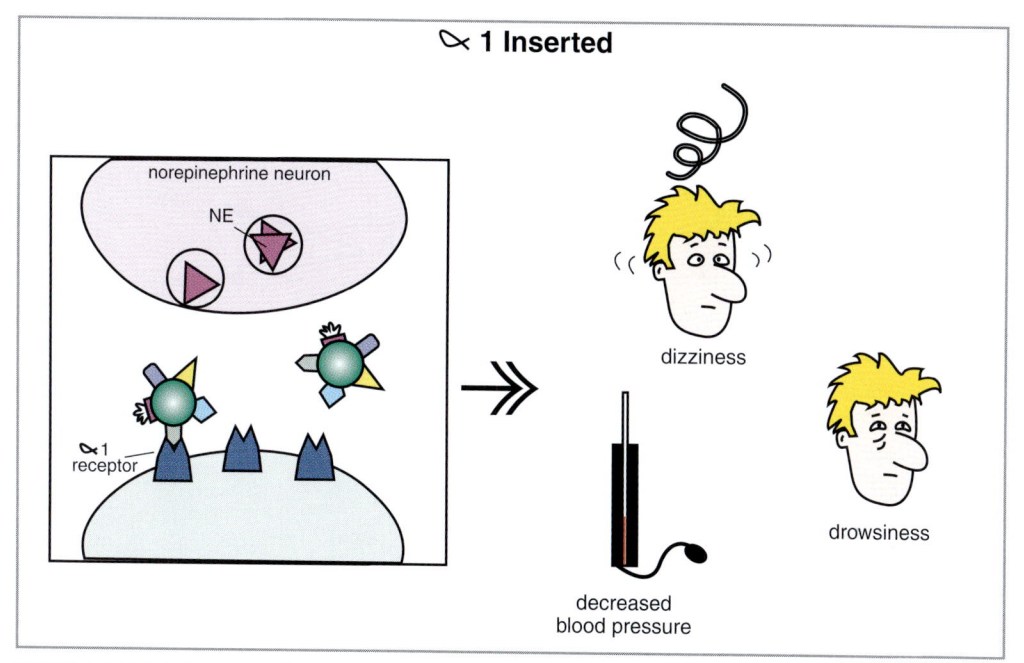

FIGURE 12-88 Side effects of tricyclic antidepressants (TCAs), part 3. In this figure, the icon of the TCA is shown with its alpha-adrenergic antagonist (alpha) portion inserted into alpha 1 adrenergic receptors, causing the side effects of dizziness, drowsiness, and decreased blood pressure.

disorder effects and others have anti-panic effects (as discussed in Chapter 14, on anxiety). Because of their side effects and potential for death in overdose, tricyclic antidepressants have fallen into second-line use for depression. However, there remains considerable use of these agents for difficult-to-treat patients, and the cost of these agents is quite low.

Antidepressant pharmacokinetics

The CYP450 enzymes and the **pharmacokinetic** actions they represent must be contrasted with the **pharmacodynamic** actions of antidepressants discussed in the previous sections of this chapter, focusing on the various mechanisms of action of antidepressants. Although most of this book deals with the **pharmacodynamics** of psychopharmacological agents, especially how drugs act on the brain, the following section provides a quick overview of the **pharmacokinetics** of antidepressants. Some of the general principles of pharmacokinetics are discussed in Chapter 10 and illustrated in Figures 10-78 through 10-80; specific issues of antipsychotic pharmacokinetics are illustrated in Figures 10-81 through 10-89.

CYP450 1A2

One CYP450 enzyme of specific relevance to antidepressants is 1A2 (Figures 12-90, 12-91, and 12-92). Certain tricyclic antidepressants (TCAs) are **substrates** for this enzyme, especially the secondary amines like clomipramine and imipramine (Figure 12-90). CYP450 1A2 demethylates such TCAs but does not thereby inactivate them. In this case, the desmethyl metabolite of the TCA is still an active drug (e.g., desmethylclomipramine, desipramine, and nortriptyline; see Figure 12-90).

CYP450 1A2 is **inhibited** by the serotonin selective reuptake inhibitor (SSRI) fluvoxamine (Figure 12-91). Thus, when fluvoxamine is given concomitantly with other drugs

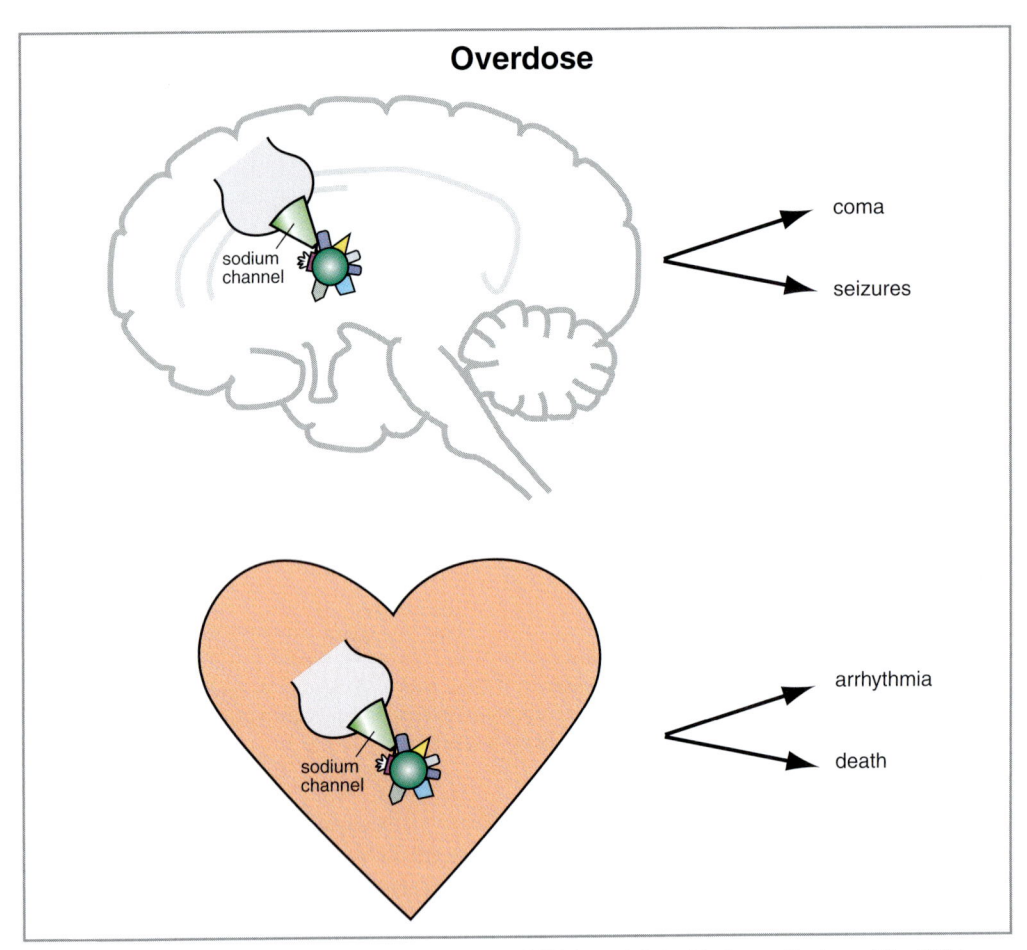

FIGURE 12-89 Side effects of tricyclic antidepressants (TCAs), part 4. In this figure, the icon of the TCA is shown with its sodium channel blocker portion blocking voltage-sensitive sodium channels in the brain (top) and heart (bottom). In overdose, this action can lead to coma, seizures, arrhythmia, and even death.

that use 1A2 for their metabolism, those drugs can no longer be metabolized as efficiently. Two instances of potentially important drug interactions are seen when fluvoxamine is given along with either duloxetine or theophyllin (Figure 12-92). In those cases, the duloxetine (or theophyllin) dose must often be lowered or else the blood levels of drug will rise and possibly cause side effects or even be toxic. The same may occur with caffeine.

CYP450 2D6

Another important CYP450 enzyme for antidepressants is 2D6. Tricyclic antidepressants are **substrates** of 2D6, which hydroxylates and thereby inactivates the TCAs. Several other antidepressants from the SSRI class are substrates of CYP2D6, and some are both substrates and inhibitors. We have already discussed venlafaxine as an important substrate of CYP2D6, as this antidepressant is converted into its active metabolite desvenlafaxine by CYP2D6, as shown in Figure 12-37. Most antidepressants that are substrates for CYP2D6, however, are converted into inactive metabolites, (e.g., the metabolites of duloxetine, paroxetine, atomoxetine, and tricyclic antidepressants are inactive) (Figure 12-93). There is a wide range of potency for 2D6 inhibition by many antidepressants, with paroxetine, fluoxetine,

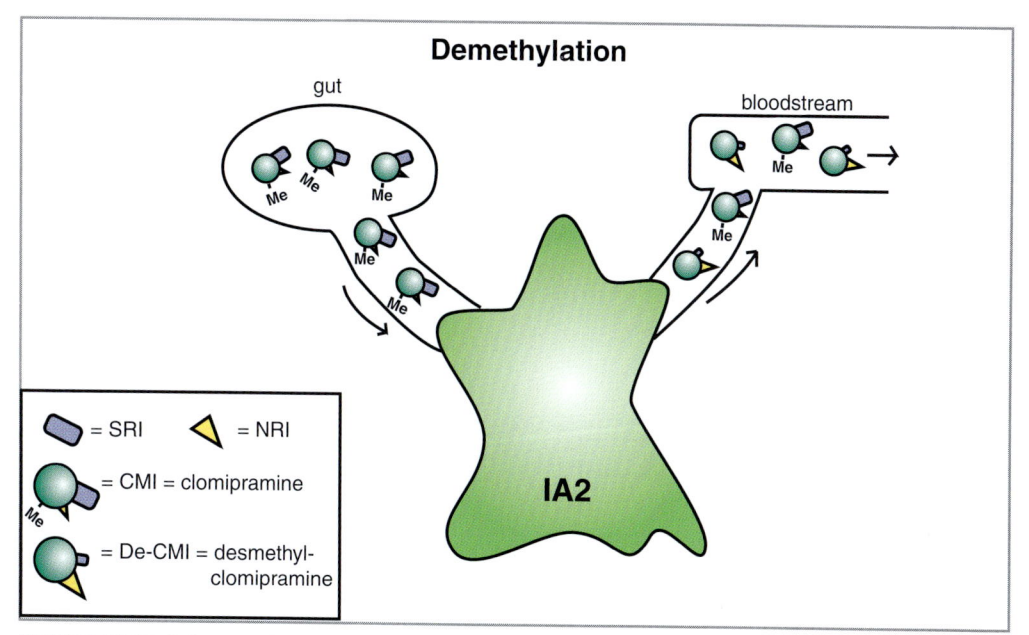

FIGURE 12-90 Substrates for CYP450 1A2. Certain tricyclic antidepressants, especially secondary amines such as clomipramine and imipramine, are substrates for CYP450 1A2. By demethylation, this enzyme converts the tricyclics into active metabolites to form desmethylclomipramine and desipramine, respectively.

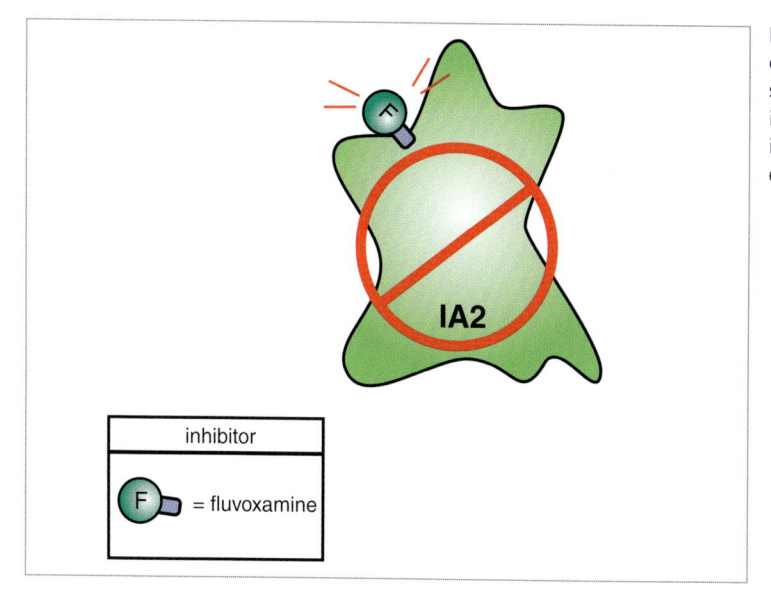

FIGURE 12-91 Inhibitors of CYP450 1A2. The serotonin selective reuptake inhibitor (SSRI) fluvoxamine is a potent inhibitor of the enzyme CYP450 1A2.

and duloxetine among the more potent inhibitors and reboxetine, bupropion, fluvoxamine, sertraline, and citalopram among those that are less potent (Figure 12-94).

One of the most important drug interactions that antidepressants can cause through inhibition of 2D6 is to raise plasma drug levels of tricyclic antidepressants (TCAs) when TCAs are given concomitantly with SSRIs or when there is switching between TCAs and SSRIs. Since TCAs are substrates for 2D6 and various antidepressants are inhibitors of

Antidepressants | 605

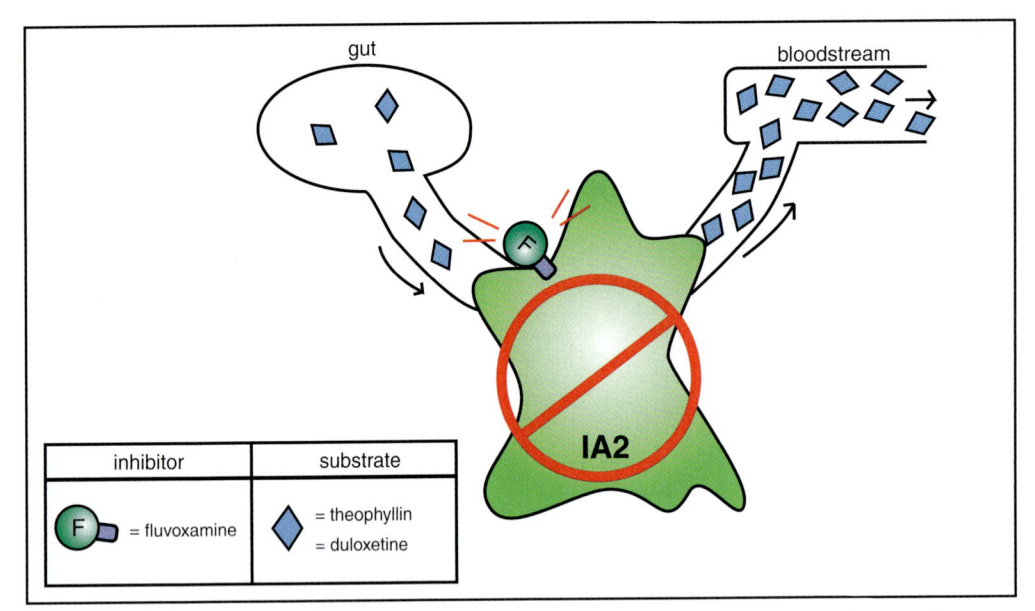

FIGURE 12-92 Consequences of CYP450 1A2 inhibition. Theophylline and duloxetine are substrates for CYP450 1A2. Thus, in the presence of the CYP450 1A2 inhibitor fluvoxamine, their levels will rise; therefore their dose must often be lowered in order to avoid side effects.

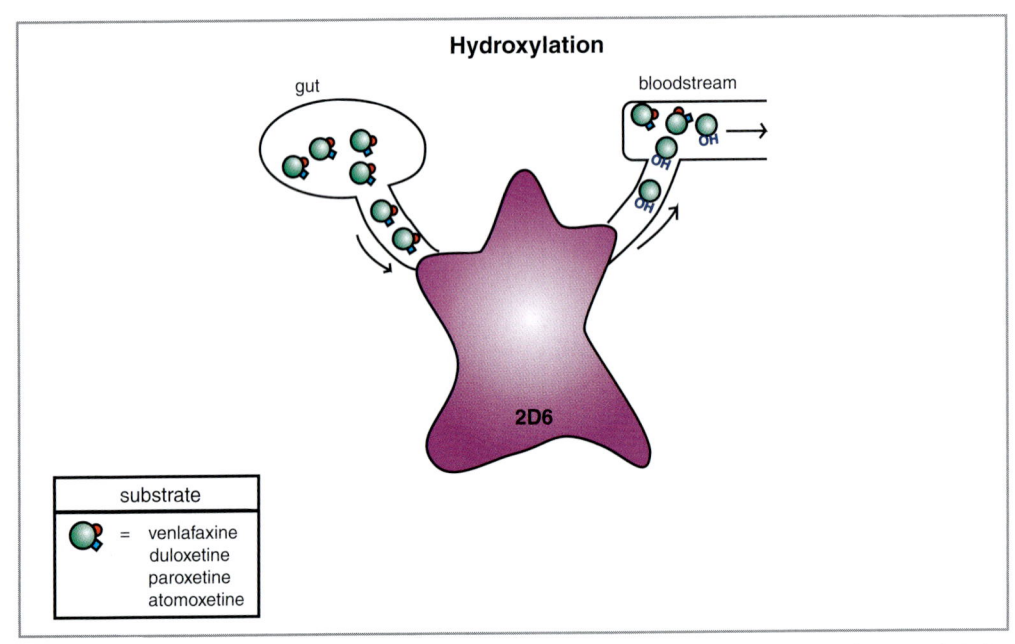

FIGURE 12-93 Substrates for CYP450 2D6. Venlafaxine, duloxetine, paroxetine, and atomoxetine are substrates for CYP450 2D6, which converts these antidepressants to active (desvenlafaxine) or inactive metabolites.

2D6 (Figure 12-94), concomitant administration will raise TCA levels, perhaps to toxic levels (Figure 12-95). Concomitant administration of an SSRI and a TCA thus requires monitoring of the plasma drug concentrations of the TCA and probably requires a dose reduction of the TCA.

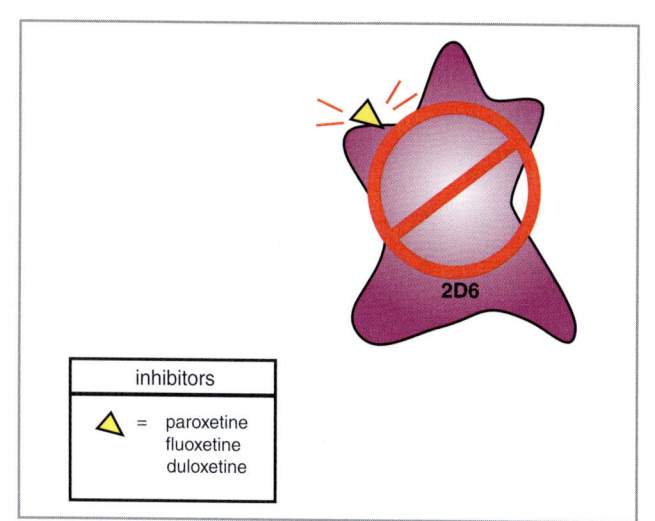

FIGURE 12-94 Inhibitors of CYP450 2D6. Some antidepressants (paroxetine, fluoxetine, duloxetine) are inhibitors of CYP450 2D6.

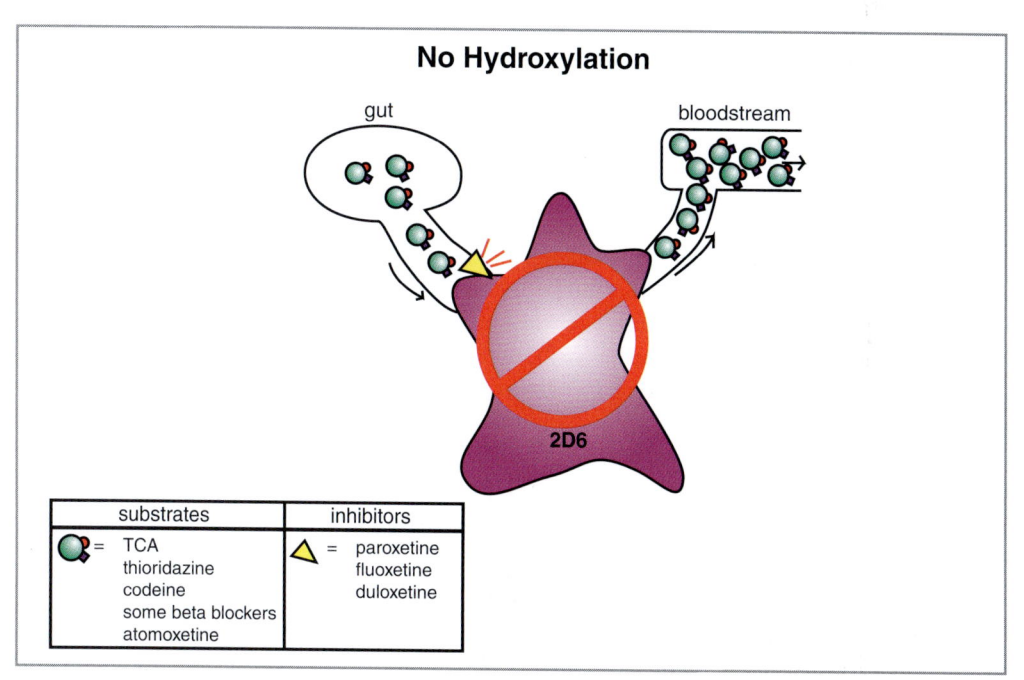

FIGURE 12-95 Consequences of CYP450 2D6 inhibition. If a tricyclic antidepressant (a substrate for CYP450 2D6) is given concomitantly with a serotonin selective reuptake inhibitor or a serotonin norepinephrine reuptake inhibitor that is an inhibitor of CYP450 2D6, this will cause the levels of the tricyclic antidepressant to increase, which can be toxic. Therefore either monitoring of tricyclic plasma concentration with dose reduction or avoidance of this combination is required.

Other substrates of 2D6 whose plasma drug levels can be raised by antidepressants that are 2D6 inhibitors include venlafaxine, duloxetine, paroxetine, and atomoxetine; however, clinical experience suggests that only atomoxetine commonly requires dosage reduction when administered with a 2D6 inhibitor. These interactions among antidepressants are important to bear in mind for prescribers who commonly use one antidepressant to augment

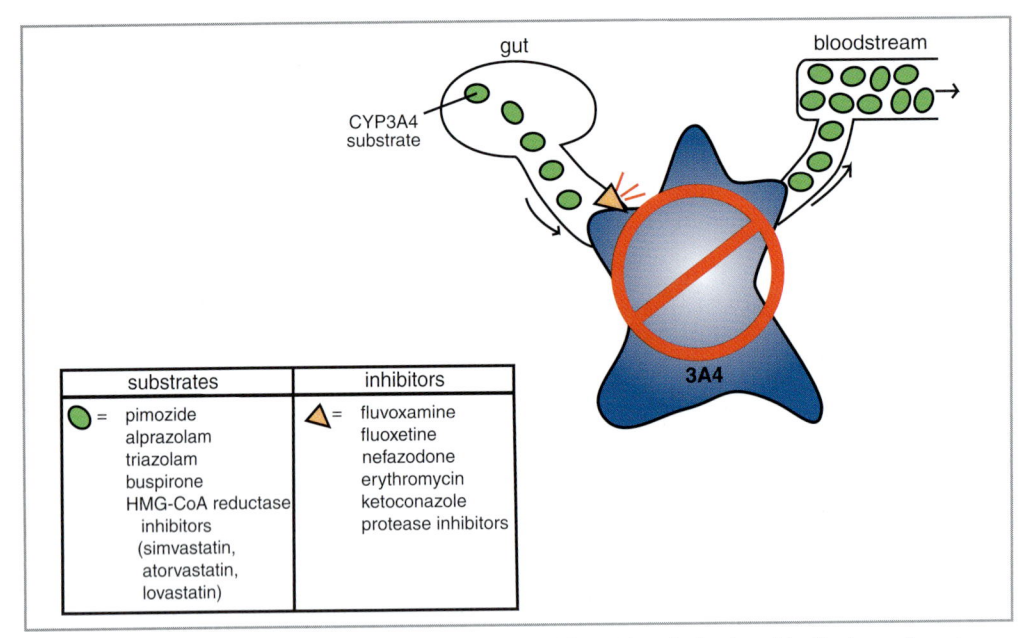

FIGURE 12-96 **Substrates and inhibitors for CYP450 3A4.** The antipsychotic pimozide, the benzodiazepines alprazolam and triazolam, the anxiolytic buspirone, and HMG-CoA reductase inhibitors are all substrates for CYP450 3A4. Fluvoxamine, fluoxetine, and nefazodone are moderate CYP450 3A4 inhibitors, as are some nonpsychotropic agents.

another or who switch patients from one antidepressant to another without a full washout of the first antidepressant. Concomitant administration of an antidepressant that is a 2D6 inhibitor could theoretically interfere with the analgesic actions of codeine (which must be converted to an active metabolite by 2D6 in order to work) and could theoretically raise the plasma drug levels of some beta blockers, as well as thioridazine, and cause dangerous arrhythmias.

CYP450 3A4

A third important CYP450 enzyme for antidepressants is 3A4 (Figure 12-96). Some antidepressants are substrates for 3A4 and others are inhibitors of this enzyme. Many drugs, including some antidepressants that are substrates for 3A4, are also substrates for several other metabolic pathways; in these cases, inhibition of 3A4 does not necessarily raise the plasma drug levels of such agents. Generally, the most important thing for a clinician to know is which drugs can have clinically important increases in their plasma drug levels when 3A4 is inhibited. It is thus important to know which of these drugs are substrates and which are inhibitors of 3A4.

Among psychotropic drugs, the antipsychotic pimozide, the anticonvulsant and mood stabilizer carbamazepine, the benzodiazepines alprazolam and triazolam, and the anxiolytic buspirone are all **substrates** of 3A4 (Figure 12-96). Among nonpsychotropic drugs, certain cholesterol-lowering HMG-CoA reductase inhibitors (e.g., simvastatin, atorvastatin, and lovastatin but not pravastatin or fluvastatin) are also **substrates** for 3A4 (Figure 12-96).

Among the antidepressants, fluvoxamine, fluoxetine, and nefazodone are moderately potent 3A4 **inhibitors**, with reboxetine and sertraline weaker 3A4 **inhibitors**

(Figure 12-96). Among nonpsychotropic drugs, certain protease inhibitors for the treatment of human immunodeficiency virus (HIV) infection, certain azole antifungals (e.g., ketoconazole), and macrolide antibiotics (e.g., erythromycin) are all potent 3A4 **inhibitors** (Figure 12-96).

Clinically important consequences of combining 3A4 substrates with 3A4 inhibitors

Combining a 3A4 inhibitor with the 3A4 substrate pimozide can result in elevated plasma pimozide levels, with consequent QTc prolongation and dangerous cardiac arrhythmias. Combining a 3A4 inhibitor with carbamazepine, alprazolam, or triazolam can cause significant sedation due to elevated plasma drug levels of the latter agents. Combining a 3A4 inhibitor with certain cholesterol-lowering drugs that are 3A4 substrates (e.g., simvastatin, atorvastatin, and lovastatin but not pravastatin or fluvastatin) can increase the risk of muscle damage and rhabdomyolysis from elevated plasma levels of these statins.

Drug interactions mediated by CYP450 enzymes are constantly being discovered; the active clinician who combines drugs must be alert to these and thus remain continually up to speed on what drug interactions are important. Here we present only the general concepts of drug interactions at CYP450 enzyme systems, but the specifics should be found in a comprehensive and up-to-date reference source before prescribing.

CYP450 inducers

Finally, drugs can not only be substrates or inhibitors for CYP450 enzymes; they can also be **inducers**. An inducer increases the activity of the enzyme over time because it induces the synthesis of more copies of the enzyme. One example of this is the effects of the anticonvulsant and mood stabilizer carbamazepine, which induces 3A4 over time (discussed in Chapter 10 and illustrated in Figure 10-88). Another example of CYP450 enzyme induction is cigarette smoking, which induces 1A2 over time (discussed in Chapter 10 and illustrated in Figure 10-82). The consequence of such enzyme induction is that substrates for the induced enzyme will be more efficiently metabolized over time, and thus their levels in the plasma will fall. Doses of such substrate drugs may therefore need to be increased over time to compensate for this.

For example, carbamazepine is both a substrate and an inducer of 3A4. Thus, as treatment becomes chronic, 3A4 is induced and carbamazepine blood levels fall (Figures 10-88 and 10-89). Failure to recognize this and to increase carbamazepine dosage to compensate may lead to a failure of anticonvulsant or mood stabilizing efficacy, with breakthrough symptoms occurring as a result.

Another important thing to remember about a CYP450 inducer is what happens if the inducer is stopped. Thus, if one stops smoking, levels of drugs that are 1A2 substrates will rise. If one stops carbamazepine, levels of drugs that are 3A4 substrates will rise.

In summary, many antidepressant drug interactions require dosage adjustment of one of the drugs. A few combinations must be strictly avoided. Many drug interactions are statistically but not clinically significant. By following the principles outlined here, the skilled practitioner will learn whether any given drug interaction is clinically relevant.

Trimonoaminergic modulators (triple monoamine modulators, or TMMs)

An increasing number of agents now appear to modulate the trimonoaminergic neurotransmitter system of 5HT, NE, and DA by mechanisms other than inhibition of monoamine transporters and in a manner that may be more effective when given with a monoamine

TABLE 12-12 Trimonoamine modulators (TMMs)

- folate
- L-MTHF (L-methyl-tetrahydrofolate)
- estrogen
- estrogen replacement therapy
- thyroid hormones (T3/T4)
- lithium
- brain stimulation
- psychotherapy

transport inhibitor rather than as a monotherapy (Tables 12-2 and 12-12). These therapeutic interventions range from hormones to vitamins, medical foods, ions, electrical and magnetic brain stimulation, and even psychotherapy (Table 12-12). A few of these key therapeutics are reviewed here very briefly to provide a quick overview of this evolving concept. All are categorized as "trimonoaminergic modulators," or TMMs (Tables 12-2 and 12-12), because their various mechanisms of action are all postulated to share in common the modulation of one or more of the monoamines. Thus, TMMs theoretically boost the action of antidepressants in the treatment of depressive episodes, particularly when given as augmenting agents for the treatment of depressive episodes that fail to remit with traditional antidepressant treatment.

Estrogen as a trimonoaminergic, GABA, and glutamate modulator

The hormone estrogen has a profound impact on mood and on the trimonoamine neurotransmitter system and thus can be considered a trimonoaminergic modulator (TMM). Estrogen also modulates the activity of other neurotransmitters, including GABA (gamma-aminobutyric acid) and glutamate, as will be discussed below. Many of estrogen's effects upon various neurotransmitter systems appear to be the result of estrogen binding to nuclear hormone receptors, known as estrogen receptors (Figure 12-97). Receptors for estrogen may also exist in neuronal cell membranes, but these are not yet well characterized. However, it is well established that nuclear ligand receptors specifically for estrogen are transformed into nuclear ligand–activated transcription factors when estrogen binds to them. This concept is discussed in Chapter 3 and illustrated in Figure 3-11, as an example of one of the major signal transduction systems for hormones.

Estrogen and nuclear hormone receptors

Estrogen modulates gene expression by binding to nuclear hormone receptors for estrogen – i.e., "estrogen receptors" (Figure 12-97A). Receptors for estrogen differ from tissue to tissue and may differ from brain region to brain region. In addition to various subtypes of estrogen receptors, there are also nuclear hormone receptors for progesterone and androgens as well as for other steroids such as glucocorticoids and mineralocorticoids (Chapter 3 and Figure 3-11; Chapter 5 and Figure 5-50). Unlike neurotransmitter receptors located on neuronal membranes, nuclear ligand–activated receptors for estrogen are located in the neuronal cell nucleus, so estrogen must penetrate the neuronal membrane and the nuclear membrane to find its receptors, which are located near the genes that estrogen influences (Figure 12-97). These genes are called estrogen response elements (Figure 12-97B). Activation of estrogen response elements by estrogen requires receptor "dimerization" (i.e., the coupling of two copies of the estrogen receptor) when estrogen binds to them; this forms an active

Estrogen Acts at Nuclear Hormone Receptors: A Nuclear Ligand–Activated Transcription Factor

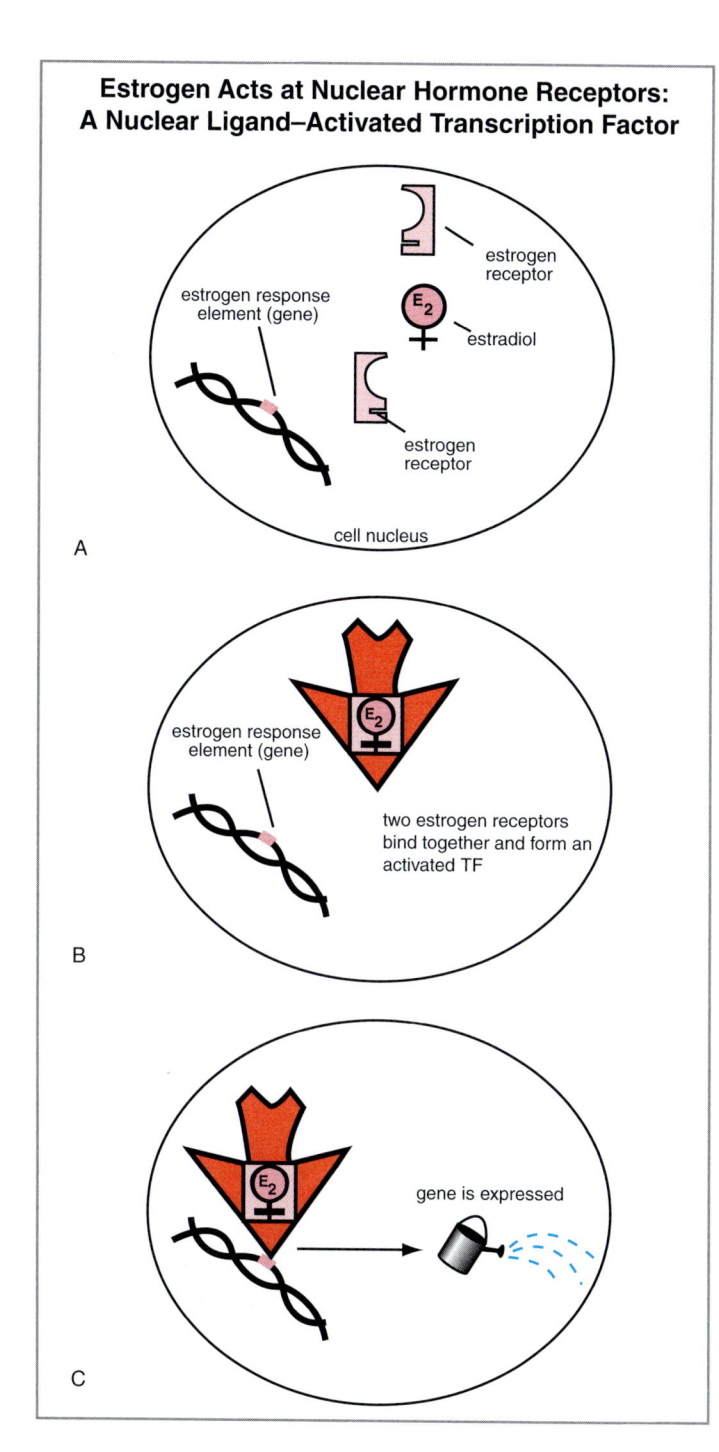

FIGURE 12-97A, B, and C Estrogen and nuclear hormone receptors. Estrogen modulates gene expression by binding to estrogen receptors. Estrogen receptors differ from tissue to tissue and may differ from brain region to brain region. (**A**) Unlike neurotransmitter receptors located on neuronal membranes, receptors for estradiol are located in the neuronal cell nucleus, so estradiol must penetrate the neuronal membrane and the nuclear membrane to find its receptors, which are therefore located near the genes to be influenced. These genes are called estrogen response elements. (**B**) The expression of estrogen response elements within the DNA of the neuron must be initiated by estrogen and its receptor. Activation of these genes by estradiol requires "dimerization" (i.e., coupling of two copies of the estrogen receptor) when estrogen binds to the receptor to form an active transcription factor (TF) capable of "turning on" the estrogen response element. (**C**) Once the estrogen receptors are activated by estradiol into transcription factors, they activate gene expression by the estrogen response elements in the neuron's DNA. The gene products expressed include direct trophic factors such as nerve growth factor (NGF) and brain-derived neurotrophic factor (BDNF), which can facilitate synaptogenesis and prevent apoptosis and neurodegeneration.

transcription factor capable of "turning on" estrogen response elements (Figure 12-97B). The formation of transcription factors is discussed in Chapter 3 and illustrated in Figures 3-22 through 3-34. Once estrogen receptors are activated as transcription factors, they activate gene expression in the neuron by binding to estrogen response elements in the neuron's DNA (Figure 12-97C).

Antidepressants | 611

Estrogen and trophic actions on dendritic spine formation
Gene products that are regulated by estrogen include trophic factors such as brain-derived neurotrophic factor (BDNF) as well as neurotransmitter synthesizing and metabolizing enzymes and various neurotransmitter receptors. Dramatic evidence of estrogen's trophic properties can be observed in hypothalamic and hippocampal neurons in adult female experimental animals within days and across a single menstrual (estrus) cycle (Figures 12-98 and 12-99). During the early phase of the cycle, estradiol levels rise, causing dendritic spines to form specifically in the ventromedial hypothalamus and on pyramidal neurons in the hippocampus of female rats. Progesterone administration rapidly potentiates this, so spine formation is at its greatest when both estrogen and progesterone peak just after the first half of the cycle (Figure 12-98). However, once estrogen levels fall significantly and progesterone continues to rise, the presence of progesterone without estrogen triggers downregulation of these spines by the end of the estrus cycle (Figure 12-98).

Estrogen as a GABA (gamma-aminobutyric acid) inhibitor
One hypothesis to explain the mechanism of this cyclical formation and then loss of dendritic spines is that estrogen regulates a type of spine formation that occurs when neurons are active and that reverses when neurons are inactive, known as "activity-dependent" dendritic spine formation (Figure 12-99). As estrogen levels rise and fall during the menstrual cycle, estrogen can cause a corresponding cyclical rather than continuous activation of neurons in certain brain areas. The cyclical activation of these neurons is explained by the fact that estrogen exerts a cyclical inhibitory influence on GABA interneurons (Figure 12-99). Inhibitory actions of GABA interneurons on pyramidal neurons are discussed in Chapter 7 and illustrated in Figure 7-23. Estrogen inhibits this inhibition. This is not psychopharmacological double talk but a well-known phenomenon called disinhibition, just a fancy way of saying "activated."

By inhibiting GABAergic inhibition, estrogen thus activates pyramidal neurons (Figure 12-99B). Estrogen does this by downregulating and thus reducing the synthesis of glutamic acid decarboxylase (GAD), the enzyme that synthesizes GABA. This, in turn, reduces the synthesis of GABA itself, which diminishes the release of GABA from GABAergic interneurons. No GABA, no inhibition; no inhibition, pyramidal neurons are activated.

Estrogen as a glutamate activator
When estrogen activates pyramidal neurons, these neurons release glutamate (Figures 12-99B and 12-99C). As estrogen levels rise during the first half of the menstrual cycle, so does pyramidal neuron activation by glutamate from other pyramidal neurons (Figure 12-99B); as estrogen levels fall during the last half of the menstrual cycle, pyramidal cells lose their activation (Figure 12-99C).

The cyclical formation of dendritic spines that is the consequence of these cyclical changes in estrogen levels is shown for a single menstrual (estrus) cycle in Figure 12-99A, B, and C. Thus, at the beginning of the cycle, estrogen levels are low, so GABA interneurons are active. When GABA interneurons are active, they inhibit pyramidal neurons (Figure 12-99A). However, as estrogen levels rise during the first half of the cycle, GABA interneurons are progressively inhibited, causing progressive disinhibition of pyramidal neurons (Figure 12-99B).

Disinhibited pyramidal neurons release glutamate (Figure 12-99B). Glutamate then interacts at a number of glutamate receptors, including postsynaptic NMDA receptors on other pyramidal neurons (Figure 12-99B). Sustained activation of NMDA receptors can

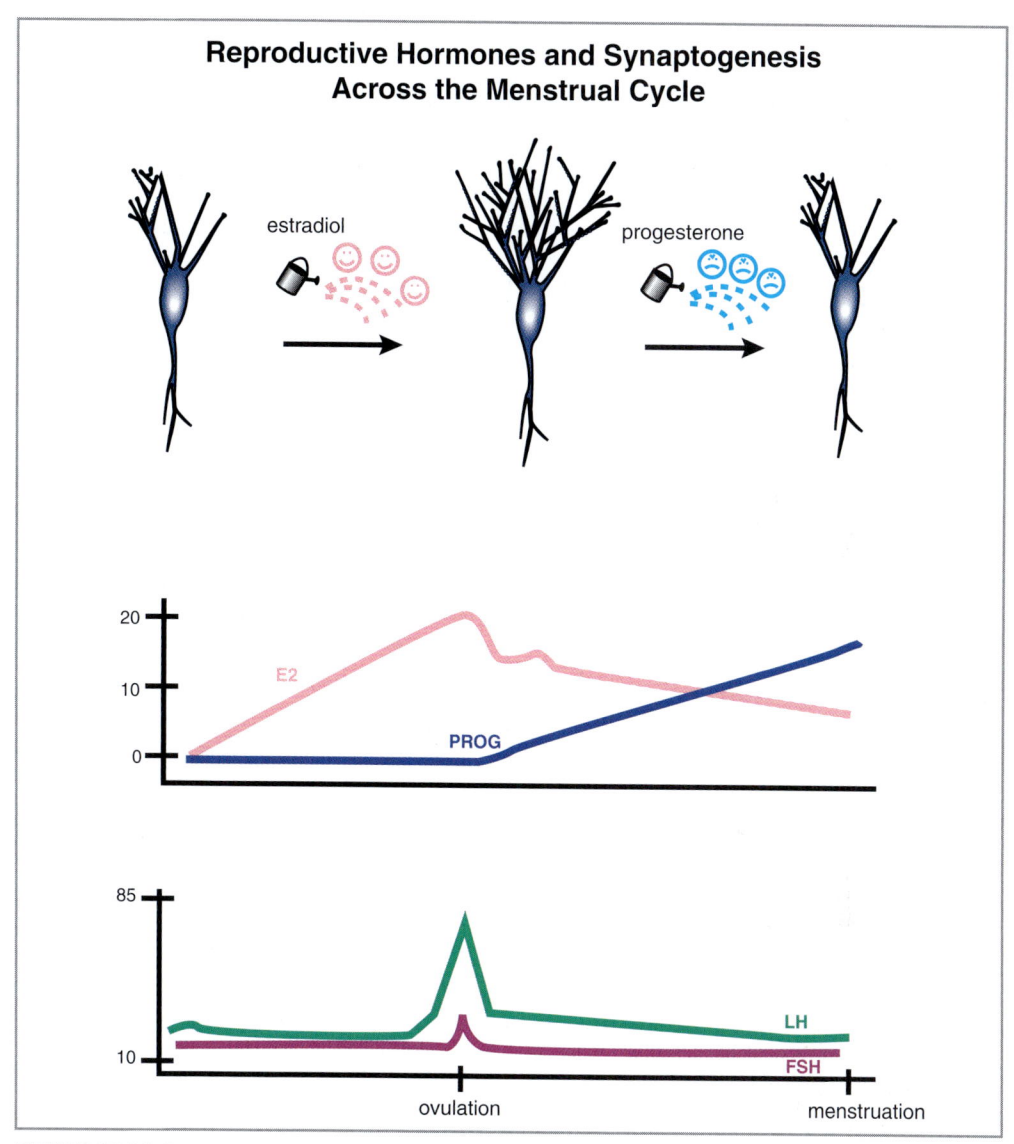

FIGURE 12-98 Reproductive hormones and synaptogenesis across the menstrual cycle. Dramatic evidence of estrogen's trophic properties can be observed in hypothalamic and hippocampal neurons in adult female experimental animals within days and across a single menstrual (estrus) cycle. During the early phase of the cycle, estradiol levels rise, and this trophic influence induces dendritic spine formation and synaptogenesis. Progesterone administration rapidly potentiates this, so spine formation is at its greatest when both estrogen and progesterone peak just after the first half of the cycle. However, once estrogen levels fall significantly and progesterone continues to rise, the presence of progesterone without estrogen triggers downregulation of these spines and removal of the synapses by the end of the estrus cycle.

trigger long-term potentiation and trophic changes in postsynaptic neurons, including the formation of dendritic spines by the middle of the cycle (Figure 12-99C). This concept of NMDA actions of glutamate upon long-term potentiation and activation of trophic changes is also discussed in Chapter 5 and illustrated in Figure 5-43. Once estrogen levels fall by the end of the cycle, glutamate neurons again become inactive, and activity-dependent dendritic spine formation is not maintained (back to Figure 12-99A).

Activity-Dependent Spine Formation by Estradiol

A — beginning of cycle: GABA inhibition

no estrogen: loss of activation and spines

estrogen: reduces GABA inhibition

C — middle to late in cycle: maximal spine formation

B — early in cycle: pyramidal cell activation by glutamate

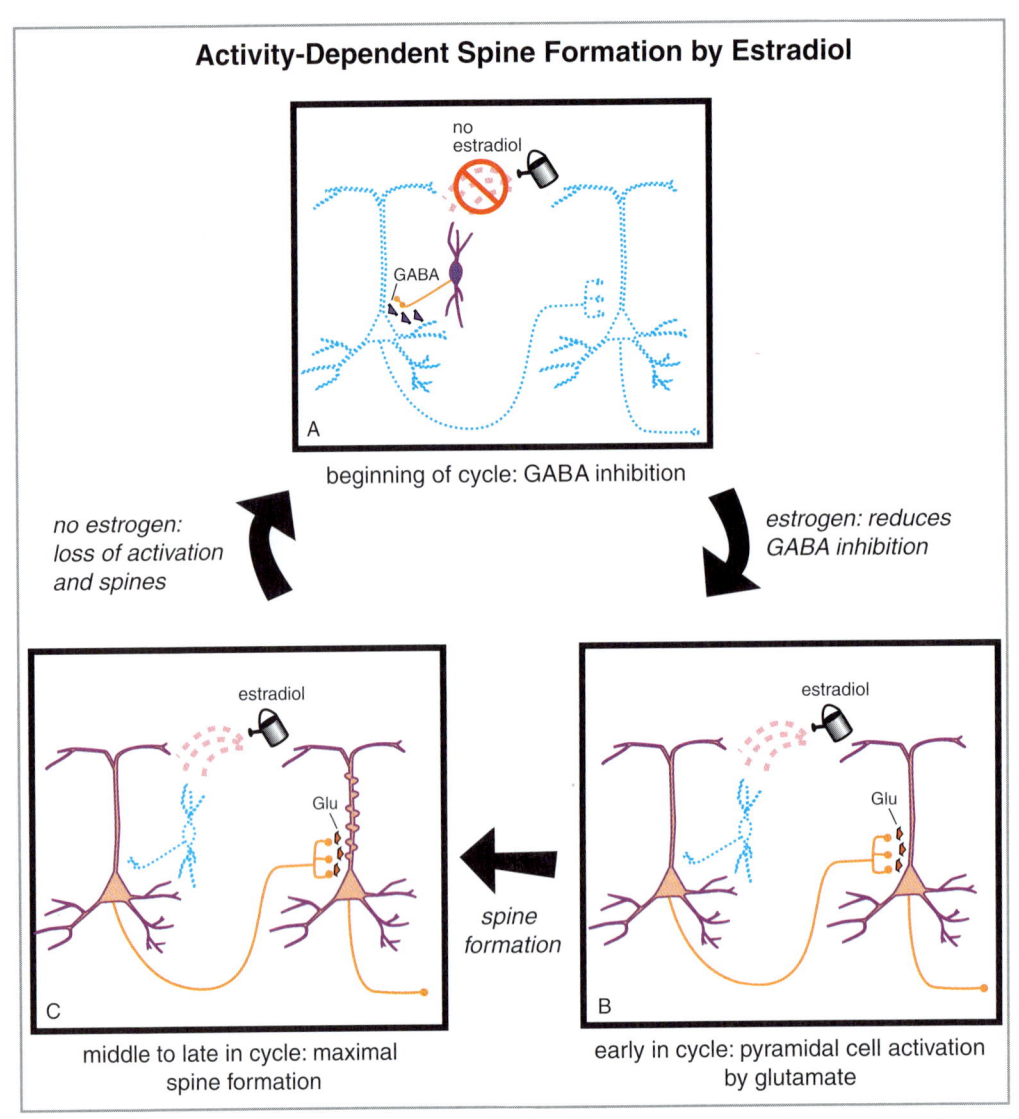

FIGURE 12-99 Activity-dependent spine formation by estradiol. Estrogen exerts a cyclical inhibitory influence on gamma-aminobutyric acid (GABA) interneurons, which in turn regulate pyramidal neurons. When estrogen levels are low, GABA interneurons are active; thus pyramidal neurons are inhibited (**A**). As estrogen levels rise early in the menstrual cycle, GABA inhibition is reduced, thus disinhibiting pyramidal neurons and leading to glutamate release (**B**). Sustained activation of N-methyl-d-aspartate (NMDA) receptors by glutamate, achieved by the middle or late cycle, can trigger long-term potentiation and trophic changes that include the formation of dendritic spines (**C**). As estrogen levels fall by the end of the menstrual cycle, GABA interneurons become active again and resume inhibition of pyramidal neurons, preventing the maintenance of dendritic spine formation (**A**).

Estrogen regulation and major depression over a woman's life cycle

Estrogen levels shift rather dramatically across the female life cycle in relation to various types of reproductive events (Figure 12-100). Such shifts are also linked to the onset or recurrence of major depressive episodes (Figures 12-100 and 12-101). In men, the incidence of depression rises in puberty and then is essentially constant throughout life, despite a slowly declining testosterone level from age twenty-five onward (Figure 12-102). By contrast, in

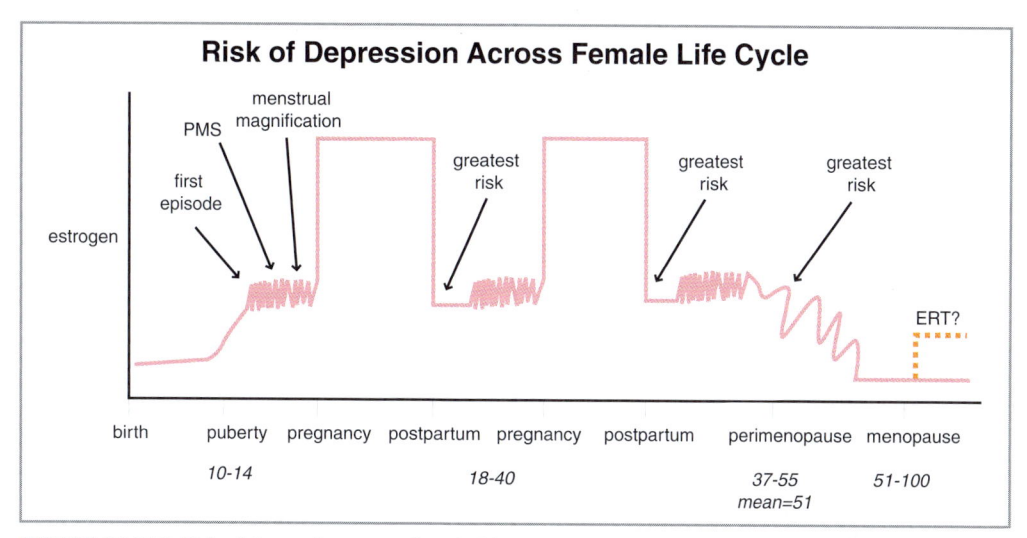

FIGURE 12-100 Risk of depression across female life cycle. Several issues of importance in assessing women's vulnerability to the onset and recurrence of depression are illustrated here. These include first onset in puberty and young adulthood, premenstrual syndrome (PMS), and menstrual magnification as harbingers of future episodes or incomplete recovery states from prior episodes of depression. There are two periods of especially high vulnerability for first episodes of depression or for recurrence if a woman has already experienced an episode, namely, the postpartum period and the perimenopausal period. ERT, estrogen replacement therapy.

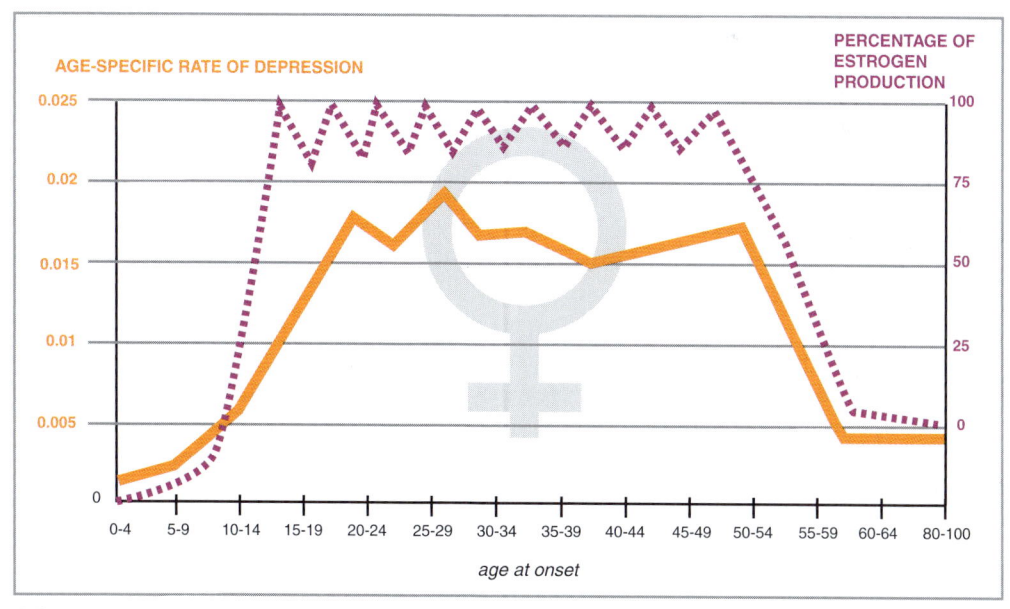

FIGURE 12-101 Incidence of depression across female life cycle. The incidence of depression in women mirrors their changes in estrogen across the life cycle. As estrogen levels rise during puberty, the incidence of depression also rises; it falls again during menopause, when estrogen levels fall. Thus before puberty and after menopause, women have the same frequency of depression as men (see Figure 12-102). During their childbearing years, however, when estrogen is high and cycling, the incidence of depression in women is two to three times as high as it is in men (see Figure 12-102).

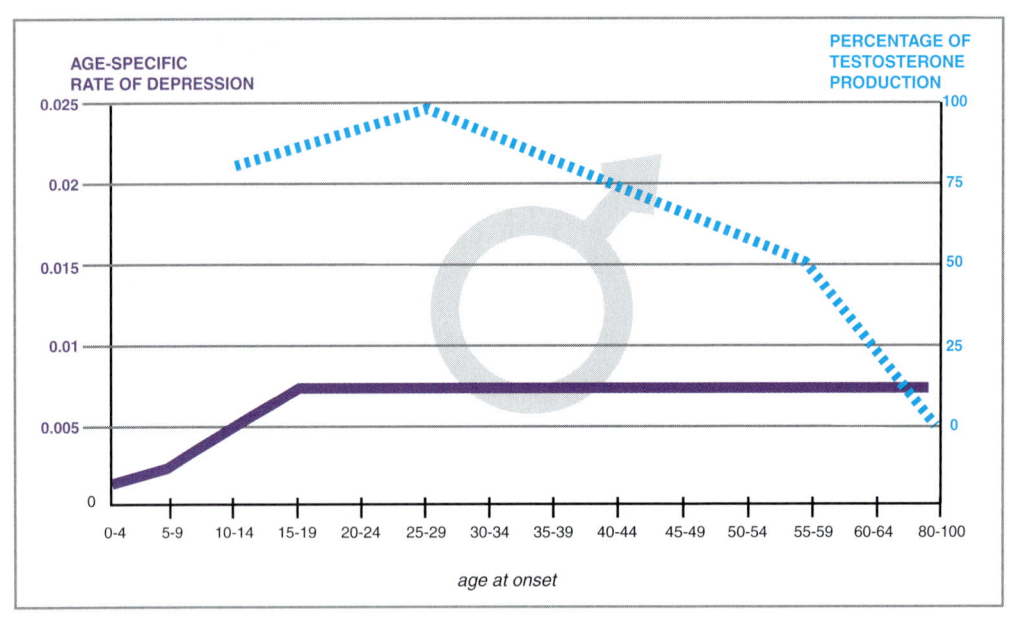

FIGURE 12-102 Incidence of depression across the male life cycle. In men, the incidence of depression rises in puberty and then is essentially constant throughout life, despite a slowly declining testosterone level from age twenty-five onward.

women, the incidence of depression in many ways mirrors their changes in estrogen across the life cycle (Figure 12-101). That is, as estrogen levels rise during puberty, the incidence of depression skyrockets in women; then, after menopause, it falls again (Figure 12-101). Thus, women have the same frequency of depression as men before puberty and after menopause. However, during their childbearing years, when estrogen is high and cycling, the incidence of depression in women is two to three times higher than it is in men (compare Figures 12-101 and 12-102).

Depression and its treatment during childbearing years and pregnancy
As estrogen levels first begin to rise and then cycle during puberty, first episodes of depression often begin (Figure 12-100). Unfortunately these episodes are frequently unrecognized and untreated. Although antidepressant efficacy is not well documented under the age of eighteen for most antidepressants and suicidality is thought to be increased in patients under the age of twenty-five for all antidepressants, treatment of first episodes of depression at any age should be seriously considered, including evaluation and initiation of treatment with antidepressants for unipolar depression or with mood stabilizers for bipolar disorder (Figure 12-103).

Throughout the childbearing years, most women experience some irritability during the late luteal phase just prior to menstrual flow of menstrual cycles; however, if this is actually incapacitating, it may be a form of mood disorder known as premenstrual dysphoric disorder (PMDD) or as premenstrual syndrome (PMS) (Figure 12-100). PMDD can be treated cyclically with oral contraceptive hormones or alternatively with antidepressants, sometimes just during the late luteal phase (Figure 12-103). In some patients, this end-of-cycle worsening is really the unmasking of a mood disorder that is actually present during the whole cycle but is sufficiently worse at the end of the cycle that it becomes obvious as a phenomenon called "menstrual magnification" (Figure 12-100). This may be a harbinger of

Integrating Use of Estrogen and/or Antidepressants Across Female Life Cycle

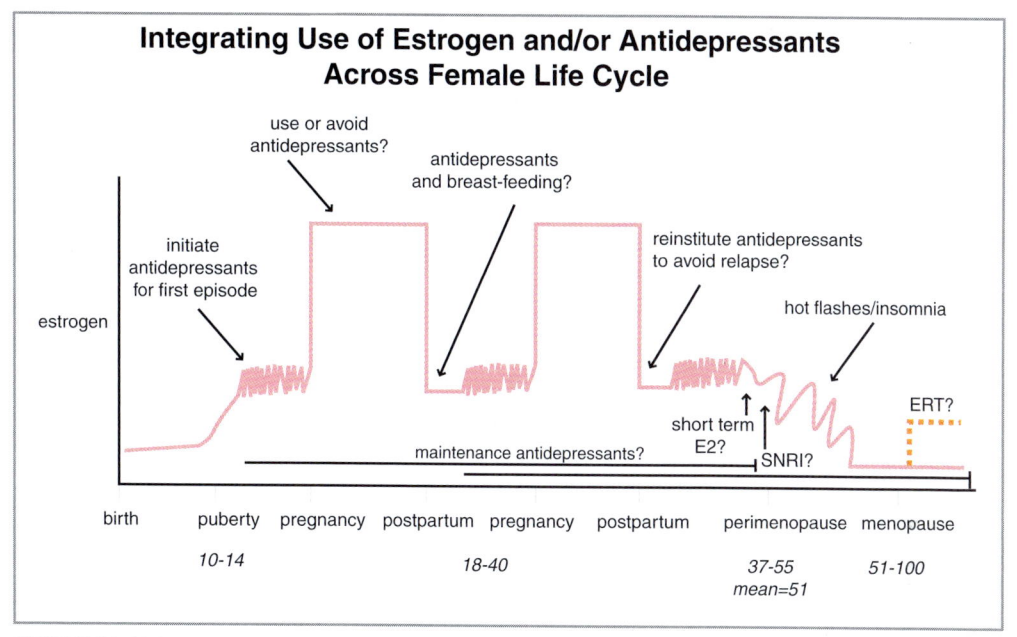

FIGURE 12-103 **Use of estrogen and/or antidepressants across the female life cycle.** This figure illustrates some of the issues involved in integrating endocrine shifts and events related to a woman's life cycle with treatment of a mood disorder with antidepressants and/or estrogen. These include use of antidepressants prior to age eighteen if necessary, calculating risks versus benefits of antidepressant maintenance during pregnancy and breast-feeding, and deciding whether to include estrogens or antidepressants in the treatment of perimenopausal symptoms or after menopause. E2, estradiol; SNRI, serotonin norepinephrine reuptake inhibitor; ERT, estrogen replacement therapy.

further worsening or may also represent a state of incomplete recovery of a previous episode of depression. Nevertheless, both PMS and menstrual magnification are important not only for the symptoms they cause in the short run but also for the risk they represent for a full recurrence in the future, signaling the potential need both for symptomatic and preventive treatment (Figure 12-103).

Regular cycling of estrogen persists during the childbearing years except during pregnancy, when a woman's estrogen levels skyrocket (Figure 12-100). Estrogen levels then plummet precipitously immediately postpartum, and regular menstrual cycles begin again once the woman stops nursing (Figure 12-100). Rapid changes in estrogen levels in the postpartum period are considered a major risk factor for the onset or recurrence of a major depressive episode, psychotic depressive episode, or bipolar manic episode (Figure 12-100).

One of the most controversial and unsettled areas of modern psychopharmacology is the selection of therapeutic interventions for the treatment of major depressive disorder and prevention of recurrence of depression in women during their childbearing years, when they may be pregnant or become pregnant (Figure 12-103).

What about risks of treatment to the girl, adolescent, or woman of childbearing potential? Antidepressants are not generally approved for the treatment of major depression and may even cause increased suicidality in girls before age eighteen, with one of the lowest benefits and highest risks for antidepressants over the female life cycle (Figure 12-11). Antidepressants, although proven effective in women between the ages of eighteen and twenty-five, may also cause increased suicidality up to the age of twenty-five, with a less than ideal benefit-to-risk ratio for antidepressant treatment (Figure 12-11).

TABLE 12-13 Risks of antidepressant use or avoidance during pregnancy

Risks: Damned if you do
Congenital cardiac malformations (especially first trimester; paroxetine)
Newborn persistent pulmonary hypertension (third trimester; SSRIs)
Neonatal withdrawal syndrome (third trimester; SSRIs)
Prematurity, low birth weight
Long-term neurodevelopmental abnormalities
Increased suicidality due to antidepressant use (up to age 25)
Medical–legal risks of using antidepressants

Risks: Damned if you don't
Relapse of major depression
Increased suicidality due to antidepressant non-use
Poor self-care
Poor motivation for prenatal care
Disruption of mother–infant bonding
Low birth weight, developmental delay in children of women with untreated depression
Self-harm
Harm to infant
Medical–legal risks of not using antidepressants

What about risks of treatment to the patient's fetus? Some antidepressants may pose risks to the fetus, including increased risk for serious congenital malformations if administered during the first trimester; increased risk for other fetal abnormalities and for fetal withdrawal symptoms after birth if administered during the third trimester; and increased risks of prematurity, low birth weight, and possibly long-term neurodevelopmental abnormalities if given any time during pregnancy (Table 12-13).

At the same time, lack of treatment during pregnancy is not without risks to mother and fetus (Table 12-13). For the mother with untreated depression, the risks include relapse or worsening of depression, poor self-care, and possible self-harm (Table 12-13). Not only is there risk of increased suicidality when young mothers are treated with antidepressants, there is also the risk of suicide when seriously depressed mothers of any age are not treated with antidepressants (Table 12-13). There are also numerous risks to the baby if the mother is not treated with antidepressants, including risk of poor prenatal care due to low motivation in the mother, risk of low birth weight and early developmental delay, disruption of maternal–infant bonding in the children of women with untreated depression, and even risk of harm to the infant by seriously depressed mothers in the postpartum period (Table 12-13).

Thus it seems that the psychopharmacologist is "damned if you do" treat pregnant patients with antidepressants, and "also damned if you don't" (Table 12-13, Figure 12-103). Without clear guidelines, clinicians are best advised to assess risks and benefits for both child and mother on a case-by-case basis. For mild cases of depression, psychotherapy and psychosocial support may be sufficient. However, in many cases, the benefits of continuing antidepressant treatment during pregnancy outweigh the risks. Since patients with unipolar or bipolar depression (especially children and adolescents) may be prone to impulsive behavior, it is a good idea for girls and women of childbearing potential who take antidepressants to receive counseling and possibly contraceptives to reduce the risk of unplanned pregnancies and first-trimester exposure of fetuses to antidepressants.

Depression and its treatment during the postpartum period and while breast-feeding

What about taking antidepressants during the postpartum period, when the mother is lactating and may be nursing (Figure 12-103)? This is a very high risk period for the onset or recurrence of a major depressive episode in women (Figure 12-100). Should a mother with depression avoid antidepressants in order to avoid risk of exposing the baby to antidepressants in the mother's breast milk (Figure 12-103)? How about a mother with past depression now in remission who is weighing the risk of her own relapse against the risk of exposing the baby to antidepressants in breast milk (Figure 12-103)? In these circumstances there are no firm guidelines that fit all cases and a risk–benefit ratio must be calculated for each situation, taking into consideration the risk of recurrence to the mother if she does not take antidepressants (given her own personal and family history of mood disorder), and the risk to her bonding to her baby if she does not breast-feed or to her baby if there is exposure to trace amounts of antidepressants in her breast milk. Although estrogen replacement therapy (ERT) has been reported to be effective in some patients with postpartum depression or postpartum psychosis, this is still considered experimental and should be reserved for use, if at all, only in patients resistant to antidepressants.

Whereas the risk to the infant of exposure to small amounts of antidepressants in breast milk is only now being clarified, it is quite clear that the mother with a prior postpartum depression who neglects to take antidepressants after a subsequent pregnancy has a 67% risk of recurrence if she does not take antidepressants, and only one-tenth of that risk of recurrence if she does take antidepressants postpartum. Also, up to 90% of all postpartum psychosis and bipolar episodes occur within the first four weeks after delivery. Such high risk patients will require appropriate treatment of their mood disorder, so the decision here is about whether to breast feed, not whether the mother should be treated.

Depression and its treatment during perimenopause

Another very high risk period for the onset or recurrence of major depression is perimenopause (Figure 12-100). Regular cycling of estrogen stops during the perimenopausal transition to menopause, when menstrual cycles are on-again, off-again, and intermittently anovulatory prior to their complete cessation (Figure 12-100). Irregular estrogen cycles may provide a trigger to new onset or recurrence of major depressive episodes in women during perimenopause. This is a long-lasting period of risk, since perimenopause can last for five to seven years until menopause begins (i.e., the complete cessation of menstruation). Hormone levels can thus be chaotic and unpredictable for many years, and these fluctuations are often experienced as both physiological and psychological stressors. Vasomotor symptoms (i.e., hot flushes or hot flashes), often accompanied by sweating and insomnia, are well-known stressors that accompany perimenopause and are a clinical signal for the presence of irregularly fluctuating estrogen levels. Vasomotor symptoms may also be a harbinger of onset or relapse of major depression, since fluctuating estrogen levels may be the physiological trigger for major depressive episodes during perimenopause.

The links between vasomotor symptoms and depression are both clinical and neurobiological. The clinical link is demonstrated by the high degree of overlap between the symptoms of depression and the symptoms of perimenopause and menopause (Figure 12-104). The neurobiological link between vasomotor symptoms and depression is that both are regulated by the trimonoamine neurotransmitter system. The specific circuits hypothesized to mediate the various symptoms of major depressive disorder have already been discussed in Chapter 11 and illustrated in Figures 11-45 to 11-55. Also mentioned in the present chapter has been the fact that estrogen affects the trimonoamine neurotransmitter system

Depression, Perimenopause, or Menopause?

depression
- depressed mood
- anhedonia
- worthlessness/guilt
- agitation/retardation
- suicidal ideation

(overlap)
- low energy
- poor concentration
- insomnia
- weight gain
- decreased libido

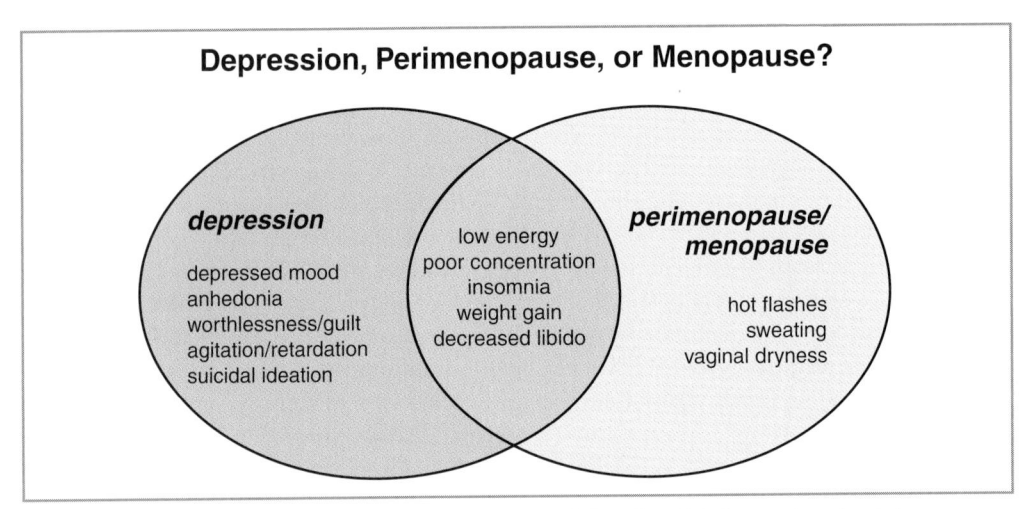

perimenopause/menopause
- hot flashes
- sweating
- vaginal dryness

FIGURE 12-104 Depression, perimenopause, or menopause? There is a high degree of overlap between symptoms of depression and those of perimenopause and menopause. Overlapping symptoms may include low energy, poor concentration, insomnia, weight gain, and decreased libido.

by regulating the expression of genes for numerous neurotransmitter receptors, synthesizing enzymes, and metabolizing enzymes (shown conceptually in Figure 12-97).

Thus, dysregulation of trimonoaminergic neurotransmitter systems within circuits that mediate the various symptoms of depression caused by irregular fluctuation of estrogen levels could lead to neurotransmitter deficiencies that trigger a major depressive episode (Figure 12-105A), consistent with the monoamine hypothesis of depression (Figure 11-42). Similarly, dysregulation of neurotransmitter systems within hypothalamic thermoregulatory centers by irregular fluctuation of estrogen levels could lead to neurotransmitter deficiencies that trigger vasomotor symptoms (Figure 12-106A). It is thus not surprising that other symptoms related to dysregulation of neurotransmitters within the hypothalamus can occur in both perimenopause and in depression (Figure 12-104), namely insomnia, weight gain, and decreased libido (Figures 11-47, 11-48, and 11-52).

How are vasomotor symptoms mediated? It appears that hypothalamic thermoregulatory centers are the homeostatic control sites for integrating internal core body temperature and peripheral temperature signals with vascular and neurochemical signals. Noradrenergic and serotonergic input to the hypothalamus are two of the key neurochemical signals. If estrogen causes dysregulation of noradrenergic and serotonergic circuits throughout the brain, it is not surprising that this could lead not only to the various symptoms of depression (Figure 12-105A and Figures 11-45 to 11-55) but also to vasomotor symptoms and other symptoms of perimenopause and menopause (Figure 12-106A), with considerable overlap between them (Figure 12-104).

The clinical and neurobiological links between vasomotor symptoms and depression predict links between the treatments for these two conditions as well. Classically, estrogen replacement therapy (ERT) has been the approved treatment for vasomotor symptoms, presumably smoothing out the chaotic fluctuations or deficient levels of estrogen that cause these symptoms in perimenopausal or postmenopausal women. Numerous studies suggest that ERT may also be effective in treating depression or may be useful in augmenting antidepressants in some women during perimenopause, although ERT has never been approved for this use (Figure 12-103). Moreover, in recent years, significant concerns have

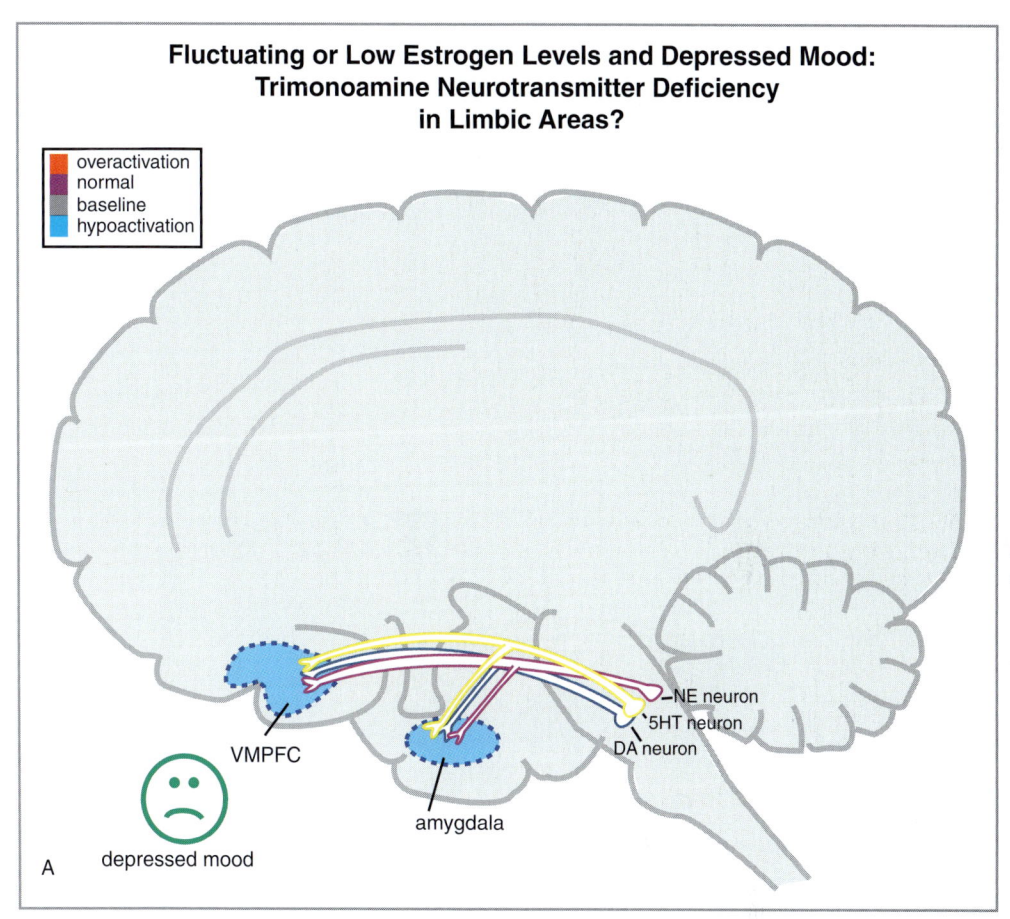

FIGURE 12-105A Estrogen interaction with monoamines may lead to depressed mood. Irregular fluctuation of estrogen levels can cause dysregulation of trimonoaminergic neurotransmitter systems within circuits mediating symptoms of depression, such as depressed mood, and thus contribute to the development of a major depressive episode.

arisen over the long-term safety of ERT, and many women and their physicians now opt out of ERT treatment.

This has created the need for a novel treatment for vasomotor symptoms, and given the clinical and neurobiological link between vasomotor symptoms and the symptoms of depression, it was logical to look at antidepressants that target the trimonoaminergic neurotransmitter system to find a treatment for vasomotor symptoms. Early studies have shown promising if inconsistent results with some SSRIs (Figure 12-106B) as well as with the alpha 2 agonist clonidine and even the anticonvulsant and chronic pain treatment gabapentin (discussed later in Chapter 15, on pain). However, the most promising results to date seem to be with SNRIs, especially the SNRI desvenlafaxine. Perhaps it is necessary to target both the profound hypothalamic regulation of temperature by norepinephrine as well as serotonin to achieve optimal efficacy in the treatment of vasomotor symptoms (Figure 12-106C) rather than targeting just serotonin regulation of temperature with an SSRI (Figure 12-106B). Studies of desvenlafaxine treatment of women with vasomotor symptoms (but not major depression) show that they achieve a 50% reduction of hot flushes

Treating Depressed Women With Fluctuating or Low Estrogen Levels: Is Boosting Serotonin With an SSRI Enough?

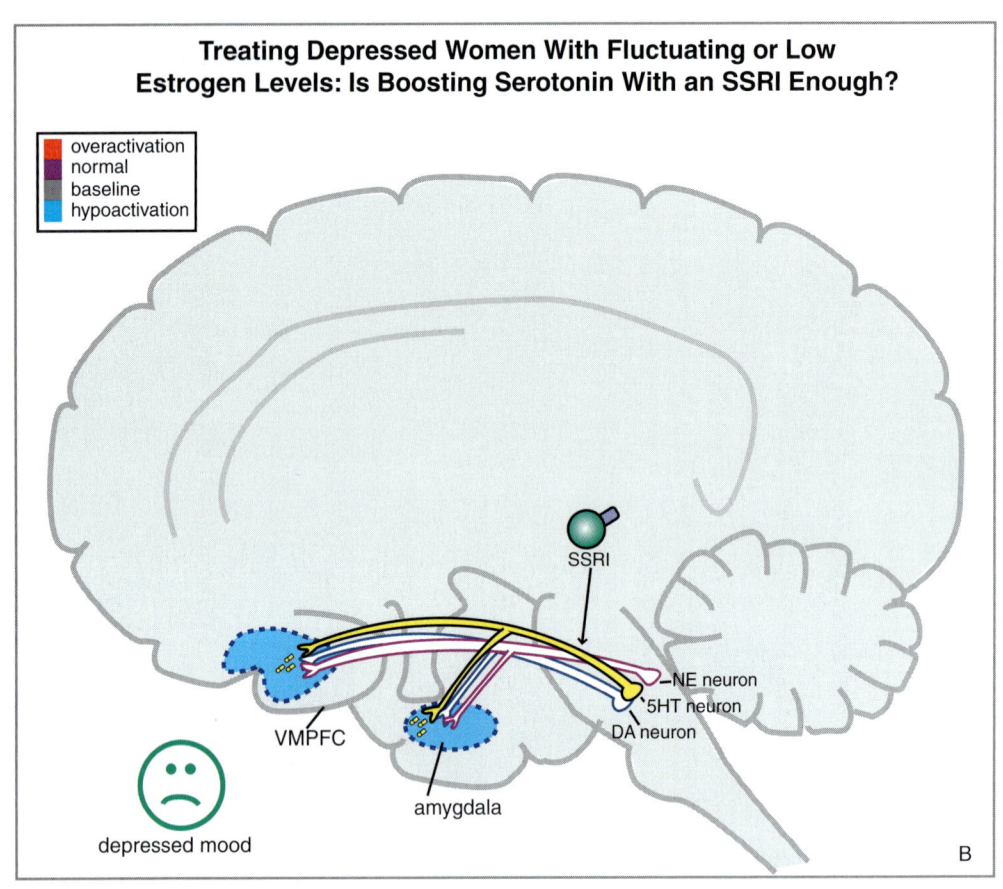

FIGURE 12-105B Treating depressed women with fluctuating estrogen: SSRI. Early studies provide inconsistent results as to the efficaciousness of serotonin selective reuptake inhibitors (SSRIs) for depressed mood in postmenopausal women who are not taking estrogen replacement therapy. This suggests that the presence of estrogen may boost the efficacy of SSRIs and the absence of estrogen may reduce the efficacy of SSRIs in some depressed women.

in about a week, with approximately half of women eventually attaining a 75% reduction in hot flushes.

The question now is whether psychopharmacologists should identify and treat vasomotor symptoms as well as the traditional symptoms of depression in perimenopausal women (Figure 12-104). Since the treatments for these two conditions overlap, this may not be difficult. Vasomotor symptoms are not only stressful to experience but their persistence can stand in the way of a perimenopausal woman reaching full remission of a major depressive episode or of sustaining that remission over the long run. Remission of the classic symptoms of depression while vasomotor symptoms persist is likely a signal that fluctuating estrogen levels are still affecting the brain, at least in hypothalamic regulatory centers. Further research is necessary to determine whether targeting vasomotor symptoms in women with depression (Figures 12-105A and 12-106A) will lead to a better chance of achieving and sustaining remission from depression and also whether targeting vasomotor symptoms in women who do not have depression but are at risk for the onset or recurrence of depression will prevent new episodes of depression. In the meantime, it makes sense for psychopharmacologists to consider taking this approach of targeting not just the classic mood symptoms

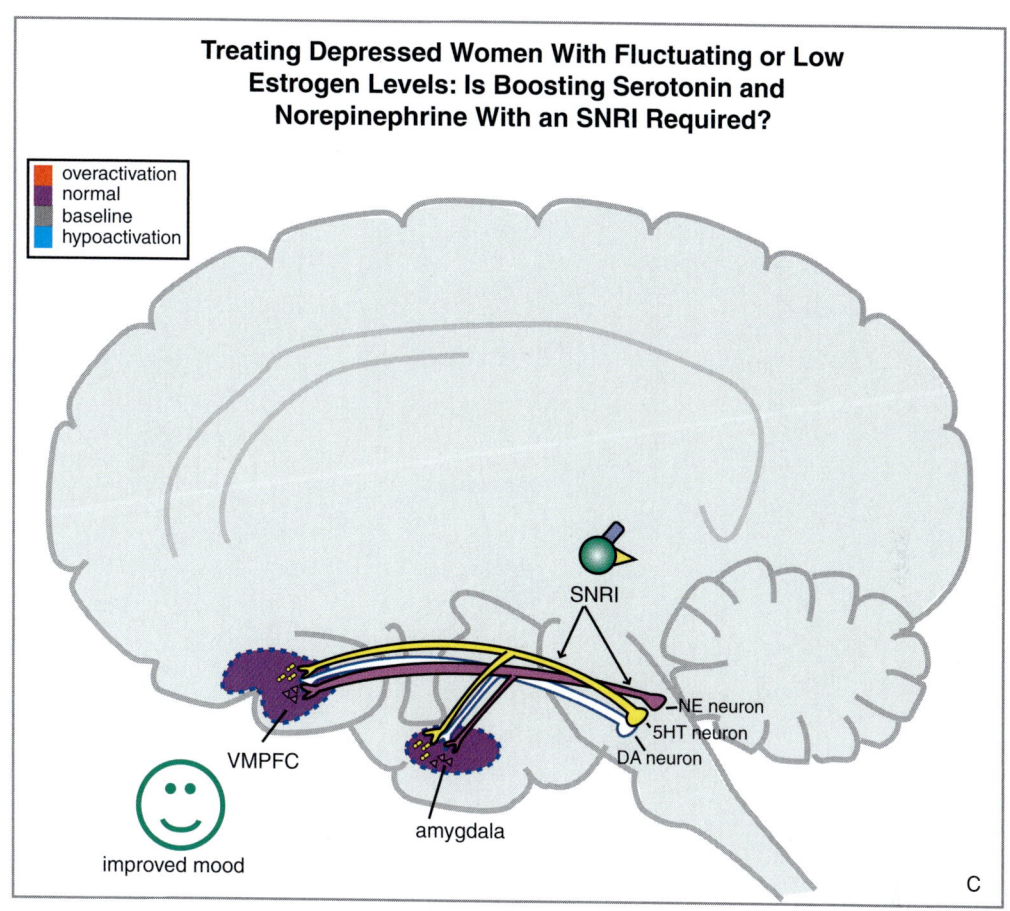

FIGURE 12-105C Treating depressed women with fluctuating estrogen: SNRI. Recent data suggest that serotonin norepinephrine reuptake inhibitors (SNRIs) may have efficacy for depressed mood in postmenopausal women whether or not they are taking estrogen. It may be that actions on both the serotonergic and noradrenergic systems are required to treat depression in some women when estrogen levels are low.

of depression (Figure 12-105A) but also vasomotor symptoms in perimenopausal women (Figure 12-106A).

Depression and its treatment during menopause

Menopause is the final stage of transition of estrogen in the female life cycle and is either a state of relative estrogen deficiency or, in a dwindling number of women, a state associated with estrogen replacement therapy (ERT). Despite the lack of chaotic estrogen fluctuations, many women continue to experience vasomotor symptoms after the onset of menopause. This may be due to the loss of expression of sufficient numbers of brain glucose transporters due to low concentrations of estrogen. Theoretically, this would cause inefficient CNS transport of glucose, which would be detected in hypothalamic centers that would react by triggering a noradrenergic alarm, with vasomotor response, increased blood flow to the brain, and compensatory increases in brain glucose transport. The situation would be potentially exacerbated in the large number of menopausal women with diabetes and prediabetes. Presumably, SNRI treatment could reduce an overreactive hypothalamus and thus minimize consequent vasomotor symptoms.

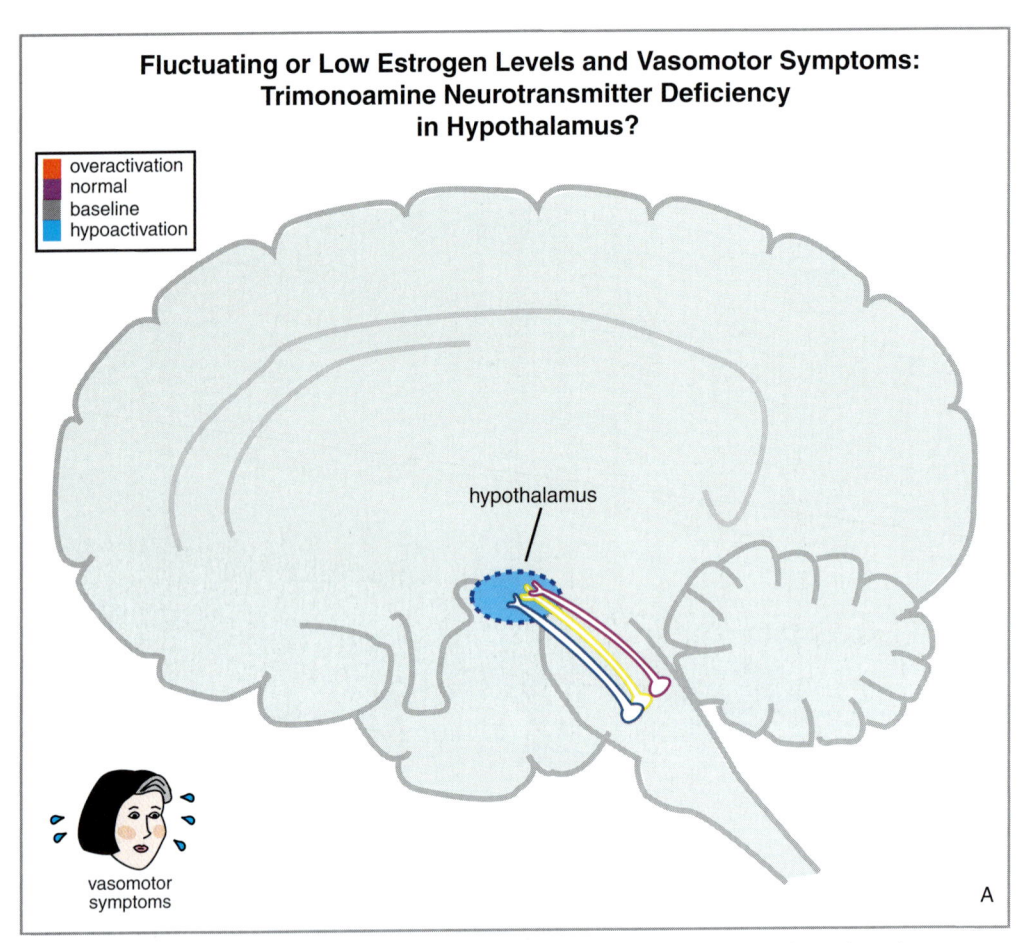

FIGURE 12-106A Estrogen interaction with monoamines may lead to vasomotor symptoms. Irregular fluctuation of estrogen levels can cause dysregulation of trimonoaminergic neurotransmitter projections to the hypothalamus and thus lead to vasomotor symptoms.

What about the treatment of depression in postmenopausal women (Figures 12-103, 12-104, 12-105B, and 12-105C)? Although depression is less of a risk after menopause than during perimenopause and all antidepressants are potentially useful, there are some special considerations for treating women with depression after menopause. One issue of note relates to the observation that SSRIs seem to work better in women in the presence of estrogen than in the absence of estrogen (Figure 12-105B). Thus, SSRIs may have more reliable efficacy in premenopausal women (who have normal cycling estrogen levels) and in postmenopausal women who are taking ERT than in postmenopausal women who are not taking ERT. By contrast, SNRIs seem to have consistent efficacy in both pre- and postmenopausal women whether they are taking ERT or not (Figure 12-105C). Furthermore, there appears to be a relative advantage of SNRIs over SSRIs for treating depression in women over the age of fifty, especially those women who are not taking ERT. Thus, the treatment of depression in postmenopausal women should take into consideration whether they have vasomotor symptoms and whether they are taking ERT before deciding whether to prescribe an SSRI (Figure 12-105B) or an SNRI (Figure 12-105C).

Treating Vasomotor Symptoms in Women With Fluctuating or Low Estrogen: Is Boosting Serotonin With an SSRI Enough?

- overactivation
- normal
- baseline
- hypoactivation

hypothalamus

SSRI

vasomotor symptoms

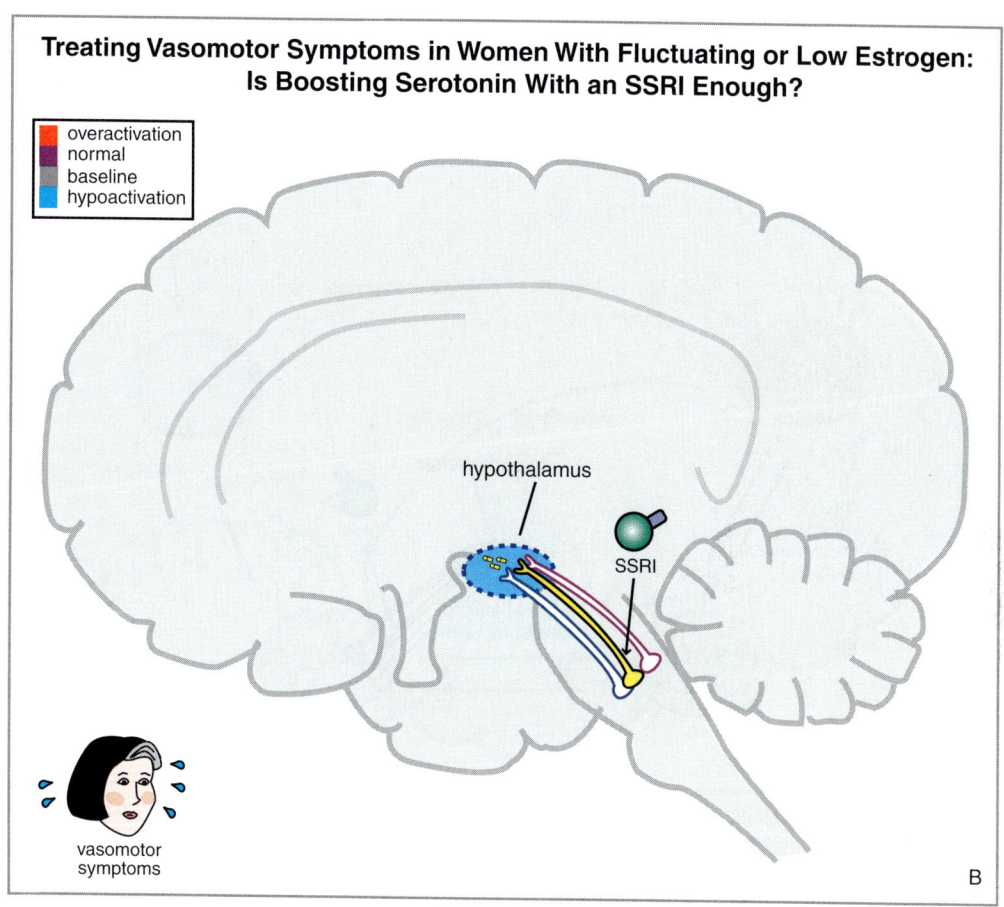

B

FIGURE 12-106B Treating vasomotor symptoms: SSRI. Early studies provide inconsistent results as to the ability of serotonin selective reuptake inhibitors (SSRIs) to improve vasomotor symptoms.

L-methylfolate (6-(S)-5-methyl-tetrahydrofolate, or MTHF) as a trimonoamine modulator (TMM)

MTHF, derived from folate (Figure 12-107), is an important regulator of a critical cofactor for trimonoamine neurotransmitter synthesis, namely tetrahydrobiopterin or BH4 (Figure 12-108A). Because BH4 is a critical enzyme cofactor, there are several mechanisms that lead to its formation, two of which are intimately entwined with MTHF metabolism (Figure 12-108).

The trimonoamine synthetic enzymes that require BH4 as a cofactor are both tryptophan hydroxylase, the rate-limiting enzyme for serotonin synthesis, and tyrosine hydroxylase, the rate-limiting enzyme for dopamine and norepinephrine synthesis (Figure 12-109). MTHF is thus considered to be a TMM (trimonoamine modulator) because of its role as an indirect regulator of trimonoamine neurotransmitter synthesis and concentrations.

Numerous studies now suggest that low plasma, red blood cell, and/or cerebrospinal fluid (CSF) levels of folate or MTHF (Figure 12-107) may be associated with depression in some patients (Figure 12-110). Since MTHF indirectly regulates monoamine levels (Figures 12-108 and 12-109), low CNS levels of MTHF could lead to reduced activity of trimonoaminergic neurotransmitter synthesizing enzymes, causing monoamine deficiency (Figure 12-110A), consistent with the monoamine hypothesis of depression (Figure 11-42).

Antidepressants

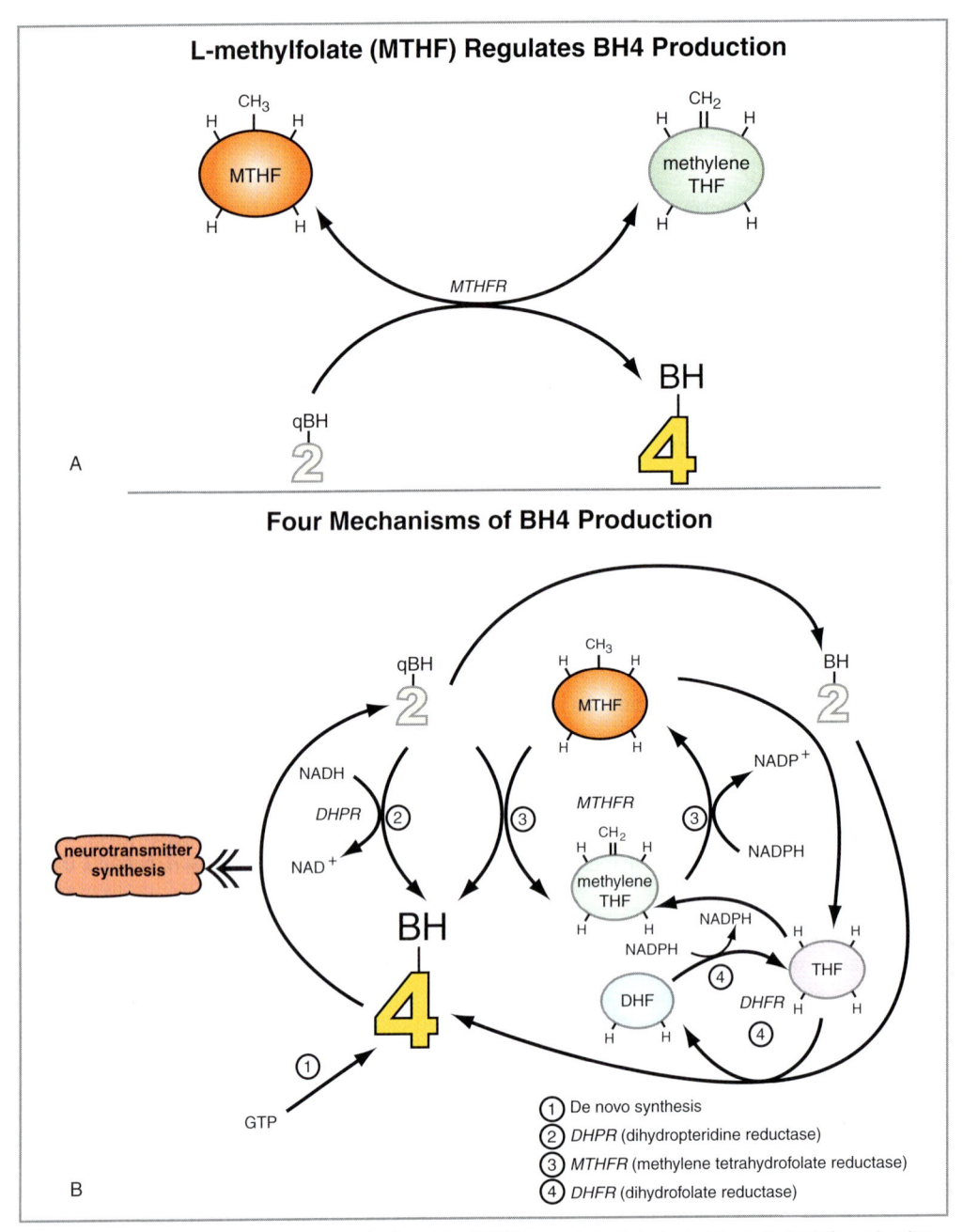

FIGURE 12-108A and B L-5-methyl-tetrahydrofolate (MTHF) regulates tetrahydrobiopterin (BH4) production. BH4 is a critical enzyme cofactor for trimonoamine neurotransmitter synthesis. There are several mechanisms that lead to its production (**B**), the most important of which may be the actions of MTHF to create BH4 (**A**).

folic acid. Thus MTHF may have significant advantages over folic acid as a TMM for depressed patients who do not respond adequately to antidepressant treatment, who may or may not be folate-deficient, who may or may not have the inefficient form of the MTHF synthesizing enzyme methylene THF reductase, and who may or may not be taking various anticonvulsant mood stabilizers that interfere with folic acid absorption.

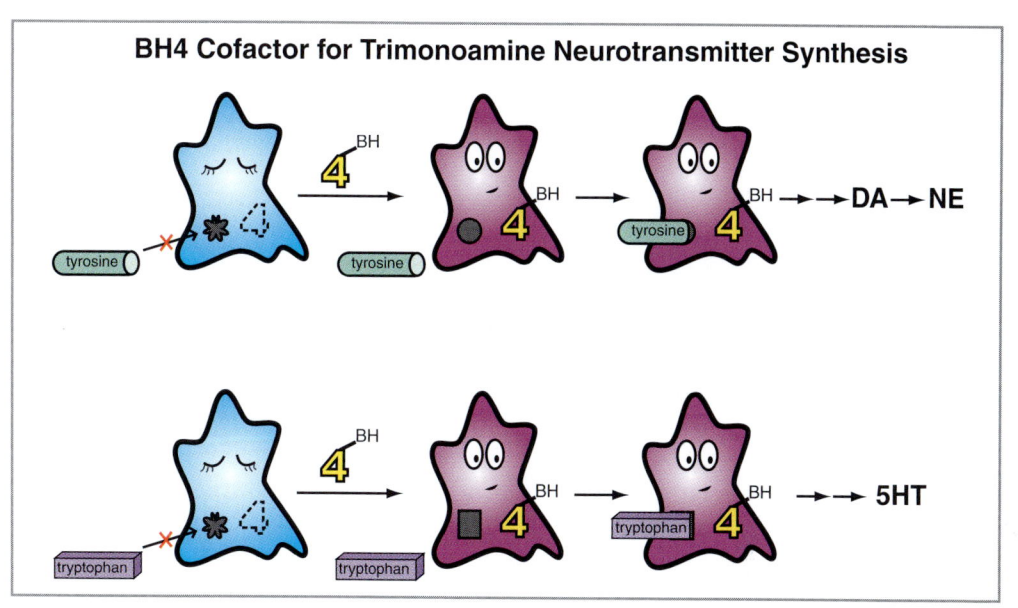

FIGURE 12-109 Tetrahydrobiopterin (BH4) cofactor for trimonoamine neurotransmitter synthesis. BH4 is a critical enzyme cofactor for tyrosine hydroxylase, the rate-limiting enzyme for dopamine and norepinephrine synthesis, and tryptophan hydroxylase, the rate-limiting enzyme for serotonin. Because L-5-methyl-tetrahydrofolate (MTHF) regulates BH4 production, it therefore plays an indirect role in regulating trimonoamine synthesis and concentrations. Thus MTHF is considered to be a trimonoaminergic modulator.

Specifically, it may take as much as 7 mg of oral folic acid to generate the same plasma levels of MTHF as giving 1 mg of oral MTHF itself. How much folic acid is this? The recommended daily allowance of folic acid from food or dietary supplements is 0.4 mg (0.8 mg for pregnant women); over-the-counter multivitamin supplements typically provide between 0.25 and 1 mg of folic acid; normal "prescription strength" folic acid is 1 mg of pure folic acid; high-dose prescription folic acid for treating pregnant women to reduce the risk of neural tube defects is between 4 and 5 mg of folic acid. By comparison, the lowest dose of MTHF studied in depression to augment antidepressant treatment is 7.5 mg, roughly equivalent to 52 mg of folic acid. Although high doses of folic acid can be administered orally, the precursors of MTHF may compete with MTHF for entry into the brain by binding to folate transport receptors and thus limit the amount of MTHF that can get into the brain (Figure 12-110B). Thus high doses of MTHF itself are likely to provide substantially more active MTHF moiety to the brain than high doses of folic acid. The exact dose of MTHF to treat depression is not fully determined, but since MTHF works indirectly to boost monoamine synthesis, high doses are likely to be necessary to optimize this action.

MTHF itself is available by prescription in the United States as a "medical food" also called L-methylfolate (Deplin) and not as an over-the-counter dietary supplement or vitamin. According to the FDA, a medical food is different both from a drug and a food and is defined as a food that is formulated to be consumed orally "under the supervision of a physician and which is intended for the specific dietary management of a disease or condition for which distinctive nutritional requirements, based on recognized scientific principles, are established by medical evaluation." Medical foods are required when dietary management cannot achieve the specific nutrient requirements. Treatment with MTHF seems to be safe,

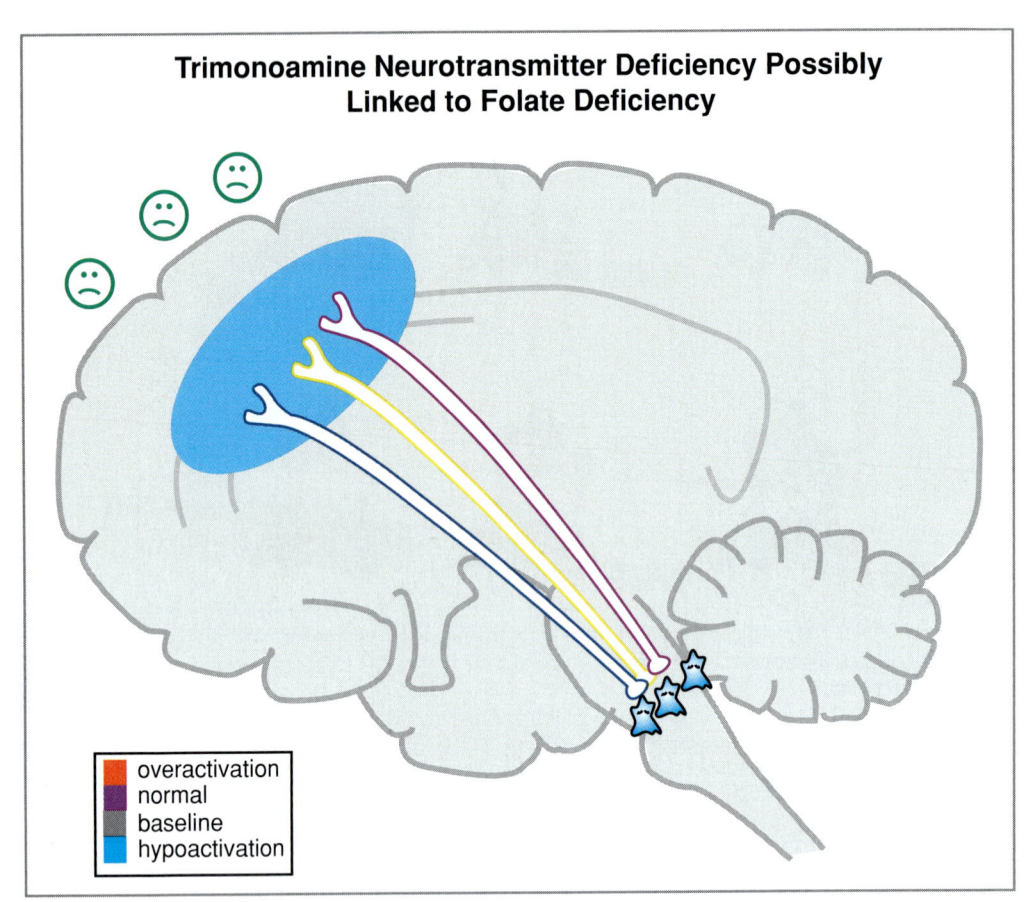

FIGURE 12-110A Folate deficiency and monoamines. Because L-5-methyl-tetrahydrofolate (MTHF) indirectly regulates trimonoamine neurotransmitter synthesis, deficiency of folate, from which it is derived, can lead to reduced monoamine levels and thus to symptoms of depression. In fact, studies show that low levels of folate or MTHF may be linked to depression in some patients.

apparently has few if any side effects, and is generally less expensive than augmenting with a second antidepressant. Further research is necessary to determine the exact priority that should be given to this approach in treatment algorithms for major depression.

S-adenosyl-methionine (SAMe), MTHF, and methylation

MTHF may have additional actions on monoamine neurotransmitter metabolism through another mechanism – namely, its well-known ability to regulate methylation reactions (Figure 12-111). Another agent possibly useful for augmenting antidepressants in patients with inadequate responses is S-adenosyl-methionine (SAMe), which shares with MTHF the ability to regulate methylation (Figure 12-111). Both MTHF and SAMe may thus affect the regulation of various critical components of monoamine neurotransmitter activity not only by indirect modulation of neurotransmitter synthesis by promoting the synthesis of BH4 enzymatic cofactor but also by modulating catabolic enzymes, monoamine transporters, and neurotransmitter receptors via methylation and its downstream effects (Figure 12-111). These complex mechanisms are under active investigation to determine how the natural products and putative TMMs MTHF and SAMe may contribute to the treatment of depression.

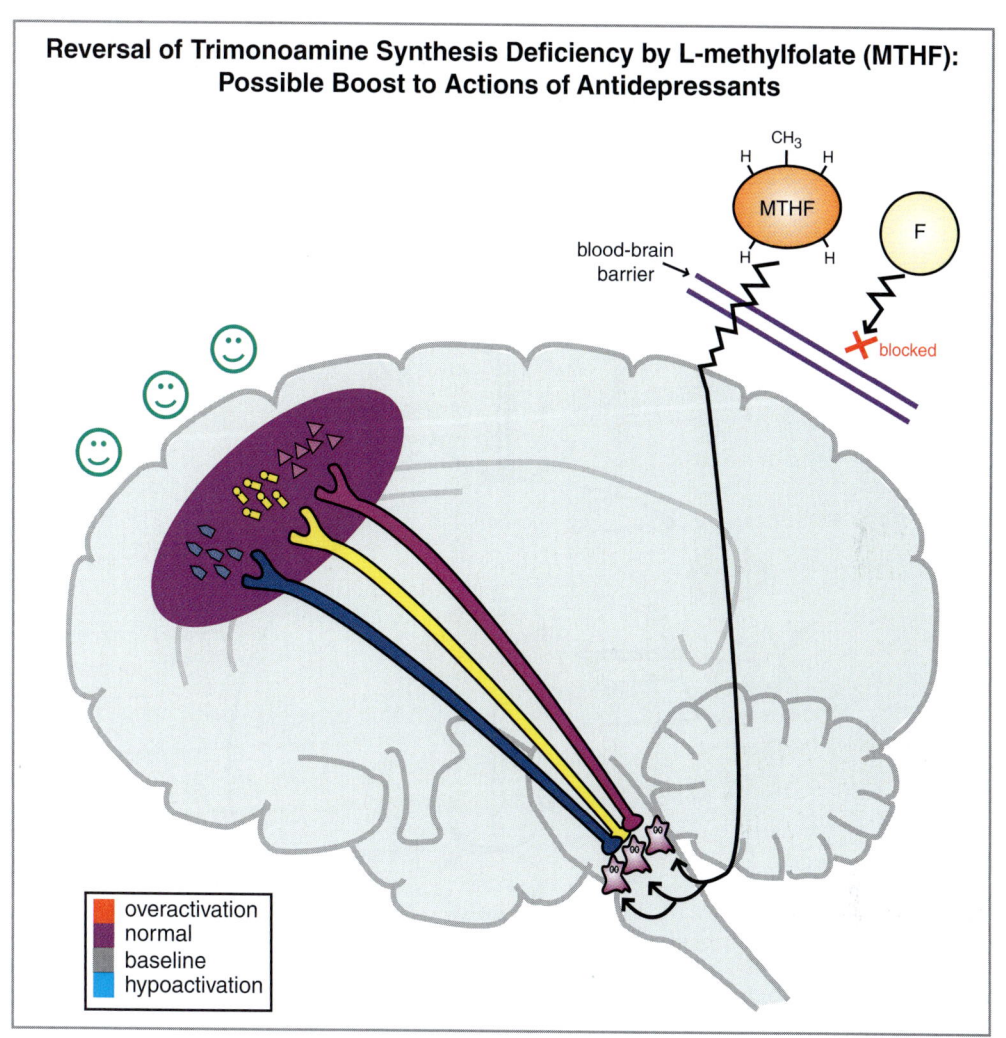

FIGURE 12-110B L-5-methyl-tetrahydrofolate (MTHF) and antidepressants. Administration of MTHF, folate, or folinic acid in conjunction with an antidepressant may boost the therapeutic effects of antidepressant monotherapy. High doses of oral MTHF may be the most efficient of these for boosting BH4 production in the central nervous system and thus enhancing brain trimonoamine neurotransmitter levels.

Thyroid

Thyroid hormones are other examples of hormones that bind to nuclear ligand receptors to form a nuclear ligand–activated transcription factor. Abnormalities in thyroid hormone levels have long been associated with depression (Figure 12-112A), and various forms and doses of thyroid hormones have long been utilized as augmenting agents to antidepressants either to boost their efficacy in patients with inadequate response or to speed up their onset of action (Figure 12-112B). Thyroid hormones have many complex cellular actions, including actions that may boost trimonoaminergic neurotransmitters as downstream consequences of thyroid's known abilities to regulate neuronal organization, arborization, and synapse formation (Figure 12-112B). Thus it may be appropriate to classify thyroid hormones as another form of trimonoaminergic modulator in order to explain their ability to enhance antidepressant action in some patients.

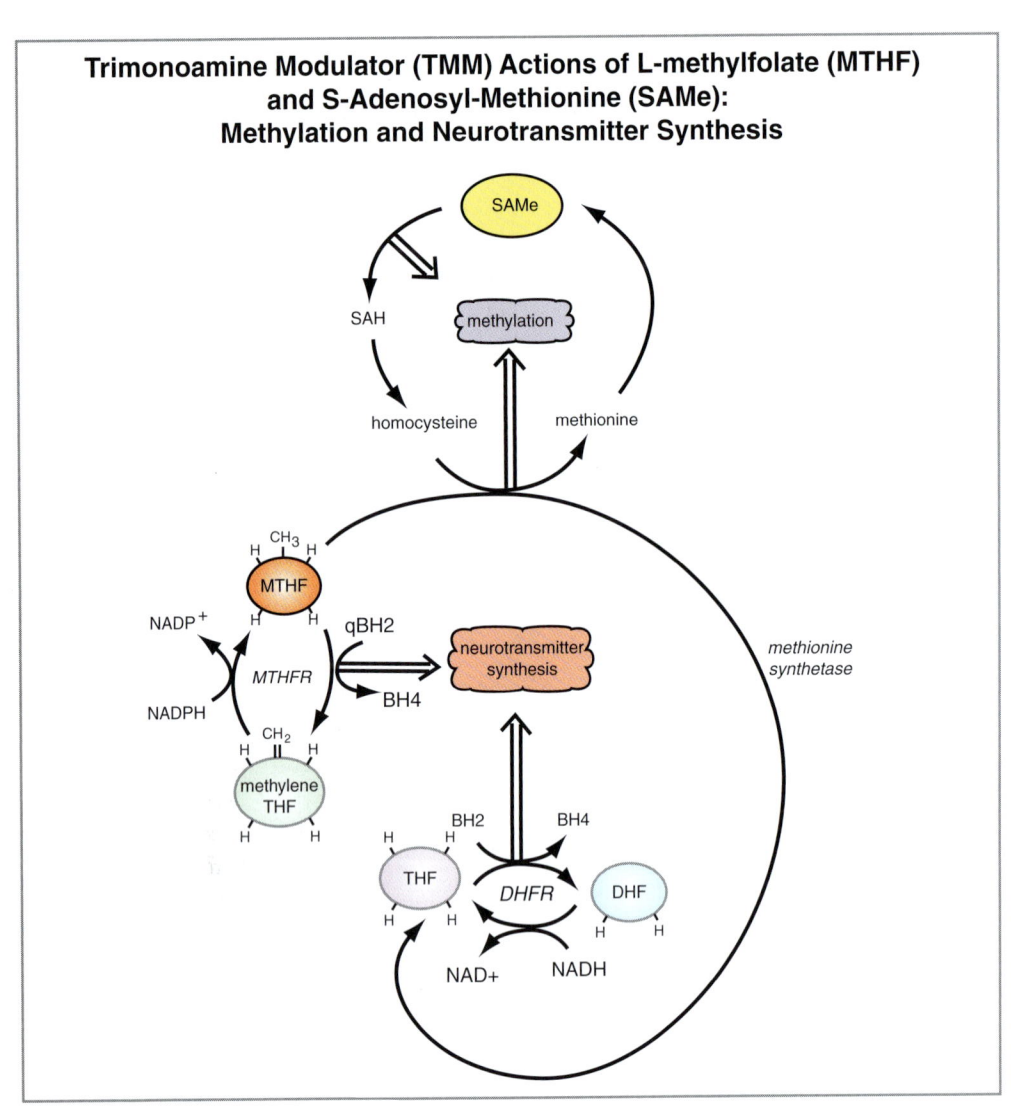

FIGURE 12-111 Trimonoamine modulation (TMM) of L-5-methyl-tetrahydrofolate (MTHF) and S-adenosyl-methionine (SAMe). MTHF regulates methylation reactions, as does SAMe, another agent that has been used to augment antidepressants. Regulation of methylation can affect modulation of catabolic enzymes, monoamine transporters, and receptors and thus is another means to regulate monoamine activity.

Lithium

The mechanism of action of lithium is still debated and not yet firmly established. Actions of lithium on the enzyme glycogen synthetase kinase (GSK) are discussed briefly in Chapter 5 and illustrated in Figure 5-51. Actions of lithium at other sites of the signal transduction cascade for neurotransmitters are discussed in Chapter 13, on mood stabilizers. In addition to these actions, lithium can boost the actions of monoamines, perhaps by one of these actions or by other mechanisms yet poorly understood (Figure 12-113). It is clear that, in addition to mood stabilizing actions, lithium can be effective as an augmenting agent to many antidepressants in patients with major depressive episodes who have inadequate responses to antidepressants, although perhaps not as a monotherapy for such patients.

Deficient Thyroid Levels and Depressed Mood: Trimonoamine Neurotransmitter Deficiency in Limbic Areas?

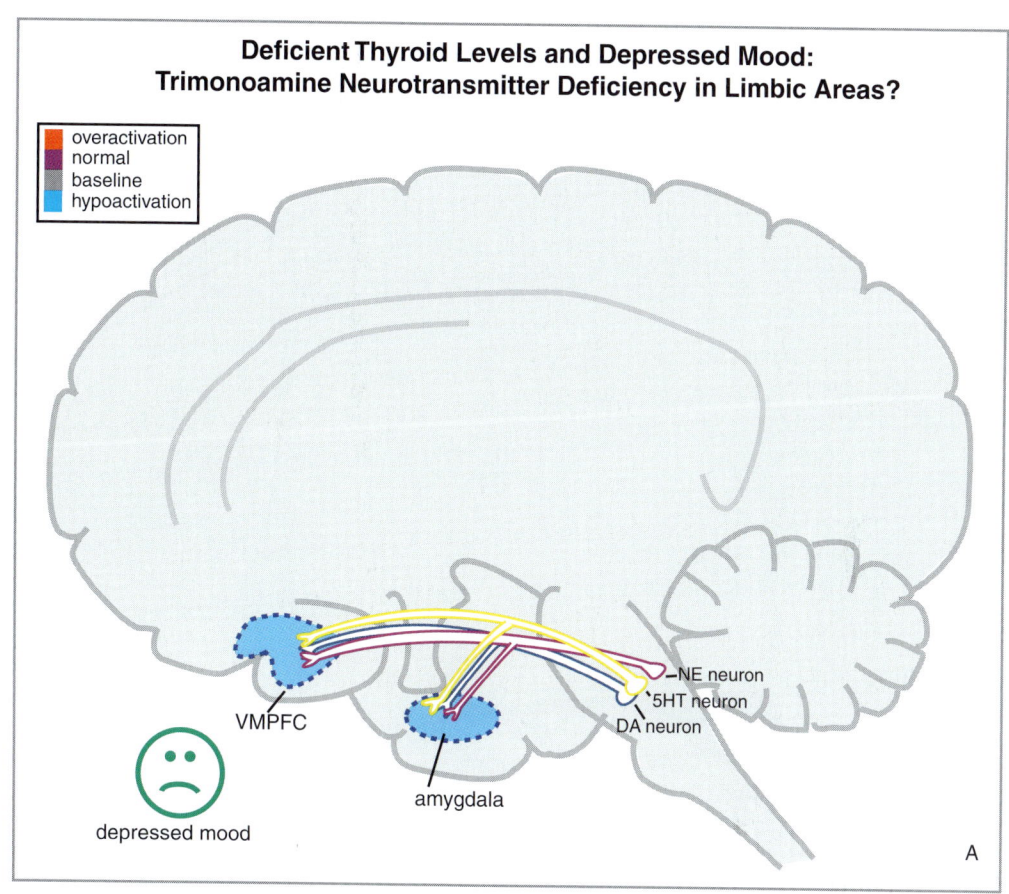

FIGURE 12-112A Thyroid levels and depressed mood. Abnormal thyroid levels have been linked to depression. This may be because thyroid hormones are involved in neuronal organization, arborization, and synapse formation, which in turn can affect levels of trimonoaminergic neurotransmitters. Deficient thyroid levels may be associated with monoamine deficiency in limbic regions and thus cause depressed mood.

Lithium as a mood stabilizing monotherapy, especially for mania, is discussed in Chapter 13, on mood stabilizers. Actions of lithium on antidepressants can be considered to be a form of trimonoaminergic modulation, and lithium should be part of the therapeutic armamentarium for unipolar depression in patients with inadequate responses to prior treatment with antidepressants (Figure 12-113).

Brain stimulation: creating a "perfect storm" in brain circuits of depressed patients
Electroconvulsive therapy (ECT) is the classic therapeutic form of brain stimulation for depression. ECT is a highly effective treatment for depression whose mechanism of action remains a mystery. Failure to respond to a variety of antidepressants, singly or in combination, is a key factor for considering ECT, although it may also be utilized in urgent and severely disabling high-risk circumstances such as psychotic, suicidal, or postpartum depressions. ECT is the only therapeutic agent for the treatment of depression that is rapid in onset; its therapeutic actions can start after even a single treatment and typically within a few days. The mechanism is unknown but thought to be related to the probable mobilization of neurotransmitters caused by the seizure; thus ECT could be considered a type of trimonoaminergic modulator. In experimental animals, ECT downregulates beta

Reversal of Trimonoamine Neurotransmitter Deficiency With Thyroid?

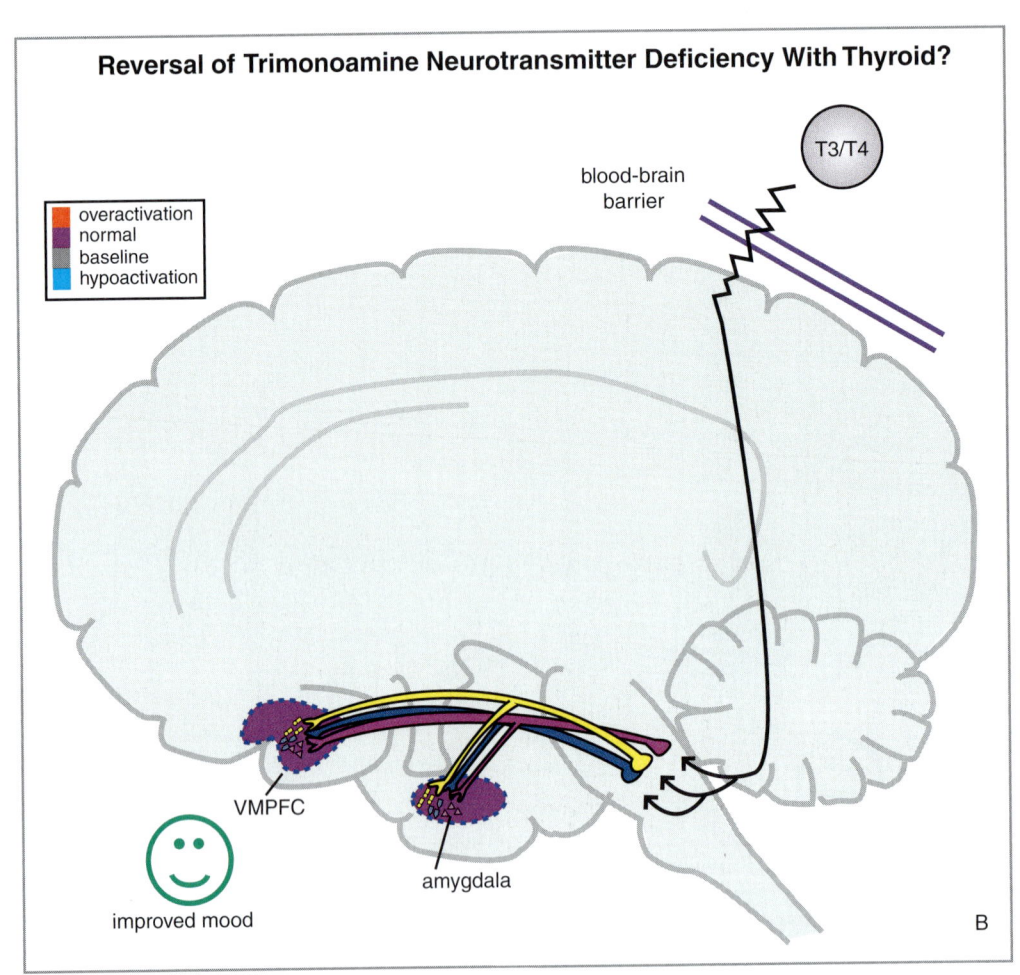

FIGURE 12-112B **Thyroid hormone as an augmenting agent.** Administration of thyroid hormone (T3/T4) in patients with thyroid deficiency may boost monoamine levels and thus contribute to improved mood in patients with depression.

1 receptors (analogous to antidepressants) but upregulates 5HT2A receptors (opposite of antidepressants). Memory loss and social stigma are the primary problems associated with ECT, which limit its use. There can also be striking regional differences across the various nations of the world in the frequency of ECT use and in ECT techniques. For example, ECT is often more commonly used in Europe and the United Kingdom and on the East Coast of the United States; it is less commonly used on the West Coast.

If the mechanism of therapeutic action of ECT could be unraveled, it might lead to new antidepressant treatments capable of rapid onset of antidepressant effects or with special value for refractory patients. More recently, at least three newer forms of therapeutic brain stimulation have emerged. These are mentioned here only in brief, as it is not the intent of this chapter, which focuses on psychopharmacological treatments, to review these promising new treatments in depth. However, these three new forms of therapeutic brain stimulation treatments are listed here as potential "trimonoaminergic modulators," and their hypothetical mechanisms of action are shown in Figures 12-114 to 12-116.

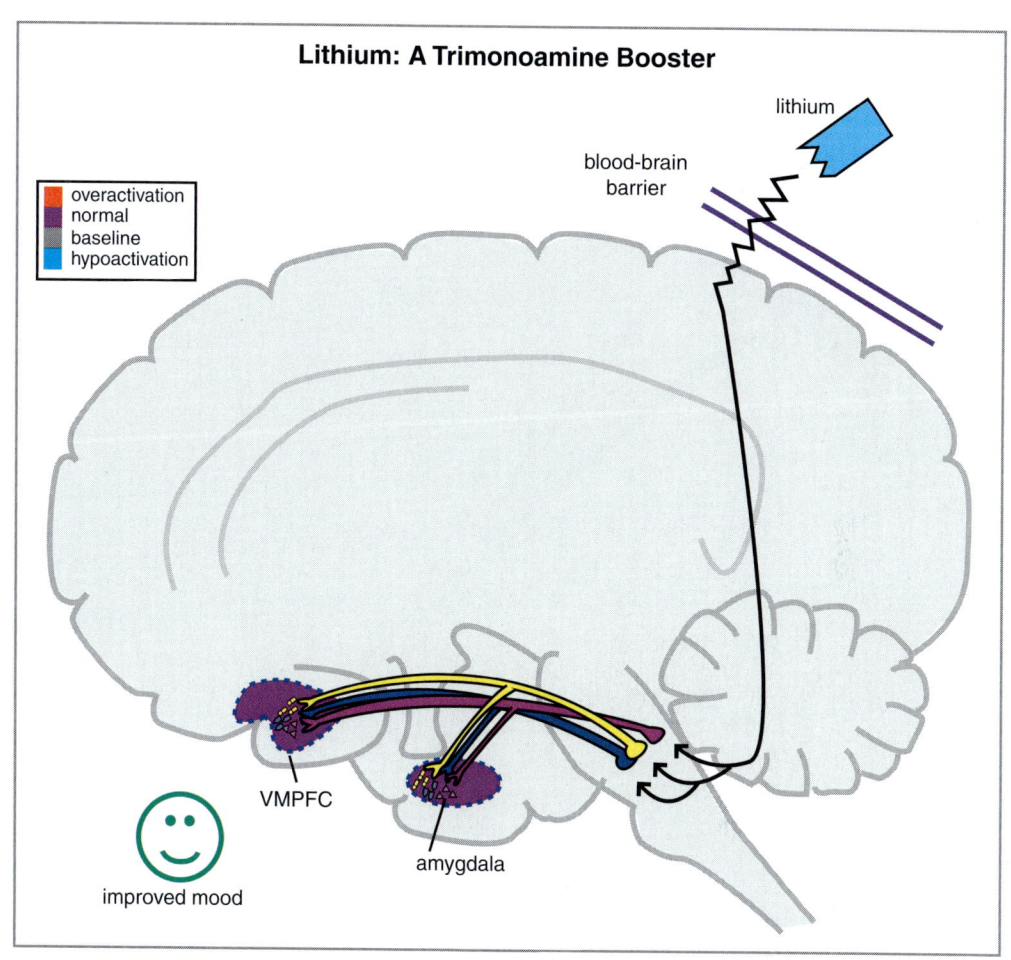

FIGURE 12-113 Lithium in depression. Although the mechanism of action of lithium is not clear, it does seem to boost the actions of monoamines, which may make it an efficacious augmenting agent in depression.

Vagus nerve stimulation, or VNS, is an approved treatment for depression in the United States and some other countries; it provides a continuous train of electrical pulses delivered from a pacemaker-like device surgically implanted in the left chest wall together with an implanted lead wrapped around the vagus nerve in the left side of the neck. The implanted pulse generator is then programmed with a telemetric wand using a computer to deliver pulses to the vagus nerve, typically for thirty seconds every five minutes twenty-four hours a day. Adjustable parameters include pulse width, signal frequency, output current, signal "on" time, and signal "off" time. The treatment thus requires a surgical implantation procedure, typically under general anesthesia. Battery life of the implanted pulse generator ranges from three to ten years.

The vagus nerve has direct and indirect anatomical connections with the trimonoaminergic neurotransmitter system in the brainstem, especially the noradrenergic locus coeruleus and the serotonergic midbrain raphe (Figure 12-114). It is possible that trans-synaptic excitation of neurotransmitter centers from input received via the vagus nerve is capable of boosting the output of neurotransmitters from these monoamine neurotransmitter centers and thereby boosting the therapeutic action of drugs in depressed patients with insufficient

Antidepressants | 635

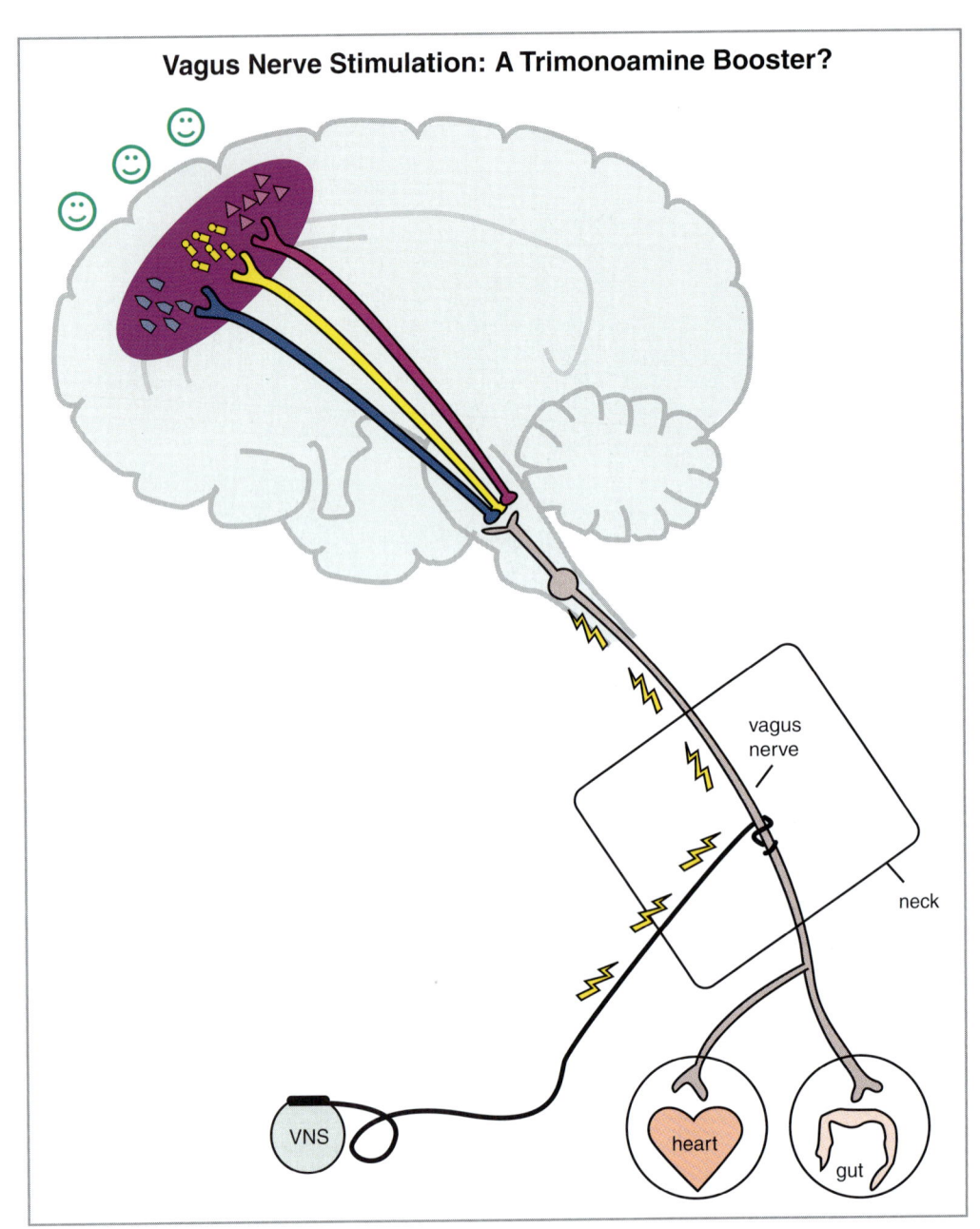

FIGURE 12-114 Vagus nerve stimulation. The vagus nerve has connections with neurotransmitter centers in the brainstem, in particular the midbrain raphe (serotonin) and the locus coeruleus (norepinephrine), and thus can modulate monoamine activity. Vagus nerve stimulation is a treatment in which a pacemaker-like device is surgically implanted in the chest wall with an implanted lead wrapped around the vagus nerve in the neck. This device delivers pulses to the vagus nerve, thus stimulating it to boost monoamine neurotransmission.

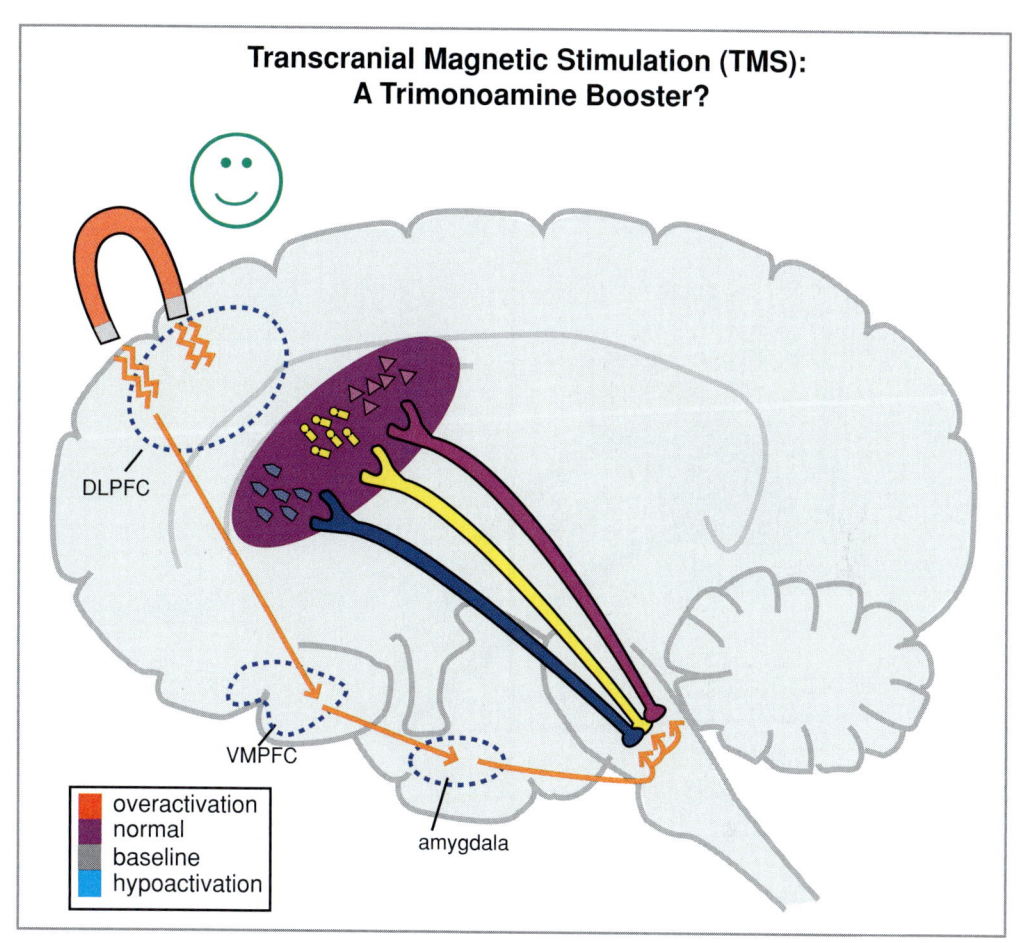

FIGURE 12-115 Transcranial magnetic stimulation. Transcranial magnetic stimulation is a treatment in which a rapidly alternating current passes through a small coil placed over the scalp. This generates a magnetic field that induces an electrical current in the underlying areas of the brain (dorsolateral prefrontal cortex, or DLPFC). The affected neurons then signal other areas of the brain. Presumably, stimulation of brain regions in which there is monoamine deficiency would lead to a boost in monoamine activity and thus alleviation of depressive symptoms.

response to antidepressants (Figure 12-114). Thus vagus nerve stimulation may be a unique form of trimonoaminergic modulator (TMM). The onset of antidepressant action by VNS is generally delayed by several weeks, and the major side effect may be hoarseness from the spread of electrical stimulation in the neck to the vocal cords.

Transcranial magnetic stimulation, or TMS, is another new brain stimulation treatment for depression in the late stages of clinical trials in several different countries; it uses a rapidly alternating current passing through a small coil placed over the scalp. TMS generates a magnetic field that induces an electrical current in the underlying areas of the brain. This electrical current depolarizes the affected cortical neurons, thereby causing nerve impulses to flow out of the underlying brain areas (Figure 12-115). During the treatment, the patient is awake and reclines comfortably in a chair while the magnetic coil is placed snugly against the scalp. There are few if any side effects except headache.

The TMS apparatus is localized so as to create an electrical impulse over the dorsolateral prefrontal cortex (Figure 12-115). Presumably, daily stimulation of this brain area

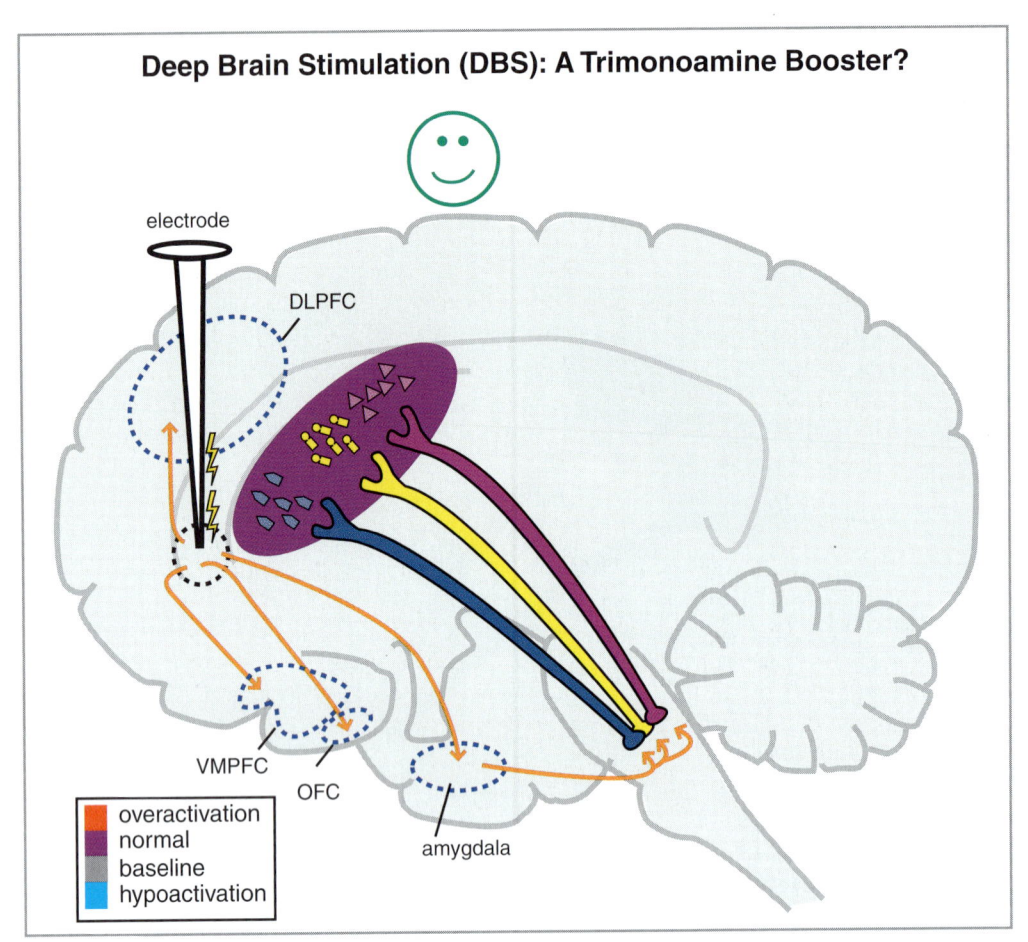

FIGURE 12-116 Deep brain stimulation. Deep brain stimulation involves a battery-powered pulse generator implanted in the chest wall. One or two leads are tunneled directly into the brain. The device then sends brief repeated pulses to the brain, which may have the result of boosting monoamine activity and thus alleviating depressive symptoms.

for up to an hour over several weeks causes activation of various brain circuits that leads to an antidepressant effect. If this procedure activates a brain circuit beginning in dorsolateral prefrontal cortex and connecting to other brain areas, such as ventromedial prefrontal cortex and amygdala, with connections to the brainstem centers of the trimonoaminergic neurotransmitter system, the net result could be trimonoaminergic modulation, especially for patients inadequately responsive to treatment with antidepressants (Figure 12-115).

Finally, a highly experimental treatment for the most severe forms of depression is known as **deep brain stimulation** (Figure 12-116). Deep brain stimulation of neurons in some brain areas has proven to be effective for the treatment of motor complications in Parkinson's disease and is now under study for treatment-resistant depression. The stimulation device is a battery-powered pulse generator implanted in the chest wall, like a pacemaker or VNS device. One or two leads are tunneled under the scalp and then into the brain, guided by neuroimaging and brain stimulation recording during the implantation procedure to facilitate the exact placement of the lead in the targeted brain area. The tip of each lead is composed of several contact areas that usually spread sequentially to cover additional parts of the intended anatomic target. The pulse generator delivers brief, repeated pulses of current, which is adjusted based on individual tissue impedance. The most common side effects are from the procedure itself. There is ongoing debate on where to place the stimulating electrodes for the treatment of depression and how such stimulation might work to treat depression in patients inadequately responsive to antidepressants. Currently, a popular location for electrodes in the treatment of depression with deep brain stimulation is in the subgenual area of the anterior cingulate cortex, part of the ventromedial prefrontal cortex (Figure 12-116). This brain area has important connections to other areas of the prefrontal cortex, including other areas of the ventromedial prefrontal cortex, orbitofrontal cortex, and dorsolateral prefrontal cortex as well as the amygdala (Figure 12-116). It is conceivable that electrical stimulation of this brain area results in the activation of circuits that lead back to brainstem monoamine centers, therefore acting as trimonoaminergic modulators in these patients. Some reports of this treatment approach are encouraging.

Psychotherapy

In recent years, modern psychotherapy research has begun to standardize and test selected psychotherapeutic approaches to treatment in a manner analogous to the way in which antidepressants are tested in clinical trials. Thus, psychotherapeutic treatments are now being tested by being administered according to standard protocols by therapists receiving standardized training and using standardized manuals as well as in standard "doses" for a fixed duration. Such uses of psychotherapies are being compared in clinical trials to placebo or antidepressants. The results have shown that brief interpersonal therapy (IPT) and cognitive behavioral therapy (CBT) for depression may be as effective as antidepressants in certain patients. Proof of efficacy of certain psychotherapies is thus beginning to evolve.

Research is only beginning to show how to combine psychotherapy with drugs. Although some of the earliest studies did not indicate any additive benefit of tricyclic antidepressants and interpersonal therapy, recent studies are now demonstrating that there can be an additive benefit of psychotherapy augmentation of antidepressants. One study of nortriptyline suggests additive benefit of interpersonal psychotherapy, particularly when looking at long-term outcomes. Another recent study of nefazodone suggests that nefazodone is particularly effective when combined with cognitive behavioral psychotherapy for patients with chronic depression. In this study, psychotherapy was an especially essential element in the treatment of patients with chronic depression who had a history of childhood trauma. It is not known whether the addition of psychotherapy in antidepressant responders who are not in full remission might lead to remission and recovery, but this is an intuitively attractive possibility, and the usefulness of this approach for selected patients is empirically obvious to practitioners.

Psychotherapy is likely a form of learning that may counteract inefficient information processing in various brain circuits, not unlike the actions attributed to the various antidepressants being discussed in this chapter. Thus, effective forms of psychotherapy may themselves be a form of trimonoaminergic modulator.

Antidepressants in clinical practice

How do you choose an antidepressant?

With so many treatment options, many questions arise not only about how to choose a first-line agent but also what to do when the first-line treatment fails to cause remission. Various treatment options are organized in Figure 12-117 as the "depression pharmacy."

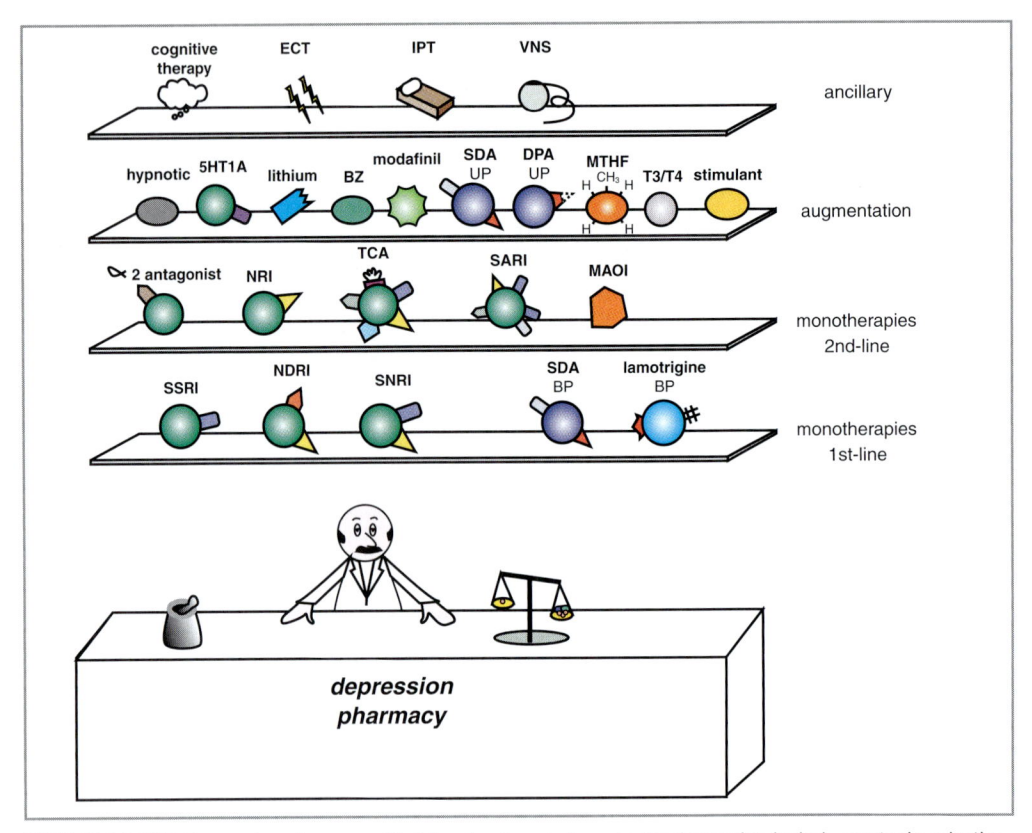

FIGURE 12-117 Depression pharmacy. First-line treatments for unipolar depression include serotonin selective reuptake inhibitors (SSRIs), norepinephrine and dopamine reuptake inhibitors (NDRIs), and serotonin norepinephrine reuptake inhibitors (SNRIs), while first-line treatments for bipolar depression include serotonin dopamine antagonists (SDAs) and lamotrigine. Second-line monotherapies include alpha 2 antagonists, selective norepinephrine reuptake inhibitors (NRIs), tricyclic antidepressants (TCAs), serotonin 2A antagonist/reuptake inhibitors (SARIs), and monoamine oxidase inhibitors (MAOIs). Potentially useful augmenting agents include hypnotics, serotonin 1A (5HT1A) agonists, lithium, benzodiazepines, modafinil, SDAs, dopamine partial agonists (DPAs), L-5-methyl-tetrahydrofolate (MTHF), thyroid hormone (T3/T4), and stimulants. Ancillary treatments to medications may include cognitive therapy, electroconvulsive therapy (ECT), interpersonal therapy (IPT), and vagus nerve stimulation (VNS).

The choices for first-line treatments for unipolar depression generally include an SSRI, SNRI, or NDRI for unipolar depression and lamotrigine or an atypical antipsychotic for bipolar depression. The treatment of bipolar depression is discussed in greater detail in Chapter 13, on mood stabilizers. Here the focus is on unipolar depression.

Generally, because of the greater side effect burden, treatments relegated to second-line choices include many of the older antidepressants, such as the alpha 2 antagonist mirtazapine, the SARI trazodone, the MAO inhibitors, and the TCAs (Figure 12-117). Selective NRIs such as reboxetine and off-label use of atomoxetine could be considered here. Agents generally used for augmentation of a first- or second-line antidepressant and not as a monotherapy are also indicated in Figure 12-117 and include a multitude of options. Finally, antidepressants can be augmented with ancillary treatments that are not drugs, including psychotherapy (such as cognitive behavior therapy or interpersonal therapy) and currently available electrical stimulation therapies (i.e., ECT and VNS).

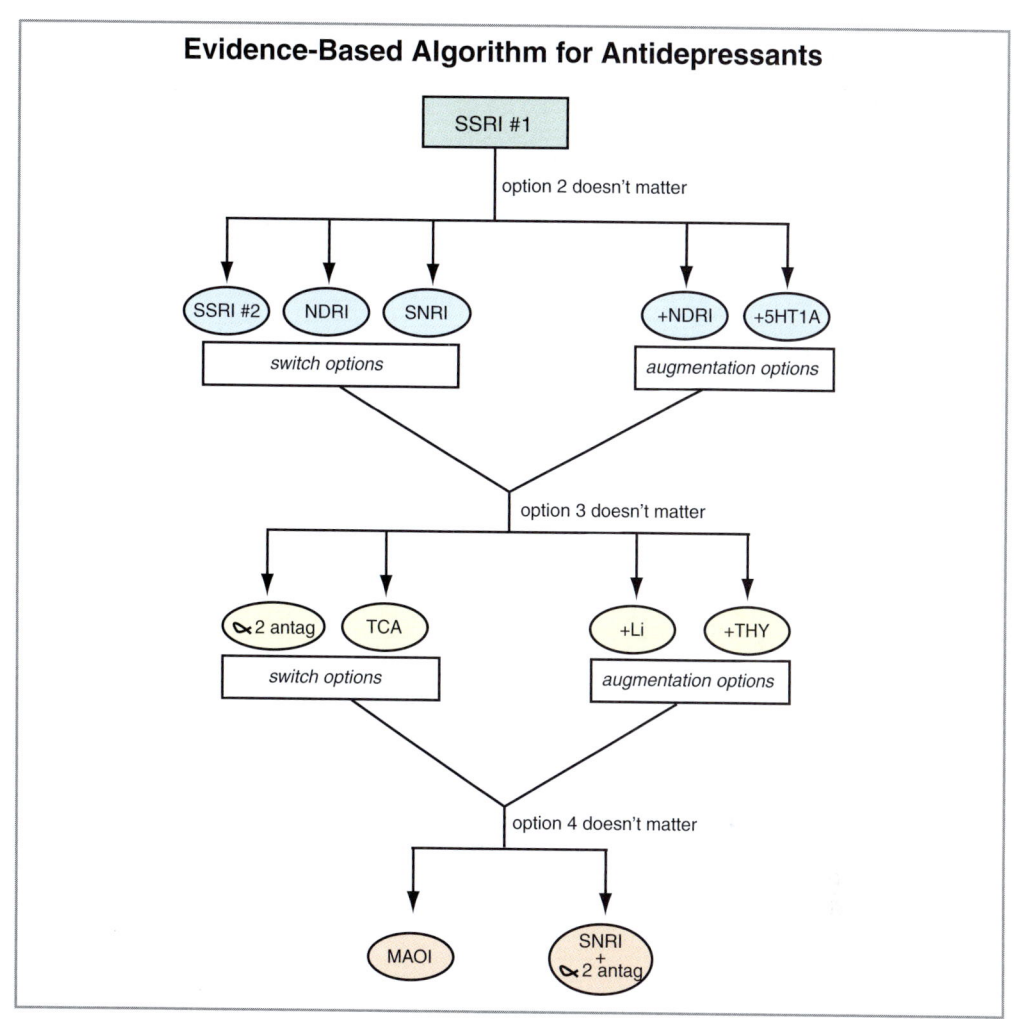

FIGURE 12-118 Evidence-based algorithm for antidepressants. Serotonin selective reuptake inhibitors (SSRIs) are generally considered the first-line treatment for depression. Patients with no response or who do not tolerate the medication may best be switched to another, while those with a partial response may do best with augmentation; however, there is little evidence to suggest which agent to switch to or which to add as an augmenting agent. Current data do not support the superiority of one over another; thus any may be a viable option.

Evidence-based antidepressant selections

One way to organize the various treatment choices for depression is to follow an evidence-based algorithm (e.g., Figure 12-118). Unfortunately there is little evidence for the superiority of one option over another. One general principle on which most patients and prescribers agree is when to switch versus when to augment. Thus there is a preference for switching when the first treatment has intolerable side effects or when there is no response whatsoever but to augment the first treatment with a second treatment when there is a partial response to the first treatment. Other than this guideline, there is little evidence that one treatment option is better than another (Figure 12-118). All treatments subsequent to the first one seem to have diminishing returns in terms of chances to reach remission (Figure 12-8) or chances to remain in remission (Figure 12-10). Thus evidence-based algorithms are not

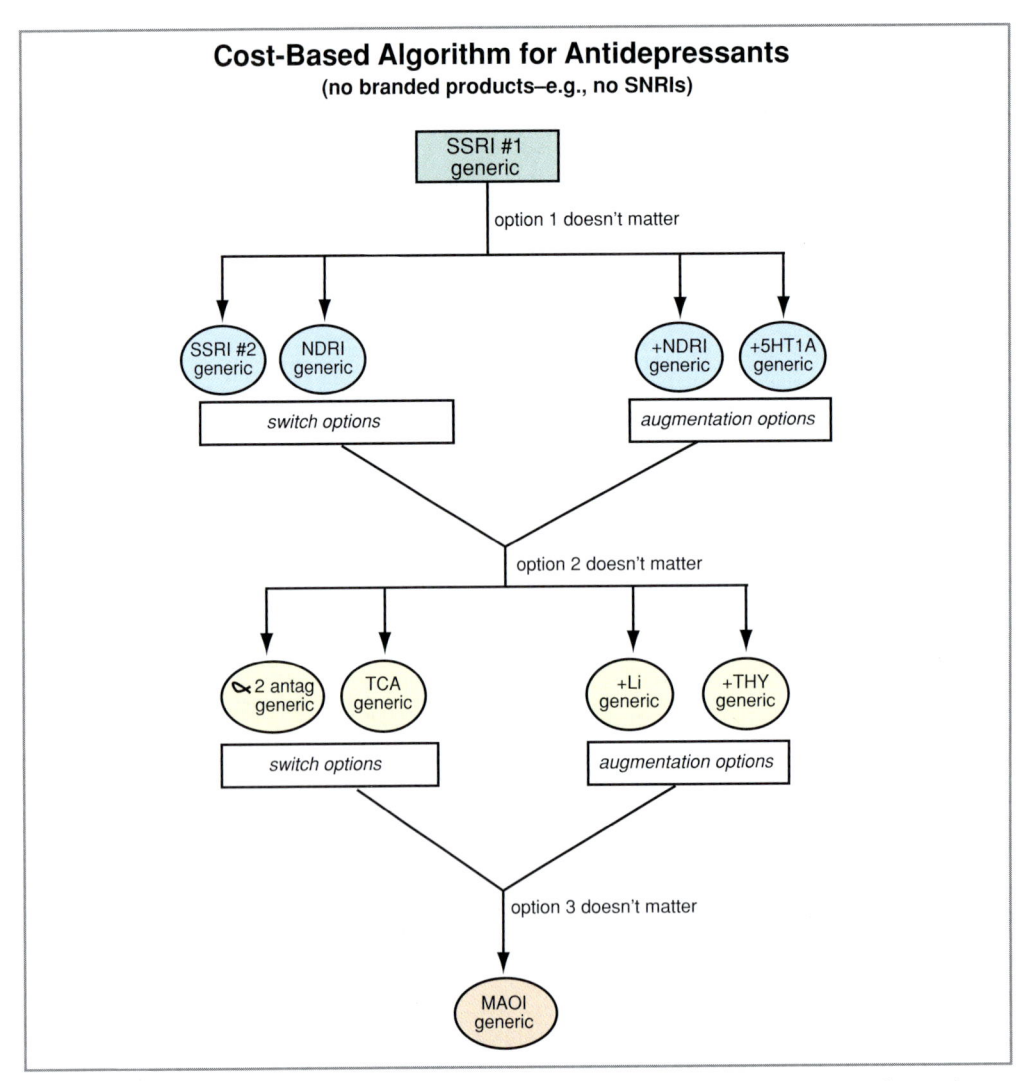

FIGURE 12-119 Cost-based algorithm for antidepressants. If a cost-based approach were taken for creating an antidepressant algorithm, as some experts and agencies have suggested, many useful options would likely be restricted, making it difficult to tailor treatment to each individual's needs.

able to provide clear guidelines on how to choose an antidepressant and what to do if an antidepressant does not work.

Cost-based antidepressant selections

In the absence of clear evidence of superiority of one option over another, some experts and agencies have suggested that payors should fund only low-cost treatments and thus follow a cost-based algorithm for antidepressants (Figure 12-119). Such an approach would guide prescribers through a series of options of inexpensive generic products and eliminate the use of branded products. That would mean different things in different countries but would essentially rule out the use of SNRIs, some SSRIs, once-daily NDRIs, atypical antipsychotics, modafinil, and most new stimulants from the depression pharmacy (Figure 12-117) until all the less expensive options were tried first and failed (Figure 12-118). This is a rather nihilistic approach to the treatment of depression and does not allow tailoring the best treatment available to an individual.

Symptom-based antidepressant selections

Finally, the neurobiologically informed psychopharmacologist may opt for adapting a symptom-based approach to selecting or combining a series of antidepressants (Figures 12-120 to 12-127). This strategy allows the construction of a portfolio of multiple agents to treat all residual symptoms of unipolar depression until the patient achieves sustained remission (Figures 12-120 to 12-127). This is the approach advocated by this book; it is based on the notion of tailoring treatments for individual patients.

First, symptoms are constructed into a diagnosis and then deconstructed into a list of specific symptoms that the individual patient is experiencing. Next, these symptoms are matched with the brain circuits that hypothetically mediate these symptoms and with the known neuropharmacological regulation of these circuits by neurotransmitters. Finally, available treatment options that target these neuropharmacological mechanisms are chosen to eliminate symptoms one by one. When symptoms persist, a treatment with a different mechanism is added or switched. No evidence proves that this is a superior approach, but it appeals not only to clinical intuition but also to neurobiological reasoning. In the absence of options that have proven superiority, the symptom-based approach is what is advocated here and what has mostly been followed throughout this book.

Reduced positive affect versus increased negative affect

For example, already discussed is how depression can be conceptualized as having symptoms either of reduced positive affect, increased negative affect, or both, with reduced positive affect hypothetically linked to dysregulation of DA (and NE) and with increased negative affect hypothetically linked to dysregulation of 5HT (and NE) (Figure 11-55). Applying this to antidepressant selection, patients with reduced positive affect may benefit from agents that boost DA activity, including NDRIs, SNRIs, selective NRIs, or MAOIs as first-line options, with the possibility of utilizing modafinil or stimulants as augmenting agents (Figure 12-120). On the other hand, patients with increased negative affect may benefit from serotonergic antidepressants such as SSRIs, SNRIs, as well as SARIs, especially in augmentation (Figure 12-120). When patients have both sets of symptoms or when symptoms of reduced positive affect emerge as side effects of SSRIs or SNRIs, putting these options together can make sense (Figure 12-120). The much neglected MAOIs may also be useful here as monotherapy.

Residual symptoms and circuits after first-line treatment of depression

The symptom-based algorithm can be taken several steps further, as most patients have more complicated or unique residual symptoms than indicated in Figure 12-120. Recall that the most common residual symptoms following antidepressant treatment are insomnia, problems concentrating, and fatigue (Figures 12-9 and 12-121). Thus it would be a good idea to have a strategy with several effective tactics available for this commonly encountered situation. The symptom-based algorithm for choosing an antidepressant suggests that one first listen to the patient to determine the specific residual symptoms that are preventing full remission and then match them to hypothetically malfunctioning brain circuits (Figure 12-122). Malfunctioning circuits tied to specific symptoms of depression are discussed extensively in Chapter 11 and illustrated as well in Figures 11-46 through 11-54. Once the specific symptoms and their circuits are determined, the idea at this point is to target the regulatory neurotransmitters for these circuits and their associated symptoms with selected

Symptom-Based Algorithm for Antidepressants: Positive or Negative Affect

NDRI, NRI, SNRI
+ modafinil/stimulant
MAOI

SSRI, SNRI, SARI

reduced positive affect

DA + NE

5HT + NE

increased negative affect

MDD

DA + NE + 5HT

both reduced positive affect and increased negative affect

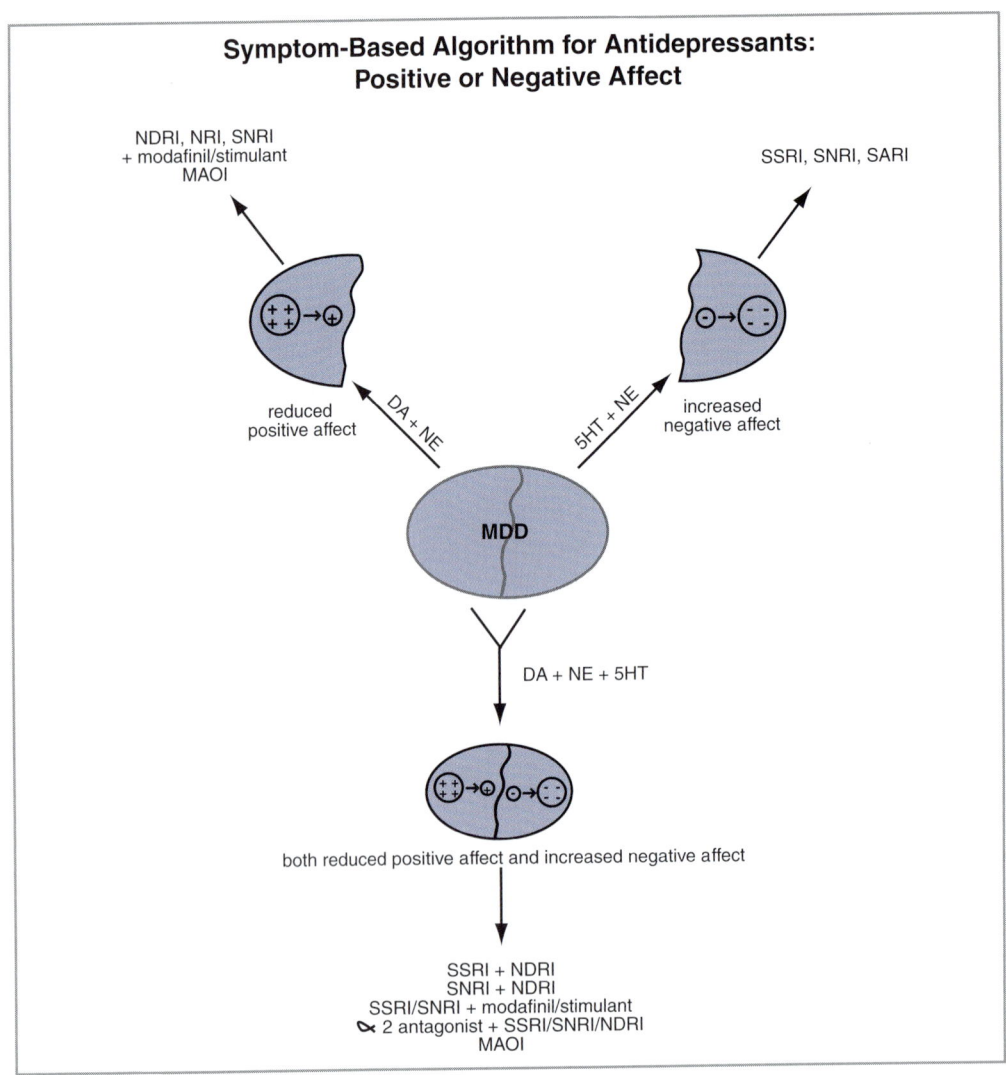

SSRI + NDRI
SNRI + NDRI
SSRI/SNRI + modafinil/stimulant
α 2 antagonist + SSRI/SNRI/NDRI
MAOI

FIGURE 12-120 Symptom-based algorithm for antidepressants. A symptom-based approach to antidepressant selection follows the theory that each of a patient's symptoms is matched with brain circuits and neurotransmitters that hypothetically mediate that symptom; this information is then used to select a corresponding pharmacological mechanism. One way to apply the symptom-based approach is to determine whether symptoms represent reduced positive affect, which is mediated by dopamine (DA) and norepinephrine (NE), or increased negative affect, which is mediated by serotonin (5HT) or NE or both. Treatment options can then be selected based on the hypothetically mediating neurotransmitters. Agents such as norepinephrine dopamine reuptake inhibitors (NDRIs), norepinephrine reuptake inhibitors (NRIs), serotonin norepinephrine reuptake inhibitors (SNRIs), and monoamine oxidase inhibitors (MAOIs) are thus options for treating reduced positive affect. On the other hand, agents such as serotonin selective reuptake inhibitors (SSRIs), SNRIs, and serotonin 2A antagonist/reuptake inhibitors (SARIs) are thus options for increased negative affect. Patients with both sets of symptoms may benefit from combination treatment or an MAOI.

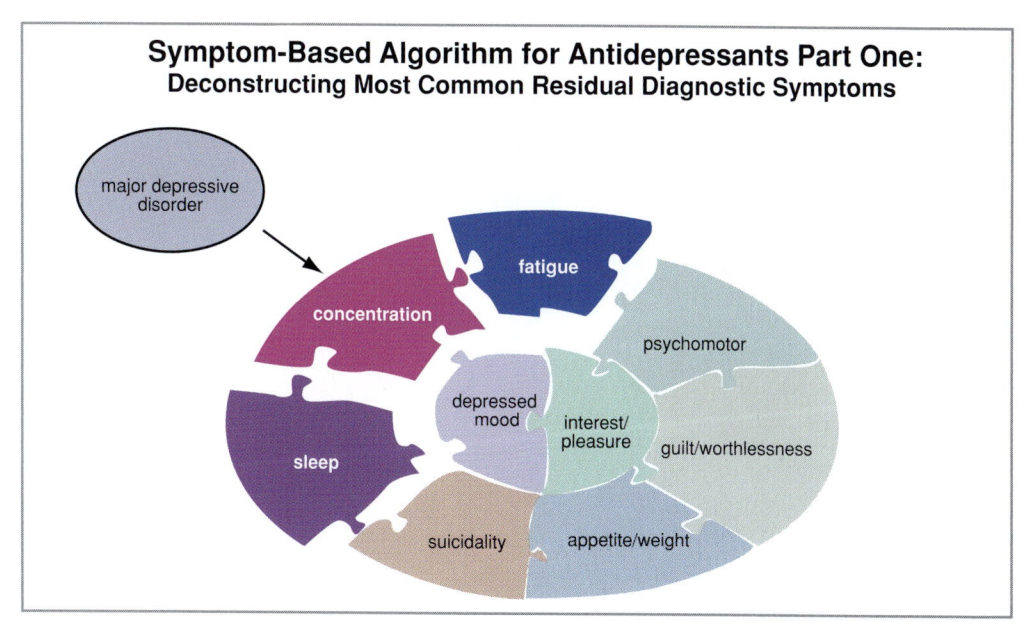

FIGURE 12-121 Symptom-based algorithm for antidepressants, part 1. Shown here is the diagnosis of major depressive disorder deconstructed into its symptoms [as defined by the *Diagnostic and Statistical Manual of Mental Disorders*, fourth edition (DSM-IV)]. Of these, sleep disturbances, problems concentrating, and fatigue are the most common residual symptoms.

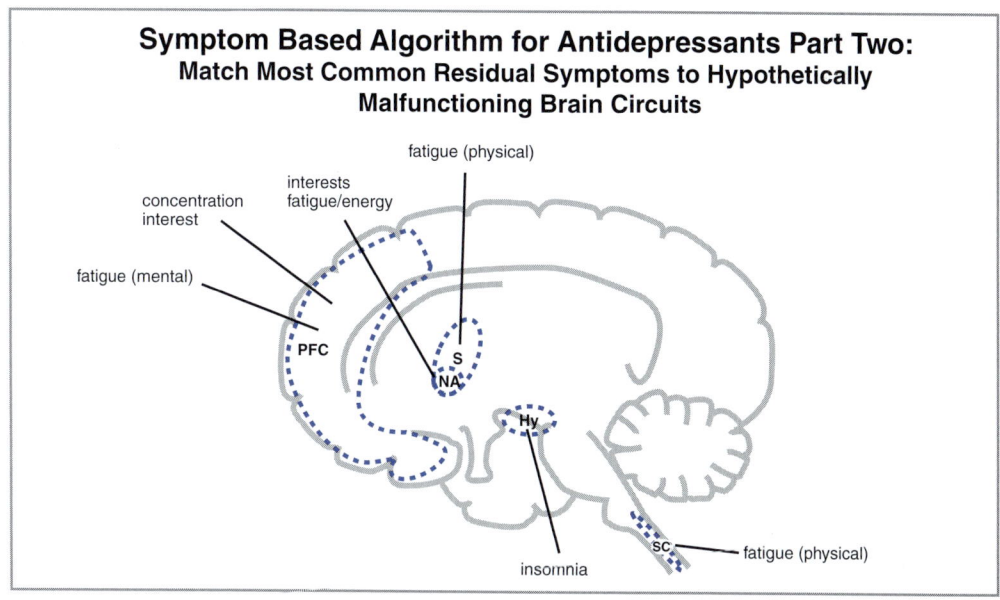

FIGURE 12-122 Symptom-based algorithm for antidepressants, part 2. In this figure the most common residual symptoms of major depression are linked to hypothetically malfunctioning brain circuits. Insomnia may be linked to the hypothalamus, problems concentrating to the dorsolateral prefrontal cortex (PFC), reduced interest to the PFC and nucleus accumbens (NA), and fatigue to the PFC, striatum (S), NA, and spinal cord (SC).

Antidepressants | 645

Symptom-Based Algorithm for Antidepressants Part Three:
Target Regulatory Neurotransmitters With Selected Pharmacological Mechanisms

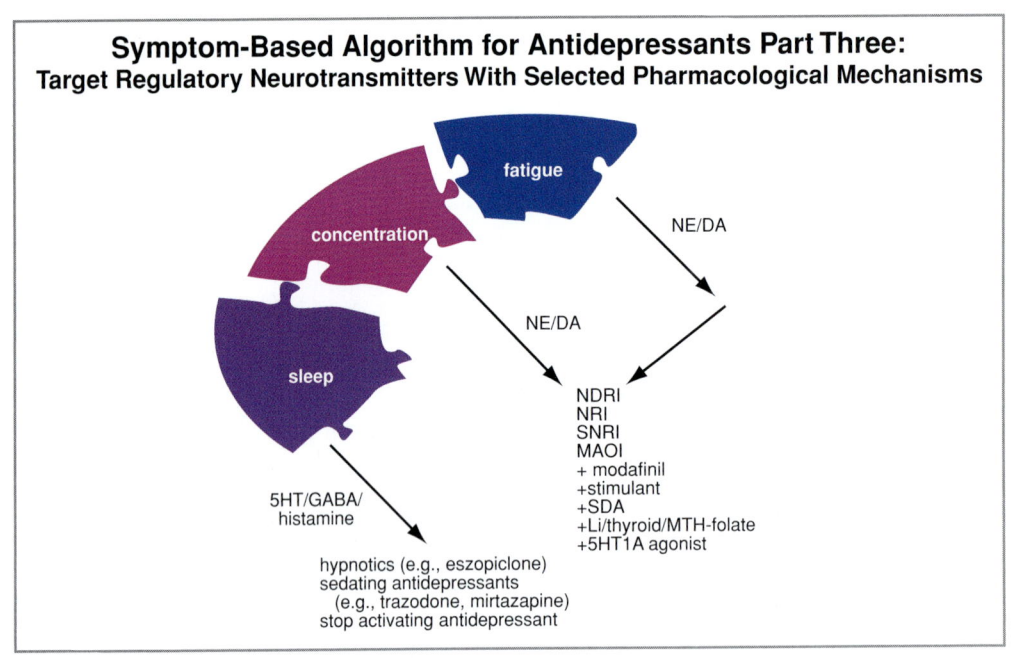

fatigue → NE/DA
concentration → NE/DA
→ NDRI
NRI
SNRI
MAOI
+ modafinil
+stimulant
+SDA
+Li/thyroid/MTH-folate
+5HT1A agonist

sleep → 5HT/GABA/histamine
→ hypnotics (e.g., eszopiclone)
sedating antidepressants
(e.g., trazodone, mirtazapine)
stop activating antidepressant

FIGURE 12-123 Symptom-based algorithm for antidepressants, part 3. Residual symptoms of depression can be linked to the neurotransmitters that regulate them and then, in turn, to pharmacological mechanisms. Fatigue and concentration are regulated in large part by norepinephrine (NE) and dopamine (DA), which are affected by many antidepressants, including norepinephrine dopamine reuptake inhibitors (NDRIs), selective norepinephrine reuptake inhibitors (NRIs), serotonin norepinephrine reuptake inhibitors (SNRIs), and monoamine oxidase inhibitors (MAOIs). Augmenting agents that affect NE and/or DA include modafinil, stimulants, serotonin dopamine antagonists (SDAs), lithium, thyroid hormone, L-5-methyl-tetrahydrofolate (MTHF), and serotonin (5HT) 1A agonists. Sleep disturbance is regulated by 5HT, gamma-aminobutyric acid (GABA), and histamine and can be treated with sedative hypnotics, sedating antidepressants such as trazodone or mirtazapine, or by discontinuing an activating antidepressant.

pharmacological mechanisms, as shown specifically for these common residual symptoms in Figure 12-123.

For problems with concentration and interest as well as for fatigue, this approach suggests targeting both NE and DA with first-line antidepressants plus augmenting agents that act on these neurotransmitters, as indicated in Figure 12-123. This can also call for stopping the SSRI if it is partially the cause of these symptoms. On the other hand, for insomnia, this symptom is hypothetically associated with an entirely different malfunctioning circuit regulated by different neurotransmitters (Figure 12-123). Therefore the treatment of this symptom calls for a different approach – namely, the use of hypnotics that act on the GABA system or sedating antidepressants that work to block rather than boost the serotonin or histamine system (Figure 12-123). It is possible that any of the symptoms shown in Figure 12-123 would respond to whatever drug is administered, but this symptom-based approach can tailor the treatment portfolio to the individual patient, possibly finding a faster way of reducing specific symptoms with more tolerable treatment selections for each patient than a purely random approach.

The symptom-based approach for selecting antidepressants may be even more important when targeting symptoms that are not components of the formal diagnostic criteria for depression but are common, bothersome, and likely to interfere with attaining remission

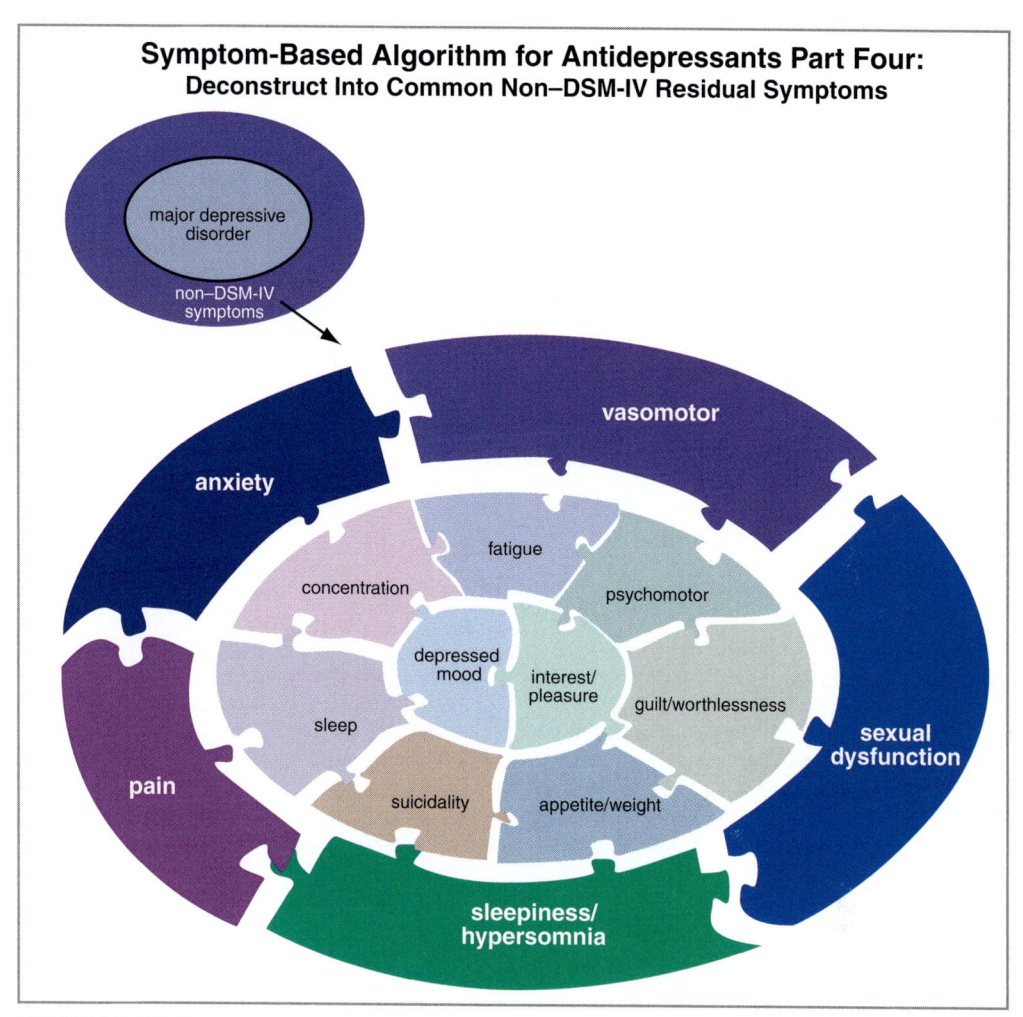

FIGURE 12-124 Symptom-based algorithm for antidepressants, part 4. There are several common symptoms of depression that are nonetheless not part of the formal diagnostic criteria for major depressive disorder. These include painful physical symptoms, excessive daytime sleepiness/hypersomnia with problems of arousal and alertness, anxiety, vasomotor symptoms, and sexual dysfunction.

if they persist (Figure 12-124). Five such symptoms commonly associated with depression which, however, are not formal components of the major depressive disorder symptom profile are highlighted in Figures 12-124 through 12-127 and include anxiety, pain, excessive daytime sleepiness/hypersomnia/problems with arousal and alertness, sexual dysfunction, and vasomotor symptoms (in women) (Figures 12-124 to 12-126).

Comorbid psychiatric illnesses distinct from major depression can also occur with a major depressive episode (Figure 12-127). Each of these comorbid conditions will likely require the elimination of all symptoms if a patient with major depression is to achieve a true remission. Treatment of each of these comorbid conditions is discussed in later chapters on sleep/wake disorders, anxiety disorders, attention deficit hyperactivity disorder, drug and alcohol abuse/dependence, and chronic pain.

In taking a history of symptoms before and after treatment with each antidepressant intervention, it is a good idea to solicit whether any of these comorbid conditions exist as

Antidepressants | 647

Symptom Based Algorithm for Antidepressants Part Five: Match Common Non-DSM-IV Residual Symptoms to Hypothetically Malfunctioning Brain Circuits

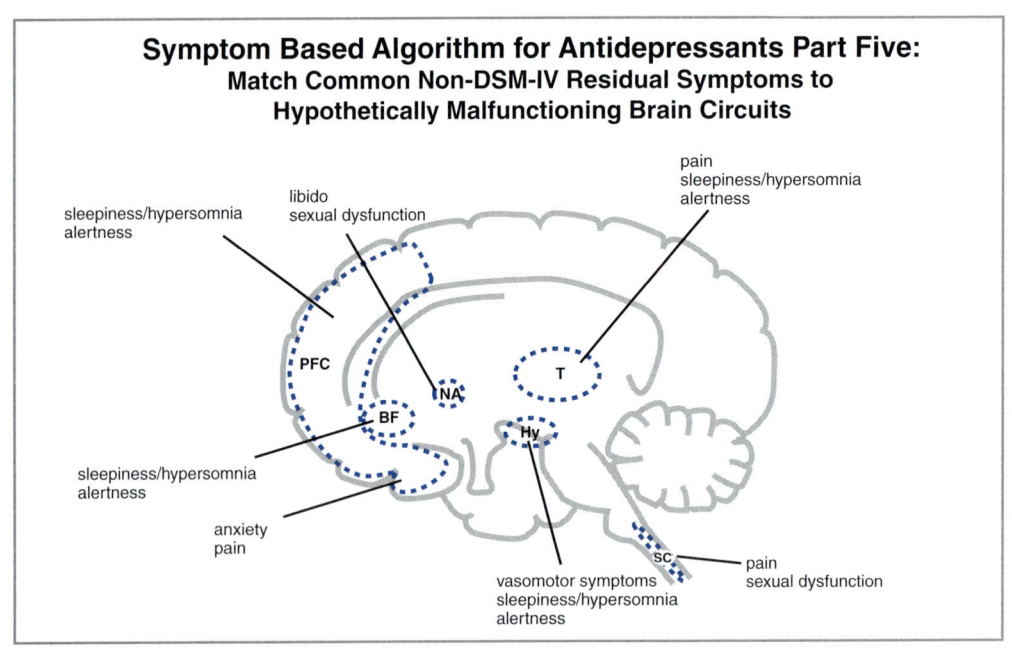

FIGURE 12-125 Symptom-based algorithm for antidepressants, part 5. In this figure common residual symptoms of major depression that are not part of formal diagnostic criteria are linked to hypothetically malfunctioning brain circuits. Painful physical symptoms are linked to the spinal cord (SC), thalamus (T), and ventral portions of the prefrontal cortex (PFC), while anxiety is associated with the ventral PFC. Vasomotor symptoms are mediated by the hypothalamus (Hy) and sexual dysfunction by the SC and nucleus accumbens (NA). Sleep symptoms that are part of the diagnostic criteria of depression involve mostly insomnia, linked to the hypothalamus; however, shown here are problems with hypersomnia and excessive daytime sleepiness, which may be beyond those symptoms included in the diagnostic criteria and be linked to problems with arousal and alertness and to arousal pathways not only in the hypothalamus but also the thalamus (T), basal forebrain (BF), and prefrontal cortex (PFC).

well as whether any of the nondiagnostic symptoms of depression are present along with the nine formal diagnostic symptoms of major depression (Figure 11-44). Each patient should have his or her major depressive episode deconstructed not only into diagnostic symptoms but also into all associated symptoms and comorbid conditions on each visit (Figure 12-124). Each and every symptom can then be mapped onto hypothetically malfunctioning brain circuits (Figure 12-125).

The pathways for the five additional nondiagnostic symptoms shown in Figure 12-126 obviously involve some differences from the pathways for the nine diagnostic symptoms shown in Figures 11-45 to 11-54 and thus often require different treatment approaches based on the unique pharmacological regulatory mechanisms that must be targeted to relieve these symptoms of depression as well. Sometimes it is said that for a good clinician to get patients with major depression into remission, he or she must target at least fourteen of the nine symptoms of depression!

Fortunately psychiatric drug treatments do not respect psychiatric disorders. Treatments that target pharmacological mechanisms in specific brain circuits do so no matter what psychiatric disorder is associated with the symptom linked to that circuit. Thus symptoms of one psychiatric disorder may be treatable with a proven agent that is known to treat the same symptom in another psychiatric disorder.

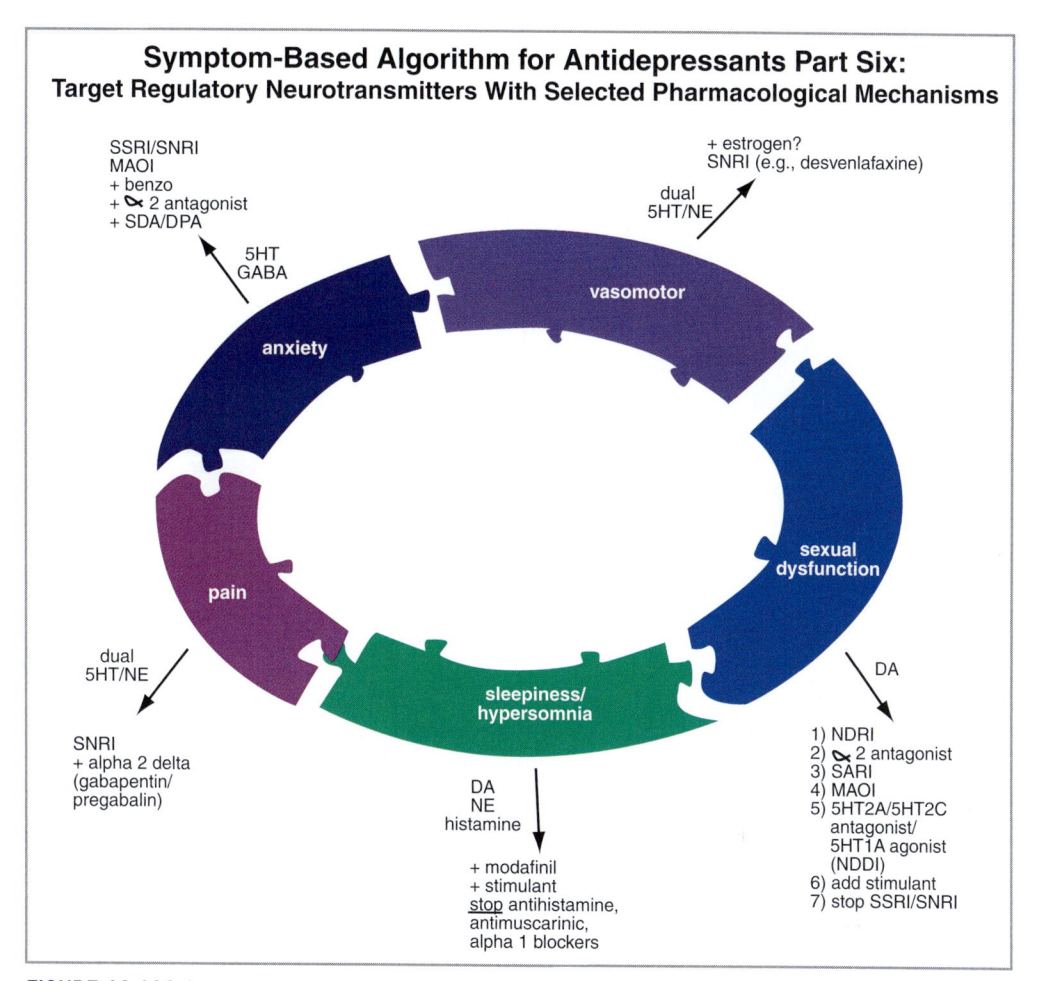

FIGURE 12-126 Symptom-based algorithm for antidepressants, part 6. Residual symptoms of depression can be linked to the neurotransmitters that regulate them and then, in turn, to pharmacological mechanisms. Painful physical symptoms are mediated by norepinephrine (NE) and to a lesser extent serotonin (5HT) and may be treated with serotonin norepinephrine reuptake inhibitors (SNRIs) or alpha 2 delta ligands (pregabalin, gabapentin). Anxiety is related to 5HT and gamma-aminobutyric acid (GABA); it can be treated with serotonin selective reuptake inhibitors (SSRIs), SNRIs, or monoamine oxidase inhibitors (MAOIs) as monotherapies as well as by augmentation with benzodiazepines, alpha 2 antagonists, serotonin dopamine antagonists (SDAs), or dopamine partial agonists (DPAs). Vasomotor symptoms may be modulated by NE and 5HT and treated with SNRIs; augmentation with estrogen therapy is also an option. Sexual dysfunction is regulated primarily by dopamine (DA) and may be treated with norepinephrine dopamine reuptake inhibitors (NDRIs), alpha 2 antagonists, serotonin 2A antagonist/reuptake inhibitors (SARIs), MAOIs, 5HT2A/5HT2C antagonists, 5HT1A agonists, addition of a stimulant, or by stopping an SSRI or SNRI. Hypersomnia and problems with arousal and alertness are regulated by DA, NE, and histamine and can be treated with activating agents such as modafinil or stimulants or by stopping sedating agents with antihistamine, antimuscarinic, and/or alpha 1 blocking properties.

For example, anxiety can be reduced in patients with major depression who do not meet full criteria for an anxiety disorder with the same serotonin and GABA mechanisms proven to work in anxiety disorders (to be discussed in more detail in Chapter 14, on anxiety disorders) (Figure 12-126).

Sleepiness/hypersomnia is a common associated symptom of depression but not all that frequently detected because patients who have this problem surprisingly do not often

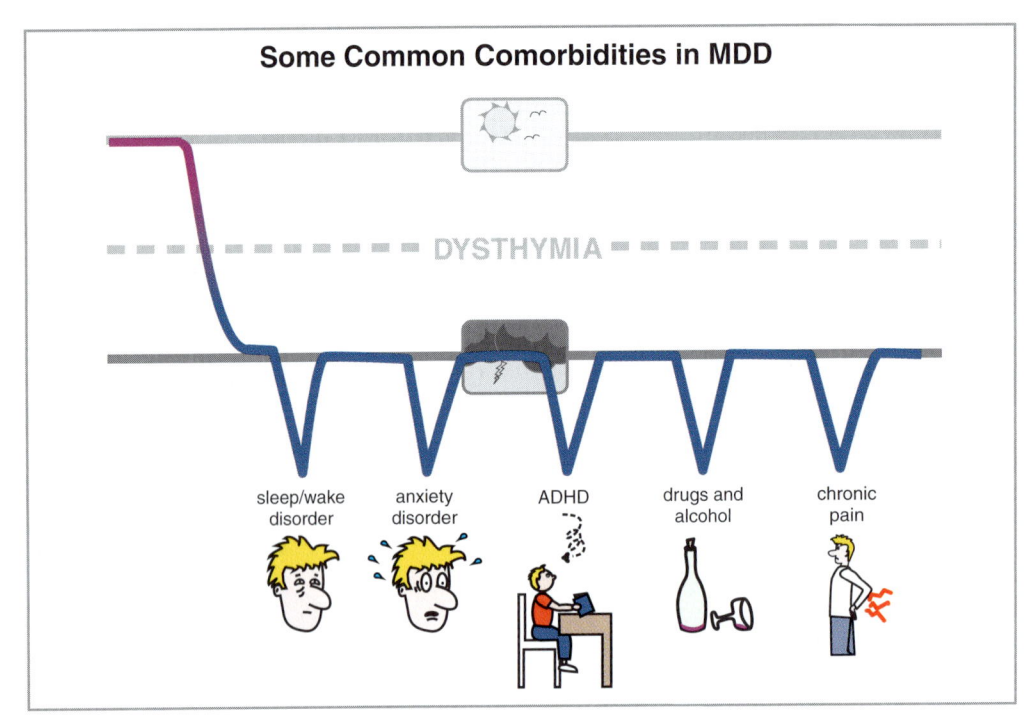

FIGURE 12-127 Common comorbidities in major depressive disorder (MDD). Some common comorbidities in MDD include sleep/wake disorders, anxiety disorders, attention deficit hyperactivity disorder (ADHD), substance use disorders, and chronic painful conditions.

complain about it. Although sleep disturbance in general is one of the diagnostic criteria for a major depressive episode (Figures 11-44 and 12-121), the specific sleep disturbance is usually insomnia. "Hypersomnia" can less commonly be one of the diagnostic criteria for a major depressive episode, but in this instance generally means oversleeping in the form of prolonged sleep episodes at night or increased daytime sleep. What is emphasized in Figures 12-124 and 12-126 is a type of hypersomnia that is frequently missed in patients with a major depressive episode because they often fail to complain about it: namely, excessive daytime sleepiness but not necessarily oversleeping. This type of hypersomnia/sleepiness is hypothetically linked to problems with arousal mechanisms and alertness as well as to problems with cognitive and executive functioning and is hypothetically linked with a different set of brain circuits (see Figure 12-125) than insomnia (Figure 12-122). Thus, excessive daytime sleepiness/hypersomnia/alertness is included here as one of the non–DSM-IV residual symptoms in Figures 12-124 and 12-125. Mechanisms to be targeted for sleepiness and hypersomnia in major depression are the same mechanisms proven effective for these same symptoms when they occur in various sleep/wake disorders, including agents that can boost DA, NE, and/or histamine (Figure 12-126). Sleepiness/hypersomnia is discussed in Chapter 16, on sleep/wake disorders.

Painful physical symptoms are present in many if not most depressed patients yet are not considered part of the diagnostic criteria for a major depressive episode. Nevertheless, it is important to relieve painful symptoms to attain remission of depression; approaches include a dual 5HT/NE strategy with possible augmentation by alpha 2 delta ligands, which is the same approach utilized in patients with chronic pain disorders (Figure 12-126). Treatment of chronic pain is discussed in Chapter 15, on pain.

Vasomotor symptoms that can accompany depression in perimenopausal and menopausal women have already been discussed. As mentioned, vasomotor symptoms in depressed women can be targeted with the same medications utilized to treat vasomotor symptoms in patients who are not depressed – namely, SNRIs.

Finally, sexual dysfunction can be a complicated problem of many causes and can range from lack of libido to problems with arousal of peripheral genitalia to lack of orgasm/ejaculation. Increasing DA or decreasing 5HT are the usual approaches to this set of problems whether the patient has major depression or not (Figure 12-126). Sexual dysfunction is discussed in more detail in Chapter 19, on reward.

In summary, the symptom-based algorithm for selecting and combining antidepressants and for building a portfolio of mechanisms until each diagnostic and associated symptom of depression is abolished is the modern psychopharmacologist's approach to major depression. This approach follows contemporary notions of neurobiological disease and drug mechanisms. The symptom-based approach to treating major depression is not the only way to select treatments for this disorder, and it is important to remember that no matter what approach is chosen, the goal of treatment is remission.

Should antidepressant combinations be the standard for treating unipolar major depressive disorder?

Given the disappointing number of patients who attain remission from a major depressive episode even after four consecutive treatments (Figure 12-8) and who can maintain that remission over the long run (Figure 12-10), the paradigm of monotherapy for major depression is rapidly changing to one of multiple simultaneous pharmacological mechanisms, often with two or more therapeutic agents. In this respect, the pattern is following that of the treatment of bipolar disorder, which usually requires administration of more than one agent, as discussed in Chapter 13, on mood stabilizers. Rather than have a simple regimen of one antidepressant and a patient who is not in remission, it now seems highly preferable to have a patient in remission without symptoms no matter how many agents this takes. Several specific suggestions of antidepressant combinations are shown in Figures 12-128 to 12-134. Many others can be constructed, but these particular combinations or "combos" have enjoyed widespread use even though there is not much in the way of actual evidence-based data from clinical trials to show that their combination results in superior efficacy. Nevertheless, these suggestions may be useful for practicing clinicians to use in some patients.

Single-action and multiple-action monotherapies have already been extensively discussed in this chapter, as have combos containing lithium, thyroid, serotonin 2A antagonists and dopaminergic agents (Figure 12-128). Several additional combos are shown in Figure 12-128; they are discussed here and illustrated as well in Figures 12-129 through 12-134.

5HT1A Combo

The serotonin 1A partial agonist (SPA) buspirone is an approved treatment for anxiety but is more commonly used to augment patients with major depressive episodes who are partial responders to SSRIs (Figures 12-128 and 12-129). The beta blocker pindolol is also a partial agonist at 5HT1A receptors and has been utilized experimentally as an augmenting agent to SSRIs (Figure 12-128). Gepirone, a new 5HT1A partial agonist, is in late clinical testing in depression and may be useful not only as an augmenting agent for partial responders to SSRIs, but also as a monotherapy for major depression.

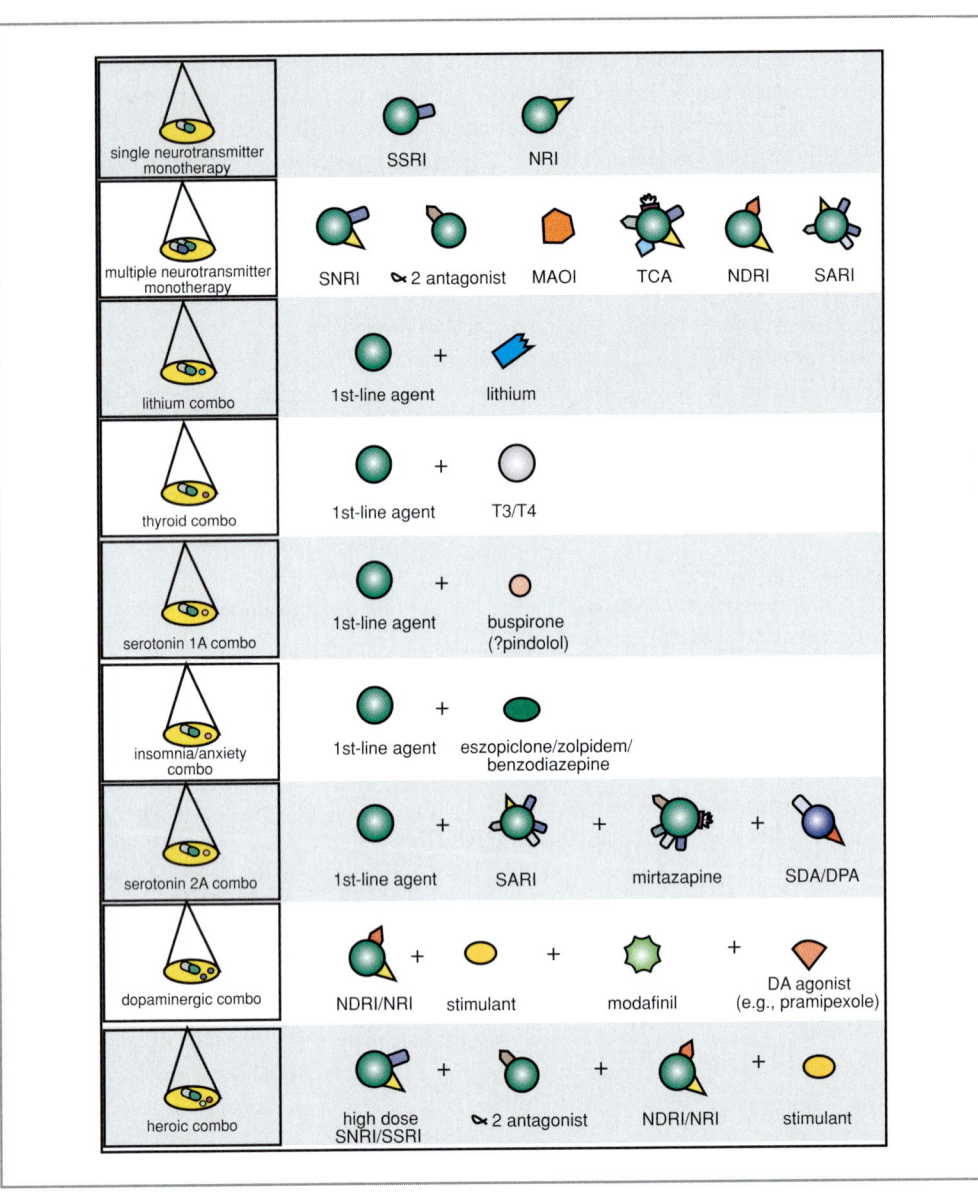

FIGURE 12-128 **Combination treatments for unipolar depression.** The treatment of depression generally begins with a single agent, called a first-line agent, as monotherapy. If single agents acting by a single neurotransmitter mechanism fail, then single agents acting by multiple neurotransmitter mechanisms may be effective. If these monotherapies also fail, antidepressants are often used in combination with other drugs or hormones or even other antidepressants. For example, a first-line agent can be paired with lithium (lithium combo). Another strategy is to augment a first-line agent with thyroid hormone (thyroid combo). Yet another approach is addition of the serotonin 1A (5HT1A) partial agonist buspirone or possibly the 5HT1A antagonist pindolol to a first-line antidepressant, especially a serotonin selective reuptake inhibitor (serotonin 1A combo). Short-term use of sedative–hypnotics or anxiolytics may be necessary if insomnia or anxiety is persistent and cannot be managed by other strategies (insomnia/anxiety combo). Another multimechanism option is to add a serotonin 2A antagonist such as a serotonin 2 antagonist/reuptake inhibitor (SARI), mirtazapine, or a serotonin dopamine antagonist (SDA) or dopamine partial agonist (DPA) (serotonin 2A combo). Patients with fatigue or cognitive symptoms may benefit from the addition of an agent that enhances dopamine neurotransmission (dopaminergic combo). Finally, patients who are not responding may need to be treated with high doses of a first-line agent in combination with an alpha 2 antagonist, norepinephrine dopamine reuptake inhibitor, or stimulant.

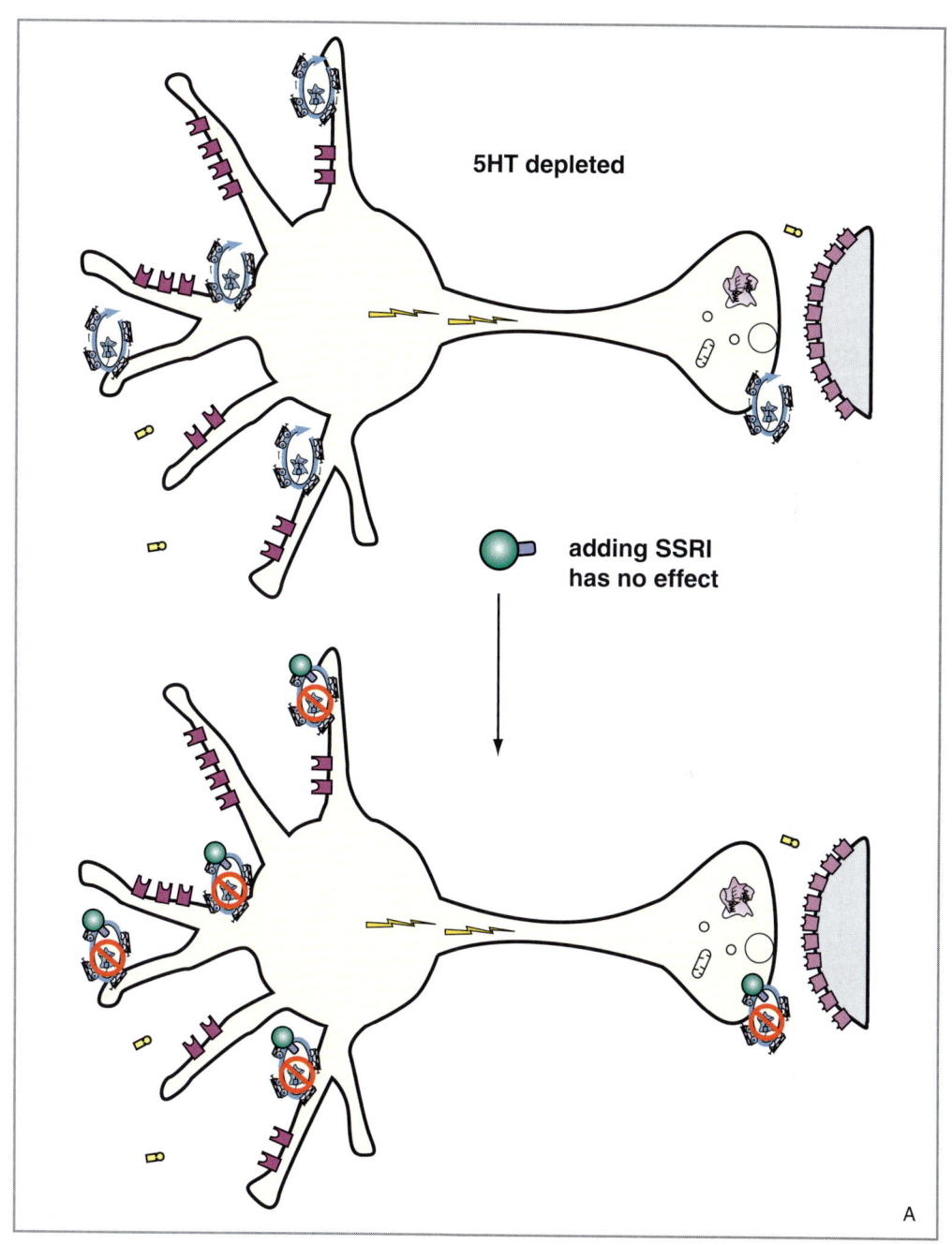

FIGURE 12-129A Mechanism of action of buspirone augmentation, part 1. Serotonin selective reuptake inhibitors (SSRIs) act indirectly by increasing synaptic levels of serotonin (5HT) that have been released there. If 5HT is depleted, there is no 5HT release and SSRIs are ineffective. This has been postulated to be the explanation for the lack of SSRI therapeutic actions or loss of therapeutic action of SSRI ("poop out") in some patients.

Antidepressants | 653

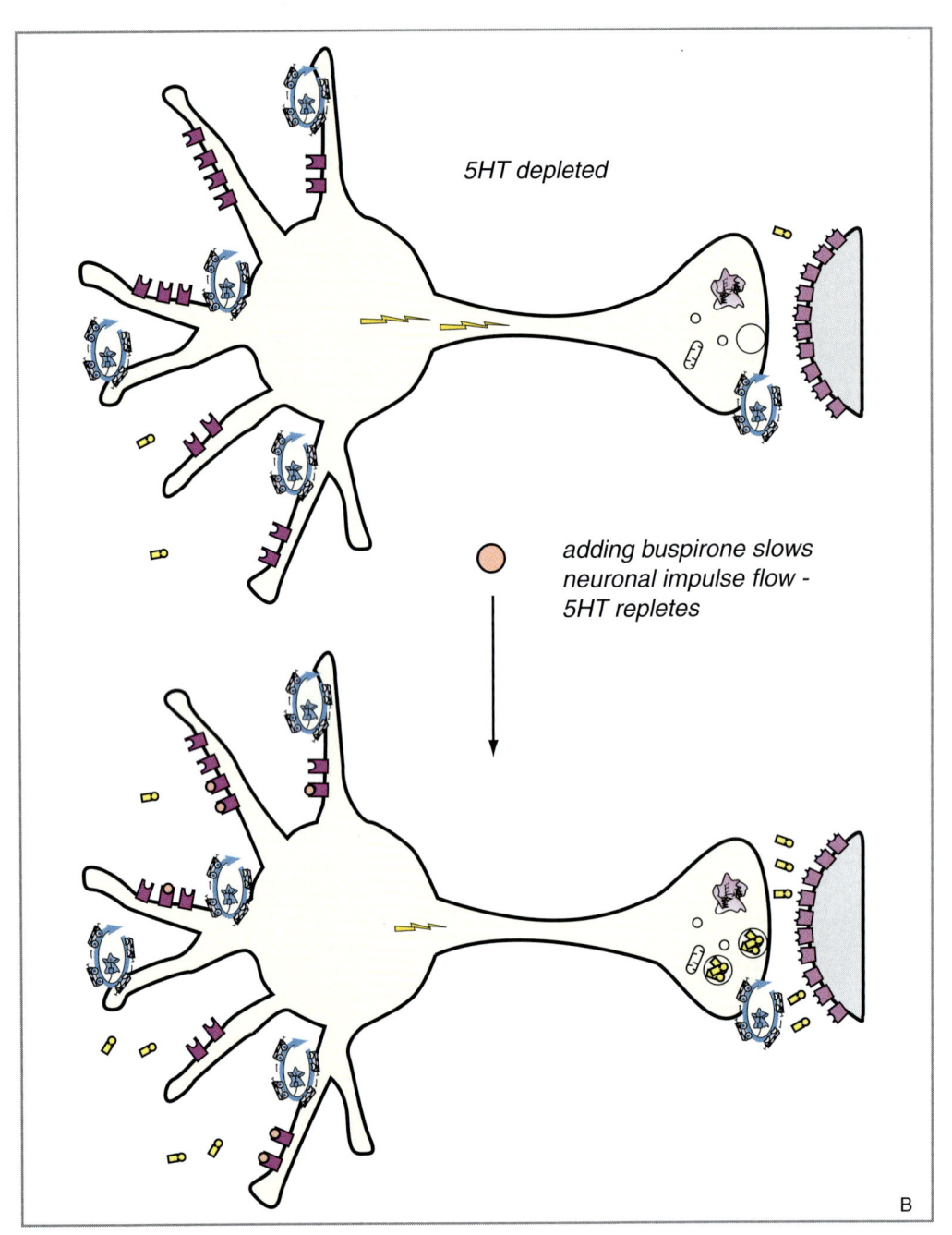

FIGURE 12-129B Mechanism of action of buspirone augmentation, part 2. Shown here is how buspirone may augment the action of serotonin selective reuptake inhibitors (SSRIs) both by repleting serotonin (5HT) and directly desensitizing 5HT1A receptors. One theoretical mechanism of how 5HT is allowed to reaccumulate in the 5HT-depleted neuron is the shutdown of neuronal impulse flow. If 5HT release is essentially turned off for a while so that the neuron retains all the 5HT it synthesizes, this may allow repletion of 5HT stores. A 5HT partial agonist such as buspirone acts directly on somatodendritic autoreceptors to inhibit neuronal impulse flow, possibly allowing repletion of 5HT stores. Also, buspirone could boost actions directly at 5HT1A receptors to help the small amount of 5HT available in this scenario accomplish the targeted desensitization of 5HT1A somatodendritic autoreceptors that is necessary for antidepressant actions.

now, SSRIs can act

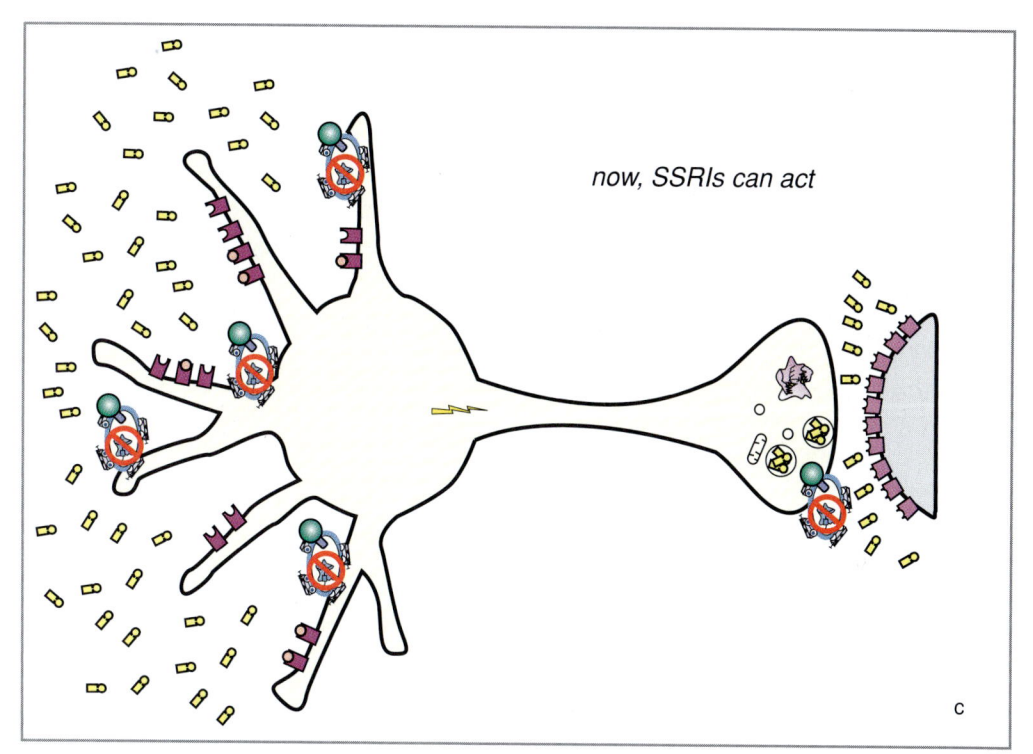

FIGURE 12-129C Mechanism of action of buspirone augmentation, part 3. Shown here is how buspirone potentiates ineffective serotonin selective reuptake inhibitor (SSRI) action at serotonin 1A (5HT1A) somatodendritic autoreceptors, resulting in the desired disinhibition of the 5HT neuron. This combination of 5HT1A agonists plus SSRIs may be more effective, not only in depression but also in other disorders treated by SSRIs, such as obsessive compulsive disorder and panic.

Heroic Combos

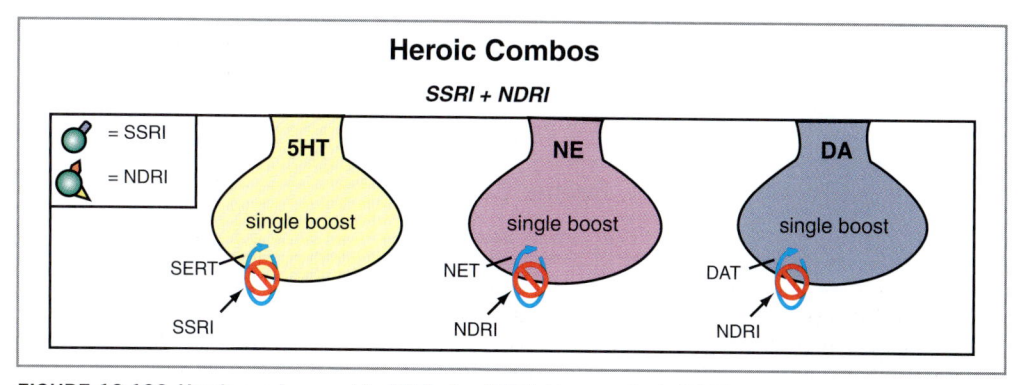

SSRI + NDRI

FIGURE 12-130 Heroic combos, part 1: SSRI plus NDRI. Here serotonin (5HT), norepinephrine (NE), and dopamine (DA) are all single-boosted.

Antidepressants | 655

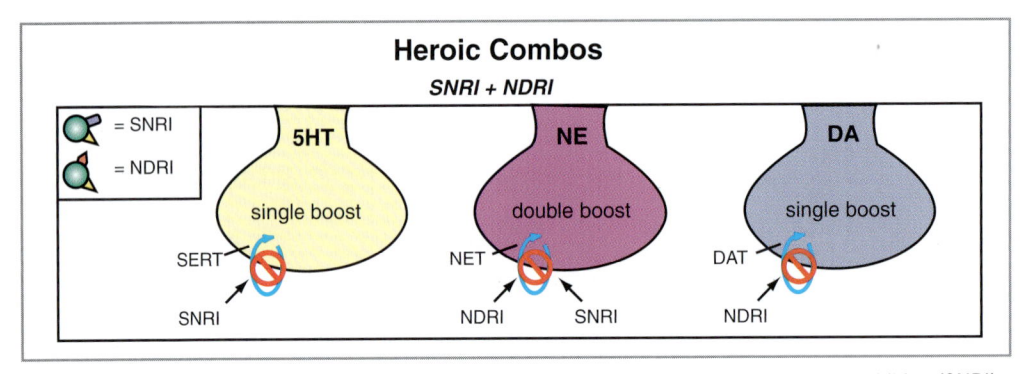

FIGURE 12-131 **Heroic combos, part 2: SNRI plus NDRI.** Serotonin norepinephrine reuptake inhibitor (SNRI) plus a norepinephrine dopamine reuptake inhibitor (NDRI) leads to a single boost for serotonin (5HT), a double boost for norepinephrine (NE), and a single boost for dopamine (DA).

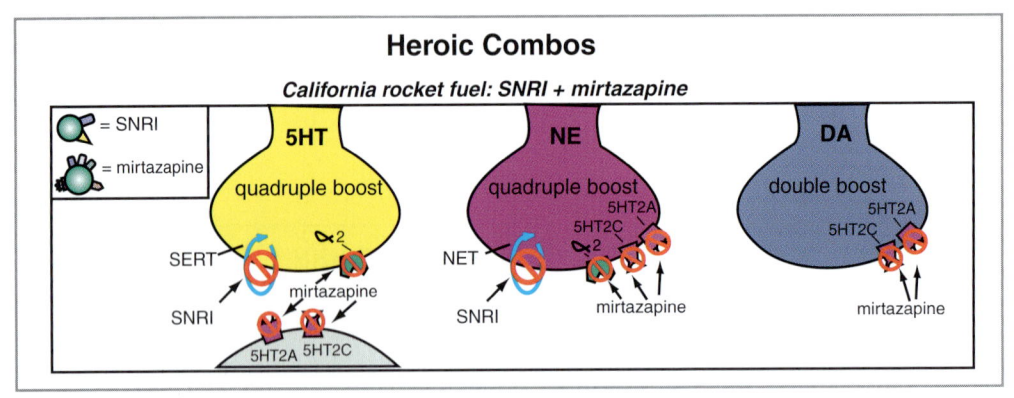

FIGURE 12-132 **Heroic combos, part 3: California rocket fuel (SNRI plus mirtazapine).** Serotonin norepinephrine reuptake inhibitor (SNRI) plus mirtazapine is a combination that has a great degree of theoretical synergy: norepinephrine reuptake blockade plus alpha 2 blockade, serotonin (5HT) reuptake plus 5HT2A and 5HT2C antagonism, and thus many 5HT actions plus norepinephrine (NE) actions. Specifically, 5HT is quadruple-boosted (with reuptake blockade, alpha 2 antagonism, 5HT2A antagonism, and 5HT2C antagonism), NE is quadruple-boosted (with reuptake blockade, alpha 2 antagonism, 5HT2A antagonism, and 5HT2C antagonism), and there may even be a double boost of dopamine (with 5HT2A and 5HT2C antagonism).

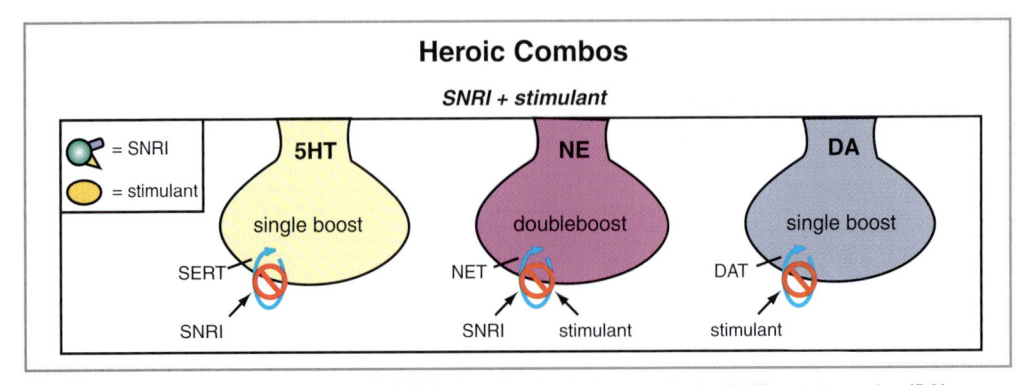

FIGURE 12-133 **Heroic combos, part 4: SNRI plus stimulant.** Here serotonin (5HT) and dopamine (DA) are single-boosted and norepinephrine (NE) is double-boosted.

Heroic Combos
SNRI + modafinil

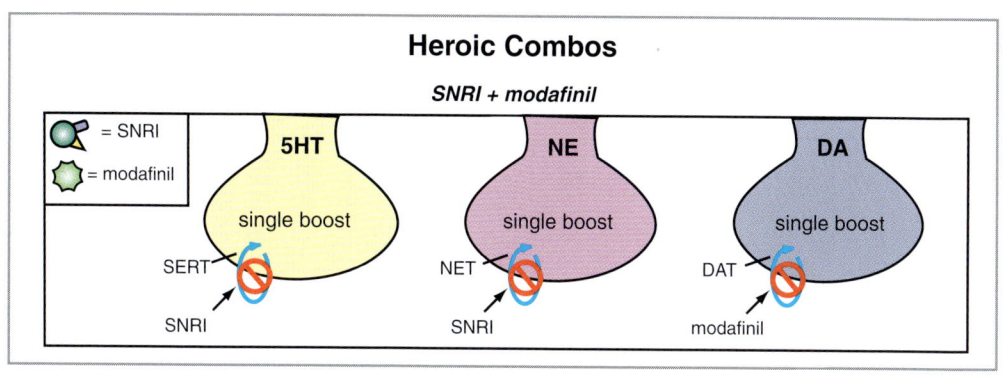

FIGURE 12-134 Heroic combos, part 5: SNRI plus modafinil. Here serotonin (5HT) and norepinephrine (NE) are single-boosted by the serotonin norepinephrine reuptake inhibitor (SNRI) while dopamine (DA) is single-boosted by modafinil.

Buspirone is a short-acting compound requiring twice- or thrice-daily administration; its peak-dose side effects of nausea and dizziness have interfered with its wide use as a monotherapy. Gepirone is being tested in a controlled-release formulation as gepirone ER and thus requires only once-daily administration, with lesser peak-dose side effects than buspirone. Possible additional advantages of gepirone ER over buspirone include being a "fuller" or "less partial" agonist than buspirone and possibly being metabolized to active metabolites, including a 5HT1A full agonist as well as another active metabolite with alpha 2 antagonist properties. The antidepressant actions of alpha 2 antagonism are discussed above, in the section on mirtazapine (see Figures 12-51 to 12-54). Unlike SSRIs and SNRIs, neither buspirone nor gepirone is associated with sexual dysfunction.

One theory for how the combination of a 5HT1A partial agonist with an SSRI can have enhanced efficacy is the notion that an SSRI monotherapy added to the regimen of a patient with severely depleted serotonin levels would have no therapeutic actions, since there is no serotonin released whose reuptake can be blocked by the SSRI (Figure 12-129A). However, adding a 5HT1A partial agonist like buspirone (or gepirone ER) would act at somatodendritic 5HT1A autoreceptors, and this would be predicted to allow serotonin levels to be repleted (Figure 12-129B). Now SSRIs would be able to act because serotonin would again be released and its reuptake could again be blocked (Figure 12-129C).

Triple-action combo: SSRI/SNRI ± NDRI

If boosting one neurotransmitter is good and two is better, maybe boosting three is best (one of the heroic combos in Figure 12-128 and also illustrated in Figures 12-130 and 12-131). Triple-action antidepressant therapy with modulation of all three of the trimonoamine neurotransmitter systems would be predicted to occur by combining either an SSRI with an NDRI, perhaps the most popular combination in U.S. antidepressant psychopharmacology (Figure 12-130), or combining an SNRI with an NDRI, providing even more noradrenergic and dopaminergic action (Figure 12-131).

California rocket fuel: SNRI plus mirtazapine

This potentially powerful combination utilizes the pharmacological synergy attained by adding the enhanced serotonin and norepinephrine release from inhibition of both dual serotonin and norepinephrine reuptake by an SNRI to the disinhibition of both

TABLE 12-14 Antidepressants in development: various monoaminergic mechanisms

Atypical antipsychotics as antidepressants for unipolar major depression
    quetiapine
    ziprasidone
    aripiprazole
    olanzapine
    risperidone
    paliperidone
    bifeprunox
    asenapine
    SX 313, 314

Triple reuptake inhibitors (TRIs): serotonin, norepinephrine and dopamine reuptake inhibitors (SNDRIs)
    DOV 216303
    DOV 21947
    GW 372475 (NS2359)
    Boehringer/NS2330
    NS2360
    Sepracor SEP 225289

TRI plus
    SRI>NRI>DRI/5HT2C, 5HT3, 5HT2A, alpha 1A
        Lu AA24530
    SRI>NRI>DRI/5HT6
        Lu AA37096
    SRI>NRI/5HT2A/alpha 1A/5HT6
        Lu AA34893

NDDIs – norepinephrine dopamine disinhibitors
    agomelatine (Valdoxan) – 5HT2C antagonist/melatonin 1/2 agonist
    flibanserin (Ectris) – 5HT2A/2C antagonist/5HT1A agonist – (for HSDD, hypoactive sexual desire disorder)

Beta 3 agonist
    amibegron (SR58611A)

---

serotonin and norepinephrine release by the alpha 2 antagonist actions of mirtazapine (Figure 12-132). It is even possible that additional pro-dopaminergic actions result from the combination of norepinephrine reuptake blockade in prefrontal cortex due to SNRI actions with 5HT2A/2C actions disinhibiting dopamine release (Figure 12-132). This combination can provide very powerful antidepressant action for some patients with unipolar major depressive episodes.

Arousal combos

The frequent complaints of residual fatigue, loss of energy, motivation, sex drive, and problems concentrating/problems with alertness may be approached by combining either a stimulant with an SNRI (Figure 12-133) or modafinil with an SNRI (Figure 12-134) to recruit triple monoamine action and especially enhancement of dopamine.

TABLE 12-15 Antidepressants in development: novel serotonin-linked mechanisms

5HT1A partial agonists
    gepirone ER
    PRX 00023
    MN 305
5HT6 agonists/antagonists
5HT1B/D antagonist
    elzasonan
SSRI plus 5HT1A PA
    vilazodone (SB 659746A)
Sigma 1/5HT1A PA>SRI
    VPI 013 (OPC 14523)
SSRI/5HT3>5HT1A
    Lu AA21004
5HT1A agonist/5HT2A antagonist
    TGW-00-AD/AA
SRI/5HT2/5HT1A/5HT1D
    TGBA-01-AD

Future treatments for mood disorders

An explosion of potential new treatments with novel mechanisms are in testing for major depression (Tables 12-14 to 12-17). This includes the use of **atypical antipsychotics** for unipolar major depression and for treatment-resistant unipolar depression (Table 12-14).

Atypical antipsychotics are discussed in greater detail in the following chapter on mood stabilizers and bipolar depression. Whether these same agents will be proven effective with a sufficiently favorable side effect and cost profile for unipolar depression is still under intense investigation.

A large number of **novel serotonin targets** are in testing and are listed in Table 12-15. The various receptors they target are discussed in Chapter 10 and illustrated in Figures 10-17 to 10-22. One particularly interesting novel serotonin target is the **5HT2C receptor**. This receptor was extensively discussed earlier in this chapter in relation to the SSRI fluoxetine (Figure 12-25) and to the SARI trazodone (Figure 12-64). Blockade of 5HT2C receptors causes release of both norepinephrine and dopamine, which is why these agents can be called **norepinephrine dopamine disinhibitors or NDDIs**. A novel antidepressant **agomelatine** (Valdoxan; Table 12-14) combines this property of 5HT2C antagonism and thus NDDI actions with additional agonist actions at melatonin receptors (MT1 and MT2) (Figure 12-135). Agomelatine also has 5HT2B antagonist properties. This portfolio of pharmacological actions predicts not only antidepressant actions due to the NDDI mechanism of 5HT2C antagonism but also sleep-enhancing properties due to MT1 and MT2 agonist actions (Figure 12-135). Another NDDI with 5HT2C antagonist properties is **flibanserin** (Ectris). This agent also has 5HT2A antagonist and 5HT1A agonist properties and, owing to its robust NDDI properties, is under investigation for sexual dysfunction linked to deficient dopamine activity, including conditions such as hypoactive sexual desire disorder (HSDD); it is discussed in Chapter 19, on reward.

TABLE 12-16 Antidepressants in development: targeting neurokinins

NK2 antagonists
    saredutant (SR48968)
    SAR 1022279
    SSR 241586 (NK2 and NK3)
    SR 144190
    GR 159897
NK3 antagonists
    osanetant (SR142801)
    talnetant (SB223412)
    SR 146977
Substance P antagonists
    aprepitant/MK869/L-754030 (Emend)
    L-758,298; L-829–165; L-733,060
    CP122721; CP99994; CP96345
    casopitant GW679769
    vestipitant GW 597599 +/− paroxetine
    LY 686017
    GW823296
    nolpitantium SR140333
    SSR240600; R-673
    NKP-608/AV608
    CGP49823
    SDZ NKT 34311
    SB679769
    GW597599
    vafopitant GR205171

TABLE 12-17 Antidepressants in development: targeting novel sites of action

MIF-1 pentapeptide analogs
    nemifitide (INN 00835)
    5-hydroxy-nemifitide (INN 01134)
Glucocorticoid antagonists
    mifepristone (Corlux)
    Org 34517; Org 34850 (glucocorticoid receptor II antagonists)
CRF1 antagonists
    R121919
    CP316,311
    BMS 562086
    GW876008
    ONO-233M
    JNJ19567470/TS041
    SSR125543
    SSR126374
Vasopressin 1B antagonists
    SSR149415

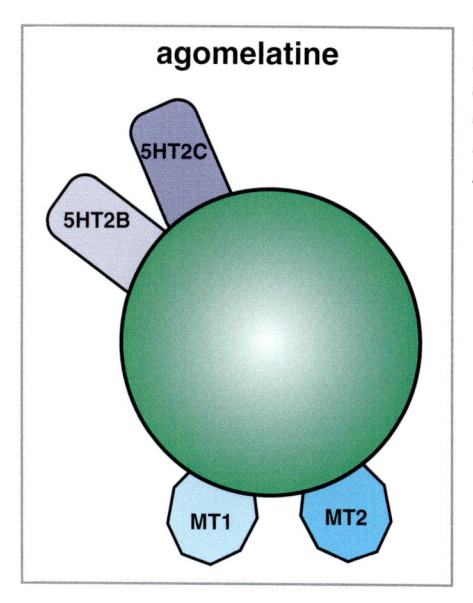

FIGURE 12-135 Icon of agomelatine. The novel antidepressant agomelatine, in testing, combines the property of serotonin (5HT) 2C antagonism (and thus indirect enhancement of norepinephrine and dopamine) with actions at melatonin 1 (M1) and melatonin 2 (M2) receptors. Agomelatine is also an antagonist at 5HT2B receptors.

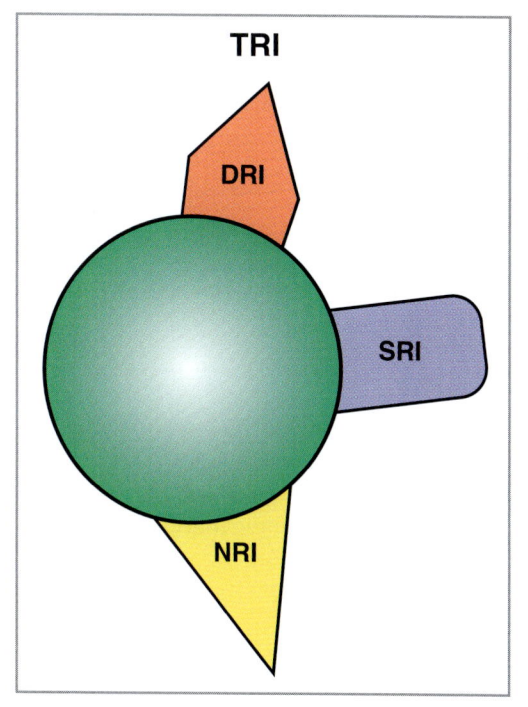

FIGURE 12-136 Icon of triple reuptake inhibitor (TRI). Several triple reuptake inhibitors (serotonin norepinephrine dopamine reuptake inhibitors) are in testing. Different agents may have different balances of serotonin to norepinephrine to dopamine reuptake blockade.

Triple reuptake inhibitors (TRIs) or serotonin-norepinephrine-dopamine-reuptake inhibitors (SNDRIs) (Figure 12-136)

These drugs are testing the idea that if one mechanism is good (i.e., SSRI) and two mechanisms are better (i.e., SNRI), then maybe targeting all three mechanisms of the trimonoamine neurotransmitter system would be the best in terms of efficacy. Several different

Beta 3 Receptors: Located in Amygdala

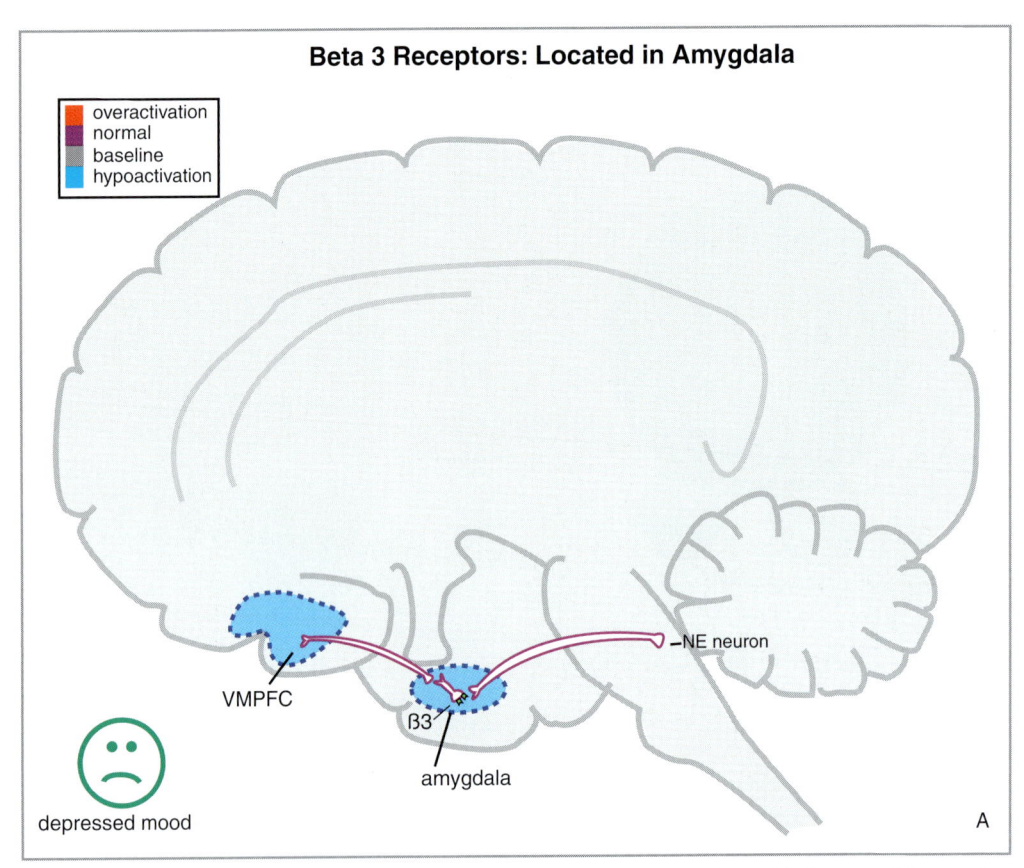

- overactivation
- normal
- baseline
- hypoactivation

VMPFC
β3
amygdala
NE neuron
depressed mood

A

FIGURE 12-137A Beta 3 receptors. Some data suggest that beta 3 receptors, located in the amygdala, may be related to depressed mood. Decreased efficiency of these receptors could lead to hypoactivation of the amygdala as well as brain regions closely connected to the amygdala, such as the ventromedial prefrontal cortex (VMPFC).

triple reuptake inhibitors (or serotonin-norepinephrine-dopamine reuptake inhibitors) are listed in Table 12-14. Some of these agents have additional pharmacological properties as well ("TRI plus" in Table 12-14). The question for TRIs is how much blockade of each monoamine transporter is desired, especially for the dopamine transporter or DAT. This was also discussed extensively in the section on NDRIs above. Too much dopamine activity can lead to a drug of abuse, and not enough means that the agent is essentially an SNRI. Perhaps the desirable profile is robust inhibition of the serotonin transporter and substantial inhibition of the norepinephrine transporter, like the known SNRI, plus a little frosting on the cake of 10% to 25% inhibition of DAT. Some testing suggests that DRI action also increases acetylcholine release, so TRIs may modulate a fourth neurotransmitter system and act as multitransmitter modulators. Further testing will determine whether the available TRIs will represent an advance over SSRIs or SNRIs in the treatment of depression.

Beta 3 agonist
A very novel mechanism for an antidepressant is posed by **amibegron**, an agonist of beta 3 receptors (Table 12-14). The role of beta 3 receptors in the brain is still being clarified, but it

**ß3 Agonist Actions in Amygdala:
Enhanced Neuronal Activity in VMPFC**

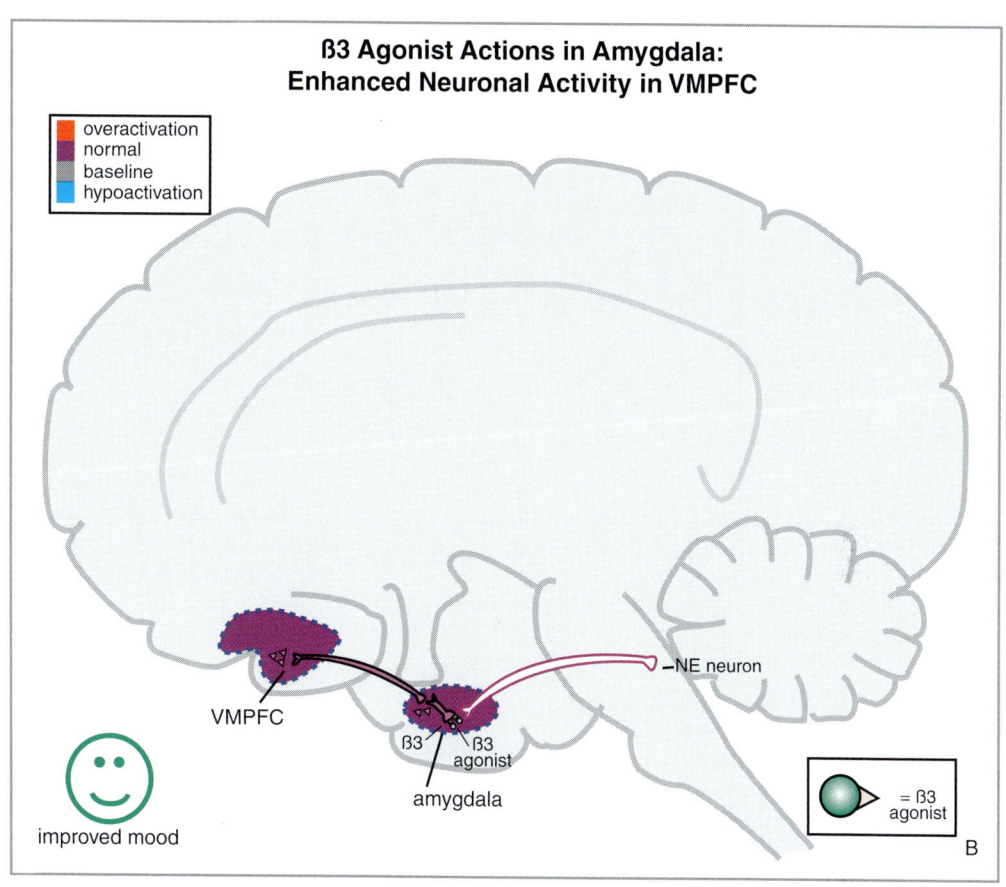

FIGURE 12-137B Beta 3 agonists. Agonists of beta 3 receptors in the amygdala may restore neurotransmission in that region, thus also restoring neurotransmission in the ventromedial prefrontal cortex (VMPFC). This may lead to improved mood. Amibegron is a beta 3 agonist currently in testing.

appears that they may be localized in high density in the amygdala, where they may regulate neuronal activity in ventromedial prefrontal cortex and thereby exert their antidepressant actions (Figure 12-137). Extensive testing in animal models of depression demonstrates the antidepressant actions of amibegron, and human testing is currently in progress.

Also, a large number of agents that act at several other novel targets are listed in Tables 12-16 and 12-17. Many of the agents listed in Table 12-17 are low-molecular-weight drugs that target stress hormone release from the hypothalamic-pituitary-adrenal (HPA) axis, including **glucocorticoid antagonists, corticotrophin releasing factor 1 (CRF1) antagonists, and vasopressin 1B antagonists**. These agents are in testing not only for depression but also for various stress-related conditions, and several of them are discussed in more detail in Chapter 14, on anxiety. **Nemifitide** is itself a novel pentapeptide modeled on the structure of melanocyte inhibitory factor (MIF-1), a tripeptide shown to be active in animal models of depression and in small clinical studies of depressed patients (Table 12-17 and Figure 12-138). MIF-1 (also known as L-prolyl-L-leucy-L-glycinamide, or PLG) is also the tripeptide tail of oxytocin and its precursor neurophysin. Nemifitide is a pentapeptide analog not only of the tripeptide MIF-1 but also of the tripeptide tail of vasopressin (Figure 12-138). Nemifitide is administered by subcutaneous injection and has been

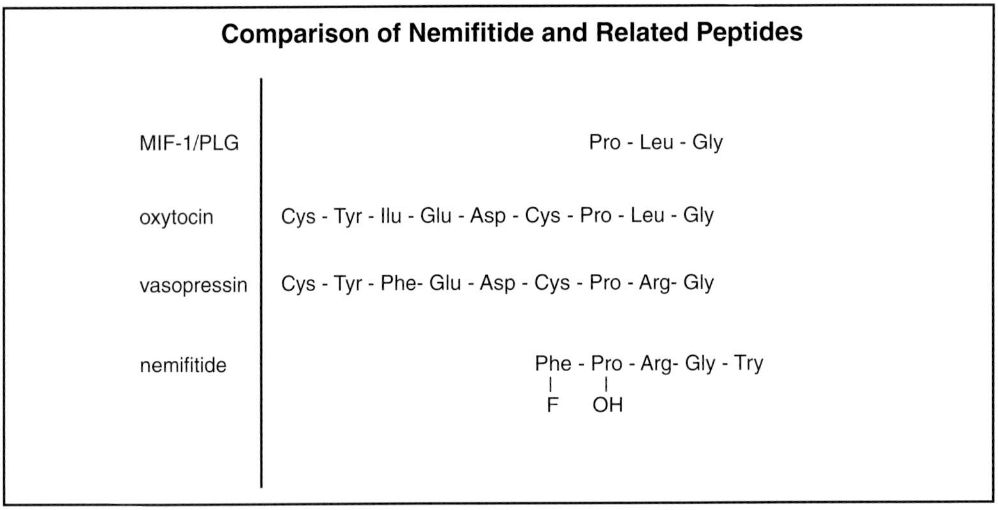

Comparison of Nemifitide and Related Peptides

MIF-1/PLG	Pro - Leu - Gly
oxytocin	Cys - Tyr - Ilu - Glu - Asp - Cys - Pro - Leu - Gly
vasopressin	Cys - Tyr - Phe - Glu - Asp - Cys - Pro - Arg - Gly
nemifitide	Phe - Pro - Arg - Gly - Try 	| F OH

FIGURE 12-138 Novel peptides. Novel peptides in testing for depression include nemifitide, an analog of melanocyte inhibitory factor (MIF-1; also known as L-prolyl-L-leucine-L-glycinamide, or PLG). PLG is also the tripeptide tail of oxytocin and its precursor neurophysin. Nemifitide's structure shows that it is also structurally related to the tripeptide tail of vasopressin. Nemifitide has shown antidepressant actions in animal models and in early clinical testing in depression.

shown to be active in animal models of depression; it is in testing in depressed patients, where early findings suggest possible efficacy with rapid onset, including effectiveness in treatment-resistant patients. Further testing in patients with major depressive episodes is ongoing.

Another class of peptide antagonists is the **neurokinin antagonists** (Table 12-16). Neurokinins belong to the family of peptides known as tachykinins (Table 12-18). Tachykinins include not only neurokinins but also newly discovered endokinins and tachykinin

TABLE 12-18 Human tachykinins

Neurokinins
    SP (substance P; neurokinin 1; NK1)
    NKA (neurokinin A)
    NPK (neuropeptide K; extended form of NKA)
    NP gamma (neuropeptide gamma; another extended form of NKA)
    NKA 3-10 (shortened form of NKA)
    NKB (neurokinin B)

Endokinins
    EKA (endokinin A)
    EKB (endokinin B)
    hHK 1 (human hemokinin 1)
    hHK 4-11 (shortened form of hHK1)

Tachykinin gene–related peptides
    EKC (endokinin C)
    EKD (endokinin D)

TABLE 12-19 Neurokinin receptors

Neurokinin 1 receptors
    Also called substance P receptors
    In brain, agonist is substance P
    In periphery, agonist is either substance P, or one of the endokinins
Neurokinin 2 receptors
    Agonist is NKA (neurokinin A, and its extended and shortened versions)
Neurokinin 3 receptors
    Agonist is NKB (neurokinin B)

gene–related peptides that act mostly outside the brain but at the same receptors where the tachykinins act (especially the NK1 receptor) (Table 12-18). Low-molecular-weight antagonists (Table 12-16) have been identified for each of the three known neurokinin receptors, NK1, NK2, and NK3 (Table 12-19). **NK1 antagonists, also known as substance P antagonists**, have been hotly pursued for many years as treatments not only for depression but also for pain, schizophrenia, and other psychiatric disorders. To date, the clinical results with substance P antagonists, from testing in major depression and in pain-related conditions, have been disappointing. However, recent evidence suggests that **saredutant**, an **NK2 antagonist**, may be effective not only in animal models of depression but also in patients with major depressive episodes (Table 12-16). Hypothetically, conditions associated with excessive release of endogenous NKA (or its extended or shortened versions) (see Tables 12-18 and 12-19), especially under conditions of stress or major depression, benefit from the blocking of NK2 receptors; that could explain why this mechanism may produce an antidepressant effect. **NK3 antagonists** are also in testing for various psychiatric disorders.

Summary

This extensive chapter began with an overview of antidepressant response, remission, relapse, and residual symptoms after treatment with antidepressants. The leading hypothesis for major depression for the past forty years, namely the monoamine hypothesis, was discussed and critiqued. The mechanisms of action of the major antidepressant drugs, including dozens of individual agents working by many unique mechanisms, were also covered. The acute pharmacological actions of these agents on receptors and enzymes were described, as well as the major hypothesis – trimonoamine modulation of serotonin, dopamine, and norepinephrine – which attempts to explain how all current antidepressants ultimately work. Pharmacokinetic concepts relating to the metabolism of antidepressants and mood stabilizers by the cytochrome P450 enzyme system were also introduced.

    Specific antidepressant agents that the reader should now understand include the serotonin selective reuptake inhibitors (SSRIs), serotonin norepinephrine reuptake inhibitors (SNRIs), norepinephrine dopamine reuptake inhibitors (NDRIs), selective norepinephrine reuptake inhibitors (selective NRIs), alpha 2 antagonists, serotonin antagonist/reuptake inhibitors (SARIs), MAO inhibitors, and tricyclic antidepressants. We have also covered numerous trimonoamine modulators (TMMs) that either have antidepressant action or boost the antidepressant action of other agents, including estrogen, 5-L-methyl-tetrahydrofolate, S-adenosyl-methionine, thyroid, lithium, therapeutic electrical modulation therapies such as electroconvulsive therapy (ECT), vagus nerve stimulation (VNS), transcranial magnetic stimulation (TMS), and deep brain stimulation (DBS) and, briefly, psychotherapy. Also provided was some guidance for how to select and combine antidepressants by following a symptom-based algorithm for patients who do not remit on their first antidepressant. Some options for combining drugs to treat such patients were illustrated and a glimpse into the future was provided by mentioning numerous novel antidepressants on the horizon.

CHAPTER 13

Mood Stabilizers

- Definition of a mood stabilizer: a labile label
- Lithium: the classic mood stabilizer
- Anticonvulsants as mood stabilizers
  - Valproic acid
  - Carbamazepine
  - Oxcarbazepine/eslicarbazepine
  - Lamotrigine
  - Riluzole
  - Topiramate
  - Zonisamide
  - Gabapentin and pregabalin
  - Levetiracetam
- Atypical antipsychotics: not just for psychotic mania
  - Putative pharmacological mechanism of action of atypical antipsychotics in mania and bipolar depression
- Other agents used in bipolar disorder
  - Benzodiazepines
  - Memantine
  - Amantadine
  - Ketamine
  - Calcium channel blockers (L-type)
  - Omega-3 fatty acids
  - Inositol
  - L-methylfolate (6-(S)-5-methyl-tetrahydrofolate, or MTHF)
  - Thyroid hormone
  - Do antidepressants make you bipolar?
- Mood stabilizers in clinical practice
  - How does one choose a mood stabilizer?
  - Symptom-based treatment algorithm for sequential treatment choices and drug combinations in bipolar disorder
  - Residual symptoms and circuits after first-line treatment of bipolar disorder
  - Bipolar disorder and women
  - Children, bipolar disorder, and mood stabilizers
  - Combinations of mood stabilizers are the standard for treating bipolar disorder
- Future mood stabilizers
- Summary

This chapter reviews pharmacological concepts underlying the use of mood stabilizers. There are many definitions of a mood stabilizer and various drugs that act by distinctive mechanisms. The goal of this chapter is to acquaint the reader with current ideas about how different mood stabilizers work. The mechanisms of action of these drugs will be explained by building on general pharmacological concepts introduced in earlier chapters. Also to be discussed are concepts about how these drugs are best used in clinical practice, including strategies for what to do if initial treatments fail and how to rationally combine one mood stabilizer with another, as well as whether and when to combine a mood stabilizer with an antidepressant. Finally, the reader is introduced to some novel mood stabilizers in clinical development that may become available in the future.

The treatment of mood stabilizers in this chapter is at the conceptual level, not at the pragmatic level. The reader should consult standard drug handbooks (such as the companion *Essential Psychopharmacology: Prescriber's Guide*) for details of doses, side effects, drug interactions, and other issues relevant to the prescribing of these drugs in clinical practice.

Definition of a mood stabilizer: a labile label

"There is no such thing as a mood stabilizer."
- FDA

"Long live the mood stabilizers."
– Prescribers

What is a mood stabilizer? Originally, a mood stabilizer was a drug that treated mania and prevented its recurrence, thus "stabilizing" the manic pole of bipolar disorder. More recently, the concept of "mood stabilizer" has been defined in a wide-ranging manner, from "something that acts like lithium" to "an anticonvulsant used to treat bipolar disorder" to "an atypical antipsychotic used to treat bipolar disorder," with antidepressants being considered as "mood destabilizers." With all this competing terminology and the number of drugs for the treatment of bipolar disorder exploding, the term "mood stabilizer" has become so confusing that regulatory authorities and some experts now suggest that it would be best to use another term for agents that treat bipolar disorder.

Rather than using the term "mood stabilizers," some would argue that there are drugs that can treat any or all of four distinct phases of bipolar disorder (Figures 13-1 and 13-2). Thus, a drug can be "mania-minded" and "treat from above" to reduce symptoms of mania and/or "stabilize from above" to prevent relapse and the recurrence of mania (Figure 13-1). Furthermore, drugs can be "depression-minded" and "treat from below" to reduce symptoms of bipolar depression and/or "stabilize from below" to prevent relapse and the recurrence of depression (Figure 13-2). This chapter discusses agents that have one or more of these actions in bipolar disorder; for historical purposes and simplification, any of these agents may be referred to as a "mood stabilizer."

Lithium, the classic mood stabilizer

Bipolar disorder has been treated with lithium for at least 50 years. Lithium is an ion whose mechanism of action is not certain. Candidates for its mechanism of action are various signal transduction sites beyond neurotransmitter receptors (Figure 13-3). This includes second messengers, such as the phosphatidyl inositol system, where lithium inhibits the enzyme inositol monophosphatase; modulation of G proteins; and, most recently, regulation of gene expression for growth factors and neuronal plasticity by interaction with downstream signal

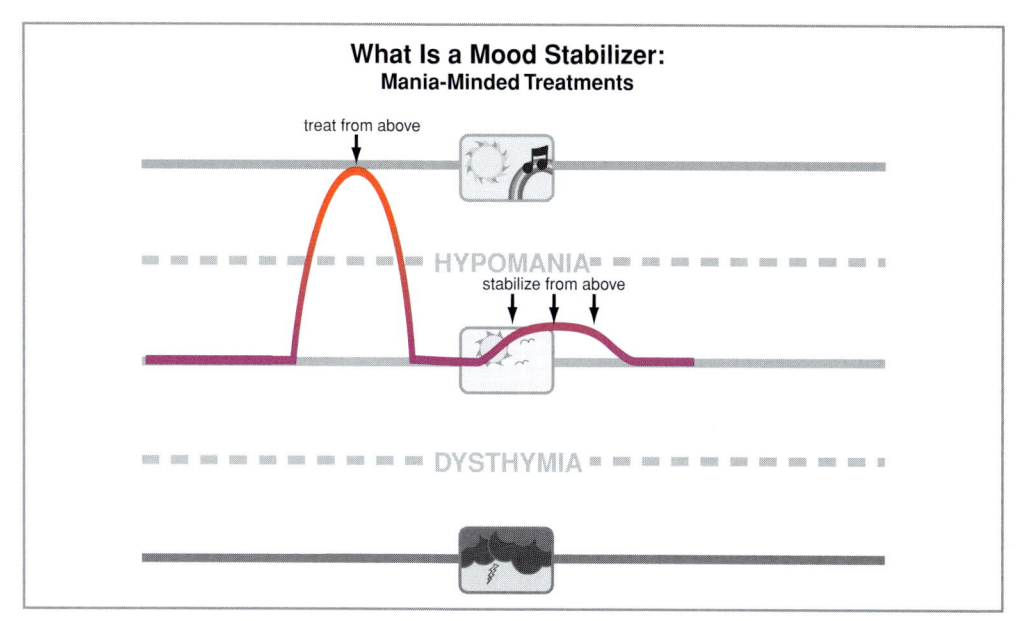

FIGURE 13-1 Mania-minded treatments. Although the ideal "mood stabilizer" would treat both mania and bipolar depression while also preventing episodes of either pole, in reality there is as yet not evidence to suggest that any single agent can achieve this consistently. Rather, different agents may be efficacious for different phases of bipolar disorder. As shown here, some agents seem to be "mania-minded" and thus able to "treat from above" and/or "stabilize from above" – in other words, to reduce and/or prevent symptoms of mania.

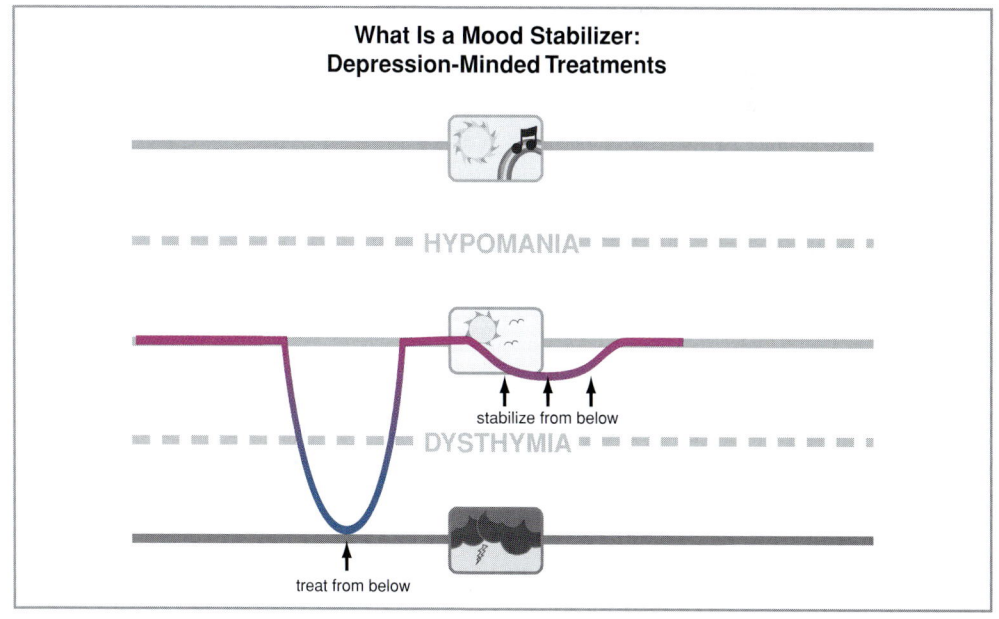

FIGURE 13-2 Depression-minded treatments. Although the ideal "mood stabilizer" would treat both mania and bipolar depression while also preventing episodes of either pole, as mentioned for the previous illustration, in reality there is as yet not evidence to suggest that any single agent can achieve this consistently. Rather, different agents may be efficacious for different phases of bipolar disorder. As shown here, some agents seem to be "depression-minded" and thus able to "treat from below" and/or "stabilize from below" – in other words, to reduce and/or prevent symptoms of bipolar depression.

Possible Mechanism of Lithium Action on Downstream Signal Transduction Cascades

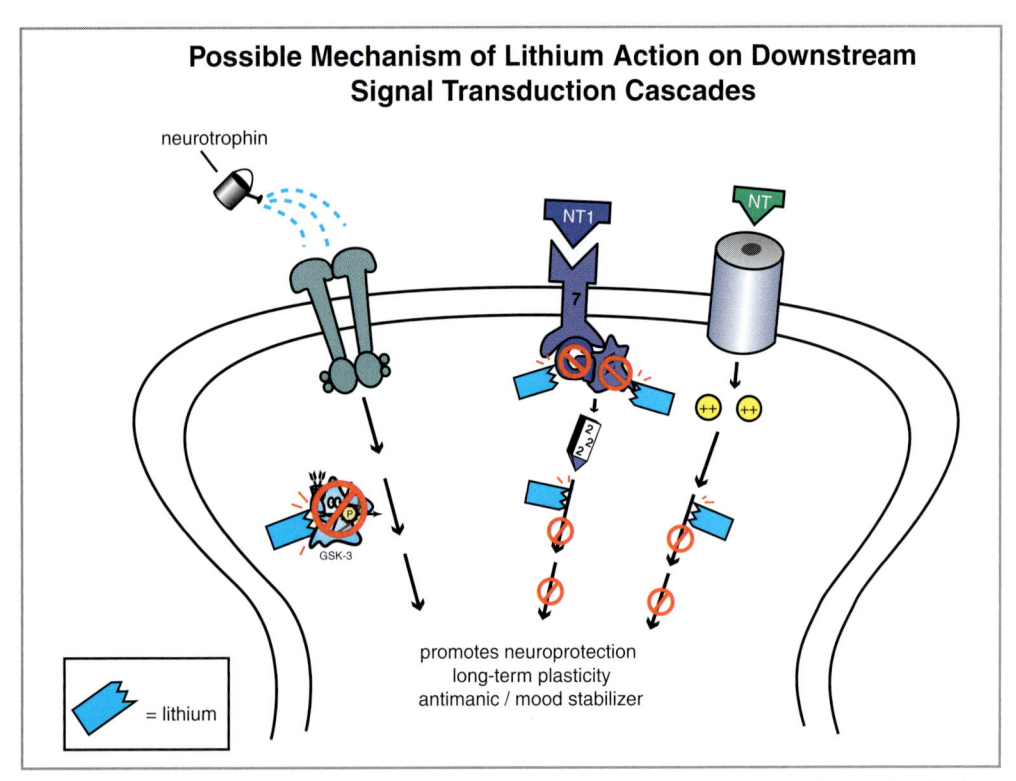

FIGURE 13-3 Lithium's mechanism of action. Although lithium is the oldest treatment for bipolar disorder, its mechanism of action is still not well understood. Several possible mechanisms exist and are shown here. Lithium may work by affecting signal transduction, perhaps through its inhibition of second messenger enzymes such as inositol monophosphatase (right), by modulation of G proteins (middle), or by interaction at various sites within downstream signal transduction cascades (left).

transduction cascades, including inhibition of glycogen synthetase kinase 3 (GSK3) and protein kinase C (illustrated in Figure 13-3; see also Figure 5–51).

However lithium works, it is proven effective in manic episodes and in the prevention of recurrence, especially for manic episodes and perhaps to a lesser extent for depressive episodes (Figure 13-4). In fact, lithium is the first psychotropic drug to be proven effective in maintenance treatment for any psychiatric disorder, and it has opened the way for maintenance claims for many other psychotropic agents over the past decades. Lithium is less well established as a robust treatment for acute bipolar depression but probably has some efficacy for this phase of the illness and certainly is well established as preventing suicide, deliberate self-harm, and death from all causes in patients with mood disorders (Figure 13-4).

Lithium was once popular as an augmenting agent to antidepressants for unipolar depression, as discussed in Chapter 12 and illustrated in Figure 12-113. In retrospect, some of the patients categorized in past decades as having unipolar depression who were treated with lithium augmentation would today be considered as fitting into the bipolar spectrum; therefore it should not be surprising that such patients have responded favorably to lithium augmentation of antidepressants (Figure 11-12). Lithium's putative mechanism as a trimonoamine modulator to boost antidepressant action is discussed in Chapter 12 (Figure 12-113).

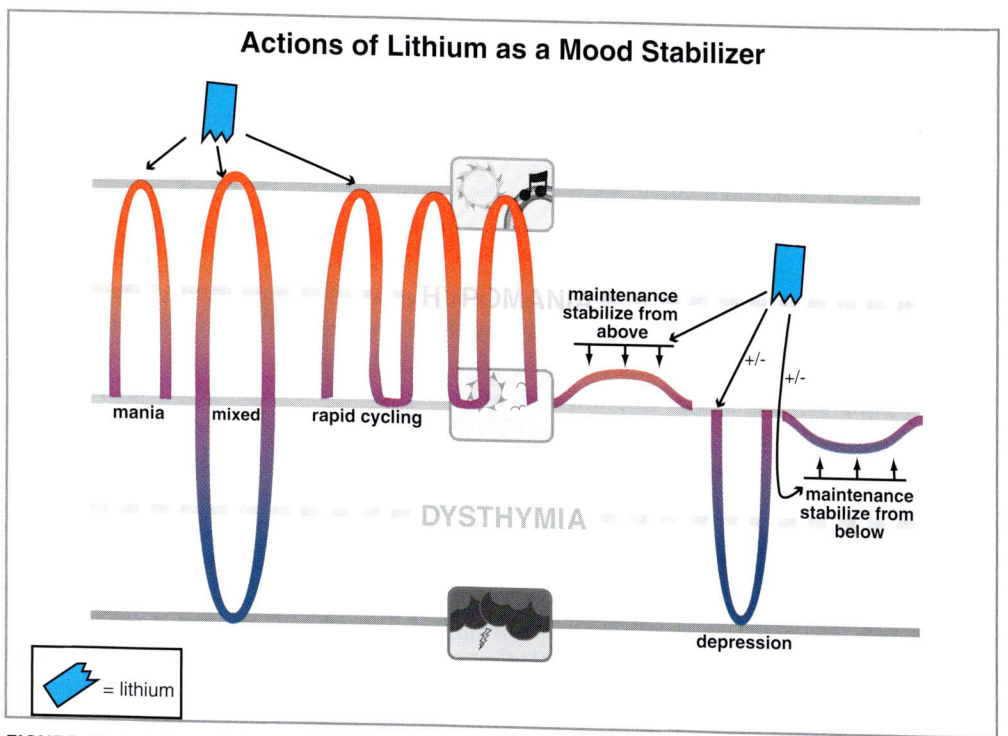

FIGURE 13-4 Actions of lithium as a mood stabilizer. Lithium has proven efficacy in mania, particularly for euphoric mania, although some experts suggest that it may not be as effective for rapid cycling or mixed episodes. Lithium is also efficacious for the prevention of manic episodes and of suicide. Lithium's efficacy for treating and preventing the depressed phase of bipolar disorder is less well established.

For many reasons, the use of lithium has declined in recent years, particularly among younger psychopharmacologists. This is due to many factors, including the entry of multiple new treatment options into the therapeutic armamentarium for bipolar disorder, to the side effects and monitoring burdens of lithium, and also to the lack of promotional marketing efforts for lithium, which is now a generic drug. Also, some experts feel that lithium is not as effective for rapid cycling and mixed episodes of bipolar disorder; they recommend it preferentially for euphoric mania but not for rapid cycling or mixed episodes. However, this selective use of lithium may not be justified, since response can be very individualized no matter what types of bipolar symptoms are being experienced.

Furthermore, lithium today is no longer used as high-dose monotherapy but rather as one member of a portfolio of treatments. Thus modern psychopharmacologists can now, in many cases, utilize lithium by treating patients with doses toward the bottom of the therapeutic range, often giving it only once daily and combining it with other mood stabilizers. This strategy of using lithium as an augmenting agent may provide incremental efficacy with acceptable tolerability.

Well-known side effects of lithium include gastrointestinal symptoms such as dyspepsia, nausea, vomiting, and diarrhea as well as weight gain, hair loss, acne, tremor, sedation, decreased cognition, and incoordination. There are also long-term adverse effects on the thyroid and kidney. Lithium has a narrow therapeutic window, requiring monitoring of plasma drug levels. Because of possible weight gain and metabolic complications, modern treatment with lithium also requires metabolic monitoring, just like that recommended

Possible Sites of Action of Valproate on GABA

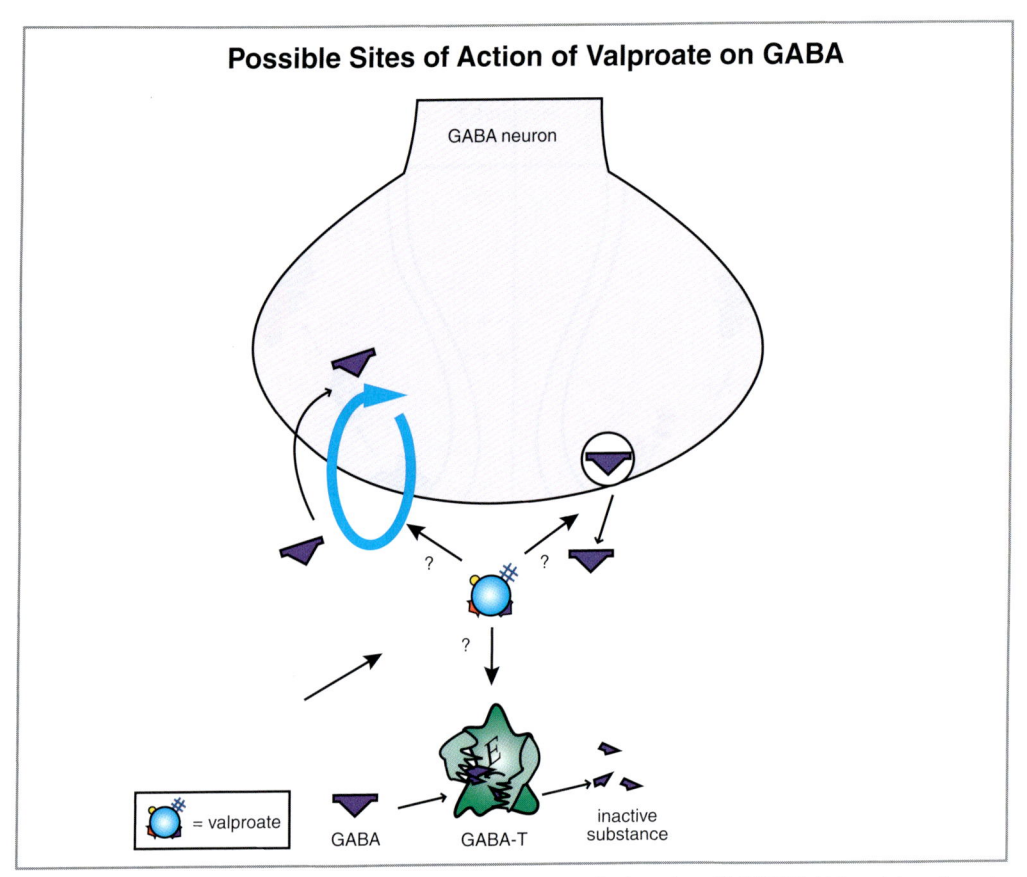

FIGURE 13-7 **Possible sites of action of valproate on gamma-aminobutyric acid (GABA).** Valproate's antimanic effects may be due to enhancement of GABA neurotransmission, perhaps by inhibiting GABA reuptake, enhancing GABA release, or interfering with the metabolism of GABA by GABA-T (GABA transaminase).

amenorrhea and polycystic ovaries in women of childbearing potential. A syndrome of menstrual disturbances, polycystic ovaries, hyperandrogenism, obesity, and insulin resistance may be associated with valproic acid therapy in such women. Thus, as mentioned for lithium, the modern psychopharmacologist must provide metabolic monitoring for patients taking valproate, just as described in detail for atypical antipsychotics in Chapter 10 and illustrated in Figures 10-60 through 10-69.

Carbamazepine

This anticonvulsant was actually the first to be shown effective in the manic phase of bipolar disorder, but it did not receive FDA approval until recently as a once-daily controlled-release formulation (Equetro). Although carbamazepine and valproate both act on the manic phase of bipolar disorder (Table 13-1), they appear to have different pharmacological mechanisms of action (Tables 13-3 and 13-4) and also different clinical actions (Tables 13-1 and 13-2), including different side effect profiles. Thus carbamazepine is hypothesized to act by blocking voltage-sensitive sodium channels (VSSCs), perhaps at a site within the channel itself, also known as the alpha subunit of VSSCs (Figure 13-10; Table 13-3). VSSCs are discussed in Chapter 5 and illustrated in Figures 5-27 through 5-42. The action of

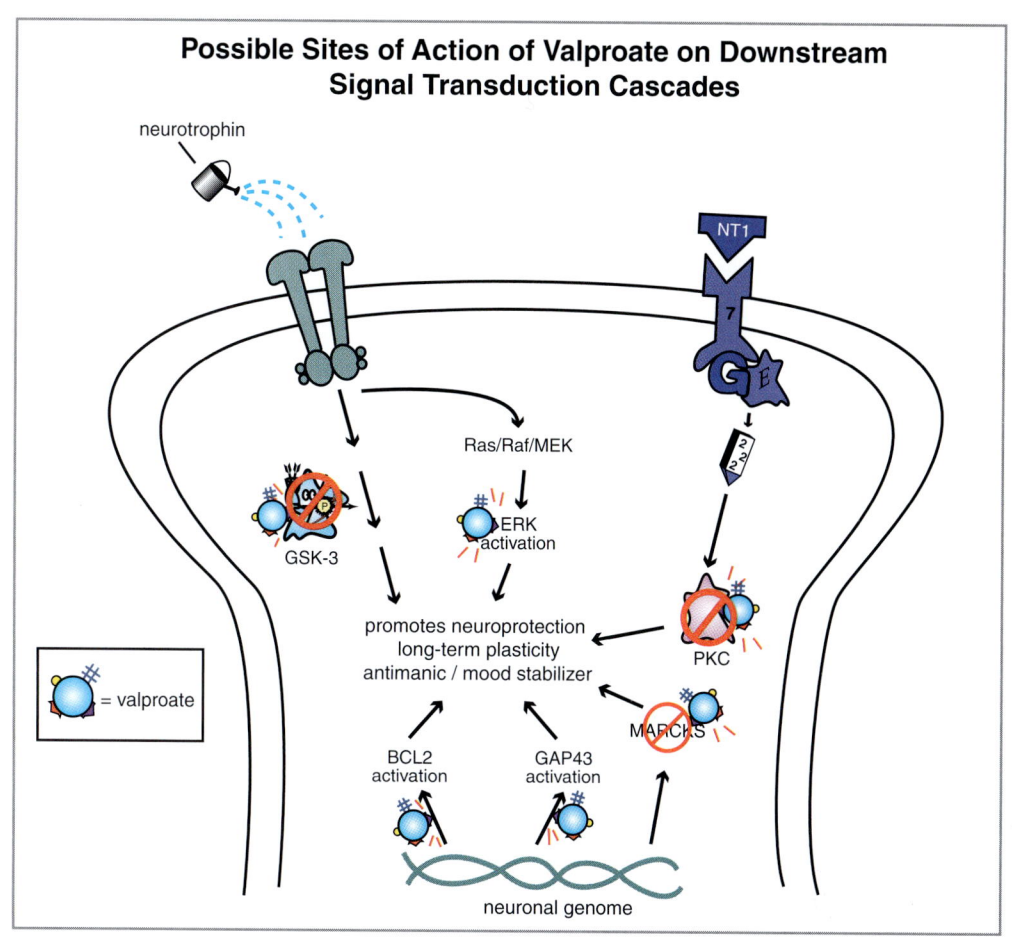

FIGURE 13-8 Possible sites of action of valproate on downstream signal transduction cascades. Valproate has been shown to have multiple downstream effects on signal transduction cascades, which may be involved in its antimanic effects. Valproate inhibits glycogen synthetase kinase 3 (GSK3), phosphokinase C (PKC), and myristolated alanine rich C kinase substrate (MARCKS). In addition, valproate activates signals that promote neuroprotection and long-term plasticity, such as extracellular signal-regulated kinase (ERK), cytoprotective protein B-cell lymphoma/leukemia-2 gene (BCL2), and GAP43.

carbamazepine on the alpha subunit of VSSCs is different from the hypothesized actions of valproate, but it is shared with the anticonvulsants oxcarbazepine and eslicarbazepine, the active metabolite of oxcarbazepine (Table 13-3; Figures 13-11 and 13-12). Although both carbamazepine and valproate are anticonvulsants and are used to treat mania from above, there are many differences between these two agents. For example, valproate is proven effective in migraine, but carbamazepine is proven effective in neuropathic pain (Table 13-1). Furthermore, carbamazepine has a different side effect profile than valproate, including suppressant effects on the bone marrow, requiring blood counts to be monitored, and notable induction of the cytochrome P450 enzyme 3A4. Carbamazepine is sedating and can cause fetal toxicity such as neural tube defects. Generally, this agent is considered a second-line mood stabilizer. It is proven effective in bipolar mania and is often utilized as maintenance treatment for preventing manic recurrences, but it has not been as extensively studied in the depressed phase of bipolar disorder (Figure 13-13).

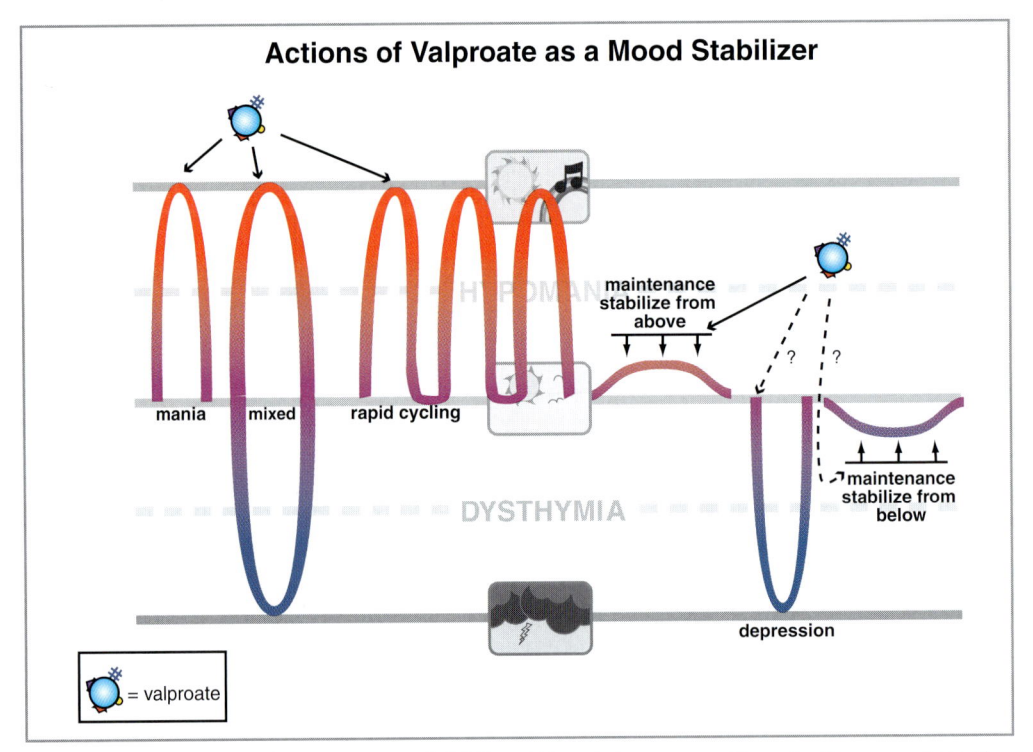

FIGURE 13-9 Actions of valproate as a mood stabilizer. Valproate has proven efficacy for the manic phase of bipolar disorder and may also prevent recurrence of mania. Valproate does not have established efficacy for treating or preventing the depressed phase of bipolar disorder, although it may be effective for the depressed phase in some patients.

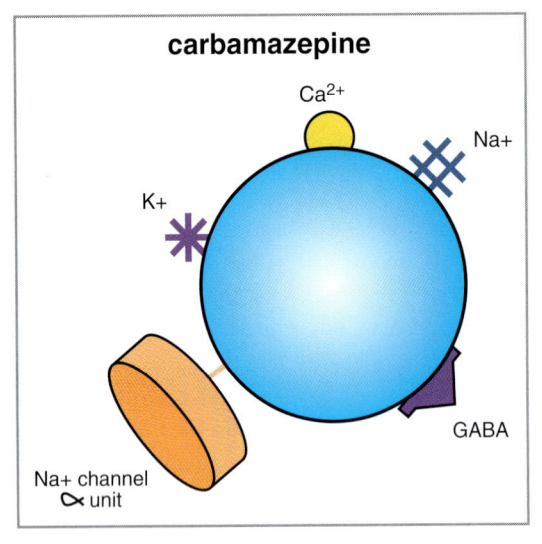

FIGURE 13-10 Carbamazepine. Shown here is an icon of the pharmacological actions of carbamazepine, an anticonvulsant used in the treatment of bipolar disorder. Carbamazepine may work by binding to the alpha subunit of voltage-sensitive sodium channels (VSSCs) and could perhaps have actions at other ion channels for calcium and potassium. By interfering with voltage-sensitive channels, carbamazepine may enhance the inhibitory actions of gamma-aminobutyric acid (GABA).

Conversion of Prodrug Oxcarbazepine Into the Active Agent Licarbazepine

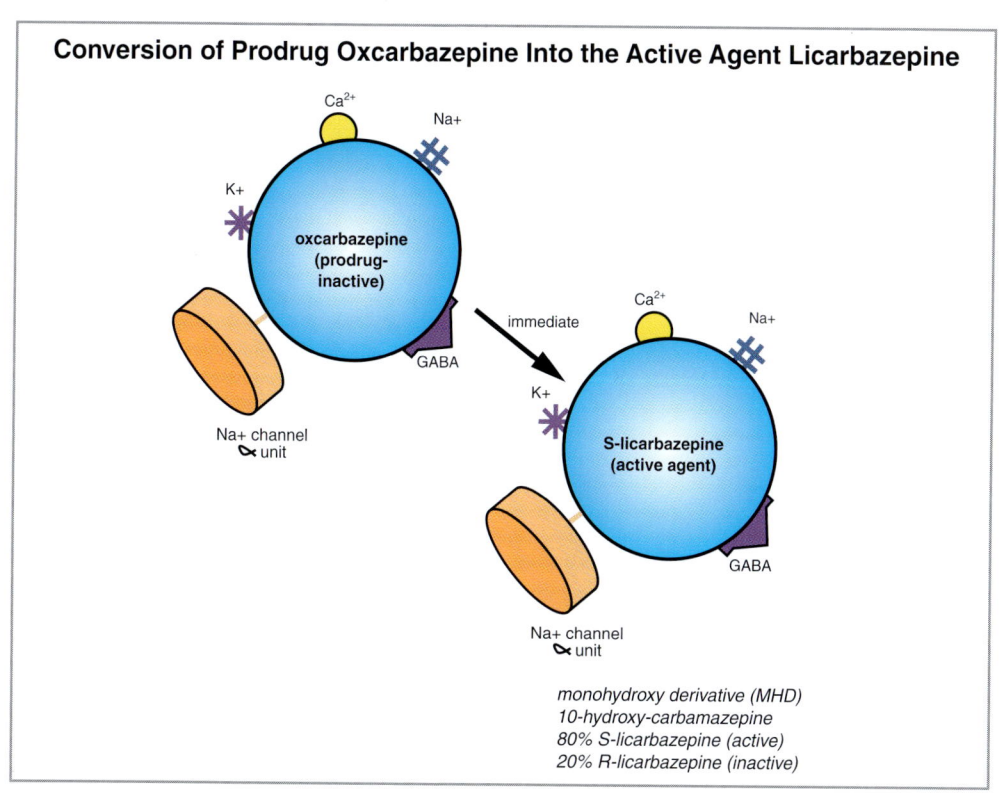

FIGURE 13-11 **Conversion of oxcarbazepine into licarbazepine.** Oxcarbazepine is a prodrug (inactive) that is converted into the active drug 10-hydroxy derivative (monohydroxyderivative), which is called licarbazepine. Licarbazepine has two enantiomers, R and S; it is specifically the S enantiomer that is active.

Oxcarbazepine/eslicarbazepine

Oxcarbazepine is structurally related to carbamazepine, but it is not a metabolite of carbamazepine. Oxcarbazepine is actually not the active form of the drug but a prodrug that is immediately converted into a 10-hydroxy derivative, also called the monohydroxyderivative; most recently it has been named licarbazepine (Figure 13-12). The active form of licarbazepine is the S enantiomer, known as eslicarbazepine. Thus oxcarbazepine really works via conversion to eslicarbazepine.

Oxcarbazepine is well known as an anticonvulsant with a presumed mechanism of anticonvulsant action the same as that for carbamazepine, namely, binding to the open channel conformation of the VSSC at a site within the channel itself on the alpha subunit (Table 13-3 and Figure 13-12). However, oxcarbazepine seems to differ in some important ways from carbamazepine, including being less sedating, having less bone marrow toxicity, and also having fewer CYP450 3A4 interactions, making it a more tolerable agent that is easier to dose. On the other hand, oxcarbazepine has never been proven to work as a mood stabilizer. Nevertheless, because of its similar postulated mechanism of action (Table 13-3 and Figure 13-2) but a better tolerability profile, oxcarbazepine has been utilized "off label" by many clinicians, especially for the manic phase of bipolar disorder (Figure 13-13). Because the patent protection has expired, the active moiety eslicarbazepine as a potential mood stabilizer is now being investigated, particularly for the manic phase and possibly for maintenance against the relapse of mania. Eslicarbazepine is not yet marketed.

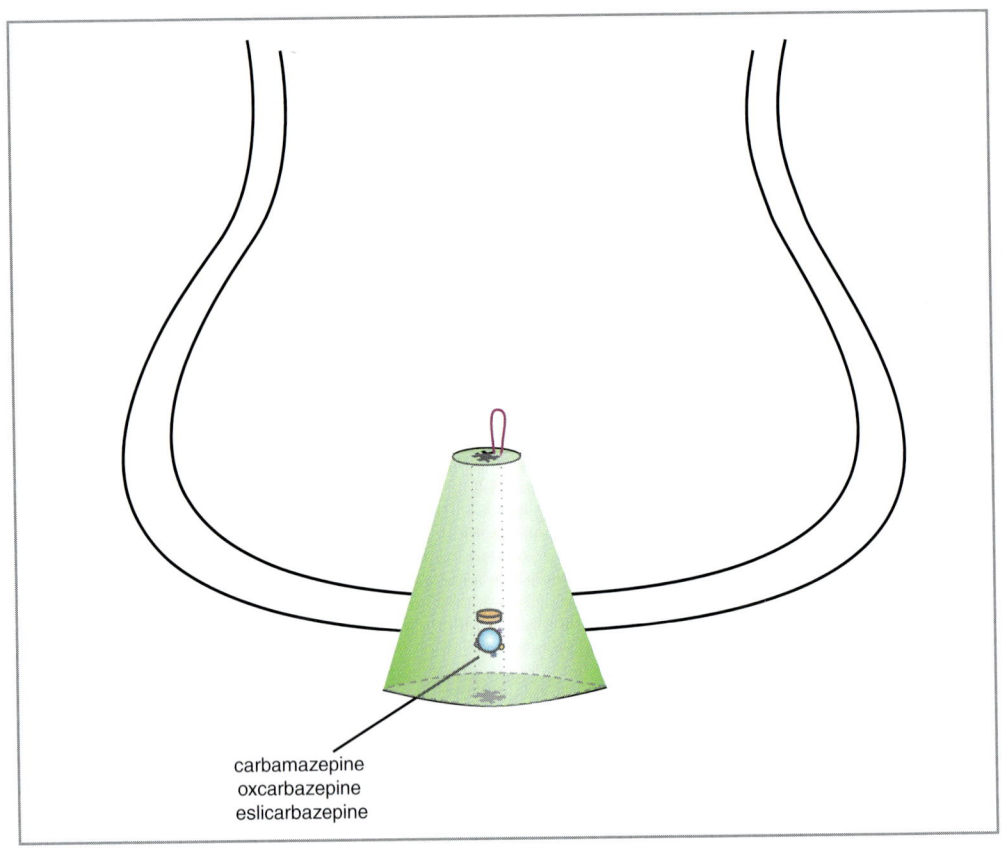

FIGURE 13-12 Binding site of carbamazepine, oxcarbazepine, and licarbazepine. Carbamazepine, oxcarbazepine, and licarbazepine are believed to share a common binding site, located within the open channel conformation of the voltage-sensitive sodium channel (VSSC) alpha subunit.

Lamotrigine

Lamotrigine (Figure 13-14) is approved as a mood stabilizer to prevent the recurrence of both mania and depression. There are many curious things about lamotrigine as a mood stabilizer. First, the FDA has not approved its use for bipolar depression, yet most experts believe lamotrigine to be effective for this indication. In fact, given the growing concern about antidepressants inducing mania, causing mood instability, and increasing suicidality in bipolar disorder, lamotrigine has largely replaced antidepressants and found its way to first-line treatment of bipolar depression. In that regard, lamotrigine has transformed the treatment of this difficult phase of bipolar disorder as one of the very few agents that seem to be effective for bipolar depression based on results seen in clinical practice rather than on evidence derived from clinical trials.

A second interesting thing about lamotrigine is that even though it has some overlapping mechanistic actions with carbamazepine – namely, binding to the open channel conformation of VSSCs (Table 13-1 and Figure 13-15) – lamotrigine is not approved for bipolar mania. Perhaps its actions at VSSCs are not potent enough (Figure 13-15), or perhaps the long titration period required in starting this drug makes it difficult to show any useful effectiveness for mania, which generally requires treatment with drugs that can work quickly.

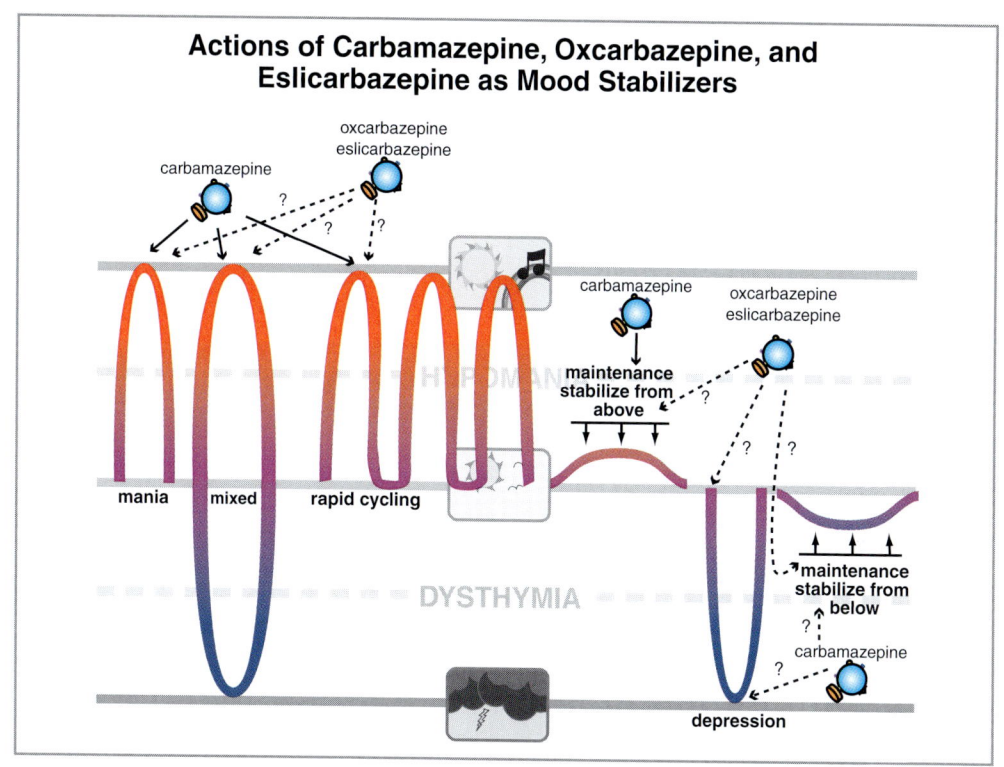

FIGURE 13-13 Actions of carbamazepine, oxcarbazepine, and eslicarbazepine as mood stabilizers. Carbamazepine has proven efficacy in the manic phase of bipolar disorder and may also be useful for preventing the recurrence of mania. Carbamazepine's efficacy for treating and/or preventing depression is not well established. The mood-stabilizing effects of oxcarbazepine and eslicarbazepine are also not established, but the similarity in proposed mechanism of action to carbamazepine's suggests they would have similar effects.

A third aspect of lamotrigine that is unusual for an antidepressant mood stabilizer is its tolerability profile. Lamotrigine is generally well tolerated for an anticonvulsant, except for its propensity to cause rashes, including (rarely) the life-threatening Stevens–Johnson syndrome (toxic epidermal necrolysis). Rashes caused by lamotrigine can be minimized by very slow uptitration of drug during the initiation of therapy, avoiding or managing drug interactions such as those with valproate that raise lamotrigine levels, and understanding how to identify and manage serious rashes, including being able to distinguish them from benign rashes (see the discussion of lamotrigine in the *Essential Psychopharmacology Prescriber's Guide*).

Finally, lamotrigine seems to have some unique aspects to its mechanism of action (Tables 13-3 and 13-4). That is, it may act to reduce the release of the excitatory neurotransmitter glutamate (Figure 13-16 and Table 13-4). It is not clear whether this action is secondary to blocking the activation of VSSCs (Figure 13-15) or to some additional synaptic action (Figure 13-16). Reduction of excitatory glutamatergic neurotransmission, especially if this is excessive in bipolar depression, may be a unique action of lamotrigine and could explain why it has such a different clinical profile as a treatment and stabilizer from below (Figure 13-17). That is, it shares some actions on VSSCs with anticonvulsants such as carbamazepine and eslicarbazepine (compare Figures 13-12 and 13-15; also Table 13-3) that are apparently effective for the manic phase of bipolar disorder (Table 13-1);

Mood Stabilizers | 683

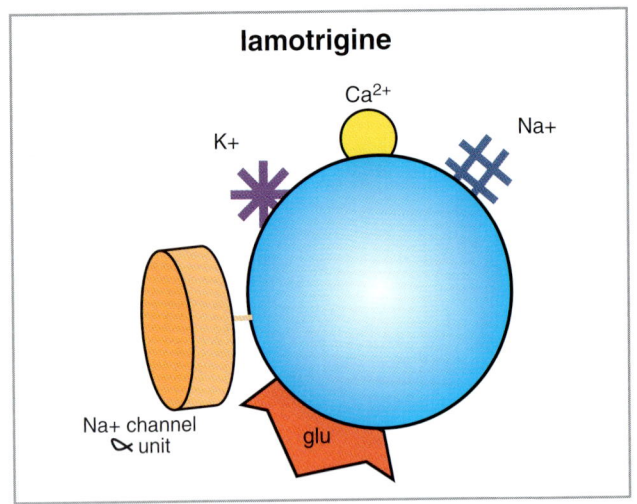

FIGURE 13-14 Lamotrigine. Shown here is an icon of the pharmacological actions of lamotrigine, an anticonvulsant used in the treatment of bipolar disorder. Lamotrigine may work by blocking the alpha subunit of voltage-sensitive sodium channels (VSSCs) and could perhaps also have actions at other ion channels for calcium and potassium. Lamotrigine is also thought to reduce the release of the excitatory neurotransmitter glutamate.

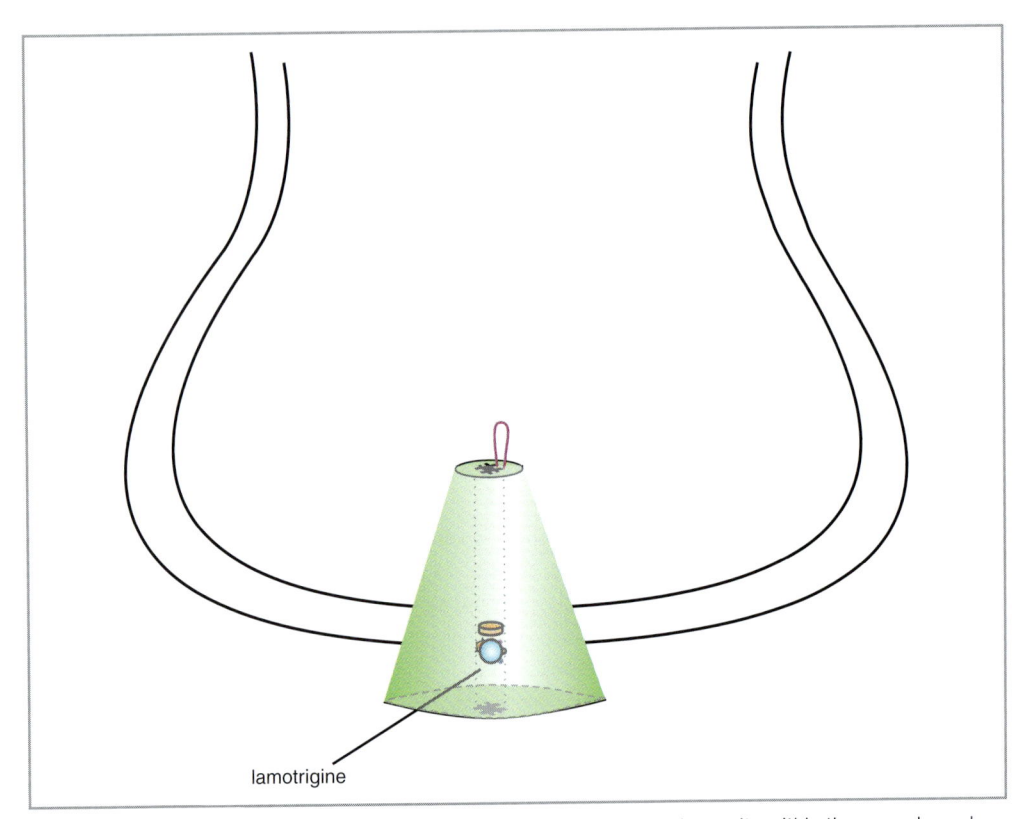

FIGURE 13-15 Binding site of lamotrigine. Lamotrigine is believed to bind to a site within the open channel conformation of the voltage-sensitive sodium channel (VSSC) alpha subunit.

yet lamotrigine has a relatively unique profile of effectiveness for the depressed phase and for preventing the recurrence of depression (compare Figures 13-13 and 13-17; also Table 13-1). The additional actions that lamotrigine may have upon glutamate release could theoretically account for this difference in clinical profile, but much further research will be necessary in order to understand those pharmacological mechanisms necessary to treat the

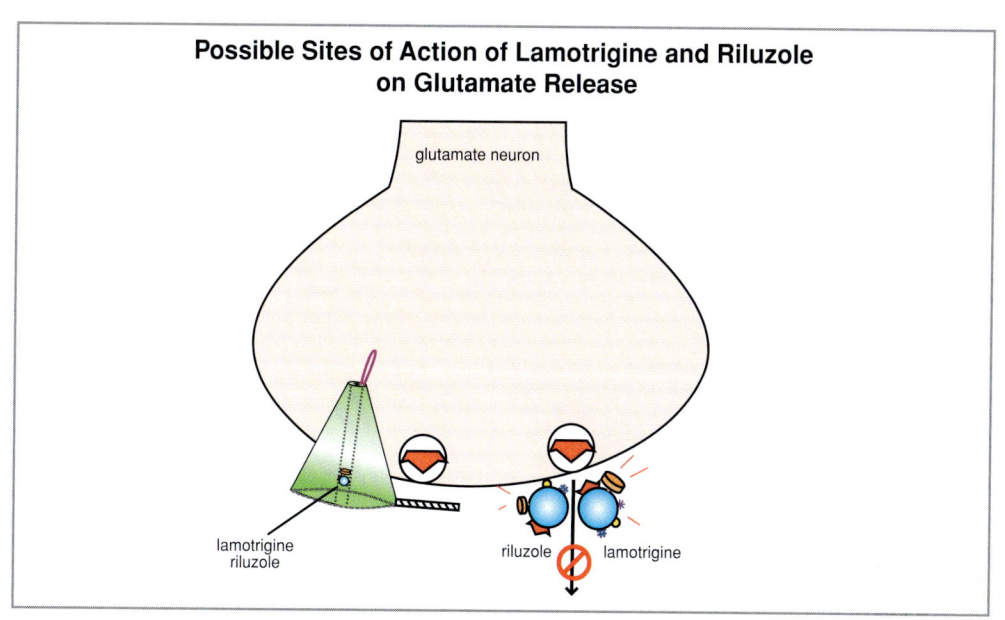

FIGURE 13-16 Possible sites of action of lamotrigine and riluzole on glutamate release. It is possible that lamotrigine reduces glutamate release through its blockade of voltage-sensitive sodium channels (VSSCs). Alternatively, lamotrigine may have this effect via an additional synaptic action that has not yet been identified. Riluzole, another anticonvulsant approved to treat amyotrophic lateral sclerosis (ALS or Lou Gehrig's disease), also reduces glutamate release and may do so via the same mechanism as lamotrigine, and may thus have therapeutic actions in bipolar disorder.

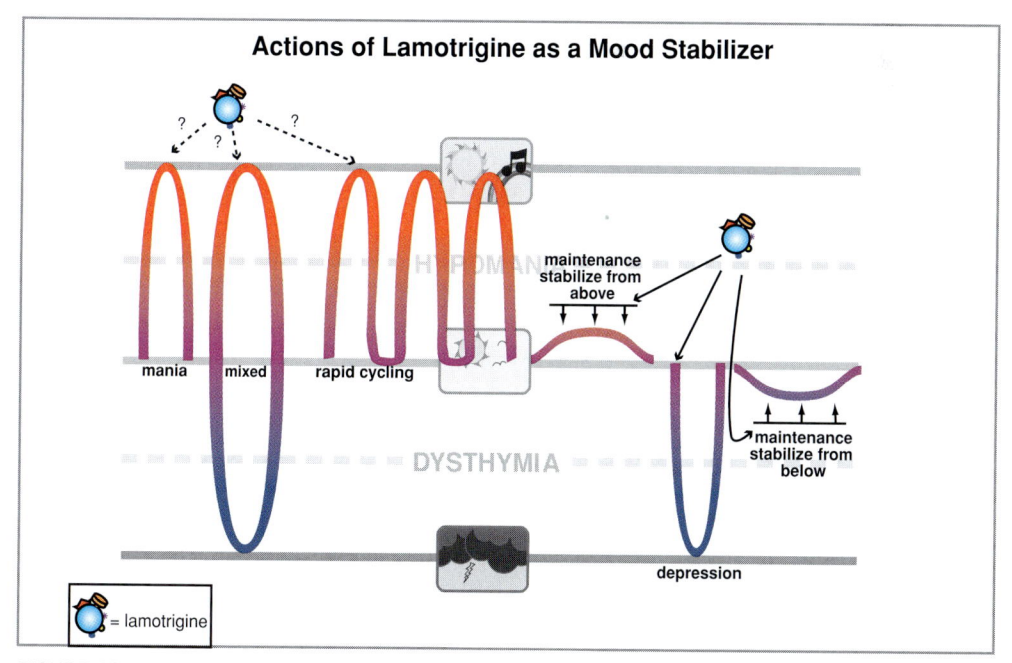

FIGURE 13-17 Actions of lamotrigine as a mood stabilizer. Lamotrigine has proven efficacy for preventing the recurrence of both manic and depressive episodes and has also demonstrated efficacy for treating the depressed phase of bipolar disorder. Lamotrigine has not demonstrated efficacy for treating mania despite a shared binding site with agents that do (e.g., carbamazepine); this may be due to differences in the manner of binding or to the dosing requirements of lamotrigine.

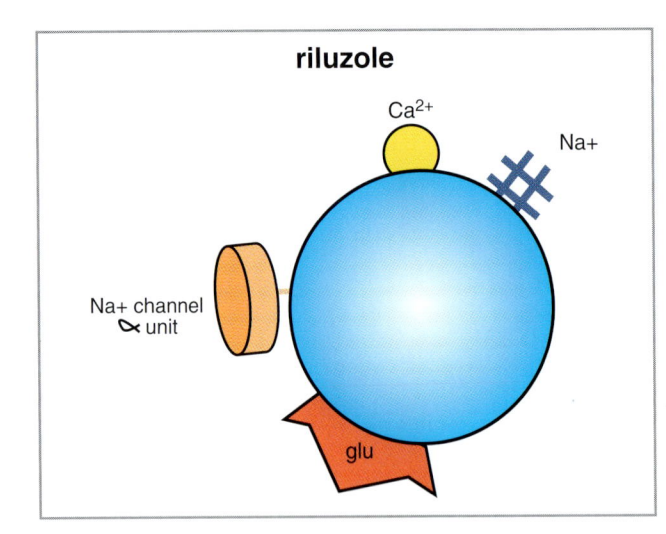

FIGURE 13-18 Riluzole. Shown here is an icon of the pharmacological actions of riluzole, an agent with anticonvulsant properties developed for use in amyotrophic lateral sclerosis (ALS). Riluzole may also be effective in bipolar disorder, as its mechanism of action appears to be similar to that of lamotrigine. Specifically, riluzole is believed to block the alpha subunit of voltage-sensitive sodium channels (VSSCs) and also to reduce the release of the excitatory neurotransmitter glutamate.

manic phase versus those necessary to treat the depressed phase of bipolar disorder. In the meantime, lamotrigine is a mainstay of treating and stabilizing recurrences of the depressed phase of bipolar disorder, and the elucidation of its mechanism of action will be critical to discovering additional agents with clinical efficacy for bipolar depression.

Riluzole

Riluzole (Figure 13-18) has anticonvulsant actions in preclinical models but was developed to slow the progression of amyotrophic lateral sclerosis (ALS, or Lou Gerhig's disease) (Table 13-2). Theoretically, riluzole binds to VSSCs and prevents glutamate release in an action similar to that postulated for lamotrigine (Figure 13-16 and Table 13-4). The idea is that diminishing glutamate release in ALS would prevent the postulated excitotoxicity that might be causing death of motor neurons in ALS. Excitotoxicity as a disease mechanism in neurodegenerative disorders is discussed in Chapter 2 and illustrated in Figures 2-36 and 2-37 as well as in Chapter 9 and illustrated in Figures 9-46 through 9-51. If ALS is caused by glutamate-mediated excitotoxicity, an agent that prevents glutamate release would theoretically prevent or slow disease progression. Excessive glutamate activity may not only be occurring in ALS but is also a leading hypothesis for the dysregulation of neurotransmission during bipolar depression, although not necessarily so severe as to cause widespread neuronal loss.

Owing to riluzole's putative action in preventing glutamate release, it has been tested in case series in a number of treatment-resistant conditions hypothetically linked to excessive glutamate activity, including not only bipolar depression but also treatment-resistant unipolar depression and anxiety disorders, with some promising results. Further research with riluzole is in progress, as it is for other agents that interfere with glutamate neurotransmission (discussed later in this chapter). There is great need for another agent that has the same clinical effects as lamotrigine. The problem with riluzole is that it is quite expensive, and has frequent liver function abnormalities associated with its use.

Topiramate

Topiramate (Figure 13-19) is another compound approved as an anticonvulsant and for migraine; it has also been tested in bipolar disorder, but with ambiguous results

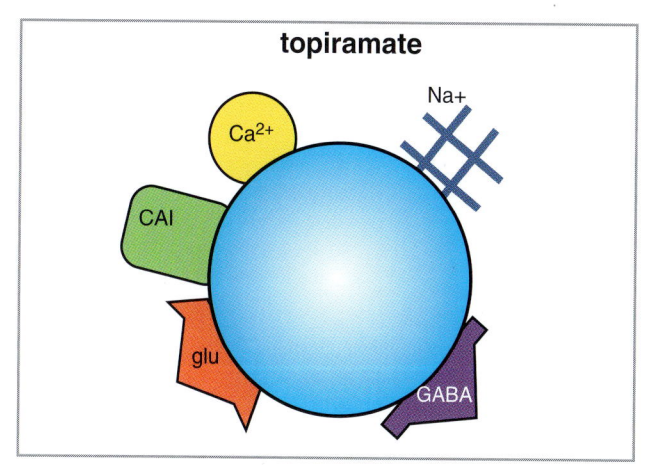

FIGURE 13-19 Topiramate. Shown here is an icon of the pharmacological actions of topiramate, an anticonvulsant that has been tested, with varying results, in the treatment of bipolar disorder. Its exact binding site is not known, but it may interfere with voltage-sensitive sodium and/or calcium channels and thereby enhance the function of gamma-aminobutyric acid (GABA) and reduce glutamate function. Topiramate is also a weak inhibitor of carbonic anhydrase.

(Table 13-1). It does seem to be associated with weight loss and is sometimes given as an adjunct to mood stabilizers that cause weight gain, but it can cause unacceptable sedation in some patients. Topiramate is also being tested in various substance abuse disorders, including stimulant abuse and alcoholism (Table 13-2). However, topiramate is not clearly effective as a mood stabilizer, either from evidence-based randomized controlled trials (which are not consistently positive) or from clinical practice.

The reason that topiramate may not have the robust efficacy of valproate or carbamazepine in the manic phase or of lamotrigine in the depressed and maintenance phases of bipolar disorder is that it has a different mechanism of action from any of these agents (Tables 13-3 and 13-4). The exact binding site for topiramate is not known, but this agent seems to enhance GABA function and reduce glutamate function by interfering with both sodium and calcium channels, but in a different way and at a different site than the previously discussed anticonvulsants (Tables 13-3 and 13-4). In addition, topiramate is a weak inhibitor of carbonic anhydrase (Figure 13-19; Table 13-3). Topiramate is now considered an adjunctive treatment for bipolar disorder, perhaps helpful for weight gain, insomnia or anxiety, or possibly for comorbid substance abuse but not necessarily as a mood stabilizer per se.

Zonisamide

Zonisamide (Figure 13-20) is another anticonvulsant that is not approved for bipolar disorder but is sometimes used to treat this condition (Table 13-1). Its mechanism of action is also unknown, as is its binding site, but its mechanism seems to be different from that of the other anticonvulsants that are proven mood stabilizers (Tables 13-3 and 13-4). Like topiramate, zonisamide may enhance GABA function and reduce glutamate function by interfering with both sodium and calcium channels. Interestingly, like topiramate, zonisamide may also cause weight loss. As a sulfonamide derivative, zonisamide can be associated with rashes, including (rarely) a serious rash (Stevens–Johnson syndrome, or toxic epidermal necrolysis). Zonisamide is considered an adjunctive treatment without, as yet, convincing evidence of efficacy in bipolar disorder.

Gabapentin and pregabalin

Gabapentin and pregabalin (Figure 13-21) seem to have little or no action as mood stabilizers, yet they are robust treatments for various pain conditions, from neuropathic pain to

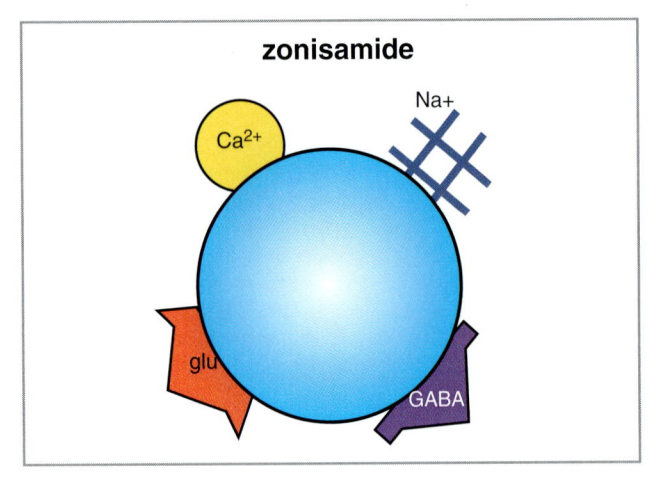

FIGURE 13-20 Zonisamide. Shown here is an icon of the pharmacological actions of zonisamide, an anticonvulsant that is not well tested in the treatment of bipolar disorder. Its mechanism of action is not known, but it may interfere with voltage-sensitive sodium and/or calcium channels and thereby enhance the function of gamma-aminobutyric acid (GABA) and reduce glutamate function.

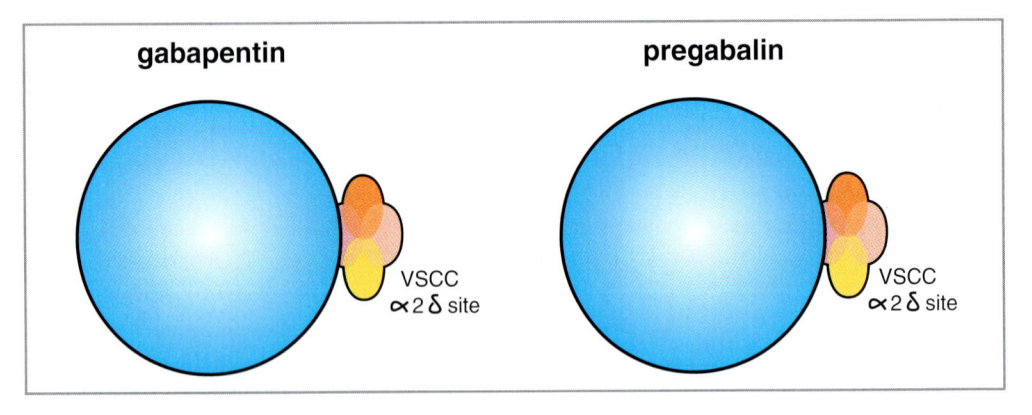

FIGURE 13-21 Gabapentin and pregabalin. Shown here are icons of the pharmacological actions of gabapentin and pregabalin, two anticonvulsants that do not appear to have efficacy in bipolar disorder. These agents bind to the alpha 2 delta subunit of voltage-sensitive calcium channels (VSCCs) and, rather than being efficacious as mood stabilizers, instead seem to have efficacy in chronic pain and anxiety.

fibromyalgia, and for various anxiety disorders (Tables 13-1 and 13-2) and are discussed in more detail in Chapters 14 and 15, on anxiety and on chronic pain, respectively. Gabapentin and pregabalin may also be useful treatments for some sleep disorders (discussed in Chapter 16, on sleep/wake disorders). However, these agents are not currently considered to be effective mood stabilizers.

Gabapentin and pregabalin are now classified as "alpha 2 delta ligands" since they are known to bind selectively and with high affinity to the alpha 2 delta site of voltage-sensitive calcium channels (VSCCs) (Table 13-3). These channels are discussed in Chapter 3 and illustrated in Figures 3-33 through 3-35 and 3-37 and also in Chapter 15, on pain. It appears that blocking these VSCCs when they are open and in use causes improvement of pain but not stabilization of mood (Figure 3-37 and Table 13-1). That is, "use-dependent" blockade of VSCCs prevents the release of neurotransmitters such as glutamate (Table 13-4) in pain and anxiety pathways and also prevents seizures, but it does not appear to affect the mechanism involved in bipolar disorder, since clinical trials of these agents in bipolar disorder show unconvincing mood stabilization (Tables 13-1 and 13-2). However, many

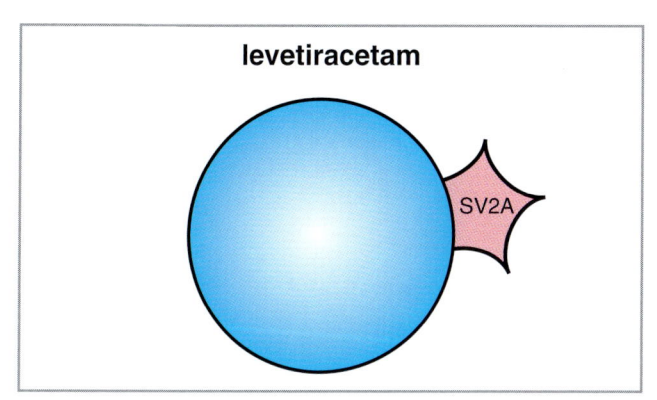

FIGURE 13-22 Levetiracetam. Shown here is an icon of the pharmacological actions of levetiracetam, an anticonvulsant that is not well tested in the treatment of bipolar disorder. Levetiracetam binds to the SV2A protein on synaptic vesicles, which should affect neurotransmitter release.

bipolar patients do experience chronic pain, anxiety, and insomnia, and gabapentin and pregabalin may be useful adjunctive treatments to effective mood stabilizers, even though they do not appear to be robustly effective as mood stabilizers themselves. This is not surprising, given the very different mechanism of action of these compounds as selective alpha 2 delta ligands, compared to the mechanisms of proven mood stabilizers such as valproate, carbamazepine, and lamotrigine discussed above (Tables 13-3 and 13-4).

Levetiracetam

Levetiracetam (Figure 13-22) is an anticonvulsant with a very novel mechanism of action: it binds to the SV2A protein on synaptic vesicles (Table 13-3). SV2A is a type of transporter; it is discussed in Chapter 5 and illustrated in Figure 5-36. Levetiracetam selectively and potently binds to this site on synaptic vesicles, presumably changing neurotransmission by altering neurotransmitter release, thereby providing anticonvulsant actions (Figure 13-23). Anecdotal use and case studies suggest some utility in bipolar disorder, but this is not yet well established. Since this is a quite different mechanism of action, there is no assurance that this agent will be an effective mood stabilizer, but its unique actions also suggest the possibility of helping some bipolar patients resistant to the other mechanisms of mood stabilization discussed here. Further research is necessary to clarify the value of this mechanism at SV2A synaptic vesicle transporter sites.

Atypical antipsychotics: not just for psychotic mania

When atypical antipsychotics were approved for schizophrenia, it was not surprising that these agents would work for psychotic symptoms associated with mania, since the D2 antagonist actions predict efficacy for psychosis in general (discussed in Chapter 10 and illustrated in Figure 10-2). However, it was somewhat surprising that these agents proved effective for the core nonpsychotic symptoms of mania and for maintenance treatment to prevent the recurrence of mania. These latter actions are consistent with those of mood stabilizers such as lithium and various anticonvulsants, which act by very different mechanisms than do the antipsychotics. Furthermore, evolving data now suggest that at least certain atypical antipsychotics are effective for bipolar depression and in preventing the recurrence of depression. The question that arises is how do atypical antipsychotics work as mood stabilizers? Also, do they act by the same pharmacological mechanism as mood stabilizers as they do as antipsychotics? Finally, do they work for the symptoms of mania by the same pharmacological mechanisms as they do for bipolar depression?

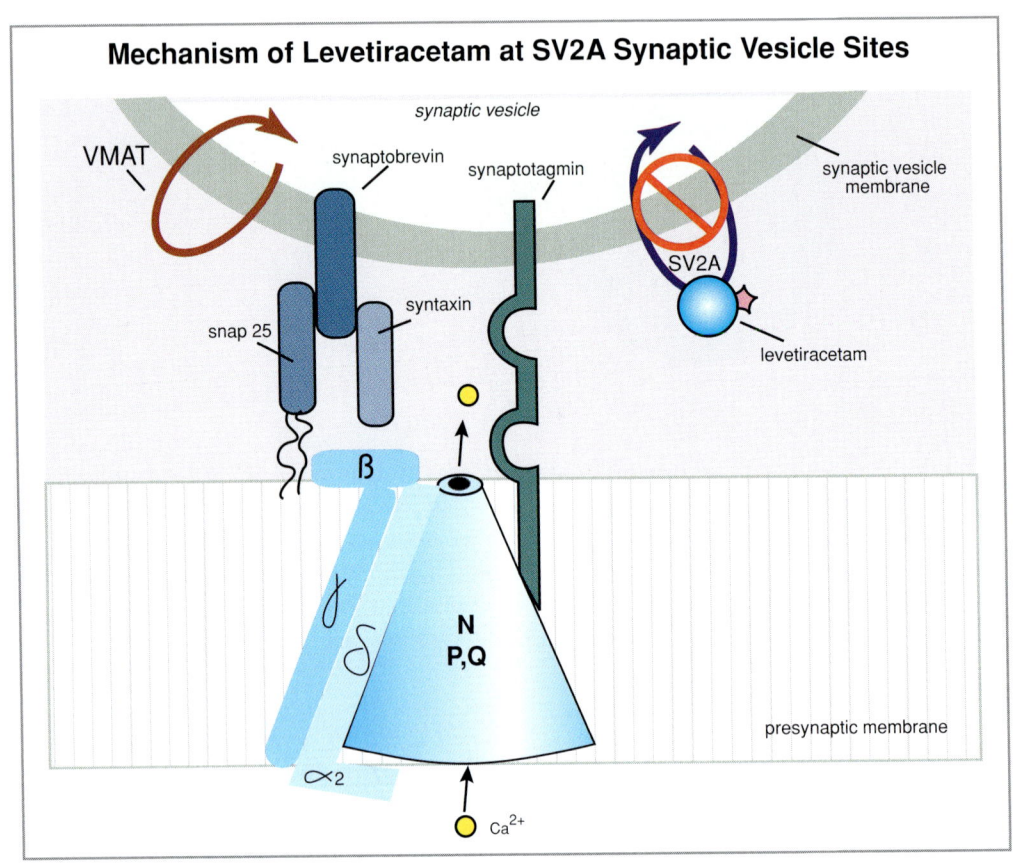

FIGURE 13-23 Mechanism of action of levetiracetam at SV2A synaptic vesicle sites. Levetiracetam selectively binds to SV2A, a type of transporter on synaptic vesicles. Actions at sites on these vesicles could have downstream effects on neurotransmitter release. VMAT, vesicular monoamine transporter.

Putative pharmacological mechanism of atypical antipsychotics in mania and bipolar depression

The answer to the question of how atypical antipsychotics work in mania is that we do not really know. In fact, theories about atypical antipsychotic pharmacological actions in bipolar disorder are less well developed than they are for schizophrenia, such as those discussed extensively in Chapter 10. Indeed, it is still a mystery how bipolar disorder itself can create seemingly opposite symptoms during various phases of the illness as well as the combination of both manic and depressive symptoms simultaneously. Ideas about dysfunctional circuits in the depressed phase of bipolar disorder (discussed in Chapter 11 and illustrated in Figures 11-45 through 11-56 and 11-65) are contrasted with different dysfunctions in both overlapping and distinctive circuits during the manic phase of the illness (discussed in Chapter 11 and illustrated for the manic phase in Figures 11-57 through 11-62 and 11-66). Rather than being conceptualized as having activity that is simply "too low" in depression and "too high" in mania, the idea is that dysfunctional circuits in bipolar disorder are "out of tune" and chaotic, as discussed in Chapter 7 and illustrated in Figures 7-25 and 7-26. According to this notion, mood stabilizers have the ability to "tune" dysfunctional circuits, increasing the efficiency of information processing in symptomatic circuits and thus decreasing symptoms, whether they are manic or depressed.

Atypical Antipsychotic Actions in Psychotic and Nonpsychotic Mania

reduces glutamate hyperactivity

blocks DA hyperactivity

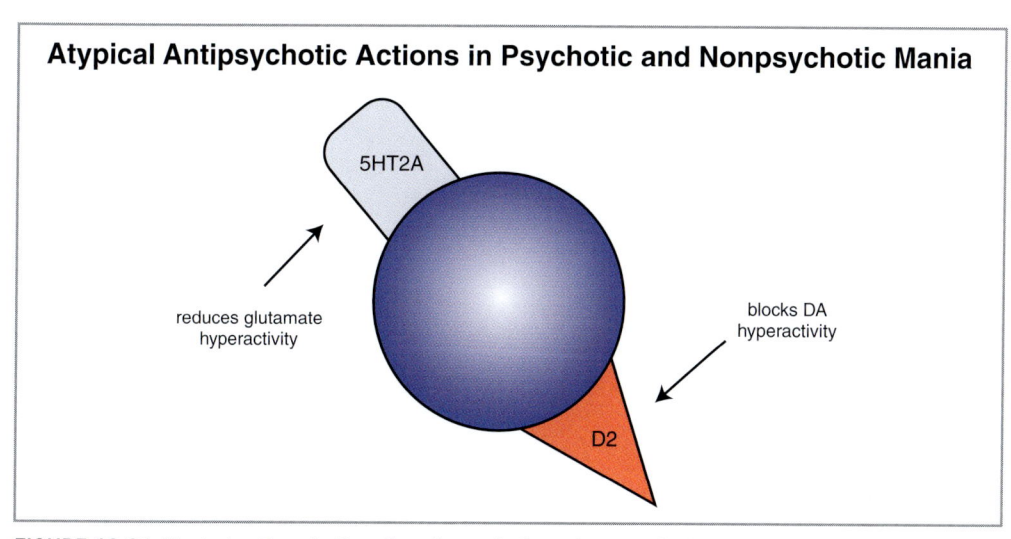

5HT2A

D2

FIGURE 13-24 Atypical antipsychotic actions in psychotic and nonpsychotic mania. Atypical antipsychotics have established efficacy not only for psychotic mania but also for nonpsychotic mania. Antagonism or partial agonism of dopamine 2 receptors, which block dopamine hyperactivity, may account for the reduction of psychotic symptoms in mania, just as these actions do for psychotic symptoms in schizophrenia. Antagonism of serotonin 2A receptors, which can indirectly reduce glutamate hyperactivity, may account for the reduction of manic symptoms.

If so, the D2 antagonist or partial agonist properties of atypical antipsychotics as well as conventional antipsychotics may account for reduction of psychotic symptoms in mania (Figure 13-24; see also Figure 10-2), but the 5HT2A antagonist properties of atypical antipsychotics may account for the reduction of nonpsychotic manic and depressive symptoms. This could occur via reduction of glutamate hyperactivity from overly active pyramidal neurons by 5HT2A antagonist actions (discussed in Chapter 10 and illustrated in Figures 10-30 and 10-31). This could reduce symptoms associated with glutamate hyperactivity, which could include both manic and depressive symptoms, depending on the circuit involved (Figures 11-45 through 11-56). Anti-glutamate actions of atypical antipsychotics (Figure 13-24) are consistent with the known pharmacological mechanisms of several anticonvulsants that are also mood stabilizers, as discussed above (Figures 13-12, 13-15, and 13-16 and Table 13-4). The combination of different mechanisms that decrease excessive glutamate activity could explain the observed therapeutic benefits of combining atypical antipsychotics with proven anticonvulsant mood stabilizers.

Several other mechanisms are feasible explanations for how certain atypical antipsychotics work to improve symptoms in the depressed phase of bipolar disorder (Figures 13-25 and 13-26). Numerous mechanisms of different atypical antipsychotics can increase the availability of the trimonoamine neurotransmitters serotonin, dopamine, and norepinephrine, known to be critical in the action of antidepressants in unipolar depression (Figure 13-25). Such actions would be predicted to have favorable effects not only on mood but also on cognition (Figure 13-25). Furthermore, some pharmacological actions of atypical antipsychotics predict favorable effects on sleep and also on neurogenesis (Figure 13-25), but by different yet potentially complementary neurotrophic mechanisms than those proposed for the actions of lithium (Figure 13-3) or valproate (Figure 13-8).

There are very different pharmacological properties of one atypical antipsychotic compared to another, which could potentially explain not only why some atypical antipsychotics

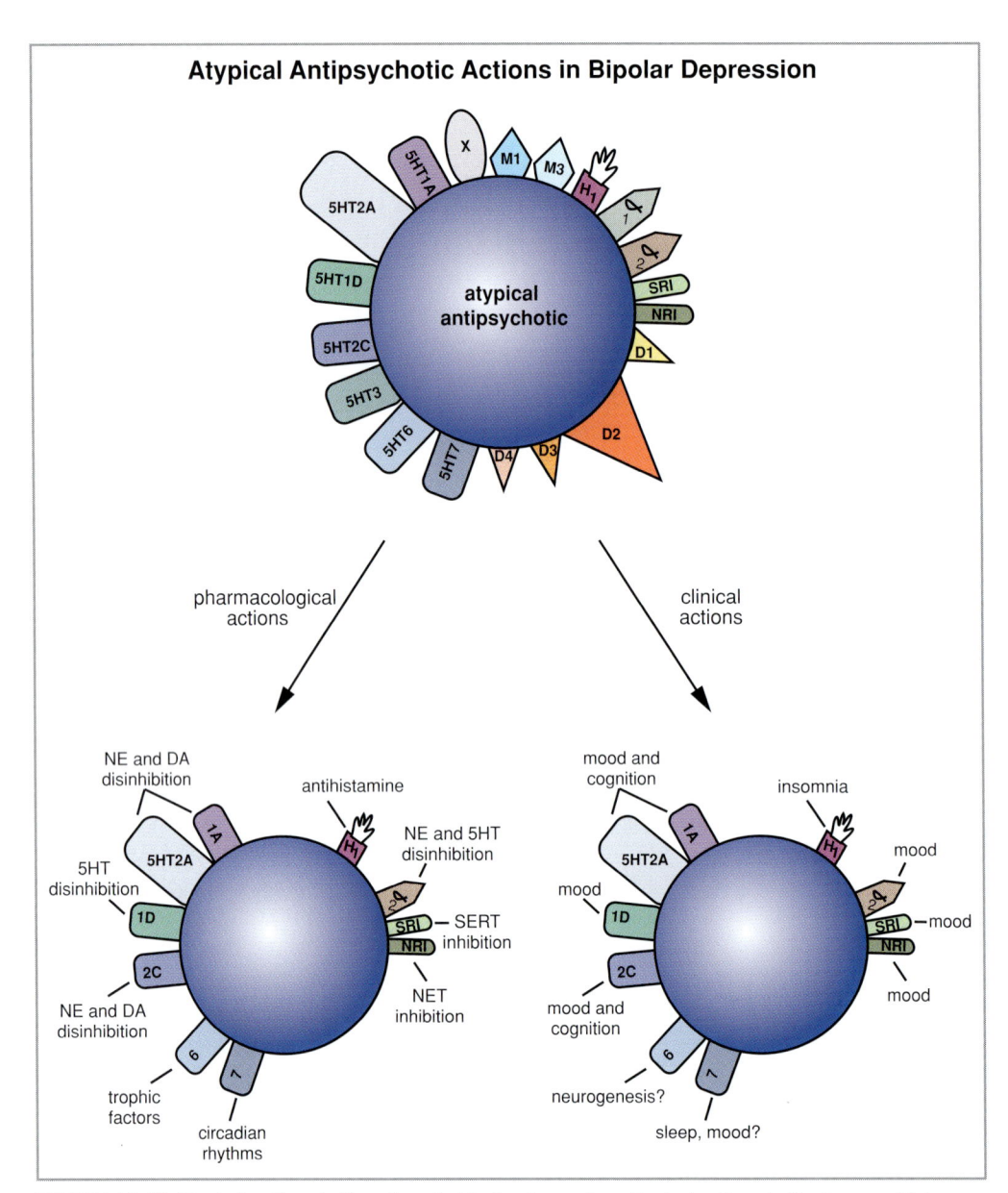

FIGURE 13-25 Atypical antipsychotic actions in bipolar depression. Atypical antipsychotics have multiple mechanisms that lead to increased availability of serotonin (5HT), norepinephrine (NE), and/or dopamine (DA), which could account for the efficacy of some of these agents in bipolar depression. Actions at 5HT2A, 5HT2C, and 5HT1A receptors indirectly lead to NE and DA disinhibition, which may improve mood and cognition. Mood may also be improved by increasing NE and 5HT via actions at alpha 2 receptors, by increasing NE via blockade of the NE transporter, and by increasing 5HT via actions at 5HT1D receptors and blockade of the 5HT transporter. Antihistamine actions could improve insomnia associated with bipolar depression. Actions at other 5HT receptors may also play a role in treating bipolar depression.

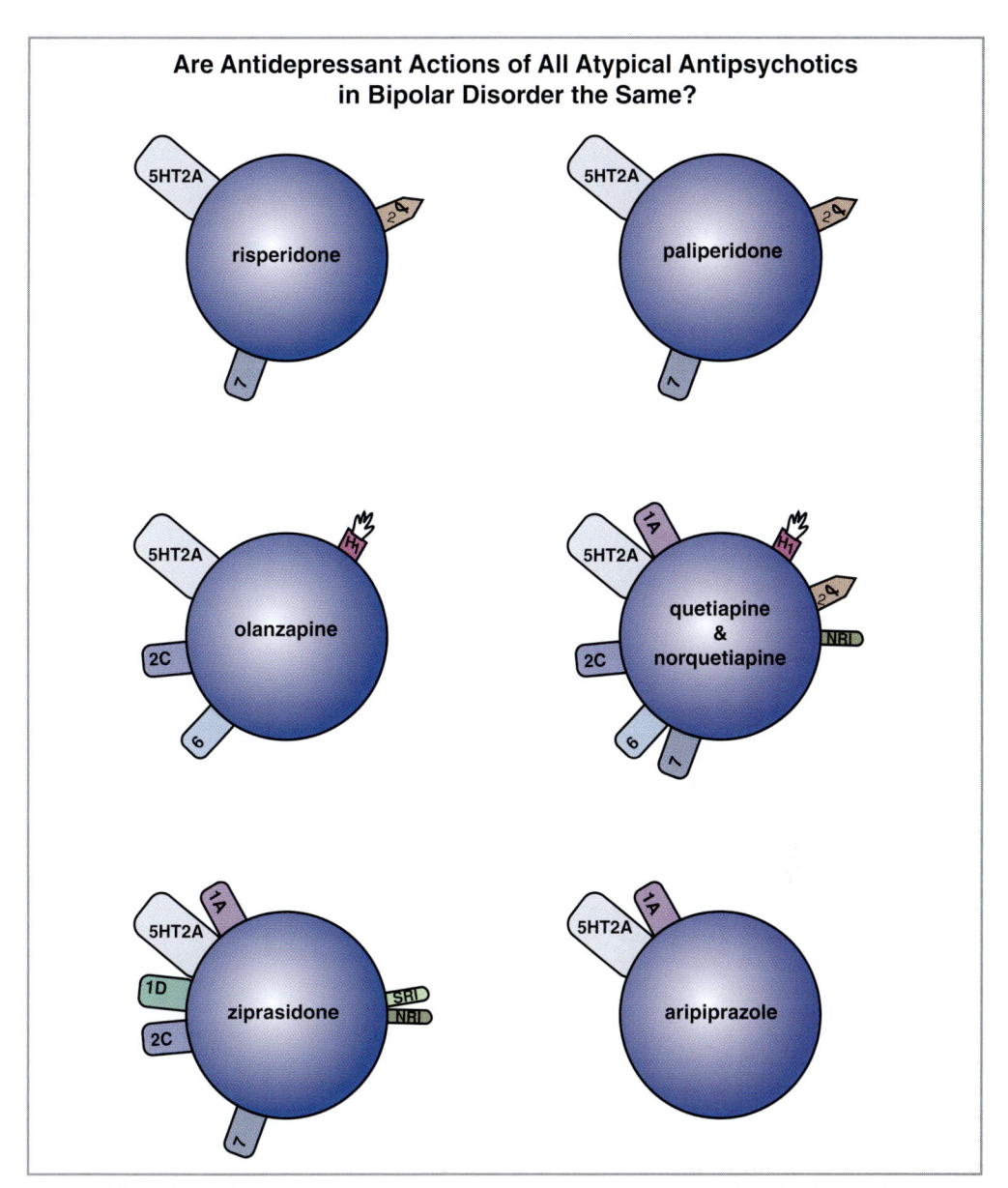

FIGURE 13-26 Atypical antipsychotics: differing portfolios of pharmacological actions for bipolar depression. As shown here, each atypical antipsychotic has a unique portfolio of pharmacological actions, which may contribute to its antidepressant actions. This may explain why these agents differ in their ability to treat the depressed phase of bipolar disorder and also why some patients respond to one of these drugs and not to another.

have different actions in bipolar disorder than other atypical antipsychotics but also why some bipolar patients respond to one atypical antipsychotic and not another (Figure 13-26). Thus, all atypical antipsychotics are approved for schizophrenia and most for mania but only a few for bipolar depression. This may be somewhat of an artifact of commercial considerations and lack of completion of clinical trials for some of the newer agents, but it may also reflect differing portfolios of pharmacological actions (Figure 13-26) among those properties that might have antidepressant effects (Figure 13-25). Much further research

Mood Stabilizers | 693

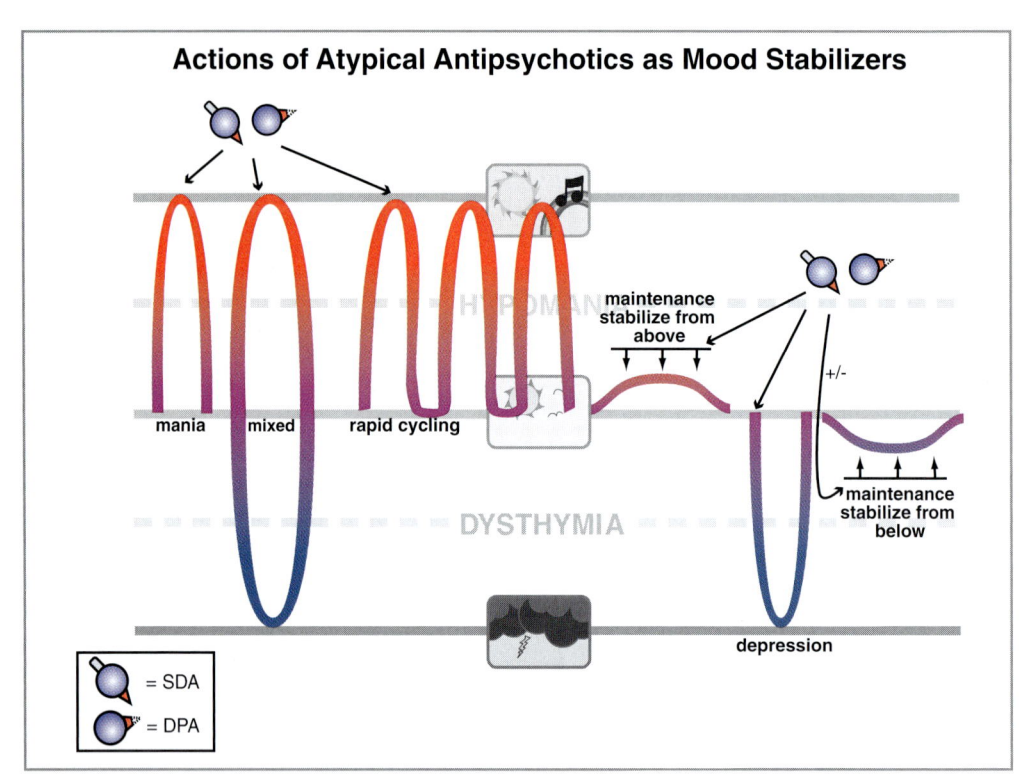

FIGURE 13-27 Actions of atypical antipsychotics as mood stabilizers. The atypical antipsychotics risperidone, olanzapine, quetiapine, ziprasidone, and aripiprazole all have established efficacy for treating the manic phase of bipolar disorder, and some (particularly aripiprazole and olanzapine) have also demonstrated efficacy for preventing the recurrence of mania. Quetiapine and olanzapine are efficacious for treating bipolar depression; other atypical antipsychotics may be effective as well but are not currently well studied. Atypical antipsychotics are not well studied in the prevention of depression recurrence.

must be completed before we will know the reason why atypical antipsychotics may work in mania or in bipolar depression. In the meantime, these agents as a class provide some of the broadest efficacy in bipolar disorder available (Figure 13-27) – indeed, broader than that for most anticonvulsants (Figures 13-9, 13-13, and 13-17; also Table 13-1) and comparable or better than that for lithium (Figure 13-4). Increasingly therefore, bipolar disorder is not only treated with two or more agents but with one of those agents as an atypical antipsychotic.

Other agents used in bipolar disorder

Benzodiazepines

Although benzodiazepines are not formally approved as mood stabilizers, they are anticonvulsants, anxiolytics, and sedative hypnotics and therefore provide valuable adjunctive treatment to proven mood stabilizers. In emergent situations, intramuscular or oral administration of benzodiazepines can have a calming action immediately and provide valuable time for mood stabilizers with a longer onset of action to begin working. Also, benzodiazepines are quite valuable for patients on an as-needed basis for intermittent agitation, insomnia, and incipient manic symptoms. Skilled intermittent use can leverage the mood-stabilizing actions of concomitant mood stabilizers and prevent eruption of more severe symptoms, possibly also avoiding rehospitalization. Of course benzodiazepines should be administered

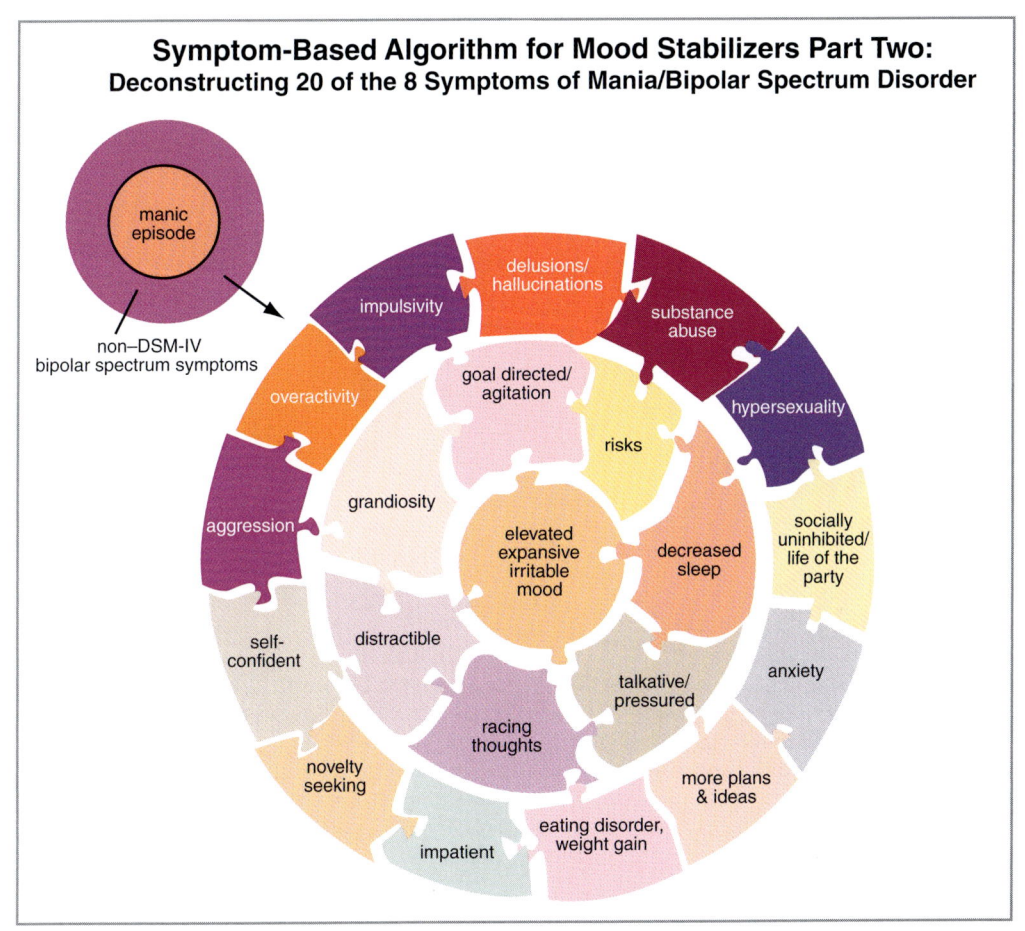

FIGURE 13-36 Symptom-based algorithm for mood stabilizers, part 2. Several common symptoms associated with mania can be disabling and prevent remission but are nonetheless not part of the formal diagnostic criteria for a manic episode. These are shown here as the outer ring.

pharmacological mechanisms in order to enhance the efficiency of information processing in these circuits and thereby reduce symptoms. This is shown specifically for the common residual symptoms of fatigue, loss of concentration, and insomnia in depression in Figure 12-123 along with the recommended treatments; this is also the same approach taken for depression in bipolar disorder as long as it is done while augmenting a mood stabilizer that protects against the possible emergence of mania, which is associated with some of the treatments suggested.

How about residual symptoms of mania that continue after treatment with a mood stabilizer? Core diagnostic symptoms of mania are shown in Figure 13-35 and discussed extensively in Chapter 11 and illustrated in Figures 11-56 through 11-62. The circuits hypothetically associated with each of these symptoms are summarized in Figure 11-57, and the regulation of numerous specific circuits by monoamine neurotransmitters is shown in Figures 11-58 through 11-62.

If this is not complicated enough, there are many other symptoms associated with a manic or mixed episode that are not considered core diagnostic criteria; these are illustrated as the outer ring in Figure 13-36. The postulated circuits associated with each of these

Symptom-Based Algorithm for Mood Stabilizers Part Three:
Match Each Symptom Associated with Mania
to Hypothetically Malfunctioning Brain Circuits

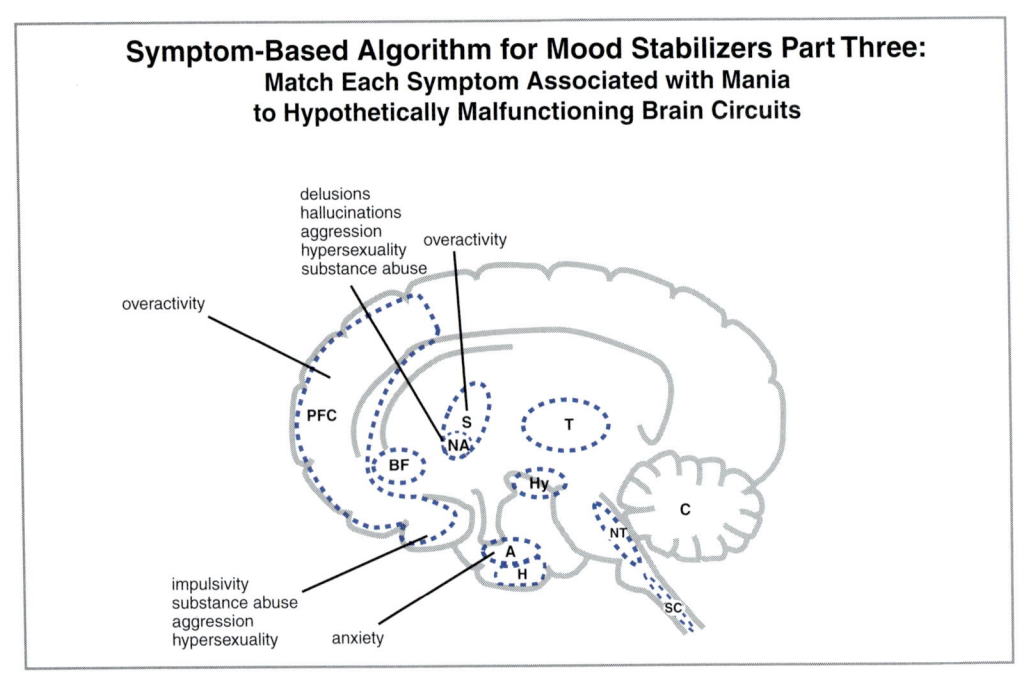

FIGURE 13-37 Symptom-based algorithm for mood stabilizers, part 3. In this figure common associated but not diagnostic symptoms of mania are linked to hypothetically malfunctioning brain circuits. Delusions and hallucinations are linked primarily to the nucleus accumbens (NA); while aggression, hypersexuality, and substance abuse are mediated not only by the NA but also by the prefrontal cortex (PFC). The PFC may also play a role in impulsivity and overactivity; overactivity is also associated with the striatum (S). Anxiety may occur in bipolar disorder and is primarily mediated by the amygdala (A).

nondiagnostic symptoms of mania are summarized in Figure 13-37. Similarly, the nondiagnostic symptoms associated with depression are discussed in chapter 12 and illustrated in Figure 12-124, with associated circuits shown in Figure 12-125 and suggested treatments in Figure 12-126. These same considerations in Figures 12-124 through 12-126 apply as well for bipolar patients in the depressed or mixed phases of the illness.

Suggested treatments for the nondiagnostic mania-related symptoms are shown in Figures 13-38 through 13-41. Differing mechanisms of action for mood stabilizers, discussed throughout this chapter, are illustrated in Figures 13-39 through 13-41. Since these mechanisms are certainly quite different, act at separate and distinct targets, and may be additive if not synergistic when combined, they provide the rationale for combining drugs with different mechanisms when ongoing treatments are associated with residual symptoms and not with complete remission.

That is, manic symptoms are largely conceptualized as the product of unstable and excessive if not chaotic neurotransmission in specific brain circuits, depending on the exact symptom being expressed (Figure 13-37). This state of unstable and excessive neurotransmission is illustrated in Figure 13-39A with a "bipolar storm" shown brewing between the two neurons in the circuit, conceptualized as too much sodium ion flow through voltage-sensitive sodium channels (VSSCs), too much calcium flow through voltage-sensitive calcium channels (VSCCs), and too much release of excitatory glutamate neurotransmitter. In reality, the problem may be that a bipolar circuit is "out of tune" and therefore acting

Symptom-Based Algorithm for Mood Stabilizers Part Four:
Target Regulatory Neurotransmitters With Selected Pharmacological Mechanisms

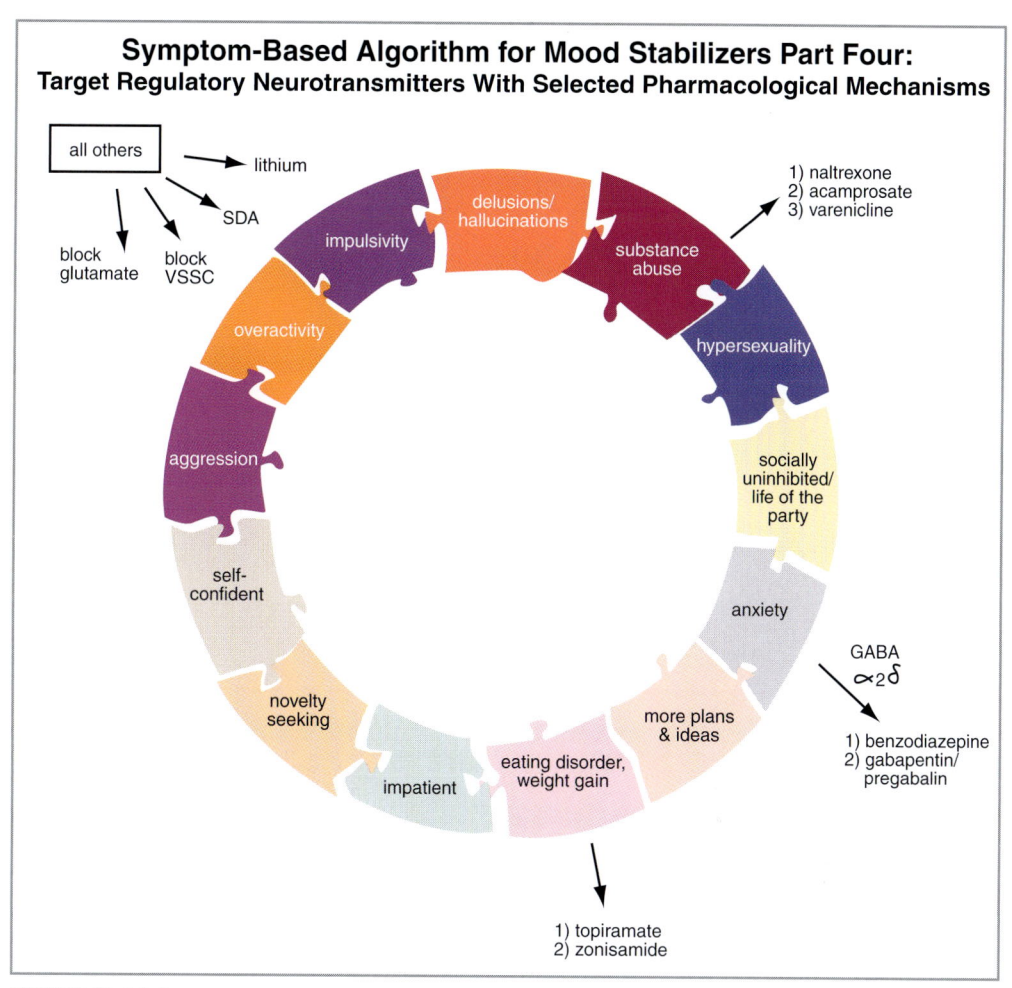

all others → lithium
→ SDA
block glutamate
block VSSC

- impulsivity
- delusions/hallucinations
- substance abuse → 1) naltrexone 2) acamprosate 3) varenicline
- hypersexuality
- overactivity
- socially uninhibited/life of the party
- aggression
- anxiety — GABA $\alpha_2\delta$ → 1) benzodiazepine 2) gabapentin/pregabalin
- self-confident
- more plans & ideas
- novelty seeking
- eating disorder, weight gain → 1) topiramate 2) zonisamide
- impatient

FIGURE 13-38 Symptom-based algorithm for mood stabilizers, part 4. Nondiagnostic symptoms of mania can be linked to the neurotransmitters that regulate them and in turn linked to pharmacological mechanisms for treatment selection. Many of these symptoms may be targeted by first-line treatments that block voltage-sensitive sodium channels (VSSCs), dopamine 2 and serotonin 2A receptors (by atypical antipsychotics), or glutamate; lithium may also treat many of these symptoms. Particular symptoms that may benefit from adjunctive treatment include substance abuse, which may be treated by naltrexone (alcohol), acamprosate (alcohol), or varenicline (smoking); anxiety, which may be related to gamma-aminobutyric acid (GABA) and voltage-sensitive calcium channels (VSCCs) and treated with benzodiazepines or gabapentin/pregabalin; and eating disorders or weight gain, which may be treated by topiramate or zonisamide.

inconsistently and chaotically in its neurotransmission rather than simply being too active as shown in Figure 13-39A.

Figures 13-39B and C through 13-41 show the various pharmacological mechanisms of action that can be selected or combined in order to attempt to reduce all symptoms and achieve remission in bipolar disorder. This starts with stabilizing and reducing neurotransmission in targeted and symptomatic circuits by blocking VSSCs with some mood stabilizers (Figure 13-39B), by reducing glutamate release or glutamate actions at NMDA receptors (Figure 13-39C) with other mood stabilizers, and/or by reducing dopamine hyperactivity with atypical antipsychotics or lithium (Figure 13-40), and/or by reducing glutamate hyperactivity by blocking 5HT2A receptors with atypical antipsychotics (Figure 13-41).

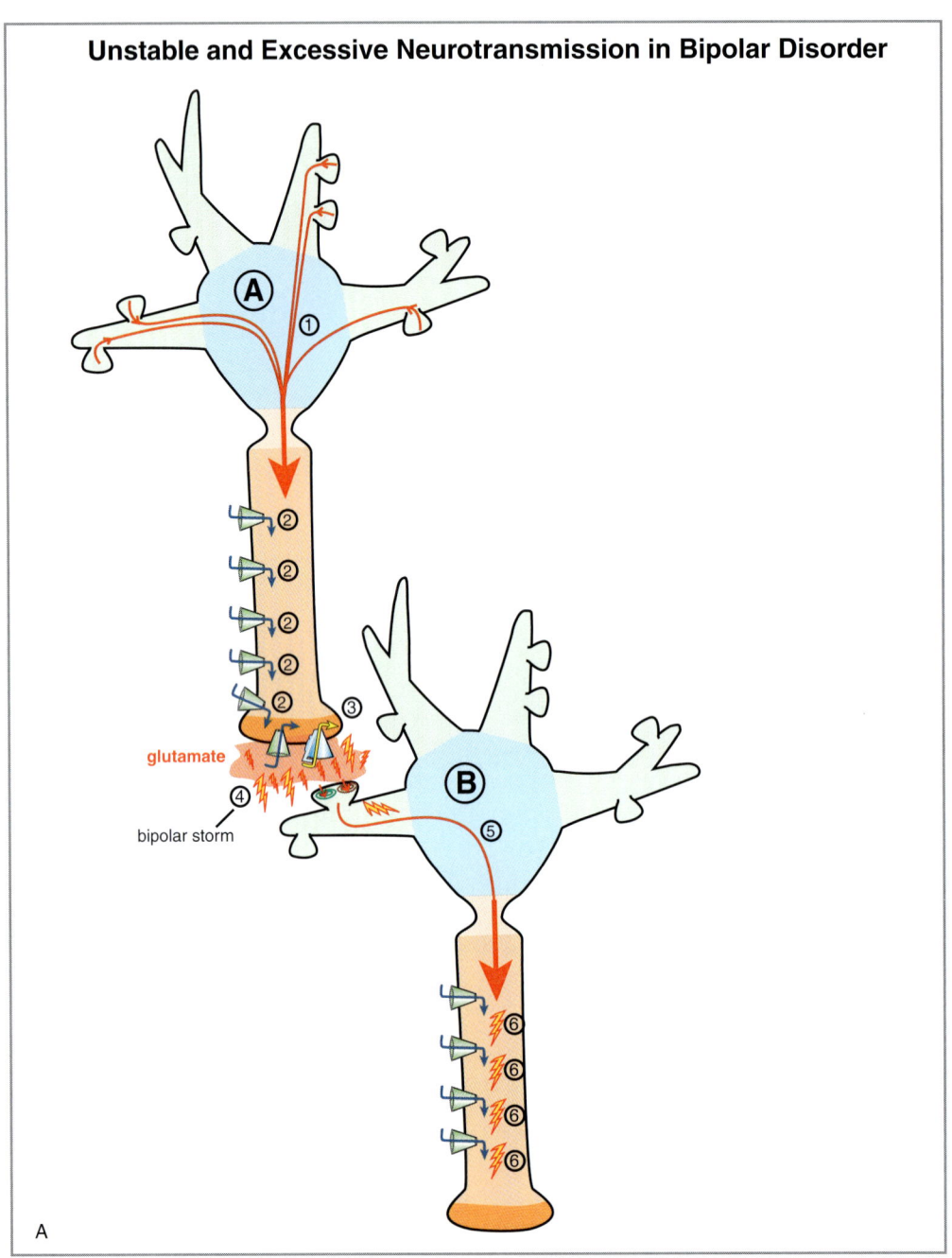

FIGURE 13-39A Unstable and excessive neurotransmission in bipolar disorder. Rather than being a function of too much or too little neurotransmission, bipolar disorder may instead occur as a result of unstable and excessive neurotransmission culminating in a "bipolar storm" at synapses. The bipolar storm is conceptualized here as too much activity of neuron A with widespread input from its dendritic tree (1) triggering too much axonal impulse flow, mediated by overly active voltage-sensitive sodium channels (2). When the nerve impulse invades the axon terminal, this, in turn, overly activates the voltage-sensitive calcium channels linked to glutamate release there (3), triggering a "bipolar storm" (4) of excessive, chaotic, or unpredictable neurotransmission from neuron A to neuron B. Postsynaptic NMDA receptors on neuron B detect this bipolar storm (4) and propagate excessive, chaotic, or unpredictable neurotransmission in neuron B (5), which in turn converts this information into its own nerve impulse, its own excessive activation of voltage-sensitive sodium channels (6), and so on.

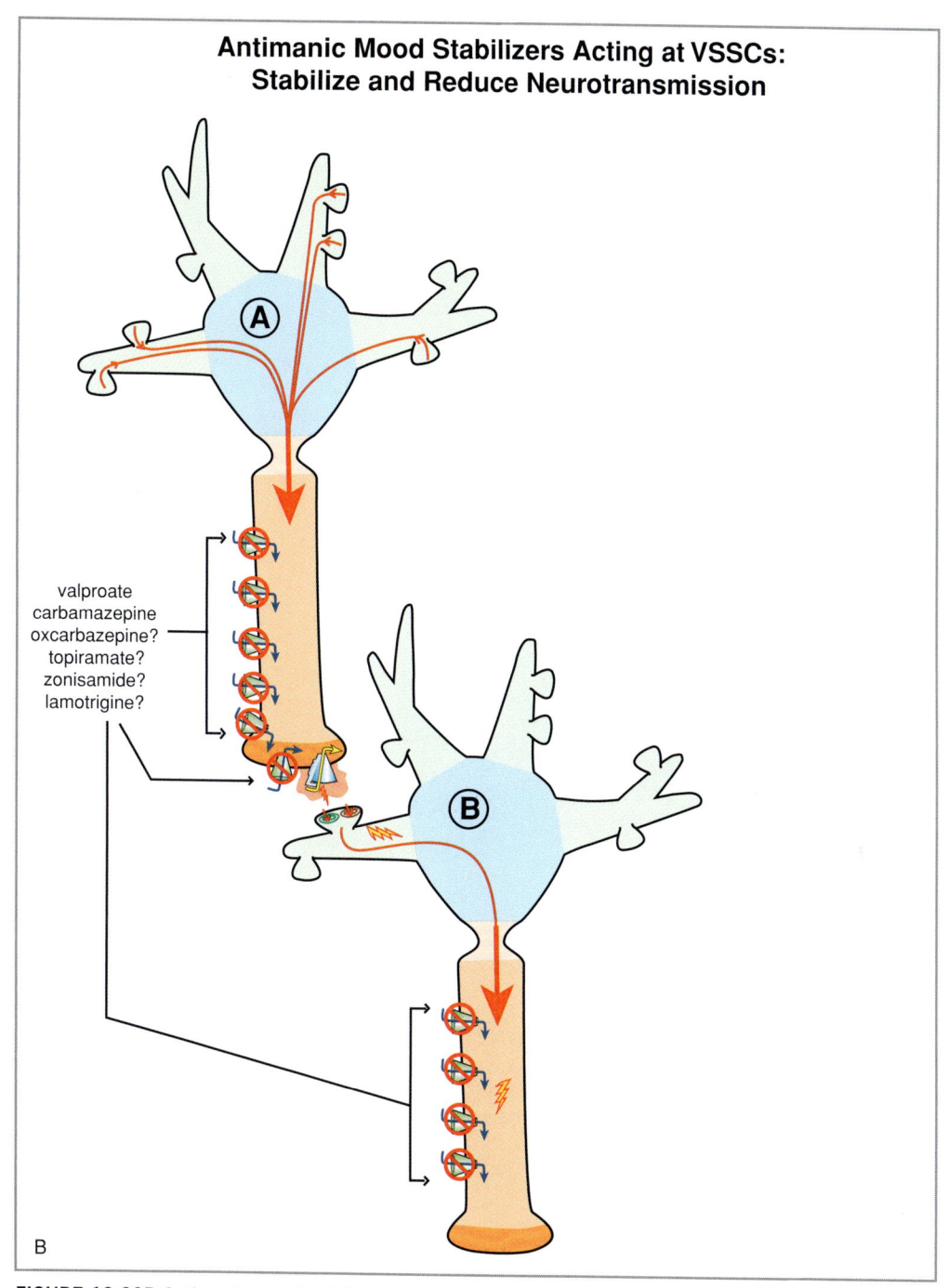

FIGURE 13-39B Antimanic mood stabilizers acting at voltage-sensitive sodium channels (VSSCs). Mood stabilizers that block VSSCs may stabilize and reduce propagation of nerve impulses and neurotransmission and thus reduce symptoms of mania. Examples of antimanic agents that act at VSSCs are valproate and carbamazepine; other VSSC blockers include oxcarbazepine, topiramate, zonisamide, and lamotrigine.

Mood Stabilizers | 707

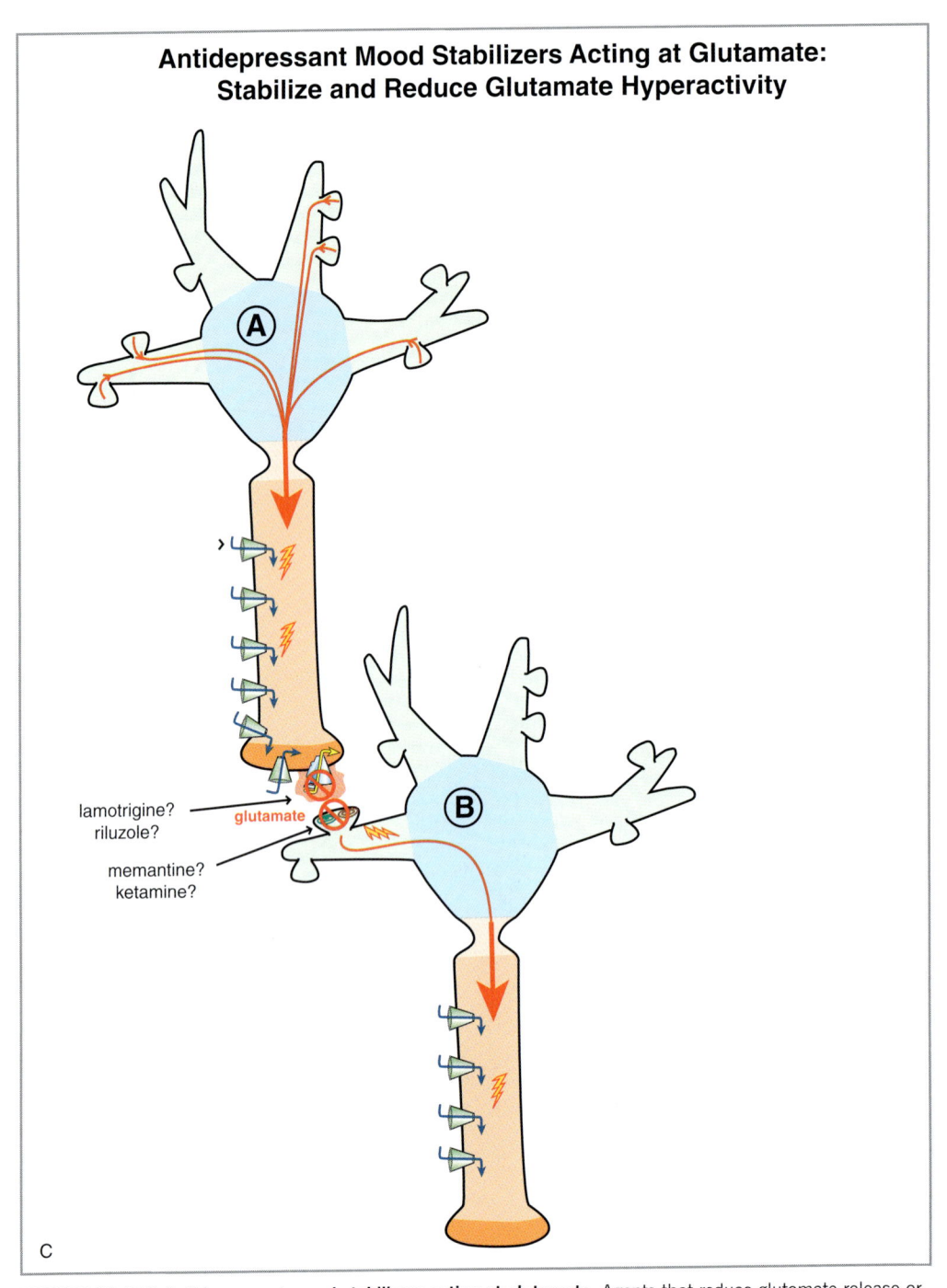

FIGURE 13-39C Antidepressant mood stabilizers acting at glutamate. Agents that reduce glutamate release or block glutamate actions at N-methyl-d-aspartate (NMDA) receptors may stabilize and reduce glutamate hyperactivity and thus have efficacy in the depressed phase of bipolar disorder. Lamotrigine and riluzole may reduce glutamate release, while memantine and ketamine act at NMDA receptors.

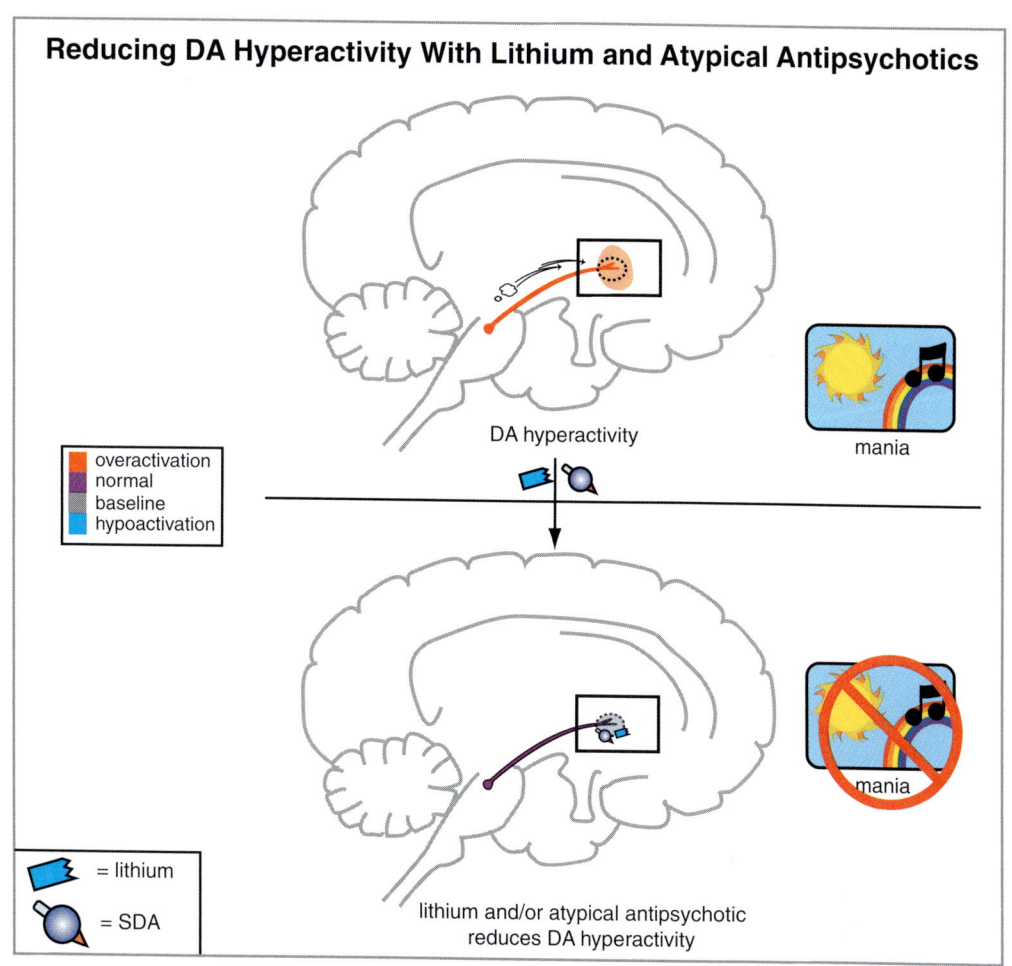

FIGURE 13-40 Reducing dopamine hyperactivity with lithium and atypical antipsychotics. Dopamine hyperactivity could play a role in the development of manic symptoms; therefore the reduction of dopamine hyperactivity, which can be achieved with lithium or atypical antipsychotics, may be an effective antimanic strategy.

If this is not sufficient, other pharmacological mechanisms may need to be recruited to suppress all symptoms. Pain and anxiety are discussed in Chapter 12 and the associated circuits illustrated in Figure 12-125 and treatment recommendations given in Figure 12-126. These concepts also apply when these same symptoms are residual in bipolar disorder. Adjunctive topiramate or zonisamide may be helpful for weight gain, and adjunctive drug abuse treatments may be helpful for substance abuse, including acamprosate and/or naltrexone for alcohol abuse and varenicline for smoking cessation (Figure 13-38).

Finally, bipolar disorder may not only have associated nondiagnostic symptoms but also many comorbid conditions, ranging from various anxiety disorders, psychosis, impulse control disorders, attention deficit hyperactivity disorder, conduct disorder, borderline personality disorder, migraine, bulimia, thyroid disorders, and many more (Figure 13-42). The point is to try to eliminate all such symptoms so as to get the patient to remission. The importance of this approach is difficult to underestimate. It has been estimated that for every residual manic/hypomanic symptom there is a 20% increase in the chance of manic

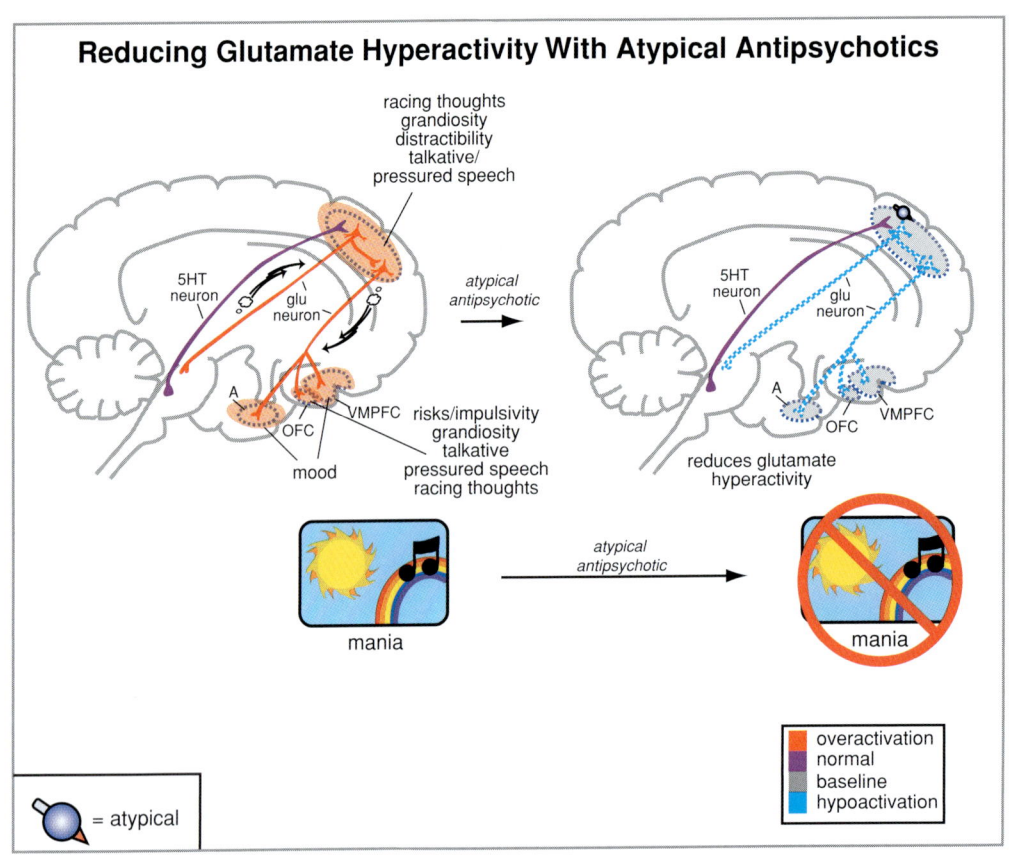

FIGURE 13-41 Reducing glutamate hyperactivity with atypical antipsychotics. Glutamate hyperactivity is proposed to contribute to development of both manic and depressive symptoms in bipolar disorder, perhaps in different pathways. Blockade of serotonin 2A (5HT2A) receptors by atypical antipsychotics can lead to reduced glutamate hyperactivity and thus may treat these symptoms. Potential sites of action for mania are shown here.

relapse, and for every residual depressive symptom a 15% increase in the chance of depressive relapse. This is why psychopharmacologists should consider treating all 20 of the 8 symptoms of a bipolar manic episode (Figure 13-36), all 14 of the 9 symptoms of a depressive episode (Figure 12-124), all comorbidities, and beyond! This requires taking a history that looks for all such symptoms not only before treatment but also after each sequential treatment. Each patient would have his or her bipolar symptoms deconstructed not only into diagnostic symptoms but also into all associated symptoms and comorbid conditions on each visit (Figures 12-124, 12-127, 13-36, and 13-42). Each and every symptom could then be mapped onto hypothetically malfunctioning brain circuits (Figures 12-125 and 13-37). The goal of treatment, of course, is not only sustained remission but also the prevention of more complicated and unstable outcomes, including the development of resistance to known treatments (Figure 11-29).

Bipolar disorder and women

The use of antidepressants in women is extensively discussed in Chapter 12 and illustrated in Figures 12-97 through 12-106. Although gender issues in bipolar disorder are less well investigated than they are in unipolar disorder, a brief discussion is in order for those special considerations known to be relevant to women with bipolar disorder.

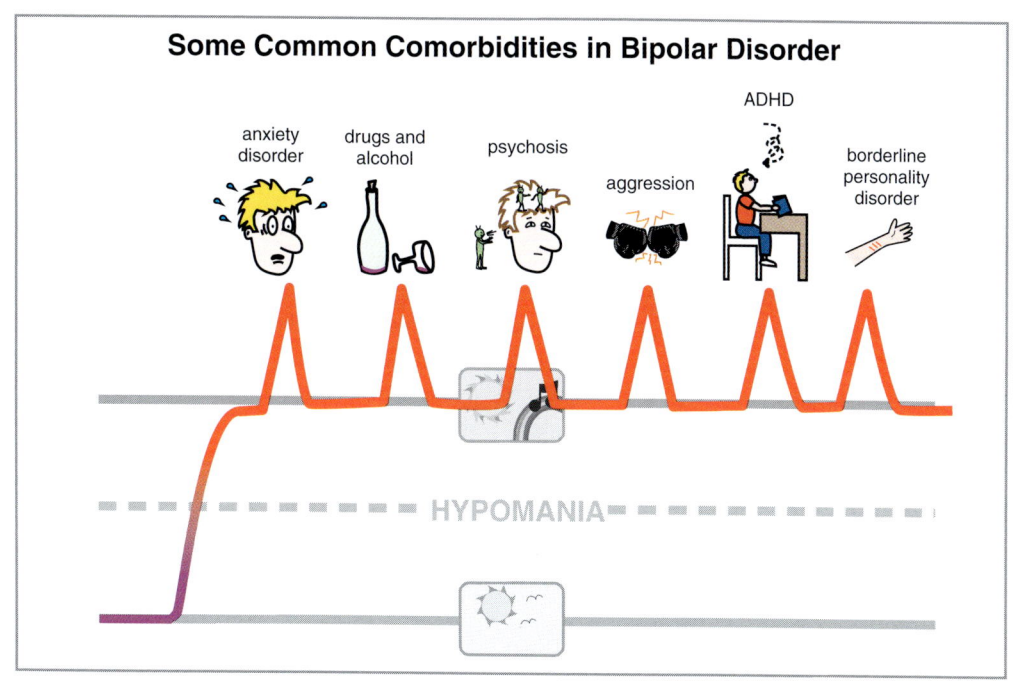

FIGURE 13-42 Common comorbidities in bipolar disorder. Many patients with bipolar disorder also have comorbid conditions. Common comorbidities include anxiety disorders, drug and alcohol abuse, psychosis, attention deficit hyperactivity disorder (ADHD), and borderline personality disorder. Aggression may also be a common symptom in patients with bipolar disorder.

For example, in women, bipolar disorder is even more depressive in nature than it is in men with this condition, with more suicide attempts, mixed mania, and rapid cycling than in men. Women have more thyroid dysfunction than men, and some experts believe that augmentation of bipolar patients with thyroid hormone (T3) – in men but particularly in women – may enhance stability even in the absence of overt thyroid dysfunction (see discussion in Chapter 12; also Figure 12-112 as well as Figure 13-34). Women are more likely than men to report atypical or reverse vegetative symptoms during the depressed phase, especially increased appetite and weight gain. Comorbid anxiety and eating disorders are more frequent in bipolar women; comorbid substance use disorders are more frequent in men.

There is limited evidence that bipolar disorder may worsen during the premenstrual phase in some women, just as unipolar major depression may worsen premenstrually (discussed in Chapter 12 as menstrual magnification and illustrated in Figure 12-100). Pregnancy is not protective against bipolar mood episodes, and the postpartum period is a very high risk time for experiencing first onset and recurrence of depressive, manic, mixed, and psychotic episodes (postpartum depressive episodes are discussed in Chapter 12 and illustrated in Figures 12-100 and 12-103).

There is little empirical study of bipolar disorder in perimenopausal or postmenopausal women, but there are suggestions that bipolar recurrence is more common during perimenopause and that estrogen may stabilize mood in perimenopausal women with bipolar disorder. No research shows what specific interventions to make for a perimenopausal bipolar woman with vasomotor symptoms or for perimenopausal or postmenopausal women who have unstable mood symptoms and do not take estrogen replacement therapy. Vasomotor symptoms in unipolar depression are discussed in Chapter 12 and illustrated in Figures 12-104 through 12-106.

No major gender differences have been consistently reported for mood stabilizers in terms of efficacy, but there are differences in side effects, including the possible risk of polycystic ovarian syndrome with amenorrhea, hyperandrogenism, weight gain, and insulin resistance from valproate in women.

During pregnancy, most anticonvulsant mood stabilizers and lithium are associated with risk for various fetal toxicities. Some may be mitigated by coadministration of folate. However, at this writing it may be prudent to consider stabilizing bipolar women with atypical antipsychotics during pregnancy. If mood stabilizers are discontinued for pregnancy, this should not be done abruptly, or it may increase the chance of recurrence. Of course, nontreatment of bipolar illness has its consequences, too, as discussed for nontreatment of unipolar depression during pregnancy in Chapter 12 with the problems outlined in Table 12-13. Many of the same considerations apply as well to the treatment of bipolar women during pregnancy, including the decision whether to continue or discontinue mood stabilizers during pregnancy, postpartum periods, and breast-feeding. Such decisions should be made on an individual basis after weighing the risks and benefits for a particular patient. Generally speaking, breast-feeding while taking lithium is not recommended, whereas breast-feeding while taking valproate, lamotrigine, carbamazepine, or atypical antipsychotics can be cautiously considered, with careful monitoring of the infant and, if necessary, obtaining infant blood drug levels.

Children, bipolar disorder, and mood stabilizers

This is one of the great controversial areas of psychopharmacology today. As this book is not focused on child psychopharmacology, only a few key issues will be mentioned here. Controversies in the treatment of unipolar depression in children and adolescents with antidepressants are mentioned in Chapter 12 and illustrated in Figure 12-11. For bipolar disorder, there is debate about whether children even get this illness and whether symptoms attributable to bipolar disorder should be treated at all with powerful psychotropic medications.

In reality, it is increasingly clear that prepubertal and adolescent manias do exist and are more common than had been appreciated in the past; however, the symptoms are different from those of "classic" adult mania. That is, prepubertal mania is characterized by severe irritability, absence of discrete episodes yet periodic "affective storms" with severe, persistent, and often violent outbursts, attacking behavior and anger. Symptoms tend to be chronic and continuous rather than episodic and acute. Moods are only rarely euphoric, but there are high levels of hyperactivity and overactivity. It seems increasingly clear that pediatric mania may not be rare so much as it is difficult to diagnose and to distinguish from attention deficit hyperactivity disorder and conduct disorder. Thus, an atypical picture of a chronic course characterized by predominantly irritable mood and mania mixed with depression looks much different than euphoric mania with a biphasic and episodic course.

Adolescent-onset mania may more frequently include euphoria but otherwise has the symptom characteristics of childhood-onset rather than adult-onset mania. In fact, "mixed mania," affecting 20% to 30% of adults with bipolar mania, may often have its onset in retrospect in childhood or adolescence, with the additional characteristics of chronic course, high rate of suicide, poor response to treatment, and early history of cognitive symptoms highly suggestive of ADHD. Thus, pediatric mania may develop into adult mixed mania.

In children, mania has considerable symptomatic overlap with ADHD, and it has been estimated that over half (and possibly up to 90%) of patients with pediatric mania also have ADHD. This is not just due to "distractibility, motoric hyperactivity, and talkativeness," diagnostic symptoms that overlap with both mania and ADHD, but to true comorbidity. In such patients, it seems to be necessary to stabilize the mania before treating the ADHD to get best results, and also to combine mood stabilizers with ADHD treatments.

In children, conduct disorder is also strongly associated with mania. Most patients with mania qualify for the diagnosis of conduct disorder, making this association quite controversial if it leads to antipsychotic treatment of essentially all children with conduct disorder. However, there are differences in symptoms between the two groups, with physical restlessness and poor judgment more common in comorbid cases of conduct disorder and mania than in cases with mania alone. Finally, anxiety disorders, especially panic disorder and agoraphobia, are frequently comorbid for mania in children.

For treatment, the best options are to use what has been proven in adults, but there is a striking paucity of evidence for how to treat bipolar disorder in children and adolescents. Much further study of mood stabilizers is required in children and adolescents.

Combinations of mood stabilizers are the standard for treating bipolar disorder

Given the disappointing number of patients who attain remission from any phase of bipolar disorder after any given monotherapy or sequence of monotherapies, who can maintain that remission over the long run, and who can tolerate the treatment, it is not surprising that the majority of bipolar patients require treatment with several medications. Rather than have a simple regimen of one mood stabilizer at high doses and a patient with side effects but who is not in remission, it now seems highly preferable to have a patient in remission without symptoms no matter how many agents this takes. Furthermore, sometimes the doses of each agent can be lowered to tolerable levels while the synergy among their therapeutic mechanisms provides more robust efficacy than single agents even in high doses.

Several specific suggestions of mood stabilizer combinations are shown in Figures 13-43 through 13-45. Many others can be constructed, but these particular combinations or "combos" have enjoyed widespread use even though for many of them there are few actual evidence-based data from clinical trials that their combination results in superior efficacy. Because of the strong role of "eminence-based medicine" (with sometimes conflicting recommendations by different experts) rather than "evidence-based medicine" for combination treatments, some of the options are discussed with whimsy and humor below and in Figures 13-43 through 13-45. Nevertheless, treatment of bipolar disorders with rational and empirically useful combinations is serious business and the reader may find that several of these suggestions are useful for practicing clinicians in the treatment of some patients.

The best evidence-based combinations are the addition of lithium or valproate to an atypical antipsychotic, especially antipsychotics such as risperidone, olanzapine, and quetiapine, which have been on the market the longest. Thus these are atypical lithium and atypical valproate combos, as shown in Figure 13-43. Probably clozapine as well as somewhat newer agents such as ziprasidone, aripiprazole, and paliperidone are generally useful as well in combination with either lithium or valproate.

Although lithium, lamotrigine, and valproate have all been available for a long time, there are remarkably few controlled studies of their use together. Nevertheless, they all have different mechanisms of action and have different clinical profiles in the various phases of bipolar illness; they can therefore usefully be combined in clinical practice due to practice-based evidence as li-do (lithium-Depakote/divalproex/valproate), la-li

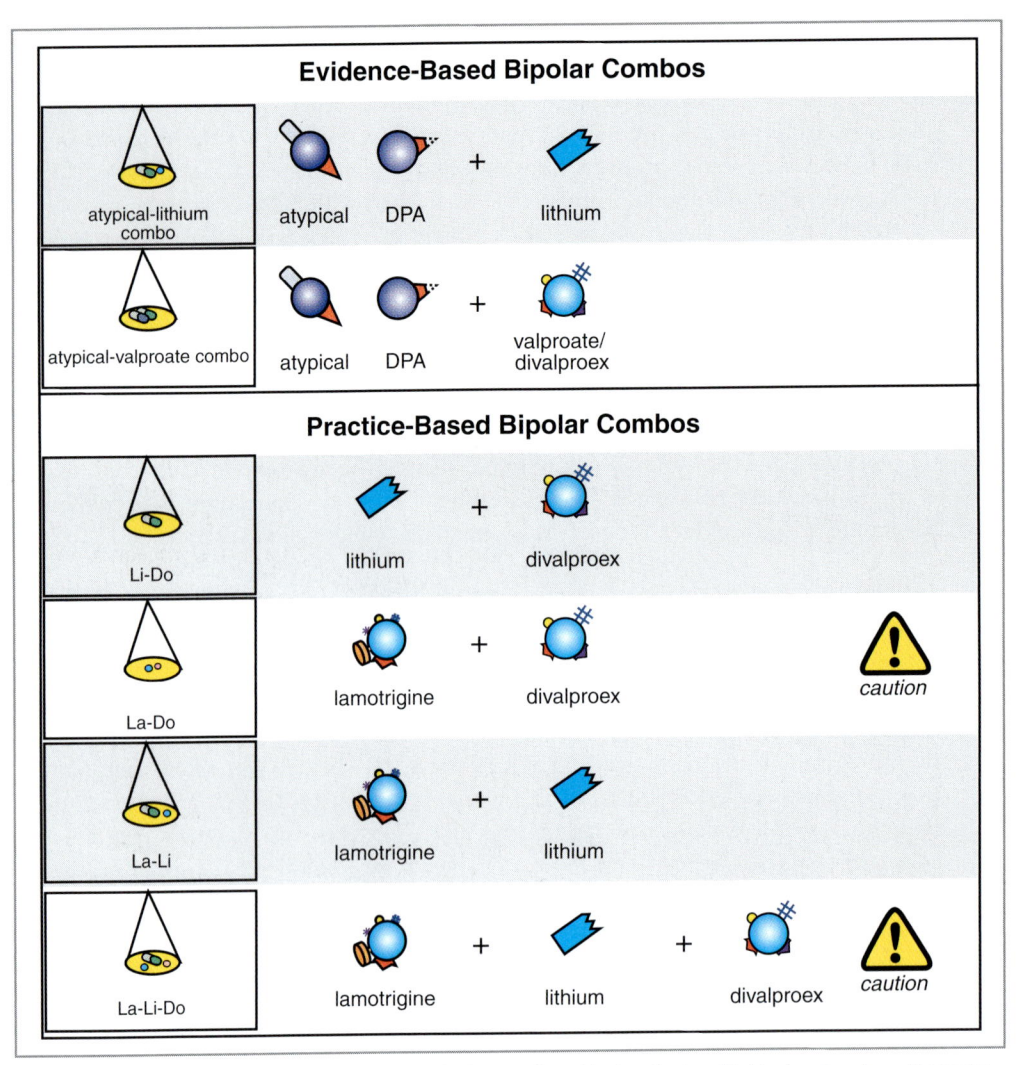

FIGURE 13-43 Evidence- and practice-based bipolar combos. Most patients with bipolar disorder will require treatment with two or more agents. The combinations with the most evidence include addition of an atypical antipsychotic to either lithium (atypical-lithium combo) or valproate/Depakote (atypical-valproate combo). Combinations that are not well studied in controlled trials but that have some practice-based evidence include lithium plus Depakote (li-do), cautious use of lamotrigine plus Depakote (la-do), lamotrigine plus lithium (la-li), and cautious combination of lamotrigine, lithium, and Depakote (la-li-do).

(lamotrigine-lithium), la-do (lamotrigine-Depakote) or even la-li-do (lamotrigine-lithium-Depakote) (Figure 13-43). Combinations of lamotrigine and valproate need to be carefully monitored for the consequences of the drug interactions between the two, especially for elevations of lamotrigine levels and the possible increased risk of rashes, including serious rash, unless the lamotrigine dose is decreased by as much as half.

Various natural products can also be added as adjuncts to any proven mood stabilizer, but these are not expected to have sudden and robust efficacy, including T3, L-methylfolate (MTHF), inositol, omega-3 fatty acids, SAMe, and others (Figure 13-34). Adjuncts are expected to help associated symptoms but not to be mood stabilizing per se, including agents for substance abuse (naltrexone, acamprosate, varenicline); weight loss (zonisamide, topiramate); pain, anxiety, and sleep (gabapentin, pregabalin); agitation (benzodiazepines); and many others (Figure 13-34).

Some of the more innovative if "eminence-based" combos are the most frequently used; several of these are shown in Figures 13-44 and 13-45.

Boston bipolar brew

Several experts, including many trained or working in Boston, are proponents of essentially *never* utilizing an antidepressant for bipolar patients. Thus, a "Boston bipolar brew" is any combination of mood stabilizers that does *not* include an antidepressant (Figure 13-44).

California careful cocktail

On the other hand, some experts in California are more laid back and are proponents of "earning" the right to add an antidepressant, carefully, once having exhausted other options for a bipolar depressed patient whose depression is not in remission. A "California careful cocktail" is the addition of an antidepressant to one or more mood stabilizers, particularly including one or more that has robust efficacy against mania and recurrence of mania (Figure 13-44).

Tennessee mood shine

Yet another option for treating bipolar depression occurs when giving an antidepressant and discovering that the patient either has activating side effects or treatment resistance or that the diagnosis is changing from unipolar to bipolar depression as the condition evolves. In this case, rather than stopping the antidepressant, an atypical antipsychotic is added. Experts in Tennessee came up with the idea to put some shine on depressed mood in patients inadequately responsive or tolerant to antidepressant monotherapy, so this approach is called "Tennessee mood shine" (Figure 13-44).

Buckeye bipolar bullets

Experts working in Ohio, the Buckeye State, have prominently proposed lamotrigine monotherapy as the magic bullet for first-line treatment of bipolar depression as well as for preventing relapse into depression (Figure 13-44). Although this can indeed be highly effective, one must remember that in many ways lamotrigine therapy is the "stealth" approach to treating bipolar depression, given the long titration times (two months or longer) and latency of onset of action once adequate dosing is reached (up to another three months). Thus, efficacy can appear to be clandestine and literally sneak up on the patient over three or four months rather than dramatically boosting mood soon after the initiation of treatment.

Rather than add an antidepressant to lamotrigine when there is inadequate response, an alternative approach would be to avoid that until several other combinations are tried first, including augmentation with an atypical antipsychotic, especially another Buckeye bipolar bullet called quetiapine (the combination is known as "Lami-quel" in Figure 13-44 – i.e., Lamictal/lamotrigine plus Seroquel/quetiapine). Any combination utilizing Seroquel/quetiapine with another mood stabilizer or antidepressant can be called a "Quel kit."

Yet another Buckeye bipolar bullet to combine with lamotrigine rather than augmenting with an antidepressant is the wake-promoting agent modafinil (modafinil combo in Figure 13-44), especially if the patient is "still sleepy after all these cures" and while monitoring

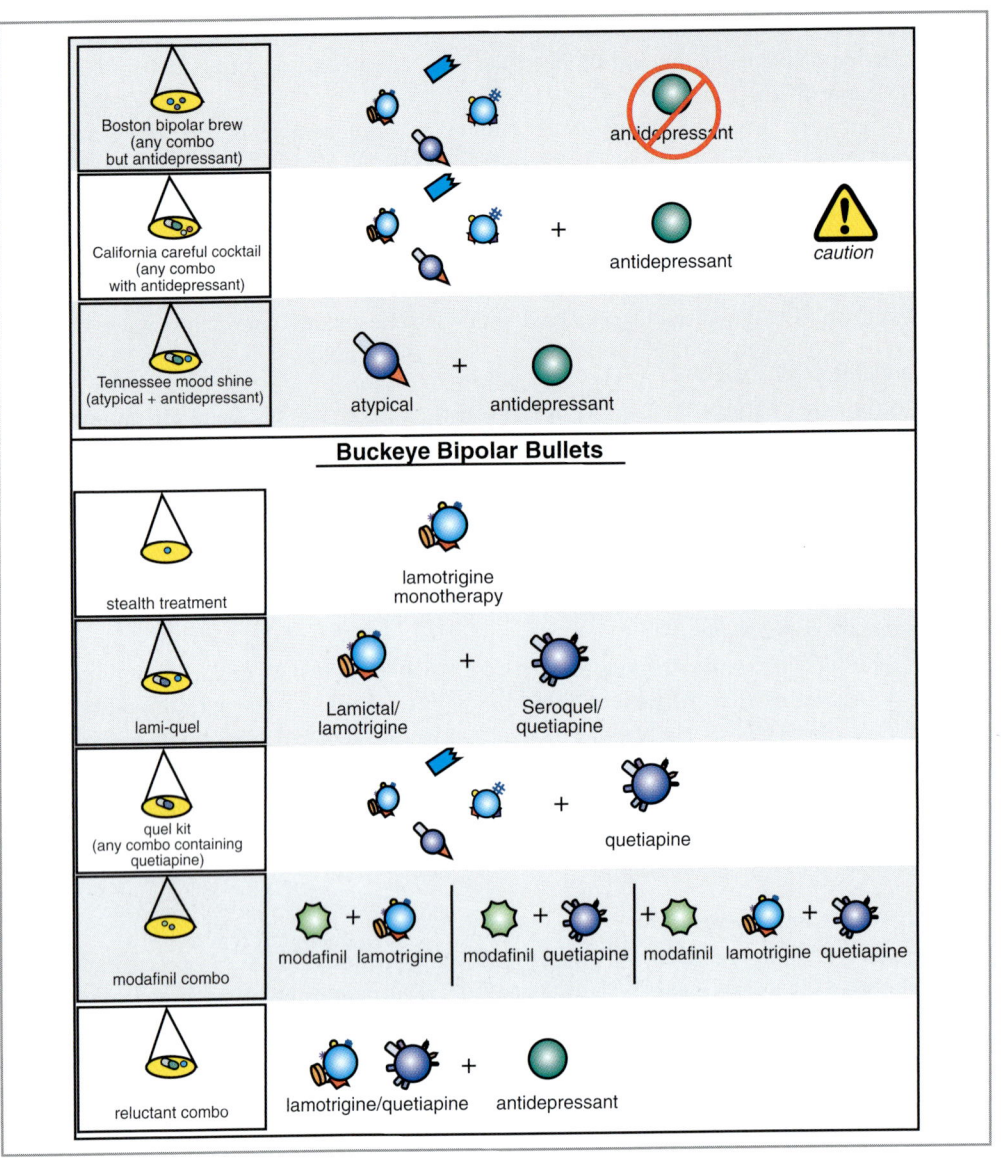

FIGURE 13-44 Bullet combos for bipolar depression. Experts diverge in their opinions of how to treat bipolar depression, particularly when it comes to antidepressants. Some believe that even when combination treatment is required, it should never involve use of an antidepressant (Boston bipolar brew), while others recommend cautious addition of an antidepressant to one or more mood stabilizers (California careful cocktail). For patients who develop symptoms of activation during treatment with an antidepressant for unipolar depression, some experts suggest adding an atypical antipsychotic rather than discontinuing the antidepressant (Tennessee mood shine). Another school of thought (Buckeye bipolar bullets) focuses on lamotrigine as the primary treatment for bipolar depression, with augmentation of other mood stabilizers (as opposed to antidepressants) when lamotrigine monotherapy is not enough. Lamotrigine may be considered a "stealth treatment," as it must be titrated slowly and can have a long latency of onset of action. Reasonable augmenting agents would include an atypical antipsychotic, particularly quetiapine (lami-quel). Quetiapine itself is an established monotherapy for bipolar depression and can be combined with many other agents as well (quel-kit). Another potential agent to add to lamotrigine, quetiapine, or lamotrigine and quetiapine is modafinil, particularly for patients with daytime sleepiness (modafinil combo). If none of these combinations produce a good response, one may consider adding an antidepressant to lamotrigine/quetiapine (reluctant combo).

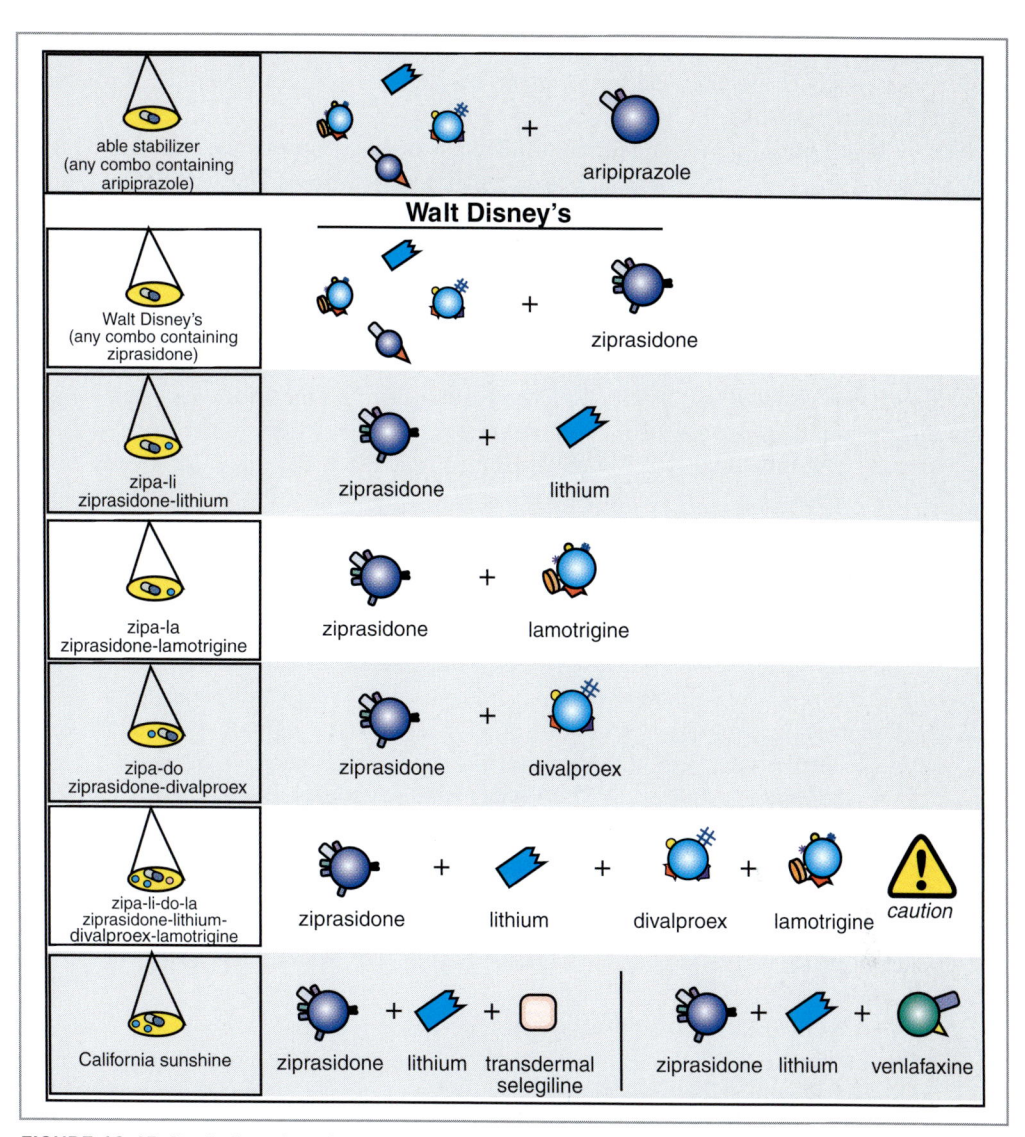

FIGURE 13-45 Atypical combos. Any combination containing the partial dopamine agonist aripiprazole may be referred to as an "able stabilizer," while any combination containing the serotonin dopamine antagonist ziprasidone may be collectively termed a "Walt Disney." These include ziprasidone plus lithium (zipa-li), ziprasidone plus lamotrigine (zipa-la), ziprasidone plus Depakote (zipa-do), and ziprasidone plus lithium, lamotrigine, and Depakote (zipa-li-do-la). California sunshine is a powerful combination for bipolar depression with full-dose ziprasidone and full-dose lithium as well as augmentation with either transdermal selegiline or high-dose venlafaxine.

for activation of mania. Modafinil's mechanism of action is discussed in further detail in Chapter 16, on sleep/wake disorders.

Finally, after trying all these options, continuing poor response in bipolar depression may require reluctant augmentation of lamotrigine or various of the lamotrigine combos described above with an antidepressant (reluctant combo in Figure 13-44).

"Able stabilizers" include any combo containing the dopamine partial agonist and dopamine system stabilizer Abilify/aripiprazole (Figure 13-45). For depressed patients, it

Mood Stabilizers | 717

may generally be advisable to use between 2 and 10 mg of aripiprazole and not more for best results in bipolar disorder and in treatment-resistant unipolar depression when combined with antidepressants.

"Walt Disney" combos refer to any mixture containing ziprasidone (Geodon) (Figure 13-45). Thus, this includes zipa-li, zipa-la, zipa-do, zipa-li-do-la. One of the Walt Disneys that may be effective for some of the most resistant of bipolar depressions is called "California sunshine" and includes ziprasidone in combination with lithium, both at full therapeutic doses, with transdermal selegiline or with high-dose venlafaxine.

Future mood stabilizers

Several new possibilities exist for novel mood stabilizers. This includes several new **atypical antipsychotics** in development, from bifeprunox to iloperidone to asenapine and others. Any **new anticonvulsant** is a potential mood stabilizer, and a few are already on the horizon, including eslicarbazepine, the active metabolite of oxcarbazepine discussed above (Figure 13-11) and a compound related to lamotrigine (JZP-4). **Dopamine agonists** such as pramipexole and related agents such as ropinirole may be useful for the depressed phase of bipolar disorder, especially in combination with mood stabilizers that could protect from the possible induction of mania.

New research is also targeting novel ways to **enhance GABA action or to block glutamate action** for new mood stabilizers, although these compounds are generally still in preclinical testing. Another novel site mentioned earlier is the **sigma 1 site**. An interesting set of observations suggests that dextromethorphan, which may act via sigma 1 receptors and secondarily as a weak NMDA antagonist, may be useful in stabilizing affect in involuntary emotional expression disorder (pseudobulbar affect) associated with various neurological conditions. One specific agent combines dextromethorphan with quinidine to enhance dextromethorphan bioavailability (AVP923, or Zenvia) and appears promising for this indication. It is possible that this combination or other agents that target sigma 1 sites may also be useful in stabilizing mood in bipolar disorder, but further research is necessary.

Clearly any antidepressant developed for unipolar depression is a candidate for cautious addition to mood stabilizers in some cases; these agents in development are discussed in Chapter 12. Agents that can reduce stress-related responses by acting at the hypothalamic pituitary adrenal (HPA) axis are also candidates for the treatment of major depressive disorder, bipolar disorder, anxiety disorders, and other conditions. These agents, including **glucocorticoid antagonists, corticotrophin releasing factor (CRF1) antagonists, and vasopressin 1b (V1b) antagonists** are discussed in Chapter 14, on anxiety.

Scientists are trying to create a future lithium mimetic by targeting actions at the same signal transduction cascades where lithium acts. Such approaches are still highly theoretical and in preclinical testing at this time, including how to activate the formation of **neurotrophic growth factors** such as BDNF or to act at relevant neurotrophic receptors.

Summary

Mood stabilizers have evolved significantly in recent years. They include agents that are mania-minded and treat mania while preventing manic relapse as well as agents that are depression-minded and treat bipolar depression while preventing depressive relapse. Numerous agents of diverse mechanisms of action are mood stabilizers, especially lithium, various anticonvulsants, and atypical antipsychotics. Numerous new agents developed for other uses are also being tested in bipolar disorder. However, because of limits to the efficacy and tolerability of current mood stabilizers, combination therapy is the rule and mood stabilizer monotherapy the exception. Evidence is evolving for how to combine agents to relieve all symptoms of bipolar disorder and prevent relapse, but the treatment of bipolar disorder today remains as much a psychopharmacological art as it does a science. New mood stabilizers of diverse novel mechanisms are also on the horizon.

CHAPTER 14

Anxiety Disorders and Anxiolytics

- Symptom dimensions in anxiety disorders
    - When is anxiety an anxiety disorder?
    - Overlapping symptoms of major depression and anxiety disorders
    - Overlapping symptoms of anxiety disorder subtypes
- The amygdala and the neurobiology of fear
- GABA, anxiety, and benzodiazepines
    - GABA-A receptor subtypes
    - Benzodiazepines as positive allosteric modulators (PAMs)
    - Novel GABA anxiolytics
- Serotonin, stress, and anxiety
- Stress sensitization
- Alpha 2 delta ligands as anxiolytics
- Noradrenergic hyperactivity in anxiety
- Fear conditioning versus fear extinction
    - Fear extinction means learning to forgive but not to forget
- Cortico-striatal-thalamic-cortical (CSTS) loops and the neurobiology of worry
- Treatments for anxiety disorder subtypes
- Summary

This chapter will provide a brief overview of anxiety disorders and their treatments. Included are descriptions of how the anxiety disorder subtypes overlap with each other and with major depressive disorder. Clinical descriptions and formal criteria for how to diagnose anxiety disorder subtypes are mentioned only in passing. The reader should consult standard reference sources for this material. The discussion here will emphasize how discoveries about the functioning of various brain circuits and neurotransmitters – especially those centered on the amygdala – affect our understanding of fear and worry, which cut across the entire spectrum of anxiety disorders.

The goal of this chapter is to acquaint the reader with ideas about the clinical and biological aspects of anxiety disorders in order to clarify the mechanisms of action of the various treatments for these disorders as they are discussed along the way. Many of these treatments are extensively discussed in previous chapters. For details of mechanisms of anxiolytic agents used also for the treatment of depression (i.e., certain antidepressants),

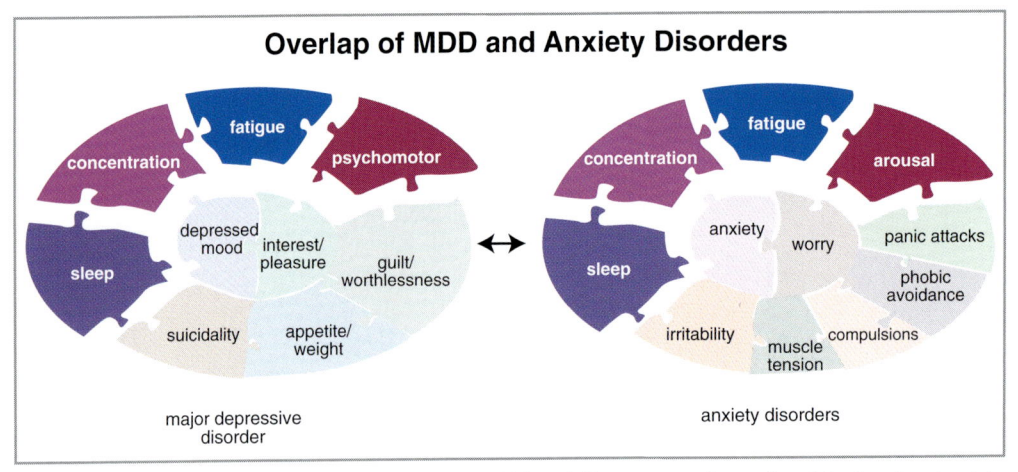

FIGURE 14-1 Overlap of MDD and anxiety disorders. Although the core symptoms of anxiety disorders (anxiety and worry) differ from the core symptoms of major depression (loss of interest and depressed mood), there is considerable overlap among the rest of the symptoms associated with these disorders (compare the "anxiety disorders" puzzle on the right to the "MDD" puzzle on the left). For example, fatigue, sleep difficulties, and problems concentrating are common to both types of disorders.

the reader is referred to Chapter 12; for those anxiolytic agents used also as mood stabilizers for the treatment of bipolar disorder (i.e., certain anticonvulsants), the reader is referred to Chapter 13; and for those anxiolytics used as antipsychotics, the place to look is Chapter 10. The discussion in this chapter is at the conceptual level, and not at the pragmatic level. The reader should consult standard drug handbooks (such as *Essential Psychopharmacology: Prescriber's Guide*) for details of doses, side effects, drug interactions, and other issues relevant to the prescribing of these drugs in clinical practice.

Symptom dimensions in anxiety disorders

When is anxiety an anxiety disorder?

Anxiety is a normal emotion under circumstances of threat and is thought to be part of the evolutionary "fight or flight" reaction of survival. Whereas it may be normal or even adaptive to be anxious when a saber-tooth tiger (or its modern-day equivalent) is attacking, there are many circumstances in which the presence of anxiety is maladaptive and constitutes a psychiatric disorder. The idea of anxiety as a psychiatric disorder is evolving rapidly. It is characterized by the concept of core symptoms of excessive fear and worry (symptoms at the center of anxiety disorders in Figure 14-1) compared to major depression, which is characterized by core symptoms of depressed mood or loss of interest (symptoms at the center of major depressive disorder in Figure 14-1).

Anxiety disorders have considerable symptom overlap with major depression (see those symptoms surrounding core features shown in Figure 14-1), particularly sleep disturbance, problems concentrating, fatigue, and psychomotor/arousal symptoms. Each anxiety disorder also has a great deal of symptom overlap with other anxiety disorders (Figures 14-2 through 14-6). Anxiety disorders are also extensively comorbid, not only with major depression but also with each other, since many patients qualify over time for a second or even third concomitant anxiety disorder (Figures 14-2 through 14-6). Finally, anxiety disorders are frequently comorbid with many other conditions such as substance abuse, attention deficit

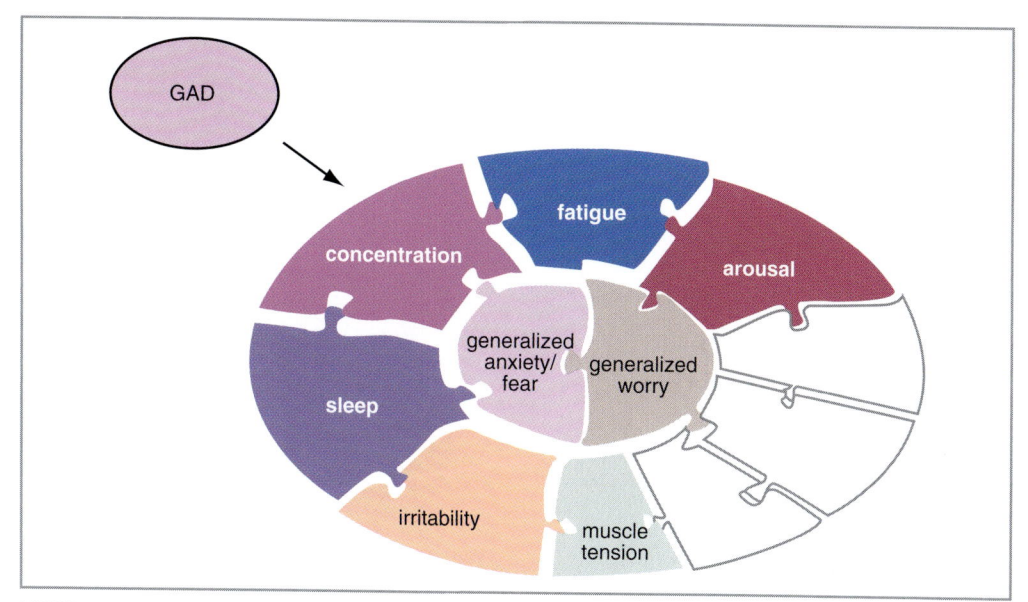

FIGURE 14-2 Generalized anxiety disorder (GAD). The symptoms typically associated with GAD are shown here. These include the core symptoms of generalized anxiety and worry as well as increased arousal, fatigue, difficulty concentrating, sleep problems, irritability, and muscle tension. Many of these symptoms, including the core symptoms, are present in other anxiety disorders as well.

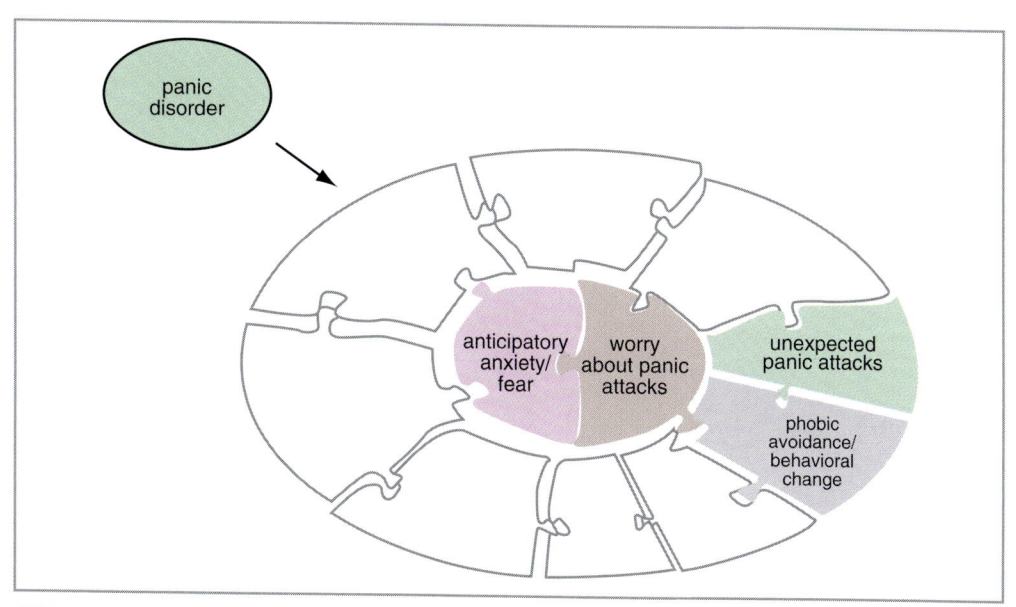

FIGURE 14-3 Panic disorder. The characteristic symptoms of panic disorder are shown here and include the core symptoms of anticipatory anxiety as well as worry about panic attacks; associated symptoms are the unexpected panic attacks themselves and phobic avoidance or other behavioral changes associated with concern over panic attacks.

Anxiety Disorders and Anxiolytics

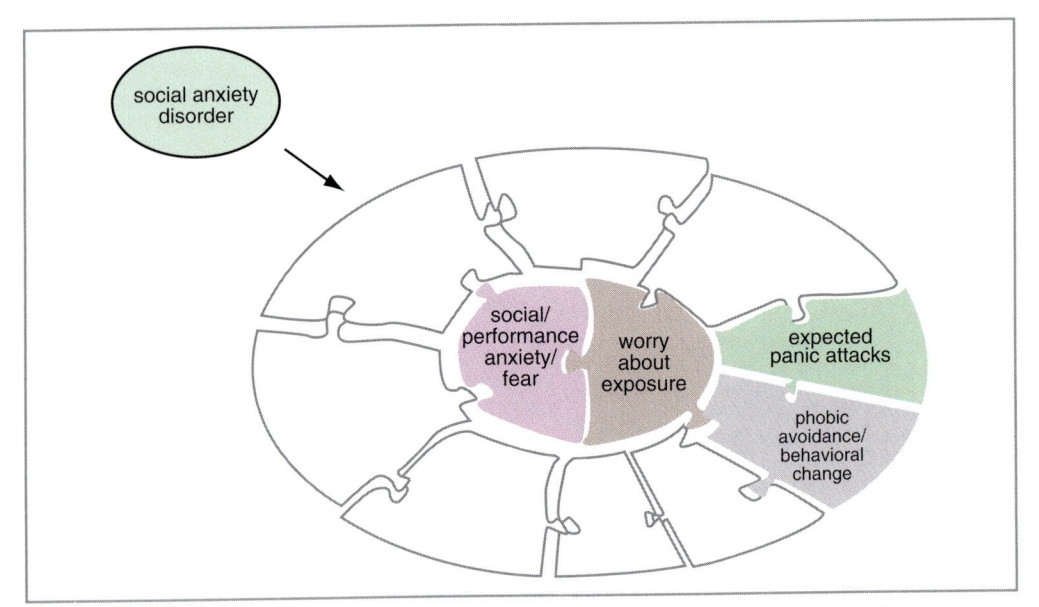

FIGURE 14-4 Social anxiety disorder. Symptoms of social anxiety disorder, shown here, include the core symptoms anxiety or fear over social performance plus worry about social exposure. Associated symptoms are panic attacks that are predictable and expected in certain social situations as well as phobic avoidance of those situations.

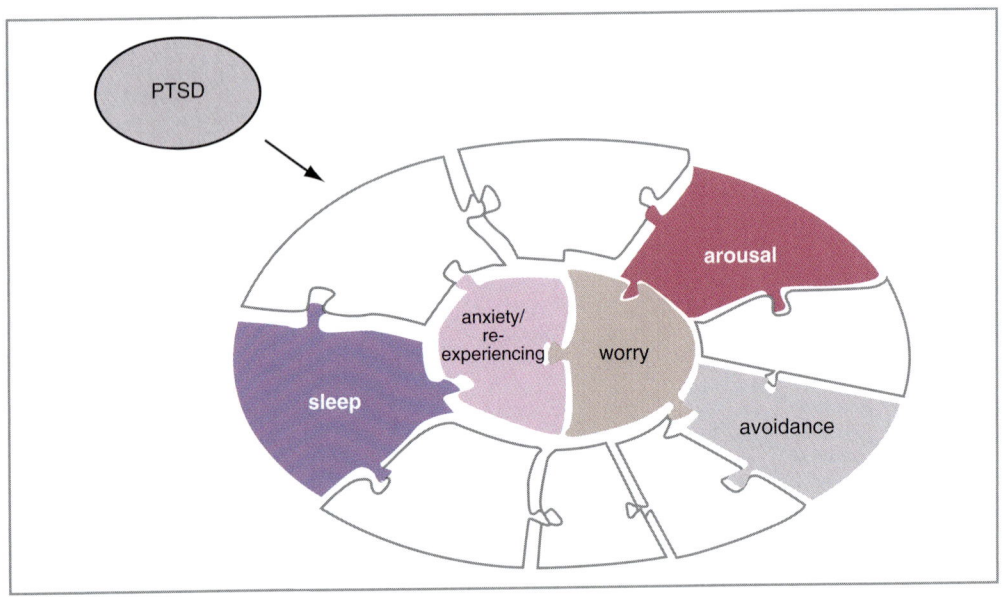

FIGURE 14-5 Posttraumatic stress disorder (PTSD). The characteristic symptoms of PTSD are shown here. These include the core symptoms of anxiety while the traumatic event is being reexperienced as well as worry about having the other symptoms of PTSD, such as increased arousal and startle responses, sleep difficulties including nightmares, and avoidance behaviors.

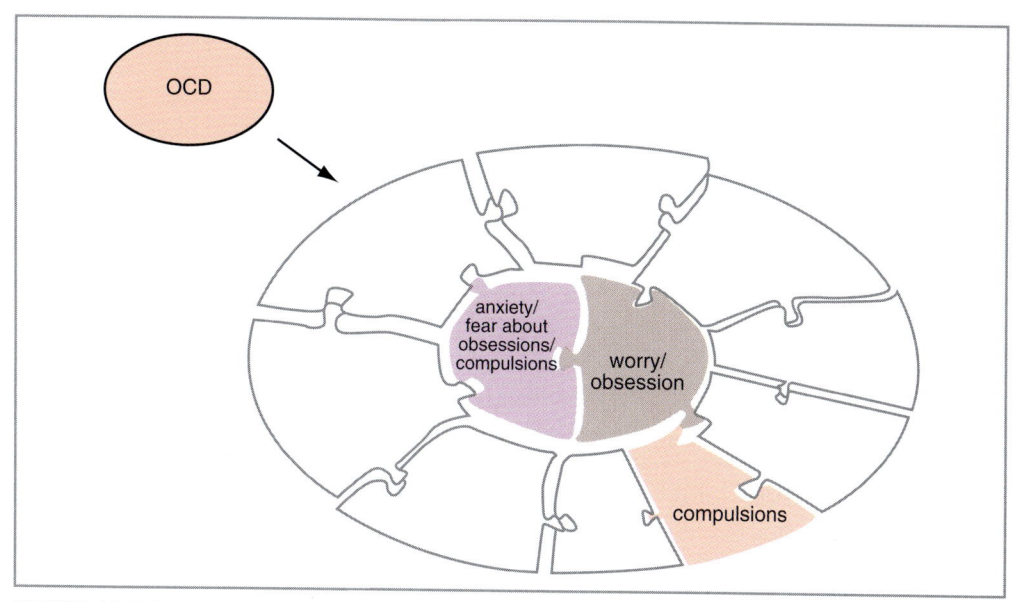

FIGURE 14-6 Obsessive compulsive disorder (OCD). Symptoms of OCD, shown here, include the core symptom of anxiety, which triggers obsessions and compulsions in attempts to reduce that worry as well as the obsessions themselves, which can be seen as a type of worry. Compulsions are a key associated feature.

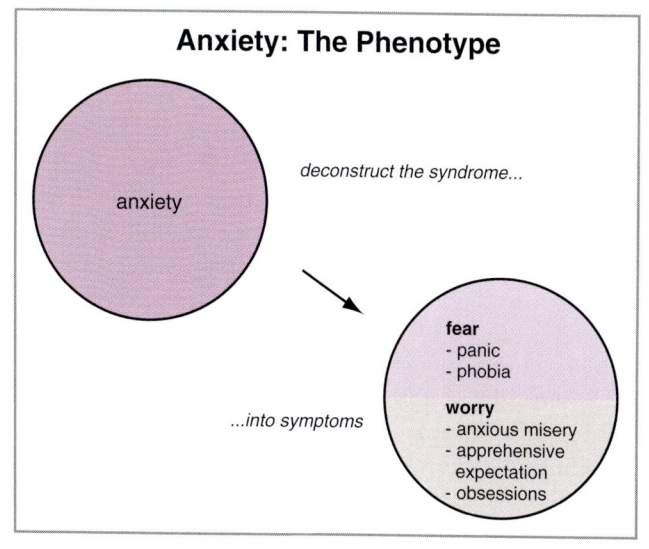

FIGURE 14-7 Anxiety: the phenotype. Anxiety can be deconstructed, or broken down, into the two core symptoms of fear and worry. These symptoms are present in all anxiety disorders, although what triggers them may differ from one disorder to the next.

hyperactivity disorder, bipolar disorder, pain disorders, sleep disorders, and more, just as in major depression (discussed in Chapter 12 and illustrated in Figure 12-127) and bipolar disorder (discussed in Chapter 13 and illustrated in Figure 13-42).

What, therefore, is an anxiety disorder? These disorders all seem to maintain the core features of some form of anxiety or fear coupled with some form of worry (Figure 14-7), but their natural history over time shows them to morph from one into another, to evolve into full-syndrome expression of anxiety disorder symptoms (Figure 14-1) and then to recede

Anxiety Disorders and Anxiolytics | 725

into subsyndromal levels only to reappear again as the original anxiety disorder, a different anxiety disorder (Figures 14-2 through 14-6), or major depression (Figure 14-1). If anxiety disorders all share core symptoms of fear and worry (Figure 14-7) and, as discussed later in this chapter, are all basically treated with the same drugs, including many of the same drugs that treat major depression, the question now arises: What is the difference between one anxiety disorder and another? Also, one could ask: What is the difference between major depression and anxiety disorders? Are all these entities really different disorders or are they just different aspects of the same illness?

Overlapping symptoms of major depression and anxiety disorders

Although the core symptoms of major depression (depressed mood or loss of interest) differ from the core symptoms of anxiety disorders (anxiety/fear and worry), there is a great deal of overlap with the other symptoms considered diagnostic for both a major depressive episode and several different anxiety disorders (Figure 14-1). These overlapping symptoms include problems with sleep, concentration, and fatigue as well as psychomotor/arousal symptoms (Figure 14-1). It is thus easy to see how the gain or loss of just a few additional symptoms can morph a major depressive episode into an anxiety disorder (Figure 14-1) or one anxiety disorder into another (Figures 14-2 through 14-6).

From a therapeutic point of view, it may matter little what the specific diagnosis is across this spectrum of disorders (Figures 14-1 through 14-6). That is, psychopharmacological treatments may not be much different for a patient who currently qualifies for a major depressive episode plus the symptom of anxiety (but not an anxiety disorder) versus a patient who currently qualifies for a major depressive episode plus a comorbid anxiety disorder with full-criteria anxiety symptoms. Although it can be useful to make specific diagnoses for following patients over time and for documenting the evolution of symptoms, the emphasis from a psychopharmacological point of view is increasingly to take a symptom-based therapeutic strategy to patients with any of these disorders. That is, specific treatments can be tailored to the individual patient by deconstructing whatever disorder the patient has into a list of the specific symptoms a given patient is experiencing (see Figures 14-2 through 14-6) and then matching these symptoms to hypothetically malfunctioning brain circuits regulated by specific neurotransmitters in order to rationally select and combine psychopharmacological treatments to eliminate all symptoms and get the patient to remission.

Discussion of this strategy for treating the symptoms of a major depressive episode to attain remission is provided in Chapter 12 and illustrated in Figures 12-120 to 12-126. Specific discussion of how to approach the overlapping symptoms of problems with sleep, concentration, and fatigue are illustrated in Figures 12-121 to 12-123.

Overlapping symptoms of anxiety disorder subtypes

Although there are different diagnostic criteria for different anxiety disorders (Figures 14-2 though 14-6), they can all be considered to have overlapping symptoms of anxiety/fear coupled with worry (Figure 14-7). Remarkable progress has been made in understanding the circuitry underlying the core symptom of anxiety/fear (Figure 14-7) based on an explosion of neurobiological research on the amygdala (Figures 14-8 through 14-42). The links between the amygdala, fear circuits, and treatments for the symptom of anxiety/fear across the spectrum of anxiety disorders are discussed throughout the rest of this chapter.

Worry is the second core symptom shared across the spectrum of anxiety disorders (Figure 14-8). This symptom is hypothetically linked to the functioning of cortico-striatal-

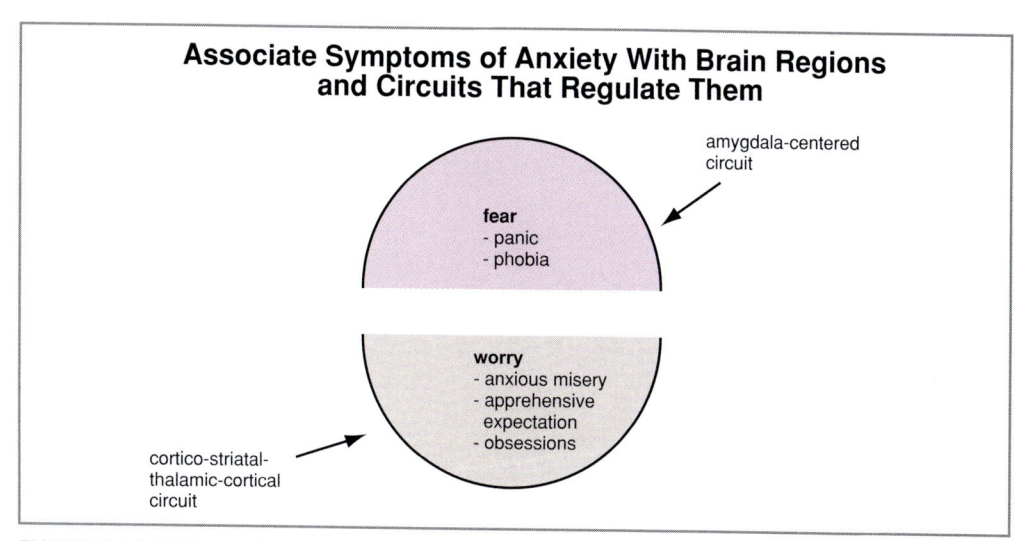

Associate Symptoms of Anxiety With Brain Regions and Circuits That Regulate Them

FIGURE 14-8 Linking anxiety symptoms to circuits. Anxiety and fear symptoms (e.g., panic, phobias) are regulated by an amygdala-centered circuit. Worry, on the other hand, is regulated by a cortico-striatal-thalamic-cortical (CSTC) loop. These circuits may be involved in all anxiety disorders, with the different phenotypes reflecting not unique circuitry but rather divergent malfunctioning within those circuits.

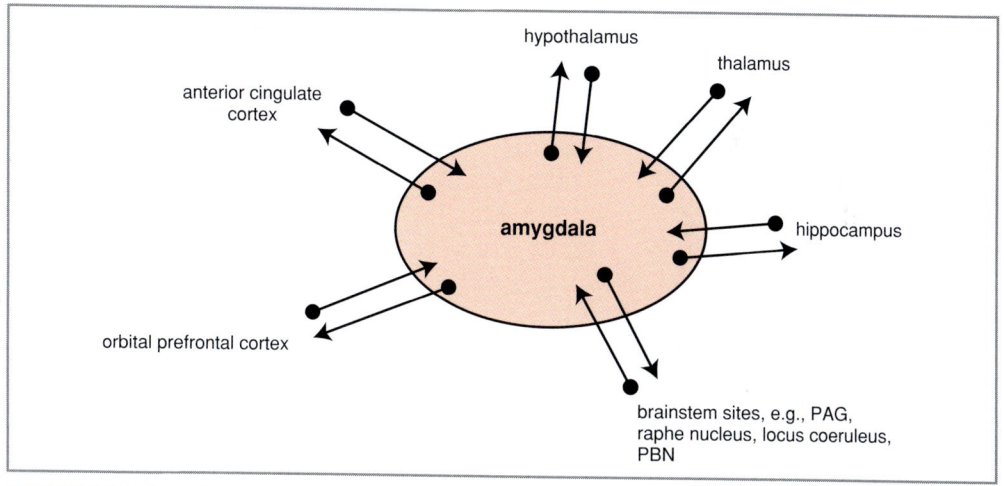

FIGURE 14-9 Amygdala. The amygdala, which plays a central role in the experience of anxiety and fear, has reciprocal connections with a wide range of other brain regions. These connections allow the amygdala to integrate both sensory and cognitive information and then use that information to trigger (or not) a fear response.

thalamo-cortical (CSTC) loops. CSTC loops were introduced in Chapter 7 and are illustrated in Figures 7-16 through 7-21. The links between the CSTC circuits, "worry and obsession loops," and treatments for the symptom of worry across the spectrum of anxiety disorders are discussed later in this chapter (see also Figures 14-43 through 14-45). We shall see that what differentiates one anxiety disorder from another may not be the anatomical localization or neurotransmitters regulating fear and worry (Figure 14-7 and Figure 14-8) but rather the specific nature of malfunctioning within these same circuits in various anxiety disorders.

Anxiety Disorders and Anxiolytics

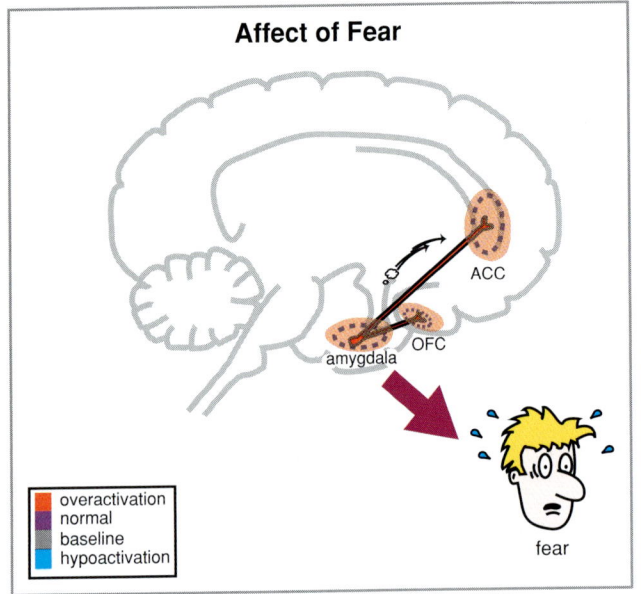

FIGURE 14-10 Affect of fear. Feelings of fear are regulated by reciprocal connections between the amygdala and the anterior cingulate cortex (ACC) and the amygdala and the orbitofrontal cortex (OFC). Specifically, it may be that overactivation of these circuits produces feelings of fear.

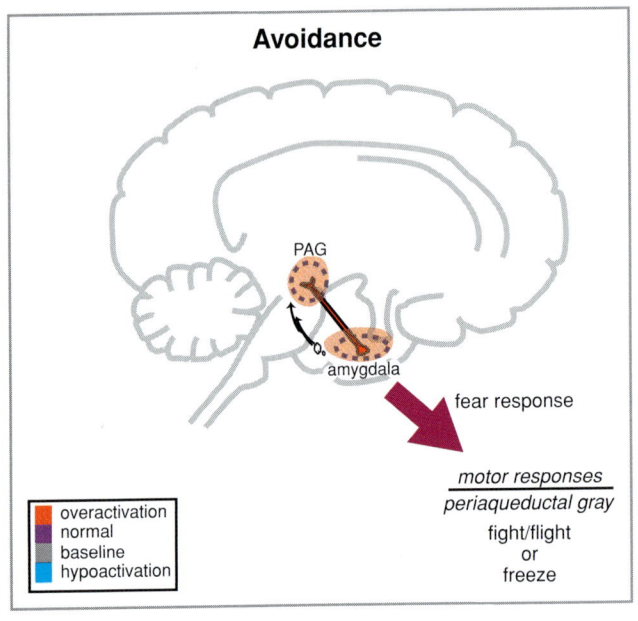

FIGURE 14-11 Avoidance. Feelings of fear may be expressed through behaviors such as avoidance, which is partly regulated by reciprocal connections between the amygdala and the periaqueductal gray (PAG). Avoidance in this sense is a motor response and may be analogous to freezing under threat. Other motor responses are to fight or to run away (flight) in order to survive threats from the environment.

That is, in generalized anxiety disorder, malfunctioning in the amygdala and CSTC loops may be persistent and unremitting yet not severe (Figure 14-2), whereas malfunctioning may be intermittent but catastrophic in an unexpected manner for panic disorder (Figure 14-3) or in an expected manner for social anxiety (Figure 14-4). Circuit malfunctioning may be traumatic in origin in posttraumatic stress disorder (PTSD) (Figure 14-5) or trapped in a redundant, repetitive loop for obsessive compulsive disorder (OCD) (Figure 14-6).

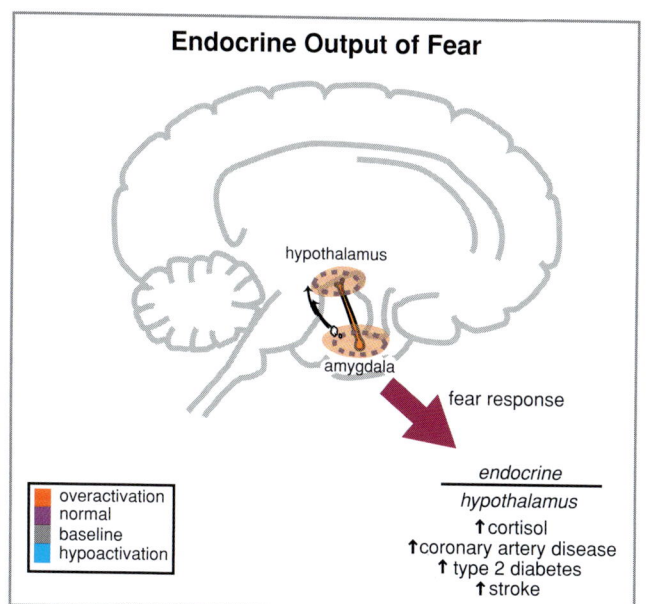

FIGURE 14-12 Endocrine output of fear. The fear response may be characterized in part by endocrine effects such as increases in cortisol, which occur because of amygdala activation of the hypothalamic-pituitary-adrenal (HPA) axis. Prolonged HPA activation and cortisol release can have significant health implications, such as increased risk of coronary artery disease, type 2 diabetes, and stroke.

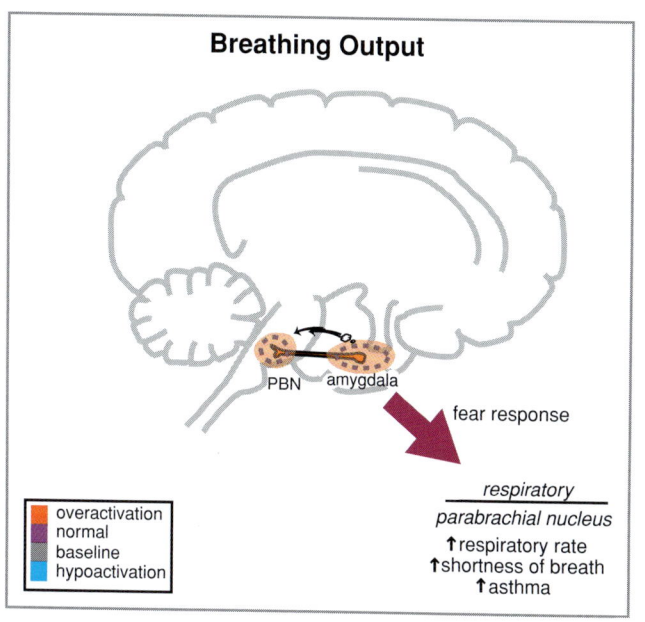

FIGURE 14-13 Breathing output. Changes in respiration may occur during a fear response; these changes are regulated by activation of the parabrachial nucleus (PBN) via the amygdala. Inappropriate or excessive activation of the PBN can lead not only to increases in the rate of respiration but also to symptoms such as shortness of breath, exacerbation of asthma, or a sense of being smothered.

The amygdala and the neurobiology of fear

The amygdala, an almond-shaped brain center located near the hippocampus (see Figure 9-63), has important anatomical connections that allow it to integrate sensory and cognitive information and then to determine whether there will be a fear response (see Figures 9-64 and 9-65 as well as Figures 7-12, 7-13, and 7-19 through 7-20). Figures 14-9 through 14-15 illustrate how the amygdala's connections relate to the signs and symptoms associated with the fear response. Specifically, the affect or feeling of fear may be regulated via the reciprocal connections the amygdala shares with key areas of prefrontal cortex that regulate emotions,

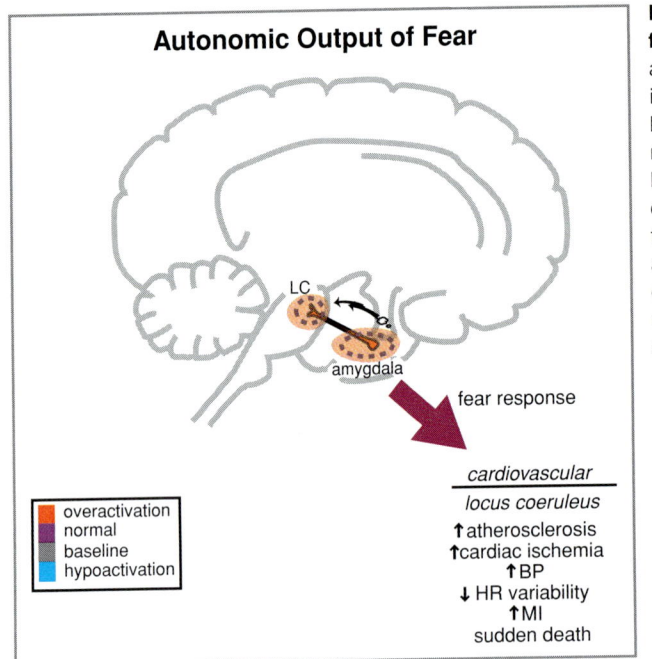

FIGURE 14-14 Autonomic output of fear. Autonomic responses are typically associated with feelings of fear. These include increases in heart rate (HR) and blood pressure (BP), which are regulated by reciprocal connections between the amygdala and the locus coeruleus (LC). Long-term activation of this circuit may lead to increased risk of atherosclerosis, cardiac ischemia, change in BP, decreased HR variability, myocardial infarction (MI), or even sudden death.

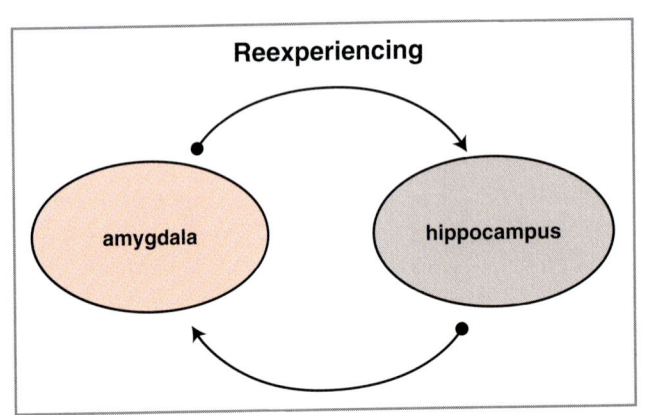

FIGURE 14-15 Reexperiencing. Anxiety can be triggered not only by an external stimulus but also by an individual's memories. Traumatic memories stored in the hippocampus can activate the amygdala, causing the amygdala, in turn, to activate other brain regions and generate a fear response. This is termed reexperiencing and is a particular feature of posttraumatic stress disorder.

namely the orbitofrontal cortex and the anterior cingulate cortex (Figure 14-10). However, fear is not just a feeling. The fear response can also include motor responses. Depending on the circumstances and one's temperament, those motor responses could be fight, flight, or freezing in place. Motor responses of fear are regulated in part by connections between the amygdala and the periaqueductal gray area of the brainstem (Figure 14-11).

There are also endocrine reactions that accompany fear, in part due to connections between the amygdala and the hypothalamus, causing changes in the hypothalamic-pituitary-adrenal (HPA) axis and thus of cortisol levels. A quick boost of cortisol may enhance survival when a person is encountering a real but short-term threat. However, chronic and persistent activation of this aspect of the fear response can lead to increased medical comorbidity, including increased rates of coronary artery disease, type 2 diabetes, and stroke (Figure 14-12). Breathing can also change during a fear response, regulated in part by the connections between amygdala and the parabrachial nucleus in the brainstem

Associate Symptoms With Brain Regions, Circuits, and Neurotransmitters That Regulate Them

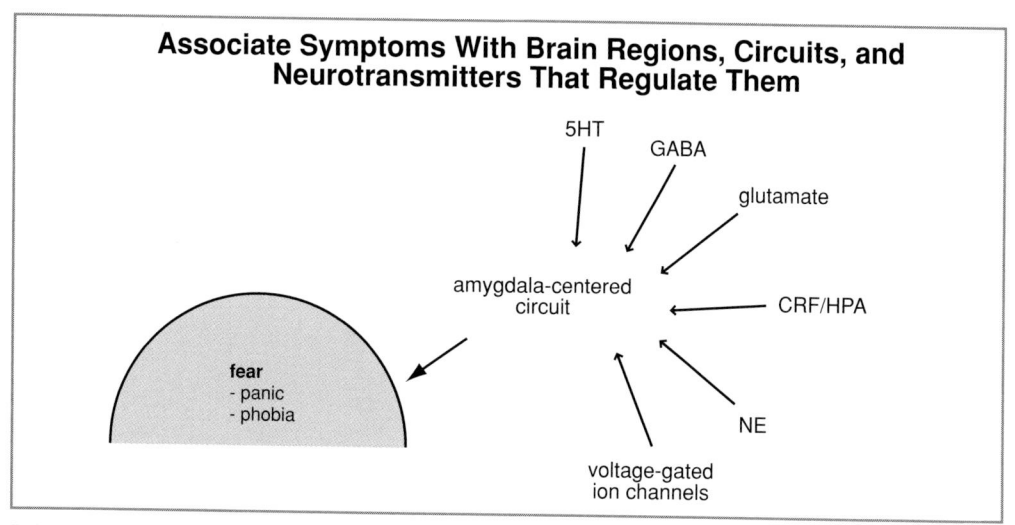

FIGURE 14-16 Linking anxiety symptoms to circuits to neurotransmitters. Symptoms of anxiety/fear are associated with malfunctioning of amygdala-centered circuits; the neurotransmitters that regulate these circuits include serotonin (5HT), gamma-aminobutyric acid (GABA), glutamate, corticotrophin releasing factor (CRF), and norepinephrine (NE), among others. In addition, voltage-gated ion channels are involved in neurotransmission within these circuits.

(Figure 14-13). An adaptive response to fear is to accelerate respiratory rate in the course of a fight/flight reaction to enhance survival; in excess, however, this can lead to unwanted symptoms of shortness of breath, exacerbation of asthma, or a false sense of being smothered (Figure 14-13) – all of which are common during anxiety and especially during attacks of anxiety such as panic attacks.

The autonomic nervous system is attuned to fear and is able to trigger responses – such as increased pulse and blood pressure for fight/flight reactions and survival during real threats – from the cardiovascular system. These autonomic and cardiovascular responses are mediated by connections between the amygdala and the locus coeruleus, home of the noradrenergic cell bodies (Figure 14-14) (noradrenergic neurons are discussed in Chapters 7 and 11 and noradrenergic pathways are illustrated in Figure 7-9). When autonomic responses are repetitive – that is, when they are inappropriately or chronically triggered as part of an anxiety disorder – this can eventually lead to increases in atherosclerosis, cardiac ischemia, hypertension, myocardial infarction, and even sudden death (Figure 14-15). "Scared to death" may not always be an exaggeration or a figure of speech! Finally, anxiety can be triggered internally from traumatic memories stored in the hippocampus and activated by connections with the amygdala (Figure 14-15), especially in conditions such as posttraumatic stress disorder.

Processing of the fear response is regulated by the numerous neuronal connections flowing into and out of the amygdala. Each connection utilizes specific neurotransmitters acting at specific receptors (Figure 14-16). Some of the key neurotransmitters acting at the amygdala are shown in Figure 14-16, although the exact anatomical connections within the amygdala and the specific receptor subtypes for these various circuits are still being clarified. What is known about these connections is that several neurotransmitters are involved in the production of symptoms of anxiety at the level of the amygdala and that numerous anxiolytic drugs have actions on these specific neurotransmitter systems to relieve the symptoms of anxiety and fear (Figure 14-16).

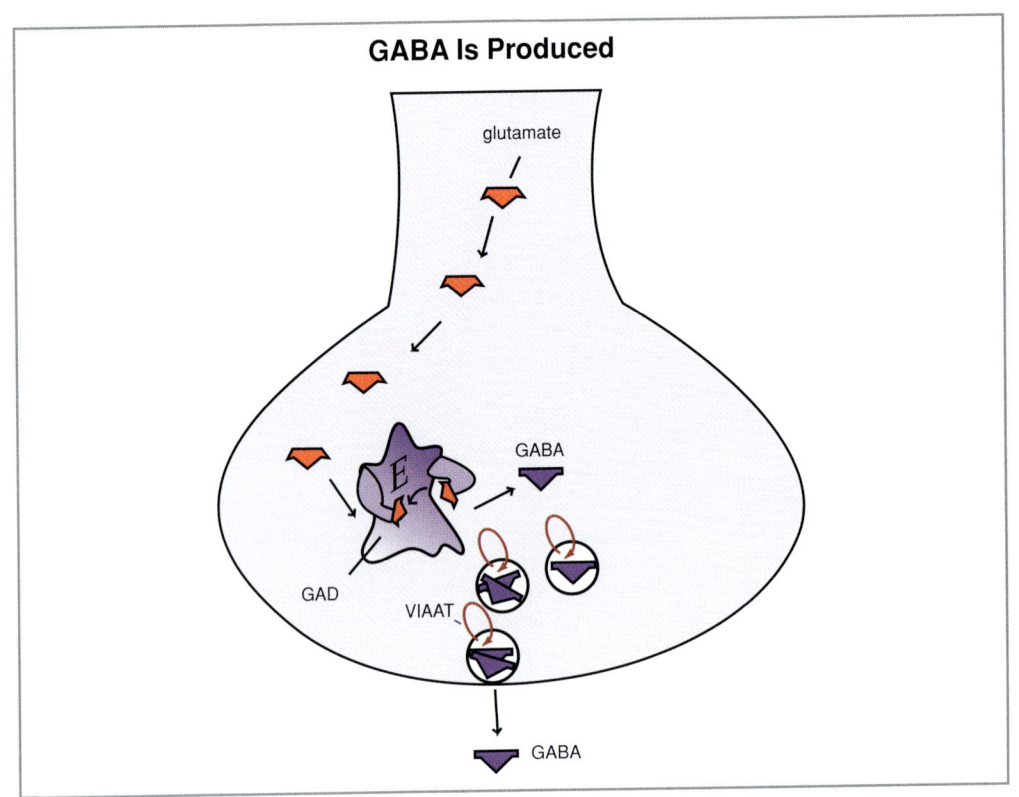

FIGURE 14-17 Gamma-aminobutyric acid (GABA) is produced. The amino acid glutamate, a precursor to GABA, is converted to GABA by the enzyme glutamic acid decarboxylase (GAD). After synthesis, GABA is transported into synaptic vesicles via vesicular inhibitory amino acid transporters (VIAATs) and stored until its release into the synapse during neurotransmission.

GABA, anxiety, and benzodiazepines

GABA is one of the key neurotransmitters involved in anxiety and in the anxiolytic action of many drugs used to treat the spectrum of anxiety disorders. GABA is the principal inhibitory neurotransmitter in the brain and normally serves an important regulatory role in reducing the activity of many neurons, including those in the amygdala and in the CSTC loops. Benzodiazepines, perhaps the best-known and most widely used anxiolytics, act by enhancing GABA actions at the level of the amygdala and the prefrontal cortex within CSTC loops to relieve anxiety. To understand how GABA regulates brain circuits in anxiety and how benzodiazepines exert their anxiolytic actions, it is important to understand the GABA neurotransmitter system, including how GABA is synthesized, how its action is terminated at the synapse, and especially the properties of GABA receptors (Figures 14-17 through 14-25).

Specifically, GABA is produced, or synthesized, from the amino acid glutamate (glutamic acid) via the actions of the enzyme glutamic acid decarboxylase (GAD) (Figure 14-17). Once formed in presynaptic neurons, GABA is transported into synaptic vesicles by vesicular inhibitory amino acid transporters (VIAATs), where GABA is stored until it is released into the synapse during inhibitory neurotransmission (Figure 14-17). GABA's synaptic actions are terminated by the presynaptic GABA transporter (GAT), also known as the GABA reuptake pump (Figure 14-18), analogous to similar transporters for other

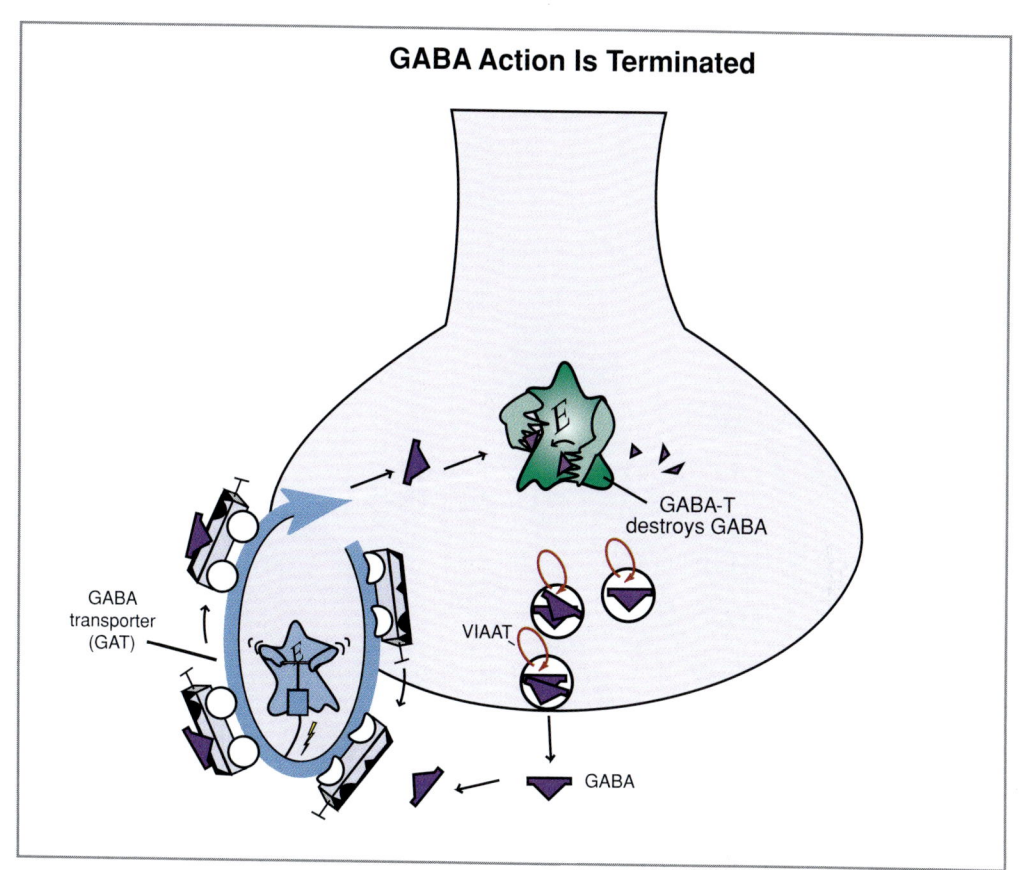

FIGURE 14-18 Gamma-aminobutyric acid (GABA) action is terminated. GABA's action can be terminated through multiple mechanisms. GABA can be transported out of the synaptic cleft and back into the presynaptic neuron via the GABA transporter (GAT), where it may be repackaged for future use. Alternatively, once GABA has been transported back into the cell, it may be converted into an inactive substance via the enzyme GABA transaminase (GABA-T).

neurotransmitters discussed throughout this text. VIAATs and GATs are introduced in Chapter 4 and illustrated in Figure 4-10. GABA's action can also be terminated by the enzyme GABA transaminase (GABA-T), which converts GABA into an inactive substance (Figure 14-18).

Classification of numerous GABA receptor subtypes has proceeded at a rapid pace. An understanding of the properties of GABA receptor subtypes is the key to grasping the role of GABA in anxiety and the mechanism of action of benzodiazepine anxiolytics. There are three major types of GABA receptors and numerous subtypes of GABA receptors. The major types are GABA-A, GABA-B and GABA-C receptors (Figure 14-19). GABA-A receptors and GABA-C receptors are both ligand-gated ion channels. This class of receptor, also known as ionotrophic receptors and as ion channel–linked receptors, is discussed in Chapter 5 and illustrated in Figures 5-2 through 5-25. Both GABA-A receptors and GABA-C receptors are part of a macromolecular complex that forms an inhibitory chloride channel (Figure 14-20). As will be explained here in detail, various subtypes of GABA-A receptors are targets of benzodiazepines, barbiturates, and/or alcohol (Figure 14-20) and are involved with either tonic or phasic inhibitory neurotransmission at GABA synapses

Anxiety Disorders and Anxiolytics | 733

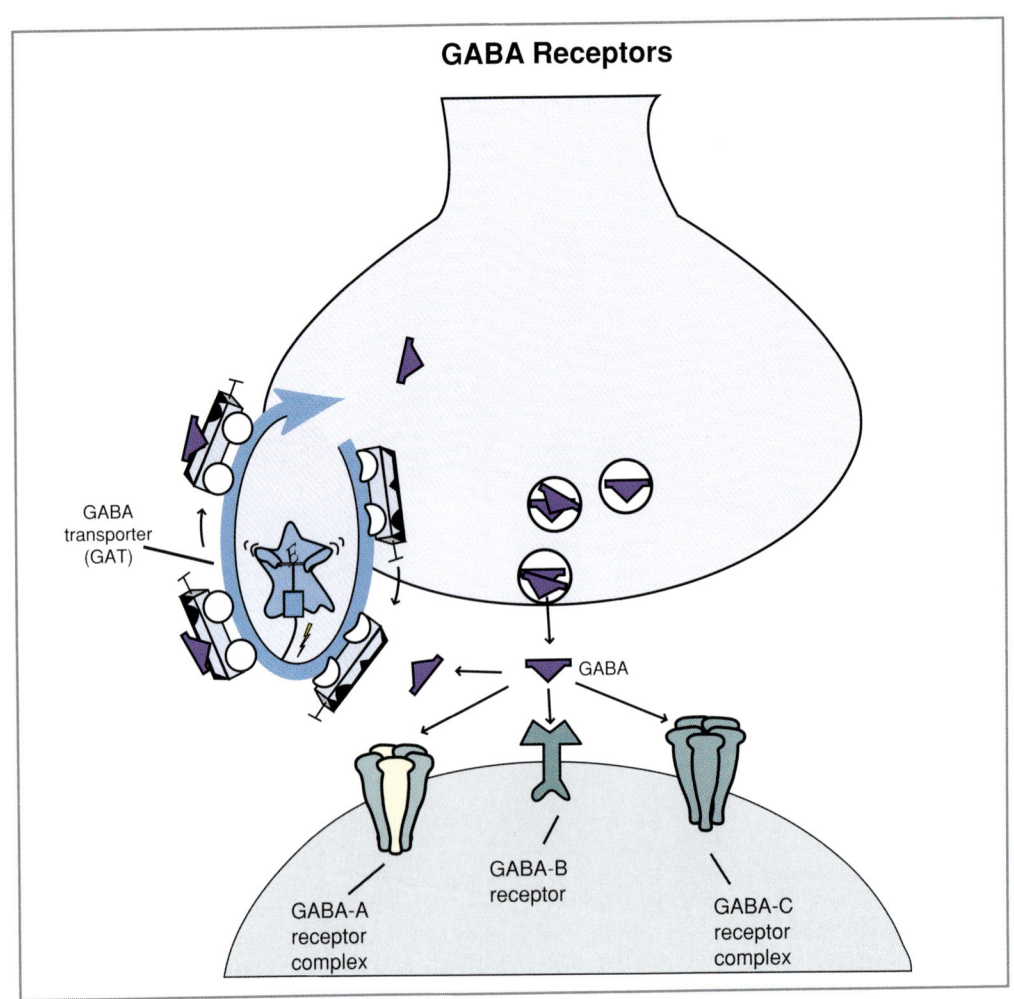

FIGURE 14-19 Gamma-aminobutyric acid (GABA) receptors. Shown here are receptors for GABA that regulate its neurotransmission. These include the GABA transporter (GAT) as well as three major types of postsynaptic GABA receptors: GABA-A, GABA-B, and GABA-C. GABA-A and GABA-C receptors are ligand-gated ion channels; they are part of a macromolecular complex that forms an inhibitory chloride channel. GABA-B receptors are G protein–linked receptors that may be coupled with calcium or potassium channels.

(Figure 14-21). The physiological role of GABA-C receptors is not well clarified as yet, but they do not appear to be targets of benzodiazepines.

GABA-B receptors, by contrast, are members of a different receptor class, namely, G protein–linked receptors. G protein–linked receptors are discussed in Chapter 4 and illustrated in Figures 4-16 through 4-28. GABA-B receptors may be coupled to calcium and/or potassium channels and may be involved in pain, memory, mood, and other CNS functions.

GABA-A receptor subtypes
Given the critical roles of various subtypes of GABA-A receptors in mediating inhibitory neurotransmission and as targets of the anxiolytic benzodiazepines, this class of receptors will be discussed in further detail. The molecular structure of GABA-A receptors is shown in

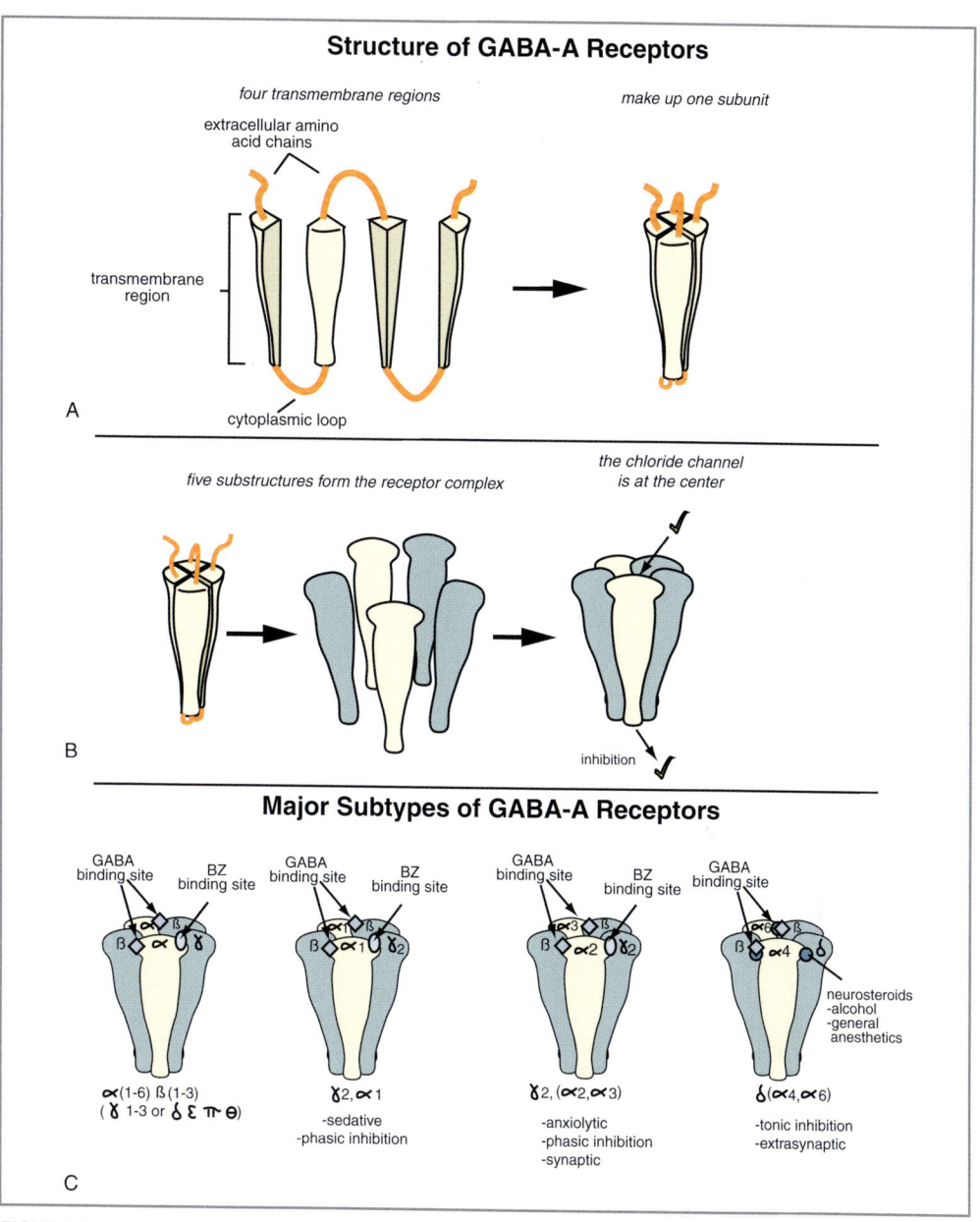

FIGURE 14-20A, B, and C Gamma-aminobutyric acid-A (GABA-A) receptors. (**A**) Shown here are the four transmembrane regions that make up one subunit of a GABA-A receptor. (**B**) There are five copies of these subunits in a fully constituted GABA-A receptor, at the center of which is a chloride channel. (**C**) Different types of subunits (also called isoforms or subtypes) can combine to form a GABA-A receptor. These include six different alpha isoforms, three different beta isoforms, three different gamma isoforms, delta, epsilon, pi, theta, and three different rho isoforms. The ultimate type and function of each GABA-A receptor subtype will depend on which subunits it contains. Benzodiazepine-sensitive GABA-A receptors (middle two) contain gamma and alpha (1 through 3) subunits and mediate phasic inhibition triggered by peak concentrations of synaptically released GABA. Benzodiazepine-sensitive GABA-A receptors containing alpha 1 subunits are involved in sleep (second from left), while those that contain alpha 2 and/or alpha 3 subunits are involved in anxiety (second from right). GABA-A receptors containing alpha 4, alpha 6, gamma 1, or delta subunits (far right) are benzodiazepine-insensitive, are located extrasynaptically, and regulate tonic inhibition.

Anxiety Disorders and Anxiolytics | 735

Two Types of GABA-A Mediated Inhibition

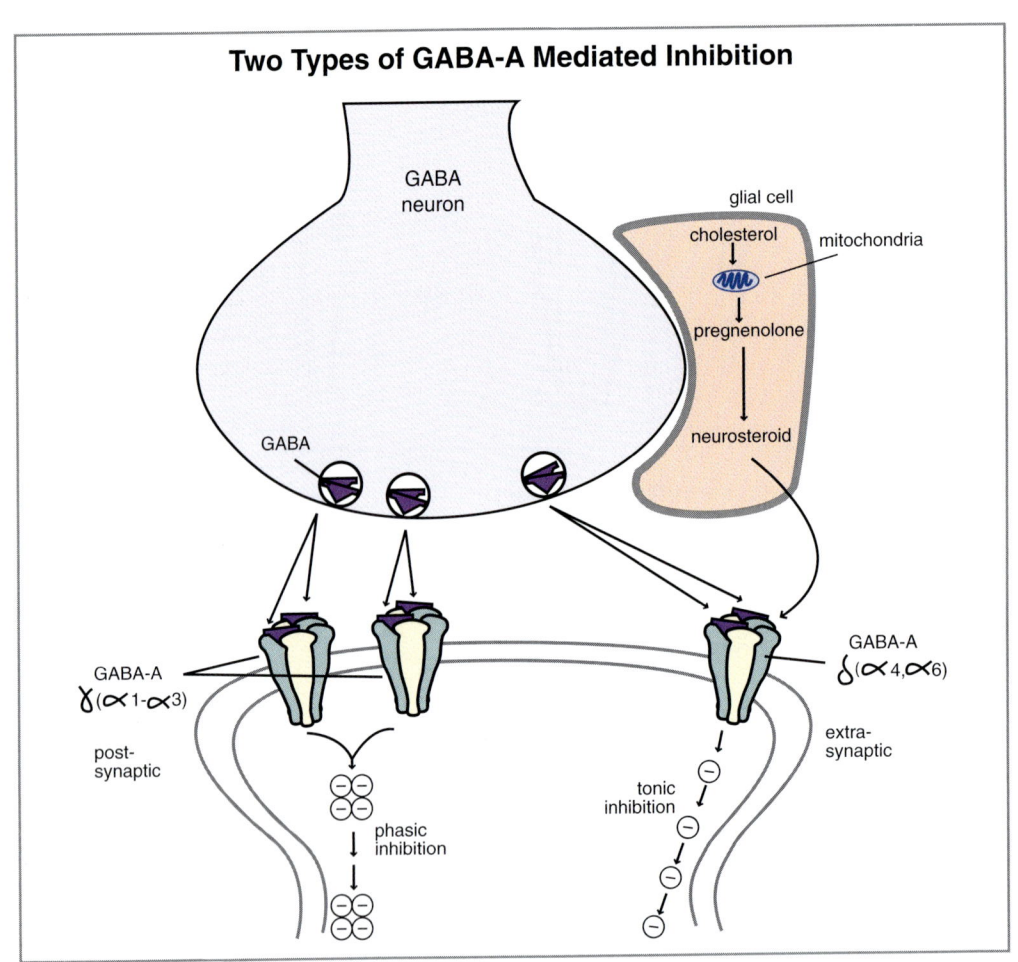

FIGURE 14-21 GABA-A mediation of tonic and phasic inhibition. Benzodiazepine-sensitive GABA-A receptors (those that contain gamma and alpha 1 through alpha 3 subunits) are postsynaptic receptors that mediate phasic inhibition, which occurs in bursts triggered by peak concentrations of synaptically released GABA. Benzodiazepine-insensitive GABA-A receptors (those containing alpha 4, alpha 6, gamma 1, or delta subunits) are extrasynaptic and capture GABA that diffuses away from the synapse as well as neurosteroids that are synthesized and released by glia. These receptors mediate inhibition that is tonic (i.e., mediated by ambient levels of extracellular GABA that has escaped from the synapse).

Figure 14-20. Each subunit of a GABA-A receptor has four transmembrane regions (Figure 14-20A). When five subunits cluster together, they form an intact GABA-A receptor with a chloride channel in the center (Figure 14-20B). This molecular structure of ligand-gated ion channels is introduced in Chapter 5 and illustrated in Figures 5-3 and 5-4.

There are many different subtypes of GABA-A receptors, depending on which subunits are present (Figure 14-20C). Subunits of GABA-A receptors are sometimes also called isoforms and include alpha (with six isoforms, alpha 1 to 6), beta (with three isoforms, beta 1 to 3), gamma (with three isoforms, gamma 1 to 3), delta, epsilon, pi, theta, and rho (with three isoforms, rho 1 to 3) (Figure 14-20C). Important for this discussion is the fact that, depending on which subunits are present, the functions of a GABA-A receptor can vary significantly.

Benzodiazepine-insensitive

GABA-A receptors are those with alpha 4, alpha 6, gamma 1, or delta subunits (Figure 14-20C). GABA-A receptors with a delta subunit rather than a gamma subunit plus either alpha 4 or alpha 6 subunits do not bind to benzodiazepines. Such GABA-A receptors do bind to other modulators, namely the naturally occurring neurosteroids, as well as to alcohol and to some general anesthetics (Figure 14-20C). The binding site for these non-benzodiazepine modulators is located between the alpha and the delta subunits, one site per receptor complex (Figure 14-20C). Two molecules of GABA bind per receptor complex at sites located between the alpha and the beta subunits, sometimes referred to as the GABA agonist site (Figure 14-20C). Since the site for the modulators is in a different location from the agonist sites for GABA, the modulatory site is often called allosteric (literally "other site"), and the agents that bind there, allosteric modulators.

Benzodiazepine-insensitive GABA-A receptor subtypes (with delta subunits and alpha 4 or 6 subunits) are located extrasynaptically, where they capture not only GABA that diffuses away from the synapse but also neurosteroids synthesized and released by glia (Figure 14-21). Extrasynaptic, benzodiazepine-insensitive GABA-A receptors are thought to mediate a type of inhibition at the postsynaptic neuron that is *tonic*, in contrast to the *phasic* type of inhibition mediated by postsynaptic benzodiazepine-sensitive GABA-A receptors (Figure 14-21). Thus tonic inhibition may be regulated by the ambient levels of extracellular GABA molecules that have escaped presynaptic reuptake and enzymatic destruction. Tonic inhibition is thought to set the overall tone and excitability of the postsynaptic neuron and to be important for certain regulatory events, such as the frequency of neuronal discharge in response to excitatory inputs.

Since the GABA-A receptors that modulate this action are not sensitive to benzodiazepines, they are not likely to be involved in the anxiolytic actions of benzodiazepines in various anxiety disorders. However, novel hypnotics as well as anesthetics have targeted these extrasynaptic benzodiazepine-insensitive GABA-A receptors, and it is possible that novel synthetic neurosteroids that also target benzodiazepine-insensitive GABA-A receptor subtypes could some day become novel anxiolytics. Indeed, anxiety itself may in part be dependent on having the right amount of tonic inhibition in key anatomic areas such as the amygdala and cortical areas of CSTC loops. Furthermore, naturally occurring neurosteroids may be important in setting that inhibitory tone in critical brain areas. If this tone becomes dysregulated, it is possible that abnormal neuronal excitability could become a factor in the development of various anxiety disorders.

Benzodiazepine-sensitive

GABA-A receptors have several structural and functional features that make them distinct from benzodiazepine-insensitive GABA-A receptors. In contrast to benzodiazepine-insensitive GABA-A receptors, for a GABA-A receptor to be sensitive to benzodiazepines and thus to be a target for benzodiazepine anxiolytics, there must be two beta units plus a gamma unit of either the gamma 2 or gamma 3 subtype, plus two alpha units of either the alpha 1, alpha 2, or alpha 3 subtype (Figure 14-20C). Benzodiazepines appear to bind to the region of the receptor between the gamma 2/3 subunit and the alpha 1/2/3 subunit, one benzodiazepine molecule per receptor complex (Figure 14-20C). GABA itself binds with two molecules of GABA per receptor complex to the GABA agonist sites in the regions of the receptor between the alpha and the beta units (Figure 14-20C).

Benzodiazepine-sensitive GABA-A receptor subtypes (with gamma subunits and alpha 1/2/3 subunits) are thought to be postsynaptic in location and to mediate a type of inhibition at the postsynaptic neuron that is phasic, occurring in bursts of inhibition triggered by peak concentrations of synaptically released GABA (Figure 14-21). Theoretically, benzodiazepines acting at these receptors, particularly the alpha 2/3 subtypes clustered at postsynaptic GABA sites, should exert an anxiolytic effect due to enhancement of phasic postsynaptic inhibition. If this action occurs at overly active output neurons in the amygdala or in CSTC loops, it would theoretically cause anxiolytic actions, with a reduction both of fear and worry.

Not all benzodiazepine-sensitive GABA-A receptors are the same. Notably, those benzodiazepine-sensitive GABA-A receptors with alpha 1 subunits may be most important for regulating sleep and are the presumed targets of numerous sedative hypnotic agents, including both benzodiazepine and nonbenzodiazepine positive allosteric modulators of the GABA-A receptor (Figure 14-20C). The alpha 1 subtype of GABA-A receptor and the drugs that bind to it are discussed further in Chapter 16, on sleep. Some of these agents are selective only for the alpha 1 subtype of GABA-A receptor.

On the other hand, benzodiazepine-sensitive GABA-A receptors with alpha 2 (and/or alpha 3) subunits may be most important for regulating anxiety and are the presumed targets of the anxiolytic benzodiazepines (Figure 14-20C). However, currently available benzodiazepines are nonselective for GABA-A receptors with different alpha subunits. Thus, there is an ongoing search for selective alpha 2/3 agents that could be utilized to treat anxiety disorders in man. Such agents would theoretically be anxiolytic without being sedating. Partial agonists selective for alpha 2/3 subunits of benzodiazepine sensitive GABA-A receptors hypothetically would cause less euphoria, be less reinforcing and thus less abusable, cause less dependence, and cause fewer problems in withdrawal. Such agents are being investigated but have not yet been introduced into clinical practice.

The concept of partial agonists for ligand-gated ion channels was introduced in Chapter 5 and is illustrated in Figures 5-9 through 5-15. Abnormal expression of gamma 2, alpha 2 or delta subunits is associated with different types of epilepsy. Receptor subtype expression can change in response to chronic benzodiazepine administration and withdrawal and could theoretically be altered in patients with various anxiety disorder subtypes.

Benzodiazepines as positive allosteric modulators (PAMs)

Since the benzodiazepine-sensitive GABA-A receptor complex is regulated not only by GABA itself but also by benzodiazepines at a highly specific allosteric modulatory binding site (Figure 14-22), this has led to the notion that there may be an "endogenous" or naturally occurring benzodiazepine synthesized in the brain (the brain's own Xanax!). However, the identity of any such substance remains elusive. Furthermore, it is now known that synthetic drugs that do not have a benzodiazepine structure also bind to the benzodiazepine receptor. These developments have led to endless confusion with terminology! Thus, many experts now call the benzodiazepine site the GABA-A allosteric modulatory site and anything that binds to this site, including benzodiazepines, an allosteric modulator.

Allosteric modulation is known to occur over a broad spectrum, from positive allosteric modulation (PAM) to neutral antagonism to negative allosteric modulation (NAM). The concepts of PAMs and NAMs and the agonist spectrum are introduced in Chapter 5 and illustrated in Figure 5-21 through Figure 5-23. These ideas are further developed in Figures 14-22 through 14-24 as applied to the modulation of GABA-A receptors by benzodiazepine anxiolytics.

Acting alone, GABA can increase the frequency of opening of the chloride channel, but only to a limited extent (compare Figures 14-22A and 14-22B). The combination of

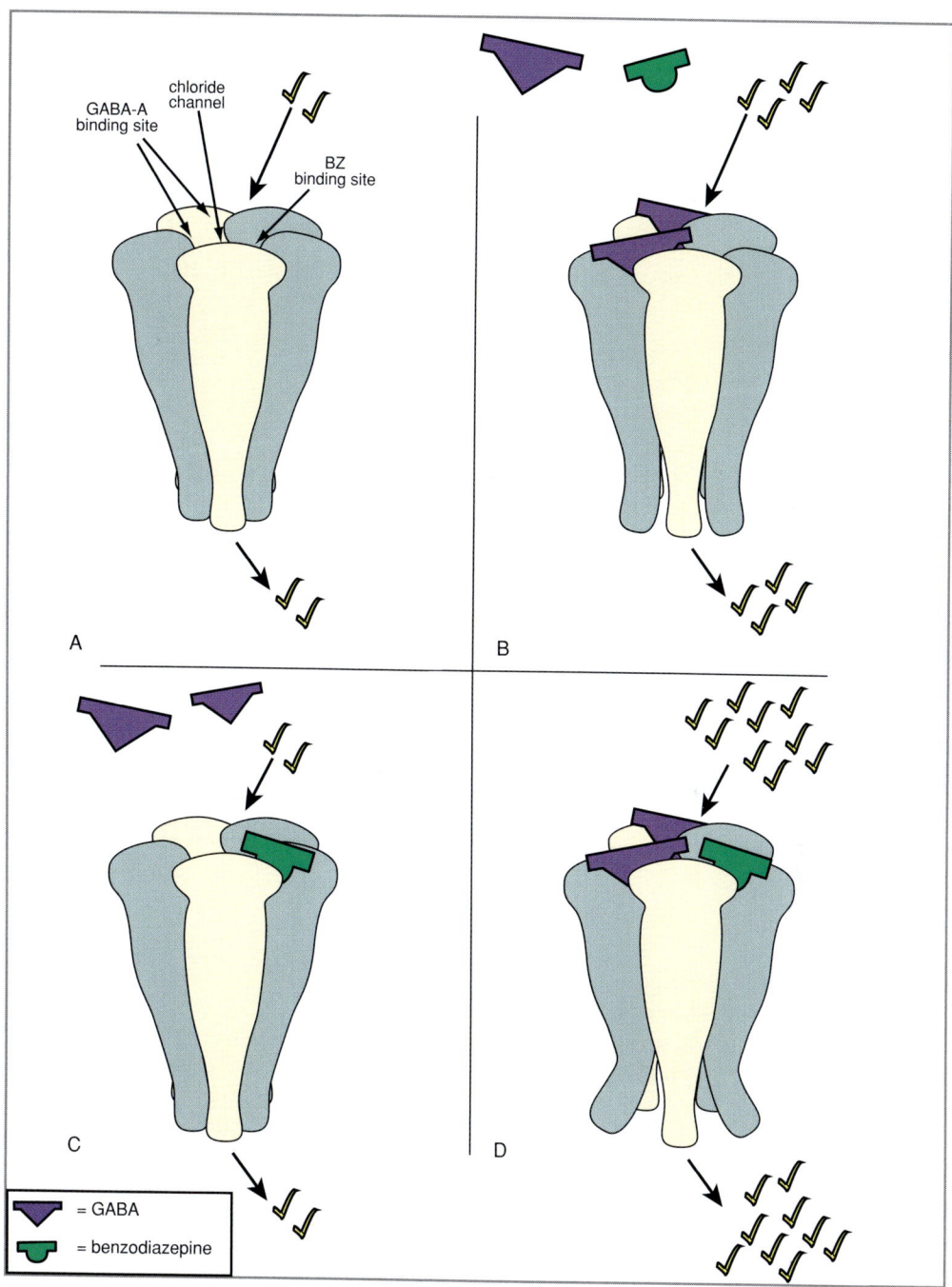

FIGURE 14-22A, B, C, and D Positive allosteric modulation of GABA-A receptors. (**A**) Benzodiazepine-sensitive GABA-A receptors, like the one shown here, consist of five subunits with a central chloride channel and have binding sites not only for GABA but also for positive allosteric modulators (e.g., benzodiazepines). (**B**) When GABA binds to its sites on the GABA-A receptor, it increases the frequency of opening of the chloride channel and thus allows more chloride to pass through. (**C**) When a positive allosteric modulator such as a benzodiazepine binds to the GABA-A receptor in the absence of GABA, it has no effect on the chloride channel. (**D**) When a positive allosteric modulator such as a benzodiazepine binds to the GABA-A receptor in the presence of GABA, it causes the channel to open even more frequently than when GABA alone is present.

Anxiety Disorders and Anxiolytics

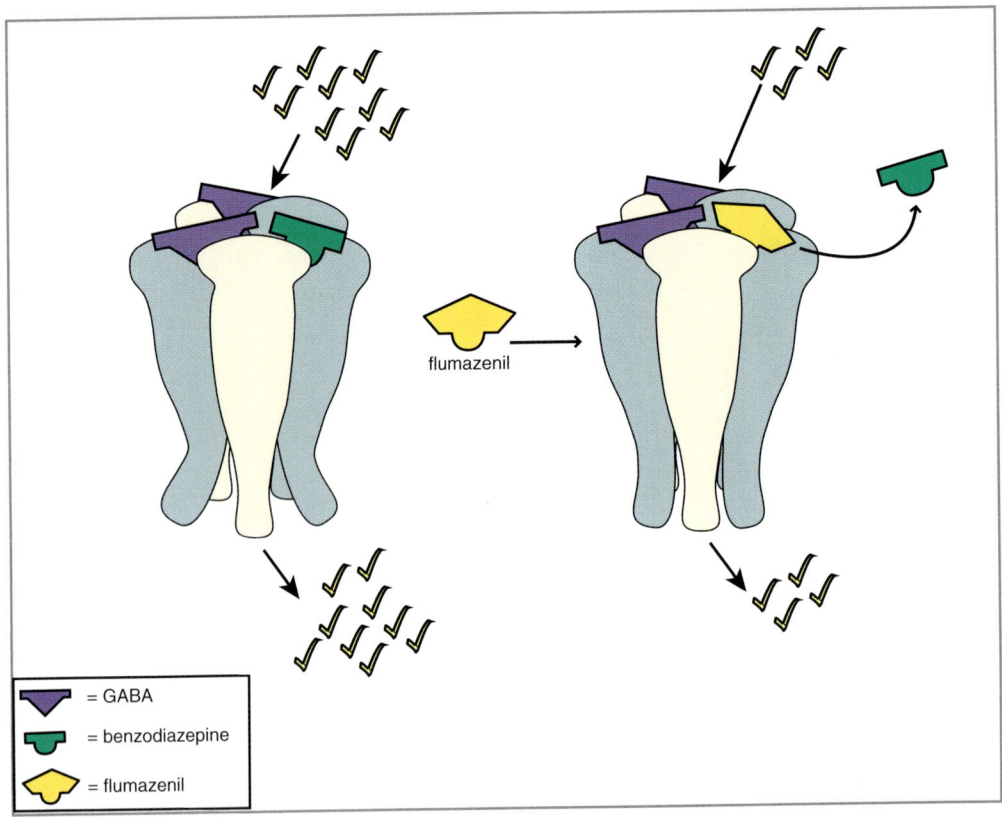

FIGURE 14-23 Flumazenil. The benzodiazepine receptor antagonist flumazenil is able to reverse a full agonist benzodiazepine acting at its site on the GABA-A receptor. This may be helpful in reversing the sedative effects of full agonist benzodiazepines when administered for anesthetic purposes or when taken in overdose by a patient.

GABA with benzodiazepines is thought to increase the frequency of opening of inhibitory chloride channels but not to increase the conductance of chloride across individual chloride channels or to increase the duration of channel opening. The end result is more inhibition. More inhibition supposedly yields more anxiolytic action. How does this happen?

The answer is that benzodiazepines act as agonists at the allosteric modulatory site of GABA binding. They are positive allosteric modulators, or PAMs, but have no activity on their own. Thus, when benzodiazepines bind to the allosteric modulatory site, they have no activity when GABA is not simultaneously binding to its agonist sites (compare Figures 14-22A and 14-22C).

So how do benzodiazepines act as PAMs? This can occur only when GABA is binding to its agonist sites. The combination of benzodiazepines at the allosteric site plus GABA at its agonist sites increases the frequency of opening of the chloride channel to an extent not possible with GABA alone (compare Figures 14-22B and 14-22D).

The agonist spectrum and a hypothetical shift in the "set point" for GABA-A allosteric modulatory sites in anxiety disorders

Agonist actions of anxiolytic benzodiazepine PAMs can be reversed by the benzodiazepine antagonist known as flumazenil (Figure 14-23). Flumazenil does little by itself, since it is mostly a "silent" antagonist, but it will reverse the positive allosteric modulation of benzodiazepines and is used clinically to reverse sedation when benzodiazepines are taken in overdose or given as adjuncts to anesthesia.

Agents that act as inverse agonists at the GABA-A allosteric modulatory site have also been synthesized (Figure 14-24). These agents have the opposite action of benzodiazepines, and are thus negative allosteric modulators (NAMs), and *cause* anxiety. Members of the agonist spectrum – including agonists, silent antagonists, and inverse agonists – are discussed in greater detail in Chapter 5 and are illustrated in Figures 5-9 through 5-23.

One theory for what goes wrong in an anxiety disorder is that the "set point" for GABA-A allosteric modulatory sites is switched, either due to abnormal regulation of these sites or chronic benzodiazepine treatment, such that the entire agonist spectrum shifts (Figure 14-25). According to this theory, allosteric sites on GABA-A receptors can detect benzodiazepines, but only as partial agonists rather than full agonists; thus they have weakened efficacy for anxiety. This notion is supported by the fact that the antagonist flumazenil is "silent" and has no effects in unmedicated normal controls but can induce mild anxiety in unmedicated patients with panic disorder. This observation is consistent with a shift in receptor set point of the agonist spectrum, such that abnormal receptors in the anxiety patient now detect an antagonist as an inverse agonist and respond with the production of anxiety rather than with a neutral response. Neuroimaging research is now exploring the possibility that GABA-A receptors have abnormal regulation of their allosteric modulatory sites in a number of anxiety disorders.

Benzodiazepines as anxiolytics

A simplified notion of how benzodiazepine anxiolytics might modulate excessive output from the amygdala during fear responses in anxiety disorders is shown in Figure 14-25. Excessive amygdala activity is theoretically reduced by enhancing the phasic inhibitory actions of benzodiazepines at postsynaptic GABA-A receptors within the amygdala to blunt fear-associated outputs (shown in Figures 14-10 through 14-15).

Novel GABA anxiolytics

Ideas about how novel anxiolytics could target the GABA neurotransmitter system are shown in Figure 14-26. We have already mentioned partial agonists selective for alpha 2/3 subtypes of benzodiazepine-selective postsynaptic GABA-A receptors, shown here as well. In addition, it is possible that positive modulation of GABA-B receptors could provide an anxiolytic action. Preliminary results with the anticonvulsant tiagabine, which blocks the presynaptic transporter for GABA (GAT1), already suggest that enhancing the synaptic availability of GABA via this mechanism may provide anxiolytic effects. Finally, there are agents, including some known anticonvulsants, that enhance GABA action either by reducing its enzymatic destruction by GABA transaminase or by enhancing the release of GABA. These may prove to be useful as anxiolytics (Figure 14-26).

Serotonin, stress, and anxiety

Since the symptoms, circuits, and neurotransmitters linked to anxiety disorders overlap extensively with those for major depressive disorder (Figure 14-1), it is not surprising that drugs developed as antidepressants have proven to be effective treatments for anxiety disorders (Figure 14-27). Indeed, the leading treatments for anxiety disorders today are increasingly drugs originally developed as antidepressants.

Serotonin is a key neurotransmitter that innervates the amygdala, and it is known that antidepressants that can increase serotonin output by blocking the serotonin transporter

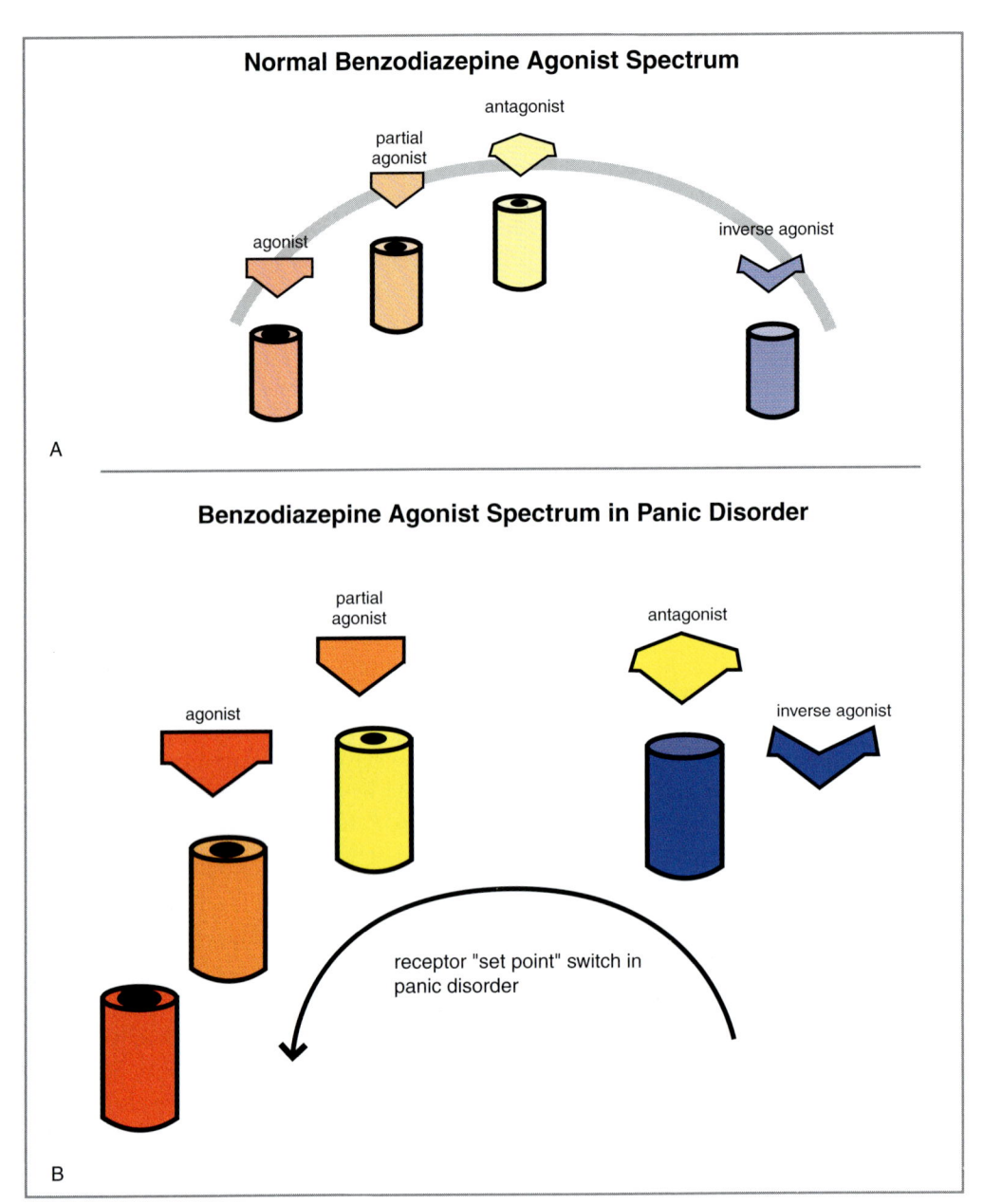

FIGURE 14-24A and B Benzodiazepine agonist spectrum in panic disorder. A theory about the biological basis of anxiety disorders, and particularly panic disorder, is that there is an abnormality in the set point for benzodiazepine receptors. Perhaps the normal sensitivity of these receptors (**A**) is switched to the left in this spectrum (**B**), rendering the receptors less sensitive to full agonists and experiencing antagonists as inverse agonists.

(SERT) are also effective in reducing symptoms of anxiety and fear in every one of the five anxiety disorders illustrated in Figures 14-2 through 14-6, namely, GAD, panic disorder, social anxiety disorder, PTSD, and OCD. Such agents include the well known SSRIs (serotonin selective reuptake inhibitors; discussed in Chapter 12; their mechanism of action is illustrated in Figures 12-17 through 12-32) as well as the SNRIs (serotonin norepinephrine

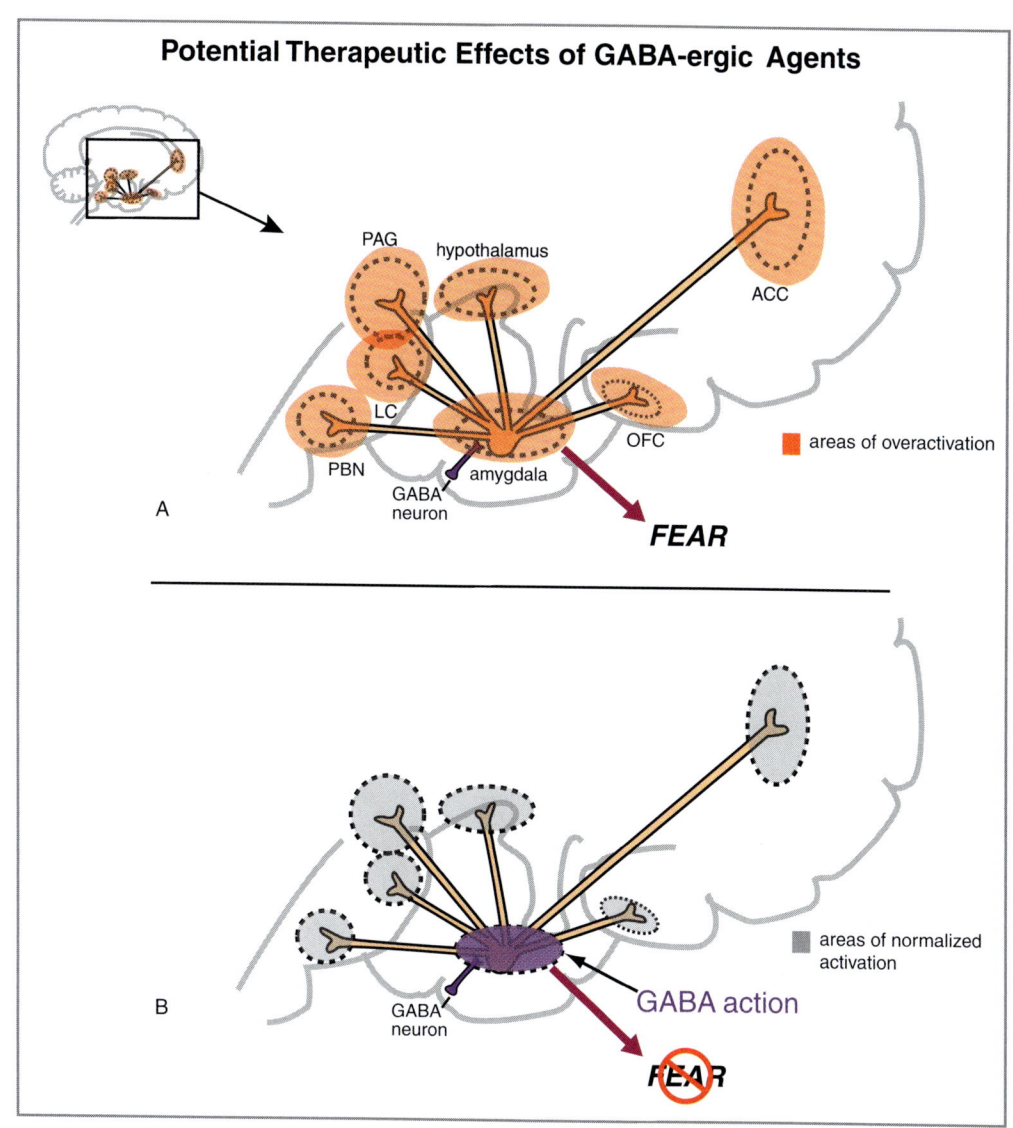

FIGURE 14-25 Potential therapeutic effects of GABA-ergic agents. (**A**) Pathological anxiety/fear may be caused by overactivation of amygdala circuits. (**B**) GABA-ergic agents such as benzodiazepines may alleviate anxiety/fear by enhancing phasic inhibitory actions at postsynaptic GABA-A receptors within the amygdala.

reuptake inhibitors; also discussed in Chapter 12; their mechanism of action is illustrated in Figures 12-33 through 12-42).

A serotonin 1A partial agonist, buspirone, is recognized as a generalized anxiolytic but not as a treatment for anxiety disorder subtypes. A related compound, gepirone ER, is in testing for major depression. Serotonin 1A partial agonists as augmenting agents to antidepressants are discussed in Chapter 12 and illustrated in Figure 12-129. Serotonin 1A partial agonist actions, also called SPA actions, which are among the mechanisms of atypical antipsychotic action, are discussed in Chapter 10 and illustrated in Figures 10-55 and 10-56.

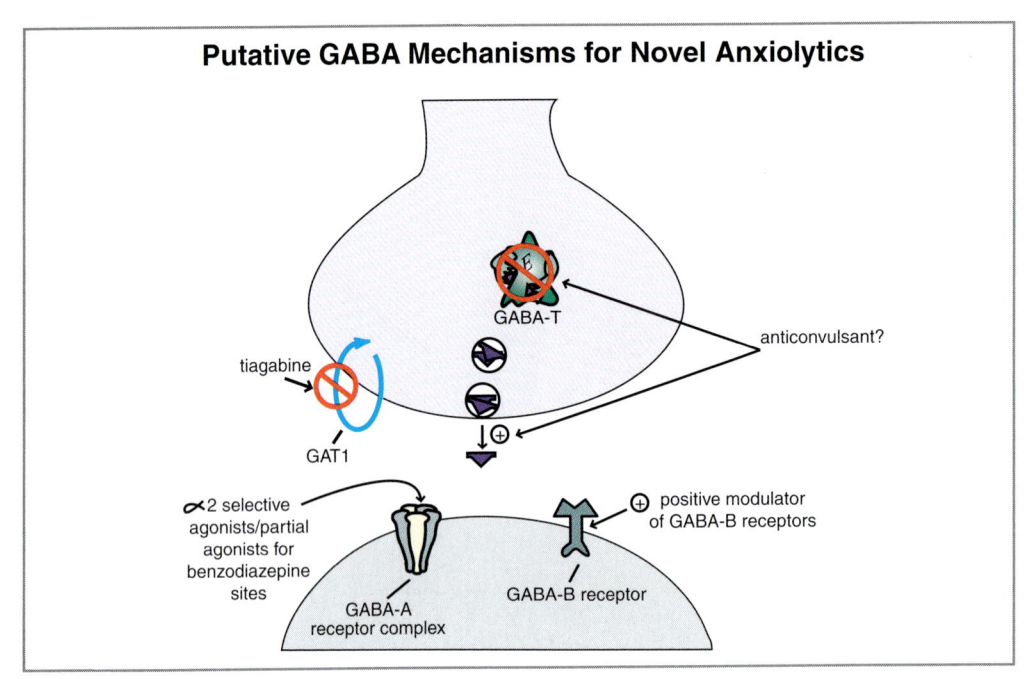

FIGURE 14-26 Putative GABA mechanisms for novel anxiolytics. There are several potential ways to modulate GABA neurotransmission that could prove to be anxiolytic. Partial agonists that are selective for the alpha 2 or 3 subunits of the GABA-A receptor may, like current benzodiazepines that bind there, be anxiolytic yet may also cause less sedation and have less abuse potential than nonselective full agonist benzodiazepines. Inhibition of the GABA transporter (GAT) – for example, by the anticonvulsant tiagabine – has been shown to provide anxiolytic effects. Some anticonvulsants may increase GABA's release or reduce its destruction via GABA transaminase (GABA-T), either of which could also have anxiolytic effects. Finally, it is possible that GABA-B receptors may play a role in anxiety; thus positive modulators of those receptors are potential therapeutic agents.

The potential anxiolytic actions of buspirone at both presynaptic and postsynaptic 5HT1A receptors are illustrated in Figure 14-28. Since the onset of anxiolytic action for buspirone is delayed, just as it is for antidepressants, this has led to the belief that 5HT1A agonists exert their therapeutic effects by virtue of adaptive neuronal events and receptor events rather than simply by the acute occupancy of 5HT1A receptors by the drug, as shown in Figure 14-28. In this way, the presumed mechanism of action of 5HT1A partial agonists is analogous to that of the antidepressants, which are also presumed to act by adaptations in neurotransmitter receptors, and different from that of the benzodiazepine anxiolytics, which act relatively acutely by occupancy of benzodiazepine receptors.

A simplified notion of how serotonergic anxiolytics might modulate excessive output from the amygdala, associated with anxiety and fear in various anxiety disorders, is shown in Figure 14-27. Excessive amygdala activity is theoretically reduced, after a delay, by enhancing the input of serotonin to key amygdala nuclei so as to blunt fear-associated outputs (see also Figures 14-10 through 14-15).

Born fearful?
Serotonin is involved not only in the therapeutic action of numerous proven anxiolytics for anxiety disorder subtypes (Figure 14-27) but also in regulating the efficiency of information processing in the amygdala and therefore the vulnerability or resilience of fear circuits

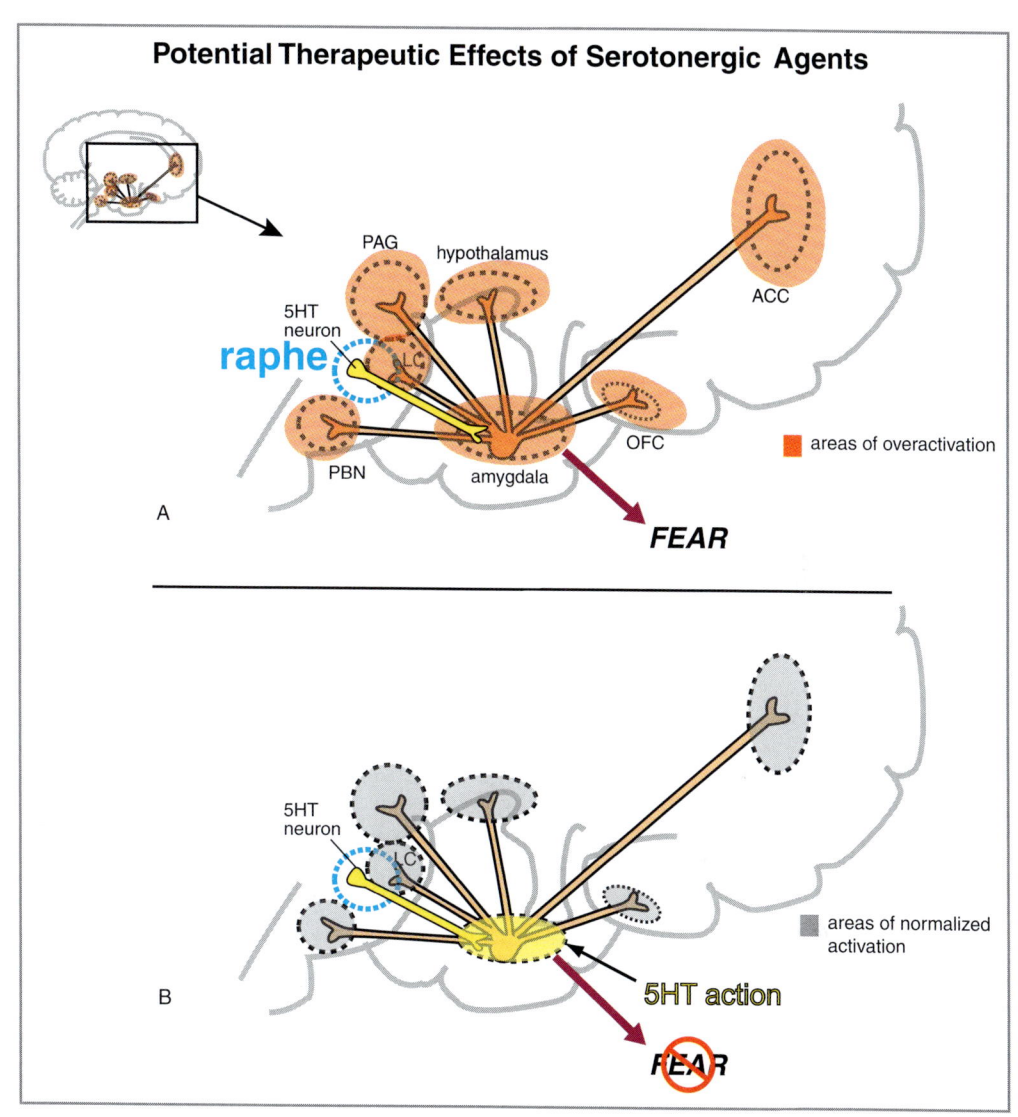

FIGURE 14-27A and B Potential therapeutic effects of serotonergic agents. (**A**) Pathological anxiety/fear may be caused by overactivation of amygdala circuits. (**B**) The amygdala receives input from serotonergic neurons, which can have an inhibitory effect on some of its outputs. Thus, serotonergic agents may alleviate anxiety/fear by enhancing serotonin input to the amygdala.

(Figure 14-29). That is, the type of serotonin transporter (SERT) with which you are born determines whether your amygdala overreacts to fearful faces (Figure 14-29). It also determines how well you respond to stress and perhaps whether your brain atrophies with exposure to chronic stress or your anxiety disorder responds well to an SSRI/SNRI (Figure 14-29). Thus, can you be born fearful?

The processing of fearful faces is discussed in Chapter 8 and illustrated in Figures 8-11 through 8-20. Specifically, the excessive reaction of the amygdala to fearful faces for normal controls who are carriers of the "s" variant of the gene for SERT is shown in Figure 8-13 and is also represented as excessive amygdala activity in Figure 14-29. Under stress, this overactivity and inefficient information processing (Figures 8-13 and 14-29) may become an

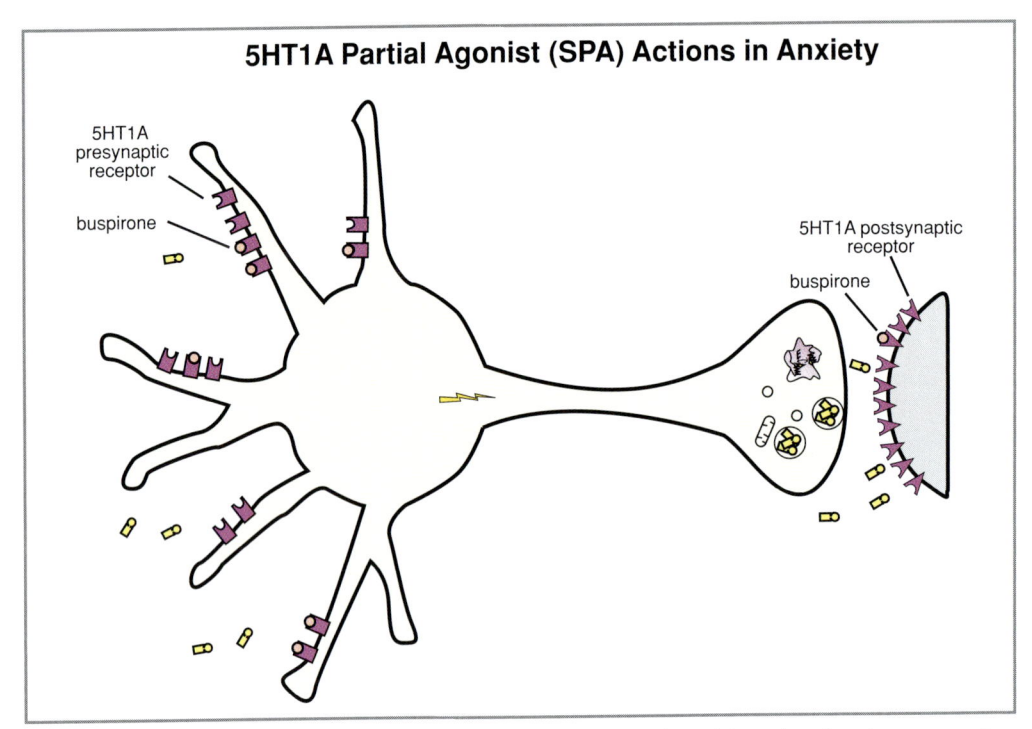

FIGURE 14-28 5HT1A partial agonist actions in anxiety. 5HT1A partial agonists such as buspirone may reduce anxiety by actions both at presynaptic somatodendritic autoreceptors (left) and at postsynaptic receptors (right). The onset of action of buspirone, like that of antidepressants, is delayed, suggesting that the therapeutic effects are actually related to downstream adaptive changes rather than acute actions at these receptors.

overt symptom of anxiety (Figure 8-18) whether that symptom is part of a major depressive episode or a component of one of the anxiety disorder subtypes (Figure 8-17). Both GABA and serotonin regulate circuits in the amygdala (Figure 8-19), and benzodiazepines, SSRIs, SNRIs, and cognitive behavioral therapy can all potentially modify this circuitry to produce anxiolytic actions (Figure 8-20).

The point is that the specific gene that you have for the serotonin transporter can alter the efficiency of affective information processing by your amygdala and consequently your risk for developing an anxiety disorder or major depression if you experience multiple life stressors as an adult (Figure 14-29). Specifically, the "l" genotype of SERT is more resilient (Figure 14-29), with less reactivity to fearful faces (Figures 8-13 and 13-29), less likelihood of breaking down into a major depressive episode or anxiety disorder when exposed to multiple life stressors (Figure 14-29), and perhaps less vulnerability to atrophy of the hippocampus (Figure 14-29) and greater likelihood of responding to treatment with SSRIs if an anxiety disorder is present.

On the other hand, the "s" genotype is apparently more vulnerable, overreacting to fearful faces (Figures 8-13 and 14-29), more likely to develop an affective disorder when exposed to multiple life stressors, and possibly associated with more hippocampal atrophy and less responsiveness to SSRI treatment (Figure 14-29). Whether you have the "l" or the "s" genotype of SERT accounts for only a small amount of the variance for whether or not you will develop an anxiety disorder under stress and thus does not totally predict who will develop an anxiety disorder and who will not. However, this example does prove

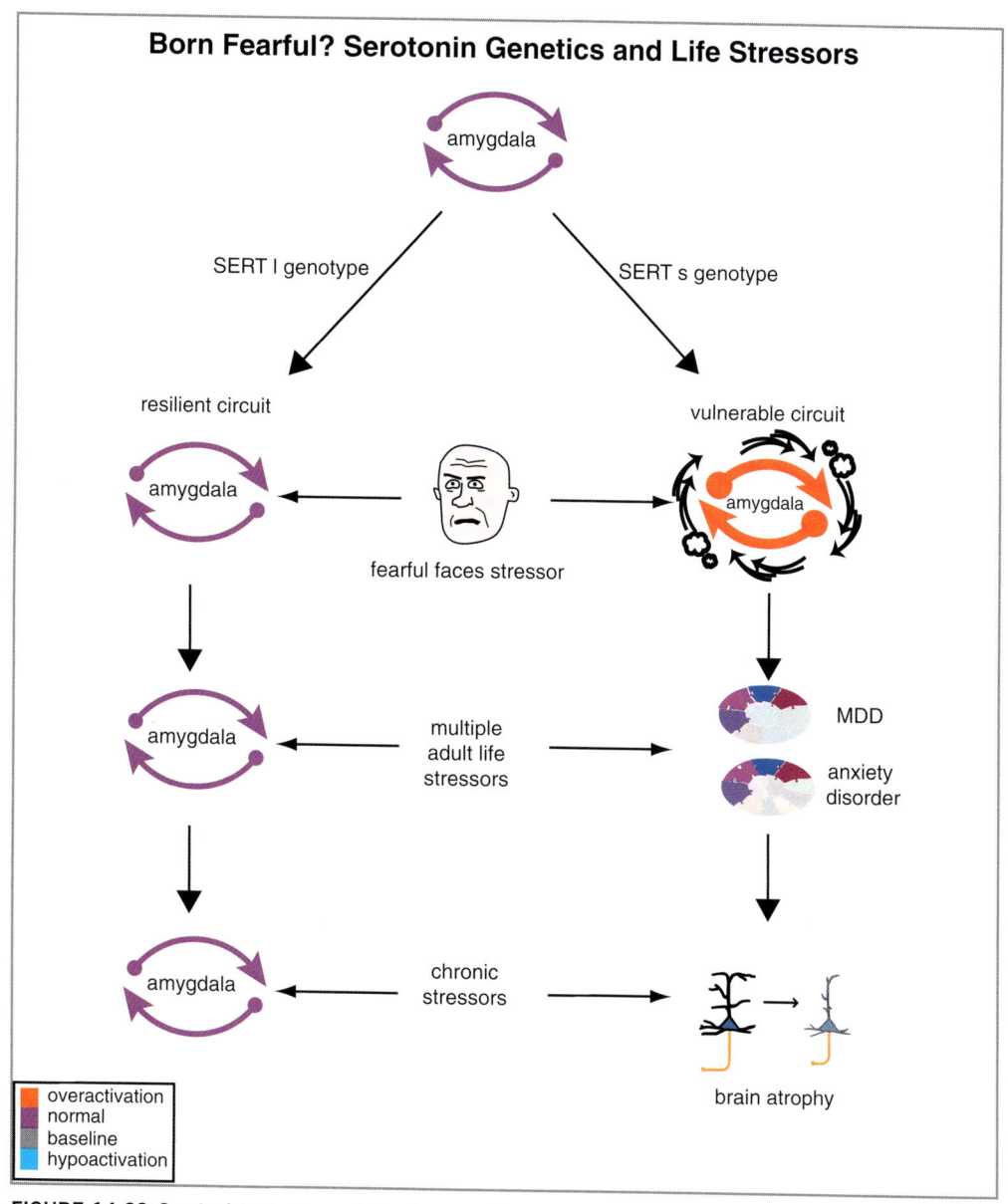

FIGURE 14-29 Serotonin genetics and life stressors. Genetic research has shown that the type of serotonin transporter (SERT) with which you are born can affect how you process fearful stimuli and perhaps also how you respond to stress. Specifically, individuals who are carriers of the s variant of the gene for SERT appear to be more vulnerable to the effects of stress or anxiety, whereas those who carry the l variant appear to be more resilient. Thus, s carriers exhibit increased amygdala activity in response to fearful faces and may also be more likely to develop a mood or anxiety disorder after suffering multiple life stressors or to have brain atrophy following exposure to chronic stress.

the importance of genes in general and those for serotonin neurons in particular in the regulation of the amygdala and in determining the odds of developing an anxiety disorder or major depression under stress. Therefore one may not be born fearful but rather born vulnerable or resilient to developing fear and an anxiety disorder or major depressive episode later on, in response to adult stressors, especially if they are chronic, multiple, and severe.

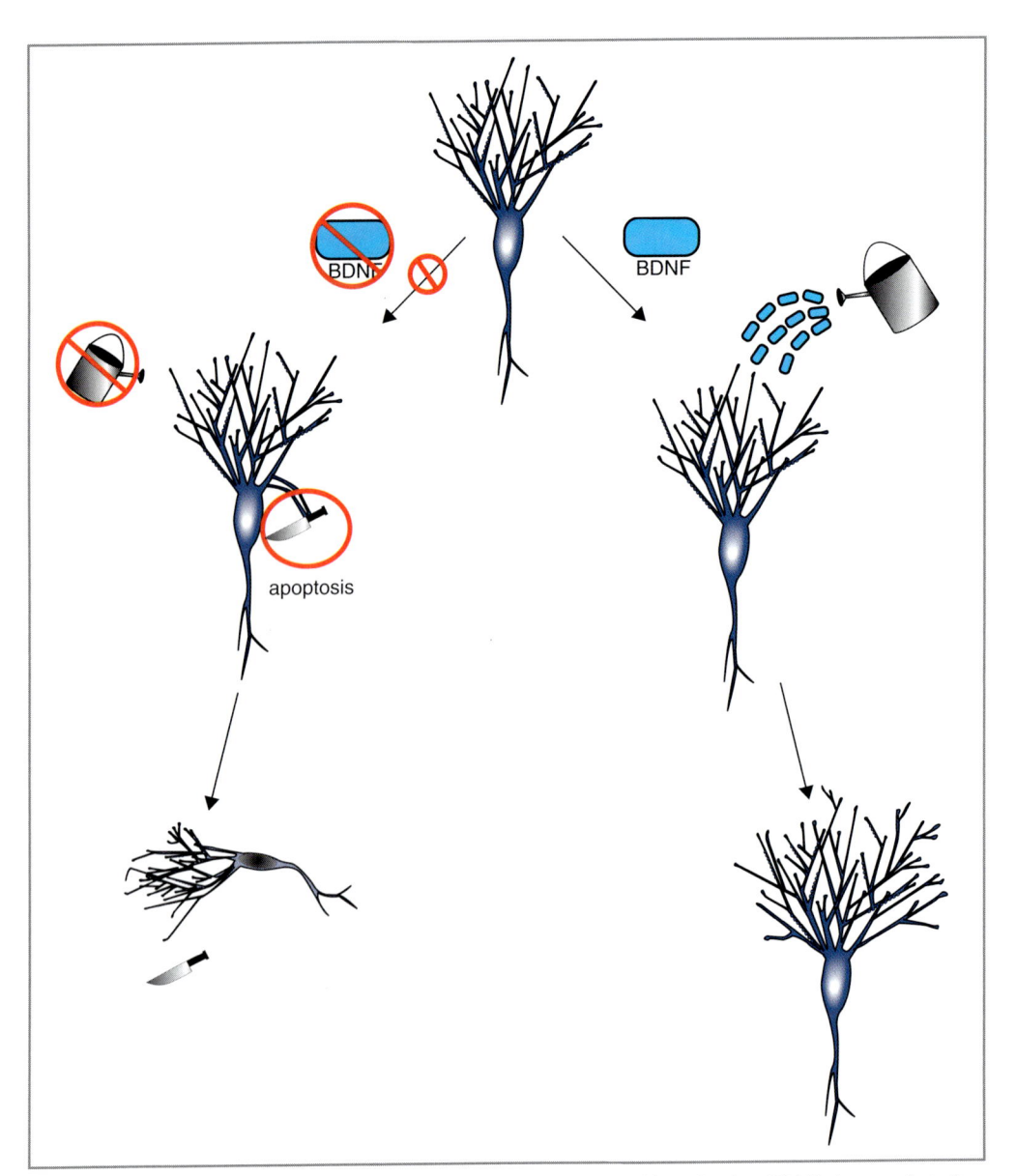

FIGURE 14-32 Suppression of brain-derived neurotrophic factor (BDNF) production. BDNF plays a role in the proper growth and maintenance of neurons and neuronal connections (right). If the genes for BDNF are turned off due to chronic stress (left), the resultant decrease in BDNF could compromise the brain's ability to create and maintain neurons and their connections. This could lead to loss of synapses or even whole neurons by apoptosis.

an anxiety disorder or depression when the individual is exposed, later in life, to multiple adult life stressors, just as vulnerability genes can increase the risk for an anxiety disorder or a major depressive episode.

Stress is not always bad
The adaptation of brain circuits to stress and the development of stress sensitization is discussed in Chapter 8 and illustrated in Figures 8-1 through 8-11. When stress is not

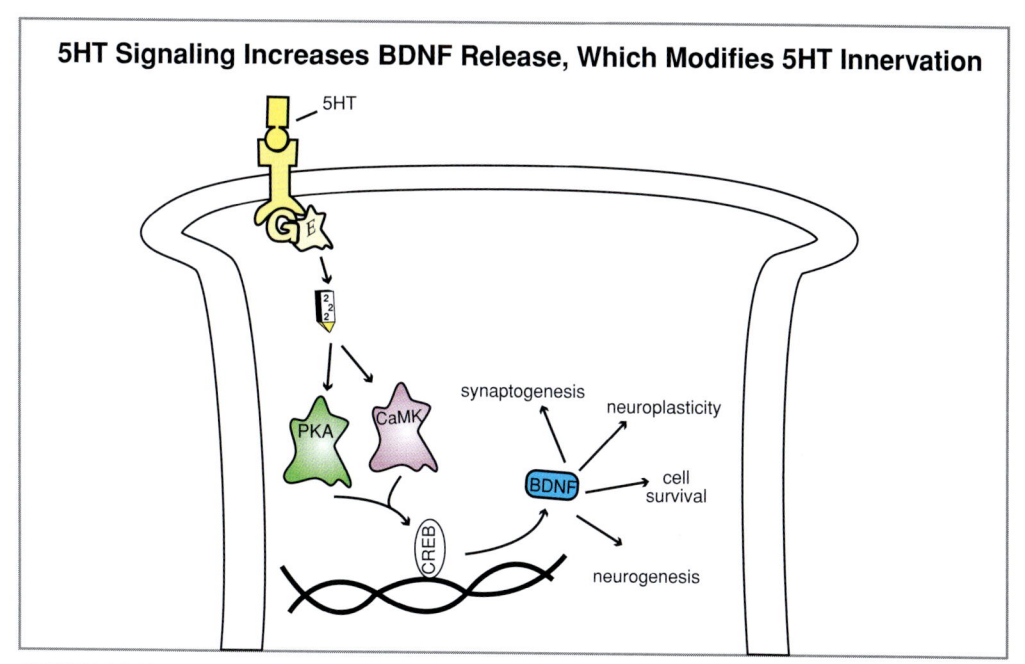

FIGURE 14-33 Serotonin (5HT) signaling and brain-derived neurotrophic factor (BDNF) release. Serotonin can increase the availability of BDNF by initiating signal transduction cascades that lead to its release. Thus, the brain has compensatory mechanisms that can reverse or prevent neuronal loss resulting from suppression of BDNF genes. These actions may be further enhanced by therapeutic agents that boost serotonin (e.g., serotonin selective reuptake inhibitors).

overwhelming, chronic, or appearing as multiple simultaneous stressors, it may activate circuits as they process the stress. But then once the emotional trauma of the stressor is withdrawn, the circuits return to normal levels of activation (Figure 8-11). In fact, all stress in childhood may not be bad (Figure 14-34). In experimental animals, it has been shown that exposure to mild stress in infancy can even render that animal less reactive to stress than another animal not exposed to stress in infancy (Figure 14-34). Thus mild stress may actually desensitize circuits to subsequent stress and produce a type of experience-based resilience.

Child abuse

On the other hand, overwhelming early life stress – such as physical, emotional, or sexual abuse – can emphatically cause a condition known as stress sensitization (Figure 14-34). The development of stress sensitization is illustrated in Figure 8-2, showing that certain types of sustained and repeated stressors from emotional trauma not only lead to activation of brain circuits while the stressor is being experienced but also cause the circuit to be irreversibly activated even when the stressor is withdrawn. In many cases, this initial activation of brain circuitry is clinically silent but represents a reduced capacity to process future stressors (Figure 8-2).

Child abuse appears to sensitize circuits to future adult stressors even if the child shows no signs of distress or mental illness at the time of the early life exposure to abusive stressors. Upon reexposure of a stress-sensitized individual to multiple stressors later in adulthood,

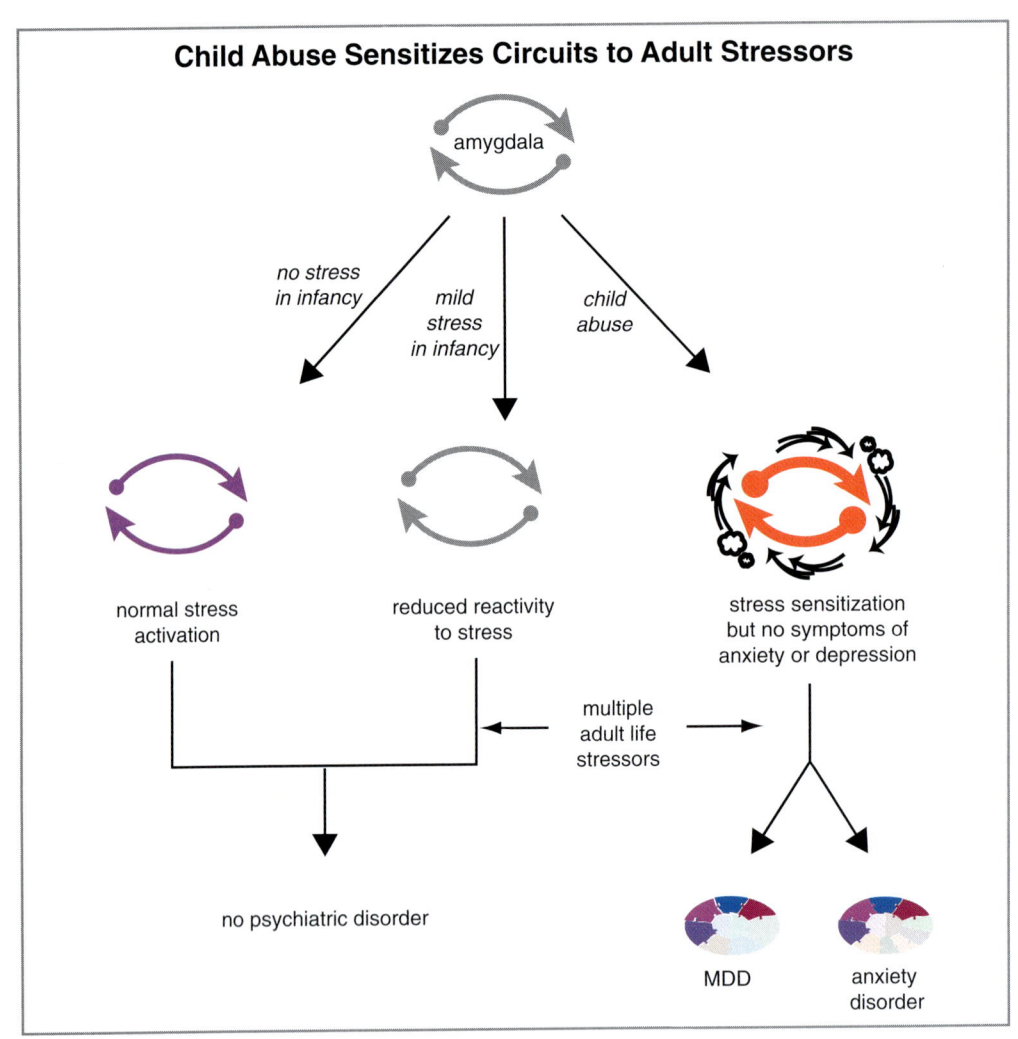

FIGURE 14-34 Early exposure to stress. It may be that the degree of stress one experiences during early life affects how the circuits develop and therefore how a given individual responds to stress in later life. No stress during infancy may lead to a circuit that exhibits "normal" activation during stress and confers no increased risk of developing a psychiatric disorder. Interestingly, mild stress during infancy may actually cause the circuits to exhibit reduced reactivity to stress in later life and provide some resilience to adult stressors. Overwhelming and/or chronic stress from child abuse, however, may lead to stress-sensitized circuits that may become activated even in the absence of a stressor. Individuals with stress sensitization may not exhibit phenotypic symptoms but may be at increased risk of developing a mental illness if exposed to future stressors.

however, the circuits now decompensate and the patient develops an anxiety disorder or a major depressive episode (Figures 8-3 and 14-34).

Stress and the hypothalamic-pituitary-adrenal (HPA) axis

Circuits involved in stress sensitization comprise not only the amygdala (Figure 14-34) but also the hypothalamic-pituitary-adrenal (HPA) axis (Figure 14-35). Sensitization of both circuits may contribute to the development of an anxiety disorder or a major depressive episode in response to stress. The normal stress response of the HPA axis is to increase the release of corticotrophin releasing factor (CRF), adrenocorticotropic hormone (ACTH),

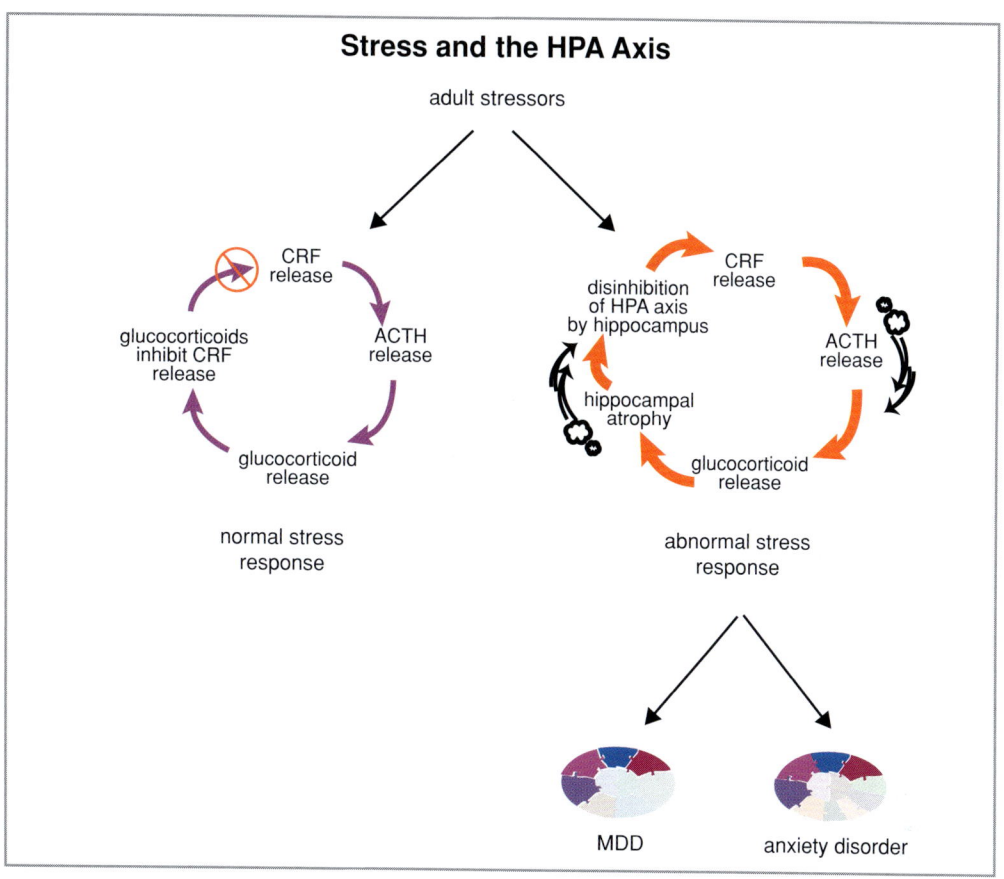

FIGURE 14-35 Stress and the hypothalamic-pituitary-adrenal (HPA) axis. The normal stress response (left) involves activation of the hypothalamus and a resultant increase in corticotrophin releasing factor (CRF), which in turn stimulates the release of adrenocorticotropic hormone (ACTH) from the pituitary. ACTH causes glucocorticoid release from the adrenal gland, which feeds back to the hypothalamus and inhibits CRF release, terminating the stress response. In situations of chronic stress, excessive glucocorticoid release may eventually cause hippocampal atrophy. Because the hippocampus inhibits the HPA axis, atrophy in this region may lead to chronic activation of the HPA axis, which may increase risk of developing a psychiatric illness.

and glucocorticoids acutely until the danger is gone, usually after a short time (Figure 14-35). In the long term, glucocorticoids exert negative feedback upon CRF release, returning the HPA system to normal.

However, an abnormal stress response may result from chronic and unremitting stress, especially in circuits that are vulnerable and already stress-sensitized from child abuse (Figure 14-35). Here, CRF, ACTH, and glucocorticoids are all released, but instead of recovering rapidly, they all remain persistently elevated. Eventually, these elevated glucocorticoids may exert a toxic effect on the hippocampus due to changes in gene expression there. Actions of glucocorticoids on nuclear hormone glucocorticoid receptors and neuronal gene expression are discussed in Chapter 5 and illustrated in Figure 5-50. Persistently elevated glucocorticoids may not only damage the hippocampus and cause it to atrophy but also prevent it from inhibiting the HPA axis, thus resulting in disinhibition of the HPA axis and chronic elevation of all HPA stress hormones (Figure 14-35). Over time, this could

Potential Sites of Action for Novel Treatments for Stress-Induced Affective Disorders

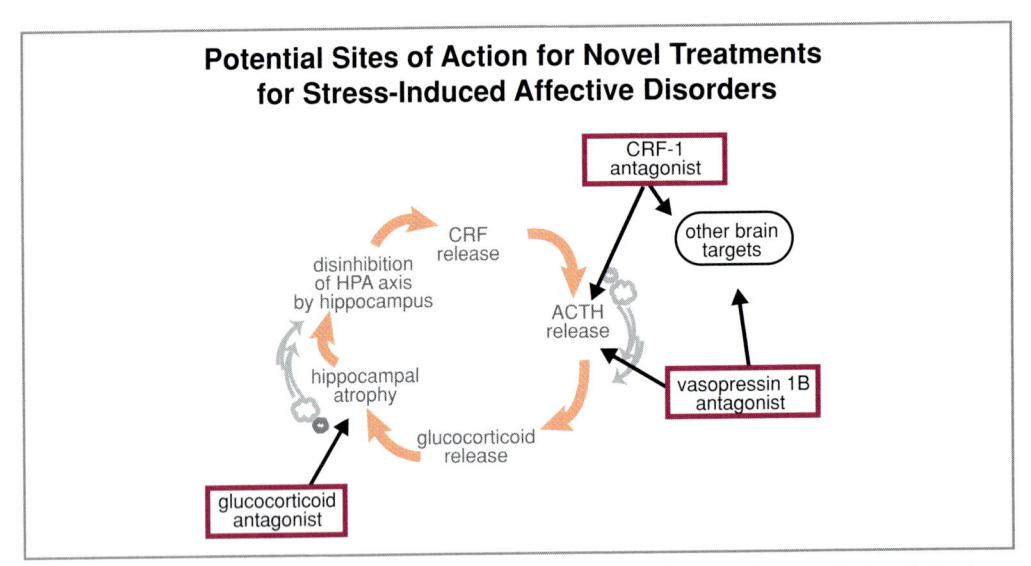

FIGURE 14-36 Potential novel treatments for stress-induced affective disorders. Because the hypothalamic-pituitary-adrenal (HPA) axis is central to stress processing, it may be that novel targets for treating stress-induced disorders lie within the axis. Mechanisms being examined include antagonism of glucocorticoid receptors, corticotrophin releasing factor 1 (CRF-1) receptors, and vasopressin 1B receptors.

lead not only to hippocampal atrophy (see Figure 14-30) but also to the onset of an anxiety disorder or major depressive episode (Figure 14-35).

Novel treatments for stress and its progression to anxiety disorders or major depression
Because of the profound influence of the HPA axis on anxiety disorders and on the processing of stress reactions, a great deal of effort has gone into identifying therapeutic interventions that could interrupt this vicious cycle and improve not only the symptoms of an anxiety disorder but also the physiological consequences of stress (Figure 14-36). The actions of glucocorticoid antagonists are discussed in Chapter 5 and illustrated in Figure 5-50. This concept is also shown in Figure 14-36, the idea being that antagonism of glucocorticoid action could prevent hippocampal atrophy and damage to the negative feedback regulation of the HPA axis hypothetically caused by elevated glucocorticoid levels.

The abnormal stress response shown in Figure 14-35 also involves elevation of CRF, and persistent CRF action at HPA CRF1 receptors leads to glucocorticoid elevation. This has led to the idea that the blocking of CRF actions at CRF1 receptors may be helpful in blunting abnormal stress responses (Figure 14-36). CRF1 receptors are also distributed outside of the HPA axis in other brain areas, and to the extent that excessive actions of CRF at these receptors lead to the development of an anxiety disorder or a major depressive episode, the blocking of CRF actions at these sites may also help to treat or prevent anxiety and depression. Thus numerous CRF1 antagonists are in clinical testing in various anxiety disorders, major depressive disorder, and other stress-linked conditions.

A novel notion now showing promise in experimental animals is to block one of the receptors for vasopressin, known as the V1b receptor. Vasopressin's actions at V1b receptors in the HPA axis are involved in ACTH release during stress reactions but not necessarily during normal physiological regulation. Theoretically, by blocking the ability of vasopressin to release ACTH and glucocorticoids during stress, it may be possible to prevent complications within the HPA axis, including the onset or progression of stress-related conditions such as anxiety disorders and major depression. Vasopressin 1b receptors in brain areas outside the HPA axis may also be involved in pathological stress reactions, and blocking these receptors could also exert therapeutic actions for preventing or treating anxiety and depression. Human testing of some V1b antagonists is now on the horizon.

Alpha 2 delta ligands as anxiolytics

Voltage-sensitive calcium channels (VSCCs) and specifically presynaptic N and P/Q subtypes of VSCCs and their role in excitatory neurotransmitter release are discussed in Chapter 5 (Figures 5-33 through 5-37, 5-41, 5-42, 5-44, and 5-45). Two proven anticonvulsants with a novel mechanism of action are gabapentin and pregabalin, also known as alpha 2 delta ligands, since they bind to the alpha 2 delta subunit of presynaptic N and P/Q VSCCs. This binding action blocks the release of excitatory neurotransmitters such as glutamate when neurotransmission is excessive (Figure 5-37). In some brain areas, this results in anticonvulsant action, but possibly in the amygdala and in cortical areas of CSTC loops, these same alpha 2 delta ligands could hypothetically bind to overly active anxiety circuits, reduce their activity, and improve the symptoms of anxiety. The alpha 2 delta ligands pregabalin and gabapentin do seem to have anxiolytic actions, especially in social anxiety disorder and panic disorder, and are already proven agents for the treatment of epilepsy and certain pain conditions, including neuropathic pain and fibromyalgia. The actions of alpha 2 delta ligands in pain conditions are discussed in Chapter 15, on pain.

An interesting aspect of alpha 2 delta ligands is that they appear to have much greater affinity for their binding site when the channel is in use and thus may be most effective in situations where neurons have excessive activity, as hypothesized for anxiety disorders in the amygdala while the patient is experiencing anxiety and fear. Ongoing research will clarify the relative efficacy and clinical utility of these agents. However, since they have clearly different mechanisms of action compared to serotonin reuptake inhibitors or benzodiazepines, alpha 2 delta ligands may be useful for patients who do not do well on SSRIs/SNRIs or benzodiazepines. Also, it may be very useful to combine alpha 2 delta ligands with SSRIs/SNRIs or benzodiazepines in patients who are partial responders and are not in remission. A simplified notion for how alpha 2 delta ligands may improve the symptoms of anxiety and fear by targeting excessive release of glutamate in the amygdala is illustrated in Figure 14-37.

Noradrenergic hyperactivity in anxiety

Norepinephrine is another neurotransmitter with important regulatory input to the amygdala (Figure 14-38) as well as to many of the projection areas of the amygdala (Figure 14-9). Excessive noradrenergic output from the locus coeruleus can result not only in numerous peripheral manifestations of autonomic overdrive, as discussed above and as illustrated in Figures 14-12 through 14-14, but can also trigger numerous central symptoms of anxiety and fear, such as nightmares, hyperarousal states, flashbacks, and panic attacks (Figure 14-38). Hypothetically, these symptoms may be mediated in part by excessive noradrenergic input to alpha 1 and beta 1 adrenergic receptors in the amygdala (Figure 14-38), because in some patients such symptoms can be reduced by treatment either with beta adrenergic blockers (Figure 14-39A) or alpha 1 adrenergic blockers such as prazosin (Figure 14-39B). Although antidepressants with prominent noradrenergic actions, such as those with noradrenergic reuptake blocking properties (i.e., inhibitors of the norepinephrine transporter, or NET), are not generally favored for the treatment of anxiety disorders compared to those with serotonin reuptake blocking properties (i.e., inhibitors of the serotonin transporter,

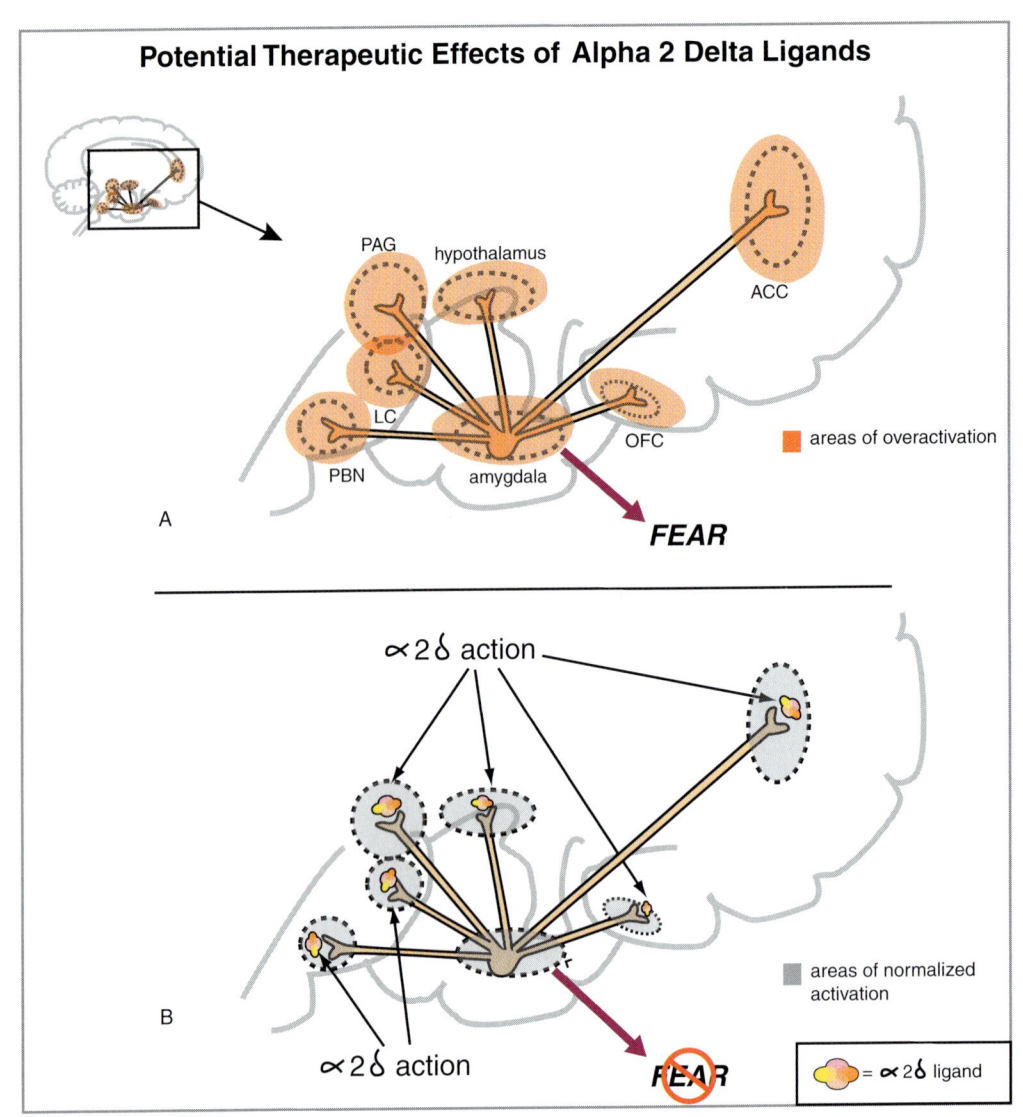

FIGURE 14-37A and B Potential therapeutic effects of alpha 2 delta ligands. (**A**) Pathological anxiety/fear may be caused by the overactivation of amygdala circuits. (**B**) Agents that bind to the alpha 2 delta subunit of presynaptic N and P/Q voltage-sensitive calcium channels can block the excessive activation of neurons in the amygdala and thereby reduce the symptoms of anxiety.

or SERT), some patients do respond to NET inhibitors, presumably due in part to their ability to desensitize postsynaptic beta and alpha 1 noradrenergic receptors over time.

Fear conditioning versus fear extinction

Fear conditioning is a concept as old as Pavlov's dogs. If an aversive stimulus such as foot shock is coupled with a neutral stimulus such as a bell, the animal learns to associate the two and will develop fear when it hears a bell. In humans, fear is learned during stressful experiences associated with emotional trauma and is influenced by genetic predisposition (stress diathesis). Often, fearful situations are managed successfully and then forgotten. Because fear of truly dangerous situations is crucial for survival, the mechanism of learned

Noradrenergic Hyperactivity in Anxiety

locus coeruleus

β1 receptor

NE

α1 receptor

amygdala

anxiety/panic attacks
tremor
sweating
tachycardia
hyperarousal
nightmares

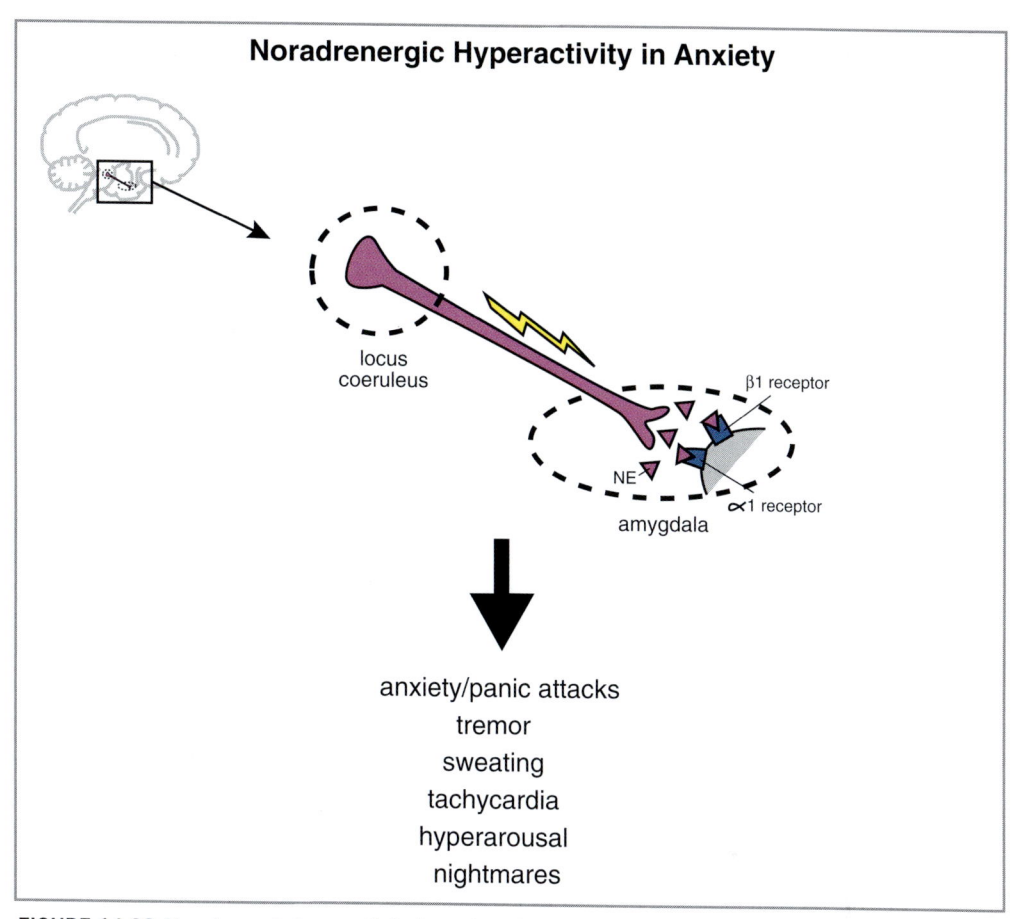

FIGURE 14-38 Noradrenergic hyperactivity in anxiety. Norepinephrine provides input not only to the amygdala but also to many regions to which the amygdala projects; thus it plays an important role in the fear response. Noradrenergic hyperactivation can lead to anxiety, panic attacks, tremors, sweating, tachycardia, hyperarousal, and nightmares. Alpha 1 and beta 1 adrenergic receptors may be specifically involved in these reactions.

fear, called fear conditioning, has been extremely well conserved across species, including man.

However, overwhelming fears can also be learned, and if they cannot be forgotten, may progress to anxiety disorders or a major depressive episode. This is a big problem, since almost 30% of the population will develop an anxiety disorder, due in large part to stressful environments, including exposure to fearful events during normal activities in today's society but in particular during war and natural disasters. Hearing an explosion, smelling burning rubber, seeing a picture of a wounded civilian, and seeing or hearing floodwaters are all sensory experiences that can trigger traumatic reexperiencing and generalized hyperarousal and fear in PTSD. Panic associated with social situations will "teach" the patient to panic in social situations in social anxiety disorder. Panic randomly associated with an attack that happens to have occurred in a crowd, on a bridge, or in shopping centers will also trigger another panic attack when the same environment is encountered in panic disorder. These and other symptoms of anxiety disorders are all forms of learning known as fear conditioning (Figure 14-40).

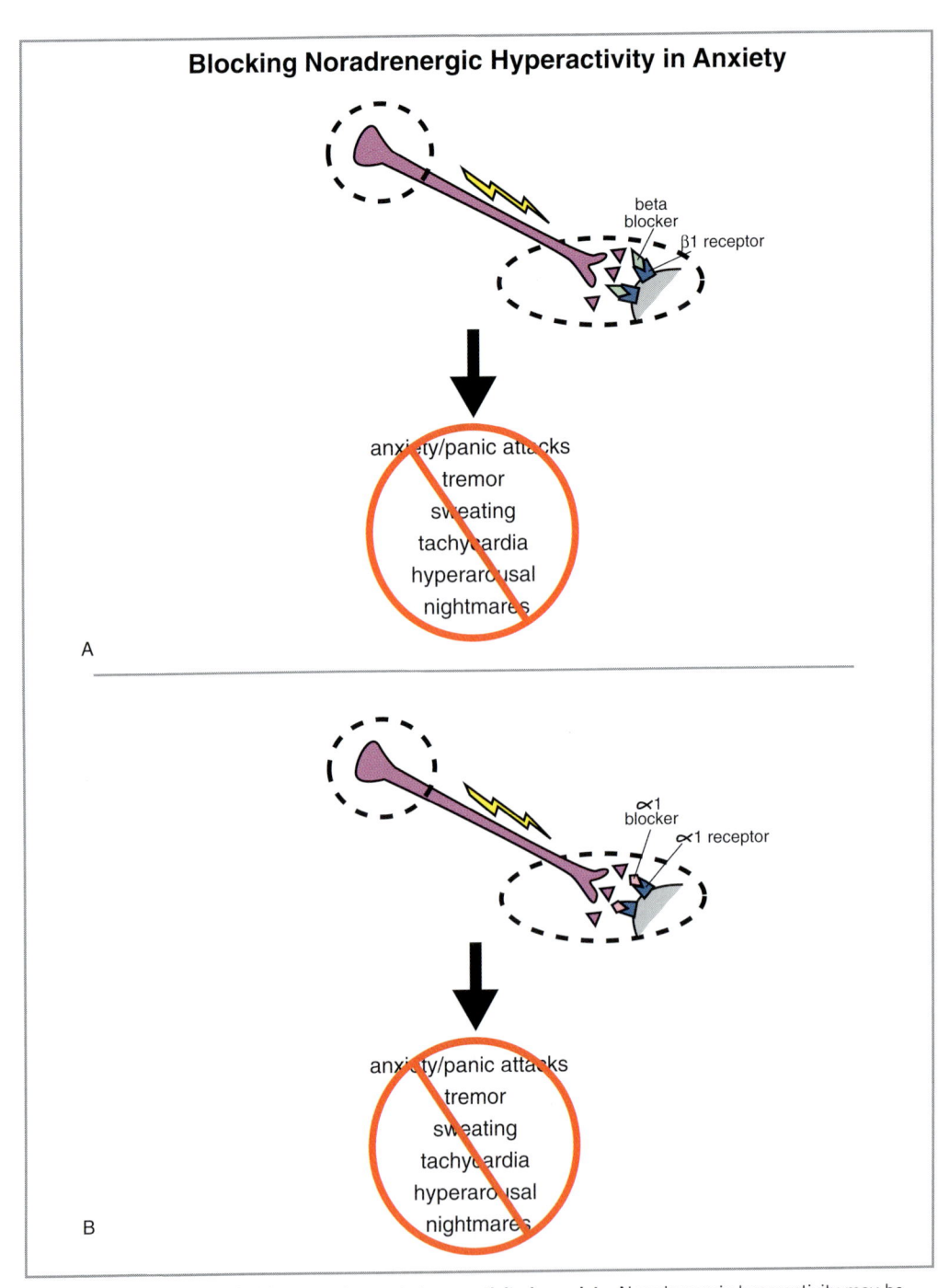

FIGURE 14-39A and B Blocking noradrenergic hyperactivity in anxiety. Noradrenergic hyperactivity may be blocked by the administration of beta adrenergic blockers (**A**) or alpha 1 adrenergic blockers (**B**), which can lead to the alleviation of anxiety and other stress-related symptoms.

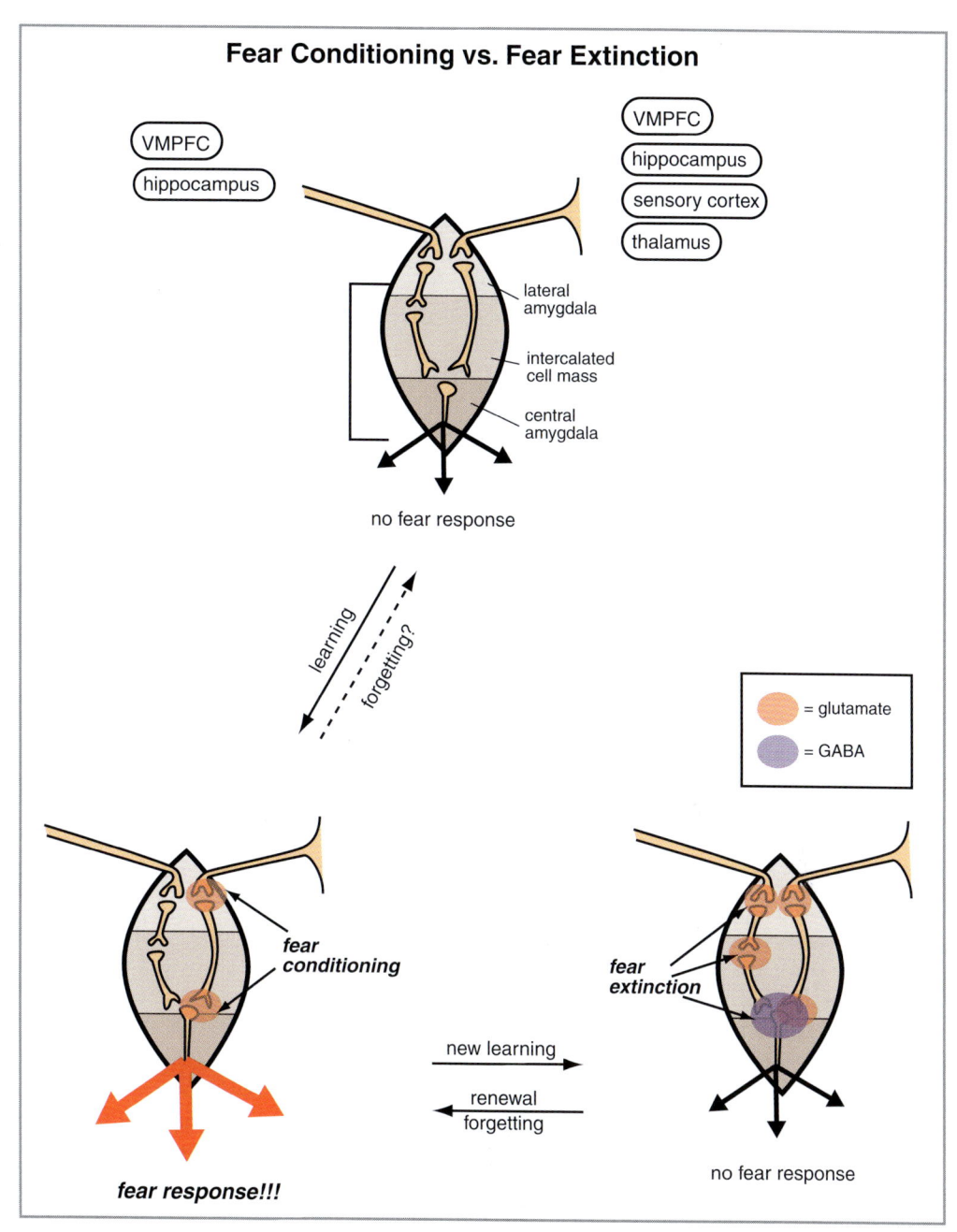

FIGURE 14-40 Fear conditioning versus fear extinction. When an individual encounters a stressful or fearful experience, the sensory input is relayed to the amygdala, where it is integrated with input from the ventromedial prefrontal cortex (VMPFC) and hippocampus, so that a fear response can be either generated or suppressed. The amygdala may "remember" stimuli associated with that experience by increasing the efficiency of glutamate neurotransmission, so that on future exposure to stimuli, a fear response is more efficiently triggered. If this is not countered by input from the VMPFC to suppress the fear response, fear conditioning proceeds. Fear conditioning is not readily reversed, but it can be inhibited through new learning. This new learning is termed fear extinction and is the progressive reduction of the response to a feared stimulus that is repeatedly presented without adverse consequences. Thus the VMPFC and hippocampus learn a new context for the feared stimulus and send input to the amygdala to suppress the fear response. The "memory" of the conditioned fear is still present, however.

The amygdala is involved in "remembering" the various stimuli associated with a given fearful situation. It does this by increasing the efficiency of neurotransmission at glutamatergic synapses in the lateral amygdala as sensory input about those stimuli comes in from the thalamus or sensory cortex (Figure 14-40). This input is then relayed to the central amygdala, where fear conditioning also improves the efficiency of neurotransmission at another glutamate synapse there (Figure 14-40). Both synapses are restructured and permanent learning is embedded into this circuit by NMDA receptors, triggering long-term potentiation and synaptic plasticity, so that subsequent input from the sensory cortex and thalamus is very efficiently processed to trigger the fear response as output from the central amygdala every time there is sensory input associated with the original fearful event (Figure 14-40; see also Figures 14-10 through 14-15).

Input to the lateral amygdala is modulated by the prefrontal cortex, especially the ventromedial prefrontal cortex (VMPFC), and by the hippocampus. If the VMPFC is unable to suppress the fear response at the level of the amygdala, fear conditioning proceeds. The hippocampus remembers the context of the fear conditioning and makes sure fear is triggered when the fearful stimulus and all its associated stimuli are encountered. Most contemporary psychopharmacological treatments for anxiety and fear act by suppressing the fear output from the amygdala (see Figures 14-25, 14-27, 14-37, and 14-39) and therefore are not cures, since the fundamental neuronal learning underlying fear conditioning in these patients remains in place.

Fear extinction means learning to forgive but not to forget

Once fear conditioning is in place, it can be very difficult to reverse. However, fear conditioning and its associated fear response can be inhibited by a process known as fear extinction. Fear extinction is the progressive reduction of the response to a feared stimulus and occurs when the stimulus is repeatedly presented without any adverse consequence.

When fear extinction occurs, it appears that the original fear conditioning is not really "forgotten" even though the fear response can be profoundly reduced over time by the active process of fear extinction. Rather than reversing the synaptic changes described above for fear conditioning, it appears that a new form of learning with additional synaptic changes in the amygdala occurs during fear extinction. These changes can suppress symptoms of anxiety and fear by inhibiting the original learning but not by removing it (Figure 14-40). Specifically, activation of the amygdala by the VMPFC occurs while the hippocampus remembers the context in which the feared stimulus did not have any adverse consequences (Figure 14-40). Fear extinction occurs when inputs from VMPFC and hippocampus activate glutamatergic neurons in the lateral amygdala that synapse on an inhibitory GABAergic interneurons located within the intercalated cell mass of the amygdala (Figure 14-40). This sets up a gate within the central amygdala, with fear output occurring if the fear conditioning circuit predominates and no fear output occurring if the fear extinction circuit predominates.

Fear extinction predominates when synaptic strengthening and long-term potentiation in the new circuit is able to produce inhibitory GABAergic drive that can overcome the excitatory glutamatergic drive produced by the pre-existing fear conditioning circuitry (Figure 14-40). Much of what is now understood about anxiety disorders and novel treatments is related to whether the fear conditioning circuit or the fear extinction circuit predominates. When fear extinction exists simultaneously with fear conditioning, memory for both is present, but the output depends on which system is stronger, better remembered, and which has the most robust synaptic efficiency. This will determine which gate will open, the one with the fear response or the one that keeps the fear response in check. Unfortunately, over time, fear conditioning may have the upper hand over fear extinction. Unlike fear conditioning, fear extinction is labile and tends to reverse over time. Also, fear conditioning can return if the old fear is presented in a context different than that of the one learned to suppress the fear during fear extinction, a process termed renewal.

Furthermore, the inability to extinguish or inhibit maladaptive fear responses by fear extinction is theoretically the hallmark of anxiety disorders, especially PTSD.

This suggests that novel therapeutic interventions for anxiety disorders would be those that facilitate and maintain fear extinction, rather than just suppressing the fear response triggered by fear conditioning, as do most current treatments for anxiety. If the fear extinction circuit in the amygdala could somehow be preferentially activated, this might lead to reduction of symptoms of anxiety. Also, activity in VMPFC neurons is necessary for the expression of fear conditioning, and the VMPFC can both excite and inhibit fear expression. Thus, pharmacological interventions aimed not only at the amygdala but also at the VMPFC and its CSTC loops may also be able to favor the recall of fear extinction rather than the recall of fear conditioning.

How could novel therapeutics favor fear extinction circuits over fear conditioning circuits?

First, cognitive behavioral therapies using exposure techniques and that require the patient to confront the fear-inducing stimuli in a safe environment may trigger the learning of fear extinction in the amygdala. Unfortunately, because the hippocampus remembers the context of this extinction, such therapies are context-specific and do not always generalize to the real world once the patient is outside the safe therapeutic environment. Current psychotherapy research is investigating how contextual cues can be used to strengthen extinction learning so that the therapeutic learning generalizes to other environments.

Also, if synapses on the fear extinction side of the amygdala gate could be strengthened disproportionately to the synapses on the fear conditioned side of the amygdala gate, perhaps extinction pathways would predominate and the symptoms of anxiety disorders would be reduced. This idea is shown in Figure 14-41, where the NMDA receptor coagonist d-cycloserine is being administered to a patient receiving systematic exposure to feared stimuli during cognitive behavioral therapy. As therapy progresses, and learning occurs, glutamate is released in the lateral amygdala and in the intercalated cell mass at inhibitory GABA neurons. If NMDA receptors at these two glutamate synapses could trigger disproportionately robust long-term potentiation and synaptic plasticity during this learning while these synapses are selectively activated by cognitive behavioral therapy, it could result in the predominance of the extinction pathway over the conditioned pathway.

How could this be done? Recall that NMDA receptors are coincidence detectors that act to trigger long-term potentiation and synaptic plasticity when three things happen at the same time: glutamate occupies the glutamate site, glycine occupies the glycine site, and depolarization of the neuron occurs. The chances of this occurring are enhanced not only by cognitive behavioral therapy and exposure, which theoretically activates glutamate release in the amygdala during the learning associated with fear extinction, but also by providing a coagonist for the glycine site. The importance of the glycine coagonist site on NMDA receptors is discussed in Chapter 5 and illustrated in Figure 5-25; it is also discussed in Chapter 9 and illustrated in Figures 9-34 and 9-35. One of the known agonists for the

Facilitating Fear Extinction: Enhancing Inhibitory Learning With the NMDA Agonist D-Cycloserine

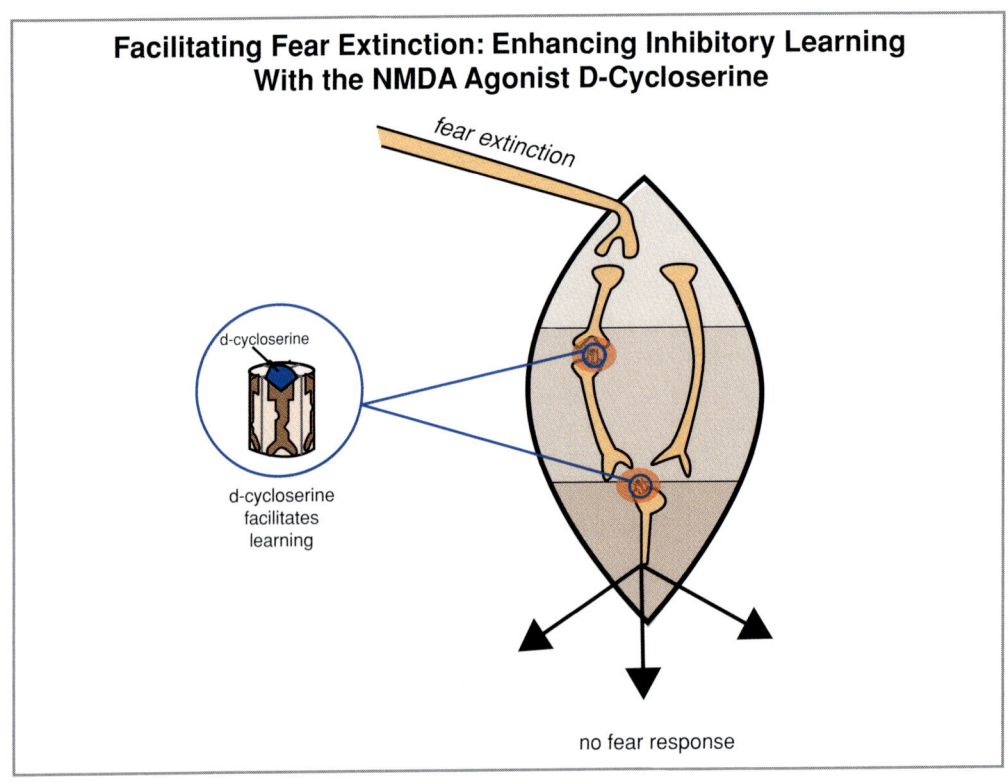

FIGURE 14-41 Facilitating fear extinction with d-cycloserine. Strengthening of synapses involved in fear extinction could help enhance the development of fear extinction learning in the amygdala and reduce symptoms of anxiety disorders. Administration of the N-methyl-d-aspartate (NMDA) coagonist d-cycloserine while an individual is receiving exposure therapy could increase the efficiency of glutamate neurotransmission at synapses involved in fear extinction. If this leads to long-term potentiation and synaptic plasticity while the synapses are activated by exposure therapy, it could result in structural changes in the amygdala associated with the fear extinction pathway and thus the predominance of the extinction pathway over the conditioned pathway.

glycine site is d-cycloserine, discussed also in Chapter 10 and illustrated in Figure 10-123. This agent has been given to experimental animals during experimental fear extinction training and has been shown to facilitate fear extinction in these models. This has led to d-cycloserine also being administered to patients with anxiety disorders while they were undergoing cognitive behavioral therapy and exposure. The results are promising in that they suggest improvement in the development of fear extinction for such patients.

If these and similar approaches continue to show promising results, it means that a whole new therapeutic strategy for anxiety disorders could be on the horizon – namely, facilitating naturally occurring fear extinction rather than just blocking the fear responses that occur in anxiety disorders due to fear conditioning, as current therapies now act. It also would mean an increasingly important role not only for cognitive behavioral therapy for anxiety disorders but also for the clever and artful combination of psychopharmacological mechanisms with appropriately timed psychotherapeutic interventions.

Preemptive or prophylactic treatments for anxiety disorders
Another novel idea for the treatment of anxiety disorders is based on blocking the formation of fear conditioning in the first place. This has been called preemptive or prophylactic

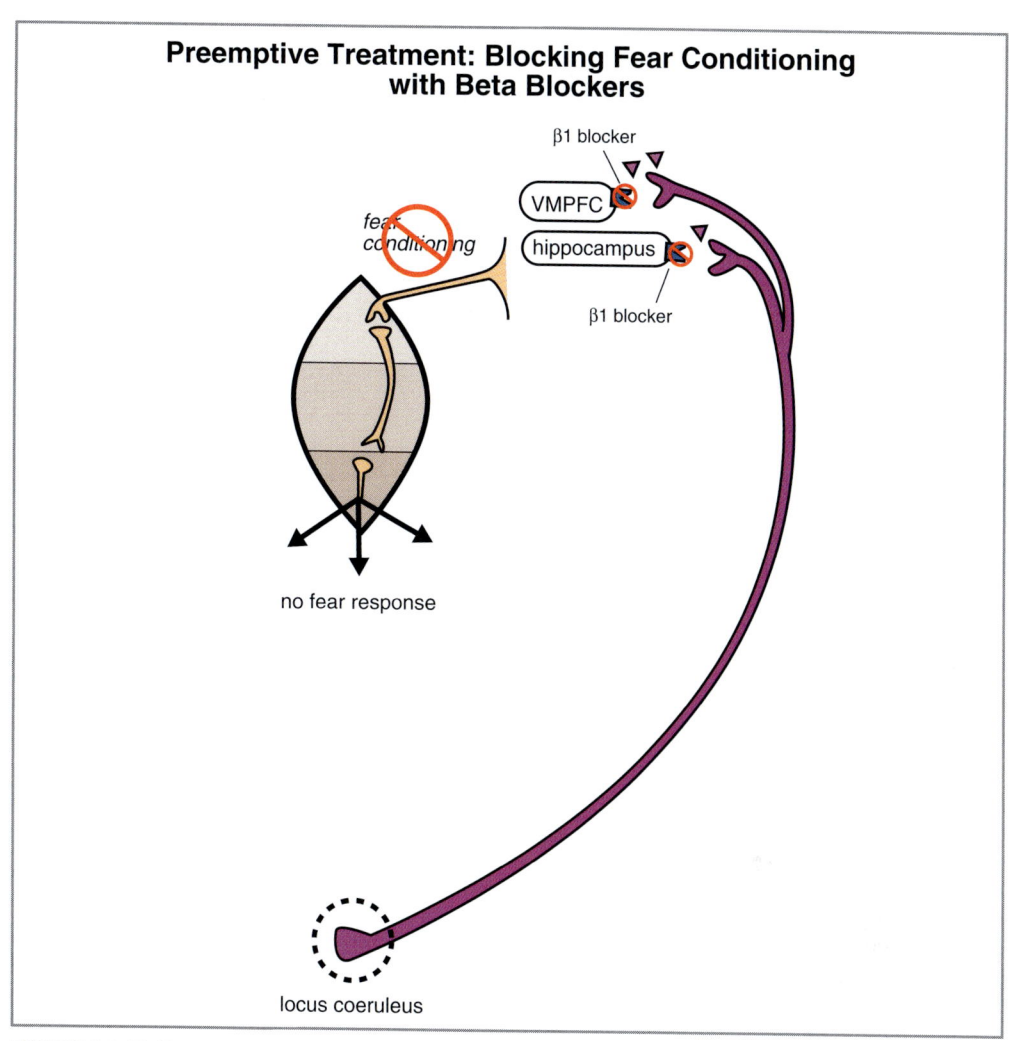

FIGURE 14-42 Preemptive treatment with beta blockers. There is some research to suggest that administration of beta adrenergic blockers immediately following exposure to trauma could block fear conditioning before it even occurs. Blockade of beta receptors in the ventromedial prefrontal cortex (VMPFC) and hippocampus may prevent input from reaching the amygdala and thus prevent synaptic changes that lead to fear conditioning.

treatment. Some even call it postexposure "inoculation." Whatever it is, the idea is to prevent the formation of permanent synaptic changes associated with fear conditioning by suppressing these changes either with drugs or with early fear extinction learning paradigms.

For example, following acute exposure to highly traumatic stimuli, there may be a window of time when fear conditioning can be blocked before it is permanently embedded into the amygdala. Promising studies with beta adrenergic blockers suggest that in some individuals at high risk for developing PTSD because of exposure to highly traumatic stimuli, PTSD might be prevented (Figure 14-42). This is an exciting avenue of research and a novel treatment approach for anxiety disorders, which are often irreversible and difficult to treat. Perhaps in the future it will be possible to clarify the pharmacology of preemptive treatments that could prevent fear conditioning following exposure to a traumatic event.

Associate Symptoms With Brain Regions, Circuits, and Neurotransmitters That Regulate Them

cortico-striatal-thalamic-cortical circuit "worry loop" — modulated by 5HT, GABA, DA, NE, glutamate, voltage-gated ion channels

worry
- anxious misery
- apprehensive expectation
- obsessions

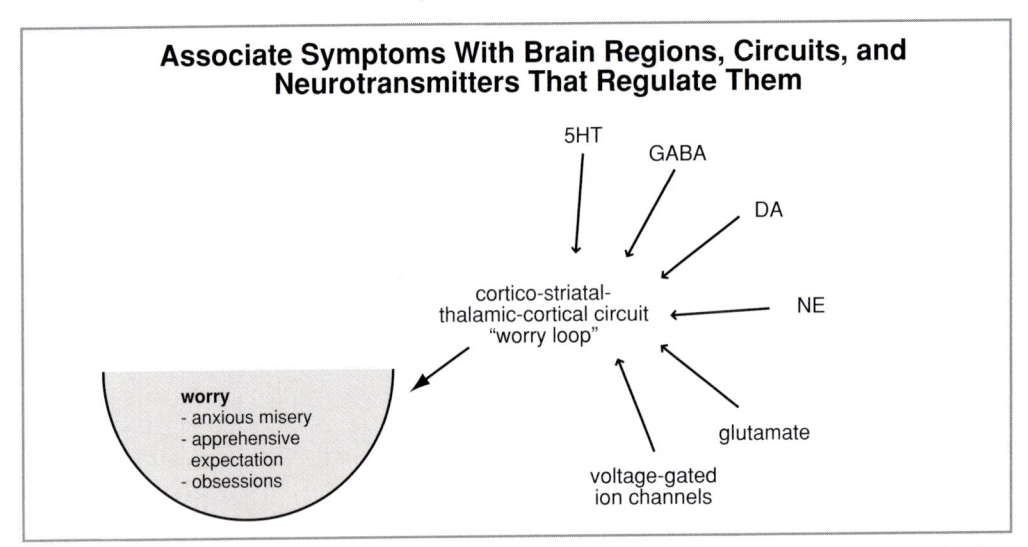

FIGURE 14-43 **Linking worry symptoms to circuits to neurotransmitters.** Symptoms of worry are associated with malfunctioning of cortico-striatal-thalamic-cortical loops, which are regulated by serotonin (5HT), gamma-aminobutyric acid (GABA), dopamine (DA), norepinephrine (NE), glutamate, and voltage-gated ion channels.

Worry/Obsessions

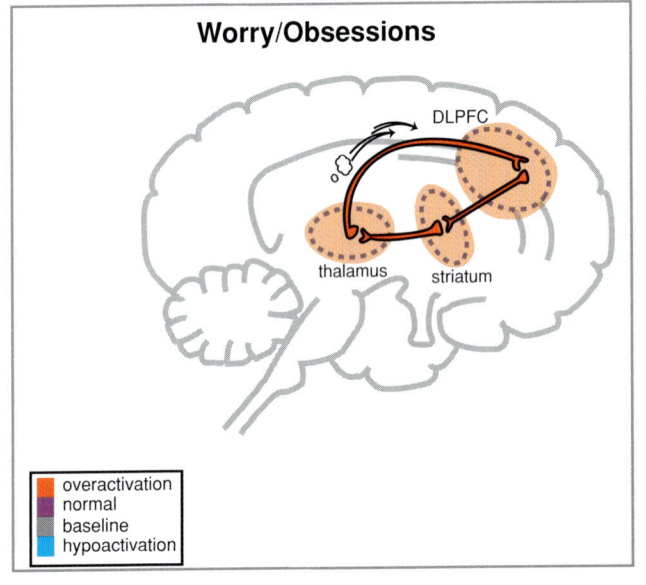

DLPFC, thalamus, striatum

overactivation
normal
baseline
hypoactivation

FIGURE 14-44 **Worry/obsessions circuit.** Shown here is a cortico-striatal-thalamic-cortical loop originating and ending in the dorsolateral prefrontal cortex (DLPFC). Overactivation of this circuit may lead to worry or obsessions.

Cortico-striatal-thalamic-cortical (CSTC) loops and the neurobiology of worry

Born worried?

Most of this chapter has focused on the amygdala and the neurobiology of fear. However, there is a second core symptom of anxiety disorders – namely, worry – and this involves another unique set of circuits to be discussed in this section (Figure 14-43). Worry, which can include anxious misery, apprehensive expectations, catastrophic thinking, and obsessions, is linked to cortico-striatal-thalamic-cortical feedback loops in the prefrontal cortex (Figure 14-44). Several neurotransmitters and regulators modulate these circuits, including serotonin, GABA, dopamine, norepinephrine, glutamate, and voltage-gated ion channels (Figure 14-43). Many of these neurotransmitters have already been discussed in the section on the amygdala and have overlapping regulatory functions in CSTC loops as well. This section discusses how different genotypes for the enzyme COMT (catechol-O-methyl-transferase) not only regulate the availability of the neurotransmitter dopamine in prefrontal cortex but also how such differences in dopamine availability may affect the risk for worry and anxiety disorder and may determine whether you can be born worried (Figure 14-45).

Warrior versus worrier

In Chapter 8, the impact of genetic variants of COMT on cognitive functioning were discussed; they are illustrated in Figure 8-10. Specifically, normal controls with the Met variant of COMT have more efficient information processing in the dorsolateral prefrontal cortex (DLPFC) during a cognitive task such as the n-back test (Figure 8-10). These subjects have lower COMT activity due to their specific genetic variant of the enzyme, higher dopamine levels, and presumably better information processing during tasks of executive functioning that recruit circuits in the DLPFC. Because of more efficient cognitive information processing, such subjects also have a lower risk of schizophrenia than subjects that are Val carriers of COMT (Figure 14-45).

At first glance, it would seem that all the biological advantages go to those with the Met variant of COMT. However, that is not necessarily true when it comes to processing stressors that cause dopamine release. With the Met genotype, low COMT activity, and high dopamine levels, stressors can produce excessive dopamine activity, which disrupts cognitive information processing and creates symptoms of anxiety in this circuit, such as worry and obsessions. Too much dopamine activity can also lead pyramidal neurons in the DLPFC to go "out of tune." This concept of optimal tuning of pyramidal neurons with dopamine, with the ideal functioning of this neuron from prefrontal cortex being neither too much nor too little, is discussed in Chapter 7 and illustrated in Figures 7-25 and 7-26. Under stress, therefore, it appears that Val carriers of COMT have dopamine activity optimized with stress, have increased COMT activity to cope with the extra dopamine, and are "warriors" who are not afraid or worried. On the other hand, those with the Met variant of COMT may decompensate with the increased availability of dopamine under stress, be unable to process this extra dopamine due to lower COMT activity, and thus are "worriers" who are afraid and worried and who also have an increased risk of developing an anxiety disorder (Figure 14-45).

Treatments for anxiety disorder subtypes

Generalized anxiety disorder

Treatments for generalized anxiety disorder overlap greatly with those for other anxiety disorders and depression (Figure 14-46). Today, first-line treatments include SSRIs and SNRIs as well as benzodiazepines and buspirone. Some prescribers are reluctant to give benzodiazepines for anxiety disorders in general and for GAD in particular owing to the long-term nature of GAD and the possibility of dependence, abuse, and withdrawal reactions with benzodiazepines.

Although it is not a good idea to give benzodiazepines to a GAD patient who is abusing other substances, particularly alcohol, benzodiazepines can be useful in initiating

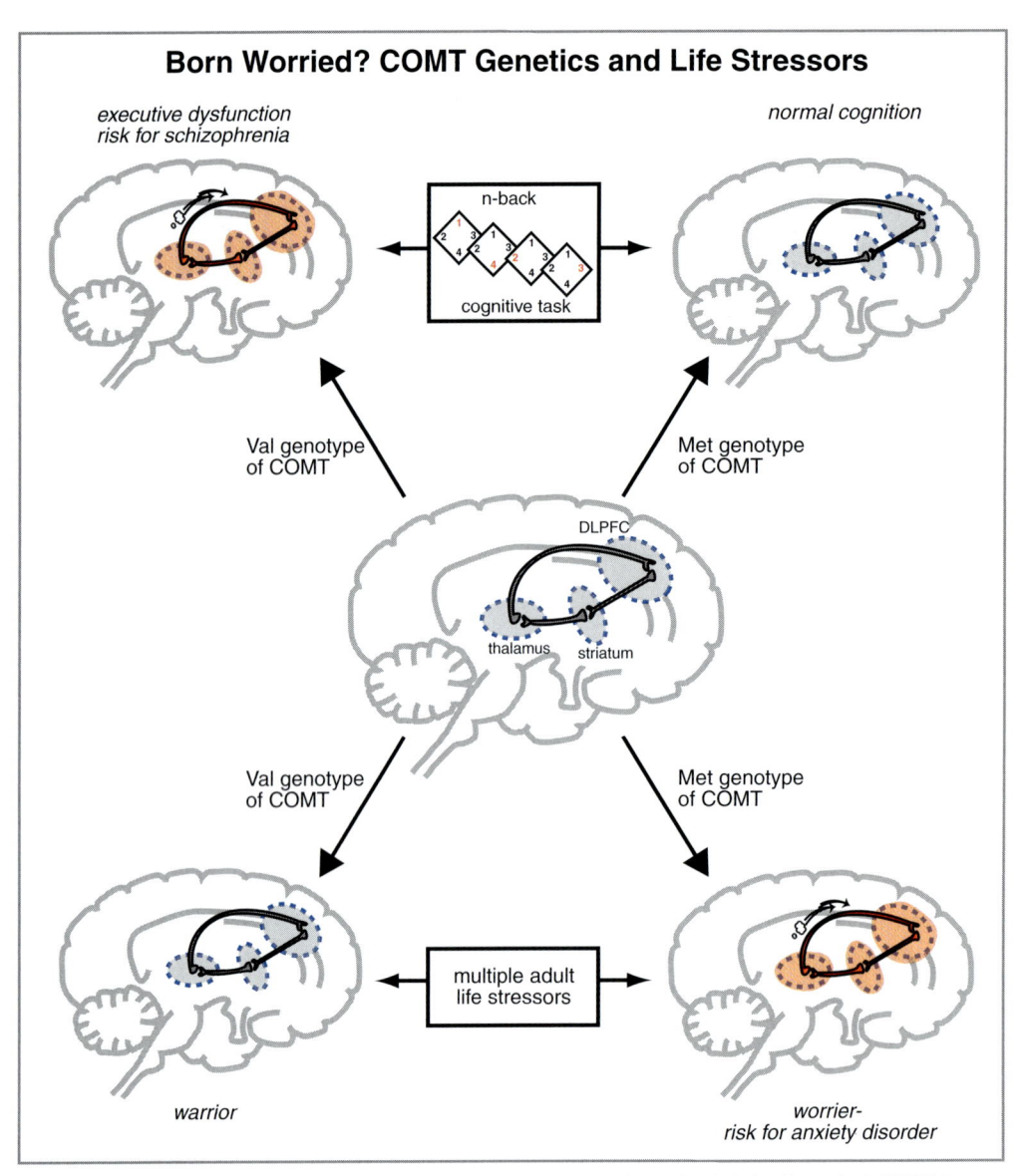

FIGURE 14-45 COMT genetics and life stressors. Activity in the cortico-striatal-thalamic-cortical (CSTC) loop may vary during cognitive tasks depending on the variant of catechol-O-methyl-transferase (COMT) that an individual has (upper portion of figure). Thus, those with the Met genotype for COMT (i.e., those that have lower COMT activity and thus higher dopamine levels) may have "normal" activation and no problems with performance during a cognitive task, whereas those with the Val genotype may exhibit inefficiency of cognitive information processing, require overactivation of this circuit, and potentially make more errors during the same task. These latter individuals may also be at increased risk for schizophrenia. Similarly, the variant of COMT that an individual has may affect response to stress, since the CSTC loop also regulates worry. In this case, however, the beneficial genotype may be reversed. That is, because individuals with the Met genotype have lower COMT activity and thus higher dopamine levels, dopamine release in response to stress may be excessive and contribute to worry and risk for anxiety disorders. Those with the Val genotype, on the other hand, may be less reactive to stress because COMT can destroy the excess dopamine.

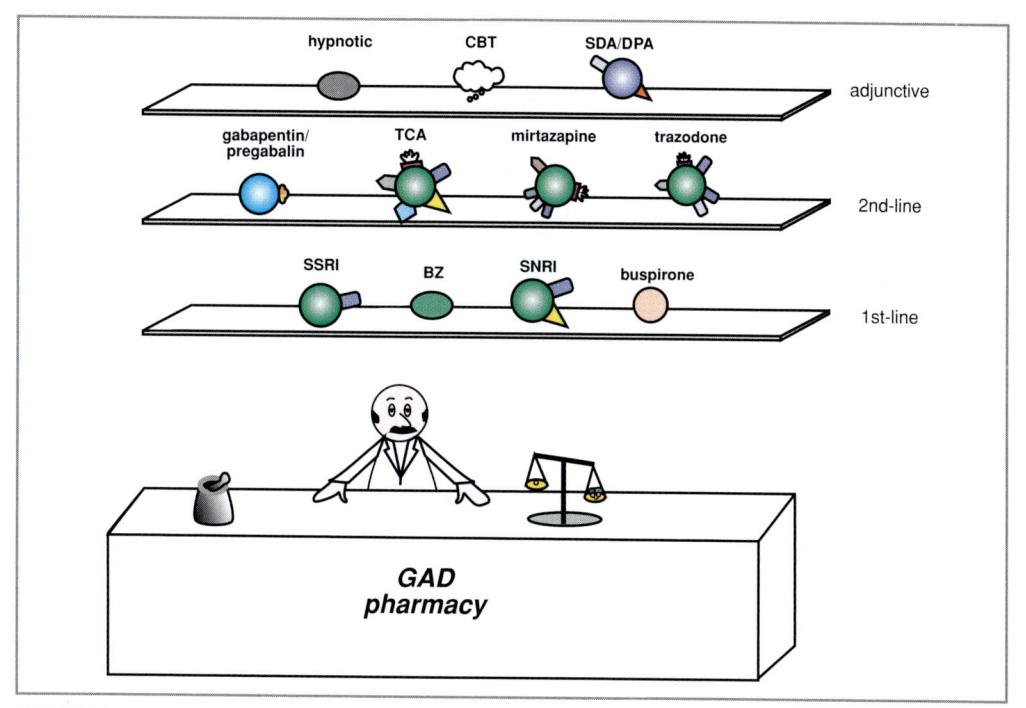

FIGURE 14-46 Generalized anxiety disorder (GAD) pharmacy. First-line treatments for GAD include serotonin selective reuptake inhibitors (SSRIs), benzodiazepines, serotonin norepinephrine reuptake inhibitors (SNRIs), and buspirone. Second-line treatments include gabapentin or pregabalin, tricyclic antidepressants (TCAs), mirtazapine, and trazodone. Adjunctive medications that may be helpful include hypnotics or an atypical antipsychotic; cognitive behavioral therapy is also an important component of anxiety treatment.

an SSRI or SNRI, since these serotonergic agents are often activating, difficult to tolerate early in dosing, and have a delayed onset of action. Benzodiazepines thus have a role in some patients at the initiation of treatment with another agent. In other patients who have experienced only partial relief of symptoms, benzodiazepines can be useful to "top up" an SSRI or SNRI. Benzodiazepines can also be useful for occasional intermittent use when symptoms surge and relief is needed quickly.

It should be noted that remission from all symptoms in patients with GAD who are taking an SSRI or SNRI may be slower in onset than it is in depression and may be delayed for 6 months or longer. If a GAD patient is not doing well after several weeks or months of treatment, switching to another SSRI/SNRI or buspirone or augmenting with a benzodiazepine can be considered. Failure to respond to first-line treatments can lead to trials of the novel alpha 2 delta ligands gabapentin or pregabalin, approved for epilepsy, neuropathic pain, and fibromyalgia but still in testing for anxiety disorders. One can also try sedating antidepressants such as mirtazapine, trazodone, or tricyclic antidepressants or even sedating antihistamines such as hydroxyzine. Adjunctive treatments that can be added to first- or second-line therapies for GAD include hypnotics for continuing insomnia; atypical antipsychotics for severe, refractory, and disabling symptoms unresponsive to aggressive treatment; and cognitive behavioral psychotherapy. Old-fashioned treatments for anxiety, such as barbiturates and meprobamate, are not considered appropriate today, given the other choices shown in Figure 14-46.

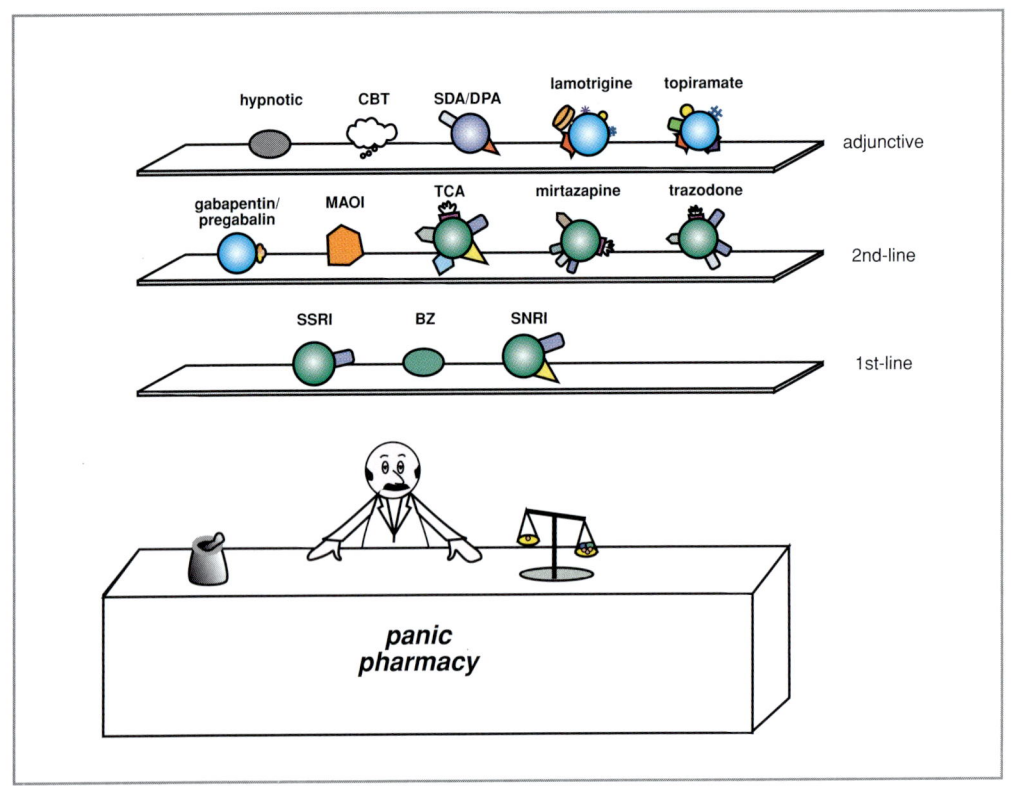

FIGURE 14-47 **Panic pharmacy.** First-line treatments for panic disorder include serotonin selective reuptake inhibitors (SSRIs), benzodiazepines, and serotonin norepinephrine reuptake inhibitors (SNRIs). Second-line treatments include gabapentin or pregabalin, monoamine oxidase inhibitors (MAOIs), tricyclic antidepressants (TCAs), mirtazapine, and trazodone. Cognitive behavioral therapy may be beneficial for many patients. In addition, adjunctive medications for residual symptoms may include hypnotics, an atypical antipsychotic, lamotrigine, or topiramate.

Panic disorder

Panic attacks occur in many conditions, not just panic disorder, and panic disorder is frequently comorbid with the other anxiety disorders and with major depression. It is thus not surprising that contemporary treatments for panic disorder overlap significantly with those for the other anxiety disorders and with those for major depression (Figure 14-47). First-line treatments include SSRIs and SNRIs as well as benzodiazepines, although benzodiazepines are often used as second-line options, during treatment initiation with an SSRI/SNRI, for emergent use during a panic attack, or for incomplete response to an SSRI/SNRI.

Second-line treatments include the novel alpha 2 delta ligands gabapentin and pregabalin as well as older agents such as the tricyclic antidepressants. Mirtazapine and trazodone are sedating antidepressants that can be helpful in some cases and are occasionally used as augmenting agents to SSRIs/SNRIs when these first-line agents elicit only a partial treatment response. The MAO inhibitors, discussed in Chapter 12 and illustrated in Figures 12-65 through 12-79, are much neglected in psychopharmacology in general and for the treatment of panic disorder in particular. However, these agents can have powerful efficacy in panic disorder and should be considered when first-line agents and various augmenting strategies fail.

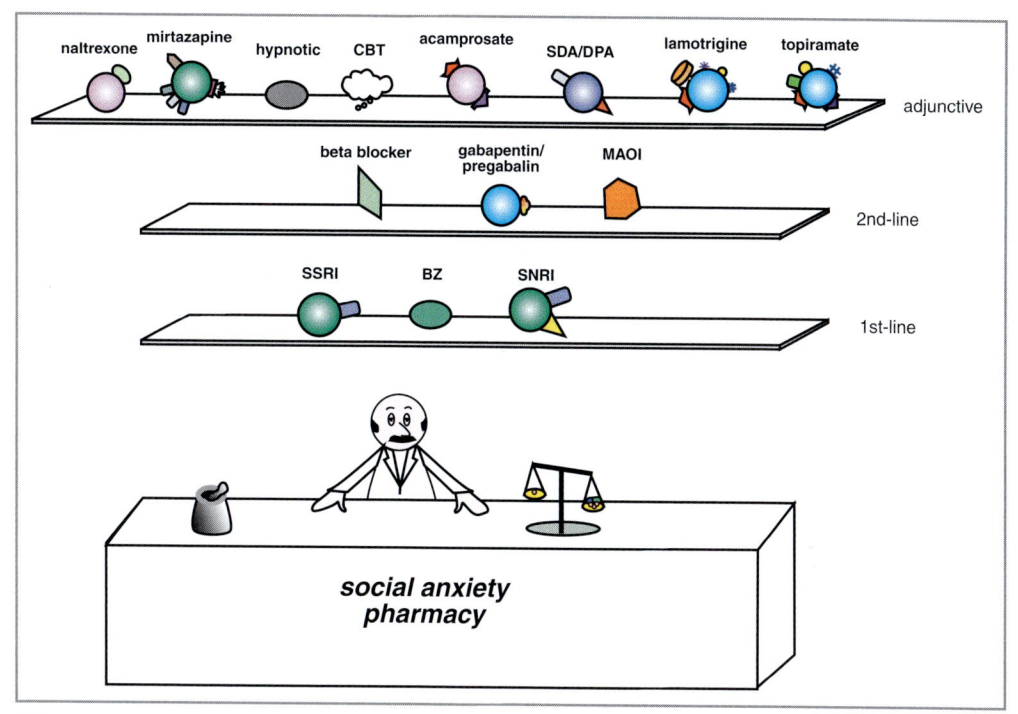

FIGURE 14-48 Social anxiety pharmacy. First-line treatments for social anxiety disorder include serotonin selective reuptake inhibitors (SSRIs), benzodiazepines, and serotonin norepinephrine reuptake inhibitors (SNRIs). Monoamine oxidase inhibitors (MAOIs) have been shown to be beneficial and may be a second-line option; other second-line options include gabapentin/pregabalin and beta blockers. Several medications may be used as adjuncts for residual symptoms; cognitive behavioral therapy may be useful as well.

Various adjunctive treatments for panic disorder include augmenting with atypical antipsychotics for severe and treatment-resistant cases, with hypnotics for patients with insomnia, with various anticonvulsants for patients resistant to first-line treatments, and with cognitive behavioral therapy to augment psychopharmacological approaches, modify cognitive distortions, and – through exposure – diminish phobic avoidance behaviors.

Social anxiety disorder
The treatment options for this anxiety disorder (Figure 14-48) are very similar to those for panic disorder (Figure 14-47), with a few noteworthy differences. The SSRIs and SNRIs are certainly first-line therapies, but the utility of benzodiazepine monotherapy for first-line treatment is not generally as widely accepted as it might be for GAD and panic disorder. There is also less evidence for the utility of older antidepressants for social anxiety disorder, particularly the tricyclic antidepressants, but also other sedating antidepressants such as mirtazapine and trazodone. A good second-line option would be one of the alpha 2 delta ligands, pregabalin or gabapentin. Beta blockers, sometimes with benzodiazepines, can be useful for some patients with very discrete types of social anxiety, such as performance anxiety.

Listed as adjunctive treatments are agents for alcohol dependence/abuse, such as naltrexone and acamprosate, since many patients may discover the utility of alcohol in relieving their social anxiety symptoms and develop alcohol dependence/abuse.

Anxiety Disorders and Anxiolytics | 769

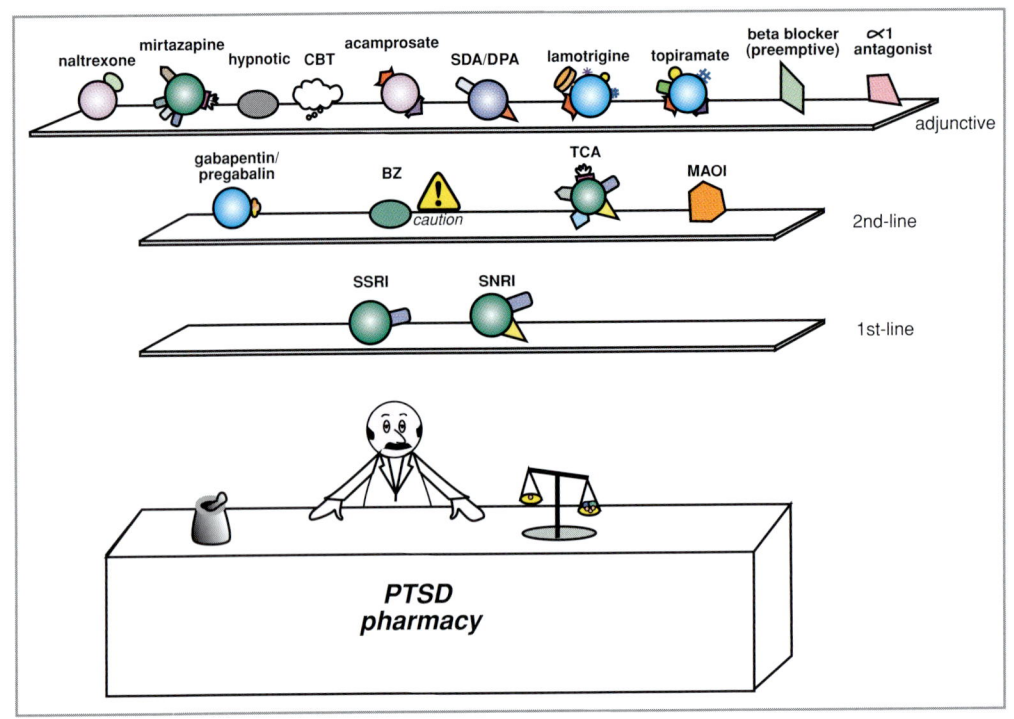

FIGURE 14-49 Posttraumatic stress disorder (PTSD) pharmacy. First-line pharmacological options for PTSD are serotonin selective reuptake inhibitors (SSRIs) and serotonin norepinephrine reuptake inhibitors (SNRIs). In PTSD, unlike other anxiety disorders, benzodiazepines have not been shown to be as helpful, although they may be considered with caution as a second-line option. Other second-line treatments include gabapentin or pregabalin, tricyclic antidepressants (TCAs), and monoamine oxidase inhibitors (MAOIs). Several medications may be used as adjuncts for residual symptoms, and cognitive behavioral therapy is typically recommended as well.

Posttraumatic stress disorder

Although many treatments are shown in Figure 14-49, treatments for PTSD in general may not be as effective as these same treatments are in other anxiety disorders. SSRIs and SNRIs are proven effective and are considered first-line treatments, but they often leave the patient with residual symptoms, including sleep problems. Thus, most patients with PTSD do not take monotherapy. Benzodiazepines are to be used with caution, not only because of limited evidence from clinical trials for efficacy in PTSD but also because many PTSD patients abuse alcohol and other substances. A unique treatment for PTSD is the administration of an alpha 1 antagonist at night to prevent nightmares. Preemptive treatment with beta blockers is discussed above but is not a proven or practical treatment option at this point. Much more effective treatments for PTSD are greatly needed.

Obsessive compulsive disorder

OCD is another condition frequently comorbid with other anxiety disorders and with major depression, and with great overlap of treatments (Figure 14-50). However, there are some unique features to OCD treatment. First-line treatment is specifically with one of the SSRIs. Although second-line treatment with the serotonergic tricyclic antidepressant clomipramine, an SNRI, or an MAO inhibitor is worthy of consideration, the best option for a patient who has failed several SSRIs is often to consider very high doses with an

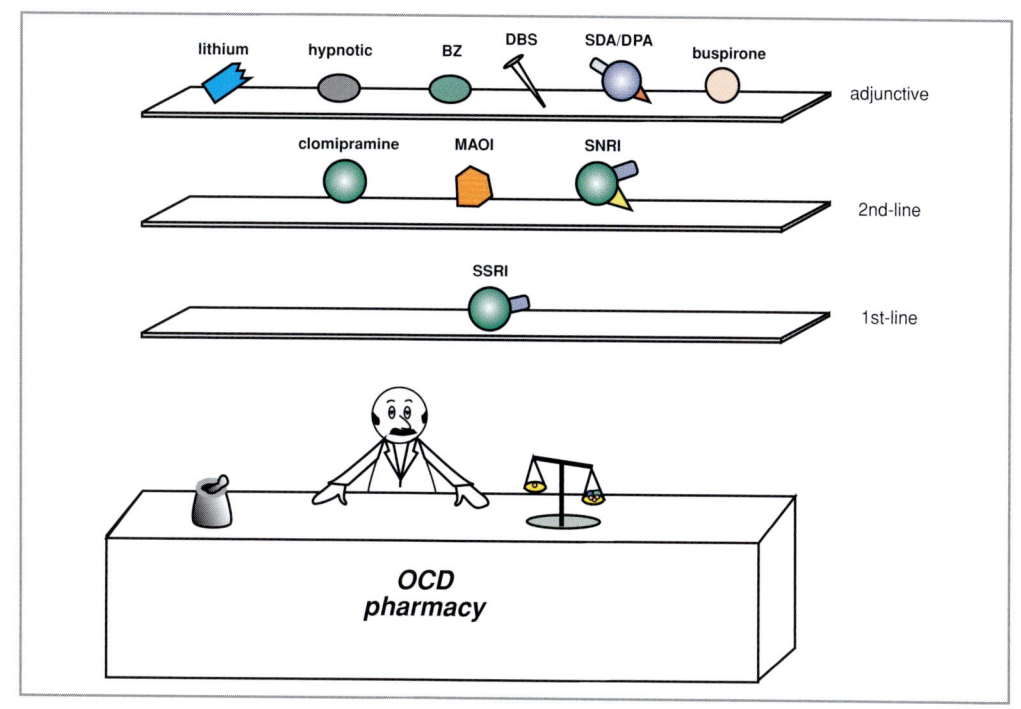

FIGURE 14-50 **Obsessive compulsive disorder (OCD) pharmacy.** Serotonin selective reuptake inhibitors (SSRIs) are the first-line recommendation for patients with OCD. Second-line treatments include clomipramine, monoamine oxidase inhibitors (MAOIs), and serotonin norepinephrine reuptake inhibitors (SNRIs). Several medications may be used as adjuncts for residual symptoms. Deep brain stimulation is an experimental option for treatment-resistant patients.

SSRI or augmentation of an SSRI with an atypical antipsychotic. Augmentation with benzodiazepines, lithium, or buspirone can also be considered. An experimental treatment for OCD is deep brain stimulation, discussed in Chapter 12 for depression and illustrated in Figure 12-116.

These same treatments can be considered for OCD spectrum disorders, sometimes known as obsessive impulsive disorders or impulsive compulsive disorders, including gambling, kleptomania, trichotillomania, body dysmorphic disorder, eating disorders, paraphilias, hypochondriasis, somatization disorder, Tourette's syndrome, autism, Asperger's syndrome, and others.

Summary

Anxiety disorders have core features of fear and worry that cut across the entire spectrum of anxiety disorder subtypes, from generalized anxiety disorder to panic disorder, social anxiety disorder, posttraumatic stress disorder, and obsessive compulsive disorder. A great deal of progress has been made in elucidating the role of the amygdala in the fear response and the role of cortico-striatal-thalamic-cortical circuits in the symptom of worry. Numerous neurotransmitters are involved in regulating the circuits that underlie the anxiety disorders. GABA is a key neurotransmitter discussed in this chapter, as well as the benzodiazepine anxiolytics that act on this neurotransmitter system. Serotonin, norepinephrine, alpha 2 delta ligands for voltage-gated calcium channels, and other regulators of anxiety circuits are also discussed as approaches to the treatment of anxiety disorders. A new concept that describes the production of anxiety symptoms as well as a possible new strategy for treating anxiety symptoms is that of the opposing actions of fear conditioning versus fear extinction within amygdala circuits. Stress is an important factor in the pathophysiology of anxiety disorders, and genetic factors impart important risks for anxiety disorders as well. Numerous treatments are available for anxiety disorders, most of which are similar for the entire anxiety disorder spectrum and are also used for the treatment of depression.

CHAPTER 15

Pain and the Treatment of Fibromyalgia and Functional Somatic Syndromes

- What is pain?
- "Normal" pain and the activation of nociceptive nerve fibers
  - Nociceptive pathways to the spinal cord
  - Nociceptive pathways from the spinal cord to the brain
- Neuropathic pain
  - Peripheral mechanisms
  - Central mechanisms
  - Incoming synapses from peripheral neurons (primary afferents)
  - Descending spinal synapses in the dorsal horn
  - Here today and not gone tomorrow: the curse of chronic pain and other central sensitization syndromes
  - Can pain gates be opened from the inside and cause pain in affective spectrum disorders and functional somatic syndromes?
- Pain in affective spectrum disorders and functional somatic syndromes
  - The spectrum of mood and anxiety disorders with pain disorders
  - Does depression or anxiety hurt?
  - Fibromyalgia
  - Gut feelings about irritable bowel syndrome
  - Pain in other functional somatic syndromes
- Summary

This chapter provides a brief overview of a relatively new area in psychopharmacology – namely, the management of various chronic pain conditions associated with different psychiatric disorders and treated with psychotropic drugs. Included here are discussions of the symptomatic and pathophysiological overlap between disorders with pain and many other disorders treated in psychopharmacology, especially those with depression and anxiety. Clinical descriptions and formal criteria for how to diagnose painful conditions are only mentioned here in passing. The reader should consult standard reference sources for this material. The discussion here emphasizes how discoveries about the functioning of various brain circuits and neurotransmitters – especially those acting upon the central processing of pain – have affected our understanding of the pathophysiology and treatment of many painful conditions that may occur with or without various psychiatric disorders. The goal of this chapter is to acquaint the reader with ideas about the clinical and biological aspects of the symptom of pain, how it can be hypothetically caused by alterations of pain processing within the central nervous system, how it can be associated with many of the symptoms of depression and anxiety, and finally, how it can be treated with several of the same agents that can treat depression and anxiety.

Many of the treatments discussed in this chapter are covered extensively in previous chapters. For details of mechanisms of pain treatments that are also used for the treatment of depression, the reader is referred to Chapter 12; for those pain treatments also used as mood stabilizers, the reader is referred to Chapter 13. The discussion in this chapter is at the conceptual level, not at the pragmatic level. The reader should consult standard drug handbooks (such as *Essential Psychopharmacology: Prescriber's Guide*) for details of doses, side effects, drug interactions, and other issues relevant to the prescribing of these drugs in clinical practice.

What is pain?

No experience rivals pain for its ability to capture our attention, focus our actions, and cause suffering (see Table 15-1 for some useful definitions regarding pain). The powerful experience of pain, especially acute pain, can serve a vital function – to make us aware of damage to our bodies and to rest the injured part until it has healed (Tables 15-1 and 15-2). Such **acute** pain is a part of our everyday lives, and when the cause is not obvious, we consult a medical professional to diagnose the underlying condition, treat it, and thereby resolve the pain (Tables 15-1 and 15-2).

However, the cause of pain cannot always be identified, or can be identified but cannot be entirely resolved with current treatments. In these circumstances, the pain continues and becomes **chronic** (Tables 15-1 through 15-3). The best-characterized chronic pain states are often peripheral in origin (i.e., they originate outside of the central nervous system) or mixed in origin (i.e., they involve peripheral mechanisms that trigger additional central pain mechanisms) (Table 15-3). In osteoarthritis, for example, the peripheral pathology cannot be entirely stopped, but disease-modifying treatments can slow progress and reduce pain (Table 15-3). Peripheral pain occurs in most patients with advanced cancer, and although the cause often cannot be treated (e.g., bone metastases), pain can be managed successfully in the majority of patients with opioid and nonopioid analgesics (Table 15-3).

By contrast, many chronic pain states that are frequently associated with psychiatric disorders, including some considered to be affective spectrum disorders (Table 15-4) or functional somatic syndromes (Table 15-5), are less well characterized and sometimes thought not to be "real." These painful conditions are now hypothesized to be forms of chronic neuropathic pain that are considered to be central or possibly mixed in origin (Table 15-3). The link of chronic pain states to the pathophysiology of numerous psychiatric disorders is established by the recent discovery that certain psychotropic agents used to treat various psychiatric disorders are also now proving to be useful in reducing the symptom of pain in various chronic pain conditions. These treatments include the SNRIs (serotonin norepinephrine reuptake inhibitors, discussed in Chapter 12 and illustrated in Figures 12-33 through 12-42), the alpha 2 delta ligands (anticonvulsants that block voltage-sensitive calcium channels, or VSCCs, discussed in Chapter 5 and illustrated in Figures 5-28, 5-33 to 5-35, and 5-37 to 5-45 and also discussed in Chapters 13 and 14 and illustrated in Figures 13-21 and 14-37), and various other psychotropic agents acting centrally at various neurotransmitter

TABLE 15-1 Pain: some useful definitions

Pain	An unpleasant sensory and emotional experience associated with actual or potential tissue damage or described in terms of such damage
Acute pain	Pain that is of short duration and resolves; usually directly related to the resolution or healing of tissue damage
Chronic pain	Pain that persists for longer than would be expected; an artificial threshold for chronicity (e.g., 1 month) is not appropriate
Neuropathic pain	Pain that arises from damage to or dysfunction of any part of the peripheral or central nervous system
Allodynia	Pain caused by a stimulus that does not normally provoke pain
Hyperalgesia	An increased response to a stimulus that is normally painful
Analgesia	Any process that reduces the sensation of pain while not affecting normal touch
Local anesthesia	Blockade of all sensation (innocuous and painful) from a local area
Noxious stimulus	Stimulus that inflicts damage or would potentially inflict damage on tissues of the body
Primary afferent neuron (PAN)	The first neuron in the somatosensory pathway; detects mechanical, thermal, or chemical stimuli at its peripheral terminals and transmits action potentials to its central terminals in the spinal cord; all PANs have a cell body in the dorsal root ganglion
Nociceptor	A primary afferent (sensory) neuron that is only activated by a noxious stimulus
Nociception	The process by which a nociceptor detects a noxious stimulus and generates a signal (action potentials) that is propagated toward higher centers in the nociceptive pathway
Dorsal root ganglion (DRG)	Contains the cell bodies of primary afferent neurons; proteins – including transmitters, receptors, and structural proteins – are synthesized here and transported to peripheral and central terminals
Interneuron	Neuron with its cell body, axon and dendrites within the spinal cord; can be excitatory (e.g., containing glutamate) or inhibitory (e.g., containing GABA)
Projection neurons	Neuron in the dorsal horn that receives input from PANs and/or interneurons, and projects up the spinal cord to higher processing centers
Spinothalamic tract	Tract of neurons that project from the spinal cord to the thalamus
Spinobulbar tracts	Several different tracts of neurons that project from the spinal cord to brainstem nuclei
Somatosensory cortex	Region of the cerebral cortex that receives input mainly from cutaneous sensory nerves; the cortex is topographically arranged, with adjacent areas receiving input from adjacent body areas; stimulation of the somatosensory cortex creates sensations from the body part that projects to it

TABLE 15-2 Acute versus chronic pain

	Causes of symptoms	Treatment	Outcome	Time course	Features
"Normal pain" (acute pain)	Known	Adequate and available	Recovery anticipated	Short-term	Essential to survival
Chronic pain	May be unknown	May be suboptimal	Complete remission often not possible	Indeterminate	Pathological

TABLE 15-3 Chronic pain: peripheral versus central

	Site	Treatments	Behavioral factors and psychiatric comorbidity	Examples
Peripheral	Primarily inflammation or damage in the periphery	NSAIDs Opiates	Minor	Osteoarthritis Rheumatoid arthritis Dental extraction Postoperative Cancer
Central	Primarily due to central disturbance in pain processing	SNRIs Alpha 2 delta ligands TCAs Anticonvulsants	Prominent	Fibromyalgia Spinal cord injury Poststroke pain Multiple sclerosis
Mixed	Both	Both, especially central treatments	Either	Diabetic peripheral neuropathy Back pain? Headache (migraine, tension)? Irritable bowel syndrome? Postherpetic neuralgia Trigeminal neuralgia Phantom limb pain Complex regional pain syndrome

TABLE 15-4 Affective spectrum disorders

Mood disorders
- Major depressive disorder
- Dysthymic disorder
- Premenstrual dysphoric disorder
- Bipolar disorder (especially bipolar depression or mixed)

Anxiety disorders
- Generalized anxiety disorder
- Panic disorder
- Obsessive compulsive disorder
- Posttraumatic stress disorder
- Social phobia/social anxiety disorder

Painful somatic disorders
- Fibromyalgia
- Irritable bowel syndrome
- Migraine

Others
- Attention deficit/hyperactivity disorder
- Bulimia nervosa
- Cataplexy

receptor sites. The chronic pain conditions that can be targeted with these interventions range from multiple painful physical complaints associated with affective and anxiety disorders to fibromyalgia, diabetic peripheral neuropathic pain, and various other conditions listed in Tables 15-4 and 15-5. These conditions and their treatments with psychotropic drugs are discussed in this chapter.

TABLE 15-5 Functional somatic syndromes: conditions with chronic pain of presumed central or mixed origin and without obvious continuing neuronal or tissue damage or pathology

Conditions with prominent painful somatic symptoms
- Major depression and other mood disorders
- Generalized anxiety disorder, panic disorder, and other anxiety disorders
- Fibromyalgia
- Chronic cervical or lumbar back pain
- Irritable bowel syndrome
- Temporomandibular joint (TMJ) disorder
- Burning mouth syndrome
- Chronic pelvic pain
  - Interstitial cystitis
  - Female urethral syndrome
  - Vulvodynia
  - Primary dysmenorrhea
- Regional musculoskeletal pain
  - Chronic cervical pain
  - Chronic lumbar pain
  - Tendinosis
  - Myofascial pain syndrome
- Chronic tension/migraine headache
- Noncardiac chest pain
- Nonulcer dyspepsia/non-GERD heartburn
- Costochondritis

Conditions with distressful and often vague somatic symptoms
- Chronic fatigue syndrome
- Somatoform disorder
- Multiple chemical sensitivity
- Exposure syndromes (Gulf War illnesses; sick-building syndrome)

GERD = gastroesophageal reflux disorder

The detection, quantification, and treatment of pain are rapidly becoming standardized parts of a psychiatric evaluation. Modern psychopharmacologists increasingly consider pain to be a psychiatric "vital sign," thus requiring routine evaluation and symptomatic treatment. In fact, elimination of pain is increasingly recognized as necessary in order to have full symptomatic remission of many psychiatric disorders.

In diagnosing pain, understanding its neurobiology, and treating pain, certain terminology should be understood and used appropriately to avoid confusion (Table 15-1). The International Association of the Study of Pain defines pain as "**An unpleasant sensory and emotional experience associated with actual or potential tissue damage, or described in terms of such damage**" (Table 15-1). This definition is very carefully worded. Notice two things: first, pain does not require actual tissue damage. This is an especially important point for the affective spectrum disorders – such as fibromyalgia – that are functional somatic syndromes as well as for other neuropathic pain states discussed in this chapter. Evolving new insights about such conditions show that if a patient describes feeling pain but you find no physical cause, it is generally a good idea to accept that they are really in pain. Second, pain is tied to **human** experience; it is a subjective experience and high-level cognitive construct, not just activity within neurons in the "pain" pathway. Such neuronal activity by itself is called nociception rather than pain.

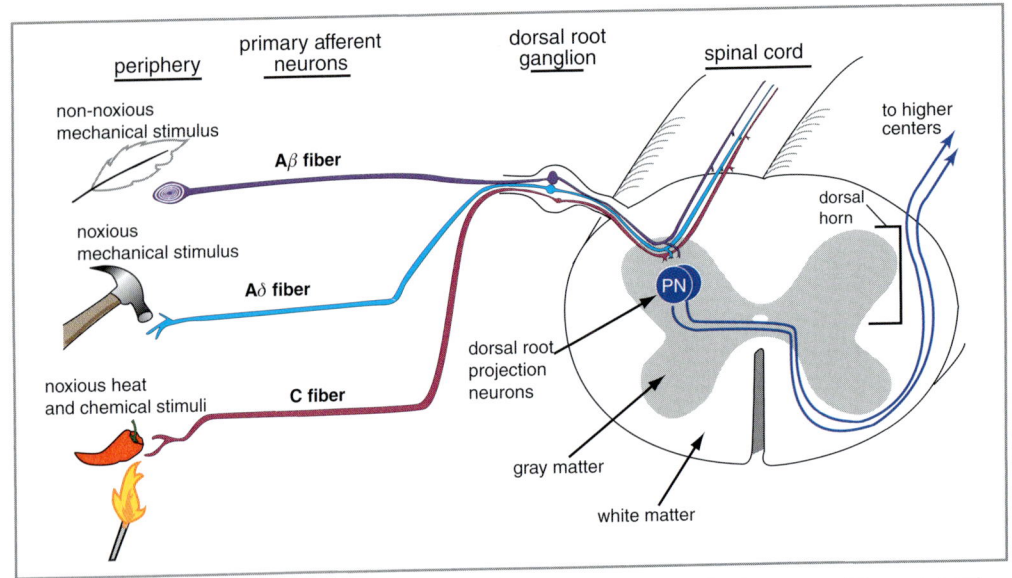

FIGURE 15-1 Activation of nociceptive nerve fibers. Detection of a noxious stimulus occurs at the peripheral terminals of primary afferent neurons. Aβ fibers respond only to non-noxious stimuli, while Aδ and C fibers respond to noxious mechanical, heat, and chemical stimuli, generating action potentials that propagate along the axon to the central terminals. Primary afferent neurons have their cell bodies in the dorsal root ganglion and send terminals into that spinal cord segment as well as sending less dense collaterals up the spinal cord for a short distance. Primary afferent neurons synapse onto several different classes of dorsal horn projection neurons (PN), which project via different tracts to higher centers.

"Normal" pain and the activation of nociceptive nerve fibers

The pain pathway is the series of neurons that begins with detection of a noxious stimulus and ends with the subjective perception of pain. This "nociceptive pathway" starts from the periphery, enters the spinal cord and projects to the brain (Figure 15-1). It is important to understand the processes by which incoming information can be modulated to increase or decrease the perception of pain associated with a given stimulus because these processes can explain not only why maladaptive pain states arise but also why drugs that work in other psychiatric conditions such as depression and anxiety can also be effective in reducing pain.

Nociceptive pathways to the spinal cord

Nociception begins with transduction – the process by which specialized membrane proteins detect a stimulus and generate a voltage change at the neuronal membrane of a sensory neuron known as a primary afferent neuron. A sufficiently strong stimulus will lower the voltage at the membrane (i.e., depolarize the membrane) enough to activate voltage-sensitive sodium channels (VSSCs) and trigger an action potential that will be propagated along the length of the axon to the central terminals of the neuron (Figure 15-2). VSSCs are introduced in Chapter 5 and illustrated in Figures 5-27 to 5-31. Targeting of these channels by some mood stabilizers is discussed in Chapter 13 and illustrated in Figures 5-32, 13-12 and 13-15. Nociceptive impulse flow from primary afferent neurons (Figure 15-3A) can be reduced or stopped (Figure 15-3B) when VSSCs are blocked by peripherally administered local anesthetics such as lidocaine (Figures 15-3 and 15-4). Preventing the flow of sodium ions through VSSCs to prevent the propagation of nociceptive nerve impulses from the

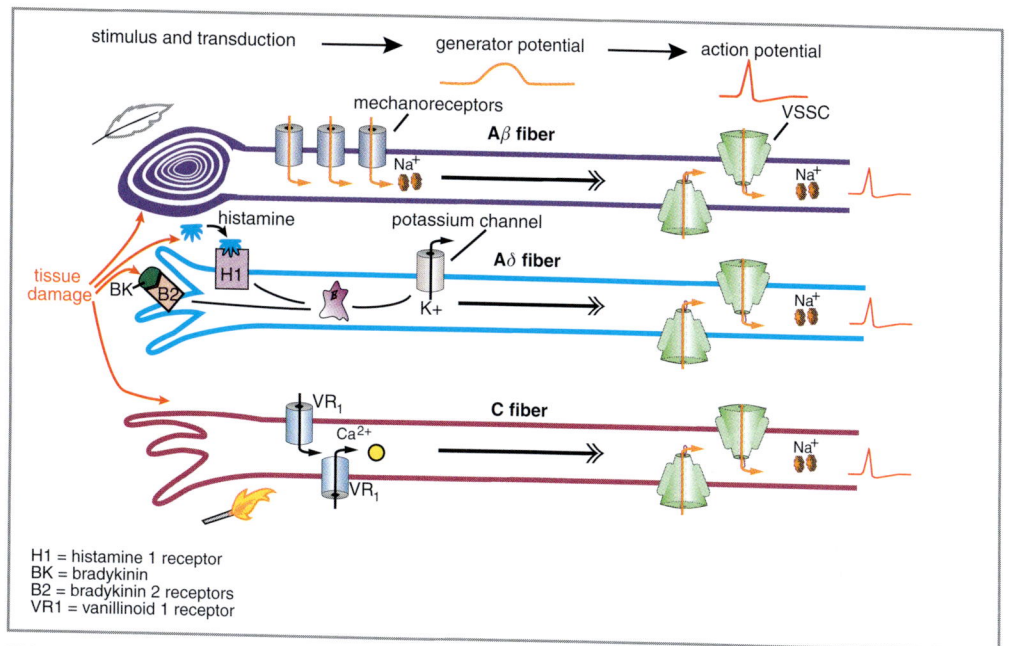

FIGURE 15-2 Nociceptive transduction. Specialized receptors transduce sensory stimuli into electrical activity by altering flow of ions (Na^+, Ca^{2+}, K^+, Cl^-) to depolarize the membrane. If this generator potential exceeds threshold, it opens voltage-sensitive sodium channels (VSSCs) to trigger an action potential. Specialized structures around Aβ fiber terminals allow low intensity stimuli to open stretch-activated ion channels and cause Na^+ influx. Noxious mechanical stimuli (tissue damage) stretch high-threshold mechanoreceptors to cause Na^+ influx. Damage also releases histamine and bradykinin (BK), which activate H1 and B2 receptors to reduce K^+ efflux and create a generator potential. Low pH (H^+ ions), heat, and capsaicin can all activate the vanillinoid 1 receptor (VR1) ion channel to allow Na^+ and Ca^{2+} influx. Firing frequency of the neuron is proportional to the intensity of the stimulus.

periphery into the CNS is presumably the mechanism of action of local anesthetics (Figures 15-3 and 15-4).

The specific response characteristics of primary afferent neurons are determined by the specific receptors and channels expressed by that neuron (Figure 15-2). For example, primary afferent neurons that express a stretch-activated ion channel are mechanosensitive; those that express the vanillinoid receptor 1 (VR1) ion channel are activated by capsaicin, the pungent ingredient in chili peppers, and also by noxious heat, leading to the burning sensation both these stimuli evoke. These functional response properties, as well as physical and phenotypic properties, are used to classify primary afferent neurons into three types: A beta, A delta, and C fiber neurons (Figures 15-1 and 15-2). A beta fibers detect small movements, light touch, hair movement, and vibrations; C fiber peripheral terminals are bare nerve endings that are only activated by noxious mechanical, thermal, or chemical stimuli; A delta fibers fall somewhere in between, sensing noxious mechanical stimuli and subnoxious thermal stimuli (Figures 15-1 and 15-2).

Primary afferent neurons thus detect changes in the outside world at their terminals in the periphery, such as those in the muscles or visceral mucosa like the digestive tract. Abnormal central processing of sensory information from these sources, for example, may create the subjective experience of pain in the muscles in fibromyalgia or depression; it may also create the subjective experience of pain in the abdomen in irritable bowel syndrome or

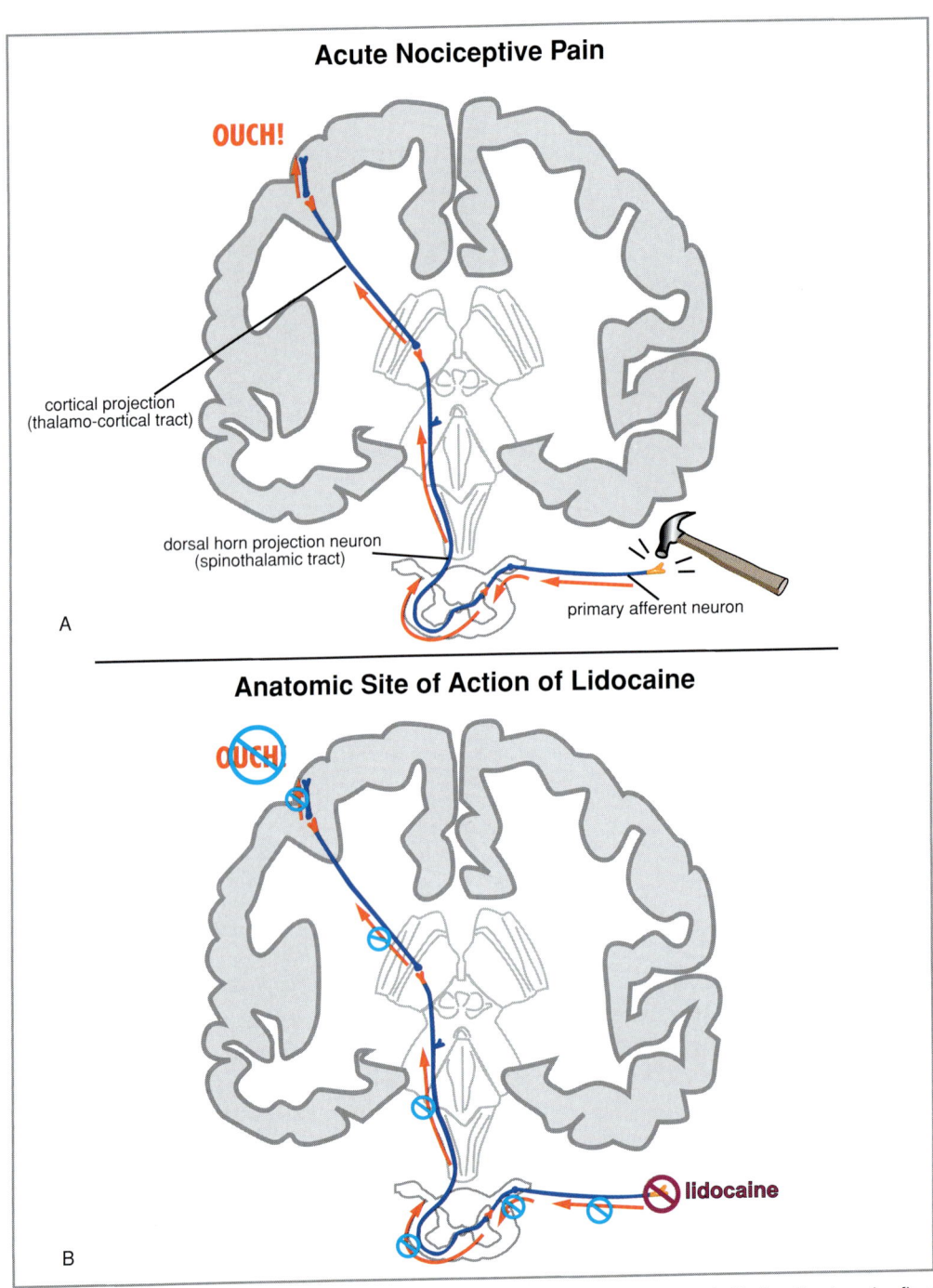

FIGURE 15-3A and B Peripheral blockade of acute nociceptive pain (anatomic view). Nociceptive impulse flow from primary afferent neurons is transmitted via dorsal horn neurons to higher brain centers, where it can ultimately be interpreted as pain (represented by the "ouch" in **A**). Local anesthetics such as lidocaine are presumed to prevent transmission of nociceptive impulse flow to the spinal cord by peripherally blocking voltage-sensitive sodium channels (VSSCs), so that the information never reaches the central nervous system (**B**).

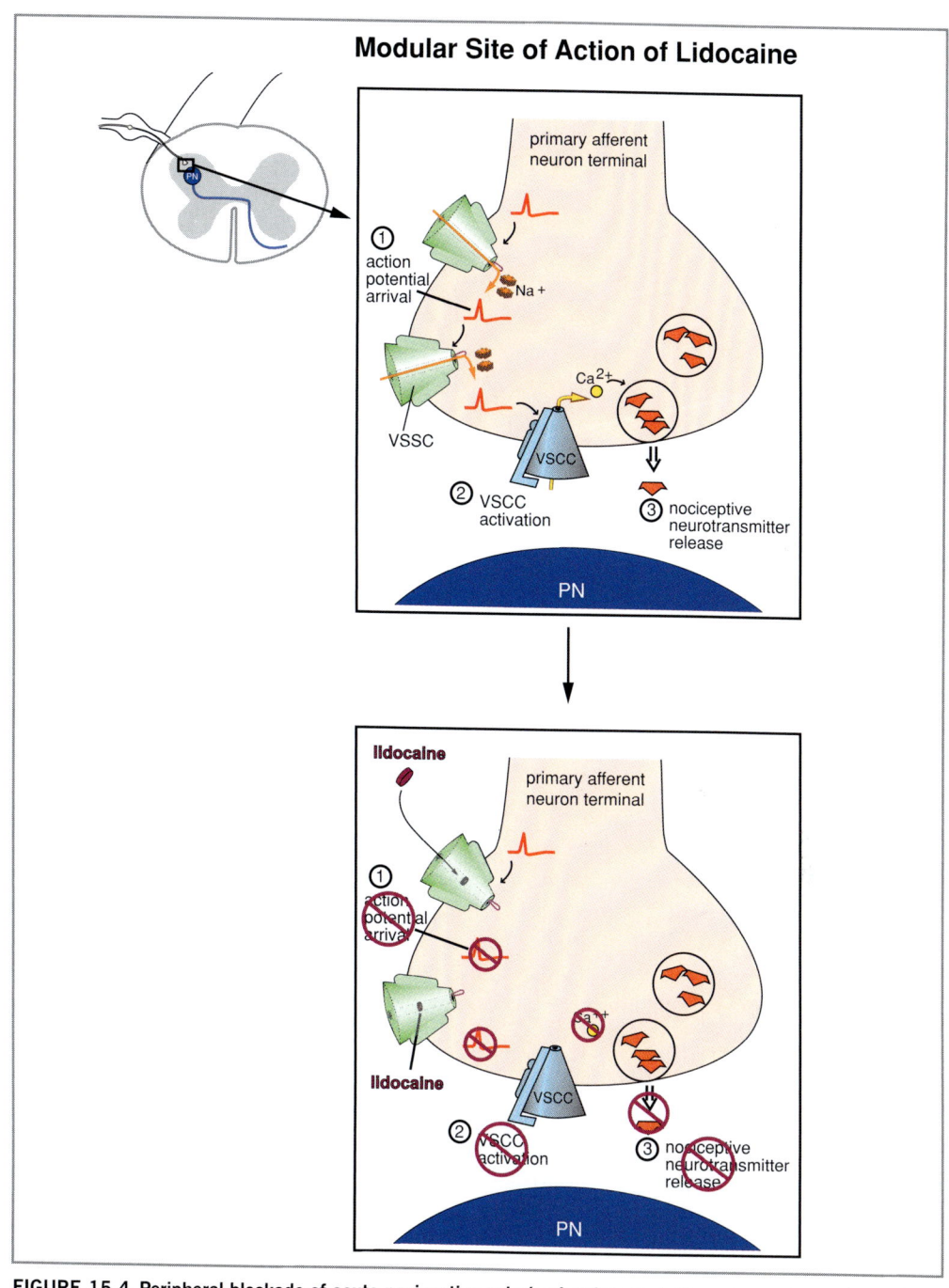

FIGURE 15-4 Peripheral blockade of acute nociceptive pain (molecular view). The release of neurotransmitters from central primary afferent nerve terminals requires activation of voltage-sensitive calcium channels (VSCCs). Top: Action potentials arriving at the primary afferent nerve terminal depolarize the membrane by their actions first on voltage-sensitive sodium channels (VSSCs in green) (1), which in turn activate VSCCs (in blue) (2). The VSCCs open to allow calcium influx into the neuron (2). Calcium influx triggers fusion of vesicles with the membrane and release of neurotransmitter into the synapse (3). Bottom: A local anesthetic such as lidocaine blocks VSSCs (in green) (1) and thus prevents propagation of the nerve impulse (1), as well as preventing activation of VSCCs (in blue) (2), so that nociceptive neurotransmitter is not released (3).

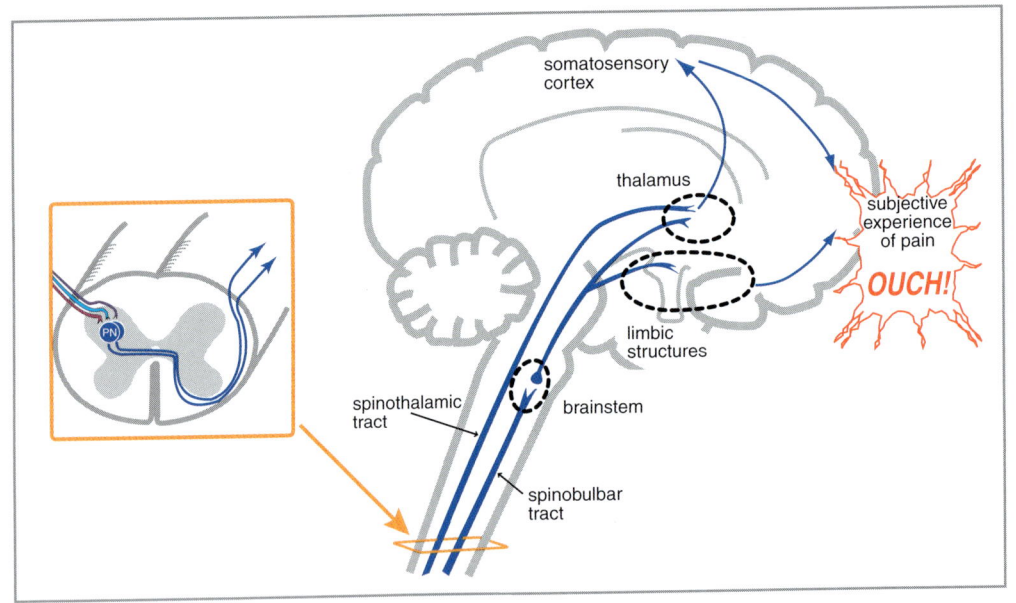

FIGURE 15-5 From nociception to pain. Dorsal horn neurons in the spinothalamic tract project to the thalamus and then to the primary somatosensory cortex. This pathway carries information about the intensity and location of the painful stimuli and is termed the discriminatory pathway. Neurons ascending in the spinobulbar tract project to brainstem nuclei and then to both the thalamus and limbic structures. These pathways convey the emotional and motivational aspects of the pain experience. Only when information from the discriminatory (thalamocortical) and emotional/motivational (limbic) pathways combine is the human subjective experience of pain formed ("ouch").

anxiety disorders; and it may do this even when there is no apparent peripheral input or damage of primary afferent neurons, as discussed below.

All primary afferent neurons have their cell bodies in the dorsal root ganglia located along the spinal column outside of the CNS; thus these neurons are peripheral and not central (Figure 15-1). Primary afferent neurons synthesize vital proteins in these cell bodies (e.g., peptide neurotransmitters, ion channels, receptors, structural proteins), and transport them not only to their peripheral terminals (Figures 15-1 and 15-2) but also to their central terminals (Figures 15-5 and 15-6).

Nociceptive pathways from the spinal cord to the brain

The central terminals of peripheral nociceptive neurons synapse in the dorsal horn of the spinal cord onto the next cells in the pathway, dorsal horn neurons, which receive input from many primary afferent neurons and then project to higher centers (Figure 15-5). For this reason, they are sometimes also called dorsal horn projection neurons (PN in Figures 15-4 and 15-6; see also dorsal horn projection neuron in the spinothalamic tract in Figure 15-3A). Dorsal horn neurons are thus the first neurons of the nociceptive pathway that are located within the central nervous system (CNS) and thus a key site for modulation of nociceptive neuronal activity as it comes into the CNS. A vast number of neurotransmitters have been identified in the dorsal horn, some of which are shown in Figure 15-6.

Neurotransmitters in the dorsal horn are synthesized not only by primary afferent neurons, but by the other neurons in the dorsal horn as well including descending neurons and various interneurons (Figure 15-6). Some neurotransmitter systems in the dorsal horn are successfully targeted by known pain relieving drugs, especially opiates, serotonin and

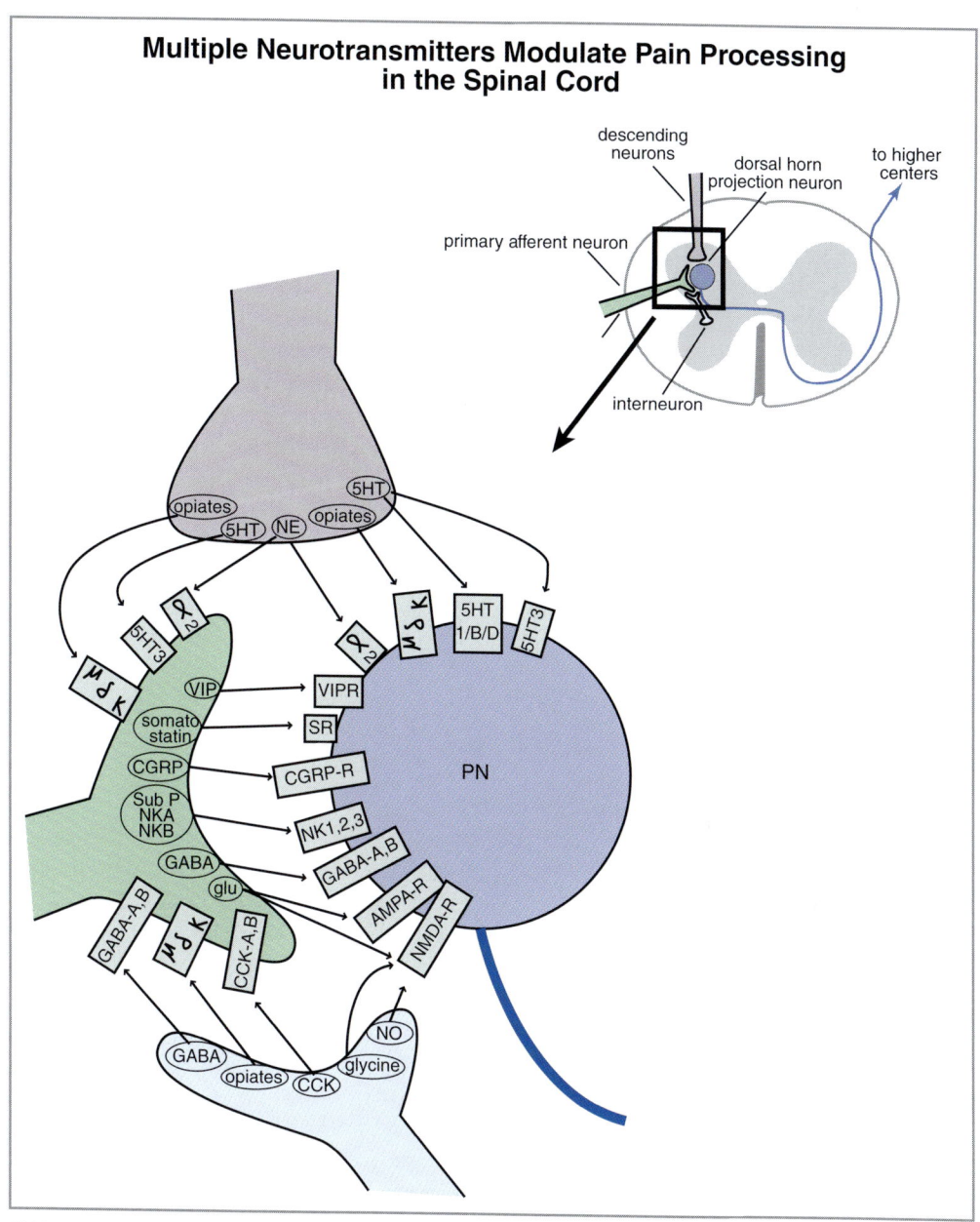

FIGURE 15-6 Multiple neurotransmitters modulate pain processing in the spinal cord. There are many neurotransmitters and their corresponding receptors in the dorsal horn. Neurotransmitters in the dorsal horn may be released by primary afferent neurons, by descending regulatory neurons, by dorsal horn projection neurons (PN) and by interneurons. Neurotransmitters present in the dorsal horn that have been best studied in terms of pain transmission include substance P (NK1, 2, and 3 receptors), endorphins (mu opioid receptors), norepinephrine (alpha 2 adrenoceptors), and serotonin (5HT1B/D and 5HT3 receptors). Several other neurotransmitters are also represented, including VIP (vasopressin inhibitory protein and its receptor VIPR); somatostatin and its receptor SR; calcitonin G related peptide (CGRP and its receptors CGRP-R); GABA and its receptors GABA-A and GABA-B); glutamate and its receptors AMPA-R (alpha-amino-3-hydroxy-5-methyl-4-isoxazole propionic acid receptor) and NMDA-R (N-methyl-d-aspartate receptors); nitric oxide (NO); cholecystokinin (CCK and its receptors CCK A and CCK B); and glycine and its receptor NMDA-R.

norepinephrine boosting SNRIs, and alpha 2 delta ligands acting at voltage-sensitive calcium channels (VSCCs) (Figures 15-4A and 15-6; see also figures below). These pain relieving agents are all discussed in further detail below. All of the neurotransmitter systems acting in the dorsal horn are potential targets for novel pain-relieving drugs (Figure 15-6) and a plethora of such novel agents is currently in clinical and preclinical development.

There are several classes of dorsal horn neurons: some receive input directly from primary sensory neurons, some are interneurons, and some project up the spinal cord to higher centers (Figures 15-5 and 15-6). There are several different tracts in which these projection neurons can ascend, which can be crudely divided into two functions: the sensory/discriminatory pathway and the emotional/motivational pathway (Figure 15-5).

In the sensory/discriminatory pathway, dorsal horn neurons ascend in the spinothalamic tract; then, thalamic neurons project to the primary somatosensory cortex (Figures 15-3 and 15-5). This particular pain pathway is thought to convey the precise location of the nociceptive stimulus and its intensity. In the emotional/motivational pathway, other dorsal horn neurons project to brainstem nuclei, and from there to limbic regions (Figure 15-5). This second pain pathway is thought to convey the affective component that nociceptive stimuli evoke. Only when these two aspects of sensory discrimination and emotions come together and the final, subjective perception of pain is created can we use the word "pain" to describe the modality (see "ouch" in Figure 15-5). Before this point, we are simply discussing activity in neural pathways, which should be described as noxious-evoked or nociceptive neuronal activity but not necessarily as pain.

Neuropathic pain

The term **neuropathic pain** describes pain that arises from damage to or dysfunction of any part of the peripheral or central nervous system, whereas "normal" pain (so-called nociceptive pain, just discussed in the section above) is caused by activation of nociceptive nerve fibers. Neuropathic pain may be acute and resolve rapidly, and may have an identified cause that can be treated to relieve the pain (Tables 15-2 and 15-3). But all too often, the cause of neuropathic pain cannot be identified, or can be identified but cannot be stopped with current treatments. Affective spectrum disorders associated with multiple unexplained painful physical symptoms (Table 15-4) or that are functional somatic syndromes such as fibromyalgia and irritable bowel syndrome (Table 15-5) may all be examples of pain syndromes with prominent central neuropathic activity.

When perceived pain is out of proportion to a physical cause or even has no identifiable physical cause, this can add an extra dimension to the patient's suffering. These people may once have been perceived as difficult or "malingerers" by healthcare professionals and may have been told that the pain was all in their minds. Those of us who treat patients with pain must generally accept that if the patient reports pain, he or she is in pain and deserves treatment, whether or not what we consider a rational cause can be identified.

Neuropathic pain thus is certainly not "all in the mind," but it may be "all in the brain" (and spinal cord), where maladaptive central processes maintain pain beyond its natural usefulness. Malingering and unconscious mechanisms that affect pain perception – especially when litigation and disability payments are involved – do exist but are not discussed further in this chapter. The reader is referred to standard reference sources for this information. Neuropathic pain states and their evolving treatments with various psychotropic drugs are emphasized here and are commonly defined in terms of the site of the presumed lesion – i.e., peripheral versus central (Table 15-3). Even in the absence of an identified lesion, the

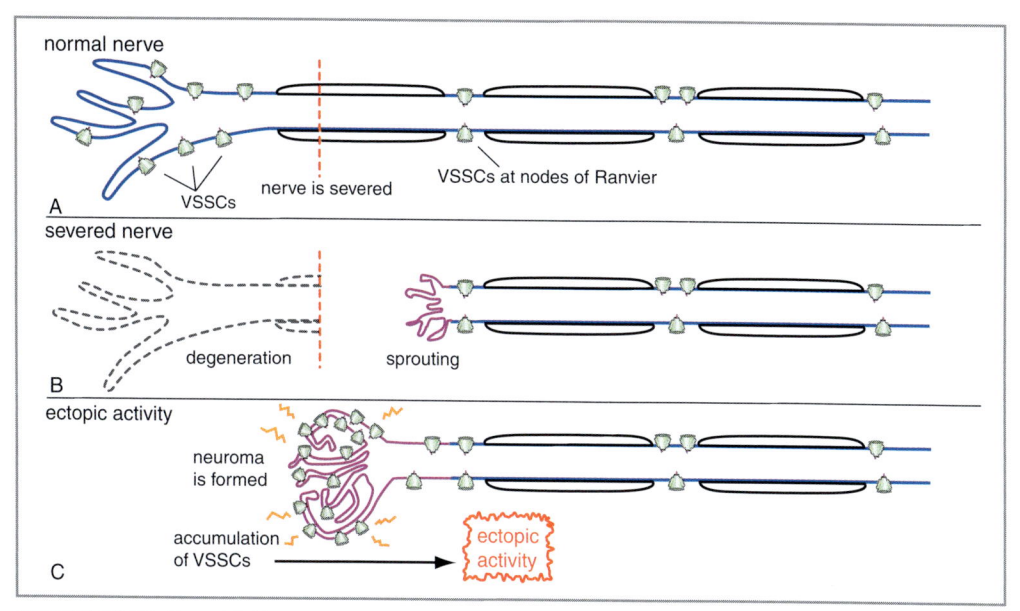

FIGURE 15-7A, B, and C Neuronal damage and ectopic activity, part 1. (**A**) A normal nerve has voltage-sensitive sodium channels (VSSCs) at its peripheral terminals and at the nodes of Ranvier, between myelinated segments. (**B**) When a nerve is severed, the distal portion degenerates; the proximal portion dies back a little and then regenerates sprouts that try to reach the previous target tissues. (**C**) The sprouts lack guidance, and form tangled neuromas. VSSCs accumulate at neuromas and generate spontaneous (ectopic) activity and heightened sensitivity to mechanical, thermal, and chemical stimuli.

tendency is to ascribe a name or label to the condition. This can be helpful in some cases, validating the patient's experience and suffering as a legitimate medical condition. However, searching for a name or a cause does not necessarily help treatment decisions. Despite the varying (and elusive) etiologies and pathologies of neuropathic pain states, some common mechanisms underlie their generation and maintenance. Understanding those mechanisms leads to an understanding of why not only opiates but also alpha 2 delta ligands and SNRIs are rational treatments to choose or combine for various types of neuropathic pain.

Peripheral mechanisms

Normal transduction and conduction in peripheral afferent neurons can be hijacked in neuropathic pain states to maintain nociceptive signaling in the absence of a relevant noxious stimulus. Neuronal damage by disease or trauma can alter electrical activity of neurons, allow cross-talk between neurons, and initiate inflammatory processes to cause "peripheral sensitization" (Figures 15-7 through 15-9).

We have already mentioned that transduction and conduction of nociception in primary afferent neurons depends on voltage-sensitive sodium channels (VSSCs) and that VSSCs exist at nerve terminals and at the nodes of Ranvier, between myelinated segments (Figure 15-7A). There is a high turnover of VSSCs, and they are continually synthesized in the cell body and transported along the axon to their destinations. Thus, in severed myelinated neurons, VSSCs accumulate at regenerating sprouts (Figure 15-7B) and at sites where a neuronal "scar" forms (i.e., neuromas; Figure 15-7C) as well as in demyelinated regions, leading to spontaneous (ectopic) nociceptive neuronal activity (Figures 15-7C and 15-8C). This is a probable cause of the ongoing pain reported in many neuropathic pain states

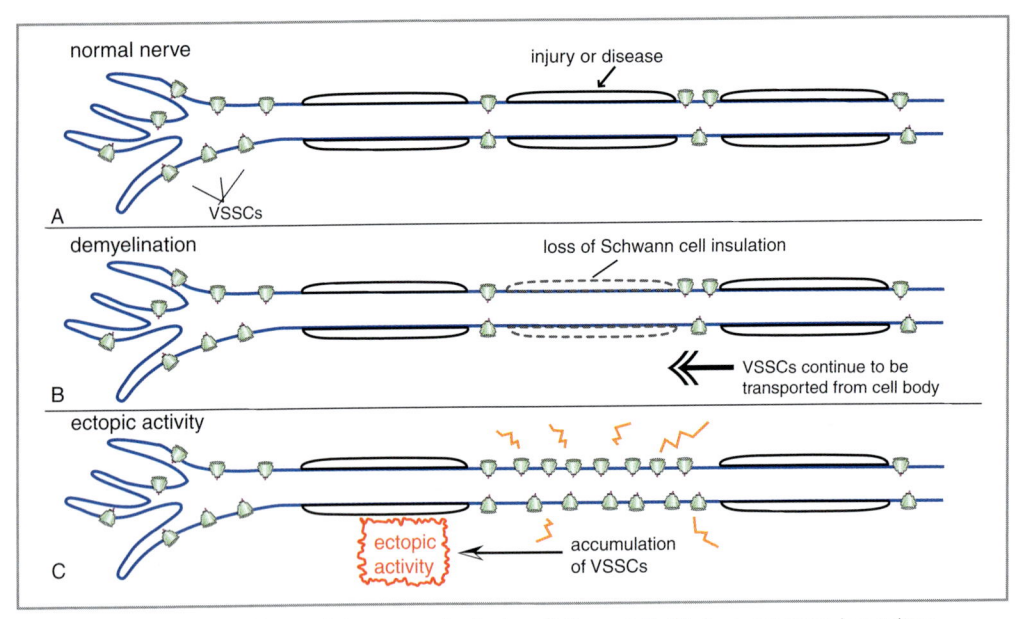

FIGURE 15-8A, B, and C Neuronal damage and ectopic activity, part 2. (A) A normal nerve has voltage-sensitive sodium channels (VSSCs) at its peripheral terminals and at the nodes of Ranvier, between myelinated segments. (B) Injury or disease can damage the Schwann cells that provide the myelination, causing cell death and loss of myelin insulation. VSSCs continue to be synthesized, and can now insert into the axon membrane where myelination is absent. (C) VSSCs accumulate in these demyelinated regions, generating spontaneous (ectopic) activity and heightened sensitivity to mechanical, thermal, and chemical stimuli.

associated with neuronal injury, such as diabetes and trauma. Ectopic sites (Figures 15-7C and 15-8C) are also hypersensitive to mechanical, thermal, and chemical stimuli. Thus, everyday innocuous stimuli (joint movement, clothing brushing the skin, a cool breeze, changes in blood gas concentrations) can cause excruciating pain (allodynia, see Table 15-1) and strange "shock-like" sensations (paresthesias). Also, any truly painful stimulus may cause exaggerated perception of pain (hyperalgesia, see Table 15-1).

Demyelination of primary afferent nerves (compare Figure 15-8A to 15-8B) can be caused by diabetes, trauma, and other diseases (Figure 15-8B) and can not only result in sites of ectopic nociceptive activity (Figure 15-8C) but even in a situation of "cross-talk" between neurons (i.e., ephaptic cross-talk in Figure 15-9) that can amplify the perception of pain (hyperalgesia).

Another drive for primary afferent neuronal nociceptive activity in neuropathic pain states may come from the sympathetic nervous system. For example, in complex regional pain syndromes (CRPSs) and other states, pain can be induced, maintained, or made worse by sympathetic activity or application of adrenaline/norepinephrine and can be relieved (often temporarily) by sympathetic block. Drive in the sympathetic nervous system is not increased in these conditions, but sprouting of sympathetic fibers allows normally released norepinephrine to come in closer contact with sensory nerves. Also, increased expression of alpha 2A adrenoceptors by primary afferent neurons may explain their increased sensitivity to norepinephrine or sympathetic activation.

Finally, "inflammatory pain" and "neuropathic pain" have classically been considered separately; one as a normal result of tissue injury, and one as a maladaptive process. However, the normal inflammatory process that underlies primary hyperalgesia (a painful response

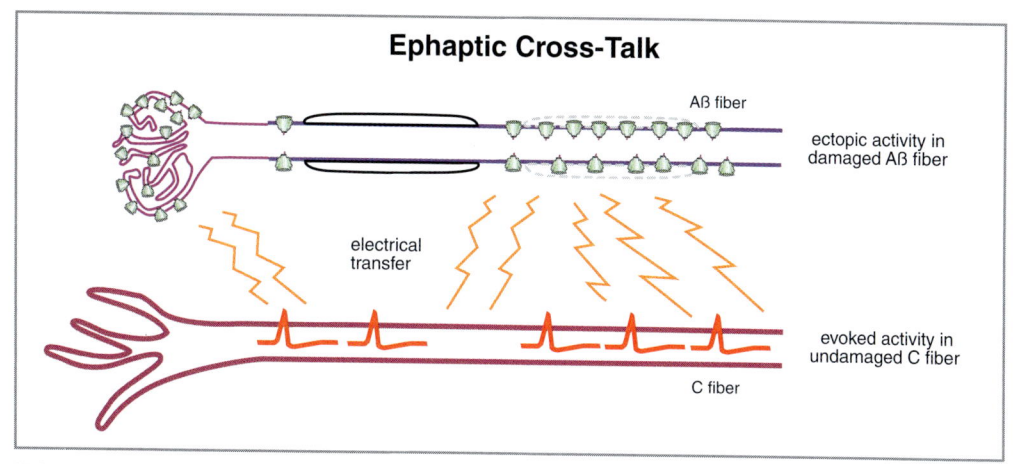

FIGURE 15-9 Ephaptic cross-talk. Disruption to myelination may also allow cross-talk between neurons. At the injury site, so-called ephaptic cross-talk can arise: ectopic activity in an Aβ fiber neuroma can electrically stimulate activity in an adjacent C fiber. Another process that can occur, both at peripheral sites of injury and in the dorsal root ganglion, is thought to be more important in development of hyperalgesia and allodynia: "crossed afterdischarge." Repetitive firing of one neuron causes accumulation of K^+ ions, and perhaps also neurotransmitter release, which can stimulate activity in neighboring neurons.

to a stimulus that is normally not painful) (Table 15-1; Figures 15-2 and 15-10A) may also contribute to peripheral sensitization in nerve damage, especially if accompanied by tissue damage. Similar inflammatory events may be initiated in the absence of tissue injury by the invasion of degenerating nerves by macrophages and the release of cytokines from myelin-synthesizing Schwann cells (Figure 15-8B). Therefore inflammatory events cannot be ignored in the pathophysiology of neuropathic pain, especially in the early stages. This may explain why anti-inflammatory agents such as the nonsteroidal anti-inflammatory drug (NSAID) cyclooxygenase (COX-2) inhibitors can be effective in a wide variety of pain states associated with inflammation, including presumably several types of neuropathic pain (Figure 15-10B).

Central mechanisms
At each major relay point in the pain pathway (Figure 15-5), the nociceptive pain signal is susceptible to modulation by endogenous processes to either dampen down the signal or to amplify it. This happens not only peripherally at primary afferent neurons, as just discussed, but also at central neurons in the dorsal horn of the spinal cord as well as in numerous brain regions. The events in the dorsal horn are better understood than those in brain regions of nociceptive pathways, but pain processing in the brain may be the key to understanding pain in affective and anxiety disorders and in fibromyalgia and other functional somatic syndromes.

Incoming synapses from peripheral neurons (primary afferents)
As we have stated, different primary afferent neurons release many different neurotransmitters at their synapses with spinal cord neurons (Figure 15-6). Each neurotransmitter's release mechanism requires presynaptic depolarization and activation of N-type and P/Q-type voltage-sensitive calcium channels (VSCCs; Figure 15-4A), often coupled to the release of glutamate but also to aspartate, substance P (SP), calcitonin-gene–related peptide (CGRP), and other neurotransmitters. VSCCs are introduced in Chapter 5 and illustrated

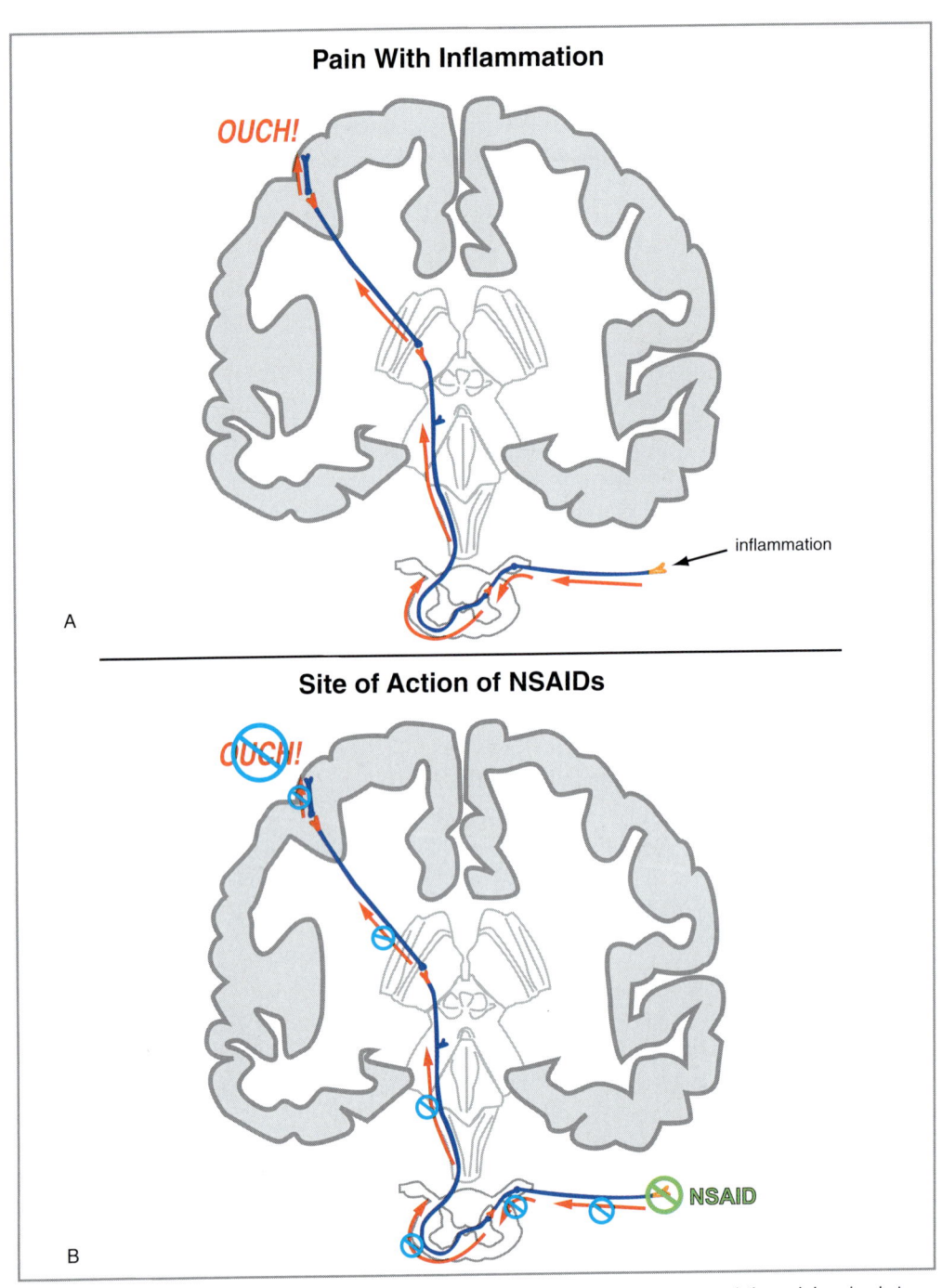

FIGURE 15-10A and B Inflammatory pain. In the normal inflammatory process, normal tissue injury leads to nociceptive impulse flow from primary afferent neurons to dorsal horn neurons and then to higher brain centers, where it can ultimately be interpreted as pain (represented by the "ouch" in **A**). Nonsteroidal anti-inflammatory drugs (NSAIDs) prevent transmission of nociceptive impulse flow associated with inflammation so that the information never reaches the central nervous system (**B**), thus there is no subjective experience of pain.

in Figures 5-27 and 5-28 as well as in Figures 5-33 to 5-45. Blocking VSCCs with alpha 2 delta ligands is discussed in Chapters 5 and 14; it is illustrated in general in Figure 5-37 and for anxiety disorders in Figure 14-37.

Surprisingly, blocking substance P actions with NK1 antagonists has not proven to be helpful in relieving pain (see Figure 15-6). However, blocking VSCCs with alpha 2 delta ligands inhibits release of various neurotransmitters in the dorsal horn (Figure 15-4A) and has indeed proven to be an effective treatment for neuropathic pain, presumably in part by disrupting transmission of nociceptive inputs from primary afferent neurons to the dorsal horn up the spinal cord to the brain (see Figure 5-37).

Descending spinal synapses in the dorsal horn

The periaqueductal gray (PAG) is the site of origin and regulation of much of the descending inhibition that projects down the spinal cord to the dorsal horn (Figures 15-6 and 15-11A). The periaqueductal gray is discussed in relation to its connections with the amygdala and the motor component of the fear response in Chapter 14 and illustrated in Figures 14-9 and 14-11. The PAG also integrates inputs from nociceptive pathways and limbic structures such as the amygdala and limbic cortex and sends outputs to brainstem nuclei and the rostroventromedial medulla to drive descending inhibitory pathways. Some of these descending pathways release endorphins, which act via mostly presynaptic mu opioid receptors to inhibit neurotransmission from nociceptive primary afferent neurons (Figures 15-6 and 15-11B). Spinal mu opioid receptors are one target of opioid analgesics; so are mu opioid receptors in the PAG itself (Figure 15-11B). Interestingly, since A beta fibers (Figure 15-1) do not express mu opioid receptors, this may explain why opioid analgesics spare normal sensory input. Enkephalins, which also act via delta opioid receptors, are also antinociceptive, whereas dynorphins, acting at kappa opioid receptors, can be either anti- or pronociceptive.

Two other important descending **inhibitory** pathways are shown in Figures 15-6, 15-12 and 15-13. One is the descending spinal norepinephrine pathway (Figure 15-12A), which originates in the locus coeruleus (LC) and especially from noradrenergic cell bodies in the lower (caudal) parts of the brainstem neurotransmitter center (lateral tegmental norepinephrine cell system) discussed in Chapter 7 and illustrated in Figure 7-9. The other important descending pathway is the descending spinal serotonergic pathway (Figure 15-13A), which originates in the nucleus raphe magnus of the rostroventromedial medulla and especially the lower (caudal) serotonin nuclei (raphe magnus, raphe pallidus, and raphe obscuris) discussed in Chapter 7 and illustrated in Figure 7-10. Descending noradrenergic neurons inhibit neurotransmitter release from primary afferents directly via inhibitory alpha 2 adrenoceptors (Figure 15-6), explaining why direct acting alpha 2 agonists such as clonidine can be useful in relieving pain in some patients. Serotonin inhibits primary afferent terminals via postsynaptic 5-HT1B/D receptors (Figure 15-6). These inhibitory receptors are G protein–coupled, and indirectly influence ion channels to hyperpolarize the nerve terminal and inhibit nociceptive neurotransmitter release. Serotonin receptors are discussed in Chapter 10 and illustrated in Figure 10-20.

Serotonin is also a major neurotransmitter in descending **facilitation** pathways to the spinal cord. Serotonin released onto some primary afferent neuron terminals in certain areas of the dorsal horn acts predominantly via excitatory 5-HT3 receptors to **enhance** neurotransmitter release from these primary afferent neurons (Figure 15-6). The combination of both inhibitory and facilitatory actions of serotonin may explain why SSRIs, with actions that increase only serotonin levels, are not consistently useful in the treatment of pain,

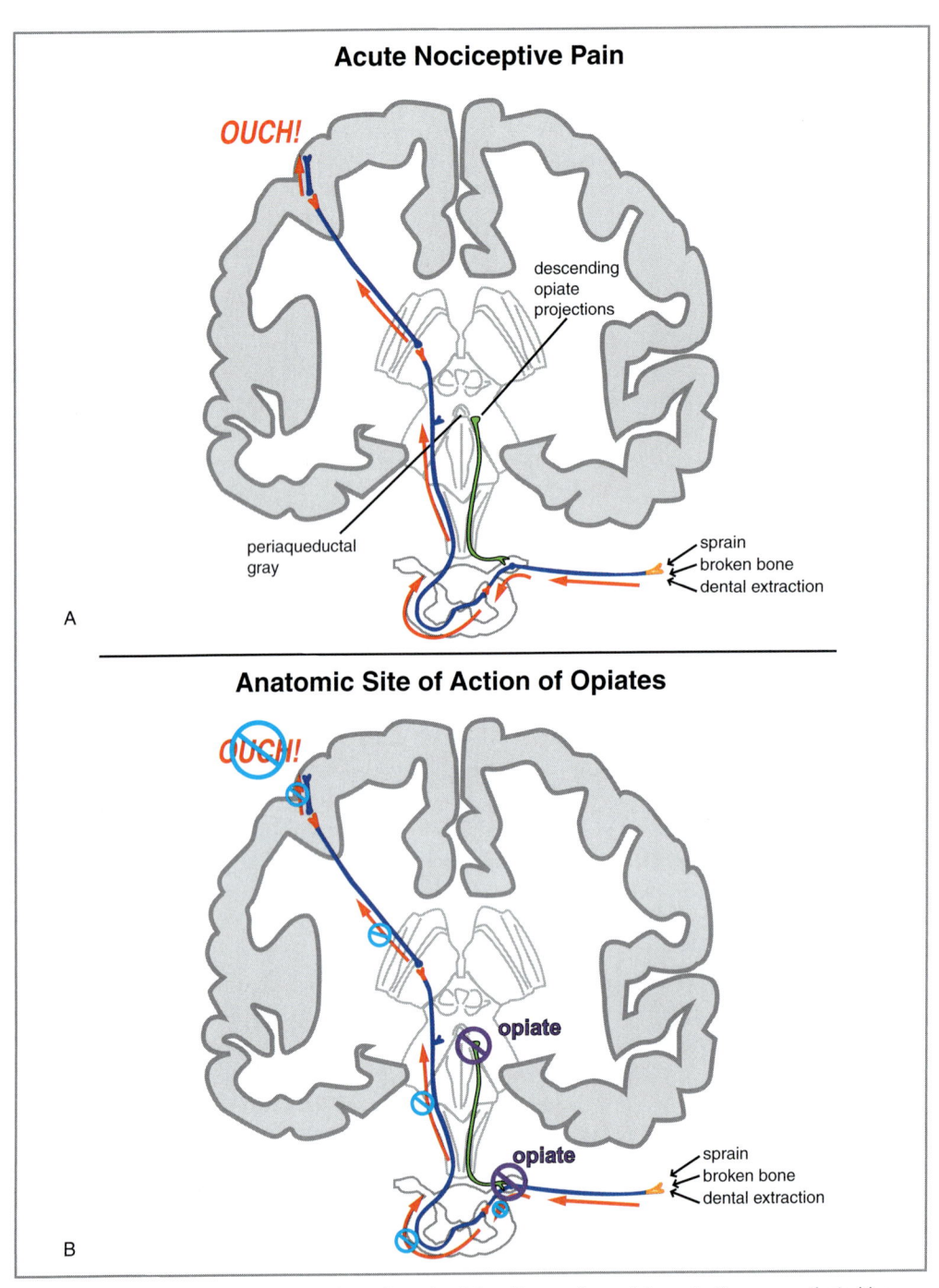

FIGURE 15-11A and B Acute nociceptive pain and opiates. Descending opiate projections are activated by severe injury or "danger" to inhibit nociceptive neurotransmission in the dorsal horn, which allows the individual to escape any immediate danger without being compromised. (**A**) Shown here is nociceptive input from a peripheral injury being transmitted to the brain and interpreted as pain. The descending opiate projection is not activated and thus is not inhibiting the nociceptive input. (**B**) Endogenous opioid release in the descending opiate projection, or exogenous administration of an opiate, can cause inhibition of nociceptive neurotransmission in the dorsal horn or in the periaqueductal gray and thus prevent or reduce the experience of pain.

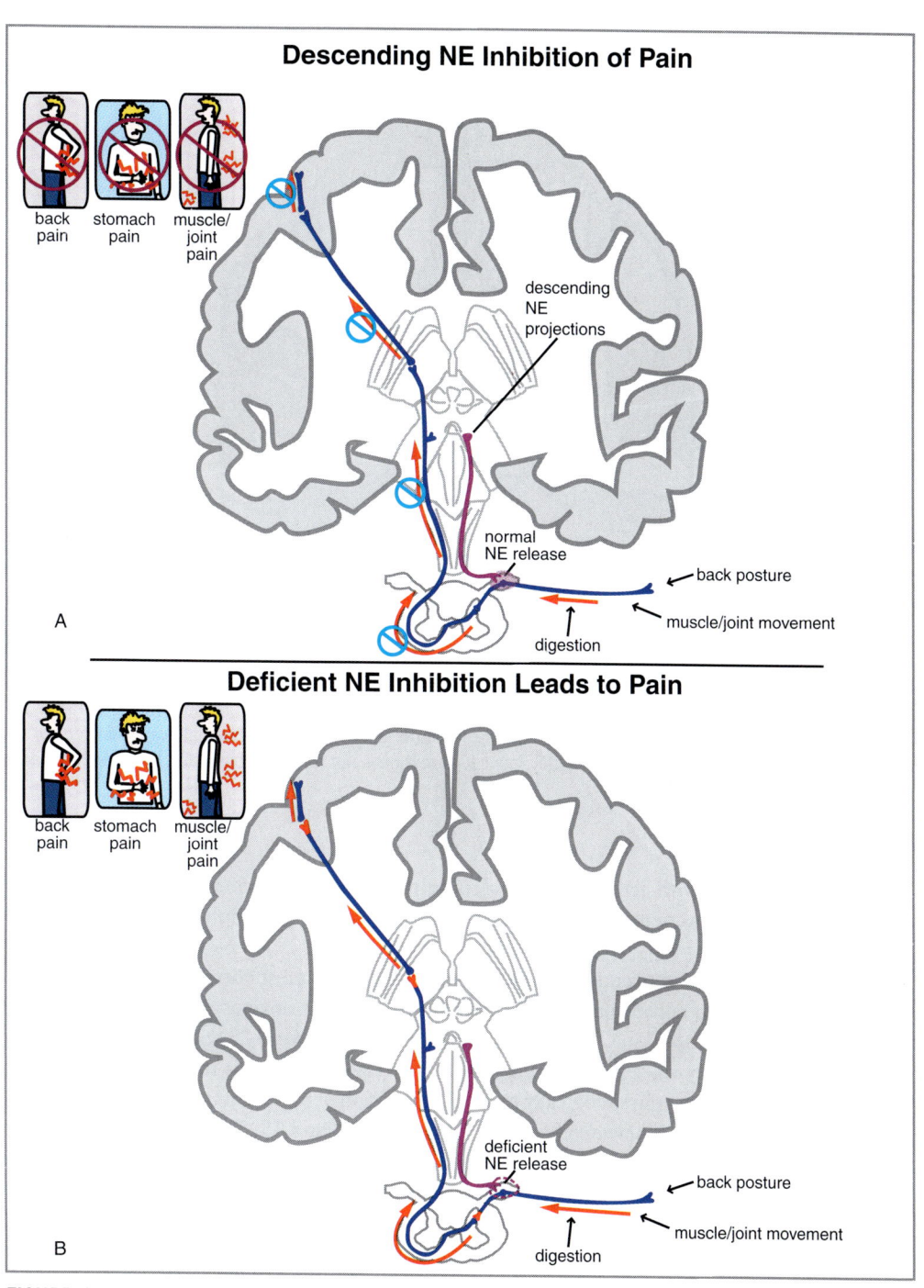

FIGURE 15-12A and B Descending noradrenergic neurons and pain. (**A**) Descending spinal noradrenergic (NE) neurons inhibit neurotransmitter release from primary afferent neurons via presynaptic alpha 2 adrenoceptors, and inhibit activity of dorsal horn neurons via postsynaptic alpha 2 adrenoceptors. This suppresses bodily input (e.g., regarding muscles/joints or digestion) from reaching the brain and thus prevents it from being interpreted as painful. (**B**) If descending NE inhibition is deficient, then it may not be sufficient to mask irrelevant nociceptive input, potentially leading to perception of pain from input that is normally ignored. This may be a contributing factor for painful somatic symptoms in fibromyalgia, depression, irritable bowel syndrome, and anxiety disorders.

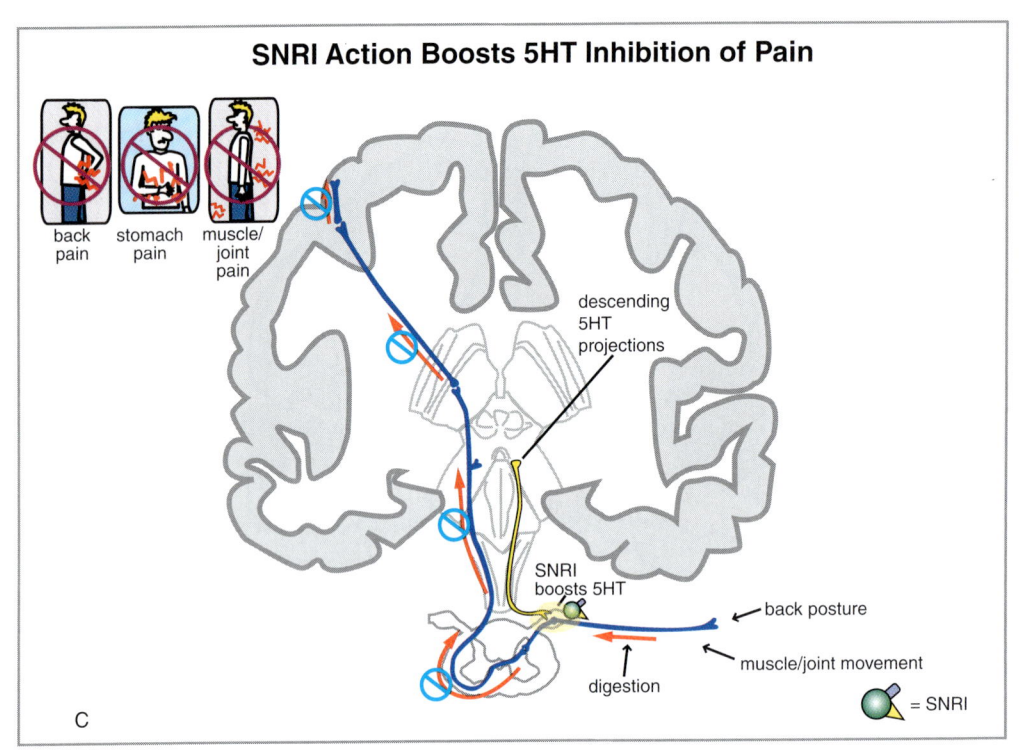

FIGURE 15-13C Enhancement of descending serotonergic inhibition. A serotonin norepinephrine reuptake inhibitor (SNRI) can increase serotonergic neurotransmission in the descending spinal pathway to the dorsal horn, and thus may enhance inhibition of bodily input so that it does not reach the brain and get interpreted as pain. However, the noradrenergic effects of SNRIs may be more relevant to suppression of nociceptive input.

Descending inhibition is also activated during severe injury by incoming nociceptive input and in dangerous "conflict" situations via limbic structures, causing the release of endogenous opioid peptides (Figure 15-11B), serotonin (Figure 15-13A), and norepinephrine (Figure 15-12A). When this happens, it reduces not only the release of nociceptive neurotransmitters in the dorsal horn (Figure 15-6) but also the transmission of nociceptive impulses up the spinal cord into the brain (Figure 15-5), thereby reducing the perception of pain, dulling it to allow escape from the situation without the injury compromising physical performance in the short run (reduction of "ouch" in Figure 15-5). On return to safety, descending facilitation replaces the inhibition to redress the balance, increase awareness of the injury, and force rest of the injured part (lots of "ouch" in Figure 15-5).

The power of this system can be seen in humans persevering through severe injury in sports and on the battlefield. The placebo effect may also involve endogenous opioid release from these descending inhibitory neurons (Figure 15-11B), since activation of a placebo response to pain is reversible by the mu opioid antagonist naloxone. These are adaptive changes within the pain pathways that facilitate survival and enhance function for the individual. However, maladaptive changes can also hijack these same mechanisms to maintain pain inappropriately without relevant tissue injury, as may occur in various forms of neuropathic pain ranging from diabetes to fibromyalgia and beyond (Table 15-3).

Here today and not gone tomorrow: the curse of chronic pain and other central sensitization syndromes

Pain may perpetuate pain if it is a marker of an irreversible sensitization process within the CNS. As already discussed, acute pain indicates a type of CNS activity that causes suffering in the "here and now." Chronic pain indicates another type of CNS activity, namely that a vicious cycle has been triggered where progressive and potentially irreversible molecular changes eventually lead to progressive and potentially irreversible pain symptoms (Figure 15-14; see also Tables 15-2 and 15-3). These changes are dependent upon neuronal activity within the pain pathway and thus are called "activity-dependent," with subthreshold nociceptive neuronal activity insufficient to cause pain (Figure 15-14A), full nociceptive neuronal activity sufficient to cause a "normal" acute pain response (Figure 15-14B), and repetitive activation of nociception causing ongoing neuronal activity that induces CNS plasticity within the pain pathway, with molecular, synaptic, and structural changes, including sprouting (Figure 15-14C). The latter condition is the theoretical substrate for various central sensitization syndromes (Figure 15-14C).

Activity-dependent nociceptive activity in the pain pathway requires release of neurotransmitters via a mechanism that involves both voltage-sensitive sodium channels (VSSCs; discussed above and illustrated in Figure 15-14A, B, C, and D) and voltage-sensitive calcium channels (also illustrated in Figure 15-14A, B, C, and D). The alpha 2 delta ligands bind potently and selectively to the alpha 2 delta subunit of VSCCs (Figure 15-14D). In fact, these agents, which include gabapentin and pregabalin, may more selectively bind the "open channel" conformation of VSCCs and thus be particularly effective in blocking those channels that are the most active, with a "use-dependent" form of inhibition (Figure 15-15). This molecular action predicts more affinity for centrally sensitized VSCCs that are actively conducting neuronal impulses within the pain pathway and thus having a selective action on those VSCCs causing neuropathic pain, ignoring other VSCCs that are not open, and thus not interfering with normal neurotransmission in central neurons uninvolved in mediating the pathological pain state (Figure 15-15).

"Segmental" central sensitization syndromes are thought to be caused when these plastic changes occur in the dorsal horn in conditions such as phantom pain and progressive worsening of diabetic peripheral neuropathic pain where there is definite peripheral injury combined with central sensitization at the spinal cord segment receiving nociceptive input from the damaged area of the body (Figure 15-16). Segmental central sensitization syndromes are thus "mixed" states where the insult of central change is added to the peripheral injury (Table 15-3; Figures 15-14C and 15-16). Activity-dependent (i.e., use-dependent) neuronal plasticity in the dorsal horn causes exaggerated (hyperalgesic) or prolonged responses to noxious inputs – sometimes called "wind-up" – as well as painful responses to normally innocuous inputs (called allodynia). Phosphorylation of key membrane receptors and channels in the dorsal horn appears to increase synaptic efficiency and thus to trip a master switch opening the gate to the pain pathway and turning on central sensitization that acts to amplify or create the perception of pain. The gate can also close, as conceptualized in the classic "gate theory" of pain, in order to explain how innocuous stimulation (e.g., acupuncture, vibration, rubbing) away from the site of an injury can close the pain gate and reduce the perception of the injury pain. Alpha 2 delta ligands may also function to close the pain gate when they close VSCCs in the overly active dorsal horn (Figure 15-16C).

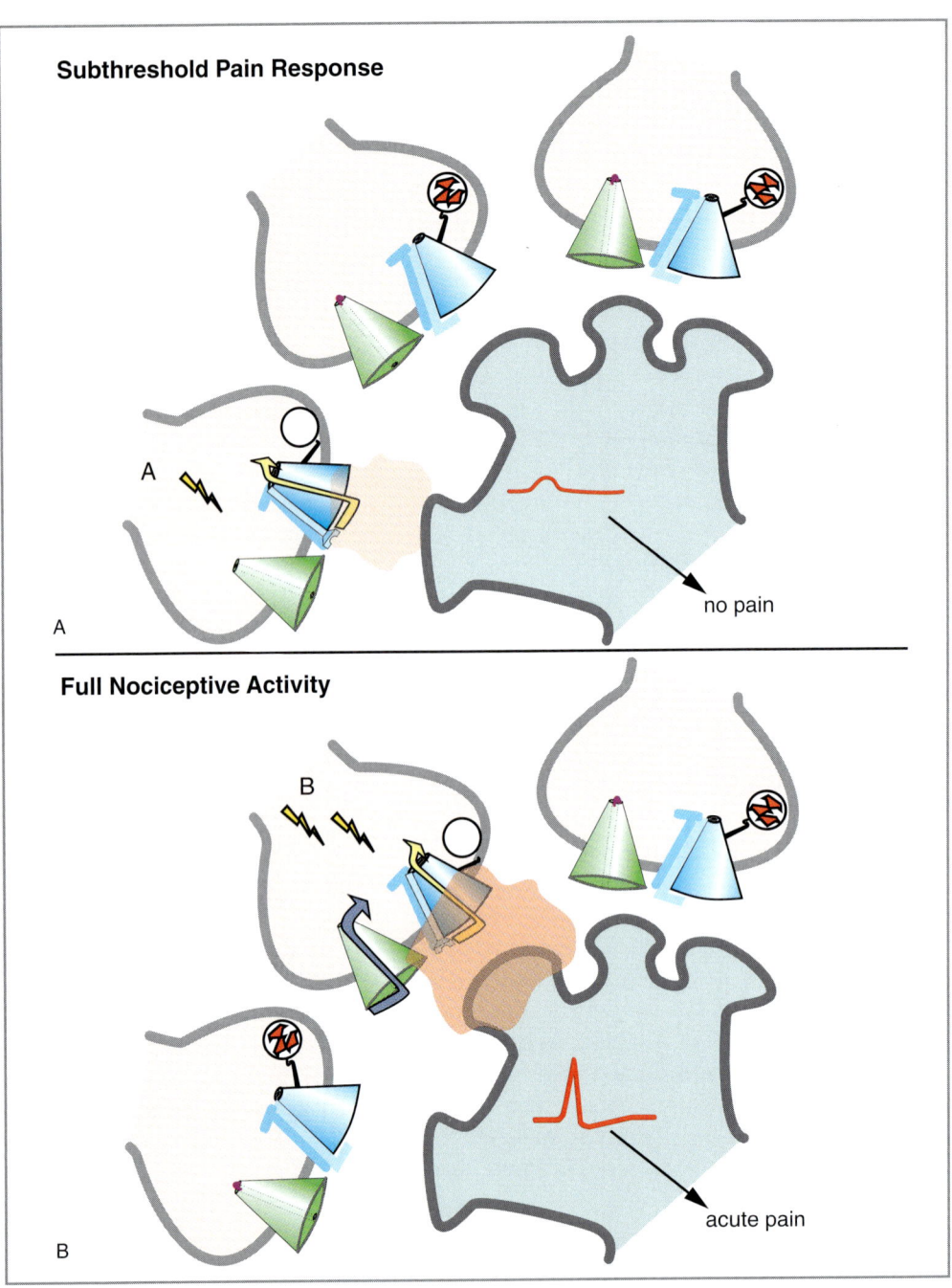

FIGURE 15-14A and B Activity-dependent nociception in pain pathways, part 1: acute pain. The degree of nociceptive neuronal activity in pain pathways determines whether one experiences acute pain. An action potential on a presynaptic neuron triggers sodium influx, which in turn leads to calcium influx and ultimately release of neurotransmitter. (**A**) In some cases, the action potential generated at the presynaptic neuron causes minimal neurotransmitter release; thus the postsynaptic neuron is not notably stimulated and the nociceptive input does not reach the brain (in other words, there is no pain). (**B**) In other cases, a stronger action potential at the presynaptic neuron may cause voltage-sensitive calcium channels to remain open longer, allowing more neurotransmitter release and more stimulation of the postsynaptic neuron. Thus, the nociceptive input is transmitted to the brain and acute pain occurs.

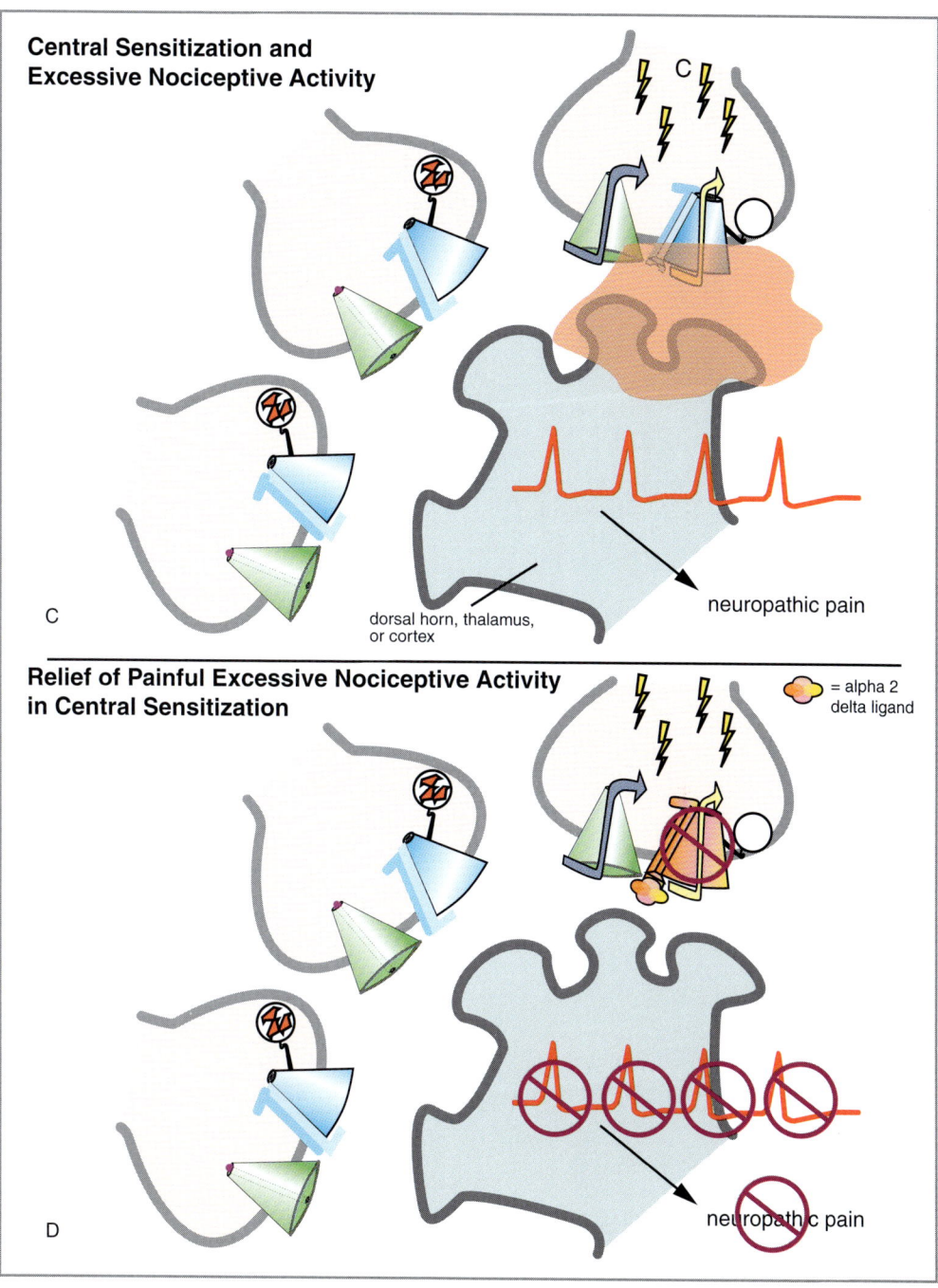

FIGURE 15-14C and D Activity-dependent nociception in pain pathways, part 2: neuropathic pain. (C) Strong or repetitive action potentials can cause prolonged opening of calcium channels, which may lead to excessive release of neurotransmitter into the synaptic cleft, and consequently to excessive stimulation of postsynaptic neurons. Ultimately this may induce molecular, synaptic, and structural changes, including sprouting, which are the theoretical substrates for central sensitization syndromes. In other words, this can lead to neuropathic pain. **(D)** Alpha 2 delta ligands such as gabapentin or pregabalin bind to the alpha 2 delta subunit of voltage-sensitive calcium channels, changing their conformation to reduce calcium influx and therefore reduce excessive stimulation of postsynaptic receptors.

Pain and the Treatment of Fibromyalgia and Functional Somatic Syndromes | 797

Molecular Action of Alpha 2 Delta Ligands

A. open conformation of VSCC

B. Alpha 2 delta ligand binding to open conformation and inhibiting VSCC

C. closed conformation of VSCC

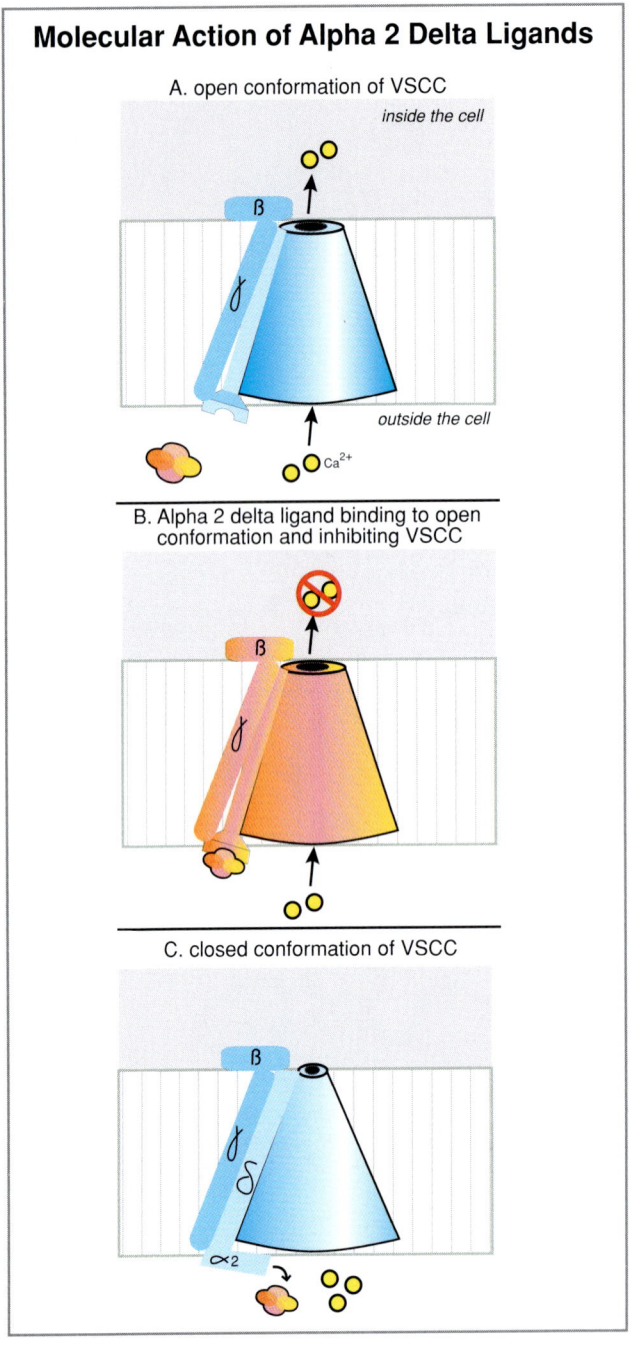

FIGURE 15-15A, B, and C Binding of alpha 2 delta ligands. (**A**) Calcium influx occurs when voltage-sensitive calcium channels (VSCCs) are in the open channel conformation. (**B**) Alpha 2 delta ligands such as gabapentin and pregabalin have greatest affinity for the open channel conformation and thus block those channels that are most active. (**C**) When VSCCs are in the closed conformation alpha 2 delta ligands do not bind and thus do not disrupt normal neurotransmission.

"Suprasegmental" central sensitization syndromes are hypothesized to be linked to plastic changes that occur in brain sites within the nociceptive pathway, especially the thalamus and cortex, even in the absence of identifiable triggering events (Figures 15-14C and 15-17A). In this case the CNS insult is added to no apparent peripheral injury. Conditions hypothesized to be suprasegmental central sensitization syndromes include fibromyalgia, painful symptoms in depression and other affective spectrum disorders, and

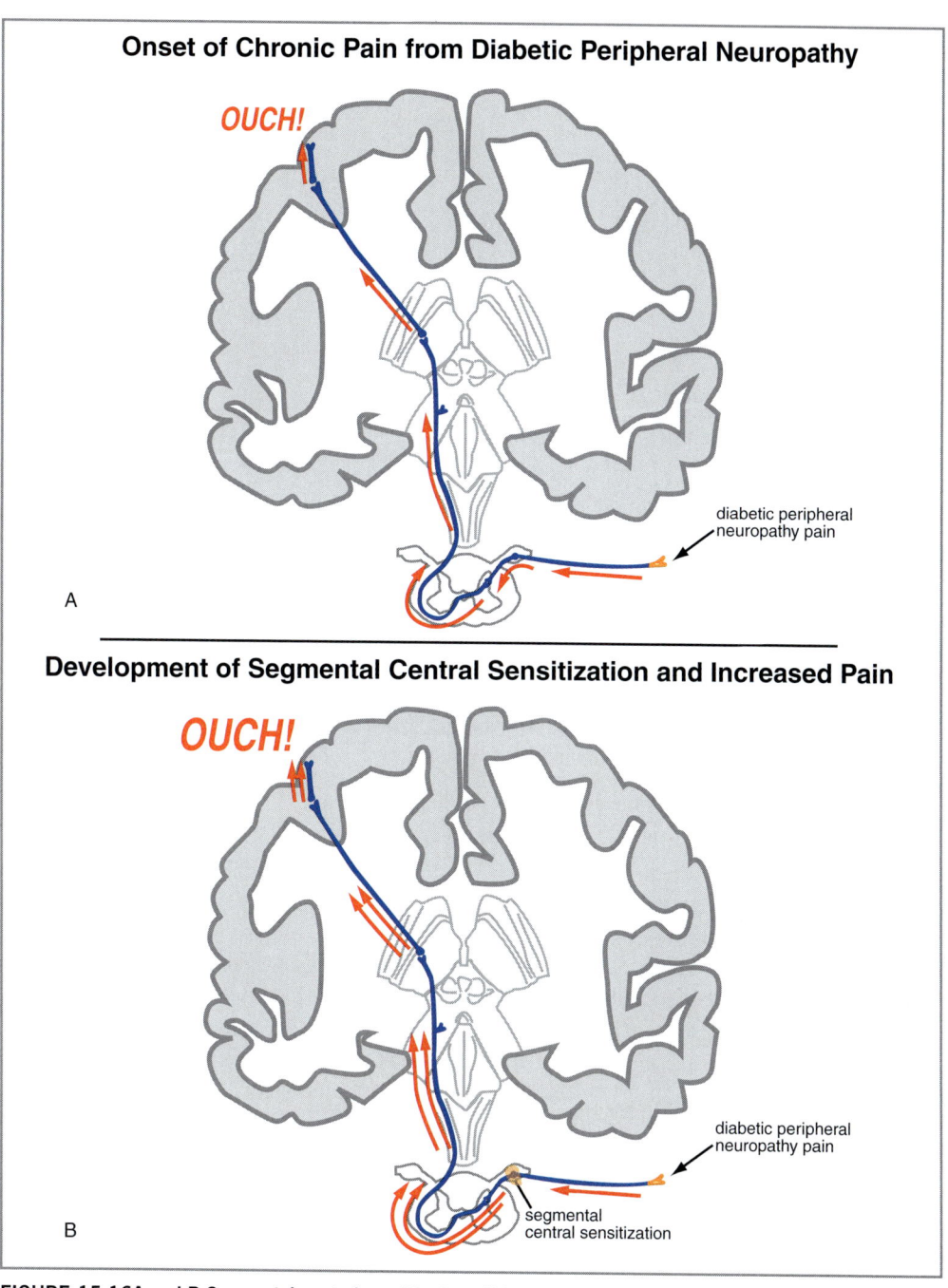

FIGURE 15-16A and B Segmental central sensitization. (A) In some cases, inflammation associated with peripheral injury can lead to a reduced threshold of nociceptive endings for pain, termed peripheral sensitization. Peripheral sensitization may cause nonpainful stimuli to be interpreted as painful, which is known as allodynia, and may also cause hyperalgesia, or increased pain in response to a painful stimulus. **(B)** In some cases, injury or disease directly affecting the nervous system may result in plastic changes that lead to sensitization within the central nervous system, such that the experience of pain continues even after tissue damage is resolved. Impulses may be generated at abnormal locations either spontaneously or via mechanical forces. At the level of the spinal cord, this process is termed segmental central sensitization. This mechanism underlies conditions such as diabetic peripheral neuropathic pain and phantom pain.

Pain and the Treatment of Fibromyalgia and Functional Somatic Syndromes | 799

Anatomic Actions of Alpha 2 Delta Ligands

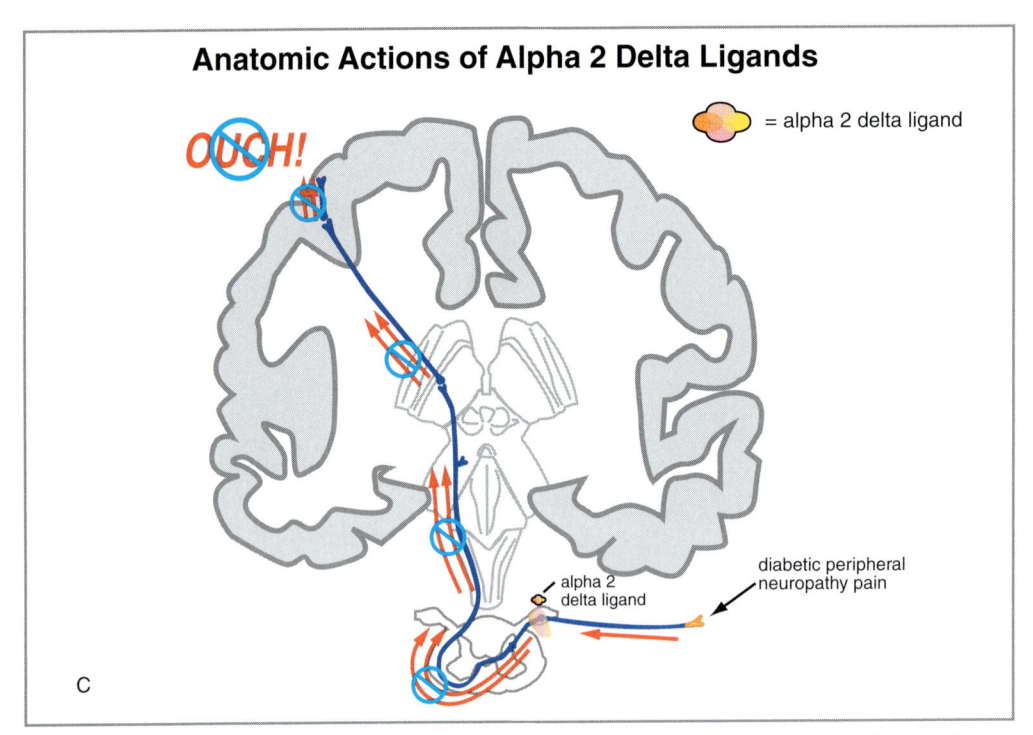

FIGURE 15-16C Alpha 2 delta ligands in the dorsal horn. Alpha 2 delta ligands may alleviate chronic pain associated with sensitization at the level of the dorsal horn. As illustrated here, alpha 2 delta ligands may bind to voltage-sensitive calcium channels in the dorsal horn to reduce excitatory neurotransmission and thus, alleviate pain.

functional somatic syndromes (Tables 15-4 and 15-5). Alpha 2 delta ligands may be attracted to wherever there are open VSCCs mediating centrally originated pain in suprasegmental central sensitization states (Figure 15-17B).

Central sensitization can also be thought of as a form of "diabolical learning" within pain circuits. The concept of diabolical learning is introduced in Chapter 8 and illustrated in Figures 8-1 through 8-6. Diabolical learning may also occur in various addictive disorders (discussed in Chapter 19, on drug abuse), stress disorders (discussed in Chapter 14 and illustrated in Figures 14-29 through 14-36), and numerous other CNS conditions.

Can pain gates be opened from the inside and cause pain in affective spectrum disorders and functional somatic syndromes?

Since the notion of central sensitization has now expanded to include affective spectrum disorders and functional somatic syndromes, it is possible that patients with fibromyalgia, noncardiac chest pain, irritable bowel syndrome, and similar conditions may have their disorders triggered centrally by a sensitizing emotional event or by residual somatic symptoms of depression or anxiety rather than from a peripheral painful input. It is as though the brain "learns" from its experience of pain and decides not only to keep the process going but also to enhance it and make it permanent. Interrupting this process and getting the CNS to "forget" its molecular memories may be one of the greatest unmet needs in psychopharmacology today, not only because this may be a therapeutic strategy for various chronic neuropathic pain conditions but also because it may be a viable approach to treating

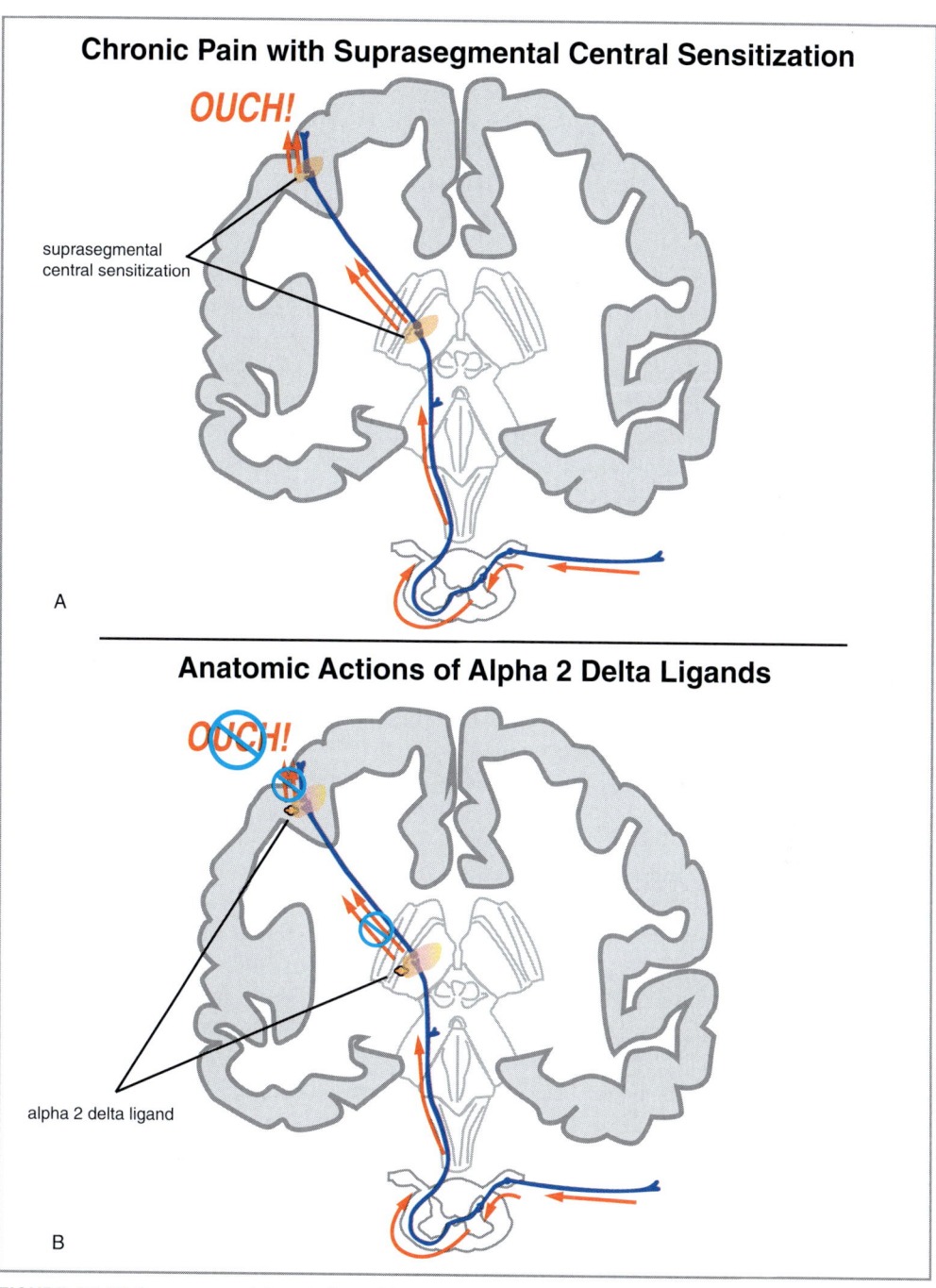

FIGURE 15-17 Suprasegmental central sensitization. (**A**) Plastic changes in brain sites within the nociceptive pathway can cause sensitization, for instance at the level of the thalamus or the sensory cortex. This process within the brain is termed suprasegmental central sensitization. This mechanism is believed to underlie conditions such as fibromyalgia, painful symptoms in depression, and other affective spectrum disorders and functional somatic syndromes. (**B**) Alpha 2 delta ligands may alleviate chronic pain associated with sensitization at the level of the thalamus or cortex. As illustrated here, alpha 2 delta ligands may bind to voltage-sensitive calcium channels in the thalamus and cortex to reduce excitatory neurotransmission and thus, alleviate pain.

the hypothesized molecular changes that may underlie psychotic disorders, stress-induced anxiety and affective disorders, and even addictive disorders.

Early innovative approaches to this problem include experimental strategies to prevent pain before it predictably occurs by administering analgesics *before* surgery to reduce the need for analgesics postoperatively. This same notion is discussed in Chapter 10, on schizophrenia, where presymptomatic/prodromal treatments for schizophrenia are conceptualized and illustrated in Figure 10-120, and in Chapter 14 on anxiety, where preemptive treatments immediately after exposure to catastrophic stressors may reduce the emergence of anxiety disorders such as posttraumatic stress disorder (see Figures 14-38 and 14-39).

Thus, just as for schizophrenia and anxiety disorders, preemptive analgesia, if proven successful, would suggest that pain is less costly when you "pay" for it in advance. The hope is that early treatment of pain could interfere with the development of chronic persistent painful conditions by blocking the ability of painful experiences to imprint themselves upon the CNS by not allowing triggering of central sensitization. Thus the mechanisms whereby symptomatic suffering of chronic neuropathic pain is relieved, such as with SNRIs or alpha 2 delta ligands, may also be the same mechanisms that could prevent disease progression to chronic persistent pain states.

Early treatment of painful symptoms with "rescue analgesia" with such agents may prevent progression to more severe levels of pain or to treatment-resistant pain states. A sensitized nervous system that has experienced pain results in more pain perception than a nonsensitized nervous system, so rescue analgesia could theoretically intercept painful physical symptoms in affective spectrum disorders and functional somatic syndromes and prevent the progression of conditions such as fibromyalgia. This notion calls for aggressive treatment of painful symptoms in these conditions that theoretically have their origin within the CNS, thus "intercepting" the central sensitization process before it is durably imprinted into angry circuits.

Thus major depression, anxiety disorders, and functional somatic syndromes can be treated with SNRIs and/or alpha 2 delta ligands to eliminate any painful physical symptoms and thereby improve the chances of reaching full symptomatic remission. The opportunity to prevent permanent pain syndromes or progressive worsening of pain is one reason why pain is increasingly being considered a psychiatric "vital sign" that must be assessed routinely in the evaluation and treatment of psychiatric disorders by psychopharmacologists. Future testing of agents capable of reducing pain should be done to determine whether eliminating painful symptoms early in the course of psychiatric and functional somatic illnesses will improve outcomes, including preventing symptomatic relapses, the development of treatment resistance, or even hippocampal atrophy (hippocampal atrophy from stress in anxiety and affective disorders is discussed in Chapter 14 and illustrated in Figure 14-30). Preemptively treating pain before it occurs – or at least rescuing centrally mediated and sensitizing pain by intercepting such pain before it becomes permanent – may be among the most promising therapeutic applications of dual reuptake inhibitors and alpha 2 delta ligands and deserves careful clinical evaluation.

Pain in affective spectrum disorders and functional somatic syndromes

The spectrum of mood and anxiety disorders with pain disorders

Affective spectrum disorders include not only disorders of mood but various other disorders that can be treated with antidepressants, such as anxiety disorders and a number of conditions characterized by symptoms of chronic pain (Table 15-4, Figure 15-18). The range

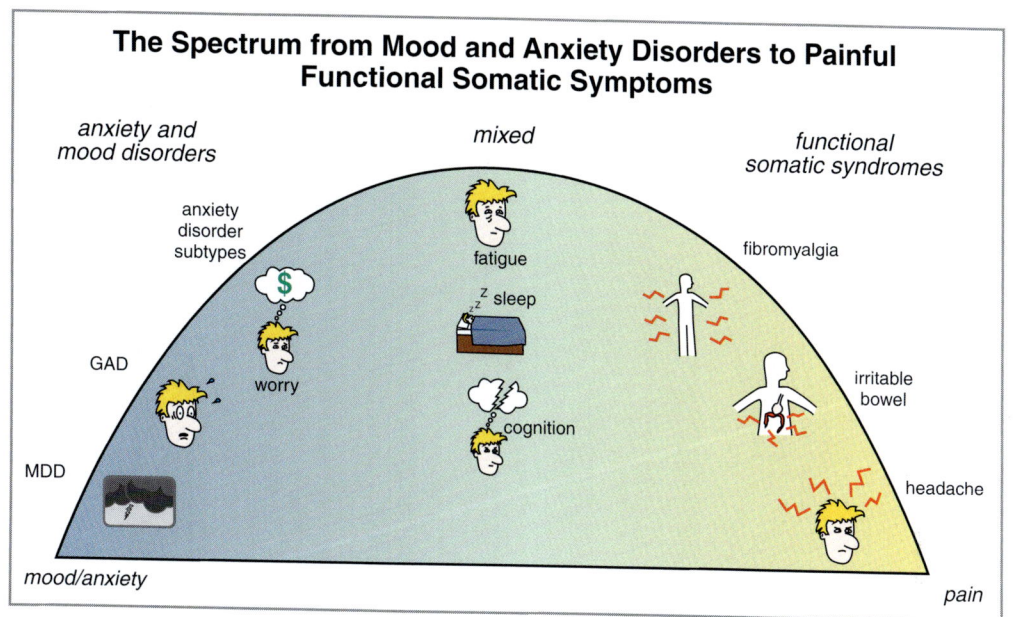

FIGURE 15-18 The spectrum from mood and anxiety disorders to painful functional somatic syndromes. Affective spectrum disorders include mood and anxiety disorders, while "functional somatic syndrome" is a term used to describe disorders such as fibromyalgia, irritable bowel syndrome, and headache. Pain, though not a formal diagnostic feature of depression or anxiety disorders, is nonetheless frequently present in patients with these disorders. Similarly, depressed mood, anxiety, and other symptoms identified as part of depression and anxiety disorders are now recognized as being common in functional somatic syndromes. Thus, rather than being discrete groups of illnesses, affective spectrum disorders and functional somatic syndromes may instead exist along the same spectrum.

of diagnostic (Figure 11-44) and nondiagnostic symptoms of major depression including pain (Figure 12-124) is discussed in Chapter 11, including the hypothetically malfunctioning pathways associated with these symptoms (Figures 11-45 to 11-54 and 12-125); the treatments proposed for these symptoms, based on targeting neurotransmitters in the malfunctioning circuits (e.g., pain in depression), are discussed in Chapter 12 and their treatment with SNRIs and alpha 2 delta ligands illustrated in Figure 12-126. Only recently have painful physical symptoms been recognized as important concomitant symptoms of depression and anxiety disorders (see left-hand portion of the spectrum in Figure 15-18); their relief is necessary in order to attain full remission. It is thus somewhat surprising that pain is nevertheless not considered to be a formal diagnostic feature of any mood or anxiety disorder.

On the other hand, many experts are now recognizing that numerous disorders that do have pain as a central and formal diagnostic feature also have important concomitant symptoms of depression and anxiety (see right-hand portion of the spectrum in Figure 15-18). Also included in numerous central pain disorders are several other symptoms that are formal diagnostic features of mood and anxiety disorders, including fatigue, sleep disturbance, and problems concentrating (see middle of spectrum in Figure 15-18). Such central neuropathic pain disorders include fibromyalgia, irritable bowel syndrome, headache, and other disorders sometimes called functional somatic syndromes (Table 15-5 and the right-hand portion of Figure 15-18). This has led to the proposal that mood and anxiety disorders may be on a diagnostic and therapeutic spectrum with certain pain disorders – namely, the functional

Dose-Response Curve for Painful Symptoms and Likelihood of a Mood or Anxiety Disorder

likelihood of MDD

likelihood of anxiety disorder

1 2 3 4 5 ≥6
number of unexplained painful physical symptoms

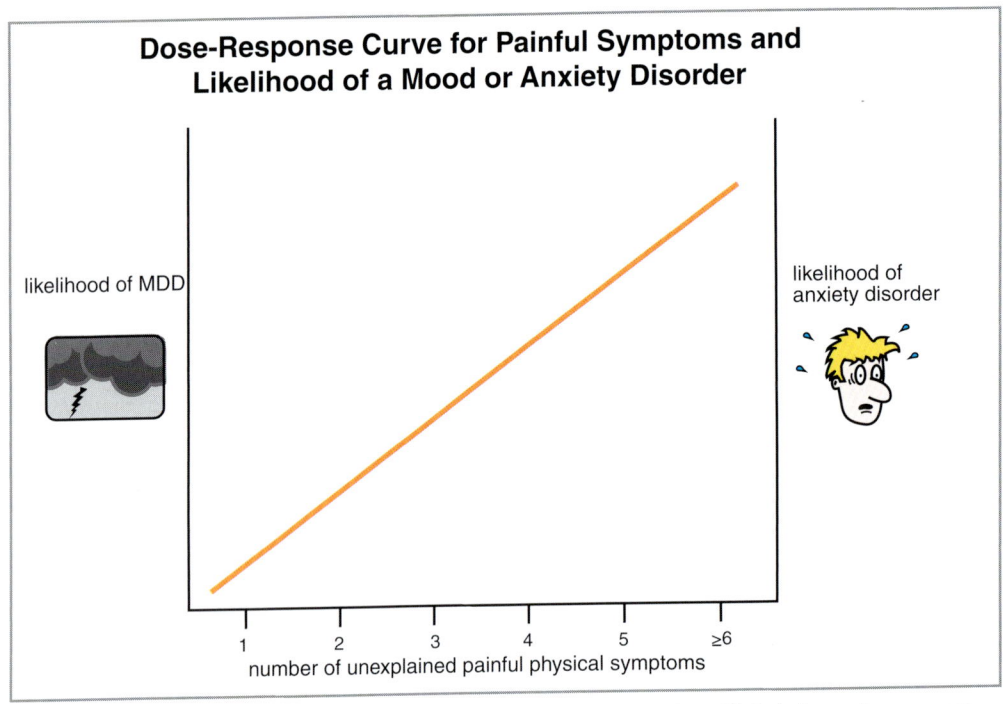

FIGURE 15-19 Association between painful symptoms and mood and anxiety. Clinical observations suggest that the higher the number of painful physical symptoms a patient has, the greater the likelihood that that patient has a mood or anxiety disorder.

somatic syndromes (see full spectrum of Figure 15-18). The powerful association between painful symptoms on the one hand and mood and anxiety on the other is demonstrated by numerous observations showing that the more unexplained painful physical symptoms a patient has, the more likely that patient is to have either a mood or anxiety disorder in a rather perverse, painful dose–response curve (Figure 15-19).

The issue is that modern psychopharmacologists can no longer ignore pain symptoms in mood and anxiety disorders, or mood and anxiety symptoms in pain disorders, or sleep disturbances, cognitive complaints, or fatigue in either type of disorder. Thus, the practitioner now must identify all symptoms associated with disorders across the spectrum shown in Figure 15-18 (not just mood and anxiety in the mood and anxiety disorders and not just pain in the pain disorders) and treat all symptoms with rational combinations of agents to relieve every symptom and thus to achieve remission of each disorder across this spectrum. As discussed throughout this chapter, it is clear that some therapeutic agents effective for mood and anxiety disorders (such as SNRIs, alpha 2 delta ligands, and others) are also proving effective for treating not only the symptoms of pain but also the overlapping symptoms common to both affective and pain disorders, such as problems concentrating, sleep disturbance, and fatigue. These therapeutic actions are easily understood as the consequences of successful targeting of neurotransmission in specific malfunctioning CNS pathways to increase the efficiency of information processing in these circuits and thus reduce symptoms.

Does depression or anxiety hurt?

In primary care practices, up to 80 percent of patients present exclusively with physical symptoms, which can include headache, abdominal pain, and musculoskeletal pains in the

TABLE 15-6 American College of Rheumatology (ACR) 1990 criteria for fibromyalgia

History of widespread pain
- Considered widespread when present in all of the following:
  – Left side of the body
  – Right side of the body
  – Above the waist
  – Below the waist
  – Axial skeleton (cervical spine, anterior chest, thoracic spine, or low back)
- Must be present for at least 3 months

Pain in 11 of 18 tender point sites on digital palpation
- Digital palpation should be performed with an approximate force of 4 kg
- For a tender point to be considered positive, the subject must state that the palpation was painful

Source: Wolfe F et al. *Arthritis Rheum.* 1990;33:160–172.

lower back, joints, and neck. If such painful physical symptoms are so common in depression and may even be the only presenting symptoms in significant numbers of patients, why are they not emphasized more in the recognition of depression? One possible reason is that such complaints, especially in primary care practices, may be interpreted as symptoms of a "real" somatic illness and lead only to a workup for medical illness. While most psychopharmacologists respond to psychological and emotional complaints with a high index of suspicion for anxiety or depression, many clinicians, especially in specialties other than mental health, may be misled into an exhaustive search for somatic causes without considering depression in patients who complain of fatigue, low energy, and painful physical ailments but not emotional or vegetative symptoms. It is now recognized, however, that all symptoms – emotional, vegetative and painful – must be eliminated in the treatment of depression in order to attain a complete remission of this illness; this is now the standard of care in managing depressed and/or anxious patients.

Fibromyalgia

> I am more seriously ill than my doctors think.
> Alfred Nobel

In the nineteenth century, the discoverer of dynamite and the founder of the Nobel prizes may have suffered from it. During that era, Freud might have seen it as neurasthenia and treated it with psychoanalysis; Charcot might have seen it as hypochondria and treated it with hypnosis. In the twentieth century, this condition became debated either as a syndrome of abnormal muscles, sleep, pain, and mood or as an entity invented by lawyers, charlatans, and disability seekers related to chronic fatigue syndrome, irritable bowel syndrome, "Yuppie flu," and multiple chemical sensitivity. Now, in the twenty-first century, as psychiatric disorders struggle to fly first class with medical and surgical disorders, fibromyalgia is finally being upgraded from cargo to coach.

Pain disorder, mood disorder, or not a disorder at all?

Fibromyalgia is thus emerging as a diagnosable and potentially treatable pain syndrome with tenderness but no structural pathology in muscles, ligaments, or joints. Fibromyalgia is recognized by rheumatologists as a chronic, widespread pain syndrome associated with fatigue, nonrestorative sleep, and tenderness at 11 or more of 18 designated "trigger points" where ligaments, tendons, and muscle attach to bone (Table 15-6 and Figure 15-20). It

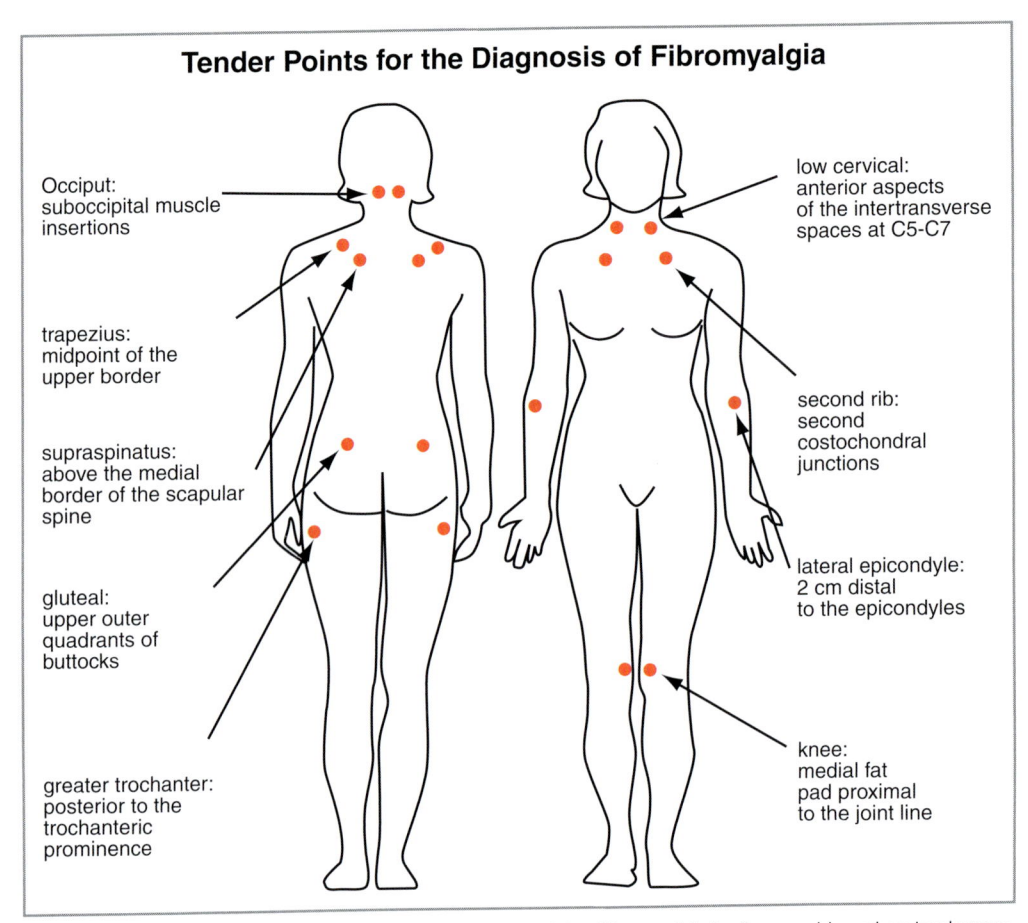

FIGURE 15-20 Tender points for the diagnosis of fibromyalgia. Fibromyalgia is diagnosed based on tenderness in at least 11 of 18 designated "trigger points" where ligaments, tendons, and muscle attach to bone. Other diagnostic features include fatigue and nonrestorative sleep.

is the second most common diagnosis in rheumatology clinics and may affect from 2 to 4 percent of the population. Although symptoms of fibromyalgia are chronic and debilitating, they are not necessarily progressive.

There is no known cause, although the condition may occur following viral infections, exposure to toxins, or physical or emotional trauma. There is no known pathology identifiable in the muscles or joints. Various hypotheses suggest that fibromyalgia may be a central sensitization syndrome linked to abnormal neurotransmission in pain pathways and to abnormalities in the hypothalamic-pituitary-adrenal (HPA) axis, but the cause and pathophysiology of fibromyalgia remain obscure. As a chronic pain state, fibromyalgia has been hypothesized to represent abnormal sensory processing at N-methyl-d-aspartate (NMDA) glutamate receptor–mediated neurotransmission in unmyelinated C fibers, which carry pain impulses. It has also been hypothesized as abnormal substance P–mediated neurotransmission. Thus, some theories conceptualize fibromyalgia as a segmental central sensitization syndrome (see Figure 15-16). Other hypotheses suggest stress-related HPA axis abnormalities in CRH-ACTH-cortisol regulation (see discussion of stress and the HPA axis in Chapter 14 and Figures 14-29 through 14-36) or abnormal pain processing in the cortex, causing exaggerated pain responses and therefore a suprasegmental central sensitization

TABLE 15-7 Comorbid mood and anxiety disorders in fibromyalgia

Disorder	Lifetime prevalence rate (%)
Any major mood disorder	**73.1**
▪ Major depressive disorder	62.0
▪ Bipolar disorder	11.1
Any anxiety disorder	**55.6**
▪ Panic disorder	28.7
▪ Posttraumatic stress disorder (PTSD)	21.3
▪ Social phobia	19.4
▪ Obsessive compulsive disorder (OCD)	6.5

Source: Adapted from Arnold LM et al. *J Clin Psychiatry*. 2006;67:1219–1225.

TABLE 15-8 Comorbid functional somatic syndromes in fibromyalgia

Disorder	Prevalence rate (%)
Chronic fatigue syndrome	21–80
Irritable bowel syndrome	32–80
Temporomandibular disorder	75
Tension and migraine headache	10–80
Multiple chemical sensitivities	33–55
Interstitial cystitis	13–21
Chronic pelvic pain	18

Source: Aaron LA and Buchwald D. *Best Pract Res Clin Rheumatol*. 2003; 17:563–574.

syndrome (see Figure 15-17). However, none of these is well established and the pathophysiology of fibromyalgia remains obscure.

Most of those diagnosed with fibromyalgia have a comorbid mood or anxiety disorder (Table 15-7), a comorbid functional somatic syndrome (Table 15-8), or both. Many also qualify for the diagnosis of a somatoform disorder. Because of this high degree of comorbidity, some have asked whether fibromyalgia is a real illness unto itself, especially considering that "normal" people have aches and pains all the time, with almost all of us experiencing a somatic symptom (e.g., headache, neckache, backache, joint ache, muscle stiffness) every 4 to 6 days. Some skeptical experts apply the logic of the baseball great and folk philosopher Yogi Berra to fibromyalgia, namely, "If I hadn't believed it, I wouldn't have seen it." Thus fibromyalgia is considered by some to be the result of unconscious conflicts manifesting themselves as physical symptoms, with pain serving as a somatic metaphor for unhappiness and a life that is not working out.

This rather unsympathetic and old-fashioned point of view has slowly given way to the idea that although fibromyalgia is not a mood disorder or an anxiety disorder per se, it is as "real" as panic disorder, obsessive compulsive disorder, social anxiety disorder, and other previously ill-defined entities that were not recognized as legitimate illnesses until proven treatments began to define them as valid disorders. Some studies suggest that 75

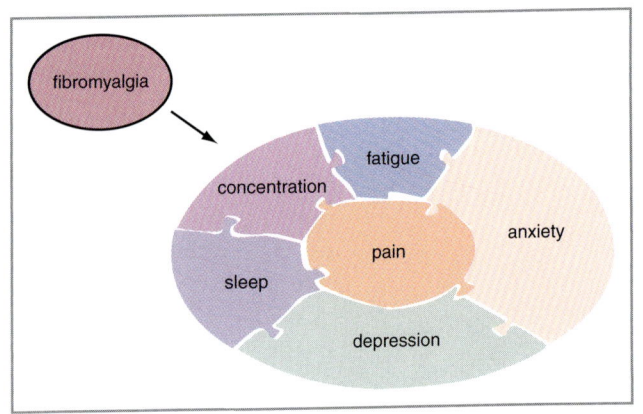

FIGURE 15-21 Symptoms of fibromyalgia. In addition to pain as a central feature of fibromyalgia, many patients experience fatigue, anxiety, depression, disturbed sleep, and problems concentrating.

to 90 percent of identified patients are women, especially Caucasian women. Is it possible that fibromyalgia has been as neglected as many other women's mental health issues? Is it no longer on the fringe because political and consumer activism are forcing a serious look at this problem? As fibromyalgia becomes more legitimate, will more men be diagnosed with it?

Fortunately, fibromyalgia has been taken seriously by an increasing cohort of investigators and clinicians, and this has led to the establishment of alpha 2 delta ligands and SNRIs as proven treatments. There are even new initiatives searching for pharmacogenomic markers of fibromyalgia. This bodes well for eventually clarifying exactly what this entity is and for the continued development of more treatments.

The most common symptoms of fibromyalgia are shown in Figure 15-21. This syndrome can be deconstructed into its component symptoms and then matched with hypothetically malfunctioning brain circuits (Figure 15-22).

Treatment of fibromyalgia
We have repeatedly mentioned the proven usefulness of the alpha 2 delta ligands gabapentin and pregabalin (Figures 15-14 through 15-17) and the SNRIs duloxetine, milnacipran, venlafaxine, and desvenlafaxine (Figures 15-12 and 15-13) for treating the painful symptoms of fibromyalgia. Thus, alpha 2 delta ligands and SNRIs are considered first-line treatments for fibromyalgia (see fibro-pharmacy in Figure 15-23). Although these two classes have not been studied extensively in combination, they are frequently used together in clinical practice and can sometimes give additive improvement in relieving pain (Figure 15-23).

Alpha 2 delta ligands are proven useful not only for treating pain (Figures 15-14D, 15-16C, and 15-17C) but also for reducing symptoms of anxiety in fibromyalgia (see discussion in Chapter 14 and Figure 14-37) and for improving the slow-wave sleep disorder of fibromyalgia (sleep disorders and their treatment are discussed in further detail in Chapter 16).

SNRIs can be useful not only for painful symptoms but also for reducing symptoms of anxiety and depression in fibromyalgia (see mechanism of action discussion for depression in Chapter 12 and Figures 12-33 through 12-42) and for treating the cognitive symptoms associated with fibromyalgia, sometimes also called "fibro-fog." Problems with executive functioning are generally linked to inefficient information processing in the dorsolateral prefrontal cortex (DLPFC), where dopamine neurotransmission is important in regulating brain circuits. This concept of dopaminergic regulation of cognition in DLPFC is

Match Each Symptom of Fibromyalgia to Hypothetically Malfunctioning Brain Circuits

- "fibro-fog"
- problems concentrating
- lack of interest/pleasure

pleasure interests fatigue/energy

psychomotor fatigue (physical)

pain

psychomotor fatigue (mental)
pain

mood

depressed mood
anxiety

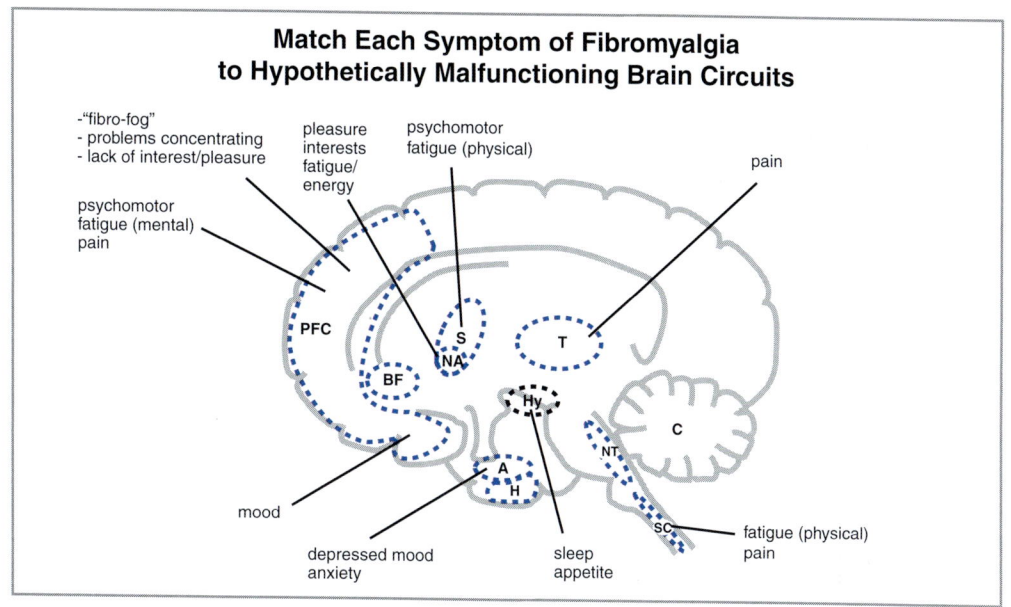

sleep
appetite

fatigue (physical)
pain

FIGURE 15-22 **Symptom-based algorithm for fibromyalgia.** A symptom-based approach to treatment selection for fibromyalgia follows the theory that each of a patient's symptoms can be matched with malfunctioning brain circuits and neurotransmitters that hypothetically mediate those symptoms; this information is then used to select a corresponding pharmacological mechanism for treatment. Pain is linked to transmission of information via the thalamus (T), while physical fatigue is linked to the striatum (S) and spinal cord (SC). Problems concentrating and lack of interest (termed "fibro-fog") as well as mental fatigue are linked to the prefrontal cortex (PFC), specifically the dorsolateral PFC. Fatigue, low energy, and lack of interest may all also be related to the nucleus accumbens (NA). Disturbances in sleep and appetite are associated with the hypothalamus (Hy), depressed mood with the amygdala (A) and orbital frontal cortex, and anxiety with the amygdala.

introduced in Chapter 7 and illustrated in Figure 7-17; in Chapter 8, it is illustrated in Figures 8-9, 8-10, and 8-18 through 8-20. This concept is also discussed in relation to major depression in Chapter 11 and illustrated in Figure 11-50; in Chapter 12, on antidepressants, it is illustrated in Figures 12-121 through 12-123. In relation to anxiety disorders, it is discussed in Chapter 14 and illustrated in Figures 14-43 through 14-45. The role of boosting dopamine neurotransmission for executive dysfunction is also discussed in Chapter 17, on attention deficit hyperactivity disorder.

In terms of fibromyalgia, this same DLPFC circuit and its regulation by dopamine seem to be involved in causing problems concentrating and mental fatigue (fibro-fog) (Figure 15-22). Some very troubling preliminary reports suggest that chronic pain may even "shrink the brain" in the DLPFC and thereby contribute to cognitive dysfunction in certain pain states. Brain atrophy is discussed in relation to stress and anxiety disorders in Chapter 14 and illustrated in Figure 14-30. It would not be surprising if stressful conditions that cause pain, as well as pain that causes distress, may all be involved in causing brain atrophy and/or cognitive dysfunction in fibromyalgia. Chronic back pain, for example, has been reported to be associated with decreased prefrontal and thalamic gray matter density. Some experts have hypothesized that, in fibromyalgia and other functional somatic syndromes, the persistent perception of pain could lead to overuse of DLPFC neurons, excitotoxic cell death in this brain region, and reduction of the cortico-thalamic "brake" on nociceptive pathways. Such an outcome could cause not only increased pain perception but also diminished executive functioning.

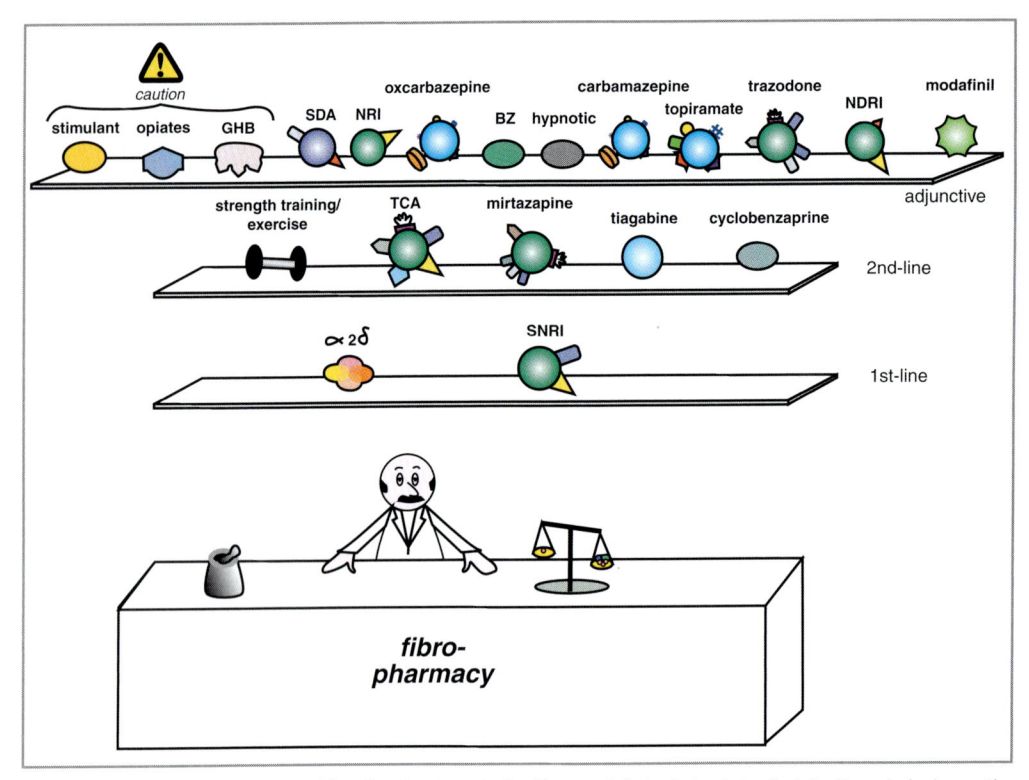

FIGURE 15-23 Fibro-pharmacy. First-line treatments for fibromyalgia include alpha 2 delta ligands (gabapentin, pregabalin) and serotonin norepinephrine reuptake inhibitors (SNRIs). Second-line treatments include strength training/exercise, tricyclic antidepressants (TCAs), mirtazapine, tiagabine (selective GABA reuptake inhibitor) and the muscle relaxant cyclobenzaprine. Adjunctive treatments may be used for the associated symptoms of fibromyalgia and are also shown here.

No matter what the cause of the cognitive dysfunction in fibromyalgia, since SNRIs increase dopamine concentrations in DLPFC (see Figure 12-36), these agents can improve symptoms of fibro-fog in fibromyalgia patients. This may be particularly so for the SNRI milnacipran, which has potent norepinephrine reuptake binding properties at all clinically effective doses (Figure 12-41), or for higher doses of the SNRIs duloxetine, venlafaxine, and desvenlafaxine, which act to increase norepinephrine reuptake blocking properties of these agents and thus act to increase concentrations of dopamine in DLPFC. Other strategies for improving fibro-fog in fibromyalgia patients include the same ones used to treat cognitive dysfunction in depression, outlined in Chapter 12 and illustrated in Figure 12-123. These approaches are also listed in the "fibro-pharmacy" illustrated in Figure 15-23 and include modafinil, selective norepinephrine reuptake inhibitors (NRIs) such as atomoxetine, norepinephrine dopamine reuptake inhibitors (NDRIs) such as bupropion, and, with caution, stimulants. SNRIs, sometimes augmented with modafinil, stimulants, or bupropion, can also be useful for symptoms of physical fatigue as well as mental fatigue in fibromyalgia patients.

Second-line treatments for pain in fibromyalgia are illustrated in the fibro-pharmacy of Figure 15-23 and can include the antidepressants mirtazapine and tricyclic antidepressants as well as the tricyclic muscle relaxant cyclobenzaprine. The anticonvulsant tiagabine can not only help pain but also enhance slow-wave sleep in some patients with fibromyalgia; however, it can be difficult to dose and may rarely cause seizures (Figure 15-23).

Adjunctive treatments for fibromyalgia pain that can augment first-line treatments include not only opiates (with caution) but also anticonvulsants such as oxcarbazepine, carbamazepine, and topiramate (Figure 15-23). Sleep aids such as benzodiazepines, hypnotics, and trazodone can be helpful in relieving sleep disturbance in fibromyalgia (Figure 15-23). Evidence is also accumulating for the efficacy of gamma hydroxybutyrate (GHB, or sodium oxybate) in fibromyalgia (to be used with extreme caution because of diversion and abuse potential) (Figure 15-23). GHB is approved for narcolepsy, enhances slow-wave sleep, and is discussed in Chapter 16, on sleep. In heroic cases, the use of GHB by experts for the treatment of severe and treatment-resistant cases of fibromyalgia may be justified. Occasionally, serotonin dopamine antagonists as augmenting agents to first-line treatments can be helpful for sleep and pain symptoms in fibromyalgia (Figure 15-23). Nondrug treatments such as strength training and exercise may also prove effective in reducing pain in fibromyalgia. Obviously, a multidisciplinary approach to the treatment of fibromyalgia may yield the best results, analogous to how psychotherapy can enhance the efficacy of antidepressants in many patients with depression or an anxiety disorder.

In summary, there are many new therapeutic vistas for fibromyalgia. The strategies that have been discussed for mood disorders and psychotic disorders in previous chapters for choosing treatments apply to the psychopharmacological approach to fibromyalgia: namely, deconstructing the symptoms of the disorder into component symptoms (Figure 15-21), then matching these symptoms to hypothetically malfunctioning brain circuits (Figure 15-22), and finally choosing and combining treatments that target neurotransmitters in these circuits to reduce all symptoms and attain remission (Figure 15-23).

Gut feelings about irritable bowel syndrome

The brain and the gut have parallel pharmacological regulatory systems that are also interlinked. Since irritable bowel syndrome may result from malfunctioning of these pharmacological systems and their regulatory mechanisms, future treatments could be directed simultaneously at both the brain and the gut. The gut is controlled peripherally by a "little brain" – namely, the enteric nervous system – derived from the same neural crest as the central nervous system. Gut motility is regulated not only by neurotransmitters of enteric neurons that innervate the bowel but also by neurotransmitters in brain regions such as the locus coeruleus and vagal nerve centers.

The diagnostic criteria for irritable bowel syndrome are given in Table 15-9. Irritable bowel syndrome may share a common pathophysiology with anxiety and affective disorders and with other functional somatic syndromes, which may also explain why it is so commonly comorbid with them (Figure 15-18). Effective treatments for anxiety and affective disorders may relieve irritable bowel syndrome, by both a central pharmacological action and a peripheral pharmacological action directly in the gut. By analogy with other functional somatic syndromes that may have a component of neuropathic pain, it seems possible that the use of SNRIs and alpha 2 delta ligands may prove useful in the pain of irritable bowel syndrome. Trials are ongoing.

Pain in other functional somatic syndromes

Charles Darwin, the nineteenth-century naturalist and author of *The Origin of Species*, suffered from multiple physical complaints for most of his adult years. His symptoms involved many organ systems; he often complained of digestive problems, insomnia, numb

TABLE 15-9 Diagnostic criteria for irritable bowel syndrome (IBS)

At least 3 months of continuous or recurrent symptoms of:
- Abdominal pain or discomfort that is:
  – relieved with defecation; and/or
  – associated with a change in frequency of stool; and/or
  – associated with a change in consistency of stool; and
- Two or more of the following, at least 25% of occasions or days:
  – altered stool frequency (>3 bowel movements each day or <3 bowel movements each week)
  – altered stool form (lumpy/hard or loose/watery stool)
  – altered stool passage (straining, urgency or feeling of incomplete evacuation)
  – passage of mucus; and/or
  – bloating or feeling of abdominal distention

TABLE 15-10 Tips for the evaluation of pain

- Location of pain
- How and when pain started
- Character of pain
- Continuous or intermittent
- Factors that cause or worsen
- Factors that relieve or lessen
- Effects of positions and activities
- Effects of stress
- Effects of alcohol, prescriptions on pain
- Presence of depression
- Presence of sleep disturbance
- Effect on work/school functioning
- Effect on quality of life: sexual, social, family
- Prior treatments, effects on pain and side effects
- Is there a lawsuit or anyone the patient blames for pain?
- Is the patient confident to pursue everyday activities despite pain?
- Does the patient believe pain will never get better?
- Coping strategies
- Psychosocial support

fingertips, and, many evenings, he vomited right after dinner. This chronic illness, which impaired his functioning, severely limited his activities, and altered the course of his life, was present during the 22-year period when Darwin was writing *The Origin of Species* (published in 1859). As a young man he had episodes of abdominal distress, especially in stressful situations, and in anticipation of his voyage on the *Beagle* he experienced cardiac palpitations and chest pain. At the age of 28 he was writing in his journal: "I have awakened in the night being slightly unwell and felt so much afraid though my reason was laughing and told me there was nothing to and tried to seize hold of objects to be frightened of." In turning down an invitation to attend a social event, he told his friends that he dreaded "going anywhere, on account of my stomach so easily failing under any excitement." Throughout the remainder of his life, Darwin experienced recurrent attacks accompanied by a variety of physical and emotional symptoms including shortness of breath, palpitations, light-headedness, trembling, and abdominal distress; he saw himself as an invalid, and medical appointments were made for his "frail condition." Within 2 years of the onset of his

TABLE 15-11 Numerical rating scale for monitoring pain during treatment

Basic requirement: measure amount of pain

Have you experienced unusual or ongoing pain recently? Yes___ No___   Location of pain_____(provide body figure drawing if necessary)

Numeric rating scale (NRS)

	No pain 0									Worst possible pain 10
Overall pain now (circle one)	0	1	2	3	4	5	6	7	8	9	10
Average over past week	0	1	2	3	4	5	6	7	8	9	10
Worst pain over past week	0	1	2	3	4	5	6	7	8	9	10
Least pain over past week	0	1	2	3	4	5	6	7	8	9	10
Acceptable level of pain	0	1	2	3	4	5	6	7	8	9	10
I would be happy with my treatment/could do the things I want/return to work, etc. if I had a pain level of	0	1	2	3	4	5	6	7	8	9	10
What medication and other treatments do you use for pain relief now?											

	No relief									Complete relief
Level of pain relief (with current medication and other treatments)	0	1	2	3	4	5	6	7	8	9	10

TABLE 15-12 Pain diaries: good or bad

Good	Bad
Patients have trouble accurately recalling pain during the previous week	Patients often don't write in it every day, so recall is still a problem
Diary gives a more reliable record of pain each day	Focuses patient's attention on the pain, perhaps making it worse
Identify pain triggers	
Identify pain relief approaches	
Can also record amount/frequency of medication, and verify compliance	
Useful for patients who believe they can conquer their pain	Detrimental for patients prone to catastrophizing or who feel pessimistic about treatment outcomes

illness, he had begun to live "the life of a hermit." His doctors considered "dyspepsia with an aggravated character," "catarrhal dyspepsia," and "suppressed gout." In his later years, many of his symptoms subsided, and he lived to the age of 73. Based on this information, historians have suggested a variety of diagnoses from arsenic poisoning to Da Costa syndrome to hyperventilation to neurasthenia. Had he lived in the twenty-first century, would Darwin's condition have been diagnosed as an affective spectrum disorder such as panic disorder or a functional somatic syndrome such as fibromyalgia?

Many of the functional somatic syndromes listed in Table 15-5 remain poorly characterized and without effective treatments and represent the frontier of pain research in psychopharmacology today. In the meantime, while diagnostic criteria are being standardized and treatments discovered, some general principles of good pain management can apply to these conditions as well as to all the other painful conditions discussed in this chapter (Tables 15-10 through 15-12). That is, evaluation of pain from any cause can be done as suggested in Table 15-10 and monitored as suggested in Table 15-11 with a numerical rating scale or in Table 15-12 with a pain diary. Having an open mind and utilizing treatments that rationally target hypothetically malfunctioning brain circuits may be the most useful approach for the modern clinical psychopharmacologist.

Summary

This chapter has defined pain and has explained the processing of nociceptive neuronal activity into the perception of pain by pathways that lead to the spinal cord and then up the spinal cord to the brain. Neuropathic pain is discussed extensively, including both peripheral and central mechanisms and the concept of central sensitization. The key role of descending inhibitory pathways that reduce the activity of nociceptive pain neurons with the release of serotonin and norepinephrine is explained and shown to be the basis for the actions of serotonin norepinephrine reuptake inhibitors (SNRIs) as agents that reduce the perception of pain in conditions ranging from major depression to fibromyalgia to diabetic peripheral neuropathy. The critical role of voltage-sensitive calcium channels is also explained, providing the basis for the actions of alpha 2 delta ligands as agents that also reduce the perception of pain in diabetic peripheral neuropathy and fibromyalgia. Finally, the spectrum of conditions from affective disorders to painful functional somatic syndromes is introduced, with emphasis on the condition of fibromyalgia and its newly evolving psychopharmacological treatments.

CHAPTER 16

Disorders of Sleep and Wakefulness and Their Treatment

- Neurobiology of sleep and wakefulness
  - The arousal spectrum
  - Sleep/wake switch
  - Histamine
- Insomnia and hypnotics
  - What is insomnia?
  - Chronic treatment for chronic insomnia?
  - Benzodiazepine hypnotics
  - GABA-A positive allosteric modulators (PAMs) as hypnotics
  - Psychiatric insomnia and the GABA-A PAMs
  - Melatonergic hypnotics
  - Serotonergic hypnotics
  - Histamine H1 antagonists as hypnotics
  - Who cares about slow-wave sleep?
  - The hypnotic pharmacy
- Excessive daytime sleepiness (hypersomnia) and wake-promoting agents
  - What is sleepiness?
  - How sleepy is sleepiness?
  - What's wrong with being sleepy?
  - Mechanism of action of wake-promoting agents
  - The wake-up pharmacy
- Summary

This chapter provides a brief overview of the psychopharmacology of disorders of sleep and wakefulness. Included here are short discussions of the symptoms, diagnostic criteria, and treatments for disorders that cause insomnia, excessive daytime sleepiness, or both. Clinical descriptions and formal criteria for how to diagnose sleep disorders are mentioned here only in passing. The reader should consult standard reference sources for this material. The discussion here emphasizes the links between various brain circuits and their neurotransmitters with disorders that cause insomnia or sleepiness. The goal of this chapter is to acquaint the reader with ideas about the clinical and biological aspects of sleep and wakefulness, how various disorders can alter sleep and wakefulness, and how many new and evolving treatments can resolve the symptoms of insomnia and sleepiness.

The detection, assessment, and treatment of sleep/wake disorders are rapidly becoming standardized parts of a psychiatric evaluation. Modern psychopharmacologists increasingly consider sleep to be a psychiatric "vital sign," thus requiring routine evaluation and symptomatic treatment whenever a sleep problem is encountered. This is similar to the earlier discussion in Chapter 15, where pain is also increasingly being considered as another psychiatric vital sign. That is, disorders of sleep (and pain) are so important, so pervasive, and cut across so many psychiatric conditions that the elimination of these symptoms – no matter what psychiatric disorder may be present – is increasingly recognized as necessary in order to achieve full symptomatic remission for the patient.

Many of the treatments discussed in this chapter are covered in previous chapters. For details of mechanisms of insomnia treatments that are also used for the treatment of depression, the reader is referred to Chapter 12; for those insomnia treatments that share the same mechanism of action with various benzodiazepine anxiolytics, the reader is referred to Chapter 14. For various hypersomnia treatments, especially stimulants, the reader is referred to Chapter 4, which introduces drugs that target monoamine transporters, and also to Chapter 17, on ADHD, and Chapter 19, on drug abuse as well as the use and abuse of stimulants. The discussion in this chapter is at the conceptual level, not at the pragmatic level. The reader should consult standard drug handbooks (such as *Essential Psychopharmacology: Prescriber's Guide*) for details of doses, side effects, drug interactions, and other issues relevant to the prescribing of these drugs in clinical practice.

Neurobiology of sleep and wakefulness

The arousal spectrum

Although many experts approach insomnia and sleepiness by emphasizing the separate and distinct *disorders* that cause them, many pragmatic psychopharmacologists approach insomnia and excessive daytime sleepiness as important *symptoms* that cut across many conditions and occur along a spectrum from deficient arousal to excessive arousal (Figure 16-1). In this conceptualization, an awake, alert, creative and problem solving person has the right balance between too much and too little arousal (baseline brain functioning in gray at the middle of the spectrum in Figure 16-1). As arousal increases beyond normal, during the day there is hypervigilance (Figure 16-1); if this increased arousal occurs at night, there is insomnia (Figure 16-1 and overactivation of the brain in red at the right hand side of the spectrum in Figure 16-2). From a treatment perspective, insomnia can be conceptualized as a disorder of excessive nighttime arousal, with hypnotics moving the patient from too much arousal to sleep (Figure 16-2).

On the other hand, as arousal diminishes, symptoms crescendo from mere inattentiveness to more severe forms of cognitive disturbance until the patient has excessive daytime sleepiness with sleep attacks (Figure 16-1 and hypoactivation of the brain in blue at the left-hand side of the spectrum in Figure 16-3). From a treatment perspective, sleepiness can be conceptualized as a disorder of deficient daytime arousal, with wake-promoting agents moving the patient from too little arousal to being awake with normal alertness (Figure 16-3).

Note in Figure 16-1 that cognitive disturbance is the product of both too little as well as too much arousal, consistent with the need of cortical pyramidal neurons to be optimally

Arousal Spectrum of Sleep and Wakefulness

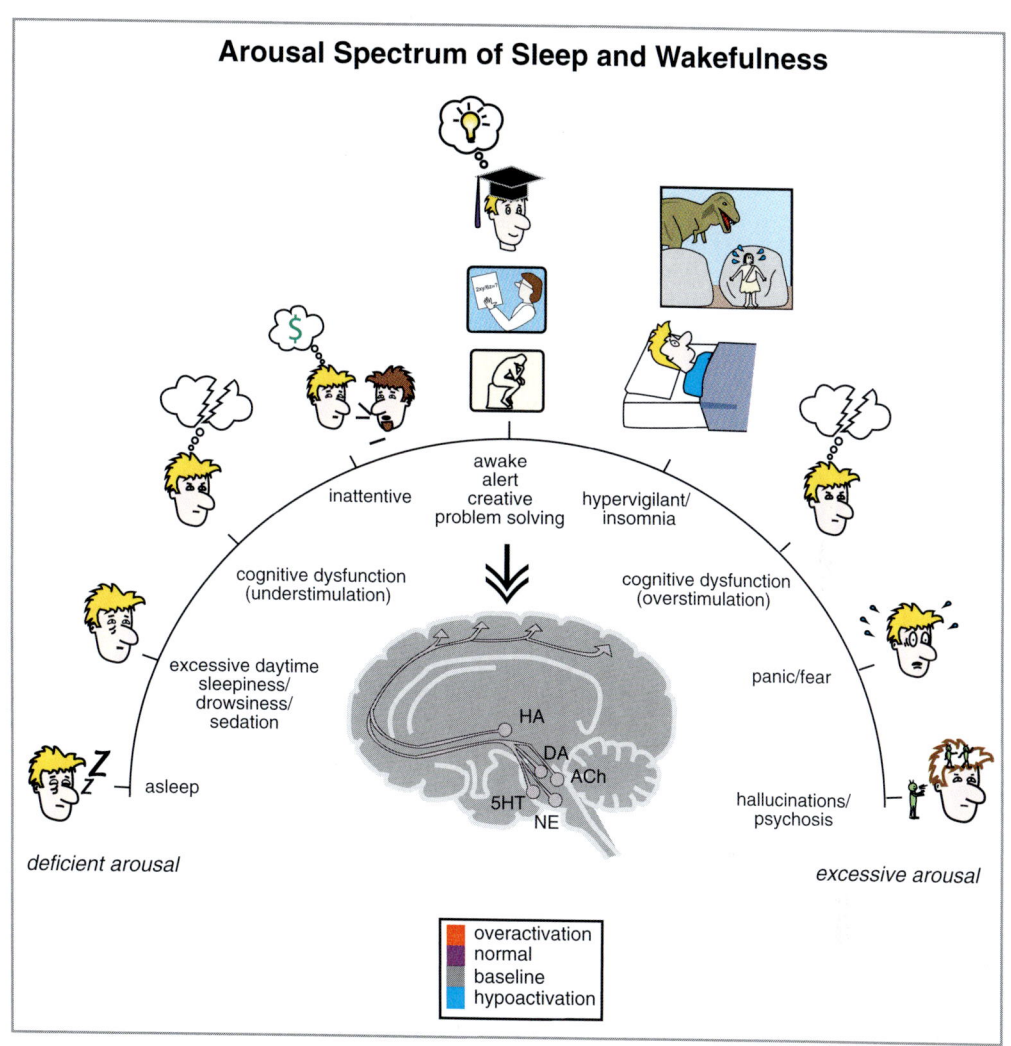

FIGURE 16-1 Arousal spectrum of sleep and wakefulness. One's state of arousal is more complicated than simply "awake" or "asleep." Rather, arousal exists as if on a dimmer switch, with many phases along the spectrum. Where on the spectrum one lies is influenced in large part by five key neurotransmitters: histamine, dopamine, norepinephrine, serotonin, and acetylcholine. When there is good balance between too much and too little arousal [depicted by the gray (baseline) color of the brain], one is awake, alert, and able to function well. As the dial shifts to the right there is too much arousal, which may cause hypervigilance and consequently insomnia at night. As arousal further increases this can cause cognitive dysfunction, panic, and in extreme cases perhaps even hallucinations. On the other hand, as arousal diminishes, individuals may experience inattentiveness, cognitive dysfunction, sleepiness, and ultimately sleep.

"tuned," with too much activity making them just as out of tune as too little. This concept is introduced in Chapter 7 and illustrated in Figures 7-25 and 7-26. Note also in Figures 16-1 through 16-3 that the arousal spectrum is linked to the actions of five neurotransmitters shown in the brains represented in these figures (i.e., histamine, dopamine, norepinephrine, serotonin, and acetylcholine). Sometimes these neurotransmitter circuits as a group are called the ascending reticular activating system, because they are known to work together to regulate arousal. The pathways for all five of these neurotransmitters are discussed in Chapter 7 and illustrated in Figures 7-8 through 7-13. This same ascending neurotransmitter system

Disorders of Sleep and Wakefulness and Their Treatment

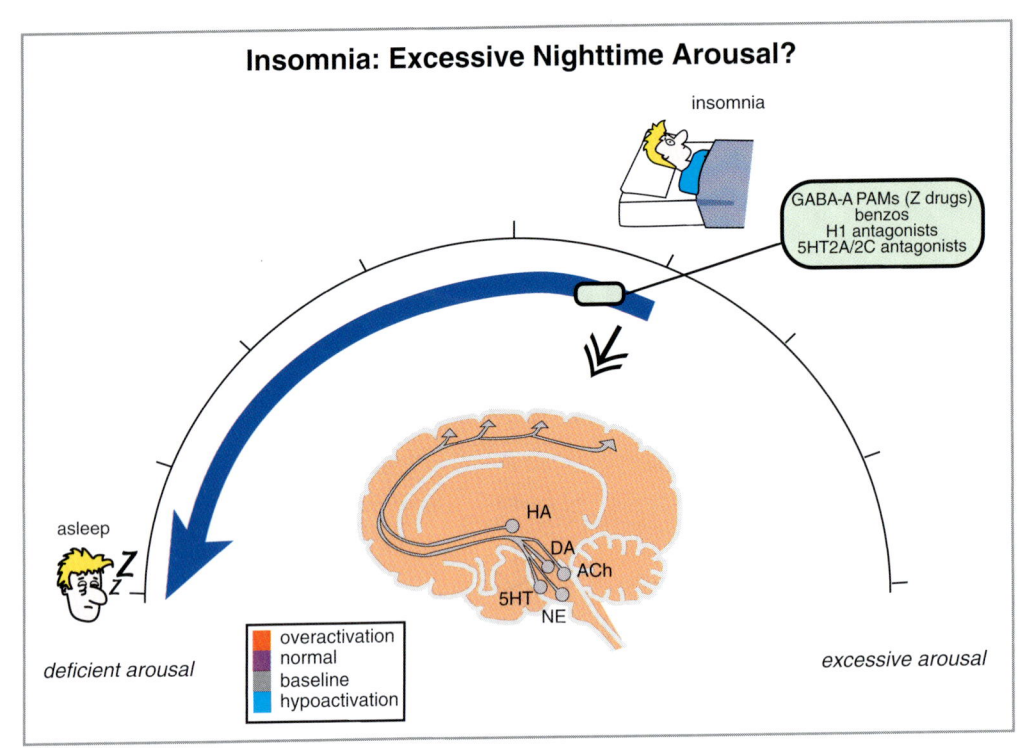

FIGURE 16-2 Insomnia: excessive nighttime arousal? Insomnia is conceptualized as hyperarousal at night, depicted here as the brain being red (overactive). Agents that reduce brain activation, such as positive allosteric modulators of GABA-A receptors (e.g., benzodiazepines, "Z-drugs"), histamine 1 antagonists, and serotonin 2A/2C antagonists, can shift one's arousal state from hyperactive to sleep.

is blocked at several sites by many agents that cause sedation. Actions of sedating drugs on these neurotransmitters are discussed in Chapter 10 on antipsychotics and illustrated in Figures 10-70 through 10-77.

A more sophisticated version of brain circuits regulating arousal is shown in Figures 16-4 and 16-5. Cortico-striatal-thalamic-cortical (CSTC) loops regulate arousal in part by controlling the size of a thalamic filter, thus regulating arousal by filtering out sensory input for normal sleep (Figure 16-4B) or by allowing sensory input to the cortex for normal wakefulness (Figure 16-5B). CSTC loops are introduced in Chapter 7 and illustrated in Figures 7-16 through 7-22.

Sleep/wake disorders can be conceptualized as a problem with the thalamic filters in these CSTC loops, causing insomnia when they fail to filter out sensory input to the cortex at night (Figure 16-4A) or daytime sleepiness when they filter out too much sensory input to the cortex during the day (Figure 16-5A). Treatment of insomnia (Figure 16-4A) is thus conceptualized as boosting the thalamic filter with GABA-enhancing agents (Figure 16-4B), whereas treatment of sleepiness (Figure 16-5A) is conceptualized as reducing the thalamic filter with dopaminergic agents (Figure 16-5B).

This same circuitry is also discussed in Chapter 9 in relation to psychosis and illustrated in Figures 9-41A through 9-41E. Note in Figure 16-1 that excessive arousal can extend past insomnia to panic, hallucinations, and all the way to frank psychosis (far right-hand side of the spectrum). In the case of psychosis, extreme arousal may be linked to a very

818 | Essential Psychopharmacology

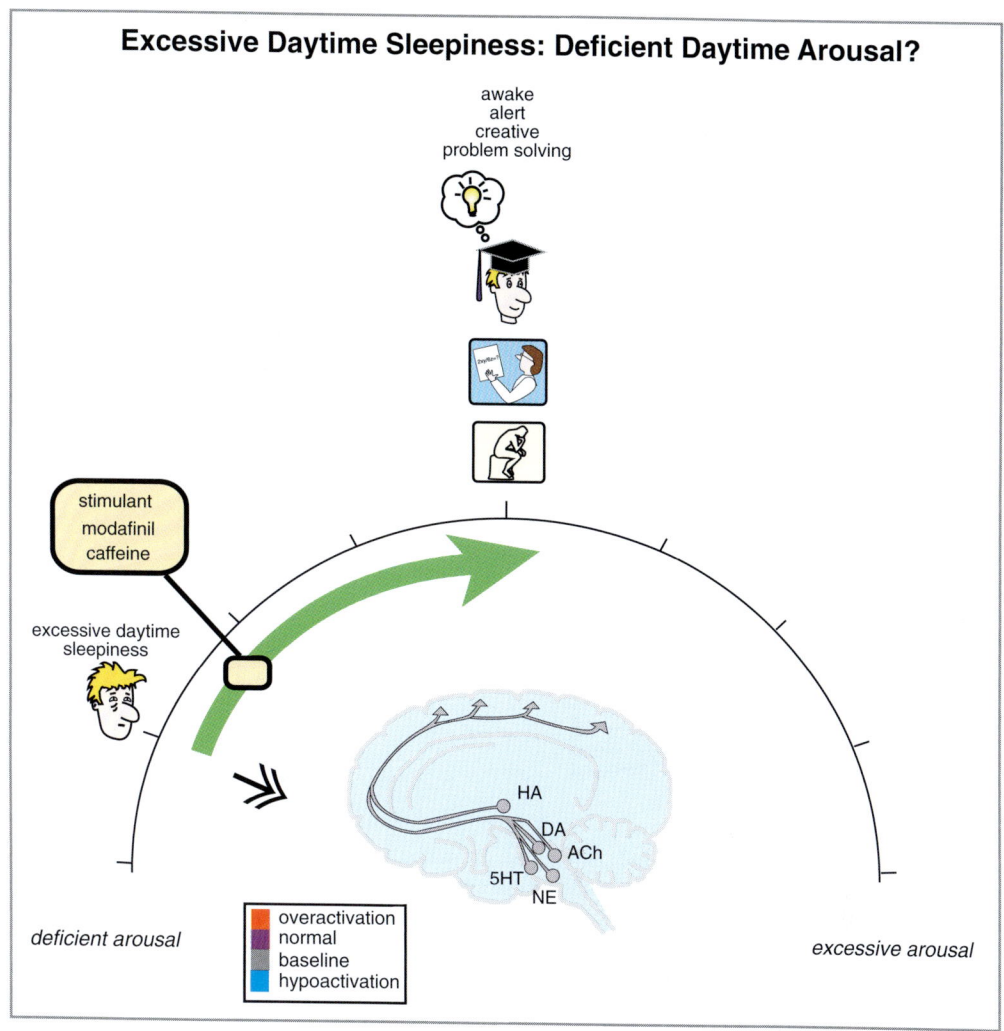

FIGURE 16-3 Excessive daytime sleepiness: deficient daytime arousal. Excessive sleepiness is conceptualized as hypoarousal during the day, depicted here as the brain being blue (hypoactive). Agents that increase brain activation, such as the stimulants, modafinil, and caffeine, can shift one's arousal state from hypoactive to awake with normal alertness.

ineffective thalamic filter that results from dopamine hyperactivity (Figure 9-41D) and glutamate hypoactivity (Figure 9-41E).

Sleep/wake switch

We have discussed how the ascending neurotransmitter systems from the brainstem regulate a cortical arousal system on a smooth continuum like a rheostat on a lighting system or a volume button on a radio. There is another set of circuits in the hypothalamus that regulate sleep and wake discontinuously, like an on–off switch. Not surprisingly, this circuitry is called the "sleep/wake switch" (Figure 16-6). The "on" switch is known as the "wake promoter" and is localized within the tuberomammillary nucleus (TMN) of the hypothalamus (Figure 16-6A). The "off" switch is known as the "sleep promoter" and is localized within the ventrolateral preoptic (VLPO) nucleus of the hypothalamus (Figure 16-6B).

Disorders of Sleep and Wakefulness and Their Treatment | 819

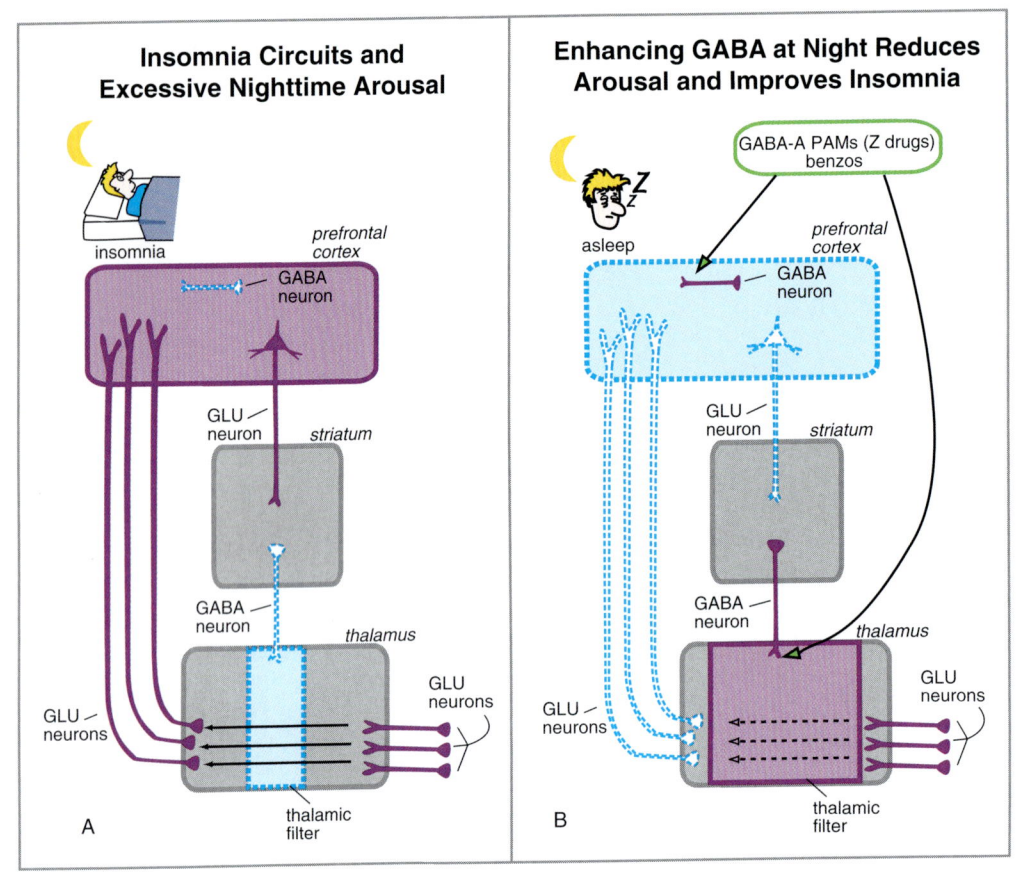

FIGURE 16-4A and B Insomnia circuits. Pyramidal glutamatergic neurons descend from the prefrontal cortex to the striatum, where they terminate on gamma-aminobutyric acid (GABA) neurons that project to the thalamus. The release of GABA in the thalamus creates a sensory filter that, when effective, filters out most sensory input arriving in the thalamus, so that only selected types of sensory input are relayed to the cortex. (**A**) In insomnia, this GABA-ergic neurotransmission may be deficient at night, thus reducing the effectiveness of the filter so that too much input reaches the cortex and the individual is hyperaroused. (**B**) Administration of GABA-ergic medications at night may restore the filter and thus reduce glutamatergic input to the cortex, allowing sleep to occur.

Two other sets of neurons are shown in Figure 16-6 as regulators of the sleep/wake switch: orexin-containing neurons of the lateral hypothalamus (LAT) and melatonin-sensitive neurons of the suprachiasmatic nucleus (SCN). The lateral hypothalamus serves to stabilize and promote wakefulness via a peptide neurotransmitter known by two different names: orexin and hypocretin. These lateral hypothalamic neurons and their orexin are lost in narcolepsy, especially narcolepsy with cataplexy. The SCN is the brain's internal clock, or pacemaker, and regulates circadian input to the sleep/wake switch in response to how it is programmed by hormones such as melatonin and by the light/dark cycle. The circadian wake drive is shown in Figure 16-7 over two full 24-hour cycles.

Also shown in Figure 16-7 is the ultradian sleep cycle [a cycle faster than a day, showing cycling in and out of rapid-eye-movement (REM) and slow-wave sleep several times during the night]. Homeostatic sleep drive is also shown in Figure 16-7, which increases the drive for sleep as the day goes on, presumably due to fatigue, and diminishes at night with rest. The novel neurotransmitter adenosine is linked to homeostatic drive and appears to

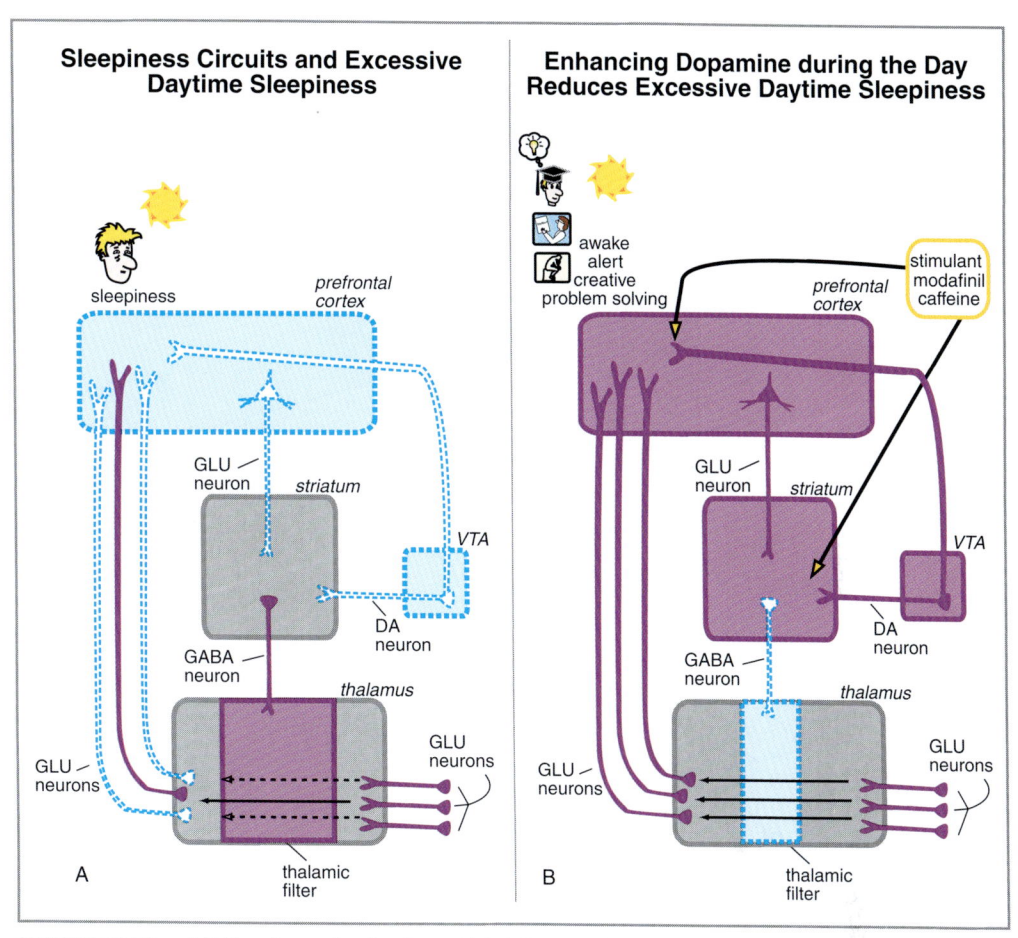

FIGURE 16-5A and B Sleepiness circuits. Pyramidal glutamatergic neurons descend from the prefrontal cortex to the striatum, where they terminate on gamma-aminobutyric acid (GABA) neurons that project to the thalamus. The release of GABA in the thalamus creates a sensory filter that, when effective, filters out most sensory input arriving in the thalamus, so that only selected types of sensory input are relayed to the cortex. Dopaminergic input to the nucleus accumbens via the mesolimbic dopamine pathway has an inhibitory effect on GABA neurons, which reduces the effectiveness of the thalamic sensory filter since less GABA is released by GABA neurons projecting from the nucleus accumbens to the thalamus. (**A**) If dopaminergic projections to the nucleus accumbens are hypoactive during the day, the filter may not allow enough sensory input to reach the cortex, and excessive daytime sleepiness can occur. (**B**) Enhancing dopaminergic neurotransmission during the day may reduce the filter and thus allow enough sensory input to reach the cortex so that normal wakefulness can occur.

accumulate as this drive increases during the day and to diminish at night. Caffeine is now known to be an antagonist of adenosine, and this may explain in part its ability to promote wakefulness and diminish fatigue by opposing endogenous adenosine's regulation of the homeostatic sleep drive.

Two key neurotransmitters regulate the sleep/wake switch: histamine from the TMN and GABA from the VLPO. Thus, when the sleep/wake switch is on, the wake promoter TMN is active and histamine is released (Figure 16-6A). This occurs both in the cortex to facilitate arousal and in the VLPO to inhibit the sleep promoter. As the day progresses, circadian wake drive diminishes and homeostatic sleep drive increases (Figure 16-7); eventually a tipping point is reached, and the VLPO sleep promoter is triggered, the sleep/wake

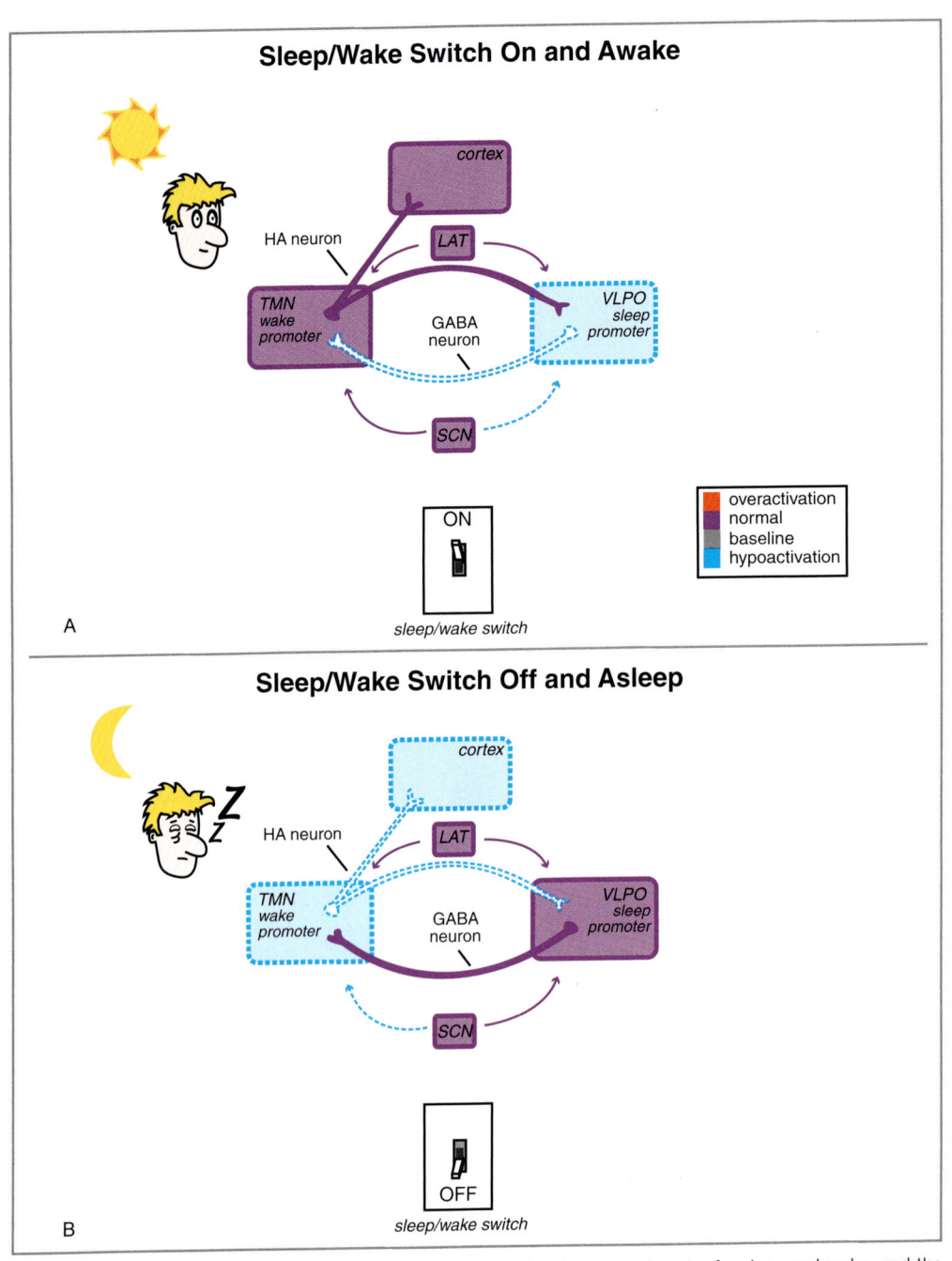

FIGURE 16-6A and B Sleep/wake switch. The hypothalamus is a key control center for sleep and wake, and the specific circuitry that regulates sleep/wake is called the sleep/wake switch. The "off" setting, or sleep promoter, is localized within the ventrolateral preoptic nucleus (VLPO) of the hypothalamus; while "on"–wake promoter – is localized within the tuberomammillary nucleus (TMN) of the hypothalamus. Two key neurotransmitters regulate the sleep/wake switch: histamine from the TMN and GABA from the VLPO. (**A**) When the TMN is active and histamine is released in the cortex and the VLPO, the wake promoter is on and the sleep promoter is inhibited. (**B**) When the VLPO is active and GABA is released in the TMN, the sleep promoter is on and the wake promoter inhibited. The sleep/wake switch is also regulated by orexin/hypocretin neurons in the lateral hypothalamus (LAT), which stabilize wakefulness, and by the suprachiasmatic nucleus (SCN) of the hypothalamus, which is the body's internal clock and is activated by melatonin, light, and activity to promote either sleep or wake.

Processes Regulating Sleep

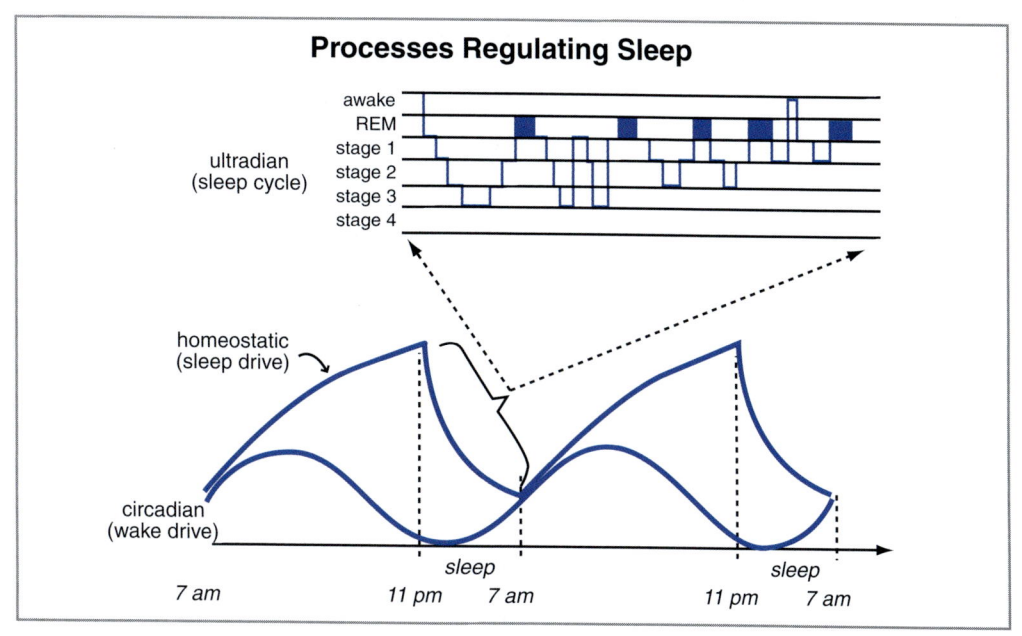

FIGURE 16-7 Processes regulating sleep. Several processes that regulate sleep/wake are shown here. The circadian wake drive is a result of input (light, melatonin, activity) to the suprachiasmatic nucleus. Homeostatic sleep drive increases the longer one is awake and decreases with sleep. As the day progresses, circadian wake drive diminishes and homeostatic sleep drive increases until a tipping point is reached and the ventrolateral preoptic sleep promoter (VLPO) is triggered to release GABA in the tuberomammillary nucleus (TMN) and inhibit wakefulness. Sleep itself consists of multiple phases that recur in a cyclical manner; this process is known as the ultradian cycle and depicted at the top of this figure.

switch is turned off, and GABA is released in the TMN to inhibit wakefulness (Figure 16-6B).

Disorders characterized by excessive daytime sleepiness can be conceptualized as the sleep/wake switch being off during the daytime (Figure 16-8A). Wake-promoting treatments such as modafinil given during the day tip the balance back to wakefulness by promoting the release of histamine from TMN neurons (Figure 16-8B). The exact mechanism of this enhancement of histamine release by modafinil or stimulants is not known but is currently hypothesized to be related in part to a downstream consequence of wake-promoting drug actions on dopamine neurons. Actions of wake-promoting drugs on dopamine are discussed later in this chapter and are also shown in Figure 16-5B.

On the other hand, disorders characterized by insomnia can be conceptualized as the sleep/wake switch being on at night (Figure 16-9A). Insomnia can be treated either by agents that enhance GABA actions, and thus inhibit the wake promoter (Figure 16-9B), or by agents that block the action of histamine released from the wake promoter and act at postsynaptic H1 receptors (Figure 16-9C).

Disorders characterized by a disturbance in circadian rhythm can be conceptualized as either "phase delayed," with the wake promoter and sleep/wake switch being turned on too late in a normal 24-hour cycle (Figure 16-10A), or "phase advanced," with the wake promoter and sleep/wake switch being turned on too early in a normal 24-hour cycle (Figure 16-11A). That is, individuals who are phase delayed, including many depressed patients and many normal adolescents, still have their sleep/wake switch off when it is time to get up (Figure 16-10A). Giving such individuals morning light with evening melatonin can

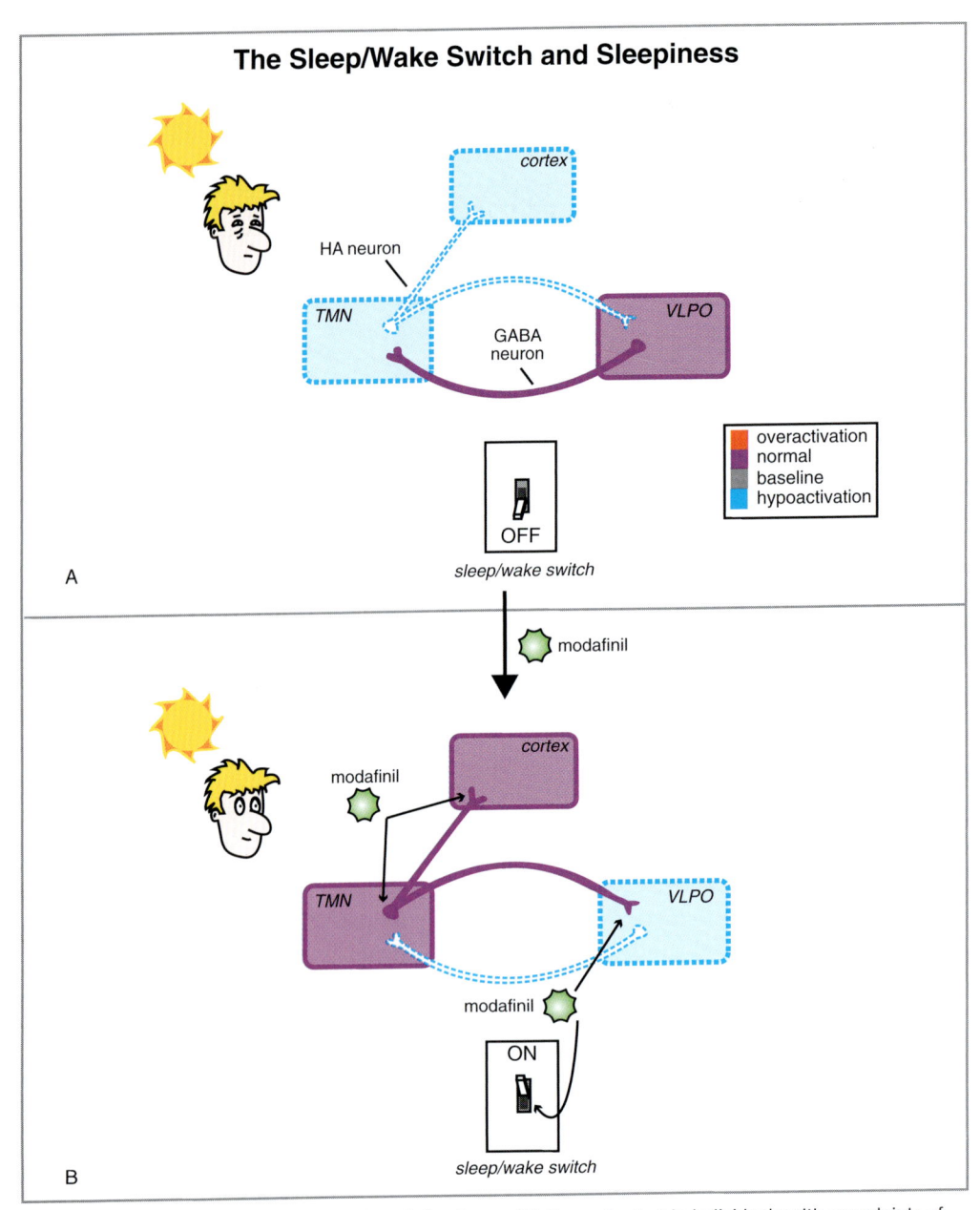

FIGURE 16-8A and B Sleep/wake switch and sleepiness. (**A**) It may be that in individuals with complaints of excessive sleepiness the sleep/wake switch is inappropriately turned "off" during the day, so that the ventrolateral preoptic area (VLPO) is active and GABA is released in the tuberomammillary nucleus (TMN) to inhibit it. (**B**) A wake-promoting treatment such as modafinil may increase histamine release, activating the TMN and inhibiting the VLPO and thus turning the sleep/wake switch "on."

reset the circadian clock in the SCN so that it wakes the person up earlier (Figure 16-10B). Other individuals may be phase advanced, including many normal elderly (Figure 16-11A). Giving these individuals evening light and morning melatonin can reset their SCNs so that the sleep/wake switch stays off a bit longer, returning the patient to a normal rhythm (Figure 16-11B).

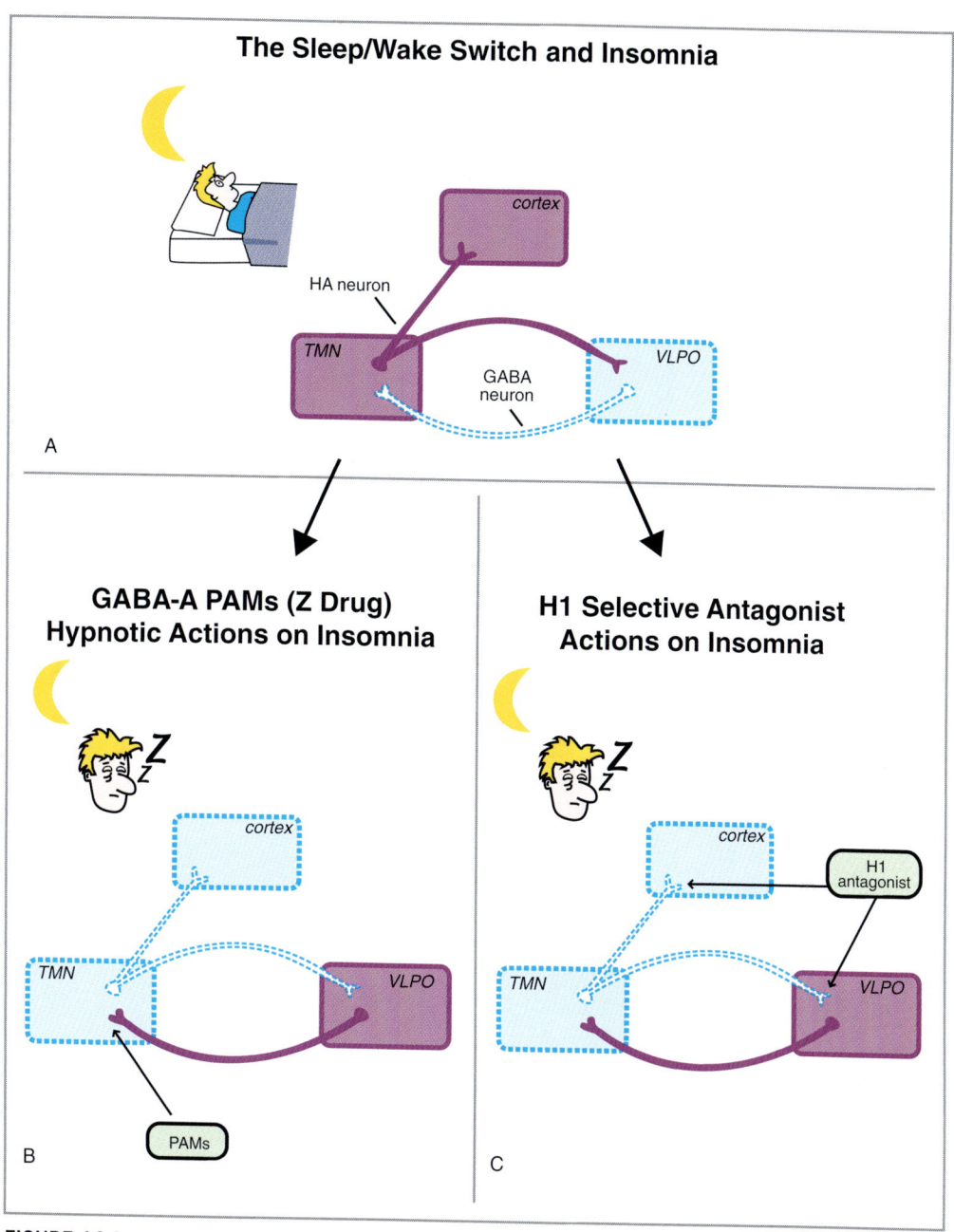

FIGURE 16-9A, B, and C Sleep/wake switch and insomnia. (A) It may be that in individuals with insomnia the sleep/wake switch is inappropriately turned "on" at night, so that the tuberomammillary nucleus (TMN) is active and histamine release inhibits the ventrolateral preoptic area (VLPO). (B) Hypnotic agents such as the "Z" drugs, which are positive allosteric modulators (PAMs) at GABA-A receptors, may increase GABA action, inhibiting the TMN and thus turning the sleep/wake switch "off." (C) Another mechanism for turning the sleep/wake switch "off" is to block histamine 1 receptors in the cortex and VLPO.

Disorders of Sleep and Wakefulness and Their Treatment

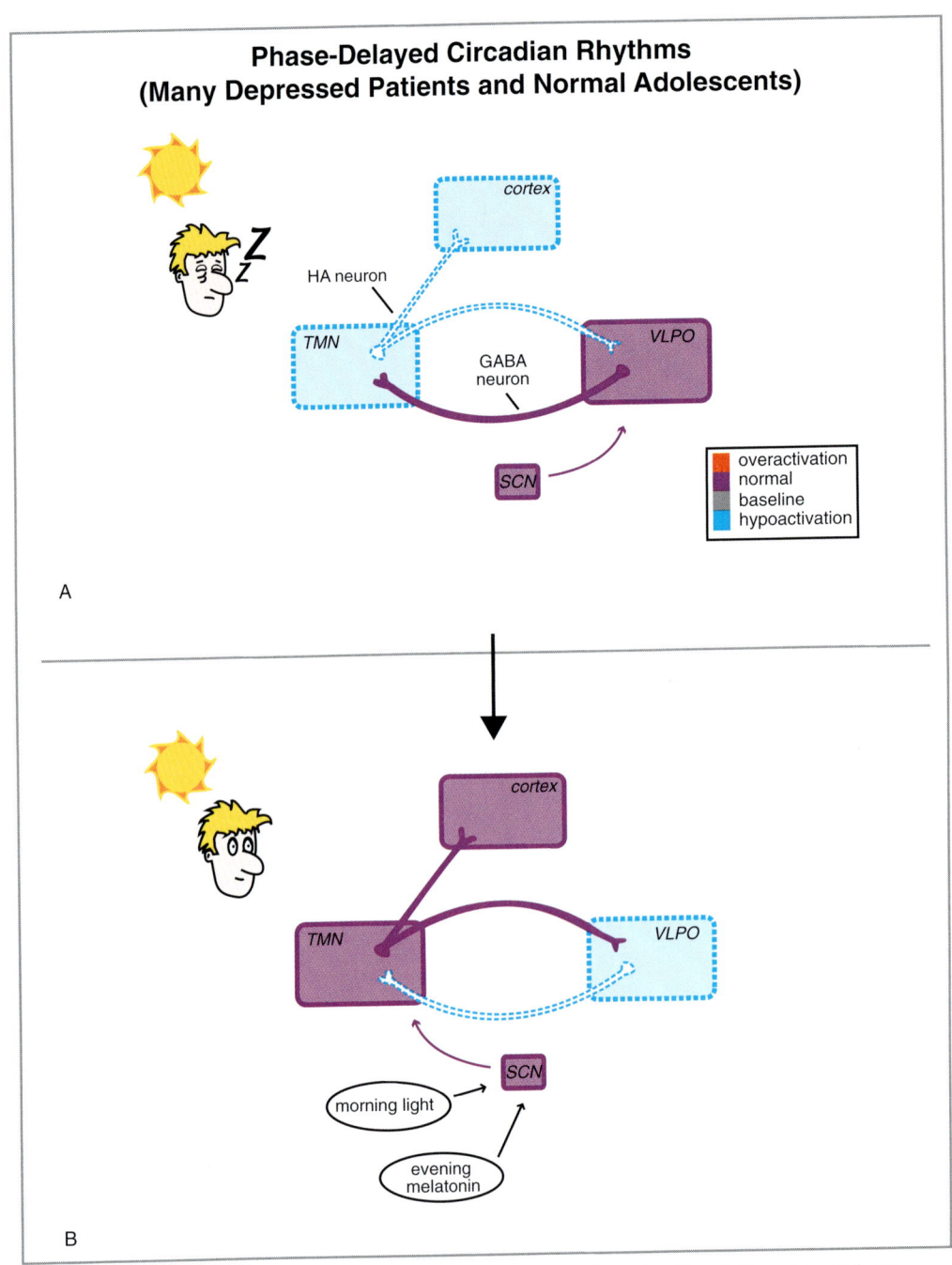

FIGURE 16-10A and B Phase delayed circadian rhythms. Shifting of the circadian rhythm of arousal can contribute to sleep/wake problems. (**A**) When the circadian rhythm is phase delayed, the sleep/wake switch is turned on too late in a normal 24-hour cycle. This is common for adolescents and for depressed patients, and causes morning sleepiness because the sleep/wake switch is still off when it is time to get up. (**B**) Individuals who have a phase delayed circadian rhythm may benefit from morning light and evening melatonin, which could help reset the suprachiasmatic nucleus (SCN) so that the sleep/wake switch turns on earlier.

826 | Essential Psychopharmacology

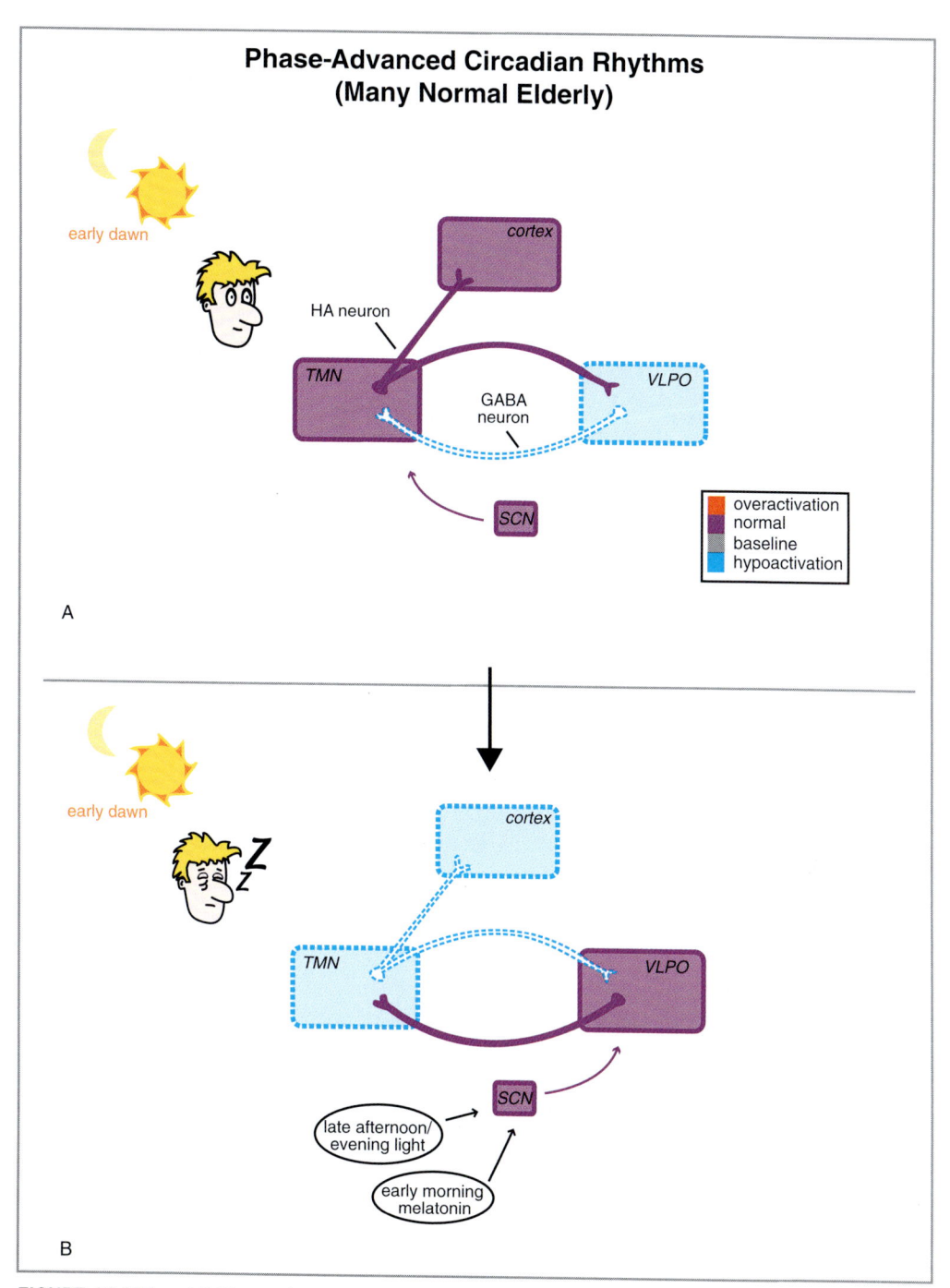

FIGURE 16-11A and B Phase advanced circadian rhythms. Shifting of the circadian rhythm of arousal can contribute to sleep/wake problems. (**A**) When the circadian rhythm is phase advanced, the sleep/wake switch is turned on too early in a normal 24-hour cycle. This is common for elderly individuals, and causes them to wake up very early in the morning. (**B**) Individuals who have a phase advanced circadian rhythm may benefit from evening light and morning melatonin, which could help reset the suprachiasmatic nucleus (SCN) so that the sleep/wake switch stays off longer.

Disorders of Sleep and Wakefulness and Their Treatment | 827

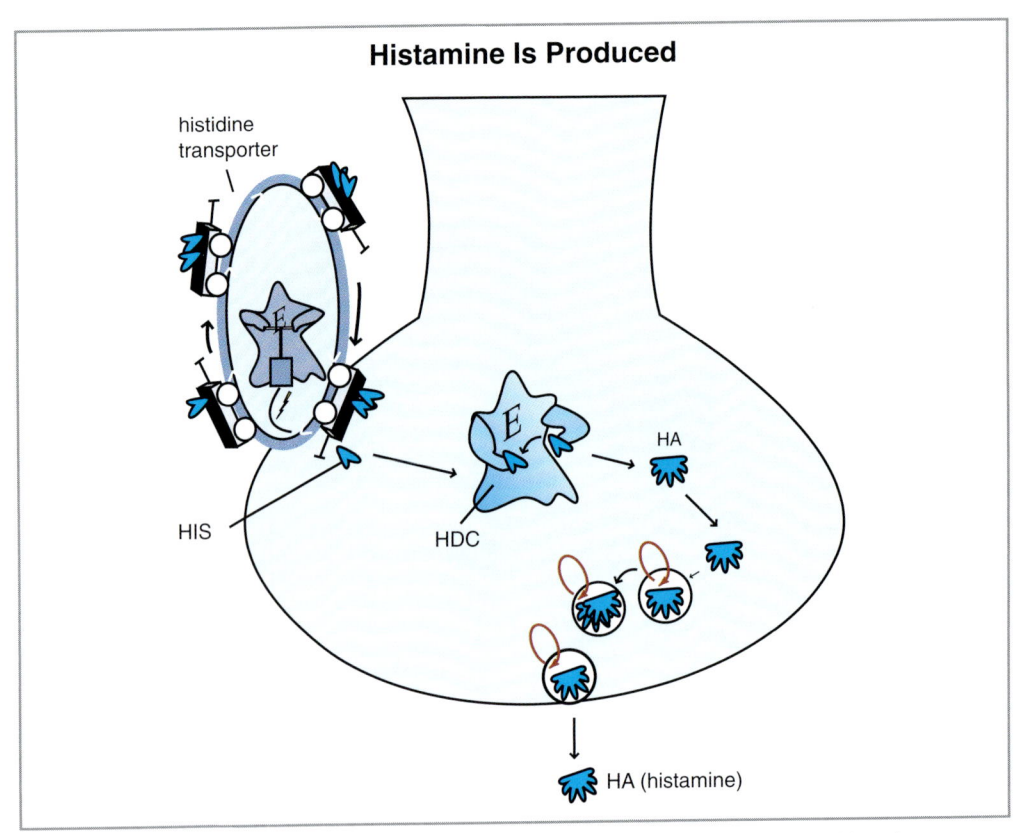

FIGURE 16-12 Histamine is produced. Histidine, a precursor to histamine, is taken up into histamine nerve terminals via a histidine transporter and converted into histamine by the enzyme histidine decarboxylase (HDC). After synthesis, histamine is packaged into synaptic vesicles and stored until its release into the synapse during neurotransmission.

Histamine

Histamine is one of the key neurotransmitters regulating wakefulness, and is the ultimate target of many wake-promoting drugs (histamine releasers) and sleep-promoting drugs (antihistamines and novel H1 selective histamine antagonists and inverse agonists). Histamine is produced from the amino acid histidine, which is taken up into histamine neurons and converted to histamine by the enzyme histidine decarboxylase (Figure 16-12). Histamine's action is terminated by two enzymes working in sequence: histamine N-methyl-transferase, which converts histamine to N-methyl-histamine, and MAO-B, which converts N-methyl-histamine into N-MIAA (N-methyl indole acetic acid), an inactive substance (Figure 16-13). Additional enzymes, such as diamine oxidase, can also terminate histamine action outside of the brain. Note that there is no apparent reuptake pump for histamine. Thus, histamine is likely to diffuse widely away from its synapse, just as dopamine does in prefrontal cortex. This concept is introduced in Chapter 3 and illustrated in Figure 3-5.

There are a number of histamine receptors (Figures 16-14 through 16-17). The postsynaptic histamine 1 receptor is best known (Figure 16-15A) because it is the target of "antihistamines" (i.e., H1 antagonists) (Figure 16-15B). When histamine itself acts at H1 receptors, it activates a G protein–linked second messenger system that activates phosphatidyl inositol and the transcription factor cFOS, resulting in wakefulness, normal alertness,

828 | Essential Psychopharmacology

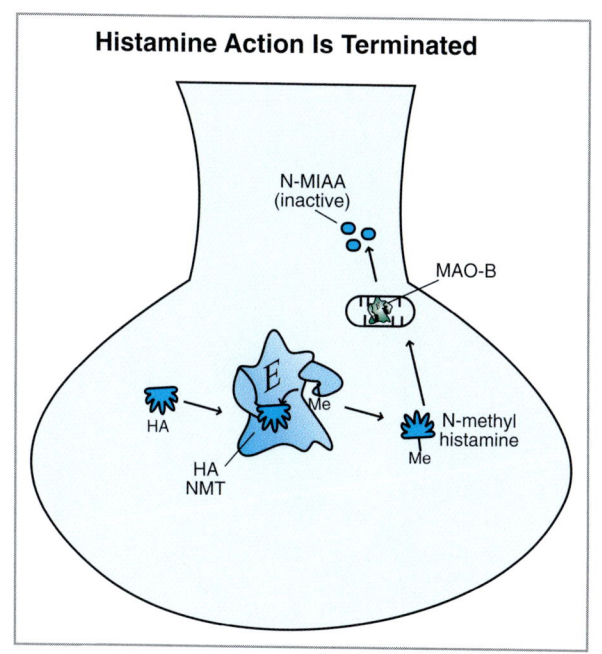

FIGURE 16-13 Histamine's action is terminated. Histamine is broken down intracellularly by two enzymes acting sequentially. Histamine N-methyl-transferase (histamine NMT) converts histamine into N-methyl-histamine, which is then converted by monoamine oxidase B (MAO-B) into the inactive substance N-methyl indole acetic acid (N-MIAA).

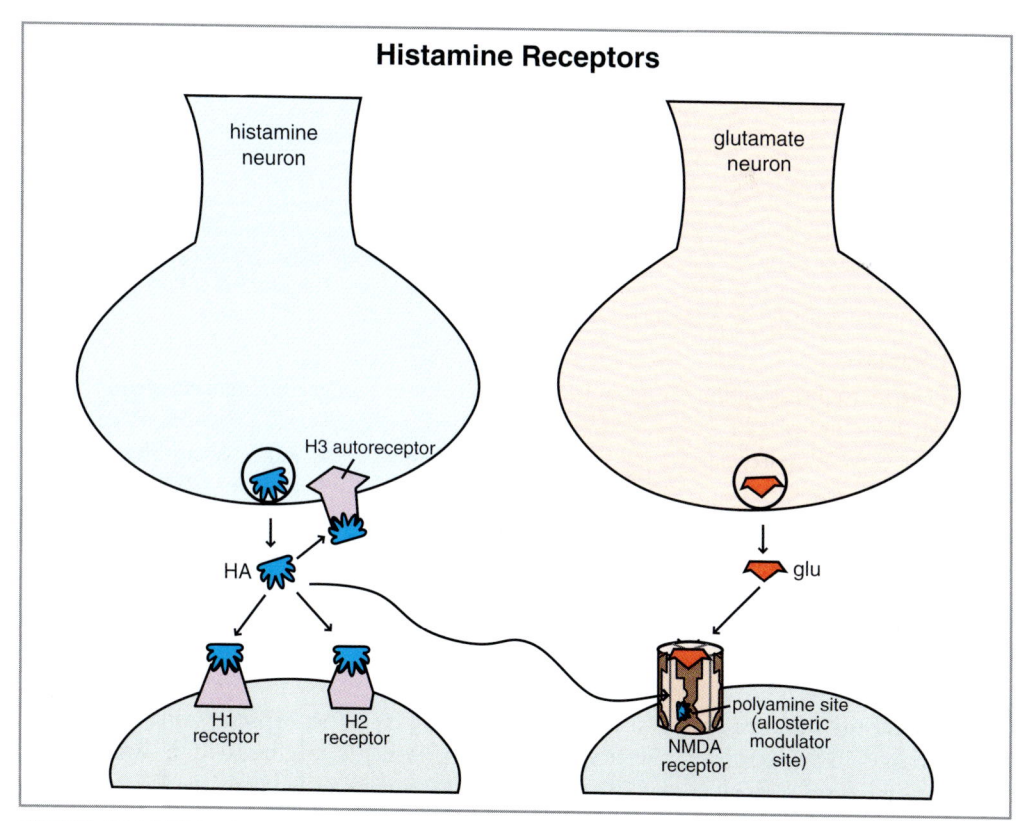

FIGURE 16-14 Histamine receptors. Shown here are receptors for histamine that regulate its neurotransmission. Histamine 1 and histamine 2 receptors are postsynaptic, while histamine 3 receptors are presynaptic autoreceptors. There is also a binding site for histamine at the polyamine site on NMDA receptors. This polyamine site is an allosteric modulatory site for glutamate action at NMDA receptors.

Disorders of Sleep and Wakefulness and Their Treatment

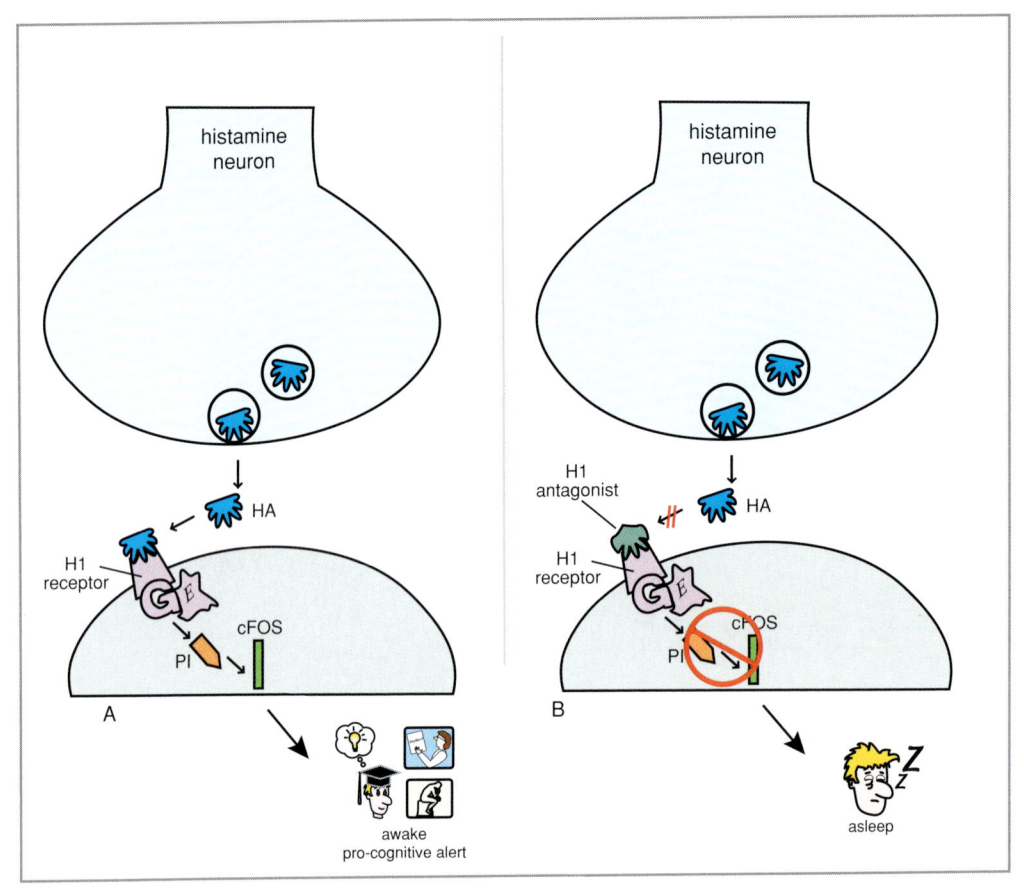

FIGURE 16-15A and B Histamine 1 receptors. (**A**) When histamine binds to postsynaptic histamine 1 receptors, it activates a G protein–linked second messenger system that produces phosphatidyl inositol and the transcription factor cFOS. This results in wakefulness and normal alertness. (**B**) Histamine 1 antagonists prevent activation of this second messenger and thus can facilitate sleep.

and pro-cognitive actions (Figure 16-15A). Second messenger cascades involving PI and cFOS are introduced in Chapter 3 and illustrated in Figures 3-22 to 3-31. When these H1 receptors are blocked in the brain, they interfere with the wake-promoting actions of histamine and thus can cause sedation, drowsiness, or sleep (Figure 16-15B).

Histamine 2 receptors, best known for their actions in gastric acid secretion and the target of a number of anti-ulcer drugs, also exist in the brain (Figure 16-16). These postsynaptic receptors also activate a G protein second messenger system with cAMP, phosphokinase A, and the gene product CREB (see Chapter 3, Figure 3-11, and Tables 3-6 and 3-7). The function of H2 receptors in brain is still being clarified but apparently is not linked directly to wakefulness.

A third histamine receptor is present in brain, namely the H3 receptor (Figure 16-14 and 16-17). Synaptic histamine H3 receptors are presynaptic (Figure 16-17A) and function as autoreceptors (Figure 16-17B). That is, when histamine binds to these receptors, it turns off further release of histamine (Figure 16-17B). One novel approach to new wake-promoting and pro-cognitive drugs is to block these receptors, thus facilitating the release of histamine and allowing histamine to act at H1 receptors to produce the desired effects (Figure 16-17C). Several H3 antagonists are in clinical development.

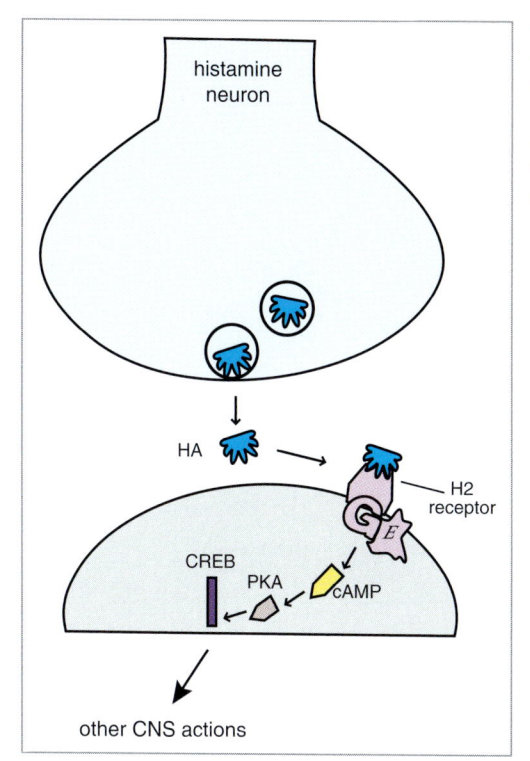

FIGURE 16-16 Histamine 2 receptors. Histamine 2 receptors are present both in the body and in the brain. When histamine binds to postsynaptic histamine 2 receptors it activates a G protein–linked second messenger system with cAMP, phosphokinase A, and the gene product CREB. The function of histamine 2 receptors in the brain is not yet elucidated.

There is a fourth type of histamine receptor, H4, but it is not known to occur in the brain. Finally, histamine also acts at NMDA receptors (Figure 16-14). Interestingly, when histamine diffuses away from its synapse to a glutamate synapse containing NMDA receptors, it can act at an allosteric modulatory site, called the polyamine site, to alter the actions of glutamate at NMDA receptors (Figure 16-14). The role of histamine and the function of this action are not well clarified.

Insomnia and hypnotics

What is insomnia?
Insomnia is defined in Table 16-1. It has many causes, including both sleep disorders (Table 16-2) and psychiatric disorders (Table 16-3). Insomnia can also contribute to the onset, exacerbation, or relapse of many psychiatric disorders (Table 16-3) and is linked to various dysfunctions in many medical illnesses (Table 16-4). Primary insomnia may be a condition with too much arousal both at night and during the day and thus may be a form of insomnia where the patient is not sleepy during the day despite having poor sleep at night (Table 16-2). Primary insomnia may also be a symptom that can progress to a first major depressive episode (Table 16-3). Is insomnia therefore a symptom or a disorder? The answer appears to be yes.

Chronic treatment for chronic insomnia?
A major reconceptualization of insomnia has recently occurred among experts, with a newly formed consensus that insomnia can be chronic and that it may need to be treated chronically. This is a departure from the position held by many sleep experts until recently, that insomnia was treated by attacking its underlying cause and not by giving symptomatically "masking" treatment with hypnotics chronically. The old guidelines recommending short-term use of

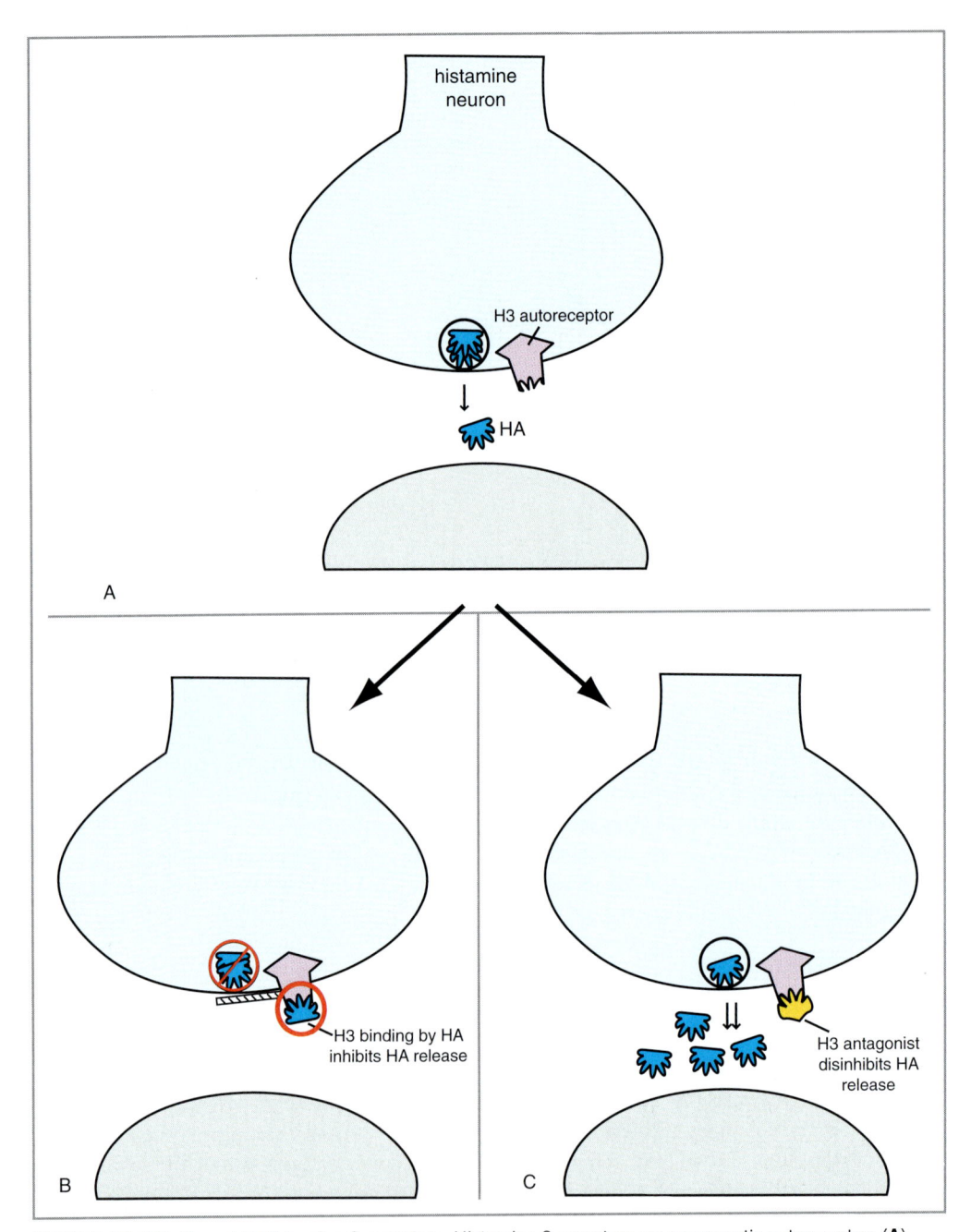

FIGURE 16-17A, B, and C Histamine 3 receptors. Histamine 3 receptors are presynaptic autoreceptors (**A**), which means that when histamine binds to these receptors it turns off further histamine release (**B**). Antagonists of these receptors, which are in development as novel wake-promoting drugs, therefore disinhibit histamine release (**C**).

TABLE 16-1 What is insomnia?

One or more of the following despite adequate opportunity to sleep:
- Difficulty initiating sleep
- Difficulty maintaining sleep
- Waking up too early
- Nonrestorative or poor quality sleep

Plus one or more daytime impairment:
- Fatigue; malaise; lack of energy, motivation, or initiative
- Daytime sleepiness
- Attention, concentration, or memory impairment
- Prone to errors or accident at work or while driving
- Mood disturbance, irritability, worries about sleep
- Physical symptoms due to sleep loss (e.g., tension headaches)

TABLE 16-2 What causes insomnia?

- Sleep disorders
  - Primary insomnia
    - Conditioned arousal at bedtime?
    - Sleep-disruptive habits?
    - Inability to sleep at night or nap during the day
    - Possible harbinger of a psychiatric disorder, especially depression
  - Restless legs syndrome
  - Periodic limb movement disorder
  - Parasomnias (nightmares, sleep terror, sleepwalking, confusional arousals, dissociative disorders, nocturnal eating disorder)
  - Circadian rhythm disorders (shift work, jet lag, delayed sleep)
  - Poor sleep hygiene
- Psychiatric illnesses
- Psychiatric and other medications
- Substance use/abuse
- Medical disorders
- Painful disorders
- Bed partner with a sleep disorder (e.g., bed partner with snoring, irregular breathing, or movements during sleep)
  - Have patient whose bed partner has a sleep disorder estimate partner's sleep quality and length and any changes in mood and performance, especially daytime sleepiness (patients complain more about fatigue and cognition than sleepiness and partners of sleepy patients complain about their partner's sleepiness)
  - Have bed partner referred for evaluation and treatment of his or her sleep disorder

hypnotics for insomnia were the product of safety concerns for hypnotics identified first during the barbiturate era and then during the benzodiazepine era.

Other problems associated with long-term use of hypnotics have to do with use of drugs whose half-lives make them not ideal for use as hypnotics (Figures 16-18A, B, and C). That is, many agents used as hypnotics have half-lives that are too long (Figure 16-18A and B). This can cause drug accumulation and hip fractures from falls, especially in the elderly, when such agents are used every night (Figure 16-18A). A long half-life can also cause next-day carryover effects and sedation as well as memory problems from residual daytime drug

TABLE 16-3 Insomnia and psychiatric illnesses

- Insomnia as a psychiatric "vital sign"
- No remission unless sleep normalized
- Increased risk of relapse unless sleep normalized
- Panic disorders and nocturnal panic: insomnia through conditioned arousal/conditioned insomnia
- PTSD: nightmares, decreased stage 3/4 sleep, increased arousal and conditioned arousal, conditioned insomnia
- Depression: increased and disrupted REM sleep, decreased stage 3/4 sleep
- Schizophrenia, mania: severe insomnia may precede relapse
- Schizophrenia: Stage 3/4 sleep decreases as negative symptoms increase

TABLE 16-4 Insomnia and medical illnesses

- The more diagnosed medical illnesses you have, the more insomnia you have
- Perimenopause: nocturnal awakenings correlate with hot flushes, hypothalamic dysregulation, and relapse/onset of major depression
- Dementia: disrupted sleep correlates with cognitive decline, especially disturbed circadian rhythm and "sundowning," nocturnal wandering, daytime sleepiness
- Parkinson's disease: nighttime pain and rigidity as meds wear off, nightmares, hallucinations, REM behavior disorder, sleep talking, and narcolepsy-like daytime symptoms
- Activation of HPA in OSA, obesity and diabetes is a risk factor for insomnia with decreased sleep associated with increased weight and appetite

TABLE 16-5 Restless legs syndrome (RLS) versus periodic limb movement disorder (PLMD)

- Clinically diagnosed as urge to move the legs, worse during inactivity, relieved in part by movement, worse in the evening
- Can prevent or delay onset of sleep; disrupt sleep if RLS returns; tiredness or sleepiness next day
- May be idiopathic or symptomatic (i.e., associated with pregnancy, end-stage renal disease, fibromyalgia, iron deficiency, arthritis, peripheral neuropathy, radiculopathy)
- Can be triggered by alcohol, nicotine, caffeine
- Majority of RLS patients have PLMD, but only a few PLMD patients have RLS; both may be linked to dopamine (DA) or iron deficiency
- RLS patients should have iron, iron stores and ferritin levels (ferritin is a cofactor of tyrosine hydroxylase, which synthesizes DA)
- RLS is not PLMD, which occurs during sleep and is diagnosed by polysomnography; there is no urge sensation to move while awake

Treatments for RLS:

Primary:
- DA agonists (ropinirole, pramipexole) (may cause somnolence, nausea)
- Iron replacement
- Levodopa (fast onset but short-acting – may just delay onset of RLS until later at night unless redosed)

Secondary:
- Gabapentin/pregabalin, especially if RLS painful; low-potency opiates (propoxyphene, codeine)
- Benzos or GABA-A PAMS

Ultralong Half-Life Hypnotics Cause Drug Accumulation (Toxicity)

A

half-lives: 24-150 hours
examples: flurazepam (Dalmane)
quazepam (Doral)

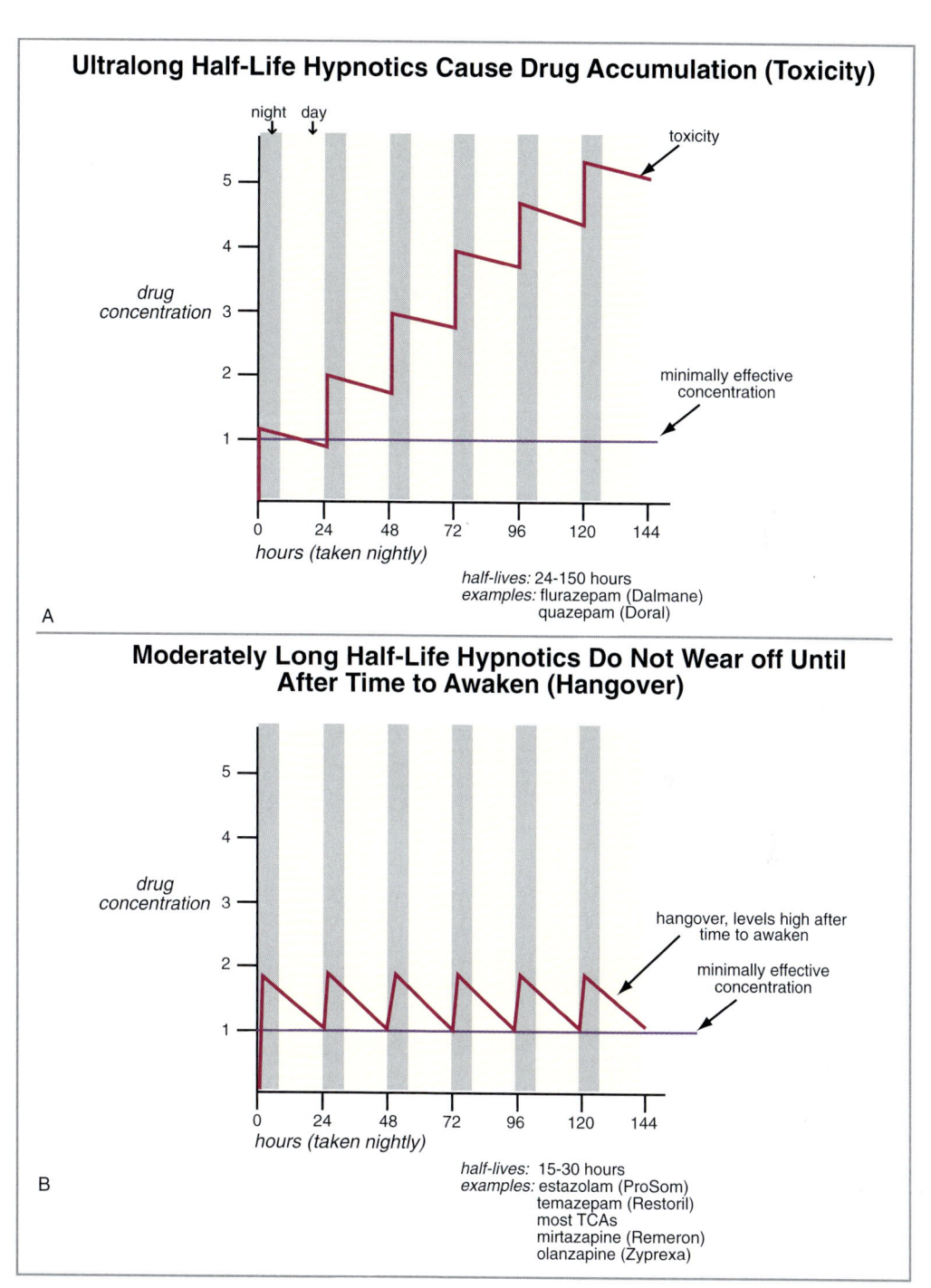

Moderately Long Half-Life Hypnotics Do Not Wear off Until After Time to Awaken (Hangover)

B

half-lives: 15-30 hours
examples: estazolam (ProSom)
temazepam (Restoril)
most TCAs
mirtazapine (Remeron)
olanzapine (Zyprexa)

FIGURE 16-18A and B Half-lives of hypnotics, part 1. The half-lives of hypnotics can have an important impact on their tolerability profiles. (**A**) Hypnotics with ultra-long half-lives (greater than 24 hours; for example, flurazepam and quazepam) can cause drug accumulation with chronic use. This can cause impairment that has been associated with increased risk of falls, particularly in the elderly. (**B**) Hypnotics with moderate half-lives (15–30 hours; estazolam, temazepam, most tricyclic antidepressants, mirtazapine, olanzapine) may not wear off until after the individual needs to awaken and thus may have "hangover" effects (sedation, memory problems).

Disorders of Sleep and Wakefulness and Their Treatment

Ultrashort Half-Life Hypnotics Wear off Before Time to Awaken (Loss of Sleep Maintenance)

hours (taken nightly)

half-lives: 1-3 hours
examples: triazolam (Halcion)
zaleplon (Sonata)
zolpidem (Ambien)
melatonin
ramelteon (Rozerem)

Optimized Duration of Action

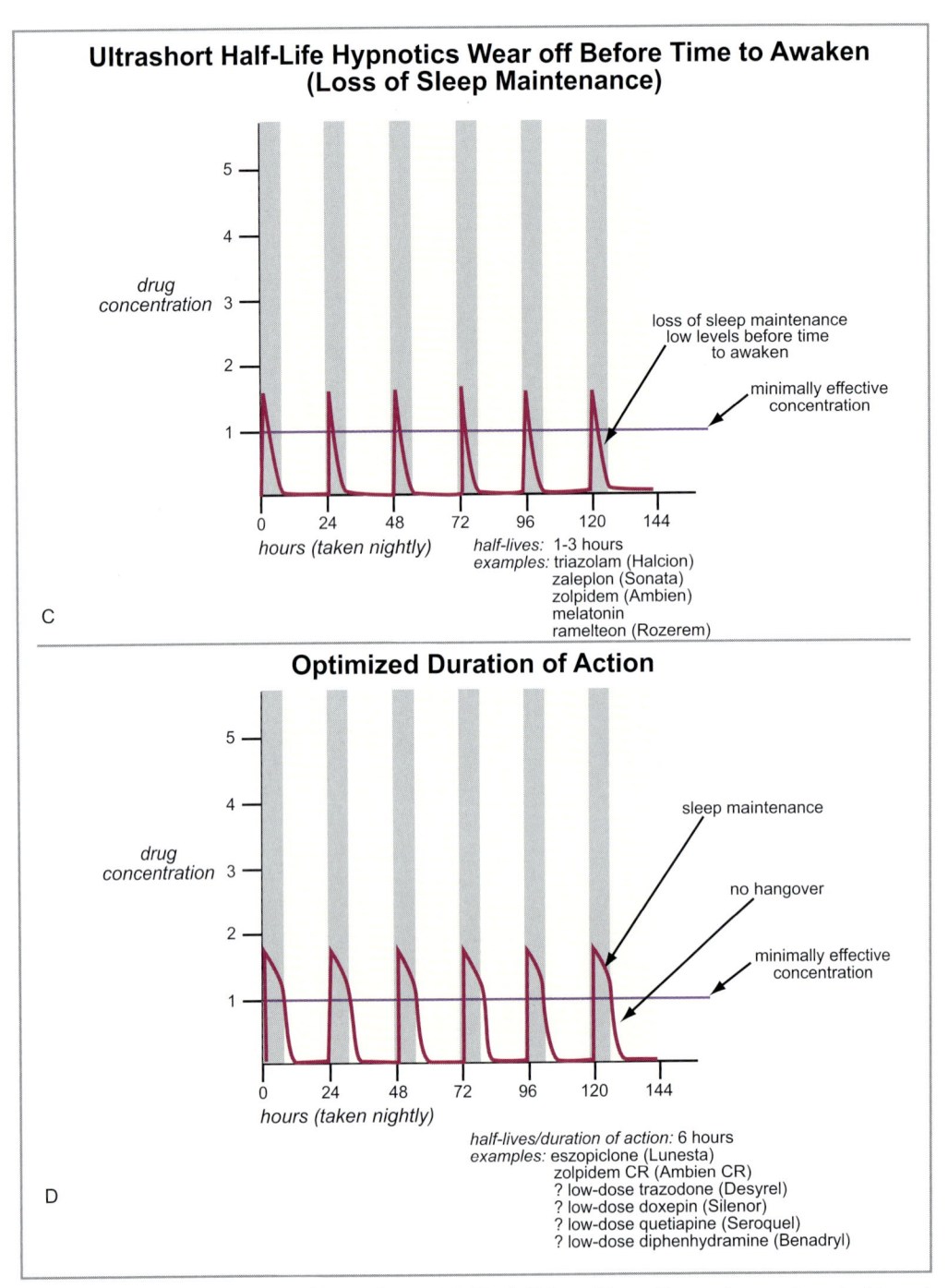

hours (taken nightly)

half-lives/duration of action: 6 hours
examples: eszopiclone (Lunesta)
zolpidem CR (Ambien CR)
? low-dose trazodone (Desyrel)
? low-dose doxepin (Silenor)
? low-dose quetiapine (Seroquel)
? low-dose diphenhydramine (Benadryl)

FIGURE 16-18C and D Half-lives of hypnotics, part 2. The half-lives of hypnotics can have an important impact on their tolerability and efficacy profiles. (**C**) Hypnotics with ultra-short half-lives (1–3 hours; triazolam, zaleplon, zolpidem, melatonin, ramelteon) can wear off before the individual needs to awaken and thus cause loss of sleep maintenance. (**D**) Hypnotics with half-lives that are short but not ultra-short (approximately 6 hours; eszopiclone, zolpidem CR, and perhaps low doses of trazodone, doxepin, quetiapine, or diphenhydramine) may provide rapid onset of action and plasma levels above the minimally effective concentration only for the duration of a normal night's sleep.

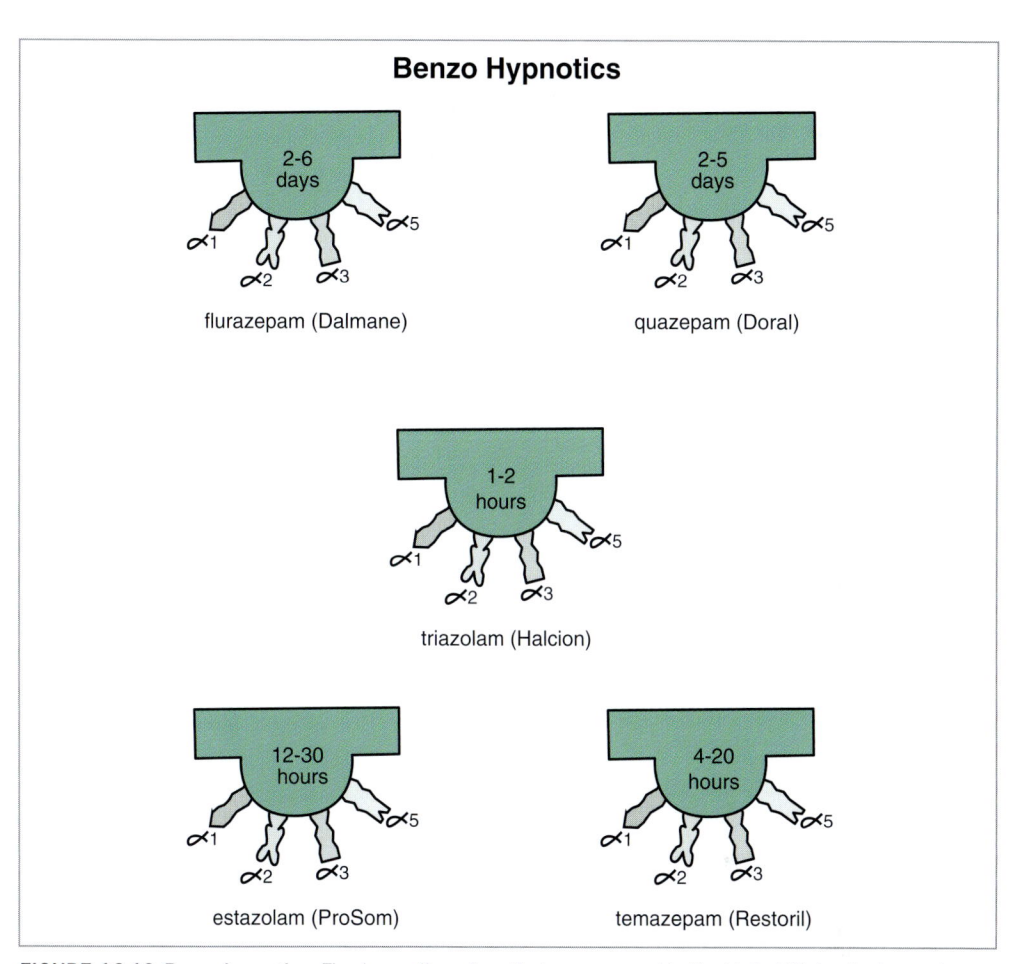

FIGURE 16-19 Benzo hypnotics. Five benzodiazepines that are approved in the United States for insomnia are shown here. These include flurazepam and quazepam, which have ultra-long half-lives; triazolam, which has an ultra-short half-life; and estazolam and temazepam, which have moderate half-lives.

levels (Figure 16-18A and B). Other agents used as hypnotics have half-lives that are too short and can wear off before it is time to wake up, causing insufficient sleep maintenance and nocturnal awakenings as well as restless and disturbed sleep in some patients (Figure 16-18C). More recently, however, the hypnotics given most often for chronic use are those that have optimized half-lives targeting rapid onset of action and plasma drug levels above the minimally effective concentration, but only until it is time to wake up (Figure 16-18D). Perhaps no therapeutic area of psychopharmacology is as critically dependent upon plasma drug levels and thus on the pharmacokinetics of the drug than is the use of hypnotics. This fact may be related to the nature of the arousal system and of the sleep/wake switch, which require pharmacologic action to a degree sufficient to reach the critical tipping point that trips the switch "off" to allow sleep, but only at night.

Other reasons for short-term restrictions on benzodiazepine hypnotics (Figure 16-19) in the past had to do with their long-term effects, including loss of efficacy over time (tolerance) and withdrawal effects, such as rebound insomnia in some patients worse than their original insomnia (Figure 16-20A). Recent investigations have shown that some nonbenzodiazepine hypnotics may not have these problems (Figure 16-20B). This includes the

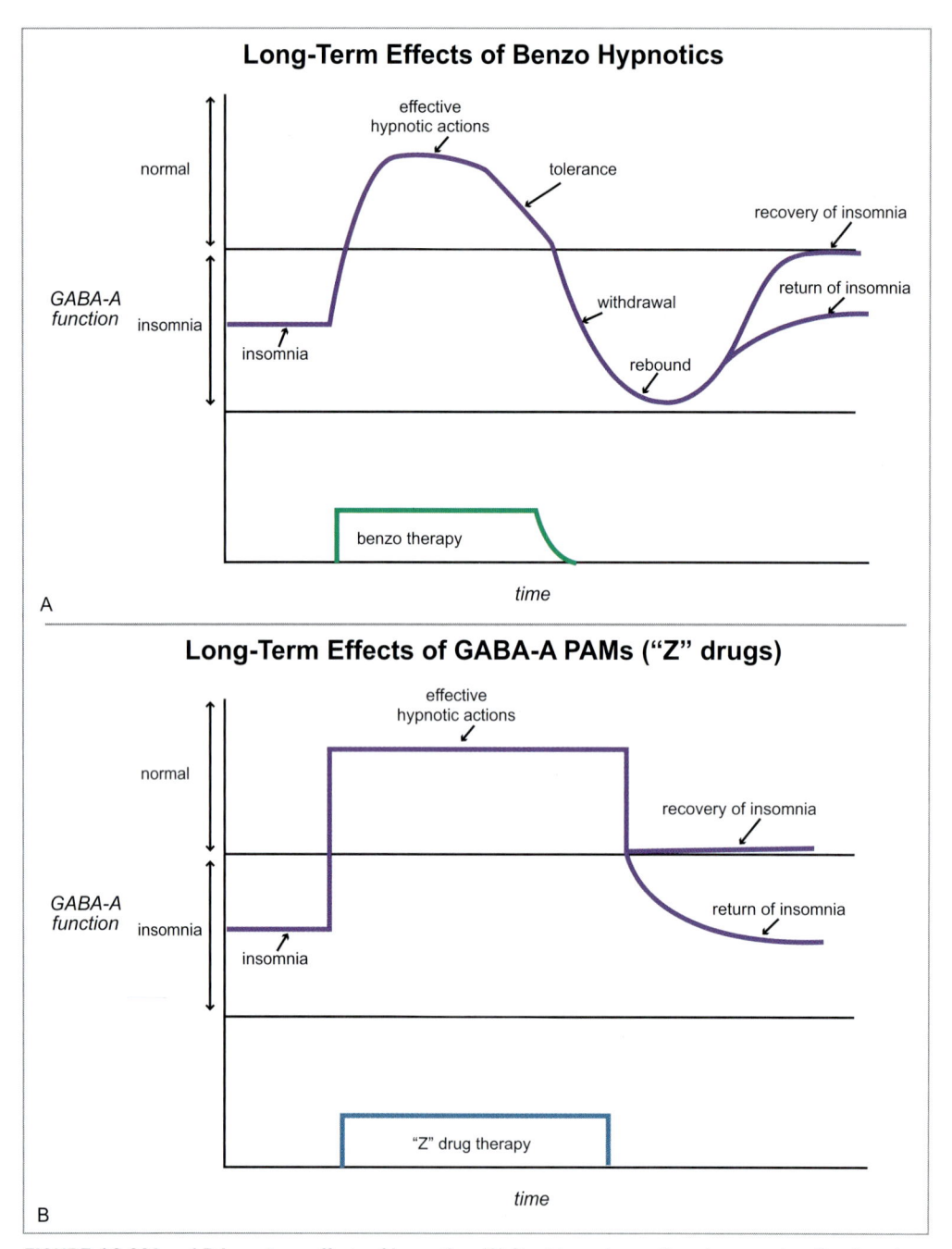

FIGURE 16-20A and B Long-term effects of hypnotics. (**A**) Short-term, benzodiazepines can be efficacious for treating insomnia. With long-term use, however, benzodiazepines may cause tolerance and, if discontinued, withdrawal effects that may include rebound insomnia. (**B**) Positive allosteric modulators (PAMs) at GABA-A receptors are efficacious for insomnia in the short-term, and in the long-term do not seem to cause tolerance or withdrawal effects.

GABA-A PAMs—"Z" Drugs

R,S-zopiclone
(Stillnox - not in U.S.)

eszopiclone
(Lunesta)

zaleplon
(Sonata)

zolpidem
(Ambien)

zolpidem CR
(Ambien CR)

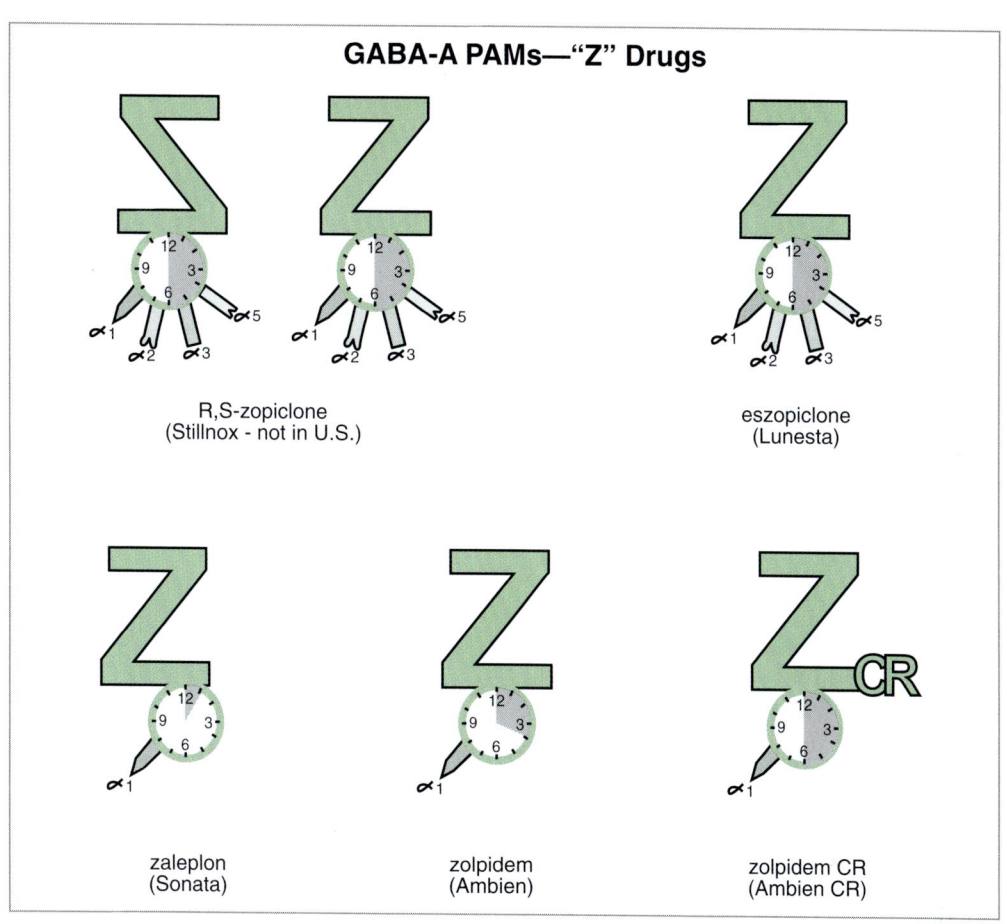

FIGURE 16-21 GABA-A positive allosteric modulators (PAMs). Several GABA-A PAMs, or "Z" drugs, are shown here. These include racemic zopiclone (not available in the United States), eszopiclone, zaleplon, zolpidem, and zolpidem CR. Zaleplon, zolpidem, and zolpidem CR are selective for GABA-A receptors that contain the alpha 1 subunit; however, zopiclone and eszopiclone do not have this selectivity.

GABA-A positive allosteric modulators (PAMs), sometimes also called "Z" drugs (because they all start with the letter Z: zaleplon, zolpidem, zopiclone) (Figure 16-21). Perhaps the best long-term studies have been done with eszopiclone, which shows little or no tolerance, dependence, or withdrawal with use for many months (Figure 16-20B). This is probably also the case for long-term use of zolpidem CR and for the melatonergic agent ramelteon as well as for "off label" use of the sedating antidepressant trazodone and the sedating atypical antipsychotic quetiapine, none of which have restrictions against chronic use. For these reasons, it is now recognized that chronic insomnia may need chronic treatment with certain hypnotics.

Benzodiazepine hypnotics

There are at least five benzodiazepines approved specifically for insomnia in the United States (Figure 16-19), although there are several others in different countries. Various benzodiazepines developed for the treatment of anxiety disorders are also frequently used to treat insomnia. Benzodiazepine anxiolytics are discussed in Chapter 14 and their mechanism of action is illustrated in Figure 14-22. Because benzodiazepines do not have ideal half-lives

Disorders of Sleep and Wakefulness and Their Treatment | 839

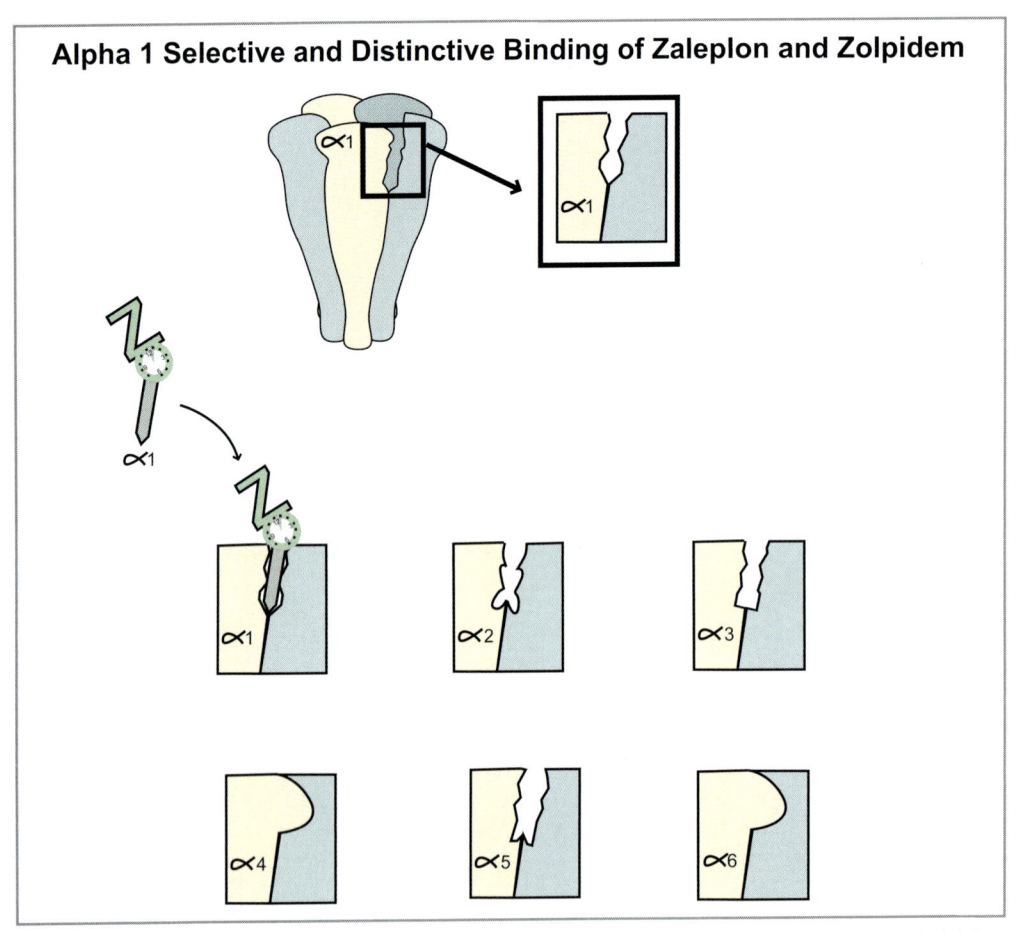

FIGURE 16-22 Alpha 1 selective hypnotics. The hypnotics zaleplon and zolpidem bind selectively to GABA-A receptors that contain the alpha 1 subunit, which is important for sedation and possibly also anticonvulsant and amnesic actions. These agents bind in a manner that does not cause tolerance, dependence, or withdrawal upon discontinuation; this is depicted as the drug having smooth edges where it binds to the GABA-A receptor.

for many patients (Figures 16-18A, B, and C) and can cause long-term problems (Figure 16-20A), they are generally considered second-line agents for use as hypnotics. However, when first-line agents fail to work, benzodiazepines still have a place in the treatment of insomnia, particularly for insomnia associated with various psychiatric and medical illnesses. These agents are also generally less expensive than newer agents.

GABA-A positive allosteric modulators (PAMs) as hypnotics
These hypnotics act at GABA-A receptors to enhance the action of GABA by binding to a site other than that where GABA itself binds to this receptor. PAMs are introduced in Chapter 5 and illustrated in Figures 5-21 and 5-23. Benzodiazepines are also a type of GABA-A PAM (discussed in Chapter 14 and illustrated in Figure 14-22). Barbiturate hypnotics are yet another type of GABA-A PAM. However, not all GABA-A PAMs are the same, as there are important differences in the ways in which various drugs bind to the GABA-A receptor, and this affects both the safety and efficacy of various classes of GABA-A PAMs (compare Figures 16-22 and 16-23).

Nonselective Actions of Benzodiazepines at GABA-A Receptors

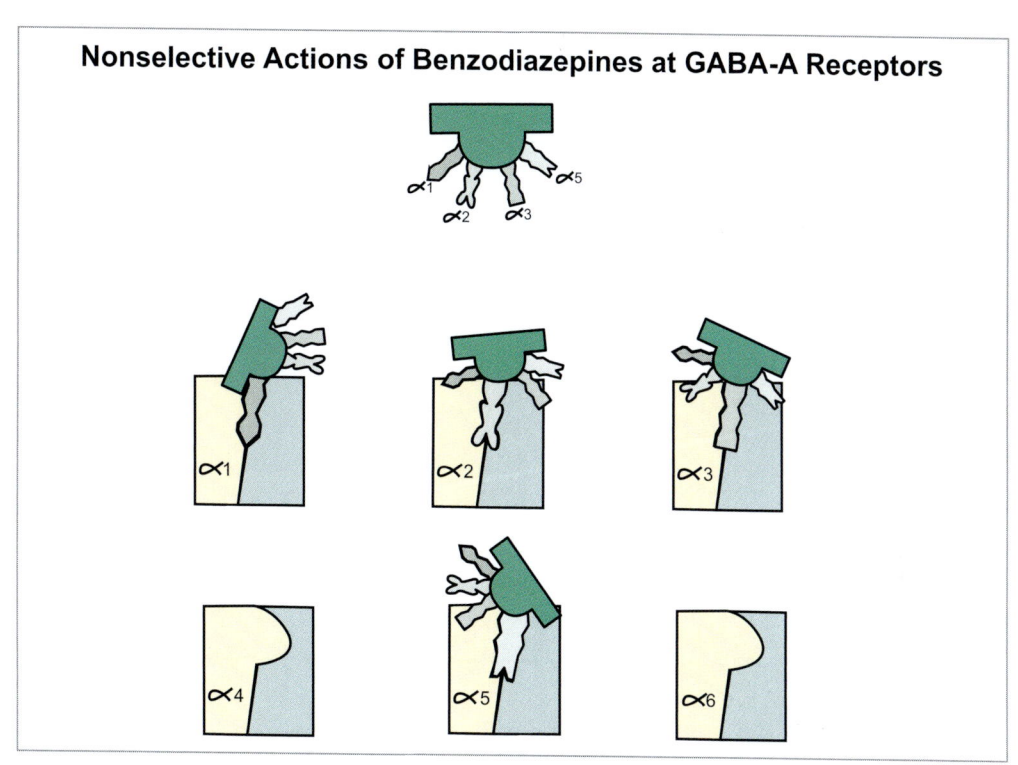

FIGURE 16-23 **Nonselective benzodiazepines.** Benzodiazepines bind to four of the six different types of GABA-A alpha subunits: alpha 1, alpha 2, alpha 3, and alpha 5. Each of these subunits is associated with different effects, and thus benzodiazepines not only cause sedation but can also be anxiolytic, cause muscle relaxation, and have alcohol potentiating actions. In addition, benzodiazepines bind in a manner that changes the conformation of the GABA-A receptor such that tolerance, dependence, and withdrawal effects can occur; this is depicted by the jagged edges where these drugs bind to the GABA-A receptor.

That is, the GABA-A PAMs zaleplon, zolpidem, and zopiclone appear to bind to the GABA-A receptor in a way that does not cause a high degree of tolerance to their therapeutic actions, dependence, or withdrawal upon discontinuation from long-term treatment (depicted as smooth edges of the binding sites for the Z drugs in Figures 16-21 and 16-22). By contrast, benzodiazepines bind in a manner that changes the conformation of the GABA-A receptor such that tolerance generally develops, as well as some degree of dependence and withdrawal, especially for some patients and for some benzodiazepines (depicted as jagged edges of the benzodiazepine binding sites of benzodiazepine hypnotics in Figures 16-19 and 16-23).

Furthermore, for some Z drugs, there is selectivity for the alpha 1 subtype of GABA-A receptor (Figures 16-21 and 16-22). GABA-A receptor subtypes are introduced in Chapter 14 and illustrated in Figure 14-20. There are six different subtypes of alpha subunits for GABA-A receptors, and benzodiazepines bind to four of them (alpha 1, alpha 2, alpha 3, and alpha 5) (Figures 16-19 and 16-23), as do zopiclone and eszopiclone (Figure 16-21). The alpha 1 subtype is known to be critical to producing sedation and thus is targeted by every effective GABA-A PAM hypnotic. The alpha 1 subtype is also linked to daytime sedation, anticonvulsant actions, and possibly to amnesia. Adaptations of this receptor with chronic hypnotic treatments that target it are thought to lead to tolerance and withdrawal. The alpha 2 and alpha 3 receptor subtypes are linked to anxiolytic, muscle relaxant, and

Disorders of Sleep and Wakefulness and Their Treatment

TABLE 16-6 Does R zopiclone interfere with eszopiclone?

R, S, zopiclone (Stilnox)	Eszopiclone (Lunesta)	Potential advantages of single isomer eszopiclone
Dose 7.5 mg	Dose 2–3 mg	Less than half the dose; could mean less hangover and fewer side effects if efficacy maintained
R isomer inhibits speed of peak plasma concentrations of S isomer (T max)	No interference – faster T max	Faster sleep onset
Active metabolites of R isomer have longer half-lives and may prolong half-life of other active metabolites	Active metabolites have shorter half-lives	Less hangover
R isomer has different pharmacological properties than S isomer	Only S isomer pharmacological properties active	Contribute to lack of tolerance to hypnotic efficacy and lack of dependence and withdrawal with long-term use?
Some positive results of genetic toxicology in preclinical cancer assays	Negative toxicology in preclinical cancer assays	Safer for long-term treatment?

alcohol potentiating actions. Finally, the alpha 5 subtype, mostly in the hippocampus, may be linked to cognition and other functions. Zaleplon and zolpidem are alpha 1 selective (Figures 16-21 and 16-22). The functional significance of selectivity is not yet proven but may contribute to the lower risk of tolerance and dependence of these agents.

There are recent modifications to two of the Z drugs, zolpidem and zopiclone. For zolpidem, there is a new controlled-release formulation known as zolpidem CR (Figure 16-21). This formulation extends the duration of action of zolpidem immediate release from about 2 to 4 hours (see Figure 16-18B) to a more optimized duration of 6 to 8 hours, improving sleep maintenance (see Figure 16-18D). For zopiclone, a racemic mixture of both R and S zopiclone, there is the introduction of the S enantiomer, better known as eszopiclone (Figure 16-21). Differences between the active enantiomer and the racemic mixture are debated, but the potential advantages of the selective enantiomer eszopiclone over the racemic mixture are listed in Table 16-6.

Indiplon is another new alpha 1 selective GABA-A PAM being developed in both immediate-release and controlled-release formulations and is in late clinical testing. Another class of GABA-A PAMs in testing as novel hypnotics are those selective for the delta subtype of GABA-A receptor (discussed in Chapter 14 and illustrated in Figures 14-20 and 14-21). Benzodiazepines and Z drugs do not bind to this site, but neurosteroids and some possibly novel hypnotics do. Gaboxadol is one such agent selective for the delta GABA-A receptors as a PAM, and thus as a modulator of extrasynaptic GABA-A receptors and the tonic inhibition they mediate (see Figure 14-21), but it has been dropped from further development at this time. Other agents that target this site might prove to be novel hypnotics.

Psychiatric insomnia and the GABA-A PAMs
In many ways, the introduction of the Z drugs has contributed to the reconceptualization of the treatment of chronic insomnia. That is, optimized pharmacokinetic durations of action

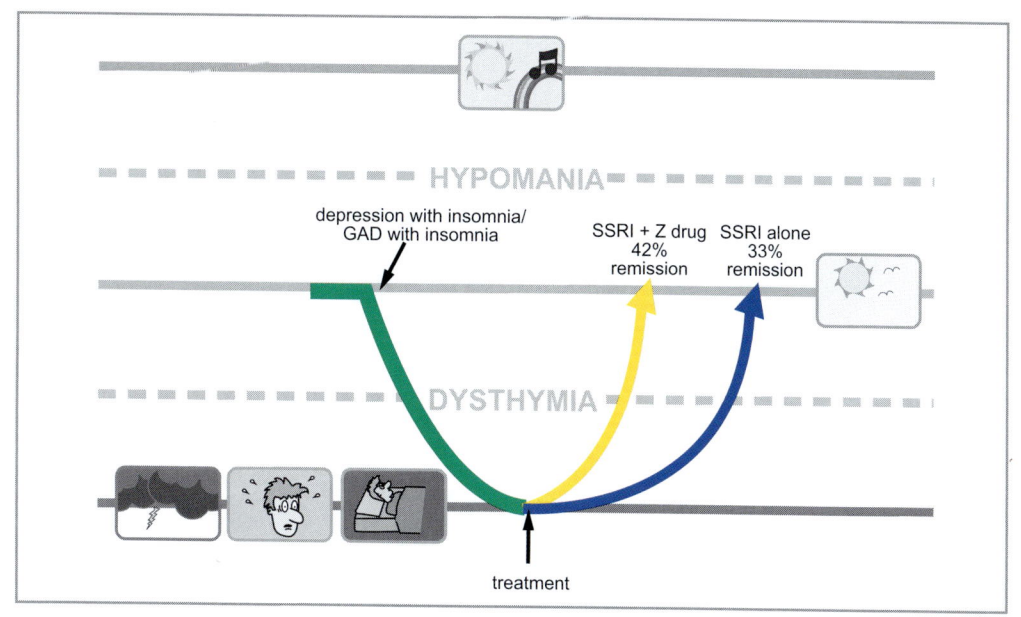

FIGURE 16-24 Treating psychiatric insomnia. Insomnia is a common residual symptom of psychiatric disorders, including depression and generalized anxiety disorder (GAD). Recent findings suggest that remission rates may be increased in depression or GAD with insomnia when a hypnotic is added to first-line antidepressant treatment, and that this is attributable not only to improvement in insomnia but also to improvement in other symptoms.

(Figure 16-18D) coupled with studies establishing safety in long-term use without a high incidence of tolerance or dependence (Figure 16-20B) have opened the door to the chronic treatment of chronic insomnia. However, most studies of hypnotics are in primary insomnia, not in insomnia associated with psychiatric disorders, leading to fewer clear guidelines as to how to use hypnotics to treat insomnia in conditions such as depression, anxiety disorders, bipolar disorder, etc.

Investigators are currently beginning to address the appropriate use, including long-term use, of concomitant hypnotics for various psychiatric disorders. For example, recent studies have shown that hypnotics may enhance remission rates both for patients with major depression who have insomnia and for those with generalized anxiety disorder (GAD) who have insomnia (Figure 16-24). Not only do the symptoms of insomnia improve as expected when patients with GAD or major depression are treated with eszopiclone added to an SSRI (e.g., fluoxetine or escitalopram), but so do the other symptoms of GAD or depression, leading to higher remission rates (Figure 16-24). Whether this applies to all Z drugs or indeed to any hypnotic of any mechanism that is successful in improving insomnia added to any antidepressant for these conditions is not yet known. Whether treating insomnia will also help prevent future episodes of depression or GAD is also not known, but considering that insomnia is perhaps the most frequent residual symptom after treating depression with an antidepressant (discussed in Chapter 12 and illustrated in Figures 12-9 and 12-121 through 12-123), it makes intuitive sense to utilize hypnotics as augmenting agents to first-line treatments for depression or anxiety disorders and if necessary to utilize hypnotics chronically to eliminate symptoms of insomnia in these conditions.

Disorders of Sleep and Wakefulness and Their Treatment

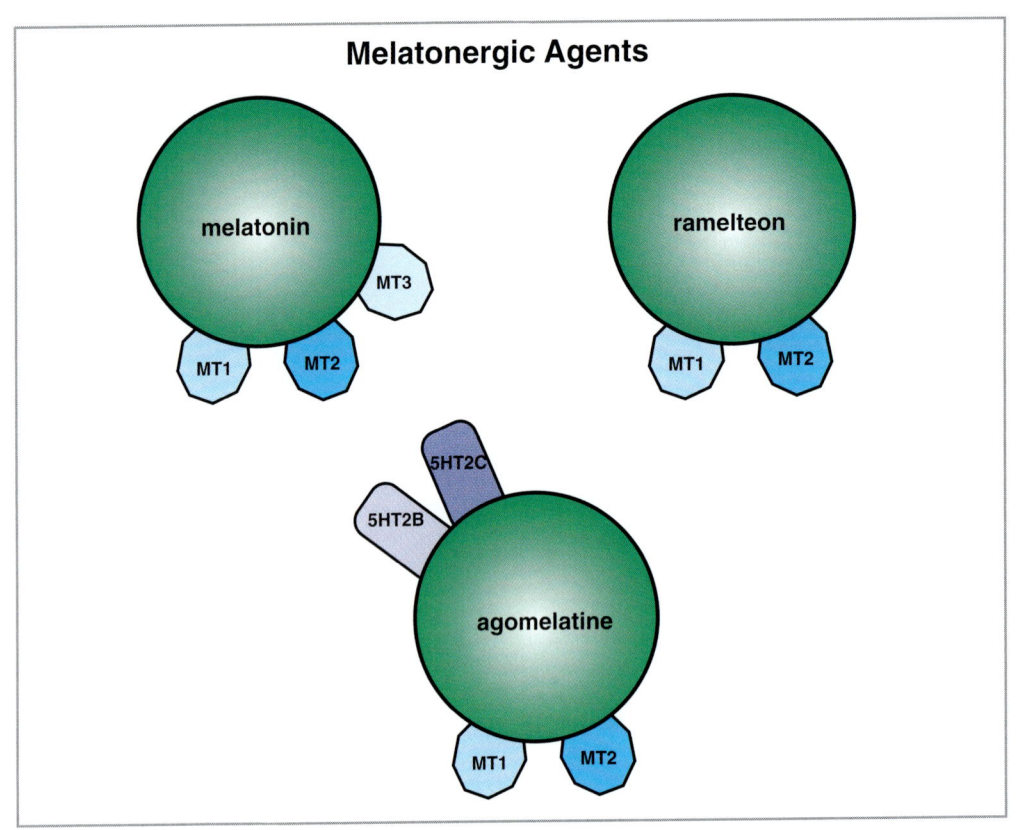

FIGURE 16-25 Melatonergic agents. Endogenous melatonin is secreted by the pineal gland and mainly acts in the suprachiasmatic nucleus to regulate circadian rhythms. There are three types of receptors for melatonin: 1 and 2, which are both involved in sleep, and 3, which is actually the enzyme NRH: quinine oxidoreductase 2 and not thought to be involved in sleep physiology. There are several different agents that act at melatonin receptors, as shown here. Melatonin itself, available over the counter, acts at melatonin 1 and 2 receptors as well as at the melatonin 3 site. Ramelteon is a melatonin 1 and 2 receptor agonist available by prescription and seems to provide sleep onset though not necessarily sleep maintenance. Agomelatine is not only a melatonin 1 and 2 receptor agonist, but is also a serotonin 2C and 2B receptor antagonist and is in development as an antidepressant.

Melatonergic hypnotics

Melatonin is the neurotransmitter secreted by the pineal gland; it acts especially in the suprachiasmatic nucleus to regulate circadian rhythms. Figures 16-10 and 16-11 show the effects of evening or morning melatonin in shifting circadian rhythms in subjects with phase delay or phase advance, respectively. It is also known that melatonin is an effective hypnotic for sleep onset. Melatonin itself is available over the counter, in doses that are not always reliable. Furthermore, research has not clearly established the efficacy of various doses of melatonin. These factors compromise the utility of melatonin itself as a hypnotic.

Melatonin acts at three different sites, not only melatonin 1 (MT1) and melatonin 2 (MT2) receptors but also at a third site, sometimes called the melatonin 3 site, which is now known to be the enzyme NRH: quinone oxidoreductase 2 and which is probably not involved in sleep physiology (Figure 16-25). MT1-mediated inhibition of neurons in the suprachiasmatic nucleus (SCN) could help to promote sleep by decreasing the wake-promoting actions of the circadian "clock" or "pacemaker" that functions there, perhaps by attenuating the SCN's alerting signals, allowing sleep signals to predominate and thus inducing sleep. Phase shifting and circadian rhythm effects of the normal sleep/wake cycle are thought to be primarily mediated by MT2 receptors, which entrain these signals in the SCN.

A proven hypnotic with an established dose is the MT1/MT2 agonist ramelteon (Figure 16-25). This agent improves sleep onset, sometimes better when used for several days in a row. It is not known to help sleep maintenance but will induce natural sleep in those subjects who suffer mostly from initial insomnia. Discussed in Chapter 12 on antidepressants is a new agent, agomelatine, that is hypothesized to act as an antidepressant at 5HT2C receptors, but it is also more potent as an MT1 and MT2 agonist, just like ramelteon (see Figures 12-135 and 16-25). Thus it is possible that agomelatine will not only be an effective hypnotic due to its melatonergic actions but may also combine synergistic actions for GAD and MDD, as shown in Figure 16-24, due to its independent actions as an antidepressant and as a hypnotic. Other melatonergic agents are also in development, including those selective for just the MT1 or the MT2 receptor.

Serotonergic hypnotics

One of the most popular hypnotics among psychopharmacologists is the antidepressant trazodone. This sedating antidepressant with a half-life of only about 6 to 8 hours was recognized long ago by clinicians as being highly effective as a hypnotic when given at a lower dose than that used as an antidepressant and by giving it just once a day, at night (see Figure 16-18D). In fact, trazodone was never approved as a hypnotic or marketed as a hypnotic, but it accounts for up to half of all prescriptions for hypnotics.

How does trazodone work? In Chapter 12, trazodone's mechanism as an antidepressant is discussed; it is illustrated in Figures 12-59 to 12-64. It is clear that to act as an antidepressant, the dose of trazodone must be sufficiently high to recruit not only its most potent 5HT2A antagonist properties but also its serotonin reuptake blocking properties (Figure 12-59; see also Figure 16-26, on the left). At these doses, trazodone can be quite sedating, because its H1 antihistamine and alpha 1 antagonist properties are also recruited (Figure 16-26 on the left). Contributions of H1 antagonism and alpha 1 adrenergic antagonism to sedation are discussed in Chapter 10 and illustrated in Figures 10-71 and 10-74.

By trial and error if not by serendipity, clinicians discovered that trazodone's half-life is actually an advantage when this drug is administered as a hypnotic (Figure 16-18D), because its daytime sedating effects, which are so evident when the drug is administered at high doses twice daily for depression (Figure 16-26, on the left), can be greatly diminished by giving this short-half-life agent only at night and by lowering its dose (Figure 16-26, on the right). Thus trazodone loses its serotonin reuptake blocking properties (Figure 16-26, on the right) and its antidepressant actions but retains alpha 1 blocking actions as well as H1 antagonist and some of its 5HT2C antagonist actions (Figure 16-26, on the right).

Perhaps because of its 5HT2C and 5HT2A antagonist actions, trazodone can increase slow-wave sleep when given as a monotherapy and can also block the slow-wave sleep disruption of SSRIs when given concomitantly with them. Selective 5HT2A/2C antagonists and inverse agonists are in testing as novel hypnotics, especially for sleep maintenance and as promoters of slow-wave sleep. 5HT2A and 5HT2C receptors are discussed in Chapter 10 as augmenting agents to antipsychotics and illustrated in Figure 10-31.

What Is Trazodone's Mechanism as a Hypnotic?

antidepressant dose (150-600 mg)   hypnotic dose (25-150 mg)

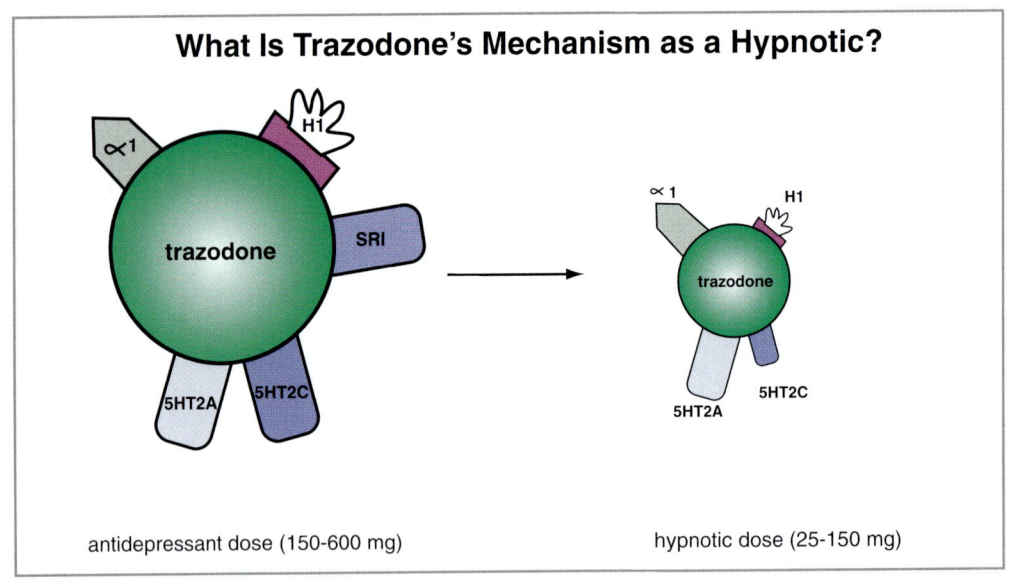

FIGURE 16-26 Trazodone. At antidepressant doses (150–600 mg/day) trazodone is a serotonin reuptake inhibitor and also has serotonin 2A and 2C antagonism. In addition, trazodone is an antagonist at histamine 1 and alpha 1 adrenergic receptors, which can make it very sedating, particularly when given at antidepressant doses during the day. At low doses (25–150 mg/day), trazodone does not adequately block serotonin reuptake but retains its other properties; thus it can still be sedating. However, because trazodone has a relatively short half-life (6–8 hours), if dosed only once daily at night it can improve sleep without having daytime effects.

Histamine H1 antagonists as hypnotics

It is widely appreciated that antihistamines are sedating. Antihistamines are popular as over-the-counter sleep aids (especially those containing diphenhydramine/Benadryl or doxylamine). Because antihistamines have been widely used for many years, there is the common misperception that the properties of classic agents such as diphenhydramine apply to any drug with antihistaminic properties. This includes the idea that all antihistamines have "anticholinergic" side effects, such as blurred vision, constipation, memory problems, dry mouth; that they cause next-day hangover effects when used as hypnotics at night; that tolerance develops to their hypnotic actions; and that they cause weight gain.

It now seems that these ideas about antihistamines are due to the fact that most agents with potent antihistamine properties, from diphenhydramine, to tricyclic antidepressants, mirtazapine, quetiapine, and many others, are not selective for H1 receptors at normal doses and that many of the undesirable properties classically associated with antihistamines are probably due to other receptor actions, not to H1 antagonism per se. In particular, diphenhydramine and many of the agents classified as antihistamines are also potent antagonists of muscarinic receptors (Figure 16-27), so it is not generally possible to separate the antihistamine actions of such agents from their antimuscarinic actions in clinical use. The same is true for most tricyclic antidepressants, which have antimuscarinic and alpha 1 adrenergic blocking properties in addition to their antihistaminic properties. Tricyclic antidepressants are discussed in Chapter 12 and their pharmacological properties are illustrated in Figures 12-81 through 12-89. The triple-action combination of antihistamine, anticholinergic, and alpha 1 adrenergic antagonism as highly sedating mechanisms for antipsychotics is discussed in Chapter 10 and illustrated in Figures 10-70, 10-71, and 10-74.

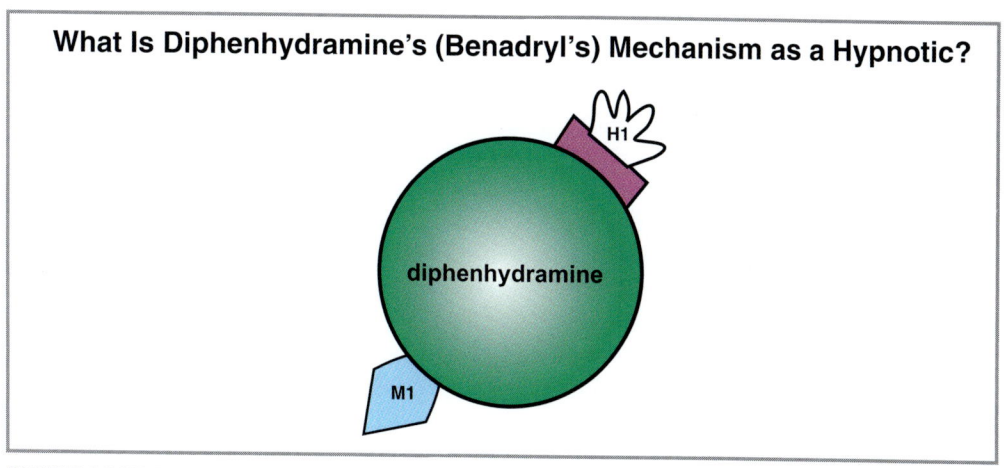

What Is Diphenhydramine's (Benadryl's) Mechanism as a Hypnotic?

FIGURE 16-27 Diphenhydramine. Diphenhydramine is a histamine 1 receptor antagonist commonly used as a hypnotic. However, this agent is not selective for histamine 1 receptors and thus also has additional pharmacologic actions. Specifically, diphenhydramine is also a muscarinic 1 receptor antagonist and thus causes anticholinergic effects (blurred vision, constipation, memory problems, dry mouth).

What Is the Mechanism of Doxepin as a Hypnotic?

antidepressant dose (150-300 mg)   hypnotic dose (1-6 mg)

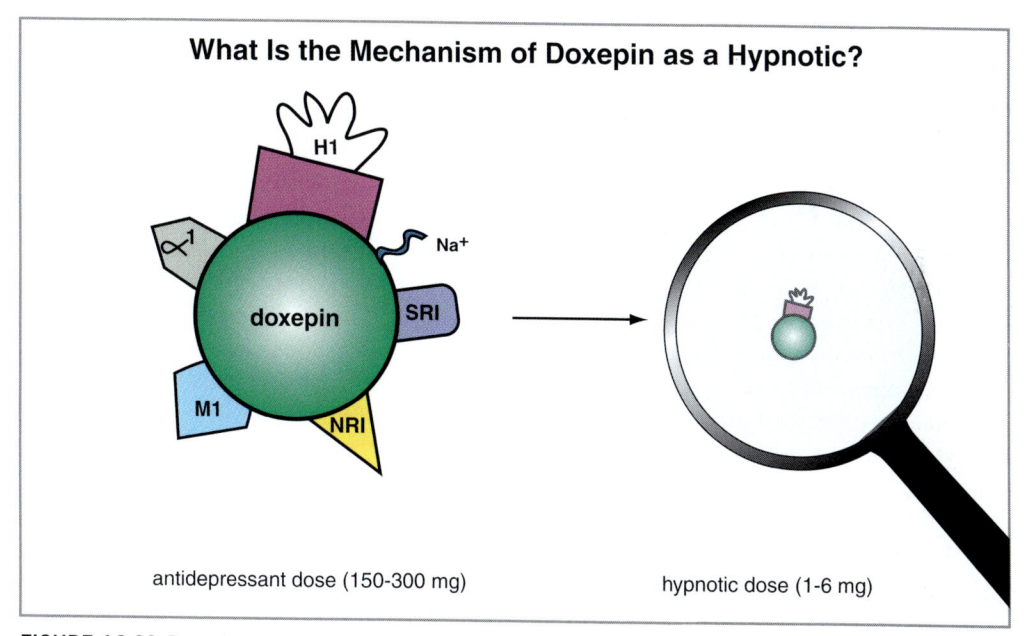

FIGURE 16-28 Doxepin. Doxepin is a tricyclic antidepressant (TCA) that, at antidepressant doses (150–300 mg/day), inhibits serotonin and norepinephrine reuptake and is an antagonist at histamine 1, muscarinic 1, and alpha 1 adrenergic receptors. At low doses (1–6 mg/day), however, doxepin is quite selective for histamine 1 receptors and thus may be used as a hypnotic.

Some very interesting findings are beginning to emerge from clinical investigations of H1 selective antagonists as hypnotics. The prototype of this approach is very low doses of the tricyclic antidepressant doxepin (Figure 16-28). Because of the very high affinity of doxepin for the H1 receptor, it is possible to make it into an H1 selective antagonist just by lowering the dose (Figure 16-28). This agent is so selective at low doses that it

Disorders of Sleep and Wakefulness and Their Treatment | 847

is even being used as a ligand in positron emission tomography (PET) to label CNS H1 receptors selectively. At doses a small fraction of those necessary for its antidepressant actions, doxepin can occupy a substantial number of CNS H1 receptors (e.g., at 1 to 6 mg of doxepin as a hypnotic compared to 150 to 300 mg of doxepin as an antidepressant) (Figure 16-28). Furthermore, doxepin is actually a mixture of two chemical forms, one of which (and its active metabolites) has a shorter half-life (8 to 15 hours) than the other, which has a traditional long tricyclic antidepressant half-life of 24 hours. Functionally, the mixture of the two agents means that nighttime administration yields substantially lower residual plasma drug levels in the morning compared to tricyclics with a 24-hour half-life, thus reducing daytime carryover effects (see Figure 16-18D).

Although it is not surprising that very low doses of doxepin that selectively antagonize H1 histamine receptors are effective hypnotics, early clinical testing is revealing that long-term administration of doxepin provides rapid sleep induction with all-night sleep maintenance but without next-day carryover effects, development of tolerance to its hypnotic efficacy, or weight gain. Eliminating alpha 1 adrenergic and muscarinic cholinergic blockade may explain the lack of anticholinergic side effects and the lack of development of tolerance to hypnotic actions. Although agents with H1 antagonist properties can cause weight gain, apparently H1 selective antagonism without 5HT2C antagonism may not be associated with weight gain. These mechanisms are discussed in relation to weight gain in Chapter 10 and illustrated in Figures 10-58 and 10-59.

There are at least two further examples of turning a psychotropic drug with many pharmacological actions into an H1 selective antagonist: mirtazapine and quetiapine. Both of these agents have long been observed to have hypnotic actions, not only at their normal clinical doses but at lower doses as well. Both agents are documented to have substantially more potent H1 antagonist actions than any other pharmacological action (see discussion of mirtazapine's pharmacology in Chapter 12 and illustrations in Figures 12-55 through 12-58; see discussion of quetiapine's pharmacology in Chapter 10 and illustration in Figure 10-94). Mirtazapine has two active enantiomers, and clinical testing is ongoing with esmirtazapine to determine whether low doses of this agent will prove to be an effective hypnotic. Quetiapine, normally effective as an antipsychotic, antimanic, and bipolar antidepressant agent in doses of 300 to 600 mg, can be effective as a hypnotic in doses 10-fold lower. Several novel H1 selective antagonists and inverse agonists are also in clinical development.

Who cares about slow-wave sleep?

The exact function of stage 3 and 4 sleep (delta or slow-wave sleep) remains under active investigation. Not all patients with insomnia have a deficiency of slow-wave sleep, and not all patients with a deficiency of slow-wave sleep have insomnia. However, some empirical clinical observations suggest that a deficiency of slow-wave sleep can contribute to a sense of lack of restorative sleep and daytime fatigue. Patients with pain syndromes and a deficiency of slow-wave sleep can have an enhanced daytime subjective experience of their pain; patients with depression and a deficiency of slow-wave sleep can have enhanced symptoms of fatigue, apathy, and cognitive dysfunction. Thus, having sufficient restorative slow-wave sleep seems intuitively like a good thing, but the proof of how much is enough or what the implications of too little or sufficient slow-wave sleep are remain elusive.

Some agents, such as serotonergic antidepressants (SSRIs, SNRIs), stimulants, and stimulating antidepressants (e.g., NDRIs) can all interfere with slow-wave sleep, and a limited number of agents are known to enhance slow-wave sleep [see hypnotic pharmacy

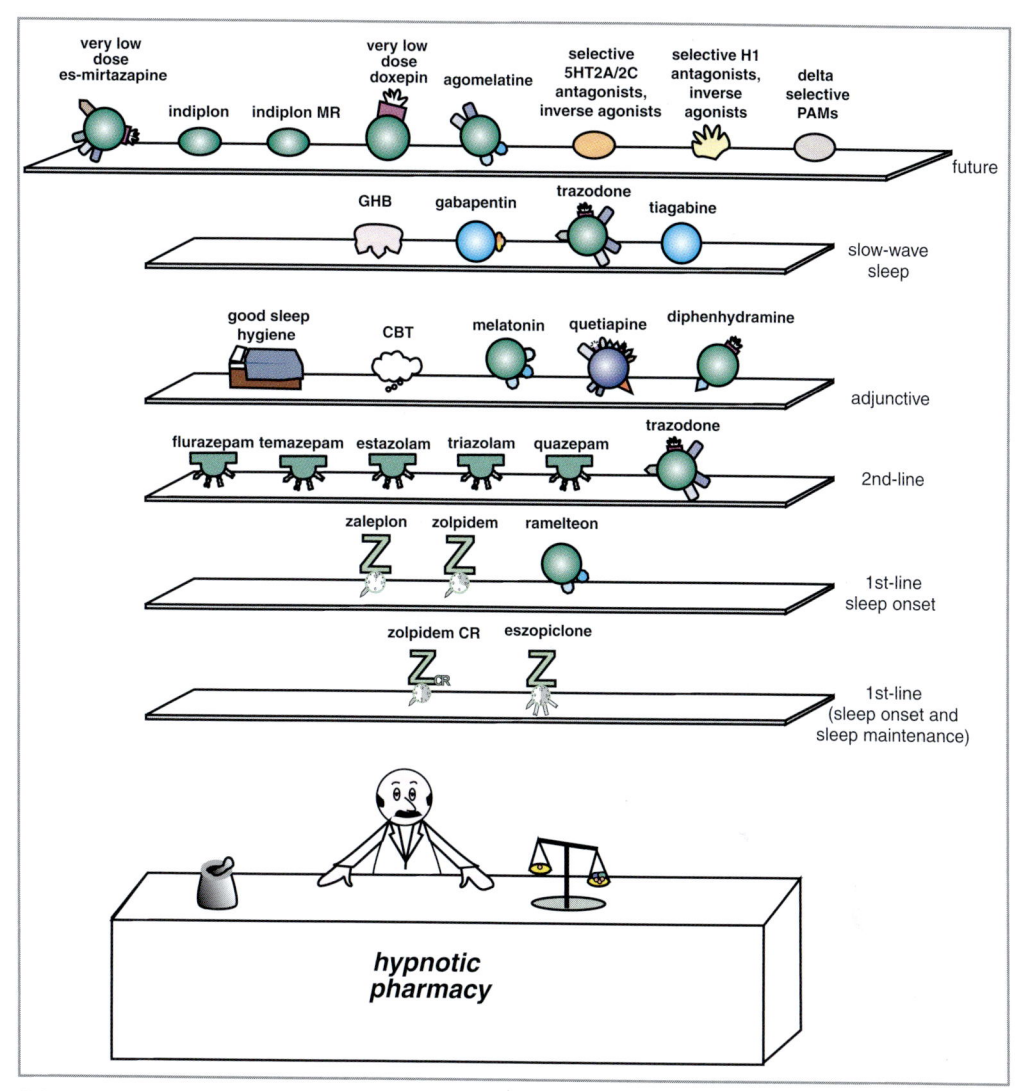

FIGURE 16-29 Hypnotic pharmacy. Treatment selection for insomnia is based on the specific sleep problems an individual has (i.e., trouble with sleep onset or sleep maintenance). For patients with sleep onset problems, zolpidem, zolpidem CR, eszopiclone, zaleplon, and ramelteon are first-line options. For patients with sleep onset and sleep maintenance problems, zolpidem CR or eszopiclone may be preferred choices. Second-line treatments can include several benzodiazepines or trazodone, while adjunctive treatments may include melatonin, quetiapine, or diphenhydramine. All patients should optimize their sleep hygiene; in addition, cognitive behavioral therapy can be beneficial. Agents that may enhance slow-wave sleep include sodium oxybate (GHB), gabapentin, trazodone, and tiagabine. Several new medications, or variations of existing medications, are also in development and may be options in the future.

in Figure 16-29 for alpha 2 delta ligands such as gabapentin and pregabalin; the GABA reuptake inhibitor tiagabine; 5HT2A/2C antagonists including trazodone and GHB (the GABA-B enhancing gamma hydroxybutyrate or sodium oxybate)]. Augmenting the treatment of fatigue and pain with slow-wave sleep–enhancing agents can sometimes reduce these symptoms, especially in patients with an affective spectrum disorder or a functional somatic syndrome (see Chapter 15 and Figure 15-18).

TABLE 16-7 Good sleep hygiene

- Avoid naps
- Use the bed for sleeping, not reading, TV, etc.
- Avoid alcohol, caffeine, and nicotine before sleep
- Avoid strenuous exercise before sleep
- Limit time in bed to sleep time (get up if not asleep within 20 minutes and return to bed when sleepy)
- Don't watch the clock
- Adopt regular sleep/wake habits
- Avoid bright light late at night and expose self to light in the morning

TABLE 16-8 What causes sleepiness?

- Sleep deprivation
- Sleep disorders
  - Narcolepsy
  - Obstructive sleep apnea
  - Restless legs
  - Periodic limb movement disorder
  - Circadian rhythm disorders (shift work, jet lag, delayed sleep)
  - Primary hypersomnia
  - Poor sleep hygiene
- Psychiatric illness
- Psychiatric and other medications
- Substance use/abuse
- Medical disorders
  - Obesity
  - Insulin resistance/diabetes

The hypnotic pharmacy

In summary, the various agents utilized as hypnotics are shown in Figure 16-29. This includes what would now be considered first-line agents approved as hypnotics (the GABA-A PAMs), the melatonergic agent ramelteon, and the second-line benzodiazepines as well as trazodone. Numerous other agents are shown, including several drugs in development. One should not forget cognitive behavioral approaches and improvement of sleep hygiene (see also Table 16-7) as adjunctive treatments, as these can be quite effective in selected patients with various types of insomnia.

Excessive daytime sleepiness (hypersomnia) and wake-promoting agents

What is sleepiness?

"Sleepiness" is a term that is sometimes used synonymously with "hypersomnia." Here we will discuss the symptom of excessive daytime sleepiness, its causes, and especially its treatment with three wake-promoting agents: caffeine, modafinil, and stimulants. The most common cause of sleepiness is sleep deprivation and the treatment is sleep, not drugs (Table 16-8). Other causes of excessive daytime sleepiness are various sleep disorders, psychiatric disorders, medications, and medical disorders (Table 16-8). Although society often devalues sleep and can imply that only wimps complain of sleepiness, it is clear that excessive daytime sleepiness is not benign and in fact can be lethal (Table 16-9). Loss of sleep causes performance decrements equivalent to intoxication with alcohol (Table 16-10), and, not

TABLE 16-9 What does sleepiness cause?

- Traffic accidents
- Errors/accidents at work
- Decreased work productivity
- Psychomotor impairment
- Deficits in cognitive function, learning, and memory
- Alcohol interactions
- Stimulant seeking
- Mood effects
- Lack of awareness
- Reduced quality of life
- Hypoxemia
- Insulin resistance
- Increased sympathetic activity
- Blunted arousal response
- Obesity associated with hypersomnia
- 46.5% of patients with hypersomnia have a psychiatric illness
- Increased body pain
- Increased health care costs

TABLE 16-10 Drunk with sleepiness?

Sleep loss	Equivalent alcohol dose in U.S. beers	Equivalent alcohol level (%)
Post-call pediatric residents	–	0.04–0.05
Normals		
2 hours (i.e., only 6 hour time in bed)	2–3	0.045
Legally drunk		
4 hours (i.e., only 4 hour time in bed)	5–6	0.095
6 hours (i.e., only 2 hour time in bed)	7–8	0.102
8 hours (i.e., no time in bed)	10–11	0.190

surprisingly, traffic accidents and fatalities. Thus, this symptom is important to assess even though patients often do not complain about it when they have it (Table 16-11). Just as discussed in Chapter 11 for bipolar disorder (see Table 11-2), assessment of patients with sleepiness requires that additional information be obtained from the patient's partner, particularly the bed partner (Table 6-11). Most conditions can be evaluated by patient and partner interviews, but sometimes subjective ratings of sleepiness (such as the Epworth Sleepiness Scale, Tables 16-11 and 16-12) as well as objective evaluations of sleepiness (i.e., overnight polysomnograms plus next-day multiple sleep latency testing and/or maintenance of wakefulness testing, Table 16-12) are required. Tips for which patients to refer for sleep studies are given in Table 16-13.

How sleepy is sleepiness?

The severity of sleepiness for a number of conditions is quantified in Figure 16-30. Patients tend to underestimate their own sleepiness when they suffer from chronic sleepiness, but they are well aware of their acute sleepiness after as little as a few hours sleep loss on a single night. Subjective ratings of sleepiness (Figure 16-30A) show that narcolepsy patients have

TABLE 16-11 Initial assessment of patients with excessive sleepiness

- Daily sleep patterns
  - Estimated total sleep time
  - Number of nocturnal awakenings
  - Prolonged sleep latency (time to sleep onset)
  - Snoring (ask partner)
  - Witnessed apneas (ask partner)
  - Symptoms of restless legs or periodic limb movements
- Drug and alcohol use
- Medication use
- Medical conditions
- Epworth Sleepiness Scale

TABLE 16-12 How is sleepiness evaluated?

Subjective method:
- Epworth Sleepiness Scale
  - 8 questions self rated on a 0–3 scale

Objective method:
- Multiple sleep latency test (MSLT)
  - Nocturnal polysomnogram
  - Five daytime nap opportunities lying in a quiet, dark room at 2-hour intervals, told not to oppose sleep
  - Score time to sleep onset defined by EEG
    - Max time 20 minutes
    - Wake patient 15 minutes from sleep onset
- Maintenance of wakefulness test (MWT)
  - Nocturnal polysomnogram
  - Five daytime nap opportunities lying in a quiet, dark room at 2-hour intervals, instructed to resist sleep
- Often the morning after an overnight PSG

TABLE 16-13 Whom do you need to refer for additional testing?

If the clinical evaluation suggests:	PSG	MSLT	MWT
Obstructive sleep apnea	Y	N	N
Narcolepsy with cataplexy*	N[†]	N[†]	For treatment assessment
Narcolepsy without cataplexy	Y	Y	For treatment assessment
Idiopathic hypersomnia	N	Y	For treatment assessment
Restless legs syndrome	N	N	N
Periodic limb movement	Y	N	N
Circadian rhythm disorder	N	N	N

PSG = polysomnography; MSLT = multiple sleep latency test; MWT = maintenance of wakefulness test; Y = typically used; N = not generally used.
*Documentation of cataplexy history may be sufficient for diagnosis.
[†]May be useful if a safety issue is suspected.

How Sleepy Is Sleepiness? Epworth Ratings

Epworth

0 — 6 — 12 — 18 — 24

- normal
- insomnia
- moderate sleep apnea
- anesthesiology residents
- narcolepsy

A

How Sleepy Is Sleepiness? MSLT Ratings

minutes

excessive daytime sleepiness — 7.7% of general population

moderate sleepiness — 29% of general population

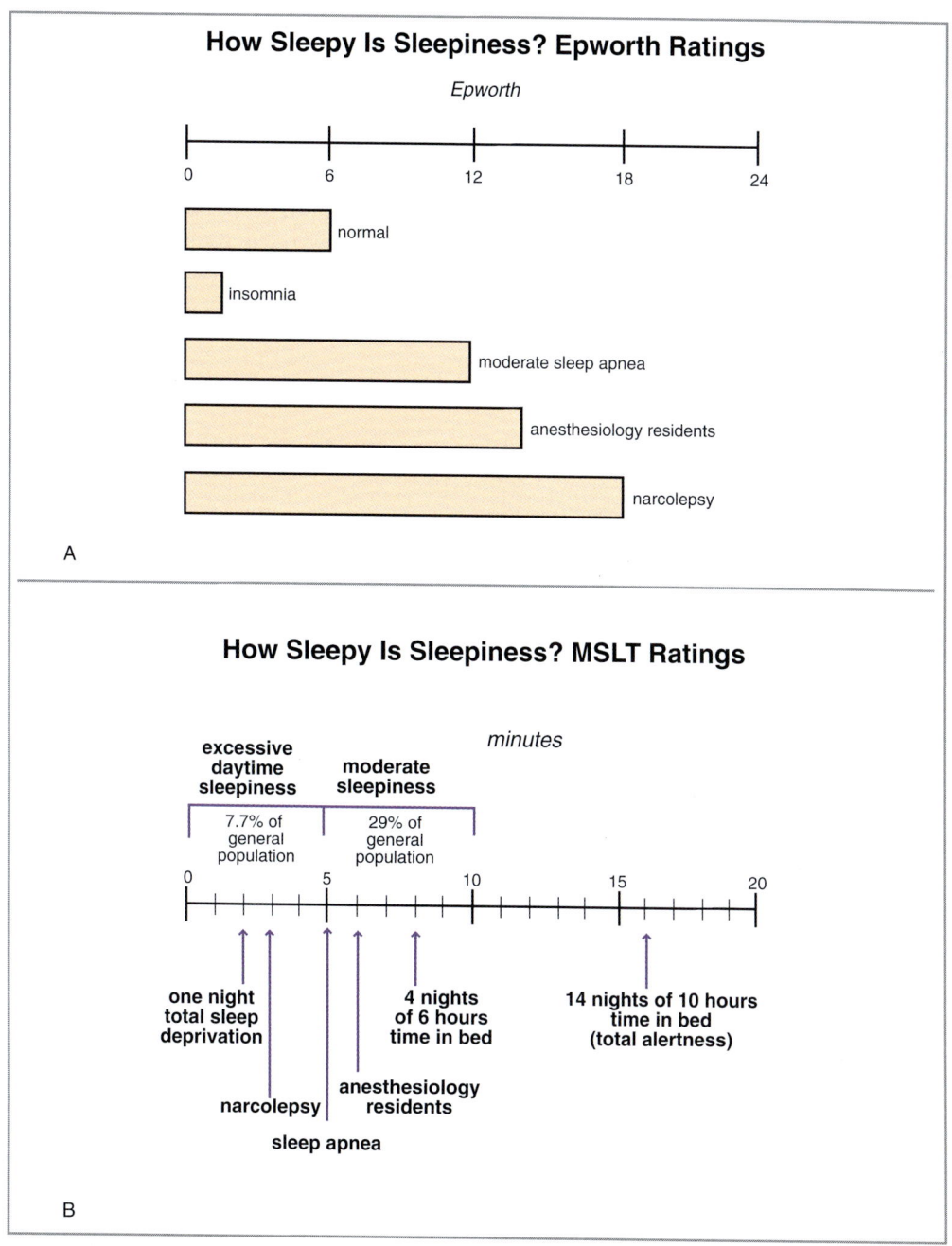

0 — 5 — 10 — 15 — 20

- one night total sleep deprivation
- narcolepsy
- sleep apnea
- 4 nights of 6 hours time in bed
- anesthesiology residents
- 14 nights of 10 hours time in bed (total alertness)

B

FIGURE 16-30A and B How sleepy is sleepiness? Subjective and objective measures. (A) The Epworth Sleepiness Scale (ESS) is a subjective, self-administered rating scale of how sleepy an individual is, with higher scores indicating a higher level of sleepiness. For the general population, the average score on the ESS may be approximately 5.9; scores over 11 indicate excessive sleepiness. Individuals who are sleep-deprived (e.g., anesthesiology residents) and those with sleep disorders generally perceive themselves as sleepy. Interestingly, those with insomnia do not, lending further weight to the theory that insomnia is a disorder of the arousal mechanisms that, as well as keeping someone awake at night, can leave someone in a state of hyperarousal during the day. **(B)** The Multiple Sleep Latencies Test (MSLT) is an objective measure of sleepiness based on how quickly one falls asleep while sitting in a dark, comfortable room. The shorter one's latency to sleep, the sleepier that individual is considered to be, with a latency of less than five minutes indicating excessive sleepiness.

the greatest amount of perceived sleepiness. However, chronically sleep-deprived anesthesiology residents are not far behind, nor are patients with moderate sleep apnea (Figure 16-30A). It is interesting to note that insomnia patients are generally not sleepy, perhaps because they experience excessive arousal in the day as well as at night, as discussed earlier in this chapter (Figure 16-30A).

Objective measures of sleepiness in the general population show that about 30 percent of us have moderate sleepiness and about 8 percent have severe sleepiness, mostly from sleep deprivation (Figure 16-30B). One night of total sleep deprivation actually causes more objective sleepiness than narcolepsy, and sleep-deprived anesthesiology residents are as sleepy as patients with sleep apnea!

What's wrong with being sleepy?

Patients with excessive daytime sleepiness have problems with cognitive functioning. For example, when patients with narcolepsy or sleep deprivation try to perform cognitive testing, they can, with great effort, often activate their dorsolateral prefrontal cortex normally, but they cannot sustain it (Figure 16-31A). When these same patients take a stimulant or modafinil, they are able to sustain the activation of their DLPFC and also to sustain their cognitive performance without decrement (Figure 16-31B). Presumably, this improvement is the result of optimizing and increasing the actions of dopamine in DLPFC (dorsolateral prefrontal cortex) brain circuits. The role of the DLPFC in cognitive functioning, the neuroimaging of DLPFC activation, and the influence of genetic variability affecting dopamine are introduced in Chapter 8 and illustrated in Figures 8-8 through 8-10.

How much dopamine is a good thing? The DLPFC must be optimally "tuned" with dopamine in order to improve cognitive functioning (see Chapter 7 and Figures 7-25 and 7-26). Sleepy patients have their DLPFC out of tune, and the pyramidal neurons there have inefficient information processing; thus cognitive symptoms such as inattentiveness, problems concentrating, and mental fatigue occur. This state of affairs is represented in Figure 16-32A as low amounts of tonic dopamine firing from dopamine neurons. When wake-promoting agents "softly" enhance dopamine, presumably in CSTC circuits of the DLPFC (see Figures 7-16 and 7-17), this leads to an enhancement of tonic dopamine firing, as shown in Figure 16-32B, and a return of alertness. However, dopamine neurons and their postsynaptic connections in CSTC circuits are temperamental, and too much dopamine released too quickly can produce sudden phasic bursts of dopamine that trigger reinforcement, reward, and ultimately stimulant abuse (Figure 16-32C). For this reason, nonstimulants such as modafinil and caffeine, which improve wakefulness but do not really cause drug abuse due to their ability to enhance tonic but not phasic dopamine firing, may be preferred for patients with sleepiness. If stimulants are used, there are ways to prescribe and dose them so that they are more likely to enhance tonic than phasic firing and thus to cause wakefulness without euphoria (compare Figure 16-32B and 16-32C). Giving stimulants orally that have slow onset and sustained action is thus preferred to high-dose, rapid-onset administration or any route of administration other than oral or transdermal.

Because of the potential of abuse of stimulants, many psychopharmacologists are hesitant to prescribe them for sleepiness. Because even modafinil can be abused in a different way by patients using it in lieu of sleep and thus perpetuating chronic sleep deprivation, some psychopharmacologists may be hesitant to prescribe this agent as well. Therefore the modern psychopharmacologist must provide an answer for the question: Who gets to have wakefulness on demand?

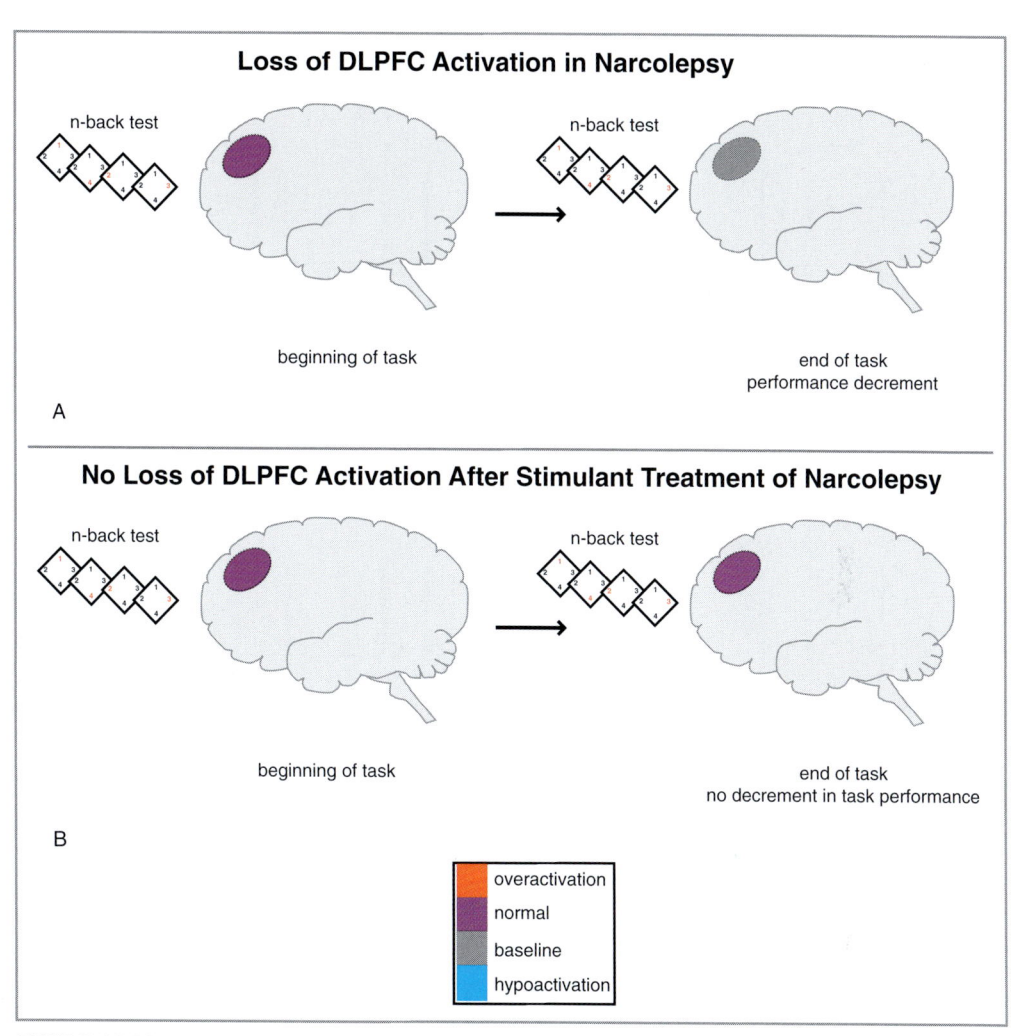

FIGURE 16-31A and B Information processing in narcolepsy. Excessive sleepiness may impair cognitive functioning, which can be demonstrated in narcolepsy patients as they perform the n-back test. Performing the n-back test normally results in activation of the dorsolateral prefrontal cortex (DLPFC). The degree of activation indicates how efficient the information processing is in DLPFC, with both overactivation and hypoactivation associated with inefficient information processing. **(A)** With effort, narcolepsy patients may be able to activate their DLPFC normally at the start of a cognitive task (indicated by the purple color); however, they cannot sustain this activation (indicated by the gray color) and thus perform poorly toward the end of the task. **(B)** Administration of a dopaminergic wake-promoting treatment such as a stimulant or modafinil may enable the individual to sustain activation of the DLPFC and thus allow for improved cognitive performance.

Is it only for patients with narcolepsy and sleep apnea? Most patients with narcolepsy are likely to come to medical attention, but with the prevalence of obstructive sleep apnea in adults estimated as between 3 and 30 percent and rising with the current epidemic of obesity, many of these people are not diagnosed and even fewer of them receive wake-promoting drugs. Perhaps more of them do receive continuous positive airway pressure (CPAP) without augmentation with modafinil. Nevertheless, an important subset of sleep apnea patients present with treatment-resistant depression and undiagnosed sleep apnea, suggesting that a higher index of suspicion for sleepiness in general and sleep apnea in particular

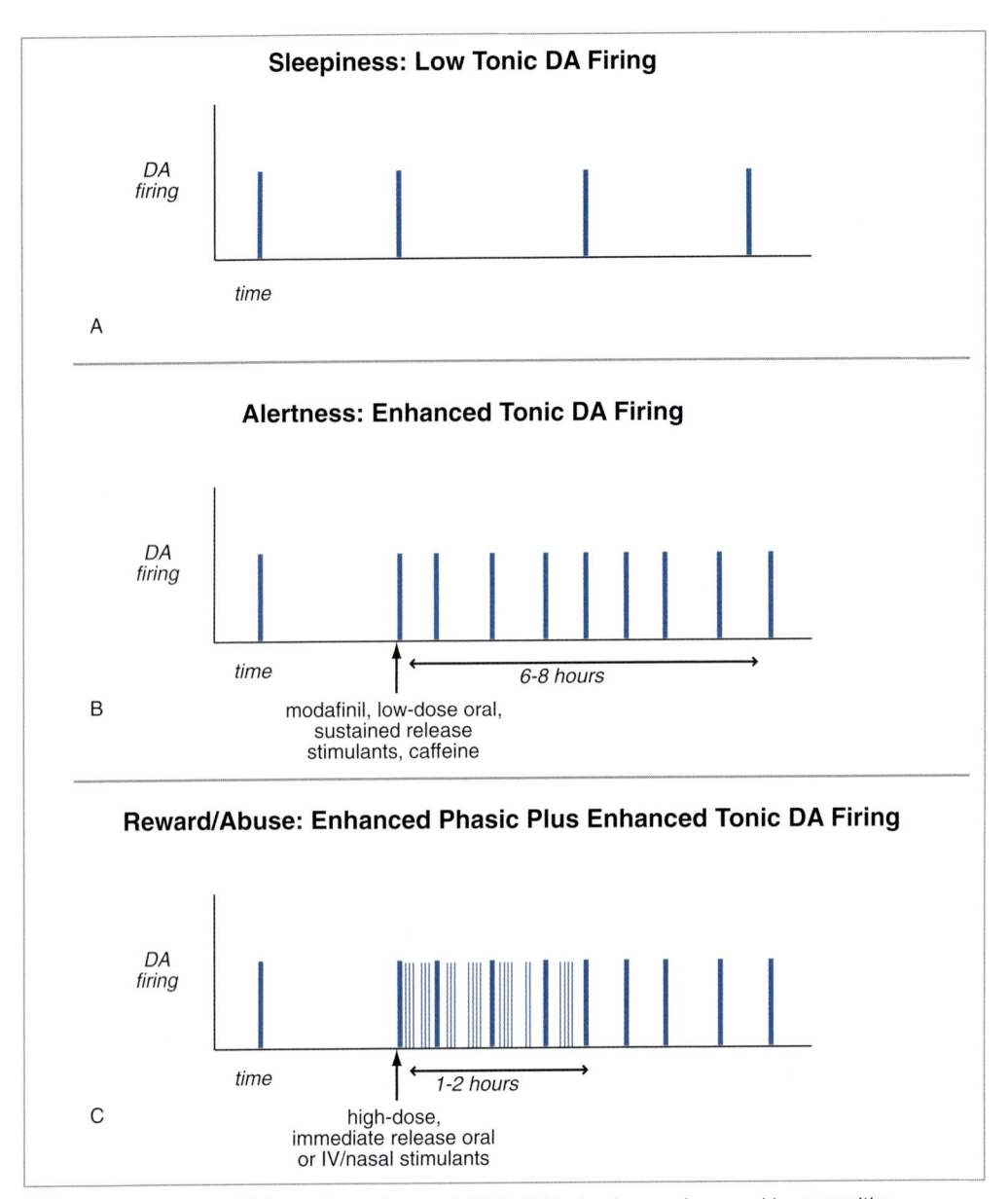

FIGURE 16-32A, B, and C Dopamine and arousal. (**A**) Individuals who are sleepy and have cognitive impairment may have low tonic dopamine firing. (**B**) "Soft" effects on dopamine, such as by modafinil or caffeine, can lead to enhancement of tonic dopamine firing and thus normal alertness. (**C**) Agents that produce sudden phasic bursts of dopamine, such as immediate-release stimulants, may carry increased risk for reward/abuse.

would be well served in psychopharmacology. CPAP and modafinil or stimulants may be more effective for the depression in such patients than combinations of antidepressants alone.

What persons with circadian rhythm disturbances get to take wake-promoting agents? Sleepy shift workers like police, firefighters, nurses? It is estimated that a third of shift workers have shift-work sleep disorder, but almost none take a wake-promoting agent other than caffeine. Should jet-lagged executives traveling internationally be provided with wake-promoting drugs? How about surgeons operating all night in an emergency and then driving home the next morning after 24 hours of sleep deprivation? Computer programmers and students pulling all-nighters and then driving? Teenagers with phase delay unresponsive to melatonin and bright-light therapy? Depressed patients with hypersomnia, fatigue, or problems concentrating but no documented sleep disorder (see Chapter 12 and Figures 12-124 through 12-126)? These situations all require prudent assessment of risks and benefits of prescribing wake-promoting agents, keeping up with the literature, and a sophisticated idea of the mechanism of action of wake-promoting agents in order to judge to whom to provide them.

Mechanism of action of wake-promoting agents
Modafinil

This drug is a proven wake-promoting agent whose exact molecular mechanism of action remains debated. It is known to activate relatively selectively neurons in the wake promoter TMN and the lateral hypothalamus, which leads to the release of both histamine and orexin. However, the activation of the lateral hypothalamus and release of orexin do not appear to be necessary for the action of modafinil, since modafinil still promotes wakefulness in patients who have loss of hypothalamic orexin neurons in narcolepsy. The activation of TMN and lateral hypothalamic neurons may be secondary and downstream actions resulting from modafinil's effects on dopamine neurons.

The most likely modafinil binding site is probably the dopamine transporter (DAT or DA reuptake pump in Figure 16-33). Although modafinil is a weak DAT inhibitor, the concentrations of the drug achieved after oral dosing are quite high and sufficient to have a substantial action on DAT. How much occupancy of DAT is required to have an effective clinical action is debated in Chapter 12 on antidepressants and illustrated in Figures 12-44 and 12-46 in relation to the weak DAT (and NET, norepinephrine transporter) inhibitor bupropion. In fact, the pharmacokinetics of modafinil suggest that this drugs acts via a slow rise in plasma levels, sustained plasma levels for 6 to 8 hours, and incomplete occupancy of DAT, all properties that could be ideal for enhancing tonic dopamine activity to promote wakefulness (Figure 12-32B) rather than phasic dopamine activity to promote reinforcement and abuse (Figure 12-32C). Once dopamine release is activated by modafinil and the cortex is aroused, this can apparently lead to downstream release of histamine from the TMN and then further activation of the lateral hypothalamus with orexin release to stabilize wakefulness. The same appears to occur after administration of the stimulants amphetamine and methylphenidate.

Since this mechanism of action of modafinil as primarily a weak and pharmacokinetically favorable DAT inhibitor (Figure 16-33) remains a theory and is not proven, it is difficult to discover and develop further modafinil-like agents. One possible therapeutic advance in the quest for novel wake-promoting agents is the R enantiomer of modafinil, called armodafinil (Nuvigil). Armodafinil has an even later time to peak levels, a longer half-life, and higher plasma drug levels 6 to14 hours after oral administration than the marketed form of modafinil, which is a racemic mixture of R plus S modafinil. The pharmacokinetic properties of armodafinil could theoretically improve the clinical profile of modafinil, with greater activation of phasic dopamine firing, possibly eliminating the need for a second daily dose, as is often required with racemic modafinil. Armodafinil is currently in late-stage clinical development as a wake-promoting agent. Another wake-promoting drug in early development that may have some similarities to modafinil is VSF-173, in testing for excessive sleepiness and for cognitive disorders.

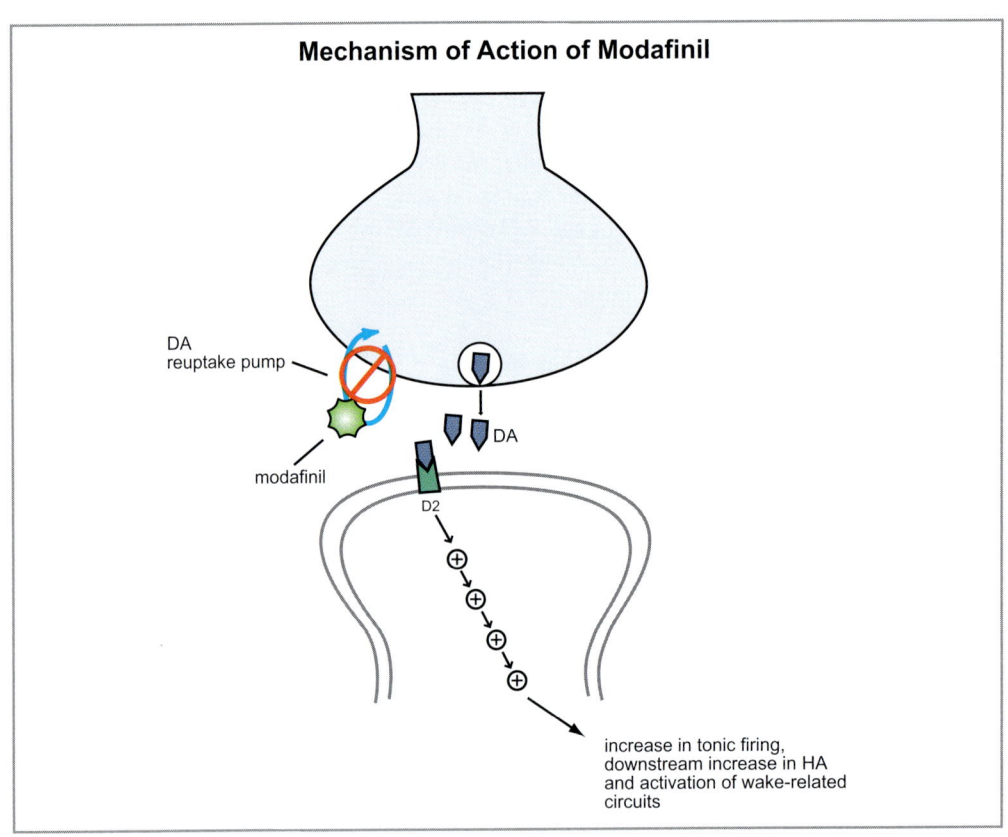

FIGURE 16-33 Modafinil. The precise mechanism of action of modafinil is yet to be fully elucidated. It is known to bind to the dopamine transporter (DAT) and in fact requires its presence. Modafinil's low affinity for the DAT has led some to question whether its binding there is relevant; however, because plasma levels of modafinil are high, this "compensates" for the low binding affinity. It is believed that the increase in synaptic dopamine following blockade of DAT leads to increased tonic firing and downstream effects on neurotransmitters involved in wakefulness, including histamine and orexin/hypocretin.

Stimulants
The two principal stimulants used as wake-promoting agents are methylphenidate and amphetamine, especially d-amphetamine. Many forms of these stimulants are now available and are reviewed in detail in Chapter 17, on attention deficit hyperactivity disorder (ADHD). Actions of amphetamine as a competitive inhibitor and substrate for DAT and also as a dopamine releaser and inhibitor of the vesicular monoamine transporter (VMAT2) are discussed in detail in Chapter 4 and illustrated in Figure 4-15. Methylphenidate is known to be an inhibitor of DAT, which acts not unlike the NDRI (norepinephrine and dopamine reuptake inhibitor) antidepressants discussed in Chapter 12 and illustrated in Figure 12-46. The mechanism of methylphenidate is also discussed in Chapter 17 on ADHD. The mechanism of action of amphetamine is also discussed in further detail in Chapter 17 and in Chapter 19, on drug abuse. Generally not emphasized are important properties of stimulants in blocking the norepinephrine transporter (NET), especially at low doses in controlled-release formulations. Basically, the stimulants enhance the synaptic availability of dopamine and norepinephrine and thereby improve wakefulness.

TABLE 16-14 Caffeine formulations

Beverage (12 oz unless otherwise noted)	Caffeine (mg)
Grande Starbucks	520!!
Coffee, drip or brewed	80–175
Red Bull (8.2 oz)	80
Jolt	71.2
Pepsi One	55.5
Mountain Dew (regular, diet, Code Red)	55
Surge	51
Iced tea	47
Diet Coke (12 oz)	45.6
Diet Pepsi	36
Coca-Cola (12 oz)	34

Caffeine

Caffeine is an incredible over-the-counter drug and popular in many beverages (Table 16-14), but how does it work? Originally thought to work as an inhibitor of the enzyme phosphodiesterase, it is now believed to act mostly as an antagonist of endogenous neurotransmitters called purines, of which an important one is adenosine, at purine receptors (Figures 16-34). Certain purine receptors are functionally coupled with dopamine receptors, such that the actions of dopamine at D2 receptors (Figure 16-34A) are antagonized when adenosine is binding to its receptor (Figure 16-34B). Not surprisingly, therefore, when an antagonist of adenosine like caffeine is present, this indirectly promotes the actions of dopamine (Figure 16-34C).

Gamma hydroxybutyrate

Gamma hydroxybutyrate, or GHB, is also known as sodium oxybate and as Xyrem. This agent is approved for the treatment of excessive daytime sleepiness associated with narcolepsy as well as for cataplexy. It is also in testing for fibromyalgia, as discussed in Chapter 15. It appears to promote wakefulness by its profound actions on slow-wave sleep at night, making the patient more rested and therefore more alert the next day. Because of its abuse potential and colorful history, it is scheduled as a controlled substance and its supplies are tightly regulated through a central pharmacy in the United States. It has been labeled a "date rape" drug by the press, as it has occasionally been used with alcohol for this purpose. Because it profoundly increases slow-wave sleep and the growth hormone surge that accompanies slow-wave sleep, it has been used (abused) by athletes as a performance-enhancing drug, especially in the 1980s, when it was sold over the counter in health food stores. GHB is used in some European countries as a treatment for alcoholism. Due to its observed enhancement of slow-wave sleep, GHB was recently developed for the treatment of narcolepsy and cataplexy.

GHB is actually a natural product present in the brain, with its own GHB receptors, upon which it acts (Figure 16-35). GHB is formed from the neurotransmitter GABA and also acts at GABA-B receptors as a partial agonist (Figure 16-35).

The wake-up pharmacy (Figure 16-36)
The major wake-promoting agents are caffeine, modafinil, and the stimulants methylphenidate and d-amphetamine.

Summary
The neurobiology of wakefulness is linked to an arousal system that utilizes the five neurotransmitters histamine, dopamine, norepinephrine, acetylcholine, and serotonin as components of the ascending reticular activating system. Sleep and wakefulness are also regulated by a hypothalamic sleep/wake switch, with wake-promoter neurons in the tuberomammillary nucleus that utilize histamine as neurotransmitter and sleep-promoter neurons in the ventrolateral preoptic nucleus that utilize GABA as neurotransmitter. The synthesis, metabolism, and receptors for the neurotransmitter histamine are reviewed in this chapter. Insomnia is also briefly reviewed, as are the mechanisms of action of several hypnotics from the benzodiazepines to the popular "Z" drugs that act as positive allosteric modulators or PAMs for GABA-A receptors. Other hypnotics include trazodone, melatonergic hypnotics, and antihistamines, including novel H1 selective antagonists.

Excessive daytime sleepiness is also briefly reviewed, as are the mechanisms of action of the wake-promoting drugs modafinil, caffeine, and stimulants. The actions of gamma hydroxybutyrate plus a number of novel sleep- and wake-promoting drugs in clinical development are also reviewed.

CHAPTER 17

Attention Deficit Hyperactivity Disorder and Its Treatment

- Symptoms and circuits: ADHD as a disorder of the prefrontal cortex
- States of deficient and excessive arousal in ADHD
  - Deficient arousal and ADHD
  - Excessive arousal and ADHD
  - Stress, comorbidities, and simultaneous deficient and excessive arousal in ADHD
  - ADHD and comorbidity: What should be treated first?
- ADHD in children versus adults
- Stimulant treatment of ADHD
- Noradrenergic treatment of ADHD
  - Atomoxetine
  - Alpha 2A adrenergic agonists
- The ADHD pharmacy
- Summary

Attention deficit hyperactivity disorder (ADHD) is an area of psychopharmacology that is changing rapidly. A myriad of new drugs, especially in new drug-delivery technologies, is entering clinical practice. ADHD is also increasingly being seen not just as a disorder of attention, nor just as a disorder of children. Paradigm shifts are altering the landscape for treatment options across the full range of ADHD symptoms, now reaching into treatment of comorbidities and being refined for the important differences involved in treating adults.

This chapter provides a brief overview of the psychopharmacology of ADHD. This includes a short discussion of the symptoms and treatments for ADHD, but information on the full clinical descriptions and formal criteria for how to diagnose and rate ADHD and its symptoms should be obtained by consulting standard reference sources. The discussion here emphasizes the links between various brain circuits and their neurotransmitters with the various symptoms and comorbidities of ADHD. The goal of this chapter is to acquaint the reader with ideas about the clinical and biological aspects of attention, impulsivity, hyperactivity, underarousal, overarousal, and stress. This chapter also covers some of the special aspects involved in treating adults, such as the impact of the frequent comorbidities of anxiety, substance abuse, and mood disorders. Emphasis is on the biological basis of symptoms and their relief by psychopharmacological agents as well as the mechanism of action of drugs that treat ADHD in children and adults. For details of doses, side effects, drug interactions, and other issues relevant to the prescribing of these drugs in clinical practice, the reader should consult standard drug handbooks (such as the *Essential Psychopharmacology: Prescriber's Guide*).

Symptoms and circuits: ADHD as a disorder of the prefrontal cortex

ADHD is noted for a trio of symptoms: inattention, hyperactivity, and impulsivity (Figure 17-1). It is currently hypothesized that all these symptoms arise in part from abnormalities in various parts of the prefrontal cortex. Specifically, symptoms of selective inattention are hypothetically linked to inefficient information processing in the anterior cingulate cortex (ACC); symptoms of executive dysfunction, particularly the inability to sustain attention and thus the inability to solve problems, are hypothetically linked to inefficient information processing in another part of the prefrontal cortex, the dorsolateral prefrontal cortex (DLPFC) (Figure 17-2). Hyperactive symptoms in ADHD are linked to the supplementary motor cortex/prefrontal motor cortex, whereas impulsive symptoms are hypothetically related to the orbital frontal cortex (Figure 17-2). Not all patients have all of these symptoms or have them all with the same severity, suggesting a topographical distribution of different prefrontal cortex abnormalities in different patients with different symptom profiles.

Each area of prefrontal cortex is linked to other brain areas via cortical circuits that connect one area of prefrontal cortex to another (see discussion in Chapter 7 and Figures 7-3, 7-14, and 7-15) and via cortico-striatal-thalamic-cortical (CSTC) loops that connect

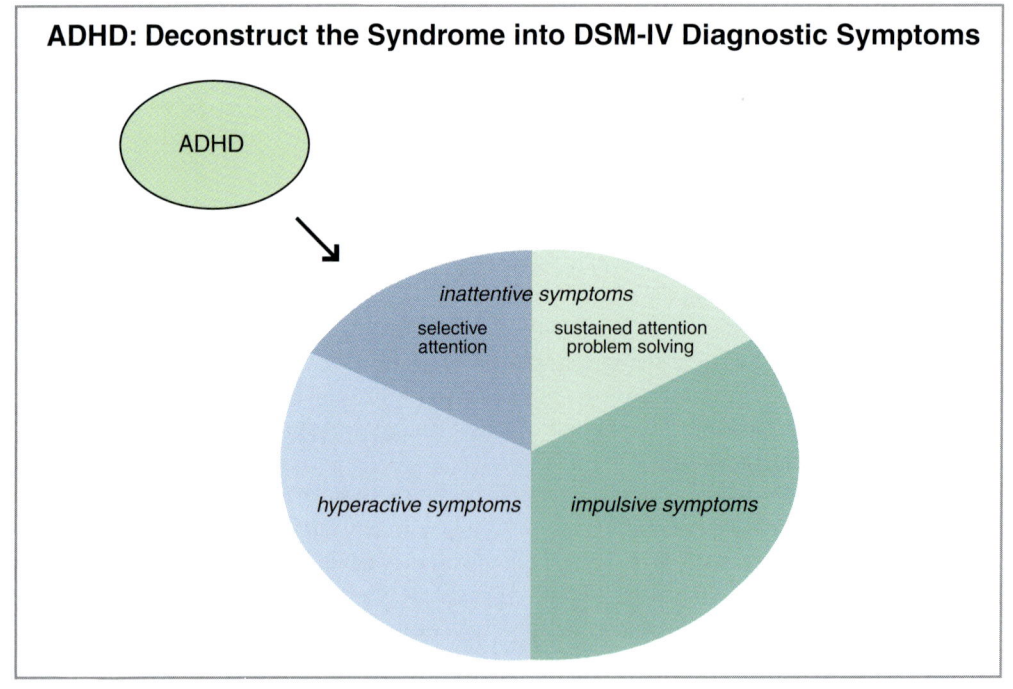

FIGURE 17-1 DSM-IV symptoms of ADHD. There are three major categories of symptoms associated with attention deficit hyperactivity disorder (ADHD): inattention, hyperactivity, and impulsivity. Inattention itself can be divided into difficulty with selective attention and difficulty with sustained attention and problem solving.

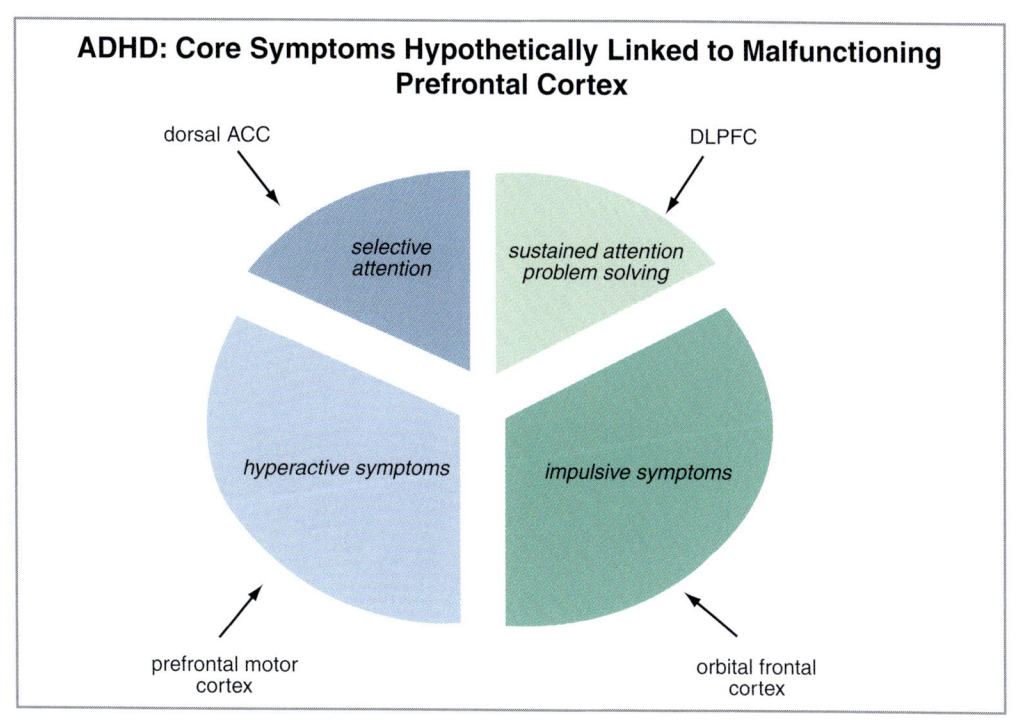

FIGURE 17-2 Matching ADHD symptoms to circuits. Problems with selective attention are believed to be linked to inefficient information processing in the dorsal anterior cingulate cortex (ACC), while problems with sustained attention are linked to inefficient information processing in the dorsolateral prefrontal cortex (DLPFC). Hyperactivity may be modulated by the prefrontal motor cortex and impulsivity by the orbital frontal cortex (OFC).

specific areas of prefrontal cortex to subcortical brain areas. CSTC loops are introduced in Chapter 7 and illustrated in Figures 7-16 through 7-21. Each area of prefrontal cortex is linked to specific topographical areas in the striatum–nucleus accumbens and in the thalamus (see Figures 7-17 through 7-21 and 17-3 through 17-6).

The specific symptoms of ADHD hypothetically linked to each of these prefrontal brain circuits are listed in Figures 17-3 through 17-6. For example, the dorsal ACC can be activated by tests of selective attention, such as the Stroop test (Figure 17-3). Hypothetically, patients who cannot focus their attention have inefficient information processing in this part of the brain, including its CSTC projections, shown in Figure 17-3. ADHD patients may either fail to activate this part of the brain when they should be focusing their attention, or they activate this part of the brain very inefficiently and only with great effort and easy fatigability. Activation of the dorsal ACC by the Stroop test is introduced in Chapter 8 and illustrated in Figures 8-14 and 8-15.

The DLPFC can be activated by tests of executive function, such as the n-back test (Figure 17-4). Hypothetically, patients who cannot sustain their attention on a task and who experience difficulties in organizing, following through, and solving problems have inefficient information processing in the DLPFC (Figure 17-5). Activation of DLPFC by the n-back test is introduced in Chapter 8 and illustrated in Figures 8-8 through 8-10 and 8-18 through 8-20. Problems activating this part of the brain cut across many syndromes that share the symptom of executive dysfunction, from schizophrenia (discussed in Chapter 9 and illustrated in Figures 9-15 through 9-17 and 9-59 through 9-61); to major depression (discussed in Chapter 11 and illustrated in Figures 11-45 and 11-50); to mania (discussed

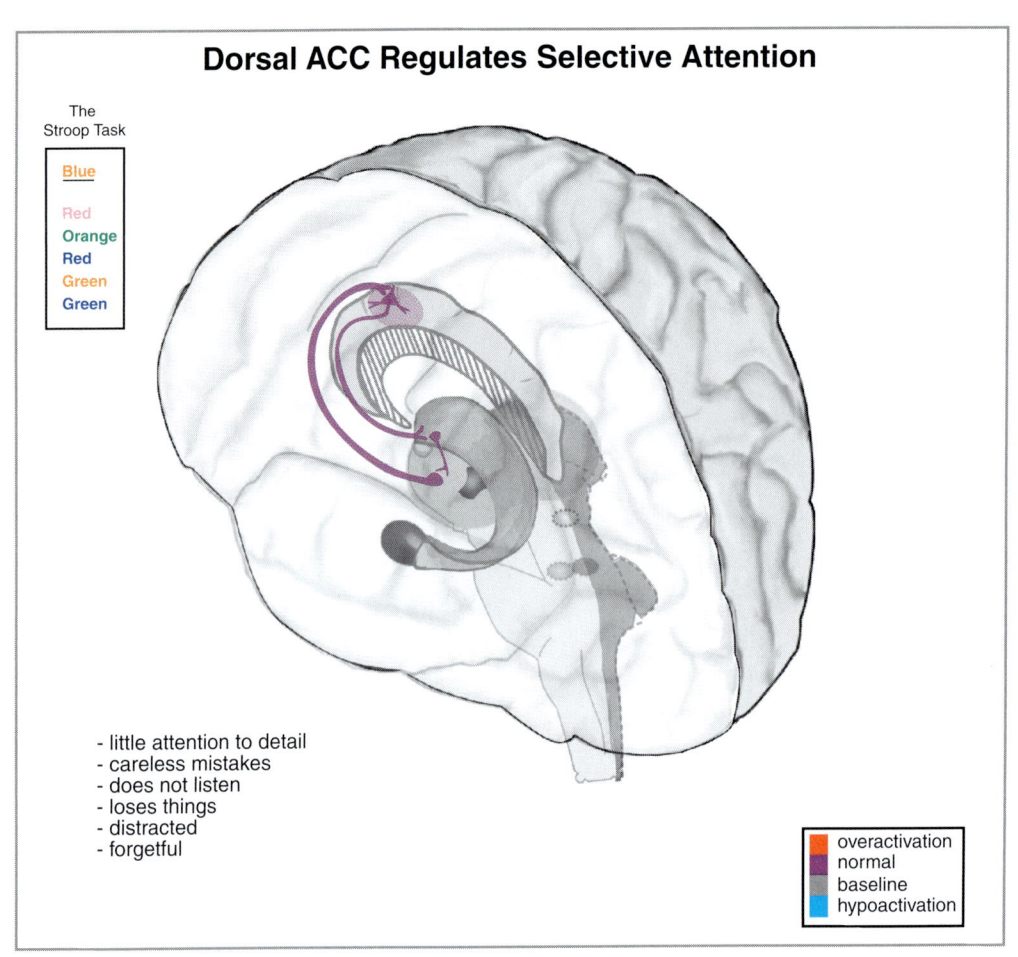

FIGURE 17-3 Selective attention circuit. Selective attention is hypothetically modulated by a cortico-striatal-thalamic-cortical loop arising from the dorsal anterior cingulate cortex (ACC) and projecting to the bottom of the striatum, then the thalamus, and back to the dorsal ACC. Deficient and/or inefficient activation of this brain region can result in symptoms such as paying little attention to detail, making careless mistakes, not listening, losing things, being distracted, and forgetting things. An example of a task that involves selective attention, and thus should activate the dorsal ACC, is the Stroop test.

in Chapter 11 and illustrated in Figures 11-56, 11-61, and 11-64); to anxiety (discussed in Chapter 14 and illustrated in Figures 14-44 and 14-45); to disorders of pain (e.g., fibromyalgia and "fibro-fog," discussed in Chapter 15 and illustrated in Figure 15-22); to disorders of sleep and wakefulness (discussed in Chapter 16 and illustrated in Figures 16-1 and 16-31).

The pervasiveness of problems with attention and concentration across psychiatric disorders is so great that it can lead one to ask: What is the difference between attention deficit and attention deficit disorder (see also Table 17-1)? Indeed, what are the differences between treatments for attention deficit in different psychiatric syndromes and those for ADHD? It turns out that the same DLPFC circuit may be involved in mediating these symptoms of executive dysfunction across many psychiatric disorders (Table 17-1), and the same empiric treatments, discussed in detail in this chapter, may be useful for executive dysfunction and inattention, whether the patient has the attention deficit of a psychiatric

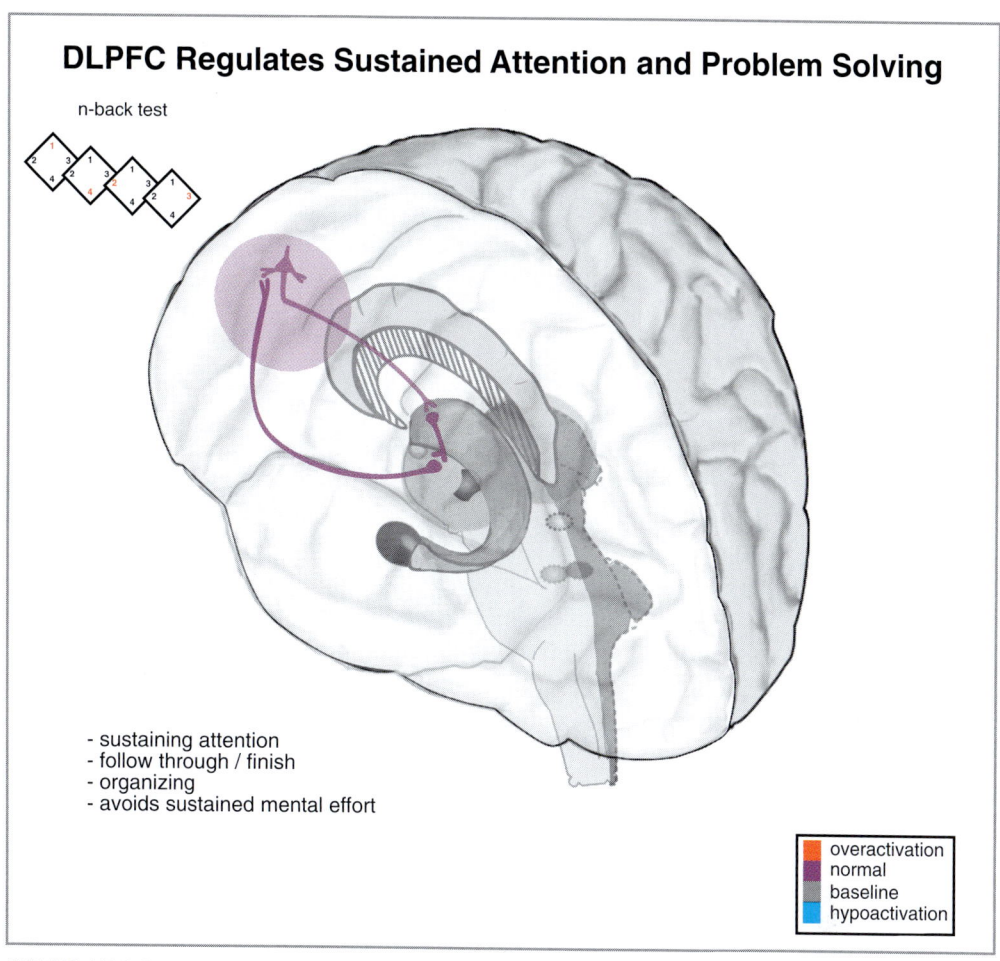

FIGURE 17-4 Sustained attention circuit. Sustained attention is hypothetically modulated by a cortico-striatal-thalamic-cortical loop that involves the dorsolateral prefrontal cortex (DLPFC) and the rostral (top) part of the caudate within the striatal complex. Deficient and/or inefficient activation of the DLPFC can lead to difficulty following through or finishing tasks, disorganization, and trouble sustaining mental effort. Tasks such as the n-back test are used to measure sustained attention and problem solving abilities.

disorder or the attention deficit of ADHD. For adults in particular, comorbidity of ADHD with other psychiatric disorders characterized by executive dysfunction is so pervasive that trying to distinguish the attention deficit of ADHD from the attention deficit of other psychiatric conditions may not be clinically useful (Table 17-1).

Other areas of prefrontal cortex that may not be functioning efficiently in ADHD are the supplementary motor area and prefrontal motor cortex, linked to symptoms of motor hyperactivity (Figure 17-5), and orbital frontal cortex, linked to symptoms of impulsivity (Figure 17-6). Orbital frontal cortex is a very important part of prefrontal cortex and has been discussed in relation to a wide variety of symptoms that cut across several psychiatric conditions, from impulsivity in schizophrenia (discussed in Chapter 9 and illustrated in Figure 9-14) to suicidality in depression (discussed in Chapter 11 and illustrated in Figure 11-53) to impulsivity in mania (discussed in Chapter 11 and illustrated in Figures 11-58, 11-59, and 11-66). Perhaps all of these symptoms of impulsivity are due to defective thalamic

Prefrontal Motor Cortex Regulates Motor Hyperactivity

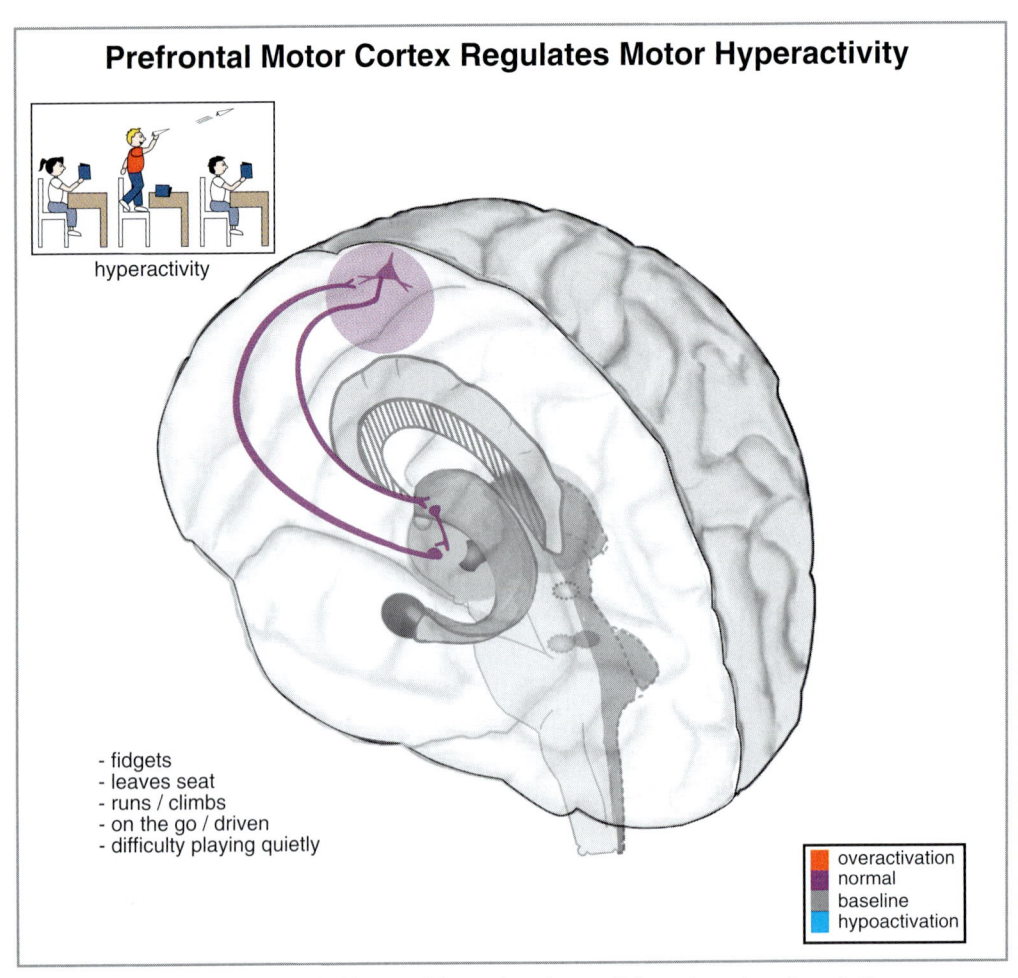

- fidgets
- leaves seat
- runs / climbs
- on the go / driven
- difficulty playing quietly

overactivation
normal
baseline
hypoactivation

FIGURE 17-5 Hyperactivity circuit. Motor activity, such as hyperactivity and psychomotor agitation or retardation, can be modulated by a cortico-striatal-thalamic-cortical loop from the prefrontal motor cortex to the putamen (lateral striatum) to the thalamus and back to the prefrontal motor cortex. Common symptoms of hyperactivity in children with ADHD include fidgeting, leaving one's seat, running/climbing, being constantly on the go, and having trouble playing quietly.

filtering of information in CSTC loops, allowing impulsive action to occur before the "governor" of the prefrontal cortex, the DLPFC, can inhibit it (see discussions of thalamic filters in Chapters 9 and 16 and Figures 9-41, 16-4, and 16-5).

The orbital frontal cortex is part of the limbic system and is linked to another important limbic area, known as the nucleus accumbens, via CSTC loops (Figures 7-20 and 17-6). This specific circuit may be responsible for linking an incoming stimulus to emotions and for transforming emotions into actions. The limbic CSTC circuit from orbital frontal cortex seems to do this by responding to various stimuli that are relevant, interesting, fascinating, or rewarding with the release of neurotransmitters such as dopamine. The features of a stimulus that can provoke dopamine release in the nucleus accumbens are sometimes also described as having "salience." Thus, salient stimuli are powerful motivators, and when received, they have the potential of being immediately transformed into action prior to the application of cognitive analysis, reflection, and judgment. That is the essence of impulsivity and might

TABLE 17-1 The same symptoms can overlap in many different syndromes and disorders

Symptom \ Disorder	ADHD	MDD/GAD	Narcolepsy	OSA	SW	Sleep deprivation
Inattention/problems concentrating	+++	++	++	++	++	+++
Mood/anxiety	–	+++	–	+	–	+/–
Sleepiness	+	+	+++	+++	+++	+++
Fatigue	+	++	++	++	++	+++

ADHD = attention deficit hyperactivity disorder; MDD = major depressive disorder; GAD = generalized anxiety disorder; OSA = obstructive sleep apnea; SW = shift-work sleep disorder.
+++Most Common
++Common
+Average
- None

Orbital Frontal Cortex Regulates Impulsivity

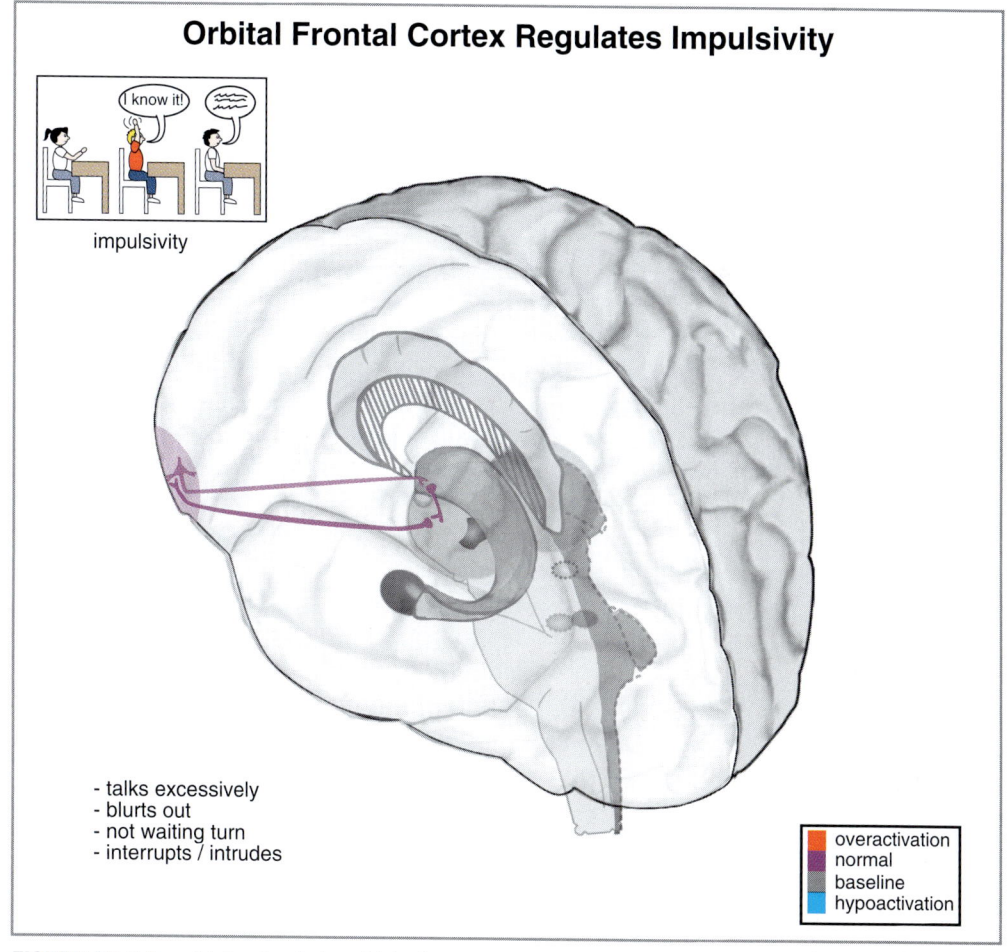

- talks excessively
- blurts out
- not waiting turn
- interrupts / intrudes

overactivation
normal
baseline
hypoactivation

FIGURE 17-6 Impulsivity circuit. Impulsivity is associated with a cortico-striatal-thalamic-cortical loop that involves the orbital frontal cortex (OFC), the bottom of the caudate, and the thalamus. Examples of impulsive symptoms in ADHD include talking excessively, blurting things out, not waiting one's turn, and interrupting.

TABLE 17-2 What causes ADHD?

Genetics	Environment
▪ ~75% of variance	▪ Fetal distress (e.g., preterm birth)
▪ As heritable or more so as schizophrenia	▪ Maternal smoking
▪ Genes implicated	▪ Iron deficiency?
– DAT (dopamine transporter)	▪ Lead exposure?
– DRD 4 (D_4 receptor)	
– DRD 5 (D_5 receptor)	
– DBH (dopamine beta hydroxylase)	
– ADRA 2A (alpha 2A receptor)	
– SNAP 25 (synaptic protein)	
– 5HTTLPR (long) (5HT transporter)	
– HTR 1B (serotonin 1B receptor)	
– FADS 2 (fatty acid desaturase 2)	

help to explain why impulsive people act in self-destructive ways that are not rational and make no sense. Perhaps their brain circuits are not capable of evaluating powerful salient stimuli before they spring into action; such brain circuits may not have the ability to inhibit the expression of feelings and forestall overt behavior. Not surprisingly, the orbital frontal cortex is also implicated in substance abuse, so it is no wonder that there is considerable abuse of nicotine, alcohol, stimulants, and other drugs in patients with ADHD. The role of the orbital frontal cortex circuits in disorders other than ADHD but that are similarly characterized by impulsivity is discussed in further detail in Chapter 19, on drug abuse.

What causes these problems in the prefrontal cortex? Currently, genetic factors are thought to be the major cause of neurodevelopmental abnormalities in the prefrontal cortex in ADHD (Table 17-2). In fact, genes that code for subtle molecular abnormalities are thought to be just as important to the etiology of ADHD as they are to the etiology of schizophrenia. Many of the ideas about the neurodevelopmental basis of schizophrenia, such as abnormal synapse formation and abnormal synaptic neurotransmission, serve as a conceptual framework and neurobiological model for ADHD. The genetic factors linked to schizophrenia are discussed extensively in Chapter 9 and illustrated in Figures 9-52 through 9-58. The major genes implicated in ADHD are those linked to the neurotransmitter dopamine (Table 17-2), although links to the genes for the alpha 2A adrenergic receptor, serotonin receptors, and some other proteins are also under intense investigation (Table 17-2). Environmental factors inevitably contribute to ADHD, as they do to so many other psychiatric disorders (Table 17-2). This includes factors such as preterm birth, maternal smoking during pregnancy, and others (Table 17-2). The stress diathesis hypothesis integrating genetics and environment to the etiology of mental illnesses is introduced in Chapter 6 and illustrated in Figures 6-7 through 6-17.

States of deficient and excessive arousal in ADHD

Deficient arousal and ADHD

ADHD is linked to the neurobiology of arousal mechanisms. Hyperactive children often seem "wired" and overstimulated. From this perspective it can seem counterintuitive that ADHD would be treated with stimulants, which actually cause normal individuals to become wired and overstimulated. As discussed above, however, we now know that defective inhibitory influences of a neurodevelopmentally compromised prefrontal cortex can

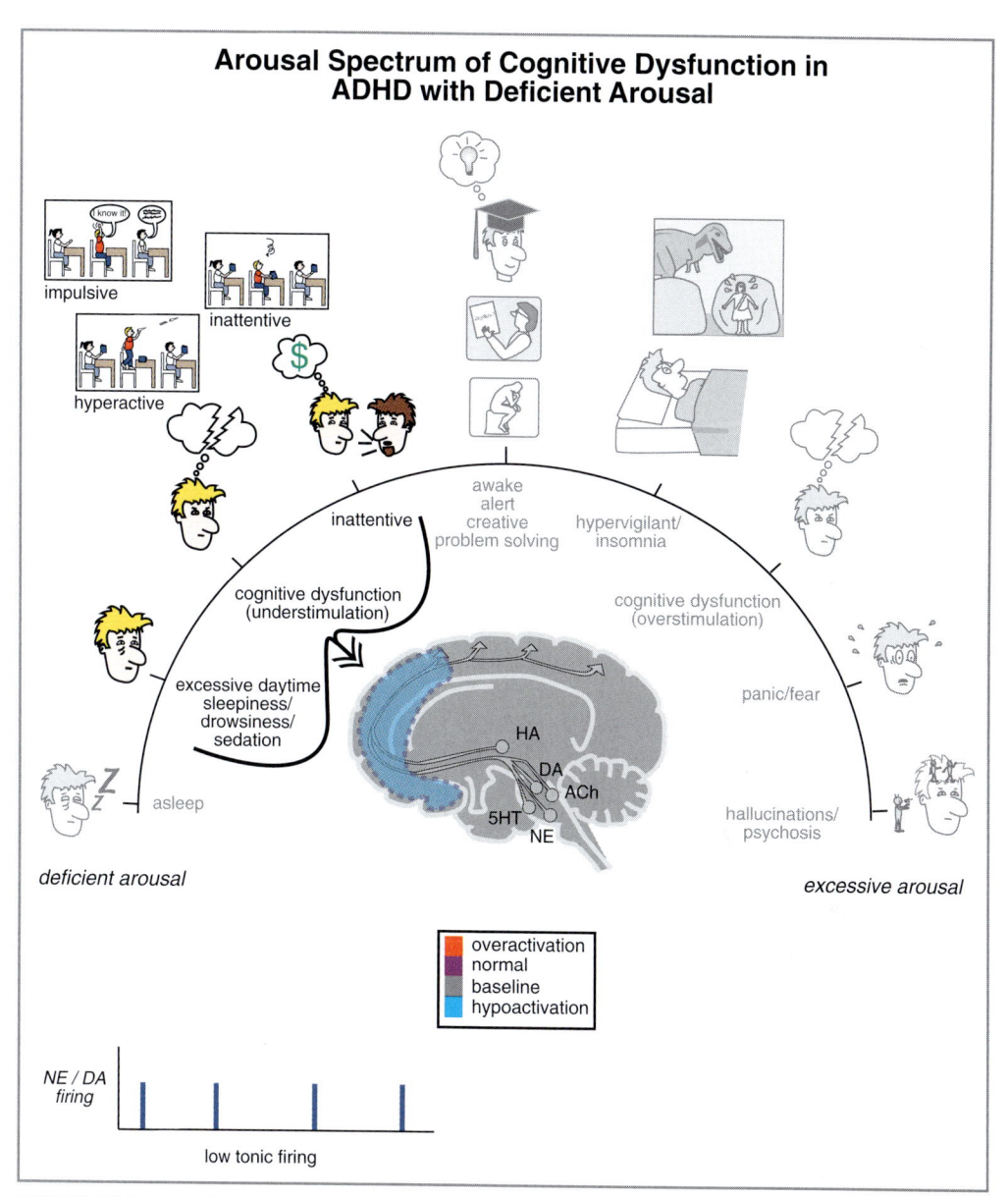

FIGURE 17-7 Arousal spectrum of cognitive dysfunction in ADHD: deficient arousal. The spectrum of arousal is shown here. Individuals in a state of hypoarousal during the day (depicted here as the prefrontal cortex being blue) may experience inattentiveness, cognitive dysfunction, and sleepiness, with impulsivity particularly associated with hypoactivation of the orbital frontal cortex. In addition, hyperactivity in ADHD patients may result from an effort to combat the state of hypoarousal that these patients are in. Hypoarousal during the day may be associated with low tonic dopamine and norepinephrine firing.

contribute to inefficient information processing, resulting in the ADHD symptoms of inattention, hyperactivity, and impulsivity (Figures 17-3 through 17-6). Specifically, this inefficient information processing is often thought to be the product of deficiencies in arousal networks (Figure 17-7 on the left). Therefore agents that increase the drive of the arousal network by enhancing the synaptic actions of dopamine (DA) and norepinephrine

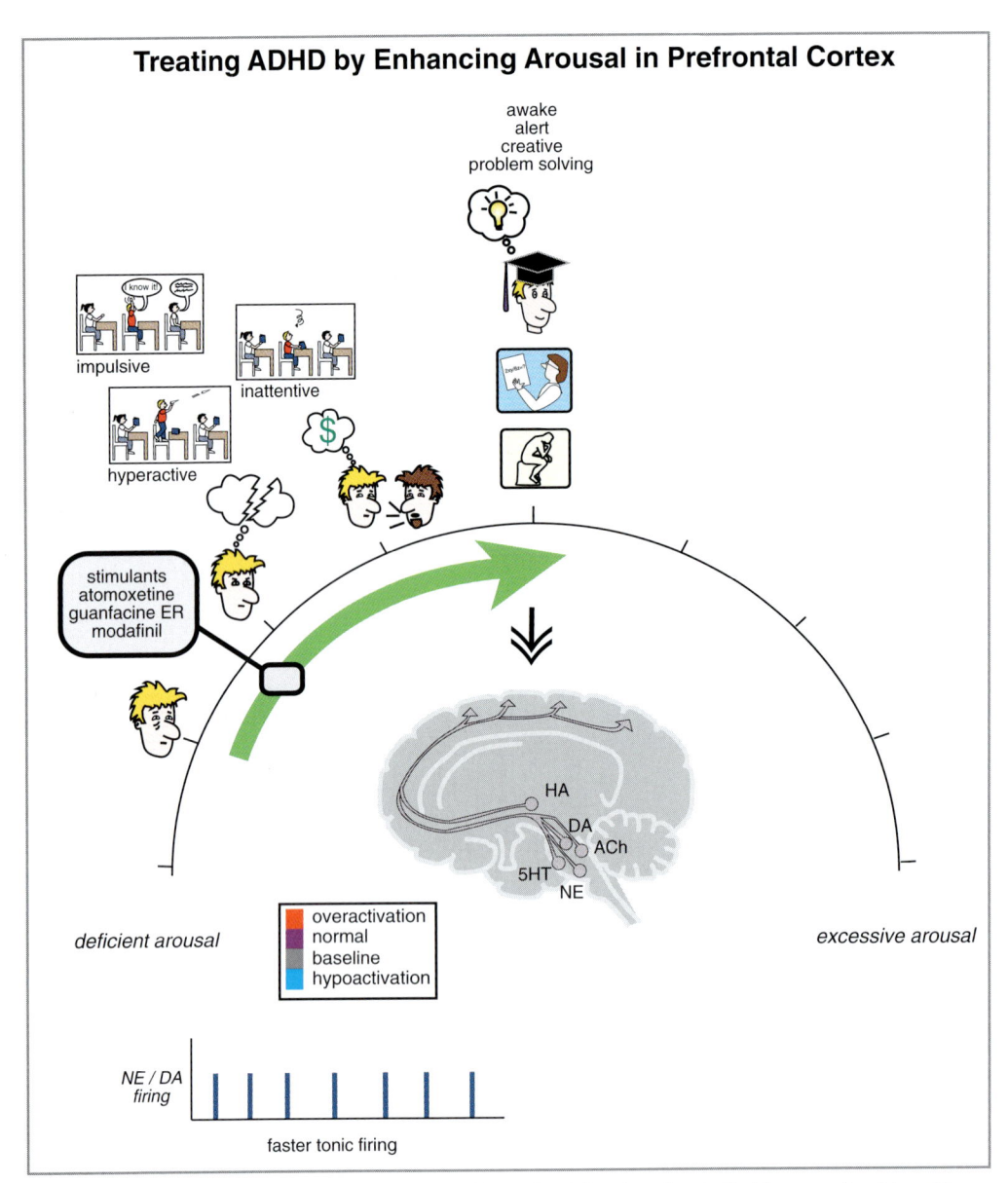

FIGURE 17-8 Treating ADHD by enhancing arousal in prefrontal cortex. Agents that increase the drive of the arousal network by enhancing arousal neurotransmitters such as dopamine and norepinephrine (and thus amplifying tonic firing rates) can increase the efficiency of information processing in prefrontal cortex and thus improve symptoms of inattention, impulsivity, and hyperactivity. Such agents include the stimulants, atomoxetine, guanfacine ER, and modafinil.

(NE) can improve the efficiency of information processing in prefrontal circuits and thus, somewhat paradoxically, improve the symptoms of inattention, impulsivity, and hyperactivity in ADHD (see Figure 17-8, moving arousal from deficient on the left in Figure 17-7 to normal in the middle of Figure 17-8).

Note that the hypoactivated brain in Figure 17-7, associated with ADHD symptoms on the left, is also associated with a decreased frequency of tonic firing of dopamine and norepinephrine neurons, shown at the bottom of the figure. Deficient arousal mechanisms, as shown in the brain in Figure 17-7, can be increased to normal levels of activation, as shown in the brain in Figure 17-8, following successful treatment with stimulants, with the norepinephrine transporter (NET) inhibitor atomoxetine, with the oral sustained-release formulation of the alpha 2A selective adrenergic agonist guanfacine ER, or with the wake-promoting agent modafinil (Figure 17-8).

Changes in brain circuitry in ADHD before and after treatment are also shown in Figure 17-9. ADHD patients generally cannot activate prefrontal cortex areas appropriately in response to cognitive tasks of attention and executive functioning. Some studies show that ADHD patients not only fail to activate the dorsal ACC in response to the Stroop test but also actually recruit brain areas that normally do not participate in this function (shown in purple in Figure 17-9, top), a process that gets the job done, but inefficiently, slowly, and with errors. When treated with agents that increase the activation of D1 dopamine receptors and/or alpha 2A adrenergic receptors in prefrontal cortex, these individuals can now activate the appropriate brain area, and perform the task accurately (Figure 17-9, bottom). A very similar phenomenon is observed in prefrontal cortex of narcolepsy patients after they are given stimulants to improve their cognitive performance (see discussion in Chapter 16 and Figure 16-31). Arousal networks are thus also linked robustly to the neurobiological basis of sleep/wake disorders and their treatments (discussed extensively in Chapter 16 and also illustrated in Figures 16-1 through 16-5).

Note in Figure 17-8 that after treatment, not only are ADHD symptoms relieved but tonic firing rates of dopamine and norepinephrine neurons are increased. Tonic versus phasic firing rates for dopamine neurons is introduced in Chapter 16 and illustrated in Figure 16-32. The normal rate of tonic firing of DA and NE neurons is hypothetically linked to being normally aroused and having efficient information processing in the prefrontal cortex and thus normal levels of attention, motor activity, and impulse control (see Figure 17-8, bottom).

When arousal mechanisms are low, not only are the tonic firing rates low in arousal neurons utilizing NE and DA (Figure 17-7 at the bottom) but pyramidal neurons in the prefrontal cortex are "out of tune" and unable to distinguish important neuronal signals from unimportant "noise" (Figure 17-10 on the left). When prefrontal pyramidal neurons are out of tune in ADHD, patients cannot focus on one thing more than another because all signals are the same; they cannot sustain attention because it is easy to be distracted from one signal to another; they may move or act impulsively, without thought. Increasing prefrontal arousal mechanisms by enhancing the activity of DA and NE can improve signal-to-noise detection in prefrontal cortex (middle of Figure 17-10) and relieve ADHD symptoms. DA acting at D1 receptors may diminish the level of the noise, whereas NE acting at alpha 2A adrenergic receptors may enhance the size of the signal (middle of Figure 17-10). This notion of malfunctioning prefrontal circuits that are "out of tune" rather than too high or too low is introduced in Chapter 7 and illustrated in Figures 7-25 and 7-26.

Excessive arousal and ADHD

There is also the possibility of too much of a good thing. Thus, when arousal mechanisms are too high, the signal-to-noise detection deteriorates and is no better than when the arousal mechanisms are too low (compare far right-hand side of the spectrum on Figure 17-10 with the far left-hand side of the spectrum). Correspondingly, some ADHD patients with excessive arousal (Figure 17-11 on the right) can have the same symptoms as other ADHD patients with deficient arousal (Figure 17-7 on the left). In the state of excessive

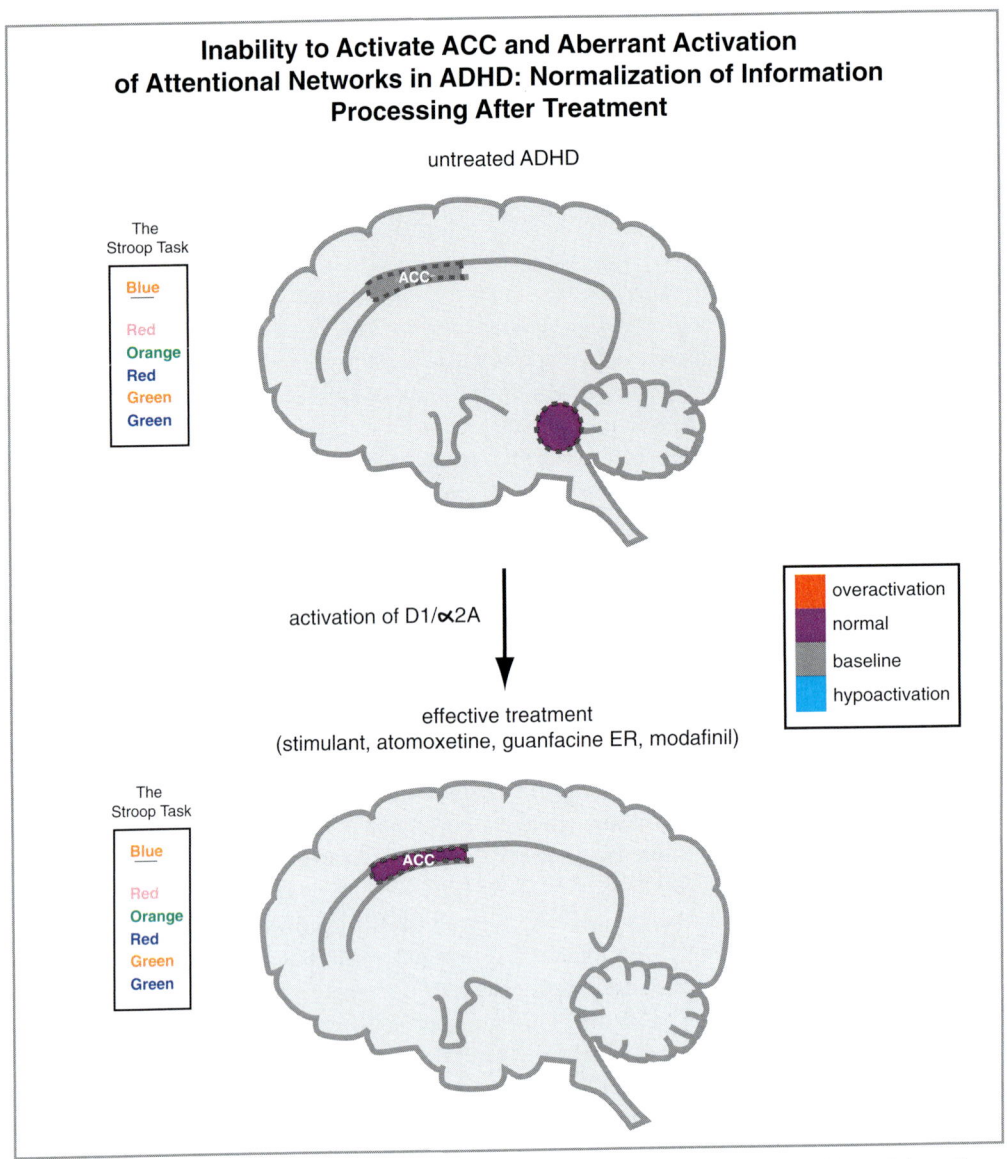

FIGURE 17-9 Information processing in ADHD. Individuals with ADHD may experience inefficient information processing during cognitive tasks. Specifically, tasks that involve selective attention, such as the Stroop test, normally recruit the dorsal anterior cingulate cortex (ACC). Individuals with ADHD appear to be unable to activate this brain region properly (depicted by the gray color of the ACC in the top brain). To compensate, these individuals recruit other brain regions not normally involved in selective attention (shown in purple in the brain at the top), which allows them to perform the task but inefficiently, slowly, and with errors. Agents that increase activation of dopamine 1 and/or alpha 2A adrenergic receptors in the prefrontal cortex (stimulants, atomoxetine, guanfacine ER, modafinil) allow proper activation of the ACC (purple in bottom brain), and thus patients can perform the task accurately.

arousal, there is often the presence of chronic stress and, in adults, a high incidence of comorbidities linked to overstimulation by NE and DA, such as anxiety states, substance abuse, and mania/mixed mood states (see right-hand side of Figure 17-11). When arousal is too high, it can also cause sleep/wake disorders, as discussed in Chapter 16 and illustrated in Figures 16-1, 16-2, and 16-4.

Tuning Cortical Pyramidal Neurons in ADHD

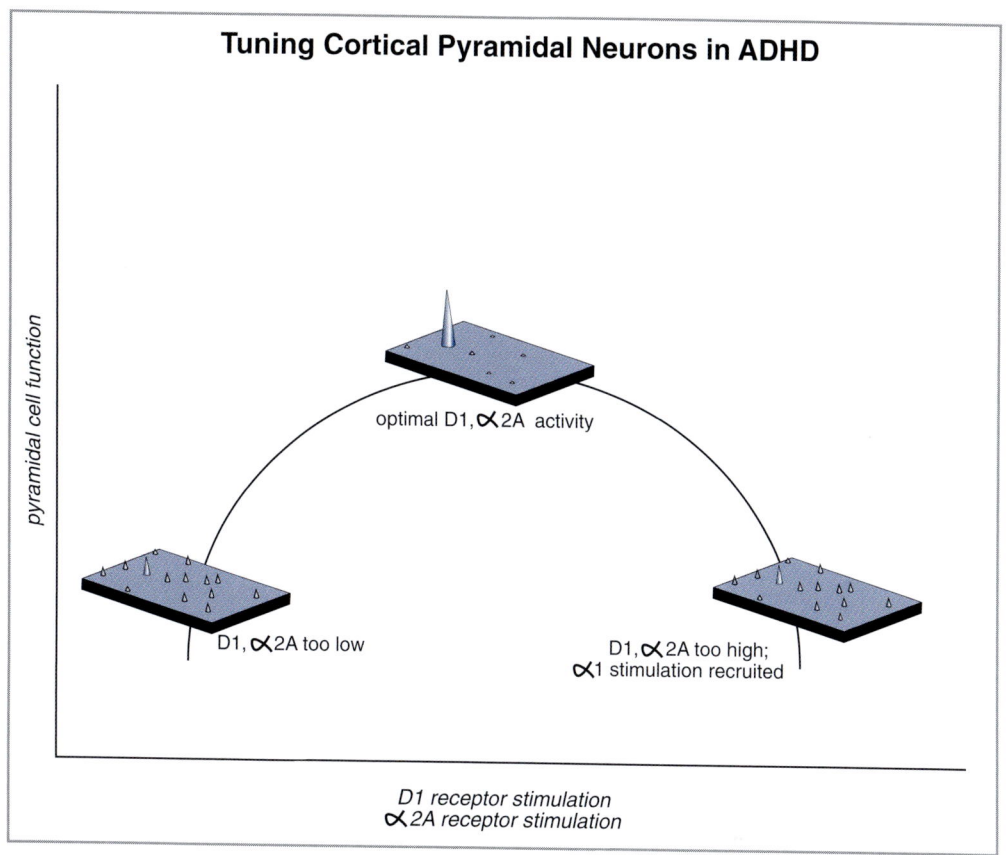

pyramidal cell function vs. *D1 receptor stimulation / α2A receptor stimulation*

- optimal D1, α2A activity
- D1, α2A too low
- D1, α2A too high; α1 stimulation recruited

FIGURE 17-10 Tuning cortical pyramidal neurons in ADHD. When stimulation of dopamine 1 and alpha 2A adrenergic receptors is too low, pyramidal neurons in prefrontal cortex are "out of tune" and unable to distinguish important signals from unimportant noise. This means that individuals are unable to focus on one thing because all signals are the same, which can manifest as problems with selective and sustained attention as well as impulsivity. Enhancing dopaminergic and noradrenergic neurotransmission in prefrontal cortex can improve the signal-to-noise ratio and thus relieve these symptoms. However, too much dopamine and norepinephrine neurotransmission in the prefrontal cortex can stimulate additional receptors and cause the signal-to-noise detection to deteriorate, again leading to symptoms of poor attention and impulsivity.

There are important differences between the functioning of NE and DA neurons when arousal is too high compared to when arousal is too low, although in either case the prefrontal cortex is out of tune and the symptoms of ADHD may be very similar. That is, in cases that are hypothetically due to excessive arousal, phasic firing of NE and DA neurons is present (see Figure 7-11, bottom). This contrasts with cases that are hypothetically due to deficient arousal, where inadequate amounts of tonic firing but no phasic firing is present (see Figure 7-7, bottom). Phasic firing of DA and NE neurons can be an indication of overstimulation; the clinical states thought to be associated with overstimulation include not just persistent ADHD symptoms but also enduring comorbid symptoms of anxiety disorders, substance abuse, and mood disorders. Furthermore, overstimulation states can theoretically result from chronic stress, which also overactivates the HPA axis. That, in turn, can cause downstream alterations in neuronal circuits, including brain atrophy. (Stress-induced changes in brain circuits including brain atrophy are discussed in Chapter 14 and illustrated in Figures 14-29 through 14-36). The last thing one might wish to do in this situation is to increase

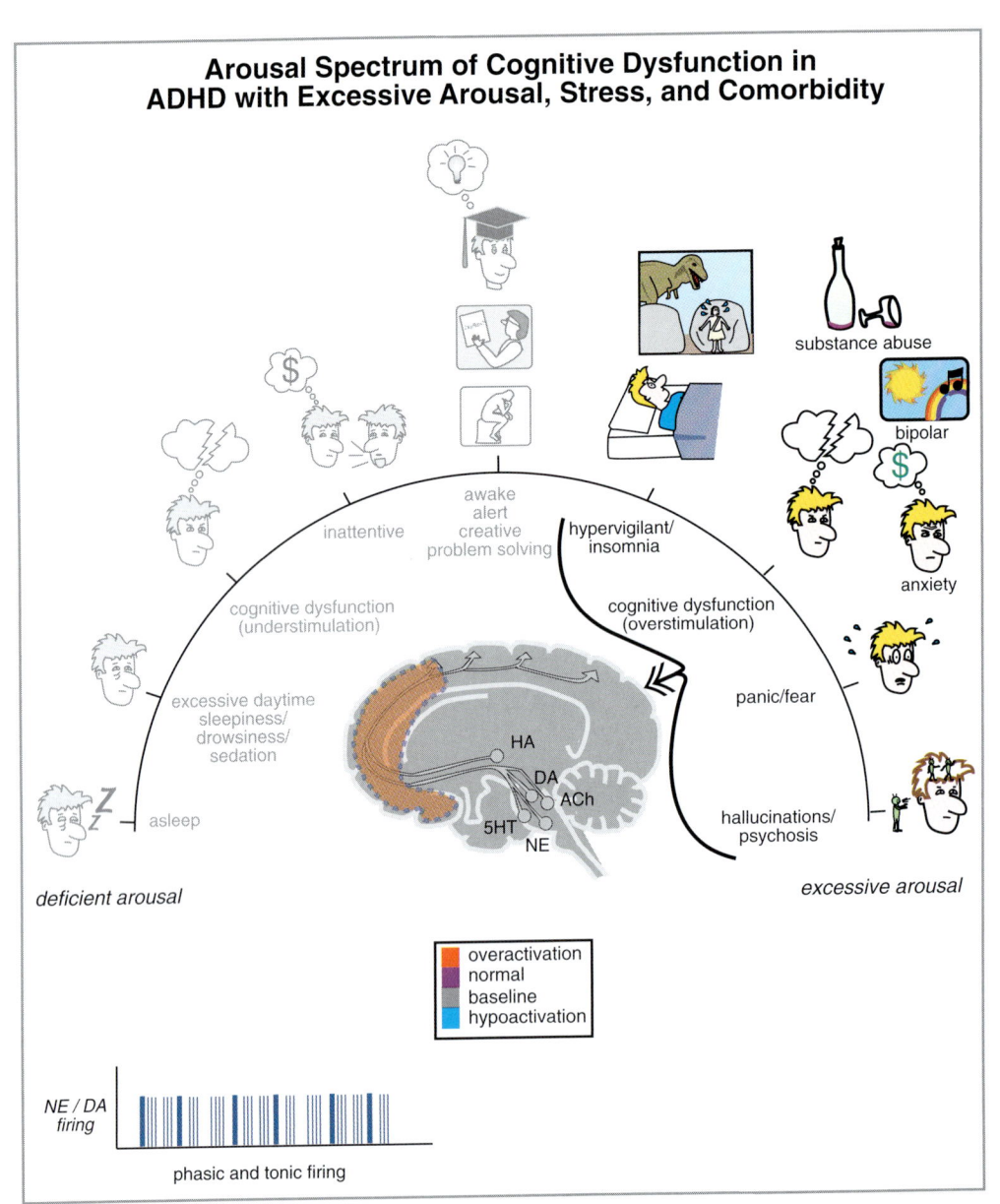

FIGURE 17-11 Arousal spectrum of cognitive dysfunction in ADHD: excessive arousal. The spectrum of arousal is shown here. Individuals in a state of hyperarousal during the day (depicted here as the prefrontal cortex being red) may experience some of the same cognitive symptoms as individuals with hypoactivation of the prefrontal cortex. However, hyperarousal is also associated with chronic stress and may be linked to additional symptoms/comorbidities such as anxiety, bipolar disorder, and substance abuse. In this case, as with hypoarousal during the day, the prefrontal cortex is "out of tune"; however, while hypoarousal is associated with low tonic dopamine and norepinephrine firing, hyperarousal is associated with phasic firing of dopamine and norepinephrine neurons.

the arousal mechanisms and DA and NE activity even more, so what is one to do, since available ADHD treatments all increase DA and/or NE activity?

The answer may be to give treatments that not only slowly reduce the excessive arousal over time by desensitizing postsynaptic NE and DA receptors but also steadily downregulate neuronal activity in order to return NE and DA neurons to normal phasic firing. Treatments that do this may be those that increase DA and/or NE actions tonically themselves rather than phasically. That is, most stimulants have powerful, sudden, but abrupt actions on DA and NE. Even controlled-release stimulants act only intermittently throughout a 24-hour period (i.e., during part of the day but not at night), and their biological actions seem to be dependent upon the moment-to-moment amount of occupancy of the dopamine transporter (DAT) and the norepinephrine transporter (NET); stimulants are also critically dependent upon the rate of change in their blockade of DAT and NET. For these reasons, they are useful in states of deficient arousal but might not be ideal in states of excessive arousal.

On the other hand, NET inhibitors (norepinephrine reuptake inhibitors, NRIs) that block NET around the clock (Figure 17-12) seem to desensitize excessive arousal systems over time and return them to faster tonic NE and DA firing (see bottom of Figure 17-12), the same endpoint as treatments that enhance deficient arousal systems (see Figure 17-8, bottom). Selective actions on alpha 2A adrenergic receptors that are persistent may also reset the sensitivity and firing rates of overactive NE neurons over time (Figure 17-12). Such actions may concomitantly reduce comorbid symptoms that are also the product of excessive arousal in prefrontal cortex, such as anxiety, substance abuse, and mania/mixed mood states (Figure 17-12, right, improving with treatment at the middle). It may seem somewhat counterintuitive at first that agents that increase DA and or NE, even tonically, could reduce excessive DA and NE activity over time. Indeed, such treatments can make conditions such as anxiety somewhat worse before they make them better. Nevertheless, the therapeutic effects of such agents in the treatment of ADHD and its comorbidities increase over the first few months as NE and DA systems theoretically desensitize. Receptor desensitization by blockers of monoamine transporters is discussed in detail in Chapter 12 and illustrated in Figures 12-13 and 12-14; long-term downstream effects of chronic treatment with such agents are illustrated in Figure 12-15.

Stress, comorbidities, and simultaneous deficient and excessive arousal in ADHD

Explanations of deficient and excessive arousal in ADHD offered here have been overly simplified, as it is likely that different circuits have different states of arousal in the various areas of prefrontal cortex. Indeed, in complex cases, some circuits may be understimulated while others are simultaneously overstimulated. This state of affairs is illustrated in Figure 17-13, where the core symptoms of ADHD are represented as either underactivated or overactivated (as also shown in Figures 17-7 and 17-11). Also illustrated in Figure 17-13 are the most common symptoms and conditions that are comorbid with ADHD; these represent both states of theoretical underactivation and states of theoretical overactivation of DA and NE neurons and more specifically of D1 receptors and alpha 2A adrenergic receptors.

Experienced clinicians are well aware that such patients can be very difficult to treat. For example, in children tics generally representing excessive DA activation can be very difficult to treat simultaneously in patients with ADHD who have deficient DA activation and require stimulants. Stimulants may help the ADHD symptoms but make the tics much worse. Children and adolescents who have conduct disorders, oppositional disorders,

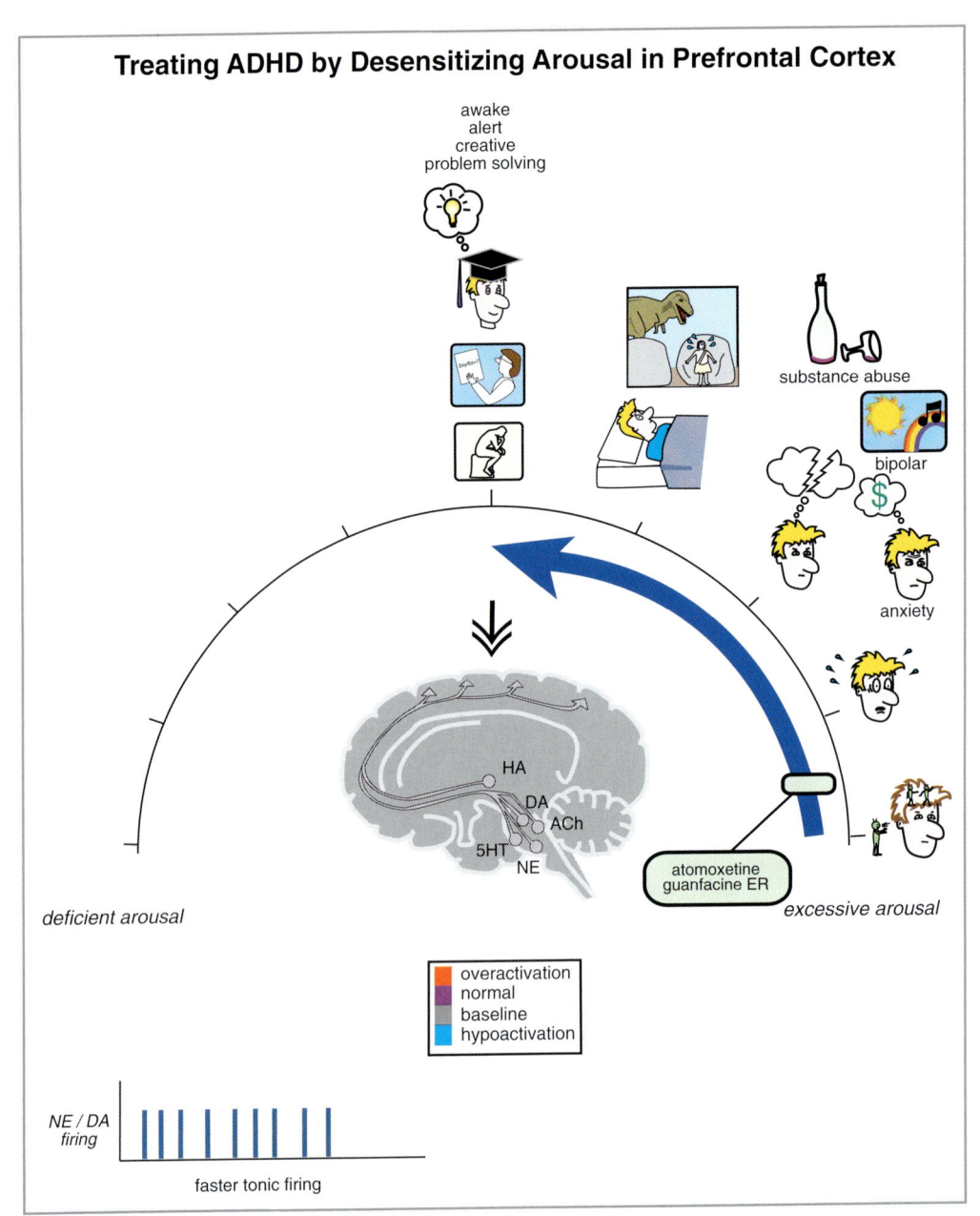

FIGURE 17-12 Treating ADHD by desensitizing arousal in prefrontal cortex. Agents that desensitize postsynaptic dopamine (DA) and norepinephrine (NE) receptors may slowly reduce excessive arousal over time and return neurons to tonic firing. Such agents may be those that themselves have tonic actions on DA and NE, such as atomoxetine, which blocks the NE transporter continuously, and guanfacine ER, which acts continuously at alpha 2A adrenergic receptors.

psychotic disorders, and/or bipolar mania or mixed conditions (theoretically associated with excessive DA activation) comorbid with ADHD (theoretically associated with deficient DA activation) are among the most challenging patients for clinicians treating young patients.

Conditions of excessive DA activation suggest treatment with an atypical antipsychotic, yet ADHD suggests treatment with a stimulant. Can these two agents be combined? In

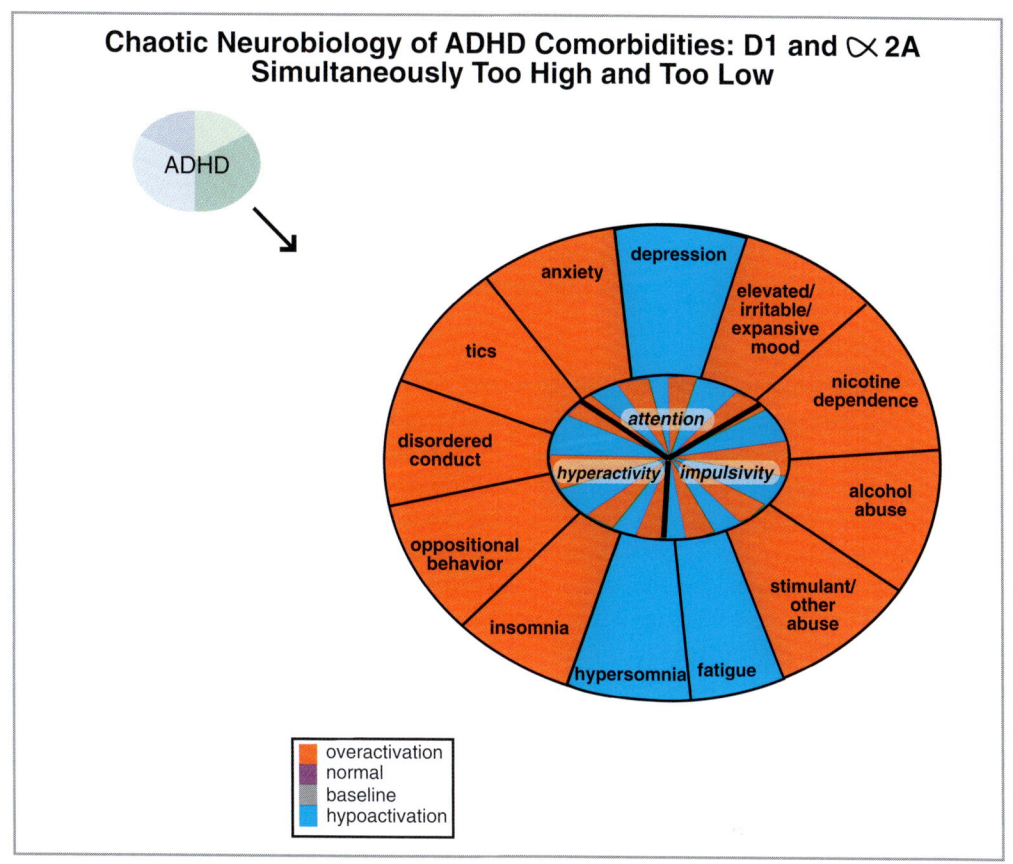

FIGURE 17-13 Simultaneous deficient and excessive arousal in ADHD. Core symptoms of ADHD (inattention, hyperactivity, and impulsivity) can be a result of either hypoactive or hyperactive circuits, depicted here as both red and blue coloring the center of the circle. Surrounding the core symptoms of ADHD are common comorbid symptoms and conditions, some of which are associated with hyperactivation and others that are associated with hypoactivation. Treatment of patients with symptoms from both ends of the arousal spectrum may be particularly difficult.

fact, in heroic cases, stimulants can be combined with atypical antipsychotics. The rationale for this combination exploits the fact that atypical antipsychotics simultaneously release DA in prefrontal cortex to stimulate D1 receptors there while acting in limbic areas to block D2 receptors there. This mechanism of action of atypical antipsychotics is discussed extensively in Chapter 10 and illustrated in Figures 10-2, 10-22, 10-28, and 10-29. In patients who may require atypical antipsychotic treatment for psychotic or manic symptoms yet still have ADHD, it is possible to augment the atypical antipsychotic cautiously with a stimulant, thereby increasing DA release to an even greater extent to act at D1 receptors in prefrontal cortex, hopefully reducing ADHD symptoms while blocking DA stimulation sufficiently in limbic areas to prevent worsening of mania or psychosis. Such an approach is controversial and best left to experts for difficult patients who fail to improve adequately on monotherapies.

For adults with ADHD and anxiety, it can be difficult or even self-defeating to try to treat anxiety with SSRIs/SNRIs or benzodiazepines while simultaneously administering a stimulant to improve the ADHD, which may only cause the anxiety to worsen. For adults with ADHD and substance abuse, it makes little sense to give stimulants to drug abusers in order to treat their ADHD. In these cases, augmenting antidepressant or anxiolytic therapies with a tonic activator of DA and/or NE systems such as a long-lasting NET inhibitor (norepinephrine reuptake inhibitors, NRIs), or alpha 2A adrenergic agonist rather than a stimulant can be an effective long-term approach for comorbid anxiety, depression, or substance abuse with ADHD. Some studies of NET inhibitors report improvement in both ADHD and anxiety symptoms, and other studies report improvement in both ADHD and heavy drinking. Further controlled trials are needed to clarify the responsiveness of both ADHD and comorbid conditions to treatment with NET inhibitors or alpha 2A adrenergic agonists.

ADHD and comorbidity: What should be treated first?
In all of these situations of simultaneous excessive and deficient arousal in the same brain at the same time, the neurobiology appears to be quite chaotic (Figure 17-13). Because of this, it can be helpful in managing such cases to prioritize which symptoms to target first with psychopharmacological treatments, even at the expense of delaying treatment for a while for some conditions or even making some of these comorbid conditions transiently worse while other symptoms are targeted for improvement first (Figure 17-14). Although there are no definitive studies on this approach, clinical experience from many experts suggests that in such complex cases, it can be very difficult to make any therapeutic progress if the patient continues to abuse alcohol or stimulants; thus substance abuse problems must be managed top line (Figure 17-14). Treating ADHD may also have to await improvement from mood and anxiety disorder treatments, with ADHD seen as more of a fine tune adjustment to a patient's symptom portfolio (Figure 17-14).

There are problems, however, with this approach of setting priorities as to which symptoms and disorders to treat first. For example, many children are treated for their ADHD first and perhaps in isolation without necessarily evaluating possible comorbidities until they fail to respond robustly to stimulant treatment (Figure 17-14). In adults, it can be so difficult to treat substance abuse, mood disorders, and anxiety disorders that the focus of therapeutic attention never gets to ADHD and certainly not to nicotine dependence. Once the mood or anxiety disorder is improving, treatment can plateau or stop. Too often the focus of psychopharmacological management is the mood or anxiety disorder to the exclusion of any comorbid ADHD (or nicotine dependence). That is, ADHD can be considered a mere afterthought to be addressed if cognitive symptoms do not remit once the primary focus of therapeutic attention – namely, the mood or anxiety disorder – is treated. It is interesting that ADHD is rarely the focus of treatment in adults unless it presents with no comorbid conditions. Since lack of comorbidity in adults with ADHD is rare, this may explain why the majority of adults with ADHD are not treated.

The modern, sophisticated psychopharmacologist keeps a high index of suspicion for the presence of ADHD in mood, anxiety, and substance abuse disorders especially in adults, always aiming for complete symptomatic remission in patients under treatment. In practice, this means exploring the use of ADHD treatments as augmenting agents to first-line treatments of mood, anxiety, and substance abuse disorders rather than the other way around. It also means, for long-term management of ADHD, to eventually address the treatment of nicotine dependence once the ADHD symptoms are under control (Figure 17-14). Adults with ADHD smoke as frequently as adults with schizophrenia, at about twice the rate of the normal adult population in the United States. This may be because nicotine subjectively improves ADHD symptoms, especially in patients who are not treated for their ADHD.

What Should Be Treated First?

- alcohol / stimulant / substance abuse
- mood disorders
- anxiety disorders
- ADHD
- nicotine dependence

order of treatment

↑ treatment in adults often ends here

↑ treatment in children/adolescents often begins here

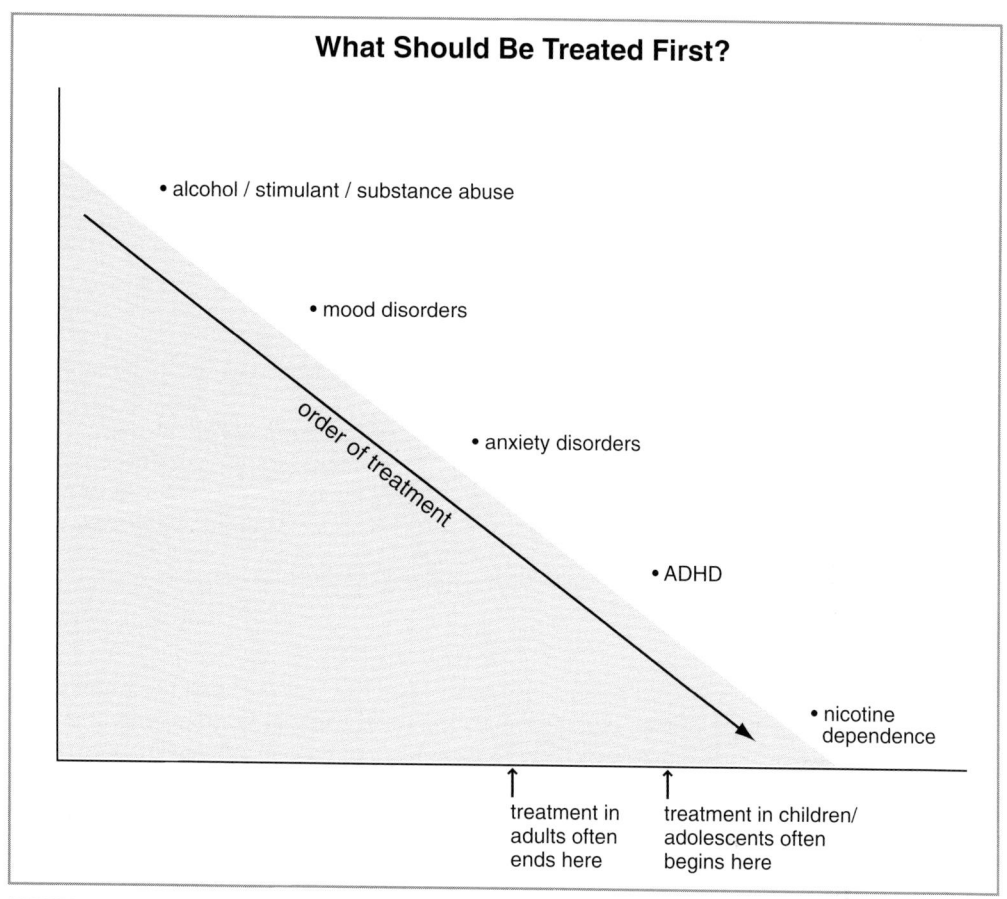

FIGURE 17-14 What should be treated first? Because ongoing substance abuse can hinder treatment progress of other disorders, it may be necessary to address this problem first. In addition, comorbid mood and anxiety disorders may require management before addressing ADHD. In the long term, ADHD patients who smoke should receive treatment for nicotine dependence once ADHD symptoms are under control. Although these are general guidelines for the ordering of treatment, one should be careful that this prioritization of symptoms/conditions does not lead to the neglect of ADHD treatment in adults. On the other end of the spectrum, children are often treated for ADHD first, prior to considering the presence of these other comorbidities.

Nicotine enhances DA release and arousal, so it is not surprising that it may be subjectively effective for ADHD symptoms. Nicotine dependence and psychopharmacological treatments for smoking cessation are discussed in more detail in Chapter 19, on drug abuse.

ADHD in children versus adults

ADHD has traditionally been considered a childhood disorder, with inclusion in adult and general psychopharmacology textbooks as a footnote for practitioners who see adults whose ADHD began in childhood. This perspective is rapidly changing, with ADHD now being seen also as a major psychiatric disorder of adults, with some major differentiating features from ADHD in children and adolescents (Table 17-3). Nevertheless, the classic form of ADHD has its onset by age 7, possibly related to abnormalities in prefrontal cortex circuits that begin before age 7 but last a lifetime (Figure 17-15). Synapses rapidly increase in prefrontal cortex by age 6, and then up to half of them are rapidly eliminated during

TABLE 17-3 Differences in ADHD in adults vs. children and adolescents

Children 6–12/Adolescents 13–17	Adults ≥18
7%–8% prevalence	4%–5% prevalence
Easy to diagnose	Hard to diagnose
	▪ Inaccurate retrospective recall of onset
	▪ Onset by age 7 too stringent
	▪ Late onset same genetics, comorbidity, and impairment
Diagnosed by pediatricians, child psychiatrists, child psychologists	Diagnosed by adult psychiatrists, adult mental/medical health professionals
High levels of identification and treatment: >50% treated	Low levels of identification and treatment: <20% treated
Stimulants prescribed first-, second-line	Nonstimulants often prescribed first-line
Two-thirds of stimulant use is under age 18, most of this under age 13	One-third of stimulant use is age 18 or over
One-third of atomoxetine use is under age 18, most of this over age 12	Two-thirds of atomoxetine use is age 18 or over

adolescence (Figure 17-15). The timing of onset of ADHD suggests that the formation of synapses and, perhaps more importantly, the selection of synapses for removal in prefrontal cortex during childhood, may contribute to the onset and lifelong pathophysiology of this condition (Figure 17-15). Those who are able to compensate for these prefrontal abnormalities by new synapse formation may be the ones who "grow out of their ADHD," and this may explain why the prevalence of ADHD in adults is only half that in children and adolescents.

The impact of development on the specific symptom patterns of ADHD is shown in Figure 17-16. Inattentive symptoms are not really seen in preschool children with ADHD, perhaps because they do not have a sufficiently mature prefrontal cortex to manifest these symptoms in a manner that is abnormal. Preschool ADHD and its treatment are current controversial concepts in the field because most studies of stimulants involve children over the age of 6. Once inattention becomes a prominent symptom of ADHD, it remains so throughout the individual's life (Figure 17-16). However, impulsivity and hyperactivity decline notably by adolescence and early adulthood, while recognized comorbidities skyrocket in frequency as ADHD patients enter adulthood (Figure 17-16).

The prevalence of ADHD in adults may be only about half that in children, but it is not recognized nearly as often as it is in children, possibly because it is much harder to diagnose and its symptoms are very often not treated. Whereas half of all children or adolescents with ADHD are thought to be diagnosed and treated, less than 1 in 5 adults with ADHD is thought to be diagnosed and treated (Table 17-3). The reasons for this are multiple, starting with the diagnostic requirement that ADHD symptoms must begin by age 7. Adults often have difficulty making accurate retrospective diagnoses, especially if the condition was not identified and treated when they were children. Furthermore, many experts now question whether it is appropriate to exclude from the diagnosis of ADHD those adults whose ADHD symptoms started after age 7, so-called late-onset ADHD. Many cases have onset up to the age of 12 and some up to the age of 45. Do these patients have ADHD? Genetic studies suggest that full-syndrome ADHD with onset after age 7

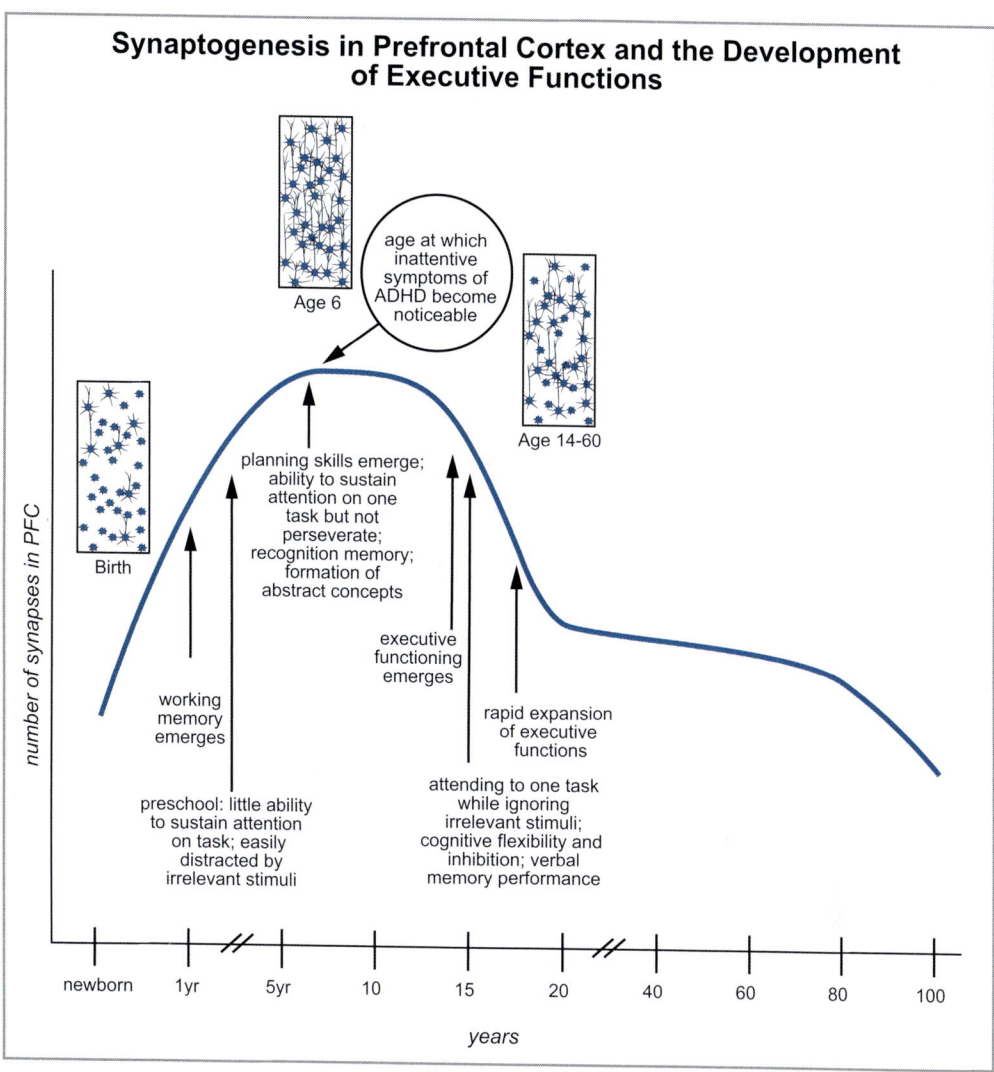

FIGURE 17-15 Synaptogenesis in prefrontal cortex and the development of executive functions. The development of executive functions occurs throughout childhood and adolescence. Working memory emerges at approximately 1 year of age. At preschool age, individuals do not yet have much ability to sustain attention and are easily distracted by irrelevant stimuli. At around age 6 or 7, children begin to be able to sustain attention and develop planning skills; it is at this time that symptoms of inattention may become noticeable. This is also the time when synapses, which until now have rapidly been increasing, begin to be rapidly eliminated, a process that occurs through early adolescence. Thus abnormalities in synapse selection may account for onset of ADHD and affect the further development of executive functions.

has psychiatric comorbidity, functional impairment, and familial transmission similar to that in ADHD with onset by age 7. Thus there is a movement to consider the DSM-IV age-of-onset criterion as too stringent for the diagnosis of ADHD in adults.

Differences in diagnostic rates in children versus adults may possibly also be explained by differences in referral patterns and in the specialties of practitioners who treat children versus those who treat adults. Most children with ADHD are diagnosed and treated by pediatricians, child psychiatrists, and child psychologists and are referred by parents and

Impact of Development on ADHD

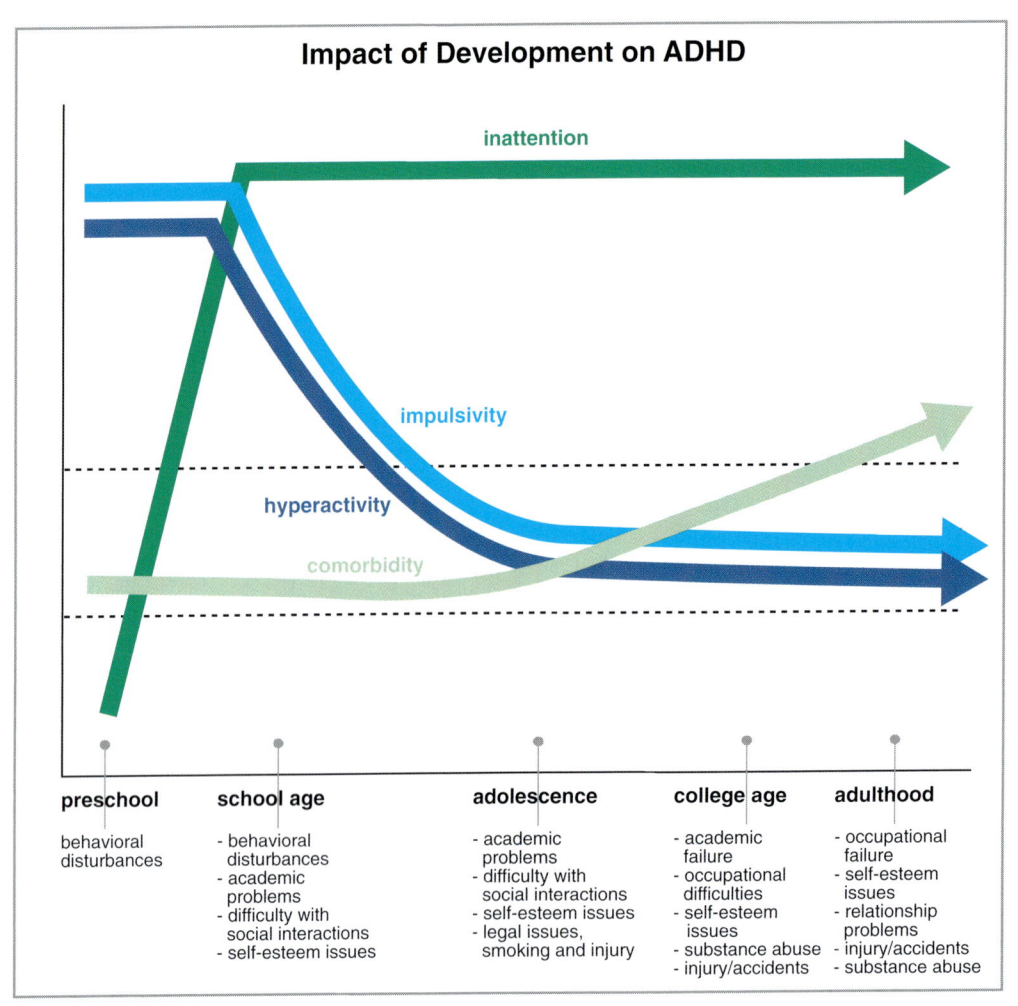

preschool	school age	adolescence	college age	adulthood
behavioral disturbances	- behavioral disturbances - academic problems - difficulty with social interactions - self-esteem issues	- academic problems - difficulty with social interactions - self-esteem issues - legal issues, smoking and injury	- academic failure - occupational difficulties - self-esteem issues - substance abuse - injury/accidents	- occupational failure - self-esteem issues - relationship problems - injury/accidents - substance abuse

FIGURE 17-16 Impact of development on ADHD. Preschool-age children with ADHD may exhibit hyperactivity and impulsivity, but inattentiveness may be difficult to identify, as normal development does not lead to sustained attention until age 6 or 7. By school age, inattentiveness becomes apparent and hyperactivity and impulsivity are frequently still present. Through adolescence, although inattentiveness remains prominent, hyperactivity and impulsivity generally decline, and by adulthood ADHD is often characterized only by attentional difficulties. Adults with ADHD also have a high rate of comorbidities, although it may be that these comorbidities were present earlier and were simply overlooked as treatment focused on ADHD.

teachers with a high degree of suspicion for the diagnosis, generally requesting a trial of a stimulant, and usually these are patients without comorbidity. On the other hand, most adults with ADHD are self-referred and seen by psychiatrists and adult mental and medical health professionals; adult cases mostly have a comorbid condition that is the focus of treatment, not the ADHD. Thus, practitioners treating adults may prioritize the treatment of these other conditions over ADHD (see Figure 17-14) to the extent that ADHD is never formally diagnosed, nor is it specifically targeted for treatment.

There are also many differences in how ADHD is treated in children and adolescents compared to adults (Table 17-3). For example two-thirds of all stimulant use for ADHD is in patients under the age of 18, most of these under the age of 13. Stimulant use falls off in adolescents and then falls way off in adults. Only one-third of all stimulant use for

ADHD involves adults. On the other hand, two-thirds of all atomoxetine use involves adults, and only one-third involves those under the age of 18, mostly adolescents (Table 17-3). Why these differences? One reason could be that many practitioners treating adults do not like to prescribe controlled substances such as stimulants. Another factor could be the differences in the rates of comorbidity in children versus adults with ADHD and in the types of comorbid conditions of children versus adults with ADHD. Thus, the frequent comorbidities of substance abuse, anxiety disorders, and bipolar or mixed states can limit the utility and tolerability of stimulants in the typical adult ADHD patient with these comorbidities. Augmenting antidepressants and anxiolytics with nonstimulants can therefore be preferable. There is also much more off-label use of the NDRI antidepressant bupropion, the various SNRIs, and the wake-promoting agent modafinil in adults than in children, often as augmenting agents in comorbid adult ADHD.

Currently, the recognition and treatment of ADHD in adults, tailoring the diagnostic and psychopharmacologic considerations to the unique features of this illness in adults, is increasing at a rapid pace. Thus there is a call for more recognition that ADHD is only half the problem in mostly comorbid adults, and that treatment of ADHD in adults generally means concomitant treatment of ADHD with one or more additional disorders, and generally with a combination of drugs for the different conditions. It is increasingly recognized that atomoxetine (or another NET inhibitor) augmentation of antidepressants and anxiolytics can not only improve cognitive symptoms of ADHD but also has the potential to improve anxiety symptoms, depressive symptoms, and perhaps even heavy drinking. It is possible that the alpha 2A selective adrenergic agonist guanfacine ER, in late-stage development for children, may also be useful for off-label treatment of adults. Long-acting stimulants may also be useful in adults, and not just those stimulants specifically approved in adults but also those newer agents first tested and approved for use in children, which can be used for off-label treatment of adults.

Stimulant treatment of ADHD

ADHD is generally conceptualized as a condition where NE and DA signals in the prefrontal cortex are weak (Figure 17-17). This is consistent with the idea that the arousal system is deficient and that tonic NE and DA firing rates are too low (Figure 17-7). Stimulants approved to treat ADHD include various preparations of methylphenidate and amphetamine, and both are considered to boost NE and DA signals in a number of different ways. The general boosting action of stimulants on NE and DA signals in ADHD is shown in Figure 17-8. More specifically, methylphenidate blocks NET and DAT, whereas amphetamine is a competitive inhibitor and pseudosubstrate for NET and DAT. Thus, methylphenidate stops the reuptake pumps so that nothing is transported, but amphetamine inhibits NE and DA reuptake so it can be transported itself. These principles of amphetamine action are introduced in Chapter 4 and illustrated in Figures 4-14 and 4-15. Methylphenidate acts differently from amphetamine in many ways; in terms of its effects on NET and DAT, it is like a much more potent and effective norepinephrine and dopamine reuptake inhibitor (NDRI) than bupropion, discussed in Chapter 12 and illustrated in Figure 12-46.

Both methylphenidate and amphetamine have d and l isomers, with the d isomer of methylphenidate being much more potent than the l isomer on both NET and DAT binding. Methylphenidate is available as the single enantiomer d-methylphenidate in both immediate-release and controlled-release preparations. Amphetamine's d isomer is more

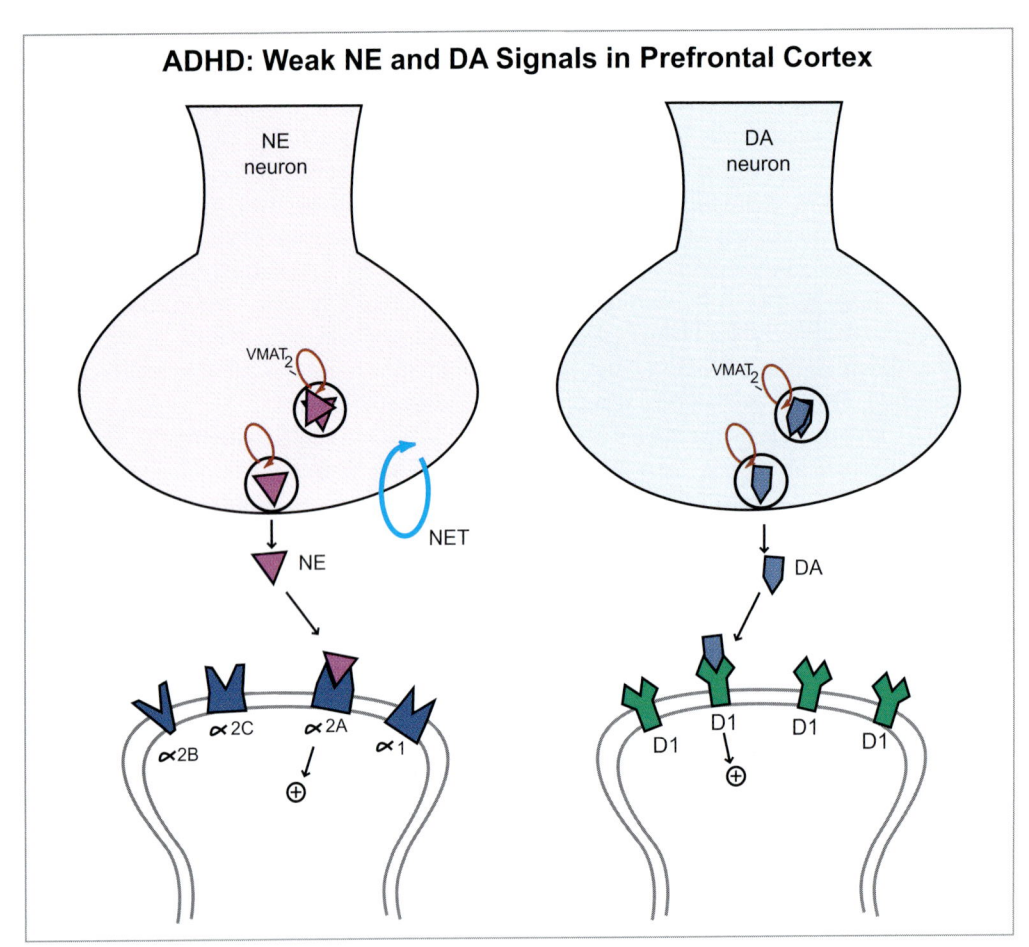

FIGURE 17-17 ADHD: weak NE and DA signals in prefrontal cortex. The idea that arousal is deficient in ADHD and that tonic NE and DA firing is low is depicted here as minimal NE and DA stimulation of postsynaptic receptors.

potent than the l isomer for DAT binding, but d and l amphetamine isomers are more equally potent in their actions on NET binding. Thus, d-amphetamine preparations will have relatively more action on DAT than NET; mixed salts of both d- and l-amphetamine will have relatively more action on NET than d-amphetamine but overall still more action on DAT than NET (Figure 17-18). These pharmacological mechanisms of action of the stimulants come into play particularly at lower therapeutic doses utilized for the treatment of ADHD. However, higher doses of these stimulants have additional actions that come into play when utilized by stimulant abusers. That is, when methylphenidate saturates DAT, this can produce substantially more synaptic DA availability in the nucleus accumbens and thus cause reinforcement, reward, euphoria, and continuing abuse (Figure 17-19). High doses of amphetamine trigger further pharmacological actions in addition to competitive inhibition of DAT and its own transport into the presynaptic DA neuron (Figure 4-15A). This includes being a competitive inhibitor of the vesicular transporter for both DA and NE, known as VMAT2, in both prefrontal cortex and in nucleus accumbens (Figure 4-15B). Once amphetamine gets into synaptic vesicles, it displaces DA there, causing a flood of DA release (Figure 14-15C). As DA accumulates in the cytoplasm of the presynaptic

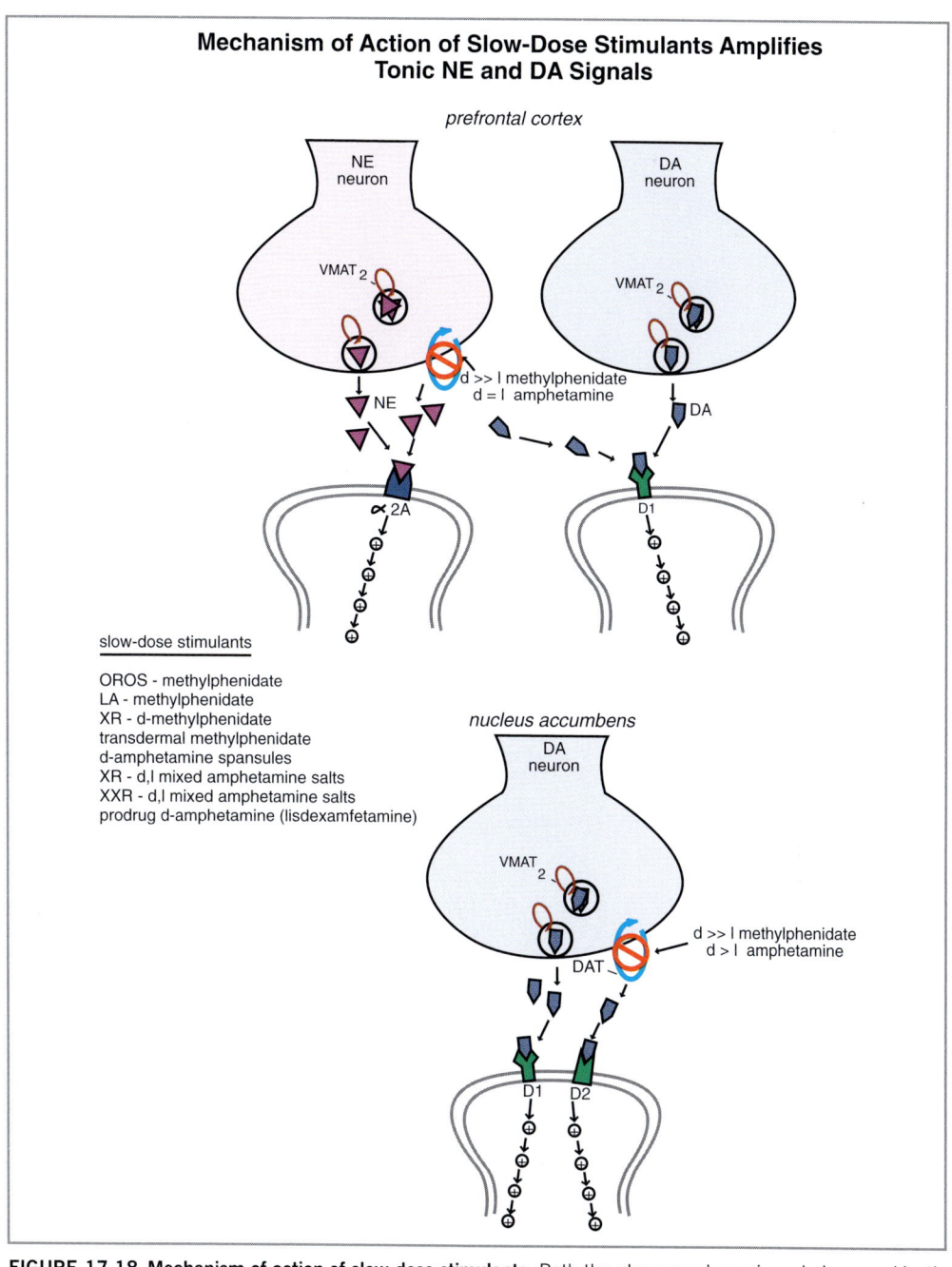

FIGURE 17-18 Mechanism of action of slow-dose stimulants. Both the pharmacodynamic and pharmacokinetic properties of stimulants affect their therapeutic and abuse profiles. Slow-dose stimulants, such as the various extended-release oral formulations as well as transdermal methylphenidate and the new prodrug d-amphetamine, may amplify tonic NE and DA signals, presumed to be low in ADHD. They do this by blocking the norepinephrine transporter (NET) in the prefrontal cortex and the dopamine transporter (DAT) in the nucleus accumbens. More specifically, the d isomers of both methylphenidate and amphetamine are more potent than the l isomers for DAT, while d-methylphenidate is more potent than l-methylphenidate for NET and both d- and l-amphetamine are equally potent for NET. The slow-dose stimulants occupy NET in prefrontal cortex with slow enough onset and for long enough duration to enhance tonic NE and DA signaling via alpha 2A and D1 receptors, respectively, but do not occupy DAT fast or long enough in the nucleus accumbens to increase phasic signaling via D2 receptors.

Attention Deficit Hyperactivity Disorder and Its Treatment

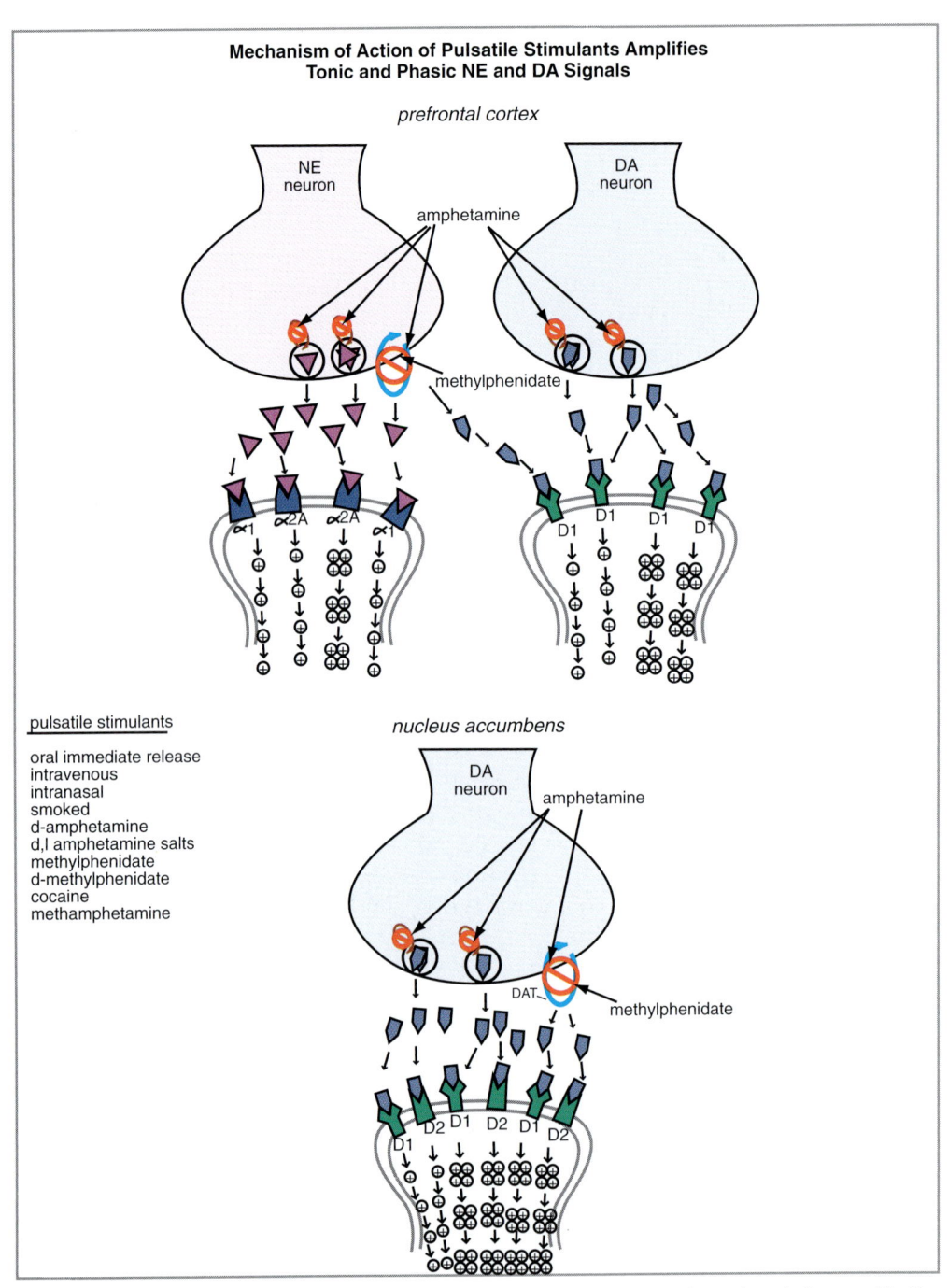

FIGURE 17-19 Mechanism of action of pulsatile stimulants. Both the pharmacodynamic and pharmacokinetic properties of stimulants affect their therapeutic and abuse profiles. Pulsatile stimulants, such as immediate-release oral formulations as well as intravenous, smoked, or snorted stimulants, cause rapid increases in NE and DA and thus may increase phasic NE and DA signals, which is associated with euphoria and abuse. In addition, at higher doses amphetamine not only blocks the dopamine transporter (DAT) but is also taken up into the neuron, where it binds to the vesicular monoamine transporter (VMAT) to displace dopamine and cause its release. This increased release of DA may also contribute to abuse potential.

neuron, it causes the DAT to reverse directions, spilling intracellular DA into the synapse and also opening presynaptic channels to further release DA in a flood into the synapse (Figure 14-15D). These pharmacological actions of high-dose amphetamine are not linked to any therapeutic action in ADHD but to reinforcement, reward, euphoria, and continuing abuse (Figure 17-19). Actions of high-dose amphetamine, methamphetamine, and cocaine, given orally in immediate-release formulations or intranasally, intravenously, or smoked, are discussed further in Chapter 19, on drug abuse.

Another insight quite relevant to a discussion of the therapeutic use of stimulants for ADHD are recent findings that pharmacokinetic considerations may be just as important to the use and abuse of stimulants as their pharmacodynamic mechanisms. The past several years have seen a flurry of new drug development activities aimed at optimizing the drug delivery characteristics of stimulants for ADHD. These are not mere patent extension gimmicks, nor are they mere convenience features, although it is certainly an advantage for a child not to have to take a second dose of a stimulant in the middle of the day at school. More importantly, the "slow-dose" stimulants, shown in Figure 17-18, optimize the rate, amount, and length of time that a stimulant occupies NET and DAT for therapeutic use in ADHD. Optimization for ADHD means occupying enough of the NET in prefrontal cortex at a slow enough onset and long enough duration of action to enhance tonic NE signaling there via alpha 2A receptors and to increase tonic DA signaling there via D1 receptors, yet occupying little enough of the DAT in nucleus accumbens so as not to increase phasic signaling there via D2 receptors (Figure 17-18). It appears that ADHD patients have their therapeutic improvement by stimulants at the mercy of how fast, how much, and how long stimulants occupy NET and DAT. When this is done in an ideal manner with slow onset, robust but subsaturating drug levels, and long duration of action before declining and wearing off, the patient benefits with improved ADHD symptoms, hours of relief, and no euphoria. Tonic drug delivery of stimulants amplifies the desired tonic increases in DA and NE action for ADHD improvement for several hours.

On the other hand, Figure 17-19 shows how *not* to treat ADHD with stimulants: namely, by frequent high-dose and pulsatile delivery of short-acting stimulants. This approximates very closely the best way to use these agents for euphoria and reinforcement, so there can be the risk of amplifying phasic NE and DA signals (Figure 17-19), just as in overly aroused ADHD patients with stress and comorbidity, as illustrated in Figure 17-11.

Contrasts between pulsatile and sustained release of stimulants are shown also in Figure 17-20, where phasic pulsatile drug delivery amplifies undesirable phasic DA and NE firing (Figure 17-20A) but slow-dose tonic drug delivery amplifies desirable tonic DA and NE firing (Figure 17-20B).

Noradrenergic treatment of ADHD

Atomoxetine

Atomoxetine is a selective norepinephrine reuptake inhibitor, or selective NRI. Selective NRIs are discussed in Chapter 12 on antidepressants and illustrated in Figure 12-49. They are also sometimes called NET inhibitors. Atomoxetine is the only such agent approved for use in ADHD, but several other agents have NRI actions, including the approved antidepressant (outside of the United States) and selective NRI reboxetine (Figure 12-48) and the various SNRIs, which not only have NRI actions but also serotonin reuptake inhibiting properties (Figures 12-33 through 12-42). Bupropion is a weak NRI and also a

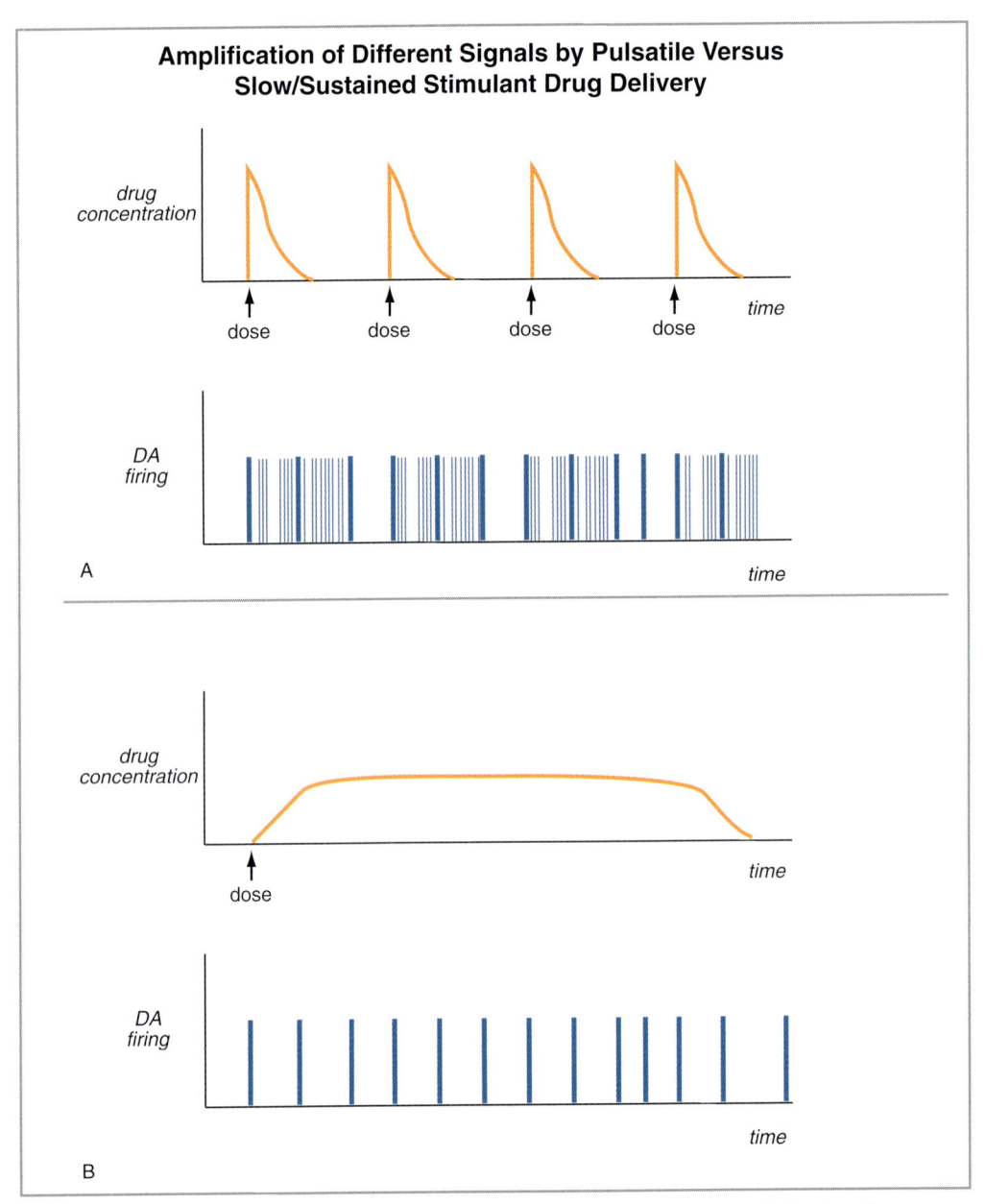

FIGURE 17-20A and B Amplification of different signals by pulsatile vs. slow/sustained stimulant drug delivery. (A) Pulsatile delivery of stimulants causes frequent, rapid increases in norepinephrine (NE) and dopamine (DA) and thus amplifies phasic firing, which is associated with reward, euphoria, and abuse. (B) Slow/sustained delivery of stimulants causes a gradual and sustained increase in NE and DA that therefore enhances tonic firing, which is associated with the therapeutic effects of stimulants in ADHD.

weak DAT inhibitor, known as a norepinephrine and dopamine reuptake inhibitor (NDRI) (Figures 12-45 through 12-47). Several tricyclic antidepressants, such as desipramine and nortriptyline, have notable NRI actions. All of these agents with NRI properties have been utilized in the treatment of ADHD with varying amounts of success, but only atomoxetine is well investigated and approved for this use in children and adults.

NRI pharmacological actions are discussed in Chapter 12 in relation to their use as antidepressants and illustrated in Figure 12-36. Since the prefrontal cortex lacks high concentrations of DAT, DA is inactivated in this part of the brain by NET. Thus, inhibiting NET increases both DA and NE in prefrontal cortex (Figures 12-36 and 17-21). However, since there are only a few NE neurons and NETs in nucleus accumbens, inhibiting NET does not lead to an increase in either NE or DA there (Figure 17-21). For this reason, in ADHD patients with deficient arousal and weak NE and DA signals in prefrontal cortex, a selective NRI such as atomoxetine increases both NE and DA in prefrontal cortex, enhancing tonic signaling of both, but it increases neither NE nor DA in the nucleus accumbens. Therefore atomoxetine has no abuse potential.

Atomoxetine's hypothetical actions in ADHD patients with stress and comorbidity states presumably linked to excessive and phasic DA and NE release are shown conceptually by comparing the untreated states in Figure 17-22 with the changes that theoretically follow chronic treatment with atomoxetine in Figure 17-23. That is, ADHD linked to conditions that are associated with chronic stress and comorbidities is theoretically caused by overly active NE and DA circuits in prefrontal cortex, causing an excess of phasic NE and DA activity (Figure 17-22). When slow-onset, long-duration and essentially perpetual NET inhibition occurs in prefrontal cortex due to atomoxetine, this theoretically restores tonic postsynaptic D1 and alpha 2A adrenergic signaling, downregulates phasic NE and DA actions, and desensitizes postsynaptic NE and DA receptors. The possible consequences of this are to reduce chronic overactivation of the HPA axis and thereby potentially reverse stress-related brain atrophy and even induce neurogenesis, which could protect the brain. Such biochemical and molecular changes could be associated with decreases in ADHD symptoms; reduction of relapse; and decreases in anxiety, depression, and heavy drinking. Unlike stimulant use where the therapeutic actions are at the mercy of plasma drug levels and momentary NET/DAT occupancies, long-term NRI actions give 24-hour symptom relief in much the same manner as SSRIs and SNRIs for the treatment of depression and anxiety. Such possibilities are already indicated by early clinical investigations of this mechanism of selective NRI action in ADHD, but much further work is necessary to establish with certainty the long-term effects of selective NRI action, the differences in outcomes (if any) compared to long-term stimulant actions, and the best ADHD patient profile to choose for the selective NRI mechanism. Selective NRIs generally have smaller effect sizes for reducing ADHD symptoms than stimulants in short-term trials, especially in patients without comorbidity. However, NRIs are not necessarily inferior in ADHD patients who have not been previously treated with stimulants or in ADHD patients who have been treated long-term (greater than 8 to 12 weeks). NRIs may actually be preferred to stimulants in patients with complex comorbidities.

Alpha 2A adrenergic agonists

Norepinephrine receptors are discussed in Chapter 11 and illustrated in Figures 11-32 to 11-34. There are numerous subtypes of alpha adrenergic receptors, from presynaptic autoreceptors, generally of the alpha 2A or 2C subtype (Figures 11-32 to 11-34), to postsynaptic alpha 2A, alpha 2B, alpha 2C, and alpha 1 subtypes (Figures 11-32 and 17-24). Alpha 2A receptors are widely distributed throughout the CNS, with high levels in the cortex and locus coeruleus. These receptors are thought to be the primary mediators of the effects of NE in prefrontal cortex regulating symptoms of inattention, hyperactivity, and impulsivity in ADHD. Alpha 2B receptors are in high concentrations in the thalamus and may be important in mediating sedating actions of NE, perhaps due to actions on the thalamic filter,

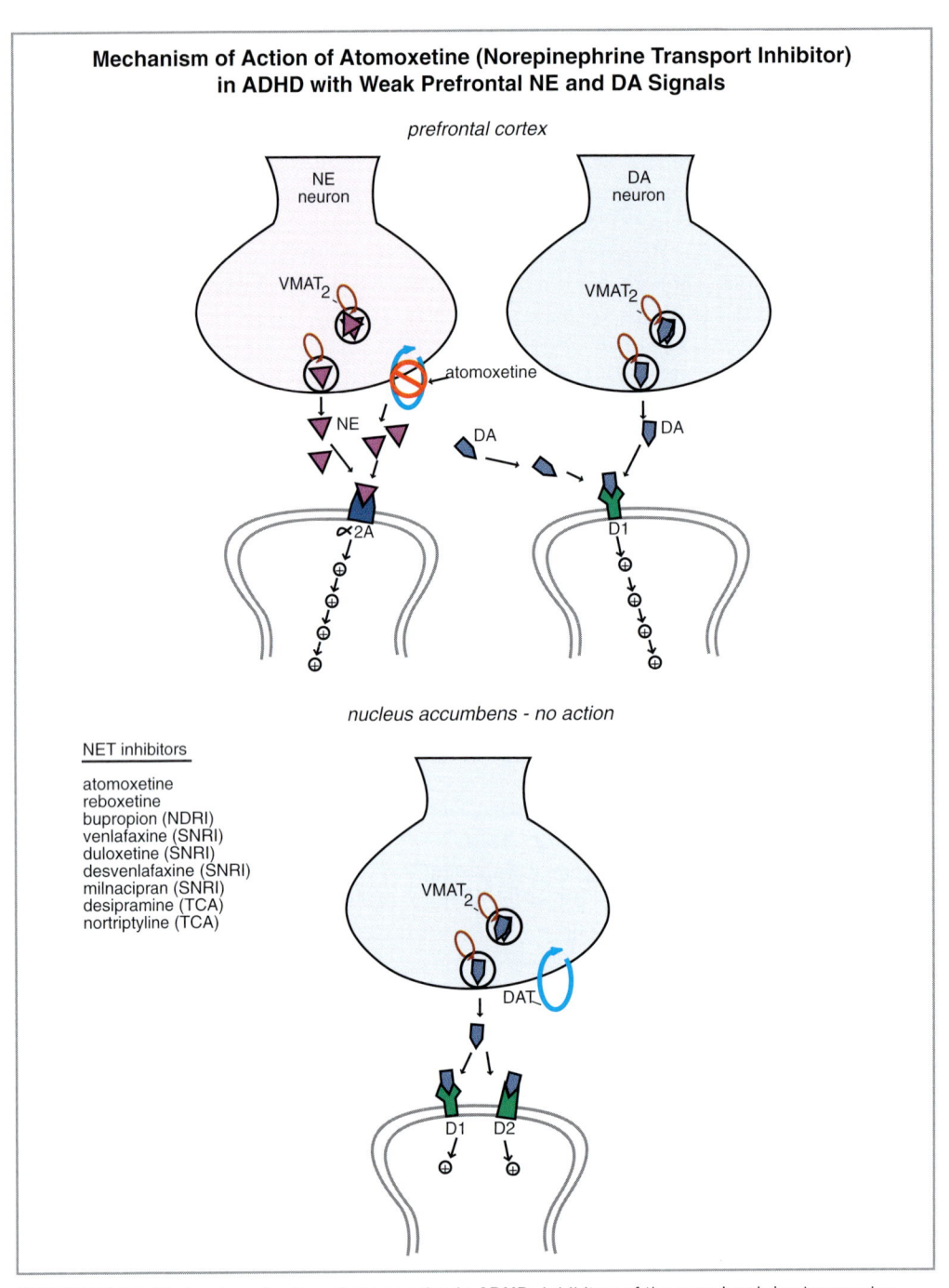

FIGURE 17-21 Mechanism of action of atomoxetine in ADHD. Inhibitors of the norepinephrine transporter (NET), such as atomoxetine, can have therapeutic effects in ADHD without abuse potential. This is because they can increase both norepinephrine (NE) and dopamine (DA) in the prefrontal cortex, where clearance of both is largely due to NET, yet they do not increase NE or DA in the nucleus accumbens because there are few NETs present there.

892 | Essential Psychopharmacology

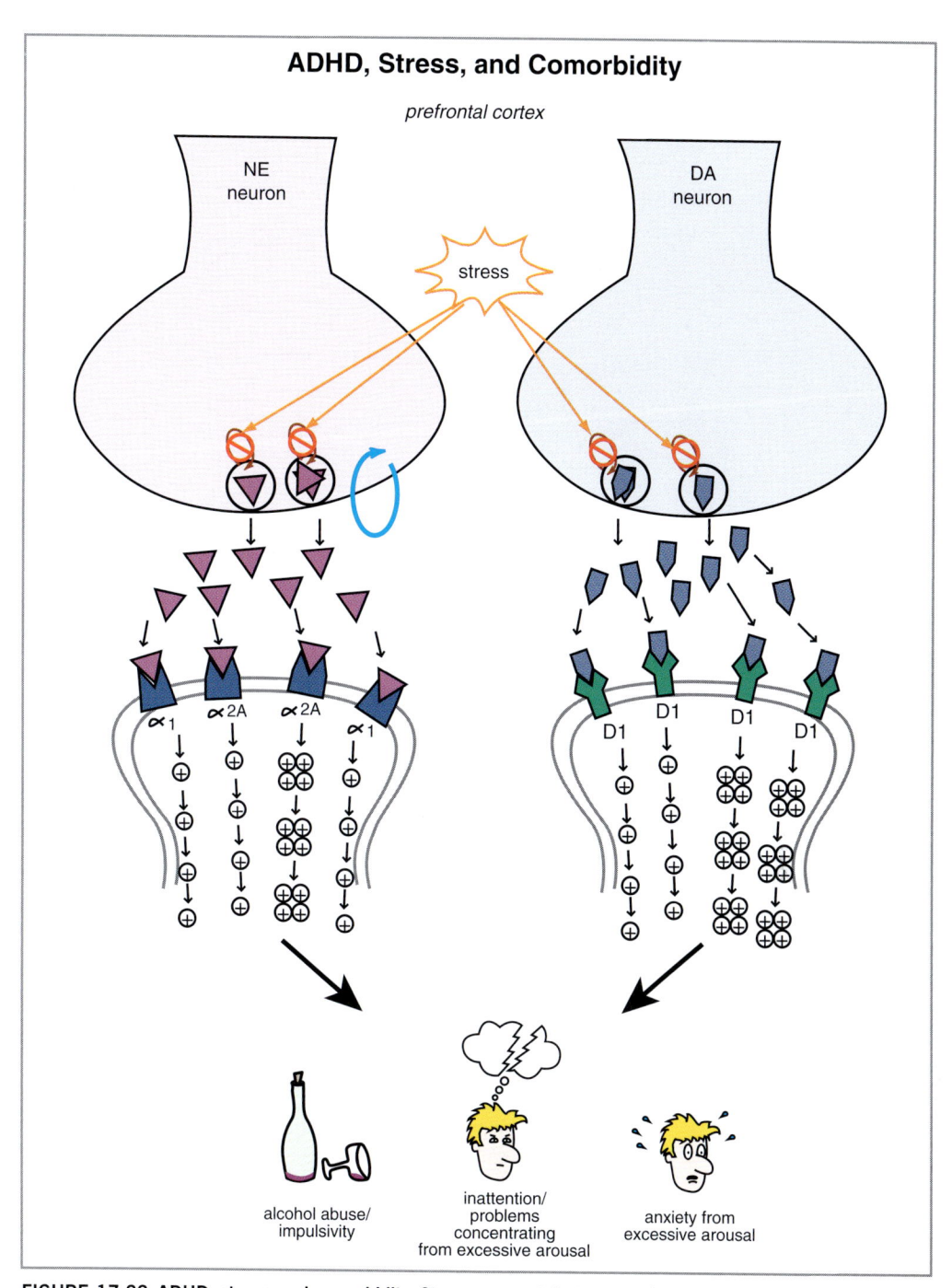

FIGURE 17-22 ADHD, stress, and comorbidity. Stress can contribute to overly active NE and DA circuits in the prefrontal cortex and thus to an excess of phasic NE and DA firing. This may contribute, in turn, to the development of drug and alcohol abuse, impulsivity, inattention, and anxiety.

Attention Deficit Hyperactivity Disorder and Its Treatment | 893

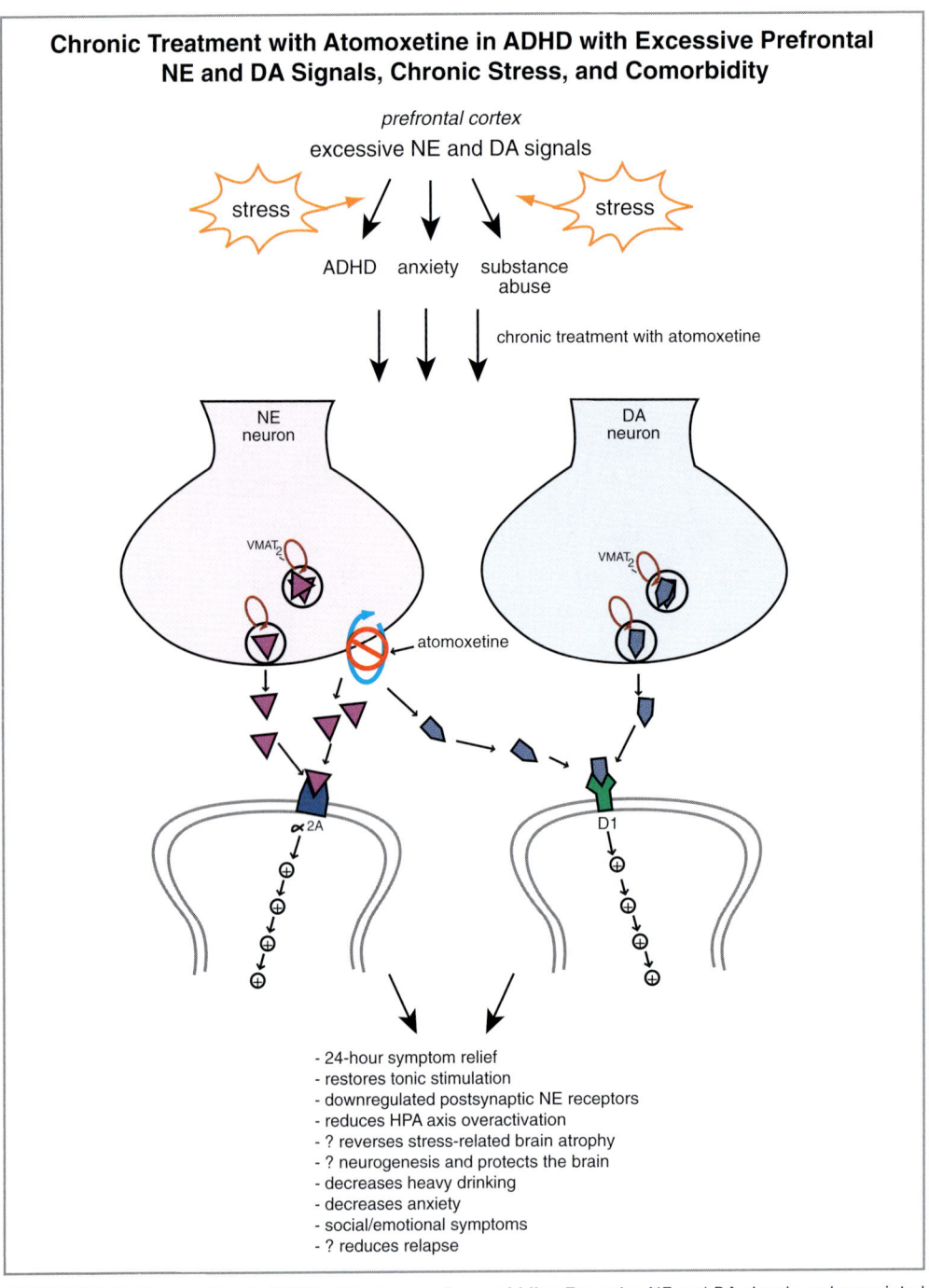

FIGURE 17-23 Atomoxetine in ADHD with stress and comorbidity. Excessive NE and DA signals and associated stress could lead to ADHD as well as to comorbid problems with anxiety or substance abuse. Agents that desensitize postsynaptic dopamine (DA) and norepinephrine (NE) receptors may slowly reduce excessive arousal over time and return neurons to tonic firing. Such agents may be those that themselves have tonic actions on DA and NE, such as atomoxetine, which blocks the NE transporter continuously. This may ultimately reduce HPA axis overactivity and could possibly reverse stress-related brain atrophy or even induce neurogenesis.

Mechanism of Action of Alpha 2A Agonists Guanfacine ER and Clonidine

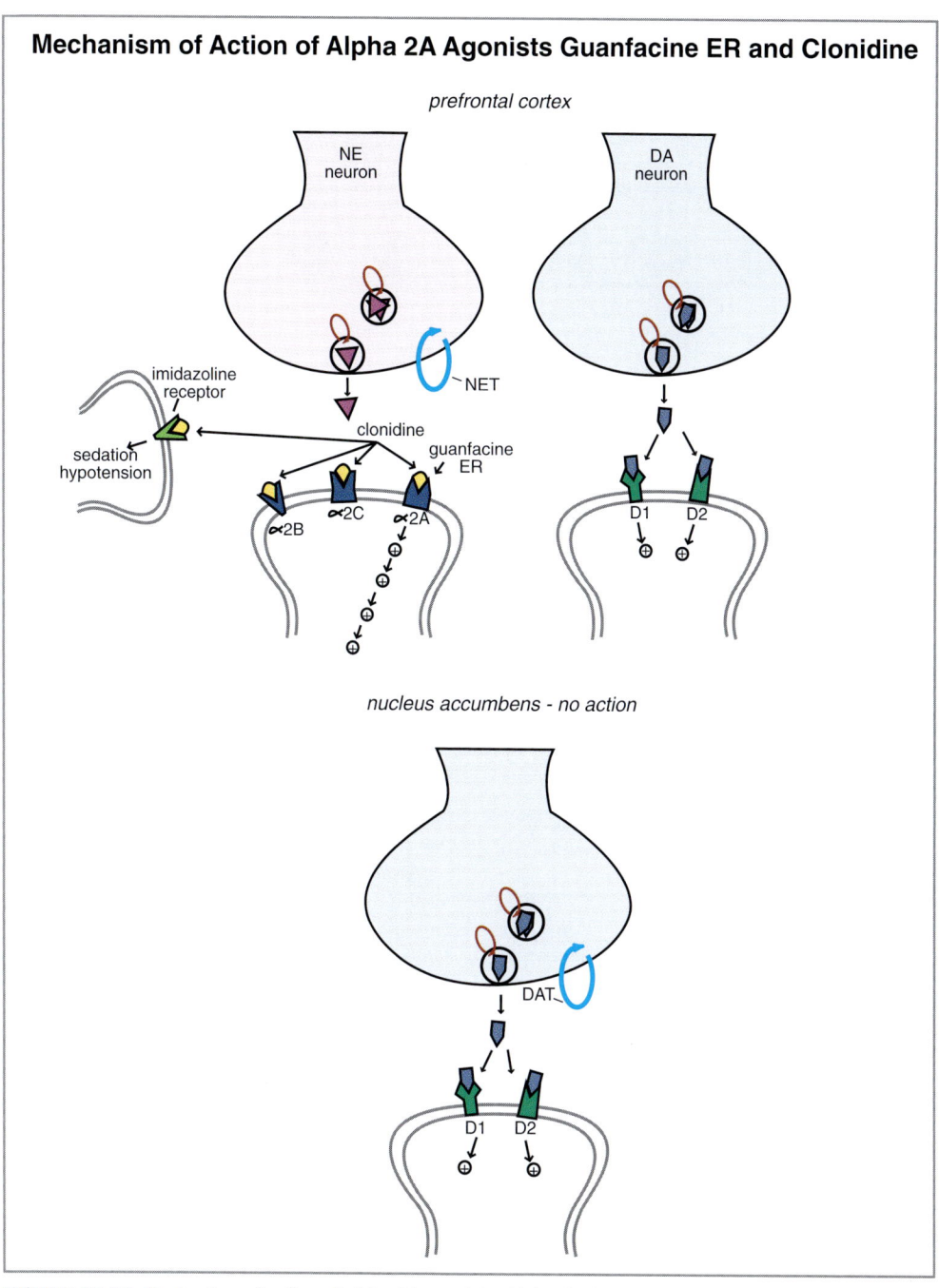

FIGURE 17-24 **Mechanism of action of alpha 2A agonists.** Alpha 2 adrenergic receptors are present throughout the CNS, including the prefrontal cortex, but do not have high concentrations in the nucleus accumbens. Alpha 2A adrenergic receptors in particular are believed to mediate the inattentive, hyperactive, and impulsive symptoms of ADHD, while other alpha 2 adrenergic receptors may have other functions. Clonidine is an alpha 2 adrenergic agonist that is nonselective and binds to 2A, 2B, and 2C receptors; it also binds to imidazoline receptors, which contribute to its sedating and hypotensive effects. Although clonidine's actions at alpha 2A receptors make it a therapeutic option for ADHD, its actions at other receptors may increase side effects. Guanfacine (immediate and extended release) is a selective alpha 2A receptor agonist and thus has therapeutic efficacy with a reduced side effect profile compared to clonidine.

Attention Deficit Hyperactivity Disorder and Its Treatment

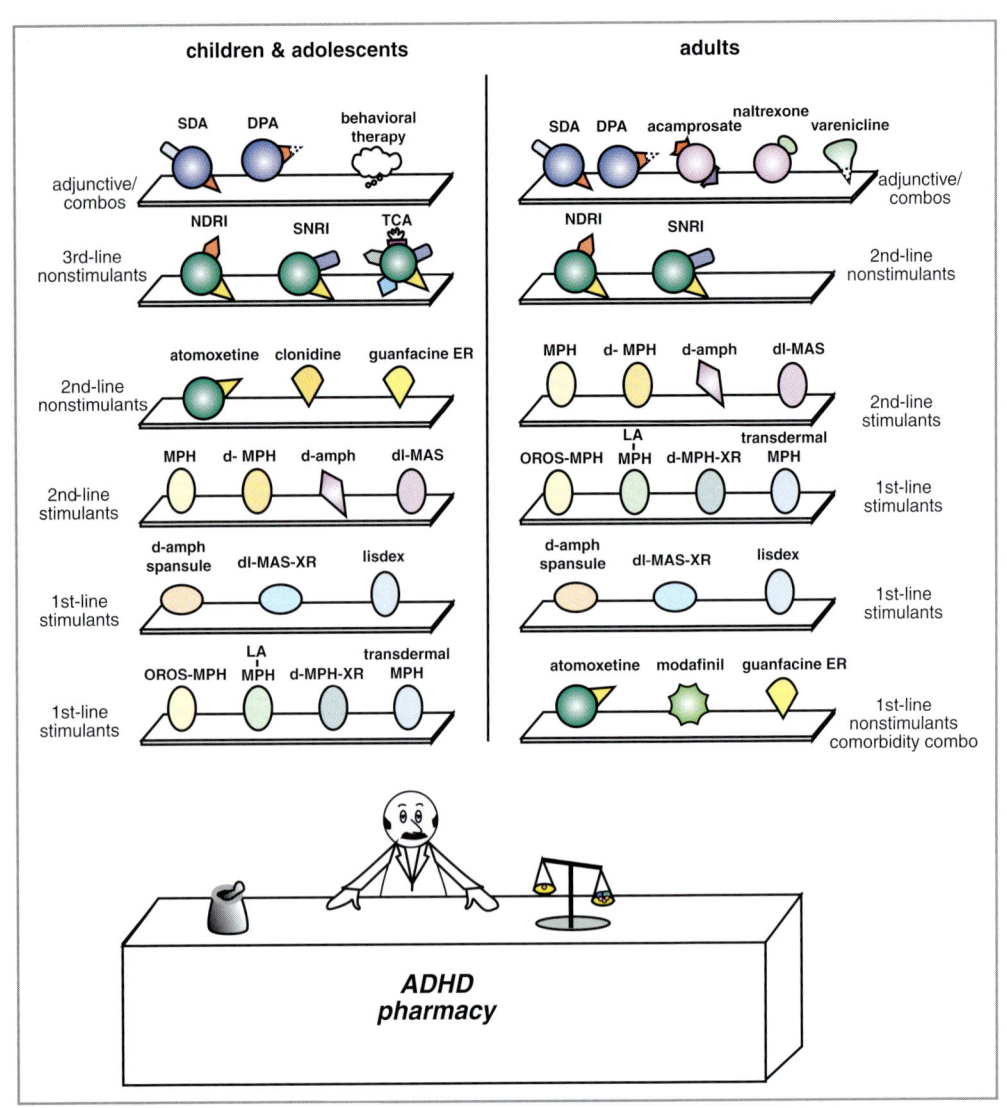

FIGURE 17-25 ADHD pharmacy. First-line treatments for ADHD in children include slow-dose stimulants, while immediate-release stimulants, atomoxetine, and alpha 2A agonists are second-line options. Third-line options include antidepressants with noradrenergic properties. Adjunctive options are atypical antipsychotics or behavioral therapy. For adults, first-line treatments include nonstimulants such as atomoxetine, guanfacine ER, or perhaps modafinil as well as slow-dose stimulants. Immediate-release stimulants and noradrenergic antidepressants are second-line options. Adjunctive options may include atypical antipsychotics or drug abuse treatments for patients with addiction/dependence.

while alpha 2C receptors are densest in striatum. Alpha 1 receptors generally have opposing actions to alpha 2 receptors, with alpha 2 mechanisms predominating when NE release is low or moderate (i.e., for normal attention), but with alpha 1 mechanisms predominating at NE synapses when NE release is high (e.g., associated with stress and comorbidity) and contributing to cognitive impairment. Thus, selective NRIs will first increase activity at alpha 2A postsynaptic receptors to enhance cognitive performance, but at high doses may swamp the synapse with too much NE and cause sedation, cognitive impairment, or both. Patients with these responses to selective NRIs may benefit from lowering the dose.

Also available are direct-acting agonists for alpha 2 receptors. Clonidine is a relatively nonselective agonist at alpha 2 receptors, with actions on alpha 2A, alpha 2B, and alpha 2C receptors (Figure 17-24). In addition, clonidine has actions on imidazoline receptors, thought to be responsible for some of clonidine's sedating and hypotensive actions (Figure 17-24). By contrast, guanfacine is a more selective alpha 2A adrenergic agonist, with less sedation and less powerful hypotensive actions (Figure 17-24). Recently, guanfacine has been formulated into a controlled-release product that allows once-daily administration and lower peak-dose side effects than immediate-release guanfacine. Guanfacine ER is in the late stages of clinical development for ADHD and could prove to be another useful noradrenergic agent for the core symptoms of ADHD in children. It is also being tested in adults, and it will be interesting to see if it has any advantages in ADHD patients with chronic stress and comorbidities.

The ADHD pharmacy

Treatments for ADHD are shown in the ADHD pharmacy in Figure 17-25. For children, slow-dose stimulants are considered first-line, with immediate-release stimulants, selective NRIs such as atomoxetine, and alpha 2A adrenergic agonists such as guanfacine ER and clonidine second-line. A number of noradrenergic antidepressants are shown for third-line treatment, as are atypical antipsychotics and behavioral therapy as adjunctive treatments.

For adults, many prescribers and ADHD patients actually prefer to begin with nonstimulants, and this may be an especially good idea for patients with comorbidities. Modafinil is also included here for adults. Slow-dose stimulants are also acceptable first-line. Immediate-release stimulants are definitely second-line, as are noradrenergic antidepressants. In addition to atypical antipsychotics, agents to assist in treating drug abuse are also very useful adjuncts.

Summary

ADHD has core symptoms of inattentiveness, impulsivity, and hyperactivity linked theoretically to specific malfunctioning neuronal circuits in prefrontal cortex. ADHD can also be conceptualized as a disorder of arousal, including some patients with deficient arousal and others with excessive arousal. Treatments theoretically return patients to normal states of arousal by improving the efficiency of information processing in prefrontal brain circuits. Important differences exist between children and adults with ADHD, and the special considerations for adults, such as treating comorbidities and using nonstimulants, are receiving increasing attention in psychopharmacology. The mechanisms of action, in terms of both pharmacodynamics and pharmacokinetics, for stimulant treatments of ADHD are discussed in detail. The goal is to amplify tonic but not phasic norepinephrine and dopamine actions in ADHD by controlling the rate of stimulant drug delivery, the degree of transporter occupancy, and the duration of transporter occupancy by stimulants. Theoretical mechanism of action of selective norepinephrine reuptake inhibitors such as atomoxetine and their possible advantages in adults with chronic stress and comorbidities are discussed. Actions of a novel alpha 2A adrenergic agonist, guanfacine ER, are also introduced. Finally, ADHD treatments are summarized for first, second- or third-line treatment selection.

CHAPTER 18

Dementia and Its Treatment

- Causes, pathology, and clinical features of dementia
- Alzheimer dementia, beta amyloid plaques, and neurofibrillary tangles
  - Amyloid cascade hypothesis
  - Apo-E and the risk of Alzheimer's disease
- Are there predementia states?
  - Amnestic mild cognitive impairment (MCI)
  - Depression: harbinger of dementia?
- Symptomatic treatments for dementia
  - Acetylcholine and the pharmacological basis of cholinesterase treatments for dementia
  - Cholinergic deficiency hypothesis of amnesia in Alzheimer's disease and other dementias
  - Cholinesterase inhibitors
  - Memantine
  - Other proposed treatments
- Future treatments
  - Marketed products with potential therapeutic actions in dementia
  - Disease-modifying agents in development that act on amyloid processing
  - Other potential disease-modifying treatment approaches
  - Symptomatic treatments in development for Alzheimer's disease and other cognitive disorders and dementias
- The dementia pharmacy
- Summary

Dementia is an area of psychopharmacology where symptomatic treatments are already available. However, the most exciting aspect to this field is the possibility of disease-modifying treatments on the horizon, particularly for Alzheimer's disease. Imagine the impact of new treatments that could halt the progression of this disorder or even partially reverse it! The goal of this chapter is to provide the biological background that will enable the reader to understand not only how currently symptomatic treatments for Alzheimer's disease work but also the rationale for current research efforts to discover truly disease-modifying treatments for this debilitating illness.

This chapter therefore provides only a very brief overview of the various causes of dementias and their pathologies. Full clinical descriptions and formal criteria for the diagnosis of the numerous known dementias should be obtained by consulting standard

TABLE 18-1 Pathological features of selected degenerative dementias

Disorder	Pathology
Alzheimer's disease	Amyloid/tau pathology
Dementia with Lewy bodies Parkinson's dementia Multisystem atrophy	Alpha-synuclein pathology
Frontotemporal dementia Progressive supranuclear palsy Corticobasilar degeneration	Tau pathology
Huntington's disease Spinocerebellar ataxia	Trinucleotide repeat
Wilson's disease (copper) Hallervorden-Spatz (iron)	Toxic/metabolic
Metachromatic leukodystrophy	Leukodystrophy
Creutzfeldt-Jakob disease Variant Creutzfeldt Jakob disease (bovine spongiform encephalopathy) Gerstmann-Straussler-Sheinker disease Fatal familial insomnia (thalamic dementia)	Prior related dementias

reference sources. The discussion here emphasizes the links between various pathological mechanisms, brain circuits, and neurotransmitters with the various symptoms of dementia, especially those of Alzheimer's disease. The goal of this chapter is to acquaint the reader with ideas about the clinical and biological aspects of dementia and its currently approved treatments as well as the many exciting treatments that are on the horizon. The emphasis here is on the biological basis of symptoms of dementia and of their relief by psychopharmacological agents as well as the mechanism of action of drugs that treat these symptoms. For details of doses, side effects, drug interactions, and other issues relevant to the prescribing of these drugs in clinical practice, the reader should consult standard drug handbooks (such as *Essential Psychopharmacology: Prescriber's Guide*).

Causes, pathology, and clinical features of dementia

Dementia consists of memory impairment (amnesia) plus deficits in either language (aphasia), motor function (apraxia), recognition (agnosia), or executive function, such as working memory and problem solving. Personality change can also be present, sometimes even before memory impairment begins. There are many causes of dementia (Tables 18-1 through 18-3). The unique pathologies associated with some of the major dementias are listed in Table 18-1. Knowing the pathology does not mean that a treatment is available, as it is often not evident how to translate information about brain pathology into pharmacological treatments. The best progress is probably occurring in the area of amyloid pathology, where new treatments are attempting to interfere with amyloid processing in Alzheimer's disease, as discussed later in this chapter.

Just because a patient develops memory disturbance does not mean it is Alzheimer's disease (Table 18-2). Alzheimer dementia is perhaps the best known and commonest dementia, but it is often the other symptoms associated with memory loss that help make the

TABLE 18-2 Not all memory disturbance is Alzheimer's disease: clinical features of selected degenerative dementias

Dementia	Clinical features
Alzheimer's disease	Memory deficit
	Aphasia
	Apraxia
	Agnosia
Dementia with Lewy bodies	Memory deficit
	Fluctuating attention
	Extrapyramidal signs
	Psychosis (hallucinations)
Frontotemporal dementia	Memory deficit
	Speech/language disorders
	Disinhibition
	Hyperorality
Huntington's disease	Memory deficit
	Executive dysfunction
	Chorea
Creutzfeldt-Jakob disease	Memory deficit
	Ataxia
	Myoclonus
	Language disturbance

clinical diagnosis (Table 18-2). Just to complicate things, many patients have mixed types of dementia, particularly Alzheimer dementia plus dementia with Lewy bodies or Alzheimer dementia plus vascular dementia (Figure 18-1). Such cases are complicated to diagnose clinically, and definitive diagnosis sometimes must await autopsy. Most dementias are really pathological diagnoses, not clinical diagnoses.

A wide variety of dementias are considered nondegenerative and are listed in Table 18-3. Many of these are treatable upon discovering the underlying cause, but others are not. Extensive clinical evaluation and laboratory testing must rule out these causes prior to concluding that a case of dementia is due to Alzheimer's disease.

Alzheimer dementia, beta amyloid plaques, and neurofibrillary tangles

According to experts, without the introduction of disease-modifying treatments, Alzheimer's disease is poised for an exponential increase throughout the world, with projections that it will quadruple over the next 40 years to affect 1 in every 85 people on earth: over 100 million people by 2050. Fortunately, major progress is being made in understanding the cause of Alzheimer's disease and new treatments are being designed to interfere with the known pathological processes in an attempt to halt them, stop disease progression, and potentially to reverse the disease before neurons are irretrievably lost.

To understand Alzheimer's disease, it is necessary to understand current concepts about how the two hallmarks of this disorder, amyloid plaques and neurofibrillary tangles, are formed in the brain. For many years, scientists have debated which of these two are more important, the beta amyloid plaques (BAPs), thought to be caused by abnormal processing

**Mixed Dementia:
Overlap of Alzheimer Disease with Other Dementias**

Alzheimer's
60-70%

dementia
with Lewy bodies
15-25%

vascular dementia
10-20%

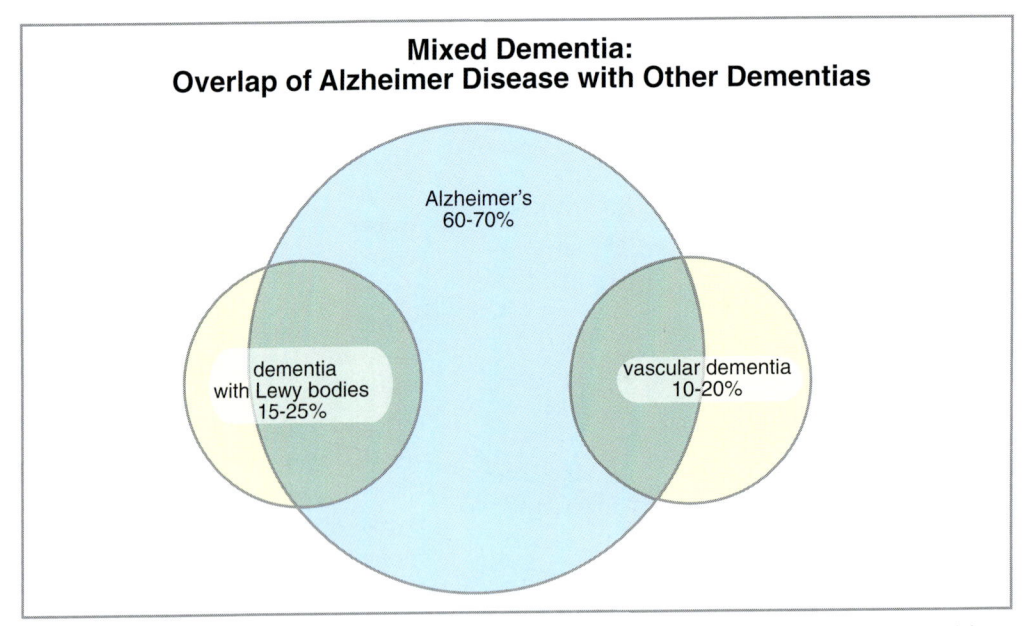

FIGURE 18-1 Mixed dementia. There are several types of dementia; they are distinguished by their underlying pathologies, of which Alzheimer's disease is the most common. It is possible to have more than one dementia, and in fact many patients have both Alzheimer's disease and either dementia with Lewy bodies or vascular dementia.

of amyloid proteins, or the tangles, thought to be caused by abnormal phosphorylation of tau proteins in neuronal microtubules. Although sometimes taking on the tone of religious fervor between these two schools (i.e., the BAP-tists versus the tau-ists), the consensus now is known as the amyloid cascade hypothesis. This theory posits that Alzheimer's disease starts with the abnormal processing of amyloid, which then leads to abnormal phosphorylation of tau proteins as a downstream consequence.

Amyloid cascade hypothesis
A leading contemporary theory for the biological basis of Alzheimer's disease centers around the formation of toxic amyloid plaques due to the abnormal processing of amyloid peptides from amyloid precursor protein (APP). Certainly amyloid plaques destroy cholinergic neurons in the basal forebrain (i.e., nucleus basalis of Meynert) relatively early in this disorder, causing memory disturbance and providing the basis for symptomatic treatment with drugs that boost the enzyme acetylcholine. The major acetylcholine projections are introduced in Chapter 7 and illustrated in Figures 7-11 and 7-12. Treatment of Alzheimer's disease with cholinesterase inhibitors is discussed later in this chapter.

Hypothetically, Alzheimer's disease is a disorder in which beta amyloid deposition eventually destroys neurons diffusely throughout the brain, somewhat analogous to how the abnormal deposition of cholesterol causes atherosclerosis. Thus, Alzheimer's disease may be essentially a problem of too much formation of beta amyloid or too little removal of it.

One idea is that neurons in some patients destined to have Alzheimer's disease have abnormalities either in genes that code for APP or in the enzymes that cut this precursor into smaller peptides. APP is a transmembrane protein with the C terminal inside the neuron and the N terminal outside the neuron. One pathway for APP processing does not produce toxic peptides and involves the enzyme alpha secretase (Figure 18-2). Alpha secretase cuts

TABLE 18-3 Nondegenerative dementias

Vascular	Multi-infarct dementia
	Strategic single-infarct dementia
	Small vessel disease
	Watershed area hypoperfusion
Infectious	HIV dementia
	Neurosyphilis
	Whipple's disease
	Progressive multifocal leukoencephalopathy
	Tuberculosis
	Fungal/protozoal
	Sarcoidosis
Demyelinating	Multiple sclerosis
Endocrine	Hypothyroidism
	Cushing's syndrome
	Adrenal insufficiency
	Hypoparathyroidism
	Hyperparathyroidism
Brain injuries	Postanoxic
	Postencephalitic
	Chronic subdural hematoma
Vitamin deficiency	B_{12}, B_1, folate, niacin
Vasculitides	Lupus erythematosus
	Sjögren's disease
Toxicities	Heavy metal (storage) disorders (arsenic, mercury, lead)
	Industrial/environmental toxins (fertilizers, pesticides)
	Medications
	Chronic alcohol/drug abuse
	Wernicke-Korsakoff syndrome
	Marchiafava-Bignami disease
Organ failure	Hepatic encephalopathy
	Uremic encephalopathy
	Pulmonary insufficiency
Other causes	Dementia syndrome of depression
	Normal-pressure hydrocephalus
	Nonconvulsive status epilepticus
	Acute intermittent poyphyria

APP close to the area where the protein comes out of the membrane, forming two peptides: a soluble fragment known as alpha APP and a smaller 83 amino acid peptide that remains embedded in the membrane until it is further cleaved by a second enzyme acting within the neuronal membrane, called gamma secretase (Figure 18-2). That enzyme produces two smaller peptides, p7 and p3, which are apparently not "amyloidogenic" and therefore not toxic (Figure 18-2).

Another pathway for APP processing can produce toxic peptides that form amyloid plaques (i.e., "amyloidogenic" peptides). In this case a different enzyme, beta secretase, cuts

Processing of Amyloid Precursor Protein into Soluble Peptides

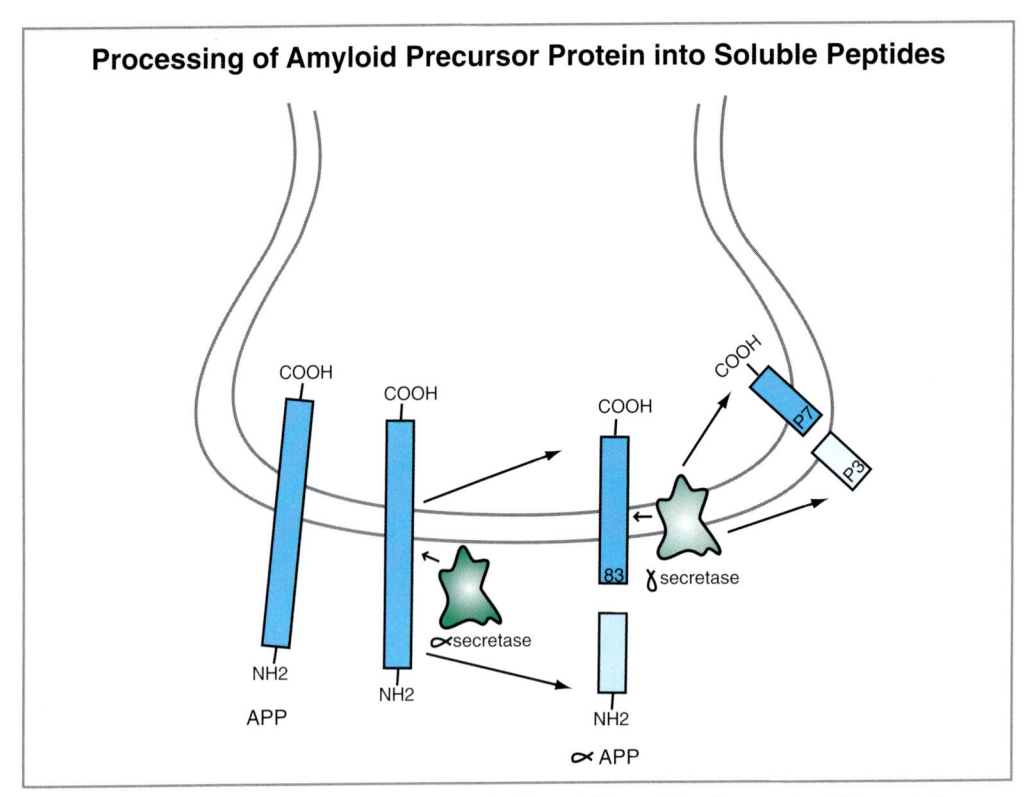

FIGURE 18-2 Processing of amyloid precursor protein into soluble peptides. The way in which amyloid precursor protein (APP) is processed may help determine whether an individual develops Alzheimer's disease or not. A nontoxic pathway for APP processing is shown here. APP is a transmembrane protein with the C terminal inside the neuron and the N terminal outside the neuron. The enzyme alpha secretase cuts APP close to where it comes out of the membrane to form two peptides: alpha-APP, which is soluble, and an 83-amino acid peptide that remains in the membrane. A second enzyme, gamma secretase, cuts the embedded peptide into two smaller peptides, p7 and p3, which are not "amyloidogenic" and thus are not toxic.

APP a little bit further away from the area where APP comes out of the membrane, forming two peptides: a soluble fragment known as beta APP and a smaller 91 amino acid peptide that remains embedded in the membrane until it is further cleaved by gamma secretase within the membrane (Figure 18-3). This releases A-beta peptides of 40, 42 or 43 amino acids, that are "amyloidogenic," especially A-beta-42 (Figure 18-3).

In Alzheimer's disease, genetic abnormalities may produce an altered APP that, when processed by this second pathway involving beta secretase, produces smaller peptides that are especially toxic. Individuals who do not get Alzheimer's disease may produce peptides that are not very toxic or may have highly efficient removal mechanisms that prevent neuronal toxicity from developing. The amyloid cascade hypothesis of Alzheimer's disease therefore begins with an APP that is hypothetically genetically abnormal; therefore, when it is processed into smaller peptides, those peptides are toxic, or amyloidogenic (Figure 18-4). Hypothetically, this triggers a lethal chemical cascade that ultimately results in Alzheimer's disease (Figures 18-3 through 18-8).

Specifically, abnormal genes cause the formation of an altered APP, which is first processed into toxic A-beta-42 peptides (Figure 18-4, amyloid cascade hypothesis part 1). Next, the A-beta-42 peptides form oligomers (a collection of a few copies of A-beta-42

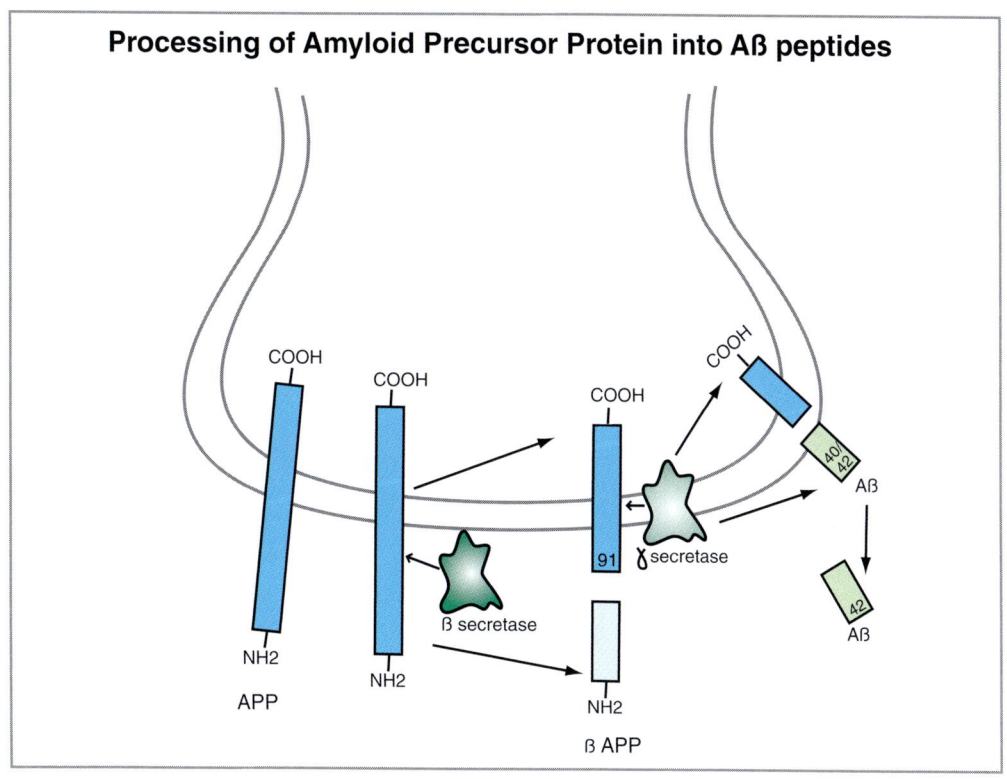

FIGURE 18-3 Processing of amyloid precursor protein into Aβ peptides. The way in which amyloid precursor protein (APP) is processed may help determine whether an individual develops Alzheimer's disease or not. A toxic pathway for APP processing is shown here. APP is a transmembrane protein with the C terminal inside the neuron and the N terminal outside the neuron. The enzyme beta secretase cuts APP at a spot outside of the membrane to form two peptides: beta-APP, which is soluble, and a 91–amino acid peptide that remains in the membrane. Gamma secretase then cuts the embedded peptide; this releases Aβ peptides of 40, 42, or 43 amino acids. These toxic (amyloidogenic) peptides form amyloid plaques.

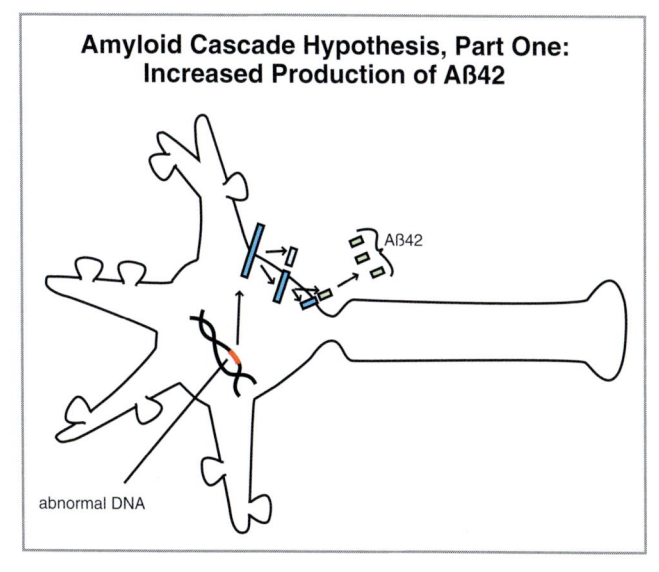

FIGURE 18-4 Amyloid cascade hypothesis, part one: increased production of Aβ42. One theory for the pathophysiology of Alzheimer's disease is that there are genetic abnormalities in amyloid precursor protein (APP), so that when it is processed by the pathway involving beta secretase, it produces smaller, toxic peptides (especially Aβ42, as shown here).

Dementia and Its Treatment

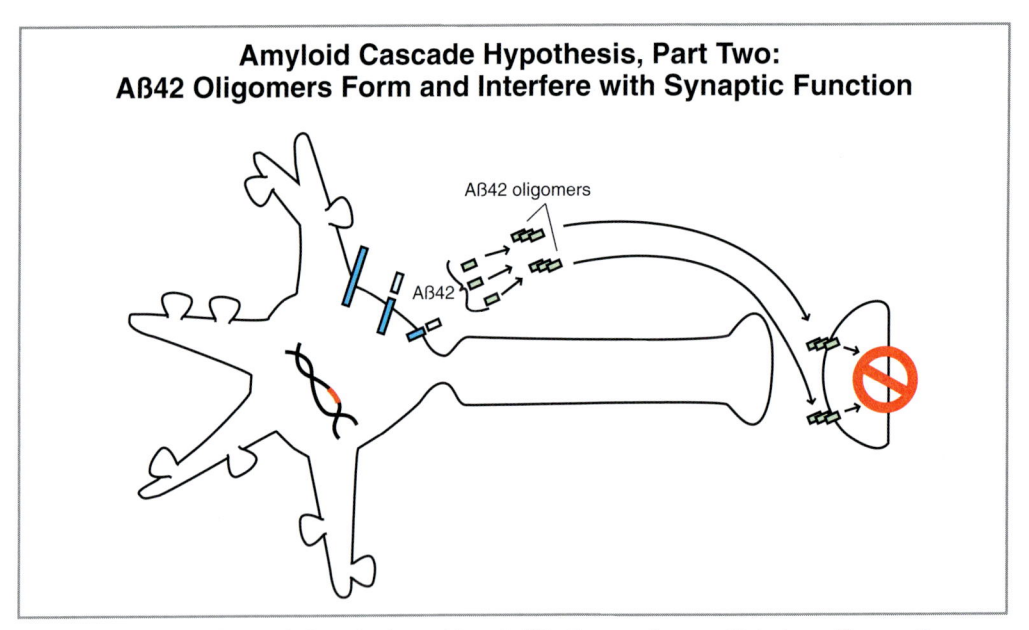

FIGURE 18-5 Amyloid cascade hypothesis, part two: Aβ42 oligomers form and interfere with synaptic function. Aβ42 peptides assemble together to form oligomers, which interfere with synaptic functioning and neurotransmitter actions but are not necessarily lethal to neurons.

assembled together; Figure 18-5, amyloid cascade hypothesis part 2). These oligomers can interfere with synaptic functioning and neurotransmitter actions such as those of acetylcholine, but they are not necessarily lethal to the neurons. Eventually, A-beta-42 oligomers form amyloid plaques, which are even larger clumps of A-beta-42 peptides stuck together with a number of other molecules (Figure 18-6, amyloid cascade hypothesis part 3). A number of nasty biochemical events then occur, including inflammatory responses, activation of microglia and astrocytes, and release of toxic chemicals including cytokines and free radicals (Figure 18-6). These chemical events then hypothetically trigger the formation of tangles within neurons by altering the activities of various kinases and phosphatases, causing hyper-phosphorylation of tau proteins, and converting neuronal microtubules into tangles. Neuronal microtubules are discussed in Chapter 1 and illustrated in Figures 1-9, 1-10, 1-13, 1-15, and 1-17 through 1-20. Finally, widespread synaptic dysfunction from A-beta-42 oligomers, and neuronal dysfunction and death from formation of amyloid plaques outside of neurons and neurofibrillary tangles within neurons, lead to diffuse neuronal death in the cortex and the relentless progression of Alzheimer symptoms of amnesia, aphasia, agnosia, apraxia, and executive dysfunction.

Support for the amyloid cascade hypothesis comes from genetic studies of those relatively rare inherited autosomal dominant forms of Alzheimer's disease. Sporadic cases (i.e., noninherited cases) are the vast majority of Alzheimer's disease cases, but inherited cases can provide clues for what is wrong in the usual sporadic cases of Alzheimer's disease.

Rare familial cases of Alzheimer's disease have an early onset (i.e., before age 65) and have been linked to mutations in at least three different chromosomes: 21, 14, and 1. The mutation on chromosome 21 codes for a defect in APP, leading to increased deposition of beta amyloid. Recall that Down's syndrome is also a disorder of this same chromosome (i.e., trisomy 21), and virtually all such persons develop Alzheimer's disease if they live past

Amyloid Cascade Hypothesis, Part Three: Formation of Amyloid Plaques Causing Inflammation

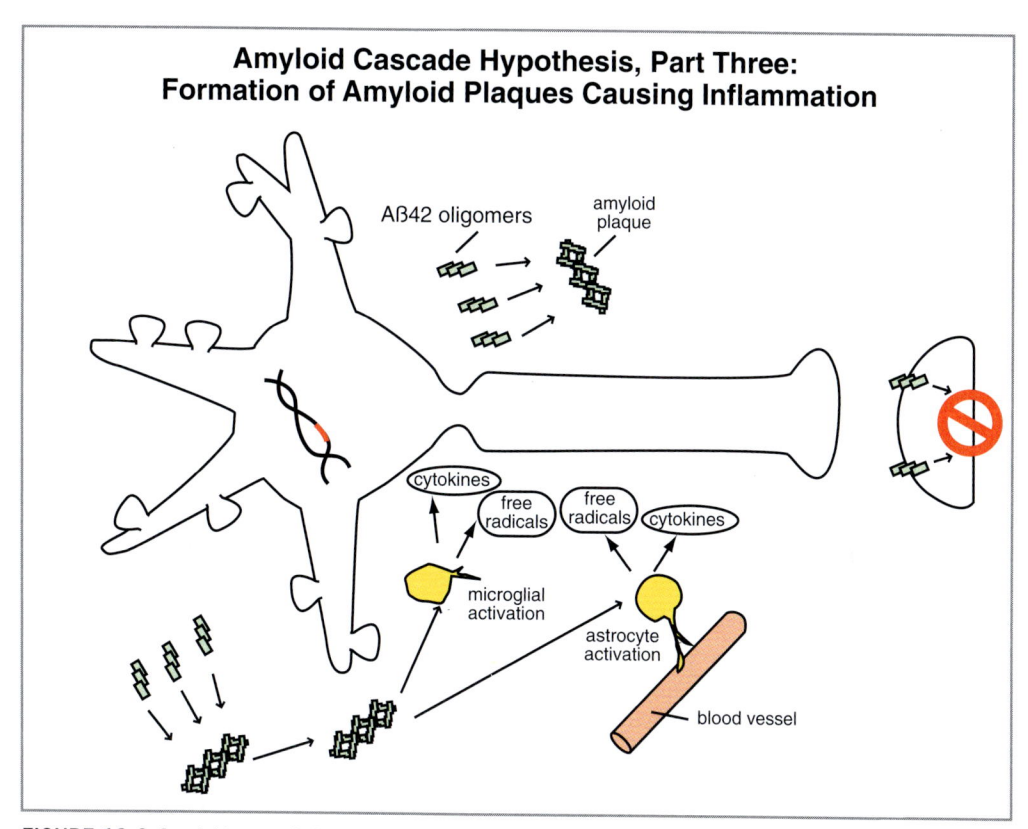

FIGURE 18-6 Amyloid cascade hypothesis, part three: formation of amyloid plaques causing inflammation. Aβ42 oligomers clump together along with other molecules to form amyloid plaques. These plaques can cause inflammatory responses, activation of microglia and astrocytes, and release of toxic chemicals such as cytokines and free radicals.

age 50. A different mutation on chromosome 14 codes for an altered form of a protein called presenilin 1, a component of the enzyme gamma secretase. A third mutation on chromosome 1 codes for an altered form of presenilin 2, a component of a different form of gamma secretase. It is not yet clear what if anything these three mutations in the rare familial cases tell us about the pathophysiology of the usual sporadic, nonfamilial, and late-onset cases of Alzheimer's disease or how cholinergic neurons are damaged. However, they all point to abnormal processing of APP into amyloidogenic beta amyloid peptides as a cause for the dementia, consistent with the amyloid cascade hypothesis.

Theoretically, different abnormalities in amyloid processing may occur in sporadic Alzheimer's disease from those identified in inherited cases, and there may even be multiple abnormalities that could be responsible for sporadic Alzheimer's disease as a final common pathway, but the evidence nevertheless suggests that something in the amyloid cascade has gone wrong in Alzheimer's disease. If so, this implies that preventing the formation of amyloidogenic peptides could prevent Alzheimer's disease.

Apo-E and the risk of Alzheimer's disease

A corollary to the amyloid cascade hypothesis is the possibility that something may be wrong with a protein that binds to amyloid in order to remove it (Figure 18-9). That protein is called Apo-E. In the case of "good" Apo-E, it binds to beta amyloid and removes

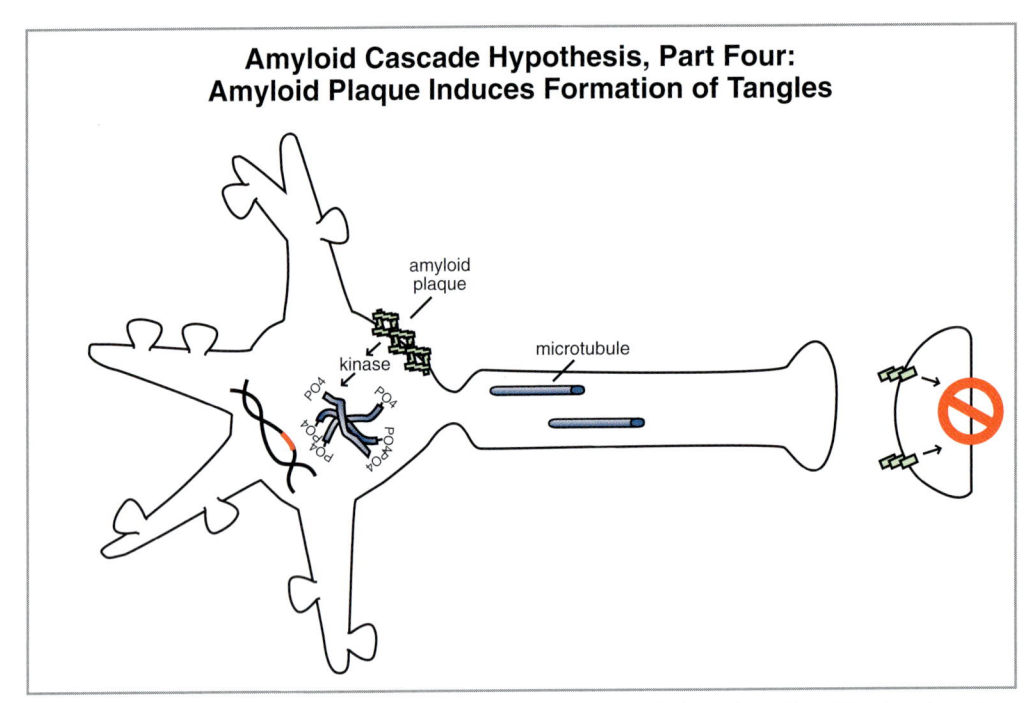

FIGURE 18-7 Amyloid cascade hypothesis, part four: amyloid plaque induces formation of tangles. Amyloid plaques and the chemical events they cause activate kinases, cause phosphorylation of tau proteins, and convert microtubules into tangles within neurons.

it, preventing the development of Alzheimer's disease and dementia (Figure 18-9A). In the case of "bad" Apo-E, a genetic abnormality in the formation of Apo-E causes it to be ineffective in how it binds to beta amyloid. This causes beta amyloid to be deposited in neurons, which then goes on to damage the neurons and cause Alzheimer's disease.

Genes coding for Apo-E are associated with different risks for Alzheimer's disease. There are three alleles (or copies) of this gene coding for this apolipoprotein called E2, E3, and E4. For example, a gene on chromosome 19 that codes of Apo-E is linked to many cases of late-onset Alzheimer's disease. Apo-E is associated with cholesterol transport and involved with other neuronal functions including repair, growth, and maintenance of myelin sheaths and cell membranes. Having one or two copies of E4 increases the risk of getting Alzheimer's disease, and Alzheimer patients with E4 have more amyloid deposits.

Are there predementia states?

Amnestic mild cognitive impairment (MCI)

MCI is a concept defined as memory impairment compared to age-matched peers, with normal cognitive function in other domains (no aphasia, apraxia, agnosia, or executive dysfunction) and no functional evidence of actual dementia. Is this a precursor to Alzheimer's disease, part of normal aging, or a mild and very slowly progressive form of Alzheimer's disease (Alzheimer light)? These questions are now being vigorously debated by experts.

What is "normal aging"? Over half of elderly residents living in the community complain of memory impairment. They have four common complaints: compared to their functioning of 5 or 10 years ago, they experience diminished ability (1) to remember names, (2) to find the correct word, (3) to remember where objects are located, and (4) to concentrate. When such

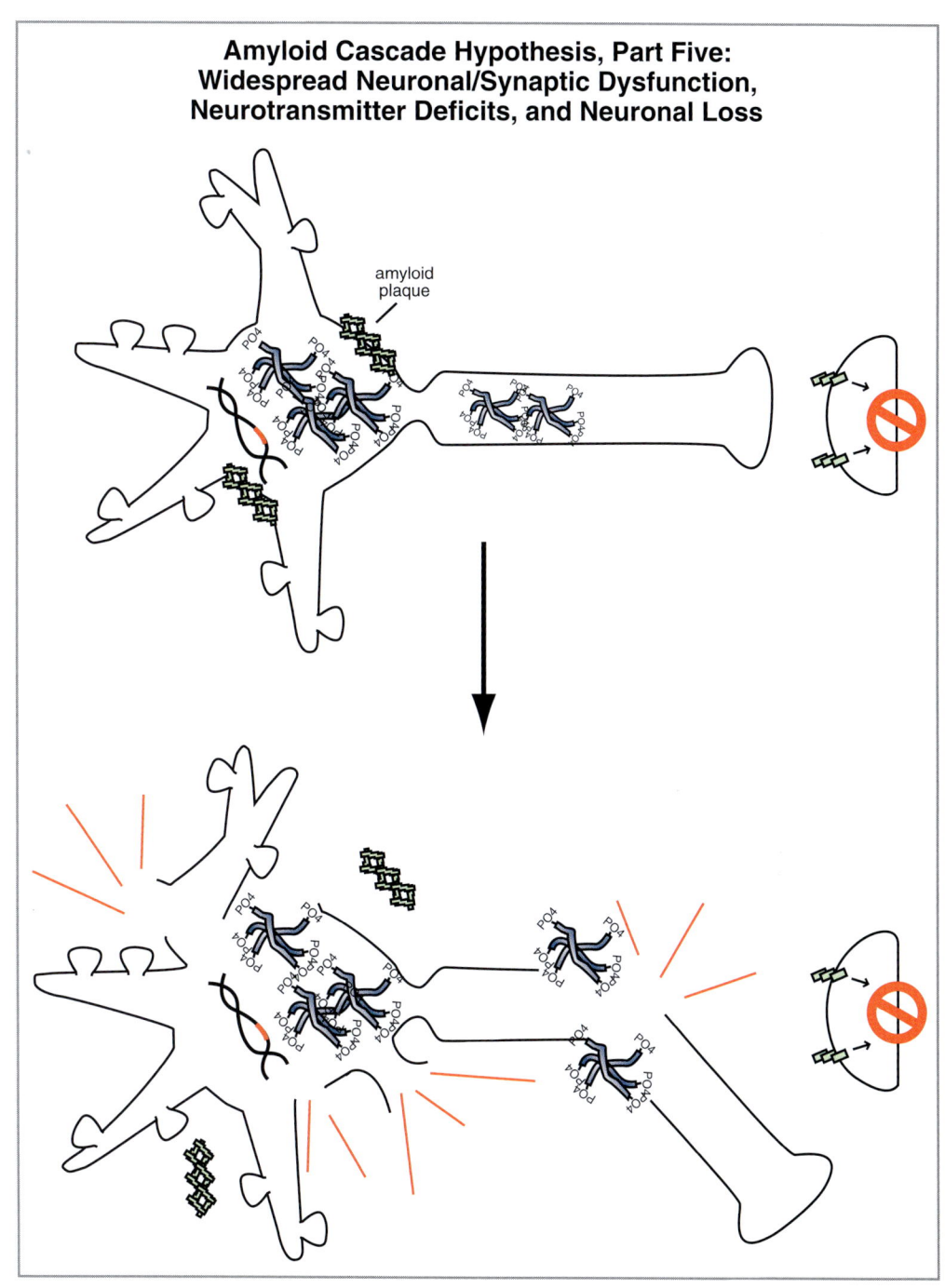

FIGURE 18-8 Amyloid cascade hypothesis, part five: neuronal dysfunction and loss. The effects of amyloid plaques and the buildup of neurofibrillary tangles can ultimately lead to neuronal dysfunction and death.

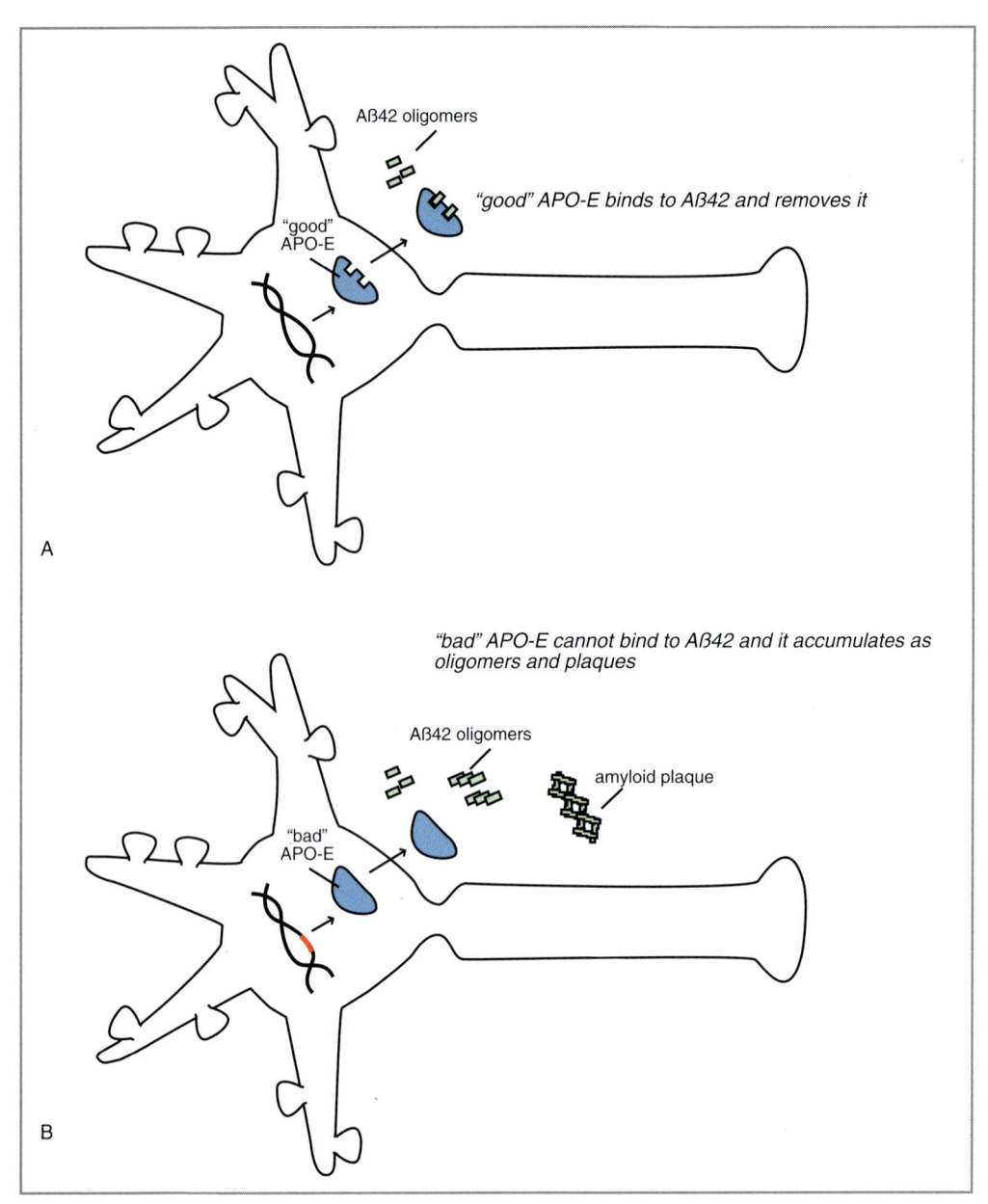

FIGURE 18-9A and B Apo-E and Alzheimer's disease. Another version of the amyloid cascade hypothesis is the possibility that something is wrong with the protein Apo-E. (**A**) Properly functioning ("good") Apo-E binds to beta amyloid and removes it, thus preventing development of Alzheimer's disease and dementia. (**B**) An abnormality in DNA could lead to the formation of a defective or "bad" version of the Apo-E protein, such that it cannot effectively bind to amyloid. This would prevent removal of amyloid, allowing it to accumulate and damage neurons, so that Alzheimer's disease develops.

Presymptomatic/Prodromal Diagnostic Goals and Disease-Modifying Treatment Strategies

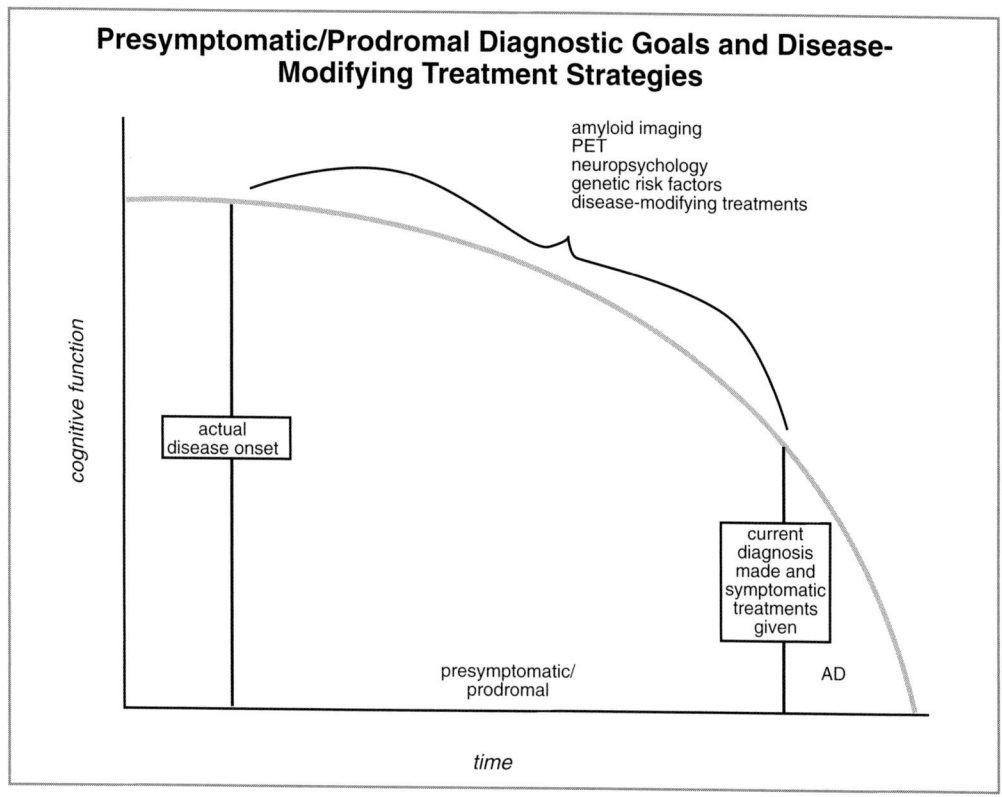

FIGURE 18-10 **Presymptomatic/prodromal diagnostic and treatment goals.** Currently, probable Alzheimer's disease is not identified or treated until it is in a later stage, generally after neurodegeneration has already begun to occur. Several new diagnostic methods are being investigated in an effort to identify Alzheimer's disease earlier, at the presymptomatic/prodromal stage. These include amyloid imaging, PET scans of neuronal activity in frontal versus temporal regions, neuropsychological evaluations, and measurement of genetic risk factors. Disease-modifying treatments are also being investigated in the hope that it may ultimately be possible to prevent, stop progression, or even reverse the neurodegeneration of dementia.

complaints occur in the absence of overt dementia, depression, anxiety disorder, sleep/wake disorder, pain disorder, or ADHD (attention deficit hyperactivity disorder), the condition is sometimes called MCI, age-associated memory impairment, or cognitive impairment no dementia (CIND). It is likely that MCI is not a benign condition, as studies show that between 6 and 15 percent of these patients convert to a diagnosis of dementia every year; after 5 years, about half meet the criteria for dementia; after 10 years or autopsy, up to 80 percent will prove to have or have had Alzheimer's disease.

Given the possibility of disease-modifying treatments on the horizon for Alzheimer's disease, there is intense interest in finding a way to recognize this illness early, at the stage of MCI or even earlier, so that treatments can begin early rather than after significant irreversible brain damage has already occurred. If such a state of pre-Alzheimer's disease or early Alzheimer's disease could be recognized, it would allow disease-modifying treatments to be administered at the stage of presymptomatic or very early symptomatic/prodromal disease (Figure 18-10). This notion is also discussed for schizophrenia in Chapters 9 and 10 and illustrated in Figures 9-44 and 10-120. The idea is not to remove current symptoms but to prevent future symptoms and deterioration.

There are many methodological and logistical problems with conducting such studies in both schizophrenia and Alzheimer's disease: deciding what subjects to enter into the study; the expense (because these studies need huge numbers of patients and take a very long time to conduct); the problems in defining satisfactory endpoints (when do you have early schizophrenia or Alzheimer's disease?, etc.); and the risks of potentially exposing those not destined to develop the disease to drugs with side effects.

A number of psychopharmacological agents have been tested for their potential as disease-modifying agents in Alzheimer's disease, but none has yet proven effective. This includes various antioxidants, anti-inflammatory agents, statins, the cholinesterase inhibitors used to treat the symptoms of patients who already have Alzheimer's disease, vitamin E, estrogen, the MAO inhibitor selegiline, and others. Currently there are a number of novel psychopharmacological agents based upon the amyloid cascade hypothesis in early testing as disease-modifying agents for Alzheimer's disease.

It is interesting to note that so far, the only intervention that has been consistently replicated as a disease-modifying treatment to diminish the risk for MCI or Alzheimer's disease and that can slow the progression of these conditions is cognitive activity. Thus, "exercising" the brain in a "use it or lose it" paradigm appears effective when leisure activities include reading, writing, crossword puzzles, board or card games, group discussions, and playing music. Even physical exercise may be effective, including tennis, golf, swimming, bicycling, dancing, group exercises, team games, walking, climbing more than two flights of stairs, and babysitting. It is now known that the brain makes new neurons throughout life, as discussed in Chapter 2 and illustrated in Figures 2-3 and 2-4. However, it appears that only if you actively engage in learning will these cells survive, whereas the mentally lazy may lose these new neurons.

In order to help identify patients with presymptomatic or prodromal/early symptomatic Alzheimer's disease, several diagnostic tests are being evaluated, from novel neuroimaging techniques capable of measuring amyloid, to PET scans of neuronal activity in frontal versus temporal cortical area, to sophisticated neuropsychological evaluations, to the measurement of genetic risk factors, including Apo E (Figure 18-10).

Depression: harbinger of dementia?
Depression can not only be mistaken for dementia but can also precede the onset of dementia (Figure 18-11). One of the difficult diagnostic and therapeutic management areas of modern psychopharmacology is depression in the elderly. In such patients, dementia and depression can be interrelated in many complex ways. When depression occurs in late life, whether it is a recurrent episode in a patient with a lifetime of episodes or a first episode with onset in late life, a major depressive episode can actually present with prominent cognitive symptoms, especially apathy, lack of interest, and slowing of information processing rather than depressed mood and sadness. Depression with lack of interest or sadness can also occur in patients with established dementia, in patients whose depression represents a prodrome to dementia (Figure 18-11), and in those who ultimately prove to have reversible cognitive impairments from "pseudodementia" or the "dementia of depression."

Late-onset depression may be a dysfunction of prefrontal circuits, including the prefrontal CSTC circuits discussed extensively in relation to executive dysfunction in Chapter 17 and illustrated in Figures 17-3 and 17-4. Some experts call the clinical syndrome associated with hypothetical prefrontal striatal dysfunction in the elderly the DED (depression-executive dysfunction) syndrome. This syndrome is characterized by psychomotor retardation, reduced interest in activities, impaired insight, and pronounced behavioral disability.

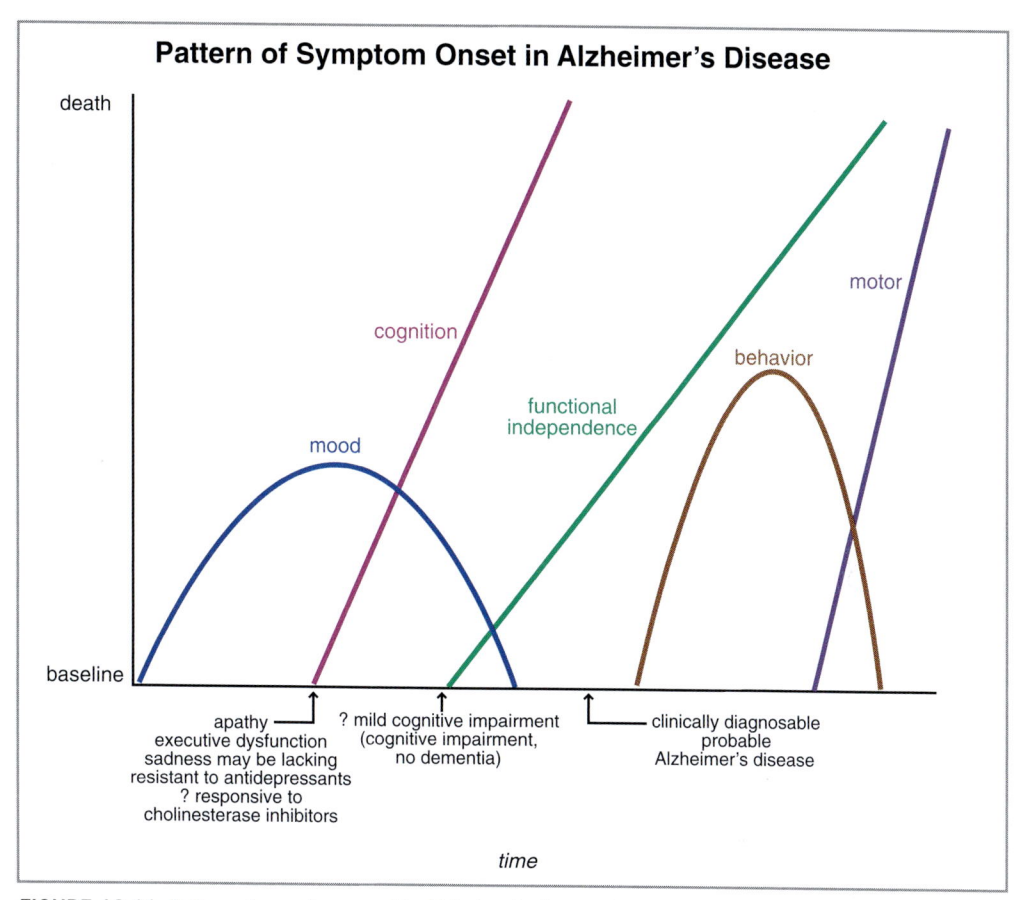

FIGURE 18-11 Pattern of symptom onset in Alzheimer's disease. In most cases, mood changes are the first symptoms of Alzheimer's disease. These mood symptoms may manifest as apathy rather than sadness and may be resistant to antidepressants but perhaps responsive to cholinesterase inhibitors. Cognitive impairment may soon follow and may be considered part of a depressive episode as opposed to indicative of developing dementia. As cognitive impairment increases, functional independence may begin to decline; it is at this stage that probable Alzheimer's disease may be clinically diagnosable. Ultimately, behavioral and motor symptoms develop and become a major management issue.

The DED syndrome may progress to a diagnosable dementia and may have a poor response to traditional antidepressants, but it may respond to dopaminergic agents (such as dopamine agonists, amantadine, modafinil, or even stimulants in selected cases) or to cholinergic agents (such as cholinesterase inhibitors).

Effective treatment of depression in the elderly can improve cognitive function, but unlike younger patients, many depressed elderly will not return to their premorbid level of cognitive performance, especially their memory and executive functioning. In such cases, the depression may be heralding the onset of Alzheimer's disease (Figure 18-11). Up to half of elderly patients who present with depression and cognitive impairment will prove within 5 years to have cognitive impairment that is irreversible. Cognitive impairment in depression of the elderly may be associated with poor or very slow antidepressant response (12 weeks or longer); however, recent findings with SNRIs are somewhat more encouraging, in that both mood and cognitive symptoms can improve notably. Patients with vascular depression may benefit by prevention of further ischemic events from treatments with antithrombotic

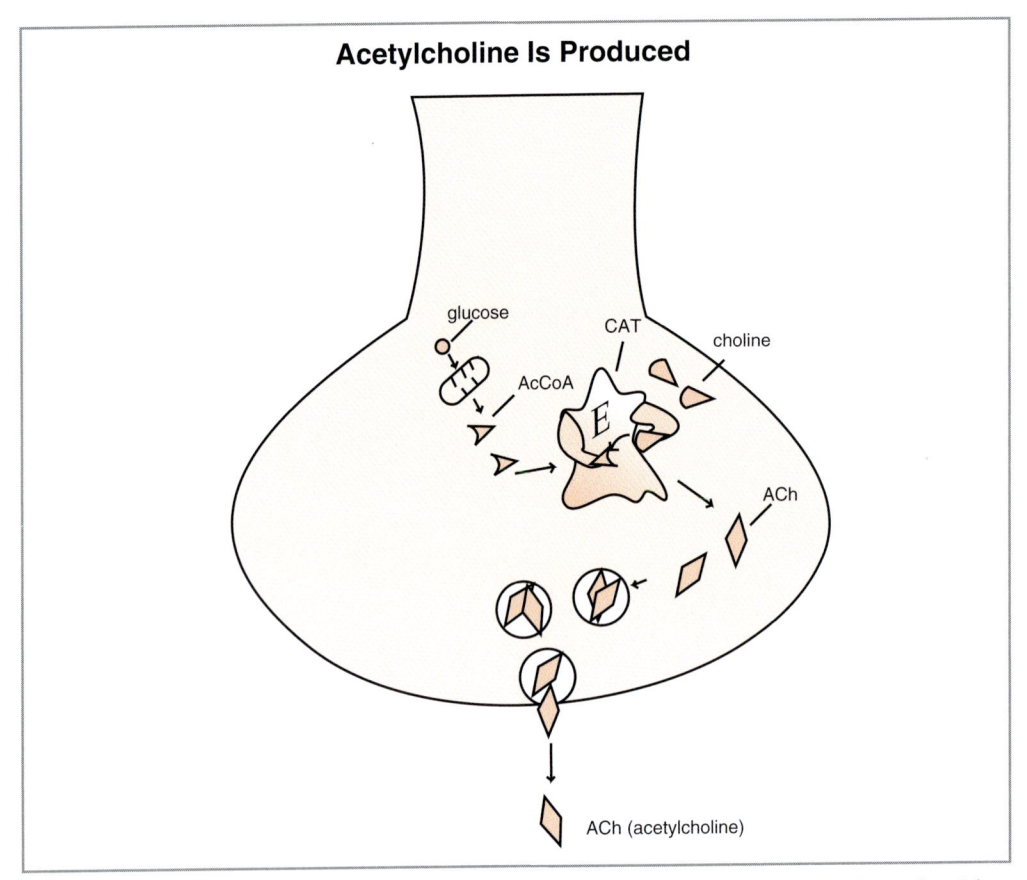

FIGURE 18-12 Acetylcholine is produced. Acetylcholine is formed when two precursors – choline and acetyl coenzyme A (AcCoA) – interact with the synthetic enzyme choline acetyl transferase (CAT). Choline is derived from dietary and intraneuronal sources and AcCoA is made from glucose in the mitochondria of the neuron.

agents such as aspirin and clopidogrel. Patients whose depression may represent a prodrome to Alzheimer's disease (Figure 18-11) may experience symptomatic benefit, such as improvement of apathy and memory as well as mood, from treatment with cholinesterase inhibitors, although these agents are not approved for this use.

Symptomatic treatments for dementia

Acetylcholine and the pharmacological basis of cholinesterase treatments for dementia

Many of the current treatments for symptoms of dementia are based upon boosting the availability of the neurotransmitter acetylcholine. Prior to discussing these treatments, we will review the pharmacology of acetylcholine. The principal cholinergic pathways are introduced in Chapter 7 and illustrated in Figures 7-11 and 7-12.

Acetylcholine is formed in cholinergic neurons from two precursors: choline and acetyl coenzyme A (AcCoA) (Figure 18-12). Choline is derived from dietary and intraneuronal sources, and AcCoA is made from glucose in the mitochondria of the neuron. These two substrates interact with the synthetic enzyme choline acetyl transferase (CAT) to produce the neurotransmitter acetylcholine (ACh).

Acetylcholine Action Is Terminated

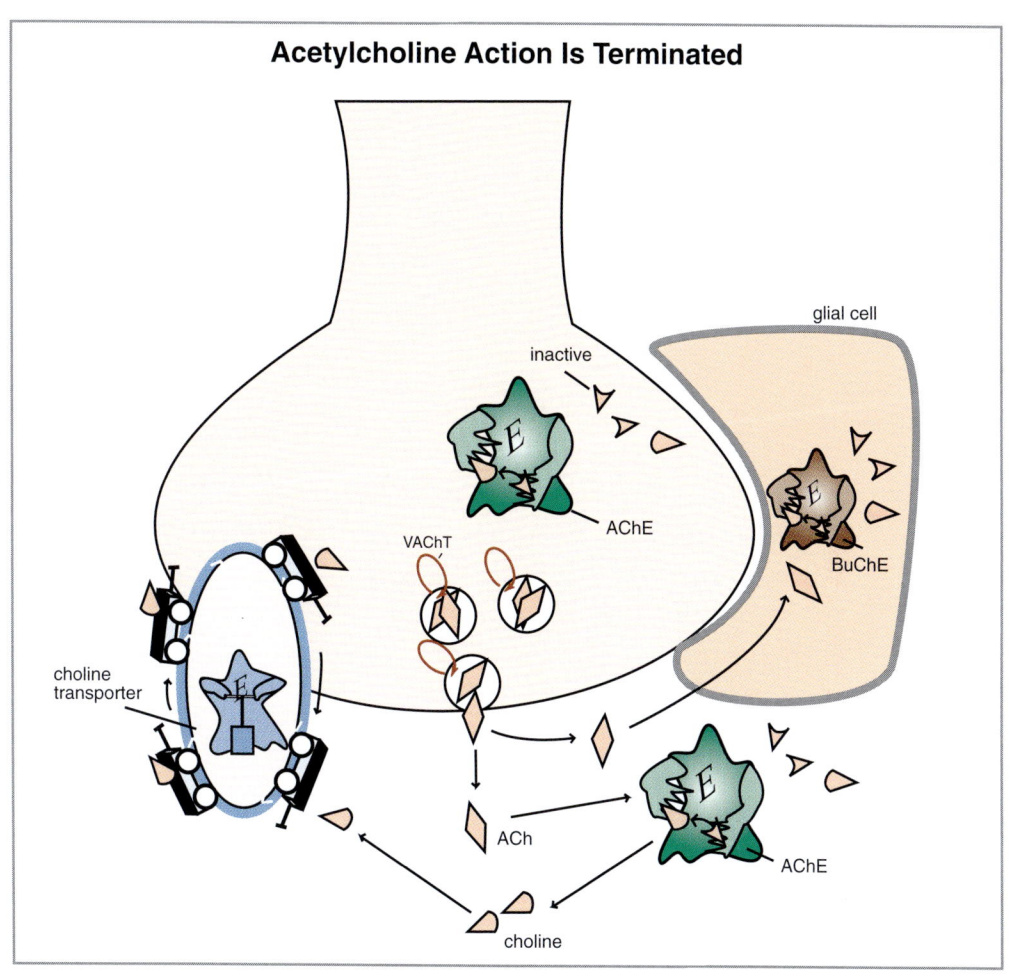

FIGURE 18-13 Acetylcholine's action is terminated. Acetylcholine's action can be terminated by two different enzymes: acetylcholinesterase (AChE), which is present both intra- and extracellularly, and butyrylcholinesterase (BuChE), which is particularly present in glial cells. Both enzymes convert acetylcholine into choline, which is then transported out of the synaptic cleft and back into the presynaptic neuron via the choline transporter. Once inside the presynaptic neuron, choline can be recycled into acetylcholine and then packaged into vesicles by the vesicular transporter for acetylcholine (VAChT).

ACh's actions are terminated by one of two enzymes, either acetylcholinesterase (AChE) or butyrylcholinesterase (BuChE), sometimes also called "pseudocholinesterase" or "nonspecific cholinesterase" (Figure 18-13). Both enzymes convert ACh into choline, which is then transported back into the presynaptic cholinergic neuron for resynthesis into ACh (Figure 18-13). Although both AChE and BuChE can metabolize ACh, they are quite different in that they are encoded by separate genes and have different tissue distributions and substrate patterns. There may be different clinical effects of inhibiting these two enzymes as well. High levels of AChE are present in brain, especially in neurons that receive ACh input (Figure 18-13). BuChE is also present in brain, especially in glial cells (Figure 18-13). As discussed below, some cholinesterase inhibitors specifically inhibit AChE, whereas others inhibit both enzymes. It is AChE that is thought to be the key enzyme for inactivating ACh at cholinergic synapses (Figure 18-13), although BuChE can take on this

Muscarinic Acetylcholine Receptors

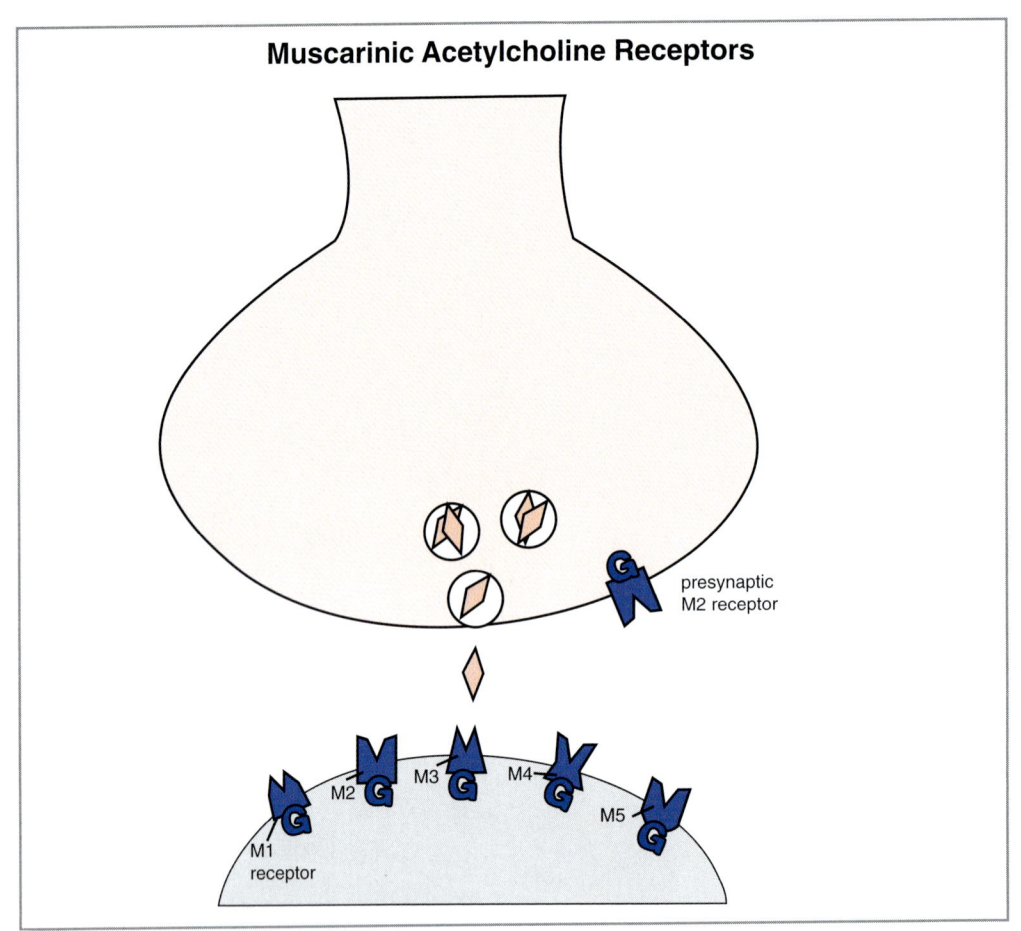

FIGURE 18-14 Muscarinic acetylcholine receptors. Acetylcholine neurotransmission can be regulated by G protein–linked muscarinic acetylcholine receptors, shown here. Muscarinic 1 (M1) receptors are postsynaptic and important for regulation of memory. Muscarinic 2 (M2) receptors exist both presynaptically as autoreceptors and postsynaptically. Other postsynaptic muscarinic receptors include M3, M4, and M5.

activity if ACh diffuses to nearby glia. AChE is also present in the gut, skeletal muscle, red blood cells, lymphocytes, and platelets. BuChE is also present in the gut, plasma, skeletal muscle, placenta, and liver. BuChE may be present in some specific neurons, and it may also be present in amyloid plaques.

ACh released from CNS neurons is destroyed too quickly and too completely by AChE to be available for transport back into the presynaptic neuron, but the choline that is formed by the breakdown of ACh is readily transported back into the presynaptic cholinergic nerve terminal by a transporter similar to the transporters for other neurotransmitters already discussed in relation to norepinephrine, dopamine, and serotonin neurons. Once back in the presynaptic nerve terminal, it can be recycled into new acetylcholine synthesis (see Figure 18-3). Once synthesized in the presynaptic neuron, ACh is stored in synaptic vesicles after being transported into these vesicles by the vesicular transporter for ACh (VAChT), analogous to the vesicular transporters for the monoamines and other neurotransmitters.

There are numerous receptors for ACh (Figures 18-14 and 18-15). The major subtypes are nicotinic and muscarinic subtypes of cholinergic receptors. Classically, muscarinic

Nicotinic Acetylcholine Receptors

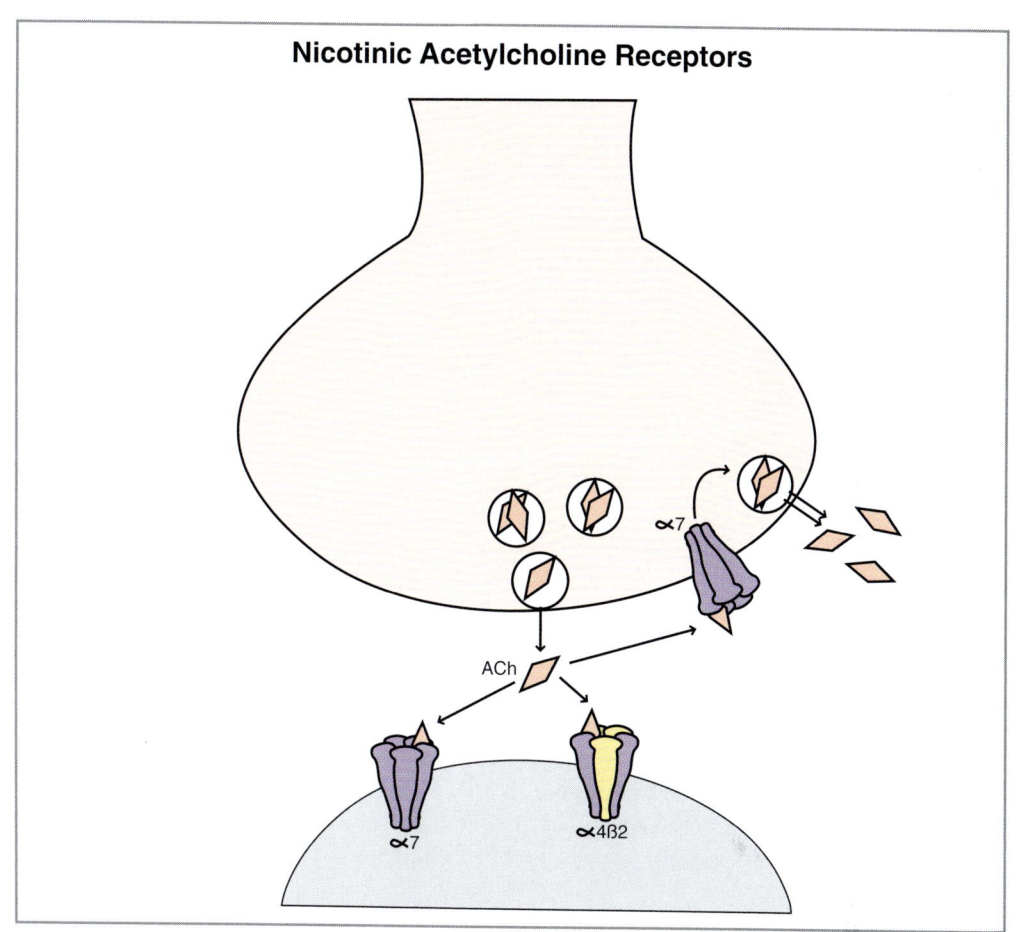

FIGURE 18-15 **Nicotinic acetylcholine receptors.** Acetylcholine neurotransmission can be regulated by ligand-gated excitatory ion channels known as nicotinic acetylcholine receptors, shown here. There are multiple subtypes of these receptors, defined by the subunits they contain. Two of the most important are those that contain all alpha 7 subunits and those that contain alpha 4 and beta 2 subunits. Alpha 7 receptors can exist presynaptically, where they facilitate acetylcholine release, or postsynaptically, where they are important for regulating cognitive function. Alpha 4 beta 2 receptors are postsynaptic and regulate release of dopamine in the nucleus accumbens.

receptors are stimulated by the mushroom alkaloid muscarine and nicotinic receptors by the tobacco alkaloid nicotine. Nicotinic receptors are all ligand-gated, rapid-onset, excitatory ion channels blocked by curare. Muscarinic receptors, by contrast, are G protein–linked and can be excitatory or inhibitory; many are blocked by atropine, scopolamine, and other well known "anticholinergics" discussed throughout this text. Both nicotinic and muscarinic receptors have been further subdivided into numerous receptor subtypes.

Subtypes of muscarinic receptors include the well-known postsynaptic M1 subtype, which appears to be key to the regulation of some of the memory functions of ACh acting at cholinergic synapses (Figure 18-14). The M2 subtype is presynaptic and serves as an autoreceptor, blocking the further release of ACh when it is activated by the buildup of synaptic levels of ACh (Figure 18-14). The M3 subtype is introduced in Chapter 10 on antipsychotics and discussed in relation to the regulation of peripheral insulin release from the pancreas and the blockade of these muscarinic receptor subtypes by some of the atypical antipsychotics (see Figure 10-64).

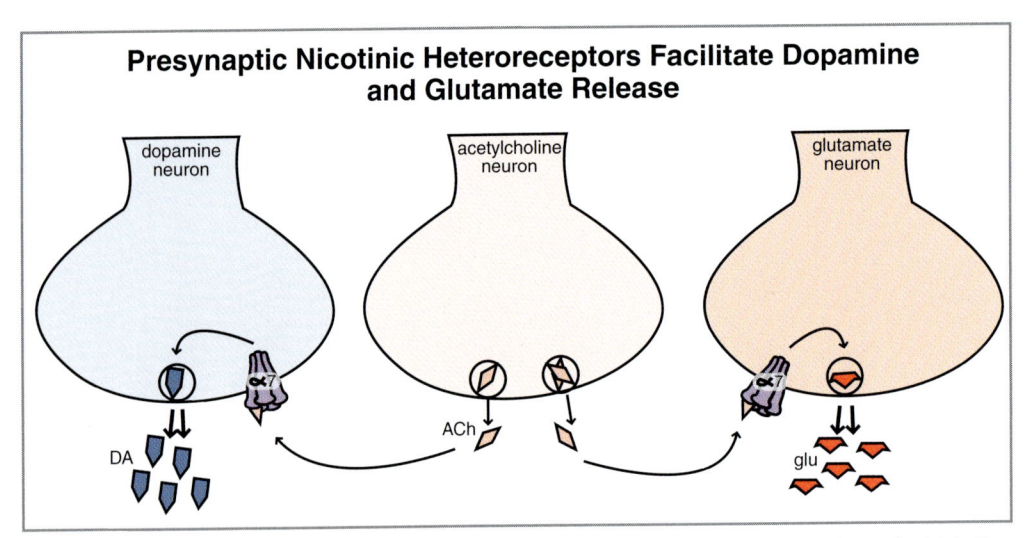

FIGURE 18-16 Presynaptic nicotinic heteroreceptors facilitate dopamine and glutamate release. Acetylcholine that diffuses away from the synapse can bind to presynaptic alpha 7 nicotinic receptors on dopamine and glutamate neurons, where it stimulates release of these neurotransmitters.

A number of nicotinic receptor subtypes also exist in the brain, with different subtypes also outside of the brain in skeletal muscle and ganglia. Two of the most important CNS nicotinic cholinergic receptors are the subtype with all alpha 7 subunits and the subtype with alpha 4 and beta 2 subunits (Figure 18-15). The alpha 4 beta 2 subtype is postsynaptic and plays an important role in regulating dopamine release in the nucleus accumbens. It is thought to be a primary target of nicotine in cigarettes and to contribute to the reinforcing and addicting properties of tobacco. Alpha 4 beta 2 subtypes of nicotinic cholinergic receptors are discussed in further detail in Chapter 19, on drug abuse.

Alpha 7 nicotinic cholinergic receptors can be either presynaptic or postsynaptic (Figures 18-15 and 18-16). When they are postsynaptic, they may be important mediators of cognitive functioning in the prefrontal cortex. When they are presynaptic and on cholinergic neurons, they appear to mediate a "feed-forward" release process where ACh can facilitate its own release by occupying presynaptic alpha 7 nicotonic receptors (Figure 18-15). Furthermore, alpha 7 nicotinic receptors are present on neurons that release other neurotransmitters, such as dopamine and glutamate neurons (Figure 18-16). When ACh diffuses away from its synapse to occupy these presynaptic heteroreceptors, it facilitates the release of the neurotransmitter there (e.g., dopamine or glutamate) (see Figure 18-16).

Just as described for other ligand-gated ion channels such as the GABA-A receptor and the NMDA receptor, it appears that ligand-gated nicotinic cholinergic receptors are also regulated by allosteric modulators (Figure 18-17). Positive allosteric modulators (PAMs) have been identified for nicotinic receptors in brain; indeed, the cholinesterase inhibitor galantamine has a second therapeutic mechanism as a PAM for nicotinic receptors, as described for this agent below.

Cholinergic deficiency hypothesis of amnesia in Alzheimer's disease and other dementias
Numerous investigators have shown that a deficiency in cholinergic functioning is linked to a disruption in memory, particularly short-term memory. For example, blockers of muscarinic cholinergic receptors (such as scolopamine) can produce a memory disturbance in normal

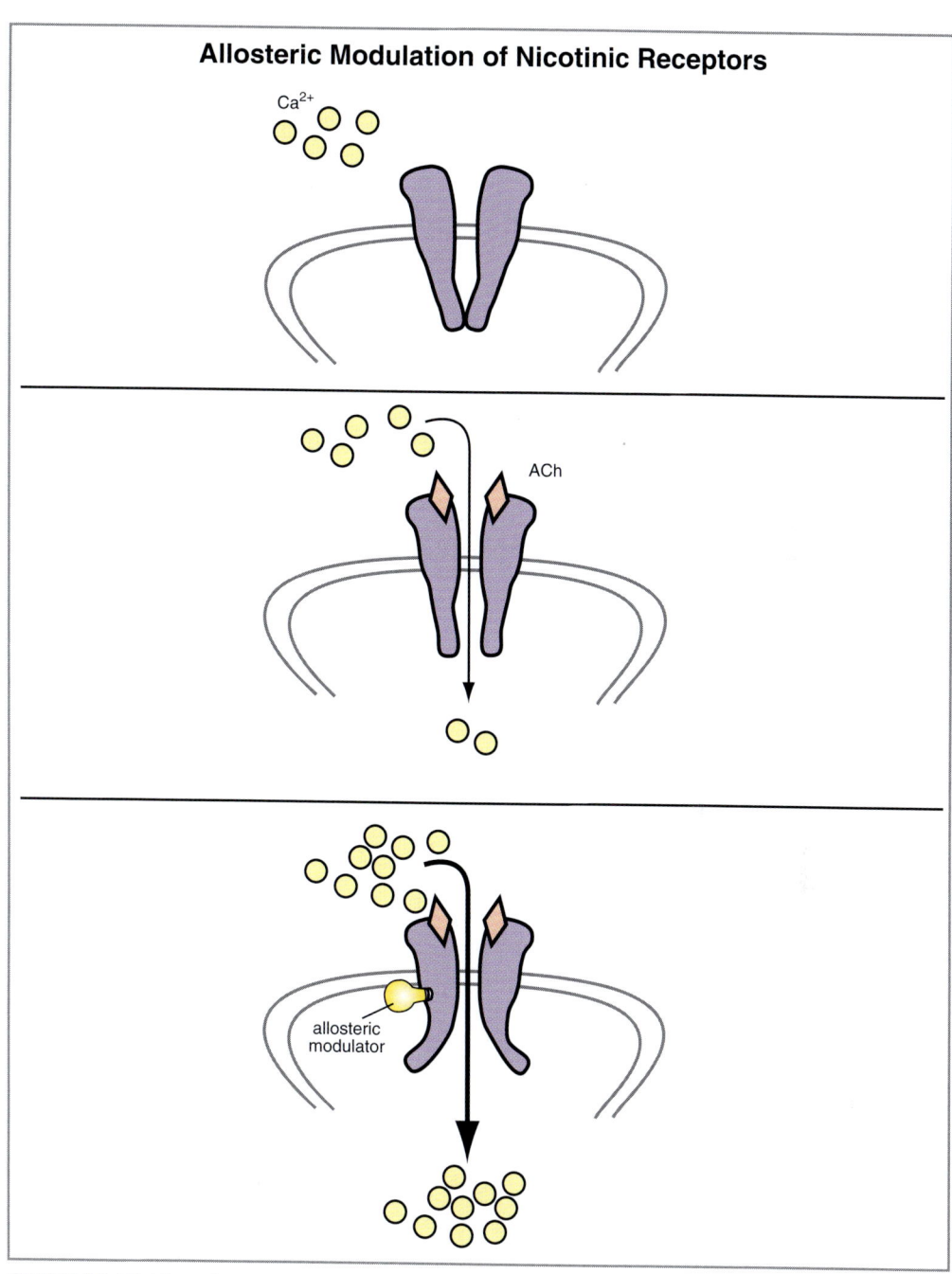

FIGURE 18-17 Allosteric modulation of nicotinic receptors. Nicotinic receptors can be regulated by allosteric modulators. These ligand-gated ion channels control the flow of calcium into the neuron (top panel). When acetylcholine is bound to these receptors, it allows calcium to pass into the neuron (middle panel). A positive allosteric modulator bound in the presence of acetylcholine increases the frequency of opening of the channel and thus can allow for more calcium to pass into the neuron (bottom panel).

human volunteers that has similarities to the memory disturbance in Alzheimer's disease. Boosting cholinergic neurotransmission with cholinesterase inhibitors not only reverses scopolamine-induced memory impairments in normal human volunteers but also enhances memory functioning in patients with Alzheimer's disease. Both animal and human studies have demonstrated that the nucleus basalis of Meynert in the basal forebrain is the major brain center for cholinergic neurons that project throughout the cortex (Figure 7-12). These neurons have the principal role in mediating memory formation. It is suspected that the short-term memory disturbance of Alzheimer patients is due to degeneration of these particular cholinergic neurons. Other cholinergic neurons, such as those in the striatum and those projecting from the lateral tegmental area (Figure 7-11), are not involved in the memory disorder of Alzheimer's disease.

A "cholinergic deficiency syndrome" due to degeneration limited to the nucleus basalis of the basal forebrain could theoretically also be responsible for the more limited short-term memory problems without other signs of dementia that define mild cognitive impairment. When vascular damage or chronic alcoholism affects cholinergic neurons, cholinergic deficiency may also be a part of vascular dementia or of alcoholic dementia. This may be why some patients with vascular dementia or alcohol-related dementias respond to cholinesterase inhibitors. When Lewy bodies damage cholinergic neurons in Lewy body dementia or Parkinson dementia, cholinergic deficiency may also become part of these dementias. In such cases, patients may respond to cholinesterase inhibitors. However, when tau pathology affects the frontal lobes and the temporal lobe in frontotemporal dementia, the memory disturbance, personality changes, disinhibition, and social inappropriateness of this dementia are not generally improved by cholinesterase inhibitors, perhaps because the pathology and these symptoms do not arise from cholinergic neurons.

Nevertheless, cholinesterase inhibitors are best documented for use in Alzheimer's disease, where cholinergic deficiency is perhaps the most pervasive, early in the course of the dementia. Although Alzheimer's disease may start with a profound cholinergic deficiency – and this is the likely cause of memory disturbances early in its course – the illness is obviously progressive and many other symptoms develop, such as difficulties in problem solving, judgment, language, and behavior. Thus it appears that degeneration of cholinergic neurons due to deposition of amyloid plaque may begin early within the nucleus basalis of the basal forebrain at the time of vague and undiagnosed memory symptoms (Figure 18-18), spreading to projection areas such as hippocampus, amygdala, and entorhinal cortex by the time of early diagnosis and then diffusely throughout neocortex by the time of nursing home placement and loss of functional independence, eventually involving the loss of a great many neurons and neurotransmitter systems by the time of death (Figure 18-18).

Cholinesterase inhibitors

Evidence that cholinergic neuronal functioning is one of the earliest neurotransmitters to change in Alzheimer's disease and that it changes dramatically during the first year of symptoms comes from findings that the synthetic enzyme for acetylcholine, choline acetyl transferase (see Figure 18-12), may already be decreased by 40 to 90 percent in cortex and hippocampus by the time of early diagnosis (Figure 18-18). The nucleus basalis of Meynert in the basal forebrain also shows a progressive neuronal loss in AD that correlates with the progressive loss of memory function in Alzheimer's disease (Figure 18-18).

The most successful approach to boosting cholinergic functioning in Alzheimer's disease patients and improving memory has been to inhibit ACh destruction by blocking the

Untreated Time Course of Alzheimer's Disease

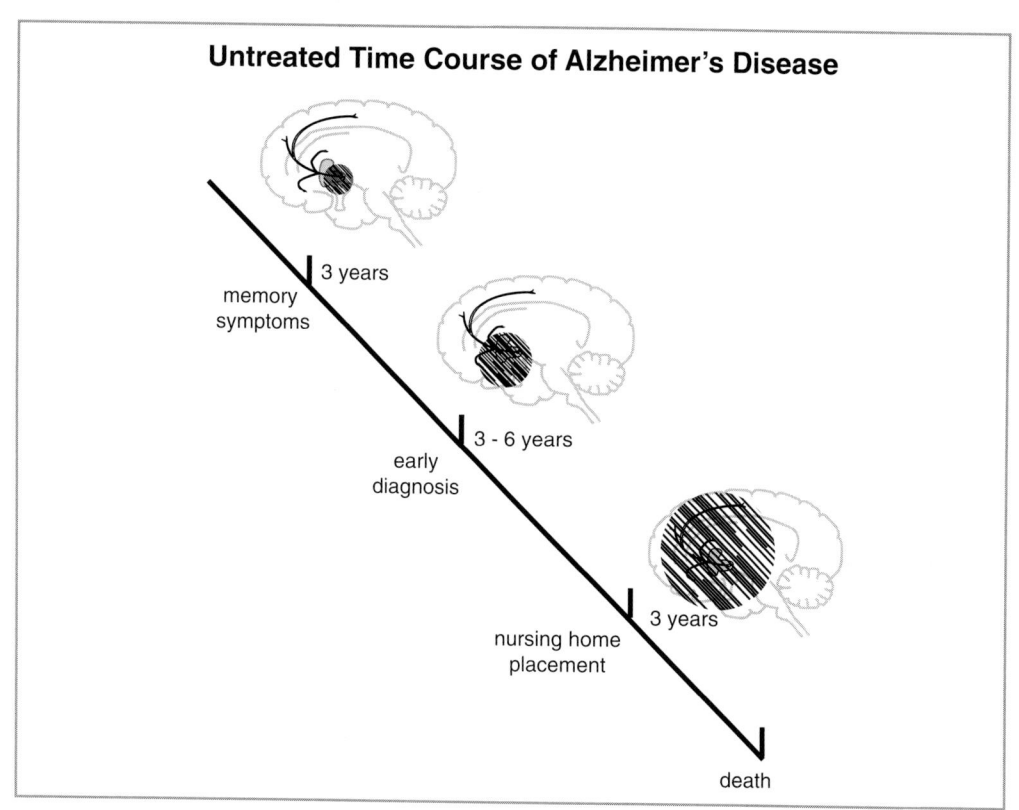

memory symptoms
3 years
early diagnosis
3 - 6 years
nursing home placement
3 years
death

FIGURE 18-18 Untreated time course of Alzheimer's disease. The untreated time course of Alzheimer's disease is progressive and downhill, beginning with very mild and nondiagnostic memory problems probably signaling the beginning of cholinergic neuron degeneration in the nucleus basalis of Meynert. After about 3 years of nonspecific symptoms, an early diagnosis of Alzheimer's disease can often be made, at which time damage to the cholinergic system has spread at least to the near projections of the nucleus basalis (i.e., to the amygdala, hippocampus, and entorrhinal cortex) and the person is losing a great deal of functional independence. In another 3 to 6 years, the neurodegenerative process spreads to the neocortex diffusely and the person requires placement in a nursing home; a further 3 years brings death.

enzyme acetylcholinesterase (Figure 18-13). This causes a buildup of ACh because it can no longer be destroyed by acetylcholinesterase. A wide range of clinical outcomes results (Figures 18-19 through 18-21). Although cholinesterase inhibitors can enhance memory in Alzheimer patients and are therefore sometimes called "cognitive enhancers" or "promnestic" (as opposed to an amnestic) agents, they often do not. They are best documented to prevent or slow the decline in function of Alzheimer patients for several months rather than to improve their functioning above baseline. Since cholinergic agents require postsynaptic cholinergic receptors to mediate the benefits of the enhanced cholinergic input, they may be most effective in the early stages of Alzheimer's disease, while postsynaptic cholinergic targets are still present. However, late in the illness, degeneration of neurons that have postsynaptic ACh receptors means that the drug may lose its benefits.

The spectrum of outcomes from treatment of Alzheimer's disease with cholinesterase inhibitors

Studies of the untreated course of Alzheimer's disease (Figure 18-18) coupled with extensive long-term experience with three cholinesterase inhibitors in clinical practice have defined

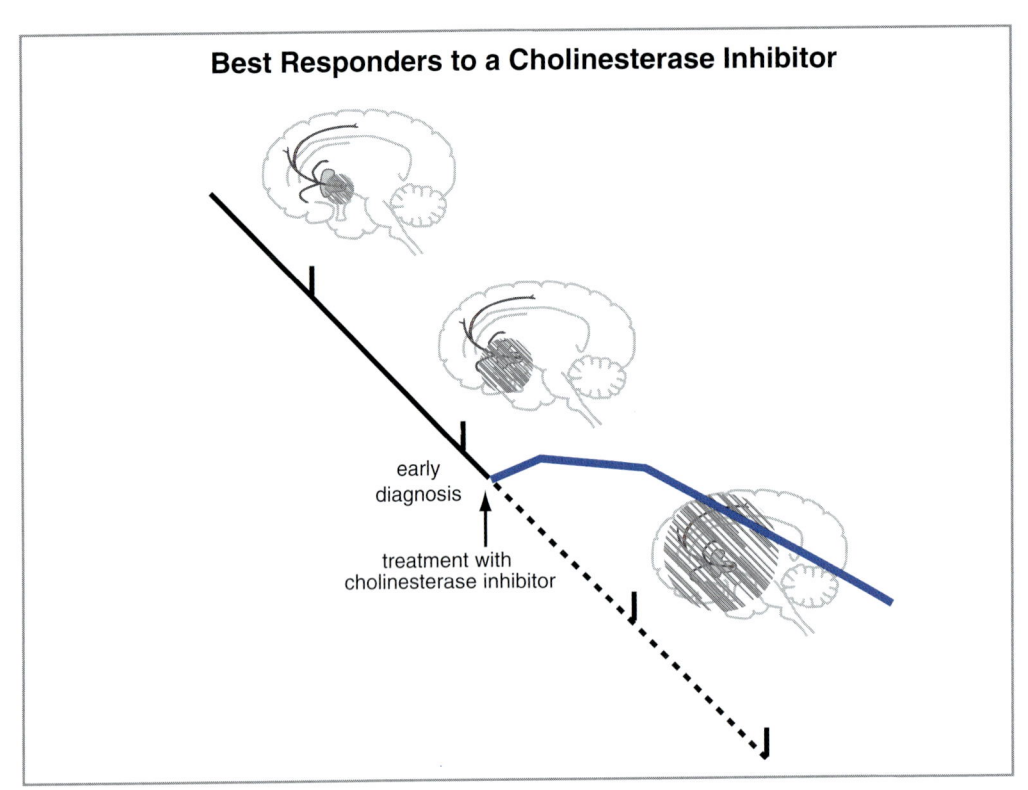

FIGURE 18-19 Best responders to a cholinesterase inhibitor. The best responses to cholinesterase inhibitor therapy in Alzheimer's disease can be substantial improvement, large enough to be noticeable to the patient and to his or her caregiver within weeks of initiation of therapy. Some of these patients sustain this robust improvement for many months or have a noticeably slower than expected decline in memory.

what to expect from treatment with these agents. As with many psychopharmacological treatments, the median response of a large group of patients often belies the range of responses exhibited by individuals, and there is no way of predicting who will experience the more robust clinical responses. Only empiric trial and error of individual patients can ultimately tell who will be helped the most by these agents. Nevertheless, the *range* of responses is well known and is summarized in Figures 18-19 through 18-21.

The *best responses* to cholinesterase inhibitors can be substantial improvement, large enough to be noticeable to the patient and to his or her caregiver within weeks of initiation of therapy (Figure 18-19). Some of these patients sustain this robust improvement for many months or have a noticeably slower than expected decline in their memory. The *usual (median) response*, however, is for the initial improvement to be statistically detectable on cognitive testing and perhaps noticeable to the caregiver but often not to the patient (Figure 18-20). Such a response usually lasts about 6 months, and then cognitive functioning as measured on cognitive testing is back to where it was before beginning the drug. This response is clearly drug-related, because if the drug is stopped, cognitive function immediately declines back to what would be expected if the patient had never been treated. Thereafter, the decline may occur at about the same rate as before taking the drug, but the drug-induced benefits sometimes are not recaptured by immediate retreatment. Yet another response to cholinesterase inhibition can be a mere *palliative response*, in which there is no immediate improvement but a definite slowing in the expected rate of decline

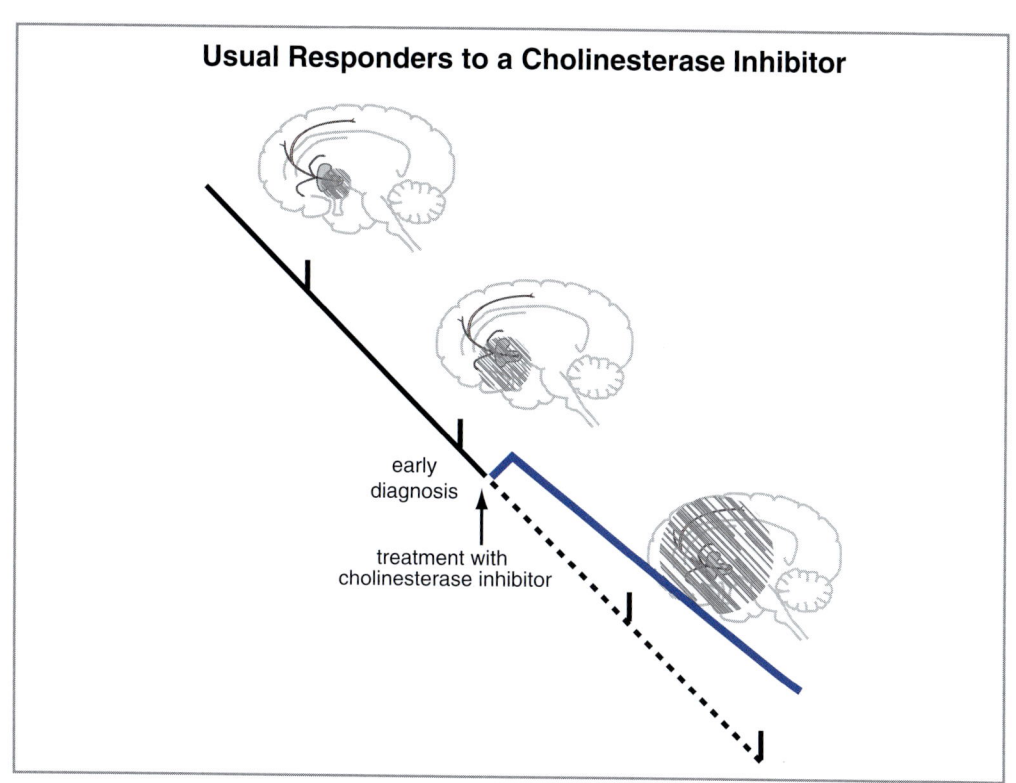

FIGURE 18-20 Usual responders to a cholinesterase inhibitor. The usual (median) response to cholinesterase inhibitor therapy in Alzheimer's disease is initial improvement that is statistically detectable on cognitive testing and perhaps noticeable to the caregiver but not necessarily to the patient. Such a response usually lasts about 6 months, at which point cognitive functioning as measured on cognitive testing is back to where it was before beginning the drug. This response is clearly drug-related, because if the drug is stopped, cognitive function declines back to what would be expected if the patient had never been treated. Thereafter the decline may occur at about the same rate as before the drug was taken.

(Figure 18-21). Of course, some patients do not respond at all, but it is distinctly rare for a patient to worsen on cholinesterase inhibitor treatment.

Tacrine

The original cholinesterase inhibitor introduced for the treatment of Alzheimer's disease was tacrine, but due to its short duration of action, difficulty in dosing, side effects, toxicities, and drug interactions, it is now rarely used.

Donepezil

This is a reversible, long-acting, selective inhibitor of acetylcholinesterase (AChE) without inhibition of butyrylcholinesterase (BuChE) (Figure 18-22). Donepezil inhibits AChE in pre- and postsynaptic cholinergic neurons and in other areas of the CNS outside of cholinergic neurons where this enzyme is widespread (Figure 18-23A). Its CNS actions boost the availability of ACh at the remaining sites normally innervated by cholinergic neurons but which are now suffering from a deficiency of ACh as cholinergic neurons die off (Figure 18-23A). Donepezil also inhibits AChE in the periphery, where its actions in the GI tract can produce gastrointestinal side effects (Figure 18-23B). Donepezil is easy to dose, has mostly gastrointestinal side effects, and these are mostly transient.

Palliative Responders to a Cholinesterase Inhibitor

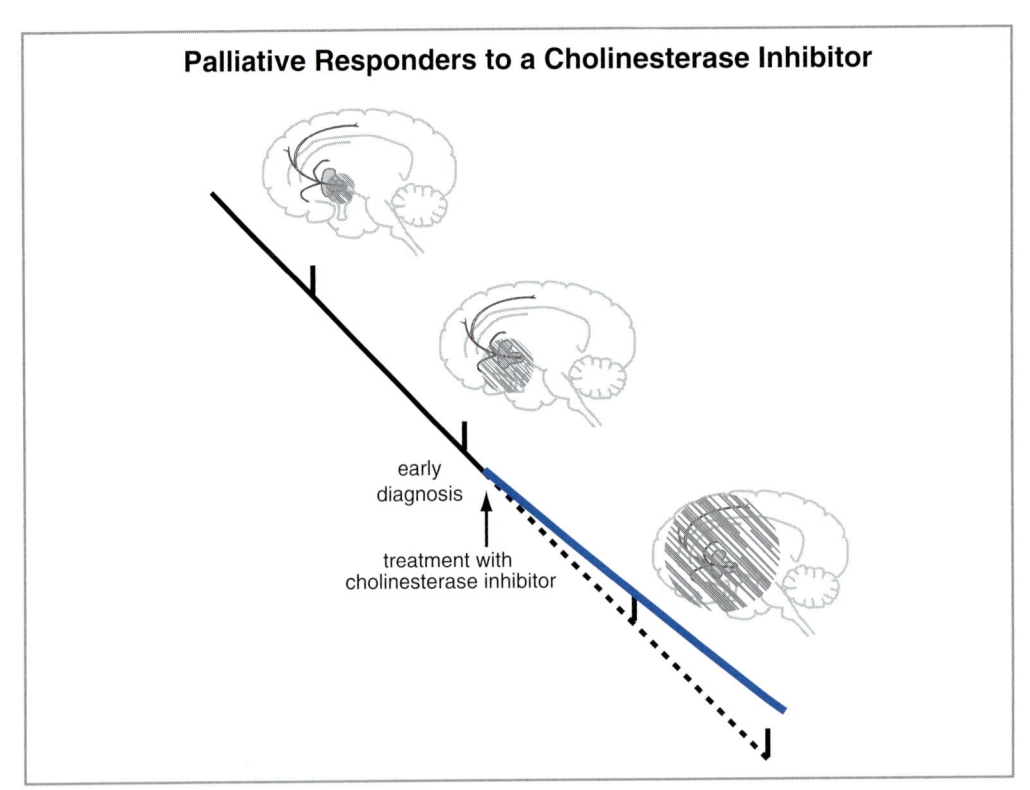

FIGURE 18-21 **Palliative responders to a cholinesterase inhibitor.** Another response to cholinesterase inhibitor therapy in Alzheimer's disease is no immediate improvement but a definite slowing in the expected rate of decline.

Donepezil

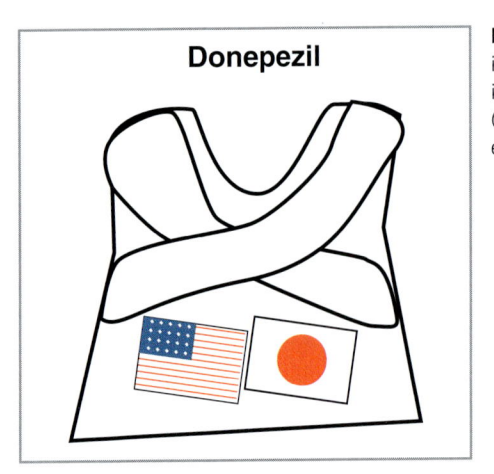

FIGURE 18-22 **Icon of donepezil.** The cholinesterase inhibitor donepezil is a reversible, long-acting, selective inhibitor of acetylcholinesterase (AChE). It is easy to dose (once daily) and has mostly transient gastrointestinal side effects.

Rivastigmine
This (Figure 18-24) is a "pseudoirreversible" (which means it reverses itself over hours) and intermediate-acting agent; it is not only selective for AChE over BuChE but perhaps for AChE in the cortex and hippocampus over AChE in other areas of brain (Figure 18-25A). Rivastigmine also inhibits BuChE within glia, which may contribute somewhat to the enhancement of ACh levels within the CNS (Figure 18-25A). Inhibition of BuChE within glia may be even more important in Alzheimer's disease patients as they develop

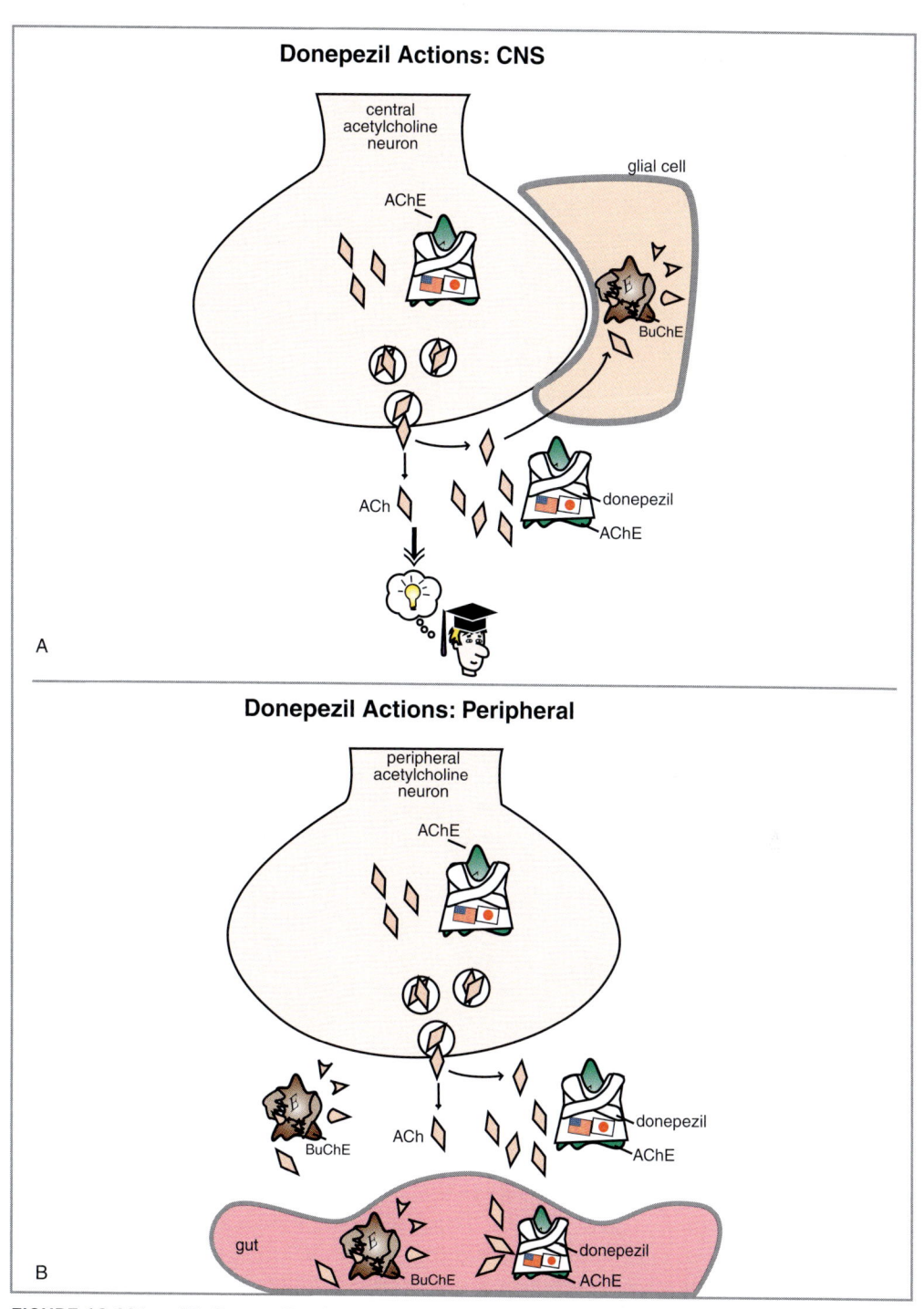

FIGURE 18-23A and B: Donepezil actions. Donepezil inhibits the enzyme acetylcholinesterase (AChE), which is present both in the central nervous system (CNS) and peripherally. (**A**) Central cholinergic neurons are important for regulation of memory; thus in the CNS, the boost of acetylcholine caused by AChE blockade contributes to improved cognitive functioning. (**B**) Peripheral cholinergic neurons in the gut are involved in gastrointestinal effects; thus the boost in peripheral acetylcholine caused by AChE blockade may contribute to gastrointestinal side effects.

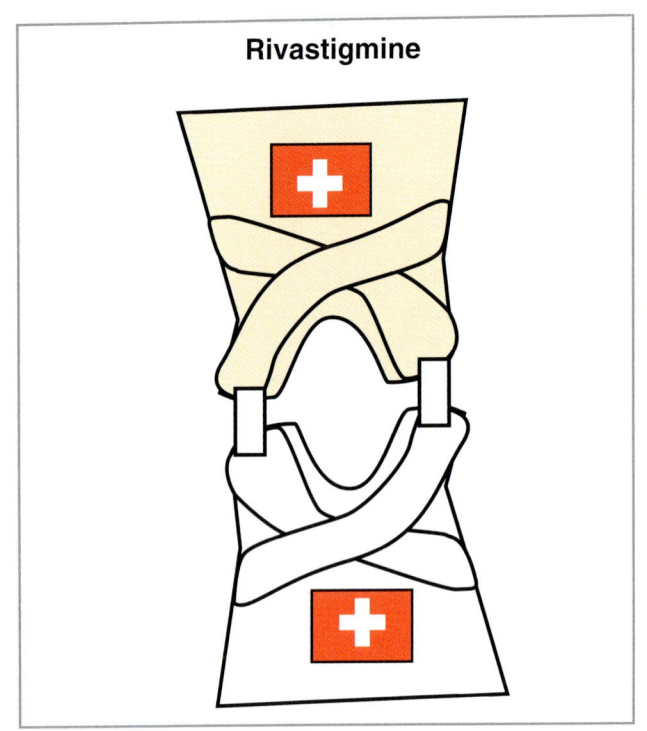

FIGURE 18-24 Icon of rivastigmine. The cholinesterase inhibitor rivastigmine is a pseudoirreversible (meaning it reverses itself over hours), intermediate-acting inhibitor of acetylcholinesterase (AChE). In addition, rivastigmine inhibits butyrylcholinesterase (BuChE) within glia. Its most common side effects are gastrointestinal, although side effects may be reduced with its recent transdermal formulation compared to the oral formulation.

gliosis when cortical neurons die, because these glia contain BuChE, and inhibition of this increased enzyme activity may have a favorable action on increasing the availability of ACh to cholinergic receptors via this second mechanism. Rivastigmine appears to have comparable safety and efficacy to donepezil, although it may have more gastrointestinal side effects when given orally (Figure 18-25B), perhaps due to its pharmacokinetic profile and perhaps owing to inhibition of both AChE and BuChE in the periphery (Figure 18-25C). However, a transdermal formulation of rivastigmine is now available that greatly reduces the peripheral side effects of oral rivastigmine, probably by optimizing drug delivery and reducing peak drug concentrations.

Galantamine

This very interesting cholinesterase inhibitor is found in snowdrops and daffodils. It has a dual mechanism of action, matching AChE inhibition with positive allosteric modulation (PAM) of nicotinic cholinergic receptors (Figure 18-26). Theoretically, the inhibition of AChE (Figure 18-27A) can be enhanced when joined by the second action of galantamine at nicotinic receptors (Figure 18-27B). Thus, raising ACh levels at nicotinic cholinergic receptors by AChE inhibition may be boosted by the PAM actions of galantamine (Figure 18-27B). However, it has not been proven that this theoretically advantageous second action as a nicotinic PAM translates into clinical advantages.

Memantine

Glutamate hypothesis of cognitive deficiency in Alzheimer's disease

We have discussed in some detail in this chapter the leading hypothesis for the etiology of Alzheimer's disease, which proposes that neuronal death is due to the production of

Rivastigmine Actions: CNS

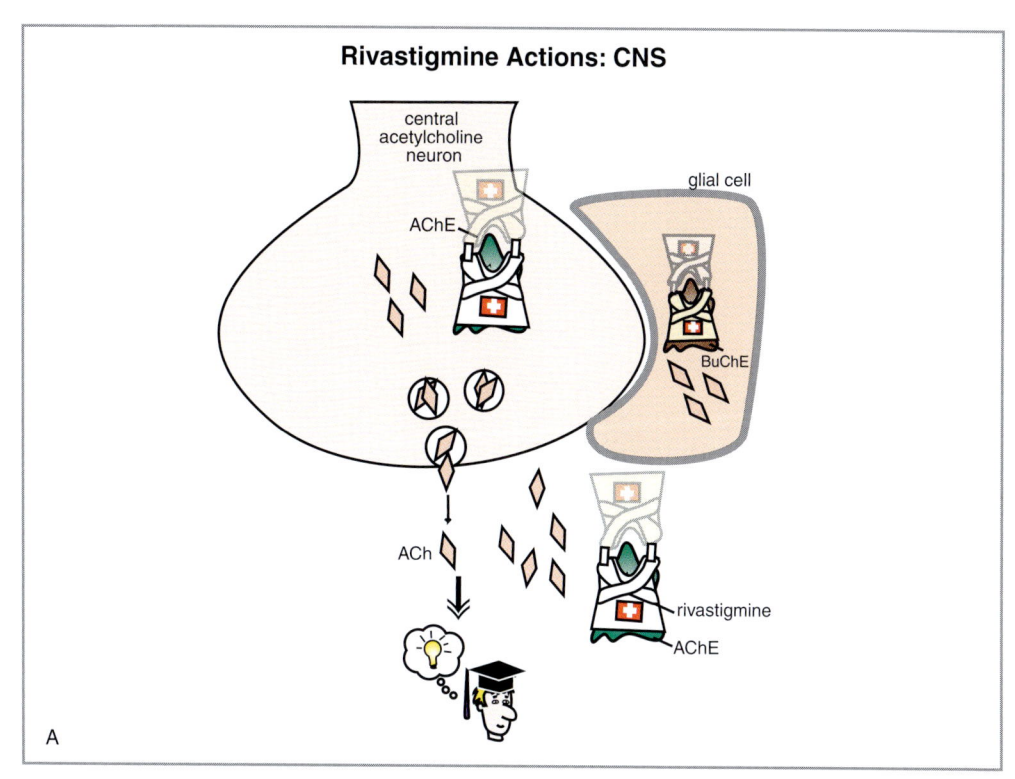

FIGURE 18-25A: Rivastigmine actions, part one. Rivastigmine inhibits the enzymes acetylcholinesterase (AChE) and butyrylcholinesterase (BuChE), which are present both in the central nervous system (CNS) and peripherally. Central cholinergic neurons are important for regulation of memory; thus in the CNS the boost of acetylcholine caused by AChE blockade contributes to improved cognitive functioning. In particular, rivastigmine appears to be selective for AChE in the cortex and hippocampus – two regions important for memory – over other areas of the brain. Rivastigmine's blockade of BuChE in glia may also contribute to enhanced acetylcholine levels.

toxic plaques from amyloid precursors (see Figures 18-4 through 18-8). The molecular mechanisms of exactly how these plaques are neurotoxic are not fully understood, but current theories suggest that this is due to triggering the formation of toxic neurofibrillary tangles as well as provoking a neurotoxic inflammatory reaction (shown in Figures 18-7 and 18-8). In addition, it is possible that amyloid plaques provoke the release of glutamate in a manner that is excitotoxic (Figure 18-28). This notion of excessive glutamate release causing neuronal excitotoxicity is introduced in Chapter 2 and illustrated in Figures 2-34 through 2-37. It is also discussed in relation to the etiology of schizophrenia in Chapter 9 and illustrated in Figures 9-43 and 9-45 through 9-52.

In the resting state, glutamate is normally quiet, and the NMDA receptor is physiologically blocked by magnesium ions (Figure 18-28A). When normal excitatory neurotransmission comes along, a flurry of glutamate is released (Figure 18-28B). The postsynaptic NMDA receptor is a "coincidence detector" and allows inflow of ions if three things happen at the same time: neuronal depolarization, often from activation of nearby AMPA receptors; glutamate occupying its binding site on the NMDA receptor; and the cotransmitter glycine occupying its site on the NMDA receptor (Figure 18-28B). Normal glutamatergic neurotransmission and the physiological role of the NMDA receptor

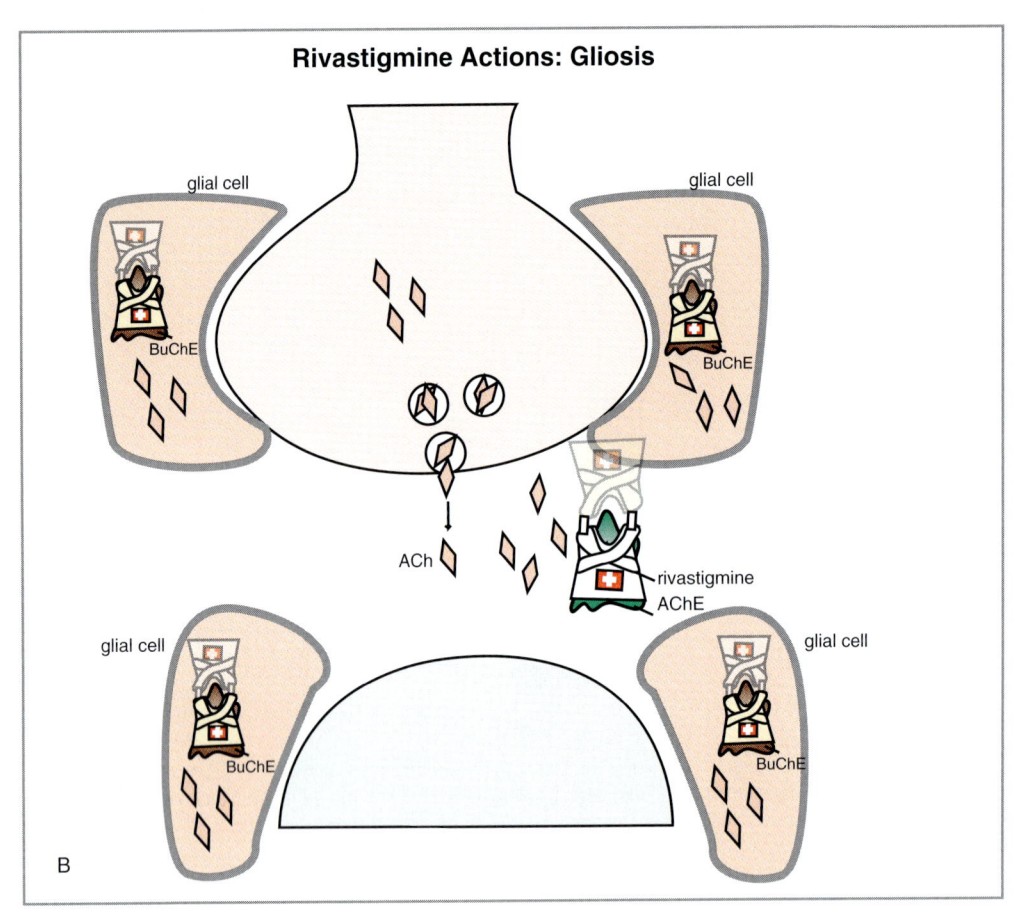

FIGURE 18-25B: Rivastigmine actions, part two. Rivastigmine inhibits the enzymes acetylcholinesterase (AChE) and butyrylcholinesterase (BuChE), which are present both in the central nervous system (CNS) and peripherally. Inhibition of BuChE may be more important in later stages of disease, because as more cholinergic neurons die and gliosis occurs, BuChE activity increases.

are introduced in Chapter 5 and illustrated in Figure 5-43, with additional discussion of glutamate neurons in Chapter 9 and illustrations in Figures 9-34 through 9-36.

If amyloid downregulates the glutamate transporter (see EAAT, the excitatory amino acid transporter in Figure 9-36), inhibits the reuptake of glutamate, and/or enhances glutamate release, it could cause a steady "leak" of glutamate that starts out as a mere nuisance, interfering with the fine tuning of glutamate neurotransmission and possibly also with memory and learning but not necessarily damaging neurons (Figure 18-28C). Hypothetically, as the disease progresses, amyloid eventually causes glutamate release to be increased to a level that is tonically bombarding the postsynaptic receptor, eventually killing off dendrites and then also full neurons (Figure 18-28C). Some experimental evidence even suggests that enhancement of postsynaptic NMDA receptor activity can increase phosphorylation of tau protein in microtubules (see Figure 18-7), possibly contributing to the formation of more neurofibrillary tangles (see Figures 18-7 and 18-8).

This formulation of cognitive deficiency and neuronal degeneration via glutamatergic mechanisms as contributors to the pathophysiology of Alzheimer's disease has been called

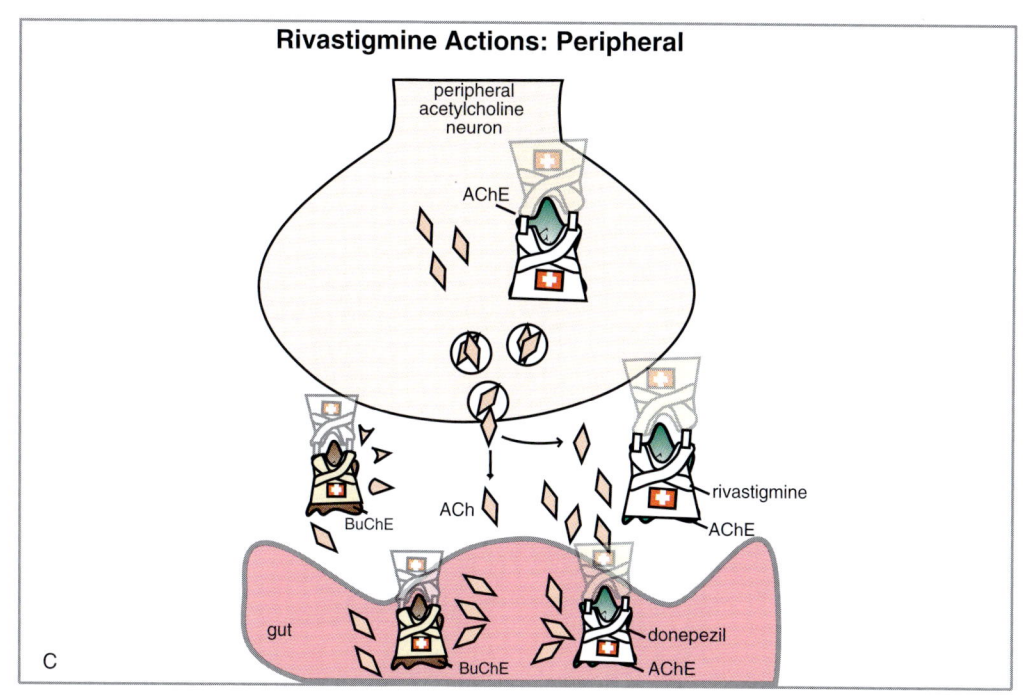

FIGURE 18-25C Rivastigmine actions, part three. Rivastigmine inhibits the enzymes acetylcholinesterase (AChE) and butyrylcholinesterase (BuChE), which are present both in the central nervous system (CNS) and peripherally. Peripheral cholinergic neurons in the gut are involved in gastrointestinal effects; thus the boost in peripheral acetylcholine caused by AChE and BuChE blockade may contribute to gastrointestinal side effects.

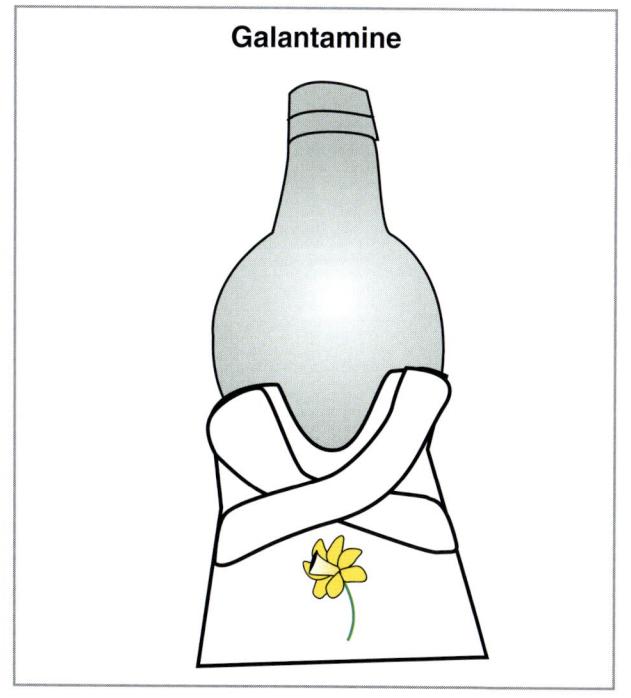

FIGURE 18-26 Icon of galantamine. The cholinesterase inhibitor galantamine inhibits the enzyme acetylcholinesterase (AChE) and also has the unique feature of being a positive allosteric modulator of nicotinic cholinergic receptors.

Dementia and Its Treatment | 929

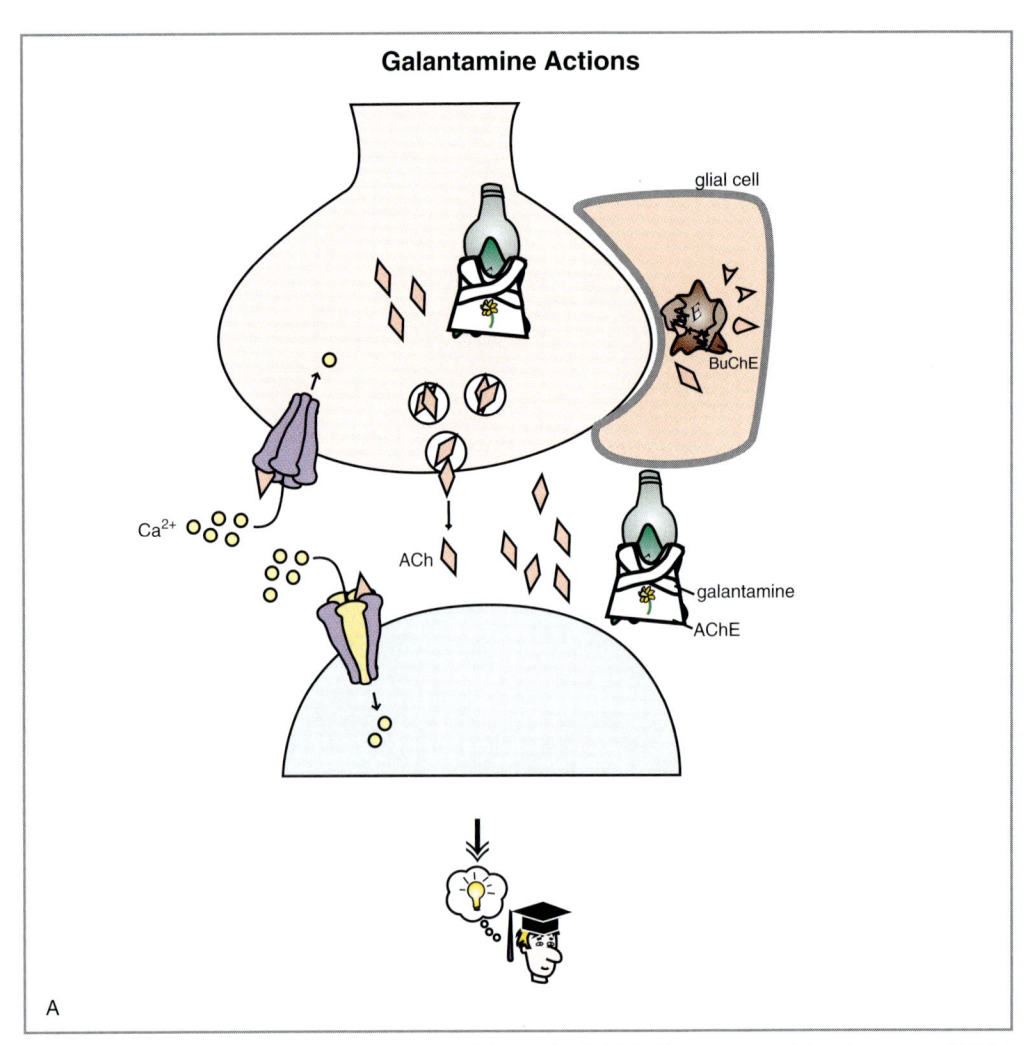

FIGURE 18-27A: Galantamine actions, part one. Galantamine inhibits the enzyme acetylcholinesterase (AChE). Central cholinergic neurons are important for regulation of memory, and thus in the CNS the boost of acetylcholine caused by AChE blockade contributes to improved cognitive functioning.

the NMDA glutamate hyperactivity hypothesis of cognitive deficiency (Figure 18-28C). The idea is that sustained low-level activation of NMDA receptors interferes with synaptic functioning at glutamate synapses and eventually leads to neuronal damage (Figure 18-28C).

Mechanism of action of memantine

The rationale for the use of memantine, a type of NMDA antagonist, is to reduce abnormal activation of glutamate neurotransmission and thus interfere with the pathophysiology of Alzheimer's disease, improve cognitive function, and slow the rate of decline over time (Figure 18-29). However, interfering with NMDA neurotransmission can cause big problems, as described in Chapter 9 for schizophrenia, where NMDA antagonists such as phencyclidine (PCP) or ketamine cause psychosis with positive and negative symptoms that very much mimic those of schizophrenia (Figures 9-39 and 9-40). Blocking of NMDA receptors

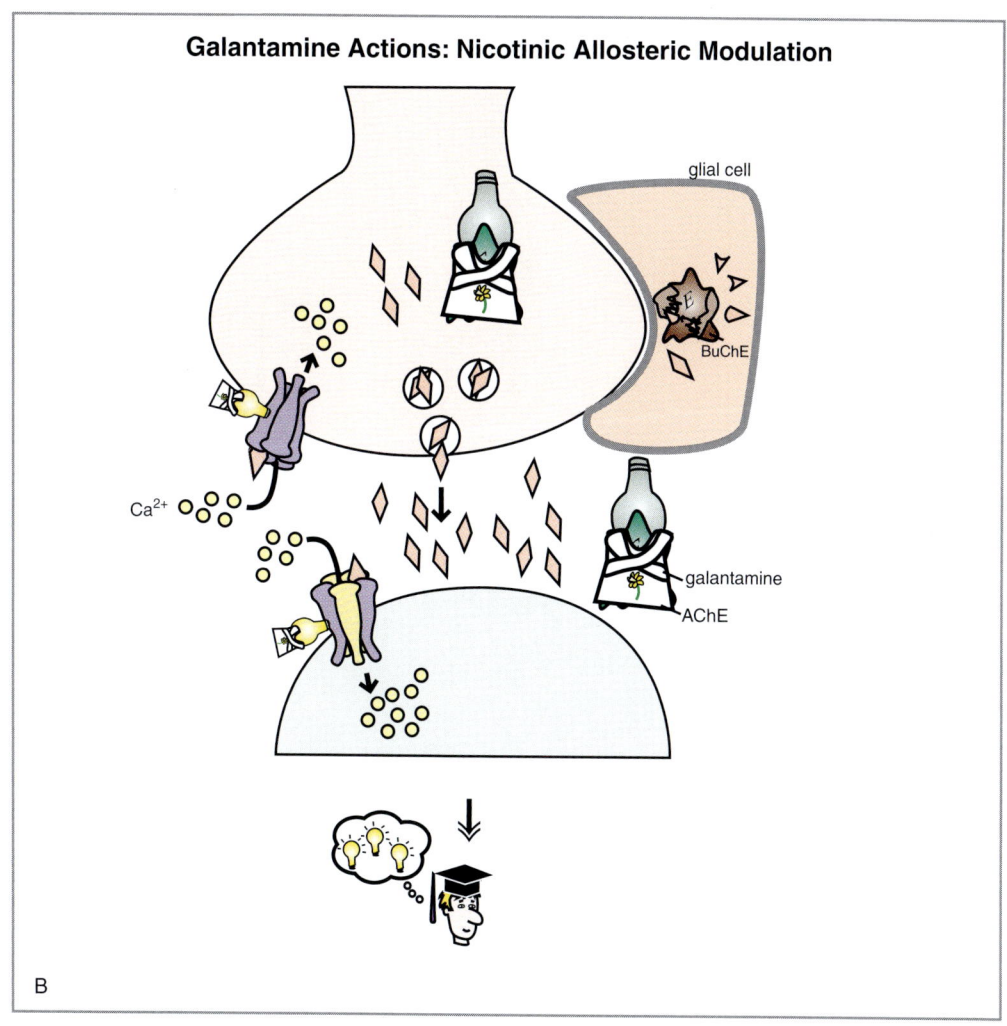

FIGURE 18-27B: Galantamine actions, part two. Galantamine is unique among cholinesterase inhibitors in that it is also a positive allosteric modulator (PAM) at nicotinic cholinergic receptors, which means it can boost the effects of acetylcholine at these receptors. Thus galantamine's second action as a PAM at nicotinic receptors could theoretically enhance its primary action as a cholinesterase inhibitor.

chronically also interferes with memory formation and neuroplasticity. So what do you do to decrease the excessive and sustained but low level of excitotoxic activation of NMDA receptors yet not interfere with learning, memory, and neuroplasticity and without inducing a schizophrenia-like state?

The answer seems to be that you interfere with NMDA-mediated glutamatergic neurotransmission with a weak (low affinity) NMDA antagonist that works at the same site, plugging the ion channel where the ion magnesium normally blocks this channel at rest (Figure 18-29). That is, memantine is an uncompetitive open channel NMDA receptor antagonist with low to moderative affinity, voltage dependence, and fast blocking and unblocking kinetics. That is a fancy way of saying that it blocks only the ion channel of the NMDA receptor when it is open. This is why it is called an open channel antagonist and why it is dependent upon voltage: namely, to open the channel. It is also a fancy way of

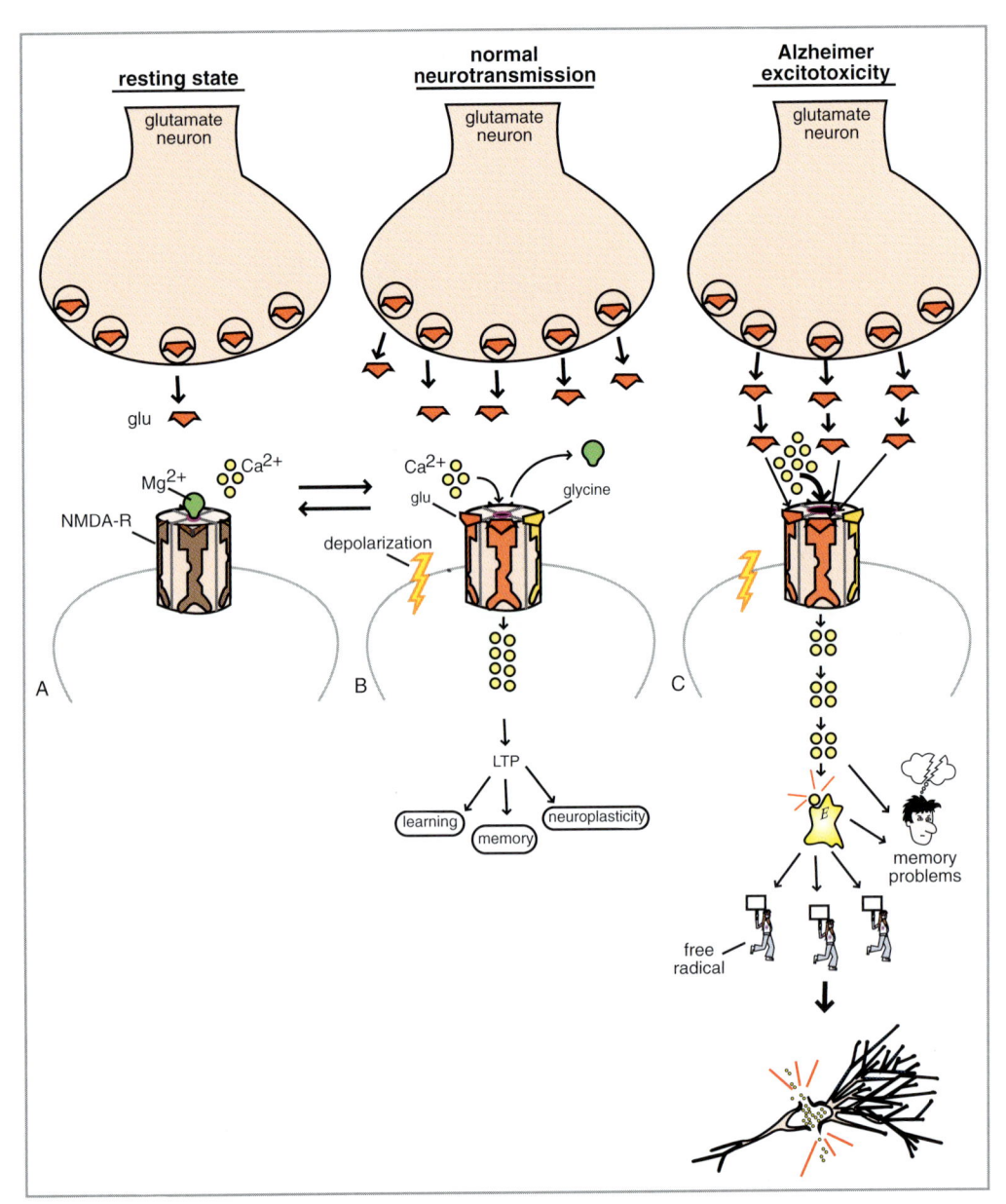

FIGURE 18-28A, B, and C: Amyloid plaques and glutamate excitotoxicity. (**A**) In the resting state glutamate is quiet and N-methyl-d-aspartate (NMDA) receptors are blocked by magnesium. (**B**) With normal neurotransmission, glutamate binds to NMDA receptors and, if the postsynaptic receptor is depolarized and glycine is simultaneously bound to the NMDA receptors, the channel opens and allows ion influx. (**C**) If amyloid's synaptic effects include downregulating the glutamate transporter, inhibiting glutamate reuptake, or enhancing glutamate release, this could cause a steady leak of glutamate and result in excessive calcium influx in postsynaptic neurons, which in the short term may cause memory problems and in the long term may cause accumulation of free radicals and thus destruction of neurons.

932 | Essential Psychopharmacology

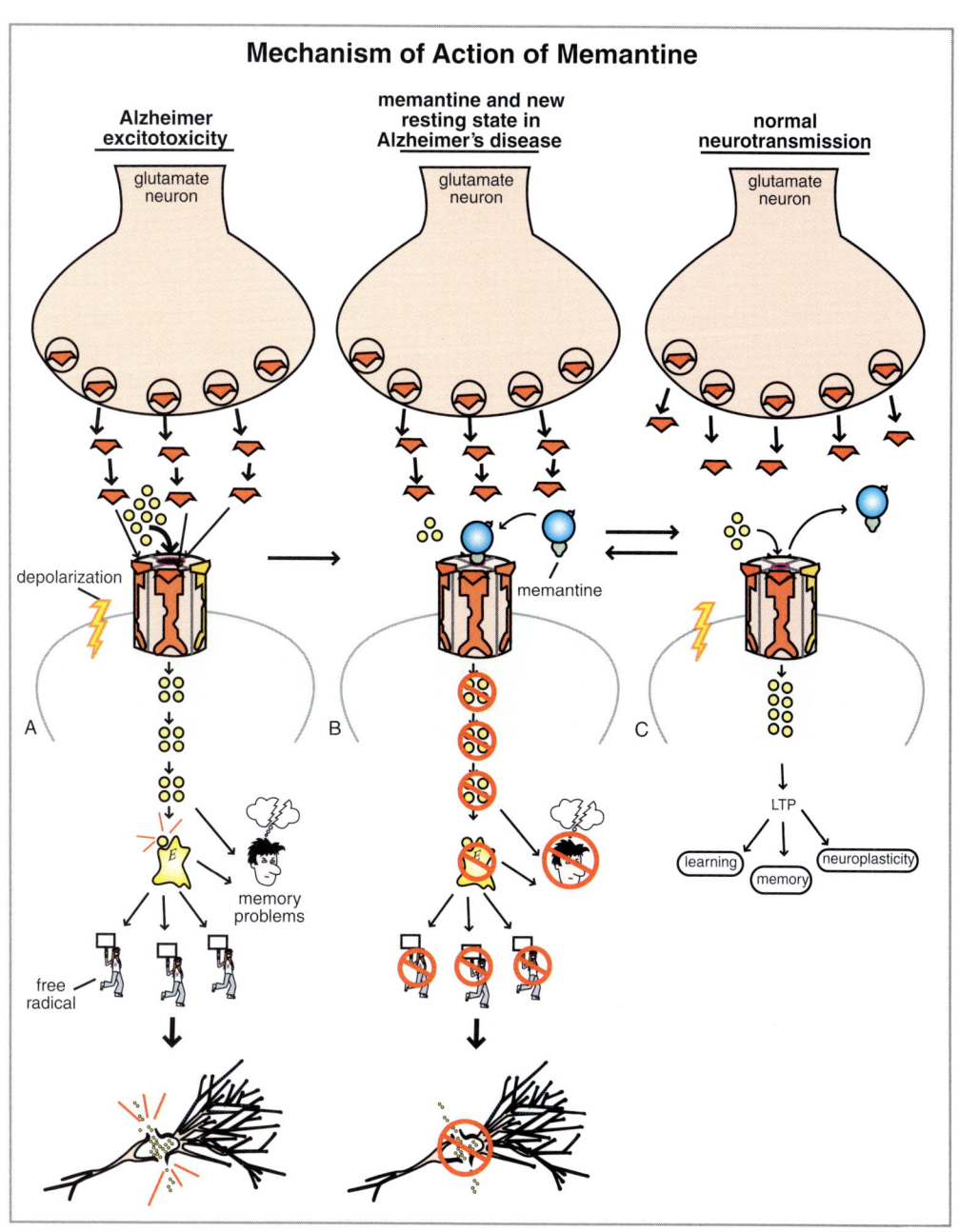

FIGURE 18-29A, B, and C: Memantine actions. Memantine is a noncompetitive low affinity N-methyl-d-aspartate (NMDA) receptor antagonist that binds to the magnesium site when the channel is open. (**A**) If amyloid's synaptic effects lead to a steady (tonic) leak of glutamate and result in excessive calcium influx in postsynaptic neurons, this could cause memory problems and, in the long term, accumulation of free radicals and thus destruction of neurons. (**B**) Memantine blocks the downstream effects of tonic glutamate release by "plugging" the NMDA ion channel and thus may improve memory and prevent neurodegeneration. (**C**) Because memantine has low affinity, when there is a phasic burst of glutamate and depolarization occurs, this is enough to remove memantine from the ion channel and thus allow normal neurotransmission.

Dementia and Its Treatment | 933

saying that memantine blocks the open channel quickly but is readily and quickly reversible if a barrage of glutamate comes along from normal neurotransmission.

This concept is illustrated in Figure 18-29. First, the hypothetical state of the glutamate neuron during Alzheimer excitotoxicity is shown in Figure 18-29A. Here, steady, tonic, and excessive amounts of glutamate are continuously released in a manner that interferes with the normal resting state of the glutamate neuron (shown in Figure 18-28A) and in a manner that interferes with established memory functions, new learning, and normal neuronal plasticity. Eventually, this leads to the activation of intracellular enzymes that produce toxic free radicals that damage the membranes of the postsynaptic dendrite and eventually destroy the entire neuron (Figure 18-29A). When memantine is given, it blocks this tonic glutamate release from having downstream effects, thus returning the glutamate neuron to a new resting state despite the continuous release of glutamate (Figure 18-29B). Hypothetically, this stops the excessive glutamate from interfering with the resting glutamate neuron's physiological activity, therefore improving memory; it also hypothetically stops the excessive glutamate from causing neurotoxicity, therefore slowing the rate of neuronal death and also the associated cognitive decline that this causes in Alzheimer's disease (Figure 18-29B).

However, at the same time, memantine is not so powerful a blocker of NMDA receptors that it stops all neurotransmission at glutamate synapses (Figure 18-29C). That is, when a phasic burst of glutamate is transiently released during normal glutamatergic neurotransmission, this causes a depolarization that is capable of reversing the memantine block until the depolarization goes away (Figure 18-29C). For this reason, memantine does not have the psychotomimetic actions of other more powerful NMDA antagonists such as PCP and ketamine and does not shut down new learning or the ability of normal neurotransmission to occur when necessary (Figure 18-29C). The blockade of NMDA receptors by memantine can be seen as a kind of "artificial magnesium," more effective than physiological blockade by magnesium which is overwhelmed by excitotoxic glutamate release but less effective than PCP or ketamine, so that the glutamate system is not entirely shut down. Sort of like having your cake and eating it too.

Memantine also has sigma antagonist properties (see Figure 13-28) and weak 5HT3 antagonist properties, but it is not clear what these contribute to the actions of this agent in Alzheimer's disease. Memantine is discussed as a potential novel mood stabilizer in Chapter 13, also illustrated in Figure 13-32. Since its mechanism of action in Alzheimer's disease is so different from cholinesterase inhibition, memantine is usually given concomitantly with a cholinesterase inhibitor to exploit the potential of both of these approaches and obtain additive results in patients.

Other proposed treatments
Treatments for psychiatric and behavioral symptoms in dementia

Dementia is not just a disturbance of memory, because many patients have a variety of behavioral and emotional symptoms as well. Treatment of agitation and aggression in dementia is a very controversial area owing to the potential for misuse of psychotropic drugs as "chemical straightjackets" to over-tranquilize patients and also new safety concerns about the use of antipsychotics in such patients. Before using medications, reversible precipitants of agitation in dementia should be managed: pain, nicotine withdrawal, medication side effects, undiagnosed medical and neurological illnesses, and provocative environments that are either too stimulating or not stimulating enough.

When use of medications is necessary, a cholinesterase inhibitor may be effective in some patients and is a first-line consideration in Alzheimer's disease, but it might work better for prevention of these symptoms than for their treatment once they have emerged. Also, frontotemporal dementia patients may be more likely to benefit from SSRIs (e.g., citalopram or escitalopram) or SNRIs. In general, first-line treatment of agitation and aggression in dementia is SSRI/SNRI therapy, which is now displacing the use of atypical antipsychotics because of current concerns that atypical antipsychotics may cause increased cardiovascular events and increased mortality in elderly patients with dementia and agitation or aggression. Second-line treatments that may help to avoid the use of atypical antipsychotics can also include beta blockers, valproate, gabapentin, pregabalin, and selegiline. Others may respond to carbamazepine/oxcarbazepine, benzodiazepines, buspirone, or trazodone.

Coupled with concerns about the safety of atypical antipsychotic are concerns about their efficacy. Recent studies such as the CATIE-AD (Clinical Antipsychotic Trial of Intervention Effectiveness in Alzheimer's Disease) have been disappointing in terms of documenting any long-lasting robust efficacy of atypical antipsychotics in probable Alzheimer's disease patients with dementia as well as psychosis, agitation, or aggression. At this time, none of the atypical antipsychotics is FDA-approved for this use and all carry warnings about the risk of cardiovascular events and increased mortality in this population. Because, in the real world, there are also risks of nontreatment, including early institutionalization and the dangers of agitated and psychotic behaviors to the patient and others around them, some patients will nevertheless require treatment with an atypical antipsychotic. In this case, risperidone is often a preferred agent at very low doses. Clinicians should be alerted to the need to distinguish Alzheimer's disease from dementia with Lewy bodies prior to prescribing an antipsychotic. Patients with dementia with Lewy bodies can look psychotic, with their prominent behavioral symptoms, dramatic fluctuations, and visual hallucinations, but they are exquisitely sensitive to the extrapyramidal side effects of even the atypical antipsychotics, which can result in very severe and potentially life-threatening reactions to such drugs.

Future treatments

Marketed products with potential therapeutic actions in dementia
Folate preparations

The use of folate (especially L-methyl-folate, also called L-5-methyl-tetrahydrofolate, or MTHF), is extensively discussed as a potential augmenting agent for major depression in Chapter 12 and illustrated in Figures 12-107 to 12-111. Folate (and MTHF) have biochemical actions that could theoretically also make them effective in Alzheimer's disease and in prodromal cases of mild cognitive impairment. For example, folate is linked to the synthesis of ACh by its ability to facilitate the methylation of ACh precursors. Low levels of folate can cause decreased availability of precursors for ACh, which can result in less efficient synthesis of ACh. Folate is also linked to the regulation of key enzymes that keep tau phosphorylation in check by the ability of folate to facilitate the methylation of various dephosphorylating enzymes. Theoretically, low folate levels could result in more tau phosphorylation, which could facilitate the formation of more neurofibrillary tangles (see Figure 18-7). Finally, folate is a key regulator of homocysteine levels by its role in converting homocysteine into S-adenyl methionine for downstream use in methylation reactions (Figure 12-111). Increased plasma homocysteine is established as an independent risk factor in the development of dementia and Alzheimer's disease. In animal models, homocysteine can damage neuronal DNA, impair the ability of neurons to repair their DNA, cause oxidative stress in neurons, enhance neurotoxicity via NMDA receptor activation, increase the toxicity of beta amyloid, and cause neuronal cell loss through apoptosis. Folate lowers homocysteine levels, especially in individuals who have low plasma folate levels (see Figure 12-111).

Because of these biochemical actions, the therapeutic actions of folate have been investigated in patients with Alzheimer's disease and in aging individuals with memory complaints. There are several reports that plasma folate levels are low in such individuals and many anecdotal reports, case reports, and even some controlled trials indicating that treatment with folate alone or in combination with vitamin B6, vitamin B12, antioxidants such as N-acetylcysteine (a precursor to glutathione), or cholinesterase inhibitors improves memory complaints in such individuals.

Selegiline
Selegiline is a selective inhibitor of MAO-B when taken orally in low doses. Selegiline's actions as a central MAO-A plus MAO-B inhibitor and peripheral MAO-B inhibitor in transdermal formulation for the treatment of depression are discussed in Chapter 12 and illustrated in Figures 12-65 through 12-79. For use in low oral doses in Alzheimer's disease or Parkinson's disease with dementia, it is presumed to boost dopamine, although there is some preclinical evidence of antioxidant and neuroprotective actions and some theoretical reasons, therefore, that selegiline could slow disease progression. However, beneficial results of selegiline treatment of dementia are modest at best.

Vitamin E (alpha tocopherol)
As an antioxidant, vitamin E has been proposed as a treatment to prevent disease progression in Alzheimer's disease and has been studied alone or in combination with selegiline or cholinesterase inhibitors. Currently, there is no convincing evidence for the efficacy of vitamin E in dementia and some concern about increased mortality from long-term high-dose treatment with vitamin E. Therefore many experts now recommend discontinuation of vitamin E treatment for dementia patients.

Ginko biloba
Effects in dementia are not well established and at best are probably not as robust as for cholinesterase inhibitors. There are also some concerns about increased bleeding and unregulated product purity.

Statins
Statins, or hydroxy-methyl-glutaryl coenzyme A (HMG-CoA) reductase inhibitors used for treating hyperlipidemia are being studied in Alzheimer's disease because cholesterol is linked to the processing of amyloid precursor protein by the more amyloidogenic pathway via beta secretase (see Figure 18-3). Trials are still under way to see whether this approach will be helpful in Alzheimer's disease.

Rosiglitazone and peroxisome proliferator activated receptor (PPAR) gamma agonists
Diabetes is a known risk factor for Alzheimer's disease. PPAR gamma agonists such as rosiglitazone are approved for the treatment of diabetes and are insulin sensitizing agents; they allow more effective utilization of insulin and thus reduce insulin resistance in diabetes. Rosiglitazone has some anti-inflammatory properties as well. Insulin and beta amyloid compete as substrates for the insulin-degrading enzyme, so reducing circulating insulin

should allow more degradation of beta amyloid by this enzyme and possibly reduce or slow down its production. Thus rosiglitazone is being tested in Alzheimer's disease.

Estrogen

As a trophic factor for neurons, estrogen might hypothetically improve cognition. See discussion in Chapter 12 on the mechanism of action of estrogen in the brain and its role in the action of antidepressants in Figures 12-97 to 12-99. However, recent studies have concluded that not only are dementia and mild cognitive impairment not reduced in estrogen treated women but they might actually be increased, along with stroke.

NSAIDs (nonsteroidal anti-inflammatory drugs)

Attempts to interfere with the inflammatory reaction caused by amyloid plaque formation (See Figure 18-6) have stimulated the testing of NSAIDs, which have so far not shown any definitive slowing of disease progression in Alzheimer's disease. Investigations are still in progress, including some with agents that act by mechanisms other than cyclooxygenase (COX) inhibition (see flurizan, below).

Omega-3 fatty acids (e.g., DHA, docosahexaenoic acid) and various antioxidants

These are being investigated in Alzheimer's disease but are not recommended for routine clinical use on the basis of available evidence.

Lithium/GSK (glycogen synthase kinase) inhibitors

Lithium inhibits the enzyme GSK. This is introduced in Chapter 5 and illustrated in Figure 5-51; it is also discussed in Chapter 13 and illustrated in Figure 13-3. Theoretically by this mechanism, lithium could block hyperphosphorylation of tau in animal models, and it as well as other GSK inhibitors could potentially have such an action in Alzheimer's disease as well. Studies are in progress.

Disease-modifying agents in development that act on amyloid processing
Vaccines and immunotherapy

The quest for an Alzheimer's vaccine has great appeal, but clinical development has had its ups and downs. Immunizing the body to beta amyloid could in concept not only slow or stop progression of cognitive decline but, by removal of plaques already formed, potentially improve cognitive function. Positive tests of amyloid vaccines in animals have led to early clinical trials that showed evidence not only of stabilization of memory in Alzheimer's patients but, perhaps more importantly, also that amyloid plaques were removed (Figure 18-30). However, the first vaccine [bapineuzumab, AN1792(QS21)] caused brain inflammation (meningoencephalitis) and the trials had to be stopped. Other immunotherapy trials include active immunization with ACC-001 and CAD106, passive immunization with AAB-001, treatment with beta amyloid–derived diffusible ligands (ADDLs), trials of a humanized monoclonal antibody, RN1219, and many more. There are even trials of intravenous immunoglobulin in the hope that it might contain naturally occurring antibodies against beta amyloid and promote the clearance of beta amyloid from the brain.

Beta amyloid antagonists

Blocking the action of beta amyloid with small molecules rather than immunotherapy is also being tested with tramiprosate and AZD 103. These agents bind to beta amyloid and may prevent the assembly of amyloid plaques (Figure 18-31).

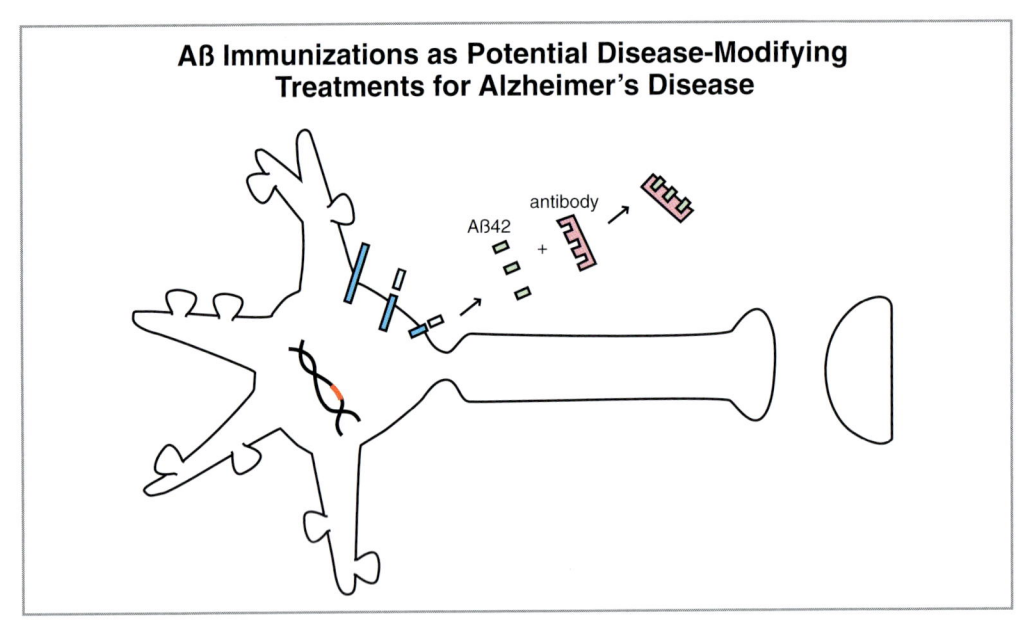

FIGURE 18-30 Future treatments: beta amyloid immunizations. One potential future treatment for Alzheimer's disease is a vaccine that immunizes against beta amyloid, which could not only slow cognitive decline but also perhaps remove already formed plaques.

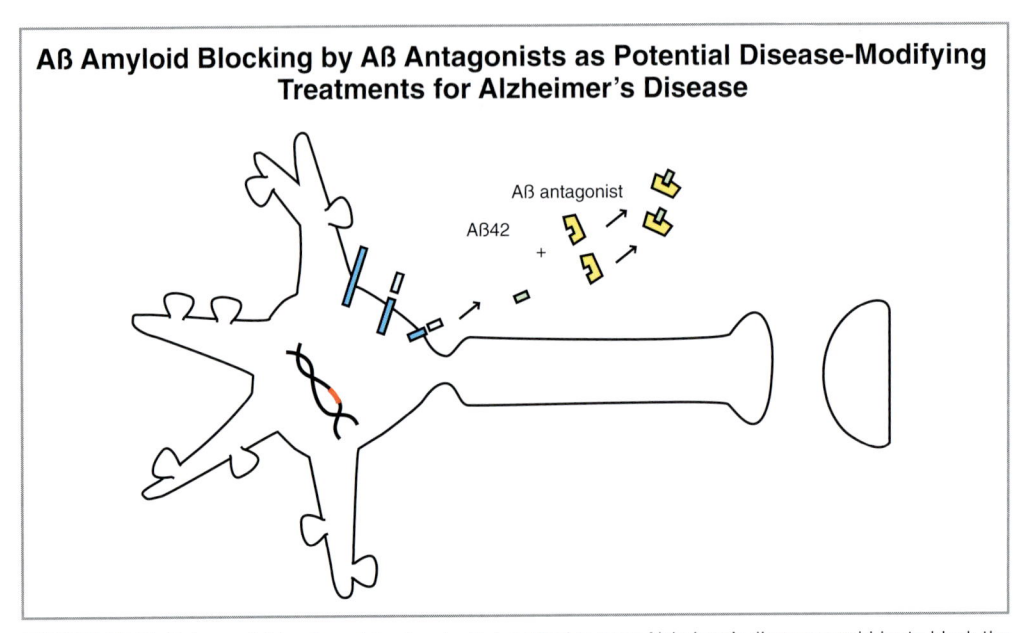

FIGURE 18-31 Beta amyloid antagonists. A potential method to treat Alzheimer's disease would be to block the actions of beta amyloid with agents that bind to it and prevent its assembly into plaques.

Gamma Secretase Inhibitors and Gamma Secretase Modulators (Selective Amyloid-Lowering Agents) as Potential Disease-Modifying Treatments for Alzheimer's Disease

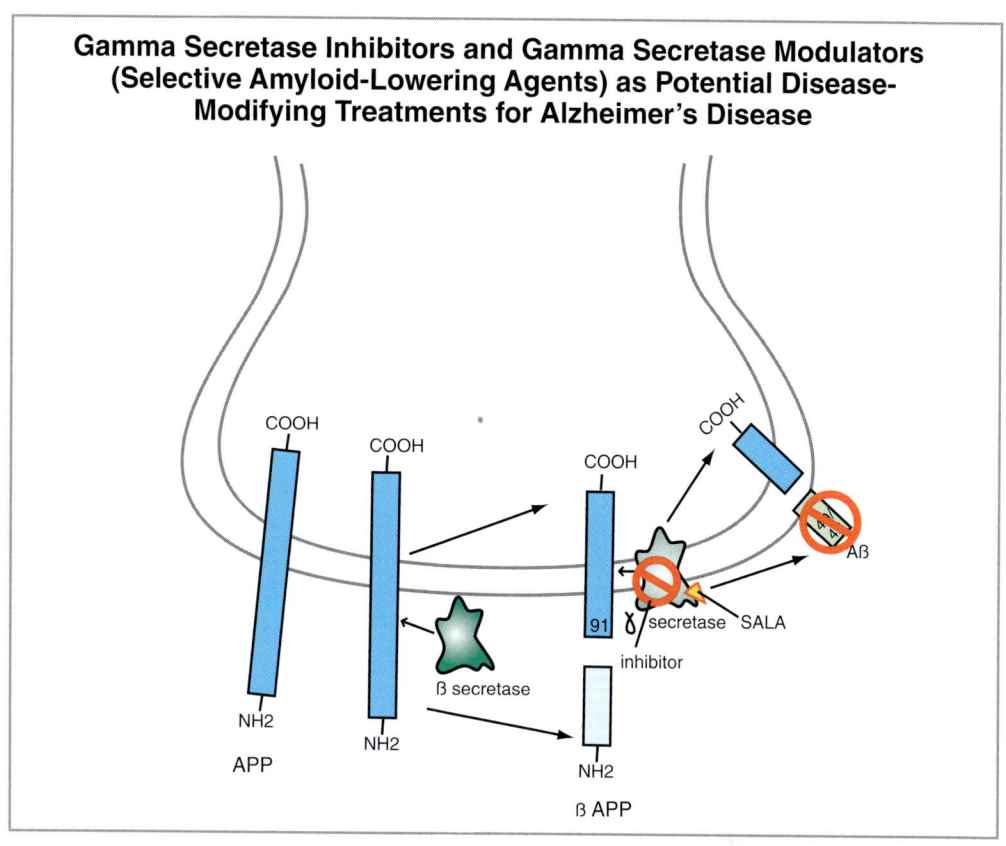

FIGURE 18-32 **Gamma secretase inhibitors and modulators.** The way in which amyloid precursor protein (APP) is processed may help determine whether an individual develops Alzheimer's disease; thus a drug that affects this process could prevent or treat Alzheimer's disease. The enzyme gamma secretase cleaves embedded peptides which in some cases leads to release of toxic peptides (particularly Aβ42). Inhibition of this enzyme could therefore prevent formation of toxic peptides, and so could modulation of this enzyme with selective amyloid lowering agents (SALAs).

Gamma secretase inhibitors and modulators

Another strategy to block amyloid plaque formation is to inhibit the enzyme gamma secretase (Figure 18-32). Several compounds are in early clinical development, including SCH 1390499, SCH 1396674, LY450139, MK0752, and GSI 953. In addition to classic inhibition of gamma secretase, it is also possible to modulate this enzyme with compounds that cause it to selectively inhibit A-beta-42 formation in favor of shorter non-amyloidogenic A-beta peptides but without affecting gamma secretase's overall physiological functions (Figure 18-32). This approach may have some safety advantages. Sometimes these types of agents are called SALAs (selective amyloid lowering agents) (see Figure 18-32).

Gamma secretase modulators (SALAs) include flurizan (the R enantiomer of flurbiprofen) and E2012. Flurizan is an interesting compound. It is the "inactive" enantiomer of R,S flurbiprofen, a known NSAID. All the NSAID properties are in the S isomer, which acts as a COX inhibitor. The R enantiomer does not inhibit COX but does seem to modulate gamma secretase without necessarily inhibiting it, resulting in a reduction of amyloid formation in animal models. Flurizan is in large-scale clinical testing in Alzheimer's disease, with some promising early results.

Beta Secretase Inhibitors as Potential Disease-Modifying Treatments for Alzheimer's Disease

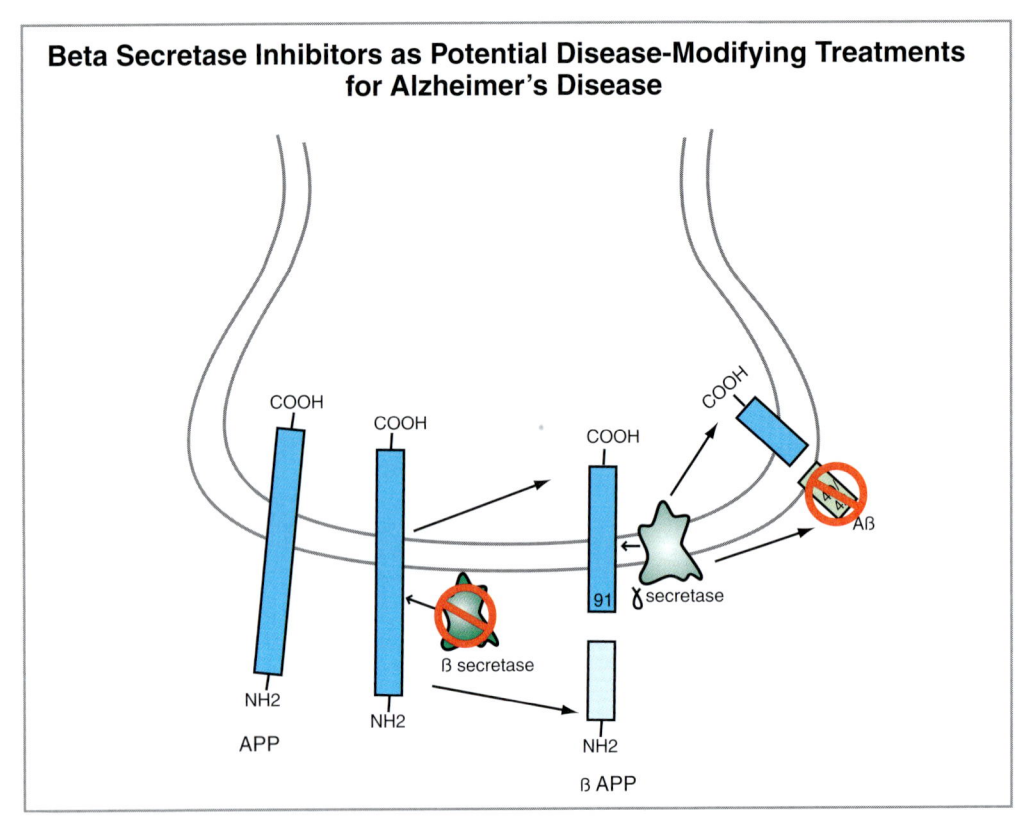

FIGURE 18-33 Beta secretase inhibitors. The way in which amyloid precursor protein (APP) is processed may help determine whether an individual develops Alzheimer's disease; thus a drug that affects this process could prevent or treat Alzheimer's disease. The enzyme beta secretase cuts APP at a spot outside of the membrane to form two peptides: beta-APP, which is soluble, and a 91–amino acid peptide that remains in the membrane. Gamma secretase then cuts the embedded peptide; this releases Aβ peptides of 40, 42, or 43 amino acids, which are toxic. Thus inhibition of beta secretase could prevent the formation of toxic peptides.

Beta secretase inhibitors

Inhibitors of the beta secretase enzyme have been difficult to synthesize, but compounds such as SCH 1381252 are poised to enter clinical development and their results are eagerly awaited because of their theoretical promise as a mechanism of preventing beta amyloid formation (Figure 18-33).

Other potential disease-modifying treatment approaches

Mem 1003 is a blocker of L type voltage-sensitive calcium channels (VSCCs) that might reduce neurotoxicity in Alzheimer's disease. Agents that mimic various growth hormones such as nerve growth factor (NGF) are also in preclinical development.

Symptomatic treatments in development for Alzheimer's disease and other cognitive disorders and dementias

While we await disease-modifying treatments, it may be possible to further improve cognition symptomatically in Alzheimer patients and other patients with various cognitive disorders including other dementias, by utilizing various neurotransmitter-directed approaches. These include additional cholinesterase inhibitors such as the Chinese herb huperzine A.

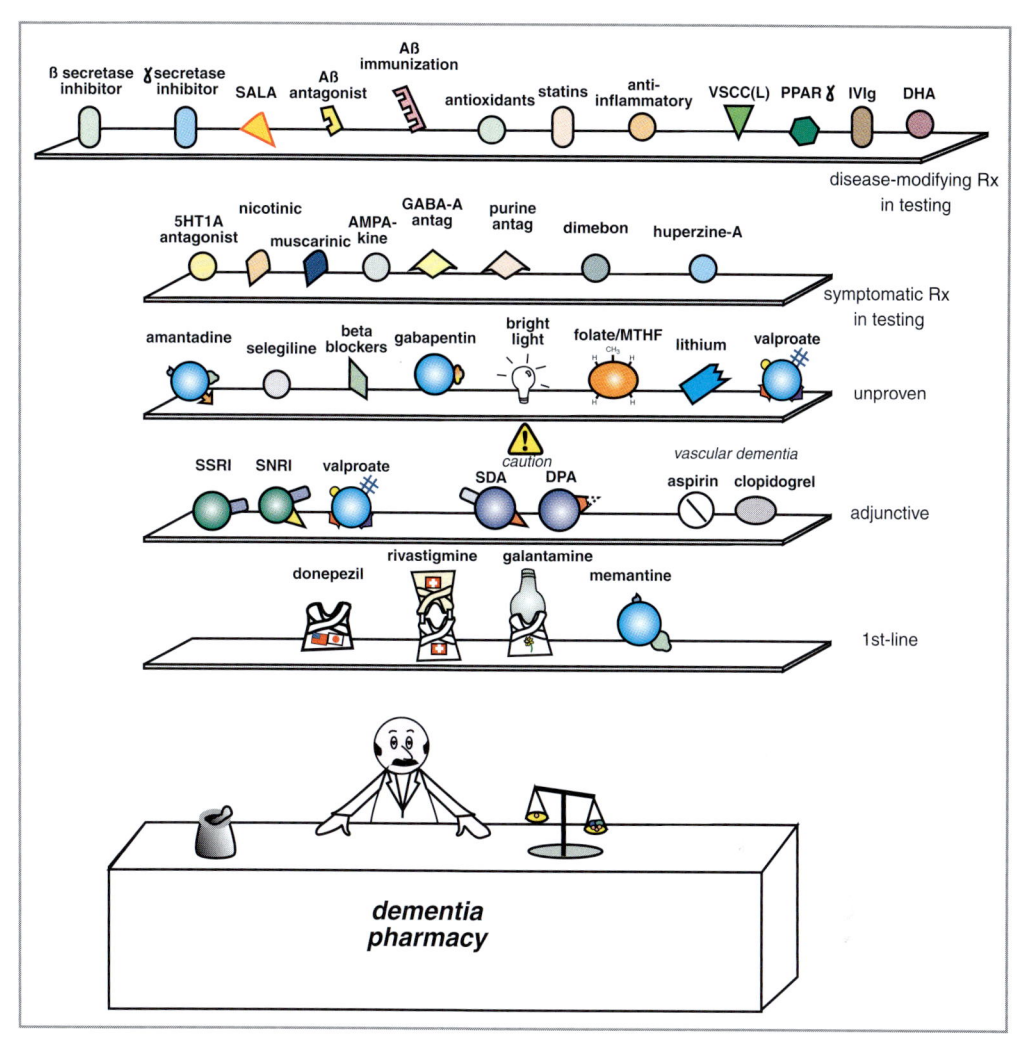

FIGURE 18-34 Dementia pharmacy. First-line treatments for dementia include donepezil, rivastigmine, galantamine, and memantine. Adjunctive treatments may include newer antidepressants, valproate, atypical antipsychotics (with caution), or, specifically for vascular dementia, aspirin and clopidogrel. Several existing treatments have been tried in dementia but are so far unproven. Agents currently under investigation include several that are symptom-focused and many others that would be disease-modifying.

Cholinesterase inhibition is also one component of the action of dimebon (Medivation), a Russian antihistamine with cholinesterase inhibitory properties, NMDA antagonist properties, potentiating actions on AMPA receptors, calcium channel blocking actions, and neuroprotective effects. Trials are in progress in Russia.

Directly stimulating muscarinic receptors or nicotinic receptors, or modulating nicotinic receptors with alpha 7 selective allosteric modulators, are approaches that exploit a procholinergic approach. One nicotinic agonist in testing is ispronicline (TC1734). Serotonergic strategies to improving cognition include blocking 5HT1A receptors with lecozotan or AV965 (also discussed in Chapter 10 in the discussion of new drugs for schizophrenia). Boosting glutamate function with the AMPA modulator CX717 is another approach, also discussed in Chapter 10 in the discussion of pro-cognitive approaches to schizophrenia.

Other approaches include GABA-A antagonists and phosphodiesterase inhibitors/purine antagonists.

The dementia pharmacy

Treatments proven, unproven, and anticipated in the future are all shown in Figure 18-34. Three cholinesterase inhibitors plus memantine are all first-line treatments for Alzheimer's disease and off label treatments for various other dementias. Adjunctive treatments can include various antidepressants and mood stabilizers for neuropsychiatric symptoms, various platelet blockers for vascular dementia, and – only with the utmost caution – atypical antipsychotics.

The "unproven" shelf could also be called the hopeful shelf and is full of agents on the market for another indication that have some theoretical appeal for Alzheimer's disease and some ongoing clinical testing. Bright light for "sundowning" is also included here. The top shelves are full of promise and discussed extensively in the sections above.

Summary

The most common dementia is Alzheimer's disease and the leading theory for its etiology is the amyloid cascade hypothesis. Other dementias are briefly discussed as well, as are their differing pathologies. Leading treatments for Alzheimer's disease today include the cholinesterase inhibitors, based upon the cholinergic hypothesis of amnesia, and memantine, an NMDA antagonist, based upon the glutamate hypothesis of cognitive decline. Major research efforts are attempting to find disease-modifying treatments that could halt or even reverse the course of this illness. Most efforts attempt to interfere with beta amyloid production and processing into toxic amyloid plaques.

CHAPTER 19

Disorders of Reward, Drug Abuse, and Their Treatment

- Reward circuits
- Nicotine
- Alcohol
- Opiates
- Stimulants
- Sedative hypnotics
- Marijuana
- Hallucinogens
- Club drugs
- Sexual disorders
    - Sexual disorders and reward
- Eating disorders
- Other impulse-control disorders
- Summary

Psychopharmacology is generally defined as the study of drugs that affect the brain. Until now, all the chapters of this book have addressed how psychotropic drugs affect the brain for therapeutic purposes. Unfortunately, psychotropic drugs can also be abused, and this has caused major public health problems throughout the world. Here we will attempt to explain how abuse of psychotropic agents affects the brain. Our approach to this problem is to discuss how nontherapeutic use, short-term abuse (intoxication), and the complications of long-term abuse affect chemical neurotransmission, particularly within reward circuits. We will also discuss the mechanism of action of agents that are now used to treat various substance abuse disorders.

Also covered briefly in this chapter are several other disorders thought to be regulated by reward circuitry, including sexual disorders, eating disorders, and various impulse disorders such as gambling. Reward circuitry has a prominent role in most psychiatric disorders, not just in drug abuse. Indeed, links to the reward circuitry can be seen not only for disorders of impulsivity such as attention deficit hyperactivity disorder (ADHD) (discussed in

TABLE 19-1 Paradigm-shifting questions for the modern treatment of substance abuse

1. Do you have to be an addict in recovery yourself to treat patients with addiction?
2. Is total abstinence the only desirable goal or is reduction in heavy use a valuable stepping stone to recovery?
3. Can drugs be used to treat drug abuse or are they really crutches?

Chapter 17), bipolar mania (discussed in Chapters 11 and 13), and anxiety disorders such as obsessive compulsive disorder (OCD) (discussed in Chapter 14), but also for disorders of motivation, such as major depression (discussed in Chapters 11 and 12), apathy in dementia (discussed in Chapter 18) and in schizophrenia (discussed in Chapters 9 and 10), use and abuse of pain medications in chronic pain syndromes (discussed in Chapter 15), and use and abuse of stimulants and sedative hypnotics in sleep/wake disorders (discussed in Chapter 16). In many ways, therefore, abnormalities in the adequate functioning of reward circuitry are key aspects to all the disorders discussed in this text. For that reason, we will discuss what is known about reward circuits in some detail.

New treatments for disorders of reward circuitry are finally entering psychopharmacology and the prospects for future therapeutics that target malfunctioning in this circuitry have never been greater. So far, psychopharmacologists have been reluctant to embrace new therapeutics for substance abuse, and thus the uptake of new treatments into clinical practice is often slow and many new treatments are still used minimally by many clinicians. Perhaps the lack of effective psychopharmacological treatments until relatively recently has allowed the field to develop therapeutic nihilism to psychopharmacological approaches. Even today, available psychopharmacological treatments for substance abuse remain few and limited in efficacy, as we shall see in this chapter.

However, the time might be right for some paradigm-shifting questions to be posed for the field of substance abuse treatment in the modern era (Table 19-1). For example, should professional psychopharmacologists be first-line treaters of substance abuse, or should this be left predominantly to lay counselors and professionals who have triumphed over their own past substance abuse? Since some treatments may blunt rather than stop all drug abuse behavior, particularly at the initiation of treatment, this leads one to ask: Is total abstinence the only desirable goal of treatment? Finally, is it rational to use drugs to treat drug abuse, or should drugs be seen mostly as crutches to be avoided?

Answers to these questions may determine whether more psychopharmacological practitioners become proactive in identifying and treating nicotine addiction; whether more practitioners start to use treatments for heavy drinking and alcoholism, including those that assure compliance for a month but are rarely used; whether more practitioners start to use opiate partial agonists for "middle class" patients dependent upon opiates who have never taken methadone. Perhaps the psychopharmacology of substance abuse and related disorders of reward is poised at the beginning of a new era, analogous to where psychopharmacology stood for the treatment of depression and psychosis in the 1950s, with major new therapeutics just around the corner.

At this point, understanding of the neuroscientific basis of reward circuitry and the pharmacological mechanism of action of substances of abuse and their drug treatments is exploding. What is known about this exciting field is summarized and reviewed briefly in this chapter. Mastering this will empower the modern psychopharmacologist to make decisions about whether to enter this field of new therapeutics.

TABLE 19-2 Nine key terms and their definitions

ABUSE: Self-administration of any drug in a culturally disapproved manner that causes adverse consequences

ADDICTION: A behavioral pattern of drug abuse characterized by overwhelming involvement with the use of a drug (compulsive use), the securing of its supply, and a strong tendency to relapse after discontinuation

DEPENDENCE: The physiological state of neuroadaptation produced by repeated administration of a drug, necessitating continued administration to prevent the appearance of the withdrawal syndrome

REINFORCEMENT: The tendency of a pleasure-producing drug to lead to repeated self-administration

TOLERANCE: Tolerance has developed when after repeated administration, a given dose of a drug produces a decreased effect, or, conversely, when increasingly larger doses must be administered to obtain the effects observed with the original use

CROSS-TOLERANCE AND CROSS-DEPENDENCE: The ability of one drug to suppress the manifestations of physical dependence produced by another drug and to maintain the physically dependent state

WITHDRAWAL: The psychologic and physiologic reactions to abrupt cessation of a dependence-producing drug

RELAPSE: The recurrence, upon discontinuation of an effective medical treatment, of the original condition from which the patient suffered

REBOUND: The exaggerated expression of the original condition sometimes experienced by patients immediately after cessation of an effective treatment

The goal of this chapter is to provide the biological background that will enable the reader to understand not only how substance abuse is thought to alter reward circuitry but also how currently available treatments for various substance abuse disorders work, including the rationale for current research efforts to discover truly novel and highly effective new treatments for these common and very debilitating illnesses. This chapter therefore provides only a very brief overview of the various substance abuse disorders. Full clinical descriptions and formal criteria for how to diagnose the numerous known diagnostic entities should be obtained by consulting standard reference sources. Some useful definitions of key terms used in this field are given in Table 19-2. The discussion here emphasizes the links between various pathological mechanisms, brain circuits, and neurotransmitters with the various symptoms of substance abuse, from nicotine to alcohol to opiates to stimulants. Brief mention is made of other drugs of abuse and other impulse disorders that do not involve drugs. Finally, a discussion of various types of sexual dysfunction that are hypothetically linked to reward circuitry is included.

Reward circuits

The mesolimbic dopamine circuit as the final common pathway of reward

The final common pathway of reinforcement and reward in the brain is hypothesized to be the mesolimbic dopamine pathway (Figure 19-1). Some even consider this to be the "pleasure center" of the brain and dopamine to be the "pleasure neurotransmitter." There are many natural ways to trigger your mesolimbic dopamine neurons to release dopamine, ranging from intellectual accomplishments, to athletic accomplishments, to enjoying a good symphony, to experiencing an orgasm. These are sometimes called "natural highs" (Figure 19-1). The inputs to the mesolimbic pathway that mediate these natural highs include a

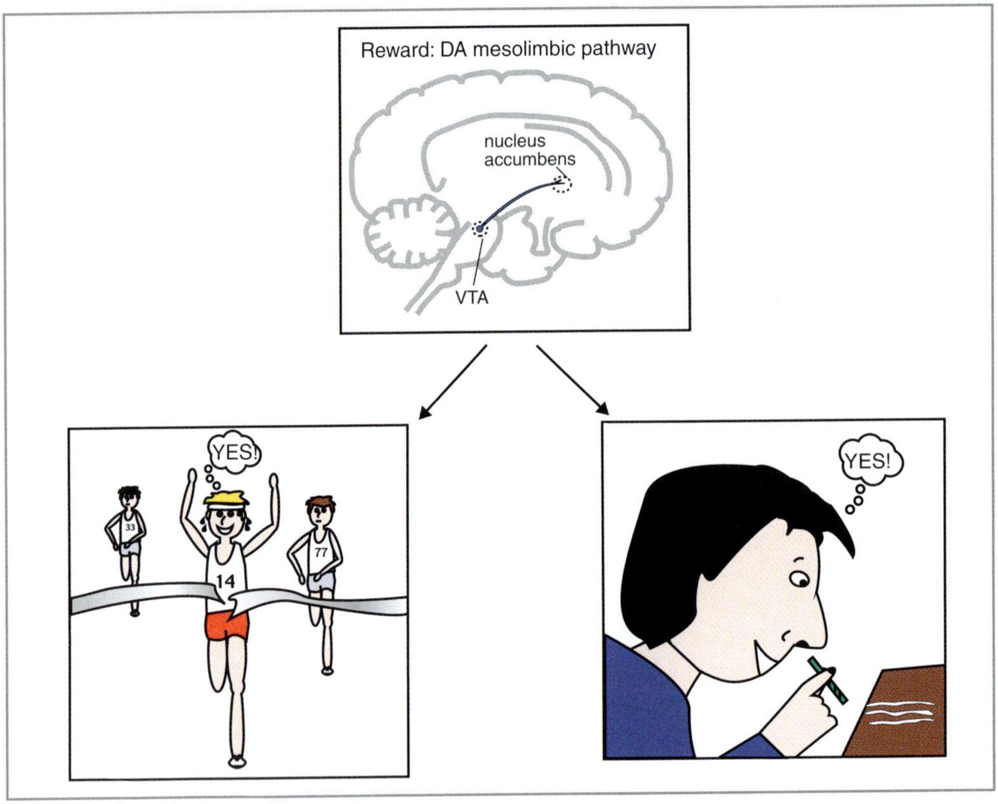

FIGURE 19-1 The final common pathway of reward. The mesolimbic dopamine pathway mediates the psychopharmacology of reward, whether that is a natural high or a drug-induced high, and is sometimes referred to as the pleasure center of the brain, with dopamine as the pleasure neurotransmitter.

most incredible "pharmacy" of naturally occurring substances ranging from the brain's own morphine/heroin (endorphins), to the brain's own marijuana (anandamide), to the brain's own nicotine (acetylcholine), to the brain's own cocaine and amphetamine (dopamine itself) (Figure 19-2).

The numerous psychotropic drugs of abuse also have a final common pathway of causing the mesolimbic pathway to release dopamine, often in a manner more explosive and pleasurable than that which occurs naturally. These drugs bypass the brain's own neurotransmitters and directly stimulate the brain's own receptors for these drugs, causing dopamine to be released. Since the brain already uses neurotransmitters that resemble drugs of abuse, it is not necessary to earn your reward naturally, since you can get a much more intense reward in the short run and upon demand from a drug of abuse than you can from a natural high with the brain's natural system. However, unlike a natural high, a drug-induced reward causes such wonderful feeding of dopamine to postsynaptic limbic dopamine receptors that they furiously crave even more drug to replenish dopamine once the drug stops working, leading one to be preoccupied with finding drug and thus beginning a vicious cycle of abuse, addiction, dependence, and withdrawal.

The reactive reward system: reward from the bottom up

Addicts act impulsively, automatically, and obligatorily to cues that lead them to seek and ingest more drug. That is the power of the reactive reward system, which functions

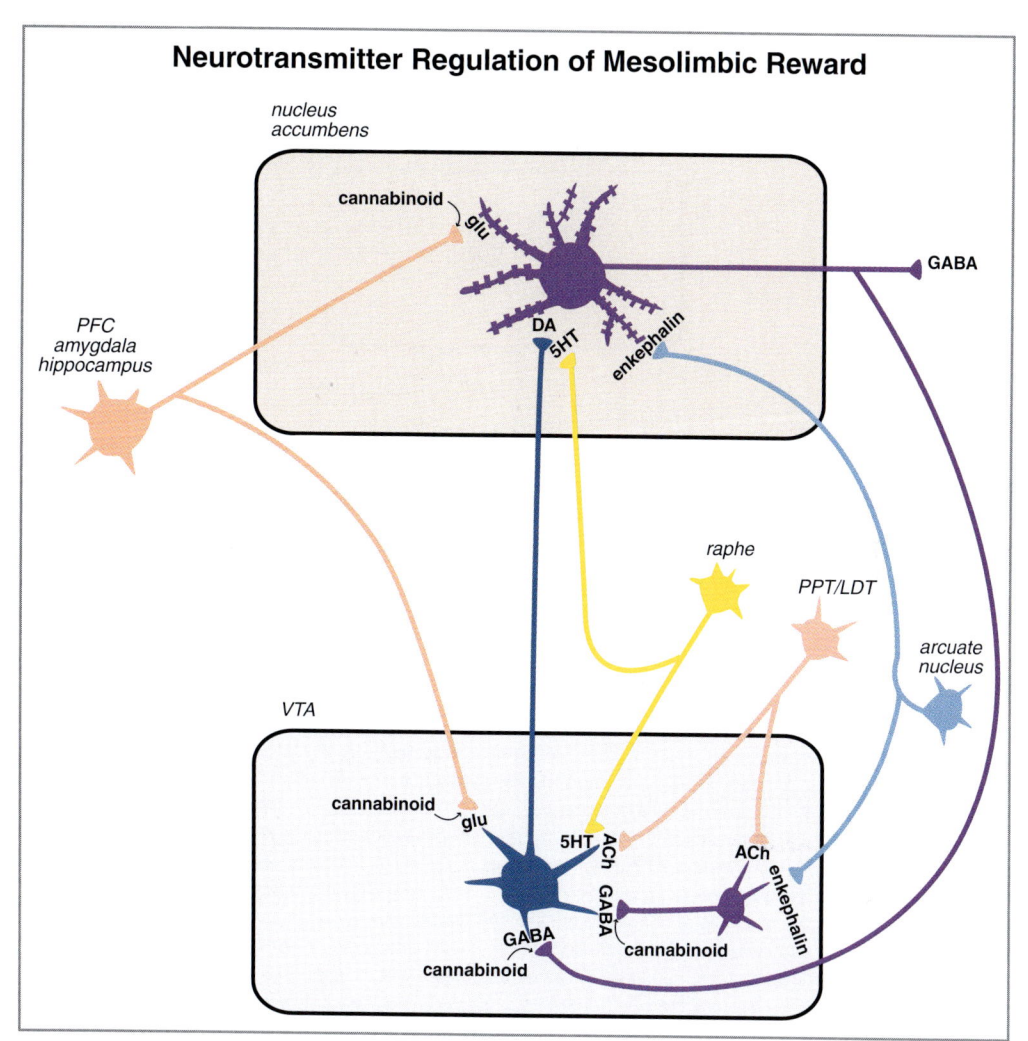

FIGURE 19-2 Neurotransmitter regulation of mesolimbic reward. The final common pathway of reward in the brain is hypothesized to be the mesolimbic dopamine pathway. This pathway is modulated by many naturally occurring substances in the brain in order to deliver normal reinforcement to adaptive behaviors (such as eating, drinking, sex) and thus to produce "natural highs," such as feelings of joy or accomplishment. These neurotransmitter inputs to the reward system include the brain's own morphine/heroin (i.e., endorphins such as enkephalin), the brain's own cannabis/marijuana (i.e., anandamide), the brain's own nicotine (i.e., acetylcholine), and the brain's own cocaine/amphetamine (i.e., dopamine itself), among others. The numerous psychotropic drugs of abuse that occur in nature bypass the brain's own neurotransmitters and directly stimulate the brain's receptors in the reward system, causing dopamine release and a consequent "artificial high." Thus alcohol, opiates, stimulants, marijuana, benzodiazepines, sedative hypnotics, hallucinogens, and nicotine all affect this mesolimbic dopaminergic system.

to signal the immediate prospects of either pain or pleasure (Figure 19-3). The reactive reward system provides motivation and behavioral drive from the "bottom up," including not only the ascending mesolimbic dopamine (DA) pathway (shown in Figures 19-1 and 19-2) but also the amygdala and its projections to both ends of the mesolimbic pathway (Figure 19-3). Shown in Figure 19-3 are the connections the amygdala makes both with DA cell bodies in the ventral tegmental area (VTA) and with spiny neurons in the nucleus

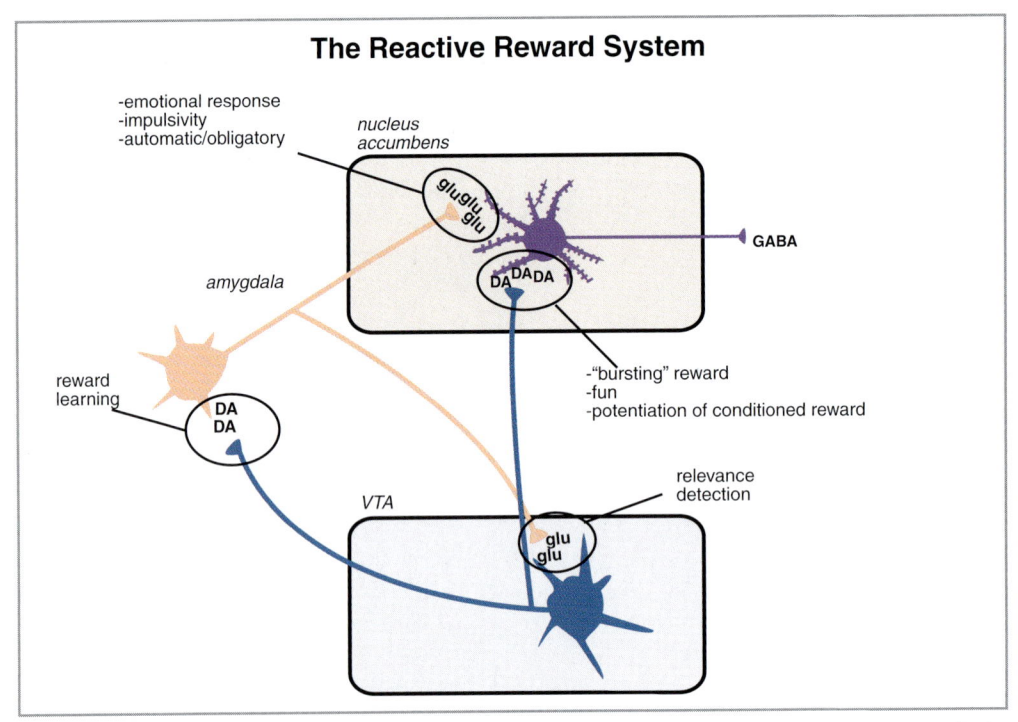

FIGURE 19-3 The reactive reward system. The reactive reward system is a "bottom up" system that signals the immediate prospect of either pleasure or pain and provides motivation and behavioral drive to achieve that pleasure or to avoid that pain. For example, internal cues such as craving and withdrawal cause the reactive reward system to trigger drug-seeking behavior. The reactive reward system consists of the ventral tegmental area (VTA), which is the site of dopamine cell bodies; the nucleus accumbens, where dopaminergic neurons project; and the amygdala, which has connections with both the VTA and the nucleus accumbens. Rewarding input to the nucleus accumbens is due to bursts of dopamine release and thus phasic dopamine firing with "fun" and potentiation of conditioned reward as the result. Connections of dopaminergic neurons with the amygdala are involved in reward learning (such as memory of pleasure associated with drug abuse), while connections of the amygdala back to the VTA communicate whether anything relevant to a previously experienced pleasure has been detected. Connections of the amygdala with the nucleus accumbens communicate that emotions have been triggered by internal or external cues and signal an impulsive, almost reflexive response to be taken.

accumbens. Spiny neurons in the nucleus accumbens also receive input from the mesolimbic DA pathway (Figure 19-3).

Upon repeated exposure to drugs of abuse, this reactive reward system pathologically "learns" to trigger drug seeking behavior and "remembers" how to do this when confronted with internal cues such as craving and withdrawal and external cues from the environment such as people, places, and paraphernalia associated with past drug use. The processes by which plastic changes modify brain circuits are introduced in Chapter 2 and illustrated in Figures 2-22 through 2-31. Substance abuse is a good example of how the normal mechanisms of learning are hijacked and built into a brain disorder. This is introduced as the concept of "diabolical learning" in Chapter 8 and illustrated in Figure 8-6. Diabolical learning may apply to different brain circuits not only in addiction but also in chronic pain (discussed in Chapter 15) and for symptoms triggered by stress (discussed in Chapter 14).

Connections of the mesolimbic dopamine system within the nucleus accumbens create bursts of dopamine release from phasic dopamine firing, pleasure, reward, and "fun," potentiating the effects of conditioned reward from previous drug abuse experiences (Figure 19-3). Connections of DA neurons with the amygdala are involved with reward learning (Figure 19-3). The amygdala is an important site of emotional learning. For example, the amygdala is involved both in learning about fear (i.e., fear conditioning) and in learning to no longer fear (i.e., fear extinction). This is discussed in Chapter 14 and illustrated in Figures 14-40 through 14-42. The amygdala is also involved in learning about reward. As shown in Figure 19-3, connections received from dopamine neurons projecting from the VTA cause the amygdala to develop adaptive changes that condition it to remember the rewards of drug abuse, including not just memory of pleasure but also memory of the environmental cues associated with the pleasurable experience.

Once reward learning has been conditioned in the amygdala, connections of the amygdala back to the VTA DA neuron later communicate whether anything relevant to the previously rewarding drug abuse experience is being detected (Figure 19-3). Connections of the amygdala with the nucleus accumbens tell the spiny neurons there that emotional memories have been triggered by internal or external cues, and instruct these spiny neurons to take action impulsively, right away, automatically, obligatorily, and without thought, almost as a reflex action, to find and take more drugs (Figure 19-3). The net result of these changes is that the reactive reward system hijacks the entire reward circuitry when addiction has developed. Individuals in this state are no longer able to base their decisions upon the long-term consequences of their behavior.

The reflective reward system: reward from the top down

A complementary and in some ways competitive component of the reactive reward system is the reflective reward system, or the "top down" component of reward circuitry (Figure 19-4). This includes important connections from prefrontal cortex down to the nucleus accumbens. These connections are the first legs of cortico-striatal-thalamic-cortical (CSTC) loops, introduced in Chapter 7 and illustrated in Figures 7-18 through 7-21. CSTC loops are discussed in relation to many different psychiatric disorders throughout this text. Particularly relevant to a discussion of impulsive drug abuse is the discussion of impulsivity in ADHD and the related CSTC loops regulating symptoms in ADHD (discussed in Chapter 17 and illustrated in Figures 17-3 through 17-6).

Prefrontal projections from the orbitofrontal cortex may be involved in regulating impulses (Figure 19-4; see also Figures 7-20 and 17-6), whereas prefrontal projections from the dorsolateral prefrontal cortex (DLPFC) may be involved in analyzing the situation, keeping some flexibility of choice in play, and regulating whether it is rational to take an action (Figure 19-4; see also Figures 7-17 and 17-4). Finally, the ventromedial prefrontal cortex (VMPFC; see Figure 7-19) may try to integrate impulsiveness from OFC with analysis and cognitive flexibility from DLPFC with its own regulation of emotions, and come up with a final decision of what to do (Figure 19-4). Additional input for such a final decision also comes from two areas not shown in Figure 19-4: the insula and sensory cortex, contributing feelings about prior experiences of reward and punishment, and the hippocampus, providing contextual information about the decision to be made. When all the inputs are integrated, the final output is either to stop the action that the reactive reward system is triggering (generally drug seeking), or to let it happen.

The reflective reward system is built and maintained over time based upon various influences including neurodevelopment, genetics, experience, peer pressure, learning social rules, and learning the benefits of suppressing current pleasure for more valuable future gain (Figure 19-4). The reflective reward system has the power to shape the final output of the

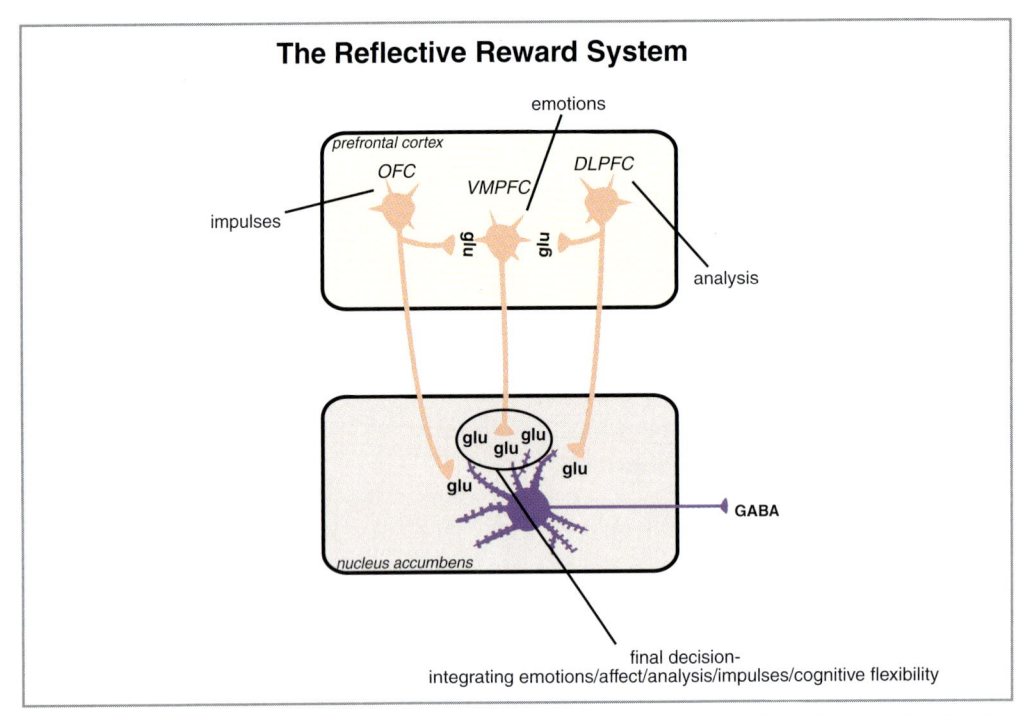

FIGURE 19-4 The reflective reward system. Stimulatory input from the "bottom up" reactive reward system is regulated by the "top down" reflective reward system, which consists of projections from the prefrontal cortex to the nucleus accumbens (the "cortico-striatal" portion of cortico-striatal-thalamic-cortical loops). Projections from the orbitofrontal cortex (OFC) are involved in regulating impulses, from the ventromedial prefrontal cortex (VMPFC) are involved in regulating emotions, and from the dorsolateral prefrontal cortex (DLPFC) are involved in analyzing situations and regulating whether an action takes place.

reward system into long-term beneficial goal-directed behaviors, such as the will power to resist drugs. When fully developed and functioning properly, the reflective reward system can also provide the motivation for pursuing more naturally rewarding experiences such as education, accomplishments, recognition, financial benefits, career development, enriching social and family connections, etc.

Turning reward into goal-directed behavior: output of the reward system

The output of the reward system (Figure 19-5) is really just the completion of CSTC loops starting in the prefrontal cortex (see the cortico-striatal leg of the CSTC loop in Figure 19-4 being completed as striatal thalamic and thalamo-cortical projections in Figure 19-5). Specifically, the striatal/accumbens component of reward circuitry has output via GABA-ergic neurons (number 1 in Figure 19-5) that travel to another part of the striatal complex, the ventral pallidum. From there, connections go to the thalamus (number 2 in Figure 19-5), and then back up to the prefrontal cortex, where behaviors are implemented, such as learning and activities resulting in long-term rewards (number 3 in Figure 19-5) or drug-seeking behavior resulting in short-term rewards (number 4 in Figure 19-5).

Determining whether the output of the reward system will be converted into short- or long-term rewards is the result of the balance between bottom up reactive reward drives and top down reflective reward decisions (Figures 19-6 through 19-8). For example, the first time you take a drug, there is immediate pharmacological action upon the mesolimbic pleasure

Turning Reward into Goal-Directed Behavior

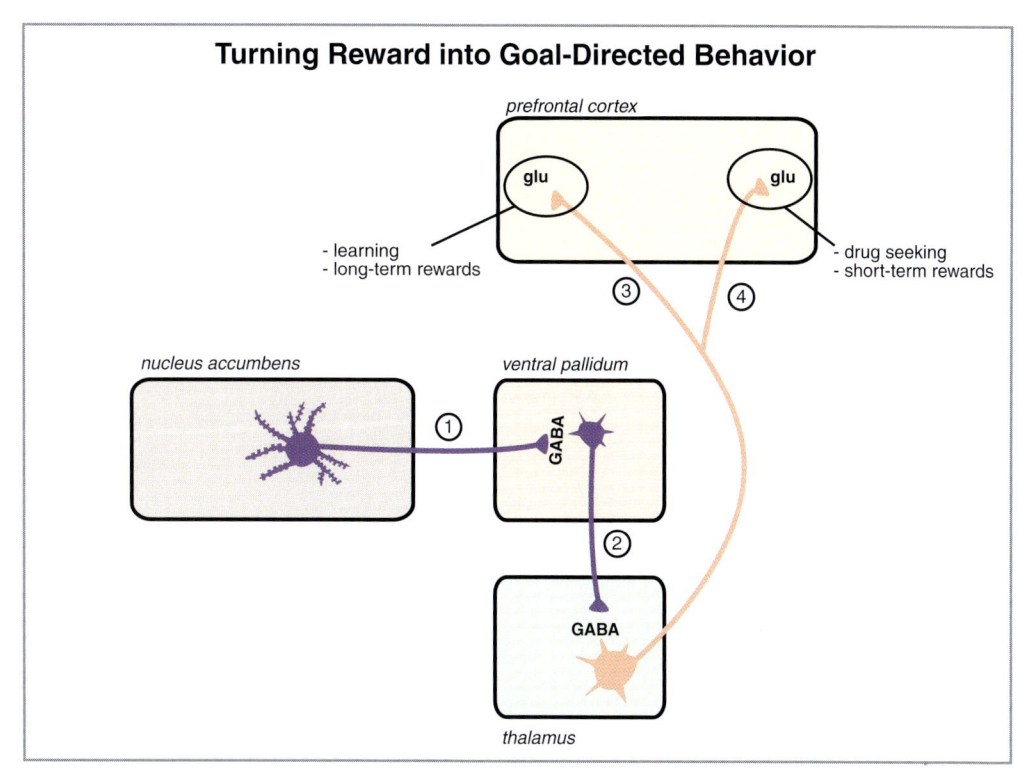

FIGURE 19-5 Turning reward into goal-directed behavior. The second half of the cortico-striatal-thalamic-cortical loop is responsible for output of the reward system (i.e., turning reward into goal-directed behavior). GABA-ergic neurons project from the nucleus accumbens to another part of the striatum, the ventral pallidum (1), from which GABA-ergic neurons project to the thalamus (2). Connections from the thalamus project back up to the prefrontal cortex, where behaviors are implemented, such as learning and activities involved in long-term reward (3) or drug-seeking behavior leading to short-term reward (4).

center, the exact site of action dependent upon the exact substance ingested (see number 1 in Figure 19-6; see also Figure 19-2). Dopamine is released, pleasure is experienced (number 2 and "wow!" in Figure 19-6), and the amygdala "learns" that this is a rewarding experience (number 3 in Figure 19-6). Reward has now been conditioned in the amygdala.

After repetitive rewarding experiences with the drug, the reward circuits become "addicted," so the next time there is an opportunity to use the drug, it is not just the ingesting of the drug that causes dopamine release and pleasure; the cues that predict hedonic pleasure already cause dopamine release (arrow 1 in Figure 19-7). The reward system has learned to anticipate the reward, and that anticipation itself becomes pleasurable. The amygdala signals the dopamine neuron in the VTA that something good is about to happen because it remembers the past drug reward; it may also signal that relief from craving is in sight. Getting the anticipated reward is a very compelling option, so there is a powerful impulse sent to the VTA (arrow 2 in Figure 19-7) triggering DA in the nucleus accumbens (arrow 3 in Figure 19-7) to transform this impulse into the action of finding some drugs and making this reward really happen (arrow 4 in Figure 19-7). Substantial reward and relief is already experienced just by anticipating the reward, but the real kick comes when the drugs are actually ingested again. In addiction, reward is overvalued and hyperactive by virtue of the "diabolical learning" that has occurred in reward circuits. This process of

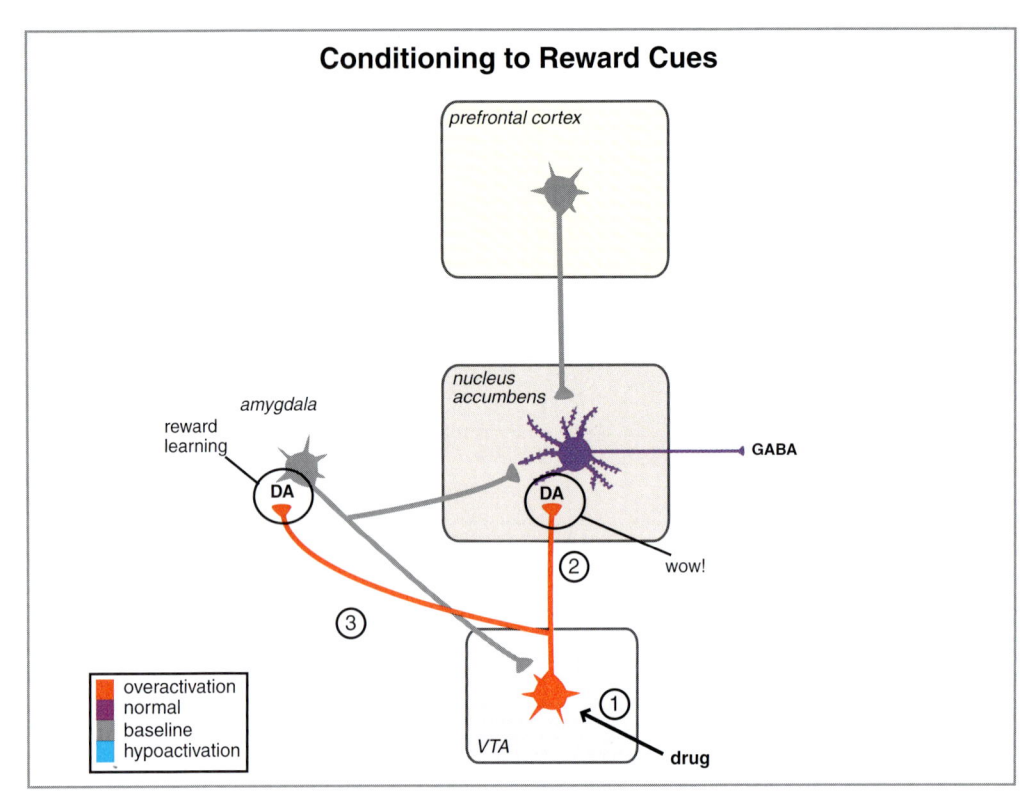

FIGURE 19-6 Conditioning to reward cues. The first time a drug is taken (1) it causes immediate release of dopamine (depicted by red color of neurons) and a corresponding experience of pleasure (2). As a result of this the amygdala "learns" that this is a rewarding experience (3).

synaptic plasticity changes the efficiency of information flow in the reactive reward circuitry to allow its neuronal activity to preempt all contradictory input coming from the reflective reward circuit in the prefrontal cortex (see hypoactive prefrontal cortex circuits in Figure 19-7).

But can impulses from the reactive reward system ever be resisted? What is the role of will power over temptation? That is explained in Figure 19-8. If temptation is bottom-up demands from the reactive reward system, will power can be seen as top down decision making by the reflective reward system. Specifically, drug seeking is not always an involuntary response to internal and external cues urging that behavior, especially before addiction sets in and when the prefrontal decision-making circuits are well developed and frequently utilized. If addiction is diabolic learning, will power may be virtuous learning within the same reward system (Figure 19-8).

Thus, when temptation occurs with the opportunity to ingest drugs arising at a party, in a bar, or when seeing or feeling drugs or their paraphernalia, the amygdala anticipates the pleasure that the drugs would bring (number 1 in Figure 19-8A) by signaling an impulsive choice to the VTA (number 2 in Figure 19-8A) to release dopamine (arrow 3 in Figure 19-8A) that urges output from the nucleus accumbens to engage in behavior that leads to ingesting the drugs again. The OFC in prefrontal cortex is signaling craving and voting for more drug ingestion as well (number 4 in Figure 19-8A). However, this is just temptation. For a split second there may be the opportunity for the DLPFC to think about whether it

952 | Essential Psychopharmacology

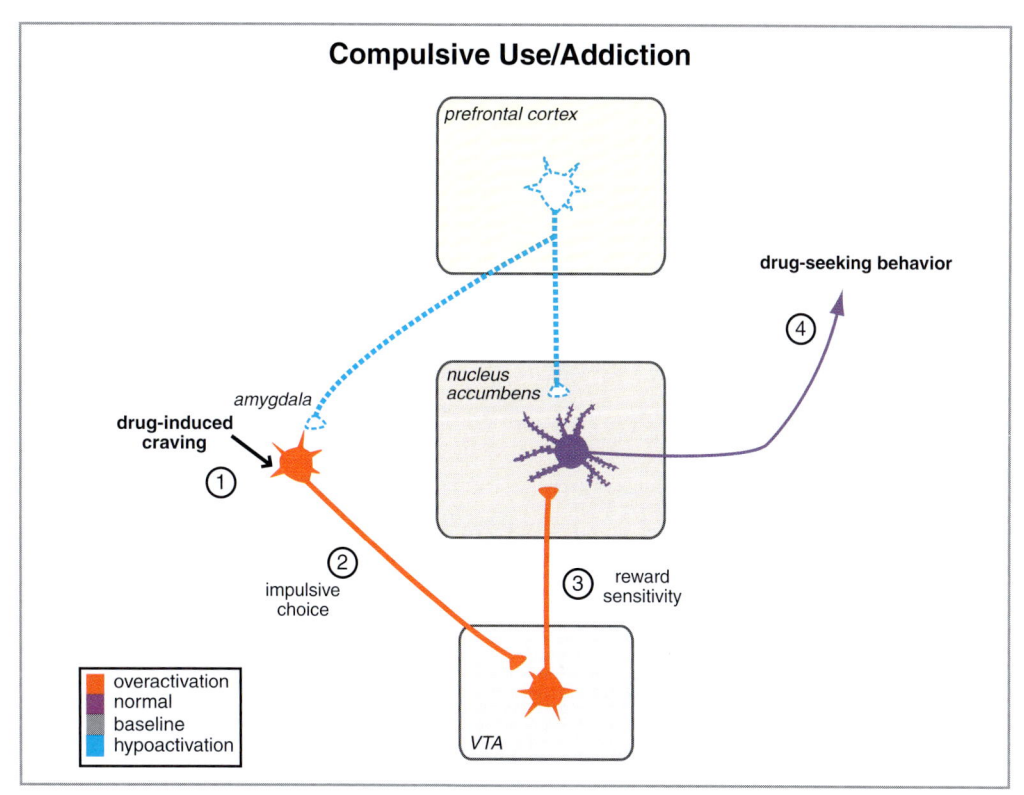

FIGURE 19-7 Compulsive use/addiction. The amygdala can not only learn that a drug causes pleasure but can also associate cues for that drug with pleasure. Thus, when cues are encountered, the amygdala signals dopamine neurons in the ventral tegmental area (VTA) that something good is coming; it may even signal relief from drug craving (1 and 2). This leads to dopamine release in the nucleus accumbens (3), which triggers GABA-ergic input to the thalamus, thalamic input to the prefrontal cortex, and, unless the reflective reward system is activated (i.e., if the prefrontal neurons were red as opposed to blue), leads to action such as drug-seeking behavior (4).

wants to take this action and to cast an opposing vote, showing cognitive flexibility (number 5 in Figure 19-8A), keeping the system from taking an immediate obligatory action just because the reactive reward system is demanding it.

Will power can be represented in the reward system as the ability of prefrontal circuits to become activated and prevent impulses being expressed as drug-seeking behavior (Figure 19-8B). Having a functioning top down reflective reward system allows the time to evaluate whether losing your driver's license, getting into an auto accident, losing your job or your relationship is worth becoming intoxicated, and if the answer is no, can trigger the choice of becoming a designated driver and not ingesting the drug (e.g., alcohol) (Figure 19-8B).

This is an overly simplistic representation of temptation and will power, but it makes the point that the balance between competing circuits can be tipped in one direction or the other. On the one hand, "diabolical learning" and changes in dominance of the reactive reward system from repeated drug ingestion that overvalues short-term rewards can result in compulsive drug-seeking behavior; on the other hand, "virtuous learning" and plastic changes that lead to dominance of the reflective reward system can produce the ability to suppress short-term rewards for long-term gains.

Disorders of Reward, Drug Abuse, and Their Treatment | 953

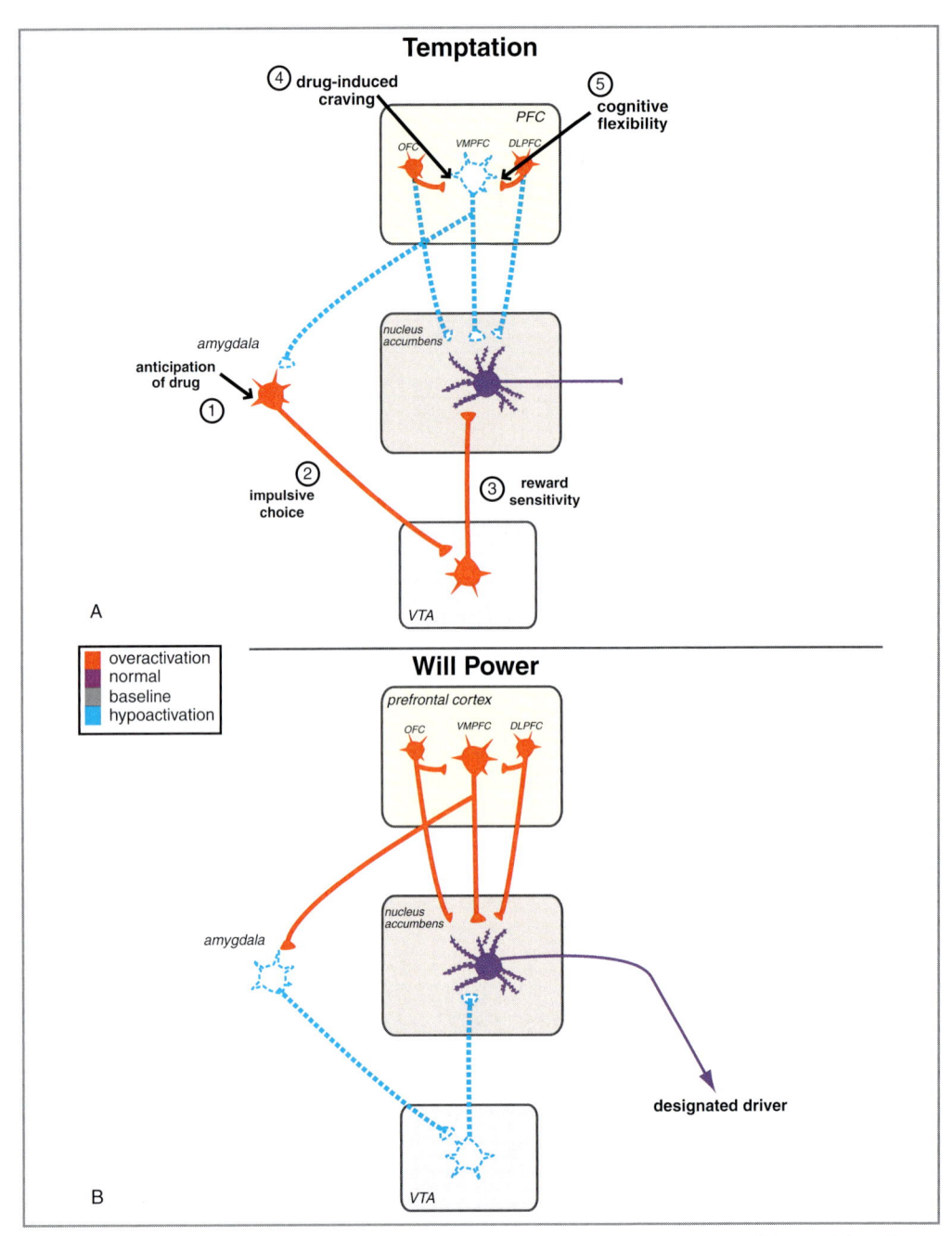

FIGURE 19-8A and B Temptation and will power. Temptation may be seen as "bottom up" demand from the reactive reward system, while will power is a result of "top down" decision making by the reflective reward system. (**A**) When drug anticipation occurs, (1) this signals an impulsive choice (2) to the ventral tegmental area (VTA) to release dopamine in the nucleus accumbens (3), which in turn produces output to engage in behavior that leads to ingesting drugs again. In the prefrontal cortex, the orbitofrontal cortex (OFC) signals drug-induced cravings and thus supports the "vote" for drug ingestion (4). The dorsolateral prefrontal cortex (DLPFC) interprets the various signals and, showing cognitive flexibility, decides whether to take the action of drug ingestion (5). (**B**) If the reflective reward system (prefrontal circuits) is activated (shown here by the prefrontal neurons turning red), this can prevent impulses (temptation) from being expressed as behavior.

Nicotine

How common is smoking in clinical psychopharmacology practices? Some estimates are that more than half of all cigarettes are consumed by patients with a concurrent psychiatric disorder and that smoking is the most common comorbidity among seriously mentally ill patients. It is estimated that about 20 percent of the general population (in the United States) smoke, about 30 percent of people who regularly see general physicians smoke, but that 40 to 50 percent of patients in a psychopharmacology practice smoke, including 60 to 85 percent of patients with ADHD, schizophrenia, and bipolar disorder.

Histories of current smoking are often not carefully taken or recorded as one of the diagnoses for smokers in mental health practices. Only about 10 percent of smokers report being offered treatment proactively by psychopharmacologists and other clinicians. Perhaps this therapeutic nihilism results from the facts that smoking is so addicting and that smoking cessation treatments are so rarely successful. It may also be because the treatment of smoking in patients with psychiatric disorders has been relatively neglected in mental health training programs. Also, companies making smoking cessation treatments tend to spend their efforts educating and marketing to that half of smokers without psychiatric disorders, who may be a more glamorous population associated with less stigma than patients with mental disorders.

Nicotine and reward

Cigarette smoking is self-administering nicotine in a clever but evil delivery system. Smoking tobacco may be the best way to maximize pleasure from nicotine. Unfortunately, dosing nicotine this way may also maximize the chances of addiction due to the effects that high-dose pulsatile delivery of nicotine has on reward circuitry. Tobacco smoking also delivers carcinogens and other toxins that damage the heart, lungs, and other tissues.

In terms of psychopharmacological mechanism of action, nicotine acts directly upon nicotinic cholinergic receptors in reward circuits (Figure 19-9 through 19-11). Cholinergic neurons and the neurotransmitter acetylcholine are discussed in Chapter 18 and illustrated in Figures 18-12 through 18-17. Nicotinic receptors are illustrated in Figures 18-15 through 18-17. There are two major subtypes of nicotinic receptors that are known to be present in the brain, the alpha 4 beta 2 subtype and the alpha 7 subtype (discussed in Chapter 18 and illustrated in Figure 18-15).

Nicotine's actions in the ventral tegmental area are those that are theoretically linked to addiction (Figure 19-9). Details of these actions are shown in Figure 19-10, namely, activation of alpha 4 beta 2 nicotinic postsynaptic receptors on DA neurons, leading to DA release in the nucleus accumbens; activation of alpha 7 nicotinic presynaptic neurons on glutamate neurons, which causes glutamate release, and, in turn, DA release in the nucleus accumbens. The release-promoting actions of presynaptic alpha 7 nicotinic receptors on glutamate neurons are discussed in Chapter 18 and illustrated in Figure 18-16. Nicotine also appears to desensitize alpha 4 beta 2 postsynaptic receptors on inhibitory GABA-ergic interneurons in the VTA (Figure 19-10); this also leads to DA release in nucleus accumbens by disinhibiting dopaminergic mesolimbic neurons.

Nicotine and addiction

Nicotine has other actions at many nicotinic receptor subtypes and in many areas of the brain. For example, actions of nicotine on postsynaptic alpha 7 nicotinic receptors in the prefrontal cortex may be linked to the pro-cognitive and mentally alerting actions of nicotine but not to addictive actions. However, it is the alpha 4 beta 2 nicotinic receptors on VTA DA neurons that are thought to be the primary targets of nicotine's reinforcing properties

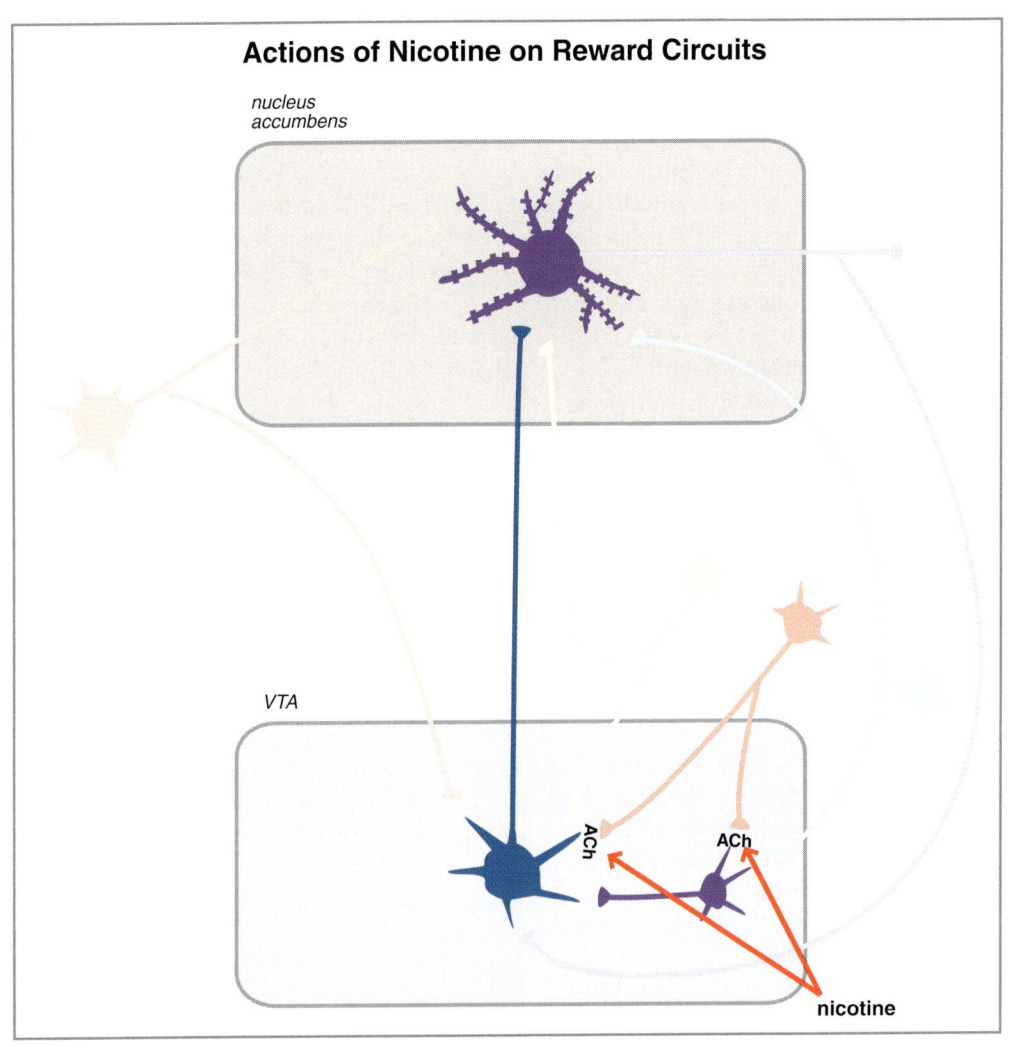

FIGURE 19-9 Actions of nicotine on reward circuits. Shown here is the site of action of nicotine on the reactive reward system. Nicotine acts directly upon nicotinic cholinergic receptors in the VTA.

(Figure 19-10). These receptors adapt to the chronic intermittent pulsatile delivery of nicotine in a way that leads to addiction (Figure 9-11).

That is, initially, alpha 4 beta 2 receptors in the resting state are opened by delivery of nicotine, which in turn leads to dopamine release and reinforcement, pleasure and reward (Figure 19-11A). By the time the cigarette is finished, these receptors become desensitized, so that they cannot function temporarily by reacting to either acetylcholine or nicotine (Figure 19-11A). In terms of obtaining any further reward, you might as well stop smoking at this point. An interesting question to ask is: How long does it take for the nicotinic receptors to desensitize? The answer seems to be: About as long as it takes to inhale all the puffs of a standard cigarette and burn it down to a butt. Thus, it is probably not an accident that cigarettes are the length that they are. Shorter does not maximize the pleasure. Longer is a waste, since by then the receptors are all desensitized anyway (Figure 19-11A).

The problem for the smoker is that when the receptors resensitize to their resting state, this initiates craving and withdrawal due to the lack of release of further dopamine

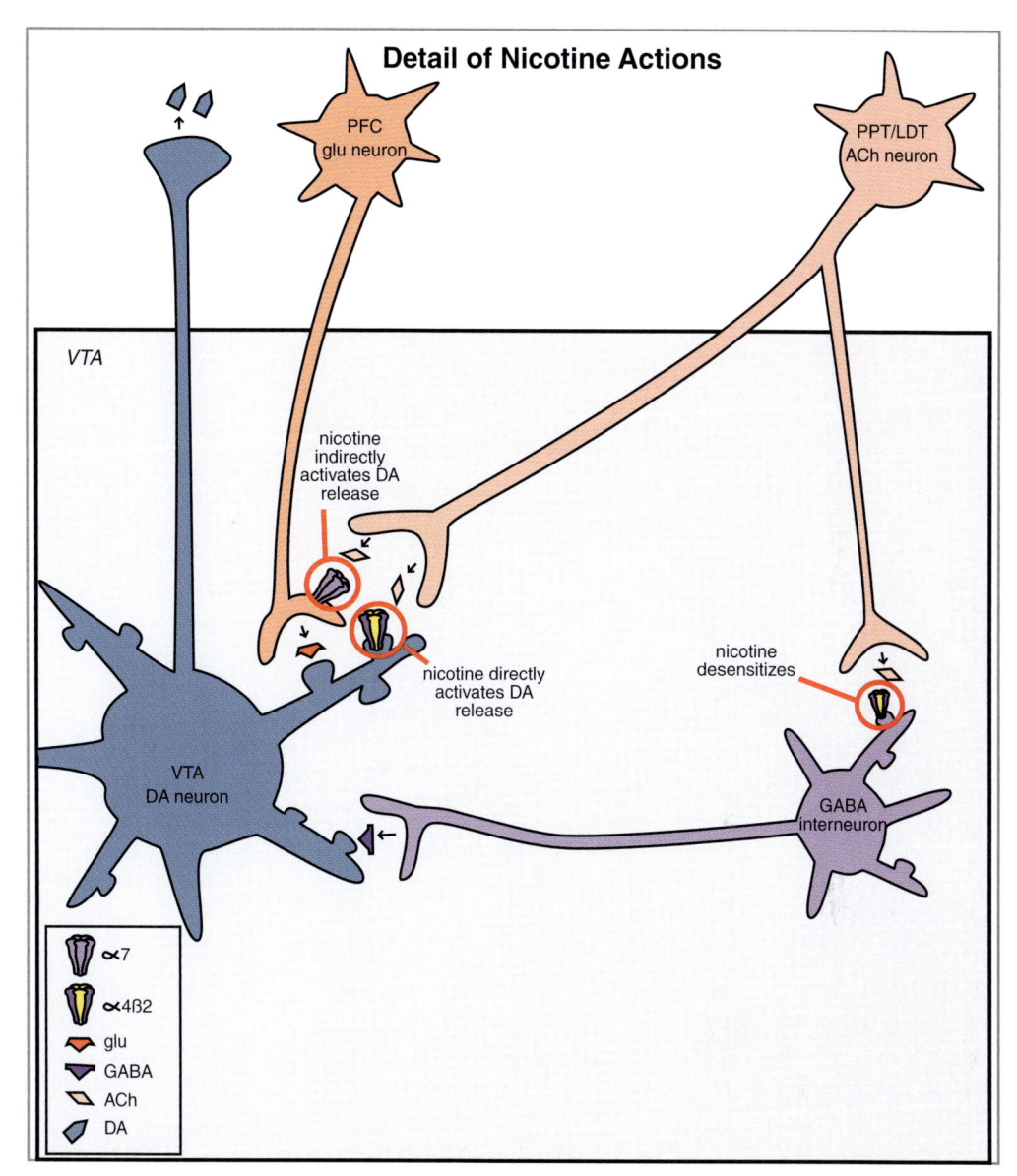

FIGURE 19-10 Detail of nicotine actions. Nicotine directly causes dopamine release in the nucleus accumbens by binding to alpha 4 beta 2 nicotinic postsynaptic receptors on dopamine neurons in the ventral tegmental area (VTA). In addition, nicotine binds to alpha 7 nicotinic presynaptic receptors on glutamate neurons in the VTA, which in turn leads to dopamine release in the nucleus accumbens. Nicotine also seems to desensitize alpha 4 beta 2 postsynaptic receptors on GABA interneurons in the VTA; the reduction of GABA neurotransmission disinhibits mesolimbic dopamine neurons and thus is a third mechanism for enhancing dopamine release in the nucleus accumbens.

(Figure 19-11A). Another interesting question is: How long does it take to resensitize nicotinic receptors? The answer seems to be: About the length of time that smokers take between cigarettes. For the average one-pack-per-day smoker awake for 16 hours, that would be about 45 minutes, possibly explaining why there are 20 cigarettes in a pack (i.e., enough for an average smoker to keep his or her nicotinic receptors completely desensitized all day long).

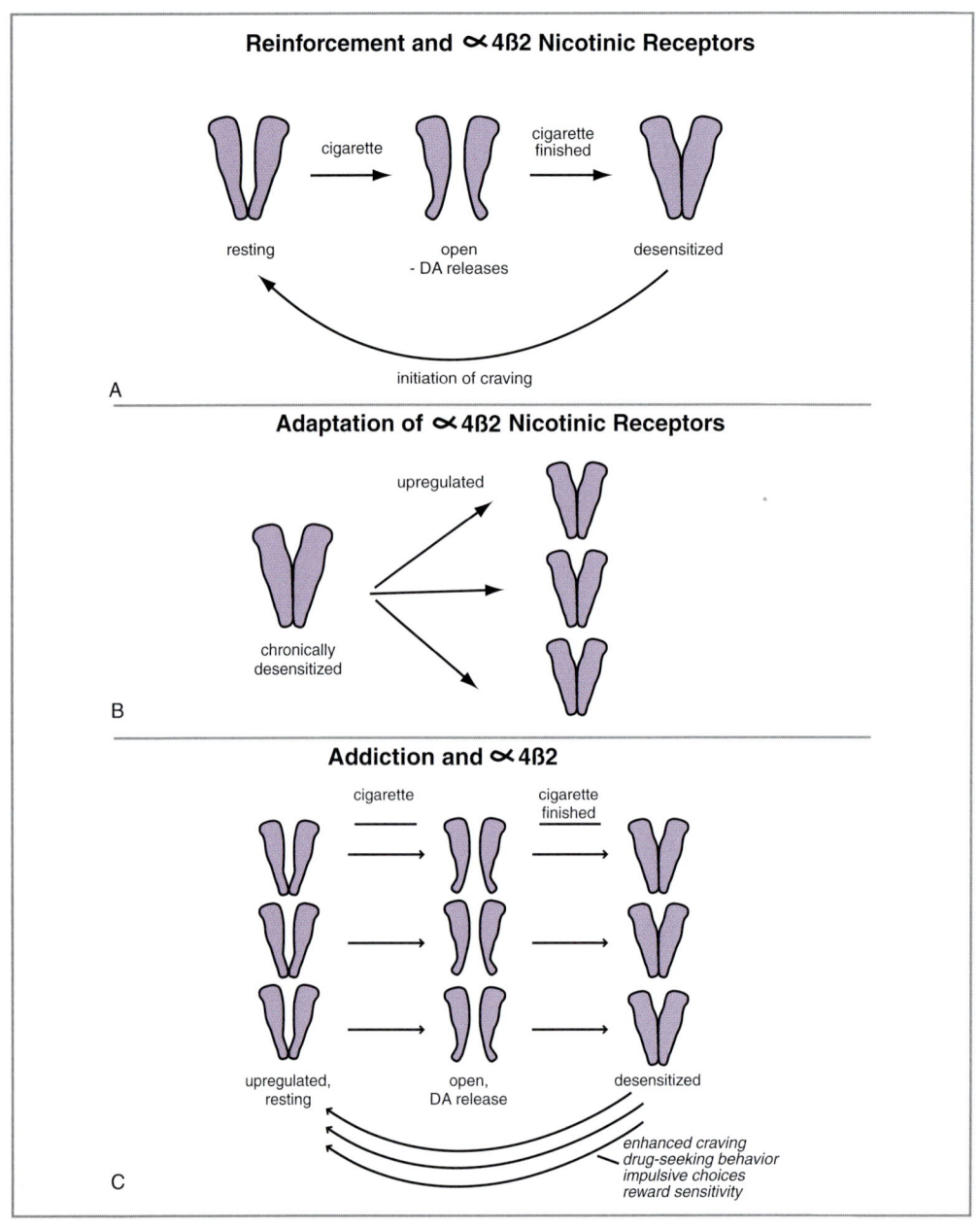

FIGURE 19-11A, B, and C Reinforcement and alpha 4 beta 2 nicotinic receptors. (**A**) In the resting state alpha 4 beta 2 nicotinic receptors are closed (left). Nicotine administration, as by smoking a cigarette, causes the receptor to open, which in turn leads to dopamine release (middle). Long-term stimulation of these receptors leads to their desensitization, such that they temporarily can no longer react to nicotine (or to acetylcholine); this occurs in approximately the same length of time it takes to finish a single cigarette (right). As the receptors resensitize, they initiate craving and withdrawal due to the lack of release of further dopamine. (**B**) With chronic desensitization, alpha 4 beta 2 receptors upregulate to compensate. (**C**) If one continues smoking, however, the repeated administration of nicotine continues to lead to desensitization of all of these alpha 4 beta 2 receptors and thus the upregulation does no good. In fact, the upregulation can lead to amplified craving as the extra receptors resensitize to their resting state.

Putting nicotinic receptors out of business by desensitizing them all the time causes neurons to attempt to overcome this lack of functioning receptors by upregulating the number of receptors (Figure 19-11B). That, however, is futile, since nicotine just desensitizes all of them the next time a cigarette is smoked (Figure 19-11C). Furthermore, this upregulation is actually self-defeating, since it serves to amplify the craving that occurs when the extra receptors are resensitizing to their resting state (Figure 19-11C).

From a receptor point of view, the goal of smoking is to desensitize all nicotinic alpha 4 beta 2 receptors, get the maximum DA release, and prevent craving. Positron emission tomography (PET) scans of alpha 4 beta 2 nicotinic receptors in human smokers confirm that nicotinic receptors are exposed to just about enough nicotine for just about long enough from each cigarette to accomplish this. Craving seems to be initiated at the first sign of nicotinic receptor resensitization. Thus, the bad thing about receptor resensitization is craving. The good thing from a smoker's point of view is that as the receptors resensitize, they are available to release more dopamine and cause pleasure again.

Treatment of nicotine addiction

Treating nicotine dependence is not easy. There is evidence that nicotine addiction begins with the first cigarette, with the first dose showing signs of lasting a month in experimental animals (e.g., activation of the anterior cingulate cortex for this long after a single dose). Craving begins within a month of repeated administration. Perhaps even more troublesome is the finding that the "diabolical learning" that occurs from substance abuse of all sorts, including nicotine, may be very, very long-lasting once exposure is stopped. Some evidence suggests that these changes even last a lifetime with a form of "molecular memory" to nicotine, even in long-term-abstinent former smokers. It is quite clear that the 4- to 12-week periods of treatment often employed in testing treatments for addiction are nowhere close to long enough to reverse the molecular changes in the reward circuitry of a nicotine addict.

Currently experts hypothesize that reward conditioning may be very similar to fear conditioning, with both occurring in the amygdala (see Figure 14-40). Just as fear conditioning may be permanently engrained in the amygdala when it occurs, so may reward conditioning. The process of getting over fear is not passive, waiting for the amygdala to "forget," but rather an active one of new learning that inhibits the old. Unfortunately the new learning does not seem to be as strong as the old, and without "practice" and reinforcement of the new learning, it is possible for that new learning to fade away in a process called "renewal forgetting" and thus renewal of fear (see Figure 14-40). By analogy, reward learning may require active learning and active reinforcement of that new learning in order to counter the craving and drug-seeking behavior, even months after the last ingestion of substance. Furthermore, the reward circuitry may always be at risk of "snapping back" into an addicted state due to engrained molecular memories, with only one "slip" and one reuse of the previously abused substance. It may be that one never forgets how to smoke or take any other substance once one is addicted to it. Thus it may not be unreasonable to predict, for substance abuse in general and for nicotine addiction in particular, that treatment periods of more than a year may be required to attain a state of sustained abstinence with reduced risk of relapse. Few available treatments for substance abuse are administered this way, and few studies are available to guide long-term use of these agents.

Thus one of the greatest unmet needs regarding currently available smoking cessation treatments is research about how long to continue treatment after smoking has stopped. Another important gap in smoking cessation therapeutics is that it is not known how

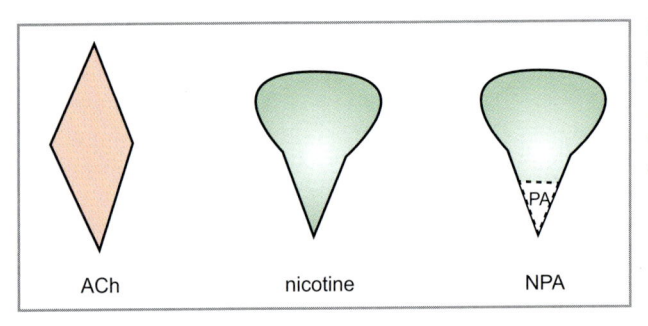

FIGURE 19-12 **Alpha 4 beta 2 agonists and partial agonists.** Shown here are icons for acetylcholine, nicotine, and nicotinic partial agonists (NPAs), all of which bind nicotinic cholinergic receptors.

effective repeat quit attempts are over time. Many patients try to quit smoking and fail. Do additional attempts to quit increase the chances of long-term success in quitting, or are they just futile? What about in psychiatric disorders such as ADHD, schizophrenia, and depression where patients may not only be addicted but also using nicotine to self-medicate their psychiatric disorder? Although many smokers try to quit and fail, the same can be said for learning how to ride a bike or a horse. There is an old saying among horse riders that it takes seven falls to make a rider, so get back up on the horse when you fall. It may also take seven (or more) quit attempts to make a substance abuser a successful quitter, but there is little research on this.

For treating nicotine dependence with psychopharmacological agents, one of the first successful agents proven to be effective is nicotine itself (Figure 19-12), but in a route of administration other than smoking: gums, lozenges, nasal sprays, inhalers, and most notably transdermal patches. Delivering nicotine by these other routes does not produce the high levels or the pulsatile blasts that are delivered to the brain by smoking, so they are not very reinforcing. However, alternative delivery of nicotine can help to reduce craving due to a steady amount of nicotine that is delivered and presumably desensitizes an important number of resensitizing and craving nicotinic receptors.

The leading treatment for nicotine dependence may be the newly introduced nicotinic partial agonist (NPA) varenicline, a selective alpha 4 beta 2 nicotinic acetylcholine receptor partial agonist (Figure 19-12). Figure 19-13 contrasts the effects of NPAs with nicotinic full agonists and with nicotinic antagonists on the cation channel associated with nicotinic cholinergic receptors. Nicotinic full agonists include acetylcholine, a short-acting full agonist, and nicotine, a long-acting full agonist. They open the channel fully and frequently (Figure 19-13, on the left). By contrast, nicotinic antagonists stabilize the channel in the closed state but do not desensitize these receptors (Figure 19-13, on the right). NPAs stabilize nicotinic receptors in an intermediate state, which is not desensitized and where the channel is open less frequently than with a full agonist but more frequently than with an antagonist (Figure 19-13, middle). Varenicline is the first NPA to be approved for smoking cessation in the United States, but it is now known that a plant alkaloid called cytisine and used in eastern Europe for over 40 years for smoking cessation is also an NPA. Its poor brain penetration may limit its efficacy. Another selective alpha 4 beta 2 NPA in clinical testing is dianicline (SSR-591813).

Within the reward circuitry, the important sites of action of the NPA varenicline are at alpha 4 beta 2 sites in the VTA, particularly those receptors located directly on mesolimbic DA neurons (Figure 19-14). These actions are contrasted with those of acetylcholine and nicotine at this same site in Figures 19-15 through 19-17. The full agonist acetylcholine (Figure 19-15) is short-acting because of the ubiquity of the enzyme acetylcholinesterase,

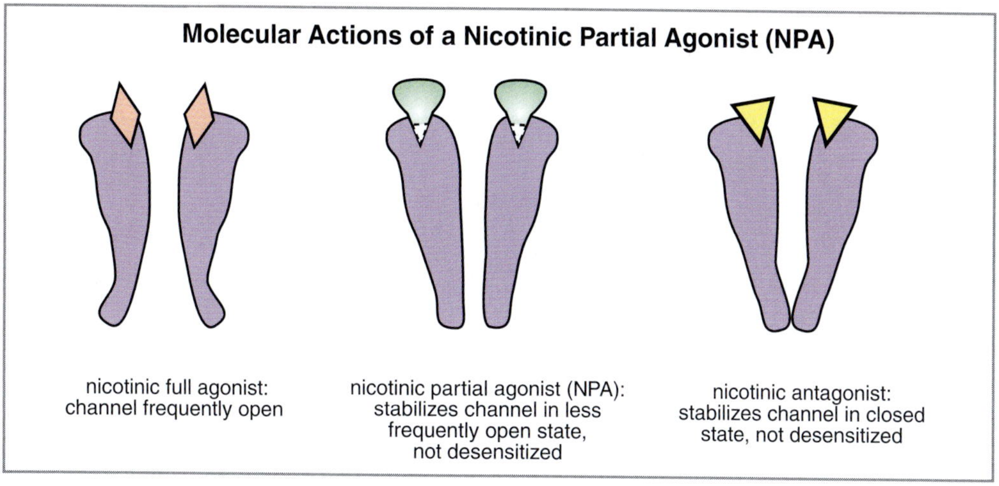

Molecular Actions of a Nicotinic Partial Agonist (NPA)

nicotinic full agonist: channel frequently open

nicotinic partial agonist (NPA): stabilizes channel in less frequently open state, not desensitized

nicotinic antagonist: stabilizes channel in closed state, not desensitized

FIGURE 19-13 Molecular actions of a nicotinic partial agonist (NPA). Full agonists at alpha 4 beta 2 receptors, such as acetylcholine and nicotine, cause the channels to open frequently (left). In contrast, antagonists at these receptors stabilize them in a closed state, such that they do not become desensitized (right). Nicotinic partial agonists (NPAs) stabilize the channels in an intermediate state, causing them to open less frequently than a full agonist but more frequently than an antagonist (middle).

always on the ready to destroy acetylcholine. The actions of acetylcholinesterase are introduced in Chapter 18 and illustrated in Figures 18-13 and 18-22 through 18-27. Because of the short-acting nature of acetylcholine at alpha 4 beta 2 nicotinic receptors on VTA DA neurons, it causes a short burst of action potentials and a similar short pulse of DA release in the nucleus accumbens (Figure 19-15). This is the physiological action of neurotransmitters regulating DA release in the reward pathway. It is the type of DA release associated with a stimulus that is novel, interesting, relevant, or fascinating to the individual. These features of a nondrug stimulus that can provoke the release of neurotransmitters such as acetylcholine and thus a short burst of DA in the nucleus accumbens are sometimes said to be "salient."

When nicotine occupies these same alpha 4 beta 2 nicotinic receptors on DA neurons in the VTA, it causes an abnormally prolonged burst of action potentials until the nicotinic receptor desensitizes (Figure 19-16). Nicotine is long-acting because it is not destroyed by acetylcholinesterase. The prolonged burst of action potentials is accompanied by an abnormally prolonged and supraphysiological release of DA in the nucleus accumbens, creating pleasure until the nicotinic receptors desensitize, and creating craving as the nicotinic receptors begin to resensitize.

Finally, when an NPA like varenicline occupies these receptors, the result is a lower-grade increase in the frequency of action potentials, with consequent sustained but small amounts of DA release (Figure 19-17). Rather than the "glare of spotlights" from the excessive DA release that occurs with nicotine, NPAs have been described as leaving a "night light" of DA on, without desensitizing nicotinic receptors, sufficient to reduce craving but not sufficient to cause euphoria.

Another way to compare the actions of nicotine and NPAs is shown in Figures 19-18 and 19-19. When a person is smoking, nicotine arterial levels and brain levels rise with each puff and fall between puffs (Figure 19-18A). Immediately following the smoking of a single cigarette, nicotine levels are sufficiently high to keep the receptors desensitized for

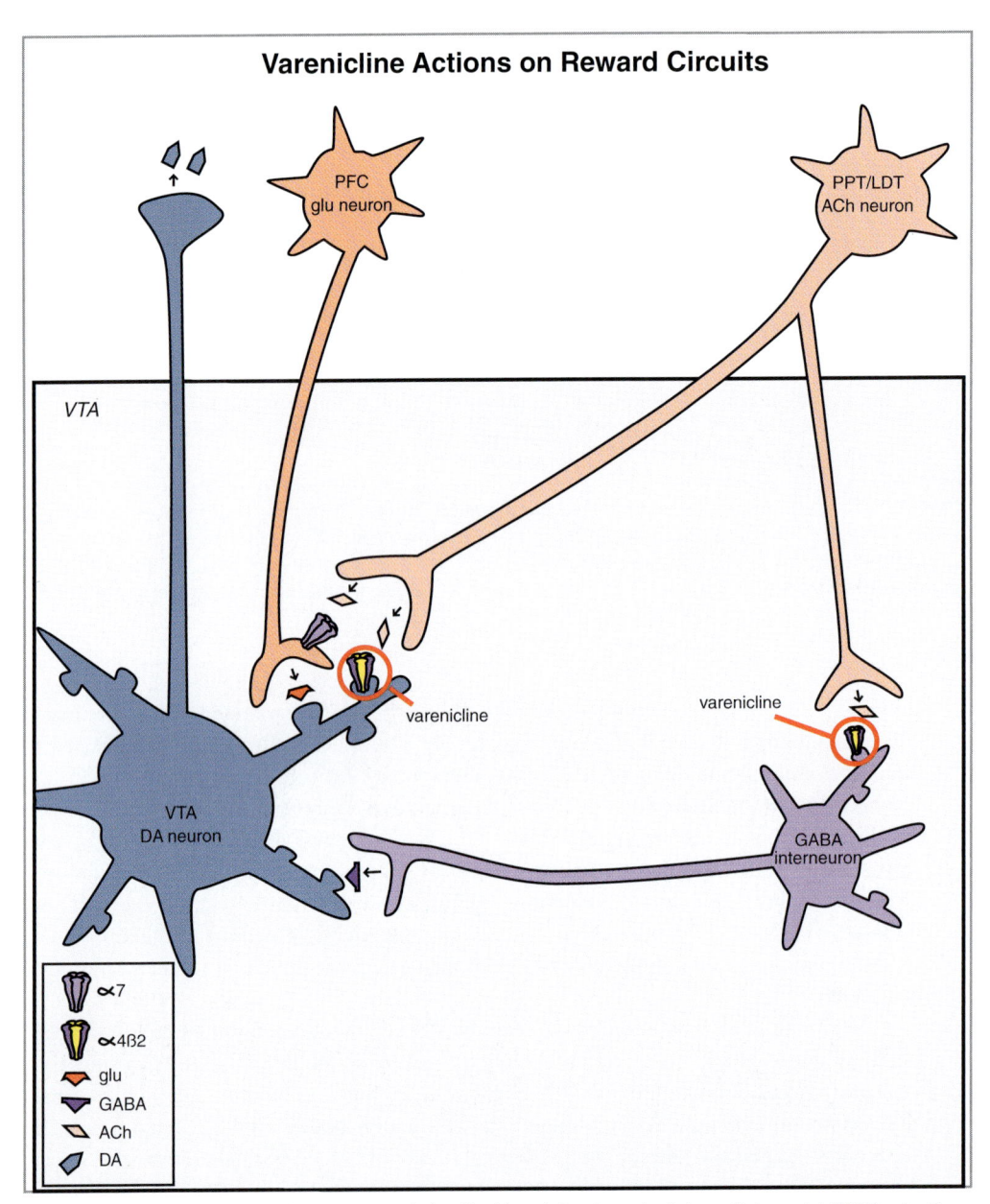

FIGURE 19-14 Varenicline actions on reward circuits. Varenicline is a nicotinic partial agonist (NPA) selective for the alpha 4 beta 2 receptor subtype. Its actions at alpha 4 beta 2 nicotinic receptors – located on dopamine neurons, glutamate neurons, and GABA interneurons in the VTA – are all shown.

a while; but when nicotine levels fall over time, nicotinic receptors begin to resensitize and cause craving. In order to treat the craving without causing euphoria, one approach is to use nicotine in a transdermal delivery system that produces steady levels of nicotine, taking the edge off of craving due to occupying and desensitizing at least some nicotinic receptors (Figure 19-18B). The problem with this approach and related approaches of nicotine gum and inhaled nicotine, etc., is that the level of nicotine achieved at VTA receptors is often not sufficient to reduce craving to a satisfactory level. This leads to impulsive smoking to relieve

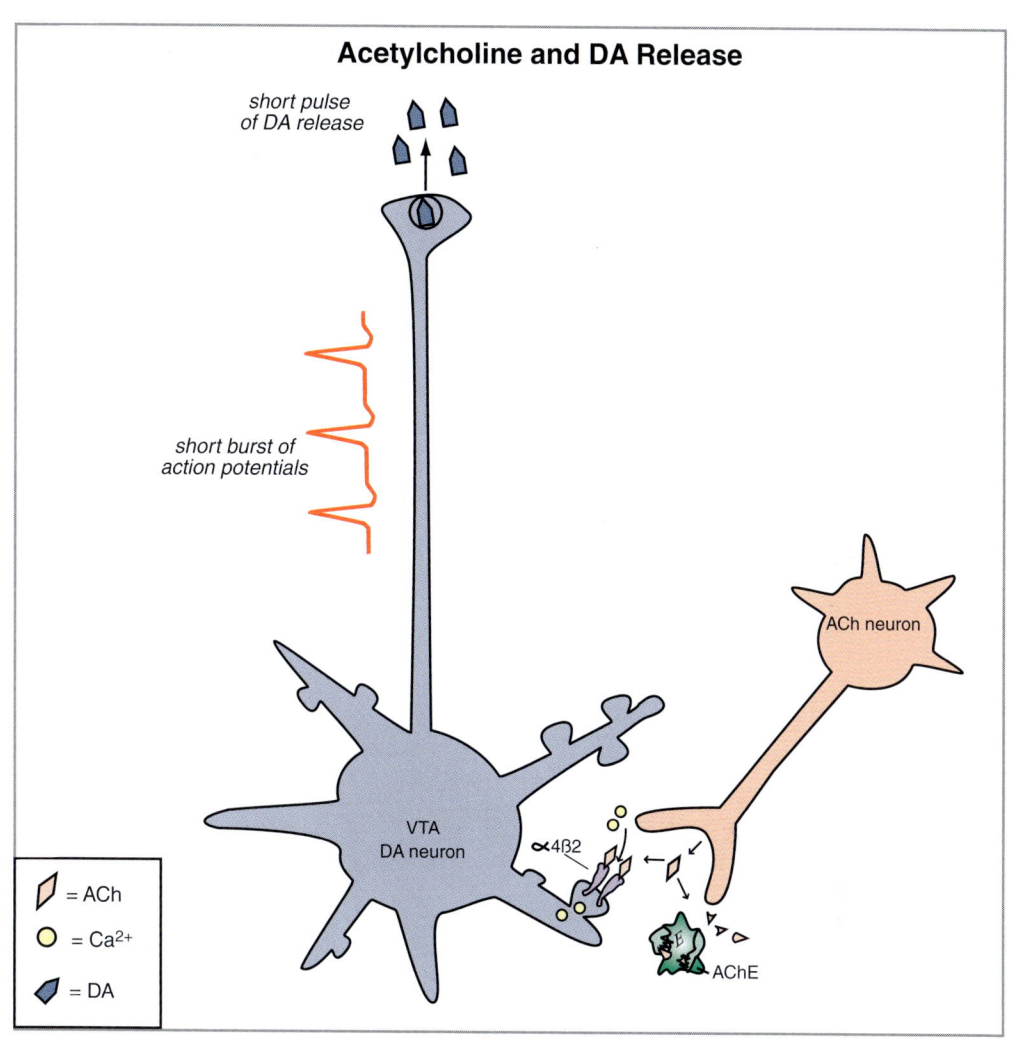

FIGURE 19-15 Acetylcholine and dopamine release. Acetylcholine is a full agonist at alpha 4 beta 2 nicotinic receptors located on dopamine neurons in the ventral tegmental area (VTA); however, it is also short-acting due to its quick breakdown by acetylcholinesterase (AChE). Thus acetylcholine triggers a short burst of action potentials and a resultant short pulse of dopamine release in the nucleus accumbens.

craving. Nicotine replacement therapies can all be "smoked over," meaning that despite receiving nicotine by an alternate route of administration, it is possible to simultaneously smoke in order to achieve pleasure and completely abolish craving (Figure 19-19B). This rather defeats the purpose of the alternate route of nicotine administration.

Contrast this to the actions of NPAs (Figure 19-19). Shown here is the response level of a smoker in withdrawal (Figure 19-19A on the far left) who then has all of his nicotinic receptors partially activated with an NPA (Figure 19-19A on the left), with generally more reduction in craving than can be achieved with subreinforcing levels of transdermal nicotine, shown in Figure 19-18B. Furthermore, when that same smoker is given an NPA while smoking, nicotine delivery via smoking is no longer rewarding, since the alpha 4 beta 2 receptors become occupied by an agent that allows only partial receptor activation. Thus, NPAs cannot be "smoked over" (Figure 19-19B). This can be an important therapeutic

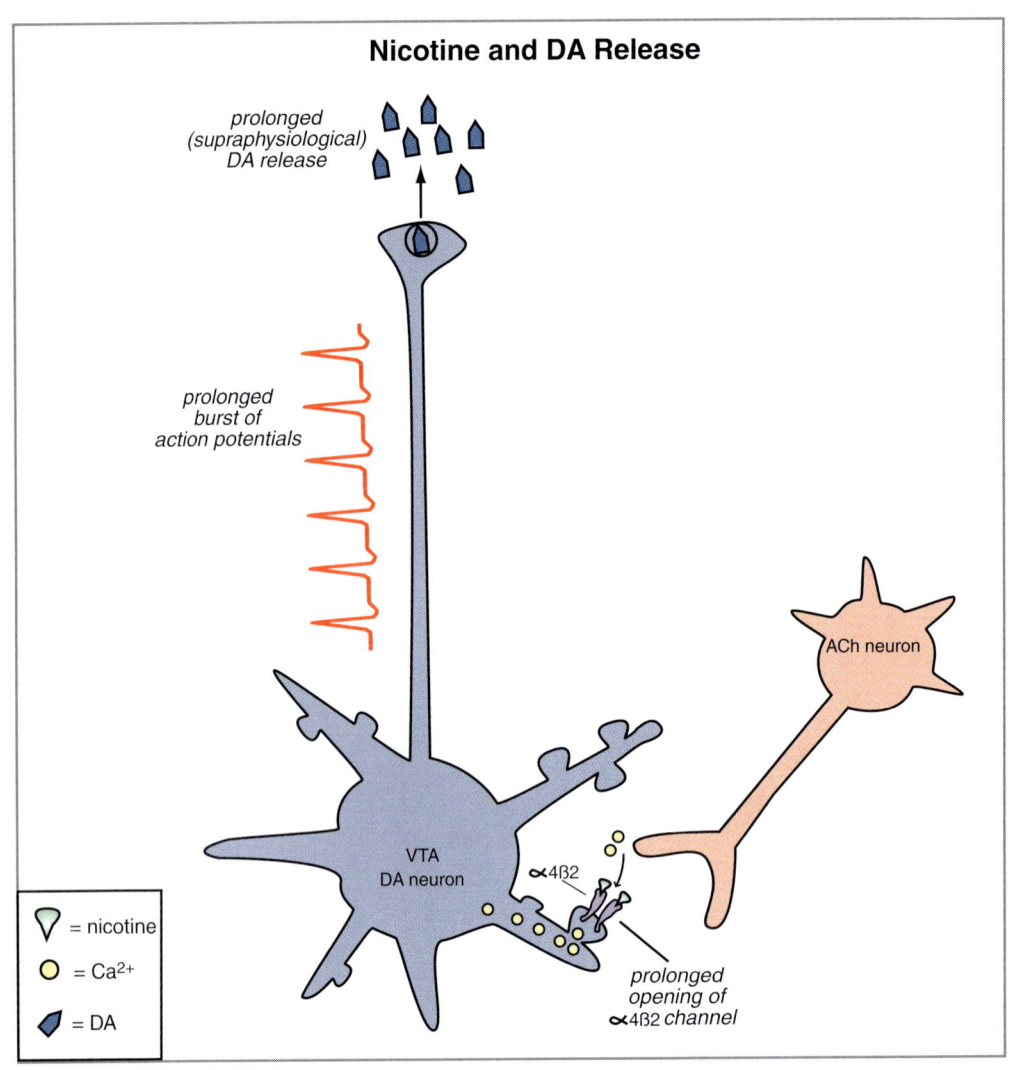

FIGURE 19-16 Nicotine and dopamine release. Nicotine is a full agonist at alpha 4 beta 2 nicotinic receptors located on dopamine neurons in the ventral tegmental area (VTA) and causes prolonged opening of these channels until they desensitize. This results in a prolonged burst of action potentials and consequently prolonged (supraphysiological) dopamine release.

benefit for those taking an NPA who have a sudden impulse to smoke, because if they "slip" and smoke while taking an NPA, they will realize that smoking is not pleasurable to them. Often, by the time the urge to smoke passes, the patient will continue to take the NPA and realize it is not worth smoking (rather than stop the NPA and start smoking).

How addicting is tobacco and how well do NPAs work to achieve cessation of smoking? Figure 19-20 shows that about two thirds of smokers want to quit, one third try, but only 2 or 3 percent succeed. Of all the substances of abuse, some surveys show that tobacco has the highest probability of causing dependency when one has tried it at least once (Table 19-3). It could be argued, therefore, that nicotine might be the most addicting substance known. The good news is that the NPA varenicline triples or quadruples the 1-month, 6-month, and 1-year quit rates compared to placebo (Figure 19-20, on the right). The bad news is that

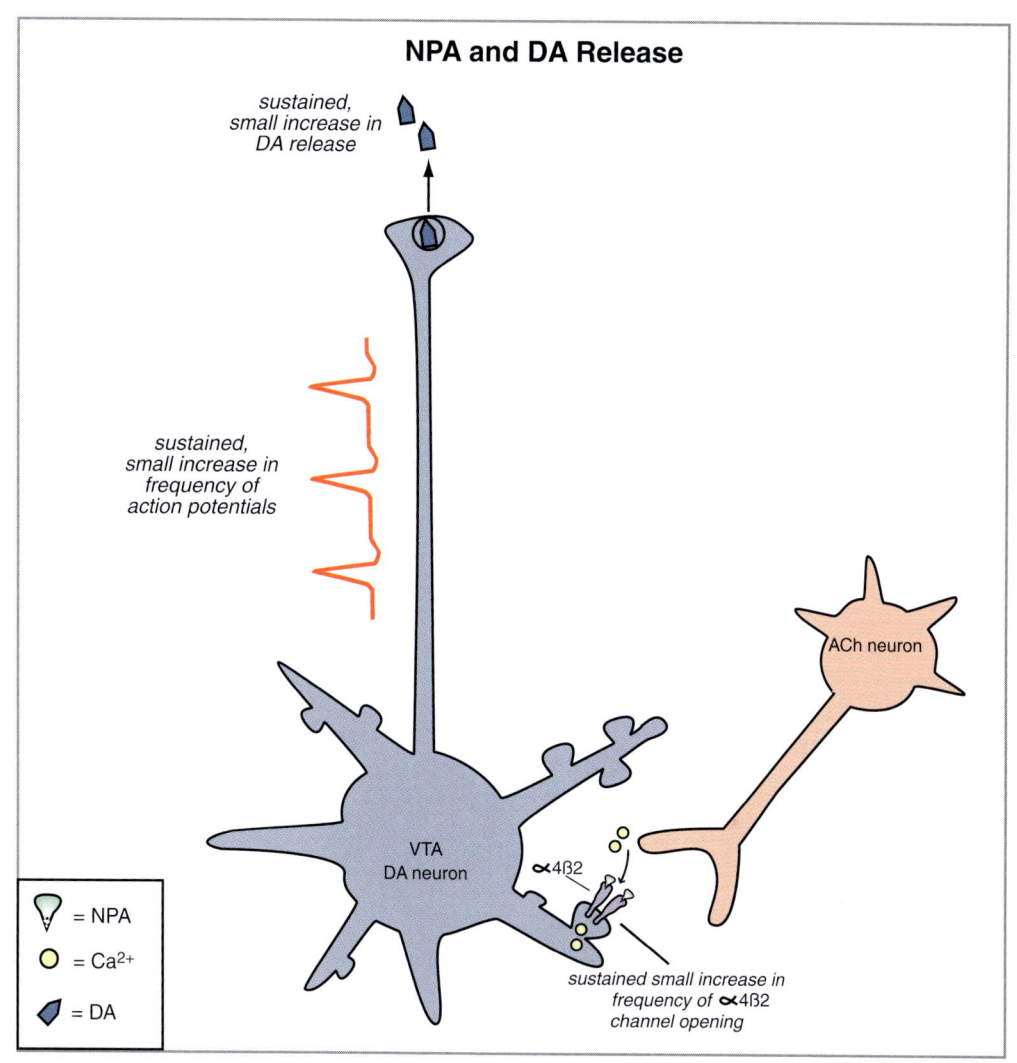

FIGURE 19-17 Nicotinic partial agonists (NPAs) and dopamine release. NPAs cause sustained small increases in the frequency of opening of alpha 4 beta 2 nicotinic receptors in the ventral tegmental area (VTA), which causes sustained small increases in frequency of action potentials and thus sustained small increases in dopamine release.

this means only about 10 percent of smokers taking varenicline are still abstinent a year later (Figure 19-20). Many of these patients are prescribed varenicline for only 12 weeks, which might be far too short a period of time for maximal effectiveness, as mentioned above.

Another approach to the treatment of smoking cessation is to try to reduce the craving that occurs during abstinence by boosting dopamine with the dopamine and norepinephrine reuptake inhibitor (NDRI) bupropion (see Chapter 12 and Figures 12-43 through 12-47). The idea is to give back some of the dopamine downstream to the craving postsynaptic D2 receptors in the nucleus accumbens while they are readjusting to the lack of getting their dopamine "fix" from the recent withdrawal of nicotine (Figure 19-21). Thus, while the individual is smoking, DA is happily released in the nucleus accumbens because of the actions of nicotine on alpha 4 beta 2 receptors on the VTA DA neuron (shown in

Disorders of Reward, Drug Abuse, and Their Treatment | 965

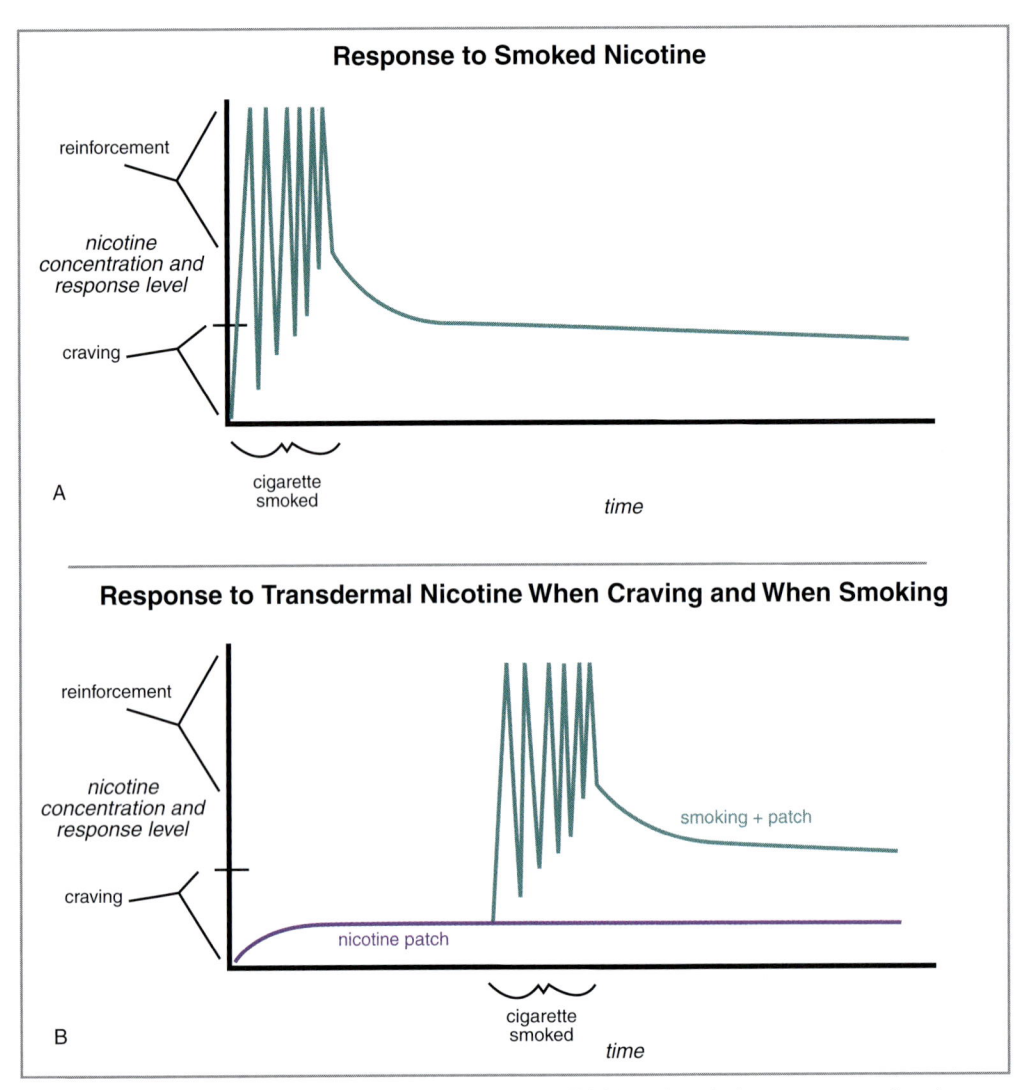

FIGURE 19-18A and B Response to nicotine administration. (A) Shown here is the response over time to nicotine administered through cigarette smoking. With each puff, the nicotine level rises to a pleasurable, reinforcing level. Between puffs, the levels fall, but progressively less so with more puffs. Following smoking a cigarette, nicotine levels are sufficiently high to keep the receptors desensitized for a while; as nicotine levels fall, however, nicotinic receptors begin to resensitize and cause craving. **(B)** Shown here is the response over time to nicotine administered transdermally while craving (i.e., while abstinent from smoking) and also while smoking on top of taking the transdermal nicotine patch. Transdermal delivery of nicotine causes steady levels of nicotine, which may desensitize some receptors and relieve some craving. It does not, however, provide the phasic bursts of dopamine release necessary to induce reinforcement or pleasure, nor is it sufficient to abolish all craving. It is, however, possible to achieve that reinforcement by smoking while using transdermal nicotine, an action that defeats the purpose of the transdermal patch.

Figure 19-21A). During smoking cessation, resensitized nicotinic receptors no longer receiving nicotine are craving due to an absence of DA release in the nucleus accumbens ("Where is my dopamine?" Figure 19-21B). When the NDRI bupropion is administered, theoretically a bit of DA is now released in the nucleus accumbens, making the craving less but usually not eliminating it (Figure 19-21C). Another possible mechanism of action of

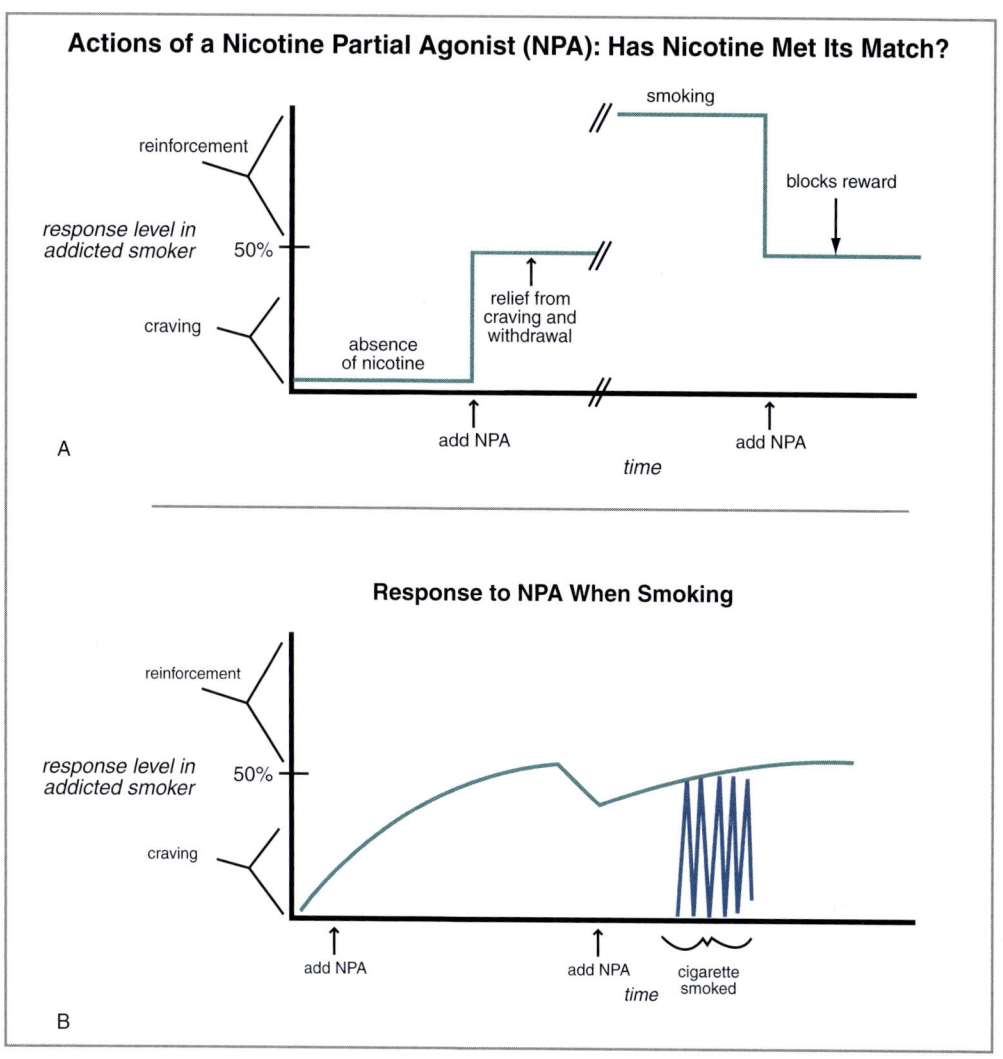

FIGURE 19-19A and B Response to nicotinic partial agonist (NPA). Administration of an NPA in the absence of nicotine causes partial activation of nicotinic receptors and thus leads to a small sustained release of dopamine; however, because the channels open less frequently than they would in the presence of nicotine, the amount and rate of dopamine release is not sufficient to cause reinforcement or pleasure but can be sufficient to significantly reduce craving (**A**). In addition, in the presence of nicotine, an NPA will compete for the nicotinic receptors and thus reduce the effects of nicotine (**A** and **B**).

bupropion that could contribute to its efficacy in smoking cessation is the observation that one of its metabolites is an antagonist of alpha 4 beta 2 nicotinic receptors. How effective is bupropion in smoking cessation? Quit rates for bupropion are about half that of the NPA varenicline (Figure 19-20). Quit rates for nicotine in alternative routes of administration such as transdermal patches are similar to those of bupropion or even less.

A number of other agents are used off label for smoking cessation with variable and usually not very impressive results: oral administration of the MAO-B inhibitor selegiline, the MAO-A inhibitor moclobemide, the opiate antagonist naltrexone, the alpha 2 agonist clonidine, the serotonin 1A partial agonist buspirone, and some tricyclic antidepressants. Novel approaches to treating nicotine addiction include the investigation of nicotine

Disorders of Reward, Drug Abuse, and Their Treatment | 967

TABLE 19-3 How addicting are different substances?

Probability of becoming dependent when you have tried a substance at least once:
Tobacco	32%
Heroin	23%
Cocaine	17%
Alcohol	15%
Stimulants	11%
Anxiolytics	9%
Cannabis	9%
Analgesics	8%
Inhalants	4%

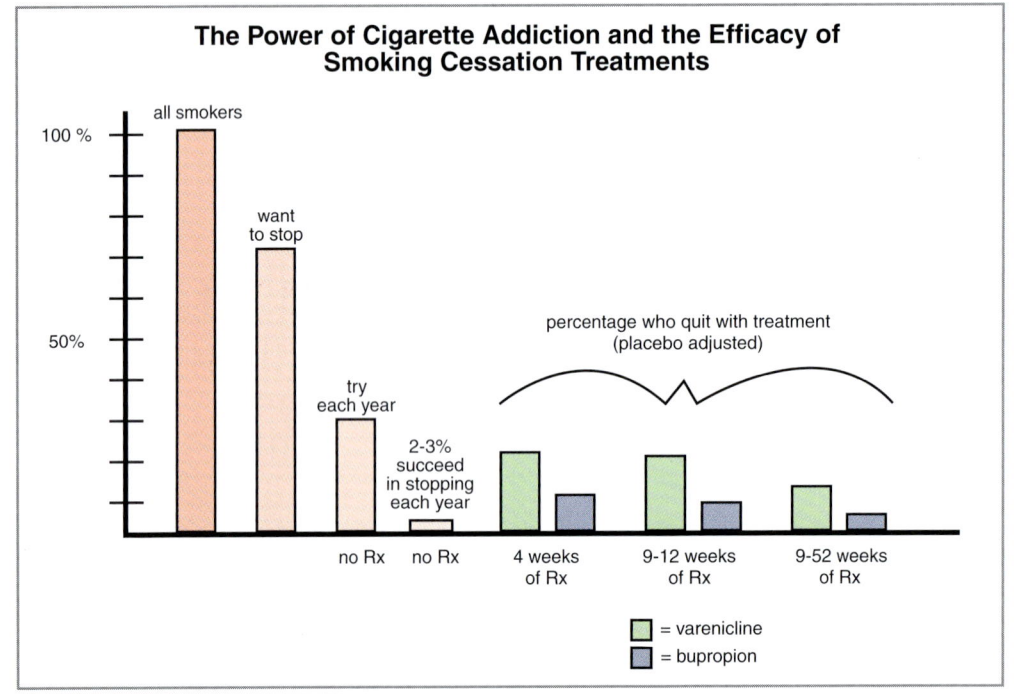

FIGURE 19-20 The power of cigarette addiction and the efficacy of smoking cessation treatments. Although approximately 70 percent of individuals who smoke report that they would like to quit, only about a third try, and only a few percent of quitters are successful in the long term. Success rates are better with treatment than without: the placebo-adjusted success rate with varenicline is about four times that without treatment, and the rate with bupropion is about double that without treatment. Success rates for nicotine replacement therapies (not shown) are the same or less than those for bupropion.

vaccines (NicVAX, TA-NIC, CYT002-NicQb); dopamine D3 receptor partial agonists (RGH188, BP987) or antagonists (NGB2904, SB277011A, ST198); the novel MAO-B inhibitor EVT302; the cannabinoid CB1 receptor antagonist rimonibant; and others.

Alcohol

The painter Vincent Van Gogh reportedly drank ruinously, some speculating that he was self-medicating his bipolar disorder in this way – a notion reinforced by his explanation, "If

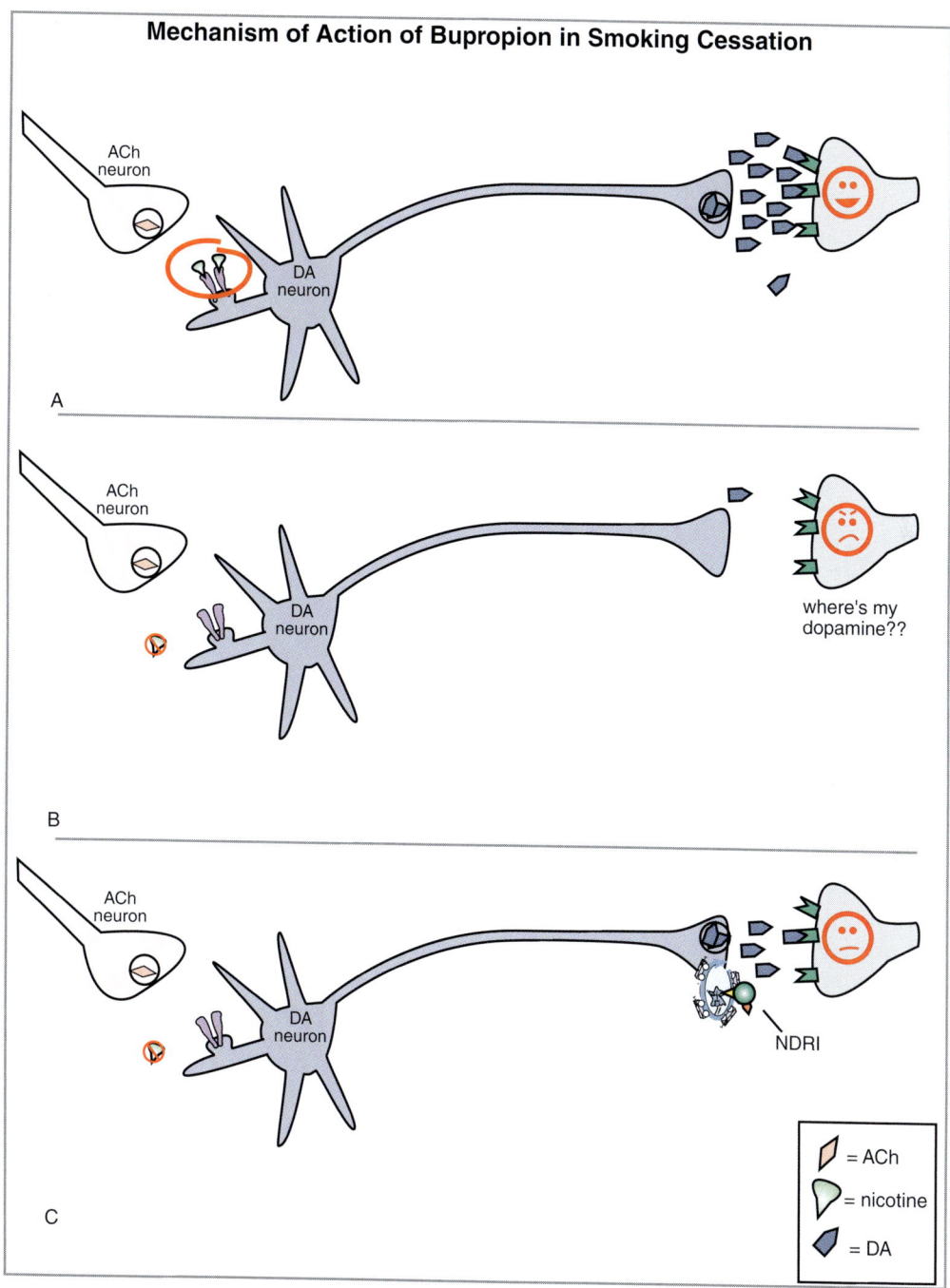

FIGURE 19-21A, B, and C Mechanism of action of bupropion in smoking cessation. (**A**) A regular smoker delivers reliable nicotine (circle), releasing dopamine in the limbic area at frequent intervals, which is very rewarding to the limbic dopamine 2 receptors on the right. (**B**) However, during attempts at smoking cessation, dopamine will be cut off when nicotine no longer releases it from the mesolimbic neurons. This upsets the postsynaptic dopamine 2 limbic receptors and leads to craving and what some call a "nicotine fit." (**C**) A therapeutic approach to diminishing craving during the early stages of smoking cessation is to deliver a bit of dopamine itself by blocking dopamine reuptake directly at the nerve terminal with bupropion. Although not as powerful as nicotine, it does take the edge off and can make abstinence more tolerable.

Disorders of Reward, Drug Abuse, and Their Treatment | 969

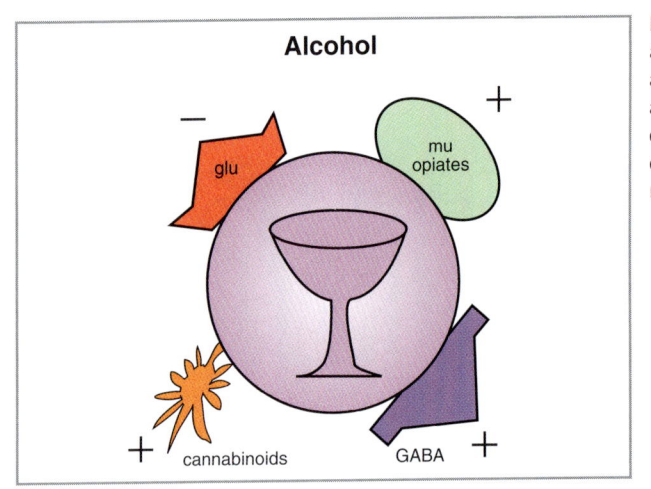

FIGURE 19-22 Icon of alcohol. In addition to enhancing GABA inhibition and reducing glutamate excitation, alcohol also enhances euphoric effects by releasing opiates and endocannabinoids, perhaps thereby mediating its "high."

the storm within gets too loud, I take a glass too much to stun myself." Alcohol may stun but it does not treat psychiatric disorders adaptively in the long term and even has been shown to enhance stress hormones such as corticotropin releasing factor (CRF) and neuropeptide Y. Unfortunately many alcoholics who have comorbid psychiatric disorders continue to self-medicate with alcohol rather than seeking treatment to receive a more appropriate psychopharmacologic agent. In addition to frequent comorbidity with psychiatric disorders, it is estimated that 85 percent of alcoholics also smoke. Usually their alcoholism is tackled first with treatment, and smoking cessation is attempted later if ever. An interesting but almost entirely unanswerable question is: How do you manage alcohol dependence that is comorbid with nicotine dependence? Does continuing to smoke sabotage or enhance the chances of success when a person tries to stop drinking? It is commonly observed anecdotally that substance abusers going through detoxification from one agent such as alcohol will furiously increase, at least in the short term, their use of cigarettes in a possibly partially successful use of a cross-tolerant substance to mitigate craving. Much further research is needed on how to manage comorbidities in alcoholism, in what order to treat them, which has highest priority, and whether different conditions should be treated concomitantly, including the place of smoking cessation in such patients.

Alcohol and reward
The pharmacology of alcohol is still relatively poorly characterized and its mechanism of action is still thought to be somewhat nonspecific, since alcohol can have effects on a wide variety of neurotransmitter systems. However, it is generally accepted that alcohol acts not only by enhancing inhibitory neurotransmission at GABA synapses but also by reducing excitatory neurotransmission at glutamate synapses (Figures 19-22 through 19-24). That is, alcohol enhances inhibition and reduces excitation, which may explain its characterization as a "depressant" of CNS neuronal functioning (Figure 19-22). These effects of alcohol may thus explain some of its intoxicating, amnestic, and ataxic effects.

Alcohol's reinforcing effects are theoretically mediated by its effects specifically on mesolimbic reward circuitry (Figures 19-23 and 19-24). This includes not only actions at GABA and glutamate synapses and receptors but also direct or indirect actions at opiate and cannabinoid synapses and receptors (Figures 19-22 and 19-23). Actions of alcohol in the VTA that both inhibit glutamate and enhance GABA effects are shown in

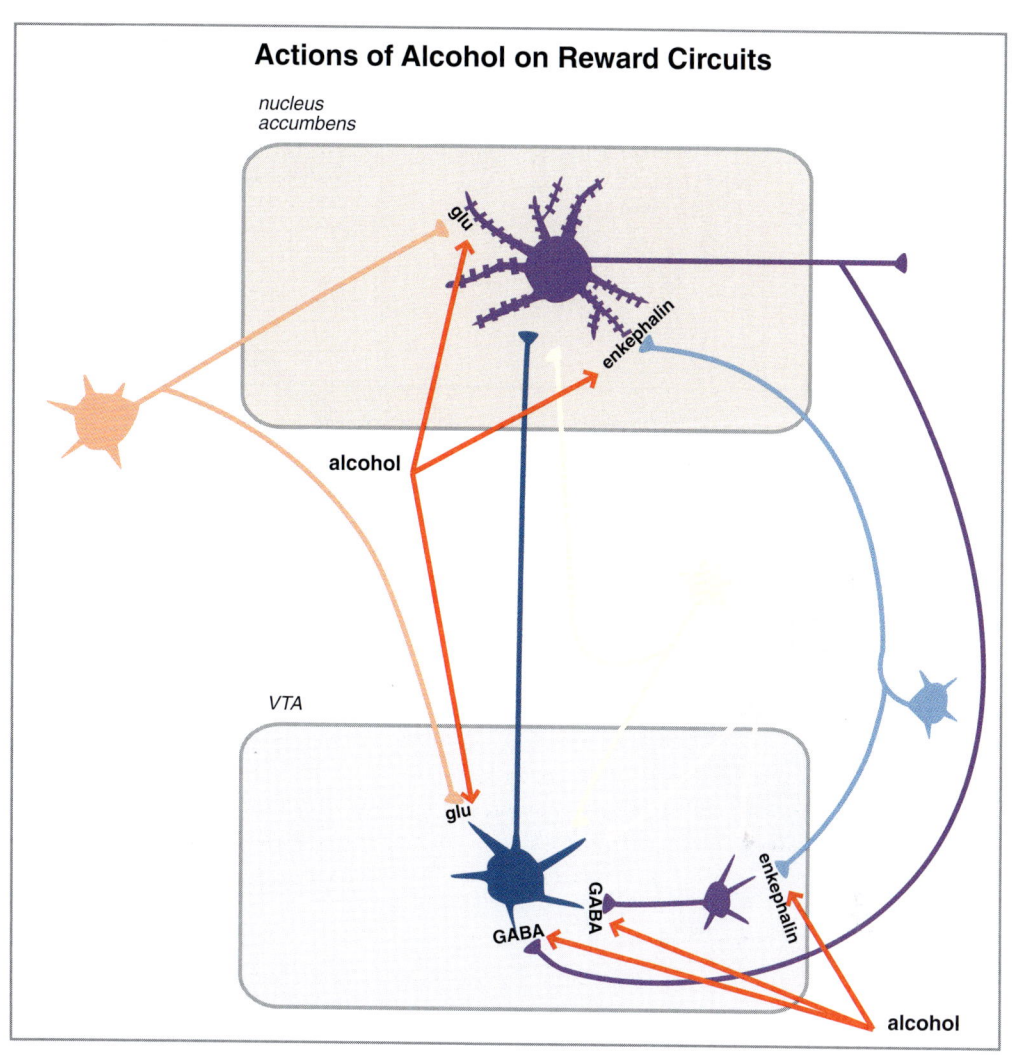

FIGURE 19-23 Actions of alcohol on reward circuits. Shown here is the reactive reward system consisting of the ventral tegmental area (VTA), site of dopamine cell bodies and area where many neurotransmitters project; the nucleus accumbens, to which dopaminergic neurons project; and the amygdala (far left), which has connections with both the VTA and the nucleus accumbens. Alcohol enhances GABA neurotransmission in the VTA and reduces glutamate neurotransmission in the VTA and nucleus accumbens. In addition, alcohol causes either direct or indirect stimulation of both opiate and cannabinoid receptors in the VTA and nucleus accumbens.

Figure 19-24. That is, alcohol acts at presynaptic metabotrophic glutamate receptors (mGluR) and presynaptic voltage-sensitive calcium channels to inhibit glutamate release (Figure 19-24). mGluRs are introduced in Chapter 9, listed in Table 9-11, and illustrated in Figure 9-36. Voltage-sensitive calcium channels and their role in glutamate release are introduced in Chapter 5 and illustrated in Figures 5-33 to 5-37 and 5-41. Alcohol may also have some direct or indirect effects on reducing the actions of glutamate at postsynaptic NMDA receptors and at postsynaptic mGlu receptors (Figure 19-24).

Alcohol's actions at GABA synapses are to enhance GABA release via blocking presynaptic GABA-B receptors; it also acts at postsynaptic GABA-A receptors, especially those of the delta subtype, which are responsive to neurosteroid modulation but not to

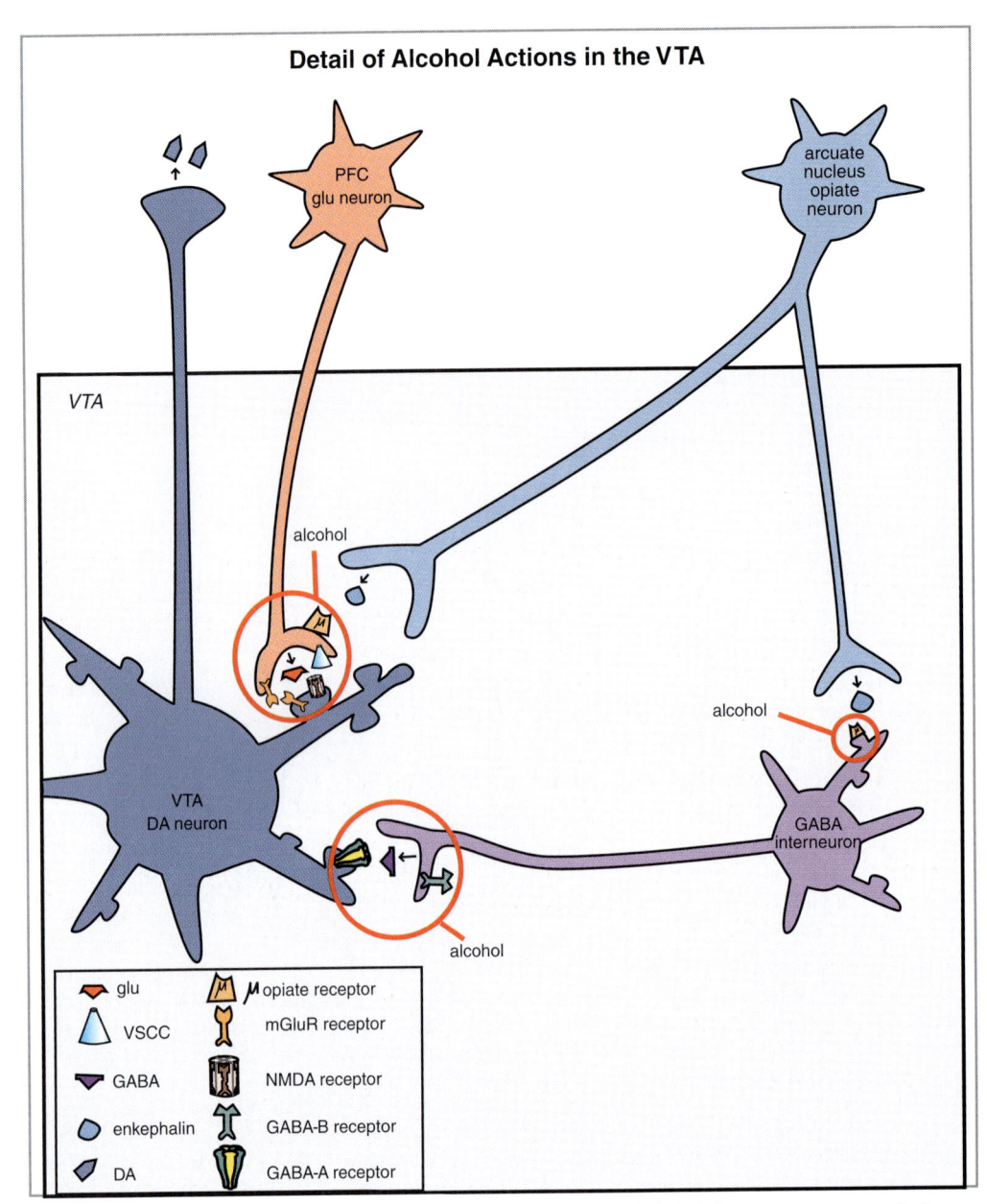

FIGURE 19-24 Detail of alcohol actions in the ventral tegmental area (VTA). Opiate neurons synapse in the VTA with GABA-ergic interneurons and with presynaptic nerve terminals of glutamate neurons. Inhibitory actions of opiates at mu opioid receptors there cause disinhibition of dopamine release in the nucleus accumbens. Alcohol either directly acts upon mu receptors or causes release of endogenous opiates such as enkephalin. Alcohol also acts at presynaptic metabotrophic glutamate receptors (mGluRs) and presynaptic voltage-sensitive calcium channels (VSCCs) to inhibit glutamate release. Finally, alcohol enhances GABA release by blocking presynaptic GABA-B receptors and through direct or indirect actions at GABA-A receptors.

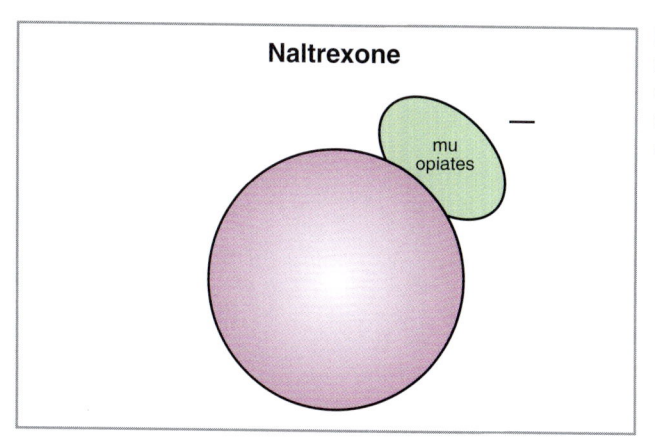

FIGURE 19-25 Icon of naltrexone. Shown here is the icon for naltrexone, which blocks mu opioid receptors and is used in the treatment of alcohol dependence.

benzodiazepine modulation, either via direct actions or by releasing neurosteroids (Figure 19-24). Delta subtypes of GABA-A receptors are discussed in Chapter 14 and illustrated in Figures 14-20 and 14-21. Delta subtypes of GABA-A receptors are also discussed later in this chapter in the section on sedative hypnotics and illustrated in Figure 19-38.

Alcohol's actions at opiate receptors are also shown in Figure 19-24. Opiate neurons arise in the arcuate nucleus and project to the VTA, synapsing on both glutamate and GABA neurons. The net result of alcohol actions on opiate synapses is thought to be the release of DA in the nucleus accumbens (Figure 19-24). Alcohol may do this either by directly acting upon mu opiate receptors or by releasing endogenous opiates such as enkephalin. These actions of alcohol create the rationale for blocking mu opiate receptors with antagonists such as naltrexone (Figures 19-25 and 19-26).

Not shown in Figure 19-24 is the presence of presynaptic cannabinoid receptors at both glutamate and GABA synapses, where alcohol may also have some actions. Presynaptic cannabinoids are represented in Figure 19-2 and the putative actions of alcohol on cannabinoid receptors are shown within the alcohol icon in Figure 19-22. Cannabinoid antagonists such as rimonabant, which blocks CB1 receptors, can reduce alcohol consumption and reduce craving in animals dependent upon alcohol; it is in testing for this use in patients with alcoholism.

Treatment of alcohol dependence, alcohol abuse, and heavy drinking

Several therapeutic agents exploit the known pharmacology of alcohol and are approved for treating alcohol dependence. One of these, naltrexone, blocks mu opiate receptors (Figures 19-25 and 19-26). As for opiate abuse, mu opiate receptors theoretically also contribute to the euphoria and "high" of heavy drinking. It is therefore not surprising that a mu opiate antagonist would block the enjoyment of heavy drinking and increase abstinence by its actions upon reward circuitry (Figure 19-26). This theory is supported by clinical trials showing that naltrexone not only increases the chances of attaining complete abstinence from alcohol but also reduces heavy drinking.

What is "heavy drinking" and how is this contrasted with the idea of "reduced-risk drinking" (Table 19-4)? The idea here is that on the road to recovery, heavy drinkers might first reduce their drinking before they become abstinent. Although this concept has been widely rejected by many alcohol experts, the pharmacology of opiate antagonists and the results from clinical trials of naltrexone in alcohol dependence suggest that the idea might deserve fresh consideration. That is, heavy drinking is defined as five or more drinks per

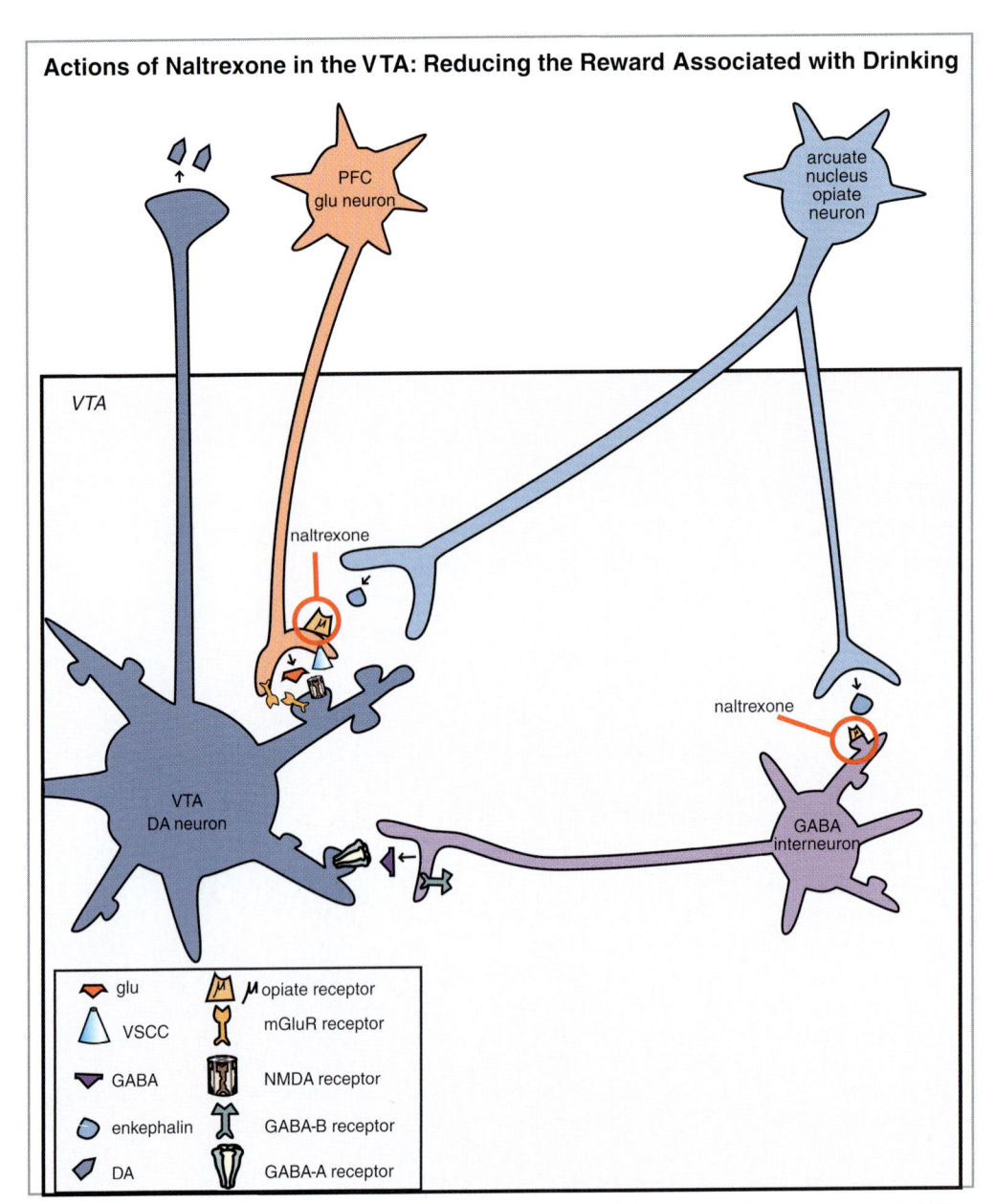

FIGURE 19-26 Actions of naltrexone in the ventral tegmental area. Opiate neurons form synapses in the VTA with GABA-ergic interneurons and with presynaptic nerve terminals of glutamate neurons. Alcohol either acts directly upon mu receptors or causes release of endogenous opiates such as enkephalin; in either case, the result is increased dopamine release to the nucleus accumbens. Naltrexone is a mu opiate receptor antagonist; thus it blocks the pleasurable effects of alcohol mediated by mu opiate receptors.

day for a man and four or more for a woman (Table 19-4). Reduced-risk drinking entails not only drinking less than this but also avoiding certain pathological behavioral patterns of drinking (Table 19-4). Some patients who drink heavily become abstinent with the mu opiate antagonist naltrexone, but others have fewer episodes of heavy drinking, and when they drink convert to reduced-risk drinking. Are these results desirable or sustainable? Will

Essential Psychopharmacology

TABLE 19-4 What is reduced-risk drinking?

Men:	3–4 drinks per day; maximum 16 drinks per week (heavy drinking is >5 drinks/day)
Women:	2–3 drinks per day; maximum 12 drinks per week (heavy drinking is >4 drinks/day)

Avoid having more than one drink in an hour
Avoid drinking patterns (same people, same location, same time of day)
Avoid drinking to deal with problems

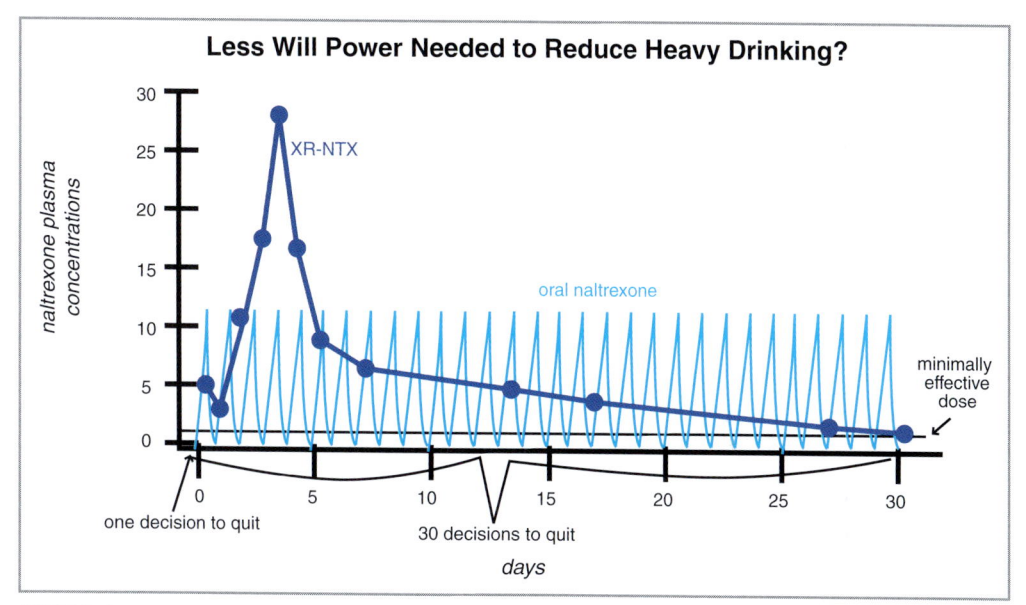

FIGURE 19-27 **Naltrexone formulations.** Naltrexone is a mu opiate receptor antagonist that can reduce the pleasurable effects of drinking and thus is used in the treatment of alcohol dependence. It is available in both an oral formulation and as a once-monthly intramuscular injection. One of the complicating factors in treating substance dependence with substances is that one has to renew the decision to quit at each dosing point. Thus, with oral naltrexone, one must decide daily whether or not to continue the attempt. Because the injection is taken only once a month, this option may require less will power to refrain from heavy drinking.

patients with reduced-risk drinking on naltrexone eventually become abstinent? Unfortunately, there are not sufficient long-term studies to answer these questions.

Outcomes for patients with alcohol dependence who take naltrexone may be more favorable when naltrexone is administered once monthly by intramuscular injection in the form of XR-naltrexone (Figure 19-27). That may be because this method of drug administration forces compliance for at least a month (Figure 19-27). Monthly rather than daily drug administration may be just what the reward circuitry needs for someone with a substance abuse problem. As discussed above and illustrated in Figure 19-7, patients addicted to various substances lose their ability to make rational decisions and instead respond immediately and impulsively to the desire to seek drugs, and they have a vast capacity for denial of the maladaptive nature of their decisions – all outcomes consistent with the notion of a hyperactive reactive reward system (Figures 19-3, 19-5 through 19-7, and 19-8A) and

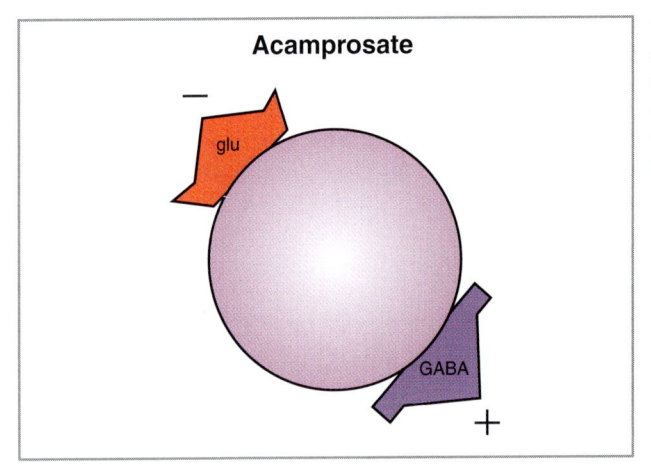

FIGURE 19-28 Icon of acamprosate. Acamprosate is a derivative of the amino acid taurine and, like alcohol, both reduces excitatory glutamate neurotransmission and enhances inhibitory GABA neurotransmission.

deficient inhibition from the reflective reward system (Figures 19-4, 19-7 and 19-8A). It is hard enough to get a patient with a substance abuse disorder to enter treatment or take medications at all, let alone making that person decide every day not only to stay abstinent but also to take a medication (Figure 19-27). Addiction and human nature being what they are, it is not surprising that patients frequently drop out of treatment and resume substance abuse.

If you drink when you take naltrexone, the opiates released do not lead to pleasure, so why bother drinking? Of course, some patients may also say why bother taking naltrexone and relapse back into drinking. However, if you have been given an injection that lasts for a month, have an irresistible impulse to drink, and you "slip" and start to drink, you are not able to discontinue your naltrexone. Thus, if you "drink over" your naltrexone, you may discover that you do not get the usual buzz or enjoyment and therefore might stop after a few drinks. You might even become abstinent again for several days. This is a bit like the situation described above for learning how to ride and falling off the horse seven times before becoming a rider.

Evidently this concept has not greatly captured the imagination of the psychopharmacology community, because there is little use of naltrexone orally or even in the monthly drug delivery system that seems tailor-made for a deficient reflective reward system. The therapeutic nihilism for treatment of alcoholism with available psychopharmacological agents is unfortunately high, just as it is for smoking. Nalmefene is another mu opioid antagonist that is also being tested in alcoholics to determine whether it increases abstinence rates.

Therapeutic nihilism also applies to a great extent to the use of other agents approved for treating alcohol dependence, including acamprosate (Figure 19-28), whose U.S. manufacturer has greatly curtailed promotional efforts due to lack of uptake of this agent by the psychopharmacology community. Acamprosate is a derivative of the amino acid taurine and interacts with both the glutamate system to inhibit it and with the GABA system to enhance it; it is somewhat like a form of "artificial alcohol" (compare Figures 19-28 and 19-22). Thus when alcohol is taken chronically and then withdrawn, the adaptive changes that it causes in both the glutamate system and the GABA system create a state of glutamate overexcitement and even excitotoxicity as well as GABA deficiency. Too much glutamate can cause neuronal damage, as discussed in Chapter 2 and illustrated in Figures 2-35 and 2-36 and also in Chapter 9 and illustrated in Figures 9-46 to 9-52.

To the extent that acamprosate can substitute for alcohol during withdrawal, the actions of acamprosate mitigate the glutamate hyperactivity and the GABA deficiency (Figure 19-29). This occurs because acamprosate appears to have direct blocking actions on certain glutamate receptors, particularly mGlu receptors (specifically mGlu5 and perhaps mGlu2). One way or another, acamprosate apparently reduces the glutamate release associated with alcohol withdrawal (Figure 19-29). Actions, if any, at NMDA receptors may be indirect, as are actions at GABA systems, both of which may be secondary downstream effects from acamprosate's actions on mGlu receptors (Figure 19-29).

Disulfiram is the classic drug for treating alcoholism. It is an irreversible inhibitor of aldehyde dehydrogenase, and when alcohol is ingested, results in the buildup of toxic levels of acetaldehyde. This creates an aversive experience, with flushing, nausea, vomiting, and hypotension, hopefully conditioning the patient to a negative rather than positive response to drinking. Obviously, compliance is a problem with this agent, and the aversive reactions it causes are occasionally dangerous.

Experimental agents that show some promise in treating alcohol dependence include the anticonvulsant topiramate (introduced in Chapter 13 and illustrated in Figure 13-19). Presumably, its actions on glutamate neurotransmission may reduce positive reinforcement and reduce craving. 5HT3 antagonists such as ondansetron have been tested with some interesting preliminary results in alcohol dependence, as has the cannabinoid CB1 receptor antagonist rimonabant. Some evidence points to the possibility that atypical antipsychotics such as olanzapine may reduce craving and alcohol consumption even in those who are alcohol dependent but not comorbid for schizophrenia.

The subject of how to treat alcohol abuse and dependence is obviously complex, and the psychopharmacological treatments are most effective when integrated with structured therapies such as 12-step programs, a topic beyond the scope of this text. Hopefully, clinicians will learn how to better leverage the various treatments for alcoholism available today and determine whether they can be used to treat this devastating illness to attain far better outcomes than are available when no treatment is provided, accepted, or sustained.

Opiates

Opiates and reward

Opiates act as neurotransmitters released from neurons that arise in the arcuate nucleus and project both to the VTA and to the nucleus accumbens and release enkephalin (Figure 19-30). Naturally occurring endogenous opiates act upon a variety of receptor subtypes. The three most important receptor subtypes are the mu, delta, and kappa opiate receptors (Figure 19-31). The brain makes a variety of its own endogenous opiate-like substances, sometimes referred to as the "brain's own morphines." These are all peptides derived from precursor proteins called POMC (pro-opiomelanocortin), proenkephalin, and prodynorphin (Figure 19-31). Parts of these precursor proteins are cleaved off to form endorphins or enkephalins, stored in opiate neurons and presumably released during neurotransmission to mediate endogenous opiate-like actions, including a role in mediating reinforcement and pleasure in reward circuitry (Figures 19-30 and 19-31).

Exogenous opiates in the form of pain relievers (such as codeine or morphine) or drugs of abuse (such as heroin) are also thought to act as agonists at mu, delta, and kappa opiate receptors, particularly at mu sites. At and above pain-relieving doses, the opiates induce euphoria, which is their main reinforcing property. Opiates can also induce a very intense but brief euphoria, sometimes called a "rush," followed by a profound sense of tranquility,

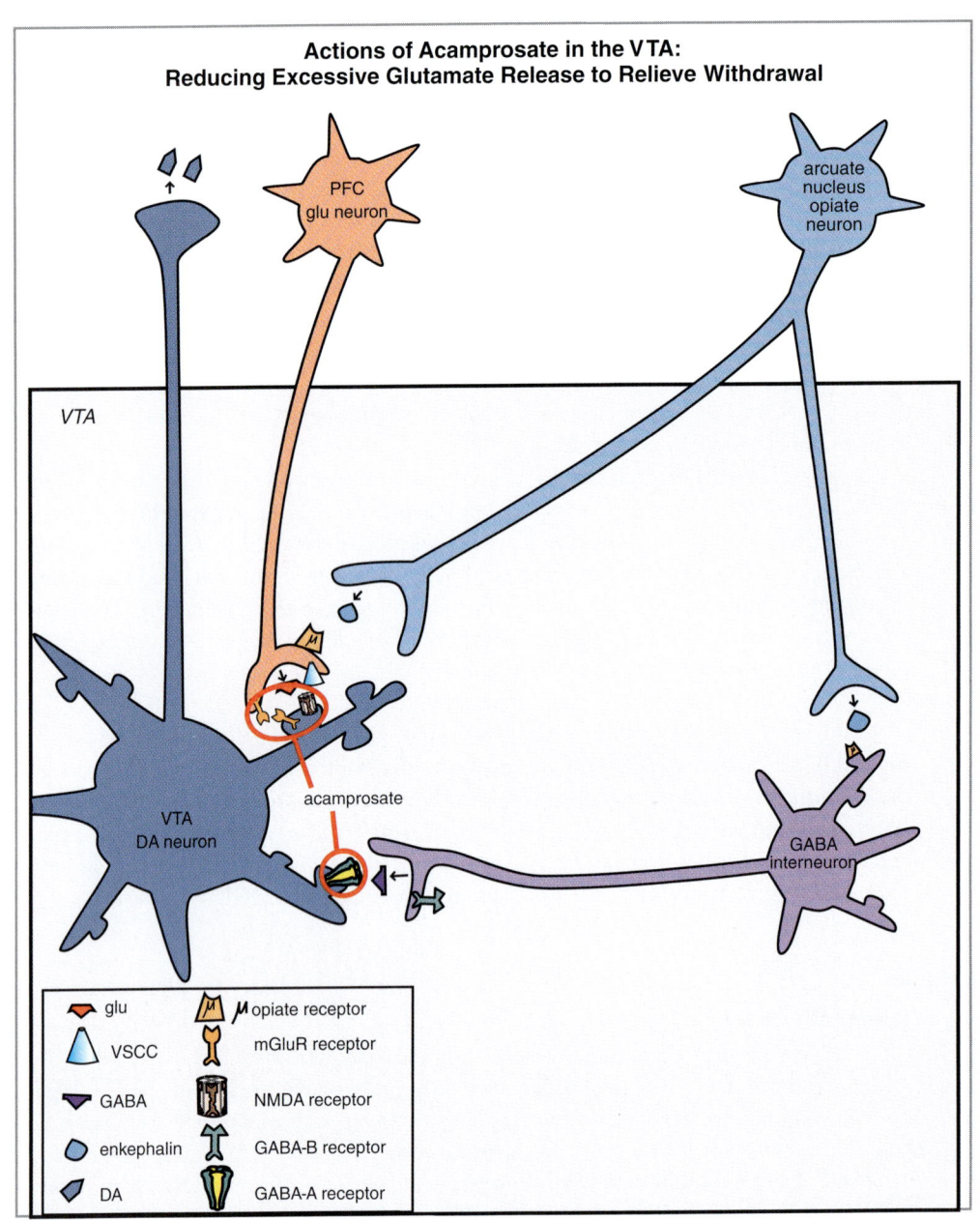

FIGURE 19-29 **Actions of acamprosate in the ventral tegmental area (VTA).** Acamprosate seems to block glutamate receptors, particularly metabotrophic glutamate receptors (mGluRs) and perhaps also N-methyl-d-aspartate (NMDA) receptors. When alcohol is taken chronically and then withdrawn, the adaptive changes that it causes in both the glutamate system and the GABA system create a state of glutamate overexcitation as well as GABA deficiency. By blocking glutamate receptors, acamprosate may thus mitigate glutamate hyperexcitability during alcohol withdrawal.

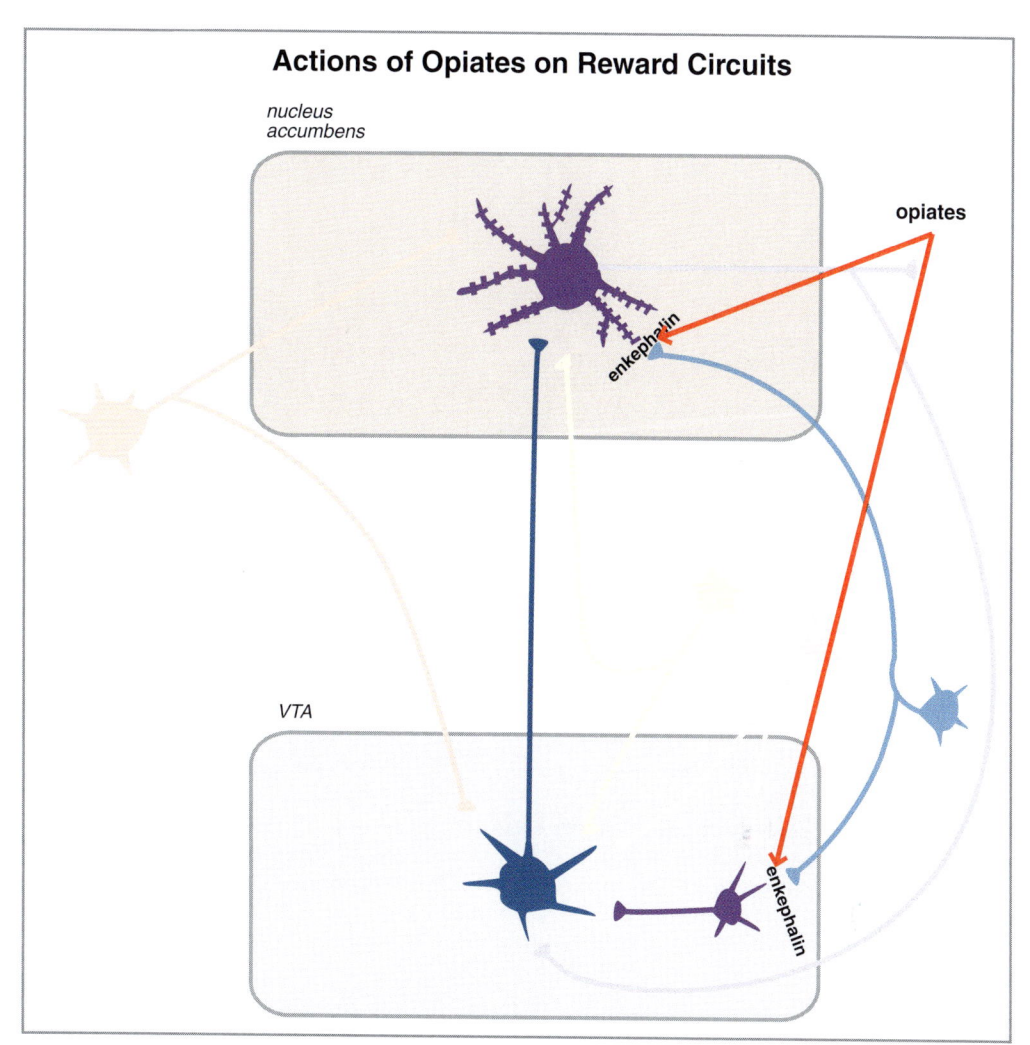

FIGURE 19-30 Actions of opiates on reward circuits. Neurons originating in the arcuate nucleus project to both the ventral tegmental area (VTA), site of dopamine cell bodies and also where many neurotransmitters project, and the nucleus accumbens, to which dopaminergic neurons project. Opiate neurons release endogenous opiates such as enkephalin.

which may last several hours, followed in turn by drowsiness ("nodding"), mood swings, mental clouding, apathy, and slowed motor movements. In overdose, these same agents act as depressants of respiration and can also induce coma. The acute actions of opiates can be reversed by synthetic opiate antagonists such as naloxone and naltrexone, which compete as antagonists at opiate receptors.

When given chronically, opiates easily cause both tolerance and dependence. Adaptation of opiate receptors occurs quite readily after chronic opiate administration. The first sign of this is the patient's need to take higher and higher doses of opiate in order to relieve pain or induce the desired euphoria. Eventually, there may be little room between the dose that causes euphoria and that which produces the toxic effects of an overdose. Another sign that dependence has occurred and that opiate receptors have adapted by decreasing their sensitivity to agonist actions is the production of a withdrawal syndrome once the

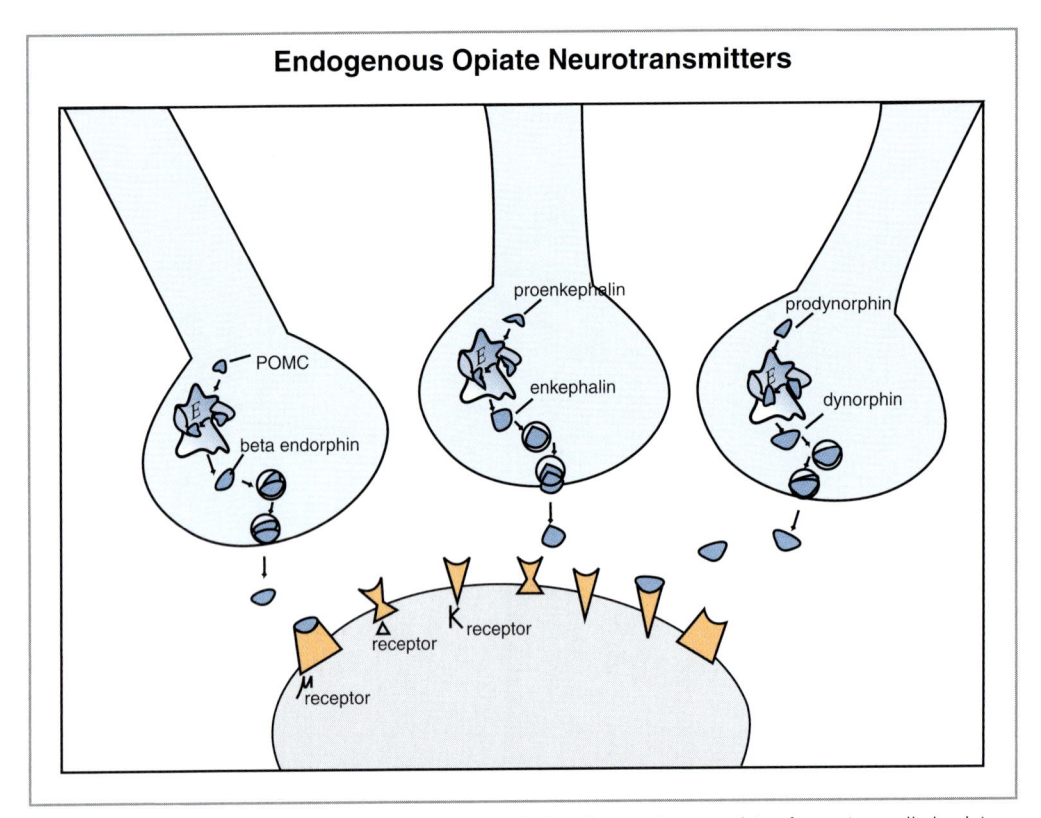

FIGURE 19-31 Endogenous opiate neurotransmitters. Opiate drugs act on a variety of receptors called opiate receptors, the most important of which are mu, delta, and kappa. Endogenous opiate-like substances are peptides derived from precursor proteins called POMC (pro-opiomelanocortin), proenkephalin, and prodynorphin. Parts of these precursor proteins are cleaved off to form endorphins, enkephalins, or dynorphin, which are then stored in opiate neurons and presumably released during neurotransmission to mediate reinforcement and pleasure.

chronically administered opiate wears off. Opiate antagonists such as naloxone can precipitate a withdrawal syndrome in opiate-dependent persons. This syndrome is characterized by feelings of dysphoria, craving for another dose of opiate, irritability, and signs of autonomic hyperactivity such as tachycardia, tremor, and sweating. Piloerection ("goose bumps") is often associated with opiate withdrawal, especially when a drug is stopped suddenly ("cold turkey"). This is so subjectively horrible that the opiate abuser will often stop at nothing in order to get another dose of opiate to relieve such symptoms. Thus, what may have begun as a quest for euphoria may end up as a quest to avoid withdrawal. Clonidine, an alpha 2 adrenergic agonist, can reduce signs of autonomic hyperactivity during withdrawal and aid in the detoxification process.

In the early days of opiate use/abuse/intoxication and prior to the completion of the neuroadaptive mechanisms that mediate opiate receptor desensitization, opiate intoxication in the abuser alternates with normal functioning. Later, after the opiate receptors adapt and the person becomes dependent, he or she may experience very little euphoria but mostly a state of lack of withdrawal alternating with the presence of withdrawal.

Treatment of opiate dependence
Opiate receptors can readapt to normal if given a chance to do so in the absence of additional intake of drug. This may be too difficult to tolerate, so reinstituting another opiate,

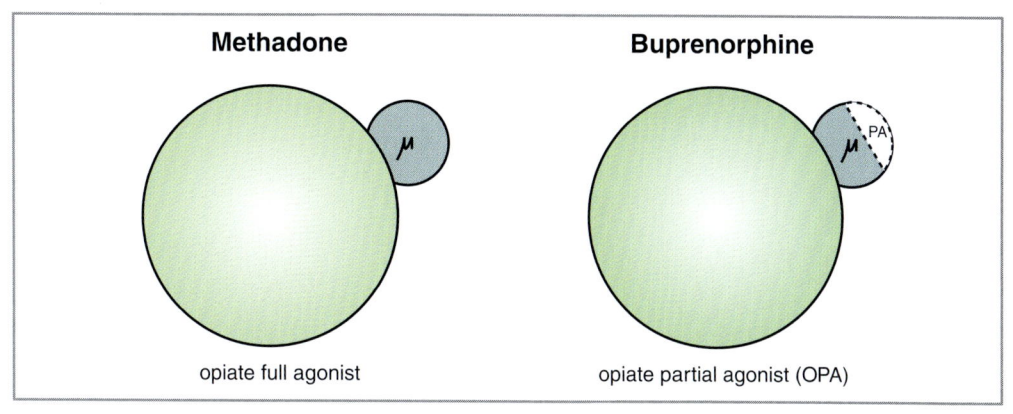

FIGURE 19-32 Icons of methadone and buprenorphine. Methadone, a full agonist at opiate receptors, and buprenorphine, a partial agonist at opiate receptors, are both used during detoxification from exogenous opiates such as codeine, morphine, and heroin.

such as methadone, which can be taken orally and then slowly tapered, may assist in the detoxification process (Figure 19-32). A partial mu opiate agonist, buprenorphine, now available in a sublingual dosage formulation combined with naloxone, can also substitute for stronger full agonist opiates and then be tapered. It is combined with the opiate naloxone, which does not get absorbed orally or sublingually but prevents intravenous abuse, since injection of the combination of buprenorphine plus naloxone results in no high and may even precipitate withdrawal. L-alpha-acetylmethodol acetate (LAAM) is a long-acting orally active opiate with pharmacological properties similar to those of methadone, but it is rarely used because of concerns over QTc prolongation. Agonist substitution treatments are best used in the setting of a structured maintenance treatment program that includes random urine drug screening and intensive psychological, medical, and vocational services. For heavy-duty opiate addicts, specialty methadone clinics may be useful.

As for other areas of drug abuse, rank-and-file office-based psychopharmacologists use very little of the agonist substitution process for treating opiate abusers or addicts, including relatively little use of buprenorphine. This situation is likely the product of therapeutic nihilism for opiate addicts and probably also the wish not to have heroin and serious intravenous opiate addicts in one's practice, since they often must live on the streets, tend to engage in criminal activities, and are highly unreliable. However, for motivated prescription opiate addicts who are still employed, reliable, and less likely to be involved with crime or living on the street and who have not taken methadone previously, buprenorphine may remain a viable option.

Stimulants

Use of stimulants as therapeutic agents is discussed extensively in several other chapters. Mechanism of action of amphetamine as an inhibitor of the dopamine transporter (DAT) and also of the vesicular monoamine transporter (VMAT) is introduced in Chapter 4 and illustrated in Figure 4-15. Therapeutic use of stimulants for sleep/wake disorders is discussed in Chapter 16 and illustrated in Figures 16-3, 16-5, 16-31, and 16-32. Therapeutic use of stimulants for ADHD is discussed in Chapter 17 and illustrated in Figures 17-8, 17-9, 17-18, 17-19, and 17-20.

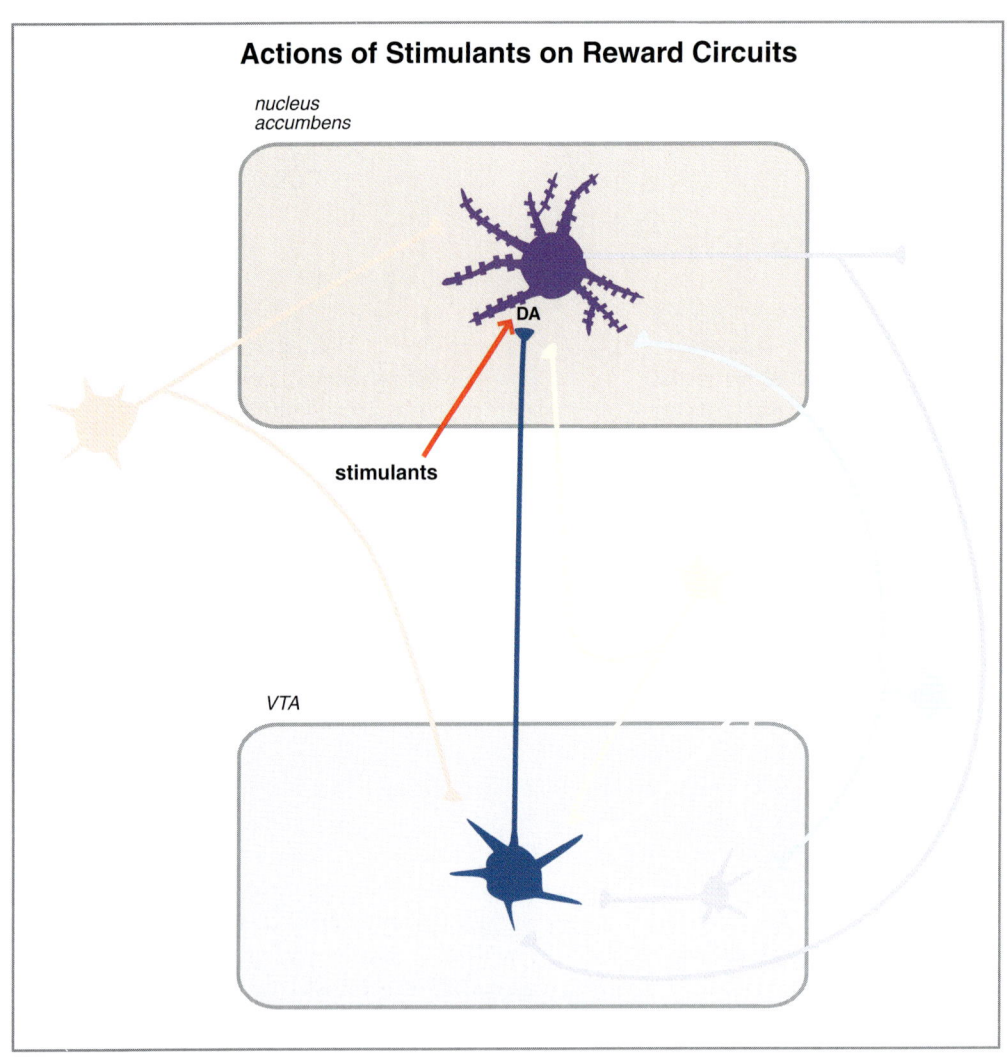

FIGURE 19-33 Actions of stimulants on reward circuits. Shown here is the reactive reward system consisting of the ventral tegmental area (VTA), site of dopamine cell bodies which also receives many neurotransmitter projections; the nucleus accumbens, to which dopaminergic neurons project; and the amygdala (far left), which has connections with both the VTA and the nucleus accumbens. The potential abuse properties of stimulants stem from their ability to enhance dopamine release in the nucleus accumbens.

Stimulants and reward

The mechanisms of enhanced reinforcement and abusability of stimulants when given in high pulsatile doses are compared and contrasted with the reduced reinforcement of stimulants when given in oral sustained release dosing in Figures 17-18 through 17-20. Although many therapeutic actions of stimulants are thought to be directed to the prefrontal cortex and also to the enhancement of both norepinephrine and dopamine neurotransmission there, the actions of stimulants that are linked to their abuse are thought to be primarily those that target reward circuits, especially dopamine release from mesolimbic dopamine neurons in the nucleus accumbens (Figure 19-33).

One stimulant without recognized therapeutic uses in psychopharmacology is cocaine (Figure 19-34). This agent has two major properties: it is both a local anesthetic and an

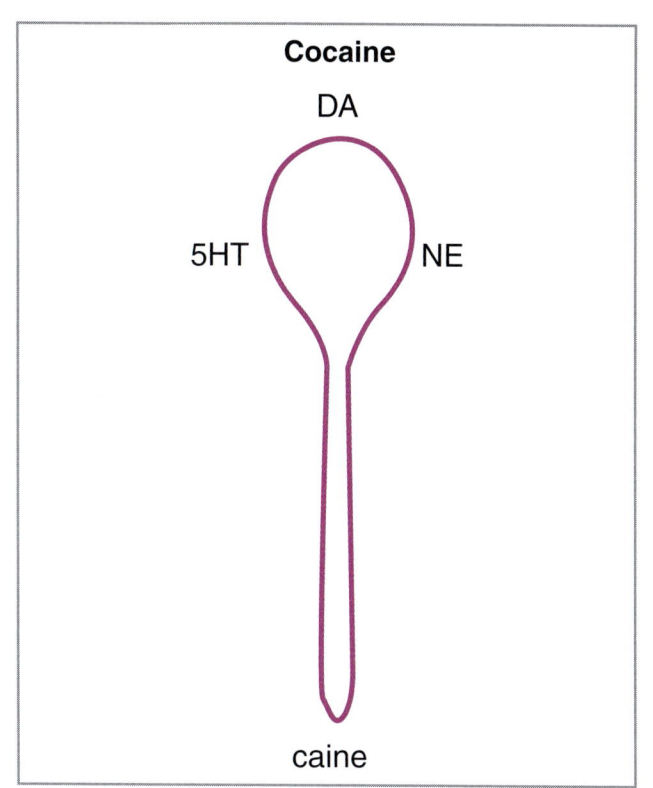

FIGURE 19-34 Icon of cocaine. The main mechanism of action of cocaine is to block reuptake and cause the release of monoamines, principally dopamine (DA) but also norepinephrine (NE) and serotonin (5HT). There is also a local anesthetic action (caine).

inhibitor of monoamine transporters, especially for dopamine (i.e., DAT, the DA transporter). But often neglected in discussions of cocaine is consideration of its ability to inhibit the serotonin transporter (SERT) and the norepinephrine transporter (NET) (Figure 19-34). Cocaine's local anesthetic properties are still used in medicine, especially by ear-nose-and-throat specialists (otolaryngologists). Freud himself exploited this property of cocaine to help dull the pain of his tongue cancer. He may have also exploited the second property of the drug, which is to produce euphoria, reduce fatigue, and create a sense of mental acuity due to inhibition of dopamine reuptake at the dopamine transporter.

Cocaine inhibits DAT in a manner similar to the action of methylphenidate. That is, cocaine is a blocker of transport of DA by DAT. Cocaine does not act upon dopamine neurons as amphetamine does, but methamphetamine (Figure 19-35) acts just like amphetamine, only faster. In addition, methamphetamine is converted to amphetamine. Amphetamine and methamphetamine are both pseudosubstrates and reverse transporters of DA via DAT and also inhibitors of VMAT. These properties of amphetamine are discussed in Chapter 4 and illustrated in Figure 4-15.

So what is the difference between methylphenidate and cocaine if they both have the same mechanism of action? Similarly, what is the difference between amphetamine for ADHD and methamphetamine for abuse? The answers are not in differences in mechanism of action but in route of administration and therefore how fast, how powerfully, and how completely DAT is blocked.

Methylphenidate is taken orally and is longer in onset and duration of action compared to stimulants that are injected, snorted intranasally, or smoked. Methylphenidate itself is

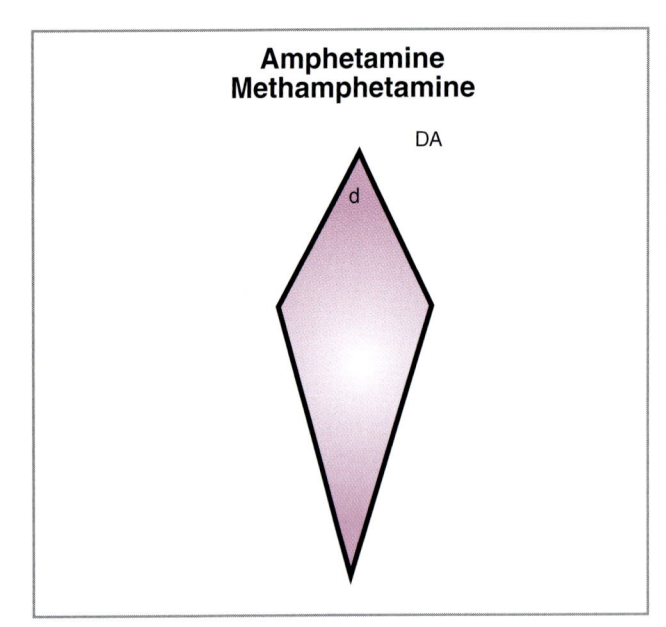

FIGURE 19-35 Icon of amphetamine/methamphetamine. Amphetamine and methamphetamine are both pseudosubstrates and reverse transporters of dopamine via the dopamine transporter (DAT) and also act as inhibitors of the vesicular monoamine transporter (VMAT).

far more abusable when injected; but even injected, methylphenidate does not seem to blast the DAT as ferociously as do other stimulants injected intravenously. Cocaine is not active orally, so users have learned over the years to take it intranasally, where the drug rapidly enters the brain directly, bypassing the heart, and thus can have a more rapid onset than even with intravenous administration. The most rapid and robust way to deliver drugs to the brain is to smoke those that are compatible with this route of administration, as this avoids first-pass metabolism through the liver and is somewhat akin to giving the drug by intra-arterial/intracarotid bolus.

As stated in previous chapters, blasting DAT in a dramatic pulsatile manner maximizes the chances for phasic DA release (see Figure 17-20), which is highly reinforcing and pleasurable when this happens in the nucleus accumbens. Taking huge oral doses of a stimulant with rapid onset, or taking it intranasally, intravenously, or smoking it can create highly intense pleasurable experiences that are often described by addicts as better than orgasm.

At intoxicating doses of cocaine or methamphetamine, however, undesirable effects can be produced, including tremor, emotional lability, restlessness, irritability, paranoia, panic, and repetitive stereotyped behavior. At even higher doses, these stimulants can induce intense anxiety, paranoia, and hallucinations, with hypertension, tachycardia, ventricular irritability, hyperthermia, and respiratory depression. In overdose, cocaine can cause acute heart failure, stroke, and seizures.

Long-term effects of stimulant abuse

Even worse for DA neurons than high doses may be effects of repetitive intoxicating doses of stimulants on these neurons. The progression of stimulant abuse is shown in Figure 19-36. First doses of stimulants cause pleasurable phasic dopamine neuronal firing (Figure 19-36A). Eventually, reward conditioning occurs, causing craving between stimulant doses and lack of pleasurable phasic dopamine firing, with only residual tonic dopamine neuronal firing (Figure 19-36B). Now that the user is addicted, higher and higher doses

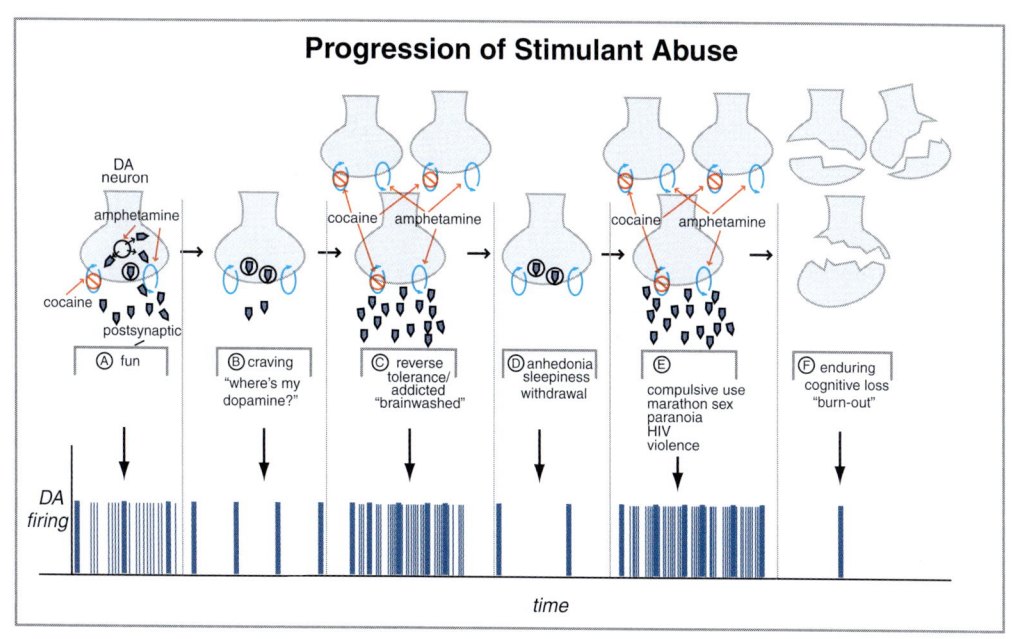

FIGURE 19-36A, B, C, D, E, and F Progression of stimulant abuse. (**A**) First doses of stimulants such as amphetamine or cocaine cause pleasurable phasic dopamine firing. (**B**) With chronic use, reward conditioning causes craving between stimulant doses and only residual tonic dopamine firing with lack of pleasurable phasic dopamine firing. (**C**) In this addicted state, higher and higher doses of stimulants are needed in order to achieve the pleasurable highs of phasic dopamine firing. (**D**) Unfortunately, the higher the high, the lower the low, and between stimulant doses the individual experiences not only the absence of a high but also withdrawal symptoms such as sleepiness and anhedonia. (**E**) The effort to combat withdrawal can lead to compulsive use and impulsive, dangerous behaviors in order to secure the stimulant. (**F**) Finally, there may be enduring if not irreversible changes in dopamine neurons, including long-lasting depletions of dopamine levels and axonal degeneration, a state that clinically and pathologically is appropriately called "burn-out."

must be taken to get better and better "highs" that accompany phasic dopamine neuronal firing (brainwashed; Figure 19-36C). Unfortunately, the higher the high, the lower the low, and between stimulant doses the experience is that of sleepiness and anhedonia, not just the absence of a high (withdrawal; Figure 19-36D). To avoid this state and get ever more satisfying highs, the situation progresses to compulsive use, often with marathon, indiscriminate, and unprotected sex, risk of HIV from shared needles and sex, with the emergence of paranoia (Figure 19-26E). Indeed, stimulants can produce a paranoid psychosis indistinguishable from acute paranoid schizophrenia, as discussed in Chapter 9 and illustrated in Figures 9-25 and 9-26. At this stage, the addict is often involved with criminal activity in order to obtain drugs and with people and situations that trigger violence (Figure 19-36E). Finally, there may be enduring if not irreversible changes in dopamine neurons, including long-lasting depletion of dopamine levels and axonal degeneration, a state that clinically and pathologically is appropriately called "burn-out" (Figure 19-36F). This can be associated with enduring cognitive loss and treatment-resistant depression, and it can take a very long time, sometimes years, to reverse if at all.

Although there are no approved treatments for stimulant abusers or stimulant addicts, there may be a cocaine vaccine (TA-CD) in the future that removes the drug before it can lead the patient along the route of progression of stimulant abuse shown in Figure 19-36. The weak DAT inhibitor modafinil is also being tested, as are various antipsychotics such as olanzapine, but particularly D2 partial agonists such as aripiprazole. Experimental treatments include dopamine D3 receptor partial agonists (RGH188, BP987) or antagonists (NGB2904, SB277011A, ST198) and long-lasting dopamine releasers such as PAL287. Naltrexone is also being investigated. N-acetyl cysteine, a precursor of the amino acid cysteine, acts on the cysteine-glutamate exchange mechanism – which may be disordered in cocaine-dependent individuals seeking drugs – to reduce craving and interest in cocaine.

Sedative hypnotics

Sedative hypnotics include barbiturates and related agents such as ethchlorvynol and ethinamate, chloral hydrate and derivatives, and piperidinedione derivatives such as glutethimide and methyprylon. Experts often include alcohol, benzodiazepines, and Z drug hypnotics in this class as well. The mechanism of action of sedative hypnotics is basically the same as that of those described in Chapter 14 and illustrated in Figures 14-20 and 14-22 for the action of benzodiazepines: namely, they are positive allosteric modulators (PAMs) for GABA-A receptors. Actions of sedative hypnotics at GABA-A receptor sites in reward circuits are shown in Figure 19-37. Molecular actions of all sedative hypnotics are similar, but benzodiazepines and barbiturates seem to work at different sites from each other and also only on some GABA-A receptor subtypes, namely those with alpha 1, alpha 2, alpha 3, or alpha 5 subunits (Figure 19-38A). Barbiturates are much less safe in overdose than benzodiazepines, cause dependence more frequently, are abused more frequently, and produce much more dangerous withdrawal reactions. Apparently the receptor site at GABA-A receptors mediating the pharmacological actions of barbiturates (Figure 19-38A) is even more readily desensitized with even more dangerous consequences than the benzodiazepine receptor (also shown in Figure 19-38). The barbiturate site must also mediate a more intense euphoria and a more desirable sense of tranquility than the benzodiazepine receptor site. Since benzodiazepines are generally an adequate alternative to barbiturates, psychopharmacologists can help to minimize abuse of barbiturates by prescribing them rarely if ever. In the case of withdrawal reactions, reinstituting and then tapering the offending barbiturate under close clinical supervision can assist the detoxification process.

Marijuana

You can indeed get stoned without inhaling (Figure 19-39)! Actions of marijuana and its active ingredient THC (delta-9-tetrahydrocannabinol) on reward circuits are shown in Figure 19-39 at sites where endogenous cannabinoids are utilized naturally as retrograde neurotransmitters. The concept of the "brain's own marijuana" is introduced in Chapter 3 and retrograde neurotransmission with these endogenous cannabinoids (or "endocannabinoids") at CB1 presynaptic cannabinoid receptors is illustrated in Figure 3-3.

Cannabis preparations are smoked in order to deliver cannabinoids that interact with the brain's own cannabinoid receptors to trigger dopamine release from the mesolimbic reward system (Figure 19-39). Marijuana can have both stimulant and sedative properties. In usual intoxicating doses, it produces a sense of well-being, relaxation, a sense of friendliness, a loss of temporal awareness including confusing the past with the present, slowing of thought processes, impairment of short-term memory, and a feeling of achieving special insights. At high doses, marijuana can induce panic, toxic delirium, and rarely psychosis. One complication of long-term use is the "amotivational syndrome" in frequent users. This syndrome is seen predominantly in heavy daily users and is characterized by the emergence of decreased drive and ambition, thus "amotivation." It is also associated

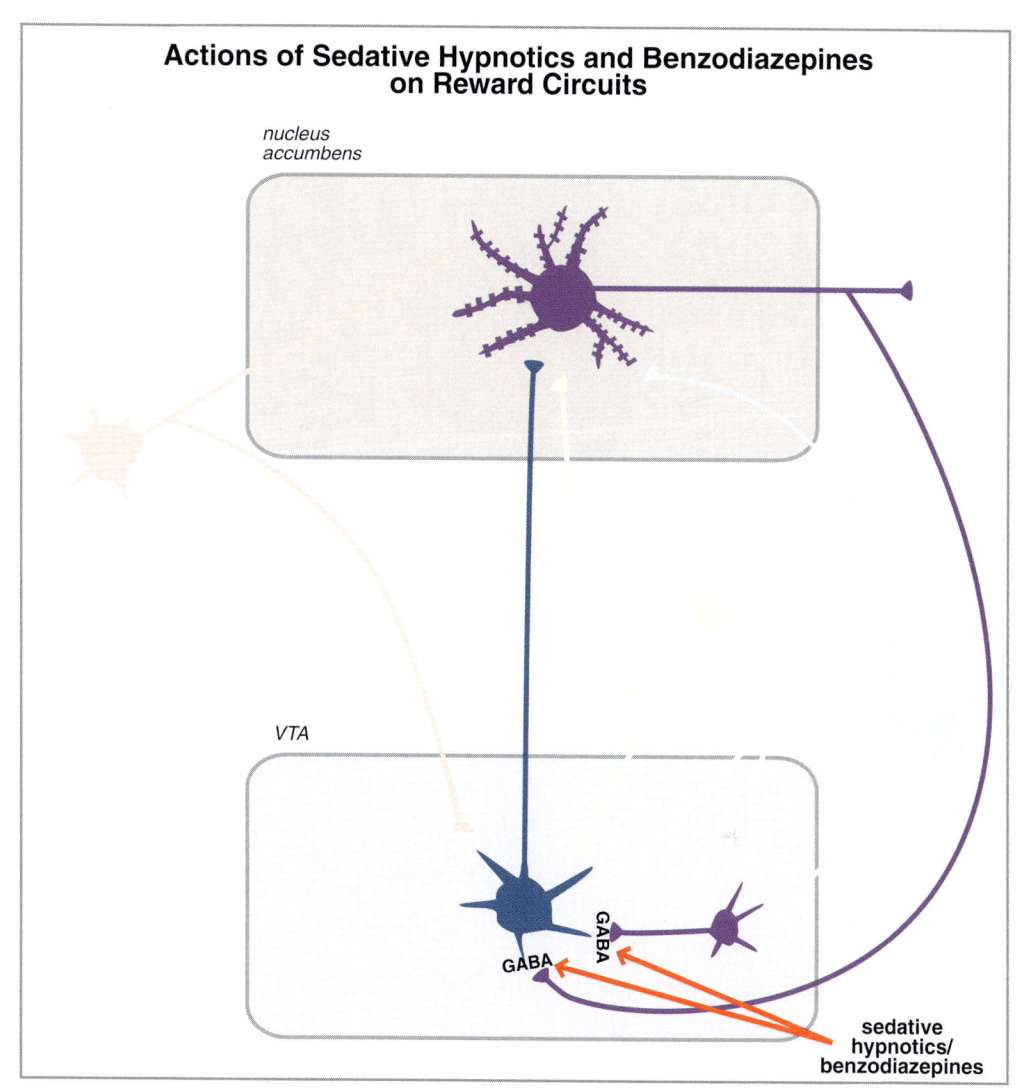

FIGURE 19-37 Actions of sedative hypnotics and benzodiazepines on reward circuits. Shown here is the reactive reward system consisting of the ventral tegmental area (VTA), site of dopamine cell bodies that receives many neurotransmitter projections; the nucleus accumbens, to which dopaminergic neurons project; and the amygdala (far left), which has connections with both the VTA and the nucleus accumbens. Sedative hypnotics and benzodiazepines are positive allosteric modulators at GABA-A receptors (such as in the VTA, as shown here).

with other socially and occupationally impairing symptoms, including a shortened attention span, poor judgment, easy distractibility, impaired communication skills, introversion, and diminished effectiveness in interpersonal situations. Personal habits may deteriorate, and there may be a loss of insight and even feelings of depersonalization. In terms of chronic administration to humans, tolerance to cannabinoids has been well documented, but the question of cannabinoid dependence has always been controversial. The discovery of the brain cannabinoid CB1 receptor antagonist rimonabant has settled this question in experimental animals because it precipitates a withdrawal syndrome in mice chronically exposed to THC. It is therefore highly likely but not yet proven that dependence also occurs in humans, presumably due to the same types of adaptive changes in cannabinoid receptors

Binding Sites for Sedative Hypnotic Drugs

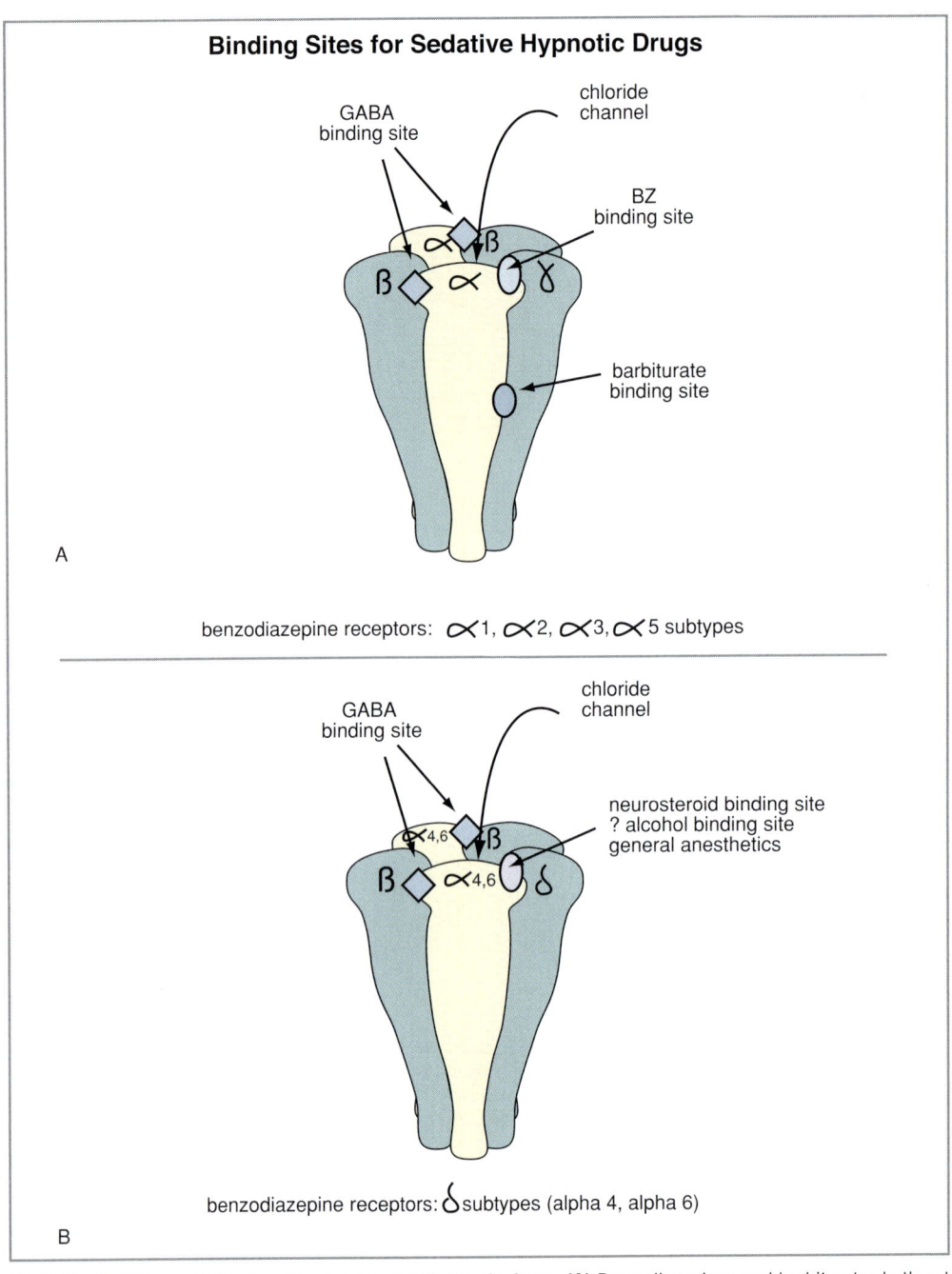

A

benzodiazepine receptors: α1, α2, α3, α5 subtypes

B

benzodiazepine receptors: δ subtypes (alpha 4, alpha 6)

FIGURE 19-38A and B Binding sites for sedative hypnotic drugs. (**A**) Benzodiazepines and barbiturates both act at GABA-A receptors, but at different binding sites. Benzodiazepines do not act at all GABA-A receptors; rather, they are selective for the alpha 1, 2, 3, and 5 subtypes. (**B**) General anesthetics, alcohol, and neurosteroids may bind to other types of GABA-A receptors.

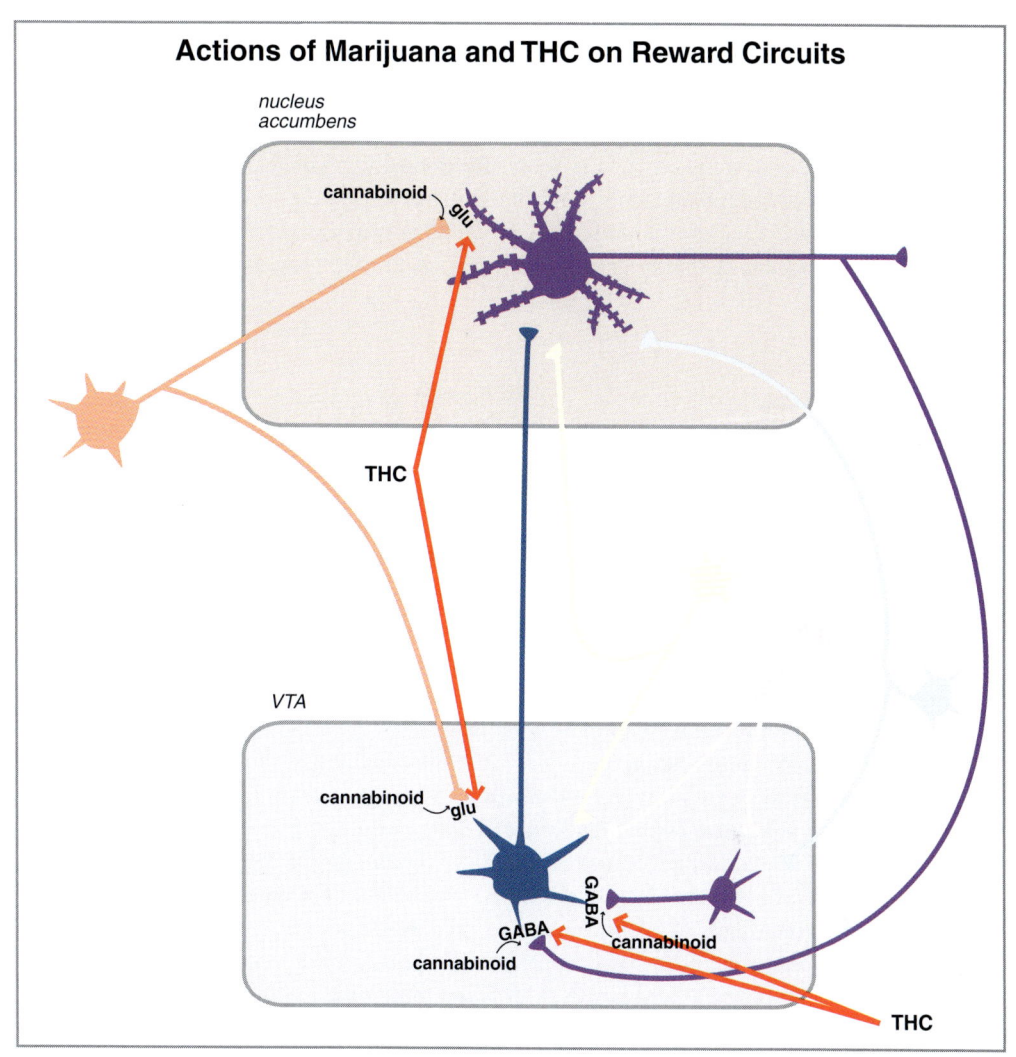

FIGURE 19-39 Actions of marijuana and THC on reward circuits. Shown here is the reactive reward system consisting of the ventral tegmental area (VTA), site of dopamine cell bodies that receives many neurotransmitter projections; the nucleus accumbens, to which dopaminergic neurons project; and the amygdala (far left), which has connections with both the VTA and the nucleus accumbens. Marijuana delivers its active ingredients, the cannabinoids (e.g., THC; delta-9-tetrahydrocannabinol), which interact with the brain's own cannabinoid receptors to trigger dopamine release in the nucleus accumbens.

that occur in other neurotransmitter receptors after chronic administration of other drugs of abuse.

There are two known cannabinoid receptors, CB1 (in brain) and CB2 (predominantly in the immune system). CB1 receptors may mediate not only marijuana's reinforcing properties but also those of alcohol and to some extent those of other psychoactive substances (including food, if sugars and fats can be considered "psychoactive"; this is discussed further on). Anandamide is one of the endocannabinoids and a member of a chemical class of neurotransmitter that is not a monoamine, not an amino acid, and not a peptide: it is a lipid, specifically a member of a family of fatty acid ethanolamides. Anandamide shares most but not all of the pharmacological properties of THC, since its actions at brain cannabinoid

Disorders of Reward, Drug Abuse, and Their Treatment

receptors are not only mimicked by THC but also antagonized in part by the selective brain cannabinoid CB1 receptor antagonist rimonabant.

The discovery of rimonabant, a "marijuana antagonist," has opened the door to using this drug as a potential therapeutic agent in various types of drug abuse, from cigarette smoking to alcoholism to marijuana abuse. Additionally, rimonabant has been extensively tested in obesity and the metabolic syndrome and has received approved for this use in some countries. However, approval in the United States has not been granted yet due to concerns about the possibility that long-term use of rimonabant might increase suicidal ideation.

Hallucinogens

The hallucinogens are a group of agents that act at serotonin synapses in the reward system (Figure 19-40). They produce intoxication, sometimes called a "trip," associated with changes in sensory experiences, including visual illusions and hallucinations and an enhanced awareness of both external and internal stimuli and thoughts. These hallucinations are produced with a clear level of consciousness and a lack of confusion and may be both **psychedelic** and **psychotomimetic**. "Psychedelic" is the term for a heightened sensory awareness and subjective experience that one's mind is being expanded, that one is in union with all humanity or the universe, and that one is having a sort of religious experience. "Psychotomimetic" means that the experience mimics a state of psychosis, but the resemblance between a trip and psychosis is superficial at best. As previously discussed, the stimulants cocaine and amphetamine much more genuinely mimic psychosis.

Hallucinogen intoxication includes visual illusions, visual "trails" where the image smears into streaks of its image as it moves across a visual trail, macropsia and micropsia, emotional and mood lability, subjective slowing of time, the sense that colors are heard and sounds are seen, intensification of sound perception, depersonalization and derealization, yet retaining a state of full wakefulness and alertness. Other changes may include impaired judgment, fear of losing one's mind, anxiety, nausea, tachycardia, increased blood pressure, and increased body temperature. Not surprisingly, hallucinogen intoxication can cause what is perceived as a panic attack, which is often called a "bad trip." As intoxication escalates, one can experience an acute confusional state (delirium) of disorientation and agitation. This can evolve further into frank psychosis, with delusions and paranoia.

Common hallucinogens include two major classes of agents. The first class resemble serotonin (indolealkylamines) and include the classic hallucinogens LSD (d-lysergic acid diethylamide), psilocybin, and dimethyltryptamine (DMT) (Figure 19-41). The second class of agents resemble norepinephrine and dopamine and are also related to amphetamine (phenylalkylamines); they include mescaline DOM (2,5-dimethoxy-4-methylamphetamine) and others. More recently, synthetic chemists have come up with some new "designer drugs" such as MDMA (3,4-methylene-dioxymethamphetamine) and "Foxy" (5-methoxy-diisopropyltryptamine). These are either stimulants or hallucinogens and produce a complex subjective state sometimes referred to as "ecstasy," which is also what abusers call MDMA itself. MDMA produces euphoria, disorientation, confusion, enhanced sociability, and a sense of increased empathy and personal insight.

Hallucinogens have rather complex interactions at neurotransmitter systems, but one of the most prominent is a common action as agonists at 5HT2A receptor sites (Figure 19-42). Hallucinogens certainly have additional effects at other 5HT receptors (especially 5HT1A somatodendritic autoreceptors and 5HT2C receptors) and also at other neurotransmitter systems, especially norepinephrine and dopamine, but the relative importance of these other

Actions of Hallucinogens on Reward Circuits

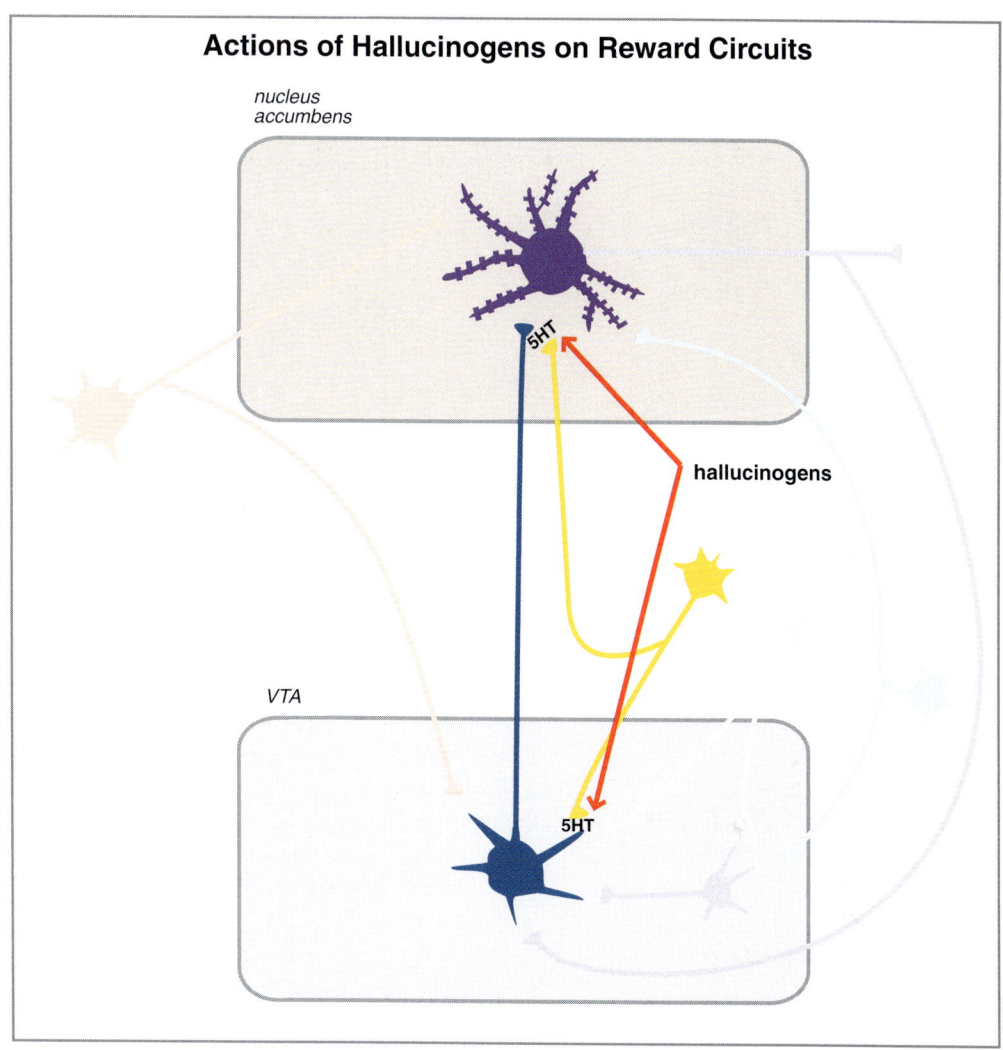

FIGURE 19-40 Actions of hallucinogens on reward circuits. Shown here is the reactive reward system consisting of the ventral tegmental area (VTA), site of dopamine cell bodies that receives many neurotransmitter projections; the nucleus accumbens, to which dopaminergic neurons project; and the amygdala (far left), which has connections with both the VTA and the nucleus accumbens. Hallucinogens act at serotonin synapses within this reward system.

actions is less well known. MDMA also appears to be a powerful inhibitor of the serotonin transporter (SERT) (Figure 19-42) and is also a releaser of 5HT. MDMA and several other drugs structurally related to it may even destroy serotonin axon terminals. However, the action that appears to explain a common mechanism for most of the hallucinogens is the stimulation of 5HT2A receptors.

Hallucinogens can produce incredible tolerance, sometimes after a single dose. Desensitization of 5HT2A receptors is hypothesized to underlie this rapid clinical and pharmacological tolerance. Another unique dimension of hallucinogen abuse is the production of "flashbacks," namely the spontaneous recurrence of some of the symptoms of intoxication that lasts from a few seconds to several hours, but in the absence of recent administration of the hallucinogen. This occurs days to months after the last drug experience and can

Disorders of Reward, Drug Abuse, and Their Treatment

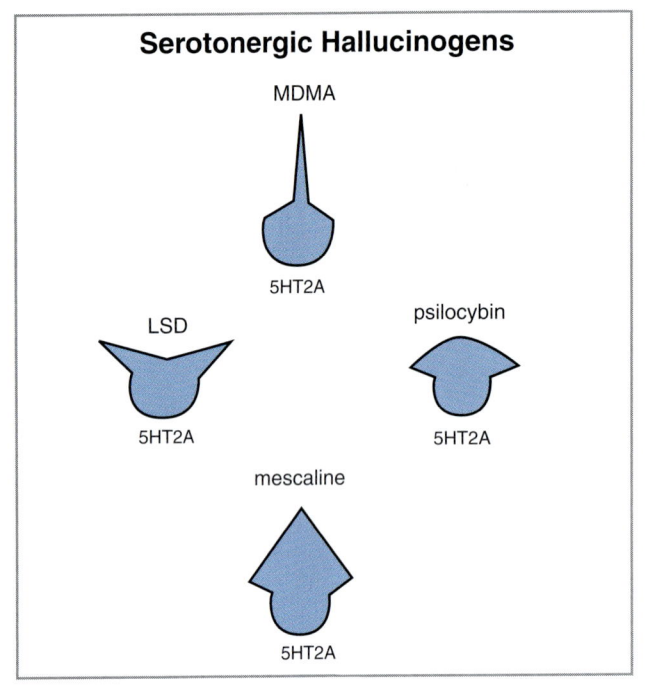

FIGURE 19-41 Icons of hallucinogens. Hallucinogens such as lysergic acid diethylamide (LSD), mescaline, psilocybin, and 3,4-methylenediosy-methamphetamine (MDMA) are agonists at serotonin 2A (5HT2A) receptors.

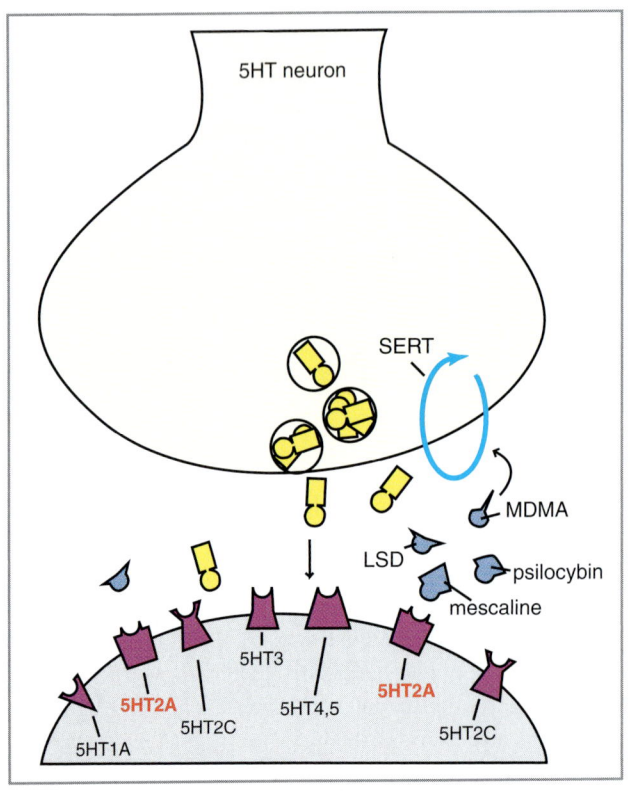

FIGURE 19-42 Actions of hallucinogens. The primary action of hallucinogenic drugs such as LSD, mescaline, psilocybin, and MDMA are shown here: namely, agonism of 5HT2A receptors. Hallucinogens may have additional actions at other serotonin receptors (particularly 5HT1A and 5HT2C) and at other neurotransmitter systems, and MDMA in particular also blocks the serotonin transporter (SERT).

apparently be precipitated by a number of environmental stimuli. The psychopharmacological mechanism underlying flashbacks is unknown, but its phenomenology suggests the possibility of a neurochemical adaptation of the serotonin system and its receptors related to reverse tolerance that is incredibly long-lasting. Alternatively, flashbacks could be a form of emotional conditioning embedded in the amygdala and then triggered when a later emotional experience, occurring when one is not taking a hallucinogen, nevertheless revives the memory of experiences that occurred during intoxication. This could precipitate a whole cascade of feelings that occurred during intoxication with a hallucinogen. This is analogous to the types of reexperiencing flashbacks that occur without drugs in patients with posttraumatic stress disorder.

Club drugs

Phencyclidine and ketamine

Phencyclidine (PCP) and ketamine both have actions at glutamate synapses within the reward system (Figure 19-43). They both act as antagonists of NMDA receptors, binding to a site in the calcium channel (see discussion in Chapter 13 and Figures 13-30 and 13-31). Both were originally developed as anesthetics. PCP proved to be unacceptable for this use because it induces a unique psychotomimetic/hallucinatory experience very similar to schizophrenia. The NMDA receptor hypoactivity that is caused by PCP has become a model for the same neurotransmitter abnormalities postulated to underlie schizophrenia (see discussion in Chapter 9 and Figures 9-39 through 9-42). Its structurally and mechanism-related analog ketamine is still used as an anesthetic, but it causes far less of the psychotomimetic/hallucinatory experience. Nevertheless, some people do abuse ketamine, one of the "club drugs" sometimes called "special K." PCP causes intense analgesia, amnesia, and delirium, stimulant as well as depressant actions, staggering gait, slurred speech, and a unique form of nystagmus (i.e., vertical nystagmus). Higher degrees of intoxication can cause catatonia (excitement alternating with stupor and catalepsy), hallucinations, delusions, paranoia, disorientation, and lack of judgment. Overdose can include coma, extremely high temperature, seizures, and muscle breakdown (rhabdomyolysis).

Gamma hydroxybutyrate (GHB)

This agent is discussed extensively in Chapter 16 as a treatment for narcolepsy/cataplexy. It is sometimes also abused (Figure 19-43). The mechanism of action of GHB is as an agonist at its own GHB receptors and at GABA-B receptors (illustrated in Figure 16-35).

Inhalants

Agents such as toluene are thought to be direct releasers of dopamine in the nucleus accumbens.

Sexual disorders

From a psychopharmacological perspective, the human sexual response can be divided into three phases, each with distinct and relatively nonoverlapping neurotransmitter functions: libido, arousal, and orgasm (Figure 19-44).

Libido

The first stage, libido, is linked to desire for sex, or sex drive, and is a complex process regulated by neurotransmitters, hormones, and past experiences. Dopamine activity in reward circuitry is thought to play a central role (Figure 19-45). In addition to the projections of

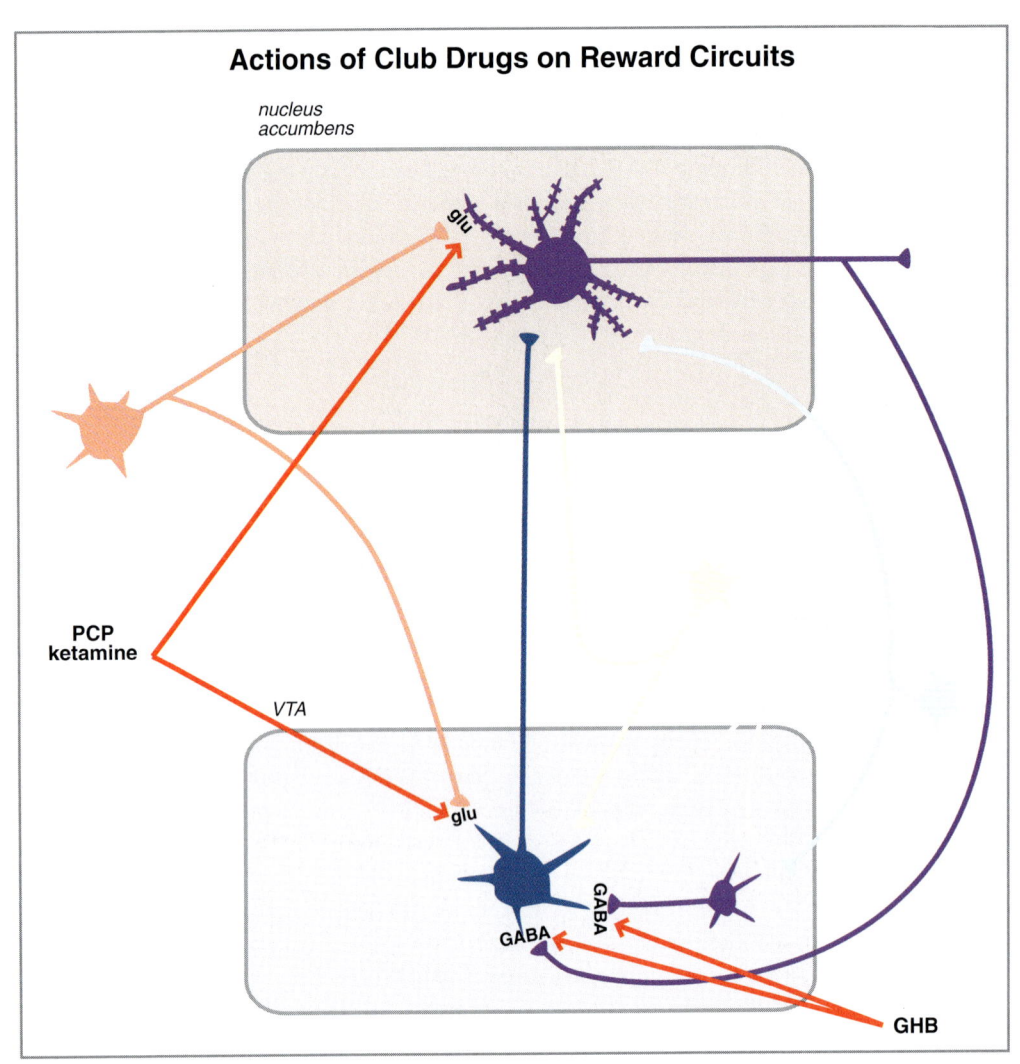

FIGURE 19-43 Actions of club drugs on reward circuits. Shown here is the reactive reward system consisting of the ventral tegmental area (VTA), site of dopamine cell bodies that receives many neurotransmitter projections; the nucleus accumbens, to which dopaminergic neurons project; and the amygdala (far left), which has connections with both the VTA and the nucleus accumbens. Club drugs such as phencyclidine (PCP) and ketamine are antagonists at N-methyl-d-aspartate (NMDA) receptors and thus cause NMDA hypoactivity, which in turn leads to disinhibition of dopamine release. Gamma hydroxybutyrate (GHB), which is an agonist at GHB and GABA-B receptors, is also sometimes abused.

dopamine to the nucleus accumbens emphasized in this chapter, dopamine also projects to the hypothalamus, where it may also have input to the regulation of sexual desire via neurons in the medial preoptic area (MPOA in Figure 19-45). The MPOA has been shown to play an important role in sexual motivation in experimental animals, whereas another area of the hypothalamus, the paraventricular nucleus, may control genital responses and a third area of the hypothalamus, the ventromedial nucleus, may regulate the expression of sexual receptivity (lordosis in animals).

Numerous agents positively regulate sexual motivation by their actions in these hypothalamic areas, including estrogen and testosterone, dopamine, as well as various

Psychopharmacology of Sex

neurotransmitter

Stage One:
Desire

DA +
melanocortin +
testosterone +
estrogen +
prolactin −
5HT −

Stage Two:
Arousal

NO +
NE +
melanocortin +
testosterone +
estrogen +
ACh +
DA +
5HT −

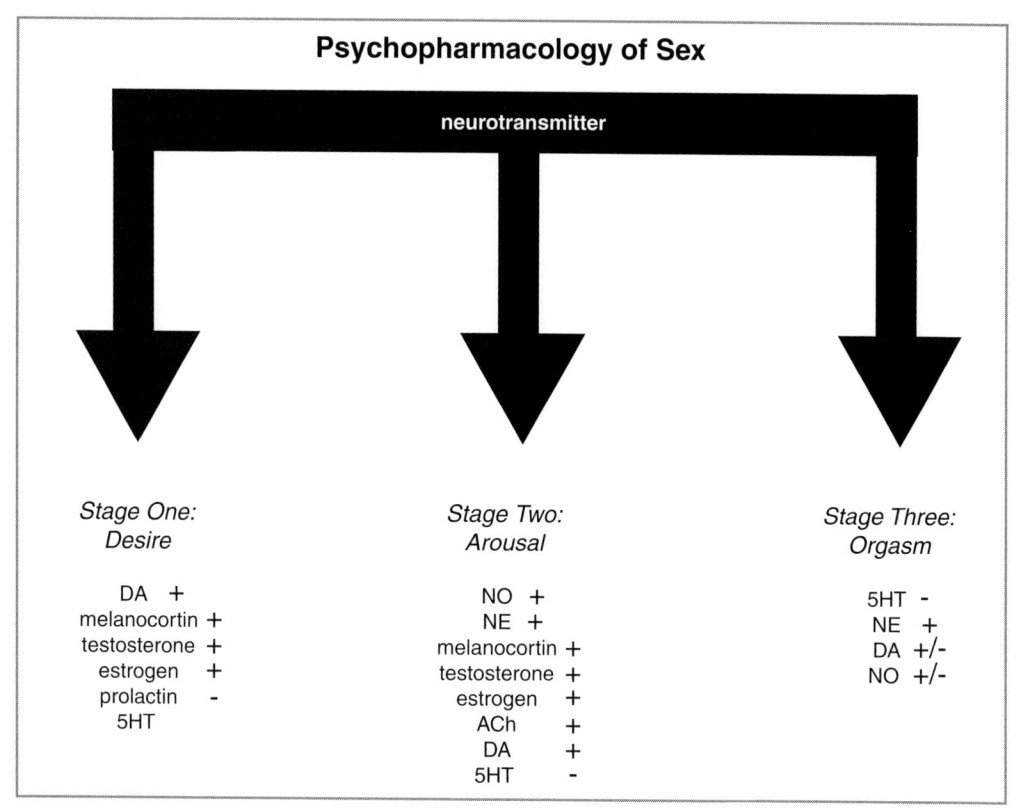

Stage Three:
Orgasm

5HT −
NE +
DA +/−
NO +/−

FIGURE 19-44 Psychopharmacology of sex. The neurotransmitters involved in the three stages of the psychopharmacology of the human sexual response are summarized here. In stage 1, desire, dopamine (DA), melanocortin, testosterone, and estrogen exert a positive influence, while prolactin and serotonin (5HT) have negative effects. In stage 2, arousal correlates with erection in men and genital swelling and lubrication in women. Several neurotransmitters facilitate sexual arousal, including nitric oxide (NO), norepinephrine (NE), melanocortin, testosterone, estrogen, acetylcholine (ACh), and DA. As with desire, 5HT has a negative effect. Stage 3, orgasm, which is associated with ejaculation in men, is inhibited by 5HT and facilitated by NE; DA and NO may have weak positive influences.

peptide neurotransmitters such as melanocortin (Figures 19-44 and 19-45). Prolactin, on the other hand, is hypothesized to have a negative influence on sexual desire (Figure 19-44). This is interesting, since there is a generally reciprocal relationship between dopamine and prolactin (as discussed in Chapter 9; see Figure 9-11). However, the relationship between prolactin and sexual dysfunction is not well documented and relatively poorly understood. Serotonin also has a negative influence on sexual motivation and desire, presumably due to its inhibitory influence on dopamine release (Figure 19-44). Serotonergic inhibition of dopamine release is discussed in Chapter 10 and illustrated in Figures 10-21 to 10-25.

Arousal

The second psychopharmacological stage of the sexual response is arousal (Figure 19-44): arousal of peripheral tissues, that is. In men, that means an erection; in women, that means genital lubrication and swelling. This type of arousal prepares the genitalia for penetration and sexual intercourse. The message of arousal starts in the brain; it is then relayed down the spinal cord and into peripheral autonomic nerve fibers that are both sympathetic and parasympathetic; next, it travels into vascular tissues and finally to the genitalia. Along

Disorders of Reward, Drug Abuse, and Their Treatment | 995

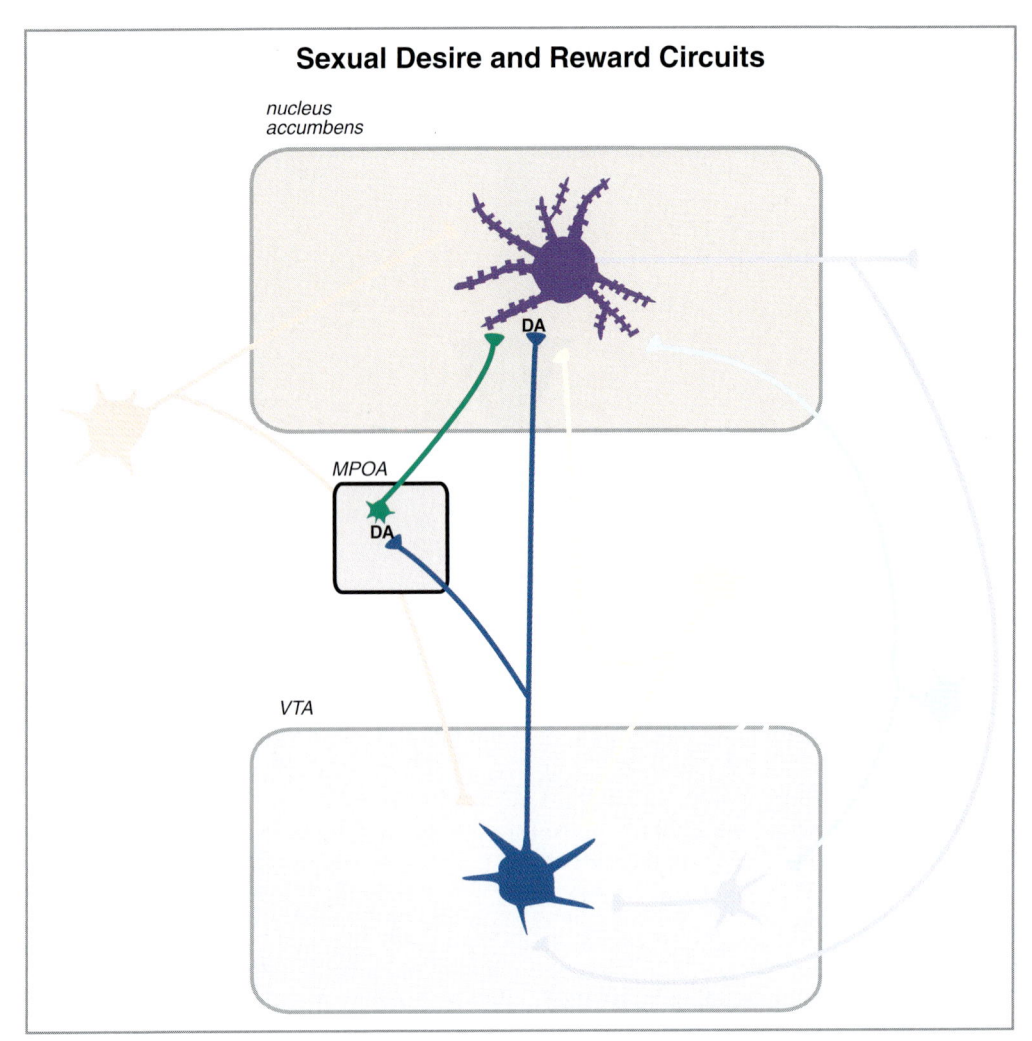

FIGURE 19-45 Sexual desire and reward circuits. Shown here is the reactive reward system consisting of the ventral tegmental area (VTA), site of dopamine cell bodies which receives many neurotransmitter projections; the nucleus accumbens, to which dopaminergic neurons project; and the amygdala (far left), which has connections with both the VTA and the nucleus accumbens. Dopamine activity in reward circuitry is thought to play a central role in sexual desire. Dopaminergic neurons also project to the hypothalamus, where they may have input to the regulation of sexual desire via neurons in the medial preoptic area (MPOA) and the projections of those neurons to the nucleus accumbens.

the way, at least two key neurotransmitters are involved, acetylcholine in the autonomic parasympathetic innervation of the genitalia and nitric oxide, which acts upon the smooth muscle of the genitalia (Figures 19-44 and 19-45). Acetylcholine and nitric oxide both promote erections in men and lubrication and swelling in women.

Nitric oxide psychopharmacology

Nitric oxide (NO), a gas, is an improbable compound for a neurotransmitter. It is not an amine, amino acid, or peptide; it is not stored in synaptic vesicles or released by exocytosis; and it does not interact with specific receptor subtypes in neuronal membranes; but it is

Sexual Arousal and Neurotransmitters

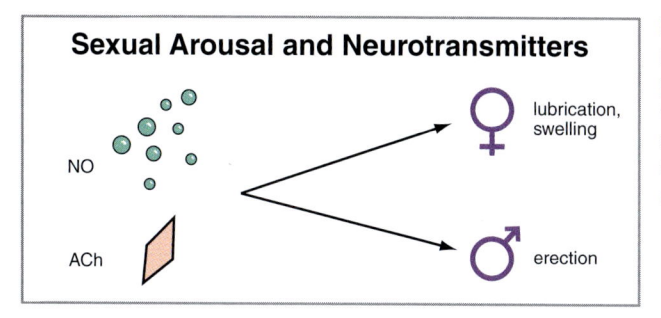

FIGURE 19-46 **Sexual arousal and neurotransmitters.** Sexual arousal in peripheral genitalia is accompanied by erections in men and lubrication and swelling in women. Both nitric oxide and acetylcholine are regulators of these actions.

"no laughing matter." Specifically, it is not nitrous oxide (N_2O) or "laughing gas," one of the earliest known anesthetics. Nitric oxide is a far different gas, although the two are often confused. It is NO that is the neurotransmitter, not N_2O. Incredible as it may seem, NO is a poisonous and unstable gas, a component of car fumes that helps to deplete the ozone layer, yet is also a chemical messenger both in the brain and in blood vessels, including those that control erections of the penis.

Yes, there is NO synthesis by neurons and the penis. Certain neurons and tissues possess the enzyme nitric oxide synthetase (NOS), which forms NO from the amino acid l-arginine (Figure 19-47A). NO then diffuses to adjacent neurons or smooth muscle and provokes the formation of the second messenger cyclic GMP (guanosine monophosphate) by activating the enzyme guanylyl cyclase (GC) (Figure 19-47B). NO is not made in advance, nor is it stored; it seems to be made on demand and released by simple diffusion. Glutamate and calcium can trigger the formation of NO by activating NOS.

No, there are no NO receptors. In striking contrast to classic neurotransmitters, which have numerous types and subtypes of membrane receptors on neurons, there are no NO membrane receptors. Rather, the target of NO is iron in the active site of GC (Figure 19-47B). Once NO binds to the iron, GC is activated and cGMP is formed. The action of cGMP is terminated by a family of enzymes known as phosphodiesterases (PDE), of which there are several forms, depending upon the tissue (Figure 19-47C).

Yes, there is NO neurotransmitter function. The first known messenger functions for NO were described in blood vessels. By relaxing smooth muscles in blood vessels of the penis, NO can regulate penile erections, allowing blood to flow into the penis. NO also can modulate vascular smooth muscle in cardiac blood vessels and mediate the ability of nitroglycerin to treat cardiac angina. NO is also a key regulator of blood pressure, platelet aggregation, and peristalsis. Its CNS neurotransmitter function remains elusive, but it may be a "retrograde neurotransmitter." That is, since presynaptic neurotransmitters activate postsynaptic receptors, it seems logical that communication in this direction should be accompanied by some form of back talk from the postsynaptic site to the presynaptic neuron. The idea is that NO formation is prompted in postsynaptic synapses by some presynaptic neurotransmitters and then diffuses back to the presynaptic neuron, carrying information in reverse. NO may also be involved in memory formation, neuronal plasticity, and neurotoxicity. The notion of retrograde neurotransmission is introduced in Chapter 3, and the role of NO as a potential retrograde neurotransmitter is illustrated in Figure 3-3.

Other neurotransmitters and hormones that affect arousal positively include norepinephrine, melanocortin, testosterone, and estrogen (Figure 19-44). Serotonin has a negative influence on sexual arousal (Figure 19-44).

Disorders of Reward, Drug Abuse, and Their Treatment

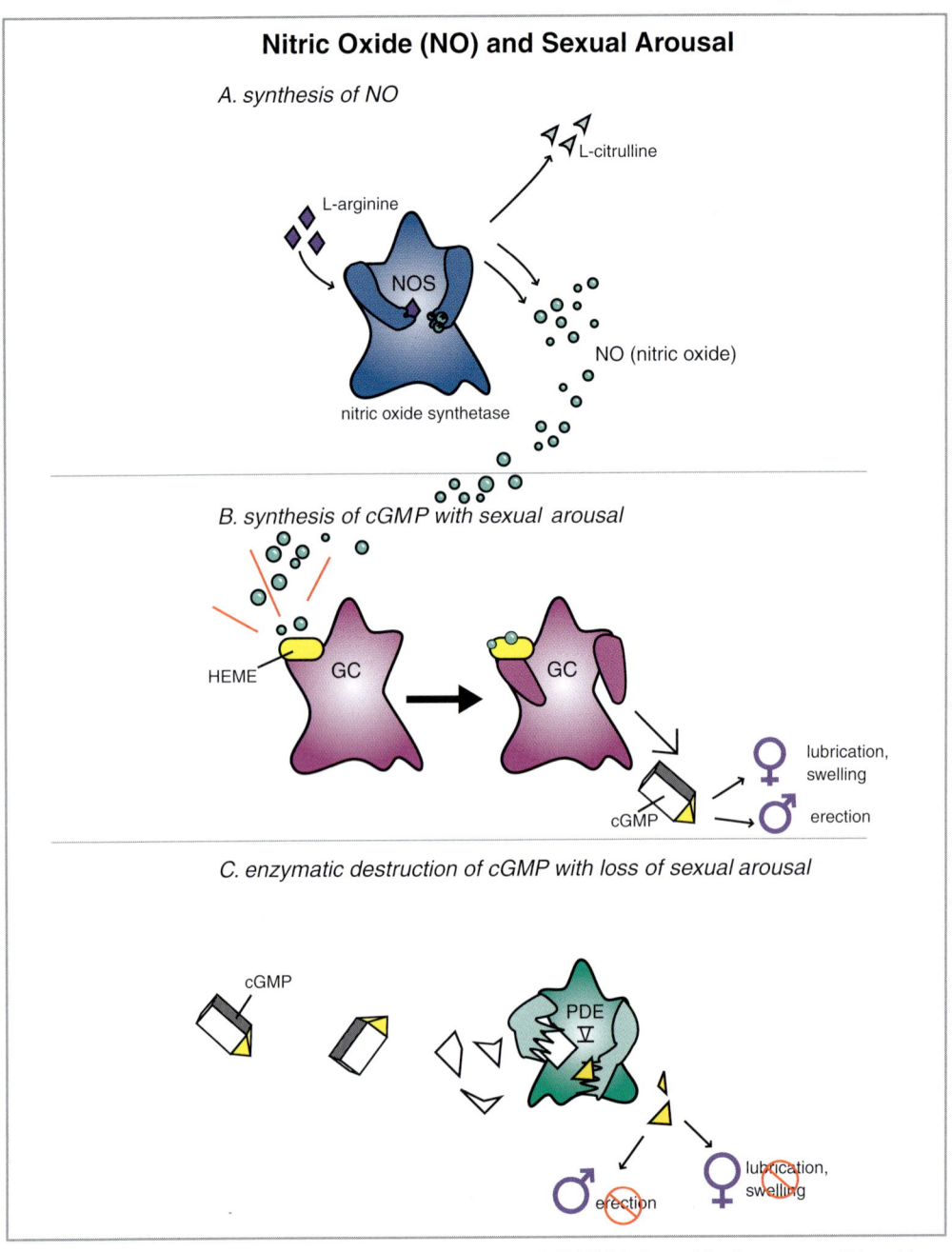

FIGURE 19-47A, B, and C Nitric oxide (NO) and sexual arousal. (**A**) NO is formed by the enzyme nitric oxide synthetase (NOS), which converts the amino acid l-arginine into NO and l-citrulline. (**B**) Once formed, NO activates the enzyme guanylyl cyclase (GC) by binding to iron (heme) in the active site of this enzyme. When activated, GC makes a messenger, cGMP (cyclic guanylate monophosphate), which relaxes smooth muscle and performs other physiological functions. In the penis, relaxation of vascular smooth muscle opens blood flow and causes an erection. (**C**) The action of cGMP is terminated by the enzyme phosphodiesterase, thus ending sexual arousal. In the penis, the type of phosphodiesterase is type V (PDE V).

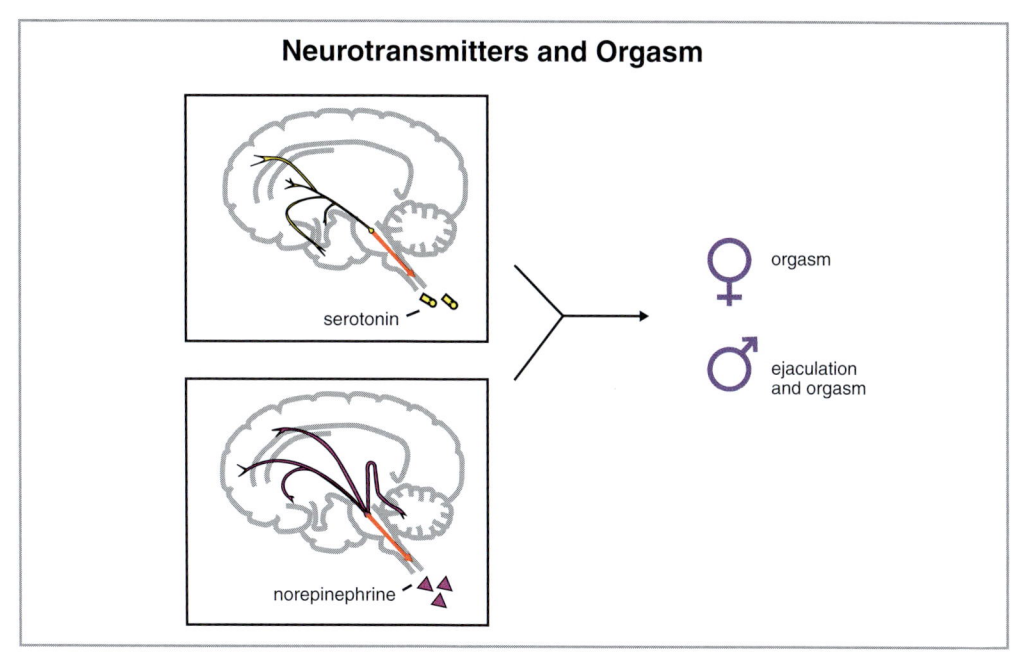

FIGURE 19-48 Neurotransmitters and orgasm. Orgasm is the third stage of the human sexual response, accompanied by ejaculation in men. Serotonin exerts an inhibitory action on orgasm and norepinephrine a facilitatory one.

Orgasm

The third stage of the human sexual response is orgasm (Figure 14-44), accompanied by ejaculation in men. Descending spinal serotonergic fibers exert **inhibitory** actions on orgasm via 5HT receptors, perhaps 5HT2A and 5HT2C receptors (Figure 19-48). Descending spinal noradrenergic fibers and noradrenergic sympathetic innervation of genitalia **facilitate** ejaculation and orgasm (Figure 19-44). Dopamine and NO may have weak positive influences on facilitating orgasm (Figure 19-44).

Sexual disorders and reward
Erectile dysfunction

The inability to maintain an erection sufficient for intercourse is called erectile dysfunction (formerly impotence). Up to 20 million men in the United States have this problem to some degree. Another way of stating the problem is that for normal men between 40 and 70 years of age living in the community, only about half do not have some degree of erectile dysfunction (Figure 19-49). The problem gets worse with age (Figure 19-50), since 39 percent of 40-year-olds have some degree of erectile dysfunction (5 percent are completely impotent); but by age 70, two thirds have some degree of erectile dysfunction (and complete impotence triples to 15 percent). The multiple causes of erectile dysfunction include vascular insufficiency, various neurological conditions, endocrine pathology (especially diabetes mellitus but also reproductive hormones and thyroid problems), drugs, local pathology in the penis, and psychological and psychiatric problems.

Until recently, psychopharmacologists were not very useful members of the treatment team for patients with erectile dysfunction other than to stop the medications they were prescribing! Effective treatment of "organic" causes of erectile dysfunction until recently was often elusive and usually involved a urological approach, such as prostheses and implants.

Prevalence of Erectile Dysfunction
Massachusetts Male Aging Study

men aged 40 to 70 years

no erectile dysfunction (48%)

some erectile dysfunction (52%)

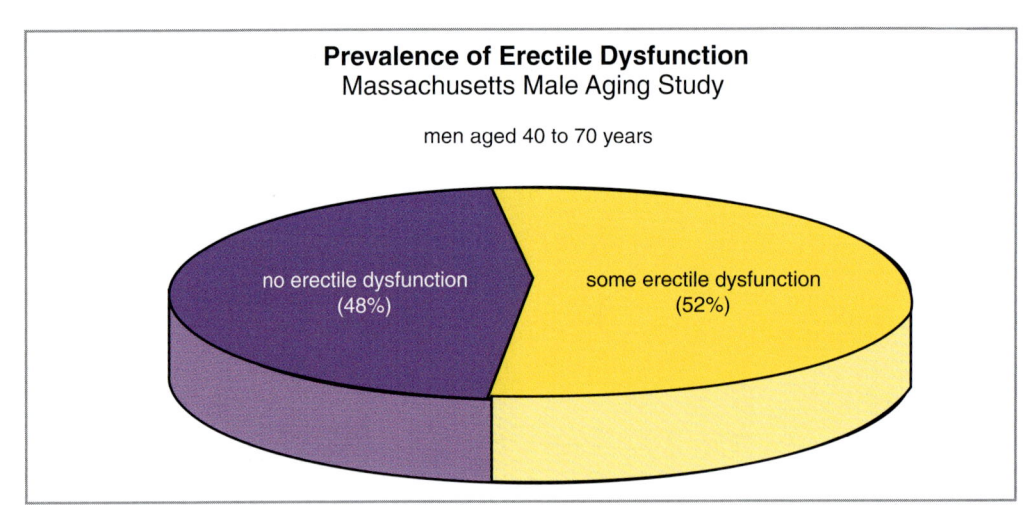

FIGURE 19-49 Prevalence of erectile dysfunction. About half of men between the ages of 40 and 70 experience some degree of erectile dysfunction (impotence).

Association between Age and Prevalence of Erectile Dysfunction (ED)
Massachusetts Male Aging Study

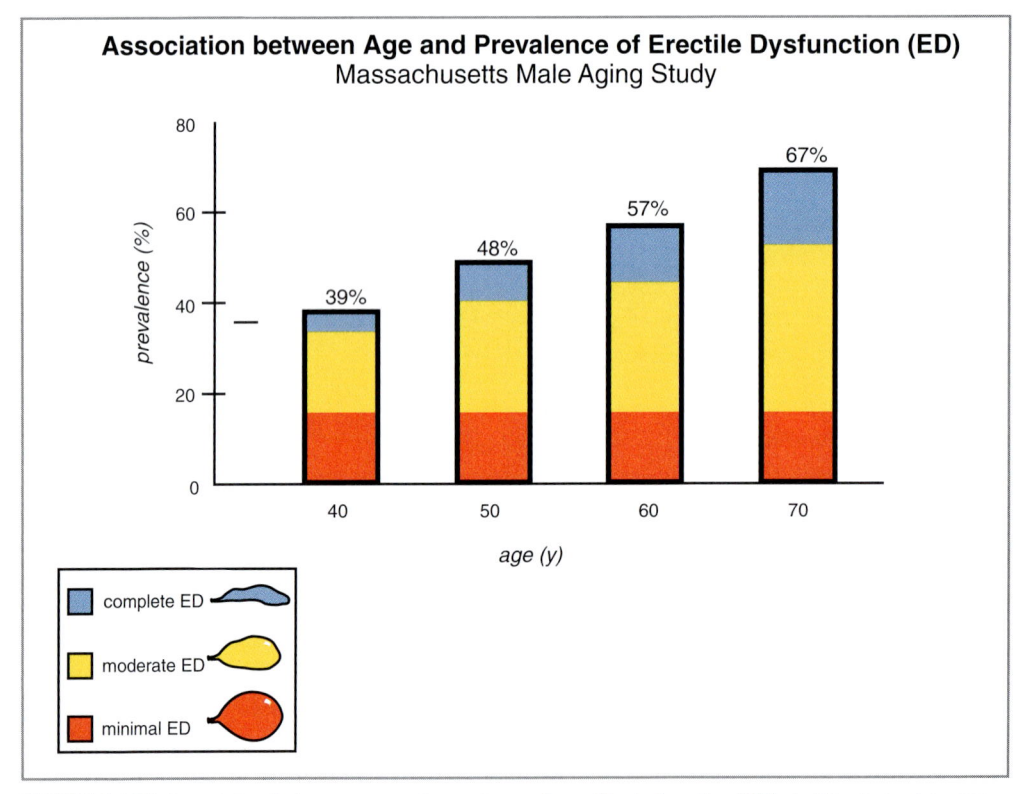

- complete ED
- moderate ED
- minimal ED

FIGURE 19-50 Association between age and prevalence of erectile dysfunction (ED). In this study of normal men between the ages of 40 and 70, the prevalence of erectile dysfunction increased with age from 39 percent at age 40 to 67 percent at age 70.

Association between Depression and Prevalence of Erectile Dysfunction
Massachusetts Male Aging Study

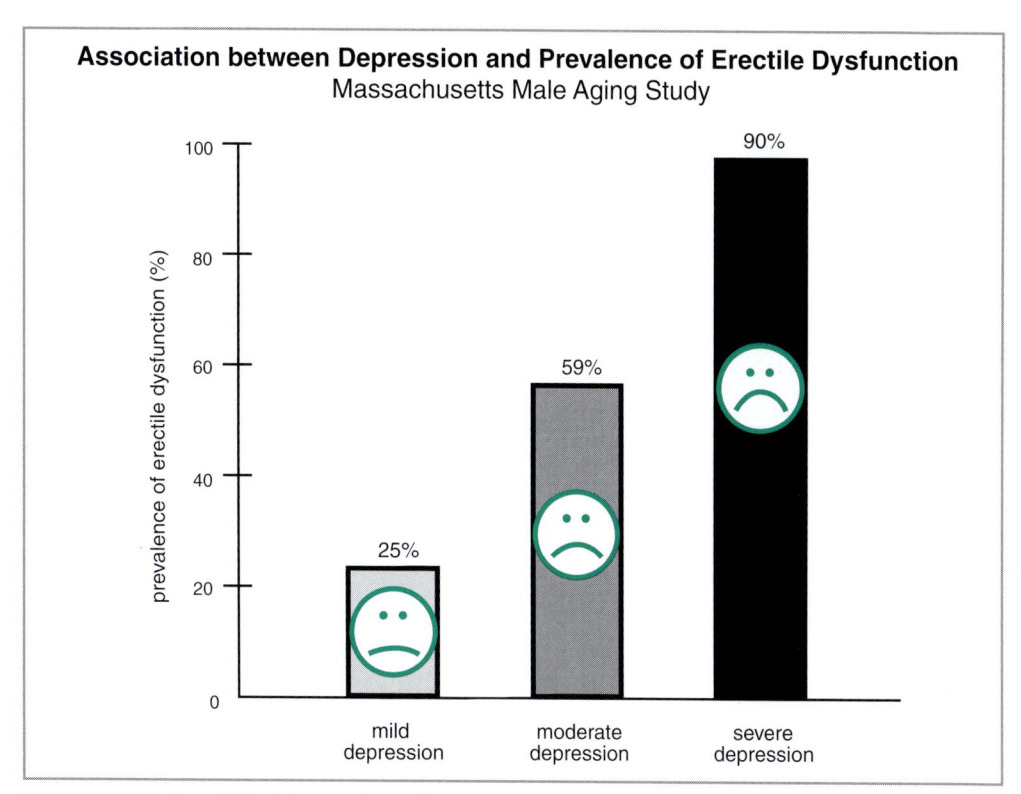

FIGURE 19-51 Association between depression and prevalence of erectile dysfunction (ED). Erectile dysfunction is associated with depression and increases in frequency as depression worsens. Some studies suggest that over 90 percent of severely depressed men have erectile dysfunction.

The old-fashioned surgical strategy bypasses diseased peripheral nerves and inadequate vascular blood supply to the penis to create erections mechanically and upon demand, but it has serious limitations in terms of patient and partner acceptability. In men who have a "functional" etiology to their erectile dysfunction, the treatment strategy has traditionally taken a psychodynamic and behavioral approach, with attention to partners and functional disorders, psychoeducation, lifestyle changes, and, where appropriate, starting (or stopping) psychotropic drugs to treat associated disorders. The typical case of erectile dysfunction, however, is due to neither a single "organic" cause nor a single "functional" cause but usually involves some combination of problems, including use of alcohol, smoking, diabetes, hypertension, antihypertensive drugs, psychotropic drugs, partner problems, performance anxiety, problems with self-esteem, and psychiatric disorder, especially depression.

The topic of erectile dysfunction has become increasingly important in psychopharmacology, not only because there are several psychotropic drugs that cause it but also because of the strikingly high incidence of erectile dysfunction in several common psychiatric disorders. For example, some studies show that more than 90 percent of men with severe depression have moderate to severe erectile dysfunction (Figure 19-51). Another reason for the importance of this topic in psychopharmacology is that several effective and simple psychopharmacological treatments based upon NO physiology and pharmacology are now available for men with erectile dysfunction.

Normal Erectile Function

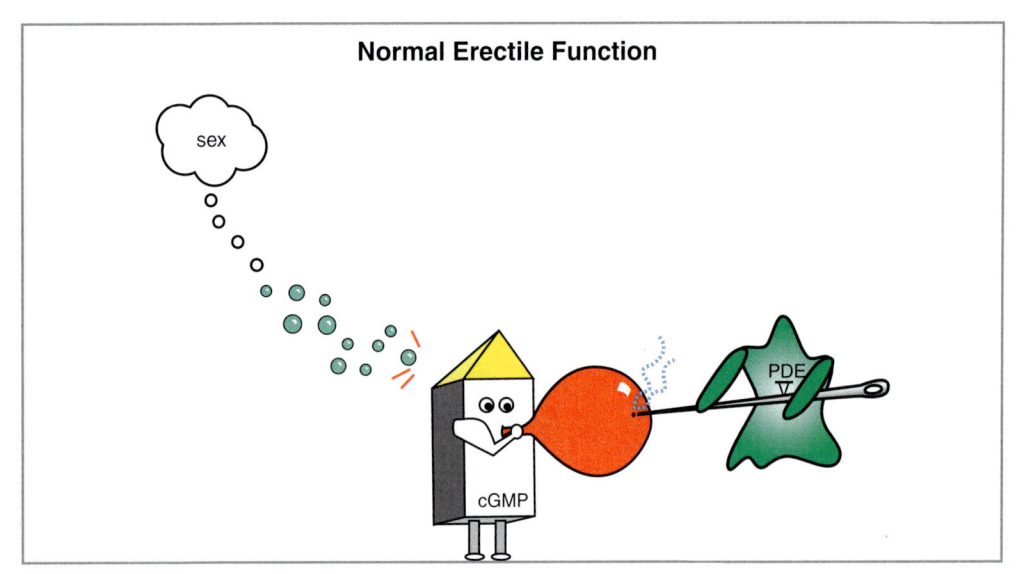

FIGURE 19-52 **Normal erectile function.** Under normal conditions, when young, healthy men are sexually aroused, nitric oxide causes cGMP to accumulate, and cGMP causes smooth muscle relaxation, resulting in a physiological erection (indicated here by an inflated balloon). The erection is sustained long enough for sexual intercourse, and then phosphodiesterase V (PDE V) metabolizes cGMP, reversing the erection (indicated here by a pin ready to prick the balloon).

Psychopharmacology of erectile dysfunction

Normally, the desire to have sex is a powerful message sent from the brain down the spinal cord and through peripheral nerves to smooth muscle cells in the penis, triggering them to produce plenty of NO to form all the cyclic GMP necessary to create an erection (Figure 19-52). The cyclic GMP lasts long enough for sexual intercourse to occur, but then phosphodiesterase (type V in the penis) eventually breaks down the cGMP (shown earlier in Figure 19-47C) and the erection is lost (called detumescence).

However, if you smoke, eat to the point of obesity, have elevated blood glucose and elevated blood pressure, your peripheral nervous system "wires" may not respond adequately to the "let's have sex" signal from the brain (i.e., neurological innervation of the penis is rendered faulty, usually by diabetes) (Figure 19-53). Furthermore, there may not be much pressure in the plumbing (i.e., atherosclerosis of the arterial supply of the penis from hypertension and hypercholesterolemia) when cGMP says "relax the smooth muscle and let the blood flow into the penis." In these cases, the desire to have sex is there, but the signal cannot get through, so insufficient cGMP is formed and therefore no erection occurs (Figure 19-53). Similarly, for a depressed patient who has the desire for sex, there is a general shutdown of neurotransmitter systems centrally and peripherally and the inability to become aroused (Figure 19-53).

Fortunately, there is a way to compensate for inadequate amounts of cGMP being formed. That compensation is to slow the rate of destruction of that cGMP that is formed. This is done by inhibiting the enzyme that normally breaks down cGMP in the penis, namely phosphodiesterase type V (Figure 19-54). There are now three inhibitors of this enzyme available: sildenafil (Viagra), tadalafil (Cialis), and vardenafil (Levitra) (Figure 19-54). These phosphodiesterase type V inhibitors will stop cGMP destruction for a time ranging from a few hours to a few days and allow the levels of cGMP to build up; therefore

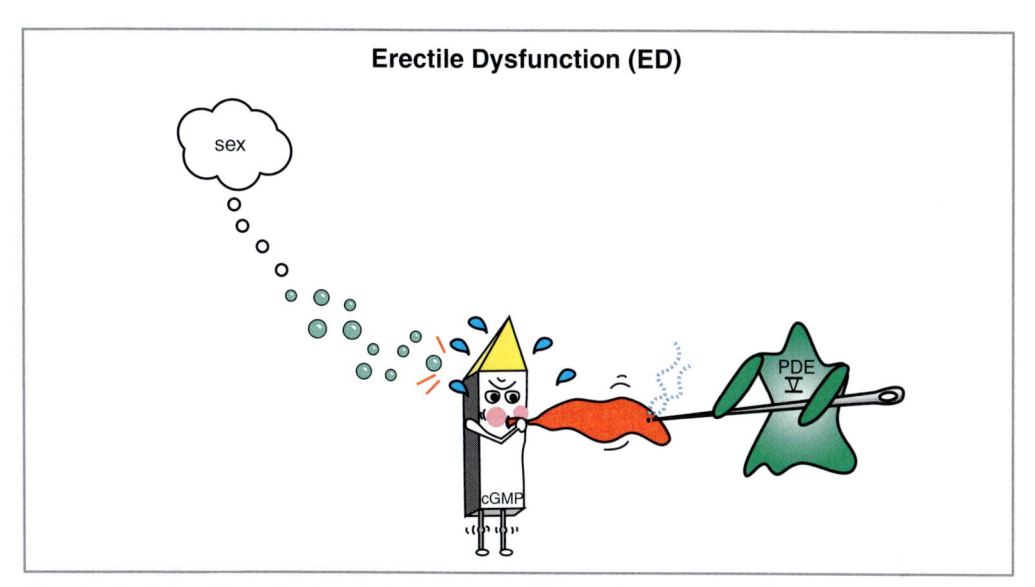

FIGURE 19-53 Erectile dysfunction. When a man has diabetes or hypertension or if he smokes, uses alcohol, takes prescription drugs, or is depressed, there is a good chance that not enough of a signal of sexual desire will be able to get through his peripheral nerves and arteries to produce sufficient amounts of cGMP to cause an erection. This leads to erectile dysfunction.

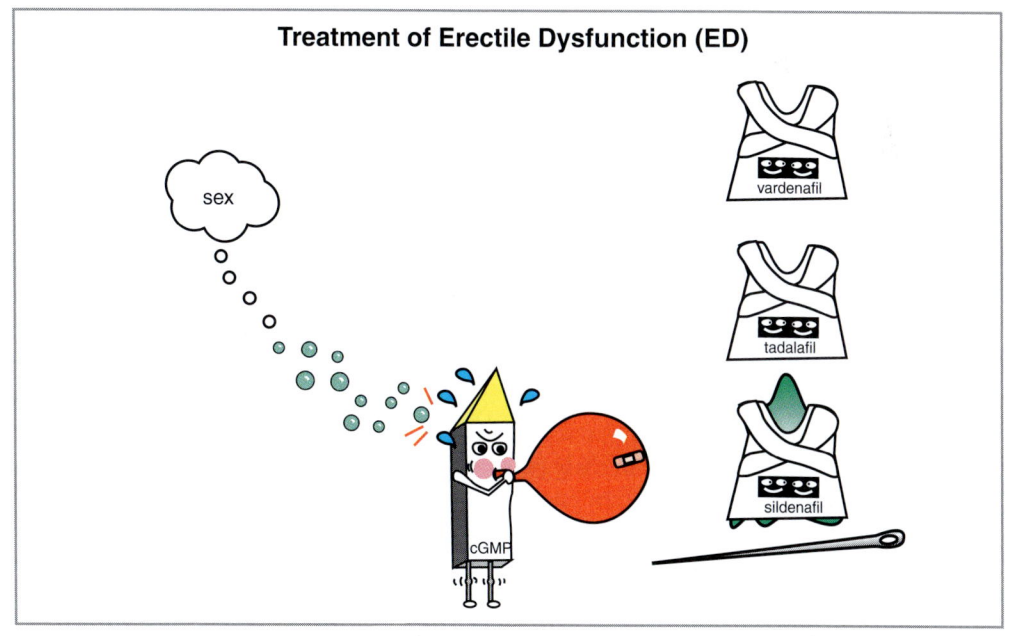

FIGURE 19-54 Treatment of erectile dysfunction. Phosphodiesterase V (PDE V) inhibitors are able to compensate for faulty signals through the peripheral nerves and arteries that produce insufficient amounts of cGMP to cause or sustain an erection. PDE V inhibitors do this by allowing cGMP to build up, since PDE V can no longer destroy cGMP for a few hours to a few days. This is indicated by a patch on the balloon in the figure. The result is that normally inadequate nerves and arteries signaling cGMP formation are now sufficient to inflate the balloon and therefore an erection can occur and sexual intercourse is possible until the drug wears off a few hours to a few days later.

Disorders of Reward, Drug Abuse, and Their Treatment | 1003

an erection can occur even though the "wires" and "plumbing" are still faulty (Figure 19-53). Interestingly, these agents work only if the patient is mentally interested in sex and attempts to become aroused, so that at least weak signals are sent to the penis (i.e., it does not work during sleep).

Smooth muscle relaxation is thus the key element in attaining an erection. Administration of prostaglandins can also relax penile smooth muscle and elicit erections in a manner that mimics typical physiological mechanisms. Thus, intrapenile injection of the prostaglandin alprostadil produces erections not only in men with organic causes of impotence but also in those with functional causes and even in the common situation of multifactorial causes. Limitations of this somewhat masochistic approach include the unacceptability of self-injection, lack of spontaneity, and the possibility of too much of a good thing, namely a prolonged and painful erection, or priapism. Prostaglandin administration will cause an erection whether the man is mentally aroused or not.

Other drugs can affect sexual arousal, including SSRIs or SNRIs in some patients. Some of these agents may inhibit NOS directly and thus can cause erectile dysfunction. On the other hand, some dopaminergic agents might boost NOS, and for this reason pro-dopaminergic agents may be useful not only in enhancing desire but also in enhancing arousal. Anticholinergic agents can interfere directly with arousal and cause erectile dysfunction. Thus, those antipsychotics, tricyclic antidepressants, and other drugs with anticholinergic properties can cause erectile dysfunction.

Hypoactive sexual desire disorder (HSDD)

Another disorder of sexual function is decreased libido, lack of sexual motivation, and decreased sexual fantasies, known as hypoactive sexual desire disorder (HSDD). This is a controversial concept, because it can be difficult to separate a chronic and disabling condition from common transient alterations in sexual behavior related to interpersonal problems, life stress, and just common fatigue, overwork, and sleep deprivation that are part of living in the modern world. Now that there are potential treatments on the horizon, is it possible that HSDD is just a "corporate sponsored creation of a new disease"? Furthermore, decreased libido is often part of major depressive disorder (see discussions in Chapters 11 and 12 and Figures 11-45, 11-55, and 12-124 through 12-126), so is it possible that decreased libido is more likely to be a residual symptom of a major depressive episode that has not gone into remission rather than an independent clinical entity (Figure 19-55)? Finally, HSDD is often considered to be mostly a disorder of females, perhaps especially by men, so is it a gender relationship issue of men rather than a true form of sexual dysfunction in women? Many women report reduction of sexual desire with the duration of a relationship, and some may have lost interest in their partner but may still feel like having sex with the guy next door. Such issues are not likely to be resolved by taking drugs to enhance sexual desire, and answers to these various questions may be forthcoming as further research is done on the symptom of decreased libido. Nevertheless, it is already clear that certain hormones and drugs can increase sexual desire in those who complain of having too little of it.

Like many of the disorders discussed in this text, to the extent that the core symptoms of decreased libido and decreased sexual fantasies define HSDD, there are frequently many associated nondiagnostic symptoms that are equally important to assess and treat (Figure 19-55). These include various symptoms of major depression, not just depressed mood and decreased libido itself but also change in appetite and weight (self-image and body-image problems can interfere secondarily with sexual desire); apathy, loss of interest and lack of

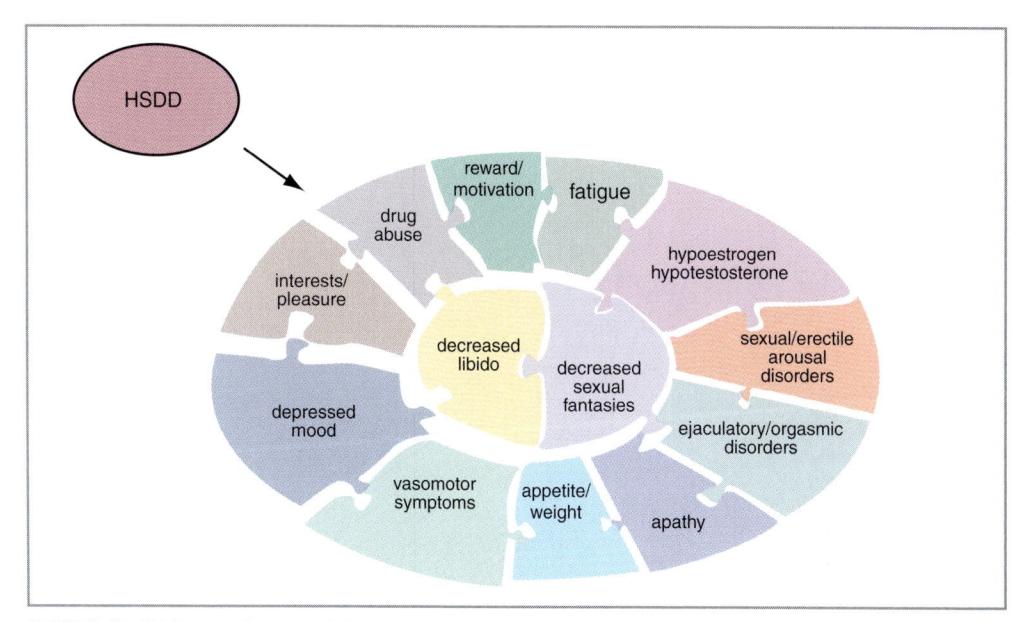

FIGURE 19-55 Hypoactive sexual desire disorder (HSDD). HSDD is a disorder of sexual function characterized by decreased libido and decreased sexual fantasies. In addition, there are many associated nondiagnostic symptoms, as shown here. These include various symptoms of major depression, vasomotor symptoms in perimenopausal women, hypoestrogen and/or hypotestosterone states in women, and hypotestosterone states in men.

experiencing pleasure globally and not just with sex; lack of motivation to do many things, not just sexual intercourse; and of course fatigue, which may be the greatest antiaphrodesiac known (Figure 19-55). Also, a number of other conditions may be associated with HSDD, including vasomotor symptoms in perimenopausal women, discussed extensively in Chapter 12 and illustrated in Figures 12-104, 12-106 and 12-124 through 12-126. Hypoestrogen and hypotestosterone states in women and hypotestosterone states in men can also be associated with lack of sexual interest as one of the symptoms (Figure 19-55).

Thus the symptom of lack of sexual interest requires in-depth evaluation and then constructing a proper diagnosis (Figure 19-55). The strategy then is to deconstruct the various symptoms of the patient's syndrome (e.g., those listed in Figure 19-55) and match them to hypothetically malfunctioning brain circuits (Figure 19-56). Knowing the neurotransmitters (and hormones) that affect neurotransmission in these circuits provides a psychopharmacological rationale for selecting and combining treatments to eliminate the patient's symptoms. Note in Figure 19-56 that the great majority of symptoms associated with HSDD (shown in Figure 19-55) are linked to the nucleus accumbens, the critical area of the brain that regulates reward (Figures 19-2, 19-3, and 19-45).

Although there are no approved treatments for HSDD, several approaches targeting neurotransmitters and hormones in reward circuitry are being tested in clinical trials. The notion is that the low sexual desire of HSDD is linked to low functioning of dopaminergic reward neurons in the mesolimbic pathway (Figure 19-57A). Indeed, anecdotal observations document that some patients taking levodopa or dopamine agonists for Parkinson's disease experience increased sex drive, as do some patients taking the pro-dopaminergic antidepressant and NDRI bupropion. Testosterone may enhance sexual interest by actions on neurons in the hypothalamus and boost the ability of dopamine to act in the hypothalamus.

Some Key HSDD Symptoms Hypothetically Linked to Specific Brain Regions

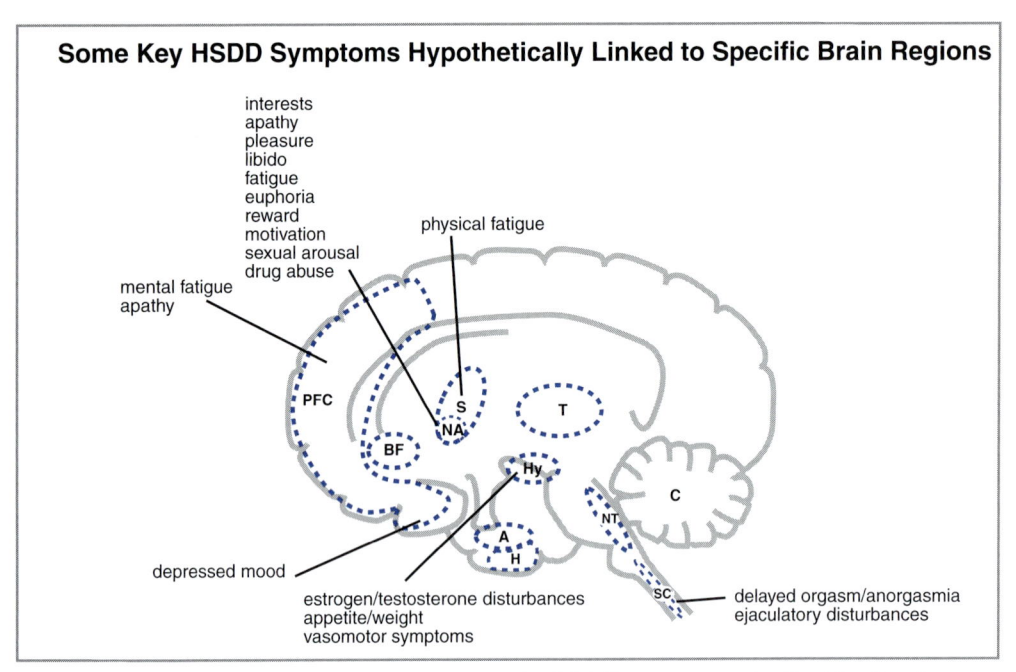

FIGURE 19-56 Matching hypoactive sexual desire disorder (HSDD) symptoms to circuits. Alterations in neurotransmission within each of the brain regions shown here can be hypothetically linked to the various symptoms associated with HSDD. Functionality in each brain region may be associated with a different constellation of symptoms. PFC: prefrontal cortex; BF: basal forebrain; S: striatum; NA: nucleus accumbens; T: thalamus; HY: hypothalamus; A: amygdala; H: hippocampus; NT: brainstem neurotransmitter centers; SC: spinal cord; C: cerebellum.

In fact, testosterone has shown positive results in women given low doses transdermally, but concerns about long-term safety led the FDA to withhold approval of this approach pending more safety studies.

One novel approach to HSDD is to administer a peptide intranasally that acts on melanocortin receptors in the hypothalamus (Figure 19-57B). Specifically, the drug bremelanotide is an agonist at melanocortin MC3 and MC4 receptors, and stimulating these receptors in the hypothalamus increases sexual behavior in animals, boosts the actions of DA in hypothalamic areas such as the medial preoptic area (MPOA) (see Figure 19-57B), and also shows preliminary evidence of efficacy in women with HSDD (and also in men with erectile dysfunction). Concerns have arisen, however, about the ability of this drug to raise blood pressure.

Another novel approach to HSDD is the serotonergic agent flibanserin, which has shown preliminary evidence of efficacy in women with HSDD. Flibanserin acts as a norepinephrine and dopamine disinhibitor (NDDI) by means of its pharmacological properties of 5HT1A agonism, plus 5HT2A and 5HT2C antagonism (Figure 19-57B). NDDI action due to 5HT2C antagonism is discussed extensively in Chapter 12 and illustrated in Figure 12-25. The enhancement of dopamine release by combining 5HT2C (and 5HT2A) antagonism with agonist actions at 5HT1A receptors is discussed in Chapter 10 and illustrated in Figure 10-21; it is also discussed in Chapter 12 and illustrated in Figures 12-61 through 12-64. Flibanserin increases dopamine (and norepinephrine) release and also reduces serotonin release, properties that would enhance reward and hypothetically increase sexual motivation when these actions occur in the MPOA and nucleus accumbens (Figure 19-57B). Ongoing

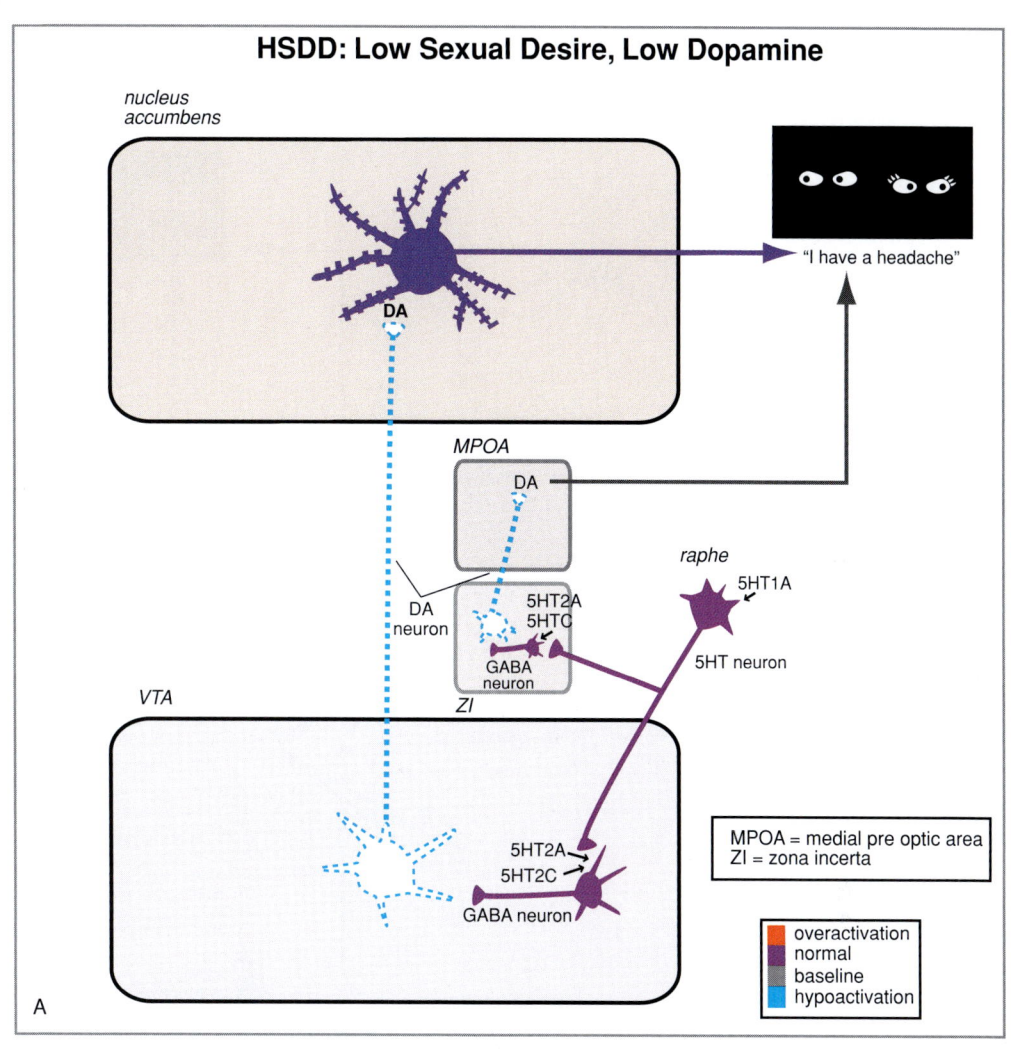

FIGURE 19-57A Hypoactive sexual desire disorder (HSDD): low dopamine? Low sexual desire in HSDD is believed to be due to hypoactivity of mesolimbic dopaminergic neurons (depicted here by the blue color and dashed lines of the neuron).

research will determine whether flibanserin has sufficient efficacy and safety in HSDD to possibly become the first approved treatment for this condition.

Compulsive sexual behavior

A number of conditions linked to sexual activity of various sorts have been categorized as disorders of impulsivity (Table 19-5). Hypothetically, some of these conditions could be linked to abnormal activity of reward circuits (Figure 19-2), analogous to an addiction, where there is deficient descending inhibitory influence from the reflective reward system in the prefrontal cortex (Figure 19-3) to stop the expression of abnormal sexual drives arising from the reactive reward system of the VTA and amygdala (Figure 19-4). These concepts are controversial if novel, and therapeutic approaches targeting neurotransmitters in reward circuitry (Figures 19-5 through 19-8) may eventually provide relief for some of these disorders (Table 19-5).

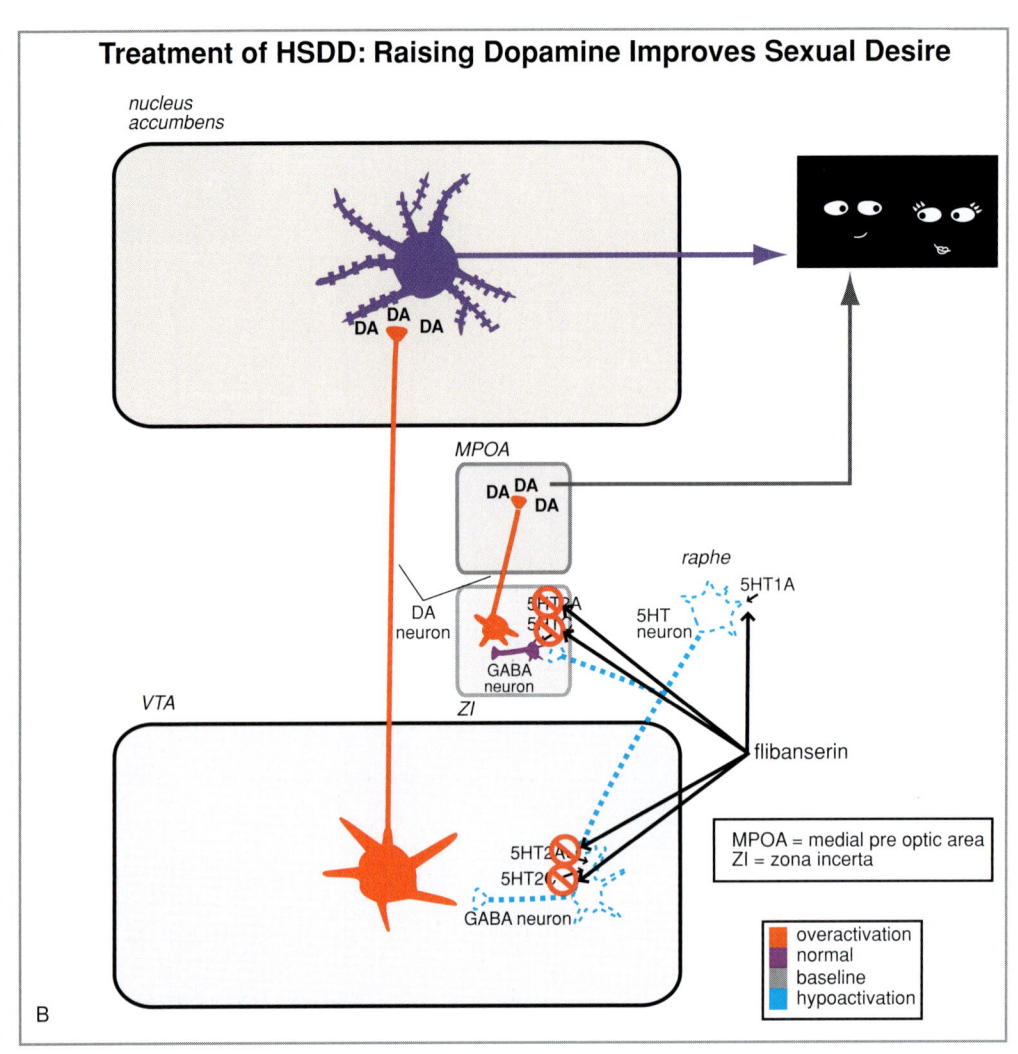

FIGURE 19-57B Treatment of hypoactive sexual desire disorder (HSDD) by raising dopamine. Potential treatments for HSDD include agents that increase dopaminergic neurotransmission in the nucleus accumbens. This may be achieved with bremelanotide, which is an agonist at melanocortin 3 and 4 (MC3 and MC4) receptors in the medial preoptic area (MPOA) of the hypothalamus, or by flibanserin, which is a 5HT1A agonist and a 5HT2A and 5HT2C antagonist.

Eating disorders

Eating disorders and reward circuits

Should obesity be included as a brain disorder? Did my receptors make me eat it? Obesity is a complex disorder, with lifestyles, diet, and exercise playing major roles in twenty-first century society. Certainly there is an ongoing epidemic of obesity and metabolic disorder in society today; this is discussed in Chapter 10 in relation to antipsychotic drugs and illustrated in Figures 10-59 through 10-69. Chapter 10 also discusses the potential roles of genes associated with various mental illnesses and drugs used to treat mental illnesses as additional risk factors for obesity, and ultimately cardiometabolic disorders.

It is also possible that some forms of obesity are driven by an excessive motivational drive for food, mediated by reward circuitry, and as such might be considered as mental

TABLE 19-5 Psychopharmacology and sexual disorder

Erectile dysfunction (ED)
Hypoactive sexual desire disorder (HSDD)
Anorgasmia/ejaculatory delay
Premature ejaculation
Sexual pain disorders
SSRI/SNRI-induced sexual dysfunctions
Sexual "addictions" – impulsivity/compulsivity disorders:
- Paraphilias
- Exhibitionism
- Fetishism
- Frotteurism
- Pedophilia
- Sexual sadism
- Sexual masochism
- Transvestic fetishism
- Voyeurism
- Compulsive cruising and multiple partners
- Compulsive fixation on an unattainable partner
- Compulsive autoeroticism
- Compulsive use of erotica
- Compulsive use of the internet
- Compulsive multiple love relationships
- Compulsive sexuality in a relationship

disorders. Can you be addicted to food with compulsive consumption and the inability to refrain from eating despite the desire to do so? Can you be addicted to carbohydrates or your "sugar fix?" Are high-fat foods "comfort foods" that relieve craving and cause pleasure because they are addicting?

These symptoms associated with obesity, overeating, and binge eating in many patients are remarkably similar to the addictions to various drugs described in this chapter. A hypothetical if oversimplified idea for how certain eating disorders could be linked to reward circuits is shown in Figure 19-58, with dopamine projections not only to the nucleus accumbens but also to the mammillary nucleus of the hypothalamus, an area of the hypothalamus that exerts important regulatory control of eating in animals. This region projects to nucleus accumbens as well, where it may regulate the motivation to eat (and addiction to food?).

Current research is attempting to clarify the role of a long list of other key regulators of hypothalamic activity in eating: leptin, ghrelin, anandamide, neurotensin, CRF, cholecystokinin, insulin, glucagon, calcitonin, amylin, bonbesin, somatostatin, cytokines, melanocortin, orexin, dynorphin, beta endorphin, galanin, neuropeptide Y and many other hormones, neurotransmitters and hypothalamic peptides. The roles of hypothalamic serotonin actions, particularly at 5HT2C receptors, and hypothalamic histamine actions, particularly at H1 receptors, are discussed in Chapter 10 and illustrated in Figure 10-59.

Treatments for compulsive eating, obesity, and "food addiction"
The prevalence and morbidity of obesity are sufficiently vast that it is important if not urgent to develop therapeutic interventions. It is possible that some patients could benefit from approaches that target hypothalamic and mesolimbic reward circuits, since obesity

Eating, Hunger, and Reward Circuits

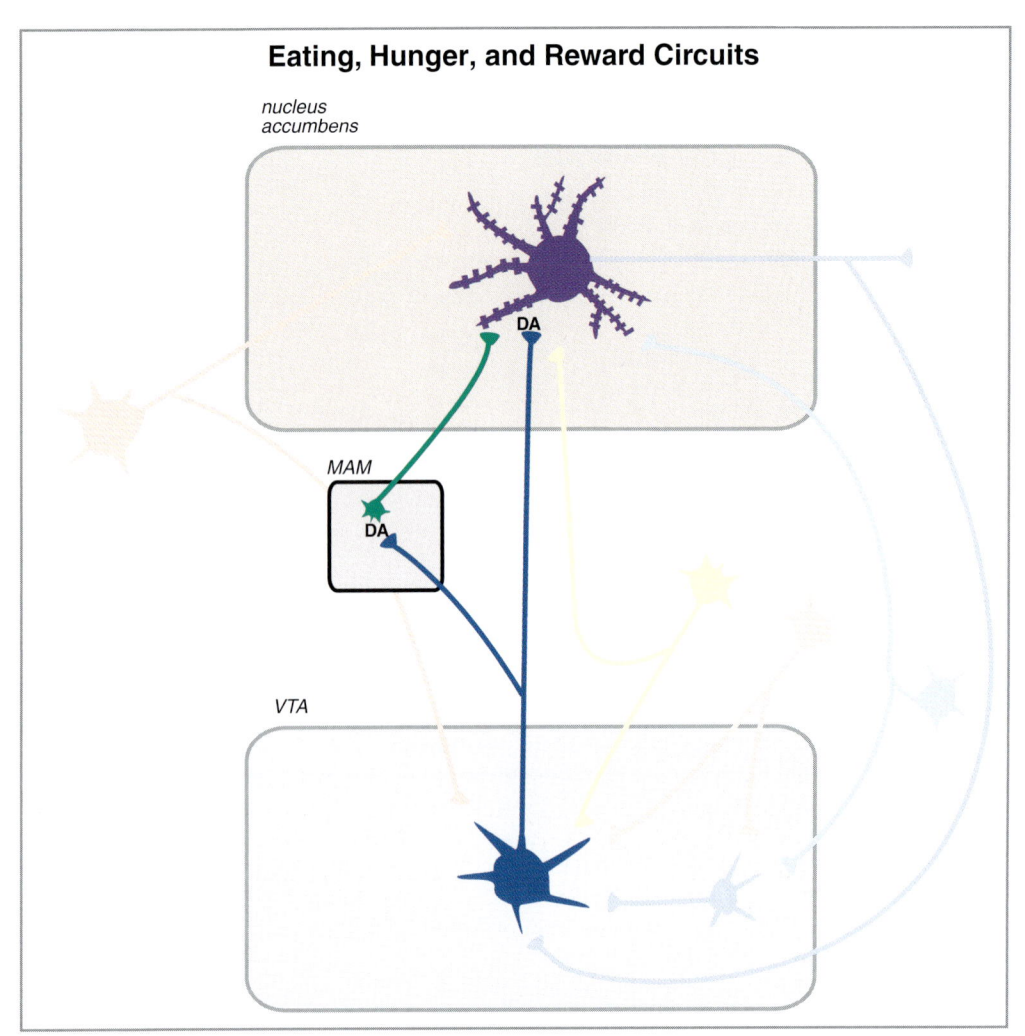

FIGURE 19-58 Eating, hunger, and reward circuits. Shown here is the reactive reward system consisting of the ventral tegmental area (VTA), site of dopamine cell bodies that receives many neurotransmitter projections; the nucleus accumbens, to which dopaminergic neurons project; and the amygdala (far left), which has connections with both the VTA and the nucleus accumbens. In addition, dopamine projections extend to the mammillary nucleus (MAM) of the hypothalamus, an area important for regulatory control of eating; projections from these regions themselves extend to the nucleus accumbens. Thus the circuitry of hunger is interconnected with the circuitry for reward.

may not always be just a metabolic disorder but, in some cases, a disorder of reward circuits or even an addiction.

Current drugs of abuse, especially stimulants and nicotine, reduce appetite. Others, such as marijuana, actually stimulate appetite, leading to the use of the cannabinoid CB1 antagonist for the treatment of obesity. As mentioned earlier, this agent is approved in some countries but not in the United States. Approved stimulants for obesity, including the SNRI sibutramine, have fallen into relative disrepute given their lack of long-term efficacy in most patients plus the risk of hypertension and the toxicity scare caused by the amphetamine derivative fenfluramine in the recent past. Orlistat, now available without prescription, inhibits fat absorption and works peripherally and not on reward circuitry except to the extent that it causes an aversive response to eating fatty foods (diarrhea and flatus). It is not highly utilized or highly palatable to many patients.

Fluoxetine is approved for bulimia and acts perhaps in part to suppress appetite via its 5HT2C antagonist properties (see Figure 12-25). Other agents active at 5HT2C sites, including both agonists (e.g., GSK 875167 and others) and antagonists (see the list at the end of Chapter 10 on new treatments for schizophrenia) are also in testing for obesity.

The anticonvulsants topiramate and zonisamide and the ADHD drug and norepinephrine reuptake inhibitor atomoxetine have anecdotally been associated with weight loss in some patients and are now in testing for obesity. Some medications approved for diabetes may hold promise for the treatment of obesity, including metformin and the injectable peptide pramlintide (Symlin; discussed in Chapter 10). Another novel agent is Axokine, or ciliary neurotrophic factor, which is in testing for obesity, since it seems to cause weight loss in humans. Cholecystolinin agonists (e.g., GSK 181771) and other agents active at various peptide receptors, including bremelanotide (MC3 and MC4 agonist discussed above for treatment of HSDD and illustrated in Figure 19-57B) are also in testing for obesity. Some analysts estimate that there are actually hundreds of agents in testing for obesity in the hope that some therapeutic intervention can be found for this epidemic. Some of the approaches target reward circuitry (Figure 12-58) and approach obesity as a disorder of reward, analogous to an addiction.

Other impulse-control disorders

A number of other conditions have been linked to reward circuitry and have been conceptualized as addictions. This includes borderline personality disorder, compulsive gambling, kleptomania, pyromania, compulsive shopping, and other related conditions. Whether these will prove to be disorders of reward and whether they will prove treatable by approaching them as addictions remains a topic of intense current interest and research.

Summary

This chapter discussed the psychopharmacology of reward and the brain circuitry that regulates reward. We have attempted to explain the psychopharmacological mechanisms of action of various drugs of abuse, from nicotine to alcohol, and also opiates, stimulants, sedative hypnotics, marijuana, hallucinogens, and club drugs. In the case of nicotine and alcohol, various novel psychopharmacological treatments are discussed, including the alpha 4 beta 2 selective nicotine partial agonist (NPA) varenicline for smoking cessation and naltrexone and acamprosate for alcohol dependence. For each of the drug classes explored, their hypothetical actions upon mesolimbic reward circuitry are explained. Disorders of sexual function hypothetically linked to dysregulation of reward mechanisms in this same circuitry are also explored. Finally, a number of disorders are discussed that are not recognized substance abuse disorders but may be forms of addiction, including obesity, gambling, and other related conditions.

Suggested Readings

General – Textbooks

Charney DS and Nestler EJ. (eds) (2004) *Neurobiology of Mental Illness*. 2nd ed. New York, Oxford University Press.

Davis KL, Charney D, Coyle JT and Nemeroff C. (eds) (2002) *Neuropsychopharmacology: The Fifth Generation of Progress*. Philadelphia, Lippincott Williams & Wilkins.

Diagnostic and Statistical Manual of Mental Disorders. (2005) 4th ed. Washington, D.C., American Psychiatric Association.

Everitt BS and Wessely S. (2004) *Clinical Trials in Psychiatry*. New York, Oxford University Press.

Jacobson SA, Pies RW and Katz IR. (2007) *Clinical Manual of Geriatric Psychopharmacology*. Washington, D.C., American Psychiatric Publishing.

Marangell LB and Martinez JM. (2006) *Psychopharmacology*. 2nd ed. Washington, D.C., American Psychiatric Publishing.

Pies RW. (2005) *Handbook of Essential Psychopharmacology*. 2nd ed. New York, Oxford University Press.

Schatzberg AF and Nemeroff CB. (eds) (2004) *Textbook of Psychopharmacology*. 3rd ed. Washington, D.C., American Psychiatric Publishing.

Schatzberg AF, Cole JO and DeBattista C. (2005) *Manual of Clinical Psychopharmacology*. 5th ed. Washington, D.C., American Psychiatric Publishing.

Stahl SM. (2005) *Essential Psychopharmacology: The Prescriber's Guide*. Cambridge, UK, Cambridge University Press.

Chapters 1–8 (Basic Science) – Textbooks

Brunton LL, Lazo JS and Parker KL. (eds) (2006) *Goodman & Gilman's The Pharmacological Basis of Therapeutics*. 11th ed. New York, McGraw Hill.

Byrne JH and Roberts JL. (eds) (2004) *From Molecules to Networks. An Introduction to Cellular and Molecular Neuroscience*. San Diego, CA, Academic Press.

Cooper JR, Bloom FE and Roth RH. (2003) *The Biochemical Basis of Neuropharmacology*. New York, Oxford University Press.

Feldman RS, Meyer JS and Quenzer LF. (1997) *Principles of Neuropsychopharmacology*. Sunderland, MA, Sinauer Associates.

Meyer JS and Quenzer LF. (2005) *Psychopharmacology: Drugs, the Brain, and Behavior*. Sunderland, MA, Sinauer Associates.

Nestler EJ, Hyman SE and Malenka RC. (2001) *Molecular Neuropharmacology: A Foundation for Clinical Neuroscience*. New York, McGraw Hill.

Nolte J and Angevine Jr JB. (2000) *The Human Brain in Photographs and Diagrams*. 2nd ed. St. Louis, Mosby.

Shepherd GM. (ed) (2004) *The Synaptic Organization of the Brain*. 5th ed. New York, Oxford University Press.

Squire LR, Bloom FE, McConnell SK, Roberts JL, Spitzer NC and Zigmond MJ. (eds) (2003) *Fundamental Neuroscience*. 2nd ed. San Diego, CA, Academic Press.

Talairach J and Tournoux P. (1988) *Co-Planar Stereotaxic Atlas of the Human Brain*. New York, Thieme Medical Publishers.

Chapters 1–8 (Basic Science)

Ackley BD and Jin Y. (2004) Genetic analysis of synaptic target recognition and assembly. *Trends Neurosci* 27; 9, 540–547.

Carlisle HJ and Kennedy MB. (2005) Spine architecture and synaptic plasticity. *Trends Neurosci* 28; 4, 182–187.

Charney DS. (2004) Psychobiological mechanisms of resilience and vulnerability: implications for successful adaptation to extreme stress. *Am J Psychiatry* 161; 2, 195–216.

Chotard C and Salecker I. (2004) Neurons and glia: team players in axon guidance. *Trends Neurosci* 27; 11, 655–690.

Cotman CW and Berchtold NC. (2002) Exercise: a behavioral intervention to enhance brain health and plasticity. *Trends Neurosci* 25; 6, 295–301.

Dean C and Dresbach T. (2006) Neuroligins and neurexins: linking cell adhesion, synapse formation and cognitive function. *Trends Neurosci* 29; 1, 21–29.

Du J, Szabo ST, Gry NA and Manji HK. (2004) CaMKII: a molecular switch in the pathophysiology and treatment of mood and anxiety disorders. *Int J Neuropsychopharmacol* 7; 243–248.

Duman RS. (2002) Synaptic plasticity and mood disorders. *Mol Psychiatry* 7; S29–S34.

Duman RS. (2004) Depression: a case of neuronal life and death? *Biol Psychiatry* 56; 140–145.

Eriksson PS and Wallin L. (2004) Functional consequences of stress-related suppression of adult hippocampal neurogenesis – a novel hypothesis on the neurobiology of burnout. *Acta Neurol Scand* 110; 275–280.

Evans RM and Zamponi GW. (2006) Presynaptic Ca^{2+} channels – integration centers for neuronal signaling pathways. *Trends in Neurosci* 29; 11, 617–624.

Garner CC, Zhai RG, Gundelfinger ED and Ziv NE. (2002) Molecular mechanisms of CNS synaptogenesis. *Trends Neurosci* 25; 5, 243–250.

Garver DL, Holcomb JA and Christensen JD. (2005) Cerebral cortical gray expansion associated with two second-generation antipsychotics. *Biol Psychiatry* 58; 62–66.

Hagg T. (2005) Molecular regulation of adult CNS neurogenesis: an integrated view. *Trends Neurosci* 28; 11, 589–595.

Henn FA and Vollmayr B. (2004) Neurogenesis and depression: etiology or epiphenomenon? *Biol Psychiatry* 56; 146–150.

Hertz L and Zielke R. (2004) Astrocytic control of glutamatergic activity: astrocytes as stars of the show. *Trends Neurosci* 27; 12, 735–743.

Horner PJ and Palmer TD. (2003) New roles for astrocytes: The nightlife of an "astrocyte." La vida loca! *Trends Neurosci* 26; 11, 597–603.

Karten YJG, Olariu A and Cameron HA. (2005) Stress in early life inhibits neurogenesis in adulthood. *Trends Neurosci* 28; 4, 171–172.

Konradi C and Heckers S. (2001) Antipsychotic drugs and neuroplasticity: insights into the treatment and neurobiology of schizophrenia. *Biol Psychiatry* 50; 729–742.

Lavretsky H, Roybal DJ, Ballmaier M, Toga AW and Kumar A. (2005) Antidepressant exposure may protect against decrement in frontal gray matter volumes in geriatric depression. *J Clin Psychiatry* 66; 8, 964–967.

Madsen TM, Yeh DD, Valentine GW and Duman RS. (2005) Electroconvulsive seizure treatment increases cell proliferation in rat frontal cortex. *Neuropsychopharmacology* 30; 27–34.

Malberg JE and Duman RS. (2003) Cell proliferation in adult hippocampus is decreased by inescapable stress: reversal by fluoxetine treatment. *Neuropsychopharmacology* 28; 1562–1571.

Malberg JE, Eisch AJ, Nestler EJ and Duman RS. (2000) Chronic antidepressant treatment increases neurogenesis in adult rat hippocampus. *J Neurosci* 20; 24, 9104–9110.

Newton SS, Collier EF, Hunsberger J, Adams D, Terwilliger R, Selanayagam E and Duman RS. (2003) Gene profile of electroconvulsive seizures: induction of neurotrophic and angiogenic factors. *J Neurosci* 23; 34, 10841–10851.

Purcell AL and Carew TJ. (2003) Tyrosinekinases, synaptic plasticity and memory: insights from vertebrates and invertebrates. *Trends Neurosci* 26; 11, 625–630.

Raig AM, Graf ER and Linhoff MW. (2006) How to build a central synapse: clues from cell culture. *Trends Neurosci* 29; 1, 8–20.

Santarelli L, Saxe M, Gross C, Surget A, Battaglia F, Dulawa S, Weisstaub N, Lee J, Duman R, Arancio O, Belzung C and Hen R. (2003) Requirement of hippocampal neurogenesis for the behavioral effects of antidepressants. *Science* 301; 8, 805–809.

Sapolsky RM. (2004) Is impaired neurogenesis relevant to the affective symptoms of depression? *Biol Psychiatry* 56; 137–139.

Suenaga T, Morinobu S, Kawano K, Sawada T and Yamawaki S. (2004) Influence of immobilization stress on the levels of CaMKII and phosphor-CaMKII in the rat hippocampus. *Int J Neuropsychopharmacol* 7; 299–309.

Tsay D and Yuste R. (2004) On the electrical function of dendritic spines. *Trends Neurosci* 27; 2, 77–83.

Zou Y. (2004) Wnt signaling in axon guidance. *Trends Neurosci* 27; 9, 528–532.

Chapters 9 (Psychosis and Schizophrenia) and 10 (Antipsychotic Agents)

Abbatecola AM, Rizzo MR, Barbieri M, Grella R, Arciello A, Laieta MT, Acampora R, Passariello N, Cacciapuoti F and Paolisso G. (2006) Postprandial plasma glucose excursions and cognitive functioning in aged type 2 diabetics. *Neurology* 67; 7, 235–240.

Agid O, Mamo D, Ginovart N, Vitcu I, Wilson AA, Zipursky RB and Kapur S. (2007) Striatal vs extrastriatal dopamine D_2 receptors in antipsychotic response – a double-blind pet study in schizophrenia. *Neuropsychopharmacology* 32; 1209–1215.

Alphs LD, Summerfelt A, Lann H and Muller RJ. (1989) The negative symptom assessment: a new instrument to assess negative symptoms of schizophrenia. *Psychopharmacol Bull* 25; 2, 159–163.

Artaloytia JF, Arango C, Lahti A, Sanz J, Pascual A, Cubero P, Prieto D and Palomo T. (2006) Negative signs and symptoms secondary to antipsychotics: a double-blind, randomized trial of a single dose of placebo, haloperidol, and risperidone in healthy volunteers. *Am J Psychiatry* 163; 3, 488–493.

Atmaca M, Kuloglu M, Tezcan E and Ustundag B. (2003) Serum leptin and triglyceride levels in patients on treatment with atypical antipsychotics. *J Clin Psychiatry* 64; 5, 598–604.

Bai YM, Lin CC, Chen JY, Lin CY, Su TP and Chou P. (2006) Association of initial antipsychotic response to clozapine and long-term weight gain. *Am J Psychiatry* 163; 1276–1279.

Bardin L, Kleven MS, Barret-Grevoz C, Depoortere R and Newman-Tancredi A. (2006) Antipsychotic-like vs cataleptogenic actions in mice of novel antipsychotics having D2 antagonist and 5-HT1A agonist properties. *Neuropsychopharmacology* 31; 1869–1879.

Bennett S and Gronier B. (2005) Modulation of striatal dopamine release in vitro by agonists of the glycine$_B$ site of NMDA receptors; interaction with antipsychotics. *Eur J Pharmacol* 527; 52–59.

Bota RG, Sagduyu K and Munro JS. (2005) Factors associated with the prodromal progression of schizophrenia that influence the course of the illness. *CNS Spectr* 10; 12, 937–942.

Bueller JA, Aftab M, Sen S, Gomez-Hassan D, Burmeister M and Zubieta JK. (2006) BDNF *Val*^{66} *Met* allele is associated with reduced hippocampal volume in healthy subjects. *Biol Psychiatry* 59; 812–815.

Cannon TD, Glahn DC, Kim J, vanErp TGH, Karlsgodt K, Cohen MS, Neuchterlein KH, Bava S and Shirinyan D. (2005) Dorsolateral prefrontal cortex activity during maintenance and manipulation of information in working memory in patients with schizophrenia. *Arch Gen Psychiatry* 62; 1071–1080.

Cannon TD, Hennah W, van Erp TGM, Thompson PM, Lonnqvist J, Huttunen M, Gasperoni T, Tuulio-Henriksson T, Pirkola T, Toga AW, Kaprio J, Mazziotta J and Peltonen L. (2005) Association of DISC1(TRAX haplotypes with schizophrenia, reduced prefrontal gray matter, and impaired short- and long-term memory. *Arch Gen Psychiatry* 62; 1205–1213.

Chiu CC, Chen KP, Liu HC and Lu ML. (2006) The early effect of olanzapine and risperidone on insulin secretion in atypical-naïve schizophrenic patients. *J Clin Psychopharmacol* 26; 5, 504–507.

Citrome L, Jaffe A, Levine J and Martello D. (2006) Incidence, prevalence and surveillance for diabetes in New York State psychiatric hospitals, 1997–2004. *Psychiatr Serv* 57; 8, 1132–1139.

Citrome L, Macher JP, Salazar DE, Mallikaarjun S and Boulton DW. (2007) Pharmacokinetics of Aripiprazole and Concomitant Carbamazepine. *J Clin Psychopharmacol* 27; 3, 279–283.

Clinton SM, Ibrahim HM, Frey KA, Davis KL, Haroutunian V and Meador-Woodruff JH. (2005) Dopaminergic abnormalities in select thalamic nuclei in schizophrenia: involvement of the intracellular signal integrating proteins calcyon and spinophilin. *Am J Psychiatry* 162; 1859–1871.

Cornblatt BA, Lencz T, Smith CW, Olsen R, Auther AM, Nakayama E, Lesser ML, Tai JY, Shah MR, Foley CA, Kane JM and Correll CU. (2007) Can antidepressants be used to treat the schizophrenia prodrome? Results of a prospective, naturalistic treatment study of adolescents. *J Clin Psychiatry* 68; 4, 546–557.

Coyle JT and Tsai G. (2004) The NMDA receptor glycine modulatory site: a therapeutic target for improving cognition and reducing negative symptoms in schizophrenia. *Psychopharmacology* 174; 32–38.

Coyle JT, Tsai G and Goff D. (2003) Converging evidence of nmda receptor hypofunction in the pathophysiology of schizophrenia. *Ann N Y Acad Sci* 1003; 318–327.

Coyle JT. (2006) Glutamate and schizophrenia: beyond the dopamine hypothesis. *Cell Mol Neurobiol* 26; 4–6, 365–384.

Cropley VL, Fujita J, Innis RB and Nathan PJ. (2006) Molecular imaging of the dopaminergic system and its association with human cognitive function. *Biol Psychiatry* 59; 898–907.

De Bartolomeis A, Fiore G and Iasevoli F. (2005) Dopamine-glutamate interaction and antipsychotics mechanism of action: implication for new pharmacological strategies in psychosis. *Curr Pharm Design* 11; 351–3594.

Detera-Wadleigh SD and McMahon FJ. (2006) G72/G30 in schizophrenia and bipolar disorder: review and meta-analysis. *Biol Psychiatry* 60; 106–114.

DiForti M, Lappin JM and Murray RM. (2007) Risk factors for schizophrenia – all roads lead to dopamine. *Eur Neuropsychopharmacol* 17; S101–S107.

Emsley R, Rabinowitz J and Medori R. (2006) Time course for antipsychotic treatment response in first-episode schizophrenia. *Am J Psychiatry* 163; 743–745.

Essock SM, Covell NH, Davis SM, Stroup TS, Rosenheck RA and Lieberman JA. (2006) Effectiveness of switching antipsychotic medications. *Am J Psychiatry* 163; 12, 2090–2095.

Fanous AH, van den Oord EJ, Riley BP, Aggen SH, Neawle MC, O'Neill FA, Walsh D and Kendler KS. (2005) Relationship between a high-risk haplotype in the DTNBP1 (dysbindin) gene and clinical features of schizophrenia. *Am J Psychiatry* 162; 10, 1824–1832.

Fenton WS and Chavez MR. (2006) Medication-induced weight gain and dyslipidemia in patients with schizophrenia. *Am J Psychiatry* 163; 1697–1704.

Gilbert F, Morissette M, St-Hilaire M, Paquet B, Rouillard C, DiPaolo T and Levesque D. (2006) *Nur77* gene knockout alters dopamine neuron biochemical activity and dopamine turnover. *Biol Psychiatry* 60; 538–547.

Glenthoj BY, Mackeprang T, Svarer C, Rasmussen H, Pinborg LH, Friberg L, Baare W, Hemmingsen R and Videbaek C. (2006) Frontal dopamine $D_{2/3}$ receptor binding in drug-naïve first-episode schizophrenia patients correlates with positive psychotic symptoms and gender. *Biol Psychiatry* 60; 621–629.

Goldberg TE, Straub RE, Callicott JH, Hariri A, Mattay VS, Bigelow L, Coppola R, Egan MF and Weinberger DR. (2006) The G72/G30 gene complex and cognitive abnormalities in schizophrenia. *Neuropsychopharmacology* 31; 2022–2032.

Green EK, Raybould R, Macgregor S, Gordon-Smith K, Heron J, Hyde S, Grozeva D, Hamshere M, Williams N, Owen MJ, O'Donovan MC, Jones L, Jones I, Kirov G and Craddock N. (2005) Operation of the schizophrenia susceptibility gene, neuregulin 1, across traditional diagnostic boundaries to increase risk for bipolar disorder. *Arch Gen Psychiatry* 62; 642–648.

Green MF, Marder SR, Glynn SM, McGurk SR, Wirshing WC, Wirshing DA, Liberman RP and Mintz J. (2002) The neurocognitive effects of low-dose haloperidol: a two-year comparison with risperidone. *Biol Psychiatry* 51; 972–978.

Harrison PJ. (2007) Schizophrenia Susceptibility Genes and Neurodevelopment. *Biol Psychiatry* 61; 1119–1120.

Harrison PJ and Law AJ. (2006) Neuregulin 1 and schizophrenia: genetics, gene expression, and neurobiology. *Biol Psychiatry* 60; 132–140.

Henderson DC, Cagliero E, Copeland PM, Louie PM, Borba CP, Fan X, Freudenreich O and Goff DC. (2007) Elevated hemoglobin A1c as a possible indicator of diabetes mellitus and diabetic ketoacidosis in schizophrenia patients receiving atypical antipsychotics. *J Clin Psychiatry* 68; 533–541.

Heresco-Levy U, Bar G, Levin R, Ermilov M, Ebstein RPand Javitt DC. (2007) High glycine levels are associated with prepulse inhibition deficits in chronic schizophrenia patients. *Schizophr Res*, in press.

Heresco-Levy U, Javitt DC, Ebstein R, Vass Ag, Lichtenbwerg P, Bar G, Catinari S and Ermilov M. (2005) D-serine efficacy as add-on pharmacotherapy to risperidone and olanzapine for treatment-refractory schizophrenia. *Biol Psychiatry* 57; 577–585.

Ho BC, Milev P, O'Leary DS, Librant A and reasen NC and Wassink TH. (2006) Cognitive and magnetic resonance imaging brain morphometric correlates of brain-derived neurotrophic factor Val66Met gene polymorphism in patients with schizophrenia and healthy volunteers. *Arch Gen Psychiatry* 63; 731–740.

Houseknecht KL, Robertson AS, Zavadoski W, Gibbs EM, Johnson DE and Rollema H. (2007) Acute effects of atypical antipsychotics on whole-body insulin resistance in rats: implications for adverse metabolic effects. *Neuropsychopharmacology* 32; 289–297.

Hoyer D, Hannon JP and Martin GR. (2002) Molecular, pharmacological and functional diversity of 5-HT receptors. *Pharmacol Biochem Behav* 71; 533–554.

Hunter MD, Ganesan V, Wilkinson ID and Spence SA. (2006) Impact of modafinil on prefrontal executive function in schizophrenia. *Am J Psychiatry* 163; 12, 2184–2186.

Ingelman-Sundberg M. (2004) Pharmacogenetics of cytochrome P450 and its applications in drug therapy: the past, present and future. *Trends in Pharmacol Sci* 25; 4, 193–200.

Ishizuka K, Paek M, Kamiya A and Sawa A. (2006) A review of disrupted-in-schizophrenia-1 (disc1): neurodevelopment, cognition, and mental conditions. *Biol Psychiatry* 59; 1189–1197.

Javitt DC. (2006) Is the glycine site half saturated or half unsaturated? Effects of glutamatergic drugs in schizophrenia patients. *Curr Opin Psychiatry* 19; 151–157.

Javitt DC, Balla A, Burch S, Suckow R, Xie S and Sershen H. (2004) Reversal of phencyclidine-induced dopaminergic dysregulation by N-methyl-d-aspartate receptor/glycine-site agonists. *Neuropsychopharmacology* 29; 300–307.

Javitt DC, Duncan L, Balla A and Sershen H. (2005) Inhibition of system A-mediated glycine transport in cortical synaptosomes by therapeutic concentrations of clozapine: implications for mechanisms of action. *Mol Psychiatry* 10; 276–286.

Jindal RD and Keshavan S. (2006) Critical role of M_3 muscarinic receptor in insulin secretion. *J Clin Psychopharmacol* 26; 5, 449–450.

Johnson DE, Yamazaki H, Ward KM, Schmidt AW, Lebel WS, Treadway JL, Gibbs, EM, Zawalich WS and Rollema H. (2005) Inhibitory effects of antipsychotics on carbachol-enhanced insulin secretion from perifused rat islets. *Diabetes* 54; 1552–1558.

Johnson MR, Morris NA, Astur RS, Calhoun VD, Mathalon DH, Kiehl KA and Pearlson GD. (2006) A functional magnetic resonance imaging study of working memory abnormalities in schizophrenia. *Biol Psychiatry* 60; 11–21.

Jones PB, Barnes TRE, Davies L, Dunn G, Lloyd H, Hayhurst KP, Murray RM, Markwick A and Lewis SW. (2006) Randomized controlled trial of the effect on quality of life of second- vs first-generation antipsychotic drugs in schizophrenia. *Arch Gen Psychiatry* 63; 1079–1087.

Kahn RS, Schulz SC, Palazov VD, Reyes EB, Brecher M, Svensson O, Andersson HM and Meulien D. (2007) Efficacy and tolerability of once daily extended release quetiapine fumarate in acute schizophrenia: a randomized, double blind, placebo controlled study. *J Clin Psychiatry* 68; 6, 832–842.

Kalkman HO, Feuerbach D, Lotscher E and Schoeffter P. (2003) Functional characterization of the novel antipsychotic iloperidone at human D_2, D_3, $Alpha_{2c}$, $5-HT_6$ and $5-HT_{1A}$ receptors. *Life Sci* 73; 1151–1159.

Kapur S and Lecrubier Y. (eds) (2003) *Dopamine in the Pathophysiology and Treatment of Schizophrenia*. London, Martin Dunitz.

Kapur S. (2003) Psychosis as a state of aberrant salience: a framework linking biology, phenomenology, and pharmacology in schizophrenia. *Am J Psychiatry* 160; 1, 13–23.

Keefe RS, Bilder RM, Davis SM, Harvey PD, Palmer BW, Gold JM, Meltzer HY, Green MF, Capuao G, Stroup TS, McEvoy JP, Swartz MS, Rosenheck RA, Perkins DO, Davis CE, Hsiao JK and Lieberman JA. (2007) Neurocognitive effects of antipsychotic medications in patients with chronic schizophrenia in the CATIE trial. *Arch Gen Psychiatry* 64; 633–647.

Keefe RS, Bilder RM, Harvey PD, Davis SM, Palmer BW, Gold JM, Meltzer HY, Green MF, Miller DD, Canive JM, Adler LW, Manschreck TC, Swartz M, Rosenheck R, Perkins DO, Walker TM, Stroup TS, McEvoy JP and Lieberman JA. (2006) Baseline neurocognitive deficits in the CATIE schizophrenia trial. *Neuropsychopharmacology* 31; 2033–2046.

Keefe RS, Seidman LJ, Christensen BK, Harner RM, Sharma T, Sitskoorn MM, Rock SL, Woolson S, Tohen M, Tollefson GD, Sanger TM and Lieberman JA. (2006) Long-Term neurocognitive effects of olanzapine or low-dose haloperidol in first episode psychosis. *Biol Psychiatry* 59; 97–105.

Kern RS, Green MF, Cornblatt BA, Owen JR, McQuade RD, Carson WH, Mirza A and Marcus R. (2006) The neurocognitive effects of aripiprazole: an open label comparison with olanzapine. *Psychopharmacology* 187; 312–320.

Kessler RM, Ansari MS, Riccardi P, Li R, Jayathilake K, Dawant B and Meltzer HY. (2006) Occupancy of striatal and extrastriatal dopamine D2 receptors by clozapine and quetiapine. *Neuropsychopharmacology* 31; 1991–2001.

Kessler RM, Ansari MS, Riccardi P, Li R, Jyathilake K, Dawant B and Meltzer JY. (2005) Occupancy of striatal and extrastriatal dopamine D2/D3 receptors by olanzapine and haloperidol. *Neuropsychopharmacology* 30; 2283–2289.

Klein DJ, Cottingham EM, Sorter M, Barton BA and Morrison JA. (2006) A randomized, double blind, placebo controlled trial of metformin treatment of weight gain associated with initiation of atypical antipsychotic therapy in children and adolescents. *Am J Psychiatry* 153; 2072–2079.

Lambert BL, Cunningham FE, Miller DR, Dalack GW and Hur K. (2006) Diabetes risk associated with use of olanzapine, quetiapine, and risperidon in Veterans health administration patients with schizophrenia. *Am J Epidemiol* 164; 672–681.

Lamberti JS, Olson D, Crilly JF, Olivares T, Williams GC, Tu X, Tang W, Wiener K, Dvorin S and Dietz MB. (2006) Prevalence of the metabolic syndrome among patients receiving clozapine. *Am J Psychiatry* 163; 1273–1276.

Lane HY, Chang YC, Liu YC, Chiu CC and Tsai GE. (2005) Sarcosine or D-Serine add-on treatment for acute exacerbation of schizophrenia. *Arch Gen Psychiatry* 62; 1196–1204.

Lane HY, Huang CL, Wu PL, Liu YC, Chang YC, Lin PY, Chen PW and Tsai G. (2006) Glycine Transporter 1 inhibitor, N-methylglycine (Sarcosine), added to clozapine for the treatment of schizophrenia. *Biol Psychiatry* 60; 645–649.

Lawler CP, Prioleau C, Lewis MM, Mak C, Jiang D, Schetz JA, Gonzalez AM, Sibley DR and Mailman RB. (1999) Interactions of the novel antipsychotic aripiprazole (OPC-14597) with dopamine and serotonin receptor subtypes. *Neuropsychopharmacology* 20; 6, 612–627.

Lencz T, Smith CW, McLaughlin D, Auther A, Nakayama E, Hovey L and Cornblatt BA. (2006) Generalized and specific neurocognitive deficits in prodromal schizophrenia. *Biol Psychiatry* 59; 863–871.

Leonard S and Freedman R. (2006) Genetics of chromosome 15q13-q14 in schizophrenia. *Biol Psychiatry* 60; 115–122.

Leucht S, Busch R, Math D, Kissling W and Kane JM. (2007) Early prediction of antipsychotic nonresponse among patients with schizophrenia. *J Clin Psychiatry* 68; 3, 352–360.

Levitt P, Ebert P, Mirnics K, Nimgaonkar VL and Lewis DA. (2006) Making the case for a candidate vulnerability gene in schizophrenia: convergent evidence for regulator of G-protein signaling 4 (RGS4). *Biol Psychiatry* 60; 534–537.

Lieberman JA, Tollefson GD, Charles, Zipursky R, Sharma T, Kahn RS, Keefe RSE, Green AI, Gur RE, McEvoy J, Perkins D, Hamer RM, Gu H and Tohen M. (2005) Antipsychotic drug effects on brain morphology in first episode psychosis. *Arch Gen Psychiatry* 62; 361–370.

Lindenmayer JP, Khan A, Iskander A, Abad MT and Parker B. (2007) A randomized controlled trial of olanzapine versus haloperidol in the treatment of primary negative symptoms and neurocognitive deficits in schizophrenia. *J Clin Psychiatry* 68; 3, 368–379.

Lipkovich I, Citrome L, Perlis R, Deberdt W, Jouston JP, Ahl J and Hardy T. (2006) Early predictors of substantial weight gain in bipolar patients treated with olanzapine. *J Clin Psychopharmacol* 26; 3, 316–320.

Liu YL, Fann SH, Liu CM, Chen WJ, Wu JY, Hung SI, Chen CH, Jou YSS, Liu SK, Hwang TJ, Hsieh MH, Ouyang WC, Chan HY, Chen JJ, Yang WC, Lin CY, Lee SFC and

Hwu HG. (2006) A single nucleotide polymorphism fine mapping study of chromosome 1q42.1 reveals the vulnerability genes for schizophrenia, GNPAT and DISC1: association with impairment of sustained attention. *Biol Psychiatry* 60; 554–562.

Lovestone S, Killick R, DiFort M and Murry R. (2007) Schizophrenia as a GSK-3 dysregulation disorder. *Trends Neurosci* 30; 4, 142–149.

Lynch G and Gall CM. (2006) Ampakines and the threefold path to cognitive enhancement. *Trends Neurosci* 29; 10.

Maeda K, Nwulia E, Chang J, Balkissoon R, Ishizuka K, Chen H, Zandi P, McInnis MG and Sawa A. (2006) Differential expression of disrupted-in-schizophrenia (DISC1) in bipolar disorder. *Biol Psychiatry* 60; 929–935.

McCreary AD, Glennon JC, Ashby Jr R, Meltzer HY, Li Z, Reinders JH, Hesselink MB, Long SK, Herremans AH, van Stuivenberg H, Feenstra RW and Kruse CG. (2007) SLV313 (1-(2,3-dihydro-benzo[1,4] dioxin-5-yl)-4-[5-(4-fluoro-phenyl)-Pyridin-3-ylmethyl]-piperazine monohydrochloride): a novel dopamine D2 receptor Antagonist and 5-HT1A receptor agonist potential antipsychotic drug. *Neuropsychopharmacology* 32; 78–94.

McEvoy JP, Lieberman JA, Sroup TS, Davis SM, Meltzer HY, Rosenheck RA, Swartz MS, Perkins DO, Keefe, RSE, Davis CE, Severe J and Hsiao JK. (2006) Effectiveness of clozapine versus olanzapine, quetiapine, and risperidone in patients with chronic schizophrenia who did not respond to prior atypical antipsychotic treatment. *Am J Psychiatry* 163; 600–610.

McGlashan TH, Zipursky RB, Perkiins D, Addington J, Miller T, Woods SW, Hawkins KA, Hoffman RE, Predaw A and Epstein I. (2006) Randomized, double-blind trial of olanzapine versus placebo in patients prodromally symptomatic for psychosis. *Am J Psychiatry* 163; 790–799.

McLaughlin T, Abbasi F, Cheal K, Chu J, Lamendola C and Reaven G. (2003) Use of metabolic markers to identify overweight individuals who are insulin resistant. *Ann Intern Med* 139; 802–809.

Melle I, Johannesen JO, Friis S, Haahr U, Joa I, Larsen TK, Opjordsmoen S and Rund BR. (2006) Early detection of the first episode of schizophrenia and suicidal behavior. *Am J Psychiatry* 163; 5, 800–804.

Meyer-Lindenberg A, Buckholtz JW, Kolachana B, Hariri AR, Pezawas L, Blasi G, Wabnitz A, Honea R, Verchinski B, Callicott JH, Egan M, Mattay V and Weinberger DR. (2006) Neural mechanisms of genetic risk for impulsivity and violence in humans. *Proc Natl Acad Sci U S A* 103; 6, 6269–6274.

Meyer-Lindenberg A, Kohn PD, Kolachana B, Kippenhan S, McInerney-Leo A, Nussbaum R, Weinberger DR and Berman KF. (2005) Midbrain dopamine and prefrontal function in humans: interaction and modulation by COMT genotype. *Nat Neurosci* 8; 5, 594–596.

Millan MJ. (2005) N-Methyl-d-aspartate receptors as a target for improved antipsychotic agents: novel insights and clinical perspectives. *Psychopharmacology* 179; 30–53.

Mizrahi R, Rusjan P, Agid O, Graff A, Mamo DC, Zipursky RB and Kapur S. (2007) Adverse subjective experience with antipsychotics and its relationship to striatal and extrastriatal D2 receptors: a PET study in schizophrenia. *Am J Psychiatry* 164; 630–637.

Murphy BP, Chung YC, Park TW and McGorry PD. (2006) Pharmacological treatment of primary negative symptoms in schizophrenia: a systematic review. *Schizophr Res* 88; 5–25.

Natesan S, Reckless GE, Barlow KBL, Nobrega JN and Kapur S. (2007) Evaluation of N-desmethylclozapine as a potential antipsychotic – preclinical studies. *Neuropsychopharmacology* 32; 1540–1549.

Natesan S, Reckless GE, Nobrega JN, Fletcher PJ and Kapur S. (2006) Dissociation between in vivo occupancy and functional antagonism of dopamine D2 receptors: comparing aripiprazole to other antipsychotics in animal models. *Neuropsychopharmacology* 31; 1854–1863.

Newman-Trancredi A, Assie MB, Leduc N, Ormiere AM, Danty N and Cosi C. (2005) Novel antipsychotics activate recombinant human and native rat serotonin 5-HT1A receptors: affinity, efficacy and potential implications for treatment of schizophrenia. *Int J Neuropsychopharmacol* 8; 341–356.

Olfson M, Blanco C, Liu L, Moreno C and Laje G. (2006) National trends in the outpatient treatment of children and adolescents with antipsychotic drugs. *Arch Gen Psychiatry* 63; 679–685.

Olfson M, Marcus SC, Corey-Lisle P, Tuomari AV, Hines P and L'Italien GJ. (2006) Hyperlipidemia following treatment with antipsychotic medications. *Am J Psychiatry* 163; 1821–1825.

Olincy A, Harris JG, Johnson LL, Pender V, Kongs S, Allensworth D, Ellis J, Zerbe GO, Leonard S, Stevens KE, Stevens JO, Martin L, Adler LE, Soti F, Kem WR and Freedman R. (2006) Proof-of-concept trial of an alpha 7 nicotinic agonist in schizophrenia. *Arch Gen Psychiatry* 63; 630–638.

Osborn DPJ, Levy G, Nazareth I, Petersen I, Islam A and King MB. (2007) Relative risk of cardiovascular and cancer mortality in people with severe mental illness from the United Kingdom's general practice research database. *Arch Gen Psychiatry* 64; 242–249.

Passamonti L, Fera F, Magariello A, Cerasa A, Gioia MC, Muglia M, Nicoletti G, Gallo O, Provinciali L and Quattrone A. (2006) Monoamine oxidase-A genetic variations influence brain activity associated with inhibitory control: new insight into the neural correlates of impulsivity. *Biol Psychiatry* 59; 334–340.

Perkins DO, Gu H, Boteva K and Lieberman JA. (2005) Relationship between duration of untreated psychosis and outcome in first episode schizophrenia: a critical review and meta-analysis. *Am J Psychiatry* 162; 1785–1804.

Pierre JM, Peloian JH, Wirshing DA, Wirshing WC and Marder SR. (2007) A randomized, double-blind, placebo-controlled trial of modafinil for negative symptoms in schizophrenia. *J Clin Psychiatry* 68; 5, 705–710.

Polsky D, Doshi JA, Bauer MS and Glick HA. (2006) Clinical trial-based cost effectiveness analyses of antipsychotic use. *Am J Psychiatry* 163; 12, 2047–2056.

Porteous DJ, Thomson P, Brandon NJ and Millar JK. (2006) The genetics and biology of DISC1 – an emerging role in psychosis and cognition. *Biol Psychiatry* 60; 123–131.

Pralong E, Magistretti P and Stoop R. (2002) Cellular perspectives on the glutamate-monoamine interactions in limbic lobe structures and their relevance for some psychiatric disorders. *Prog Neurobiol* 67; 173–202.

Reaven G. (2004) The metabolic syndrome or the insulin resistance syndrome: different names, different concepts, and different goals. *Endocrinol Metab Clin North Am* 33; 283–303.

Reist C, Mintz J, Albers LJ, Jamas MM, Szabo S and Ozdemir V. (2007) Second-generation antipsychotic exposure and metabolic-related disorders in patients with schizophrenia. *J Clin Psychopharmacol* 27; 46–51.

Remington G, Mamo D, Labelle A, Reiss J, Shammi C, Mannaert E, Mann S and Kapur S. (2006) A PET study evaluating dopamine D_2 receptor occupancy for long-acting injectable risperidone. *Am J Psychiatry* 163; 3, 396–401.

Reyes M, Buitelaar J, Toren P, Augustyns I and Eerdekens M. (2006) A randomized, double-blind, placebo-controlled study of risperidone maintenance treatment in children and adolescents with disruptive behavior disorders. *Am J Psychiatry* 163; 402–410.

Reynolds GP, Yao Z, Zhang XB, Sun J and Zhang ZJ. (2004) Pharmacogenetics of treatment in first-episode schizophrenia: D3 and 5-HT2C receptor polymorphisms separately associate with positive and negative symptom response. *Eur Neuropsychopharmacol* 15; 143–151.

Rosenheck RA, Leslie DL, Sindelar J, Miller EA, Lin H, Stroup TS, McEvoy J, Davis SM, Keefe, RSE, Swartz M, Perkins DO, Hsiao JK and Lieberman J. (2006) Cost-effectiveness of second generation antipsychotics and perphenazine in a randomized trial of treatment for chronic schizophrenia. *Am J Psychiatry* 163; 12, 2080–2089.

Sacco KA, Termine A, Seyal A, Dudas MM, Vessicchio JC, Krishnan-Sarin S, Jatlow PI, Wexler BE and George TP. (2005) Effects of cigarette smoking on spatial working memory and attentional deficits in schziophrenia. *Arch Gen Psychiatry* 62; 649–659.

Sarafidis PA and Nilsson PM. (2006) The metabolic syndrome: a glance at its history. *J Hypertens* 24; 621–626.

Sarter M. (2006) Preclinical research into cognition enhancers. *Trends Pharmacol Sci* 27:11.

Scarr E, Beneyto M, Meador-Woodruff JH and Dean B. (2005) Cortical glutamatergic markers in schizophrenia. *Neuropsychopharmacology* 30; 1521–1531.

Sepehry AA, Potvin S, Elie R and Stip E. (2007) Selective serotonin reuptake inhibitor (SSRI) add-on therapy for the negative symptoms of schizophrenia: A meta-analysis. *J Clin Psychiatry* 68; 4, 604–610.

Shayegan DK and Stahl SM. (2005) Emotion processing, the amygdala, and outcome in schizophrenia. *Prog Neuropsychopharmacol Biol Psychiatry* 29; 840–845.

Simonson GD and Kendall DM. (2005) Diagnosis of insulin resistance and associated syndromes: the spectrum from the metabolic syndrome to type 2 diabetes mellitus. *Coron Artery Dis* 16; 465–472.

Smid P, Coolen HKAC, Keizer HG, van Hes R, de Moes JP, den Hartog AP, Stork B, Plekkenpol RH, Niemann LC, Stroomer CNJ, Tulp MTM, van Stuivenberg HH, McCreary AC, Hesselink M, Herremans AHJ and Kruse CG. (2005) Synthesis, structure-activity relationships, and biological properties of 1-heteroaryl-4-[ω-(1H-indol-3-yl) alkyl] piperazines, novel potential antipsychotics combining potent dopamine D2 receptor antagonism with potent serotonin reuptake inhibition. *J Med Chem* 48; 6855–6869.

Snitz BE, MacDonald III A, Cohen JD, Cho RY, Becker T and Carter CS. (2005) Lateral and medial hypofrontality in first-episode schizophrenia: functional activity in a medication-naïve state and effects of short-term atypical antipsychotic treatment. *Am J Psychiatry* 162; 12, 2322–2329.

Spurling RD, Lamberti JS, Olsen D, Tu X and Tang W. (2007) Changes in metabolic parameters with switching to aripiprazole from another second-generation antipsychotic: a retrospective chart review. *J Clin Psychiatry* 68; 3, 406–409.

Stahl SM. (2004) Prophylactic antipsychotics: do they keep you from catching schizophrenia? *J Clin Psychiatry* 65; 11, 1445–1446.

Stephan KE, Baldeweg T and Friston KJ. (2006) Synaptic plasticity and dysconnection in schizophrenia. *Biol Psychiatry* 59; 929–939.

Straub RE and Weinberger DR. (2006) Schizophrenia genes – famine to feast. *Biol Psychiatry* 60; 81–83.

Stroup TS, Lieberman JA, McEvoy JP, Swartz MS, Davis SM, Capuano GA, Rosenheck RA, Keefe RSE, Miller AL, Belz I and Hsiao JK. (2007) Effectiveness of olanzapine, quetiapine, and risperidone in patients with chronic schizophrenia after discontinuing perphenazine: a CATIE study. *Am J Psychiatry* 164; 415–427.

Surguladze S, Russell T, Kucharska-Pietura K, Travis MJ, Giampietro V, David AS and Philips ML. (2006) A reversal of the normal pattern of parahippocampal response to neutral and fearful faces is associated with reality distortion in schizophrenia. *Biol Psychiatry* 60; 423–431.

Takahashi H, Higuchi M and Suhara T. (2006) The role of extrastriatal dopamine D2 receptors in schizophrenia. *Biol Psychiatry* 59; 919–928.

Talkowski ME, Mansour H, Chowdari KV, Wood J, Butler A, Varma PG, Prasad S, Semwal P, Bhatia T, Deshpande S, Devlin B, Thelma BK and Nimgaonkar VL. (2006) Novel, replicated associations between dopamine D3 receptor gene polymorphisms and schizophrenia in two independent samples. *Biol Psychiatry* 60; 570–577.

Tarazi FI, Baldessarini RJ, Kula NS and Zhang K. (2003) Long-term effects of olanzapine, risperidone, and quetiapine on ionotropic glutamate receptor types: implications for antipsychotic drug treatment. *J Pharmacol Exp Ther* 306; 3, 1145–1151.

Tenback DE, van Harten PN, Sloof CJ and van Os J. (2006) Evidence that early extrapyramidal symptoms predict later tardive dyskinesia: a prospective analysis of 10,000 patients in the European schizophrenia outpatient health outcomes (SOHO) study. *Am J Psychiatry* 163; 1438–1440.

Tran-Johnson TK, Sack DA, Marcus RN, Auby P, McQuade RD and Oren DA. (2007) Efficacy and safety of intramuscular aripiprazole in patients with acute agitation: a randomized, double-blind, placebo-controlled trial. *J Clin Psychiatry* 68; 1, 111–119.

Tremeau F, Malaspina D, Duval F, Correa H, Hager-Budny M, Coin-Bariou L, Macher JP and Gorman JM. (2005) Facial expressiveness in patients with schizophrenia compared to depressed patients and nonpatient comparison subjects. *Am J Psychiatry* 162; 1, 92–101.

Tsai G, Lane HY, Chong MY and Lange N. (2004) Glycine transporter 1 inhibitor, N-methylglycine (sarcosine), added to antipsychotics for the treatment of schizophrenia. *Biol Psychiatry* 55; 452–456.

Tsai GE, Yang P, Chang YC and Chong MY. (2006) D-alanine added to antipsychotics for the treatment of schizophrenia. *Biol Psychiatry* 59; 230–234.

Tunbridge EM, Harrison PJ and Weinberger DR. (2006) Catechol-o-methyltransferase, cognition, and psychosis: Val^{158} Met and beyond. *Biol Psychiatry* 60; 141–151.

Vestri HS, Maianu L, Moellering DR and Garvey WT. (2007) Atypical antipsychotic drugs directly impair insulin action in adipocytes: effects on glucose transport, lipogenesis, and antilipolysis. *Neuropsychopharmacology* 32; 765–772.

Vidalis AA.(2006) *Psychopharmacology Issues in Pregnancy and Lactation.* Thessasloniki, Greece, Contemporary Editions.

Voruganti Land Awad AG. (2004) Neuroleptic dysphoria: towards a new synthesis. *Psychopharmacology* 171; 121–132.

Walss-Bass C, Liu W, Lew DF, Villegas R, Montero P, Dassori A, Leach RJ, Almasy L, Escamilla M and Rawventos H. (2006) A novel missense mutation in the transmembrane domain of neuregulin 1 is associated with schizophrenia. *Biol Psychiatry* 60; 548–553.

Weissman EM, Zhu CW, Schooler NR, Goetz RR and Essock SM. (2006) Lipid monitoring in patients with schizophrenia prescribed second generation antipsychotics. *J Clin Psychiatry* 67; 9, 1323–1326.

Wezenberg E, Verkes RJ, Ruigt GSF, Hulstijn W and Sabbe BGC. (2007) Acute effects of the ampakine farampator on memory and information processing in healthy elderly volunteers. *Neuropsychopharmacology* 32; 1272–1283.

Williams NM, Green EK, Macgregor S, Dwyer S, Norton N, Williams H, Raybould R, Grozeva D, Hamshere M, Zammit S, Jones L, Cardno A, Kirov G, Jones I, O'Donovan MC, Owen MJ and Craddock N. (2006) Variation at the DAOA/G30 locus influences susceptibility to major mood episodes but not psychosis in schizophrenia and bipolar disorder. *Arch Gen Psychiatry* 63; 366–373.

Winterer G, Egan MF, Kolachana BS, Goldberg TE, Coppola R and Weinberger DR. (2006) Prefrontal electrophysiologic noise and catechol-O-methyltransferase genotype in schizophrenia. *Biol Psychiatry* 60; 578–584.

Yaeger D, Smith HG and Altshuler LL. (2006) Atypical antipsychotics in the treatment of schizophrenia during pregnancy and the postpartum. *Am J Psychiatry* 163; 12, 2064–2070.

Zaboli G, Jonsson EG, Gizatullin R, Asberg M and Leopardi R. (2006) Tryptophan hydroxylase-1 gene variants associated with schizophrenia. *Biol Psychiatry* 60; 563–569.

Zhang M, Ballard ME, Kohlhaas KL, Browmna KE, Jongen-Relo AL, Unger LV, Fox GB, Gross G, Decker MW, Drescher KU and Rueter LE. (2006) Effect of dopamine D3 antagonists on PPI in DBA/2J mice or PPI deficit induced by neonatal ventral hippocampal lesions in rats. *Neuropsychopharmacology* 31; 1382–1392.

Chapters 11 (Mood Disorders), 12 (Antidepressants), and 13 (Mood Stabilizers)

Agjakamoam GK and Marek GJ. (2000) Serotonin model of schizophrenia: emerging role of glutamate mechanisms. *Brain Res Rev* 31; 302–312.

Akiskal Hand Tohen M. (eds) (2006) *Bipolar Psychopharmacotherapy.* West Sussex, England, Wiley and Sons.

Akiskal HS, Akiskal KK, Perugi G, Toni C, Ruffolo G and Tusini G. (2006) Bipolar II and anxious reactive "comorbidity": toward better phenotypic characterization suitable for genotyping. *J Affective Disord* 96; 239–247.

Altshuler LL, Bookheimer SY, Townsend J, Proenza MA, Eisenberger N, Sabb F, Mintz J and Cohen MS. (2005) Blunted activation in orbitofrontal cortex during mania: a functional magnetic resonance imaging study. *Biol Psychiatry* 58; 763–769.

Amargos-Bosch M, Bortolozzi A, Puig MV, Serrats J, Adell A, Celada P, Toth M, Mengod G and Artigas F. (2004) Co-expression in vivo interaction of serotonin 1A and serotonin 2A receptors in pyramidal neurons of prefrontal cortex. *Cereb Cortex* 14; 281–299.

Amargos-Bosch M, Lopez-Gil X, Artigas F and Adell A. (2006) Clozapine and olanzapine, but not haloperidol, suppress serotonin efflux in the medial prefrontal cortex elicited by phencyclidine and ketamine. *Int J Neuropsychopharmacol* 9; 565–573.

Angst J. (2007) The bipolar spectrum. *Br J Psychiatry* 190; 189–191.

Avery DH, Holtzheimer III PE, Fawaz W, Russo J, Neumaier J, Dunner DL, Haynor DR, Claypoole KH, Wajdik C and Roy-Byrne P. (2006) A controlled study of repetitive transcranial magnetic stimulation in medication-resistant major depression. *Biol Psychiatry* 59; 187–194.

Barone P, Scarzella L, Marconi R, Antonini A, Morgante L, Bracco F, Zappia M and Musch B. (2006) Pramipexole versus sertraline in the treatment of depression in Parkinson's disease. *J Neurol* 253; 601–607.

Barsky AJ, Orav EJ and Bates DW. (2005) Somatization increases medical utilization and costs independent of psychiatric and medical comorbidity. *Arch Gen Psychiatry* 62; 903–910.

Baumer FM, Howe M, Gallelli K, Simeonova DI, Hallmayer J and Chang KD. (2006) A pilot study of antidepressant-induced mania in pediatric bipolar disorder: characteristics, risk factors, and the serotonin transporter gene. *Biol Psychiatry* 60; 1005–1012.

Berman RM, Marcus RN, Swanink R, McQuade RD, Carson WH, Corey-Lisle PK and Khan A. (2007) The efficacy and safety of aripiprazole as adjunctive therapy in major depressive disorder: a multicenter, randomized, double-blind, placebo-controlled study. *J Clin Psychiatry* 68; 843–853.

Biederman J. (2006) The evolving face of pediatric mania. *Biol Psychiatry* 60; 901–902.

Biederman J, Mick E, Hammerness P, Harpold T, Aleardi M, Dougherty M and Wozniak J. (2005) Open-label, 8 week trial of olanzapine and risperidone for the treatment of bipolar disorder in preschool age children. *Biol Psychiatry* 58; 589–594.

Bowden CL, Calabrese JR, Ketter TA, Sachs GS, White RL and Thompson TR. (2006) Impact of lamotrigine and lithium on weight in obese and nonobese patients with bipolar I disorder. *Am J Psychiatry* 163; 1199–1201.

Bridge JA, Iyengar S, Salary CB, Barbe RP, Birmaher B, Pincus HA, Ren L and Brent DA. (2007) Clinical response and risk for reported suicidal ideation and suicide attempts in pediatric antidepressant treatment. *JAMA* 297; 15, 1683–1696.

Calabrese JR, Goldberg JF, Ketter TA, Suppes T, Frye M, White R, DeVeaugh-Geiss A and Thompson TR. (2006) Recurrence in bipolar I disorder: a post hoc analysis excluding relapses in two double blind maintenance studies. *Biol Psychiatry* 59; 1061–1064.

Calabrese JR, Shelton MD, Rapport DJ, Youngstrom EA, Jackson K, Bilali S, Ganocy SJ and Findling RL. (2005) A 20-month, double-blind, maintenance trial of lithium versus divalproex in rapid cycling bipolar disorder. *Am J Psychiatry* 162; 2152–2161.

Carli M, Vaviera M, Invernizzi RW and Balducci C. (2006) Dissociable contribution of 5-HT1A and 5-HT 2A receptors in the medial prefrontal cortex to different aspects of executive control such as impulsivity and compulsive perseveration in rats. *Neuropsychopharmacology* 31; 757–767.

Cavanagh J, Patterson J, Pimlott S, Dewar D, Eersels J, Dempsey MF and Wyper D. (2006) Serotonin transporter residual availability during long term antidepressant therapy does not differentiate responder and nonresponder unipolar patients. *Biol Psychiatry* 59; 301–308.

Cipriani A, Barbui C, Brambilla P, Furukawa TA, Hotopf M and Geddes JR. (2006) Are all antidepressants really the same? The case of fluoxetine: a systematic review. *J Clin Psychiatry* 67; 6, 850–864.

Cipriani A, Pretty H, Hawton K and Geddes JR. (2005) Lithium in the prevention of suicidal behavior and all-cause mortality in patients with mood disorders: a systematic review of randomized trials. *Am J Psychiatry* 162; 1805–1819.

Cooper Kazaz R, Apter JT, Cohen R, Karagichev L, Muhammed-Moussa S, Grupper D, Drori T, Newman ME, Sackeim HA, Glaser B and Lerer B. (2007) Combined treatment with sertraline and liothyronine in major depression. *Arch Gen Psychiatry* 64; 679–688.

Cousins DA and Young AH. (2007) The armamentarium of treatments for bipolar disorder: a review of the literature. *Int J Neuropsychopharmacol* 10; 411–431.

Crossley NA and Bauer M. (2007) Acceleration and augmentation of antidepressants with lithium for depressive disorders: two meta-analyses of randomized, placebo-controlled trials. *J Clin Psychiatry* 68; 935–940.

deBartolomeis A, Fiore G and Iasevoli F. (2005) Dopamine-glutamate interaction and antipsychotics mechanism of action: implication for new pharmacological strategies in psychosis. *Curr Pharm Des* 11; 3561–3594.

DelBello MP, Adler CM, Whitsel RM, Stanford KE and Strakowski SM. (2007) A 12-week single blind trial of quetiapine for the treatment of mood symptoms in adolescents at high risk for developing bipolar I disorder. *J Clin Psychiatry* 68; 5, 789–795.

DelBello MP, Hanseman D, Adler CM, Fleck DE and Strakowski SM. (2007) Twelve-month outcome of adolescents with bipolar disorder following first hospitalization for a manic or mixed episode. *Am J Psychiatry* 164; 582–590.

DelBello MP, Kowwatch RA, Adler CM, Stanford KE, Welge JA, Barzman DH, Nelson E and Strakowski SM. (2006) A double-blind randomized pilot study comparing quetiapine and divalproex for adolescent mania. *J Am Acad Child Adolesc Psychiatry* 45; 3, 305–313.

DeMartinis NA, Yeung PP, Entsuah R and Manley AL. (2007) A double-blind, placebo-controlled study of the efficacy and safety of desvenlafaxine succinate in the treatment of major depressive disorder. *J Clin Psychiatry* 68; 677–688.

Dew MA, Whyte EM, Lenze EJ, Houck PR, Mulsant BH, Pollock BG, Stack JA, Ensasi S and Reynolds III CF. (2007) Recovery from major depression in older adults receiving augmentation of antidepressant pharmacotherapy. *Am J Psychiatry* 164; 892–899.

Dickstein DP, Milham MP, Nugent AC, Drevets WC, Charney DS, Pine DS and Leibenluft E. (2005) Frontotemporal alterations in pediatric bipolar disorder. *Arch Gen Psychiatry* 62; 734–741.

Dording CM, Mischoulon D, Peterson TJ, Kornbluh R, Gordon J, Nierenberg AA, Rosenbaum JE and Fava M. (2002) The pharmacologic management of SSRI-induced side effects: a survey of psychiatrists. *Ann Clin Psychiatry* 14; 3, 143–147.

Drabant EM, Hariri AR, Meyer-Lindenberg A, Munoz KE, Mattay VS, Kolachana BS, Egan MF and Weinberger DR. (2006) Catechol O-methyltransferase Val 158 Met genotype and neural mechanisms related to affective arousal and regulation. *Arch Gen Psychiatry* 63; 12, 1396–1406.

Du J, Suzuki K, Wei Y, Wang Y, Blumental R, Chen Z, Falke C, Zarate Jr CA and Manji HK. (2007) The anticonvulsants lamotrigine, riluzole, and valproate differentially regulate AMPA receptor membrane localization: relationship to clinical effects in mood disorders. *Neuropsychopharmacology* 32; 793–802.

Emslie GJ, Yeung PP and Kunz NR. (2007) Long-term, open-label venlafaxine extended release treatment in children and adolescents with major depressive disorder. *CNS Spectr* 12; 3, 223–233.

Epstein J, Pan H, Kocsis JH, Yang Y, Butler T, Chusid J, Hochberg H, Murrough J, Strohmayer E, Stern E and Silbersweig DA. (2006) Lack of ventral striatal response to positive stimuli in depressed versus normal subjects. *Am J Psychiatry* 163; 1784–1790.

Fava M. (2007) Augmenting antidepressants with folate: a clinical perspective. *Clin Psychiatry* 68; Suppl 10, 4–7.

Fava M, Graves LM, Benazzi F, Scaia MJ, Iosifescu DV, Alpert JE and Papakostas GI. (2006) A cross-sectional study of the prevalence of cognitive and physical symptoms during long-term antidepressant treatment. *J Clin Psychiatry* 67; 11, 1754–1758.

Findling RL, Frazier TW, Youngstrom EA, McNamara NK, Stansbrey RJ, Gracious BL, Reed MD, Demeter CA and Calabrese JR. (2007) Double-blind, placebo-controlled trial of divalproex monotherapy in the treatment of symptomatic youth at high risk for developing bipolar disorder. *J Clin Psychiatry* 68; 5, 781–788.

Frank E, Kupfer DJ, Buysse DJ, Swartz HA, Pilkois PA, Houck PR, Rucci P, Novick DM, Grochocinski VJ and Stapf DM. (2007) Randomized trial of weekly, twice monthly and monthly interpersonal psychotherapy as maintenance treatment for women with recurrent depression. *Am J Psychiatry* 164; 761–767.

Fu CHY, Williams SCR, Brammer MJ, Suckling J, Kim J, Cleawre AJ, Walsh ND, Mitterschiffthaler MT and rew CM, Pich EM and Bullmore ET. (2007) Neural responses to happy facial expressions in major depression following antidepressant treatment. *Am J Psychiatry* 164; 599–607.

Gibbons RD, Hur K, Bhumik DK and Mann JJ. (2006) The relationship between antidepressant prescription rates and rate of early adolescent suicide. *Am J Psychiatry* 163; 1898–1904.

Goodwin FK and Jamison KR. (eds) (1990) *Manic Depressive Illness*. New York, Oxford University Press.

Gould GG, Altamirano AV, Javors MA and Frazer A. (2006) A comparison of the chronic treatment effects of venlafaxine and other antidepressants on serotonin and norepinephrine transporters. *Biol Psychiatry* 59; 408–414.

Guzzetta F, Tondo L, Centorrino F and Baldessarini RJ. (2007) Lithium treatment reduces suicide risk in recurrent major depressive disorder. *J Clin Psychiatry* 68; 380–383.

Hasler G, Drevets WC, Gould TD, Gottesman II and Manji HK. (2006) Toward constructing an endophenotype strategy for bipolar disorders. *Biol Psychiatry* 60; 93–105.

Hedlund PB and Sutcliff JG. (2004) Functional, molecular and pharmacological advances in 5-HT7 receptor research. *Trends Pharmacol Sci* 25; 9, 481–486.

Hedlund PB, Huitron-Resendiz S, Henriksen SJ and Sutcliffe JG. (2005) 5-HT7 receptor inhibition and inactivation induce antidepressant like behavior and sleep pattern. *Biol Psychiatry* 58; 831–837.

Hirschfeld RMA, Weisler RH, Rawines SR and Macfadden W. (2006) Quetiapine in the treatment of anxiety in patients with bipolar I or II depression: a secondary analysis from a randomized, double-blind, placebo-controlled study. *J Clin Psychiatry* 67; 3, 355–362.

Houston JP, Ahl J, Meyers AL, Kaiser CJ, Tohen M and Baldessarini RJ. (2006) Reduced suicidal ideation in bipolar I disorder mixed episode patients in a placebo-controlled trial of olanzapine combined with lithium or divalproex. *J Clin Psychiatry* 67; 8, 1246–1252.

Hoyer D, Hannon JP and Martin GR. (2002) Molecular, pharmacological and functional diversity of 5-HT receptors. *Pharmacol Biochem Behav* 71; 533–554.

Joffe H, Cohen LS, Suppes T, McLaughlin WL, Lavori P, Adams JM, Hwang CH, Hall JE and Sachs GS. (2006) Valproate is associated with new onset oligoamenorrhea with hyperandrogenism in women with bipolar disorder. *Biol Psychiatry* 59; 1078–1086.

Judd LL, Akiskal HS, Schettler PJ, Coryell W, Endicott J, Maser JD, Solomon DA, Leon AC and Keller MB. (2003) A prospective investigation of the natural history of the long-term weekly symptomatic status of bipolar II disorder. *Arch Gen Psychiatry* 60; 261–269.

Keedwell PA, Andrew C, Williams SCR, Brammer MJ and Phillips ML. (2005) The neural correlates of anhedonia in major depressive disorder. *Biol Psychiatry* 58; 843–853.

Keedwell PA, Andrew C, Williams SCR, Brammer MJ and Phillips ML. (2005) A double dissociation of ventromedial prefrontal cortical responses to sad and happy stimuli in depressed and healthy individuals. *Biol Psychiatry* 58; 495–503.

Kellner CH, Knapp RG, Petrides G, Rummans TA, Husain MM, Rasmussen K, Mueller M, Bernstein HJ, O'Connor K, Smith G, Biggs M, Bailine SH, Malur C, Yim E, McClintock S and Sampson S. (2006) Continuation electroconvulsive therapy vs pharmacotherapy for relapse prevention in major depression. *Arch Gen Psychiatry* 63; 1337–1344.

Kennedy SH, Konarski JZ, Segal ZV, Lau MA, Bieling PJ, McIntyre RS and Mayberg HS. (2007) Differences in brain glucose metabolism between responders to CBT and venlafaxine in a 16-week randomized controlled trial. *Am J Psychiatry* 164; 778–788.

Kessing LV, Sondergard L, Kvist K and Andersen PK. (2005) Suicide risk in patients treated with lithium. *Arch Gen Psychiatry* 62; 860–866.

Kruger S, Alda M, Young LLT, Goldapple K, Parikh S and Mayberg HS. (2006) Risk and resilience markers in bipolar disorder: brain responses to emotional challenge in bipolar patients and their healthy siblings. *Am J Psychiatry* 163; 257–264.

Krystal JH, Perry Jr EB, Gueorguieva R, Belger A, Madonick SH, Abi-Dargham AA, Cooper TB, MacDougall L, Abi-Saab W and D'Souza DC. (2005) Comparative and interactive human psychopharmacologic effects of ketamine and amphetamine. *Arch Gen Psychiatry* 62; 985–995.

Kuala A and Sanatoria G. (2005) Beyond monoamines: glutamatergic function in mood disorders. *CNS Spectr* 10; 10, 808–819.

Lemke MR, Brecht HM, Koester J and Reichmann H. (2006) Effects of the dopamine agonist pramipaxole on depression, anhedonia and motor functioning in Parkinson's disease. *J Neurol Sci* 248; 266–270.

Leverich GS, Altshuler LL, Rye MA, Suppes T, Keck Jr. PE, Kupka RW, Denicoff KD, Nolen WA, Grunze H, Martinez MI and Post RM. (2006) Risk of switch in mood polarity to hypomania or mania in patients with bipolar depression during acute and continuation trials of venlafaxine, sertraline, and bupropion as adjuncts to mood stabilizers. *Am J Psychiatry* 163; 232–239.

Levinson DF. (2006) The genetics of depression: a review. *Biol Psychiatry* 60; 84–92.

Lieben CKJ, Blokland AR, Sik A, Sung E, van Nieuwenhuizen P and Schreiber R. (2005) The selective 5-HT6 receptor antagonist Ro4368554 restores memory performance in cholinergic and serotonergic models of memory deficiency in the rat. *Neuropsychopharmacology* 30; 2169–2179.

Mah L, Zarate Jr CA, Singh J, Duan YF, Luckenbaugh DA, Manji HK and Drevets WC. (2007) Regional cerebral glucose metabolic abnormalities in bipolar II depression. *Biol Psychiatry* 61; 765–775.

Marcus MM, Jardemark KE, Wadenberg ML, Langlois X, Hertel P and Svensson TH. (2004) Combined alpha 2 and delta 2/3 receptor blockade enhances cortical glutamatergic transmission and reverses cognitive impairment in the rat. *Int J Neuropsychopharmacol* 8; 315–327.

Marek GJ, Martin-Ruis R, Abo A and Artigas F. (2005) The selective 5-HT2A receptor antagonist M100907 enhances antidepressant-like behavioral effects of the SSRI fluoxetine. *Neuropsychopharmacology* 30; 2205–2215.

Mayberg HS. (2007) Defining the neural circuitry of depression: toward a new nosology with therapeutic implications. *Biol Psychiatry* 61; 729–730.

Mayberg HS, Lozano AM, Von V, McNeely HE, Seminowicz D, Hamani C, Schwalb JM and Kennedy SH. (2005) Deep brain stimulation for treatment resistant depression. *Neuron* 45; 651–660.

McGrath PJ, Stewart JW, Fava M, Trivedi MH, Wisniewski SR, Nierenberg AA, Thase ME, Davis L, Biggs MM, Shores-Wilson K, Luther JF, Niederehe G, Warden D and Rush AJ. (2006) Tranylcypromine versus venlafaxine plus mirtazapine following three failed antidepressant medication trials for depression: a STAR*D report. *Am J Psychiatry* 163; 1531–1541.

McMahon FJ, Buervenich S, Charney D, Lipsky R, Rush AJ, Wilson AF, Sorant AJM, Papanicolaou J, Laje G, Fava M, Trivedi MH, Wisniewski SR and Manji H. (2006) Variation in the gene encoding the serotonin 2A receptor is associated with outcome of antidepressant treatment. *Am J Hum Genetics* 78; 804–814.

Meyer JH, McNeely HE, Sagrati S, Boovariwla A, Martin K, Verhoeff NPLG, Wilson AA and Houle S. (2006) Elevated putamen D2 receptor binding potential in major depression with motor retardation: an [^{11}C] raclopride positron emission tomography study. *Am J Psychiatry* 163; 1594–1602.

Michelson D, Adler LA, Amsterdam JD, Dunner DL, Nierenberg AA, Reimherr FW, Schatzberg AF, Kelsey DK and Williams DW. (2007) Addition of atomoxetine for depression incompletely responsive to sertraline: a randomized, double-blind placebo-controlled study. *J Clin Psychiatry* 68; 4, 582–587.

Millan M. (2004) The role of monoamines in the actions of established and "novel" antidepressant agents: a critical review. *Eur J Pharmacol* 500; 371–384.

Mitchell ES and Neumaier JF. (2005) 5-HT6 receptors: a novel target for cognitive enhancement. *Pharmacol Ther* 108; 320–333.

Mitchell ES, Sexton T and Neumaier JF. (2007) Increased expression of 5-HT6 receptors in the rat dorsomedial striatum impairs instrumental learning. *Neuropsychopharmacology* 32; 1520–1530.

Montgomery SA and Andersen HF. (2006) Escitalopram versus venlafaxine XR in the treatment of depression. *Int J Clin Psychopharmacol* 21; 297–309.

Najt P, Perez J, Sanches M, Peluso MAM, Glahn D and Soares JC. (2006) Impulsivity and bipolar disorder. *Eur Neuropsychopharmacol* 17; 313–320.

Narendran R, Frankle WG, Keefe R, Gil R, Martinez D, Slifsein M, Kegeles LS, Talbot PS, Huang Y, Hwang DR, Khenissi L, Cooper TB, Laruelle M and Abi-Dargham A. (2005) Altered prefrontal dopaminergic function in chronic recreational ketamine users. *Am J Psychiatry* 162; 2352–2359.

Nemeroff CB, Mayberg HS, Krahl SE, McNamara J, Frazer A, Henry TR, George MS, Charney DS and Brannan SK. (2006) VNS therapy in treatment resistant depression: clinical evidence and putative neurobiological mechanisms. *Neuropsychopharmacology* 31; 1345–1355.

Nickel MK, Muehlbacher M, Nickel C, Kettler C, Gil FP, Bachler E, Buschmann W, Rother N and Fartacek R. (2006) Aripiprazole in the treatment of patients with borderline personality disorder: a double-blind, placebo-controlled study. *Am J Psychiatry* 163; 833–838.

Nierenberg A, Bronwyn RK, Leslie VC, Alpert JE, Pava JA, Worthington JJ, Rosenbaum JF and Fava M. (1999) Residual symptoms in depressed patients who respond acutely to fluoxetine. *J Clin Psychiatry* 60; 221–225.

Nierenberg AA, Adler LA, Peselow E, Zornberg G and Rosenthal M. (1994) Trazodone for antidepressant-associated insomnia. *Am J Psychiatry* 151; 7, 1069–1072.

Nierenberg AA, Cole JO and Glass L. (1992) Possible trazodone potentiation of fluoxetine: a case series. *J Clin Psychiatry* 53; 3, 83–85.

Nierenberg AA, Farabaugh AH, Alpert JA, Gordon J, Worthington JJ, Rosenbaum JF and Fava M. (2000) Timing of onset of antidepressant response with fluoxetine treatment. *Am J Psychiatry* 157; 1423–1428.

Nierenberg AA, Fava M, Trivedi MH, Wisniewski SR, Thase ME, McGrath PJ, Alpert JE, Warden D, Luther JF, Niederehe G, Lebowitz B, Shores-Wilson K and Rush AJ. (2006) A comparison of lithium and t3 augmentation following two failed medication treatments for depression: a STAR*D report. *Am J Psychiatry* 163; 1519–1530.

Nierenberg AA, Ostacher M, Calabrese JR, Ketter TA, Marangell LB, Miklowitz DJ, Miyahara S, Bauer MS, Thase ME, Wisniewski SR and Sachs GS. (2006) Treatment-resistant bipolar depression: a STEP-BD equipoise randomized effectiveness trial of antidepressant augmentation with lamotrigine, inositol, or risperidone. *Am J Psychiatry* 163; 210–216.

Oquendo MA, Currier D and Mann JJ. (2006) Prospective studies of suicidal behavior in major depressive and bipolar disorders: what is the evidence for predictive risk factors? *Acta Psychiatr Scand* 114; 151–158.

O'Rourke H and Fudge JL. (2006) Distribution of serotonin transporter labeled fibers in amygdaloid subregions: implications for mood disorders. *Biol Psychiatry* 60; 479–490.

Pace TWW, Mletzko TC, Alagbe O, Musselman DL, Nemeroff CB, Miler AH and Heim CM. (2006) Increased stress-induced inflammatory responses in male patients with major depression and increased early life stress. *Am J Psychiatry* 163; 9, 1630–1633.

Papakostas GI and Fava M. (2007) A meta-analysis of clinical trials comparing milnacipran, a serotonin-norepinephrine reuptake inhibitor, with a selective serotonin reuptake inhibitor for the treatment of major depressive disorder. *Eur Neuropsychopharmacology* 17; 32–36.

Papakostas GI, Shelton RC, Smith J and Fava M. (2007) Augmentation of antidepressants with atypical antipsychotic medications for treatment-resistant major depressive disorder: a meta-analysis. *J Clin Psychiatry* 68; 6, 826–831.

Parsey RV, Kent JM, Oquendo MA, Richards MC, Pratap M, Cooper TB, Arawngo V and Mann JJ. (2006) Acute occupancy of brain serotonin transporter by sertraline as measured by [^{11}C] DASB and positron emission tomography. *Biol Psychiatry* 59; 821–828.

Patkar AA, Masand PS, Pae CU, Peindl K, Hooper-Wood C, Mannelli P and Ciccone P. (2006) A randomized, double-blind, placebo-controlled trial of augmentation with an extended release formulation of methylphenidate in outpatients with treatment resistant depression. *J Clin Psychopharmacol* 26; 653–656.

Perlis RH, Ostacher MJ, Pael JK, Marangell LB, Zhang H, Wisniewski SR, Keter TA, Miklowitz DJ and Otto MW, Gyulai L, Reilly-Harrington NA, Sachs GS and Thase ME. (2006) Predictors of recurrence in bipolar disorder: primary outcomes from the systematic treatment enhancement program for bipolar disorder (STEP-BD). *Am J Psychiatry* 163; 217–224.

Pitchot W, Hansenne M, Pinto E, Reggers J, Fuchs S and Ansseau M. (2005) 5-hydroxytryptamine 1A receptors, major depression and suicidal behavior. *Biol Psychiatry* 58; 854–858.

Rapaport MH, Gharabawi GM, Canuso CM, Mahmoud RA, Keller MB, Bossie CA, Turkos I, Lasser RA, Loescher A, Bouhours P, Dunbar F and Nemeroff CB. (2006) Effects of risperidone augmentation in patients with treatment resistant depression: results of open label treatment followed by double blind continuation. *Neuropsychopharmacology* 31; 2505–2513.

Roberson-Nay R, McClure EB, Monk CS, Nelson EE, Guyer AE, Fromm SJ, Charney DS, Leibenluft E, Blair J, Ernst M and Pine DS. (2006) Increased amygdala activity during successful memory encoding in adolescent major depressive disorder: a fMRI study. *Biol Psychiatry* 60; 966–973.

Robertson B, Wang L, Diaz MT, Aiello M, Gersing K, Beyer J, Mukundan Jr S, McCarthy G and Doraiswamy PM. (2007) Effect of bupropion extended release on negative emotion processing in major depressive disorder: a pilot functional magnetic resonance imaging study. *J Clin Psychiatry* 68; 261–267.

Rush AJ, Trivedi MH, Wisniewski SR, Stewart JW, Nierenberg AA, Thase ME, Ritz L, Biggs MM, Warden D, Luther JF, Shores-Wilson K, Niederehe G and Fava M. (2006) Bupropion-SR, sertraline, or venlafaxine XR after failure of SSRIs for depression. *N Engl J Med* 354; 12, 1231–1242.

Sanacora G, Kendell SF, Levin Y, Simen AA, Fenton LR, Coric V and Krystal JH. (2007) Preliminary evidence of riluzole efficacy in antidepressant-treated patients with residual depressive symptoms. *Biol Psychiatry* 61; 822–825.

Santana N, Bortolozzi A, Serrats J, Mengod G and Artigas F. (2004) Expression of serotonin 1A and serotonin 2A receptors in pyramidal and GABAergic neurons of the rat prefrontal cortex. *Cereb Cortex* 14; 1100–1109.

Schaefer HS, Putnam KM, Benca RM and Davidson RJ. (2006) Event-related functional magnetic resonance imaging measures of neural activity to positive social stimuli in pre- and post-treatment depression. *Biol Psychiatry* 60; 974–986.

Schechter LE, Ring RH, Beyer CE, Hughes ZA, Khawaja X, Malberg JE and Rosenzweig-Lipson S. (2005) Innovative approaches for the development of antidepressant drugs: current and future strategies. *NeuroRx* 2; 4, 590–611.

Schramm E, van Calker D, Dykierek P, Lieb K, Kech S, Zobel I, Leonhart R and Berger M. (2007) An intensive treatment program of interpersonal psychotherapy plus pharmacotherapy for depressed inpatients: acute and long-term results. *Am J Psychiatry* 164; 768–777.

Schreiber R, Vivian J, Hedley L, Szczepanski K, Secchi RL, Zuzow M, van Laarhoven V, Moreau JL, Martin JR, Sik A and Blokland A. (2007) Effects of the novel 5-HT6 receptor antagonist RO4368554 in rat models or cognition and sensorimotor gating. *Eur Neuropsychopharmacol* 17; 277–288.

Shang Y, Gibbs MA, Marek GJ, Stiger T, Burstein AH, Marek K, Seibyl JP and Rogers JF. (2007) Displacement of serotonin and dopamine transporters by venlafaxine extended release capsule at steady state. *J Clin Psychopharmacol* 27; 1, 71–75.

Shelton RC, Haman KL, Rapaport MH, Kiev A, Smith WT, Hirschfeld RMA, Lydiard RB, Zajecka JM and Dunner DL. (2006) A randomized, double-blind, active control study of sertraline versus venlafaxine XR in major depressive disorder. *J Clin Psychiatry* 67; 11, 1674–1681.

Siegle GJ, Thompson W, Carter CS, Steinhauer SR and Thase ME. (2007) Increased amygdala and decreased dorsolateral prefrontal BOL responses in unipolar depression: related and independent features. *Biol Psychiatry* 61; 198–209.

Skidmore FM, Rodriguez RL, Fernandez HH, Goodman WK, Foote KD and Okun MS. (2006) Lessons learned in deep brain stimulation for movement and neuropsychiatric disorders. *CNS Spectr* 11; 7, 521–537.

Takano A, Suzuki K, Kosaka J, Ota M, Nozaki S, Ikoma Y, Tanada S and Suhara T. (2005) A dose finding study of duloxetine based on serotonin transporter occupancy. *Psychopharmacology* 185; 395–399.

Talbot PS and Laruelle M. (2002) The role of in vivo molecular imaging with PET and SPECT in the elucidation of psychiatric drug action and new drug development. *Eur Neuropsychopharmacol* 12; 503–511.

Tarazi FI, Baldessarini RJ, Kula NS and Zhang K. (2003) Long-term effects of olanzapine, risperidone, and quetiapine on ionotropic glutamate receptor types: implications for antipsychotic drug treatment. *J Pharmacol Exp Ther* 306; 1145–1151.

Thase ME. (2006) The failure of evidence based medicine to guide treatment of antidepressant nonresponders. *J Clin Psychiatry* 67; 12, 1833–1855.

Thase ME, Clayton AH, Haight BR, Thompson AH, Modell JG and Johnston JA. (2006) A double-blind comparison between bupropion XL and venlafaxine XR. *J Clin Psychopharmacol* 25; 5, 482–488.

Thase ME, Corya SA, Osuntokun O, Case M, Henley DB, Sanger TM, Watson SB and Dube S. (2007) A randomized, double-blind comparison of olanzapine/fluoxetine combination, olanzapine, and fluoxetine in treatment resistant major depressive disorder. *J Clin Psychiatry* 68; 2, 224–236.

Thase ME, Friedman ES, Biggs MM, Wisniewski SR, Trivedi MH, Luther JF, Fava M, Nierenberg AA, McGrath PJ, Warden D, Niederehe G, Hollon SD and Rush AJ. (2007) Cognitive therapy versus medication in augmentation and switch strategies as second step treatments: a STAR*D report. *Am J Psychiatry* 164; 739–752.

Thase ME, Macfadden W, Weisler RH, Chang W, Paulsson B, Khan A and Calabrese JR. (2006) Efficacy of quetiapine monotherapy in bipolar I and II depression. *J Clin Psychopharmacol* 26; 600–609.

Trivedi MH, Fava M, Wisniewski SR, Thase ME, Quitkin F, Warden D, Ritz L, Nierenberg AA, Lebowitz BD, Biggs MM, Luther JF, Shores-Wilson K and Rush AJ. (2006) Medication augmentation after the failure of SSRIs for depression. *N Engl J Med* 354; 1243–1252.

Trivedi MH, Rush AJ, Wisniewski SR, Nierenberg AA, Wawrden D, Ritz L, Norquist G, Howland RH, Lebowitz B, McGrath PJ, Shores-Wilson K, Biggs MM, Balasubramani GK and Fava M. (2006) Evaluation of outcomes with citalopram for depression using measurement based care in STAR*D: implications for clinical practice. *Am J Psychiatry* 163; 28–40.

Valenstein M, McCarthy JF, Austin KL, Greden JF, Young EA and Blow FC. (2006) What happened to lithium? Antidepressant augmentation in clinical settings. *Am J Psychiatry* 163;1219–1225.

Vanover KE, Weiner DM, Makhay M, Veinbergs I, GardellLR, Lameh J, Del Tredici AL, Piu F, Schiffer HH, Ott TR, Burstein ES, Uldam AK, Thygesen MB, Schlienger N, Andersson CM, Son TY, Harvey SC, Powell SB, Geyer MA, Tolf BR, Brann MR and Davis RE. (2006) Pharmacological and behavioral profile of ACP-103, a novel 5-HT2A receptor inverse agonist. *J Pharmacol Exp Ther* 317; 910–918.

Wagner KD, Kowtch RA, Emslie GJ, Findling RL, Wilens TE, McCague K, D'Souza J, Wamil A, Lehman RB, Berv D and Linden D. (2006) A double-blind, randomized, placebo-controlled trial of oxcarbazepine in the treatment of bipolar disorder in children and adolescents. *Am J Psychiatry* 163; 1179–1186.

Weisler RH, Cutler AJ, Ballenger JC, Post RM and Ketter TA. (2006) The use of antiepileptic drugs in bipolar disorders: a review based on evidence from controlled trials. *CNS Spectr* 11; 10, 788–799.

Weissman MM. (2007) Cognitive therapy and interpersonal psychotherapy: 30 years later. *Am J Psychiatry* 164; 5, 693–696.

West AR, Floresco SB, Charara A, Rosenkranz JA and Grace AA. (2003) Electrophysiological interactions between striatal glutamatergic and dopaminergic systems. *Ann N Y Acad Sci* 1003; 53–74.

Wisniewski SR, Fava M, Trivedi MH, Thase ME, Warden D, Niederehe G, Friedman ES, Biggs MM, Sackeim HA, Shores-Wilson K, McGrath PJ, Laori PW, Miyahara S and Rush AJ. (2007) Acceptability of second-step treatments to depressed outpatients: a STAR* D report. *Am J Psychiatry* 164; 753–760.

Wozniak J, Biederan J, Mick E, Waxmonsky J, Hantsoo L, Best C, Cluette-Brown JE and Laposata M. (2007) Omega-3 fatty acid monotherapy for pediatric bipolar disorder: A prospective open-label trial. *Eur Neuropsychopharmacol* 17; 440–447.

Yatham LN, Goldstein JM, Vieta E, Bowden CL, Grunze H, Post RM, Suppes T and Calabrese JR. (2005) Atypical antipsychotics in bipolar depression: potential mechanisms of action. *J Clin Psychiatry* 66; Suppl 5, 40–48.

Zarate CA, Singh JB, Carlson PJ, Brutsche NE, Ameli R, Luckenbaugh DA, Charney DS and Manji HK. (2006) A randomized trial of an N-methyl-D-aspartate antagonist in treatment resistant major depression. *Arch Gen Psychiatry* 63; 856–864.

Zarate CA, Singh JB, Quiroz JA, DeJesus G, Denicoff KK, Luckenbaugh DA, Manji HK and Charney DS. (2006) A double-blind, placebo-controlled study of memantine in the treatment of major depression. *Am J Psychiatry* 163; 153–155.

Zimmerman M, McGlinchey JB, Posternak MA, Friedman M, Attiullah N and Boerescu D. (2006) How should remission from depression be defined? The depressed patient's perspective. *Am J Psychiatry* 163; 148–150.

Chapter 14 (Anxiety Disorders and Anxiolytics)

Anderson KC and Insel TR. (2006) The promise of extinction research for the prevention and treatment of anxiety disorders. *Biol Psychiatry* 60; 319–321.

Arzt E and Holsboer F. (2006) CRF signaling: molecular specificity for drug targeting in the CNS. *Trends Pharmacol Sci* 27; 531–538.

Atkinson BN, Bell SC, DeVivo M, Kowalski LR, Lechner SM, Ognyanov VI, Tham CS, Tsai C, Jia J, Ashton D and Klitenick MA. (2001) ALX 5407: a potent, selective inhibitor of the hGlyT1 glycine transporter. *Mol Pharmacol* 60, 6; 1414–1420.

Bak M, Krabbendam L, Janssen I, deGraaf R, Vollebergh W and van Os J. (2005) Early trauma may increase the risk for psychotic experiences by impacting on emotional response and perception of control. *Acta Psychiatr Scand* 112; 360–366.

Barad M, Gean PW and Lutz B. (2006) The role of the amygdala in the extinction of conditioned fear. *Biol Psychiatry* 60; 322–328.

Benarroch EE. (2007) GABA$_A$ receptor heterogeneity, function, and implications for epilepsy. *Neurology* 68; 612–614.

Benarroch EE. (2007) Neurosteroids: endogenous modulators of neuronal excitability and plasticity. *Neurology* 68; 945–947.

Betz H, Gomeza J, Armsen W, Scholze P and Eulenburg V. (2006) Glycine transporters: essential regulators of synaptic transmission. *Biochem Soc Trans* 34; Pt 1, 55–58.

Birbaumer N, Veit R, Lotze M, Erb M, Hermann C, Grodd W and Flor H. (2005) Deficient fear conditioning in psychopathy. *Arch Gen Psychiatry* 62; 799–805.

Bouton ME, Westbrook RF, Corcoran KA and Maren S. (2006) Contextual and temporal modulation of extinction: behavioral and biological mechanisms. *Biol Psychiatry* 60; 352–360.

Branchi I, D'Andrea I, Fiore M, DiFausto V, Aloe L and Alleva E. (2006) Early social enrichment shapes social behavior and nerve growth factor and brain-derived neurotrophic factor levels in the adult mouse brain. *Biol Psychiatry* 60; 690–696.

Cohen RA, Grieve S, Hoth KF, Paul RH, Sweet L, Tate D, Gunstad J, Stroud L, McCaffery J, Hitsman B, Niaura R, Clark CR, MacFarlane A, Bryant R, Gordon E and Williams LM. (2006) Early life stress and morphometry of the adult anterior cingulate cortex and caudate nuclei. *Biol Psychiatry* 59; 975–982.

Conti F and Weinberg RJ. (1999) Shaping excitation at glutamatergic synapses. *Trends Neurosci* 22; 10, 451–458.

Corcoran KA and Quirk GJ. (2007) Recalling safety: cooperative functions of the ventromedial prefrontal cortex and the hippocampus in extinction. *CNS Spectr* 12; 3, 200–206.

Cortese BM and Phan KL. (2005) The role of glutamate in anxiety and related disorders. *CNS Spectr* 10; 820–830.

Coyle JT and Duman RS. (2003) Finding the intracellular signaling pathways affected by mood disorder treatments. *Neuron* 38; 157–160.

Cryan JF and Kaupmann K. (2005) Don't worry "B" happy!: a role for GABA$_B$ receptors in anxiety and depression. *Trends Pharmacol Sci* 26; 1, 36–43.

Czeh B, Muller-Keuker JIH, Rygula R, Abumaria N, Hiemke C, Domenici E and Fuchs E. (2007) Chronic social stress inhibits cell proliferation in the adult medial prefrontal cortex: hemispheric asymmetry and reversal by fluoxetine treatment. *Neuropsychopharmacology* 32; 1490–1503.

Davis M, Ressler K, Rothbaum BO and Richardson R. (2006) Effects of D-cycloserine on extinction: translation from preclinical to clinical work. *Biol Psychiatry* 60; 369–375.

DeBattista C, Belanof J, Glass S, Khan A, Horne RL, Blasey C, Carpenter LL and Alva G. (2006) Mifepristone versus placebo in the treatment of psychosis in patients with psychotic major depression. *Biol Psychiatry* 60; 1343–1349.

deQuervain DJF, Aerni A and Roozendaal B. (2007) Preventive effect of beta adrenoceptor blockade on glucocorticoid induced memory retrieval deficits. *Am J Psychiatry* 6; 967–969.

Floresco SB, Todd CL and Grace AA. (2001) Glutamatergic afferents from the hippocampus to the nucleus accumbens regulate activity of ventral tegmental area dopamine neurons. *J Neurosci* 21; 13, 4915–4922.

Greenberg BD, Malone DA, Friehs GM, Rezai AR, Kubu CS, Malloy PF, Salloway SP, Okun MS, Goodman WK and Rasmussen SA. (2006) Three-year outcomes in deep brain stimulation for highly resistant obsessive-compulsive disorder. *Neuropsychopharmacology* 31; 2384–2393.

Hariri AR, Drabant EM, Munoz KE, Kolachana BS, Mattay VS, Egan MF and Weinberger DR. (2005) A susceptibility gene for affective disorders and the response of the human amygdala. *Arch Gen Psychiatry* 62; 146–152.

Hariri AR, Drabant EM and Weinberger DR. (2006) Imaging genetics: perspectives from studies of genetically driven variation in serotonin function and corticolimbic affective processing. *Biol Psychiatry* 59; 888–897.

Harsing Jr LG, Gacsalyi I, Szabo G, Schmidt E, Sziray N, Sebban C, Tesolin-Decros B, Matyus P, Egyed A, Spedding M and Levay G. (2003) The glycine transporter-1 inhibitors NFPS and Org 24461: a pharmacological study. *Pharmacol Biochem Behav* 74; 811–825.

Harsing Jr LG, Juranyi Z, Gacsalyi I, Tapolcsanyi P, Czompa A and Matyus P. (2006) Glycine transporter type 1 and its inhibitors. *Curr Med Chem* 13; 1017–1044.

Hermans D, Craske MG, Mineka S and Lovibond PF. (2006) Extinction in human fear conditioning. *Biol Psychiatry* 60; 361–368.

Hofmann SG, Meuret AE, Smits JAJ, Simon NM, Pollack MH, Eisenmenger K, Shiekh M and Otto MW. (2006) Augmentation of exposure therapy with D-cycloserine for social anxiety disorder. *Arch Gen Psychiatry* 63; 298–304.

Hu AQ, Wang ZM, Lan DM, Fu YM, Zhu YH, Dong Y and Zheng P. (2007) Inhibition of evoked glutamate release by neurosteroid allopregnanolone via inhibition of L-type calcium channels in rat medial prefrontal cortex. *Neuropsychopharmacology* 32; 1477–1489.

Huizinga D, Haberstick BC, Smolen A, Menard S, Young SE, Corley RP, Stallings MC, Grotpeter J and Hewitt JK. (2006) Childhood maltreatment, subsequent antisocial behavior, and the role of monoamine oxidase A genotype. *Biol Psychiatry* 60; 677–683.

Jiang X, Xu K, Hoberman J, Tian F, Marko AJ, Waheed JF, Harris CR, Marini Am, Enoch MA and Lipsky RH. (2005) BDNF variation and mood disorders: a novel functional promoter polymorphism and Val66Met are associated with anxiety but have opposing effects. *Neuropsychopharmacology* 30; 1353–1361.

Judge SJ, Young RL and Gartside SE. (2005) GABA$_A$ receptor modulation of 5-HT neuronal firing in the median raphe nucleus: implications for the action of anxiolytics. *Eur Neuropsychopharmacol* 16; 612–619.

Kaufman J. (2006) Stress and its consequences: an evolving story. *Biol Psychiatry* 60; 669–670.

Kilts CD, Kelsey JE, Knight B, Ely TD, Bowman FD, Gross RE, Selvig A, Gordon A, Newport DJ and Nemeroff CB. (2006) The neural correlates of social anxiety disorder and response to pharmacotherapy. *Neuropsychopharmacology* 31; 2243–2253.

Kodama M, Russell DS and Duman RS. (2005) Electroconvulsive seizures increase the expression of ma kinase phosphatases in limbic regions of rat brain. *Neuropsychopharmacology* 30; 360–371.

Krystal AD and Davidson JRT. (2007) The use of prazosin for the treatment of trauma nightmares and sleep disturbance in combat veterans with posttraumatic stress disorder. *Biol Psychiatry* 61; 925–927.

Larson CL, Schaefer HS, Siegle GJ, Jackson CAB, Anderle MJ and Davidson RJ. (2006) Fear is fast in phobic individuals: amygdala activation in response to fear-relevant stimuli. *Biol Psychiatry* 60; 410–417.

Liu GX, Cai GQ, Cai YQ, Sheng ZJ, Jiang J, Mei Z, Zhu-Gang W, Guo L and Fei J. (2007) Reduced anxiety and depression like behaviors in mice lacking GABA transporter subtype I. *Neuropsychopharmacology* 32; 1531–1539.

Mathew SJ, Amiel JM, Coplan JD, Fitterling HA, Sackeim HA and Gorman JM. (2005) Open-label trial of riluzole in generalized anxiety disorder. *Am J Psychiatry* 162; 2379–2381.

McArthur S, McHale E and Gillies G. (2007) The size and distribution of midbrain dopaminergic populations are permanently altered by perinatal glucocorticoid exposure in a sex-region and time-specific manner. *Neuropsychopharmacology* 32; 1462–1476.

McClure EB, Monk CS, Nelson EE, Parrish JM, Adler A, Blair RJ, Fromm S, Charney DS, Leibenluft E, Ernst M and Pine DS. (2007) Abnormal attention modulation of fear circuit function in pediatric generalized anxiety disorder. *Arch Gen Psychiatry* 64; 97–106.

Mody I and MacDonald JF. (1995) NMDA receptor dependent excitotoxicity: the role of intracellular Ca^2 release. *Trends Pharmacol Sci* 16; 356–359.

Mody I and Pearce RA. (2004) Diversity of inhibitory neurotransmission through $GABA_A$ receptors. *Trends Neurosci* 27; 9, 569–575.

Monk S, Nelson EE, McClure EB, Mogg K, Bradley BP, Leibenluft E, Blair RJ, Chen G, Charney DS, Ernst M and Pine DS. (2006) Ventrolateral prefrontal cortex activation and attentional bias in response to angry faces in adolescents with generalized anxiety disorder. *Am J Psychiatry* 163; 1091–1097.

Montgomery JM and Madison DV. (2004) Discrete synaptic states define a major mechanism of synapse plasticity. *Trends Neurosci* 27; 12, 744–750.

Nair A, Vadodaria KC, Banerjee SB, Benekareddy M, Dias BG, Duman RS and Vaidya VA. (2007) Stressor-specific regulation of distinct brain-derived neurotrophic factor transcripts and cyclic AMP response element binding protein expression in the postnatal and adult rat hippocampus. *Neuropsychopharmacology* 32; 1504–1519.

Orr SP, Milad MR, Metzger LJ, Lasko NB, Gilbertson MW and Pitman RK. (2006) Effects of beta blockade, PTSD diagnosis, and explicit threat on the extinction and retention of an aversively conditioned response. *Biol Psychol* 732; 262–271.

Otto, MW, Basden SL, Leyro TM, McHugh K and Hofmann SG. (2007) Clinical Perspectives on the combination of D-cycloserine and cognitive behavioral therapy for the treatment of anxiety disorders. *CNS Spectr* 12; 1, 51–66, 59–61.

Parsey RV, Hastings RS, Oquendo MA, Hu X, Goldman D, Huang YY, Simpson N, Arcement J, Huang Y, Ogden RT, Van Heertum RL, Arango V and Mann JJ. (2006) Effect of a triallelic functional polymorphism of the serotonin-transporter-linked promoter region on expression of serotonin transporter in the human brain. *Am J Psychiatry* 163; 48–51.

Parsey RV, Hastings RS, Oquendo MA, Huang YY, Simpson N, Arcement J, Huang Y, Ogden RT, Van Heertum RL, Arango V and Mann JJ. (2006) lower serotonin transporter binding potential in the human brain during major depressive episodes. *Am J Psychiatry* 163; 52–58.

Paulus MP and Stein MB. (2006) An insular view of anxiety. *Biol Psychiatry* 60; 383–387.

Pezawas L, Meyer-Lindenberg A, Drabant EM, Verchinski BA, Munoz KE, Kolachana BS, Egan MF, Mattay VS, Hariri AR and Weinberger DR. (2005) 5-HTTLPR polymorphism impacts human cingulated-amygdala interactions: a genetic susceptibility mechanism for depression. *Nat Neurosci* 8; 6, 828–834.

Pitman RK, Sanders KM, Zusman RM, Healy AR, Cheema F, Lasko NB, Cahill L and Orr SP. (2002) Pilot study of secondary prevention of post-traumatic stress disorder with propranolol. *Biol Psychiatry* 51; 189–192.

Pollack MH, Simon NM, Zalta AK, Worthinton JJ, Hoge EA, Mick E, Kinrys G and Oppenheimer J. (2006) Olanzapine augmentation of fluoxetine for refractory generalized anxiety disorder: a placebo controlled study. *Biol Psychiatry* 59; 211–215.

Pralong E, Magistretti P and Stoop R. (2002) Cellular perspectives on the glutamate-monoamine interactions in limbic lobe structures and their relevance for some psychiatric disorders. *Prog Neurobiol* 67; 173–202.

Quirk GJ, Garcia R and Gonzalez-Lima F. (2006) Prefrontal mechanisms in extinction of conditioned fear. *Biol Psychiatry* 60; 337–342.

Raskind MA, Peskind ER, Hoff DJ, Hart KL, Holmes HA, Warren D, Shofer J, O'Connell J, Taylor F, Gross C, Rohde K and McFall ME. (2007) A parallel group placebo-controlled study of prazosin for trauma nightmares and sleep disturbance in combat veterans with post-traumatic stress disorder. *Biol Psychiatry* 61; 928–934.

Rauch SL, Shin LM and Phelps EA. (2006) Neurocircuitry models of posttraumatic stress disorder and extinction: human neuroimaging research – past, present and future. *Biol Psychiatry* 60; 376–382.

Reist C, Duffy JG, Fujimoto K and Cahill L. (2001) Beta adrenergic blockade and emotional memory in PTSD. *Int J Neuropsychopharmacol* 4; 377–383.

Rickels K, Pollack MH, Feltner DE, Lydiard RB, Zimbroff DL, Bielski RJ, Tobias K, Brock JD, Zornberg GL and Pande AC. (2005) Pregabalin for treatment of generalized anxiety disorder. *Arch Gen Psychiatry* 62; 1022–1030.

Rothe C, Koszycki D, Bradwejn J, King N, Deluca V, Tharmalingam S, Macciardi F, Deckert J and Kennedy JL. (2006) Association of the Va1158Met catechol O-methyltransferase genetic polymorphism with panic disorder. *Neuropsychopharmacology* 31; 2237–2242.

Sanacora G, Fenton LR, Fasula MK, Rothman DL, Levin Y, Krystal JH and Mason GF. (2006) Corcical alpha-aminobutyric acid concentrations in depressed patients receiving cognitive behavioral therapy. *Biol Psychiatry* 59; 284–286.

Scharfman HE and Hen R. (2007) Is more neurogenesis always better? *Science* 315; 336–338.

Schulkin J, Morgan MA and Rosen JB. (2005) A neuroendocrine mechanism for sustaining fear. *Trends Neurosci* 28; 12, 629–635.

Sibille E and Lewis DA. (2006) SERT-ainly involved in depression, but when? *Am J Psychiatry* 163; 1, 8–11.

Simmons A, Strigo I, Matthews SC, Paulus MP and Stein MB. (2006) Anticipation of aversive visual stimuli is associated with increased insula activation in anxiety-prone subjects. *Biol Psychiatry* 60; 402–409.

Skapinakis P, Papatheodorou T and Mavreas V. (2007) Antipsychotic augmentation of serotonergic antidepressants in treatment resistant obsessive – compulsive disorder: a meta-analysis of the randomized controlled trials. *Eur Neuropsychopharmacol* 17; 79–93.

Sotres-Bayon F, Cain CK and LeDoux JE. (2006) Brain mechanisms of fear extinction: historical perspectives on the contribution of prefrontal cortex. *Biol Psychiatry* 60; 329–336.

Spooren W, Ballard T, Gasdparini F, Amalric M, Mutel V and Schreiber R. (2003) Insight into the function of Group 1 and Group 11 metabotropic glutamate (mGlu) receptors: behavioural characterization and implications for the treatment of CNS disorders. *Behav Pharmacol* 14; 257–277.

Swanson CJ, Bures M, Johnson MP, Linden AM, Monn JA and Schoepp DD. (2005) Metabotropic glutamate receptors as novel targets for anxiety and stress disorders. *Nat Rev* 4; 131–144.

Tamminga CA (2006) The anatomy of fear extinction. *Am J Psychiatry* 163; 6; 961.

Tamminga CA. (2006) Serotonin. *Am J Psychiatry* 163; 1, 12.

Taylor SE, Way BM, Welch WT, Hilmert CJ, Lehman BJ and Eisenberger NI. (2006) Early family environment, current adversity, the serotonin transporter promoter polymorphism, and depressive symptomatology. *Biol Psychiatry* 60; 671–676.

Triller A and Choquet D. (2005) Surface trafficking of receptors between synaptic and extrasynaptic membranes: and yet they do move! *Trends Neurosci* 28, 3; 133139.

Vaiva G, Ducrocq F, Jezequel K, Averland B, Lestavel P, Brunet A and Marmar CR. (2003) Immediate treatment with propranolol decreases posttraumatic stress disorder two months after trauma. *Biol Psychiatry* 54; 947–949.

van Balkom AJLM, van Oppen P and Van Dyck R. (2005) Disorder specific neuroanatomical correlates of attentional bias in obsessive compulsive disorder, panic disorder and hypochondriasis. *Arch Gen Psychiatry* 62; 922–933.

West AR, Floresco SB, Charara A, Rosenkranz JA and Grace AA. (2003) Electrophysiological interactions between striatal glutamatergic and dopaminergic systems. *Ann N Y Acad Sci* 1003; 53–74.

Whalen PJ, Kagan J, Cook RG, Davis FC, Kim H, Polis S, McLaren DG, Somerville LH, McLean AA, Maxwell JS and Johnstone T. (2004) Human amygdala responsivity to masked fearful eye whites. *Science* 306;17, 2061.

Widom CS, DuMOnt K and Czaja SJ. (2007) A prospective investigation of major depressive disorder and comorbidity in abused and neglected children grown up. *Arch Gen Psychiatry*, 64; 49–56.

Zarate CA, Singh J and Manji HK. (2006) Cellular plasticity cascades: targets for the development of novel therapeutics for bipolar disorder. *Biol Psychiatry* 59; 1006–1020.

Chapter 15 (Pain and the Treatment of Fibromyalgia and Functional Somatic Syndromes)

Benarroch EE. (2007) Sodium channels and pain. *Neurology* 68; 233–236.

Davies A, Hendrich J, Van Minh AT, Wratten J, Douglas L and Dolphin AC. (2007) Functional biology of the alpha 2 beta subunits of voltage gated calcium channels. *Trends Pharmacol Sci* 28; 5, 220–228.

Dooley DJ, Taylor CP, Donevan S and Feltner D. (2007) Ca^{2+} channel alpha 2 beta ligands: novel modulators of neurotransmission. *Trends Pharmacol Sci* 28; 75–82.

Farrar JT. (2006) Ion channels as therapeutic targets in neuropathic pain. *J Pain*, No 1, Suppl 1.

McLean SA, Williams DA, Stein PK, Harris RE, Lyden AK, Whalen G, Park KM, Liberzon I, Sen A, Gracely RH, Baraniuk JN and Clauw DJ. (2006) Cerebrospinal fluid corticotropin-releasing factor concentration is associated with pain but not fatigue symptoms in patients with fibromyalgia. *Neuropsychopharmacology* 31; 2776–2782.

Miljanich GP. (2004) Ziconotide: neuronal calcium channel blocker for treating severe chronic pain. *Curr Med Chem* 11; 3029–3040.

Wall PD and Melzack R. (eds) (1999) *Textbook of Pain*. 4th ed. London, Harcourt Publishers.

Chapter 16 (Disorders of Sleep and Wakefulness and Their Treatment)

Abadie P, Rioux P, Scatton B, Zarifian E, Barré L, Patat A and Baron JC. (1996) Central benzodiazepine receptor occupancy by zolpidem in the human brain as assessed by positron emission tomography. *Science* 295; 35–44.

Aloia MS, Arnedt JT, Davis JD, Riggs RL and Byrd D. (2004) Neuropsychological sequelae of obstructive sleep apnea-hypopnea syndrome: A critical review. *J Int Neuropsychol* 10; 772–785.

Bateson AN. (2004) The benzodiazepine site of the $GABA_A$ receptor: an old target with new potential? *Sleep Med* 5; S9–S15.

Carney CE and Edinger JD. (2006) Identifying critical beliefs about sleep in primary insomnia. *Sleep* 29; 444–453.

Carney CE, Segal ZV, Edinger JD and Krystal AD. (2007) A comparison of rates of residual insomnia symptoms following pharmacotherapy or cognitive-behavioral therapy for major depressive disorder. *J Clin Psychiatry* 68; 254–260.

Carter LP, Richards BD, Mintzer MZ and Griffiths RR. (2006) Relative abuse liability of GHB in humans: a comparison of psychomotor, subjective, and cognitive effects of supratherapeutic doses of triazolam, pentobarbital, and GHB. *Neuropsychopharmacology* 31; 2537–2551.

Cauter EV, Plat L, Scharf MB, Leproult R, Cespedes S, L'Hermite-Balériaux M, Copinschi G. (1997) Simultaneous stimulation of slow-wave sleep and growth hormone secretion by gamma-hydroxybutyrate in normal young men. *J Clin Invest* 100; 745–753.

Chahine LM and Chemali ZN. (2006) Restless legs syndrome: a review. *CNS Spectr* 11; 511–520.

Cook H et al. (2003) A 12-month, open-label, multicenter extension trial of orally administered sodium oxybate for the treatment of narcolepsy. *Sleep* 26; 31–35.

Czeisler CA, Walsh JK, Roth T, Hughes RJ, Wright KP, Kingsbury L, Arora S, Schwartz JRL, Niebler GE and Dinges DF. (2005) Modafinil for excessive sleepiness associated with shift-work sleep disorder. *N Engl J Med* 353; 476–486.

Davies M, Newell JG, Derry JMC, Martin IL and Dunn SM. (2000) Characterization of the interaction of zopiclone with γ-aminobutyric acid type A receptors. *Mol Pharmacol* 58; 756–762.

Dawson GR, Collinson N and Atack JR. (2005) Development of subtype selective $GABA_A$ modulators. *CNS Spectr* 10; 21–27.

Deldin PJ, Phillips LK and Thomas RJ. (2006) A preliminary study of sleep-disordered breathing in major depressive disorder. *Sleep Med* 7; 131–139.

Demyttenaere K, DeFruyt J and Stahl SM. (2005) The many faces of fatigue in major depressive disorder. *Int J Neuropsychopharmacol* 8; 93–105.

Dinges DF, Arora S, Darwish M and Niebler GE. (2006) Pharmacodynamic effects on alertness of single doses of modafinil in healthy subjects during a nocturnal period of acute sleep loss. *Curr Med Res Opin* 22; 159–167.

Dinges DF and Weaver TE. (2003) Effects of modafinil on sustained attention performance and quality of life in OSA patients with residual sleepiness while being treated with CPAP. *Sleep Med* 4; 393–402.

Drover DR. (2004) Comparative pharmacokinetics and pharmacodynamics of short-acting hypnosedatives – zaleplon, zolpidem and zopiclone. *Clin Pharmacokinet* 43; 227–238.

Durmer JS and Dinges DF. (2005) Neurocognitive consequences of sleep deprivation. *Semin Neurol* 25; 117–129.

Ellis CM, Monk C, Simmons A, Lemmens G, Williams SCR, Brammer M, Bullmore E and Parkes JD. (1999) Functional magnetic resonance imaging neuroactivation studies in normal subjects and subjects with the narcoleptic syndrome. Actions of modafinil. *J Sleep Res* 8; 85–93.

España RA and Scammell TE. (2004) Sleep neurobiology for the clinician. *Sleep* 4; 811–820.

Fava M. (2004) Daytime Sleepiness and Insomnia as Correlates of Depression. *J Clin Psychiatry* 65; 27–32.

Fava M, McCall WV, Krystal A, Wessel T, Rubens R, Caron J, Amato D and Roth T. (2006) Eszopiclone co-administered with fluoxetine in patients with insomnia coexisting with major depressive disorder. *Biol Psychiatry* 59; 1052–1060.

Fleck MW. (2002) Molecular actions of (S)-desmethylzopiclone (SEP-174559), an anxiolytic metabolite of zopiclone. *J Pharmacol Exp Ther* 302; 612–618.

Hart CL, Haney M, Vosburg SK, Comer SD, Gunderson E and Foltin RW. (2006) Modafinil attenuates disruptions in cognitive performance during simulated night-shift work. *Neuropsychopharmacology* 31; 1526–1536.

Harvey AG, Schmidt DA, Scarnà A, Semler CN and Goodwin GM. (2005) Sleep-related functioning in euthymic patients with bipolar disorder, patients with insomnia, and subjects without sleep problems. *Am J Psychiatry* 162; 50–57.

Hening W, Walters AS, Allen RP, Montplaisir J, Myers A and Ferini-Strambi L. (2004) Impact, diagnosis and treatment of restless legs syndrome (RLS) in a primary care population: the REST (RLS epidemiology, symptoms, and treatment) primary care study. *Sleep Med* 5; 237–246.

Jacobs GD, Pace-Schott EF, Stickgold R and Otto MW. (2004) Cognitive behavior therapy and pharmacotherapy for insomnia – a randomized control trial and direct comparison. *Arch Intern Med* 164; 1888–1896.

Jefferson JW, Rush AJ, Nelson JC, VanMeter SA, Krishen A, Hampton KD, Wightman DS and Modell JG. (2006) Extended-release bupropion for patients with major depressive disorder presenting with symptoms of reduced energy, pleasure, and interest: findings from a randomized, double-blind, placebo-controlled study. *J Clin Psychiatry* 67; 865–873.

Jindal RD, Buysse DJ and Thase ME. (2004) Maintenance treatment of insomnia: what can we learn from the depression literature? *Am J Psychiatry* 161; 19–24.

Krystal AD, Walsh JK, Laska E, Caron J, Amato DA, Wessel TC and Roth T. (2003) Sustained efficacy of eszopiclone over 6 months of nightly treatment: results of a randomized, double-blind, placebo-controlled study in adults with chronic insomnia. *Sleep* 7; 793–799.

Landrigan CP, Rothschild JM, Cronin JW, Kaushal R, Burdick E, Katz JT, Lilly CM, Stone PH, Lockley SW, Bates DW and Czeisler CA. (2004) Effect of reducing interns work hours on serious medical errors in intensive care units. *N Engl J Med* 351; 1838–48.

Madras BK, Xie Z, Lin Z, Jassen A, Panas H, Lynch L, Johnson R, Livni E, Spencer TJ, Bonab AA, Miller GM and Fischman AJ. (2006) Modafinil occupies dopamine and norepinephrine transporters in vivo and modulates the transporters and trace amine activity in vitro. *J Pharmacol Exp Ther* 319; 561–569.

Makris AP, Rush CR, Frederich RC and Kelly TH. (2004) Wake-promoting agents with different mechanisms of action: comparison of effects of modafinil and amphetamine on food intake and cardiovascular activity. *Appetite* 42; 185–195.

Mignot E, Taheri S and Nishino S. (2002) Sleeping with the hypothalamus: emerging therapeutic targets for sleep disorders. *Nat Neurosci* Suppl 5; 1071–1075.

Morgenthaler TI and Silber MH. (2002) Amnestic sleep-related eating disorder associated with zolpidem. *Sleep Med* 3; 323–327.

Nofzinger EA, Buysse DJ, Germain A, Price JC, Miewald JM and Kupfer DJ. (2004) Functional neuroimaging evidence for hyperarousal in insomnia. *Am J Psychiatry* 161; 2126–2129.

Nofzinger EA. (2005) Neuroimaging and sleep medicine. *Sleep Med Rev* 9; 157–172.

Nutt DJ and Malizia AL. (2001) New insights into the role of the $GABA_A$–benzodiazepine receptor in psychiatric disorder. *Br J Psychiatry* 179; 390–396.

Papakostas GI, Nutt DJ, Hallett LA, Tucker VL, Krishen A and Fava M. (2006) Resolution of sleepiness and fatigue in major depressive disorder: a comparison of bupropion and the selective serotonin reuptake inhibitors. *Biol Psychiatry* 60; 1350–1355.

Peppard PE, Szklo-Coxe M, Hla KM and Young T. (2006) Longitudinal association of sleep-related breathing disorder and depression. *Arch Intern Med* 166; 1709–1715.

Perlis ML, McCall WV, Krystal AD and Walsh JK. (2004) Long-term, non-nightly administration of zolpidem in the treatment of patients with primary insomnia. *J Clin Psychiatry* 65; 1128–1137.

Petroski RE, Pomery JE, Das R, Bowman H, Yang W, Chen A and Foster AC. (2006) Indiplon is a high-affinity positive allosteric modulator with selectivity for $\alpha 1$ subunit-containing $GABA_A$ receptors. (2006) *J Pharmacol Exp Ther* 317, 369–377.

Rosen IM. (2005) Driving while sleepy should be a criminal offense. *J Clin Sleep Med* 1; 337–343.

Saper CB, Chou TC and Scammell TE. (2001) The sleep switch: hypothalamic control of sleep and wakefulness. *Trends Neurosci* 24; 726–731.

Saper CB, Lu J, Chou TC and Gooley J. (2005) The hypothalamic integrator for circadian rhythms. *Trends Neurosci* 3; 152–157.

Saper CB, Scammell TE and Lu J. (2005) Hypothalamic regulation of sleep and circadian rhythms. *Nature* 437; 1257–1263.

Scharf MB, Baumann M and Berkowitz DV. (2003) The effects of sodium oxybate on clinical symptoms and sleep patterns in patients with fibromyalgia. *J Rheumatol* 30; 5, 1070–1074.

Schwartz JRL, Nelson MT, Schwartz ER and Hughes RJ. (2004) Effects of modafinil on wakefulness and executive function in patients with narcolepsy experiencing late-day sleepiness. *Clin Neuropharmacol* 27; 74–79.

Sheikh JI, Woodward SH and Leskin GA. (2003) Sleep in post-traumatic stress disorder and panic: convergence and divergence. *Depress Anxiety* 18; 187–197.

Spence SA, Green RD, Wilkinson ID and Hunter MD. (2005) Modafinil modulates anterior cingulate function in chronic schizophrenia. *Br J Psychiatry* 187; 55–61.

Stahl SM. (2002) Psychopharmacology of wakefulness: pathways and neurotransmitters. *J Clin Psychiatry* 63; 551–552.

Stahl SM. (2002) Awakening to the psychopharmacology of sleep and arousal: novel neurotransmitters and wake-promoting drugs. *J Clin Psychiatry* 63; 467–468.

Szubu MP, Kloss JD and Dinges DF. (2003) *Insomnia Principles and Management*. Cambridge, UK, Cambridge University Press.

Taylor DJ, Lichstein KL, Durrence HH, Reidel BW and Bush AJ. (2005) Epidemiology of insomnia, depression, and anxiety. *Sleep* 28; 1457–1464.

Thase ME, Fava M, DeBattista C, Arora S and Hughes RJ. (2006) Modafinil augmentation of SSRI therapy in patients with major depressive disorder and excessive sleepiness and fatigue: a 12-week, open-label, extension study. *CNS Spectr* 11; 93–102.

Thomas RJ. (2005) Fatigue in the executive cortical network demonstrated in narcoleptics using functional magnetic resonance imaging – a preliminary study. *Sleep Med* 6; 399–406.

Thomas RJ and Kwong K. (2006) Modafinil activates cortical and subcortical sites in the sleep-deprived state. *Sleep* 29; 1471–1481.

Thomas RJ, Rosen BR, Stern CE, Weiss JW and Kwong KK. (2005) Functional imaging of working memory in obstructive sleep-disordered breathing. *J Appl Physiol* 98; 2226–2234.

Walsh JK, Randazzo AC, Stone K, Eisenstein R, Feren S, Kajy SD, Dickey P, Roehrs T, Roth T and Schweitzer PK. (2006) Tiagabine is associated with sustained attention during sleep restriction: evidence for the value of slow-wave sleep enhancement? *Sleep* 29; 433–443.

Walsh JK, Randazzo AC, Stone KL and Schweitzer PK. (2004) Modafinil improves alertness, vigilance, and executive function during simulated night shifts. *Sleep* 27; 434–439.

Willie JT, Chemelli RM, Sinton CM, Tokita S, Williams SC, Kisanuki YY, Marcus JN, Lee C, Elmquist JK, Kohlmeier KA, Leonard CS, Richardson JA, Hammer RE and Yanagisawa M. (2003) Distinct narcolepsy syndromes in *Orexin Recepter-2* and *Orexin* null mice: molecular genetic dissection of non-REM and REM sleep regulatory processes. *Neuron* 38; 715–730.

Wong CGT, Gibson KM and Snead III OC. (2004) From the street to the brain: neurobiology of the recreational drug γ-hydroxybutyric acid. *Trends Pharmacol Sci* 25; 29–34.

Wu JC, Gillin JC, Buchsbaum MS, Chen P, Keator DB, Wu NK, Darnall LA, Fallon JH and Bunney WE. (2006) Frontal lobe metabolic decreases with sleep deprivation not totally reversed by recovery sleep. *Neuropsychopharmacology* 31; 2783–2792.

Xyrem International Study Group. (2005) A double-blind, placebo-controlled study demonstrates sodium oxybate is effective for the treatment of excessive daytime sleepiness in narcolepsy. *J Clin Sleep Med* 1; 391–397.

Zeitzer JM, Morales-Villagran A, Maidment NT, Behnke EJ, Ackerson LC, Lopez-Rodriguez F, Fried I, Engel J and Wilson CL. (2006) Extracellular adenosine in the human brain during sleep and sleep deprivation: an in vivo microdialysis study. *Sleep* 29; 455–461.

Chapter 17 (Attention Deficit Hyperactivity Disorder and Its Treatment)

Allen AJ, Kurlan RM, Gilbert DL, Coffey BJ, Linder SL, Lewis DW, Winner PK, Dunn DW, Dure LS, Sallee FR, Milton DR, Mintz MI, Ricardi RK, Erenberg G, Layton LL, Feldman PD, Kelsey DK and Spencer TJ. (2005) Atomoxetine treatment in children and adolescents with ADHD and comorbid tic disorders. *Neurology* 65; 1941–1949.

Arnsten AFT. (2006) Fundamentals of attention deficit/hyperactivity disorder: circuits and pathways. *J Clin Psychiatry* 67; Suppl 8, 7–12.

Arnsten AFT. (2006) Stimulants: therapeutic actions in ADHD. *Neuropsychopharmacology* 31; 2376–2383.

Arnsten AFT and Li BM. (2005) Neurobiology of executive functions: catecholamoine influences on prefrontal cortical functions. *Biol Psychiatry* 57; 1377–1384.

Avery RA, Franowicz JS, Phil M, Studholme C, Van Dyck CH and Arnsten AFT. (2000) The alpha 2A adrenoceptor agonist, guanfacine, increases regional cerebral blood flow in dorsolateral prefrontal cortex of monkeys performing a spatial working memory task. *Neuropsychopharmacology* 23; 240–249.

Bellgrove MA, Hawi Z, Kirley A, Fitzgerald M, Gill M and Robertson IH. (2005) Association between dopamine transporter (DAT1) genotype, left-side inattention, and an enhanced response to methylphenidate in attention deficit hyperactivity disorder. *Neuropsychopharmacology* 30; 2290–2297.

Berridge CW, Devilbiss DM and rzejewski ME, Arnsten AFT, Kelley AE, Schmeichel B, Hamilton C and Spencer RC. (2006) Methylphenidate preferentially increases catecholamine neurotransmission within the prefrontal cortex at low doses that enhance cognitive function. *Biol Psychiatry* 60; 1111–1120.

Biederman J. (2004) Impact of comorbidity in adults with attention deficit/hyperactivity disorder. *J Clin Psychiatry* 65; Suppl 3, 3–7.

Biederman J, Mick E, Surman C, Doyle R, Hammerness P, Harpold T, Dunkel S, Dougherty M, Aleardi M and Spencer T. (2006) A Randomized, placebo-controlled trial of OROS methylphenidate in adults with attention deficit/hyperactivity disorder. *Biol Psychiatry* 59; 829–835.

Biederman J, Monuteaux MC, Mick E, Spencer T, Wilens TE, Klein KL, Price JE and Faraone SV. (2006) Psychopathology in females with attention deficit/hyperactivity disorder: a controlled, five year prospective study. *Biol Psychiatry* 60; 1098–1105.

Biederman J, Monuteaux MC, Mick E, Wilens TE, Fontanella JA, Poetzl KM, Kirk T, Masse J and Faraone SV. (2006) Is cigarette smoking a gateway to alcohol and illicit drug use disorders? A study of youths with and without attention deficit hyperactivity disorder. *Biol Psychiatry* 59; 258–264.

Biederman J, Petty CR, Fried R, Doyle AE, Spencer T, Seidman LJ, Gross L, Poetzl K and Faraone SV. (2007) Stability of executive function deficits into young adult years: a prospective longitudinal follow-up study of grown up males with ADHD. *Acta Psychiatr Scand* 116; 129–136.

Biederman J, Swanson JM, Wigal SB, Boellner SW, Earl CQ and Lopez FA. (2006) A comparison of once daily and divided doses of modafinil in children with attention deficit/hyperactivity disorder: a randomized, double blind and placebo controlled study. *J Clin Psychiatry* 67; 727–735.

Bush G, Valera EM and Seidman LJ. (2005) Functional neuroimaging of attention-deficit/hyperactivity disorder: a review and suggested future directions. *Biol Psychiatry* 57; 1273–1284.

Cabeza Rand Kingston A. (eds) (2001) *Handbook of Functional Neuroimaging of Cognition*. Cambridge, MA, MIT Press.

Carpenter LL, Milosavljevic N, Schecter JM, Tyrka AR and Price LH. (2005) Augmentation with open label atomoxetine for partial or nonresponse to antidepressants. *J Clin Psychiatry* 66; 10, 1234–1238.

Cortese S, Konofal E, Yateman N, Mouren MC and Lecendreux M. (2006) Sleep and alertness in children with attention deficit/hyperactivity disorder: a systematic review of the literature. *Sleep* 29; 4, 504–511.

Coull JT, Nobre AC and Frith CD. (2001) The noradrenergic alpha 2 agonist clonidine modulates behavioural and neuroanatomical correlates of human attentional orienting and alerting. *Cereb Cortex* 11; 73–84.

Evans DL, Foa EB, Gur RE, Hendin H, O'Brien CP, Seligman MEP and Walsh BT. (eds) (2005) *Treating and Preventing Adolescent Mental Health Disorders*. New York, Oxford University Press.

Faraone SV. (2006) Advances in the genetics and neurobiology of attention deficit hyperactivity disorder. *Biol Psychiatry* 60; 1025–1027.

Faraone SV, Biederman J, Doyle A, Murray K, Petty C, Adamson JJ and Seidman L. (2006) Neuropsychological studies of late onset and subthreshold diagnoses of adult attention-deficit/hyperactivity disorder. *Biol Psychiatry* 60; 1081–1087.

Faraone SV, Biederman J, Spencer T, Mick E, Murray K, Petty C, Adamson JJ and Monuteaus MC. (2006) Diagnosing adult attention deficit hyperactivity disorder: are late onset and subthreshold diagnoses valid? *Am J Psychiatry* 163; 10, 1720–1729.

Fischman AJ and Madras BK. (2005) The neurobiology of attention-deficit/hyperactivity disorder. *Biol Psychiatry* 57; 1374–1376.

Franowicz JS and Arnsten AFT. (2002) Actions of alpha 2 noradrenergic agonists on spatial working memory and blood pressure in rhesus monkeys appear to be mediated by the same receptor subtype. *Psychopharmacology* 162; 304–312.

Franowicz JS, Phil M and Arnsten AFT. (1999) Treatment with the noradrenergic alpha-2 agonist conidine, but not diazepam, improves spatial working memory in normal young rhesus monkeys. *Neuropsychopharmacology* 21; 611–621.

Gibbs SE and Depositor M. (2005) Individual capacity differences predict working memory performance and prefrontal activity following dopamine receptor stimulation. *Cogn Affective Behav Neurosci* 5; 2, 212–221.

Green WH. (2001) *Child and Adolescent Clinical Psychopharmacology*. 3rd ed. Philadelphia, Lippincott Williams & Wilkins.

Hazell P. (2005) Do adrenergically active drugs have a role in the first-line treatment of attention-deficit/hyperactivity disorder? *Expert Opin Pharmacother* 12; 1989–1998.

Jakala P, Riekkinen M, Sirvio J, Koivisto E, Kejonen K, Vanhanen M and Riekkinen Jr P. (1999) Guanfacine, but not clonidine, improves planning and working memory performance in humans. *Neuropsychopharmacology* 20; 460–470.

Jakala P, Riekkinen M, Sirvio J, Koivisto E and Riekkinen Jr P. (1999) Clonidine, but not guanfacine, impairs choice reaction time performance in young healthy volunteers. *Neuropsychopharmacology* 21; 495–502.

Jakala P, Sirvio J, Riekkinen M, Koivista E, Kejonen K, Vanhanen M and Riekkinen Jr P. (1999) Guanfacine and clonidine, alpha 2 agonists, improve paired associates learning, but not delayed matching to sample, in humans. *Neuropsychopharmacology* 20; 119–130.

Kessler RC, Adler L, Barkley R, Biederman J, Conners CK, Demler O, Fawraone SV, Greenhill LL and Howes MJ. (2006) The prevalence and correlates of adult ADHD in the United States: results from the National Comorbidity Survey replication. *Am J Psychiatry* 163; 716–723.

Kollins SH, McClernon JM and Fuemmeler BF. (2005) Association between smoking and attention deficit/hyperactivity disorder symptoms in a population based sample of young adults. *Arch Gen Psychiatry* 62; 1142–1147.

Lagace DC, Yee JK, Bolanos CA and Eisch AJ. (2006) Juvenile administration of methylphenidate attenuates adult hippocampal neurogenesis. *Biol Psychiatry* 60; 1121–1130.

Lahey BB, Pelham WE, Loney J, Lee SS and Willcutt E. (2005) Instability of the DSM-IV subtypes of ADHD from preschool through elementary school. *Arch Gen Psychiatry* 62; 896–902.

Levy R and Goldman-Rakic PS. (1999) Association of storage and processing functions in the dorsolateral prefrontal cortex of the nonhuman primate. *J Neurosci* 19; 12, 5149–5158.

Lu J, Jhou T and Saper CB. (2006) Identification of wake active dopaminergic neurons in the ventral periaqueductal gray matter. *J Neurosci* 26; 1, 193–202.

Ma CL, Arnsten AFT and Li BM. (2005) Locomotor hyperactivity induced by blockade of prefrontal cortical alpha 2 adrenoceptors in monkeys. *Biol Psychiatry* 57; 192–195.

Madras BK, Miller GM and Fischman AJ. (2005) The dopamine transporter and attention deficit/hyperactivity disorder. *Biol Psychiatry* 57; 1397–1409.

Marrs W, Kuperman J, Avedian T, Roth RH and Jentsch JD. (2005) Alpha-2 adrenoceptor activation inhibits phencyclidine-induced deficits of spatial working memory in rats. *Neuropsychopharmaoclogy* 30; 150–1510.

Martin A, Scahill L, Charney DS and Leckman JF. (2003) *Pediatric Psychopharmacology.* New York, Oxford University Press.

Mattay VS, Callicott JH, Bertolino A, Heaton I, Frank JA, Coppola R, Berman KF, Goldberg TE and Weinbreger DR. (2000) Effects of dextroamphetamine on cognitive performance and cortical activation. *NeuroImage* 12; 268–275.

McGough JJ, Wigal SB, Abikoff H, Turnbow JM, Posner K and Moon E. A randomized, double-blind, placebo-controlled, laboratory classroom assessment of methylphenidate transdermal system in children with ADHD. *J Atten Disord* 9; 3, 476–485.

Pliszka SR. (2005) The neuropsychopharmacology of attention deficit/hyperactivity disorder. *Biol Psychiatry* 57; 1385–1390.

Pliszka SR, Glahn DC, Semrud-Clikeman M, Franklin C, Perez III R, Xiong J and Liotti M. (2006) Neuroimaging of inhibitory control areas in children with attention deficit hyperactivity disorder who were treatment naïve or in long-term treatment. *Am J Psychiatry* 163; 1052–1060.

Polanczyk G, Zeni C, Genro JP, Guimaraes AP, Roman T, Hutz MH and Rohd LA. (2007) Association of the adrenergic alpha 2A receptor gene with methylphenidate improvement of inattentive symptoms in children and adolescents with attention deficit/hyperactivity disorder. *Arch Gen Psychiatry* 64; 218–224.

Posey DJ, Aman MG, McCracken JT, Scahill L, Tierney E, Arnold LE, Vitiello B, Chuang SZ, Davies M, Ramadan Y, Witwer AN, Swiezy NB, Cronin P, Shah B, Carroll DH, Young C, Wheeler C and McDougle CJ. (20007) Positive effects of methylphenidate on inattention and hyperactivity in pervasive developmental disorders: an analysis of secondary measures. *Biol Psychiatry* 61; 538–544.

Randall DC, Fleck NL, Shneerson JM and File SE. (2004) The cognitive enhancing properties of modafinil are limited in non-sleep deprived middle-aged volunteers. *Pharmacol Biochem Behav* 77; 547–555.

Randall DC, Shneerson JM and File SE. (2005) Cognitive effects of modafinil in student volunteers may depend on IQ. *Pharmacol Biochem Behav* 82; 133–139.

Randall DC, Shneerson JM, Plaha KK and File SE. (2003) Modafinil affects mood, but not cognitive function, in healthy young volunteers. *Hum Psychopharmacol* 18; 163–173.

Randall DC, Viswanath A, Bharania P, Elsabagh SM, Hartley DE, Shneerson JM and File SE. (2005) Does modafinil enhance cognitive performance in young volunteers who are not sleep deprived? *J Clin Psychopharmacol* 25; 2, 175–179.

Reimherr FW, Williams ED, Strong RE, Mestas R, Soni P and Marchant BK. (2007) A Double-blind, placebo-controlled crossover study of osmotic release oral system methylphenidate in adults with ADHD with assessment of oppositional and emotional dimensions of the disorder. *J Clin Psychiatry* 68; 1, 93–101.

Research Units on Pediatric Psychopharmacology Autism Network. (2005) Randomized, controlled, crossover trial of methylphenidate in pervasive developmental disorders with hyperactivity. *Arch Gen Psychiatry* 62; 1266–1274.

Riccardi P, Li R, Ansari MS, Zald D, Park S, Dawant B and erson S, Doop M, Woodward N, Schoenberg E, Schmidt D, Baldwin R and Kessler R. (2006) Amphetamine-induced displacement of [^{18}F] fallypride in striatum and extrastriatal regions in humans. *Neuropsychopharmacology* 31; 1016–1026.

Rutter M and Taylor E. (eds.) (2002) *Child and Adolescent Psychiatry*. 4th ed. Malden, MA, Blackwell Publishing.

Scahill L, Barloon L and Farkas L. (1999) Alpha-2 agonists in the treatment of attention deficit hyperactivity disorder. *J Child Adolesc Psychiatr Nurs* 12; 4, 168–172.

Scheffer RE, Kowatch RA, Carmody T and Rush AJ. (2005) Randomized, placebo-controlled trial of mixed amphetamine salts for symptoms of comorbid ADHD in pediatric bipolar disorder after mood stabilization with divalproex sodium. *Am J Psychiatry* 162; 58–64.

Schmitz M, Denardin D, Silva TL, Pianca T, Roman T, Hutz MH, Faraone SV and Rohde LA. Association between alpha-2a-adrenergic receptor gene and ADHD inattentive type. *Biol Psychiatry* 60; 1028–1033.

Seidman LJ, Valera EM, Makris N, Monuteaus MC, Boriel DL, Kelkar K, Kennedy DN, Caviness VS, Bush G, Aleardi M, Faraone SV and Biederman J. (2006) Dorsolateral prefrontal and anterior cingulate cortex volumetric abnormalities in adults with attention-deficit/hyperactivity disorder identified by magnetic resonance imaging. *Biol Psychiatry* 60; 1071–1080.

Shafritz KM, Marchione KE, Gore JC, Shaywitz SE and Shaywitz BA. (2004) The effects of methylphenidate on neural systems of attention in attention deficit hyperactivity disorder. *Am J Psychiatry* 161; 11, 1990–1997.

Shaw P, Gornick M, Lerch J, Addington A, Seawl J, Greenstein D, Sharp W, Evans A, Giedd JN, Castellanos FX and Rapoport JL. (2007) Polymorphisms of the dopamine D4 receptor, clinical outcome, and cortical structure in attention deficit/hyperactivity disorder. *Arch Gen Psychiatry* 64; 8, 921–931.

Smith AB, Taylor E, Brammer M, Toone B and Rubia K. (2006) Task-specific hypoactivation in prefrontal and temporoparietal brain regions during motor inhibition and task switching in mediation naïve children and adolescents with attention deficit hyperactivity disorder. *Am J Psychiatry* 163; 1044–1051.

Solanta MV. (2002) Dopamine dysfunction in AD/HD: integrating clinical and basic neuroscience research. *Behav Brain Res* 130; 65–71.

Spencer TJ, Biederman J, Madras BK, Faraone SV, Dougherty DD, Bonab AA and FIschman AJ. (2005) In vivo neuroreceptor imaging in attention deficit/hyperactivity disorder: a focus on the dopamine transporter. *Biol Psychiatry* 57; 1293–1300.

Spencer TJ, Faraone SV, Michelson D, Adler LA, Reimherr FW, Glatt SJ and Biederman J. (2006) Atomoxetine and adult attention deficit/hyperactivity disorder: the effects of comorbidity. *J Clin Psychiatry* 67; 3, 415–420.

Steere JC and Arnsten AFT. (1997) The alpha 2A noradrenergic receptor agonist guanfacine improves visual object discrimination reversal performance in aged rhesus monkeys. *Behav Neurosci* 111; 5, 883–891.

Surman CGH, Thomas RJ, Aleardi M, Pagano C and Biederman J. (2006) Adults with ADHD and sleep complaints. *J Atten Disord* 9; 3, 550–555.

Swanson JM, Greenhill LL, Lopez FA, Sedillo A, Earl CQ, Jiang JC and Biederman J. (2006) Modafinil film coated tablets in children and adolescents with attention deficit/hyperactivity disorder: results of a randomized, double-blind, placebo-controlled fixed dose study followed by abrupt discontinuation. *J Clin Psychiatry* 67; 137–147.

Tamm L, Menn V and Reiss AL. (2006) Parietal attentional system aberrations during target detection in adolescents with attention deficit hyperactivity disorder: event-related fMRI evidence. *Am J Psychiatry* 163; 1033–1043.

Taylor FB and Russo J. (2000) Efficacy of modafinil compared to dextroamphetamine for the treatment of attention deficit hyperactivity disorder in adults. *J Child Adolesc Psychopharmacol* 10; 4, 311–320.

Turner DC, Clark L, Dowson J, Robbins TW and Sahakian BJ. (2004) Modafinil improves cognition and response inhibition in adult attention deficit hyperactivity disorder. *Biol Psychiatry* 55; 1031–1040.

Turner DC, Robbins TW, Clark L, Aron AR, Dowson J and Sahakian BJ. (2003) Cognitive enhancing effects of modafinil in healthy volunteers. *Psychopharmacology* 165; 260–269.

Vaidya CJ, Bunge SA, Dudukovic NM, Zalecki CA, Elliott GR and Gabrieli JDE. (2005) Altered neural substrates of cognitive control in childhood ADHD: evidence from functional magnetic resonance imaging. *Am J Psychiatry* 162; 1605–1613.

Valera EM, Faraone SV, Biederman J, Poldrack RA and Seidman LJ. (2005) Functional neuroanatomy of working memory in adults with attention deficit/hyperactivity disorder. *Biol Psychiatry* 57; 439–447.

Volkow ND, Wang GJ, Newcorn J, Teland F, Solanto MV, Fowler JS, Logan J, Ma Y, Schulz K, Pradhan K, Wong C and Swanson JM. (2007) Depressed dopamine activity in caudate and preliminary evidence of limbic involvement in adults with attention deficit/hyperactivity disorder. *Arch Gen Psychiatry* 64; 8, 932–940.

Walsh BT (ed) (1998) *Child Psychopharmacology.* Washington, D.C., American Psychiatric Press.

Wilens TE and Dodson W. (2004) A clinical perspective of attention deficit/hyperactivity disorder into adulthood. *J Clin Psychiatry* 65; 10, 1301–1313.

Wilens TE. (2007) Lisdexamfetamine for ADHD. *Curr Psychiatry* 6; 96–98, 105.

Wilson MC, Wilman AH, Bell EC, Asghar SJ and Silverstone PH. (2004) Dextroamphetamine causes a change in regional brain activity in vivo during cognitive tasks: a functional magnetic resonance imaging study of blood oxygen level dependent response. *Biol Psychiatry* 56; 284–291.

Zang YF, Jin Z, Weng XC, Zhang L, Zeng YW, Yang L, Wang YF, Seidman LJ and Faraone SV. (2005) Functional MRI in attention deficit hyperactivity disorder: evidence for hypofrontality. *Brain Dev* 27; 544–550.

Zuvekas SH, Vitiello B and Norquist GS. (2006) Recent trends in stimulant medication use among US children. *Am J Psychiatry* 163; 579–585.

Chapter 18 (Dementia and Its Treatment)

Alexopoulos GS. (2003) Role of executive function in late life depression. *J Clin Psychiatry* 64; Suppl 14, 18–23.

Ballard C, Ziabreva I, Perry R, Larsen JP, O'Brien J, McKeith I, Perry E and Aarsland D. (2006) Differences in neuropathologic characteristics across the Lewy body dementia spectrum. *Neurology* 67; 1931–1934.

Citron M. (2004) β-secretase inhibition for the treatment of Alzheimer's disease – promise and challenge. *Trends Pharmacol Serv* 25; 2, 92–97.

Deakin JB, Rahman S, Nestor PJ, Hodges JR and Sahakian BJ. (2004) Paroxetine does not improve symptoms and impairs cognition in frontotemporal dementia: a double-blind randomized controlled trial. *Psychopharmacology* 172; 400–408.

Deutsch SI, Rosse RB and Deutsch LH. (2006) Faulty regulation of tau phosphorylation by the reelin signal transduction pathway is a potential mechanism of pathogenesis and therapeutic target in Alzheimer's disease. *Eur Neuropsychopharmacology* 16; 547–551.

Dominguez DI and De Strooper B. (2002) Novel therapeutic strategies provide the real test for the amyloid hypothesis of Alzheimer's disease. *Trends in Pharmacol Sci* 23; 7, 324–330.

Doraiswamy PM. (2003) Alzheimer's disease and the glutamate NMDA receptor. *Psychopharmacol Bull* 37; 2, 41–49.

Ercoli L, Siddarth P, Huang SC, Miller K, Bookheimer SY, Wright BC, Phelps ME and Small G. (2006) Perceived loss of memory ability and cerebral metabolic decline in persons with the apoplipoprotein E-IV genetic risk for Alzheimer disease. *Arch Gen Psychiatry* 63; 442–448.

Evans JG, Wilcock G and Birks J. 9 (2004) Evidence based pharmacotherapy of Alzheimer's disease. *Int J Neuropsychopharmacol* 7; 351–369.

Huey ED, Putnam KT and Grafman J. (2006) A systematic review of neurotransmitter deficits and treatments in frontotemporal dementia. *Neurology* 66; 17–22.

Lane RM, Potkin SG and Enz A. (2006) Targeting acetylcholinesterase and butyrylcholinesterase in dementia. *Int J Neuropsychopharmacol* 9; 101–124.

Mudher A and Lovestone S. (2002) Alzheimer's disease – do tauists and Baptists finally shake hands? *Trends Neurosci* 25; 1, 22–26.

Nichols L, Pike VW, Cai L and Innis RB. (2006) Imaging and in vivo quantitation of beta-amyloid: an exemplary biomarker for Alzheimer's disease? *Biol Psychiatry* 59; 940–947.

Ondo WG, Tintner R, Voung KD, Lai D and Ringholz G. (2005) Double-blind, placebo-controlled unforced titration parallel trial of quetiapine for dopaminergic induced hallucinations in Parkinson's disease. *Mov Disord* 20; 8, 958–963.

Padala PR, Petty F and Bhatia SC. (2006) Methylphenidate may treat apathy independent of depression. *Ann Pharmacother* 39; 1947–1949.

Raskin J, Wiltse CG, Siegal A, Sheikh J, Xu J, Dinkel JJ, Rotz BT and Mohs RC. (2007) Efficacy of duloxetine on cognition, depression, and pain in elderly patients with major depressive disorder: an 8-week, double-blind, placebo-controlled trial. *Am J Psychiatry* 164; 900–909.

Reisberg B, Doody R, Stoffler A, Schmitt F, Ferris S, Mobius HJ, Memantine Study Group. (2003) Memantine in moderate to severe Alzheimer's disease. *N Engl J Med* 348; 14, 1333–1341.

Rosenberg RN. (2005) Translational research on the way to effective therapy for Alzheimer's disease. *Arch Gen Psychiatry* 62; 1186–1192.

Rundek T and Bennett DA. (2006) Cognitive leisure activities, but not watching TV, for future brain benefits. *Neurology* 66; 794–795.

Salloway S, Ferris S, Kluger A, Goldman R, Griesing T, Kumar D and Richardson S. (2004) Efficacy of donepezil in mild cognitive impairment. *Neurology* 63; 651–657.

Schneider LS, Dagerman KS and Insel P. (2005) Risk of death with atypical antipsychotic drug treatment for dementia. *JAMA* 294; 15, 1935–1943.

Sink KM, Holden KF and Yaffe K. (2005) Pharmacological treatment of neuropsychiatric symptoms of dementia. *JAMA* 293; 5, 596–608.

Tariot PN, Farlow MR, Grossberg GT, Graham SM, McDonald S and Gergel I. (2004) Memantine treatment in patients with moderate to severe Alzheimer's disease already receiving donepezil. *JAMA* 291; 3, 317–324.

Verghese J, LeValley A, Derby C, Kuslansky G, Ktz M, Hall C, Buschke H and Lipton RB. (2006) Leisure activities and the risk of amnestic mild cognitive impairment in the elderly. *Neurology* 66; 821–827.

Williams MM, Xiong C, Morris JC and Galvin JE. (2006) Survival and mortality differences between dementia with Lewy bodies vs Alzheimer's disease. *Neurology* 67; 1935–1941.

Wishart HA, Saykin AJ, McAllister TW, Rabin LA, McDonald BC, Flashman LA, Roth RM, Mamourian AC, Tsongalis GJ and Rhodes CH. (2006) Regional brain atrophy in cognitively intact adults with a single APOE ε4 allele. *Neurology* 67; 1221–1224.

Chapter 19 (Disorders of Reward, Drug Abuse, and Their Treatment)

Anton RF, O'Malley SS, Ciraulo DA, Cisler RA, Couper D, Donovan DM, Gastfriend DR, Hosking JD, Johnson BA, LoCastro JS, Longabaugh R, Mason BJ, Mattson ME,

Miller WR, Pettinati HM, Randall CL, Swift R, Weiss RD, Williams LD and Zweben A. (2006) Combined pharmacotherapies and behavioral interventions for alcohol dependence. The COMBINE study: a randomized controlled trial. *JAMA* 295; 2003–2017.

Berlin HA, Rolls ET and Iversen SD. (2005) Borderline personality disorder, impulsivity, and the orbitofrontal cortex. *Am J Psychiatry* 162; 2360–2373.

Berridge CW. (2006) Neural substrates of psychostimulant-induced arousal. *Neuropsychopharmacology* 31; 2332–2340.

Boileau I, Dagher A, Leyton M, Gunn RN, Baker GB, Diksic M and Benkelfat C. (2006) Modeling sensitization to stimulants in humans. *Arch Gen Psychiatry* 63; 1386–1395.

Bradberry CW. (2002) Dose-dependent effect of ethanol on extracellular dopamine in mesolimbic striatum of awake rhesus monkeys: comparison with cocaine across individuals. *Psychopharmacology* 165; 67–76.

Brady KT and Sinha R. (2005) Co-occurring mental and substance use disorders: the neurobiological effects of chronic stress. *Am J Psychiatry* 162; 1483–1493.

Breitenstein C, Korsukewitz C. Flöel A, Kretzschmar T, Diederich Kand Knecht S. (2006) Tonic dopaminergic stimulation impairs associative learning in healthy subjects. *Neuropsychopharmacology* 31; 2552–2564.

Carai MAM, Colombo G and Gessa GL. (2005) Rimonabant: the first thereapeutically relevant cannabinoid antagonist. *Life Sci* 1–12.

Cervo L, Carnovali F, Stark JA and Mennini T. (2003) Cocaine-seeking behavior in response to drug-associated stimuli in rats: involvement of D_3 and D_2 dopamine receptors. *Neuropsychopharmacology* 28; 1150–1159.

Chambers RA, Taylor JR and Potenza MN. (2003) Developmental neurocircuitry of motivation in adolescence: a critical period of addiction vulnerability. *Am J Psychiatry* 160; 1041–1052.

Changeus JP and Edelstein SJ. (eds) (2005) *Nicotinic Acetylcholiine Receptors*. New York, Odile Jacob Publishing.

Dackis CA and Miller NS. (2003) Neurobiological effects determine treatment options for alcohol, cocaine, and heroin addiction. *Psychiatr Ann* 33; 585–592.

Dahchour A and DeWitte P. (2003) Effects of acamprosate on excitatory amino acids during multiple ethanol withdrawal periods. *Alcohol Clin Exp Res* 3; 465–470.

Daoust M, Legrand E, Gewiss M, Heidbreder C, DeWitte P, Tran G and Durbin P. (1991) Acamprosate modulates synaptosomal GABA transmission in chronically alcoholised rats. *Pharmacol Biochem Behav* 41; 669–674.

DeVries TJ and Schoffelmeer ANM. (2005) Cannabinoid CB_1 receptors control conditioned drug seeking. *Trends Pharmacol Sci* 26; 420–426.

DeWitte P. (2004) Imbalance between neuroexcitatory and neuroinhibitory amino acids causes craving for ethanol. *Addict Behav* 29; 1325–1339.

DeWitte P, Littleton J, Parot P and Koob G. (2005) Neuroprotective and Abstinence-Promoting Effects of Acamprosate. Elucidating the Mechanism of Action. *CNS Drugs* 6; 517–537.

Fong TW. (2004) Why aren't more psychiatrists prescribing buprenorphine? *Curr Psychiatry* 3; 46–56.

Gadde KM, Franciscy DM, Wagner II HR and Krishnan KR. (2003) Zonisamide for weight loss in obese adults. *JAMA* 289; 1820–1825.

Galanter M and Kleber HD. (eds) (2004) *Textbook of Substance Abuse Treatment*. 3rd ed. Washington, D.C., American Psychiatric Publishing.

Garbutt JC, Kranzler HR, O'Malley SS, Gastfriend DR, Pettinati HM, Silverman BL, Loewy JW and Ehrich EW. (2005) Efficacy and tolerability of long-acting injectable naltrexone for alcohol dependence: a randomized controlled trial. *JAMA* 293; 1617–1625.

Grace AA, Floresco SB, Goto Y and Lodge DJ. (2007) Regulation of firing of dopaminergic neurons and control of goal-directed behaviors. *Trends Neurosci* 5; 220–227.

Grant JE, Brewer JA and Potenza MN. (2006) The neurobiology of substance and behavioral addictions. *CNS Spectr* 11; 924–930.

Gravan H, Pankiewicz J, Bloom A, Cho JK, Sperry L, Ross TJ, Salmeron BJ, Risinger R, Kelley D and Stein EA. (2000) Cue-induced cocaine craving: neuroanatomical specificity for drug users and drug stimuli. *Am J Psychiatry* 157; 1789–1798.

Heinz A, Reimold M, Wrase J, Hermann D, Croissant B, Mundle G, Dohmen BM, Braus DH, Schumann G, Machulla HJ, Bares R and Mann K. (2005) Correlation of stable elevations in striatal μ-opioid receptor availability in detoxified alcoholic patients with alcohol craving: a positron emission tomography study using carbon 11-labeled carfentanil. *Arch Gen Psychiatry* 62; 57–64.

Heinz A, Siessmeier T, Wrase J, Buchholz HG, Gründer G, Kumakura Y, Cumming P, Schreckenberger M, Smolka MN, Rösch F, Mann K and Bartenstein P. (2005) Correlation of alcohol craving with striatal dopamine synthesis capacity and $D_{2/3}$ receptor availability: a combined [^{18}F]DOPA and [^{18}F]DMFP PET study in detoxified alcoholic patients. *Am J Psychiatry* 162; 1515–1520.

Hyman SE. (2005) Addiction: a disease of learning and memory. *Am J Psychiatry* 162; 1414–1422.

Ivanov IS, Schulz KP, Palmero RC and Newcorn JH. (2006) Neurobiology and evidence-based biological treatments for substance abuse disorders. *CNS Spectr* 11; 864–877.

Johnson BA. (2006) New weapon to curb smoking: no more excuses to delay treatment. *Arch Intern Med* 166; 1547–1550.

Kalivas PW and Volkow ND. (2005) The neural basis of addiction: a pathology of motivation and choice. *Am J Psychiatry* 162; 1403–1413.

Kessler RC. (2004) Impact of substance abuse on the diagnosis, course, and treatment of mood disorders: the epidemiology of dual diagnosis. *Biol Psychiatry* 56; 730–737.

Kiefer F, Jahn H, Tarnaske T, Helwig H, Briken P, Holzbach R, Kämpf P, Stracke R, Baehr M, Naber D and Wiedemann K. (2003) Comparing and combining naltrexone and acamprosate in relapse prevention of alcoholism. *Arch Gen Psychiatry* 60; 92–99.

Kiefer F and Wiedemann K. (2004) Combined therapy: what does acamprosate and naltrexone combination tell us? *Alcohol Alcohol* 39; 542–547.

King PJ. (2005) The hypothalamus and obesity. *Curr Drug Targets* 6; 225–240.

Koob G and Moal ML. (eds.) (2006) *Neurobiology of Addiction*. San Diego, CA, Academic Press.

Kranzler HR and Ciraulo DA. (eds.) (2005) *Clinical Manual of Addiction Psychopharmacology*. Washington, D.C., American Psychiatric Publishing.

Kuczenski R and Segal DS. (2005) Stimulant actions in rodents: implications for attention-deficit/hyperactivity disorder treatment and potential substance abuse. *Biol Psychiatry* 57; 1391–1396.

LeMoal M and Koob GF. (2006) Drug addiction: pathways to the disease and pathophysiological perspectives. *Eur Neuropsychopharmacol* 17; 377–393.

Leyton M, Boileau I, Benkelfat C, Diksci M, Baker G and Dagher A. (2002) Amphetamine-induced increases in extracellular dopamine, drug wanting, and novelty seaking: a PET/[^{11}C]raclopride study in healthy men. *Neuropsychopharmacology* 27; 1027–1035.

Lindsey KP, Wilcox KM, Votaw JR, Goodman MM, Plisson C, Carroll FI, Rice KC and Howell LL. (2004) Effect of dopamine transporter inhibitors on cocaine self-administration in rhesus monkeys: relationship to transporter occupancy determined by positron emission tomography neuroimaging. *J Pharmacol Exp Ther* 309; 959–969.

Little KY, Krolewski DM, Zhang L and Cassin BJ. (2003) Loss of striatal vesicular monomaine transporter protein (VMAT2) in human cocaine users. *Am J Psychiatry* 160; 47–55.

Lobo DSS and Kennedy JL. (2006) The genetics of gambling and behavioral addictions. *CNS Spectr* 11; 931–939.

Lodge DJ and Grace AA. (2006) The hippocampus modulates dopamine neuron responsivity by regulating the intensity of phasic neuron activation. *Neuropsychopharmacology* 31; 1356–1361.

Martinez D, Gil R, Slifstein M, Hwan DR, Huang Y, Perez A, Kegeles L, Talbot P, Evans S, Krystal J, Laruelle M and Abi-Dargham A. (2005) Alcohol dependence is associated with blunted dopamine transmission in the ventral striatum. *Biol Psychiatry* 58; 779–786.

Martinez D, Narendran R, Foltin RW, Slifstein M, Hwan DR, Broft A, Huang Y, Cooper TB, Fischman MW, Kleber HD and Laruelle M. (2007) Amphetamine-induced dopamine release: markedly blunted in cocaine dependence and predictive of the choice to self-administer cocaine. *Am J Psych* 164; 622–629.

Mason BJ. (2003) Acamprosate and naltrexone treatment for alcohol dependence: an evidence-based risk-benefits assessment. *Eur Neuropsychopharmacol* 13; 469–475.

Mason BJ. (2005) Acamprosate in the treatment of alcohol dependence. *Expert Opin Pharmacother* 6; 2103–2115.

Mason BJ, Goodman AM, Chabac S and Lehert P. (2006) Effect of oral acamprosate on abstinence in patients with alcohol dependence in a double-blind, placebo-controlled trial: the role of patient motivation. *J Psychiatr Res* 40; 382–392.

McElroy SL, Hudson JI, Capece JA, Beyers K, Fisher AC and Rosenthal NR. (2007) Topiramate for the treatment of binge-eating disorder associated with obesity: a placebo-controlled study. *Biol Psychiatry* 61; 1039–1048.

Nestler EJ. (2005) Is there a common molecular pathway for addiction? *Nat Neurosci* 11; 1445–1449.

Nestler EJ and Carlezon WA. (2006) The mesolimbic dopamine reward circuit in depression. *Soc Biol Psychiatry* 59; 1151–1159.

Netzeband JG and Gruol DL. (1995) Modulatory effects of acute ethanol on metabotropic glutamate responses in cultured Purkinje neurons. *Brain Res* 688; 105–113.

Noël X, Van Der Linden M and Bechara A. (2006) The neurocognitive mechanisms of decision-making, impulse control, and loss of willpower to resist drugs. *Psychiatry* 30–41.

O'Brien CP. (2005) Anticraving medications for relapse prevention: a possible new class of psychoactive medications. *Am J Psychiatry* 162; 14231431.

Petrakis IL, Poling J, Levinson C, Nich C, Carroll K, Rounsaville B and the VA New England VISN I MIRECC Study Group. (2005) Naltrexone and disulfiram in patients with alcohol dependence and comorbid psychiatric disorders. *Biol Psychiatry* 57; 1128–1137.

Pettinati HM, O'Brien CP, Rabinowitz AR, Wortman SM, Oslin DW, Kampman KM and Dackis CA. The status of naltrexone in the treatment of alcohol dependence. specific effects on heavy drinking. *J Clin Psychopharmacol* 26; 610–625.

Roozen HG, deWaart R, van der Windt DAW, van den Brink W, de Jong CAJ and Kerkhof AJFM. (2005) A systematic review of the effectiveness of naltrexone in the maintenance treatment of opioid and alcohol dependence. *Eur Neuropsychopharmacology* 16; 311–323.

Salamone JD, Correa M, Mingote S and Weber SM. (2002) Nucleus accumbens dopamine and the regulation of effort in food-seeking behavior: implications for studies of natural motivation, psychiatry, and drug abuse. *J Pharmacol Exp Ther* 305; 1–8.

Selzer J. (2006) Buprenorphine: reflections of an addictions psychiatrist. *Am Soc Clin Psychopharmacol* 9; 1466–1467.

Solinas M and Goldberg SR. (2005) Motivational effects of cannabinoids and opioids on food reinforcement depend on simultaneous activation of cannabinoid and opioid systems. *Neuropsychopharmacology* 30; 2035–2045.

Spencer TJ, Biederman J, Ciccone PE, Madras BK, Dougherty DD, Bonab AA, Livni E, Parasrampuria DA and Fischman AJ. (2006) PET study examining pharmacokinetics, detection and likeability, and dopamine transporter receptor occupancy of short- and long-acting oral methylphenidate. *Am J Psychiatry* 163; 387–395.

Tanda G and Goldberg SR. (2003) Cannabinoids: reward, dependence, and underlying neurochemical mechanisms – a review of recent preclinical data. *Psychopharmacology* 169; 115–134.

Tipper CM, Cairo TA, Woodward TS, Phillips AG, Liddle PF and Ngan ETC. (2005) Processing efficiency of a verbal working memory system is modulated by amphetamine: an fMRI investigation. *Psychopharmacology* 180; 634–643.

VanGaal LF, Rissanen AM, Scheen AJ, Ziegler O and Rössner S. (2005) Effects of the cannabinoid-1 receptor blocker rimonabant on weight reduction and cardiovascular risk factors in overweight patients: 1-year experience from the RIO-Europe study. *Lancet* 365; 1389–1397.

Vocci FJ, Acri J and Elkashef A. (2005) Medication development for addictive disorders: the state of the science. *Am J Psychiatry* 162; 1432–1440.

Volkow ND. (2006) Stimulant medications: how to minimize their reinforcing effects? *Am J Psychiatry* 163; 359–361.

Volkow ND, Fowler JS, Wang GJ, Ding YS and Gatley SJ. (2002) Role of dopamine in the therapeutic and reinforcing effects of methylphenidate in humans: results from imaging studies. *Eur Neuropsychopharmacol* 12; 557–566.

Volkow ND and O'Brien CP. (2007) Issues for DSM-V: should obesity be included as a brain disorder? *Am J Psychiatry* 164; 708–710.

Volkow ND, Wang GJ, Fowler JS, Telang F, Maynard L, Logan J, Gatley SJ, Pappas N, Wong C, Vaska P, Zhu W and Swanson JM. (2004) Evidence that methylphenidate enhances the saliency of a mathematical task by increasing dopamine in the human brain. *Am J Psychiatry* 161; 1173–1180.

Wilding J, Van Gaal L, Rissanen A, Vercruysse F and Fitchet M. (2004) A randomized double-blind placebo-controlled study of the long-term efficacy and safety to topiramate in the treatment of obese subjects. *Int J Obes* 28; 1399–1410.

Xi ZX, Newman AH, Gilbert JG, Pak AC, Peng XQ, Ashby Jr CR, Gitajn L and Gardner EL. (2006) The novel dopamine D_3 receptor antagonist NGB 2904 inhibits cocaine's rewarding effects and cocaine-induced reinstatement of drug-seeking behavior in rats. *Neuropsychopharmacology* 31; 1393–1405.

Index

Page numbers followed by '*f*' indicate figures; page numbers followed by '*t*' indicate tables.

3PPP, 380*f*
5HIAA (5-hydroxy-indole acetic acid), 483
   in cerebrospinal fluid, 488

AAADC (aromatic amino acid decarboxylase), 343, 344*f*
AAB-001, 937
"able stabilizers", 717, 717*f*
ABT089, 449
abuse, 945
acamprosate, 769
   actions, in ventral tegmental area (VTA), 978*f*
   for alcohol dependency, 976
   in combos for bipolar disorder, 715
   icon, 976*f*
ACC-001, 937
acetyl coenzyme A (AcCoA), as acetylcholine precursor, 914
acetylcholine (ACh), 139, 902
   in arousal pathways, 396, 398*f*
   and arousal spectrum, 817, 817*f*
   and blocked dopamine receptors, 339*f*
   overactivity, 341
   production, 914, 914*f*
   projections, 206, 207*f*
      via basal forebrain, 208*f*
   psychotropic drugs and, 53, 99, 128, 129
   reciprocal relationship with dopamine, 338*f*
   and reward, 946, 947*f*
   termination of action, 915*f*
   for treating nicotine dependence, 960
   vesicular transporter for, 102
acetylcholine-linked mechanisms, 448

acetylcholine neurotransmitter, 128*t*
   as psychotropic drug target, 115, 117
acetylcholine receptors, TCA and, 602*f*
acetylcholine transporters, 94*t*, 99*f*
acetylcholinesterase (AChE), 112, 170, 915, 915*f*
   donepezil to inhibit, 925*f*
   galantamine to inhibit, 930*f*
   rivastigmine to inhibit, 928*f*
ACh. *See* acetylcholine (ACh)
ACP 103, 446
ACP-104, 375, 380*f*
ACR16, 380*f*
ACTH (adrenocorticotropic hormone), 752, 753*f*
actin, 36, 42*f*
action potential, 145, 159, 160*f*
   control over firing, 217
   encoding of, 162*f*
   ionic components of, 147*f*
activity-dependent nociception, 795
   acute pain, 796*f*
   neuropathic pain, 797*f*
activity-dependent spine formation, by estradiol, 614*f*
acute pain, 774, 775, 796*f*
   vs. chronic, 775*t*
acute stress reaction, 193
Adapin. *See* doxepin (Sinequan, Adapin)
adaptive states, 138
adatanserin, 574
addiction, 945, 953*f*. *See also* substance abuse
   nicotine and, 955–959
   overvalued reward in, 951

1057

adenosine, 820, 859
adenylate cyclase, binding to G protein, 70
ADHD. *See* attention deficit hyperactivity disorder (ADHD)
adhesion molecules, 31
  and neuronal migration, 30*f*
adipose tissue, insulin resistance in, 387, 390*f*
adolescence
  aggressiveness in, 425
  antidepressants for, 519*f*
  brain restructuring in, 22, 22*f*, 44
  mania in, 712
  removal of synaptic connections, 42, 314
  risperidone for treating psychotic disorders, 412
adrenocorticotropic hormone (ACTH), 752, 753*f*
affective blunting, 251
affective disorders, 454. *See also* mood disorders
  stress-induced, novel treatments, 754*f*
affective flattening, as SSRI side effect, 356
affective spectrum disorders, 556, 776*t*
  norepinephrine and, 546
  pain in, 802
"affective storms", in children, 712
affective symptoms
  dorsal vs. ventral regulation, 322*f*
  mesolimbic dopamine pathway role in, 274
  multiple disorders impacting, 261*f*
  pharmacy, 428, 430*f*
  in schizophrenia, shared with other disorders, 260
afferent neurons, peripheral, neuropathic pain and, 785
age. *See also* adolescence; children; elderly
  synapse formation by, 49*f*
aggressive symptom pharmacy, 425, 427*f*
aggressiveness, 256, 704*f*
  in dementia patients, 935
  multiple disorders impacting, 261*f*
  in schizophrenic patients, 259
Agilect/Azilect (rasaligine), 579*t*
  for Parkinson's disease, 582
aging. *See also* elderly
  erectile dysfunction and, 1000*f*
  hippocampus sensitivity to, 24, 24*f*
  normal, 908
  and synapse loss, 25*f*
agitation, 547
  benzodiazepines for, 434
  in dementia patients, 935
agnosia, 900
agomelatine (Valdoxan), 574, 658, 844*f*
  icon, 661*f*

agonists
  absence of, 108, 112*f*
  actions on ion channel, 133*f*
  antagonist acting in presence of, 135*f*
  and G protein-linked receptor, 110–112
  impact on ligand-gated ion channels, 143*f*
  spectrum, 111*f*
  and receptor conformation, 378*f*
agoraphobia, in children, 713
agranulocytosis, clozapine and, 410
akathisia
  from aripiprazole, 421
  nigrostrial pathway dopamine deficiencies and, 277
  from paroxetine withdrawal, 537
  from SSRIs, 531
alanine-serine-cysteine transporter (ASC-T), glial, 280
alcohol,
  actions
    on reward circuits, 971*f*
    in ventral tegmental area (VTA), 972*f*
  consumption, vs. sleepiness, 851*t*
  dependency/abuse
    by ADHD patients, 870
    social anxiety and, 769
    treatment, 973–977
  GABA-A receptor binding to, 737
  heavy drinking
    vs. reduced-risk, 973
    will power to reduce, 975*f*
  icon, 970*f*
  probability of dependence, 968*t*
  reduced-risk drinking, 975*t*
  and reward, 970
alcoholics, smoking by, 970
aldehyde dehydrogenase, 977
alertness, 650
  loss
    bupropion for, 556
    as SSRI side effect, 530
allodynia, 775, 786, 795, 799*f*
allosteric modulation, 140, 737, 738
alogia, 251, 252*t*
alpha 1 adrenergic receptors
  atypical antipsychotic agents and, 385*f*
  and sedation, 397*f*
  TCA and, 599, 603*f*
alpha 1 antagonist, for posttraumatic stress disorder, 770
alpha-1 receptor, antagonism, 340*f*
alpha 1 selective hypnotics, 840*f*
alpha-1 unit, 153, 154*f*

alpha-2 adrenergic receptors, atypical
    antipsychotic agents and, 385f
alpha 2 antagonists, 414
    icon, 559f
    and norepinephrine, 560f
    and serotonin, 560f
    as serotonin norepinephrine disinhibitors,
        558, 562f
alpha 2 delta ligands, 156, 158f
    for anxiety disorders, 755
    binding of, 798f
    for chronic pain, 801f
    in dorsal horn, 800f
    for fibromyalgia, 808
    and pain gate, 795
    potential therapeutic effects, 756f
alpha-2 delta protein, 153
    gabapentin and pregabalin binding to,
        158
alpha-2 delta unit, 155f
alpha 2 receptors
    on axon terminal, 478f
    blockade of, 559f
    somatodendritic, 475, 479f
alpha 2A agonists, 891
    mechanism of action, 895f
alpha-4 beta-2 nicotinic acetylcholine receptor,
    449
alpha 4 beta 2 nicotinic receptors, 959, 960f
    reinforcement and, 958f
alpha-7-nicotinic cholinergic agonists, 448
alpha 7 nicotinic cholinergic receptors, 918
alpha amino-3-hydroxy-5-methyl-4-
    isoxazolepropionic acid (AMPA)
    receptors, 286, 286f
    synapses with, 313f
alpha APP, 903
alpha heliz, 109f
alpha-L-glutamyl transferace, 627
alpha pore
    of voltage-sensitive calcium channels, 154f
    of voltage-sensitive sodium channels, 151f
        anticonvulsant binding, 151
alpha secretase, 902
alpha subunit, 147, 148f
alprazolam (Xanax), 53
    and CYP 450 3A4, 608
    and sedation, 609
alprostadil, 1004
ALS (amyotrophic lateral sclerosis)
    excitotoxicity and, 48f
    riluzole for, 685f
Alzheimer's disease, 426, 900
    amyloid cascade hypothesis, 902

Aβ42 oligomer interference with synaptic
    function, 906, 906f
Aβ42 production, 905f
    inflammation from plaque formation,
        907f
    neuronal dysfunction and loss, 909f
    tangle formation, 908f
amyloid plaques in, 901
Apo-E protein and, 907, 910f
cholinergic deficiency, 920
cholinesterase inhibitors
    best responders, 922, 922f
    donepezil, 923, 924f
    galantamine, 926
    palliative responders, 924f
    rivastigmine, 924, 926f
    tacrine, 923
    treatment outcomes, 921
    usual responders, 923f
clinical features, 901t
cognitive symptoms, 259
excitotoxicity and, 48f, 302, 303f
expected exponential increase, 901
familial cases early onset, 906
folate for depression, 935
glutamate hypothesis of cognitive deficiency,
    926–930
identifying at presymptomatic/prodromal
    stage, 911f
neurofibrillary tangles in, 901
problems with studies of, 912
symptom pattern onset, 913f
symptomatic treatments in development, 940
symptoms shared with schizophrenia, 258,
    259, 259f
treatment, 128, 129
untreated time course, 921f
amantadine, 440
    for bipolar disorder, 695
    icon, 696f
    mechanism of action
        on GABA, glutamate, sigma, and
            dopamine, 676t
        VSSCs, synaptic vesicles, and carbonic
            anhydrase, 675t
    possible actions in bipolar disorder, 698f
    putative clinical actions, 673t
amenorrhea, 278, 336
American College of Rheumatology, criteria for
    fibromyalgia, 805t
American Psychiatric Association, 178
amibegron, 662
amines, 52t
d-amino acid oxidase (DAO), 284f

Index | 1059

amino acid transporters, 94t
  inhibitory, 94t
amino acids, 52t
  to close VSSC, 148
  for ligand-gated ion channels, 126
  regulation of calcium channels, 153
  in voltage-gated ion channels, 147
amisulpride, 376, 380f
  and cardiometabolic risk, 386t
  clinical actions of, 371
  and diabetes, 417
  for negative symptoms in schizophrenia, 428f
  pharmacological icon, 423f
  and QTc prolongation, 417
amitriptyline (Elavil, Endep, Tryptizol, Loroxyl), 53, 572, 597t
amnesia, 900
amotivational syndrome, 986
amoxapine (Asendin), 419, 420f
AMPA (alpha-amino-3-hydroxy-5-methyl-4-isoxazole-priopionic acid) glutamate receptors, 130, 164f
  glutamate at, 147f
  and synaptogenesis, 308
AMPA-kines, 445
amphetamines, 99t, 290, 576, 579t
  action
    in ADHD, 885
    MAO inhibitors with, 579t
  and dopamine displacement, 107f
  and dopamine release, 272
  dopamine transporter (DAT) and, 94, 103, 105f
  icon, 984f
  with MAOIs, and hypertension, 593t
  pharmacological actions, 889
  VMAT transport fo, 106f
  for wakefulness, 857, 858
amygdala, 199f
  activation, 234
    by VMPFC, 760
  and anxiety/fear, 704f
  and avoidance, 728f
  beta-3 receptors in, 662
  connection with locus coeruleus, 731
  and depressed mood, 490
  and emotional learning, 949
  and fear neurobiology, 729
  and fearful faces, 236f
  impact on suicidal ideation, 493
  information processing
    and depressed mood, 492f
    serotonin and, 744

manic episode symptoms linked to, 506
noradrenergic receptor simulation in, 547
overactive circuits, 745f
regulating anxiety in, 241
response to emotional input, 324
and schizophrenia symptoms, 262f
serotonin and fear processing by, 234
amylin, 450
amyloid, and glutamate steady leak, 928
amyloid cascade hypothesis for Alzheimer's disease, 902, 905f
  neuronal dysfunction and loss, 909f
amyloid plaques, 903
  in Alzheimer's disease, 901
  and glutamate excitotoxicity, 932f
  and glutamate release, 927
  treatment development to act on, 937
amyloid precursor protein (APP), 902
  processing into Aβ peptides,
  processing into soluble peptides, 904f
amyotrophic lateral sclerosis (ALS)
  excitotoxicity and, 48f
  riluzole for, 685f
Anafranil. See clomipramine (Anafranil)
analgesics, 775
  probability of dependence, 968t
anandamide, 53, 946, 947f
anatomic G protein-linked receptors, 110t
anatomically addressed nervous system, 21
  neurodevelopment in, 22
"angel dust", 144
anhedonia, 251, 252t
anorexia, fluoxetine for, 533
antagonists, 112–115
  acting alone, 134f
  acting in presence of inverse agonist, 140f
  acting in presence of partial agonist, 138f
  action in presence of agonists, 135f
  vs. inverse agonist, 351
  inverse agonist action reversed by, 141f
  for ligand-gated ion channels, 130
  vs. partial agonists, 378f
  presynaptic, 445f
anterior cingulate cortex (ACC), 198, 199f
anterograde motor, 8f
  localization of, 9f
anterograde transport, 14
  fast, 16f
antiaptotic receptors (TrkA), 29t
anticholinergic agents
  D2 antagonism and, 339f
  side effects, 341
anticholinergic effects, from diphenhydramine (Benadryl), 847f

1060 | Index

anticonvulsants, 129, 149. *See also specific agents*
   carbamazepine (Equetro), 678
   as mood stabilizers, 672
      gabapentin, 687
      lamotrigine, 682–686
      levetiracetam, 689
      oxcarbazepine/eslicarbazepine, 681
      pregabalin, 687
      riluzole, 686
      topiramate, 686
      zonisamide, 687
   sodium channels as action site, 150
   valproic acid, 672
antidepressant "poop out", 461
antidepressants. *See also* heroic combos; serotonin norepinephrine reuptake inhibitors (SNRIs)
   allosteric site for binding, 97
   bipolar depression response to, 472f
   brain MAO-A inhibition for efficacy, 579
   in clinical practice, 639
      cost-based algorithm, 642, 642f
      evidence-based algorithm, 641f
      evidence-based selections, 641
      reduced positive affect vs. increased negative affect, 643
      selection process, 639
      symptom-based algorithm, 645f
      symptom-based selection, 643, 644f
   clinical trials, 514
   combinations for major depressive disorder, 651
   combinations for unipolar depression, 652f
   continuation, 515f
   CYP450 2D6 impact on plasma levels, 607
   delay in relief from depression, 528f
   in development, 658t
      targeting neurokinins, 660t
      targeting novel sites of action, 660t
   effectiveness in clinical practice, 514
   enhancement of serotonin and/or norepinephrine, 98
   general principles, 512–520
   impact on mixed states of depression and mania, 467
   increase in monoamines, 520f
   interaction with MAOIs, 595t
   interference with slow-wave sleep, 848
   "intramolecular polypharmacy" of, 542
   manic or hypmanic episode on, 463
   L-5-methyltetrahydrofolate (MTHF) and, 631f
   monoamine oxidase inhibitors (MAOIs), 574–597
   monoamine transporters as targets, 99t
   and neurogenesis in hippocampus, 24f
   norepinephrine and dopamine reuptake inhibitors (NDRIs), 99t, 552–556. *See also* norepinephrine dopamine reuptake inhibitors (NDRIs)
   over life cycle, 519, 519f
   pharmacokinetics, 603
   prior responses to, and bipolar diagnosis, 470
   putative mechanisms, 533t
   response rates, 514f
   risks of use or avoidance during pregnancy, 618t
   risks to fetus, 618
   role in bipolar disorder, 699
   serotonin norepinephrine reuptake inhibitors (SNRIs), 541. *See also* serotonin norepinephrine reuptake inhibitors (SNRIs)
   sites on transporter for, 95
   suicidality in adolescent females, 617
   symptoms persisting after treatment with, 516
   time course of effects, 521f
   trimonoaminergic modulators (TMMs) and, 610
   triple-action combo, 657
   two mechanisms vs. one, 542, 542f
antihistamines, 328
   sedation by, 846
   side effects of, 846
antipsychotic agents
   as antidepressants, 658
   atypical, 342
      administration frequency, 368
      cardiometabolic risk and, 386t
      cardiometabolic risk management, 391
      hit-and-run receptor binding properties, 370f
      hypothetical action over time, 371f
      to improve schizophrenia symptoms, 355
      pharmacological properties, 385f
      and prolactin, 364f
      properties, 365, 381f
      and weight gain risk, 386t
   avoiding sedation and enhancing long-term outcome, 401f
   benzodiazepines to lead in or top off, 434f
   best practices for monitoring and managing, 395f
   cardiometabolic risk and, 383–396
   combining two, 437
   conventional, 337f
      vs. atypical, 358f

antipsychotic agents (*Contd.*)
    D2 binding of, 369*f*
    D2-receptor antagonist, 329
    hypothetical action over time, 369*f*
        muscarinic cholinergic blocking properties, 337–341
        pharmacological properties, 328–342
        and prolactin, 364*f*
        risk and benefits of long-term, 341
        in use, 331*t*
    as D2 dopamine receptor blockers, 273
    first-generation, 329*f*
    high doses, 437*f*
    links between binding properties and clinical actions, 382
    low-potency, and dissociation, 370
    "off-label" uses, 328
    patient toleration of, 409
    pharmacokinetics, 402–408
    pharmacological properties, 408–425
    prescribing information, 328
    prophylactic, 438
    receptor interactions for, 380
    sedation as short-term tool, 398*f*
    side effects and compliance, 399*f*
    switching, 431, 433*f*
        process to avoid, 433*f*
        from sedating to nonsedating, 435*f*
antisocial personality disorder, 259
anxiety
    5HT1A partial agonist actions in, 746*f*
    amygdala and, 704*f*
    GABA and, 732–741
    gabapentin for, 688
    linking symptoms to circuits, 731*f*
    memories and, 730*f*
    noradrenergic hyperactivity in, 755, 757*f*
        blocking, 758*f*
    pregabalin for, 688
    reduced, 649
    serotonin, stress and, 741–749
anxiety disorders
    5HT1A receptors and, 349*f*
    alpha 2 delta ligands for, 755
    amygdala and fear neurobiology, 729
    brain component regulating, 200
    in children, 713
    comorbid with fibromyalgia, 807*t*
    CSTC loops and worry neurobiology, 764
    diabolical learning hypothesis and, 230
    drug treatment action at ionotrophic receptors, 124
    fear conditioning, vs. fear extinction, 756, 759*f*
    fear extinction, 760
    fluvoxamine for, 537
    GABA-A allosteric modulatory sites, hypothetical shift in set point, 740
    GABA and, 241, 732–741
    generalized anxiety disorder (GAD), 723*f*
        pharmacy, 767*f*
        treatment, 765
    inability to extinguish maladaptive fear responses, 761
    linking symptoms to circuits, 727*f*
    MAO inhibitors for, 575
    NET inhibition and, 558
    noradrenergic hyperactivity in, 755
        blocking, 758*f*
    obsessive compulsive disorder, 725*f*
        pharmacy, 771*f*
        treatment, 770
    overlap with depression, 722*f*
    pain linked to, 802, 803*f*
    painful somatic symptoms in, 791*f*
    panic disorder, 723*f*
        pharmacy, 768*f*
        treatment, 768
    paroxetine for patients with, 536
    phenotype, 725*f*
    posttraumatic stress disorder, 724*f*
        pharmacy, 770*f*
        treatment, 770
    preemptive or prophylactic treatments, 762
        with beta blockers, 763*f*
    prevalence of, 757
    quetiapine for, 414*f*
    serotonin for regulating in amygdala, 241
    serotonin projections regulation of, 205, 206*f*
    social anxiety disorder, 724*f*
        pharmacy, 769*f*
        treatment, 769
    stress progression to, treatment, 754
    symptom dimensions, 722–728
    symptom overlap in subtypes, 726
    symptom overlap with depression, 726
    treating insomnia in, 843
    venlafaxine for, 549
anxiolytics
    benzodiazepines as, 741
    GABA, 741
    probability of dependence, 968*t*
anxious misery, 764
anxious mood, 260
anxious self-punishment, 249
apathetic recovery, 530, 546
apathetic temperament, 460*f*

apathy, 249
　circuits, 493f
　in depression, 491
aphasia, 900
apical dendrites, 2, 219f
　in pyramidal cell, 3f
apnea, obstructive sleep, 855
　symptoms shared with other disorders, 869t
Apo-E protein, and Alzheimer's disease, 907, 910f
apoptosis, 27, 750f
　from gene expression, 78
　and necrosis, 28f
　programmed into genome, 28
APP. See amyloid precursor protein (APP)
appetite
　changes in, 493
　circuits, 498f
　histamine-1 with 5HT2C antagonism, 387f
　reduced, 1010
appetite suppressants, interaction with MAOIs, 595t
apprehensive expectations, 764
apraxia, 900
arborization, of neurons, 35f
arcuate nucleus, 977
aripiprazole, 375, 376, 380f
　actions as mood stabilizer, 693f
　and cardiometabolic risk, 386t
　in combos for bipolar disorder, 713, 717, 717f
　as CYP 2D6 substrate, 404, 405f
　and diabetes, 417
　dosage with carbamazepine, 407f
　pharmacological actions, 693f
　pharmacological icon, 422f
　raising levels of, 406f
　and sedation, 430, 432f
　switching from sedating agent to, 435
　testing for cocaine abuse treatment, 986
　and weight gain risk, 386t
armodafinil (Nuvigil), for wakefulness, 857
aromatic amino acid decarboxylase (AAADC), 343, 344f
arousal
　deficient daytime, 819f
　desensitization in prefrontal cortex, 878f
　and dopamine, 856f
　excessive, and ADHD, 873–877
　mechanisms, 870
　norepinephrine projections regulation of, 205
　simultaneous deficient and excessive, in ADHD, 879f
　spectrum of cognitive dysfunction in ADHD
　　ADHD treatment, 872

　　deficit arousal, 871f
　　excessive arousal, 876f
arousal combos, 658
arousal spectrum, 816, 817f
ascending reticular activating system, 817
asenapine, 368f
Asendin (amoxapine), 419, 420f
asociality, 251, 252t
Asperger's syndrome, 771
assaultiveness, 256
astrocytes, and Alzheimer's disease, 906
atherosclerosis, from repetitive autonomic responses, 731
atomoxetine, 99t, 557, 604, 606f
　for ADHD, 885, 889
　mechanism of action, 892f
　with stress and comorbidity, 894f
　CYP450 2D6 impact on plasma levels, 607
　for fibromyalgia, 810
　for weight loss, 1011
atorvastatin
　and CYP 450 3A4, 608
　risk of muscle damage, 609
ATPase, 170f
attention
　in ADHD patients, 873
　CSTC loop to regulate, 213f
　impaired, in schizophrenia, 257
　provoking circuits for, 235
attention deficit hyperactivity disorder (ADHD), 103, 235, 426, 863
　adults with, 880
　　vs. children, 881, 882t
　　prevalence of, 882
　treatment, 880, 897
　arousal spectrum of cognitive dysfunction
　　ADHD treatment, 872
　　deficit arousal, 871f
　　excessive arousal, 876f
　atomoxetine for, 557, 558
　　mechanism of action, 892f
　brain restructuring and, 44
　causes, 870t
　and comorbidity, priority for treatment, 880
　deficit arousal and, 870
　desensitizing arousal in prefrontal cortex, 878f
　dopamine signals in prefrontal cortex, 886f
　how not to treat, 888f
　impact of development, 884f
　from improper neuronal migration, 29
　information processing, 874f
　mania vs., 712, 713

attention deficit hyperactivity disorder
    (ADHD) (Contd.)
  noradrenergic treatment, 889–897
    atomoxetine, 889
  norepinephrine signals in prefrontal cortex, 886f
  pharmacy, 896f
  selective attention circuit, 866f
  simultaneous deficient and excessive arousal, 879f
  stimulants for, 884, 885–889
    mechanism of action, 887f
  stress
    comorbidities and arousal levels, 877
    and comorbidity, 893f
  sustained attention circuit, 867f
  symptoms and circuits, 864–870
    DSM-IV, 864f
    matching, 865f
  symptoms shared with schizophrenia, 260
  timing of onset, 882
  tuning cortical pyramidal neurons, 875f
attention deficit, vs. attention deficit disorder, 866
attitudes, hostile, 249
atypical antipsychotic agents, 342
  for ADHD, with stimulants, 879
  administration frequency, 368
  in bipolar depression, 692f
    pharmacological actions, 693f
  cardiometabolic risk and, 386t
  cardiometabolic risk management, 391
  clozapine as, 409
  vs. conventional, 358f
  hit-and-run receptor binding properties, 370f
  hypothetical action over time, 371f
  for mania, actions, 691f
  for mania and bipolar depression, mechanism of action, 690
  as mood stabilizers, 694f
  for nonpsychotic mania symptoms, 689
  properties, 365, 385f
  and weight gain risk, 386t
auditory association cortex, 196f
auditory hallucinations, 251
Aurorix. See moclobemide (Aurorix, Manerix)
autism, 426, 771
  cognitive symptoms, 259
  irritability in children with, 427
  risperidone for irritability, 412
autonomic nervous system, 731
autoreceptors, 475
autosomal dominant pattern, classic, 178f

AV965, 941
Aventyl. See nortriptyline (Pamelor, Endep, Aventyl)
avoidance, 728f
avolution, 251, 252t
"awakening", 410, 437
axoaxonic synapses, 5, 6f, 36, 37f
axodendritic synapses, 36, 37f
Axokine, 1011
axon hillock, 7f, 8
  of pyramidal neuron, 217
axon terminals. See also presynaptic axon terminals
  alpha 2 receptors on, 478f
axonal growth cone, 31, 32f
  docking, 32f
axons, 1, 2, 2f
  in basket neurons, 4f
  in double bouquet cells, 4f
  growth of, 31
    in mature brain, 31
  myelination of fibers, 22
  neurotrophins control of growth, 31
  in pyramidal cell, 3f
  for transport function, 10
axosomatic synapses, 36, 37f
Azilect. See rasaligine (Agilect/Azilect)
Azilect/Agilect (rasaligine), 579t
  for Parkinson's disease, 582

bapineuzumab, AN1792(QS21), 937
barbiturates
  and anxiety, 767
  dependency/addiction, 986
  as hypnotics, 840
basal dendrites, 2
  in pyramidal cell, 3f
basal forebrain, 203f
  acetylcholine projections via, 208f
  cholinergic cell bodies in, 206
  inefficient information processing, and sleep disturbances, 503f
  nerve destruction, 902
  and sleep disturbances, 491, 494f
basal nucleus, 206
basilar dendrites, 219f
basket neurons, 2, 4f
  icon drawing, 4f
  realistic drawing, 4f
BDNF. See brain-derived neurotrophic factor (BDNF)
behavior
  in dementia, 934
  genes impact on, 88

hypothetical path from gene to, 182f
linked to key brain regions, 203f
repetition, and brain restructuring, 32
Benadryl (diphenhydramine), 846, 847f
  half-life of, 836f
benzamide antipsychotics, clinical actions of, 371
benzodiazepines, 244f
  actions on reward circuits, 987f
  for aggression management, 427f
  for agitation, 434
  agonist spectrum in panic disorder, 742f
  as anxiolytics, 741
  for bipolar disorder, 694
  in combos for bipolar disorder, 715
  for enhancing GABA actions, 732
  for fibromyalgia, 811
  GABA-A receptors and, 736f
  for generalized anxiety disorder, 765, 767
  injectable, 425
  for insomnia, 837f
    restrictions, 837
  to lead in or top off antipsychotics, 434f
  long-term effects, 838f
  nonselective, 841f
  as PAMs, 142
  for panic disorder, 768
  as positive allosteric modulators, 146f
  for posttraumatic stress disorder, 770
  for social anxiety disorder, 769
  when switching antipsychotics, 435f
beta 3 agonists, as antidepressants, 658, 662, 663f
beta 3 receptors, 662f
beta amyloid antagonists, 937, 938f
beta amyloid, Apo-E protein ineffective binding to, 908
beta amyloid immunizations, 938f
beta amyloid plaques, 901
beta blockers
  and CYP450 2D6 inhibitors, 608
  preemptive treatments, 763f
  for social anxiety disorder, 769
beta endorphin, 53
beta secretase, 903
  inhibitors, 940f
beta units, 155f
  of voltage-sensitive sodium channels, 149, 152f
BH4. See tetrahydrobiopterin (BH4)
bicifidine, 552, 552f
bifeprunox (DU 127090), 375, 376, 380f
  and cardiometabolic risk, 386t
  and diabetes, 417

in metabolic pharmacy, 429
metabolized by CYP 3A4, 404
for obesity, 448
pharmacological icon, 424f
and sedation, 432f
sedation risk with, 430
binary neurotransmitter receptor complex, binding to G protein, 69f
binge eating, 1009
biological endophenotype, 182, 182f
  for executive dysfunction, 233f
  in path between gene and mental illness, 185
  vs. symptom endophenotype, 229
bipolar 1/2 disorder, 461, 462f
bipolar 1/4 disorder, 461, 462f
bipolar disorder. See also mood stabilizers
  bifeprunox for treating, 424
  in children, 712
  common comorbidities, 711f
  comorbid conditions and, 709
  depressed phase of, 415
    atypical antipsychotic agents in, 692f
    bullet combos for, 716f
    history, 471f
    lamotrigine as first-line treatment, 682
    response to antidepressants, 472f
    symptoms, 471f
    vs. unipolar depression, 468, 469t
  impact of antidepressant treatment on unrecognized, 468
  olanzapine and, 411
  pharmacological mechanisms to achieve remission, 705
  postpartum, 619
  progressive nature of, 473f
  rapid cycling, 458f
  residual symptoms after first-line treatment, 702–710
  risperidone effectiveness for, 413
  spectrum, 461, 461f
  symptoms shared with schizophrenia, 258, 259, 259f
  treating insomnia in, 843
  treatment, 454, 455f
    amantadine for, 695
    benzodiazepines for, 694
    calcium channel blockers for, 697
    inositol for, 699
    ketamine for, 695
    memantine for, 695
    L-methylfolate (Deplin) for, 699
    with mood stabilizer, 668
    omega-3 fatty acids for, 698
    thyroid hormones for, 699

bipolar disorder (*Contd.*)
   unstable and excessive neurotransmission, 706*f*
   and women, 710
   ziprasidone for, 416
Bipolar I disorder, 456, 457*f*
bipolar I 1/2 disorder, 463*f*
Bipolar II disorder, 456, 459*f*
bipolar II 1/2 disorder, 463, 464*f*
bipolar III disorder, 463, 464*f*
Bipolar III 1/2 disorder, 463, 465*f*
Bipolar IV disorder, 465, 466*f*
bipolar mania, neurons mediating, 151
"bipolar storm", 704, 706*f*
Bipolar V disorder, 465, 466*f*
Bipolar VI disorder, 467, 467*f*
birth
   "apoptotic suicide" before, 27
   neuronal migration before, 22
blame, 249
blonanserin, 368*f*
blood oxygenation, measuring with fMRI scan, 232*f*
blood pressure
   L channel and, 155
   monitoring, 392, 396*f*
   noradrenergic receptor simulation and, 547
   tyramine and, 582, 589
blunted affect, 252*t*
blurred vision, from conventional antipsychotics, 337, 338*f*
BMI. *See* body mass index (BMI)
BMS181, 101, 574
BMY-14802, 446
body dysmorphic disorder, 771
body mass index (BMI), 388*f*
   baseline measurement, 395*f*
   monitoring, 396*f*
bone marrow, carbamazepine impact, 679
borderline personality disorder, 259, 426, 1011
Boston bipolar brew, 715, 716*f*
bouquet cells, double, 2
   icon drawing, 4*f*
   realistic drawing, 4*f*
BP987, testing for cocaine abuse treatment, 986
bradykinin, 779*f*
brain. *See also* circuits
   activity in depression, 490
   areas impacting sleep, 491
   areas regulating functions, 213
   axonal growth in matrue, 31
   behaviors linked to key regions, 203*f*
   as "chemical soup", 58
   damage, and mental illness, 228

deep brain stimulation, 638, 638*f*
development process, 23*f*
development time course, 22, 22*f*
dopamine pathways in, 268, 272*f*
fetal
   excitotoxicity in early development, 308*f*
   insult and schizophrenia, 303
   survival of wrong neurons, 305
focus on malfunctioning areas, 262
functional areas, 197–201
   within left hemisphere, 202*f*
glutamate pathways in, 287, 289*f*
imaging, 223
inefficient information processing, and psychiatric disorders, 201
key regions, 196*f*
mapping mania symptoms onto circuits, 505
neuroimaging of activation in depression, 507*f*
neurons in, 1
neurotransmitters in, 52*t*
neurotrophins and growth factors in, 174*t*
nociceptive pathways from spinal cord to, 782
nucleus accumbens as pleasure center, 329
planes for visualizing, 200*f*
restructuring through lifetime, 22, 22*f*, 44
symptom localization in, 241
three-dimensional perspective, 201
brain atrophy
   from chronic pain, 809
   reversing stress-related, 891
   from stress, 748
brain circuits, and schizophrenia symptoms, 260
brain damage, 426
brain-derived neurotrophic factor (BDNF), 29*t*, 304, 612
   5HT6 receptors and, 447
   genes coding for, 309*f*
   and long-term memory formation, 345
   serotonin signaling and release of, 751*f*
   stress and, 748
   suppression of production, 750*f*
   and synapse formation, 308, 311*f*
   target gene for, 489
brain imaging, 195
brain MAO-A, 579
brain stimulation, of depressed patients, 633
brainstem
   5HT3 receptor stimulation, and nausea or vomiting, 531
   cell bodies for acetylcholine in, 206
   dopamine projections originating in, 204*f*
   monoamine centers, 202*f*

brainstem neurotransmitter centers, 203f
breast-feeding
    depression and treatment during, 619
    lithium and, 712
breathing, output during fear response, 729f
bremelanotide, 1006, 1011
Brief Psychiatric Rating Scale, 253t
Brodmann areas, 197, 198f
Buckeye bipolar bullets, 715, 716f
bulimia, fluoxetine (Prozac) for, 533, 1011
buprenorphine, 981
    icon, 981f
bupropion, 99t, 103, 105, 244f
    action at dopamine transporter, 105f
    for adult ADHD, 885
    for fibromyalgia, 810
    mechanism of action, in smoking cessation, 969f
    metabolites, 553, 554f
    potency for CYP450 2D6 inhibition, 605
    to reduce nicotine craving, 965
    with sertraline, 536
burnout
    of neuronal systems, 274
    in schizophrenic patients, 300, 301f
    stimulants and, 985, 985f
buspirone, 447, 651, 657
    and anxiety disorders, 743
    and CYP 450 3A4, 608
    for generalized anxiety disorder, 765
    mechanism of action augmentation, 653f
    for treating nicotine dependence, 967–968, 977
butyrylcholinesterase (BuChE), 915, 915f
    rivastigmine to inhibit, 928f

CAD106, 937
cadherins, 32
caffeine, 821, 854, 859, 860f
    formulations, 859t
    interactions with fluvoxamine, 604
calcineurin
    activation, 72
    calcium binding to, 74f
calcium
    activation of kinases and phosphatases, 74
    activation of phosphatase, 64
    excessive
        and cell death, 48f
        and excitotoxicity, 304f
    flux through NMDA ligand-gated ion channels, 144
    influx through NMDA receptors, 164f

calcium/calmodulin kinase (CaMK), 66f
calcium-calmodulin–dependent protein kinases, 74
calcium channel blockers
    dihydropyridine, 155
    L-type, 697, 698f
    mechanism of action
        on GABA, glutamate, sigma, and dopamine, 676t
        VSSCs, synaptic vesicles, and carbonic anhydrase, 675t
    putative clinical actions, 673t
calcium channels, 61, 145
    glutamate to open, 47f
    overexcitation and dangerous opening of, 301
    voltage-sensitive (VSCCs), 60, 148
        ionic filter of, 150f
calcium ions, 124f
calcyon, genes for, 319f
California careful cocktail, 715, 716f
California rocket fuel, 656f
California sunshine, 717f
calmodulin, 74
CaMK (calcium/calmodulin kinase), 66f
cAMP response-element binding protein, 74
CAMs (cellular adhesion molecules), 36, 41f
cannabinoid 1 receptor (CB1), 57
cannabinoid antagonists, 449
cannabinoid receptors, 989
cannabis, 986
    probability of dependence, 968t
capsaicin, 779
carbamazepine (Equetro), 153f
    actions as mood stabilizer, 683f
    binding site of, 682f
    and CYP 450 3A4, 608
    CYP450 3A4 and discontinuation, 408f
    CYP450 3A4 induced by, 407f
    for fibromyalgia, 811
    icon, 680f
    interaction with MAOIs, 595t
    for manic phase of bipolar disorder, 672
    mechanism of action
        on GABA, glutamate, sigma, and dopamine, 676t
        VSSCs, synaptic vesicles, and carbonic anhydrase, 675t
    putative clinical actions, 673t
    and sedation, 609
    vs. valproate, 679
    and VSSCs, 707f
carbonic anhydrase, topiramate and, 687

cardiac arrhythmias
    from combining 3A4 substrates with
        inhibitors, 609
    as tricyclic antidepressant side effect, 604f
cardiac ischemia, from repetitive autonomic
    responses, 731
cardiometabolic risk
    antipsychotic agents and, 389f
    atypical antipsychotic agents and, 385, 386t
    clozapine and, 410
    low risk antipscychotic agents, 386t
    olanzapine and, 411
    receptors mediating, 385f
cardiovascular disease
    atypical antipsychotic agents and, 383
    risk of, 388f
cardiovascular side effects, of antipsychotic
    drugs, 341
catabolic enzymes, 36
    for prehemisynapse, 43f
cataplexy, gamma hydroxybutyrate for, 859
catastrophic thinking, 764
catechol-O-methyl transferase (COMT), 221f
    and dopamine breakdown, 267, 267f
    and dorsolateral prefrontal cortex, 265f
    genes for, 233, 319f
CATIE (Clinical Antipsychotic Trials of
    Intervention Effectiveness), 399f
CATIE-AD (Clinical Antipsychotic Trials of
    Intervention Effectiveness in
    Alzheimer's Disease), 935
caudate, 202f
CBT. *See* cognitive behavioral therapy (CBT)
CCK. *See* cholecystokinin (CCK)
cell body. *See* soma
cell nucleus, transcription factor in, 75
cellular adhesion molecules (CAMs), 36, 41f
central growth plates, neuron formation in, 30f
central nervous system, 21
    sensitization process in, 795
central sensitization syndromes
    affective spectrum disorders, 800
    fibromyalgia as, 806
    segmental, 795, 799f
    "suprasegmental", 798, 801f
central sulcus, 196f
cerebellum, 203f
    Purkinje cells from, 3, 5f
cerebral cortex, 196
    antipsychotic agent binding to postsynaptic
        5HT2A receptors, 360f
    neurons in, 3f
cerebrospinal fluid, 5HIAA in, 488
cFos gene, 81f, 83, 83f

cGMP (cyclic guanosine monophosphate), 57
chandelier neurons, 3, 5, 6f
"cheese reaction", tyramine and, 585
cheese, tyramine content of, 587f
chemical integrator, somatic zone as, 6
chemical messengers
    activation in signal transduction cascade,
        66f
    conversion of electrical impulse to, 161f
chemical neurotransmission, 51
    principles, 51–61
chemical neurotransmitters, 38f, 51–54
chemical signals
    cascades of incoming, 7
    and electrical signals, in neurotransmission,
        61
    genome encoding of, 7f
    for neuronal migration, 29
"chemical soup", brain as, 58
chest pain, noncardiac, triggers for, 800
child abuse, 749, 751
    chronic stress from, 752f
childbearing years, depression during, 616
childhood, benefits of mild stress, 750
children. *See also* autism
    "affective storms" in, 712
    aggressiveness in, 425
    antidepressants for, 519f
    bipolar disorder and mood stabilizers, 712
    brain restructuring in, 22, 22f, 44
    negative experiences, and synaptogenesis, 34
    psychotic illness, symptoms shared with
        schizophrenia, 258, 259, 259f
    risperidone for, 412
    tics in, 877
chloride
    cotransport of, 95
    reduced conductance, inverse agonists and,
        142
chloride channel, in GABA-A receptor, 735f
chloride ions, 124f
chlorpromazine (Thorazine), 328, 331t
cholecystokinin (CCK), 450
cholecystolinin agonists, 1011
choline, as acetylcholine precursor, 914
choline acetyl transferase (CAT), 914, 920
choline transporters, 99, 99f
cholinergic deficiency hypothesis, for dementia,
    918
cholinergic neurons, 206
    and memory formation, 920
cholinergic projections, and prefrontal cortex
    activity, 210f
cholinergic receptors, nicotine action on, 955

cholinesterase inhibitors
    and Alzheimer's disease, 920–926
    best responders, 922, 922f
    palliative responders, 924f
    treatment outcomes, 921
    usual responders, 923f
chorea, dopamine hyperactivity in nigrostriatal
        pathway and, 277
CHRNA (alpha-7 nicotinic cholinergic
        receptor), 318f
chromosomes, and Alzheimer's disease, 906
chronic insomnia, 831–839
chronic pain, 151, 774, 775, 795
    vs. acute, 775t
    and brain atrophy, 809
    diabolical learning hypothesis and, 229
    hypothesis for pain perception, 792
    peripheral vs. central, 776t
cigarettes. See nicotine
ciliary neurotrophic factor (CNTF), 29t
    and weight loss, 1011
CIND (cognitive impairment nodementia),
        911
circadian rhythms
    5HT7 receptors and, 349f
    disturbance in, 823
    input to sleep/wake switch, 820
    melatonin to regulate, 844, 844f
    phase advanced, 827f
    phase delayed, 826f
    wake drive, 823f
circuits, 195
    and anxiety disorders, 727f
    apathy, 493f
    appetite, 498f
    for attention, 235
    depressed mood, 492f
    in depression, 489–496
    elevated/irritable mood, 501f
    for executive functioning, genetic influence
        on, 235f
    fatigue, 495f
    functioning, 56f
    goal-directed activity, 505f
    guilt, 499f
    linking worry symptoms to, 764f
    malfunctioning, 224–231
        and depression symptoms, 643
        imaging of, 231–237
        psychiatric symptoms and, 229
    for mania, 496–507
    mania symptom, 502f
    mapping mania symptoms onto, 505
    matching mania symptoms to, 500f

    matching neurotransmitters to, 243f
    matching symptoms to, 242f
    matching to neurotransmitters, 243f
    psychomotor symptoms, 497f
    sleep, 494f
    suicide, 498f
    treatment based on, 244f
    weight, 498f
    worry/obsessions, 764f
    worthlessness, 499f
circulating hormones, 52t
citalopram, 99t, 538
    icon, 538f
    potency for CYP450 2D6 inhibition, 605
cJun gene, 81f, 83, 83f
Cl1007, 380f
classic autosomal dominant pattern, 178f
classic neurotransmission, 54, 55f
Clinical Antipsychotic Trials of Intervention
        Effectiveness (CATIE), 399f
clinical practice
    antidepressants in, 639
    vs. clinical trials, 424
    symptom treatment, vs. disease treatment,
        425
clomipramine (Anafranil), 597t
    inhibition of serotonin reuptake pump, 598
    for obsessive compulsive disorder, 770
clonidine, 621
    for ADHD, 895f
    for opiate detoxification, 980
    for treating nicotine dependence, 967–968,
        977
Clopixol (zuclopenthixol), 331t
closed state, of voltage-sensitive sodium
        channels, 152f
clozapine, 382f
    5HT6-antagonist properties of, 447
    for affective symptoms in schizophrenia, 429
    for aggression management, 426, 427f
    and antagonism of muscarinic cholinergic
        receptor, 392f
    augmenting, 437
    binding properties, 409f
    and cardiometabolic risk, 386t
    in combos for bipolar disorder, 713
    as CYP 2D6 substrate, 404, 405f
    dosage with carbamazepine, 407f
    M3 receptors blocked by, 392f
    for negative symptoms in schizophrenia,
        428f
    pharmacological icon, 409f
    pharmacological properties, 409
    potency, and dissociation, 370

Index | 1069

clozapine (*contd.*)
  raising levels of, 406*f*
  rebound psychosis from discontinued, 431
  for sedation, 431
  for suicide reduction, 410, 430*f*
  for symptom reduction in psychosis, 425
  and weight gain risk, 386*t*
club drugs, 993
  actions on reward circuits, 994*f*
CNTF (ciliary neurotrophic factor), 29*t*
Coaxil (tianeptine, Stablon), 597*t*
cocaine, 99*t*, 103, 982
  DAT blocking by, 103
  and dopamine release, 272
  icon, 983*f*
  probability of dependence, 968*t*
  undesirable effects, 984
  vaccines for, 985
codeine, 977
  and CYP450 2D6 inhibitors, 608
coding region of DNA, 79*f*, 80
cognitive behavioral therapy (CBT), 639, 761
cognitive blunting
  as antipsychotic side effect, 341
  from conventional antipsychotics, 337, 338*f*
  as SSRI side effect, 356
cognitive circuits, provoking, 233
cognitive functioning, 804
  5HT1A receptors and, 349*f*
  5HT2C receptors and, 349*f*
  arousal spectrum in ADHD, deficit arousal, 871*f*
  constant synaptic revision and, 45
  in depression, 552
  dopamine for regulating, 241
  dorsolateral prefontal cortex (DLPFC) and, 264*f*
  enhancers, 921
  histamine for regulating, 241
  impaired, 399
    in depressed elderly, 913
    mild in predementia, 908
    NMDA glutamate hyperactivity hypothesis, 930
    sedation and somnolence and, 400
    slowing progression, 912
  mesocortical prefrontal cortex and, 263*f*
  neurons regulating, 204
  norepinephrine projections regulation of, 205
  quantifying, 257
  in schizophrenia, shared with other disorders, 259, 260*f*
  serotonin receptors and, 345
  sleepiness and, 854

cognitive impairment no dementia (CIND), 911
cognitive symptom pharmacy, 428, 429*f*
cold turkey, 980
collapsins, 31
colony stimulating factors, 174
coma, from opiates, 979
combat, stress vulnerability, 193, 194*f*
"combos" (combination of medications)
  for bipolar disorder treatment, 713
  for schizophrenia, 436, 450
  for symptom reduction in psychosis, 425
communication
  dysfunction of, 251
  between neurons, 55*f*, 57*f*
competitive elimination, 22, 22*f*, 41–49, 49*f*
"complex genetics", 180
complex regional pain syndromes (CRPSs), 786
compulsions, 198
  CSTC loop to regulate, 213, 215*f*
compulsive sexual behavior, 1007
compulsive shopping, 1011
compulsive use of drugs, 953*f*
COMT (catechol-O-methyl transferase), 221*f*
  and dopamine degradation, 544
  genetics, 233
    and life stressors, 766*f*
  genotypes regulating dopamine, 765
  inhibitors, 448
  Met variant, 765
  and norepinephrine, 474
  subtle molecular abnormalities and, 235*f*
concentration, 646
  and malfunctioning circuits, 645*f*
  treatment options for difficulties, 244*f*
conceptual disorganization, 249
conduct disorder, 425
  in children and adolescents, 877
  mania vs., 712, 713
connectivity, genes affecting, 304
constipation
  from conventional antipsychotics, 337, 338*f*
  from NET inhibition, 547
"constitutive activity", 108, 112*f*
coping skills, 191*f*
coronal plane, for brain visualization, 200*f*
coronary artery disease, from cortisol in fear response, 730
cortex. *See also* dorsolateral prefontal cortex (DLPFC); orbitofrontal cortex; prefrontal cortex; ventromedial prefrontal cortex
  basket neurons in, 4*f*
  dorsal anterior cingulate, 198
  Stroop task and, 238*f*

inhibitory interneurons in, 4f, 6f
interneurons in, 2
limbic, noradrenergic receptor stimulation in, 547
mesocortical prefrontal
   and emotion and cognitive symptoms, 263f
   and schizophrenia symptoms, 261, 262f
somatosensory, 775
somatosensory association, 196f
spiny neuron input from, 3
visual association, 196f
cortex-to-cortex circuit, 207
cortical arousal, neurotransmitters of, 398f
cortical brainstem glutamate projection, 289f
cortical circuits
   malfunctioning, 224–231
   normal
      stress and, 224f
      stress sensitization, 225, 225f
   normal, stress and, 224
   and pyramidal cells, 214–221
cortical pyramidal neurons
   inhibition by 5HT1A receptors, 349f
   interneuron input to, 218f
   tuning, in ADHD, 875f
cortico-cortical interactions, 210f
cortico-striatal-thalamic-cortical (CSTC) loops, 209, 211f
   for arousal regulation, 818
   attention, 213f
   emotion, 214f
   executive functioning, 212f
   for hyperactivity, 868f
   impulses, 215f
   motor activity, 216f
   and reward, 949
   and selective attention, 866f
   and worry, 726, 727f
corticoaccumbens projections, NMDA glutamate receptor hypofunction in, 297f
corticobrainstem glutamate pathways
   neurons, 291
   and NMDA receptor hypofunction hypothesis of schizophrenia, 288–291
corticocortical circuits, 207–209
corticocortical glutamate pathways, 289f
   NMDA receptor regulation of, 299f
corticostriatal glutamate pathways, 289f
corticothalamic glutamate pathways, 289f
corticotrophin release factor 1 (CRF1)
   antagonists, 663
corticotrophin releasing factor (CRF), 754
   in stress response of HPA axis, 752, 753f

cortisol, 172, 172f
   in fear response, 730
   impact on cytoplasmic receptors, 75
cost-based selection of antidepressants, 642, 642f
cotransmitters, 143
   pairs, 53t
   at synapses, 54
craving nicotine, 959
   treatment, 962
      with bupropion, 965, 969f
CREB (cyclic AMP response element–binding protein), 66f
Creutzfeldt-Jakob disease, 901t
CRF. See corticotrophin releasing factor (CRF)
cross-dependence, 945
cross titration, 432, 433f
   getting caught in, 434f
cross-tolerance, 945
CRPSs (complex regional pain syndromes), 786
"CSTC loop". See cortico-striatal-thalamic-cortical (CSTC) loops
CX516, 445
CX546, 446
CX619/Org 24448, 446
cyamemazine (Tercian), 331t
   pharmacological icon, 421f
cyclic AMP (adenosine monophosphate), 66f
   disruptions in, 316f
   synthesis, 70
cyclic AMP response element–binding protein (CREB), 66f
cyclic guanosine monophosphate (cGMP), 57, 997, 998f
cyclobenzapine
   for fibromyalgia, 810
   interaction with MAOIs, 595t
d-cycloserine, 441, 443f
   and cognitive behavioral therapy, 761
cyclothymic temperament, 456, 459f
   with major depressive episodes, 463, 464f
Cymbalta. See duloxetine (Cymbalta, Xeristar)
cystic fibrosis, 178
cytisine, 960
cytochrome P450 (CYP450) enzyme systems, 402, 402f
   CYP450 1A2 substrates, 403, 403f
      inhibition, 605f
      inhibition consequences, 606f
      and smoking, 404, 404f
   CYP450 2C9, 404
   CYP450 2C19, 403

cytochrome P450 (CYP450) enzyme systems (*Contd.*)
  CYP450 2D6, 403, 404, 405*f*
    antidepressants as inhibitors, 406*f*
    genetic polymorphism for, 403, 403*f*
    inhibition, 539, 607*f*
    inhibition consequences, 607*f*
    paroxetine as substrate and inhibitor, 537
    in risperidone conversion to paliperidone, 405*f*
    substrates, 606*f*
    and venlafaxine conversion, 548, 548*f*
  CYP450 3 A/3, 4, 406*f*
    inhibitors, 407*f*
  CYP450 3A4, 404, 608
    combining inhibitors with substrates, 609
    substrates and inhibitors, 608*f*
  inducers, 406, 609
  pharmacokinetic actions, 603
  types, 402
cytokines, 32, 174
  and Alzheimer's disease, 906
cytoplasmic proteins, 13*f*
  transport of, 12
cytoskeleton, 8*f*
  localization of, 9*f*
  and slow transport of proteins, 13*f*
  support proteins, 10

d-amino acid oxidase activator (DAOA), 315*f*
  and NMDA receptor regulation, 314, 314*f*
d-amino acid oxidase (DAO), 314, 315*f*
Darwin, Charles, 811
DAT. *See* dopamine transporter (DAT)
"date rape" drug, 859
daytime sleepiness, 816. *See also* sleepiness/hypersomnia in daytime
  excessive, 819*f*
DBH (dopamine beta hydroxylase), 474
DDC (DOPA decarboxylase), 266, 266*f*
death. *See also* neurons, cell death
  premature
    atypical antipsychotic agents and, 383
    risk of, 388*f*
decongestants
  and blood pressure, 593
  interaction with MAOIs, 594*f*
  interactions with drugs boosting sympathomimetic amines, 591
DED (depression-executive dysfunction) syndrome, 912
deep brain stimulation, 638, 638*f*
deficit arousal, in ADHD, 870
delta opiate receptors, 977

delta sleep, 848
delusions, 248, 250
  antipsychotic action to reduce, 425
  diabolical learning hypothesis and, 230
  link to nucleus accumbens, 704*f*
  mesolimbic dopamine pathway role in, 272
  reduction with mesolimbic D2 receptor block, 336
dementia. *See also* Alzheimer's disease
  behavioral disturbances, 427
  bipolarity in, 467, 467*f*
  causes, pathology and clinical features, 900
  cholinergic deficiency hypothesis, 918
  clinical features, 901*t*
  depression as predecessor, 912
  future treatments, 935
  with Lewy bodies, 901*t*
  mild cognitive impairment preceding, 908
  mixed, 902*f*
  nondegenerative, 903*t*
  pharmacy, 941*f*
  poststroke, cognitive symptoms, 259
  psychosis with, 412
  selective degenerative, pathological features, 900*t*
  symptoms shared with schizophrenia, 258, 259*f*
  treatment, 914
    acetylcholine increase, 914
    for psychiatric and behavioral symptoms, 934
demethylation, 605*f*
dendrites, 1, 2*f*
  apical, 2, 219*f*
    in pyramidal cell, 3*f*
  basal, 2, 219*f*
    in pyramidal cell, 3*f*
  in basket neurons, 4*f*
  death from excessive neurotransmission, 48*f*
  in double bouquet cells, 4*f*
  loss of, sustained symptoms and, 230
  protein synthesis in, 12*f*
  and soma, 6
  spine formation, estrogen and trophic actions on, 612
  for transport function, 10
dendritic spines, 2*f*
dendritic tree, 2*f*
  branch growth, 34*f*
  in double bouquet cells, 4*f*
  excitotoxicity for pruning, 302
  normal pruning, 46*f*
  out of control pruning, 46*f*

of Purkinje cells, 3
in pyramidal cell, 3f
Depakote. *See* divalproex (Depakote)
dependence, 945
dephosphorylation, 73, 149
Depixol (flupenthixol), 331t
Deplin (L-methylfolate), 629
   for bipolar disorder, 699
depressed mood, 260
   circuits, 492f
   thyroid hormones and, 633f
depression
   5HT1A receptors and, 349f
   anxiety disorder symptom overlap with, 726
   in bipolar disorder
      history, 471f
      response to antidepressants, 472f
      sleep disturbances in, 503f
      symptoms, 471f
      vs. unipolar depression, 468, 469t
   bipolar vs. unipolar, treatment, 701
   chronic pain with
      duloxetine for, 551
      as suprasegmental central sensitization syndrome, 798
   comorbid psychiatric illness with, 647
   CSTC loop to regulate, 212
   as dementia predecessor, 912
   diabolical learning hypothesis and, 230
   disease progression in, 519
   and erectile dysfunction prevalence, 1001, 1001f
   estrogen interaction with monoamines, 621f
   in females
      during childbearing years and pregnancy, 616
      during menopause, 620f
      over life cycle, estrogen and, 614
      during perimenopause, 619, 620f
      during postpartum period, 619
      SNRIs for, 623f
      SSRIs for, 622f
   folate for, in Alzheimer's disease, 935
   hippocampus sensitivity to, 24, 24f
   hypotheses for etiology, 488–489
   hypothesis for pain perception, 792
   incidence across female life cycle, 615f
   incidence across male life cycle, 616f
   major, 455f
      antidepressant combinations as standard, 651
      common comorbidities, 650f
      genes for, 192
      progressive nature of, 472f

      relapse rates, 518f
      remission rates, 517f
      symptom-based algorithm, 645f
   with mixed hypomania, 465
   mixed states of mania and, 467t
   monoamine hypothesis, 520
      normal monoamine neurotransmitter activity, 487f
      reduced monoamine neurotransmitter activity, 487f
   monoamine receptor hypothesis, 488f
   on mood chart, 454, 454f
   mood stabilizers for treating, 669f
   neuroimaging of brain activation in, 507f
   neuronal response to sadness vs. happiness, 508f
   neurotransmitter receptor hypothesis, 488
   overlap with mania, 507
   pain in, 779, 804
   painful somatic symptoms in, 791f
   risk across female life cycle, 615f
   stress progression to, treatment, 754
   subtle molecular abnormalities and, 193f
   symptoms, 489, 490f
      matching to circuits, 491f
      residual, 517f
   and synapse loss, 25f
   treating insomnia in, 843
   treatment
      combination of medications, 652f
      MTHF vs. folic acid, 627
      residual symptoms after, 643
   unipolar, distinguishing from bipolar depression, 468, 469t
depression-executive dysfunction syndrome (DED), 912
depression pharmacy, 639, 640f
depressive psychosis, 249
depressive temperament, 460f
Deprimyl (Llofepramine, Gamanil), 597t
descending inhibition, and endogenous opioid peptides,
descending noradrenergic inhibition, enhancement of, 792f
descending serotonergic neurons, and pain, 793f
desensitization
   of ligand-gated ion channel, 138, 143f
   of somatodendritic 5HT1A autoreceptors, 526, 527f
"designer drugs", 990
desipramine (Norpramin, Pertofran), 597t
   inhibition of serotonin reuptake pump, 598
   NRI actions, 890
desmethylclomipramine, 605f

desvenlafaxine, 549, 621
   for fibrofog, 810
   for fibromyalgia, 808
   icon, 549*f*
   for neuropathic pain, 792
   venlafaxine conversion to, 548, 548*f*
desvenlafaxine XR (Pristiq), 541*t*
detoxification, 980, 981*f*
detumescence, 1002
dextromethorphan, 593, 718
   interaction with MAOIs, 595, 595*t*
DHA (docosahexanoic acid), as mood stabilizer, 698
DHF (dihydrofolate), 627, 627*f*
diabetes mellitus, 180
   atypical antipsychotic agents and, 383
   from cortisol in fear response, 730
   neuropathy with, 550, 795
   zotepine and, 418
diabetic ketoacidosis (DKA), 389, 393*f*
   clozapine and, 410
   olanzapine and, 411
   risperidone and, 413
diabolical learning, 229–231, 473
   central sensitization as, 800
   circuit breakdown and worsening symptoms, 231*f*
   circuit changes, new symptoms and treatment resistance, 232*f*
   psychiatric symptom persistence and circuit breakdown, 230*f*
   substance abuse and, 948, 951, 953, 959
diagnosis, categorical approach to constructing, 240*f*
Diagnostic and Statistical Manual of Mental Disorders (DSM), 178, 645*f*
   bipolar spectrum, 461*f*
   on depression symptoms, 490*f*
   on mania symptoms, 500*f*
diamine oxidase, and histamine termination, 828
dianicline (SSR-591813), 960
diarrhea, for serotonin receptor stimulation, 531
diazepam (Valium), 53
diet, tyramine modifications for MAO inhibitors, 584*t*
dihydrofolate (DHF), 627, 627*f*
dihydrofolate reductase (DHFR), 627*f*
dihydropyridine "calcium channel blockers", 155, 158
   binding to calcium channel, 159*f*
dimebon (Medivation), 941
dimerization, 611*f*

3-[(2, 4-dimethoxy) benzylidene] anabaseine (DMXB-A), 449
dimethyltryptamine (DMT), 990
diphenhydramine (Benadryl), 846, 847*f*
   half-life of, 836*f*
direct-acting agonists, 112
"dirty drugs", 542, 542*f*
DISC-1 (disrupted in schizophrenia-1), 305, 307, 310*f*
   genes for, 309*f*
   and glutamate synapses strengthening, 308, 312*f*
   and NMDA receptor regulation, 314*f*
   and NMDA regulation, 317
   and synapse formation, 308, 311*f*
   and synaptic vesicle transport, 317
discriminatory pathway, 782*f*
disease progression, in depression, 519
disinhibition, 346, 612
disorganized/excited psychosis, 249
disorientation, 249
distractibility, 506
distractibility circuit, 504*f*
disulfiram, for alcoholism, 977
divalproex (Depakote), 157*t*
   for schizophrenia, 436
      adding to antipsychotic, 437*f*
divine mission, 249
dizziness, from paroxetine withdrawal, 537
DKA. *See* diabetic ketoacidosis (DKA)
DLPFC. *See* dorsolateral prefontal cortex (DLPFC)
DMT (dimethyltryptamine), 990
DMXB-A {3-[(2, 4-dimethoxy) benzylidene] anabaseine}, 449
DNA, 78
   regulation of synthesis rate of neurotransmitter receptors, 86, 86*f*
   regulatory regions of, 79*f*, 83
DNA of neuron, 8
   damage from virus or toxin, 28
docosahexaenoic acid (DHA), as mood stabilizer, 698
Dolmatil (sulpiride), 331*t*
   clinical actions of, 371
   pharmacological icon, 423*f*
donepezil, 923
   actions, 925*f*
   icon, 924*f*
dopa, 474, 475*f*
dopa decarboxylase (DDC), 266, 266*f*
dopamine, 103, 220, 264, 318*f*
   5HT2A antagonists stimulation of release, 351

5HT2A receptors regulation of, 484f
5HT2A regulation of, 563
5HT2C receptors regulation of, 486f
and acetylcholine activity, 339f
acetylcholine release inhibition, 340
agonist actions at 5HT1A receptors and, 377
amphetamine displacement of, 107f
antidepressants impact on synaptic action, 520
antipsychotic agents and, 691, 692f
and arousal, 856f
in arousal pathways, 396
and arousal spectrum, 817, 817f
brain pathways, 268, 272f
and cognition regulation, 241
for cognitive function improvement, 854
COMT gene and, 235f
deficit in mesocortical projections to dorsolateral prefrontal cortex, 274
depression from deficiency, 520f
disinhibition, 578f
  at serotonin 1A receptors, 571–574
diverse levels in brain subsections, 275
dopa conversion to, 474, 475f
dorsolateral prefontal cortex regulation by, 265f
fluoxetine and release of, 534f
genes influencing, 265f
hit-and-run theory, 373f
increase in prefrontal cortex, NET and, 544
and information processing in prefrontal cortex, 233
interaction with serotonin, in nigrostriatal dopamine pathway, 353f
levels in untreated schizophrenia, 373f
major projections, 204f
massive intracellular amount, consequences, 104
mesolimbic pathway to release, 946
and mood disorders, 474
neuronal tuning, 275
neurotransmission, in prefrontal cortex, 59
neurotransmission spectrum, 374f
norepinephrine transporter (NET) and, 94
output
  untreated schizophrenia and after pure D2 antagonist,
  untreated schizophrenia and after serotonin dopamine antagonist, 366f
pharmacologic mechanisms influencing, 265f
as pleasure neurotransmitter, 945
in prefrontal cortex, NET and, 545f
projections, 202
prolactin inhibition by, 363f

psychotropic drugs and, 53
reciprocal relationship with acetylcholine, 338f
reducing hyperactivity with lithium, 709f
release
  5HT1A and 5HT2A receptor regulation, 345, 346
  5HT2C receptors and, 349f
  nicotine and, 964f
  nicotinic partial agonists and, 965f
  presynaptic nicotinic heteroreceptors and, 918f
  serotonin inhibition of, 352f
  serotonin receptors influence on, 351f
  serotonin regulation of, 354f
reuptake, 104f
and sexual motivation, 994
synthesis, 266f
termination of action, 267f
and thalamic filter, 294f
tuning output with serotonin 2A/dopamine-2 antagonists, 365
volume neurotransmission and, 59f
dopamine agonists, for bipolar disorder, 718
dopamine beta hydroxylase (DBH), 474
dopamine D1-selective agonists, 448
dopamine D2 partial agonists, 342, 374f
  aripiprazole as, 421
dopamine D2 receptor agonists, 374f
dopamine D2 receptors, 267
  antagonists, 329, 329f
    and anticholinergic agents, 339f
    integrated theory of schizophrenia and, 334f
    mesocortical dopamine pathway and, 331f
    nigrostrial dopamine pathway and, 332f
    rapid dissociation of, 368f
    tuberoinfundibular dopamine pathway and, 334f
  blockade in nucleus accumbens, 353
  continuous occupancy, 415
  conventional antipsychotic binding to, 365
  dilemma of blocking in all dopamine pathways, 336
  output, 375f
  presynaptic, 267, 269f
  rapid dissociation from, 365, 367
  side effects of unwanted blockade, 382
  somatodendritic, 271f
dopamine D3 antagonists, 448
"dopamine deficiency syndrome", 546
  bupropion for, 556
"dopamine hypothesis of schizophrenia", 273

Index | 1075

dopamine neurons, 351
   normal rate of tonic firing, 873
   phasic firing of, 875
dopamine neurotransmitter
   as psychotropic drug indirect target, 116
   as psychotropic drug target, 114
dopamine partial agonists (DPAs), 371, 373*f*
   for aggression management, 427*f*
   for cognitive function improvement, 428*f*
   in development, 380*f*
   development of new, 448
   for first-line treatment of schizophrenia positive symptoms, 425
   integrated theory of schizophrenia and, 378*f*
   on market, 380*f*
   in mesolimbic pathway, 376*f*
   for negative symptoms in schizophrenia, 428*f*
   and nigrostriatal pathway, 377*f*
   spectrum, 381*f*
   switching from SDA to, 436*f*
dopamine receptors, 267, 268*f*
dopamine transporter (DAT), 93, 94, 95*f*, 266, 267*f*
   and amphetamines transport, 94, 105*f*
   blocking, 103
   cocaine inhibition of, 983
   and dorsolateral prefrontal cortex, 265*f*
   excessive occupancy, 554
   modafinil and, 857, 858*f*
   reversal of, 108*f*
   sertaline for inhibiting, 535
dopaminergic combo, 652*f*
dopaminergic neurons, 266–268
   MAO subtypes in, 577
dopaminergic projections, and prefrontal cortex activity, 210*f*
dorsal anterior cingulate cortex, 198
   and Stroop task, 238*f*
dorsal anterior cingulate gyrus, 211
dorsal horn
   alpha 2 delta ligands in, 800*f*
   descending spinal synapses, 789
dorsal horn projection neurons, 782
   classes, 784
dorsal raphe, 205
dorsal root ganglion (DRG), 775
   primary afferent neuron cell bodies in, 782
dorsolateral prefrontal cortex (DLPFC), 198, 202*f*
   activation by executive function tests, 865
   activation of kinases and phosphatases, 233
   cognition regulation by, 273, 854

cognitive symptoms and, 264*f*
connections, 208
dopamine deficit in mesocortical projections to, 274
dopaminergic regulation of cognition, 808
executive dysfunction localization in, 491
and executive function, 212*f*
genes influencing, 265*f*
inefficient information processing, and distractibility, 504*f*
information processing involving, 319
interactions with ACC, 210*f*
mesocortical dopamine pathway, 275*f*
mesolimbic dopamine pathways in schizophrenia, 331*f*
and n-back test, 234*f*
regulation by dopamine and serotonin, 265*f*
and schizophrenia symptoms, 261, 262*f*
and situation analysis of reward, 949
dothiepin (Prothiaden), 597*t*
double bouquet cells, 2, 4*f*
   icon drawing, 4*f*
   realistic drawing, 4*f*
double depression, 456, 457*f*
downregulation, 87
Down's syndrome, 906
doxepin (Sinequan, Adapin), 572, 597*t*
   half-life of, 836*f*
   as hypnotic, 847, 847*f*
doxylamine, 846
DPAs. *See* dopamine partial agonists (DPAs)
drowsiness. *See also* sleepiness/hypersomnia in daytime
   from histamine-1 receptor blockade, 341
drug abuse, 425
   by schizophrenic patients, 336
   symptoms shared with schizophrenia, 259
drug-induced parkinsonism, 332
drug-induced psychoses, symptoms shared with schizophrenia, 258
drug-induced reward, 946
drug interactions, 408
dry mouth
   from conventional antipsychotics, 337, 338*f*
   from NET inhibition, 547
DSM. *See Diagnostic and Statistical Manual of Mental Disorders* (DSM)
DU 127090. *See* bifeprunox (DU 127090)
"dual action" serotonin-norepinephrine agents, 544
duloxetine (Cymbalta, Xeristar), 99*t*, 541*t*
   CYP450 2D6 impact on plasma levels, 607
   as CYP450 2D6 inhibitor, 607*f*

for fibrofog, 810
for fibromyalgia, 808
icon, 550f
interactions with fluvoxamine, 604
for neuropathic pain, 792
potency for CYP450 2D6 inhibition, 605
dynorphins, 789
dysbindin, 305
genes coding for, 309f
and glutamate synapses strengthening, 308, 312f
and NMDA receptor regulation, 314f
and NMDA regulation, 317
and synapse formation, 308, 311f
vGluT regulated by, 317
dysconnectivity, 305
dyskinesias, dopamine hyperactivity in nigrostriatal pathway and, 277, 278f
dyslipidemia, 385
aripiprazole and, 422
atypical antipsychotic agents and, 383
blood pressure monitoring, 392
ziprasidone and, 417
zotepine and, 418
dysphoria, in withdrawal syndrome, 980
dysphoric mania, 465
dysthymia, 456, 456f
on mood chart, 454, 454f
unremitting, 457f
dystonia, nigrostriatal pathway dopamine deficiencies and, 277
dystrobrevin-binding protein 1, 305

EAAT. See excitatory amino acid transporters (EAAT)
eating disorders, 771, 1008–1011
and reward circuits, 1010f
SSRIs for, 522
"ecstacy", 990
SERT transport of, 95
ECT (electroconvulsive therapy), 633
ectopic sites, hypersensitivity to stimuli, 786
Effexor XR. See venlafaxine XR (Effexor XR; Efexor XR)
efficacy, path to, 401f
efficacy profile, 400f
EGF (epidermal growth factor), 29t
eicosapentanoic acid (EPA), as mood stabilizer, 698
Elavil (amitriptyline, Endep, Tryptizol, Loroxyl), 53, 572, 597t
elderly
antidepressants for, 519, 519f
circadian rhythms of, 824, 827f
depression, 912
citalopram for, 539
treatment, 913
risperidone for, 412
electrical integrator, axon hillock as, 7f, 8
electrical signals
axon for propagating, 7f, 8
and chemical signals, in neurotransmission, 61
conversion to chemical message, 161f
electroconvulsive therapy (ECT), 633
elevated mood circuits, 501f
EMD128130 (sarizotan), 380f
emotion
amygdala response to input, 324
brain component regulating, 200, 262
CSTC loop to regulate, 212, 214f
depressed patient neuronal response, 508f
mesocortical prefrontal cortex and, 263f
mesolimbic dopamine pathway role in, 274
processing, 199f
brain areas impacting, 321
emotional abuse, and synaptogenesis, 34
emotional learning, amygdala and, 949
emotional maturity, constant synaptic revision and, 45
emotional/motivation pathway, 784
emotional symptoms, of dementia, 934
emotional trauma, circuit response to, 224
en passant presynaptic axon terminals, 2f
enantiomers, for citalopram, 538
Endep (amitriptyline, Elavil, Tryptizol, Loroxyl), 53, 572, 597t. See also nortriptyline (Pamelor, Endep, Aventyl)
endocannabinoids (ECs), 57, 57f
endocrine reactions, to fear, 730
endogenous growth factors
and neurogenesis in hippocampus, 24, 24f
promoting production, 24, 26f
"endogenous marijuana", 57
endogenous opiate neurotransmitters, 980f
endogenous opioid peptides, and descending inhibition,
endokinins, 664
endophenotypes, 181, 182f
endorphins, 789, 946, 947f
energy
loss
bupropion for, 556
as SSRI side effect, 530
for neurotransmission, 38f
enhancer element, of gene regulatory region, 83
enkephalins, 789, 977
enteric nervous system, 811

Index | 1077

enthusiasm, loss
    bupropion for, 556
    as SSRI side effect, 530
environment, 185
    factors in ADHD, 870
environmental stress, 187f
    genetic abnormalities and, 192–193
enzymes
    activation in signal transduction cascade, 64
    binding to G protein, 70
    fast transport of, 15f
    function of, 170f
    inhibitors of, 167
    as possible indirect target by psychotropic drugs, 171t
    as psychopharmacological drug action site, 167–170
    substrate binding to, 168f
    targeted by psychotropic drugs, 170t
EPA (eicosapentanoic acid), as mood stabilizer, 698
ephaptic cross-talk, 786, 787f
ephedrine, 593
    with MAOIs, and hypertension, 593t
epidermal growth factor (EGF), 29t, 174
epilepsy, from improper neuronal migration, 29
epileptic neurons, 151
eplivanserin (SR 46349), 447
EPS. *See* extrapyramidal symptoms (EPS)
Epworth Sleepiness Scale, 851, 852t
ERB signaling system, neuregulin activation of, 317
erectile dysfunction, 999, 1003f
    age and, 1000f
    pharmacology, 1002
    prevalence of, 1000f
        depression and, 1001, 1001f
    treatment, 1003f
erectile function, 1002f
ERK (extracellular signal-regulated kinase), 76
ERT (estrogen replacement therapy), 619, 620, 623
erythromycin, and CYP 450 3A4, 609
escitalopram, 99t, 539
    icon, 541f
eslicarbazepine, 681, 718
    actions as mood stabilizer, 683f
essential amino acids, 285
Essential Psychopharmacology: The Prescriber's Guide (Stahl), 408, 409
estazolam
    half-life of, 835f
    for insomnia, 837f

estradiol
    activity-dependent spine formation by, 614f
    receptors for, 611f
estrogen, 66f, 610
    for Alzheimer's disease, 937
    as GABA inhibitor, 612
    as glutamate activator, 612
    impact on cytoplasmic receptors, 75
    interaction with monoamines
        and depressed mood, 621f
        vasomotor symptoms from, 524f
    and nuclear hormone receptors, 610, 611f
    regulation and major depression, over female life cycle, 614
    and sexual motivation, 994
    and trophic actions, on dendritic spine formation, 612
    tropic properties, 613f
estrogen receptors, 610
estrogen replacement therapy (ERT), 619, 620, 623
estrogen response elements, 610, 611f
eszopiclone, 839, 839f
    and R zopiclone, 842t
euphoria, from opiates, 977
euthymia, on mood chart, 454, 454f
evidence-based selection of antidepressants, algorithm, 641, 641f
excitation-secretion coupling, 60–61, 156, 159, 161f
excitatory amino acid transporters (EAAT), 94t, 100, 101f
    for glutamate takeup, 281f
excitatory neurotransmission, 42
"excitotoxic hypothesis of schizophrenia", 300
excitotoxicity, 42, 46f, 48f, 298, 303f
    in ALS,
    cellular events during, 304f
    in early fetal brain development, 308f
    and glutamate systems, 301, 440
    and neuronal insult, 303
executive dysfunction, 257, 496f
    in ADHD, 864
    biological endophenotype for, 233f
    localization in dorsolateral prefrontal cortex, 491
    symptoms of, 241
executive functioning, 198, 650
    in ADHD patients, 873
    genetic influence on circuits regulating, 235f
    impaired
        in dementia, 900
        in schizophrenia, 257
    prefrontal cortex synaptogenesis and, 883f

regulation
    by CSTC loop, 212f
    by mesocortical dopamine pathway, 273
    tests of, 865
exercise
    and endogenous growth factors, 26f
    and neurogenesis in hippocampus, 24, 24f
"exercising" the brain, 912
extracellular portion of receptor, 109f
extrapyramidal symptoms (EPS), 367, 369f
    5HT2A antagonist to reduce, 351–353
    absence with atypical antipsychotics, 371f
    D2 receptor blockage and, 332
    dopamine partial agonism and, 378f
    risperidone and, 412
    SDAs and,
    from unwanted D2 receptor blockade, 382
extroversion, in hyperthymic temperament, 460f
exuberance, in hyperthymic temperament, 460f

facilitation pathways, serotonin as transmitter, 789
family history, and bipolar diagnosis, 469f
fast transport, 13–15
    anterograde, 16f
    low-molecular-weight neurotransmitter machinery, 18f
    of materials, 15f
    neuropeptide machinery, 19f
    retrograde, 17f
fasting triglycerides
    antipsychotic agents and, 391f
    baseline measurement, 391, 395f
    monitoring, 396f
    quetiapine and, 415
    rapid elevation of, 387
    risperidone and, 413
    ziprasidone and, 417
fatigue, 804
    circuits, 495f
    link to prefrontal cortex, 491
    and malfunctioning circuits, 645f
    slow-wave sleep deficiency and, 848
fear. See also anxiety disorders
    affect of, 728f
    autonomic output, 730f
    CSTC loop to regulate, 212
    endocrine output of, 729f
    neurobiology, and amygdala, 729
    processing, 201
    processing by amygdala, 323f
        serotonin and, 234
    processing response, 731
fear circuits, provoking, 234

fear conditioning, vs. fear extinction, 756, 759f
fear extinction, 760
fearful faces
    and amygdala, 236f
        serotonin transporter and, 745
    processing, 236f
females. See women
fetus
    brain
        excitotoxicity in early development, 308f
        insult and schizophrenia, 303
        survival of wrong neurons, 305
    insults in neurodegenerative theories of schizophrenia, 300f
    risks of antidepressants to, 618
    risks of mood stabilizers and lithium to, 712
    valproic acid toxicity, 677
fibro pharmacy, 810f
fibroblast growth factor (FGF), 29t, 174
"fibrofog", 552, 808
    improving symptoms of, 810
fibromyalgia, 777, 784, 805–811
    American College of Rheumatology criteria, 805t
    comorbid mood and anxiety disorders, 807t
    desvenlafaxine for, 550
    duloxetine for, 551
    functional somatic syndromes in, 807t
    gabapentin for, 688
    hypothesis for, 806
    hypothesis for pain perception, 792
    milnacipran for, 551
    pain in muscles, 779
    pain triggers, 800
    painful somatic symptoms in, 791f
    pregabalin for, 688
    as suprasegmental central sensitization syndrome, 798
    symptom-based algorithm, 809f
    symptoms, 808f
    tender points for diagnosis, 806f
    treatment, 808
"fight or flight", 722, 731
first-generation antipsychotic agents, 329f
flashbacks, from hallucinogens, 991
flibanserin (Ectris), 574, 1006
flight of ideas, 506
flumazenil, 740, 740f
fluoxetine (Prozac), 53, 99t, 532–536, 604
    for bulimia, 1011
    and CYP 450 3A4, 608
    as CYP450 2D6 inhibitor, 607f
    half-life of, 534
    icon, 533f

Index | 1079

fluoxetine (Prozac) (*Contd.*)
   impact on norepinephrine and dopamine release, 534*f*
   metabolite of, 405
   olanzapine and, 411
   SERT and serotonin binding prevention by, 97, 98*f*
flupenthixol (Depixol), 331*t*
fluphenazine (Prolixin), 331*t*
flurazepam
   half-life of, 835*f*
   for insomnia, 837*f*
flurizan, 939
fluvastatin, 609
   and CYP 450 3A4, 608
fluvoxamine, 99*t*, 405, 446, 537
   and CYP 450 3A4, 608
   and CYP450 1A2 inhibition, 603, 605*f*
   icon, 538*f*
   potency for CYP450 2D6 inhibition, 605
fMRI (functional magnetic resonance imaging), 231
   Stroop task for, 235
folate, 627*f*
   deficiency and monoamines, 630*f*
   for depression, in Alzheimer's disease, 935
folic acid, 627*f*
   vs. MTHF, for depression, 627
folinic acid (Leucovorin), 626
food addiction, treatment, 1009
Fos-Jun combination protein, 81*f*, 83*f*
Fos protein, 81*f*, 83*f*, 85–87
"Foxy" (5-methoxy-diisopropyltryptamine), 990
free polysomes, 10*f*, 11
free radicals, 306*f*
   and Alzheimer's disease, 906
   and neuron death, 302, 934
   scavengers for excitotoxicity, 442*f*
Freud, Sigmund, 983
frontal lobe, 197
frontotemporal dementia, 901*t*
full agonists, 110, 113*f*
   for ligand-gated ion channels, 130
function, topographical representation of, 211
functional G protein-linked receptors, 110*t*
functional magnetic resonance imaging (fMRI), 184, 231
   blood oxygenation measurement with, 232
   Stroop task for, 235
functional somatic syndromes, 777*t*
functioning circuits, 56*f*

G protein, binding to receptor-neurotransmitter complex, 70

G protein-linked receptors, 92*f*, 105, 109*f*
   chemical neurotransmission, 70
   psychotropic drug action on, 107
   as psychotropic drug indirect target, 116*t*
   as psychotropic drug target, 107, 114*t*
      with agonists, 110–112
      with antagonists,
      inverse agonists, 121
      light and dark as analogy for partial agonists, 120
      with no agonist, 108
      with partial agonists, 115–119
   structure and function, 105–107
   superfamily, 110*f*
G protein-linked signal-transduction cascades, 65, 66*f*
   binary neurotransmitter receptor complex binding to G protein, 69*f*
   elements of, 69*f*
   first messengers, 67, 69*f*
   functional outcome of neurotransmission, 68*f*
   later messengers, 71
   second messenger, 65, 67
      key elements, 70
      release, 70*f*
GABA (gamma-aminobutyric acid), 93, 94*t*, 290*f*
   alcohol actions at synapses, 971
   anxiety and, 732–741
   and anxiety disorders, 732–741
   and anxiety regulation in amygdala, 241
   anxiolytics, 741
   binding sites, 142
   estrogen and, 610
   production, 732, 732*f*
   as psychotropic drug indirect target, 117
   as psychotropic drug target, 114, 128, 129
   psychotropic drugs and, 53
   sleep/wake switch regulation, 821, 822*f*
   in thalamus, and insomnia, 820*f*
   topiramate and, 687
   transporters, 100*f*
   valproate and, 674
GABA-A allosteric modulatory sites, hypothetical shift in set point, 740
GABA-A PAMs, and psychiatric insomnia, 842
GABA agonist site, 737
GABA-ergic agents, potential therapeutic effects, 743*f*
GABA (gamma-aminobutyric acid)
   possible valproate sites of action, 678*f*
GABA (gamma-aminobutyric acid) A receptors, pentameric structure, 126

GABA (gamma-aminobutyric acid) inhibitor, estrogen as, 612
GABA (gamma-aminobutyric acid) interneurons, estrogen and, 614f
GABA (gamma-aminobutyric acid) neurons, 292, 293f
  for connecting serotonin and dopamine neurons, 351
  dopamine impact on, 294f
  release, 351f
  and sleepiness circuits, 821f
GABA neurotransmitter, 128t
GABA receptors
  GABA-A subtypes, 734–741
    mediation of tonic and phasic inhibition, 736f
    positive allosteric modulation, 739f
  subtypes, 733, 734f
GABA reuptake pump, 732
GABA transaminase (GABA-T), 733, 733f
GABA transporter (GAT), 732
GABA vesicular transporter, 102
GABAergic inhibitory interneurons, 216, 218f
gabapentin, 156, 157t
  for anxiety disorders, 767
  binding to alpha-2 delta protein, 158
  channel blocking by, 798f
  in combos for bipolar disorder, 715
  for fibromyalgia, 808
  icon, 688f
  mechanism of action
    on GABA, glutamate, sigma, and dopamine, 676t
    VSSCs, synaptic vesicles, and carbonic anhydrase, 675t
  for panic disorder, 768
  putative clinical actions, 673t
  for social anxiety disorder, 769
gaboxadol, 842
GAD (glutamic acid decarboxylase), 612, 732
galactorrhea, 278, 336
galantamine, 926
  actions, 930f
  icon, 929f
Gamanil. *See* Llofrepramine (Deprimyl, Gamanil)
gambling, 771
  compulsive, 1011
gamma-aminobutyric acid (GABA). *See* GABA (gamma-aminobutyric acid)
gamma hydroxybutyrate (GHB), 861f
  for fibromyalgia, 811
  for wakefulness, 859

gamma secretase, 903
  inhibitors and modulators, 939, 939f
gamma units, 153, 155f
gases, as neurotransmitters, 52t
gastrointestinal cramps, for serotonin receptor stimulation, 531
gastrointestinal upset, from paroxetine withdrawal, 537
GAT, transporters for, 100
"gate theory" of pain, 795
GC (guanylyl cyclase), 997, 998f
GDNF (glial cell line–derived neurotrophic factors), 29, 29t
gene expression
  enzymes regulating, 170f
  messenger triggering of, 64
  neurotransmission regulation of, 78
  signal-transduction cascades influence, 73–88
generalized anxiety disorder (GAD), 723f
  insomnia with, 843
  pharmacy, 767f
  symptoms shared with other disorders, 869t
  treatment, 765
genes
  5HT2A antagonists and expression, 570
  activation
    early, impact on late, 81f
    factors affecting, 85
    with gene turned on, 79f
    late, 82f, 83f
    products, 80f
    when gene is off, 79f
  encoding of proteins, 179, 181f
  hypothetic regulation of mood networks, 506f
  hypothetical path to behavior, 182f
  hypothetical path to mental illness, 183f
  immediate-early, 80f, 83
  monoamine hypothesis of antidepressant action on expression, 523f
  in mood disorders, 507–509
  quantitative methods measuring abnormal, 185
  regulation by neurotransmitters, 82f
  as signal-transduction target, 71, 76, 77
  susceptibility, 304
    for schizophrenia, 309t
genetic abnormalities, degrees, and environmental stressors, 192–193
genetic G protein-linked receptors, 110t
genetic programming, in neurodegenerative theories of schizophrenia, 300f

genetics in psychiatry, 177
   classic theory, 178, 178*f*
   imaging, 223, 233
   new paradigm, 179
   and prefrontal cortex abnormalities in ADHD, 870
genomes, 7
   apoptosis programmed into, 28
   decoding of incoming signals, 7*f*
   neurotransmitter signaling between, 61, 63*f*
   protein orders from, 11
gepirone, 651, 657
   and anxiety disorders, 743
GHB (gamma hydroxybutyrate), for fibromyalgia, 811
ginko biloba, for Alzheimer's disease, 936
glial alanine-serine-cysteine transporter (ASC-T), 280
glial cell line–derived neurotrophic factor (GDNF), 29, 29*t*
glial cells, 31
   glutamine release from, 282*f*
   glycine from, 284
   and neuronal migration, 30*f*
glial d-serine transporter, 284*f*
glial derived neurotrophic factor, 174
glial SNAT, 280, 282*f*
glucocorticoid antagonists, 171, 172*f*
   potential for clinical use, 172
glucocorticoid receptors, 172
glucocorticoids, release as stress response, 753, 753*f*
glucose
   monitoring fasting, 392
   PET scan to measure uptake, 232
glutamate, 42, 167
   5HT2A antagonists and inhibitory action of HT1A on release, 571
   agonist actions at 5HT1A receptors and, 377
   at AMPA and kainite receptors, 147*f*
   antipsychotic agents and, 691
   binding to NMDA complex, 143
   calcium channels associated with, 154
   conversion to glutamine, 100, 280, 281*f*
   as cortical pyramidal neuron output, 217*f*
   estrogen as activator, 612
   excitotoxicity
      amyloid plaques and, 932*f*
      system overactivity, 274, 301
   GABA synthesis from, 732
   key pathways in brain, 287, 289*f*
      NMDA hypofunction hypothesis of schizophrenia and, 288–291
   mood stabilizers action on, 708*f*
   NMDA receptor excitation spectrum by, 303*f*
   for open calcium channel, 47*f*
   pharmacology, 440
   preventing release, 445*f*
   psychotropic drugs and, 53, 128, 129
   recycled and regnerated, 281*f*
      conversion to glutamine, 282*f*
      glutamine release from glial cells, 282*f*
   reducing hyperactivity, with atypical antipsychotics, 710*f*
   release
      5HT1A and 5HT2A receptor effect, 361*f*
      amyloid plaques and, 927
      of excessive, 47*f*
      lamotrigine impact on, 683
      from presynaptic neuron, 164
      presynaptic nicotinic heteroreceptors and, 918*f*
      regulation with 5HT1A, 359, 362
      riluzole to prevent,
      serotonin inhibition of, 576*f*
      serotonin stimulation of, 575*f*
   role in schizophrenia pathophysiology, 279
   signal transduction of, 163*f*
   susceptibility gene effect on, 317
   synapses, convergence of susceptibility genes for schizophrenia on, 314
   synthesis, 279
   topiramate and, 687
glutamate receptors, 285, 286*f*
   metabotropic, 285, 288*f*
   signal propagation, 164*f*
   types, 287*t*
glutamate transporters, 94*t*, 100, 101*f*
   structure, 101*f*
   as trimers, 101
glutamatergic corticostriatal projections, NMDA glutamate receptor hypofunction in, 297*f*
glutamatergic excitatory projections, from thalamus, 219*f*
glutamic acid decarboxylase (GAD), 612, 732
glutaminase, 280, 282*f*
glutamine
   glutamate conversion to, 100, 280, 281*f*
   release from glial cells, 282*f*
glutamine synthetase, 280
glycine, 93, 167, 443*f*
   binding to NMDA complex, 143
   from glial cells, 284
   from l-serine, 285
   production, 283
glycine agonists, 441

glycine receptors, 128*t*
    pentameric structure, 126
glycine transporters (GlyT1), 94*t*, 100, 442
    inhibitors, 444*f*
glycogen synthetase kinase 3 (GSK3), 66*f*, 173, 173*f*
glycogen synthetase kinase (GSK)
    inhibitors for Alzheimer's disease, 937
    lithium and, 632
goal-directed activity
    circuit, 505*f*
    turning reward into, 950, 951*f*
"God's pharmacopeia", 53
"Goldilocks" solution, 118, 133
Golgi apparatus, 8*f*, 84*f*
    localization of, 9*f*
    protein modification, 11*f*, 12
grandiose expansiveness, 249
grandiosity, 506
    in hyperthymic temperament, 460*f*
    inefficient information processing and, 502*f*
growth cone, axonal, 31, 32*f*
    docking, 32*f*
growth factor
    in brain, 174*t*
    fast transport of, 15*f*
    restoration of neurons by, 26*f*
    transport to soma, 15, 17*f*
GSI 953, 939
GSK. *See* glycogen synthetase kinase (GSK)
GSK-3 (glycogen synthase kinase 3), 66*f*, 173, 173*f*
guanfacine, for ADHD, 873, 895*f*
guanosine monophosphate (cGMP), 997, 998*f*
guanylyl cyclase (GC), 997, 998*f*
guilt, 260
    circuits, 499*f*
    serotonin and, 493
gut, 811
    CYP450 enzymes in wall, 402
gut hormones, 52*t*
GW742457, 447

H1 histamine receptor, and weight gain, 383
hair loss, as valproic acid side effect, 677
Haldol. *See* haloperidol (Haldol)
hallucinations, 248, 251, 990
    5HT2A receptors and, 349*f*
    5HT2A receptors effect on glutamate release and, 359
    antipsychotic action to reduce, 425
    link to nucleus accumbens, 704*f*
    mesolimbic dopamine pathway role in, 272
    reduction with mesolimbic D2 receptor block, 336
    serotonin receptors and, 345
    voices in, 248
hallucinogens, 990–993
    actions, 992*f*
    actions on reward circuits, 991*f*
    icons, 992*f*
haloperidol (Haldol), 331*t*
happiness
    depressed patient neuronal response, 508*f*
    loss
        bupropion for, 556
        as SSRI side effect, 530
HDC (histidine decarboxylase), 828*f*
heat-shock protein 90 (HSP90), 172*f*
heavy drinking, 973
    will power to reduce, 975*f*
hemipostsynapse, 39*f*
hemipresynapse, 39*f*
hemisynapse, 36, 39*f*
heroic combos,
    California rocket fuel, 656*f*
    SNRI plus modafinil, 657, 657*f*
    SNRI plus NDRI, 656*f*
    SNRI plus stimulant, 656*f*
    SSRI plus NDRI, 652*f*
heroin, probability of dependence, 968*t*
HHS. *See* hyperglycemic hyperosmolar syndrome (HHS)
hippocampal dentate gyrus, 24
hippocampus, 199*f*
    adult neurogenesis in dentate region, 23*f*, 24*f*
    atrophy from excessive glucocorticoid release, 753*f*
    blockade of beta receptors in, 763*f*
    fear extinction and, 760
    and input to lateral amygdala, 760
    neurons in, and BDNF, 489
    orbital frontal cortex interactions with, 210*f*
    and stress, 759*f*
    volume reduction with stress, 748*f*
histamine, 828–831
    in arousal pathways, 396, 398*f*
    and arousal spectrum, 817, 817*f*
    and cognition regulation, 241
    modafinil for promoting release, 823
    neurotransmitter pathways for, 207
    production, 828*f*
    projections, 209*f*
    release, 779*f*
    sleep/wake switch regulation, 821, 822*f*
    termination of action, 828, 829*f*
    transporters, 102

histamine 1 receptors, 830*f*
  antagonism, 340*f*
  atypical antipsychotic agents and, 385*f*
  blockade of, 341
  and sedation, 397*f*
  and sedation, drowsiness or sleep, 830
  TCA blockade of, 599
histamine-1, with serotonin-2C antagonist, and appetite stimulation, 387*f*
histamine 2 receptors, 830, 831*f*
histamine 3 receptors, 830, 832*f*
histamine 4 receptors, 831
histamine H1 antagonists, as hypnotics, 846–848
histamine N-methyl-transferase, 828, 829*f*
histamine neurotransmitter, as psychotropic drug target, 115
histamine receptors, 829*f*
  TCA antihistamine portion in, 602*f*
histidine, 828, 828*f*
histidine decarboxylase (HDC), 828, 828*f*
"hit and run" binding, 367
homeostatic sleep drive, 820, 823*f*
horizontal plane, for brain visualization, 200*f*
hormone-linked signal-transduction cascades, 65, 66*f*
  first messengers, 67
  second messenger, 65, 67
  later messengers, 71
hormone nuclear receptor complex, 75
hormone response elements (HREs), 66*f*, 75
hormone–nuclear receptor complex, 66
hostile belligerence, 249
hostility. *See* aggressiveness
HPA axis. *See* hypothalamic-pituitary-adrenal (HPA) axis
HSDD (hypoactive sexual desire disorder), 1004, 1005*f*
  dopamine and, 1007*f*
  matching to circuits, 1006*f*
  treatment, 1008*f*
human brains. *See* brain
human genome, 78
human sexual response. *See also* sexual dysfunction
  phases, 993–1007
    arousal, 995
    libido, 993
    orgasm, 999
hunger, and reward circuits, 1010*f*
Huntington's disease, 178, 901*t*
5-hydroxy-indole acetic acid (5HIAA), 483
  in cerebrospinal fluid, 488

hydroxy-methyl-glutaryl coenzyme A (HMG-CoA) reductase inhibitors, for Alzheimer's disease, 936
hydroxy-pyruvate (OH-pyruvate), 284*f*
9-hydroxy-risperidone, 413. *See also* paliperidone
hydroxylation, 606*f*
5-hydroxytryptamine. *See* serotonin (5HT)
5-hydroxytryptophan (5HTP), 343, 344*f*
hydroxyzine, for anxiety disorders, 767
hypchondriasis, 771
hyperactivity, 882
  in ADHD, 864, 865*f*
  circuit, 868*f*
  CSTC loop to regulate, 213, 216*f*
  of mesolimbic dopamine pathway, 273
hyperalgesia, 775, 786, 799*f*
  inflammatory process in, 786
hyperarousal, 876*f*
hyperglycemic hyperosmolar syndrome (HHS), 389, 393*f*
  clozapine and, 410
  olanzapine and, 411
  risperidone and, 413
hyperinsulinemia, 383
hyperprolactinemia, 336
  5HT2A antagonists and reduction of, 362
  from unwanted D2 receptor blockade, 382
hypersexuality, 704*f*
hypersomnia, 650
hypertension, 180
  agents combined with MAOIs causing, 593*t*
  from repetitive autonomic responses, 731
hypertensive crisis, 582, 584, 586*t*
  reducing risk, 586
hyperthermia, 595, 597
hyperthermia/serotonin syndrome, from MAOIs and other agents, 595*t*
hyperthymic temperament, 460*f*
  with depressive episode, 466*f*
hypervigilance, 816
hypnotics
  alpha 1 selective, 840*f*
  benzodiazepines, 839
  doxepin as, 847, 847*f*
  for fibromyalgia, 811
  half-lives, 833, 835*f*
  histamine H1 antagonists as, 846–848
  long-term effects, 838*f*
  pharmacy, 849*f*
  serotonergic, 845
hypoactive sexual desire disorder (HSDD), 1004, 1005*f*
  dopamine and, 1007*f*

matching to circuits, 1006f
treatment, 1008f
hypoarousal, 871f
hypocretin, and narcolepsy, 820
hypomania, 454
   on antidepressant, 463
   mixed, depression with, 465
   on mood chart, 454, 454f
   protracted or recurrent, 461
hypotension, MAO inhibitors and, 593
hypothalamic nuclei, 204
   dopamine pathway from, 272f
hypothalamic-pituitary-adrenal (HPA) axis, 752, 753f
hypothalamic releasing hormones, 52t
hypothalamus, 202f
   5HT3 receptor stimulation, and nausea or vomiting, 531
   inefficient information processing, and sleep disturbances, 503f
   orexin-containing neurons in, 820
   and sleep disturbances, 491, 494f
   tuberomammillary nucleus (TMN) of, 819, 822f
   ventrolateral preoptic (VLPO) nucleus of, 819, 822f
hypthalamic thermoregulatory centers, 620

icon drawing, ligand-gated, 126f
   structure and function, 125
ILGF (insulinlike growth factors), 29t
iloperidone, 368f
imaging genetics, 223, 233
   future, 236
   "seeing" ancestors in brain, 236
   serotonin role in fear processing by amygdala, 234
imaging, of malfunctioning circuits, 231–237
imipramine (Tofranil), 597t
immediate-early gene, 80f, 83
impulsivity, 198, 259, 882
   in ADHD, 864
   circuit, 869f
   CSTC loop to regulate, 213, 215f
   diabolical learning hypothesis and, 230
   in hyperthymic temperament, 460f
   regulating, 949
   in sexual behavior, 1007
inactivated state, of voltage-sensitive sodium channels, 152f
inactivation, 138, 139
inattention, 882
incertohypothalamic pathway, 204
indiplon, 842

indolealkylamines, 990
inflammatory pain, 786, 788f
inflammatory response, in necrotic cell death, 28f, 29
information processing
   in ADHD, 874f
   in amygdala
      and depressed mood, 492f
      serotonin and, 744
   by brain, and psychiatric disorders, 201
   improving, 239
      in ADHD, 872, 872f
   inefficient
      in ADHD, 864, 865f
      in mania, 502f
      and sleep disturbances, 503f
   in narcolepsy, 855f
   NMDA receptor hypofunction affect, 292
   in prefrontal cortex, dopamine and, 233
   schizophrenia and, 257, 319, 320f
information transfer, abnormal, 33f
inhalants, 993
   probability of dependence, 968t
inherited disease, classic autosomal dominant pattern, 178f
inhibitors, of enzymes, 167
inhibitory amino acid transporters, 94t
inhibitory interneurons, 2
   chandelier neurons as, 3
   double bouquet cells as, 4f
inhibitory pathways, 789
inositol, for bipolar disorder, 699
   in combos, 714
insomnia, 816, 818f
   benzodiazepines for, 837f
   causes, 833t
   chronic, 831–839
   circuits, 820f
   defined, 833t
   diabolical learning hypothesis and, 230
   drug treatment action at ionotrophic receptors, 124
   and malfunctioning circuits, 645f
   and medical illnesses, 834t
   psychiatric
      and GABA-A PAMs, 842
      treatment, 843f
   and psychiatric disorders, 834t
   quetiapine for treating, 415
   rebound, 837
   sleep/wake switch and, 825f
   and sleepiness, 853f
   trazodone for, 566
   treatment, 128, 646, 823

insomnia/anxiety combo, 652f
insulin, blocking M3-cholinergic receptors to
         reduce, 392f
insulin family, 174
insulin resistance, 385
    atypical antipsychotic agents and, 390f
    psychopharmacologist options for, 397f
    quetiapine and, 415
    risperidone and, 413
    ziprasidone and, 417
    zotepine and, 418
insulinlike growth factors (ILGF), 29t
integral proteins, 11f, 12
integrated dopamine hypothesis of
         schizophrenia, 279, 281f
integrins, 32
interest, loss
    bupropion for, 556
    as SSRI side effect, 530
interferons, 174
interleukins, 174
"intermediate phenotypes", 182, 182f
International Association of the Study of Pain,
         777
International Classification of Diseases (ICD), 178
interneurons, 775
    in cortex, 2
    inhibitory, 2
        GABAergic, 216, 218f
interpersonal functioning, impaired, in
         schizophrenia, 324
interpersonal therapy (IPT), 639
intracellular portion of receptor, 109f
intracellular scaffolding proteins, 36, 42f
intracellular synaptic vesicle transporters, 93
inverse agonists, 111f
    actions of, 139f
    antagonist to reverse actions of, 141f
    vs. antagonists, 351
    antagonists acting in presence of, 140f
    reversal by antagonist, 115
ion channel-linked receptors, 123–125, 286
    CREB activation by, 74
ion channel-linked signal-transduction
         cascades, 65, 66f
    first messengers, 67
    second messenger, 65, 67
    later messengers, 71
ion channels, 36
    activation, 64f
    fast transport of, 15f
    ligand-gated, 92f, 123–144
        different states, 137
        pentameric subtypes, 126

as psychotropic drug target, 128t
    structure and function, 127f
    tetrameric structure, 131f
    tetrameric subunit, 129f
    tetrameric subunit, top view, 130f
and neurotransmission, 158–167
opening, 64
for prehemisynapse, 43f
third messenger opening, 77f
voltage-sensitive, 92f, 145–158
ionic components, of action potential, 147f
ionic filter, 149f
    of voltage-sensitive calcium channels, 150f
ionotrophic glutamate receptors, 130
ionotrophic receptors, 123–125, 154, 286, 733
    glutamate, structure, 128
ions, 123
iproniazid, 574
IPT (interpersonal therapy), 639
irreversible enzyme inhibitors, 167, 168f
irritability, 260
irritable bowel syndrome, 779, 784, 811
    diagnostic criteria, 812t
    pain triggers, 800
    painful somatic symptoms in, 791f
irritable mood circuits, 501f
isocarboxazid (Marplan), 575, 579t
isoforms, in GABA-A receptor, 735f
ispronicline (TC1734), 941
Ixel. *See* milnacipran (Ixel, Toledomin)

joy, loss
    bupropion for, 556
    as SSRI side effect, 530
judgment, distortions in schizophrenia,
         324
Jun proteins, 81f, 83f, 85–87
"junk" DNA, 78

kainate glutamate receptors, 130
kainite receptors, 286, 286f
    glutamate at, 147f
kappa opiate receptors, 977
ketamine, 144, 993
    for bipolar disorder, 695
    icon, 696f
    mechanism of action
        on GABA, glutamate, sigma, and
             dopamine, 676t
        VSSCs, synaptic vesicles, and carbonic
             anhydrase, 675t
    and NMDA receptor regulation, 708f
    possible actions in bipolar disorder, 698f
    putative clinical actions, 673t

and schizophrenia symptoms, 289, 440
   site of action, 697f
ketoconazole, 405
   and CYP 450 3A4, 609
kinase enzymes, 66f
kinases
   activation by receptor activation, 87
   activation in signal transduction cascade, 64, 65f, 72
   calcium activation of, 74
   clash with phosphatase, 73
kleptomania, 771, 1011

l-alpha-acetylmethodol acetate (LAAM), 981
L channel, 154, 155t
la-do (lamotrigine-Depakote), 714, 714f
la-li-do (lamotrigine-lithium-Depakote), 714, 714f
la-li (lamotrigine-lithium), 713, 714f
lactation, 278
Lami-quel, 715, 716f
lamotrigine, 153f
   actions as mood stabilizer, 685f
   binding site of, 684f
   for bipolar disorder, 701
      with depression, 700
   combination of medications with, 715, 716f
   and glutamate reduction, 708f
   icon, 684f
   mechanism of action
      on GABA, glutamate, sigma, and dopamine, 676t
      VSSCs, synaptic vesicles, and carbonic anhydrase, 675t
   putative clinical actions, 673t
   rashes from, 683
   for schizophrenia, 436
      adding to antipsychotic, 437f
   sites of action, on glutamate release, 685f
   and VSSCs, 707f
language, odd use of, 257
late gene, 81f
lateral fissure, 196f
lateral parabrachial nucleus, 204
lazaroids, as free radical scavenger, 442f
learning
   and brain restructuring, 32
   constant synaptic revision and, 45
   and endogenous growth factors, 26f
   gene expression and, 78
   long-term, 167
   and neurogenesis in hippocampus, 24, 24f
learning disabilities, from improper neuronal migration, 29

learning model, and circuit inefficiency, 230
lecozotan, 941
leptin, 174
leucine zipper transcription factor, 81f, 83, 83f, 85–87
Leucovorin (folinic acid), 626
levetiracetam, 156, 157f
   icon, 689f
   mechanism of action
      on GABA, glutamate, sigma, and dopamine, 676t
      at SV2A synaptic vesicle sites, 690f
      VSSCs, synaptic vesicles, and carbonic anhydrase, 675t
   putative clinical actions, 673t
   and seizure reduction, 102
levodopa, for Parkinson's disease, MAO-B inhibition and, 579
Lewy bodies
   damage to cholinergic neurons, 920
   dementia with, 901t
li-do (lithium-Depakote/divalproex/valproate), 713, 714f
libido, decreased, 1004
licarbazepine, 681
   binding site of, 682f
   mechanism of action
      on GABA, glutamate, sigma, and dopamine, 676t
      VSSCs, synaptic vesicles, and carbonic anhydrase, 675t
   oxcarbazepine conversion to, 681f
   putative clinical actions, 673t
lidocaine
   anatomic site of action, 780f
   molecular site of action, 781f
   and VSSC block, 778
life cycle, antidepressants over, 519, 519f
life expectancy, of schizophrenic patients, 250
lifestyle, and stress, 191f
ligand-gated ion channels, 92f, 123, 126f
   agonists impact on, 143f
   different states, 137
   GABA receptors as, 733
   pentameric subtypes, 126
   as psychotropic drug target, 128t
   states, 142f
   structure and function, 125, 127f
   subunit of tetrameric, 129f
   top view, 130f
   tetrameric structure, 131f
limbic cortex, noradrenergic receptor simulation in, 547
limbic CSTC circuit, 868

lipid neurotransmitter, 52*t*
lithium, 173, 173*f*
    for affective symptoms in schizophrenia, 429
    for Alzheimer's disease, 937
    for bipolar disorder, 701
    in combos
        for bipolar disorder, 713
        for depression, 562*f*
    for depression, 635*f*
        in bipolar disorder, 700
    for dopamine hyperactivity reduction, 709*f*
    and fetal toxicity risk, 712
    GSK-3 inhibition by, 173
    mechanism of action, 670*f*
        as mood stabilizer, 671*f*
    side effects of, 671
    for suicide reduction, 429, 430*f*
liver
    CYP450 enzymes in, 402
    insulin resistance in, 387, 390*f*
    riluzole impact,
    valproic acid toxicity, 677
local anesthesia, 775, 780*f*
    and VSSC block, 778
locus coeruleus (LC), 202*f*
    connection with amygdala, 731
    excessive noradrenergic output from, 755
lofepramine (Deprimyl, Gamanil), 597*t*
long-term outcomes, symptom exacerbation and, 230
long-term potentiation (LTP), 144, 308, 312*f*
Loroxyl (amitriptyline, Elavil, Endep, Tryptizol), 53, 572, 597*t*
Lou Gehrig's disease. *See* amyotrophic lateral sclerosis (ALS)
lovastatin
    and CYP 450 3A4, 608
    risk of muscle damage, 609
low-potency antipsychotic agents, and dissociation, 370
loxapine (Loxitane), 331*t*
    5HT6-antagonist properties of, 447
    pharmacological icon, 420*f*
Loxitane. *See* loxapine (Loxitane)
LSD (d-lysergic acid diethylamide), 990
    actions, 992*f*
LTP. *See* long-term potentiation (LTP)
LuAA34893, 552, 552*f*
Ludiomil (maprotiline), 597*t*
    inhibition of serotonin reuptake pump, 598
luxapine, 419
LY 293558, 446
LY354740, 443
LY379268, 443

LY450139, 939
d-lysergic acid diethylamide (LSD), 990
    actions, 992*f*
lysosomes, 8*f*, 84*f*
    localization of, 9*f*
    organelle and protein destruction by, 15, 17*f*

macrolide antibiotics, and CYP 450 3A4, 609
magnesium, 142
    as negative allosteric modulators, 146*f*
    removing block, 167
    removing from calcium channel, 164*f*
magnetic resonance imaging, functional (fMRI), 184
Maintenance of Wakefulness Test (MWT), 852*t*
major depressive disorder (MDD), 455*f*. *See also* depression
    antidepressant combinations as standard, 651
    common comorbidities, 650*f*
    genes for, 192
    overlap with anxiety disorders, 722*f*
    progressive nature of, 472*f*
    relapse rates, 518*f*
    remission rates, 517*f*
    symptom-based algorithm, 645*f*
    symptoms shared with other disorders, 869*t*
malingering, 784
Manerix (moclobemide, Aurorix), 579*t*
mania, 499*f*
    on antidepressant, 463
    cognitive symptoms, 504*f*
    core symptoms of episode, 506
    excess neurotransmission and, 47*f*
    mapping symptoms to circuits, 500*f*
    mixed states of depression and, 467*t*
    on mood chart, 454, 454*f*
    mood stabilizers for treating, 669*f*
    neurotransmission instabililty and, 704
    overlap with depression, 507
    patient response to no-go task, 509*f*
    prepubertal and adolescent, 712
    residual symptoms after first-line treatment, 703
    sleep disturbances in, 503*f*
    symptoms and circuits, 496, 502*f*
    treatment
        with atypical antipsychotic agents, 689, 691*f*
        with mood stabilizer, 668
MAOIs. *See* monoamine oxidase inhibitors (MAOIs)
MAPK (MAP kinase), 66*f*, 76

maprotiline (Ludiomil), 597t
　inhibition of serotonin reuptake pump, 598
marijuana, 986
　actions on reward circuits, 989f
Marplan (isocarboxazid), 575, 579t
"master switch", 287
MDL 100907, 447
MDMA (3, 4-methylene-dioxymethamphetamine), 990
　actions, 992f
medial preoptic area (MPOA), and sexual drive, 994
medial raphe, 205
"medical food", 629
medical illnesses, and insomnia, 834t
Medivation (dimebon), 941
mefipristone, 172
MEK (mitogen-activated protein kinase/extracellular signal–regulated kinase), 66f
melanocortin, and sexual desire, 995
melanocyte inhibitory factor (MIF-1), 663, 664f
melatonergic agents, 844, 844f
melatonin, 844f
　half-life of, 836f
melatonin neurotransmitter, as psychotropic drug target, 114
melatonin-sensitive neurons, in suprachiasmatic nucleus (SCN), 820
Mellaril (thioridazine), 331t
　and CYP450 2D6 inhibitors, 608
Mem 1003, 940
MEM3454, 449
memantine, 440, 926–934
　for bipolar disorder, 695
　　possible actions, 698f
　mechanism of action, 930, 933f
　　on GABA, glutamate, sigma, and dopamine, 676t
　　VSSCs, synaptic vesicles, and carbonic anhydrase, 675t
　and NMDA receptor regulation, 708f
　putative clinical actions, 673t
memory, 201
　cholinergic fibers and, 206
　formation process, cholinergic neurons and, 920
　gene expression and, 78
　long-term formation, 144
　　BDNF and, 345
　loss
　　age and, 908

　　in dementia, 900
　　electroconvulsive therapy and, 634
men, depression incidence across life cycle, 616f
menopause, depression and treatment during, 620f
menstrual cycle, reproductive hormones and synaptogenesis, 613f
"menstrual magnification", 616
"mental exercise", 45
mental illness
　and brain damage, 228
　genes and risk for, 177
　hypothetical path from gene to, 183f
　model of remission from episode, 228f
　and smoking, 955
mental retardation, 426
　from improper neuronal migration, 29
　neuron wiring and, 33f
mental stimulation, value of, 49
meperidine, interaction with MAOIs, 595, 595t
meprobamate, and anxiety, 767
mescaline DOM, 990
　actions, 992f
mesocortical dopamine neurons, 291
mesocortical dopamine pathway, 272f
　and D2 antagonists, 331f
　dopamine output and, 366f
　secondary dopamine deficiency in, 356
　and serotonin-dopamine antagonism, 359f
　to ventromedial prefrontal cortex, 276f
mesocortical prefrontal cortex
　and emotion and cognitive symptoms, 263f
　and schizophrenia symptoms, 261, 262f
mesolimbic circuits
　malfunctioning, and positive symptoms of schizophrenia, 261, 262, 262f
　and positive symptoms of schizophrenia, 263f
mesolimbic dopamine hypothesis, 274f
mesolimbic dopamine pathway, 272, 272f
　blockade of D2 receptor antagonists, 330, 330f
　blockade of D2 receptors, 329
　dopamine output and, 366f
　hyperactivity of, 281f
　and thalamus, 297f
　neurotransmitter regulation, 947f
　as pleasure center, 945, 946f
mesolimbic pathway, dopamine partial agonist in, 376f
mesoridazine (Serentil), 331t
messenger RNA, 84f
met-met carriers, 233
metabolic highway, 388f
　monitoring on, 395f

Index | 1089

metabolic pharmacy, 429, 431f
metabotropic glutamate receptors (mGluRs), 285, 288f
metformin, 1011
methadone, 981
   icon, 981f
   interaction with MAOIs, 595, 595t
methamphetamine, 983
   icon, 984f
   undesirable effects, 984
methionine, 233
5-methoxy-diisopropyltryptamine ("Foxy"), 990
6-(S)-5-methyl-tetrahydrofolate (MTHF), 699
methylation, MTHF regulation of, 630
3, 4-methylene-dioxymethamphetamine (MDMA), 990
   actions, 992f
methylene tetrahydrofolate reductase (THF-R), 627f
L-methylfolate (Deplin), 629
   for bipolar disorder, 699
   in combos, 714
methylphenidate, 99t, 103, 105
   action at dopamine transporter, 105f
   action in ADHD, 885
   and blood pressure, 593
   vs. cocaine, 983
   DAT blocking by, 103
   with MAOIs, and hypertension, 593t
   for wakefulness, 857, 858
L-5-methyltetrahydrofolate (MTHF), 625, 627f
   and antidepressants, 631f
   vs. folic acid, for depression, 627
   and methylation reactions, 630
   trimonoamine modulation of, 632f
mGluRs (metabotropic glutamate receptors), 285, 288f
mianserin, 559f
microglia, and Alzheimer's disease, 906
microtubules, 8f, 10
   localization of, 9f
   slow transport of, 14f
   transport of, 13
mild cognitive impairment, 908
milnacipran (Ixel, Toledomin), 99t, 541t
   for fibrofog, 810
   for fibromyalgia, 808
   icon, 551f
   for neuropathic pain, 792
mirtazapine, 446, 559f
   actions at serotonin synapses, 564f
   actions overview, 566f
   for anxiety disorders, 767
   for fibromyalgia, 810
   H1 antihistamine actions, 564, 565f
   half-life of, 835f
   hypnotic actions, 848
   icon, 563f
   for panic disorder, 768
   SNRI plus, 656f
   for social anxiety disorder, 769
mitochondria, 8f, 307f
   energy for neurotransmission from, 38f
   fast transport of, 14, 15f
   localization of, 9f
mixed hypomania, depression with, 465
mixed mood state, 454
MK0752, 939
Moban. *See* perphenazine (Trilafon)
moclobemide (Aurorix, Manerix), 579t
   for treating nicotine dependence, 967
modafinil, 99t, 244f
   for ADHD, 873
   in adults, 885
   combining with lamotrigine, 715, 716f
   for fibromyalgia, 810
   mechanism of action, 858f
   for promoting histamine release, 823
   SNRI plus, 657f
   testing for cocaine abuse treatment, 985
   for wakefulness, 857
molecular cascades, neurotransmitter-induced, impact on postsynaptic proteins, 88
molecular components, for synapse formation, 36, 40f
molecular G protein-linked receptors, 110t
molecular memories, and addiction, 959
molecules
   conversion by enzyme activity, 167
   subtle abnormalities
      and depression, 193f
      and schizophrenia, 192f
      and SERT, 237f
   variable impact of abnormalities, 185
molindone (Moban), 331t
monoamine autoreceptors, 60
   volume neurotransmission and, 60f
monoamine neurotransmitters, 453
monoamine oxidase inhibitors (MAOIs), 574–597
   with amphetamine actions, 579t
   currently approved, 579t
   drug interactions, 591
   interaction with decongestants, 594f
   interaction with SRIs, 596f
   irreversible, dangerous tyramine levels with, 592f

new developments, 585
for panic disorder, 768
tyramine dietary modifications for, 584t
monoamine oxidase (MAO), 112, 170, 221f
and dopamine breakdown, 267, 267f
enzymes, 579t
and norepinephrine, 474, 476f
subtype A inhibition, 580f
combined with subtype B inhibition, 583f
and dietary tyramine management, 582
and tyramine, 586f
subtype A, norepinephrine destruction by, 584f
subtype B inhibition, 581f
transdermal delivery, 588–591
subtypes, 577
monoamine transporters, 15, 94, 94t, 95f, 99, 219f
binding sites, 96f, 97f
presynaptic, 93t
as targets of antidepressants and stimulants, 99t
monoamines, 15
coupled with neuropeptide, 54
estrogen interaction with, and depressed mood, 621f
"fine-tuning" action on pyramid cells, 220
folate deficiency and, 630f
input to enhance signal, 220f
interaction with estrogen, vasomotor symptoms from, 524f
molecular sites for regulating, 221f
regulating "tuners", 221
monohydroxyderivative, 681
mood
5HT2C receptors and, 349f
norepinephrine projections regulation of, 205
serotonin projections regulation of, 205, 206f
serotonin receptors and, 345
mood chart, 454f
mood disorders
comorbid with fibromyalgia, 807t
description, 454
future treatments for, 659–664
genes and neuroimaging in, 507–509
mapping, 454f
neurotransmitters and circuits in, 474–480
with pain, 802, 803f
pain linked to, 804, 804f
prevalence of, 468f
progressive nature of, 470–473
treatment-resistant, 473
mood episodes, 455f

mood networks, genes hypothetically regulating, 506f
mood stabilizers, 406, 426, 668. *See also* lithium
for aggression management, 427f
anticonvulsants, 672. *See also specific agents*
atypical antipsychotic agents, 689, 694f
in clinical practice, 700–718
pharmacy, 700, 701f
residual symptoms after first-line treatment, 702–710
selection process, 700
symptom-based algorithm for sequential treatment, 700
combinations for bipolar disorder, 713
definition, 668
and fetal toxicity risk, 712
future options, 718
gender differences, 712
and glutamate, 708f
mechanism of action
on GABA, glutamate, sigma, and dopamine, 676t
VSSCs, synaptic vesicles, and carbonic anhydrase, 675t
putative clinical actions, 673t
for schizophrenia, 436
adding to antipsychotic, 437f
symptom-based algorithm
deconstructing mania/bipolar spectrum disorder symptoms, 703f
deconstructing mania diagnostic symptoms, 702f
symptom matching to circuits, 704f
targeting neurotransmitters, 705f
for treating depression, 669f
for treating mania, 669f
and VSSCs, 707f
morphine, 977
brain production of, 53
motivation
mesolimbic dopamine pathway role in, 272
reduction in, 251, 276
motor activity
as antipsychotic side effect, 341
CSTC loop to regulate, 216f
disturbances, 248
dopamine and prevention of side effects, 370
in fear, 730
nigrostrial dopamine pathway to control, 277
motor behavior, CSTC loop to regulate, 213
motor skills, constant synaptic revision and, 45
movement, neurons regulating, 204
mRNA, and peptide production, 11f

MTHF. *See* L-5-methyltetrahydrofolate (MTHF)
mu opioid receptors, 789, 977
　alcohol actions on, 973
Multiple Sleep Latency Test (MSLT), 852*t*
muscarinic-1 agonists, 449
muscarinic-1 receptors
　atypical antipsychotic agents and, 385*f*
　and sedation, 397*f*
muscarinic 3 (M3) antagonism, and antipsychotic agents, 393*f*
muscarinic cholinergic receptors, 547, 916*f*
　antagonism of, 390
　blockade from conventional antipsychotics, 337, 338*f*
　blocking to reduce insulin release, 392*f*
　subtypes, 917
　TCA blockade of, 599
myelination, of axon fibers, 22
myocardial infarction
　antipsychotic agents and, 417
　from repetitive autonomic responses, 731
myocarditis, clozapine and, 410
myoclonus, from SSRIs, 531

N-acetyl cysteine, 986
n-back test, 233, 233*f*
　and dorsolateral prefrontal cortex, 234*f*
　by narcolepsy patients, 855*f*
　in schizophrenia, 321*f*
N channels, 154, 155*t*
　inhibitors of, 158*f*
　and neurotransmitter release, 156
　neurotransmitter release regulation, 155, 156*f*
N-methyl-d-aspartate (NMDA) glutamate receptors, 130, 142, 164*f*
　cotransmitter binding to, 143
N-methyl-d-aspartate (NMDA) glutamate system, development abnormalities, 274
N-methyl-glycine, 442
N-methyl -histamine, 829*f*
N-methyl indole acetic acid (N-MIA), 828, 829*f*
N-methyl loxapine, 419
N-MIA (N-methyl indole acetic acid), 828, 829*f*
nalmefene, for alcohol dependency, 976
naloxone
　in detoxification process, 981
　for reversing opiate action, 979
naltrexone, 769
　actions, in ventral tegmental area (VTA), 974*f*
　for blocking mu opiate receptors, 973
　in combos for bipolar disorder, 715
　formulations, 975*f*
　icon, 973*f*
　for reversing opiate action, 979
　testing for cocaine abuse treatment, 986
　for treating nicotine dependence, 967
NAMs (negative allosteric modulators), 145*f*
narcolepsy, 820, 873
　gamma hydroxybutyrate for, 859
　information processing in, 855*f*
　symptoms shared with other disorders, 869*t*
Nardil (phenelzine), 575, 579*t*
natural disaster, stress vulnerability, 193, 194*f*
"natural highs", 945, 947*f*
nausea
　from 5HT3 receptor stimulation, 531
　bifeprunox and, 424
　from venlafaxine, 549
Navane (thiothixene), 331*t*
NCAMs (neuronal cell adhesion molecules), 31*t*, 32
NDDIs (norepinephrine dopamine disinhibitors), 658
NDRIs. *See* norepinephrine and dopamine reuptake inhibitors (NDRIs)
NE. *See* norepinephrine (NE)
NE reuptake pump, 474
NE transporter (NET). *See* norepinephrine transporter (NET)
necrosis, and apoptosis, 28*f*
nefazodone, 405, 572, 639
　and CYP 450 3A4, 608
　icon, 567*f*
negative affect, 499*f*
　increased, 495
　vs. reduced positive affect, 643
negative allosteric modulators (NAMs), 141, 145*f*
　magnesium as, 146*f*
negative feedback regulatory signal, 476
Negative Symptom Assessment, 253*t*
negative symptom pharmacy, 427, 428*f*
nemifitide, 663, 664*f*
nemonapride, 368*f*
nerve growth factor (NGF), 29, 29*t*, 57*f*
nerve impulse propagation, in presynaptic neuron, 160*f*
nerves, normal, and severed, 785*f*
NET. *See* norepinephrine transporter (NET)
net agonists, 134
net antagonists, 134
netrins, 32
neurasthenia, 805
neuregulin, 305, 310*f*
　genes coding for, 309*f*

and glutamate synapses strengthening, 312f
and NMDA receptor regulation, 314f
and NMDA regulation, 317
and synapse formation, 308, 311f
neuroanatomy, 196
neurodegeneration, 34f
　and synapse loss, 25f
neurodegenerative disorders, 35
neurodevelopment, 34f
　disorders, 34
　　neuron wiring and, 33f
　and neuronal selection, 27f
　process, 23f
　time course of, 22, 22f
neurofibrillary tangles, in Alzheimer's disease, 901
　formation process, 906, 927
neurofilaments, 8f, 10
　localization of, 9f
　slow transport of, 14f
　transport of, 13
neurogenesis, 24
　adult, in hippocampus dentate region, 23f, 24f
　from gene expression, 78
neuroimaging
　in depression, 507f
　in mood disorders, 507–509
neurokinin antagonists, 449, 664
neurokinin receptors, 665t
neurokinins, 52t
　targeting with antidepressants in development, 660t
neurolepsis, 276, 329, 396
neuroleptic-induced deficit syndrome, 330
neuroleptic-induced tardive dyskinesia, 277
neuroleptic malignant syndrome, 342
neuroleptics, 329
neuromas, 785
neuronal cell adhesion molecules (NCAMs), 31t, 32
neuronal circuitry, and psychiatric disorders, 223
neuronal migration, 29, 30f
neuronal presynaptic reuptake pump, 285
neuronal selection, 27–29
　and neurodevelopment, 27f
neuronal transport, 12–20
neurons, 21
　anatomic zones of, 7f
　arborization, 35f
　basket, 2
　branching or arborization of, 22
　cell death, 29
　　excitotoxic mechanism and, 304f
　　glutamate activity and, 301

neurotransmission and, 48f
　preventing in schizophrenia, 440
chandelier, 3
communication between, 55f, 57f
components, 8, 8f
　fast transport of, 16f
　localization of, 9f
cyclical activation, estrogen and, 612
damage from virus or toxin, 28
dopaminergic, 266–268
double bouquet cells, 2
electrical impulse in, 145
formation during prenatal gestation, 22
generic structure, 2f
internal operations, subcellular organelles, 6–10
loss of, sustained symptoms and, 230, 232f
noradrenergic, 474–476
postsynaptic, signal propagation, 163f
presynaptic, nerve impulse propagation in, 160f
restoration by growth factor, 26f
sensitivity to calcium, 305f
spiny, 2–3
structural and regulatory molecules of, 10f
structure of unique, 1–6
　pyramidal cells, 2–6
varieties of, 1–6
wiring of
　correct, 33f
　wrong, 33f
neuropathic pain, 775, 784, 797f
　peripheral mechanisms, 785
　and sympathetic nervous system, 786
neuropeptides
　coupled with monoamines, 54
　fast transport of machinery for, 19f
　function in neurotransmission, 15
　transporters, 102
neuropoietic cytokines, 174
neuropsychological assessment batteries, 257
neurosteroids, targeting
　benzodiasepine-insensitive GABA-A receptors, 737
neurotensin antagonists, 450
neurotransmission. *See also* chemical neurotransmission
　anatomical basis, 21
　and cell death, 48f
　chemical basis, 21
　classic, 54, 55f
　energy for, 38f
　excess, 47f

Index | 1093

neurotransmission (*Contd.*)
  functional outcome in G protein-linked system, 68*f*
  and ion channels, 158–167
  nonsynaptic diffusion, 58
  preventing, 156
  retrograde, 57*f*, 61
  sensitivity of, 88
  unstable and excessive in bipolar disorder, 706*f*
  volume, 58, 58*f*
neurotransmitter-induced molecular cascades, impact on postsynaptic proteins, 88
neurotransmitter nodes, 201–207
neurotransmitter receptor hypothesis of depression, 488
neurotransmitter receptors
  binding to, 70
  change in number of pre- and postsynaptic, 38
  regulation of, 85*f*
  subtypes, 111*f*
neurotransmitters, 8*f*, 36, 51–54
  activation of signal-transduction cascades, 66*f*
  and arousal spectrum, 817, 817*f*
  changes in receptor sensitivity, 521
  for circuit regulation, 241
  of cortical arousal, 398*f*
  in depression treatment, 652*f*
  in dorsal horn, 782, 783*f*
  fast transport for, 14, 15, 15*f*
  fast transport of machinery for, 18*f*
  gene regulation by, 82*f*
  glutamate as, 279
  influence on CTSC loops, 210
  ion channels opened by, 124
  linking symptoms to circuits to, 731*f*
  linking worry symptoms to circuits to, 764*f*
  listing, 52*t*
  matching to circuits, 243*f*
  naturally occurring, 53
  and orgasm, 999*f*
  for prehemisynapse, 43*f*
  presynaptic release of, 161*f*
  reception of released, 164
  receptor hypothesis of antidepressant action, 522*f*
  sexual arousal and, 997*f*
  slow-onset signaling
    A to B, 62*f*
    B to A, 63*f*
  transporters, 93*f*
    classification and structure, 92, 93
    vesicular, 94*t*

neurotrophic factors, 29, 29*t*, 57*f*
  5HT6 receptors and, 349*f*
  and axonal traffic direction, 32*f*
  constant synaptic revision and, 45
neurotrophin-linked signal-transduction cascades, 65, 66*f*
  first messengers, 67
  later messengers, 71
  second messenger, 67
neurotrophins (NT), 29*t*, 75
  and axon sprouting, 32*f*
  in brain, 174*t*
  control of axon growth, 31
  second messenger, 66
NGB2904, testing for cocaine abuse treatment, 986
NGF (nerve growth factor), 29, 29*t*, 57*f*
nicotine, 955, 960*f*
  abuse by ADHD patients, 870, 880
  actions, 957*f*
  dependence/addiction, 955–959
    alternate delivery to treat, 960
    probability of developing, 964
    treatment, 959–968
  dependency/addiction, properties, 918
  and dopamine release, 964*f*
  probability of dependence, 968*t*
  response to administration, 966*f*
nicotinic full agonists, 960
nicotinic partial agonists (NPA), 449
  and dopamine release, 965*f*
  molecular actions, 961*f*
  response to, 967*f*
nicotinic receptors
  acetylcholine, 917, 917*f*
    allosteric modulation, 919*f*
  alpha 4 beta 2, 959, 960*f*
    reinforcement and, 958*f*
  cholinergic, 139, 955
    calcium channels associated with, 154
    pentameric structure, 126
  desensitization, 956
  presynaptic, 918*f*
nigrostriatal dopamine pathway, 272*f*
  antipsychotic agent binding to postsynaptic D2 receptors, 358*f*
  and D2 antagonists, 332*f*
  dopamine output and, 366*f*
  and dopamine partial agonists (DPAs), 377*f*
  serotonin 2A antagonists in,
  serotonin-dopamine interaction, 353*f*
  serotonin regulation of dopamine release, 354*f*
"Nissl substance", 11

nitric oxide (NO), 57, 57f
  psychopharmacology, 996
  and sexual arousal, 998f
nitric oxide synthetase, inhibiting, 537
nitric oxide synthetase (NOS), 997
NK1 antagonists (substance P antagonists), 665
NK3 antagonists, 665
NMDA glutamate hyperactivity hypothesis, 930
NMDA (N-methyl-d-aspartate) antagonists, 440, 441f
NMDA (N-methyl-d-aspartate) receptors, 286, 286f
  blocking glutamate actions at, 708f
  enhancement of activity, 444f
  excitation spectrum by glutamate, 303f
  genes affecting, 304
  and glutamate systems, 283, 284f
  histamine action at, 831
  hypofunction, 446
  hypofunction hypothesis of schizophrenia, 290f
    and corticobrainstem glutamate pathways, 288–291
  hypofunction in glutamatergic corticostriatal and corticoaccumbens projections, 297f
  ketamine binding to, 697f
  long-term potentiation (LTP) triggered by, 312f
  normal excitatory neurotransmission of, 302f
  production, 283
  regulation of corticocortical glutamate pathways, 299f
  requirements for active, 443f
  susceptibility gene regulation of, 317
  synapses with, 313f
  and synaptogenesis, 308
NNDI. See norepinephrine and dopamine disinhibitors (NDDI)
nociception, 775, 777
  activity-dependent, 795
    acute pain, 796f
    neuropathic pain, 797f
    pathway to pain, 782f
nociceptive nerve fibers
  activation, 778f
    normal pain and, 778
nociceptive pain
  acute, and opiates, 790f
  peripheral blockade of acute, 780f
nociceptive pathways
  to spinal cord, 778
  from spinal cord to brain, 782
nociceptive transduction, 779f
nociceptor, 775

node, 197
nodes of Ranvier, 785, 786f
nondegenerative dementias, 903t
nonsteroidal anti-inflammatory drug (NSAID) cyclooxygenase (COX-2) inhibitors, 787
nonsteroidal anti-inflammatory drugs (NSAIDs), for Alzheimer's disease, 937
nonsynaptic diffusion neurotransmission, 58
noradrenaline. See norepinephrine (NE)
noradrenergic and specific serotonergic antidepressant (NaSSA), mirtazapine as, 563f
noradrenergic inhibition, descending, enhancement of, 792f
noradrenergic neurons, 474–476
  descending, and pain, 791f
  MAO subtypes in, 577
norepinephrine and dopamine reuptake inhibitors (NDRIs), 99t, 552–556
  action, 553f
  actions in prefrontal cortex and striatum, 555f
  icon, 553f
  SNRI plus, 656f
  SSRIs plus,
"norepinephrine deficiency syndrome", 546
norepinephrine dopamine disinhibitors (NDDIs), 658
  mirtazapine as, 563
norepinephrine dopamine inhibitors (NDRIs), for fibromyalgia, 810
norepinephrine (NE), 220, 453. See also serotonin norepinephrine reuptake inhibitors (SNRIs)
  5HT2A receptors regulation of, 484f
  and alpha 2 antagonists, 560f
  antidepressants' enhancement of, 98
  antidepressants impact on synaptic action, 520
  antipsychotic agents and, 691, 692f
  in arousal pathways, 396, 398f
  and arousal spectrum, 817, 817f
  autoreceptors as gatekeepers, 478f
  depression from deficiency, 520f
  and depression symptoms, 546
  disinhibition, 562f
    at serotonin 1A receptors, 571–574
  fluoxetine and release of, 534f
  hyperactivity in anxiety, 755, 757f
    blocking, 758f
  and mood disorders, 474
  normal destruction by MAO-A, 584f
  projections, 204, 205f
  psychotropic drugs and, 53
  regulation of serotonin release, 476, 480, 480f

Index | 1095

norepinephrine (NE) (Contd.)
   as accelerator, 482f
   bidirectional control, 483f
   as brake, 481f
   release
      5HT2C receptors and, 349f
      presynaptic alpha 2 receptor regulation, 475
      serotonin regulation of, 477
      tyramine and, 585f
   synthesis, 474, 475f
   termination of action, 474, 476f
   transport pump, 474
   tricyclic antidepressant to block reuptake pump, 598
   turning off its own release, 558
norepinephrine neurons
   normal rate of tonic firing, 873
   phasic firing of, 875
norepinephrine neurotransmitter
   as psychotropic drug indirect target, 116
   as psychotropic drug target, 114
norepinephrine receptors, 477f
norepinephrine reuptake inhibition (NRI), 420f
   to desensitize excessive arousal systems, 877
norepinephrine reuptake pump, 544
norepinephrine selective reuptake inhibitors (NRIs), 99t, 448
   actions, 558f
   for fibromyalgia, 810
   icon, 557f
   plus mirtazapine, 656f
   plus modafinil, 657f
   plus NDRI, 656f
   plus stimulant, 656f
norepinephrine transporter (NET), 93, 94, 95f, 474, 475, 476f
   cocaine ability to inhibit, 983
   inhibition, 557
      and dopamine in prefrontal cortex, 544, 545f
      high degrees of, and sedation, 558
      by norquetiapine, 415
      potential side effects, 546
      therapeutic actions of, 546
norfluoxetine, 405
Norpramin. See desipramine (Norpramin, Pertofran)
norquetiapine, 414, 414f
   actions as mood stabilizer, 693f
   pharmacological actions, 693f
nortriptyline, 572
nortriptyline (Pamelor, Endep, Aventyl), 597t
   inhibition of serotonin reuptake pump, 598

   with interpersonal psychotherapy, 639
   NRI actions, 890
"not otherwise specified" (NOS), 461
novel peptides, 664f
noxious stimulus, 775
NRA0562, 368f
NRI. See norepinephrine selective reuptake inhibitors (NRIs)
NSAIDs (nonsteroidal anti-inflammatory drugs), for Alzheimer's disease, 937
NT (neurotrophins), 29t
nuclear hormone receptors, 67, 171, 172f
   and estrogen, 610, 611f
   as possible target by psychotropic drugs, 171t
nuclear ligand–activated transcription factors, 610, 611f
nucleus raphe magnus, 789
nucleus, 8, 8f
   localization of, 9f
nucleus accumbens, 202f
   5HT2C receptors regulation of dopamine, 486f
   D2 receptor blockade in, 353
   and delusions and hallucinations, 704f
   as pleasure center, 329
   rewarding input to, 948f
   and schizophrenia symptoms, 262, 262f
nucleus basalis (of Meynert), 206, 920
nucleus linearis, 205
"number needed to harm", 333, 417

obesity, 1008
   5HT2C receptors and, 349f
   atypical antipsychotic agents and, 383
   blood pressure monitoring, 392
   peptide treatments for, 450
   serotonin receptors and, 345
   treatment, 1009
observation, for negative symptom identification in schizophrenia, 252, 254f
obsessions, 764
   diabolical learning hypothesis and, 230
obsessive compulsive disorder, 725f
   fluvoxamine for, 537, 538
   pharmacy, 771f
   treatment, 770
obstructive sleep apnea, 855
   symptoms shared with other disorders, 869t
occipital lobe, 196f
OH-pyruvate. See hydroxy-pyruvate (OH-pyruvate)
olanzapine, 403, 403f
   5HT6-antagonist properties of, 447
   actions as mood stabilizer, 693f

for alcohol dependency, 977
and antagonism of muscarinic cholinergic receptor, 392f
and cardiometabolic risk, 386t
in combos for bipolar disorder, 713
as CYP 2D6 substrate, 404, 405f
and diabetes, 417
fluoxetine with, 533
half-life of, 835f
M3 receptors blocked by, 392f
pharmacological actions, 693f
pharmacological icon, 411f
potency, and dissociation, 371
raising levels of, 406f
for sedation, 431
testing for cocaine abuse treatment, 986
and weight gain risk, 386t
olfactory bulb, 23f, 24
omega-3 fatty acids
for Alzheimer's disease, 937
for bipolar disorder, 698
in combos for bipolar disorder, 714
ondansetron, 977
OPC 4293, 375
open state, of voltage-sensitive sodium channels, 152f
opiate receptors, 980f
opiates, 977–981
actions on reward circuits, 979f
acute nociceptive pain and, 790f
dependency/addiction, treatment, 980
for fibromyalgia, 811
interaction with MAOIs, 595, 595t
reward and, 977
withdrawal, 979
opioid peptides, 52t
oppositional defiant disorder, 425
in children and adolescents, 877
optimism, in hyperthymic temperament, 460f
Orap. See pimozide (Orap)
orbitofrontal cortex, 198, 199f
CSTC loop from, 212
and impulsivity, 869f
interactions with ACC, 210f
manic episode symptoms linked to, 506
prefrontal projections from, 949
risk taking and, 502f
and schizophrenia symptoms, 261, 262f
orexin, and narcolepsy, 820
orexin-containing neurons
in hypothalamus, 820
sleep/wake switch regulation, 822f
Org 24292, 446
Org 25271, 446

Org 25501, 446
Org 25573, 446
organelles. See also subcellular organelles
destruction of discarded, 15
retrograde transport of discarded, 17f
orgasm, 999
and neurotransmitters, 999f
orlistat, 1010
osanetant (SR142801), 450
overconfidence, in hyperthymic temperament, 460f
oxcarbazepine, 153f
actions as mood stabilizer, 683f
binding site of, 682f
converion to licarbazepine, 681f
for fibromyalgia, 811
mechanism of action
on GABA, glutamate, sigma, and dopamine, 676t
VSSCs, synaptic vesicles, and carbonic anhydrase, 675t
putative clinical actions, 673t
and VSSCs, 707f

P/Q channels, 154, 155t
inhibitors of, 158f
and neurotransmitter release, 155, 156, 156f
P75 (proaptotic receptors), 29t
pain, 775. See also chronic pain; fibromyalgia
acute vs. chronic, 775t
in affective spectrum disorders, 802
definitions, 775
from Internaional Association of the Study of Pain, 777
in depression, 650
descending noradrenergic neurons and, 791f
diabolical learning hypothesis and, 229
in disorder diagnosis, depression and anxiety with, 803
evaluating, 812t
excessive excitatory neurotransmission and, 43
explained, 774
gabapentin for, 687
"gate theory", 795
link to mood and anxiety, 804, 804f
nociception to, 782f
numerical rating scale for monitoring, 813t
opening gate from inside, 800
pregabalin for, 687
preventing permanent syndromes, 802
preventing progression to chronic persistent, 802
psychopharmacologists view of, 777

pain diaries, 813t
pain relievers, opiates as, 977
paliperidone, 404, 405f
    actions as mood stabilizer, 693f
    in combos for bipolar disorder, 713
    pharmacological actions, 693f
    pharmacological icon, 413f
    and sedation, 432f
    sedation risk with, 430
Pamelor. See nortriptyline (Pamelor, Endep, Aventyl)
pancreas, valproic acid toxicity, 677
panic attacks, 731
    excess neurotransmission and, 47f
    from hallucinogens, 990
panic disorder, 723f
    benzodiazepine agonist spectrum in, 742f
    in children, 713
    MAO inhibitors for, 575
    pharmacy, 768f
    treatment, 768
panic, excessive excitatory neurotransmission and, 43
parabrachial nucleus (PBN)
    dopamine pathway from, 272f
    lateral, 204
    and respiratory changes, 729f
paranoia, 324
paranoid projection, 249
paranoid psychosis, 249
    from stimulants, 985
paraphilias, 771
paraventricular nucleus, and sexual drive, 994
paresthesias, 786
parietal lobe, 196f
parkinsonism
    drug-induced, 332
    from SSRIs, 531
Parkinson's disease, 638
    dementia, 920
    dopamine agonists for treatment, 267
    excitotoxicity and, 48f
    levodopa for, MAO-B inhibition and, 579
    nigrostriatal pathway dopamine deficiencies and, 277, 278f
    protoxins and, 582
    quetiapine for, 415
    transplantation of fetal substantia nigra cells for,
Parnate. See tranylcypromine (Parnate)
paroxetine, 99t, 536, 604, 606f
    CYP450 2D6 impact on plasma levels, 607
    as CYP450 2D6 inhibitor, 607f
    icon, 537f

partial agonists, 111f
    actions on ion channel, 136f
    antagonist acting in presence of, 138f
    vs. antagonists, 378f
    light and dark as analogy for, 120
    net effect, 137f
    reversal by antagonist, 115
PBN. See parabrachial nucleus (PBN)
PCP. See phencyclidine (PCP)
peptides, 8f, 12, 52t
    novel, 664f
    synthesis, 11f
perceptual distortions, 248
periaqueductal gray matter, 204, 789
    and avoidance, 728f
    dopamine pathway from, 272f
    and motor responses to fear, 730
perimenopause
    depression and treatment during, 619, 620f
    depression risk during, 615f
    desvenlafaxine for reducing symptoms, 550
periodic limb movement disorder (PLMD), 834t
peripheral afferent neurons
    incoming synapses from, 787
    neuropathic pain and, 785
peripheral pain, 774
    vs. central pain, 776t
peripheral proteins, 12
perospirone, 419, 559f
    pharmacological icon, 419f
peroxisome proliferator activated receptor (PPAR) gamma agonists, for Alzheimer's disease, 936
perphenazine (Trilafon), 331t
personality
    change in dementia, 900
    and stress, 191f
    as stress buffer or amplifier, 190–191
Pertofran. See desipramine (Norpramin, Pertofran)
PET (positron emission tomography), 231
    to measure glucose uptake, 232
phantom pain, 795
pharmacodynamics, 402
pharmacokinetics, 402
pharmacologic G protein-linked receptors, 110t
phase advanced circadian rhythms, 827f
phase delayed circadian rhythms, 826f
phencyclidine (PCP), 144, 696, 993
    and schizophrenia symptoms, 289, 290, 440
phenelzine (Nardil), 575, 579t
phenethylamine, 577

phentermine, with MAOIs, and hypertension, 593*t*
phenylalkylamines, 990
phenylephrine, 592
   with MAOIs, and hypertension, 593*t*
phenylpropanolamine, 593
   with MAOIs, and hypertension, 593*t*
phosphatase, 170*f*
   activation in signal transduction cascade, 65*f*, 74*f*
   calcium activation of, 74
   clash with kinase, 73
   as messenger in cascade, 64
   removal of phosphates from proteins, 76*f*
phosphates
   kinase activation to add to phosphoproteins, 75*f*
   removal from proteins, 76*f*
phosphodiesterases (PDE), 997, 1002
phosphoproteins, 64*f*, 149, 173*f*
   creation, 64, 65*f*
   phosphates added to, 75*f*
   removing phosphatase from, 64, 65*f*
   as signal-transduction target, 71
phosphorylation, 73–78, 149, 795
   abnormal, and neurofibrillary tangles, 902
physical abuse, and synaptogenesis, 34
Pick's disease, cognitive symptoms, 259
piloerection, opiate withdrawal and, 980
pimozide (Orap), 331*t*
   combining 3A4 inhibitor with, 609
   and CYP 450 3A4, 608
pindolol, 651
pineal gland, melatonin secretion from, 844
pipothiazine (Piportil), 331*t*
pituitary
   regulation of prolactin secretion, 362
   SPA action in, 377
pituitary peptides, 52*t*
pizza, tyramine content of commercial-chain, 588*f*
placebo, 514
   response rates, 515*f*
   substitution, 516*f*
plasma membrane transporters, 93
pleasure
   loss
      bupropion for, 556
      as SSRI side effect, 530
      mesolimbic dopamine pathway role in, 272, 276
   reduce ability to experience, 251
pleasure center
   mesolimbic dopamine pathway as, 945, 946*f*
   nucleus accumbens as, 329
PLG (L-prolyl-L-leucy-L-glycinamide), 663
PLMD (periodic limb movement disorder), 834*t*
PMDD (premenstrual dysphoric disorder), 616
   SSRIs for, 522
PMS (premenstrual syndrome), 616
PNU 9639/OSU 6162, 380*f*
polyamine site, 831
polypharmacy, 436, 438*f*
polysialic acid–neuronal cell adhesion molecules (PSA-NCAM), 31*t*
polysomes, 8*f*
   in dendrites, 12
   free, 10*f*, 11
   localization of, 9*f*
POMC (pro-opiomelanocortin), 977, 980*f*
pore, for VSCCs, 153
positive affect, 499*f*
   reduced, 495
      vs. increased negative affect, 643
positive allosteric modulators (PAMs), 130, 141, 144*f*
   benzodiazepines as, 146*f*
   for insomnia, 838*f*
Positive and Negative Syndrome Scale, 253*t*
positron emission tomography (PET), 231
   to measure glucose uptake, 232
posthemisynapse, required elements for, 43*f*
postpartum period
   and bipolar mood episodes, 711
   depression and treatment during, 619
   depression risk during, 615*f*
postpartum psychosis, 619
poststroke dementia, cognitive symptoms, 259
postsynaptic dendrites, 37*f*
   incoming signals from, 7, 7*f*
postsynaptic density proteins, 10
postsynaptic elements, 36
postsynaptic neurons
   nerve impulse propagation, 165*f*
   presynaptic neuron genome communication to genome, 61
   signal propagation, 166*f*
   "talk back" to presynaptic neurons, 54, 57*f*
postsynaptic receptors
   and norepinephrine, 475
   for posthemisynapse, 43*f*
   for synaptic formation, 36
postsynaptic response, increasing, 41
postsynaptic serotonin receptors, excessive stimulation of, 597

postsynaptic site, formation of separate and adjacent, 45f
posttraumatic stress disorder, 193, 194f
   pharmacy, 770f
   reexperiencing in, 730f
   treatment, 770
potassium, 146
   countertransport of, 95
   glutamate transport and, 100
potassium ions, 124f
potentiation, long-term, 167
   calcium influx through NMDA receptors and, 164f
pramipexole, 718
pramlintide, 450, 1011
pravastatin, 609
   and CYP 450 3A4, 608
precursor stem cell
   potential for transplant, 27
   transplantation of,
prefrontal cortex, 2, 196f
   5HT2A receptor activation, in schizophrenia, 360
   and ADHD, 864–870
   areas within, 197–200
   and CSTC loop, 211f
   desensitizing arousal in, 878f
   dopamine increase from NET inhibition, 544, 545f
   dopamine neurotransmission in, 59
   dopaminergic projections and, 210f
   fatigue and, 491
   fetal development, and schizophrenia, 303
   impact on suicidal ideation, 493
   information processing in, dopamine and, 233
   NDRI actions in, 555f
   regulatory importance of dopamine, 544
   and schizophrenia symptoms, 261, 262f
   and sleep disturbances, 491, 494f
   SPA action in, 377
   synaptogenesis, and executive function development, 883f
prefrontal motor cortex, supplemental motor area, 213
prefrontal pyramidal neurons, in ADHD, 873
pregabalin, 156, 157t
   for anxiety disorders, 767
   binding to alpha-2 delta protein, 158
   channel blocking by, 798f
   in combos for bipolar disorder, 715
   for fibromyalgia, 808
   icon, 688f
   mechanism of action

   on GABA, glutamate, sigma, and dopamine, 676t
   VSSCs, synaptic vesicles, and carbonic anhydrase, 675t
   for panic disorder, 768
   putative clinical actions, 673t
   for social anxiety disorder, 769
pregnancy
   antidepressant risks or avoidance during, 618t
   and bipolar mood episodes, 711
   depression during, 616
   estrogen levels during, 617
prehemisynapse, required elements for, 43f
premenstrual dysphoric disorder (PMDD), 616
   SSRIs for, 522
premenstrual phase, bipolar disorder during, 711
premenstrual syndrome (PMS), 616
prenatal gestation, neuron formation, 22
preschool ADHD, 882
presenilin 1, 907
presenilin 2, 907
presynaptic 5HT1A receptors, 348f
presynaptic 5HT1B/D receptors, 347f
presynaptic antagonists, 445f
presynaptic axon terminals, 2f, 5f, 524
   in basket neurons, 4f
   in double bouquet cells, 4f
   in pyramidal cell, 3f
presynaptic D2 receptors, 268, 269f
presynaptic density proteins, 10
presynaptic elements, 36
presynaptic monoamine transporters, 93t
   antidepressants that block, 98
presynaptic nerve, sodium in, 61
presynaptic neurons
   genome communication to postsynaptic neuron genome, 61
   nerve impulse propagation in, 160f
   postsynaptic neurons "talk back" to, 54, 57f
   signal propagation, 166f
   stimulation of, 55f
presynaptic transporters, for monoamines, 95f
presynaptic voltage-sensitive calcium channels (VSCCs), 154
presynaptic zone, 7f
primary afferent neurons (PANs), 775
   cell bodies in dorsal root ganglia, 782
   demyelination of, 786
   response characteristics, 779
   types, 779
primary auditory cortex, 196f
primary insomnia, 831
primary motor cortex, 196f
primary somatosensory cortex, 196f

Pristiq. *See* desvenlafaxine XR (Pristiq)
proapoptotic receptors (P75), 29*t*
pro-opiomelanocortin (POMC), 977, 980*f*
problem solving, 198
procognitive agents, D1-selective agonists as, 448
prodrome
   negative symptoms, 252, 256*f*
   preventing progression to, 227
prodynorphin, 977, 980*f*
proenkephalin, 977, 980*f*
progesterone, 612
projection neurons, 775
prolactin
   amisulpride and, 423
   atypical antipsychotic agents and, 364*f*
   clozapine and, 409
   conventional antipsychotic agents and, 364*f*
   elevation, 336
   inhibiting release, 278
   inhibition by dopamine, 363*f*
   olanzapine and, 411
   quetiapine and, 415
   rise in levels, 334*f*
   risperidone and, 413
   secretion regulation, 362
   serotonin stimulation of, 363*f*
   and sexual desire, 995
   zotepine and, 418
Prolixin (fluphenazine), 331*t*
L-prolyl-L-leucy-L-glycinamide (PLG), 663, 664*f*
promotor element, of gene regulatory region, 83
propoxyphene, interaction with MAOIs, 595, 595*t*
prostaglandins, 1004
protease inhibitors, 405
   and CYP 450 3A4, 609
protein kinase A, G protein-linked receptor activation of, 74
protein kinases, 170*f*
   activation in signal transduction cascade, 73*f*
   and gene activation, 79*f*
   inactive, 72
protein phosphatase, formation, 72
proteins, 8*f*
   and alpha-1 pore-forming unit of VSCC, 153
   cytoplasmic, 13*f*
      transport of, 12
   cytoskeletal support, 10
   destruction of discarded, 15
   functional changes due to activation, 64*f*

   gene encoding of, 179, 181*f*
   glutamate for biosynthesis, 279
   intracellular scaffolding, 42*f*
   ion channel subunits, 126
   peripheral, 12
   phosphates removal from, 76*f*
   postsynaptic density, 10
   presynaptic density, 10
   retrograde transport of discarded, 17*f*
   roles of, 11
   slow transport, 13*f*
   synthesis, 10*f*, 11–12, 78
      in dendrites, 12*f*
Prothiaden (dothiepin), 597*t*
"proton pump", 102
protoxins, and Parkinson's disease, 582
protriptyline (Vivactil), 597*t*
   inhibition of serotonin reuptake pump, 598
Prozac (fluoxetine). *See* fluoxetine (Prozac)
PSA-NCAM (polysialic acid–neuronal cell adhesion molecules), 31*t*
"pseudo anticholinergic" syndrome, 547
pseudocholinesterase, 915
pseudodementia, 912
pseudoephedrine, 593
   with MAOIs, and hypertension, 593*t*
psilocybin, 990
   actions, 992*f*
psychedelic, 990
psychiatric disorders
   abnormal neuronal migration and, 30*f*
   chronic pain link to pathophysiology, 774
   gene expression factors and, 78
   and insomnia, 834*t*
   remission of, risk for relapse, 229
   reward and, 943
   stress diathesis hypothesis, 749
psychiatric insomnia
   and GABA-A PAMs, 842
   treatment, 843*f*
psychiatric symptoms
   and malfunctioning circuits, 229
   progression from stress sensitization to, 226, 226*f*
   sustained and neuron loss, 232*f*
psychomotor agitation, CSTC loop to regulate, 213
psychomotor retardation
   CSTC loop to regulate, 213
   from SSRIs, 531
psychomotor symptoms
   circuits, 497*f*
   in depression, 491

psychopharmacological agents
  and endogenous growth factors, 26f
  gene expression factors and, 78
  major targets, 92f
psychopharmacologic agents, and neurogenesis in hippocampus, 24
psychopharmacologist, symptoms and circuits for, 239–245
psychopharmacology, 943
psychosis, 247
  acute, ziprasidone for, 416
  antipsychotic action to reduce symptoms, 425
  as associated feature in disorders, 249t
  disorders requiring presence as defining feature, 248, 248t
  excess neurotransmission and, 47f
  extreme arousal in, 818
  from improper neuronal migration, 29
  mesolimbic dopamine pathway role in, 272
  neurons regulating, 204
  positive symptoms, 251t
  postpartum, 619
  quetiapine for, 415
  rebound, from discontinued clozapine, 431
psychotherapy, 49, 639
  and brain restructuring, 32
  and endogenous growth factors, 26f
  and neurogenesis in hippocampus, 24, 24f
psychotic depression, symptoms shared with schizophrenia, 258, 259f
psychotic episode, 250
psychotic illness
  combination chemotherapies for, 450
  misconceptions, 247
psychotomimetic, 990
psychotropic drugs
  enzymes as possible indirect targets, 171t
  G protein-linked receptors as target, 107, 114t
    with agonists, 110–112
    with antagonists,
    inverse agonists, 121
    light and dark as analogy for partial agonists, 120
    with no agonist, 108
    with partial agonists, 115–119
  neurotransmitter transporters as targets, 99
  nuclear hormone receptors as potential target, 171t
  selecting based on topographic location of function, 241
  sites of action, 91, 149
    molecular, 91
  transduction cascade as target, 65
  voltage-sensitive ion channels as target, 157t

purines, 52t, 859
Purkinje cells, 5f
  from cerebellum, 3
pyramidal cells, 2, 3f, 6
  axon hillock of, 217
  concept of optimal tuning, 765
  and cortical circuits, 214–221
  excitatory inputs, 219
  excitatory outputs, 215
  fine tuning, 220
  inhibitory contacts close to axons of, 3
  inhibitory inputs, 216
  interneuron input to, 218f
  malfunctioning glutamate input into, 298
  output and input, 295
  output from, 217f
pyramidal neurons
  cortical, tuning, in ADHD, 875f
  prefrontal, in ADHD, 873
pyromania, 1011

QTc prolongation, ziprasidone and, 417
quazepam
  half-life of, 835f
  for insomnia, 837f
Quel kit, 715, 716f
questioning, for negative symptom identification in schizophrenia, 254f
quetiapine, 382f
  5HT6-antagonist properties of, 447
  actions as mood stabilizer, 693f
  binding properties, 414f
  and cardiometabolic risk, 386t
  in combos for bipolar disorder, 715, 716f
  and diabetes, 417
  dosage with carbamazepine, 407f
  half-life of, 836f
  hypnotic actions, 848
  pharmacological actions, 693f
  pharmacological icon, 414f
  potency, and dissociation, 370
  for sedation, 431
  switching to nonsedating agent, 435
  and weight gain risk, 386t
quinidine, 718
quinone oxidoreductase 2, 844

R channels, 155, 155t
R enantiomer
  for citalopram, 538
  at serotonin transporter, 540f
R zopiclone, and eszopiclone, 842t
racemic citalopram, 538
racemic zopiclone, 839, 839f

racing thoughts, 506
  inefficient information processing and, 502f
radafaxine, 554, 556f
RAGS (repulsive axon guidance signals), 31
ramelteon, 839, 844f
  half-life of, 836f
rape, stress vulnerability, 193, 194f
raphe magnus, 205
raphe obscurus, 205
raphe pallidus, 205
raphe pontis, 205
rapid cycling, 454, 456, 458f
  switches, 458f
rapid dissociation, 365, 367, 368f
rapid "off" time, 365
rapid "poop out", 462f
Ras, kinase cascade activation by, 76
rasaligine (Agilect/Azilect), 579t
  for Parkinson's disease, 582
rashes
  from lamotrigine, 683
  from zonisamide, 687
reasoning. *See also* cognitive functioning
  distortions in schizophrenia, 324
rebound, 945
rebound insomnia, 837
rebound psychosis, from discontinued
    clozapine, 431
reboxeine, 99t
reboxetine, 557, 889
  and CYP 450 3A4, 608
  potency for CYP450 2D6 inhibition, 605
recapture, of neurotransmitter, 92
receptor-ion channel complex, other molecules
    binding to, 140
receptor tyrosine kinases, 67, 171, 171t
receptors
  downregulation, 86f
  life cycle, 84f, 87
  optimal amount of stimulation, 221f
  synthesis, 85f
  upregulation, 87f, 88
recognition molecules, 31, 31t, 32f
  for synapse repair and regeneration, 32
recovery, 513f
recurrence of depression, 513f
recurrent collateral, in pyramidal cell, 3f
reduced-risk drinking, 973, 975t
reexperiencing, 730f
regulatory proteins
  of voltage-sensitive sodium channels, 149
  for VSCCs, 155f
regulatory regions of DNA, 79f, 80, 83
reinforcement, 945

relapse, 516, 945
  after antipsychotic treatment, vs. side effects, 341
  after psychiatric disorder remission
    preventing, 230
    risk for, 229
  of depression, 513f
  frequency with drug continuation, 515f
  rates in major depressive disorders, 518f
remission
  antidepressant combinations for, 651
  of psychiatric disorders, risk for relapse, 229
  rates for SNRIs vs. SSRIs, 543
  rates in major depressive disorders, 517f
  by schizophrenic patient, 300
  of symptoms, 513f
  as treatment goal, 512
renewal forgetting, 959
reproductive hormones, across menstrual cycle, 613f
repulsive axon guidance signals (RAGS), 31
"rescue analgesia", 802
resentment, 249
residual symptoms, in depression, 517f
resilience
  from exposure to mild stress, 751
  loss from stress overload, 225
response, to depression treatment, 512, 512f
restless leg syndrome (RLS), 834t
restlessness, from paroxetine withdrawal, 537
retardation, 249
retrograde motor, 8f
  localization of, 9f
retrograde neurotransmission, 57f, 61
retrograde transport, 14–15
  fast, 17f
retrograde vesicle, 8f
  localization of, 9f
reuptake, of neurotransmitter, 92
reuptake pumps, 15
  absence, and dopamine diffusion, 59f
  fast transport of, 15f
reuptake transporters, 36
  for prehemisynapse, 43f
reversal, of dopamine transporter (DAT), 108f
reverse signaling, 61
reversible enzyme inhibitors, 167, 168, 169f
reversible inhibitor of MAO-A (RIMA), 587, 590f
reward
  alcohol and, 970
  blocking mechanisms, 330
  in mesolimbic dopamine system, 336
  conditioning to cues, 952f

reward (*Contd.*)
  mesolimbic dopamine pathway role in, 272, 276
  neurons regulating, 204
  nicotine and, 955
  opiates and, 977
  output, 950, 951*f*
  overvalued in addiction, 951
  reactive bottom-up system, 946, 948*f*
    exposure to drugs, 948
  reflective top-down system, 949, 950*f*
  will power vs. temptation, 952, 954*f*
reward circuits, 945–953
  alcohol and, 971*f*
  disorders of, treatment, 944
  eating disorders and, 1008
  eating, food and, 1010*f*
  hallucinogen action on, 991*f*
  mesolimbic dopamine pathway for, 945, 946*f*
  nicotine action on, 956*f*
  opiate action in, 979*f*
  and psychiatric disorders, 943
  sedative-hypnotics and benzodiazepines actions, 987*f*
  sexual desire and, 996*f*
  stimulants action on, 982*f*
  varenicline actions on, 962*f*
reward conditioning, 959
RGH188, 380*f*
  testing for cocaine abuse treatment, 986
RGS4 (regulator of G-protein signaling), 317
  genes for, 318*f*
ribosomes, 10*f*
  protein synthesis in, 11
riluzole, 686
  and glutamate reduction, 708*f*
  icon, 686*f*
  mechanism of action
    on GABA, glutamate, sigma, and dopamine, 676*t*
    VSSCs, synaptic vesicles, and carbonic anhydrase, 675*t*
  possible actions in bipolar disorder, 698*f*
  putative clinical actions, 673*t*
  sites of action, on glutamate release, 685*f*
RIMA (reversible inhibitor of MAO-A), 587, 590*f*
rimonabant, 449, 973, 990
  for alcohol dependency, 977
  for marijuana dependency, 987
risk gene, with no symptoms, 187*f*
risk taking, orbital frontal cortex and, 502*f*
risperidone, 412, 429, 559*f*
  actions as mood stabilizer, 693*f*

and cardiometabolic risk, 386*t*
in combos for bipolar disorder, 713
conversion to paliperidone, 405*f*
as CYP 2D6 substrate, 404, 405*f*
and diabetes, 417
pharmacological actions, 693*f*
pharmacological icon, 412*f*
potency, and dissociation, 370
raising levels of, 406*f*
and sedation, 430, 432*f*
for treating irritability, 427
and weight gain risk, 386*t*
rivastigmine, 924
  actions, 928*f*
  icon, 926*f*
RLS (restless leg syndrome), 834*t*
RNA, 10*f*
RNA polymerase, 80, 170*f*
  and gene activation, 79*f*
ropinirole, 718
rosiglitazone, for Alzheimer's disease, 936
rough endoplasmic reticulum, 8*f*, 10*f*, 11*f*
  localization of, 9*f*
  peptide synthesis in, 11, 12
RSK (ribosomal S6 kinase), 66*f*, 76
rush, from opiates, 977

S-adenosyl-methionine (SAMs), 630
  in combos for bipolar disorder, 714
  trimonoamine modulation of, 632*f*
S enantiomer
  for citalopram, 538
  in escitalopram, 539
  at serotonin transporter, 540*f*
sad temperament, 460*f*
sadness, depressed patient neuronal response, 508*f*
sagittal plane, for brain visualization, 200*f*
SALAs (selective amyloid lowering agents), 939
salience of stimulus, 868
SAMs. *See* S-adenosyl-methionine (SAMs)
sarcosine, 442
saredutant, 665
SARIs. *See* serotonin antagonist/reuptake inhibitors (SARIs)
sarizotan (EMD128130), 380*f*
SB277011A, testing for cocaine abuse treatment, 986
Scale for Assessment of Negative Symptoms, 253*t*
"scared to death", 731
scary faces, schizophrenic patient response to, 323*f*
SCH1390499, 939

SCH1396674, 939
Schedule for the Deficit Syndrome, 253*t*
schizoaffective disorder, 461, 462*f*
   symptoms shared with schizophrenia, 258, 259*f*
schizophrenia
   5HT2A receptors activation in prefrontal cortex, 360
   acquired vs. inherited, 302
   atypical antipsychotics to improve symptoms, 355
   best long-term outcomes, 400*f*
   bifeprunox for treating, 424
   brain restructuring and, 44
   cognitive symptoms, 259, 259*t*
   combination chemotherapies for, 450
   diagnosis, value of deconstructing, 264
   excessive excitatory neurotransmission and, 43
   excitotoxicity and, 48*f*, 302, 303*f*
   fetal brain insult and, 303
   free radical scavengers, 442*f*
   genetic basis, 304
   glutametergic treatments for, 442*f*
   ideal treatment of, 358
   integrated dopamine hypothesis, 279, 281*f*
   integrated theory
      and dopamine partial agonists, 378*f*
      and hit-and-run actions, 373*f*
      and serotonin-dopamine antagonists, 367*f*
   mesocortical dopamine hypothesis of negative, cognitive, and affective symptoms of, 277*f*
   as more than psychosis, 249–253
   negative symptoms, 251, 251*t*
      causes, 260*f*
      observation to identify, 252, 254*f*
      primary and secondary, 253*t*
      in prodomal phase, 252, 256*f*
      questioning to identify, 254*f*
      reasons to measure, 253*t*
      scales for assessing, 253*t*
      shared with other disorders, 258
   neurodegenerative hypothesis, 298, 300*f*
   neurodevelopmental hypothesis, 308*f*
   neuroimaging circuits in, 319
   neuron wiring and, 33*f*
   neutral stimuli and, 324*f*
   NMDA receptor hypofunction hypothesis of, 288, 290*f*
   patient responsiveness to antipsychotic treatment, 300
   positive and negative symptoms, 250*f*

positive symptom pharmacy, 425, 426*f*
positive symptoms, 250, 251*t*
   link to mesolimbic/nucleus accumbens area, 262
   shared with other disorders, 259*f*
presymptomatic and prodromal treatment, 438, 439*f*
progressive nature of, 298
rapid clinical assessment, 255*t*
risperidone effectiveness for, 413
stages, 301*f*
substance abuse incidence in, 276
subtle molecular abnormalities and, 192*f*
susceptibility genes for, 309*t*
symptoms, 248, 257*f*
   overlap, 258*f*
   shared with other illnesses, 258–264
   treatment, vs. disease treatment, 425
ziprasidone for, 416
schizophrenic patients
   life expectancy of, 250
   siblings of, 320
      n-back test in, 322*f*
   smoking and drug abuse by, 336, 449
   suicide in, 250
Schwann cells, cytokines from, 787
SCN (suprachiasmatic nucleus), melatonin-sensitive neurons in, 820
scolopamine, and memory disturbance, 918
SDA. *See* serotonin-dopamine antagonists (SDA)
second messenger G protein-linked receptors, 110*t*
secretory granule, 8*f*
   localization of, 9*f*
secretory proteins, 11*f*, 12
   fast transport of, 14, 16*f*
secretory vesicles, fast transport of, 14, 15*f*
sedation, 818
   antipsychotic agents and, 396–400
   avoiding, 399, 401*f*
   as goal, 398
   histamine 1 receptors and, 830
   long-term avoidance, 399*f*
   NET inhibition and, 558
   quetiapine and, 415
   receptors mediating, 397*f*
   as short-term therapeutic tool, 398*f*
   vs. somnolence, 400*f*
   as valproic acid side effect, 677
   zotepine and, 418
sedation pharmacy, 430, 432*f*

sedative-hypnotics
  actions on reward circuits, 987f
  binding site of, 988f
  dependency/addiction, 986
segmental central sensitization syndromes, 795, 799f
seizures
  clozapine or zotepine and increased risk, 404, 410
  excess neurotransmission and, 47f
  excessive excitatory neurotransmission and, 43
  reduction with Levetiracetam, 102
  zotepine and, 418
selective amyloid lowering agents (SALAs), 939
selective attention, 211
  circuits, 866f
selective norepinephrine reuptake inhibitors (NRIs). *See* norepinephrine selective reuptake inhibitors (NRIs)
selegiline, 576, 579t
  for Alzheimer's disease, 936
  for Parkinson's disease, 582
  transdermal delivery system for, 587, 588, 591f
    MAO inhibitors, 591
  for treating nicotine dependence, 967
self-confidence, loss
  bupropion for, 556
  as SSRI side effect, 530
self-esteem, 506
self-mutilation, 425
semaphorins, 31
sensitization
  in central nervous system, 795, 797f
  to stress, 749–755
    child abuse, 751
    in normal circuits, 225, 225f
    preemptive treatments, 226
    presymptomatic and prodromal treatment, 227f
    progression to psychiatric symptoms, 226, 226f
sensory/discriminatory pathway, 784
SEP 227, 229, 556f
Sequenced Treatment Alternatives to Relieve Depression (STAR-D) trial, 516
Serentil (mesoridazine), 331t
serial learning, impaired, in schizophrenia, 257
d-serine, 441, 443f
  production, 283, 284f
serine hydroxyl methyl transferace (SHMT), 627f
d-serine racemase, 285

l-serine, glycine synthesis from, 285
serotonergic agents, therapeutic effects, 745f
serotonergic hypnotics, 845
serotonergic neurons, descending, and pain, 793f
serotonin 1A combo, for depression, 652f
serotonin 2A combo, 652f
serotonin-2C antagonist, histamine-1 with, and appetite stimulation, 387f
serotonin (5HT), 220, 318f
  1A agonists or antagonists, 447
  5HT1A agonist, mirtazapine action, 561
  5HT1A partial agonist, and anxiety, 746f
  5HT1A receptors
    effect on gluatmate release, 361f
    SARIs action at, 570f
  5HT1D antagonist action by ziprasidone, 418
  5HT2A antagonist binding to 5HT2A receptor, and dopamine release, 358
  5HT2A antagonists
    and D2 antagonists, 365
    hyperprolactinemia reduction, 362
    and inhibitory action of serotonin 1A on glutamate release, 571
    reduction of positive symptoms, 362f
  5HT2A receptors
    blockade at, 574f
    effect on gluatmate release, 361f
    and gene expression from 5HT1A receptors, 573f
    hallucinogen stimulation, 991
    NE and DA disinhibition at HT1A receptors, 571–574
    and positive symptoms improvment, 359, 362
    regulation of NE and DA release, 484f
    SARIs action at, 569, 569f
  5HT2A-selective antagonists/inverse agonists, 446
  5HT2C antagonist, mirtazapine action, 563
  5HT2C receptors, 659
    agonists or antagonists, 447
    fluoxetine blockade of, 534f
    functions, 349f
    NE and DA disinhibition at HT1A receptors, 571–574
    olanzapine and, 411
    regulation of dopamine in nucleus accumbens, 486f
    regulation of NE and DA release, 485f
    serotonin action, 532
    and weight gain, 383

5HT3 antagonists, 563
5HT3 receptors
　pentameric structure, 126
　stimulation of, 531
5HT6 antagonists, physiological role, 447
5HT7 antagonists, 447
5HT21 receptors, agonism of, 381*f*
and alpha 2 antagonists, 560*f*
antagonists synergy with SERT inhibition, 568–574
antidepressants' enhancement of, 98
antidepressants impact on synaptic action, 520
antipsychotic agents and, 691, 692*f*
and anxiety regulation in amygdala, 241
and arousal spectrum, 817, 817*f*
depression from deficiency, 520*f*
disinhibition, 562*f*
dorsolateral prefontal cortex regulation by, 265*f*
and fear processing by amygdala, 234
genes, expression stimulation through 5HT1A receptors, 572*f*
genetics, and life stressors, 747*f*
glutamate release stimulation, 575*f*
increasing release after alpha 2 antagonist, 559
information processing in amygdala and, 744
interaction with dopamine, in nigrostriatal dopamine pathway, 353*f*
mirtazapine actions at synapses, 564*f*
and mood disorders, 474
norepinephrine regulation of, 480, 480*f*
　as accelerator, 482*f*
　bidirectional control, 483*f*
　as brake, 481*f*
novel targets, 659
production, 344*f*
projections, 205, 206*f*
prolactin stimulation of, 363*f*
as psychotropic drug target, 128
psychotropic drugs and, 53
regulation of dopamine release, 354*f*
regulation of NE and DA release, 477
release
　within CSTC loop, 211
　norepinephrine regulation of, 476
reuptake, 98*f*
synthesis and termination of action, 343
termination of action, 345*f*
tricyclic antidepressant to block reuptake pump, 598
serotonin agonists, and 5HT2A antagonists, 378

serotonin antagonist/reuptake inhibitors (SARIs), 565, 567*f*
　actions at serotonin synapses, 567*f*
　mechanism of action
　　5HT2A antagonism and inhibitory action at 5HT1A, 577*f*
　　baseline postsynaptic actions, 568*f*
　　disinhibition of norepinephrine and dopamine, 578*f*
　　gene expression, 573*f*
　　glutamate release inhibition, 576*f*
　　glutamate release stimulation, 575*f*
　　serotonin excitatory at 5HT2A receptors, 569*f*
　　serotonin inhibitory at 5HT1A receptors, 570*f*
　　synergy between 5HT1A and 5HT2A, 571*f*
serotonin deficiency syndrome, 530
serotonin-dopamine antagonists (SDA), 342, 343*f*
　for aggression management, 427*f*
　for cognitive function improvement, 428*f*
　in development, 368*f*
　for first-line treatment of schizophrenia positive symptoms, 425
　integrated theory of schizophrenia and, 367*f*
　and mesocortical dopamine pathway, 359*f*
　for negative symptoms in schizophrenia, 428*f*
　new options, 446
　switching to DPA, 436*f*
serotonin neuron, somatodendritic area of, 526, 527*f*
serotonin neurotransmitter, 128*t*
　as psychotropic drug indirect target, 116
　as psychotropic drug target, 114
serotonin norepinephrine disinhibitors (SNDIs), 558
serotonin-norepinephrine-dopamine-reuptake inhibitors (SNDRIs), 661
serotonin norepinephrine reuptake inhibitors (SNRIs), 99*t*, 541, 793*f*
　actions, 543*f*
　bicifidine, 552, 552*f*
　for chronic pain, 774
　for dementia, 935
　for depressed women with fluctuating estrogen, 623*f*
　desvenlafaxine, 549
　　icon, 549*f*
　duloxetine (Cymbalta, Xeristar), 550
　　icon, 550*f*
　for fibromyalgia, 808
　for generalized anxiety disorder, 765

Index | 1107

serotonin norepinephrine reuptake inhibitors
 (SNRIs) (*Contd.*)
 icon, 541*f*
 interference with slow-wave sleep, 848
 listing, 541*t*
 LuAA34893, 552, 552*f*
 milnacipran (Ixel, Toledomin), 551
  icon, 551*f*
 for neuropathic pain, 792
 for panic disorder, 742, 768
 potential side effects of NET inhibition, 546
 remission rates compared with SSRIs, 543
 serotonergic, noradrenergic and
  dopaminergic pathways and, 544–547
 sibutramine, 552, 552*f*
 for social anxiety disorder, 769
 for vasomotor symptom treatment, 626*f*
 venlafaxine XR (Effexor XR; Efexor XR),
  547–549
   conversion to desvenlafaxine, 548, 548*f*
   icon, 548*f*
serotonin partial agonists (SPAs), 342, 382*f*
 atypical antipsychotic agents and, 377
serotonin receptors, 343, 346*f*
 5HT1A and 5HT2A, 345
 5HT1A autoreceptors, 348*f*
 5HT1A receptors, 351*f*
 5HT1B/D autoreceptors, 347*f*
 5HT2A antagonist reduction of EPS,
  351–353
 5HT2A receptors, 351, 351*f*
  antagonist reduction of negative
   symptoms, 354–358
 5HT3 receptors, 349*f*
 5HT6 receptors, 349*f*
 5HT7 receptors, 349*f*
 postsynaptic, 343–351
  excessive stimulation of, 597
  impact of, 344
  possible functions, 349*f*
 presynaptic, 343–351
serotonin reuptake inhibitor (SRI), 543*f*
 interaction with MAOIs, 595, 596*f*
serotonin reuptake pump. *See* serotonin
  transporter (SERT)
serotonin selective reuptake inhibitors (SSRIs),
  99*t*, 244*f*
 action potential, 524*f*
 citalopram, 538
  icon, 538*f*
 common features, 524
 for dementia, 935
 for depressed women with fluctuating
  estrogen, 622*f*

escitalopram, 99*t*, 539
 icon, 541*f*
 and estrogen impact, 624
fluoxetine (Prozac), 532–536. *See also*
  fluoxetine (Prozac)
fluvoxamine, 99*t*, 405, 446, 537
 icon, 538*f*
 for generalized anxiety disorder, 765
 interference with slow-wave sleep, 848
 listing, 523*t*
 mechanism of action, 525*f*
 and pain treatment, 789
 for panic disorder, 742, 768
paroxetine, 99*t*, 536
 icon, 537*f*
patient response to different, 532
pharmacological and molecular mechanism of
  action, 524–528
plus NDRI,
remission rates compared with SNRIs, 543
secondary pharmacological properties, 531*f*
serotonin pathways and receptors that
  hypothetically mediate actions, 529–531
sertraline, 535
 icon, 536*f*
side effects of, 530
for social anxiety disorder, 769
tolerance to side effects, 527
for vasomotor symptom treatment, 625*f*
serotonin, stress and anxiety disorders, 741–749
serotonin syndrome, 595
serotonin transporter (SERT), 93, 94, 95*f*, 221*f*
 and amygdala overreaction to fearful faces,
  745
 cocaine ability to inhibit, 983
 gene for, 319*f*
 inhibition of, 524
 MDMA as inhibitor, 991
 R vs. S enantiomer at, 540*f*
 SSRI block of, 529*f*
 subtle molecular abnormalities and, 237*f*
 transport of "ecstacy", 95
SERT. *See* serotonin transporter (SERT)
sertindole, 404, 419
 5HT6-antagonist properties of, 447
 dosage with carbamazepine, 407*f*
 pharmacological icon, 420*f*
 and QTc prolongation, 417
sertraline, 99*t*, 535
 and CYP 450 3A4, 608
 icon, 536*f*
 potency for CYP450 2D6 inhibition, 605
setiptilene, 565
sexual desire, and reward circuits, 996*f*

sexual dysfunction, 537, 651, 993–1007
  compulsive sexual behavior, 1007
  erectile dysfunction, 999, 1003f
    age and, 1000f
    prevalence of, 1000f
    psychopharmacology, 1002
    treatment, 1003f
  hypoactive sexual desire disorder (HSDD), 1004, 1005f
    dopamine and, 1007f
    matching to circuits, 1006f
    treatment, 1008f
  mirtazapine to avoid, 562
  pharmacology and, 1009t
  from SSRIs, 531
sexual response phases, 993–1007
  arousal, 995
    neurotransmitters and, 997f
    nitric oxide (NO) and, 998f
  libido, 993
  orgasm, 999
  psychopharmacology of, 995f
shift-work sleep disorder, 856
  symptoms shared with other disorders, 869t
SHMT (serine hydroxyl methyl transferase), 627f
shopping, compulsive, 1011
siblings of schizophrenic patients, 320
  n-back test in, 322f
sibutramine, 552, 552f
  interaction with MAOIs, 595t
  with MAOIs, and hypertension, 593t
sigma-1 agonists/antagonists, 446
sigma-1 receptor binding
  of fluvoxamine, 537
  of sertraline, 535
sigma 1 site, 718
"sigma enigma", 446, 537
signal cascade molecules, 36
  for posthemisynapse, 43f
signal propagation, from presynaptic to postsynaptic, 166f
signal-to-noise ratio, 220f
  enhancing, 220
  in prefrontal cortex, 873, 875f
signal transduction cascades, 61–88
  biological responses to long term effects of late gene products, 78
  first messengers, 67
  gene expression, 73–88
  gene products targeted by, 77
  later messengers, 71–73
  as psychotropic drug target, 65
  second messenger, 67

second messenger formation, 65–71
  slow onset, 62f, 63f
  time course of, 64f, 65f
  types, 65, 66f
  ultimate target, 71
  valproate and, 674, 679f
signals, neuron reception of, 6
sildenafil (Viagra), 1002
"silent" agonists, 111f
  vs. inverse agonist, 121
simvastatin
  and CYP 450 3A4, 608
  risk of muscle damage, 609
Sinequan. See doxepin (Sinequan, Adapin)
skeletal muscle, insulin resistance in, 387, 390f
SLC 1 gene family, 100
  as psychotropic drug target, 99
SLC 6 gene family, 94–99, 100
  as psychotropic drug target, 99
SLC 18 gene family, 93
  vesicular monoamine transporters (VMATs) in, 102
sleep
  5HT2A receptors and, 349f
  benzodiasepine-sensitive GABA-A receptors for regulating, 738
  circuits, 494f
  histamine 1 receptors and, 830
  histamine and, 209f
  neurobiology of, 816–831
  processes regulating, 823f
  quetiapine for improving, 414f
  serotonin projections regulation of, 205, 206f
  serotonin receptors and, 345
  slow-wave, 848
  trazodone to improve, 566
  as vital sign, 816
sleep aids, for fibromyalgia, 811
sleep disturbances, 506, 804
  brain areas impacting, 491
  gabapentin for, 688
  pregabalin for, 688
sleep hygiene, 850t
sleep promoter, 819, 822f
sleep/wake disorders, arousal networks and, 873
sleep/wake switch, 207, 819, 822f
  delayed turn on, 826f
  in elderly, 824, 827f
  insomnia and, 825f
  neurotransmitters regulating, 821
  and sleepiness, 824f

Index | 1109

sleepiness/hypersomnia in daytime, 650
  vs. alcohol consumption, 851*t*
  causes, 850*t*
  in depression, 649
  evaluating, 852*t*
  explained, 850
  impact of, 851*t*
  initial assessment, 852*t*
  problems from, 854
  quantifying severity, 851, 853*f*
  sleepiness circuits, 821*f*
  treatment
    agents for, 857
    decision process, 854
slow transport motor, 13*f*
  for microtubules and neurofilaments, 14*f*
slow-wave sleep, 848
SLV313, 375, 380*f*
SLV314, 375, 380*f*
SM13493/lurasidone, 368*f*
"smoked over", 962
smoking. *See also* nicotine
  by ADHD patients, 880
  CYP450 1A2 and, 404, 404*f*
  as CYP450 inducer, 609
  power of addiction,
  by schizophrenic patients, 336, 449
  vs. transdermal nicotine administration, 966*f*
smoking cessation, treatment, 128
smooth muscle
  L channel and, 155
  relaxation, and erection, 1004
SNAP 25, 157*f*
snare proteins, 155, 157*f*
  for prehemisynapse, 43*f*
SNDRIs (serotonin-norepinephrine-dopamine-reuptake inhibitors), 661
SNRIs. *See* serotonin norepinephrine reuptake inhibitors (SNRIs)
social anxiety disorder, 724*f*
  fluvoxamine for, 538
  pharmacy, 769*f*
  treatment, 769
social phobia, MAO inhibitors for, 575
social stigma, of electroconvulsive therapy, 634
sodium
  and monoamine transporter affinity for substrates, 95
  in presynaptic nerve, 61
sodium channels, 145
  voltage-sensitive (VSSCs), 60, 148, 149*f*
sodium/chloride-coupled transporters, 93

sodium-dependent cotransporters, monamine transporters as, 95
sodium ions, 124*f*
sodium oxybate, 859. *See also* gamma hydroxybutyrate (GHB)
sodium potassium ATPase (adenosine triphosphatase), 95, 96*f*
"sodium pump", 95, 96*f*
solute carrier SLC6 gene family, 93
soma, 1, 2*f*
  in basket neurons, 4*f*
  cell nucleus in, 8
  and dendrites, 6
  in double bouquet cells, 4*f*
  genome in, 7
  in pyramidal cell, 3*f*
  synapse formation on, 36
somatic syndromes, functional, 777*t*
somatic zone, 7*f*
somatization disorder, 771
somatodendritic alpha 2 receptors, 475, 479*f*
somatodendritic autoreceptor, 344, 348*f*
somatodendritic dopamine D2 receptors, 271*f*
somatodendritic receptors, 60
somatodendritic zone, 6, 7*f*
somatosensory association cortex, 196*f*
somatosensory cortex, 775
somnolence, vs. sedation, 400*f*
SPAs. *See* serotonin partial agonists (SPAs)
"special K", 993
spinal cord, 203*f*
  facilitation pathways, 789
  neurotransmitters modulating pain processing in, 783*f*
  nociceptive pathways to, 778
  nociceptive pathways to brain from, 782
spinal norepinephrine pathway, descending, 789
spinal serotenergic pathway, descending, 789
spines, in double bouquet cells, 4*f*
spinobulbar tracts, 775
spinophylin, genes for, 319*f*
spinothalamic tract, 775
spiny dendrites, 5*f*
spiny neurons, 5*f*
sprouting, 797*f*
SR 147778, 449
SR 241586, 450
SR141716 A, 449
SR31742A, 446
SSR 146977, 450
SSR-591813 (dianicline), 960
SSR125047, 446
SSR180711, 449

SSR181507, 380f
SSR591813, 449
SSRIs. *See* serotonin selective reuptake inhibitors (SSRIs)
ST198, testing for cocaine abuse treatment, 986
stabilizers, 111f
   partial agonists as, 134, 135
Stablon (tianeptine, Coaxil), 597t
Stahl, S.M., *Essential Psychopharmacology: The Prescriber's Guide*, 408, 409
STAR-D (Sequenced Treatment Alternatives to Relieve Depression) trial, 516
statins, for Alzheimer's disease, 936
Stelazine (trifluoperazine), 331t
stem cells
   embryonic, differentiation, 24
   precursor
      potential for transplant, 27
      transplantation of,
steroids, 66f
Stevens-Johnson syndrome, 683, 687
stimulants
   abuse, 981
      by ADHD patients, 870
      long-term effects, 984
      progression, 985f
   actions, on reward circuits, 982f
   for ADHD, 884
      with atypical antipsychotics, 879
      mechanism of action, 887f
      pulsatile vs. slow/sustained, 890f
   and blood pressure, 593
   interference with slow-wave sleep, 848
   mechanism of action, 103
   monoamine transporters as targets, 99t
   paranoid psychosis from, 985
   probability of dependence, 968t
   and reward, 982
   SNRI plus, 656f
   for wakefulness, 858
stimulus, salience of, 868
stress
   and ADHD and comorbidity, 893f
   benefits of mild, in childhood, 750
   brain atrophy from, 748
   comorbidities, and arousal levels in ADHD, 877
   development of psychiatric symptoms, 186f
   early exposure to, 752f
   genetics and response to, 747f
   hippocampal volume reduction with, 748f
   hippocampus sensitivity to, 24, 24f
   and hypothalamic-pituitary-adrenal axis, 752, 753f

and mental illness, 185
and normal circuits, 224, 224f
and personality, 190–191, 191f
progression to anxiety disorders, treatment, 754
sensitization, 749–755
   child abuse, 751
   in normal circuits, 225, 225f
   preemptive treatments, 226
   presymptomatic and prodromal treatment, 227f
   progression to psychiatric symptoms, 226, 226f
and synapse loss, 25f
stress diathesis hypothesis, 185, 186f
   breaking point, 190
   multiple risk genes with breakdown, 189f
   multiple risk genes with no breakdown, 189f
   no risk gene and normal function, 188f
   one risk gene and normal function, 189f
   with psychiatric symptoms, 188f
stress-induced affective disorders, novel treatments, 754f
stress-related brain atrophy, reversing, 891
striatal complex
   and CSTC loop, 211f
   and executive function, 212f
striatum, 3, 203f
   cell bodies for acetylcholine in, 206
   dopamine reuptake pumps in, 59
   interaction with cortex, 210
   NDRI actions in, 555f
   SPA action in, 377
   spiny neurons in, 5f
stroke, 426
   from cortisol in fear response, 730
   excitotoxicity and, 48f, 302, 303f
Stroop test, 235, 238f
   and dorsal anterior cingulate cortex, 238f
subcellular organelles,b 6–10
   localization of, 9f
subgenual area, 200, 212
substance abuse, 704f. *See also specific substance types*
   with ADHD, 880
      as treatment priority, 880, 881f
   bipolar disorder associated with, 463
   diabolical learning and, 948, 951, 953, 959
   incidence in schizophrenia, 276
   orbital frontal cortex and, 870
   overvalued reward in addiction, 951
   probability after use, 968t
   questions for treating, 944t

substance abuse (*Contd.*)
 topiramate and, 687
 treatment, 959
 will power vs. temptation, 952, 954*f*
"substance-induced mood disorder", 463
substance P antagonists, 449, 665
substantia nigra, 277
 spiny neuron input from, 3
 transplantation of fetal cells,
substrates, 167
subsyndromal states, 227
suicidal ideation, 493
 in young adults, from antidepressants, 520
suicidality
 circuits, 498*f*
 in female adolescents, from antidepressants, 617
 in schizophrenic patients, 250
  attempts, 425
  clozapine to reduce, 410, 429, 430*f*
  unrecognized bipolar disorder and, 468
"suicide inhibitor", 168, 168*f*
suicide, risk in depressed mothers, 618
sulpiride (Dolmatil), 331*t*
 clinical actions of, 371
 pharmacological icon, 423*f*
sundowning, 942
superiority, attitude of, 249
supplemental motor area, 197
suprachiasmatic nucleus (SCN),
  melatonin-sensitive neurons in, 820
"suprasegmental" central sensitization
  syndromes, 798, 801*f*
Surmontil (trimipramine), 597*t*
susceptibility genes, 304
 for schizophrenia, 309*t*
sustained attention circuit, 867*f*
SV2A transporter, 102, 156, 157*f*
switching antipsychotic agents, 431, 433*f*
 process to avoid, 433*f*
sympathetic nervous system
 and neuropathic pain, 786
 noradrenergic receptor simulation in, 547
sympathomimetic amines, decongestant
  interaction with drugs boosting, 591
symptom-based selection of antidepressants, 643, 644*f*
 algorithm for, 645*f*
symptom domains, localization of, 261, 262*f*
symptom endophenotypes, 180*f*
 vs. biological endophenotype, 229
 in path between gene and mental illness, 185
symptoms
 clinical strategy to reduce, 239

deconstructing syndromes into, 240*f*
localization in brain, 241
matching to circuits, 242*f*
overlapping among many syndromes, 869*t*
treatment based on, 244*f*
synapses, 1
 communication between neurons at, 54
 competitive elimination, 41–49
 enlarged, 38*f*
 formation by age, 49*f*
 formation failure, 34
 formation process, 36, 39*f*, 45*f*
  decorating, 43*f*
  intraneuronal scaffolding, 42*f*
  ordering supplies, 40*f*
  scaffolding, 41*f*
 loss of, 24, 25*f*, 35
  sustained symptoms and, 230
 many vs. few connections, 35*f*
 maximum in brain, at age 6, 41
 normal connection, 25*f*
 removal of connections during adolescence, 42
 strength of, and survival or elimination, 313
 strengthening, 44*f*
synaptic cleft, 38*f*
synaptic flexibility, 44*f*
synaptic plasticity, 35–41, 144
synaptic vesicles, 8*f*
 fast transport of, 14, 15*f*
 levetiracetam mechanism of action at SV2A sites, 690*f*
 localization of, 9*f*
 for prehemisynapse, 43*f*
synaptobrevin, 157*f*
synaptogenesis, 22, 31–35, 167
 abnormal, 307
  genes causing, 311*f*
 from gene expression, 78, 304
 messenger triggering of, 64
synaptotagmin, 157*f*
syndromes, 178
 deconstructing into symptoms, 240*f*
syntaxin, 157*f*
synthetic enzymes, 36
 for prehemisynapse, 43*f*

T channels, 155, 155*t*
T3, in combos for bipolar disorder, 714
tachykinins, 52*t*, 664, 664*t*
tacrine, 923
tadalafil (Cialis), 1002
talnetant, 450
tandospirone, 447

tangles. *See* neurofibrillary tangles
tardive dyskinesia, 88, 332, 333*f*
   clozapine and, 409
   neuroleptic-induced, 277
   reversal, 333
   SDAs and,
   from unwanted D2 receptor blockade, 382
tau proteins, hyper-phosphoylation, 906
taurine, 976
TC1734 (ispronicline), 941
TC1827, 449
TCAs. *See* tricyclic antidepressants (TCAs)
temazepam
   half-life of, 835*f*
   for insomnia, 837*f*
temperament, 190, 456
   depressive, 460*f*
   hyperthymic, 460*f*
   with depressive episode, 466*f*
temporal lobe, 196*f*
temptation, vs. will power, 952, 954*f*
Tennessee mood shine, 715, 716*f*
tension, 260
Tercian (cyamemazine), 331*t*
   pharmacological icon, 421*f*
terminal autoreceptor, 344
testosterone, 1006
   and sexual motivation, 994
tetrahydrobiopterin (BH4), 625
   cofactor for trimonoamine neurotransmitter synthesis, 629*f*
   MTHF regulation of, 628*f*
delta-9-tetrahydrocannabinol (THC), 986
   actions on reward circuits, 989*f*
tetrahydrofolate (THF), 627*f*
thalamic dopamine pathway, 204, 279
thalamocortical glutamate pathways, 289*f*
thalamus, 202*f*
   and CSTC loop, 211*f*
   filters and sleep/wake disorders, 818
   dopamine pathway to, 272*f*
   dopamine projections to, 204*f*
   GABA in, and insomnia, 820*f*
   glutamatergic excitatory projections from, 219*f*
   inefficient information processing, and sleep disturbances, 503*f*
   interaction with cortex, 210
   mesolimbic dopamine hyperactivity and, 296*f*
   sensory filter from GABA neurons, 292, 293*f*
   dopamine and, 294*f*
   sensory input inhibition from, 295*f*
   and sleep disturbances, 491, 494*f*
   spiny neuron input from, 3

THC (delta-9-tetrahydrocannabinol), 986
   actions on reward circuits, 989*f*
theophyllin, interactions with fluvoxamine, 604
theophylline, 606*f*
therapeutic nihilism, 976
thermoregulation, disruption in, 597
THF-R (methylene tetrahydrofolate reductase), 627*f*
THF (tetrahydrofolate), 627*f*
thioridazine (Mellaril), 331*t*
   and CYP450 2D6 inhibitors, 608
thiothixene (Navane), 331*t*
Thorazine (chlorpromazine), 328, 331*t*
thyroid
   dysfunction, men vs. women, 711
   impact on cytoplasmic receptors, 75
thyroid hormones, 631
   as augmenting agent, 634*f*
   for bipolar disorder, 699
   in combination treatments for depression, 652*f*
   and depressed mood, 633*f*
tiagabine, 100
   for fibromyalgia, 810
tianeptine (Coaxil, Stablon), 597*t*
tics
   in children, 877
   dopamine hyperactivity in nigrostriatal pathway and, 277, 278*f*
tingling, from paroxetine withdrawal, 537
tissue damage, 779*f*
tissue growth factors, in brain, 174
TMMs (trimonoaminergic modulators), 609–639
   estrogen as, 610
   L-5-methyltetrahydrofolate (MTHF) as, 625
TMS (transcranial magnetic stimulation), 637, 637*f*
tobacco. *See* nicotine
Tofranil. *See* imipramine (Tofranil)
TOH (tyrosine hydroxylase), 266, 266*f*
Toledomin (milnacipran, Ixel), 99*t*, 541*t*
tolerance, 945
tonic inhibition, 737
topiramate, 686, 709
   in combos for bipolar disorder, 715
   for fibromyalgia, 811
   icon, 687
   mechanism of action
      on GABA, glutamate, sigma, and dopamine, 676*t*
      VSSCs, synaptic vesicles, and carbonic anhydrase, 675*t*

topiramate (*Contd.*)
   putative clinical actions, 673*t*
   and VSSCs, 707*f*
   and weight loss, 1011
topographical representation of function, 211
Tourette's syndrome, 771
toxic epidermal necrolysis, 683, 687
toxins, neuron or DNA damage from, 28
tramadol, interaction with MAOIs, 595, 595*t*
transcranial magnetic stimulation (TMS), 637, 637*f*
transcription factor, 87
   and gene activation, 79*f*
transdermal nicotine administration, vs. smoking, 966*f*
transmembrane region receptors, 109*f*
   top view, 110*f*
transmembrane segments, of alpha pore-forming protein, 147
transport function. *See also* fast transport
   axons and dendrites for, 10
tranylcypromine (Parnate), 575, 576, 579*t*
trazodone, 565, 839, 846*f*
   5HT2A inhibition by, 569
   for anxiety disorders, 767
   for fibromyalgia, 811
   half-life of, 836*f*
   as hypnotic, 845
   icon, 567*f*
   for insomnia, 566
   for panic disorder, 768
   for social anxiety disorder, 769
treatment-resistant mood disorders, 473
treatment, symptoms and circuits for approach to selecting, 239*t*
tremor
   as antipsychotic side effect, 341
   nigrostrial pathway dopamine deficiencies and, 277
triazolam
   and CYP 450 3A4, 608
   half-life of, 836*f*
   for insomnia, 837*f*
   and sedation, 609
trichotillomania, 771
tricyclic antidepressants (TCAs), 99*t*, 542, 597–603
   for anxiety disorders, 767
   archaic terminology, 602
   chemical structure, 598*f*
   development, 597
   for fibromyalgia, 810
   icons, 599*f*
   listing of those still in use, 597*t*
   major limitation, 598
   for panic disorder, 768
   side effects
      coma, seizures, arrhythmia, death, 604*f*
      constipation, blurred vision, dry mouth, and drowsiness, 602*f*
      dizziness, drowsiness, decreased blood pressure, 603*f*
      weight gain and drowsiness, 602*f*
   therapeutic actions of
      5HT2A receptor block, 601*f*
      5HT2C receptor block, 601*f*
      norepinephrine reuptake inhibition (NRI), 600*f*
      serotonin reuptake inhibitor (SRI), 600*f*
trifluoperazine (Stelazine), 331*t*
triglycerides, elevated, atypical antipsychotic agents and, 390*f*
trimers, glutamate transporters as, 101
trimipramine (Surmontil), 597*t*
trimonoamine neurotransmitter synthesis, tetrahydrobiopterin (BH4) cofactor for, 629*f*
trimonoaminergic modulators (TMMs), 609–639
   estrogen as, 610
   L-5-methyltetrahydrofolate (MTHF) as, 625
trimonoaminergic neurotransmitter system, 453, 474
   antipsychotic agents and, 691
   dysregulation of, 620
trip, 990
triple monoamine modulators (TMMs). *See* trimonoaminergic modulators (TMMs)
triple reuptake inhibitors (TRIs), 658, 661
   icon, 661*f*
TrkA (antiaptotic receptors), 29*t*
trophic actions, and estrogen, on dendritic spine formation, 612
trophic factors, 28
Tryptizol (amitriptyline, Elavil, Endep, Loroxyl), 53, 572, 597*t*
tryptophan, 343, 344*f*
tryptophan hydroxylase (TRY-OH), 343, 344*f*
tuberoinfundibular dopamine pathway, 272*f*
   and D2 antagonists, 334*f*
   dopamine output and, 366*f*
   hypoactivity of, 281*f*
tuberomammillary nucleus (TMN), 207
   of hypothalamus, 819, 822*f*
   and insomnia, 825*f*
tumor growth factor beta, 174
tumor necrosis factor, 174

tyramine
    and blood pressure, 589
    cheese content, 587f
    dangerous levels with irreversible MAO-A inhibitors, 592f
    MAO-A inhibition and, 586f
    MAO-A inhibitor and, 590f
    and norepinephrine release, 585f
    pizza chain content of, 588f
    reactions and dietary restrictions, 582, 584t
    wine content, 589f
tyrosine, 266, 266f
    norepinephrine synthesis from, 474, 475f
tyrosine hydroxylase (TOH), 266, 266f
    genes for, 319f

ultradian sleep cycle, 820, 823f
undeveloped neuron, 34f
unipolar depression, 454
    distinguishing from bipolar depression, 468, 469t
    impact of chronic and widespread undertreatment, 473
    misdiagnosis, 468
    unstable form of, 461
upregulation, 87f, 88
urinary hesitancy, from milnacipran, 552
urinary retention, from NET inhibition, 547

vabicaserin, 447
vaccines, for Alzheimer's disease, 937
VAChT (vesicular acetylcholine transporter), 94
vagus nerve stimulation (VNS), 634, 636f
val carriers, 233
valine, 233
Valium (diazepam), 53
valproate
    actions as mood stabilizer, 680f
    for bipolar disorder, 701
    vs. carbamazepine, 679
    in combos for bipolar disorder, 713
    GABA and, 674
    for manic phase of bipolar disorder, 672
    mechanism of action
        on GABA, glutamate, sigma, and dopamine, 676t
        VSSCs, synaptic vesicles, and carbonic anhydrase, 675t
    possible sites of action on GABA, 678f
    possible sites of action on VSSCs, 677f
    putative clinical actions, 673t
    and VSSCs, 707f

valproic acid, 157t
    icon, 676t
    side effects, 677
vanilloid 1 receptor (VR1) ion channel, 779, 779f
vardenafil (Levitra), 1002
varenicline, 449
    actions on reward circuits, 962f
    in combos for bipolar disorder, 715
    for nicotine addiction, 960, 964
vasomotor symptoms, 620
    from estrogen interaction with monoamines, 524f
    link to depression, 650
        in perimenopause, 619
    treatment, 621
        with desvenlafaxine, 550
        with SNRIs, 626f
        with SSRIs, 625f
vasopressin 1B antagonists, 663
vasopressin, blocking receptors for, 754
venlafaxine XR (Effexor XR; Efexor XR), 99t, 541t
    conversion to desvenlafaxine, 548, 548f
    CYP450 2D6 impact on plasma levels, 607
    for fibrofog, 810
    for fibromyalgia, 808
    icon, 548f
    for neuropathic pain, 792
ventral mesencephalon, 204
    dopamine pathway from, 272f
ventral tegmental area (VTA), 202f
    alcohol actions in, 972f
    naltrexone actions in, 974f
    opiate action in, 978f
ventrolateral preoptic (VLPO) nucleus, of hypothalamus, 819, 822f
ventromedial nucleus, and sexual drive, 994
ventromedial prefrontal cortex (VMPFC), 199f
    amygdala activation by, 760
    blockade of beta receptors in, 763f
    dopamine deficit in mesocortical projections to, 274
    emotional symptom regulation by, 508f
    fear extinction and, 760
    and input to lateral amygdala, 760
    manic episode symptoms linked to, 506
    mesocortical dopamine pathway to, 276f
    and schizophrenia symptoms, 261, 262f
    and stress, 759f
verbal abuse, 425
verbal fluency, impaired, in schizophrenia, 257
vesicles, 12, 474
vesicular acetylcholine transporter (VAChT), 94

Index | 1115

vesicular glutamate transporters (vGluT), 102, 282f
   dysbindin regulation of, 317
vesicular inhibitory amino acid transporters (VIAATs), 100f
vesicular monoamine transporters (VMATs), 93, 94, 95f, 157f
   and dopamine, 268f
   transport of amphetamine, 106f
vesicular neurotransmitter transporters, 94t
vesicular transporters, 103f
   as psychotropic drug target, 102–105
   subtypes and function, 102
VIAATs (vesicular inhibitory amino acid transporters), 100f
violence, 256
virtuous learning,
viruses
   neuron or DNA damage from, 28
   transport to soma, 15, 17f
visual association cortex, 196f
visual illusions, from hallucinogens, 990
vital sign, sleep as, 816
Vitamin E
   for Alzheimer's disease, 936
   as free radical scavenger, 442f
Vivactil (protriptyline), 597t
   inhibition of serotonin reuptake pump, 598
VMATs (vesicular monoamine transporters), 93, 157f
   transport of amphetamine, 106f
VMPFC. *See* ventromedial prefrontal cortex (VMPFC)
VNS (vagus nerve stimulation), 634, 636f
voltage-sensitive calcium channels (VSCCs), 60, 148, 151–158, 755
   amino acids' regulation of, 153
   ionic filter of, 150f
   multiple associated regulatory proteins, 155f
   and nontransmission, 159
   proteins linking to, 157f
   subtypes, 153, 155t
   TCA blockade of, 599
voltage-sensitive ion channels, 92f, 124, 145–151, 158
   alpha pore, 148f
   different states, 150
   psychotropic drugs targeting, 157t
   structure and function, 145
voltage-sensitive sodium channels (VSSCs), 60, 148, 149f
   alpha pore, 151f
   anticonvulsant action at, 153f
   carbamazepine acton on, 678
   mood stabilizers action on, 707f
   and nontransmission, 159
   oxcarbazepine and, 681
   states, 152f
   structure, 152f
   subtypes, 150
   valproate and, 672
volume neurotransmission, 58, 58f
   dopamine and, 59f
   monamine autoreceptors, 60f
vomiting
   from 5HT3 receptor stimulation, 531
   5HT3 receptors and, 349f
   bifeprunox and, 424
   serotonin receptors and, 345
VSF-173, for wakefulness, 857
VSSCs. *See* voltage-sensitive sodium channels (VSSCs)

waist circumference, monitoring, 392
"wake promoter", 819
wake-up pharmacy, 861f
wakefulness. *See also* daytime sleepiness; sleep
   histamine and, 209f
   modafinil for, 857
"Walt Disney", 717f
weight
   baseline measurement, 395f
   changes in, 493
   circuits, 498f
weight gain
   from 5HT2C antagonists and/or mirtazapine, 563
   antipsychotic agents and, 389f
   aripiprazole and, 422
   atypical antipsychotic agents and, 383, 386t
   clozapine and, 410
   from histamine-1 receptor blockade, 341
   low risk antipsycyhotic agents, 386t
   from mirtazapine, 564
   monitoring, 396f
   olanzapine and, 411
   quetiapine and, 415
   as valproic acid side effect, 677
   ziprasidone and, 417
   zotepine and, 418
weight loss
   topiramate and, 687, 1011
   zonisamide and, 1011
"Well-oft" (Wellbutrin with Zoloft), 536
will power, vs. temptation, 952, 954f
"wind-up", 795
wine, tyramine content, 589f

withdrawal, 945
  opiates and, 979
women
  bipolar disorder and, 710
  life cycle
    depression incidence across, 615f
    depression risk across, 615f
    estrogen and/or antidepressant use across, 617f
    estrogen regulation and major depression over, 614
  reduction in sexual desire, 1004
  suicidality in adolescents, from antidepressants, 617
  thyroid dysfunction, 711
worry, 260, 726. *See also* anxiety
  diabolical learning hypothesis and, 230
  linking symptoms to circuits, 764f
worry/obsessions circuit, 764f
worthlessness
  circuits, 499f
  serotonin and, 493

Xanax (alprazolam), 53
Xeristar. *See* duloxetine (Cymbalta, Xeristar)
Xyrem, 859. *See also* gamma hydroxybutyrate (GHB)

Y931, 368f
YM992, 573
yohimbine, 565

"Z" drugs, for insomnia, 838f
zaleplon, 839f
  half-life of, 836f
zipa-do, 717f
zipa-la, 717f
zipa-li, 717f
zipa-li-do-la, 717f
ziprasidone, 382f
  with 5HT1D antagonist actions, 418
  actions as mood stabilizer, 693f
  and cardiometabolic risk, 386t
  in combos for bipolar disorder, 713, 717f
  dosage with carbamazepine, 407f
  pharmacological actions, 693f
  pharmacological icon, 416f
  and sedation, 430, 432f
  and weight gain risk, 386t
zolpidem, 839, 839f
  half-life of, 836f
zolpidem CR, 839, 839f
  half-life of, 836f
zona incerta, 204
zonisamide, 157t
  in combos for bipolar disorder, 715
  icon, 688f
  mechanism of action
    on GABA, glutamate, sigma, and dopamine, 676t
    VSSCs, synaptic vesicles, and carbonic anhydrase, 675t
  putative clinical actions, 673t
  and VSSCs, 707f
  and weight loss, 1011
zopiclone, 842
zotepine, 403, 403f
  5HT6-antagonist properties of, 447
  binding properties, 418f
  dosage with carbamazepine, 407f
  pharmacological icon, 418f
  and QTc prolongation, 417
zuclopenthixol (Clopixol), 331t